Workbook for
Saunders Essentials of
MEDICAL ASSISTING

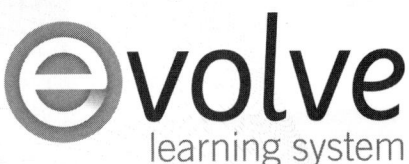
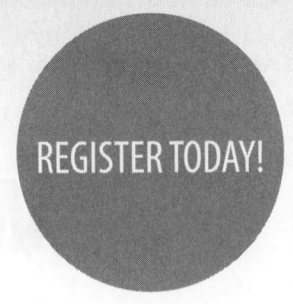

To access your Student Resources, visit the web address below

http://evolve.elsevier.com/klieger/medicalassisting

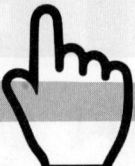

Evolve® Student Learning Resources for *Klieger: Saunders Essentials of Medical Assisting, Second Edition*, offer the following features:

- **Medical Assisting Competency Challenge**
  Interactive guided practice and application activities that allow you to experience real-world scenarios

- **Chapter Quizzes**
  Scored quizzes can serve as a valuable study tool

- **Archie Animations**
  Detailed anatomy and physiology videos

- **Body Spectrum**
  Fun and interactive coloring book that helps you study anatomy and physiology

- **Spanish-English Pronunciation Glossary**
  A pronunciation glossary to prepare you for medical office situations

- **CMA and RMA Review Questions**
  Practice questions to help you prepare for your examinations

- **Medisoft Exercises**
  Software exercises can prepare you for realistic office scenarios

- **Math Review**
  Various interactive quizzes refresh simple math knowledge, to aid you in your future career

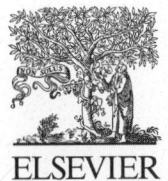

Workbook for Saunders Essentials of MEDICAL ASSISTING

Second Edition

Diane M. Klieger
RN, MBA, CMA (AAMA)
Retired Program Director, Medical Assisting
Adjunct Medical Assisting Instructor
Pinellas Technical Educational Centers (PTEC)
St. Petersburg, Florida

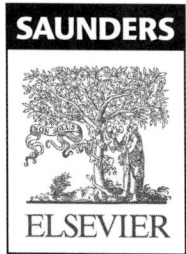

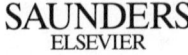

3251 Riverport Lane
St. Louis, Missouri 63043

WORKBOOK TO ACCOMPANY
SAUNDERS ESSENTIALS OF MEDICAL ASSISTING   ISBN: 978-1-4160-5675-1
Copyright © 2010, 2005 by Saunders, an imprint of Elsevier Inc.

All rights reserved. No part of this publication may be reproduced or transmitted in any form or by any means, electronic or mechanical, including photocopying, recording, or any information storage and retrieval system, without permission in writing from the publisher, except that, until further notice, instructors requiring their students to purchase WORKBOOK TO ACCOMPANY SAUNDERS ESSENTIALS OF MEDICAL ASSISTING, Second Edition by Diane M. Klieger, may reproduce the contents or parts thereof for instructional purposes, provided each copy contains a proper copyright notice as follows: Copyright © 2010, 2005 by Saunders, an imprint of Elsevier Inc. Permissions may be sought directly from Elsevier's Rights Department: phone: (+1) 215 239 3804 (US) or (+44) 1865 843830 (UK); fax: (+44) 1865 853333; e-mail: healthpermissions@elsevier.com. You may also complete your request on-line via the Elsevier website at http://www.elsevier.com/permissions.

Notice

Neither the Publisher nor the Author assumes any responsibility for any loss or injury and/or damage to persons or property arising out of or related to any use of the material contained in this book. It is the responsibility of the treating practitioner, relying on independent expertise and knowledge of the patient, to determine the best treatment and method of application for the patient.

The Publisher

978-1-4160-5675-1

Publisher: Michael S. Ledbetter
Developmental Editor: Jennifer Bertucci
Publishing Services Manager: Catherine Jackson
Project Managers: Jennifer Boudreau and David Stein

Printed in the United States of America

Last digit is the print number: 9 8 7 6 5 4 3 2

To the Student

This workbook is designed to help you apply and master key concepts and skills presented in *Saunders Essentials of Medical Assisting*, Second Edition so that you can spring into your new medical assisting career! Completing the variety of exercises in each workbook chapter will help reinforce the material you have studied in the textbook and learned in class.

You'll find exercises specially tailored to help you master the learning objectives in both theory and practice of medical assisting:

- A **vocabulary review** begins each chapter. This includes a comprehensive list of key terms in each chapter and tests your knowledge of their definitions.

- The **theory recall** section consists of true/false, multiple choice, matching, and short answer questions, as well as sentence completions.

- **Critical thinking** exercises take information presented in the textbook to the next level and prepare you for the real world through patient case scenarios.

- The **Practical Applications** section guides you through the real-world examples provided in your textbook, and ask you to analyze the situation at hand.

- The **Application of Skills** encourage you to put concepts into practice.

- **Chapter Quizzes** help reinforce what you learned from the textbook.

Also, in the anatomy and physiology chapters, there are **labeling** exercises to help you quiz yourself, as well as **word part** practice, which help you break apart words into prefixes, roots, combining forms, and suffixes, so that you can truly form a better understanding of anatomy terms.

The best feature of this workbook is the comprehensive appendix, which provides you with all the **supplemental chapter material** that you will need! This appendix is logically separated by chapter and procedure, so it's easy to use. This all-inclusive resource includes:

- **Work papers and forms**, which will provide you with important practice for your future careers

- **Procedure checklists,** which help you monitor your progress and can be used by your instructor to evaluate your competency with the variety of skills necessary to be a successful medical assistant. These are designed to accompany the skills presented in the textbook.

Best wishes as you spring into your new career as a medical assistant!

Copyright © 2010, 2005 by Saunders, an imprint of Elsevier, Inc. All rights reserved.

Contents

Section One • Strategies for Success

1 **Successful Learning, 1**
2 **Becoming a Professional, 13**

Section Two • Foundational Concepts

3 **Diversity in Health Care Delivery, 24**
4 **Law and Ethics in Health Care, 34**
5 **Understanding Human Behavior, 45**
6 **Understanding Patient Behavior, 56**
7 **Effective Communication, 67**
8 **Communicating with Patients, 78**
9 **Nutrition, 88**
10 **Understanding Medical Terminology, 98**

Section Three • Anatomy and Physiology

11 **Basic Anatomy and Physiology, 110**
12 **Cardiovascular System, 127**
13 **Blood, Lymphatic, and Immune Systems, 142**
14 **Respiratory System, 153**
15 **Digestive System, 167**
16 **Nervous System, 182**
17 **Sensory System, 195**
18 **Skeletal System, 206**
19 **Muscular System, 223**
20 **Urinary System, 236**
21 **Reproductive System, 250**
22 **Endocrine System, 264**
23 **Integumentary System, 278**

Section Four • Administrative Medical Assisting

24 **The Medical Office, 293**
25 **Computers in the Medical Office, 306**
26 **Medical Office Communication, 317**
27 **Medical Records and Chart Documentation, 332**
28 **Financial Management, 346**
29 **Medical Coding, 359**
30 **Medical Insurance, 372**

Copyright © 2010, 2005 by Saunders, an imprint of Elsevier, Inc. All rights reserved.

Section Five • Clinical Medical Assisting

31 **Infection Control and Asepsis,** 385
32 **Preparing the Examination Room,** 398
33 **Body Measurements and Vital Signs,** 407
34 **Obtaining the Medical History,** 418
35 **Assisting with the Physical Examination,** 427
36 **Electrocardiography,** 439
37 **Radiography and Diagnostic Testing,** 454
38 **Therapeutic Procedures,** 463
39 **Specialty Diagnostic Testing,** 474
40 **Introduction to the Physician's Office Laboratory,** 489
41 **Phlebotomy,** 501
42 **Laboratory Testing in the Physician's Office,** 510
43 **Understanding Medications,** 523
44 **Administering Medications,** 541
45 **Minor Office Surgery,** 552
46 **Basic First Aid and Medical Office Emergencies,** 563

Section Six • Employment and Beyond

47 **Beginning Your Job Search,** 576

Appendix

A. **Supplemental Chapter Materials,** 587

Appendix A: Supplemental Chapter Materials

Chapter 2
Procedure 2-1 Checklist: Being a Professional, 589

Chapter 4
Work Papers: Consent for Surgery, 593
    Patient Consent Forms, 595

Chapter 24
Procedure 24-1 Checklist: Prepare, Send, and Receive a Fax, 599
Procedure 24-2 Checklist: Maintain Office Equipment, 601
    Work Paper: Equipment Inventory—Sample, 603
    Work Paper: Equipment Maintenance Log—Sample, 603
Procedure 24-3 Checklist: Inventory Control: Ordering and Restocking Supplies, 605
    Work Paper: Inventory Supply List Sample, 607
Procedure 24-4 Checklist: Develop and Maintain a Current List of Community Resources, 609
    Work Paper: Agency Resource List, 610
    Work Papers: Purchase Order, 611

Chapter 26
Procedure 26-1 Checklist: Give Verbal Instructions on How to Locate the Medical Office, 613
Procedure 26-2 Checklist: Create a Medical Practice Information Brochure, 615
Procedure 26-3 Checklist: Answer a Multiline Telephone System, 617
    Work Paper: Telephone Message, 619
Procedure 26-4 Checklist: Prepare and Maintain an Appointment Book, 621
    Work Paper: Appointment Book Schedule, 623
Procedure 26-5 Checklist: Schedule a New Patient, 627
    Work Paper: Appointment Book Schedule, 629
Procedure 26-6 Checklist: Schedule Outpatient and Inpatient Appointments, 631
    Work Papers: Surgical Request Forms, 635
Procedure 26-7 Checklist: Compose Business Correspondence, 637
    Work Paper: Letterhead, 639
Procedure 26-8 Checklist: Compose a Memo, 641
    Work Paper: Memo, 643

Chapter 27
Procedure 27-1 Checklist: Pull Patient Records for a Manual Record System, 645
Procedure 27-2 Checklist: Register a New Patient, 647
    Work Paper: Patient Information Form, 649
Procedure 27-3 Checklist: Initiate a Patient File for a New Patient Using Color-Coded Tabs, 651
    Work Paper: Patient Health History Form, 653
    Work Paper: Patient Consent Form, 655
    Work Paper: Consent for Surgery, 657
    Work Paper: Progress Notes, 659
    Work Paper: Patient Information Form, 661

Copyright © 2010, 2005 by Saunders, an imprint of Elsevier, Inc. All rights reserved.

Work Paper:	Visit Log, 663
Work Paper:	Prescription Flow Sheet, 665
Procedure 27-4 Checklist:	Add Supplementary Items to an Established Patient File, 667
Procedure 27-5 Checklist:	Maintain Confidentiality of Patients and Their Medical Records, 669
Work Paper:	Patient Consent Form, 671
Procedure 27-6 Checklist:	File Medical Records Using the Alphabetical System, 673
Procedure 27-7 Checklist:	File Medical Records Using the Numerical System, 675

Chapter 28

Procedure 28-1 Checklist:	Manage an Account for Petty Cash, 677
Work Papers:	Petty Cash Vouchers, 679
Work Papers:	Checks, 681
Work Paper:	Voucher Table, 683
Procedure 28-2 Checklist:	Post Service Charges and Payments to the Patient's Account, 685
Work Papers:	Patient Ledgers, 689
Work Paper:	Day Sheet, 695
Work Paper:	Journal of Daily Charges and Payments, 697
Work Paper:	Fee Schedule, 699
Work Papers:	Encounter Forms, 701
Work Papers:	Receipts, 707
Procedure 28-3 Checklist:	Record Adjustments and Credits to the Patient's Account, 711
Work Paper:	Day Sheet, 715
Work Paper:	Journal of Daily Charges and Payments, 717
Work Papers:	Checks, 719
Work Paper:	Day Sheet, 721
Procedure 28-4 Checklist:	Prepare a Bank Deposit, 723
Work Paper:	Deposit Slip, 725
Procedure 28-5 Checklist:	Reconcile a Bank Statement, 727
Work Paper:	Balance Worksheet, 729
Procedure 28-6 Checklist:	Explain Professional Fees Before Services Are Provided, 731
Procedure 28-7 Checklist:	Establish Payment Arrangements on a Patient Account, 733
Work Paper:	Federal Truth in Lending Statement, 734
Procedure 28-8 Checklist:	Explain a Statement of Account to a Patient, 735
Work Paper:	Statement, 737
Procedure 28-9 Checklist:	Prepare Billing Statements and Collect Past-Due Accounts, 739

Chapter 29

Procedure 29-1 Checklist:	Diagnostic Coding, 743
Procedure 29-2 Checklist:	Procedural Coding, 745

Chapter 30

Procedure 30-1 Checklist:	Apply Managed Care Policies and Procedures, 747
Work Paper:	Pre-Certification Request, 749
Work Paper:	Preauthorization Request Form, 751
Procedure 30-2 Checklist:	Complete the CMS-1500 Claim Form, 753
Work Papers:	CMS-1500 Claim Forms, 757

Chapter 31

Procedure 31-1 Checklist:	Practice Standard Precautions, 761
Procedure 31-2 Checklist:	Properly Dispose of Biohazardous Materials, 763
Procedure 31-3 Checklist:	Perform Proper Handwashing for Medical Asepsis, 765
Procedure 31-4 Checklist:	Perform Alcohol-Based Hand Sanitization, 767

Procedure 31-5 Checklist:	**Apply and Remove Clean, Disposable (Nonsterile) Gloves,** 769	
Procedure 31-6 Checklist:	**Sanitize Instruments,** 771	
Procedure 31-7 Checklist:	**Perform Chemical Sterilization,** 773	
Procedure 31-8 Checklist:	**Wrap Instruments for the Autoclave,** 775	
Procedure 31-9 Checklist:	**Sterilize Articles in the Autoclave,** 777	

Chapter 33

Procedure 33-1 Checklist:	**Measure Weight and Height of an Adult,** 779
Procedure 33-2 Checklist:	**Measure Weight and Length of an Infant,** 781
Procedure 33-3 Checklist:	**Measure Head and Chest Circumference of an Infant,** 785
Work Paper:	**Growth Chart for Girls,** 789
Work Paper:	**Growth Chart for Boys,** 790
Procedure 33-4 Checklist:	**Measure Oral Body Temperature Using a Mercury-Free Glass Thermometer,** 791
Procedure 33-5 Checklist:	**Measure Oral Body Temperature Using a Rechargeable Electronic or Digital Thermometer,** 793
Procedure 33-6 Checklist:	**Measure Rectal Body Temperature Using a Rechargeable Electronic or Digital Thermometer,** 795
Procedure 33-7 Checklist:	**Measure Axillary Body Temperature Using a Rechargeable Electronic or Digital Thermometer,** 797
Procedure 33-8 Checklist:	**Measure Body Temperature Using a Tympanic Thermometer,** 799
Procedure 33-9 Checklist:	**Measure Body Temperature Using a Disposable Oral Thermometer,** 801
Procedure 33-10 Checklist:	**Measure Radial Pulse,** 803
Procedure 33-11 Checklist:	**Measure Apical Pulse,** 805
Procedure 33-12 Checklist:	**Measure Respiratory Rate,** 807
Procedure 33-13 Checklist:	**Measure Blood Pressure,** 809
	Charting for Procedures 33-1 through 33-13, 811

Chapter 34

Procedure 34-1 Checklist:	**Complete a Medical History Form,** 815
Work Paper:	**Patient Health History Form,** 817
Procedure 34-2 Checklist:	**Recognize and Respond to Verbal and Nonverbal Communication,** 821
	Charting for Procedures 34-1 and 34-2, 823

Chapter 35

Procedure 35-1 Checklist:	**Assist with the Physical Examination,** 825
Procedure 35-2 Checklist:	**Sitting Position,** 829
Procedure 35-3 Checklist:	**Recumbent Position,** 831
Procedure 35-4 Checklist:	**Lithotomy Position,** 833
Procedure 35-5 Checklist:	**Sims' Position,** 835
Procedure 35-6 Checklist:	**Prone Position,** 837
Procedure 35-7 Checklist:	**Knee-Chest Position,** 839
Procedure 35-8 Checklist:	**Fowler's Position,** 841
Procedure 35-9 Checklist:	**Assess Distance Visual Acuity Using a Snellen Chart,** 843
Procedure 35-10 Checklist:	**Assess Color Vision Using the Ishihara Test,** 845
Procedure 35-11 Checklist:	**Assess Near Vision Using a Jaeger Card,** 847
	Charting for Procedures 35-1 through 35-11, 849

Chapter 36

Procedure 36-1 Checklist:	**Obtain a 12-Lead ECG Using a Single-Channel Electrocardiograph,** 853
Procedure 36-2 Checklist:	**Obtain a 12-Lead ECG Using a Three-Channel (Multichannel) Electrocardiograph,** 857
Procedure 36-3 Checklist:	**Apply and Remove a Holter Monitor,** 861
	Charting for Procedures 36-1 through 36-3, 865

Copyright © 2010, 2005 by Saunders, an imprint of Elsevier, Inc. All rights reserved.

Chapter 38

Procedure 38-1 Checklist:	Perform an Ear Irrigation, 867
Procedure 38-2 Checklist:	Perform an Ear Instillation, 871
Procedure 38-3 Checklist:	Perform an Eye Irrigation, 873
Procedure 38-4 Checklist:	Perform an Eye Instillation, 875
Procedure 38-5 Checklist:	Apply a Tubular Gauze Bandage, 877
Procedure 38-6 Checklist:	Apply an Ice Bag, 879
Procedure 38-7 Checklist:	Apply a Cold Compress, 881
Procedure 38-8 Checklist:	Apply a Chemical Cold Pack, 883
Procedure 38-9 Checklist:	Apply a Hot Water Bag, 885
Procedure 38-10 Checklist:	Apply a Heating Pad, 887
Procedure 38-11 Checklist:	Apply a Hot Compress, 889
Procedure 38-12 Checklist:	Apply a Hot Soak, 891
Procedure 38-13 Checklist:	Administer an Ultrasound Treatment, 893
Procedure 38-14 Checklist:	Measure for Axillary Crutches, 895
Procedure 38-15 Checklist:	Instruct the Patient in Crutch Gaits, 897
Procedure 38-16 Checklist:	Instruct the Patient in the Use of a Walker, 899
Procedure 38-17 Checklist:	Instruct the Patient in the Use of a Cane, 901
Procedure 38-18 Checklist:	Assist in Plaster-of-Paris or Fiberglass Cast Application, 903
	Charting for Procedures 38-1 through 38-18, 905

Chapter 39

Procedure 39-1 Checklist:	Teach Breast Self-Examination, 911
Procedure 39-2 Checklist:	Assist with a Gynecological Examination, 915
Procedure 39-3 Checklist:	Assist with a Follow-up Prenatal Examination, 919
Procedure 39-4 Checklist:	Instruct the Patient in Obtaining a Fecal Specimen, 921
Procedure 39-5 Checklist:	Test for Occult Blood, 923
Procedure 39-6 Checklist:	Assist with Sigmoidoscopy, 925
Procedure 39-7 Checklist:	Perform Spirometry (Pulmonary Function Testing), 927
Procedure 39-8 Checklist:	Instruct the Patient in the Use of a Peak Flow Meter, 929
Procedure 39-9 Checklist:	Perform Pulse Oximetry, 931
	Charting for Procedures 39-1 through 39-9, 933

Chapter 40

Procedure 40-1 Checklist:	Use Methods of Quality Control (QC), 937
Work Paper:	hCG Control Log, 939
Procedure 40-2 Checklist:	Focus the Microscope, 941
Procedure 40-3 Checklist:	Complete a Laboratory Requisition, 943
Work Paper:	Patient Laboratory Log Sheet, 945
Procedure 40-4 Checklist:	Collect a Specimen for Transport to an Outside Laboratory, 947
Work Paper:	Patient Laboratory Log Sheet, 949
Procedure 40-5 Checklist:	Screen and Follow-up on Patient Test Results, 951
Procedure 40-6 Checklist:	Collect a Specimen for CLIA-Waived Throat Culture and Strep A Test, 953
Work Paper:	Patient Laboratory Log Sheet, 957
Work Paper:	Quickvue Control Log, 959
Procedure 40-7 Checklist:	Obtain a Urine Specimen from an Infant Using a Pediatric Urine Collector, 961
Work Paper:	Patient Laboratory Log Sheet, 963
Procedure 40-8 Checklist:	Instruct a Patient in the Collection of a Midstream Clean-Catch Urine Specimen, 965
Procedure 40-9 Checklist:	Instruct a Patient in the Collection of a 24-Hour Urine Specimen, 967
	Charting for Procedures 40-1 through 40-9, 969

Copyright © 2010, 2005 by Saunders, an imprint of Elsevier, Inc. All rights reserved.

Chapter 41

Procedure 41-1 Checklist:	Use a Sterile Disposable Microlancet for Skin Puncture,	973
Procedure 41-2 Checklist:	Collect a Blood Specimen for a Phenylketonuria (PKU) Screening Test,	975
Procedure 41-3 Checklist:	Perform Venipuncture Using the Evacuated-Tube Method (Collection of Multiple Tubes),	977
Procedure 41-4 Checklist:	Perform Venipuncture Using the Syringe Method,	981
Procedure 41-5 Checklist:	Perform Venipuncture Using the Butterfly Method (Collection of Multiple Evacuated Tubes),	985
Procedure 41-6 Checklist:	Separate Serum from a Blood Specimen,	989
	Charting for Procedures 41-1 through 41-6,	991

Chapter 42

Procedure 42-1 Checklist:	Urinalysis Using Reagent Strips,	993
Work Paper:	Urine Strip/Analyzer Control Log,	997
Work Paper:	Patient Laboratory Log Sheet,	999
Work Paper:	Urinalysis Results,	1000
Procedure 42-2 Checklist:	Prepare a Urine Specimen for Microscopic Examination,	1001
Work Paper:	Patient Laboratory Log Sheet,	1003
Procedure 42-3 Checklist:	Perform a Urine Pregnancy Test,	1005
Work Paper:	Pregnancy Control Log,	1007
Work Paper:	Patient Laboratory Log Sheet,	1009
Procedure 42-4 Checklist:	Determine a Hemoglobin Measurement Using a HemoCue,	1011
Work Paper:	Patient Laboratory Log Sheet,	1013
Work Paper:	HemoCue Control Log,	1015
Procedure 42-5 Checklist:	Perform a Microhematocrit Test,	1017
Work Paper:	Patient Laboratory Log Sheet,	1021
Procedure 42-6 Checklist:	Determine Erythrocyte Sedimentation Rate (ESR, Nonautomated) Using the Westergren Method,	1023
Work Paper:	Patient Laboratory Log Sheet,	1025
Procedure 42-7 Checklist:	Prepare a Blood Smear,	1027
Procedure 42-8 Checklist:	Perform Cholesterol Testing,	1029
Work Paper:	Cholesterol Control Log,	1031
Work Paper:	Patient Laboratory Log Sheet,	1033
Procedure 42-9 Checklist:	Perform Glucose Testing,	1035
Work Paper:	Glucometer Control Log,	1037
Work Paper:	Patient Laboratory Log Sheet,	1039
Procedure 42-10 Checklist:	Obtain a Bacterial Smear from a Wound Specimen,	1041
	Charting for Procedures 42-1 through 42-10,	1043

Chapter 43

Procedure 43-1 Checklist:	Prepare and File an Immunization Record,	1047
Work Paper:	Vaccine Administration Record,	1049
Work Paper:	Immunization Record,	1051
	Charting for Procedure 43-1,	1053

Chapter 44

Procedure 44-1 Checklist:	Administer Oral Medication,	1055
Procedure 44-2 Checklist:	Apply a Transdermal Patch,	1057
Procedure 44-3 Checklist:	Instruct a Patient in Administering Medication Using a Metered-Dose Inhaler with the Closed-Mouth Technique,	1059
Procedure 44-4 Checklist:	Reconstitute a Powdered Drug,	1061
Procedure 44-5 Checklist:	Prepare a Parenteral Medication from a Vial,	1063
Procedure 44-6 Checklist:	Prepare a Parenteral Medication from an Ampule,	1065

Copyright © 2010, 2005 by Saunders, an imprint of Elsevier, Inc. All rights reserved.

Procedure 44-7 Checklist:	**Administer an Intradermal Injection,** 1067
Procedure 44-8 Checklist:	**Administer a Subcutaneous Injection,** 1071
Procedure 44-9 Checklist:	**Administer an Intramuscular Injection to a Pediatric Patient,** 1073
Procedure 44-10 Checklist:	**Administer an Intramuscular Injection to an Adult,** 1077
Procedure 44-11 Checklist:	**Administer an Intramuscular Injection Using the Z-Track Technique,** 1079
	Charting for Procedures 44-1 through 44-11, 1081

Chapter 45

Procedure 45-1 Checklist:	**Perform Handwashing for Surgical Asepsis,** 1085
Procedure 45-2 Checklist:	**Apply a Sterile Gown and Gloves,** 1087
Procedure 45-3 Checklist:	**Apply Sterile Gloves,** 1089
Procedure 45-4 Checklist:	**Remove Contaminated Gloves,** 1091
Procedure 45-5 Checklist:	**Open a Sterile Package,** 1093
Procedure 45-6 Checklist:	**Pour a Sterile Solution,** 1095
Procedure 45-7 Checklist:	**Assist with Minor Office Surgery,** 1097
Work Paper:	**Consent for Surgery,** 1101
Procedure 45-8 Checklist:	**Remove Sutures or Staples and Change a Wound Dressing Using a Spiral Bandage,** 1103
Procedure 45-9 Checklist:	**Apply and Remove Adhesive Skin Closures,** 1107
	Charting for Procedures 45-1 through 45-9, 1111

Copyright © 2010, 2005 by Saunders, an imprint of Elsevier, Inc. All rights reserved.

NAME: _____   DATE: _____

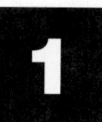 Successful Learning

VOCABULARY REVIEW

Matching: Match each term with the correct definition.

A. attitude

B. concept map

C. day planner

D. goals

E. habit

F. mnemonic device

G. prioritize

H. short-term memory

I. time management

J. Venn diagram

_____ 1. Diagram using circles to represent concepts; overlapping areas of the circles represent similarities between concepts, whereas the other areas represent differences

_____ 2. Memory that holds a small amount of information for a short time

_____ 3. Set of beliefs one holds about something

_____ 4. Organizational system for planning and recording deadlines, tasks to be completed, events, and other activities

_____ 5. Established pattern of thinking or behaving

_____ 6. To decide which situation requires the most attention; to organize tasks or activities according to their level of importance

_____ 7. Drawing that uses words to describe and define a main idea. Relationships between items are shown by connecting them with lines or arrows.

_____ 8. Organization of time to accomplish your goals; the choices that are made about how time is used

_____ 9. Plans that are developed to reach one's mission in life; includes long-term plans and short-term plans

_____ 10. Creative device used to aid memory

Copyright © 2010, 2005 by Saunders, an imprint of Elsevier, Inc. All rights reserved.

THEORY RECALL

True/False

Indicate whether the statement is true or false.

_____ 1. Information stored in long-term memory can be recalled throughout your lifetime.

_____ 2. If you manage your time efficiently, you will not need to delegate tasks to others.

_____ 3. Planning one's time to meet established goals is a skill. It takes patience and practice.

_____ 4. Being organized is often an accident.

_____ 5. A 20-minute break after 3 hours of study is most effective and prepares your mind to retain more information.

Multiple Choice

Identify the letter of the choice that best completes the statement or answers the question.

1. One way to start setting your goals is to develop a(n) _____.
   A. mind map
   B. personal mission statement
   C. anticipation guide
   D. learning log

2. SQ3R is a method used to increase reading comprehension. The second *R* stands for _____.
   A. recite
   B. read
   C. review
   D. recover

3. To determine your background knowledge of a subject, do all of the following *except* _____.
   A. use an anticipation guide
   B. take a pretest
   C. surf the Internet
   D. read the chapter objectives and see how many you know or are able to do

4. Answering questions such as "What do I want to know about a subject?" and "What have I learned about the subject?" is an example of _____.
   A. SQ3R
   B. KWL
   C. LAB RAT
   D. matrixing

5. _____ is (are) a simplified method of outlining that help(s) you make connections between the concepts presented in lecture or reading material.
   A. KWL
   B. SQ3R
   C. Venn diagram
   D. power notes

6. The use of a (an) _____ is an example of a mnemonic device.
   A. KWL
   B. acronym
   C. learning log
   D. SQ3R

7. One of the most common methods of _____ learning is simply asking questions.
   A. actively
   B. memorization
   C. inadequate
   D. repetitive

8. The use of _____ can help you learn and can prove to be beneficial discussion time.
   A. partnered reading
   B. prediction questions
   C. learning logs
   D. concept maps

9. Step 1 of preparing effectively for a test is to _____.
   A. get adequate sleep and rest the night before the examination
   B. take a deep breath and relax
   C. start early
   D. review how you did on your last examination

10. _____ is most essential to a well-functioning brain.
    A. Breakfast
    B. Protein
    C. Water, exercise, and fresh air
    D. Sugar

11. Feedback comes from your instructor in several ways, including all of the following *except* _____.
    A. study habits
    B. grades
    C. written/oral communication
    D. facial expressions

12. To change or break a habit, the habit must be replaced and consistently repeated for _____.
    A. 10 to 15 days
    B. 21 to 28 days
    C. 1 to 2 weeks
    D. 6 to 8 weeks

13. One method for choosing goals is by being _____.
    A. SMART
    B. BUFF
    C. YOUNG
    D. GOOD

14. Which of the following is *not* a reason some students may find it hard to say "No"?
    A. I do not want to be selfish.
    B. I want to be liked.
    C. I do not want to look like I cannot handle a challenge.
    D. All of the above reasons may make it difficult to say "No."

Copyright © 2010, 2005 by Saunders, an imprint of Elsevier, Inc. All rights reserved.

15. When answering multiple-choice questions, the word _____ requires the question to be studied a little more carefully because the question may be confusing.
    A. "challenge"
    B. "option"
    C. "not"
    D. "topic"

Sentence Completion

Complete each sentence or statement.

study skills	short-term
power notes	practice
coaching	experience
study	repetition
instruction	

1. _____ represents a note-taking strategy in which main concepts and subconcepts are identified and recorded in a simple format.

2. When we first encounter a new concept or piece of information, it goes into our _____ memory.

3. There are several ways to learn: through _____, through _____, and through _____, _____, and _____.

4. _____ are the tools you use to put knowledge into your long-term memory.

5. The most beneficial feedback to you as a student is _____ feedback.

Short Answer

1. Describe the four phases of preparing for a test.

2. Describe three negative and three positive effects of stress.

3. List three values of good study habits.

4. List nine tips for successful test taking.

CRITICAL THINKING

1. Susan has recently enrolled in a medical assistant program at her local community college. She wants to do well in school so she can graduate and get a good job, but she is starting to wonder if she is going to be able to make it. Susan is a single parent with a 4-year-old daughter and a 6-month-old son, and she does not have a solid support system. Susan took her first examination on Monday morning. She tried to study the night before the test, but the baby is teething and was fussy most of the night. Her daughter does not like the idea that mom is suddenly busy with homework and does everything she can to get Susan's attention. Susan did not have time to make flash cards, and when she tried to read the chapter and review the information before the examination, it just would not stick. She looked at her class notes a day or so before the examination, but they did not make a lot of sense to her when she tried to create an outline. She is really worried that she did not pass.

Copyright © 2010, 2005 by Saunders, an imprint of Elsevier, Inc. All rights reserved.

CHAPTER 1 Successful Learning

A. What suggestions do you have for Susan?

B. How can she schedule her time more efficiently?

C. What should Susan do in the future regarding her class notes?

2. What suggestions would you give Susan specifically regarding how to prepare for examinations?

3. Explain to Susan two mnemonic devices that might help her when studying.

A.

B.

4. Describe the SQ3R method to Susan to help build her reading comprehension.

PRACTICAL APPLICATIONS

If you have accomplished the objectives in this chapter, you will be able to make better choices as a medical assistant. Take a look at this situation and decide what you would do.

Alex is a student enrolled in a medical assisting class at her local vocational school. The program provides the opportunity to complete the program of study, then take the credentialing examination within 2 weeks.

Alex likes to study with others, but has experienced situations in which the others in her study group wanted to play rather than study. She wants to be well prepared to take the examination without having to do a lot of cramming. She notices two other students, Jake and Mary Lou, studying together and approaches them to see if she can join them. They welcome her, and a new study group is formed. As she talks with them, she learns that their study methods are to memorize, pass the test, and move on to the next assignment.

Because they seem to be serious students, Alex decides to stay with them and will try to teach them some new tricks. She also decides that she will schedule some study time on her own.

Do you think this arrangement will be helpful to Alex? What would you do in this situation?

1. What are some advantages to Alex trying to stay with a study group whose skills are not as refined as hers?

   _____

   _____

   _____

2. What are three study skills you would suggest that Alex teach Mary Lou and Jake?

   _____

   _____

   _____

3. How will these suggested study skills help to take the fear out of taking the examination?

   _____

   _____

   _____

4. Alex, Mary Lou, and Jake will need to set priorities as they determine how to use their time. What steps would you suggest they follow?

   _____

   _____

   _____

Copyright © 2010, 2005 by Saunders, an imprint of Elsevier, Inc. All rights reserved.

5. What are some advantages for Alex to have study time alone, away from her new friends?

_____

_____

_____

6. How will working on a study team help Alex to be better prepared to work on a medical team?

_____

_____

_____

APPLICATION OF SKILLS

1. List three short-term goals for this week. At the end of the week, evaluate how well the goals were met.

   _____

   _____

   _____

2. List three long-term goals—one to be accomplished in the next 6 months, one to be achieved within 1 year, and one you wish to achieve within the next 5 years.

   _____

   _____

   _____

3. On the first 5-day planner provided, outline your schedule for the upcoming week, using the guidelines described in the chapter. At the end of the week, evaluate where your schedule changed and where your schedule can be adjusted for more efficient use of time. After evaluation of the first week, using the second 5-day planner provided, outline your schedule for a second week, making adjustments as necessary. At the end of the second week, evaluate your use of time.

20XX

Monday

6:00 a.m.	11:30	5:00	10:30
6:30	12:00 p.m.	5:30	11:00
7:00	12:30	6:00	Notes
7:30	1:00	6:30	
8:00	1:30	7:00	
8:30	2:00	7:30	
9:00	2:30	8:00	
9:30	3:00	8:30	
10:00	3:30	9:00	
10:30	4:00	9:30	
11:00	4:30	10:00	

Tuesday

6:00 a.m.	11:30	5:00	10:30
6:30	12:00 p.m.	5:30	11:00
7:00	12:30	6:00	Notes
7:30	1:00	6:30	
8:00	1:30	7:00	
8:30	2:00	7:30	
9:00	2:30	8:00	
9:30	3:00	8:30	
10:00	3:30	9:00	
10:30	4:00	9:30	
11:00	4:30	10:00	

Wednesday

6:00 a.m.	11:30	5:00	10:30
6:30	12:00 p.m.	5:30	11:00
7:00	12:30	6:00	Notes
7:30	1:00	6:30	
8:00	1:30	7:00	
8:30	2:00	7:30	
9:00	2:30	8:00	
9:30	3:00	8:30	
10:00	3:30	9:00	
10:30	4:00	9:30	
11:00	4:30	10:00	

20XX

Thursday

6:00 a.m.	11:30	5:00	10:30
6:30	12:00 p.m.	5:30	11:00
7:00	12:30	6:00	Notes
7:30	1:00	6:30	
8:00	1:30	7:00	
8:30	2:00	7:30	
9:00	2:30	8:00	
9:30	3:00	8:30	
10:00	3:30	9:00	
10:30	4:00	9:30	
11:00	4:30	10:00	

Friday

6:00 a.m.	11:30	5:00	10:30
6:30	12:00 p.m.	5:30	11:00
7:00	12:30	6:00	Notes
7:30	1:00	6:30	
8:00	1:30	7:00	
8:30	2:00	7:30	
9:00	2:30	8:00	
9:30	3:00	8:30	
10:00	3:30	9:00	
10:30	4:00	9:30	
11:00	4:30	10:00	

Saturday / Sunday

Saturday A.M.	Saturday P.M.	Sunday A.M.	Sunday P.M.
Notes		Notes	

20XX

Monday

6:00 a.m.	11:30	5:00	10:30
6:30	12:00 p.m.	5:30	11:00
7:00	12:30	6:00	Notes
7:30	1:00	6:30	
8:00	1:30	7:00	
8:30	2:00	7:30	
9:00	2:30	8:00	
9:30	3:00	8:30	
10:00	3:30	9:00	
10:30	4:00	9:30	
11:00	4:30	10:00	

Tuesday

6:00 a.m.	11:30	5:00	10:30
6:30	12:00 p.m.	5:30	11:00
7:00	12:30	6:00	Notes
7:30	1:00	6:30	
8:00	1:30	7:00	
8:30	2:00	7:30	
9:00	2:30	8:00	
9:30	3:00	8:30	
10:00	3:30	9:00	
10:30	4:00	9:30	
11:00	4:30	10:00	

Wednesday

6:00 a.m.	11:30	5:00	10:30
6:30	12:00 p.m.	5:30	11:00
7:00	12:30	6:00	Notes
7:30	1:00	6:30	
8:00	1:30	7:00	
8:30	2:00	7:30	
9:00	2:30	8:00	
9:30	3:00	8:30	
10:00	3:30	9:00	
10:30	4:00	9:30	
11:00	4:30	10:00	

20XX

Thursday

6:00 a.m.	11:30	5:00	10:30
6:30	12:00 p.m.	5:30	11:00
7:00	12:30	6:00	Notes
7:30	1:00	6:30	
8:00	1:30	7:00	
8:30	2:00	7:30	
9:00	2:30	8:00	
9:30	3:00	8:30	
10:00	3:30	9:00	
10:30	4:00	9:30	
11:00	4:30	10:00	

Friday

6:00 a.m.	11:30	5:00	10:30
6:30	12:00 p.m.	5:30	11:00
7:00	12:30	6:00	Notes
7:30	1:00	6:30	
8:00	1:30	7:00	
8:30	2:00	7:30	
9:00	2:30	8:00	
9:30	3:00	8:30	
10:00	3:30	9:00	
10:30	4:00	9:30	
11:00	4:30	10:00	

Saturday / Sunday

Saturday A.M.	Saturday P.M.	Sunday A.M.	Sunday P.M.
Notes		Notes	

Copyright © 2010, 2005 by Saunders, an imprint of Elsevier, Inc. All rights reserved.

4. Investigate other study strategies by logging onto http://www.how-to-study.com. Write a paragraph about a new strategy you learned from this Internet site.

_____

_____

_____

_____

_____

_____

_____

CHAPTER QUIZ

Multiple Choice

Identify the letter of the choice that best completes the statement or answers the question.

1. Consistent study habits will prevent you from feeling the need to cram and will store information in your _____ memory.
   A. short-term
   B. long-term
   C. quick-term
   D. action-term

2. _____ on a test will help you prepare for the next examination, and for learning the next block of material.
   A. Cheating
   B. A passing grade
   C. Feedback
   D. Writing in ink

3. Which of the following is *not* a successful test-taking tip?
   A. Answer the easiest questions first.
   B. Arrive early and be prepared.
   C. Never guess at an answer.
   D. Briefly outline essay questions.

4. Who is primarily responsible for a student learning new information?
   A. Parent
   B. Teacher
   C. Administrator
   D. Student

5. A prereading guide that presents questions and statements about what will be presented in the text and what you will be learning is called a(n) _____.
   A. concept map
   B. anticipation guide
   C. road map
   D. day planner

6. _____ is the process of talking with others about a concept or information for the purpose of understanding or clarification.
   A. Partnered reading
   B. Prioritizing
   C. Learning log
   D. Discussion

7. _____ are plans you develop to reach your mission in life.
   A. Mission statements
   B. Goals
   C. To-do lists
   D. Organizational skills

8. A _____ is a drawing that depicts what an individual or a group knows about a subject.
   A. mind map
   B. learning log
   C. partnered reading
   D. habit

9. A _____ is a list of tasks to be completed in a given time period; items are crossed off as they are completed.
   A. learning log
   B. mind map
   C. to-do list
   D. study list

10. Learning logs are a _____ study strategy.
    A. writing
    B. verbal
    C. reading
    D. mathematical

11. Developing additional study skills will help you be more efficient with your time.
    A. True
    B. False

12. Good study habits are like riding a bicycle; you will never forget them.
    A. True
    B. False

13. When setting goals, it is important to set goals we do not think we can ever achieve. This is to keep our goals challenging.
    A. True
    B. False

Copyright © 2010, 2005 by Saunders, an imprint of Elsevier, Inc. All rights reserved.

14. _____ is a process in which we decide which situations require the most attention, and then list each in descending order of importance.
    A. Goal setting
    B. Prioritizing
    C. Creating to-do lists
    D. Venn diagramming

15. When setting priorities, a "Want to Do" item is also classified as a Priority _____.
    A. "A"
    B. "B"
    C. "C"
    D. "D"

16. During study time, effective breaks could include *all* of the following *except* _____.
    A. exercise
    B. water
    C. fresh air
    D. television programs

17. Short-term memory can hold information for approximately _____.
    A. 15 to 20 seconds
    B. 2 minutes
    C. 15 to 20 minutes
    D. 2 days

18. Short-term memory can typically hold _____ pieces, or "chunks," of information.
    A. 2
    B. 4
    C. 7
    D. 12

19. Paying attention to the format of the textbook can give you important clues about the main points and concepts you need to understand. Which one of the following is *not* something to which you should pay attention?
    A. Text boxes
    B. Objectives
    C. Print that is underlined, boldfaced, or italicized
    D. Page numbers

20. Which one of the following is *not* a method of actively reading?
    A. Taking notes
    B. Reading aloud
    C. Reading silently
    D. Telling someone else about what you have read

2 Becoming a Professional

VOCABULARY REVIEW

Matching: Match each term with the correct definition.

A. AAMA

B. ABHES

C. AMT

D. CAAHEP

E. clinical

F. competence

G. confidential

H. dexterity

I. diplomacy

J. empathy

K. ethical standards

L. integrity

M. professional

N. revalidation

O. tactful

_____ 1. Acting with sensitivity when dealing with people

_____ 2. Accrediting Bureau of Health Education Schools

_____ 3. Understanding how someone else feels by placing yourself in his or her place

_____ 4. Private

_____ 5. American Association of Medical Assistants

_____ 6. Ability to be tactful

_____ 7. Having to do with hands-on patient care

_____ 8. Person who conforms to the technical and ethical standards of a profession

_____ 9. Proficiency in identified skills

_____ 10. American Medical Technologists organization

_____ 11. Recertification

_____ 12. Commission on Accreditation of Allied Health Education Programs

_____ 13. Ability to move with skill and ease

_____ 14. Guidelines for professional decisions and conduct

_____ 15. Quality of being honest and straightforward

Copyright © 2010, 2005 by Saunders, an imprint of Elsevier, Inc. All rights reserved.

THEORY RECALL

True/False

Indicate whether the statement is true or false.

_____ 1. A professional is someone who displays positive characteristics and demonstrates competence when performing tasks.

_____ 2. First impressions often take a few hours.

_____ 3. The American Association of Medical Assistants and the American Medical Technologists are nationally recognized associations for medical assistant participation and for credentialing opportunities.

_____ 4. A person who has integrity is dishonest and deceitful.

_____ 5. Reliability means that you do your job well, and that others can rely on you.

Multiple Choice

Identify the letter of the choice that best completes the statement or answers the question.

1. Being a dependable employee includes all of the following characteristics *except* _____.
   A. deceitfulness
   B. punctuality
   C. efficiency
   D. reliability

2. Giving that "extra push" to get the job done in any situation exhibits _____.
   A. loyalty
   B. punctuality
   C. efficiency
   D. reliability

3. Being capable of looking at the "big picture" demonstrates _____.
   A. dependability
   B. empathy
   C. a positive attitude
   D. diplomacy

4. _____ helps build good relationships between people through tact and empathy.
   A. Compromise
   B. Diplomacy
   C. Confidentiality
   D. Consensus

5. A person who has _____ is honest and straightforward.
   A. integrity
   B. compassion
   C. empathy
   D. consensus

6. _____ is the ability to get things done on time and correctly.
   A. Compassion
   B. Competence
   C. Dexterity
   D. Loyalty

7. The ability to move with skill and ease is called _____.
   A. sympathy
   B. discretion
   C. trustworthiness
   D. dexterity

8. _____ is an appropriate way to greet patients and co-workers.
   A. Reservedly
   B. Compassionately
   C. Smiling
   D. Tersely

9. Your _____ can influence people's final opinion of you as a medical assistant.
   A. nonverbal communication skills
   B. personal appearance
   C. confidence
   D. all of the above

10. One advantage of a career in medical assisting is the _____ in administrative and clinical skills.
    A. lack of training
    B. cross-training
    C. limited training
    D. superficial training

11. There are many types of training programs for medical assistants, and they vary in length. Some training programs have gone through a process of _____, establishing standards and guidelines for postsecondary education.
    A. counseling
    B. peer review
    C. accreditation
    D. audit

12. Some states require that medical assistants _____ with their state for a small fee.
    A. register
    B. certify
    C. file an endorsement
    D. declare loyalty

13. The American Medical Technologists credential for medical assistants is _____.
    A. AAMA
    B. CMA
    C. AMT
    D. RMA

14. All medical assistants practice under a physician's direct supervision nationwide whether or not they have received a(n) _____.
    A. letter of recognition
    B. statement of intent
    C. assignment
    D. credential

Copyright © 2010, 2005 by Saunders, an imprint of Elsevier, Inc. All rights reserved.

16 CHAPTER 2 Becoming a Professional

15. Confidentiality is a key element of _____.
    A. competency
    B. integrity
    C. diplomacy
    D. loyalty

16. The ability of a medical assistant to adjust to change, set goals, and be a team player reflects _____.
    A. competence
    B. integrity
    C. positive attitude
    D. diplomacy

17. The certified medical assistant must revalidate his or her credentials every _____ year(s) by either examination or continuing education.
    A. 1
    B. 3
    C. 5
    D. 7

18. Making ethical decisions demonstrates _____.
    A. confidence
    B. diplomacy
    C. loyalty
    D. integrity

19. The RMA examination is offered all over the United States at testing sites _____.
    A. when an appointment has been scheduled
    B. monthly
    C. three times a year
    D. five times a year

20. The credentialing examinations for medical assistants are _____ to work in the profession.
    A. voluntary, not required,
    B. voluntary, required,
    C. mandated, not required,
    D. mandated, required,

Sentence Completion

Complete each sentence or statement.

diplomacy	certification	dependable
reliability	ethically	integrity
ethical statutes	ethical standards	
continuing education	confidentiality	

1. _____ is a term used to describe education after a credential is received.

2. _____ means that you do your job well, and that others can count on you.

3. Professionals are expected to behave according to the _____ of their chosen profession.

4. Many employers would not hire a person who has a reputation for not being _____.

5. Integrity is _____ doing the right thing, even when it is difficult. It means choosing to do what is right for all people even though it may not be what you personally want to do.

Short Answers

1. List six characteristics of a professional medical assistant, and briefly describe the importance of each.

2. State 10 things you can do to have a professional appearance at work.

3. Explain the importance of maintaining professional competence through continuing education other than recertification of credentials.

4. List four administrative duties and four clinical duties of a medical assistant.

CRITICAL THINKING

1. Susan has been working for Dr. Howard as an extern for the past 2 weeks. She is hoping that she will be given the opportunity to work at the clinic on completion of her hours. She enjoys the patients; the staff is incredible and has been so helpful. Dr. Howard has allowed Susan to assist with almost every procedure, and always finds her when something "interesting" occurs.

   A. If you were Dr. Howard, what traits would you look for in an employee?

   B. What professional characteristics do you think Susan possesses?

   C. Do you think that Dr. Howard values the job Susan is doing? If so, what gives you that impression?

   D. What would you do if you were in Susan's place?

PRACTICAL APPLICATIONS

If you have accomplished the objectives in this chapter, you will be able to make better choices as a medical assistant. Take a look at this situation and decide what you would do.

Robert is a medical assistant in a medical office. His responsibility is to draw blood samples at 8:00 A.M., but he often does not show up until 8:15 A.M. or later. The scheduled patients must wait and be late for work or must reschedule their appointment. When Robert does arrive, often his uniform is blood-stained and wrinkled, and he has not shaved or bathed before coming to work. Even if another staff member has started drawing blood, the daily operation of the office is already behind schedule. Robert also has a habit of taking a break between patients.

As the office slips even further behind with more patients waiting, Robert draws the blood, but does not take time to label the tubes with the patient's name or complete the laboratory request forms. When Robert makes mistakes, the office staff must make the corrections, resulting in even more delays and confusion about which tube of blood belongs to which patient.

One day Robert is sick and stays home, but does not call the office. By 8:30 A.M., patients have filled the waiting room, and patients coming to see the physicians have no place to sit. The office has insufficient staff, and the patients and the office personnel are stressed.

Robert's lack of professionalism is affecting patients and staff. What would you do differently from Robert?

1. **Medical assistants who are respected for their professionalism have certain personality characteristics. Which of these characteristics is Robert lacking? How is Robert's lack of professionalism affecting patients? How is it affecting co-workers? How is it affecting the office as a whole?**

   _____
   _____
   _____
   _____

2. **If you were a patient in this office, how would you feel if Robert was going to draw your blood?**

   _____
   _____
   _____
   _____

3. **How could Robert be liable for mislabeling blood samples?**

   _____
   _____
   _____
   _____

Copyright © 2010, 2005 by Saunders, an imprint of Elsevier, Inc. All rights reserved.

4. What actions have shown that Robert does not meet the ethical standards of a medical assistant?

5. How does the daily schedule fall behind in a medical office? Who is affected by this? What other potential problems and mistakes can you think of that might occur as a result of Robert being late?

6. If you were Robert's immediate supervisor, what would you say to Robert? How would you help him meet the professional and ethical standards expected of a medical assistant? What are some things he can do to arrive at work on time?

APPLICATION OF SKILLS

1. Have you ever completed a customer satisfaction survey? In health care, the patients will be your customers. If you were employed right now, how would your physician-employer and patients score your professional qualities? Complete the checklist provided and review with your instructor. Professional qualities must be evaluated constantly and developed further while in the classroom. Your instructors will use these tools to evaluate your progress during your schooling.

2. Describe one time when you were treated unprofessionally and one time when you were treated professionally by a service provider. Identify specific behaviors, how you felt as the recipient of such behavior, how you handled the situation, and, in the case of unprofessional behavior, what could have been done to improve the service.

3. Begin to gather information for your resume by providing information to the following headings:

    - Career Objective:

- Education:

  _____

  _____

- Skills and Capabilities:

  _____

  _____

- Strengths:

  _____

  _____

- Achievements or Accomplishments:

  _____

  _____

- Community Activities:

  _____

  _____

- Professional Organizations:

  _____

  _____

- Employment Experience:

  _____

  _____

CHAPTER QUIZ

Multiple Choice

Identify the letter of the choice that best completes the statement or answers the question.

1. "_____" describes having to do with general front office and financial activities.
   A. Clinical
   B. Administrative
   C. Ambulatory
   D. Theoretical

2. Proficiency in identified skills is called _____.
   A. empathy
   B. dexterity
   C. competence
   D. integrity

3. The ability to be on time is _____.
   A. punctuality
   B. reliability
   C. revalidation
   D. diplomacy

4. A person who displays certain positive characteristics and demonstrates competence when performing tasks is thought of as (a) _____.
   A. dexterous
   B. diplomatic
   C. professional
   D. good Samaritan

5. You are _____ when you perform your tasks on time and accurately, to the best of your ability.
   A. ethical
   B. punctual
   C. dependable
   D. loyal

6. Supporting team leaders and members by accepting decisions and behaving according to the ethics of the profession demonstrates _____.
   A. empathy
   B. compassion
   C. punctuality
   D. loyalty

7. Over time, as you prove you are dependable, competent, and _____, the employer will become more loyal to you as an employee.
   A. private
   B. likable
   C. trustworthy
   D. outspoken

8. Which one of the following is *not* a quality of a professional with a positive attitude?
   A. Flexible
   B. Goal-oriented
   C. Enthusiastic
   D. Fanatical

9. Wearing excessive jewelry to work as a medical assistant is unacceptable because it _____.
   A. can injure patients
   B. distracts co-workers and patients
   C. harbors pathogens
   D. A and C

10. A(n) _____ is a title that signifies a person has attained certain competency standards.
    A. credential
    B. associate degree
    C. diploma
    D. letter of recommendation

11. When taking a certification examination, select answers that are _____ centered.
    A. medical assistant
    B. nursing
    C. physician
    D. patient

12. The CMA examination consists of 200 questions within each of the following areas *except* _____.
    A. general
    B. laboratory
    C. administrative
    D. clinical

13. One advantage of a career in medical assisting is _____ in administrative and clinical duties.
    A. ambulatory training
    B. surgical training
    C. cross-training
    D. political training

14. _____ are (is) guideline(s) for professional decisions and conduct.
    A. Diplomatic standards
    B. Recertification
    C. Ethical standards
    D. Consensus standards

15. To make a decision based on mutual agreement is _____.
    A. to compromise
    B. to use tact
    C. to use revalidation
    D. to be efficient

16. A(n) _____ passes a certification examination with an accredited certifying agency.
    A. CAAHEP
    B. AMA
    C. MAT
    D. RMA

17. Formal training is a requirement for employment as a medical assistant.
    A. True
    B. False

18. One way to promote professionalism is by joining your professional organization and becoming credentialed after taking an examination.
    A. True
    B. False

19. All medical assistants practice under a physician's direct supervision nationwide whether or not they have received a credential.
    A. True
    B. False

20. Even though you are a member of a professional organization, you will not always have a voice in public policy concerning the practice of medical assisting.
    A. True
    B. False

Copyright © 2010, 2005 by Saunders, an imprint of Elsevier, Inc. All rights reserved.

3 Diversity in Health Care Delivery

VOCABULARY REVIEW

Matching: Match each term with the correct definition.

A. corporation

B. diversity

C. entity

D. group practice

E. management service organization (MSO)

F. partnership

G. sole proprietorship

H. specialization

_____ 1. Particular type of business

_____ 2. Business owned by one person who is legally responsible for the debts and taxes of the business

_____ 3. Large business entity that has incorporated to avoid personal liability from the company's debts and taxes

_____ 4. Occurs when additional training and educational requirements have been met in a specific area of medicine

_____ 5. Having a variety of skills or types

_____ 6. Organization (e.g., hospital) that handles patient services (e.g., billing and payment services) for a medical practice

_____ 7. Business owned by two people who are held legally responsible for the debts and taxes of the business

_____ 8. Practice that is owned by three or more people who are held legally responsible for the debts and taxes of the business

THEORY RECALL

True/False

Indicate whether the statement is true or false.

_____ 1. In corporate practices that are handled by an MSO, the physician is technically an employee of the MSO.

_____ 2. Most medical practices today are sole proprietorships.

_____ 3. Nationally, many physicians are general practitioners.

_____ 4. A specialist is a physician who has completed additional training and educational requirements.

_____ 5. Hippocrates is known as the "Father of Inventions."

Multiple Choice

Identify the letter of the choice that best completes the statement or answers the question.

1. The health care team member solely responsible for diagnosing and treating patients is a _____.
   A. certified medical assistant
   B. physician
   C. certified nursing assistant
   D. registered nurse

2. The medical specialty that provides treatment for patients with heart and vascular disease is _____.
   A. internal medicine
   B. emergency medicine
   C. aerospace medicine
   D. cardiology

3. A(n) _____ treats disorders of the female reproductive system.
   A. gynecologist
   B. dermatologist
   C. obstetrician
   D. urologist

4. A(n) _____ treats diseases with the use of radionuclides.
   A. aerospace medical specialist
   B. radiologist
   C. nuclear medicine specialist
   D. nephrologist

5. Holistic treatment that focuses on disease prevention and natural treatments is called _____.
   A. nuclear medicine
   B. naturopathy
   C. naprapathy
   D. neurology

6. The field of _____ involves the treatment of myofascial disorders.
   A. chiropractic medicine
   B. orthopedic medicine
   C. naprapathy
   D. naturopathy

7. A(n) _____ provides inpatient care and treatment for acute conditions.
   A. home health care agency
   B. hospice
   C. hospital
   D. assisted living facility

8. A(n) _____ provides 24-hour-a-day nursing services to individuals who are unable to function on their own on a long-term basis.
   A. ambulatory surgery center
   B. assisted living center
   C. skilled nursing home
   D. hospice

9. A _____ is a practice owned by one person who is legally responsible for the debts and taxes of the business.
   A. partnership
   B. group practice
   C. sole proprietorship
   D. corporate practice

10. Physicians are considered board certified after they have _____.
    A. completed additional training and examination by the board of their specialty
    B. performed 3 years of additional training and 2 years of board certification training
    C. completed a state registry examination and performed 2 years of board certification training
    D. performed 2 years of board certification training only

Sentence Completion

Complete each sentence or statement.

medical assistant	dermatologist
AAMA	obstetrician
AMA	infertility specialist
JCAHO (The Joint Commission)	allergist
urologist	optometrist

1. A(n) _____ is a multiskilled professional who is knowledgeable about administrative and clinical procedures.

2. _____ is a not-for-profit organization that is responsible for promoting specific improvements in patient safety.

3. A(n) _____ treats diseases of the skin.

4. A(n) _____ treats problems of conception and maintaining pregnancy.

5. A(n) _____ tests vision and prepares lenses to correct refractive problems.

Short Answers

1. Explain the importance of being knowledgeable about the various health care delivery settings in your community.

   _____
   _____
   _____
   _____

2. List seven health care delivery settings other than a medical office.

   _____
   _____
   _____
   _____

3. Describe the differences between a long-term care facility and a short-term care facility.

   _____
   _____
   _____

4. Explain the difference between a group practice and a corporation.

   _____
   _____
   _____
   _____

CRITICAL THINKING

1. Janet has been studying the different types of medical practices in her medical assistant program. She never realized there were so many different specialties. Janet has seen the same family physician from the time she was born for everything from tonsillitis to her yearly physicals. She always thought she would work for a general practitioner when she graduated, but now she is unsure. She has enjoyed studying the cardiovascular system and thinks working for a cardiologist might be interesting. She also has been intrigued with naturopathy and maybe emergency medicine. She could go back to school after she graduates and obtain her RN degree and become a flight nurse.

   A. What suggestions do you have for Janet?

   _____

   _____

   B. How can she learn more about each specialty?

   _____

   _____

2. What specialties are you considering for employment? (List a minimum of two specialties.)

   _____

   _____

   _____

   _____

3. Describe why you believe you may be suited for the specialties you are considering.

   _____

   _____

   _____

   _____

4. If you are unsure of the type of practice you would like to pursue for employment, what steps can you take to narrow your choices?

   _____

   _____

   _____

   _____

PRACTICAL APPLICATIONS

If you have accomplished the objectives in this chapter, you will be able to make better choices as a medical assistant. Take a look at this situation and decide what you would do.

Jade is a recent graduate of a medical assisting program. She is looking for a job that fits her credentials. She has not taken the credentialing examinations for medical assisting and has not had any experience in the medical field except her externship in a pediatric clinic.

Jade finds two ads in the local paper for a medical assistant. One ad specifically asks for a certified medical assistant for a group practice in a management service organization. The other ad asks for a medical assistant for a solo practice for an internist; no medical assisting credentials are specified, but applicants should have experience appropriate to the internal medicine setting. In the solo practice, Jade would be the only clinical employee for the practice. Jade decides to apply for both positions. Jade thinks that the job of a medical assistant is the same in each setting, and that she is prepared for both employment opportunities.

While reading the same paper, Jade also sees an ad for a nurse for a physician partnership in obstetrics-gynecology. She decides to apply for this position as well.

What advice would you give Jade if she asked for your input?

1. Does Jade have the credentials for these employment opportunities? If so, which ones? If not, why are some or all inappropriate?

   _____

   _____

   _____

2. What advantages would a new graduate have in a group practice rather than a solo practice in which he or she is the only clinical medical assistant? What experiences should Jade expect to find in each setting? What are the advantages and disadvantages of each?

   _____

   _____

   _____

3. Should Jade assume that she could take a nursing position? What are the implications of using that title? In what scope of practice does the title "nurse" place Jade?

   _____

   _____

   _____

4. What would be the legal implications for the physicians in each setting if Jade is hired?

   _____

   _____

   _____

Copyright © 2010, 2005 by Saunders, an imprint of Elsevier, Inc. All rights reserved.

5. What influence could Jade have on the community's perception of the physician's abilities or the scope of practice if she does not understand her own abilities and scope of training? Would her scope of practice have any effect on the physician's office? If so, how?

6. Is the physician legally responsible for Jade's actions? Explain why or why not.

APPLICATION OF SKILLS

1. Contact a health care facility in your area. Ask and then answer the following questions.

   A. What type of business entity is the facility?

   B. What types of health care providers compose the health care team?

   C. What is the name, address, and telephone number of the medical practice?

   D. What are the hours of operation?

   E. What is the practice's specialty?

   F. How many years has the practice been in operation?

CHAPTER QUIZ

Multiple Choice

Identify the letter of the choice that best completes the statement or answers the question.

1. A _____ can perform certain procedures under the supervision of a physician, examine and treat patients, order and interpret laboratory tests and radiographs, and make diagnoses.
    A. registered nurse
    B. physician assistant
    C. certified medical assistant
    D. licensed practical nurse

2. A(n) _____ provides services and assistance to people who require minimal help, such as cooking, laundry, and help with medications.
    A. hospice
    B. home health agency
    C. ambulatory surgery center
    D. assisted living facility

3. A(n) _____ assists and meets the needs of terminally ill patients and their families.
    A. hospice
    B. home health agency
    C. ambulatory surgery center
    D. assisted living facility

4. A(n) _____ is *not* a type of medical practice setting.
    A. independent contractor
    B. sole proprietorship
    C. partnership
    D. corporate practice

5. _____ treat all patients, from the newborn to the elderly.
    A. Internists
    B. Gerontologists
    C. Family practitioners
    D. Pediatricians

6. A(n) _____ requires a license to work.
    A. certified medical assistant
    B. registered nurse
    C. insurance specialist
    D. phlebotomy technician

7. Advantages of a _____ practice are the greater potential for profit; shared decision making; and shared facilities, equipment, and employees.
    A. private
    B. partnership
    C. group
    D. corporate

8. The liability of a _____ practice includes being responsible for all debts of the practice.
   A. private
   B. partnership
   C. group
   D. corporate

9. A _____ medical practice has more than three practitioners and several employees.
   A. private
   B. partnership
   C. group
   D. corporate

10. During surgery, this practitioner administers and maintains the medications given to the patient to keep him or her unconscious during the procedure.
    A. Immunologist
    B. Hematologist
    C. Anesthesiologist
    D. Oncologist

11. A(n) _____ treats conditions and disorders of the male reproductive system.
    A. urologist
    B. gynecologist
    C. oncologist
    D. neurologist

12. A(n) _____ treats disorders of the eyes.
    A. optician
    B. ophthalmologist
    C. neurologist
    D. optometrist

13. A(n) _____ counsels patients with stress or emotion-related disorders.
    A. neurologist
    B. psychologist
    C. physiologist
    D. psychiatrist

14. A(n) _____ examines tissue samples for signs of disease.
    A. pathologist
    B. oncologist
    C. internist
    D. radiologist

15. A(n) _____ treats diseases and disorders of the teeth and gums.
    A. oral surgeon
    B. orthodontist
    C. dental hygienist
    D. dentist

16. A _____ treats the patient through manipulation of the spine to relieve musculoskeletal disorders.
    A. certified medical assistant
    B. family practitioner
    C. chiropractor
    D. podiatrist

17. Which one of the following does *not* need a 4-year degree to practice their profession?
    A. MD
    B. DPM
    C. DO
    D. CMA

18. A _____ is a health care professional who works in a laboratory and performs venipunctures.
    A. radiology technician
    B. pharmacy technician
    C. phlebotomy technician
    D. histology technician

19. In a _____, the practice ends when the owner dies or closes the practice.
    A. sole proprietorship
    B. corporate practice
    C. group practice
    D. partnership

20. A(n) _____ treats disorders of the blood.
    A. anesthesiologist
    B. hematologist
    C. cardiologist
    D. internist

4 Law and Ethics in Health Care

VOCABULARY REVIEW

Matching: Match each term with the correct definition.

A. age of majority

B. contract

C. damages

D. euthanasia

E. Good Samaritan Act

F. infraction

G. noncompliance

H. reciprocity

I. subpoena

J. vicarious liability

_____ 1. Liability of an employer for the wrongdoing of an employee while on the job

_____ 2. Legislation that provides protection from lawsuits for an individual providing lifesaving or emergency treatment

_____ 3. Occurs when one state accepts another state's licensing requirements

_____ 4. Failure of a patient to comply with the physician's treatment plan; grounds for dismissal of a patient from a practice

_____ 5. Person who is considered by law to have acquired all the rights and responsibilities of an adult (age 18 in most states)

_____ 6. Payment used to compensate for physical injury, damaged property, or a loss of personal freedom; or used as a punishment

_____ 7. Violation of a law, resulting in a fine

_____ 8. Legal document that requires a person to appear in court or be available for a deposition

_____ 9. Intentional ending of life for a terminally ill patient

_____ 10. Agreement between two or more persons resulting in a consideration

THEORY RECALL

True/False

Indicate whether the statement is true or false.

_____ 1. Certification is the strongest form of professional regulation because it is a legal document.

_____ 2. Under the "Good Samaritan Act," implied consent applies if no one is available to consent for the patient, and if a "reasonable" person would consent under similar circumstances.

_____ 3. Under the Uniform Anatomical Gift Act, incompetent individuals may donate their body or body parts after they die.

_____ 4. Confidentiality breaches occur most often as a result of carelessness in elevators or hallways and over lunches in medical facilities.

_____ 5. It is the medical assistant's responsibility to know the laws and to follow them to the letter.

_____ 6. Information about a patient can be shared with another health care team member when it is directly related to the patient's treatments.

_____ 7. HIPAA bans the calling of a patient's name in the waiting room.

Multiple Choice

Identify the letter of the choice that best completes the statement or answers the question.

1. The failure to make arrangements for a patient's medical coverage is termed _____.
   A. battery
   B. gross negligence
   C. abandonment
   D. implied contract

2. _____ is a written form of defamation.
   A. Libel
   B. Felony
   C. Slander
   D. Misfeasance

3. _____ is the performance of an unlawful act causing harm.
   A. Abandonment
   B. Malfeasance
   C. Misfeasance
   D. *Quid pro quo*

4. A branch of law that deals with offenses or crimes against the welfare or safety of the public is _____.
   A. public law
   B. administrative law
   C. criminal law
   D. international law

Copyright © 2010, 2005 by Saunders, an imprint of Elsevier, Inc. All rights reserved.

5. _____ is the science of understanding the complete genetic inheritance of an organism.
   A. Fiduciary
   B. Naturopathy
   C. Naprapathy
   D. Genomics

6. The document that was formulated by the American Hospital Association in 2001 that provides information concerning expectations, rights, and responsibilities of patients is the _____.
   A. Patient Care Partnership
   B. Patient Rights Contract
   C. Private law
   D. Good Samaritan Act

7. Which one of the following is *not* a means of obtaining licensure?
   A. Examination
   B. On-the-job training
   C. Reciprocity
   D. Endorsement

8. Physicians are required to renew their license every _____ years.
   A. 2
   B. 3
   C. 4
   D. 5

9. The doctrine _____ places the liability on the physician for his or her employee's actions.
   A. *quid pro quo*
   B. *res ipsa loquitur*
   C. *respondeat superior*
   D. *subpoena duces tecum*

10. _____ is a voluntary process that professionals can go through to earn certification and other proof of their knowledge and skills.
    A. Endorsement
    B. Reciprocity
    C. Continuing education
    D. Credentialing

11. _____ deals with the rights and responsibilities of the government to the people and the people to the government.
    A. Administrative law
    B. Public law
    C. Criminal law
    D. Civil law

12. A(n) _____ is one that is specifically stated aloud or written and is understood by all parties.
    A. implied contract
    B. illegal contract
    C. breach of contract
    D. expressed contract

13. A(n) _____ is a negligent, wrongful act committed by a person against another person or property that causes harm.
    A. tort
    B. implied contract
    C. slander
    D. fiduciary

14. A threat or the perceived threat of doing bodily harm by another person is _____.
    A. slander
    B. libel
    C. assault
    D. battery

15. Ordinary _____ is not doing (or doing) something that a reasonable person would do (or would not do).
    A. negligence
    B. malfeasance
    C. misfeasance
    D. nonfeasance

16. _____ is the failure to do what is expected, resulting in harm to the patient.
    A. Negligence
    B. Malfeasance
    C. Misfeasance
    D. Nonfeasance

17. Which one of the following is *not* a component that must be present before an attorney pursues a case for professional negligence?
    A. Duty
    B. Dereliction of duty
    C. Direct cause or proximate cause
    D. Payment for services rendered

18. The _____ of 1990 requires health care institutions to give patients written information about advance directives before life-sustaining measures become necessary.
    A. Patient Bill of Rights
    B. Patient Care Partnership
    C. Patient Self-Determination Act
    D. Uniform Anatomical Act

19. The _____ provides guidelines for collecting money owed.
    A. Bankruptcy Act
    B. Fair Debt Collection Practices Act
    C. Consumer Debt Act
    D. Occupational Safety and Health Act

20. The phrase _____ refers to "this for that" or the "something for something" issues that may occur in the workplace.
    A. *quid pro quo*
    B. *res ipsa loquitur*
    C. *respondeat superior*
    D. *subpoena duces tecum*

CHAPTER 4 Law and Ethics in Health Care

Sentence Completion

Complete each sentence or statement.

contract	tort
statute	vital statistics
Occupational Safety and Health Administration (OSHA)	material safety data sheets (MSDS)
	workers' compensation
felony	insurance
emancipated minor	infraction
agreement	American Medical Association (AMA)

1. A(n) _____ is an agreement between two or more people promising to work toward a specific goal for adequate consideration.

2. A(n) _____ is an underage person who has legally separated from parents for various reasons and is legally capable of consent to treatment.

3. All states require the reporting of _____ including births, deaths, and communicable diseases.

4. Each chemical used on the job must have a(n) _____ from the manufacturer on file.

5. Employers, by law, must carry _____. This plan covers medical care and rehabilitation costs, and offers temporary or permanent pay for the injured employee.

6. The Council on Ethical and Judicial Affairs (CEJA) develops ethics policy for the _____.

Short Answers

1. List three bioethical situations and briefly explain the considerations for each.

_____

_____

_____

_____

_____

2. Explain the purpose of the ADA Amendments Act of 2008 and the National Childhood Vaccine Injury Act of 1986. (Conduct a Web search for the latest information.)

3. Create a scenario involving a breach of confidentiality that might occur in a medical office.

4. Compare and contrast licensure and certification.

5. Describe the purpose of the Medical Practice Acts.

6. What does it mean to practice within your scope of training? How is a medical assistant's standard of care different from a physician's?

7. What is the Stark Law? How does it apply to the medical office? (Conduct a Web search.)

CRITICAL THINKING

1. On externship, Terry overheard two employees of the medical clinic discussing the specifics of a patient's case in the clinic's break room. The comment that caught Terry's attention was that the patient had been physically abused by her spouse. Terry knew this patient personally; the patient was married to Terry's cousin. Terry could not believe what she had overheard and was appalled that the medical assistants would be making such claims.

   A. Did the two employees in the medical clinic breach confidentiality?

   B. Should Terry say anything to the patient or to her cousin?

   C. Legally and ethically, did the two employees violate any laws or regulations? If so, what are the violations?

   D. What would you do if you were in Terry's place?

PRACTICAL APPLICATIONS

If you have accomplished the objectives in this chapter, you will be able to make better choices as a medical assistant. Take a look at this situation and decide what you would do.

Jill is a medical assistant with on-the-job training in a medical office setting. She always strives to be caring, courteous, and respectful of patients and co-workers. Because of her caring attitude, the patients with whom Jill works all appreciate her attitude and her work. One of Jill's favorite patients, Shandra, a 24-year-old mother of two young children, has been diagnosed with cancer and recently was told by the

Copyright © 2010, 2005 by Saunders, an imprint of Elsevier, Inc. All rights reserved.

physician that her condition is terminal. Shandra is at the office for an appointment; feeling very upset about her terminal illness, she pours out her feelings and fears to Jill. Wanting to comfort Shandra, Jill tells her, "Don't worry. You'll be just fine. You know the doctor will make you better."

Shandra is comforted by her words and tells Jill how much she means to her. Shandra has so much faith in Jill that she believes that she will be fine and tells her family what Jill has said. A few months later, Shandra dies. Believing she would be fine, Shandra had not made any plans for her children and family. Her family is upset with the physician and with Jill. The family thinks they have been betrayed because they believed that Shandra would be fine. The family is discussing what to say to the physician about this betrayal and whether to bring a lawsuit because Shandra did not have a will.

How might this situation have been avoided? What are the possible implications for Shandra's family, Jill, the physician, and the practice?

1. **Jill has been trained on the job and is uncredentialed. What are the disadvantages to Jill of not having a formal medical assisting education? Would having credentialing and an education make a difference in what Jill said to Shandra?**

2. **Would credentialing make a difference if Shandra's family decides to bring a lawsuit? If so, what are the benefits to the physician if the medical assistant is credentialed?**

3. **Why was it important for Shandra to have an advance directive?**

4. **What are the legal ramifications of Jill telling Shandra not to worry and that she would be fine? What ethical guidelines should be considered in this situation? Did Jill do something illegal, something unethical, neither, or both? Explain why or why not.**

Copyright © 2010, 2005 by Saunders, an imprint of Elsevier, Inc. All rights reserved.

APPLICATION OF SKILLS

1. Contact your local Public Health Department and request a list of reportable diseases in your area and state. Conduct a Web search using the key words "reportable diseases, notifiable diseases." Which diseases require mandatory written reporting? Which require mandatory reporting by telephone? Which diseases must also be reported to the CDC?

   _____

   _____

   _____

2. Clip one current newspaper, magazine, or Internet article pertaining to medical legal or ethical issues. Summarize the article by writing a paragraph describing your impression of the article and the issue's impact on the medical community. Cite the specific legal or ethical implications.

   _____

   _____

   _____

3. Complete the forms "Consent for Surgery" and "Patient Consent" on yourself. (Forms are located in the "Supplemental Chapter Materials" section at the back of this workbook.)

   _____

   _____

   _____

CHAPTER QUIZ

Multiple Choice

Identify the letter of the choice that best completes the statement or answers the question.

1. A legal document that requires a person to appear in court and bring the records is (a) _____.
   A. subpoena
   B. *res ipsa loquitur*
   C. *subpoena duces tecum*
   D. Patient Bill of Rights

2. A legal document that allows a person to offer their skills and knowledge to the public for compensation is a(n) _____.
   A. certification
   B. license
   C. MSDS
   D. diploma

3. The intentional act of touching another person in a socially unacceptable manner without their consent is called _____.
   A. libel
   B. breach of duty
   C. battery
   D. assault

Copyright © 2010, 2005 by Saunders, an imprint of Elsevier, Inc. All rights reserved.

4. _____ is legislation that regulates patients' rights and federal regulation that mandates the protection of privacy and holds information to be confidential.
   A. Health Insurance Portability and Accountability Act
   B. Patient Care Partnership Act
   C. Standard of Care Act
   D. Good Samaritan Act

5. A person of trusted responsibility is a(n) _____.
   A. emancipated minor
   B. fiduciary
   C. dependent
   D. custodian

6. Laws, or _____, are general rules and standards designed to regulate conduct.
   A. torts
   B. medical practice acts
   C. rights
   D. statutes

7. _____ regulates business practices.
   A. Private law
   B. Partnership law
   C. Administrative law
   D. Public law

8. Not making arrangements for a substitute physician to take patient calls if the physician is unavailable could be grounds for a lawsuit and termed as _____.
   A. misfeasance
   B. battery
   C. breach of contract
   D. abandonment

9. For there to be a valid physician-patient contract, the patient must meet or perform all of the following except _____.
   A. truthfully disclose past and present medical information
   B. having reached the age of 14 years old
   C. take all medications
   D. be responsible with an appropriate reimbursement plan

10. For a physician to withdraw from patient care, all of the following must be achieved except _____.
    A. notify the patient in writing
    B. give a date when this is to take effect (minimum of 30 days)
    C. provide a personal telephone call from the physician
    D. provide for transfer of medical records

11. A(n) _____ contract is one that is specifically stated aloud or written and is understood by all parties.
    A. expressed
    B. implied
    C. invalid
    D. assumed

12. A _____ is a negligent, wrongful act committed by a person against another person or property that causes harm.
    A. fiduciary
    B. tort
    C. liability
    D. fraud

13. _____ is intentional negligence, or a wrongful act done (or not done) on purpose.
    A. Malfeasance
    B. Minor negligence
    C. Gross negligence
    D. Nonfeasance

14. _____ is defamation of character in writing.
    A. Slander
    B. Battery
    C. Libel
    D. Assault

15. If a patient were to receive a burn during ultrasound therapy, the charge may be _____.
    A. misfeasance
    B. malfeasance
    C. nonfeasance
    D. none of the above

16. _____ occurs when a health care professional fails to meet accepted standards of care.
    A. Breach of contract
    B. Dereliction of duty
    C. Fraud
    D. All of the above

17. Each state has laws that limit the length of time a person has to take legal action. This is called the _____.
    A. duration of care
    B. expressed contractual agreement
    C. standard of care requirements
    D. statute of limitations

18. The best way to avoid a lawsuit is to _____.
    A. keep the lines of communication open
    B. listen to patient's concerns or complaints; chart the facts
    C. keep patient information confidential
    D. all of the above

19. Not providing a child with clothing for the weather could be considered _____.
    A. abandonment
    B. neglect
    C. good parenting
    D. false imprisonment

20. An employer must provide every employee with the opportunity to receive a hepatitis B vaccination. The second dose in the series of three should be given _____ after the first dose.
    A. 10 days
    B. 30 days
    C. 90 days
    D. 120 days

NAME: _____ DATE: _____

5 Understanding Human Behavior

VOCABULARY REVIEW

Matching: Match each term with the correct definition.

A. anger

B. compensation

C. defense mechanism

D. depression

E. empathy

F. homeostasis

G. perception

H. phobias

I. physiological

J. psychiatry

K. psychology

L. self-esteem

M. stress

N. subconscious

O. sympathy

_____ 1. Having to do with the body's responses to its internal and external environment

_____ 2. Filtering tactic used by the unconscious to avoid unpleasant situations

_____ 3. Understanding how someone else feels by placing yourself in his or her place

_____ 4. Body in balance

_____ 5. Reaction resulting from the feeling of loss of control

_____ 6. Feeling of self-worth

_____ 7. Body's response to any demand put on it, whether it be positive or negative

_____ 8. Individual's view of a situation based on the environment

_____ 9. Having concern for a patient's situation

_____ 10. Overall feeling of hopelessness

_____ 11. Irrational fears of objects, activities, or situations

_____ 12. Scientific study of the mind and the behavioral patterns of humans and animals

_____ 13. Defense mechanism in which a strength is emphasized to cover up a weakness in another area

_____ 14. Part of the conscious that is not fully aware

_____ 15. Medical specialty that deals with the treatment and prevention of mental illness

THEORY RECALL

True/False

Indicate whether the statement is true or false.

_____ 1. The study of human behavior helps us understand how people learn, feel emotions, and establish relationships.

_____ 2. The id is the part of the personality that is aware of reality and of the consequences of different behaviors.

_____ 3. Sigmund Freud, a German psychologist, was interested in the understanding of dreams.

_____ 4. The superego is concerned with the internalization of values and standards designed to promote proper social balance.

_____ 5. Knowing how to manage stress in the short-term provides long-term rewards.

Multiple Choice

Identify the letter of the choice that best completes the statement or answers the question.

1. Of the following statements, which response *best* describes factors that influence the development of personality?
   A. Events in early development form all of a person's personality.
   B. Psychological factors such as poverty or wealth do not contribute to an individual's personality.
   C. Genetic factors are the only true markers of personality.
   D. None of the above statements is correct.

2. In Maslow's Hierarchy of Needs, _____ needs are being met when we feel loved and appreciated.
   A. safety
   B. physical
   C. social
   D. self-actualization

3. When the _____ level of Maslow's hierarchy is achieved, an individual has a sense of being in control.
   A. physical
   B. self-esteem
   C. social
   D. self-actualization

4. _____ is the process of interpreting information gathered from our surroundings.
   A. Expectation
   B. Perception
   C. Self-esteem
   D. Consensus

5. _____ is one of the primary levels of Maslow's hierarchy.
   A. Hunger
   B. Fatigue
   C. Past experiences
   D. Age

6. _____ are (is) a psychological influence on how we perform.
   A. Senses
   B. Number of experiences
   C. Expectations
   D. Health

7. Young adults are moving from the _____ concept concerning education, job, home, and family.
   A. us to them
   B. I to we
   C. you to them
   D. them to them

8. Fear is a(n) _____ reaction to _____ danger.
   A. abnormal, perceived
   B. normal, perceived
   C. abnormal, genuine
   D. normal, genuine

9. An emotional response that alerts the body to take appropriate action to protect itself from danger is _____.
   A. fight or flight
   B. fright or freeze
   C. flee or be
   D. none of the above

10. Of the following, which is *not* a phobia category?
    A. Interference
    B. Simple
    C. Social
    D. Agoraphobia

11. _____ is the feeling of apprehension, uneasiness, or uncertainty about a situation.
    A. Fear
    B. Anxiety
    C. Phobia
    D. Stress

12. Symptoms of anxiety include all of the following *except* _____.
    A. inability to sleep
    B. self-doubt
    C. difficulty breathing
    D. direct eye contact

13. During periods of _____, our natural body defense systems weaken, fatigue takes over, and we become more susceptible to disease.
    A. fear
    B. stress
    C. anxiety
    D. elation

14. Research has proved that many _____ disorders are caused by the effects of stress.
    A. psychosomatic
    B. physiological
    C. psychiatric
    D. terminal

15. Long-term stress can cause any or all of the following disorders *except* _____.
    A. headache
    B. ulcers
    C. muscle tension
    D. hypertension

16. If a person cannot recognize a real problem or situation, or chooses not to face it head-on, a _____ may be used to cope with it.
    A. psychosomatic disorder
    B. defense mechanism
    C. phobia
    D. terminal illness

17. _____ is a defense mechanism that allows a patient to deal with the shock of death.
    A. Denial
    B. Anger
    C. Bargaining
    D. All of the above

18. _____ is the process of making deals with anyone in sight, including the physician, a higher power, and family members, when dealing with grief.
    A. Denial
    B. Anger
    C. Bargaining
    D. All of the above

19. _____ is coming to terms with dying or the loss of a loved one
    A. Denial
    B. Acceptance
    C. Depression
    D. Anger

20. Putting yourself in another person's situation is called (a) _____.
    A. defense mechanism
    B. empathy
    C. sympathy
    D. socialism

21. _____ is considered daydreaming inappropriately.
    A. Displacement
    B. Projection
    C. Fantasy
    D. Compensation

22. Inventing excuses or reasons for one's behavior is called _____.
    A. compensation
    B. rationalization
    C. repression
    D. sublimation

23. A co-worker who feels shy may talk too much or too loudly in an attempt to be seen as not shy. This is called _____.
    A. rationalization
    B. aggression
    C. displacement
    D. overcompensation

24. Physically or emotionally pulling away from people or conflict is called _____.
    A. conversion reaction
    B. sublimation
    C. withdrawal
    D. repression

25. An example of a simple phobia includes _____.
    A. fear of being ridiculed
    B. fear of snakes
    C. fear of public speaking
    D. fear of crowds

Sentence Completion

Complete each sentence or statement.

hospice	middle age	rationalization
acceptance	spiritual	anger
physical	CDC	past experiences
homeostasis	stress	
self-esteem	empathy	

1. _____ is a package of services and a team of people helping patients and their families during the last months of a terminal illness.

2. Studies have shown that if a family's psychological and _____ needs are met in addition to the treatment of the patient's disease, the dying process is less distressing for all concerned.

3. _____ is a change for many people because their children are independent and often leaving home, and a void is created.

4. We recall _____ when we perform similar tasks: "I've never been very good at it" versus "With some help, I am ready to tackle this."

5. Physical needs are met when the body is in _____.

Short Answers

1. List in order of importance for survival Maslow's Hierarchy of Needs.

   _____
   _____
   _____
   _____

2. Explain why it is important to *you* to have a good self-esteem.

   _____
   _____
   _____
   _____

3. Contrast the differences between fear, phobia, anxiety, and stress.

   _____
   _____
   _____
   _____

4. List and describe six defense mechanisms.

   _____
   _____
   _____
   _____

CRITICAL THINKING

1. Tanya was hired by Dr. Ortega, an oncologist, 2 months ago. Many of Dr. Ortega's patients are terminally ill, and four patients have passed away this week. Tanya is unsure that she can cope personally with so many terminally ill patients. Tanya's mother died of breast cancer last year, which was one of the reasons that Tanya originally wanted to work for an oncologist. After a particularly upsetting day, Dr. Ortega asked Tanya to meet with her in her office, after the last appointment of the day. Dr. Ortega asked Tanya how she is handling the loss of the patients. "It has been very difficult. I am not sure that I am working through it. We talked about death and dying in school, but other than my mother passing away from cancer last year, I have never been around anyone else who has died." Dr. Ortega and Tanya talked for a long time about ways for Tanya to work through the loss of her mother and come to terms with her overall feelings about death, and then how she can best be supportive of the clinic's patients and families. Dr. Ortega gave Tanya a list of books on death and dying to read on her own and a homework assignment to write her own obituary if she were to die tomorrow and a second one if she were to die of old age at 93. Tanya thanked Dr. Ortega for being so understanding and promised to read the books, and even though she was extremely uncomfortable with writing her own obituary, she agreed to try.

   A. Write your own obituary as if you were to die tomorrow.

   _____

   _____

   B. Write your own obituary as if you were to die of old age at 93.

   _____

   _____

PRACTICAL APPLICATIONS

If you have accomplished the objectives in this chapter, you will be able to make better choices as a medical assistant. Take a look at this situation and decide what you would do.

Sara Ann is a 22-year-old single mother and a medical assistant. She has no assistance at home with child care or with any of the chores necessary to keep up a household. Sara Ann works as many hours as she can to support herself and her two children in the best way possible. On top of all of this, going to school has added major financial problems for Sara Ann.

On many days, Sara Ann is tired and frustrated, and wonders just how she will get through the day. Because of her lack of self-esteem and the lack of help, anxiety and stress are affecting the way Sara Ann deals with co-workers. Sara Ann's anxiety level often leads her to label patients. In addition, Sara Ann has difficulty adapting to any variation in the daily schedule.

Because Sara Ann feels close to some patients with whom she has spent time in the medical office, she often discusses her personal problems with these patients. Also, Sara Ann must handle some of her personal business (banking, errands) while at work because she does not leave work early enough to do these things when the businesses are open.

Sara Ann is experiencing a lot of stress, which is having an impact on her performance at work. If you were in Sara Ann's situation, what would you do to reduce stress?

Copyright © 2010, 2005 by Saunders, an imprint of Elsevier, Inc. All rights reserved.

1. How are Sara Ann's reactions to her work understandable under the circumstances? What reactions are related to anxiety and loss of self-esteem?

2. How are Sara Ann's reactions typical for someone who is not coping with personal or professional worlds?

3. What are some of the reactions that you would expect from Sara Ann's fellow employees about her behavior?

4. Where on Maslow's Hierarchy of Needs would you place Sara Ann? Why did you place her at that level?

5. Because Sara Ann has no one at home for emotional or financial support, how would you, as a patient, feel if she told you about her problems? Are her actions of involving patients ethical? Why?

APPLICATION OF SKILLS

1. Select one defense mechanism from Table 5-5 and create a situational example of how a patient may exhibit the behaviors associated with the mechanism regarding an illness (two-paragraph minimum, single spaced).

2. Based on Maslow's Hierarchy of Needs, describe how best to respond to the following situations addressing physical and emotional needs.

   A. Angry patient: self-esteem

   _____

   _____

   _____

   B. Newly diagnosed terminal illness: safety

   _____

   _____

   _____

   C. Positive pregnancy test: survival and self-actualization

   _____

   _____

   _____

CHAPTER QUIZ

Multiple Choice

Identify the letter of the choice that best completes the statement or answers the question.

1. Coming to terms with an issue (e.g., impending death or loss) is _____.
   A. depression
   B. anxiety
   C. acceptance
   D. compensation

2. The body's response to threat is called _____.
   A. fight or flight
   B. bargaining
   C. rationalization
   D. overcompensation

3. The part of the personality that includes values and standards designed to promote proper behavior is called (the) _____.
   A. id
   B. ego
   C. superego
   D. self-esteem

4. _____ is a defense mechanism in which there is an unconscious rejection of an unacceptable thought, desire, or impulse, and placing blame on someone else.
   A. Rationalization
   B. Denial
   C. Subconscious
   D. Projection

5. The _____ is the part of the brain associated with basic unconscious biological drives.
   A. id
   B. ego
   C. superego
   D. self-esteem

6. _____ was an Austrian physician who was interested in the development of the mind to treat psychological problems.
   A. Maslow
   B. Jung
   C. Hippocrates
   D. Freud

7. _____ is a medical specialty that deals with the treatment and prevention of mental illness.
   A. Psychology
   B. Psychiatry
   C. Physiology
   D. Oncology

8. The first level of Maslow's hierarchy and the foundation of a person's motivational drive is _____.
   A. security needs
   B. social needs
   C. physical needs
   D. self-esteem

9. The need to be all that you can be is called _____.
   A. social
   B. self-esteem
   C. self-defeating
   D. self-actualization

10. Self-esteem can fluctuate throughout the day based on the challenges a person faces.
    A. True
    B. False

11. _____ is (are) the process of interpreting information gathered from our surroundings.
    A. Subconscious
    B. Perception
    C. Assumptions
    D. Past experiences

12. Physiological influences of what we sense and feel and how we perform include all of the following *except* _____.
    A. fatigue
    B. age
    C. gender
    D. senses

13. _____ are irrational fears of objects, activities, or situations.
    A. Phobias
    B. Defense mechanisms
    C. Rationalizations
    D. Psychiatric responses

14. _____ is the fear of blood.
    A. Agoraphobia
    B. Hemophobia
    C. Claustrophobia
    D. Arachnophobia

15. _____ is the fear of water.
    A. Apiphobia
    B. Hydrophobia
    C. Agoraphobia
    D. Phagophobia

16. Glossophobia is the fear of speaking in public.
    A. True
    B. False

17. Physical symptoms of stress include all of the following *except* _____.
    A. forgetfulness
    B. chronic upset stomach
    C. headaches
    D. chills or heavy sweating

18. Depression is a psychological symptom of stress.
    A. True
    B. False

19. Behaving aggressively toward someone who cannot fight back as a substitute for anger toward the source of frustration is called _____.
    A. compensation
    B. displacement
    C. fantasy
    D. projection

20. Exaggerated and inappropriate behavior of a person in one area to handle inadequacy in some other area is called _____.
    A. aggression
    B. intellectualization
    C. sublimation
    D. overcompensation

Copyright © 2010, 2005 by Saunders, an imprint of Elsevier, Inc. All rights reserved.

6 Understanding Patient Behavior

VOCABULARY REVIEW

Matching: Match each term with the correct definition.

A. adulthood

B. childhood

C. cultural diversity

D. infancy

E. mental growth

F. physical growth

G. psychosocial growth

H. development

I. adolescence

J. heredity

_____ 1. Part of the human life span including birth through the first year

_____ 2. Individual's emotional and social development

_____ 3. Individual's cognitive development

_____ 4. Part of the human life span concerned with an individual during early, middle, and later years in life

_____ 5. Mix of ethnicity, race, and religion in a given population

_____ 6. Individual's growth and development in physical size and motor and sensory skills

_____ 7. Part of human life span dealing with toddlers, preschoolers, school-age children, and adolescents

_____ 8. Progressive increases in the function of the body throughout a lifetime

_____ 9. Genetics

_____ 10. Developmental stage between childhood and early adulthood

THEORY RECALL

True/False

Indicate whether the statement is true or false.

_____ 1. Growth and change occur only throughout a human's adolescent years.

_____ 2. Medical assistants have a responsibility to their profession and to their patients to accept and respect the cultural beliefs of others even if they differ from their own.

_____ 3. Fear of pain and death are two very strong emotions for most people.

_____ 4. When a patient is fearful, talkative, withdrawn, or angry, the medical assistant should get the physician immediately to take care of the problem.

_____ 5. As a patient ages, the gastrointestinal tract slows down, learning is possible but slower, and drugs are processed more slowly.

Multiple Choice

Identify the letter of the choice that best completes the statement or answers the question.

1. There is a potential for ineffective communication when all of the following occur *except* when _____.
   A. English is a second language
   B. the patient is angry, frightened, or in pain
   C. there are cultural differences
   D. direct eye contact is made

2. Which one of the following is *not* a category of change during growth and development of the human life span?
   A. Physical
   B. Socioeconomic
   C. Mental
   D. Psychosocial

3. Cognitive development occurs during _____ growth.
   A. physical
   B. socioeconomic
   C. mental
   D. psychosocial

4. During infancy, a baby who coos when happy or smiles at age 6 weeks is showing _____ growth.
   A. physical
   B. socioeconomic
   C. mental
   D. psychosocial

5. When caring for an infant (birth to 3 months) in the office or clinic, the medical assistant should _____.
   A. make eye contact when speaking to the infant
   B. focus on eating and sleeping habits
   C. encourage grasping toys and toys with sounds
   D. encourage playing with large blocks for stacking

Copyright © 2010, 2005 by Saunders, an imprint of Elsevier, Inc. All rights reserved.

6. A toddler (13 months to 3 years) typically grows slowly, gaining only _____ pounds and growing only 3 inches.
   A. 1 to 2
   B. 3 to 4
   C. 5 to 10
   D. 10 to 15

7. An infant 8 to 12 months old is capable of which of the following task(s)?
   A. Shaking head "no"
   B. Waving "bye-bye"
   C. Both A and B
   D. Neither A nor B

8. A 19- to 23-month-old is capable of which of the following task(s)?
   A. Kicking a ball
   B. Hopping
   C. Coloring within the lines
   D. None of the above

9. The medical assistant should engage a child 24 to 36 months old by _____.
   A. encouraging cooing and happy sounds
   B. encouraging grasping toys and toys with sound
   C. encouraging play with large blocks for stacking
   D. none of the above

10. Wrinkles typically first appear on patients in the age range of _____ years.
    A. 19 to 45
    B. 45 to 59
    C. 70 to 79
    D. 80 and older

11. In some _____ cultures, direct eye contact is considered to be disrespectful.
    A. Asian
    B. Latin
    C. African American
    D. European

12. _____ can cause more misunderstandings than any other form of communication.
    A. Foods
    B. Clothing
    C. Gestures
    D. Physical space

13. A(n) _____ is a universal gesture accepted by every culture.
    A. wave
    B. OK sign
    C. cry
    D. smile

14. Which one of the following can be an area of cultural difference?
    A. Eye contact
    B. Emotions
    C. Nontraditional/traditional health care
    D. All of the above

15. _____ is *not* a common response patients have toward illness, injury, or pain.
    A. Joy
    B. Anger
    C. Talkativeness
    D. Withdrawing

16. When dealing with an angry patient, it would *not* be productive to _____.
    A. remain calm and professional
    B. mimic the patient's level of anger
    C. listen because some patients just need to vent
    D. agree with the patient; after all, you may be wrong

17. In the United States, the color black is a sign of mourning; in certain Asian cultures, the color _____ indicates mourning.
    A. yellow
    B. blue
    C. white
    D. purple

18. Bone mass begins to decrease in which age group?
    A. 20 to 25 years
    B. 30 to 35 years
    C. 40 to 45 years
    D. 45 to 59 years

19. Muscle efficiency peaks in the late _____.
    A. teens
    B. 20s
    C. 30s
    D. 40s

20. Minor motor skills greatly improve in which age group?
    A. Birth to 8 months
    B. 8 to 12 months
    C. 13 to 18 months
    D. 19 to 23 months

Sentence Completion

Complete each sentence or statement.

6, 7	friends
8, 12	parents/guardian
4, 5	cognitive/mental
adult	affective/behavior
preschooler	psychosocial

1. As a toddler becomes a(n) _____, expectations about physical, mental, and psychosocial characteristics and abilities are raised.

CHAPTER 6 Understanding Patient Behavior

2. A(n) _____ development in infancy is a reaction to sound, motion, and light.

3. Involve _____ when demonstrating procedures for home care, and have them practice the procedures.

4. A child of _____ to _____ months old will smile at himself or herself in the mirror.

5. A child of _____ to _____ years old can learn to print his or her name.

Short Answers

1. List and describe the three areas of change during growth and development that occur in a lifetime.

   _____
   _____
   _____
   _____

2. Explain why the medical assistant must understand the various body system changes involved in the aging process.

   _____
   _____
   _____
   _____

3. List five things a medical assistant can do when a patient becomes angry.

   _____
   _____
   _____
   _____

4. Explain the importance of being knowledgeable about the cultural background of a patient.

   _____
   _____

5. Why is it important to understand a culture's value on time management? How do cultures that are monochronic differ from those that are polychronic? (Search the Web using key words "time management," "polychronic," and "monochronic.")

CRITICAL THINKING

1. Simon lives in a large city and works as a medical assistant for a free health clinic with 15 physicians, 6 physician assistants, and 3 nurse practitioners on staff. Simon loves the fast pace of the practice. He enjoys working with the patients and their families, and knows in his heart at the end of the day that he has given back to the community in which he grew up. The patient population is very diverse. Patients are from numerous ethnic backgrounds, with different religious beliefs, medical traditions, educational levels, and age groups. The patients are very poor, and many are homeless. The practice's philosophy states that any person in need of medical attention who comes through the door will receive treatment to the best of the facility's abilities. Some of the patients are on state-assisted programs or Medicare; many more of them pay on a sliding fee scale or do not pay at all. Simon speaks fluent Spanish and has learned several medical phrases in five languages, such as "Where does it hurt?" "How long have you been sick?" "Have you had this happen before?" "How long ago?" He cannot always understand the answers, but by watching the patient's nonverbal communication, he is able to form a basic understanding of what is going on. Simon has been able to learn the basics of many of the different cultures of his patients, and the patients respect Simon for his dedication.

    A. Learn the medical phrases in Spanish for:

    - "Where does it hurt?"

    - "How long have you been sick?"

    - "Have you had this happen before?"

    - "How long ago?"

    (If Spanish is your primary language, learn these phrases in another language that is prevalent in your area. Write them down and be able to repeat them verbally in class.)

B. How do you think Simon learned about his patients' cultures?

C. List five nonverbal communication techniques for understanding "I am in pain, here."

PRACTICAL APPLICATIONS

If you have accomplished the objectives in this chapter, you will be able to make better choices as a medical assistant. Take a look at this situation and decide what you would do.

Juan, 40 years old, has moved to the United States. His family is still in Mexico, but he hopes to find a good job soon and pay for them to come to the United States. Because Juan does not speak English well, he has had difficulty finding employment and a place to live. Lately, he has been staying at a shelter for homeless people. His educational background is limited, and his broken English makes communicating difficult. Few Hispanic people live in the area where he has settled. Juan has lost 10 pounds, his vision is declining, and he has noticed that he is not hearing as well as he used to. Because of his constant weight loss and the vision problems, he decided to visit the local medical office. He has heard the office provides services to individuals who cannot pay.

When Juan arrives at the office, his clothing is worn and torn. The new medical assistant tells Juan that he cannot be seen at the office unless he can pay for his visit before he is seen. She does not explain her statement, and because of his broken English, Juan does not ask further questions. He thinks that the physician will not see him and leaves the office very upset. He decides to start taking herbal medications and to try home remedies. He now believes that seeing a physician in America just is not worth the trouble and embarrassment. Several weeks later, Juan is hospitalized with dehydration, starvation, and severe reactions to the herbal drugs.

This situation did not have to result in Juan's being hospitalized. If you were the new medical assistant, what would you have done differently?

1. **What part does age play in the symptoms that Juan is experiencing? Could the symptoms be related to the illnesses as well? Explain.**

2. **What influence did differing cultural backgrounds have in this situation?**

3. How would the situation have turned out if the new medical assistant had studied cultural differences? What activities would help the medical assistant in understanding diversity?

4. What factors led to Juan's withdrawal from medical care until he was hospitalized?

5. As the medical assistant, how would you approach Juan differently?

APPLICATION OF SKILLS

1. Select one age group of growth and development. Interview two individuals (or parents or guardians, depending on the age group selected) that fall within the age group you selected. Using the development charts in the textbook, ask or assess whether each individual has met or accomplished each guideline listed in all three categories: physical, mental, and psychosocial.

2. On the Internet or at a local library research a culture other than your own. (You may ask an individual of that culture to provide you with information.) Write two or three sentences addressing the following areas. Cite your source(s) of information.

    A. History

    B. Food

C. Music

D. Medical traditions

E. Clothing

F. One holiday celebration unique to their culture

CHAPTER QUIZ

Multiple Choice

Identify the letter of the choice that best completes the statement or answers the question.

1. _____ is the part of the human life span concerned with an individual during early, middle, and later years in life.
    A. Physical growth
    B. Adulthood
    C. Infancy
    D. Mental growth

2. An individual's emotional and social development is called _____.
   A. cultural diversity
   B. physical growth
   C. psychosocial growth
   D. mental growth

3. _____ is the mix of ethnicity, race, and religion in a given population.
   A. Social standards
   B. Cultural diversity
   C. Socioeconomic status
   D. Self-esteem

4. _____ is *not* a common patient response to illness.
   A. Anger
   B. Talkative
   C. Withdrawn
   D. Calmness

5. Dexterity decreases in patients _____ old.
   A. 10 to 12 months
   B. 20 to 15 years
   C. 40 to 49 years
   D. 60 to 69 years

6. Toilet training should be completed by age _____ months.
   A. 6
   B. 12 to 18
   C. 20 to 24
   D. 24 to 36

7. A child _____ months old explores by banging, dropping, and throwing.
   A. 0 to 3
   B. 4 to 7
   C. 10 to 12
   D. 24 to 36

8. At what age should the medical assistant start to observe a child's behavior and interaction with peers?
   A. 13 to 18 months
   B. 19 to 23 months
   C. 24 to 36 months
   D. At no age is this appropriate

9. At what age should a child be able to drink from a cup?
   A. 10 to 12 months
   B. 13 to 18 months
   C. 19 to 23 months
   D. 24 to 36 months

10. During what age is a child most susceptible to unfavorable experiences that can lead to mistrust and hamper attempts at new things?
    A. 1 to 2 years
    B. 3 to 5 years
    C. 6 to 8 years
    D. 10 to 12 years

Copyright © 2010, 2005 by Saunders, an imprint of Elsevier, Inc. All rights reserved.

11. During the years of _____, peer pressure becomes a major issue in the child's life.
    A. childhood
    B. adolescence
    C. early adulthood
    D. geriatrics

12. Wrinkles typically first appear during the ages of _____ years.
    A. 20 to 29
    B. 30 to 39
    C. 45 to 59
    D. 64 to 69

13. The psychosocial occurrence of retirement typically occurs during what age group?
    A. 35 to 39 years
    B. 40 to 50 years
    C. 50 to 55 years
    D. 60 to 69 years

14. Does a feeling of self-worth have any impact on how a person approaches life span changes?
    A. Yes
    B. No

15. Religion, race, ethics, economics, and social upbringing have little, if any, impact on a patient's behavior.
    A. True
    B. False

16. In some cultures, it is believed that poor health is a punishment from a higher power.
    A. True
    B. False

17. Typically, financial and employment concerns do *not* contribute to the overall wellness of an individual.
    A. True
    B. False

18. A medical assistant must become very proficient in stereotyping patients as quickly as possible to ensure they receive the best health care.
    A. True
    B. False

19. In the United States, the color _____ is a sign of mourning, whereas in certain cultures, the color white signifies mourning.
    A. black
    B. yellow
    C. white
    D. purple

20. Cognitive development occurs during _____ growth.
    A. physical
    B. socioeconomic
    C. mental
    D. psychosocial

NAME: _____ DATE: _____

7 Effective Communication

VOCABULARY REVIEW

Matching: Match each term with the correct definition.

A. active listening

B. adjective

C. adverb

D. conjunction

E. distracter

F. feedback

G. grammar

H. interjection

I. noun

J. preposition

K. pronoun

L. punctuation

M. sentence

N. subject

O. verb

_____ 1. Verbal or nonverbal indication that a message was received

_____ 2. Word used to describe a noun or pronoun

_____ 3. Word used to begin a prepositional phrase

_____ 4. Word used to express strong feelings or emotion

_____ 5. Word in a sentence that expresses action or a state of being

_____ 6. Occurs when a listener maintains eye contact and provides responses to the speaker

_____ 7. Word used to join words or groups of words

_____ 8. Marks within and between sentences that separate, emphasize, and clarify the different ideas within a sentence or group of sentences

_____ 9. Study of words and their relationship to other words in a sentence

_____ 10. Something that prevents the sender or receiver from giving full attention to the message

_____ 11. Word used to name things, including people, places, objects, and ideas

____ 12. Word used to describe a verb, an adjective, or an another adverb

____ 13. Word used to take the place of a noun

____ 14. Group of words that express a complete thought

____ 15. Part of a sentence that identifies who or what is being discussed

THEORY RECALL

True/False

Indicate whether the statement is true or false.

____ 1. The goal of communication is to exchange information clearly between a sender and a receiver.

____ 2. Public space is considered to be 2 to 4 feet apart.

____ 3. Active listening involves hearing what the speaker is saying, but not listening with enough effort to become personally, intensely involved in what is being said.

____ 4. To express a complete thought, a sentence must contain at least one noun and one pronoun.

____ 5. A fax machine converts written material or pictures into electronic impulses that are transmitted by telephone lines to other locations with similar equipment.

Multiple Choice

Identify the letter of the choice that best completes the statement or answers the question.

1. Nonverbal communication comprises approximately _____ % of all communication.
   A. 10
   B. 40
   C. 75
   D. 90

2. Which one of the following is *not* an important part of delivering messages?
   A. Not using slang terms
   B. Rate of speech that is neither too fast nor too slow
   C. Voice inflection
   D. Ability to multitask while delivering the message

3. _____ is a communication distracter.
   A. Quiet environment
   B. Incorrect use of grammar
   C. Climate-controlled temperature
   D. Quiet music in the background

4. When communicating with a patient, it is best to ask _____ questions.
   A. open-ended
   B. closed-ended

5. Interpreting body language is an important part of _____ communication.
   A. verbal
   B. nonverbal

6. Two typical nonverbal signals that our eyes send are pupil size and _____.
   A. iris color
   B. direction of gaze
   C. posture
   D. A and B

7. _____ is *not* a nonverbal response.
   A. Singing
   B. Smiling
   C. Physical appearance
   D. B and C

8. Numbers may be used as nouns or _____.
   A. verbs
   B. adjectives
   C. adverbs
   D. pronouns

9. _____ is an automated answering device.
   A. Voice mail system
   B. Facsimile
   C. E-mail
   D. None of the above

10. Which of the following is a disadvantage of voice mail?
    A. People can call all day or at any hour to leave a message.
    B. Length of message is reduced because communication is one-way.
    C. Some people want to speak to a person immediately.
    D. Messages can be retrieved from other locations.

11. Which of the following is *not* an item that can be included on a website?
    A. Practice philosophy
    B. Hours of operation
    C. Billing and insurance information
    D. All of the above could be included

12. Advantages of a website include all of the following *except* that _____.
    A. it saves patients the time and effort of calling the office
    B. a website can be quickly updated
    C. it can provide answer to FAQs (frequently asked questions)
    D. patients may not have access to the Internet

13. Faxes (are or are not) considered forms of original and legal documents.
    A. are
    B. are not

Copyright © 2010, 2005 by Saunders, an imprint of Elsevier, Inc. All rights reserved.

14. A disadvantage of e-mail messages is that _____.
    A. e-mail is available 24 hours a day
    B. messages are sent and received rapidly
    C. messages once sent are often not retrievable
    D. verification can be made that a message was sent and received

15. A _____ sentence expresses only one thought.
    A. subject
    B. simple
    C. complex
    D. compound

16. Numbers that begin a sentence should be spelled out even if they are greater than _____.
    A. 3
    B. 5
    C. 7
    D. 9

17. Which one of the following is correctly spelled?
    A. Abcess
    B. Abscess
    C. Absces
    D. Abbscess

18. Which one of the following is correctly spelled?
    A. Negligence
    B. Nagligance
    C. Negligance
    D. Neglligence

19. Which one of the following is correctly spelled?
    A. Theif
    B. Percieve
    C. Concieve
    D. Believe

20. Always use a _____ when sending a fax.
    A. typewriter
    B. letter of introduction
    C. cover sheet
    D. reference page

Sentence Completion

Complete each sentence or statement.

STOP	it's	WATCH
a while	LISTEN	confidential
awhile	always	vital
its	all ways	

1. Do not send _____ information via e-mail.

2. The acronym _____ outlines the six steps to becoming a better listener.

3. I (always/all ways) _____ go to the park after school.

4. In (awhile/a while) _____ we will go to the beach.

5. (Its/It's) _____ not likely the order will arrive today.

Short Answers

1. State the goal of the communication process.

   _____
   _____
   _____

2. List and describe the three components of the communication process.

   _____
   _____
   _____

3. List the three components of effective listening.

   _____
   _____
   _____

4. Explain the importance of choosing the correct words.

   _____
   _____
   _____

CHAPTER 7 Effective Communication

CRITICAL THINKING

1. Cassandra brought her mother, Elizabeth Seneca, to her doctor's appointment this morning. Mrs. Seneca has been feeling poorly for the past 4 days. Cassandra does not know what exactly is wrong. Kym, the medical assistant, takes Cassandra and her mother into the examination room and notices bruises on Mrs. Seneca's arm. Mrs. Seneca glances quickly around the room and sits with a sigh in the chair. She straightens her skirt and brushes at an invisible speck repeatedly. Kym asks Mrs. Seneca how she is feeling today. Cassandra answers immediately, "She is not eating, she barely sleeps, and she won't even go outside for some fresh air." Mrs. Seneca twists an almost shredded tissue in her hands. Kym looks directly at Mrs. Seneca and asks again how she is feeling. Mrs. Seneca looks up briefly. Kym notices that her pupils are large and that her mouth is set in a firm, thin line. Mrs. Seneca mumbles a response almost under her breath. Kym moves closer to Mrs. Seneca to hear her better, and Mrs. Seneca moves back farther on her chair. Kym steps away. "Are you in pain?" Kym asks. There still is no response. Kym washes her hands and gathers the equipment together to take Mrs. Seneca's pulse, respiration, and blood pressure. When she reaches out to take Mrs. Seneca's arm to help her roll up her sleeve, Mrs. Seneca quickly looks at her daughter and then back at the floor and at the same time bats away Kym's hand.

   A. In your opinion, what do you think is going on with Mrs. Seneca?

   _____
   _____

   B. What verbal communication leads you to your opinion?

   _____
   _____

   C. What nonverbal communication leads you to your opinion?

   _____
   _____

   D. What should be Kym's next step? Why?

   _____
   _____

PRACTICAL APPLICATIONS

If you have accomplished the objectives in this chapter, you will be able to make better choices as a medical assistant. Take a look at this situation and decide what you would do.

Panina is a former resident of the Middle East who moved to the United States with her husband, Abed, 6 months ago. Naturally, she brings with her the cultural and ethnic contexts of her homeland. Panina awakens one morning with a pain in her breast. She becomes concerned and calls a physician's office for an appointment. Because she has difficulty understanding the English language, she misunderstands the appointment time, and Panina and Abed arrive at the office an hour late. Abed demands to accompany his wife to the examination room. Therese, the medical assistant, tells Abed that they are late for the appointment and that he must stay in the waiting room while Panina is being examined. Panina, refusing eye contact with Therese, begins to cry. Abed becomes upset and tells Therese that the only way Panina will be examined is if he accompanies her to the room to explain to the male doctor what is wrong with her. Therese refuses, and Panina and Abed leave the office, threatening to tell all their friends how this office "just does not care about patients at all."

Effective communication helps eliminate misunderstandings. If you were the medical assistant in this situation, how could you have used your understanding of effective communication skills to help?

1. What role did Panina and Abed's cultural and ethnic background play in the misunderstandings in the physician's office? What role did communication skills play in the misunderstandings?

2. What distracters may have caused the lack of communication between Panina and Therese?

3. What nonverbal communication between Panina and Therese could have been recognized and used to diffuse the negative situation that occurred in the physician's office?

4. Why is an understanding of ethnicity and cultural differences so important in the medical field?

5. What body parts are involved in the communication of body language?

APPLICATION OF SKILLS

1. Underline the *subject* in each of the following sentences.
   A. <u>We</u> will open the office at 8:00 A.M.
   B. The <u>physician</u> is in a meeting at the hospital.
   C. <u>Sharon</u> stayed late to inventory the supplies.
   D. The <u>committee</u> will adjourn and reconvene tomorrow.

2. Underline the *verb* in each of the following sentences.
   A. Sam <u>ran</u> quickly down the hall to grab the crash cart.
   B. Tomorrow, we <u>will begin</u> the new research project.
   C. Chelsea <u>booked</u> the reservations for the medical conference.
   D. Mrs. Jones <u>seems to be</u> unconscious.

3. Underline the *pronoun(s)* in each of the following sentences.
   A. <u>She</u> looked nauseated.
   B. Please pass <u>me</u> the stapler.
   C. Will <u>they</u> be done in the examination room soon?
   D. <u>I</u> would like to go over the end-of-month reports this afternoon.

4. Underline the *adjective(s)* in each of the following sentences.
   A. This <u>new</u> brand of <u>antibacterial</u> soap smells like <u>fresh</u> lemons.
   B. The physician ordered <u>two new oak</u> computer desks for his office and <u>two black leather</u> chairs.
   C. The <u>medical</u> assistant just hired has <u>exceptional</u> skills.
   D. The <u>casting</u> room was left in a <u>huge</u> mess.

5. Underline the *adverb(s)* in each of the following sentences.
   A. Mrs. Thompson <u>carefully</u> removed the bandages from Lincoln's infected toe.
   B. We <u>nearly</u> didn't make the 1 o'clock flight.
   C. Angela <u>lazily</u> thumbed through an old magazine in the waiting room.
   D. Next year we are <u>certainly</u> going to need a larger office.

6. Underline the *preposition(s)* in each of the following sentences.
   A. The new clinic is just <u>around</u> the corner.
   B. Henry will have to go <u>over</u> to the hospital <u>before</u> he can file the insurance forms.
   C. Mickey reached <u>across</u> the minor surgery tray and contaminated the sterile field.
   D. Tressa, please go <u>behind</u> the curtain and change <u>into</u> the patient gown I left <u>for</u> you.

7. Underline the *conjunction(s)* in each of the following sentences.
   A. I ordered three pairs of turquoise scrubs <u>and</u> two of the raspberry ones as well.
   B. He could change Mr. Crinshaw's medication, <u>but</u> he is concerned that it will not be as effective.
   C. <u>Since</u> Sara stopped eating fast food, she has lost 15 pounds, <u>but</u> she is still 50 pounds overweight.
   D. The biopsy was delayed <u>because</u> the patient was not fasting.

8. Underline the *interjection(s)* in each of the following sentences.
   A. <u>Stop!</u> That really hurts.
   B. <u>Perfect!</u> Just a few more stitches and we will be all done.
   C. <u>Oh</u>, we will need a second opinion before we operate.
   D. <u>Wonderful</u>, Diane, you did a great job today; thank you.

9. Using Table 7-4 as a guideline, punctuate the following sentences.
   A. Where are my new scrubs I wanted to wear them today and if I cant find them were going to be late
   B. Have you seen their lab equipment theyre going to be hiring next week I would really like to work there
   C. Dr Xaxon the world renowned physician performed the procedure impeccably
   D. Katherine has given up smoking about five times but she cannot seem to break the habit

CHAPTER QUIZ

Multiple Choice

Identify the letter of the choice that best completes the statement or answers the question.

1. _____ is *not* a component of the communication process.
   A. Organization
   B. Message
   C. Sender
   D. Receiver

2. Based on statistics, _____% of all communication is nonverbal.
   A. 10
   B. 25
   C. 75
   D. 90

3. The way a message is delivered is *not* as important as the message itself.
   A. True
   B. False

4. A _____ is anything that causes the sender or receiver of a message not to give full attention to the message.
   A. detractor
   B. distracter
   C. distortion
   D. deformation

5. Assessing _____ from the receiver allows you to determine if the message was understood the way it was intended.
   A. opinions
   B. responses
   C. feedback
   D. all of the above

6. _____ involves hearing what the speaker is saying, but not listening with enough effort to become personally involved in what is being said.
   A. Passive listening
   B. Active listening
   C. Aggressive listening
   D. Unconscious listening

7. Acceptable personal space is used for times of closeness and is typically _____ feet apart.
   A. 12 to 25
   B. 10 to 15
   C. 1½ to 2½
   D. 1 to 1½

8. _____ help(s) separate, emphasize, and clarify the different ideas within sentences and between groups of sentences.
   A. Capitalization
   B. Punctuation marks
   C. Proofreading marks
   D. Adjectives

9. A word that shows action in a sentence is a(n) _____.
   A. subject
   B. noun
   C. adverb
   D. verb

10. A(n) _____ converts written material or pictures into electronic impulses that are transmitted by telephone lines and recorded magnetically and can be printed as a hard copy.
    A. voice mail
    B. e-mail
    C. facsimile
    D. telephone call

11. "The hemostats fell to the floor with a clang." Select the *verb*.
    A. fell
    B. to the
    C. hemostats
    D. with

12. "The three medical assistants all went to lunch together yesterday." Select the *subject*.
    A. yesterday
    B. three
    C. medical assistants
    D. lunch

13. "Dr. Xaxon, the world-renowned physician, performed the procedure impeccably." Select the *adjective*.
    A. Dr. Xaxon
    B. world-renowned physician
    C. performed
    D. procedure

14. "Good grief! What now?" Select the *interjection*.
    A. Good grief
    B. What
    C. now
    D. All of the above

15. "Quickly! We are very nearly there, Thom." Select the *adverb*.
    A. Quickly
    B. are
    C. very nearly
    D. Thom

16. Which one of the following sentences is punctuated correctly?
    A. In 3 weeks' time we'll have to begin school again.
    B. After surviving this ordeal the patient felt relieved.
    C. He replied "I have no idea what you mean."
    D. Its such a beautiful day that Ive decided to take the day off.

17. Which one of the following sentences is punctuated correctly?
    A. The problems involved in this operation are I think numerous.
    B. Yes Helen did mention that all three of you were coming to the medical conference.
    C. The patient used to live at 1721 Gretchen Avenue Kansas City Missouri but has since moved to 3rd Street West Holland Way Dubuque Iowa.
    D. Chris did not see how he could organize, write, and proofread the paper in only 2 hours.

18. Which one of the following sentences is punctuated incorrectly?
    A. Having cut the roses she decided to bring them to her friend in the hospital.
    B. Jillian, who had worked in the dress shop all summer, hoped to work there again during the Christmas holidays.
    C. "Oh no" Max exclaimed, "I think that Dr. Holmes wanted Mrs. Jenson's file immediately."
    D. I hope that someday, we can redecorate the reception area.

19. Which statement is correctly written?
    A. Wear are my new scrubs? I wanted to where them today, and if I can't find them wear going to be late.
    B. Were are my new scrubs? I wanted to wear them today, and if I can't find them where going to be late.
    C. Where are my new scrubs? I wanted to wear them today, and if I can't find them we're going to be late.
    D. Where are my new scrubs? I wanted to we're them today, and if I can't find them we're going to be late.

20. Which statement is correctly written?
    A. Have you seen their lab equipment? They're going to be hiring next week. I would really like to work there.
    B. Have you seen there lab equipment? Their going to be hiring next week. I would really like to work their.
    C. Have you seen they're lab equipment? Their going to be hiring next week. I would really like to work there.
    D. Have you seen their lab equipment? Their going to be hiring next week. I would really like to work they're.

8 Communicating with Patients

VOCABULARY REVIEW

Matching: Match each term with the correct definition.

A. litigation

B. holistic

C. maturation

D. rapport

E. affective

F. cognitive

G. psychomotor

_____ 1. A growth and development process involving a patient's physical, social, and emotional functioning

_____ 2. Lawsuit

_____ 3. Effective relationship that considers physical and emotional needs

_____ 4. Involving all health needs of the patient, including physical, emotional, social, economic, and spiritual needs

_____ 5. Type of learning based on motor skills to perform tasks

_____ 6. Type of learning based on feelings and emotions

_____ 7. Type of learning based on what the patient already knows and has experienced

THEORY RECALL

True/False

Indicate whether the statement is true or false.

_____ 1. Communicating effectively with patients is a key factor in providing quality care.

_____ 2. Patient complaints should be handled directly by the physician.

_____ 3. Patients with disabilities expect sympathy and special considerations.

_____ 4. When communicating with children, use wording and methods that are appropriate to their age.

_____ 5. Use verbal and nonverbal clues to assess a patient's ability to read and comprehend information.

_____ 6. Effective patient education is the key to helping patients understand the situation and the need for change.

Multiple Choice

Identify the letter of the choice that best completes the statement or answers the question.

1. _____ does *not* apply when expecting a patient to comply with treatment plans.
   A. Patient's physical state
   B. Patient's emotional state
   C. Patient's educational background
   D. None of the above because all do apply

2. Which one of the following is *not* important in effective communication for patient teaching?
   A. Assessing a patient's readiness to learn
   B. Including a patient's family or support group in treatment plans
   C. A patient's dietary habits
   D. Providing time for questions

3. Developmentally delayed patients are individuals who are behind in _____.
   A. maturation
   B. intelligence
   C. education
   D. physical abilities

4. When communicating with children, do all of the following *except* _____.
   A. use technical terms to explain all procedures
   B. use dolls and pictures to enhance communication
   C. allow children to handle "safe" medical equipment
   D. encourage them to talk about themselves

5. The ability to process new information and to apply it appropriately in a given setting reflects a patient's _____ functioning.
   A. verbal
   B. nonverbal
   C. mental
   D. emotional

Copyright © 2010, 2005 by Saunders, an imprint of Elsevier, Inc. All rights reserved.

6. Which one of the following is *not* an effective means of communicating with a patient who is hearing impaired?
   A. Directly face the patient when speaking
   B. Speak louder and more quickly
   C. Use visual examples
   D. A and B

7. All of the following are appropriate ways to communicate effectively with patients *except* to _____.
   A. involve the patient's family in decision making
   B. argue with the patient about his or her beliefs that conflict with the medical treatment
   C. provide honest feedback
   D. B and C

8. _____ health care deals with all of the health needs of the patient.
   A. Allopathic
   B. Holistic
   C. Generic
   D. Western

9. Three of the following statements pertain to considerations that should be made when accommodating patients with physical disabilities. Which one does *not* pertain?
   A. Restate directions and instructions frequently
   B. Do not rush special needs patients
   C. Special needs patients may require assistance in the bathroom
   D. Be careful ushering a special needs patient through doorways

10. Which one of the following does *not* apply when working with patients who are visually impaired?
    A. Use written material with large print
    B. Face the patient directly when speaking
    C. Give verbal clues when necessary
    D. Alert patients before touching them

11. _____ is a type of learning.
    A. Affective
    B. Cognitive
    C. Psychomotor
    D. All of the above

Sentence Completion

Complete each sentence or statement.

tactful	clinical complaints
affective	complain
psychomotor	administrative complaints
communicate	cognitive
rapport	

1. The medical assistant must use the skills he or she has learned about human relations and behavior to develop a working _____ with patients.

2. Finding better ways to _____ with patients results in quality service and patient care.

3. A patient may _____ if he or she perceives the quality of the service to be unsatisfactory.

4. _____ occurs when the patient is unhappy with the performance of the support staff in a medical facility.

5. Use _____ language when responding to a complaint, and reassure the patient that the complaint will be investigated.

Short Answers

1. Explain the concept of holistic care.
   _____
   _____

2. Explain the importance of handling patient complaints effectively.
   _____
   _____

3. List seven ways to communicate effectively with a patient who has a hearing impairment.
   _____
   _____
   _____
   _____

4. List six considerations for communicating effectively with elderly patients.
   _____
   _____
   _____
   _____

5. What questions should a medical assistant ask when doing an inventory of the patient's readiness to follow a new health treatment plan?

CRITICAL THINKING

1. Using the paragraphs written in the Application of Skills section, exchange papers with your partner.

   A. How did your partner feel about you as the caregiver and your ability to communicate effectively?

   B. What did you learn from performing this activity that will help you to become a better medical assistant?

   C. Have you ever assisted a physically challenged individual in the past? If so, what have you learned from that experience? If not, look for an opportunity to do so within the next 2 days and then answer this question.

PRACTICAL APPLICATIONS

If you have accomplished the objectives in this chapter, you will be able to make better choices as a medical assistant. Take a look at this situation and decide what you would do.

   Mr. Joplin is a spry 82-year-old and still lives in his own home. His wife died about a year ago, but Mr. Joplin has no severe medical problems and is able to care for himself. He does have visual problems caused by cataracts in his left eye, and joint stiffness related to his age. John, the medical assistant, approaches Mr. Joplin to escort him to the examining room. John shouts at Mr. Joplin as if he has a hearing difficulty, then walks away without assisting Mr. Joplin from the chair. When John reaches the door, he looks over his shoulder, rolls his eyes, and shouts, "Do you need some help?" Mr. Joplin looks away and refuses any assistance. Dr. Smith examines Mr. Joplin and asks John to explain the treatment so that Mr. Joplin will comply. John hurriedly tells Mr. Joplin one time what is expected, then returns him to the waiting room. Several days later, Mr. Joplin calls the office to tell the receptionist to cancel his next appointment because he is going to find a new physician.

John's poor communication skills caused Dr. Smith to lose Mr. Joplin as a patient. If you were the medical assistant in this situation, what would you have done to communicate more effectively with Mr. Joplin?

1. Did John need to speak in a loud voice to Mr. Joplin, or did he stereotype Mr. Joplin because of his age and visual impairments?

   _____
   _____
   _____
   _____

2. Did John show professionalism? List three ways that John could have improved his interaction with Mr. Joplin.

   _____
   _____
   _____
   _____
   _____

3. What body language did John display that exhibited negative thoughts about Mr. Joplin?

   _____
   _____
   _____
   _____
   _____

4. What role did Mr. Joplin's age play in this interaction?

   _____
   _____
   _____
   _____

5. What steps could John have taken to show that he really wanted Mr. Joplin to comply with the physician's treatment plan?

_____

_____

_____

_____

6. What role did the receptionist play in this scenario? What should she have done when Mr. Joplin canceled his appointment?

_____

_____

_____

_____

APPLICATION OF SKILLS

1. Select a partner in class for this activity. Partner A should be blindfolded, while Partner B navigates Partner A through a 10-minute period. Then they switch places for an additional 10 minutes. Pay particular attention to communicating effectively with the blindfolded partner. Write one paragraph each journaling the experience from both perspectives, being the caregiver and being the visually impaired individual.

2. Using cotton balls or earplugs, perform the same activity as a hearing-impaired person.

CHAPTER QUIZ

Multiple Choice

Identify the letter of the choice that best completes the statement or answers the question.

1. The growth and development process involving the patient's physical, social, and emotional functioning is called _____.
   A. holistic health care
   B. litigation
   C. Americans with Disabilities Act
   D. maturation

2. Communicating ineffectively with patients is a key factor in providing quality care.
   A. True
   B. False

3. All of a patient's needs influence his or her behavior and compliance with treatment.
   A. True
   B. False

4. Which one of the following is *not* a means of assessing a patient's understanding or a method to improve communication?
   A. Communicating in technical/medical terms
   B. Asking patients to write down questions
   C. Identifying any communication barriers
   D. Not being afraid to say, "I don't know"

5. Which one of the following is *not* a category of reasons for which patients complain?
   A. Administrative complaints
   B. Medical complaints
   C. Laboratory complaints
   D. All of the above are complaint categories

6. Take all complaints seriously, but write down only the facts that feel important to you.
   A. True
   B. False

7. Always inform the physician or office manager of any statements made by the patient that reflect a negative attitude.
   A. True
   B. False

8. Numerous _____ result from careless actions or comments made by physicians and office staff when patients complain.
   A. warnings
   B. threats
   C. lawsuits
   D. thank-you cards

9. All treatment plans must allow patients to maintain their _____ and help establish trust in the health care team.
   A. self-esteem
   B. modesty
   C. confidence
   D. all of the above

10. You must get rid of all positive beliefs so that they do not affect your communication with or care for patients.
    A. True
    B. False

11. A medical assistant must answer only questions within his or her scope of training. With the physician's guidance, he or she may explain the reasons for the needed changes and the importance of compliance.
    A. True
    B. False

12. A medical assistant must never accept the patient's decisions regarding medical care if they are not in alignment with his or her personal beliefs.
    A. True
    B. False

13. When working with patients with special needs, it is important to ask if they would like assistance before assuming they are incapable of performing a task.
    A. True
    B. False

14. In working with visually impaired patients, you must *never* _____.
    A. provide verbal directions
    B. yell so they will hear you more clearly
    C. alert the patient before touching them
    D. all of the above

15. Patients with disabilities do *not* expect sympathy or special considerations.
    A. True
    B. False

16. A person is diagnosed as mentally challenged when he or she functions at a higher than normal intellectual level.
    A. True
    B. False

17. Patients with developmental delays are behind in maturation.
    A. True
    B. False

18. Very few communities have support groups or special day care centers equipped to handle mentally handicapped or developmentally delayed individuals.
    A. True
    B. False

19. A medical assistant is expected to be an active listener and to understand and anticipate the patient's needs.
    A. True
    B. False

20. An unhappy patient is more likely to sue.
    A. True
    B. False

21. To ensure that the patient understands what the medical assistant is trying to teach, the medical assistant should use the technique called _____.
    A. retention
    B. internalization
    C. interaction
    D. feedback

22. Information that is expressed primarily in words is covered in which domain?
    A. Associative
    B. Cognitive
    C. Affective
    D. Reasoning
    E. Psychological

23. The three important areas of learning are _____.
    A. associative, cognitive, and psychological
    B. cognitive, affective, and psychomotor
    C. affective, psychological, and reasoning
    D. effective, psychological, and cognitive

24. The type of learning based on what a person knows or has experienced is part of the _____ domain.
    A. psychological
    B. reasoning
    C. affective
    D. cognitive
    E. associative

25. The domain that refers to feelings, emotions, values, and attitudes is the _____.
    A. associative
    B. cognitive
    C. affective
    D. psychomotor
    E. psychological

26. The domain that must take physical barriers such as tremor, paralysis, or decreased hearing into account is the _____.
    A. psychomotor
    B. affective
    C. cognitive
    D. associative
    E. psychological

27. Teaching modalities planned for Mrs. Jones should include all of the following *except* _____.
    A. verbal explanation
    B. relying on only one teaching method
    C. demonstrating a procedure
    D. watching a videotape with the patient

28. For the medical assistant to be sure that Mrs. Jones has understood what she has been taught, the medical assistant should _____.
    A. give Mrs. Jones a written quiz
    B. ask open-ended questions to evaluate Mrs. Jones' understanding
    C. ask Mrs. Jones' family how she is doing
    D. give Mrs. Jones an oral quiz

9 Nutrition

VOCABULARY REVIEW

Matching: Match each term with the correct definition.

A. amino acids

B. anorexia

C. antioxidant

D. beriberi

E. bulimia

F. cellulose

G. cholesterol

H. dermatitis

I. display panel

J. fad diet

K. glossitis

L. goiter

M. hydrogenated

N. major minerals

O. malabsorption

P. monounsaturated fats

Q. night blindness

R. osteomalacia

_____ 1. Minerals used by the body in small amounts

_____ 2. Chief part of a cell wall

_____ 3. Minerals used in significant amounts by the body

_____ 4. Condition caused by the body's inability to absorb vitamin B_{12}

_____ 5. Building blocks

_____ 6. Polyunsaturated fats are made solid

_____ 7. Vitamins not stored in the body

_____ 8. Panel on a label used for marketing purposes

_____ 9. Disease caused by a deficiency of niacin in the body

_____ 10. Condition caused by a lack of vitamin C in the diet

_____ 11. Condition caused by a deficiency of thiamine

_____ 12. Condition caused by a deficiency of vitamin A

_____ 13. Dietary fats that have been broken down into fatty acids and glycerol

_____ 14. Diet that is structured to cause quick loss of weight

S. pellagra

T. pernicious anemia

U. rickets

V. scurvy

W. synthesize

X. trace minerals

Y. triglycerides

Z. water-soluble vitamins

_____ 15. Inability of the digestive system to absorb required nutrients

_____ 16. Condition in children caused by vitamin D deficiency

_____ 17. Psychological fear of gaining weight; also lack of appetite

_____ 18. Inflammation of the tongue

_____ 19. Inflammation of the skin caused by irritation or riboflavin deficiency

_____ 20. To make or take in

_____ 21. Disorder characterized by compulsive overeating followed by self-induced vomiting or use of laxatives or diuretics

_____ 22. Abnormal bone softening caused by vitamin D deficiency

_____ 23. Type of fat necessary for vitamin D and bile acid production

_____ 24. Enlarged thyroid

_____ 25. Substance that acts against oxidizing agents

_____ 26. Fats that are liquid at room temperature and help reduce total cholesterol

THEORY RECALL

True/False

Indicate whether the statement is true or false.

_____ 1. The information on the food label is considered a legal document.

_____ 2. Foods that have been fortified with vitamins and minerals take the place of a well-balanced diet.

_____ 3. Sodium is found naturally in many foods.

_____ 4. Effective dietary patient education is the key to helping patients understand the situation and the need for change.

_____ 5. It is okay for the medical assistant to tell the patient that reading food labels is unnecessary.

Multiple Choice

Identify the letter of the choice that best completes the statement or answers the question.

1. The food guide pyramid was developed by the _____.
   A. DHHS
   B. FDA
   C. RDA
   D. USDA

2. Honey is composed of _____% sugar.
   A. 10
   B. 25
   C. 50
   D. 75

3. _____ are organic substances that enhance the breakdown of proteins, carbohydrates, and fat.
   A. Carbohydrates
   B. Minerals
   C. Nutrients
   D. Vitamins

4. Complex carbohydrates supply the _____ with energy.
   A. heart and lungs
   B. muscles and brain
   C. brain and heart
   D. lungs and muscles

5. Signs and symptoms of poor nutrition include _____.
   A. dry and brittle hair
   B. cracked lips
   C. dry and scaling skin
   D. all of the above

6. RDAs are the nutritional guidelines that are published as the recommended dietary allowances whose name has been changed to read _____.
   A. recommended daily allowances
   B. daily allowances
   C. daily values
   D. has not been changed and still reads the same

7. _____ is an example of a fat-soluble vitamin.
   A. Vitamin B
   B. Vitamin C
   C. Vitamin K
   D. All of the above

8. The recommended intake of sodium is _____ mg per day.
   A. 1200
   B. 1500
   C. 2000
   D. 2400

9. _____ are liquid at room temperature and may help reduce blood cholesterol.
   A. Saturated fats
   B. Monounsaturated fats
   C. Polyunsaturated fats
   D. Fatty acids

10. There are _____ amino acids in protein.
    A. 10
    B. 15
    C. 22
    D. 24

11. The recommended amount of water to ingest is _____ daily.
    A. 16 ounces
    B. 1 quart
    C. 2 quarts
    D. 3 quarts

12. _____ is(are) a group of substances composed of many amino acids linked together.
    A. Proteins
    B. Carbohydrates
    C. Cholesterol
    D. Minerals

13. High-protein diets are often used _____.
    A. before surgery
    B. when an infection is present
    C. with hypothermia
    D. all of the above

14. The daily allowance of saturated fats is _____ g.
    A. 10
    B. 20
    C. 25
    D. 30

15. A diet low in saturated fats and cholesterol helps to maintain the blood cholesterol at levels less than _____ mg/dL.
    A. 100
    B. 200
    C. 250
    D. 300

16. Fad diets can result in _____.
    A. revised eating habits
    B. slowed weight loss
    C. rapid weight loss
    D. long-term weight loss

17. Dietary fats break down into fatty acids and are passed into the blood to form _____.
    A. phospholipids
    B. enzymes
    C. hormones
    D. all of the above

Copyright © 2010, 2005 by Saunders, an imprint of Elsevier, Inc. All rights reserved.

18. The Mayo Clinic considers a person overweight when the body mass index is _____.
    A. 10 to 19.9
    B. 20 to 25.9
    C. 25 to 29.9
    D. 30 to 35.9

19. Which one of the following is *not* affected by proper nutrition?
    A. hair
    B. teeth
    C. reproduction
    D. all of the above are affected

20. _____ produces quick energy.
    A. Carbohydrates
    B. Protein
    C. Fatty acids
    D. Unsaturated fats

Sentence Completion

Complete each sentence or statement.

minerals	fat-soluble
scurvy	monounsaturated
nutrition	cellulose
saturated fats	cholesterol
water-soluble	simple proteins
protein	enzymes

1. _____ are complex proteins that break down amino acids.

2. _____ is the scientific study of how different food groups affect the body.

3. _____ vitamins are not stored in the body.

4. _____ are inorganic substances used in the formation of hard and soft body tissue.

5. _____ are usually solid at room temperature.

6. The primary function of _____ is to build and repair tissue and the formation of enzymes.

7. _____ is necessary for vitamin D and bile acid production.

8. _____ are liquid at room temperature and are thought to raise HDL and LDL cholesterol levels.

9. _____ is important for elimination.

10. _____ are found in whole grains, beans, nuts, and seeds.

Short Answers

1. List the two main panels of a food label and explain each.

   _____
   _____
   _____
   _____
   _____

2. List and explain the five tips for a balanced diet.

   _____
   _____
   _____
   _____
   _____
   _____
   _____

3. Explain three conditions a medical assistant should be looking for when doing an inventory of the patient's readiness to follow a new diet plan.

   _____
   _____
   _____
   _____
   _____

CRITICAL THINKING

1. Select one of the four following diets and make a plan for three meals a day with a morning and afternoon snack for 7 days. Each plan should include a calorie count, fat count, carbohydrate count, and salt intake, regardless of which diet is selected.
   - A 1200-calorie diet
   - Low-fat diet
   - Low-carbohydrate diet
   - High-fiber diet

Copyright © 2010, 2005 by Saunders, an imprint of Elsevier, Inc. All rights reserved.

CHAPTER 9 Nutrition

PRACTICAL APPLICATIONS

If you have accomplished the objectives in this chapter, you will be able to make better choices as a medical assistant. Take a look at this situation and decide what you would do.

Josephine, age 52, has just been diagnosed with type 2 diabetes mellitus related to obesity. Living at home with Josephine are her mother, Susie, who is 80 years old; Josephine's daughter Jessie, who is 24 and pregnant; and Jessie's two very active children, ages 6 and 2. Susie has been diagnosed with a heart condition and must be on a soft diet that is low in cholesterol and sodium restricted.

Josephine's concern today is how she can maintain a diet acceptable for all the medical conditions in the household while ensuring the other family members eat what is prepared. She thinks the children need sugar, but her mother needs to watch her sugar and salt intake to remain in a stable condition and not gain weight. Susie also needs her meals to be soft and easily chewable because of her decreased intestinal motility. However, Jessie and her 2-year-old child need a diet that allows the necessary fiber for adequate bowel activity.

If you were the medical assistant, how might you educate Josephine about nutrition and answer her questions?

1. Why are learning styles important for the medical assistant to understand when teaching medical knowledge to the patient?

2. Why is it now so important for Josephine to read food labels? What information is found on these?

3. Why is diet so important for Josephine to follow in the treatment of type 2 diabetes mellitus? Why does she need to know the glycemic index of foods?

4. What are the special requirements for Susie to maintain a low-cholesterol diet?

5. Jessie's children want to eat pizza and French fries like their friends. How does this affect the dietary changes of Josephine, Susie, and Jessie?

6. Because Jessie has elevated blood pressure and early signs of edema in the legs and feet, what type of diet would you expect her to maintain for the remainder of her pregnancy?

7. What foods are found in a diabetic diet? What foods are found in a low-sodium diet?

8. What effect would low income have on this family?

9. What effect would culture have in planning this diet if the family were of Greek or Italian ethnicity?

10. Why is body mass index (BMI) a better guide for obesity than height and weight charts?

11. Why is it important that Josephine include a variety of foods in the diet for all members of the family?

CHAPTER QUIZ

Multiple Choice

Identify the letter of the choice that best completes the statement or answers the question.

1. _____ are building blocks, byproducts of protein breakdown by enzymes.
    A. Amino acids
    B. Carbohydrates
    C. Major minerals
    D. *Trans*-fatty acids

2. Saturated fats come mostly from _____.
   A. plant fat
   B. animal fat
   C. organ meat
   D. egg yolks

3. Honey is _____% sugar.
   A. 20
   B. 40
   C. 60
   D. 75

4. _____ are chemical substances within food that are released and absorbed during the digestive process.
   A. Minerals
   B. Nutrients
   C. Vitamins
   D. Carbohydrates

5. _____ are in liquid form at room temperature and may help lower total blood cholesterol.
   A. Monounsaturated fats
   B. Polyunsaturated fats
   C. *Trans*-fatty acids
   D. None of the above

6. Mineral oil interferes with the body's ability to absorb vital nutrients.
   A. True
   B. False

7. The acceptable level of saturated fats daily is _____ g.
   A. 10
   B. 15
   C. 20
   D. 25

8. An adult should consume a minimum of _____ of water a day.
   A. 16 ounces
   B. 32 ounces
   C. 1 quart
   D. 2 quarts

9. Sodium is found naturally in foods.
   A. True
   B. False

10. Cholesterol is necessary for vitamin _____ and bile production.
    A. A
    B. C
    C. D
    D. E

11. A patient undergoing chemotherapy for cancer must have a diet high in _____.
    A. carbohydrates
    B. fats
    C. vitamins
    D. all of the above

12. A body mass index of greater than _____ is considered to be obese.
    A. 20
    B. 30
    C. 40
    D. 50

13. _____ is a condition caused by the body's inability to absorb vitamin B_{12}.
    A. Beriberi
    B. Night blindness
    C. Pellagra
    D. Pernicious anemia

14. The key to patient teaching is not to focus on how to make a patient do something, but to create a situation in which the patient will want to do what is needed.
    A. True
    B. False

15. Vitamin _____ is a fat-soluble vitamin.
    A. B_6
    B. B_{12}
    C. C
    D. K

16. _____ are inorganic substances used in the formation of soft and hard tissues.
    A. Amino acids
    B. Carbohydrates
    C. Minerals
    D. Vitamins

17. _____ are the building blocks of fat that produce oil.
    A. Fatty acids
    B. Saturated fats
    C. Unsaturated fats
    D. None of the above

18. An infant should be fed _____ times in a 24-hour period.
    A. 6 to 8
    B. 8 to 12
    C. 10 to 14
    D. 12 to 15

19. A food label is a legal document.
    A. True
    B. False

20. With a diagnosis of cancer, the patient should eat a _____ diet.
    A. full liquid diet
    B. high protein
    C. regular diet
    D. soft diet

10 Understanding Medical Terminology

VOCABULARY REVIEW

Matching: Match each term with the correct definition.

A. combining form

B. combining vowel

C. consonant

D. diagnostic

E. diminutive

F. eponym

G. homonym

H. operative

I. plural

J. prefix

K. root word

L. suffix

M. symptomatic

N. synonym

O. vowel

_____ 1. Core meaning of a word

_____ 2. Name of a specific person, place, or thing for which something is being named

_____ 3. Speech sound used to pronounce words (a, e, i, o, u, and sometimes y)

_____ 4. Vowel added to a root word before any prefixes or suffixes

_____ 5. Root word with a vowel added to make pronunciation easier

_____ 6. Word that has the same pronunciation, but a different spelling and meaning than another word

_____ 7. Noun that refers to two or more

_____ 8. Having to do with the characteristics of a particular disease

_____ 9. Having to do with recognizing or identifying diseases in the body

_____ 10. Root word, prefix, or suffix that has the same or nearly the same meaning as a given word, prefix, or suffix

_____ 11. Having to do with an action or operation

_____ 12. Speech sound used to pronounce words that include all letters except a, e, i, o, u, and sometimes y

_____ 13. Word part placed at the beginning of a root word to change its meaning

_____ 14. Word part or series of word parts added to the end of a root word to change the meaning

_____ 15. Small; a small version of something

THEORY RECALL

True/False

Indicate whether the statement is true or false.

_____ 1. Most medical terms have German and French origins.

_____ 2. We use medical terminology because we can use one word for something that might otherwise take many words to describe.

_____ 3. All medical terms have at least one root word.

_____ 4. All medical terms must contain at least one prefix.

_____ 5. Phonetics help make the pronunciation of medical terms easier.

Multiple Choice

Identify the letter of the choice that best completes the statement or answers the question.

1. Generally, when a medical term has a vowel followed by a _____, the vowel receives a short pronunciation and a breve is placed over the vowel.
   A. second vowel
   B. consonant
   C. y
   D. All of the above apply

2. Some consonants are referred to as having a _____ or _____ sound.
   A. short, long
   B. quick, sharp
   C. soft, hard
   D. None of the above

3. When forming a plural of most English words, add a(n) _____.
   A. s
   B. 's
   C. es
   D. 'es

4. For nouns ending in a y preceded by a consonant, change the y to a(n) _____ and add es.
   A. a
   B. e
   C. i
   D. o

5. The synonym meaning "lung" is _____.
   A. plur/o; -pleura
   B. pulmon/o; -pneumo
   C. respirat/o; -respirata
   D. lung/o; -lunga

6. _____ is an example of an eponym.
   A. Pinkeye
   B. Athlete's foot
   C. McBurney point
   D. All of the above

7. The suffix that means "the study of" is _____.
   A. -ologist
   B. -oscopy
   C. -ic
   D. -ology

8. The term that means "the heart is located in the right hemothorax" is _____.
   A. cardiomegaly
   B. dextrocardia
   C. cardiopathy
   D. cardiac

9. _____ means "feverish" or "having a fever."
   A. Febrile
   B. Afebrile
   C. Disfebrile
   D. Anafebrile

10. "Death of cells or tissues through injury or disease" is called _____.
    A. macrosis
    B. narcolepsy
    C. necrosis
    D. cryptorchidism

11. The term meaning "above the pubis" is _____.
    A. suprapubic
    B. supranasal
    C. supracostal
    D. supraventricular

12. Bluish discoloration of the skin and mucous membranes from lack of oxygen is called _____.
    A. erythroderma
    B. cyanosis
    C. chromatoderma
    D. leukoplakia

13. "Xanthroderma" means _____.
    A. blue skin
    B. white skin
    C. yellow skin
    D. none of the above

14. "Ferrous" means _____.
    A. nitrogenous waste in the blood
    B. relating to or containing iron
    C. excretion of excessive amounts of sodium in the urine
    D. colorless, odorless gas formed from carbon and oxygen

15. Muscular tissue of the heart is _____.
    A. adipose tissue
    B. epithelium
    C. myocardia
    D. epicardia

16. The prefix meaning "half, one side, or partial" is _____.
    A. bi-
    B. milli-
    C. multi-
    D. hemi-

17. The prefix of the word "multicellular" is _____.
    A. multi-
    B. cell
    C. cellular
    D. -ar

18. A condition or disease affecting a large population is called a(n) _____.
    A. pandemic
    B. epidemic
    C. endemic
    D. peridemic

19. The process of removing the calcium from bones is called _____.
    A. deactivation
    B. catabolism
    C. decalcification
    D. endocalcification

20. A person who specializes in the study of diseases is called a(n) _____.
    A. endocrinologist
    B. pathologist
    C. anesthesiologist
    D. cardiologist

Completion

Write the correct term in the blank for each prefix, suffix, or word root.

1. _____ hemat/o

2. _____ chem/o

3. _____ aden/o

4. _____ crypt/o

5. _____ carcin/o

6. _____ dipl/o

7. _____ exo-

8. _____ hydro-

9. _____ scler/o

10. _____ noct/o

11. _____ super-

12. _____ therm/o

13. _____ glauc/o

14. _____ leuk/o

15. _____ chromat/o

16. _____ xanth/o

17. _____ cirrh/o

18. _____ chlori-

19. _____ ox-

20. _____ adip/o

21. _____ my/o

22. _____ sarc/o

23. _____ epi-

24. _____ neur/o

25. _____ bi-

26. _____ centi-

27. _____ kilo-

28. _____ micro-

29. _____ milli-

30. _____ multi-

31. _____ nulli-

32. _____ primi-

33. _____ tri-

34. _____ mono-

35. _____ ab-

36. _____ ana-

37. _____ endo-

38. _____ inter-

39. _____ para-

40. _____ post-

41. _____ sub-

42. _____ hypo-

43. _____ trans-

44. _____ anti-

45. _____ dys-

46. _____ tachy-

47. _____ -ic

48. _____ -ism

49. _____ -logist

50. _____ -stasis

51. _____ -algia

52. _____ -oid

53. _____ -lysis

54. _____ -megaly

55. _____ -pnea

56. _____ -rrhea

57. _____ -stenosis

58. _____ -gram

59. _____ -graphy

60. _____ -itis

61. _____ -iasis

Copyright © 2010, 2005 by Saunders, an imprint of Elsevier, Inc. All rights reserved.

62. _____ -malacia

63. _____ -oma

64. _____ -osis

65. _____ -plasia

66. _____ -rrhagia

67. _____ -scopy

68. _____ -rrhexis

69. _____ -centesis

70. _____ -ectomy

71. _____ -pexy

72. _____ -plasty

73. _____ -rrhaphy

74. _____ -stomy

75. _____ -tomy

76. _____ -tripsy

77. _____ -ist

78. _____ -gen

79. _____ -emia

80. _____ -lith

Short Answers

1. Explain the importance of using correct medical terminology.

2. List and define the four word parts used in medical terminology.

3. Define and give an example of an antonym, a homonym, and a synonym.

4. Explain why it is not important to memorize every medical term.

CRITICAL THINKING

1. Underline the medical terms and medical abbreviations in the following paragraph. (Underline a word or an abbreviation only once, for a total of 28 terms.)

   Susan Simmons, a 52-year-old woman, was transported by ambulance to the hospital in acute abdominal distress, severe pain in the RLQ, with guarding. Patient's vital signs were BP 140/76 P 92 R 20 all WNL. An HCG, Hct, Hgb, and sed rate were ordered by the physician. The HCG test was negative, Hct and Hgb were WNL, and the sed rate was slightly elevated. The patient affirms nausea, but denies vomiting. On further examination, the physician noted rebound tenderness over the RLQ. An abdominal ultrasound was ordered to rule out appendicitis, and a KUB was ordered to rule out renal calculi, or cystitis. The ultrasound revealed an enlarged appendix.
   An ECG and IV were performed, and a bleeding time was performed by the phlebotomist. The anesthesiologist and surgeon met with the patient, and it was determined the patient would be scheduled for an appendectomy STAT. The surgery was successful and proceeded without incident. The patient tolerated the procedure well and was sent to recovery.

PRACTICAL APPLICATIONS

If you have accomplished the objectives in this chapter, you will be able to make better choices as a medical assistant. Take a look at this situation and decide what you would do.

   Dr. Smith has a medical assistant who does the medical transcription of her patient notes. The following is a note the medical assistant has transcribed on Susie Ramos:

CHAPTER 10 Understanding Medical Terminology

"Seen in the office today for arteriaslcerosis and hipertension. Mrs. Ramos complained of feeling dizzy with some fertigo for 3 days. On questioning, Mrs. Ramos did state that she was febrille 2 days ago with some gastroentestinal symptoms such as darhea and nausea. She also complained of aralgia and laryngetes. On examination, the toncils are red and swollen. Her blood pressure is controlled by medication. There are no complaints of chest pain or anjina, nor does she have dispnea, although she does have some orthapnea. She does have some syanosis of the hands and feet, but does not complain of pain in these areas. Her sinuses are painful. Her current diagnosisses are sinisitus, athuroscleroisis, possible streptocokki infection, gastrointeritis, and faringitis."

1. There are 20 mistakes in the use of medical terminology in this dictation. Find and underline the mistakes, and then choose 10 to correct the spelling and define.

2. Explain why using and spelling the correct medical term is important in the medical record.

3. Why does the medical assistant need to study medical terminology? How does a solid understanding of medical terminology benefit the care that patients receive?

APPLICATION OF SKILLS

1. Label the word parts of the following terms. Use *P* to indicate a prefix, *CF* to indicate a combining form, *R* to indicate a root, and *S* to indicate a suffix. (Example: abnormal—ab *P* norm *R* al *S*)
    A. cytology _____
    B. oncology _____
    C. dehydrate _____
    D. android _____
    E. mesomorph _____
    F. topical _____
    G. pinocytosis _____
    H. microscope _____
    I. homeostasis _____
    J. microorganism _____

2. Write the definitions for the following medical terms.
    A. cardiopathy _____
    B. echocardiogram _____
    C. endoscope _____
    D. intrabronchial _____
    E. osteomalacia _____
    F. homeostasis _____
    G. adipose _____
    H. neuropathology _____
    I. tracheostenosis _____
    J. adenopathy _____
    K. diplococcus _____

3. Change the following from singular to plural or vice versa.
    A. anastomosis _____
    B. bulla _____
    C. diverticula _____
    D. anomaly _____
    E. ganglion _____

CHAPTER QUIZ

Multiple Choice

Identify the letter of the choice that best completes the statement or answers the question.

1. A word root, prefix, or suffix that has the opposite meaning of another word is a(n) _____.
    A. eponym
    B. antonym
    C. diminutive
    D. synonym

2. A word that has the same pronunciation, but a different spelling and meaning than another word is a(n) _____.
    A. homonym
    B. eponym
    C. diminutive
    D. synonym

3. The medical term for inflammation of a joint is _____.
   A. arthralgia
   B. arthrodynia
   C. arthritis
   D. arthroscopy

4. A(n) _____ is added to the root word before any prefix or suffix to make pronunciation easier.
   A. consonant
   B. e
   C. i
   D. combining vowel

5. A _____ is a word part that is sometimes placed at the beginning of a root word to change its meaning.
   A. combining vowel
   B. prefix
   C. suffix
   D. none of the above

6. When analyzing medical words, begin with the suffix, then proceed to the root and prefix.
   A. True
   B. False

7. Which one of the following is the correct pleural for the word "lumen"?
   A. luminol
   B. lumina
   C. lumines
   D. luminia

8. Which one of the following is the correct pleural for the word "sarcoma"?
   A. carinoma
   B. sarcomita
   C. sarcomitis
   D. sarcomata

9. Part of the small intestine is the _____.
   A. ileum
   B. ilium
   C. ilaum
   D. iloum

10. _____ is an eponym.
    A. Catheter
    B. Babinski reflex
    C. Rake retractor
    D. Forceps

11. The correct medical term for the study of blood is _____.
    A. hematopoiesis
    B. circulatology
    C. cardiology
    D. hematology

12. A pair of cocci bacteria are called _____.
    A. monococci
    B. diplococci
    C. streptococci
    D. staphylococci

13. The outermost layer of a developing embryo is called an _____.
    A. exoderm
    B. ectoderm
    C. endoderm
    D. ergoderm

14. A disorder with sudden attacks of deep sleep is _____.
    A. nyctophobia
    B. noctophobia
    C. narcolepsy
    D. all of the above

15. An accumulation of fluid in a body cavity is called hydrocele.
    A. True
    B. False

16. The medical term for "blood poisoning" is _____.
    A. uremia
    B. choloremia
    C. streptemia
    D. septicemia

17. The medical term for "an abnormal redness of the skin" is _____.
    A. erythroderma
    B. leukoderma
    C. xanthoderma
    D. cyanosis

18. The medical term for "low potassium in the blood" is _____.
    A. hypercalcium
    B. hyperkalemia
    C. hypocalcium
    D. hypokalemia

19. The medical term for "fat tissues" is _____.
    A. lipase
    B. adipose
    C. adapose
    D. lipose

20. Therapy based on the theory "like cures like" is called _____.
    A. isotonic
    B. homeostasis
    C. homeopathy
    D. isostasis

Copyright © 2010, 2005 by Saunders, an imprint of Elsevier, Inc. All rights reserved.

NAME: _____ DATE: _____

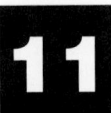 Basic Anatomy and Physiology

VOCABULARY REVIEW

Matching: Match each term with the correct definition.

A. anatomy

B. physiology

C. anterior

D. inferior

E. posterior

F. supine position

G. midsagittal plane

H. membrane

I. viscera

J. abdominopelvic cavity

K. pelvic

L. quadrants

M. mediastinum

N. thoracic cavity

O. cranial cavity

P. cervical

Q. meninges

R. spinal cord

S. vertebra

_____ 1. Recessive gene disorder of the exocrine glands causing the excretion of thick mucus into the lungs

_____ 2. Specialized tissue that covers an organ surface or lines a body cavity or is located between a space

_____ 3. Condition or anomaly that an infant is born with; is not necessarily inherited from the parents

_____ 4. Back, behind

_____ 5. Muscle of the heart

_____ 6. Study of the function of an organism

_____ 7. Having the same amount of solutes as another

_____ 8. Organs of any cavity

_____ 9. Bony structure of the spinal column

_____ 10. Quality of a membrane that allows some materials to pass through and not others

_____ 11. Threadlike strand inside the nucleus that contains genetic information

_____ 12. That which is below

_____ 13. Area located behind the sternum and in front of the lungs; houses trachea, esophagus, and large blood vessels

110

Copyright © 2010, 2005 by Saunders, an imprint of Elsevier, Inc. All rights reserved.

T. axial

U. appendicular

V. molecule

W. cell

X. organelle

Y. anabolism

Z. chromosomes

AA. genes

BB. mitochondria

CC. nucleus

DD. semipermeable

EE. diffusion

FF. hemolyze

GG. isotonic

HH. phagocytosis

II. mitosis

JJ. malignant

KK. gametes

LL. congenital

MM. familial

NN. hereditary

OO. sign

PP. symptom

QQ. Down syndrome

RR. cystic fibrosis

SS. dyspnea

TT. muscular dystrophy

_____ 14. Tissue that carries electrical impulses to body structures

_____ 15. Vertical cut through the body that divides the body into equal right and left sections

_____ 16. Cavity between the diaphragm and the pelvic floor

_____ 17. Having to do with the area of the body that includes the head, neck, and torso

_____ 18. To burst open because of taking on too much water

_____ 19. Organelle that functions as the control center of a cell and contains the chromosomes

_____ 20. Study of the structure of an organism

_____ 21. Clinical division of the abdominal area into four parts

_____ 22. Cellular activity of combining simple substances to form more complex substances

_____ 23. Cell division of body cells

_____ 24. Chromosomal disease that occurs because of a duplication of number 21 chromosome

_____ 25. Tissues that provide a protective covering for the brain and the spinal cord

_____ 26. Tissue that covers the body and internal cavities

_____ 27. Having to do with the area of the pelvis

_____ 28. Describes the body when lying on the back with the face up

_____ 29. Sex cells

_____ 30. X-linked recessive muscular wasting disease

_____ 31. Chest area

UU. sickle cell anemia

VV. epithelial tissue

WW. nervous tissue

XX. exocrine gland

YY. myocardium

ZZ. matrix

_____ 32. Substance within a cell that provides strength from which it develops

_____ 33. In or referring to the front

_____ 34. Cavity that holds the brain and is formed by the skull

_____ 35. Organelles that produce the energy within the cell called ATP

_____ 36. Nerve tissue surrounded by the spinal column

_____ 37. Movement of a substance from an area of higher concentration to one of lower concentration

_____ 38. Two or more atoms

_____ 39. Having to do with the spinal area in the neck

_____ 40. Gland that secretes its substance through a duct

_____ 41. Condition passed to an infant by its parents

_____ 42. Fundamental unit of living tissue; made up of atoms and molecules

_____ 43. Something that the patient can tell you about, but that cannot be measured or seen

_____ 44. Cancerous

_____ 45. Structure contained within the cytoplasm of a cell; each one has a specific function

_____ 46. Cellular process of taking in or digesting waste material

_____ 47. Hereditary unit containing inherited material and carried within chromosomes

_____ 48. Something that can be seen or measured

_____ 49. Difficulty in breathing; shortness of breath

_____ 50. Having to do with the area of the body that includes the upper and lower extremities

_____ 51. Occurring within a family

_____ 52. Inherited disease that causes the red blood cells to be crescent shaped

THEORY RECALL

True/False

Indicate whether the statement is true or false.

_____ 1. The body is assumed to be in a correct or true anatomical position when the individual is standing erect and facing forward.

_____ 2. The anterior and lateral cavities are the two main spaces that contain the internal organs of the human body.

_____ 3. The diaphragm is the structure dividing the abdominal and pelvic cavities.

_____ 4. Bone tissue has fibers and a hard mineral substance that provides for protection and support of the body.

_____ 5. The final organizational level in the human body consists of the body systems.

Multiple Choice

Identify the letter of the choice that best completes the statement or answers the question.

1. A vertical cut through the body that divides the body into anterior and posterior sections is called the _____.
   A. frontal plane
   B. midsagittal plane
   C. transverse plane
   D. horizontal plane

2. The _____ position describes the body lying on the belly with the face down.
   A. supine
   B. prone
   C. transverse
   D. recumbent

3. The _____ cavity contains organs that maintain homeostasis when the body is exposed to internal and external stimuli.
   A. thoracic
   B. pleural
   C. ventral
   D. pericardial

4. What is the third phase of mitosis?
   A. metaphase
   B. telophase
   C. anaphase
   D. interphase

5. The center square of the abdominal region is _____.
   A. hypochondriac
   B. iliac
   C. epigastric
   D. umbilical

6. Which quadrant contains part of the small and large intestines, left ureter, and left ovary and left fallopian tube in the female?
   A. RUQ
   B. LUQ
   C. RLQ
   D. LLQ

7. Which one of the following is *not* a division of the spinal column?
   A. Cranial
   B. Cervical
   C. Lumbar
   D. Coccygeal

8. The _____ skeleton consists of the upper and lower extremities.
   A. afferent
   B. axial
   C. appendicular
   D. appendable

9. The smallest part of the body is a(n) _____.
   A. molecule
   B. compound
   C. chemical
   D. atom

10. The fundamental unit of all living things is (the) _____.
    A. cell
    B. molecules
    C. chemicals
    D. atom

11. Red blood cells live for approximately _____.
    A. 12 hours
    B. 120 days
    C. 12 months
    D. 120 minutes

12. Which one of the following is *not* one of the three main parts of a cell?
    A. cytoplasm
    B. organelles
    C. nucleus
    D. cell membrane

13. Organelles carry out several life functions that include all of the following *except* _____.
    A. immune response and hormone replacement
    B. growth and reproduction
    C. nourishment and waste removal
    D. reacting and adapting to change

14. The cell membrane is composed of _____.
    A. acids and bases
    B. salts and sugars
    C. proteins and lipids
    D. none of the above

15. Each chromosome contains thousands of _____.
    A. nucleoli
    B. mitochondria
    C. ribosomes
    D. genes

16. Which one of the following is an example of passive transport?
    A. Diffusion
    B. Osmosis
    C. Filtration
    D. All of the above

17. _____ is the random movement of dissolved particles that move from an area of higher concentration to an area of lower concentration.
    A. Diffusion
    B. Osmosis
    C. Filtration
    D. None of the above

18. _____ occurs when particles are pushed through a membrane by a mechanical pressure.
    A. Diffusion
    B. Osmosis
    C. Filtration
    D. None of the above

19. _____ is when a stationary cell engulfs and digests droplets of a fluid ("cell drinking").
    A. Phagocytosis
    B. Pinocytosis
    C. Mitosis
    D. Meiosis

20. A person has a total of _____ chromosomes.
    A. 23
    B. 46
    C. 92
    D. an unlimited amount

CHAPTER 11   Basic Anatomy and Physiology

Sentence Completion

Complete each sentence or statement.

Klinefelter syndrome	epithelial	muscle
gametes	exocrine glands	myoma
endocrine glands	papilloma	hyaline
visual	dense	cartilage
auditory	cardiac tissue	organ
nerve tissue	meninges	
metastasis	hemophilia	

1. The brain and spinal cord are one continuous structure that is covered by _____.

2. _____ occurs when cancer cells break away from the tumor and travel to other parts of the body.

3. _____ are sex cells.

4. _____ is an example of a chromosomal disease that occurs in males when an extra X chromosome is present at birth.

5. _____ is an X-linked recessive bleeding disorder caused by a missing coagulation factor.

6. Cells of _____ tissue fit tightly together and have only small amounts of intercellular substance holding them.

7. _____ are ductless and discharge their hormones into the tissue fluid to be absorbed by the capillaries in the body.

8. _____ tissue contracts, or shortens, allowing movement.

9. _____ is a benign tumor of the epithelium.

10. Smooth or _____ muscles form the walls of hollow organs.

11. A _____ is a tumor usually found in involuntary muscles.

12. _____ tissue helps anchor muscle to bone, or connects bone to bone.

13. _____ supports the rings of the bronchi, which aid in keeping open the airway.

14. _____ is the most highly organized tissue in the body.

15. An _____ is composed of two or more types of tissues that allow it to perform a specific function or functions.

Short Answers

1. Describe the progression from an atom to a system.

2. List five things that can cause genes to mutate.

3. List the 10 body systems and describe the functions of each.

4. List the four main types of body tissues and describe the functions of each.

___

CRITICAL THINKING

1. There are many mechanisms for moving substances across the cell membrane. List the various types of movement that do not require cellular energy and the types of movement that do require cellular energy. Provide an example for each type.

PRACTICAL APPLICATIONS

If you have accomplished the objectives in this chapter, you will be able to make better choices as a medical assistant. Take a look at this situation and decide what you would do.

John Choi is a medical assistant in a primary care facility. Barb Quinn arrives and complains of pain that she thinks is in her stomach. She states that she has had vomiting with blood and diarrhea. She also complains of difficulty in eating, stating that she just does not want anything to eat, "I have to force myself to eat." After the examination, Dr. Elory tells Ms. Quinn that based on her symptoms, he is suspicious of a cancer in her abdomen. Dr. Elory orders several diagnostic tests that will be completed the next day. Dr. Elory tells Ms. Quinn that he will call as soon as he has her test results.

John needs to chart the pain using the correct cavity for the stomach, the region of the abdominopelvic area, and the correct quadrant of the abdominal area. In what body system would John know the stomach is found?

1. **How might John explain to Ms. Quinn what her symptoms mean in relation to anatomy and physiology?**

___

Basic Anatomy and Physiology **CHAPTER 11**

2. What is cancer?

3. What does cell division have to do with cancer?

4. If Ms. Quinn had complained of pain in the left upper quadrant, what organs might have been involved?

5. If the pain was in the umbilical region, what could this mean?

6. What does pain in the right lower quadrant indicate as a possible organ involvement?

7. If Ms. Quinn had complained of shortness of breath, in what cavity would you expect the discomfort to be? What organ systems would be found in this cavity? What separates this cavity from the abdominopelvic cavity?

Copyright © 2010, 2005 by Saunders, an imprint of Elsevier, Inc. All rights reserved.

8. What is the difference between a sign and a symptom when discussing illness? What are the symptoms in the above-described scenario? What is a subjective finding, and what is an objective finding in the patient's medical history?

___

9. What symptoms indicate a disturbance of the homeostasis of Ms. Quinn's body?

___

APPLICATION OF SKILLS

1. Label the word parts of the following terms. Use *P* to indicate a prefix, *CF* to indicate a combining form, *R* to indicate a root, and *S* to indicate a suffix. (Example: abnormal—ab *P* norm *R* al *S*)
    A. anatomy ___
    B. caudal ___
    C. diffusion ___
    D. physiology ___
    E. visceral ___

2. Change the following from singular to plural or vice versa.
    A. viscera ___
    B. nuclei ___
    C. mitochondria ___
    D. thoraces ___
    E. vertebrae ___

3. Write out the meaning of each the following abbreviations.
    A. RUQ ___
    B. RLQ ___
    C. LUQ ___
    D. LLQ ___
    E. A&P ___

Basic Anatomy and Physiology CHAPTER 11   121

4. Label the following diagrams.

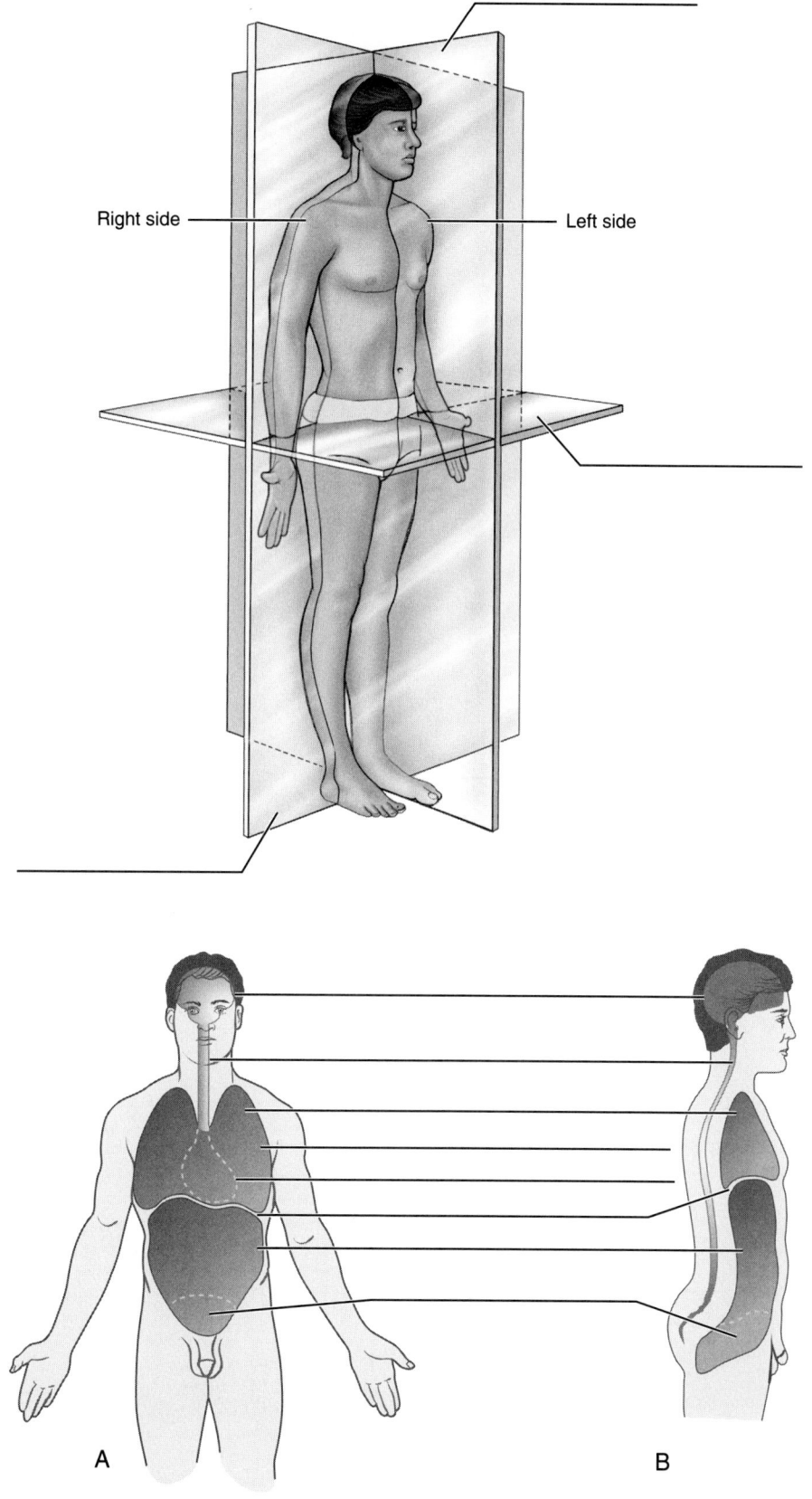

Right side — Left side

A   B

CHAPTER 11 Basic Anatomy and Physiology

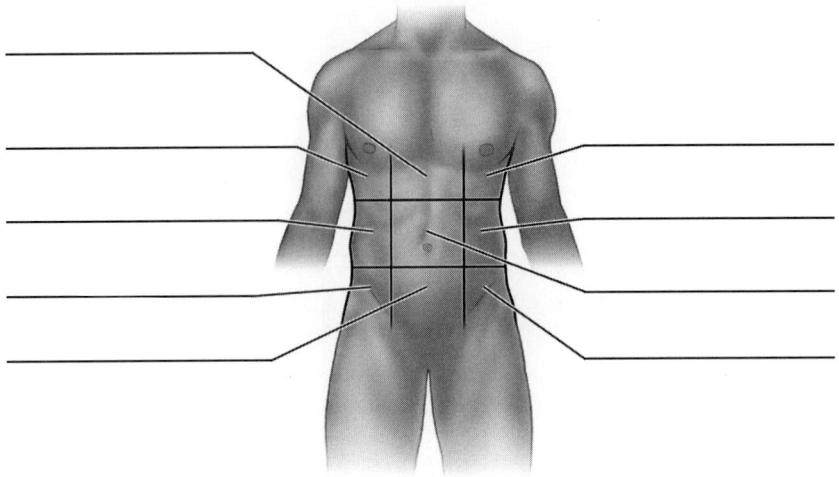

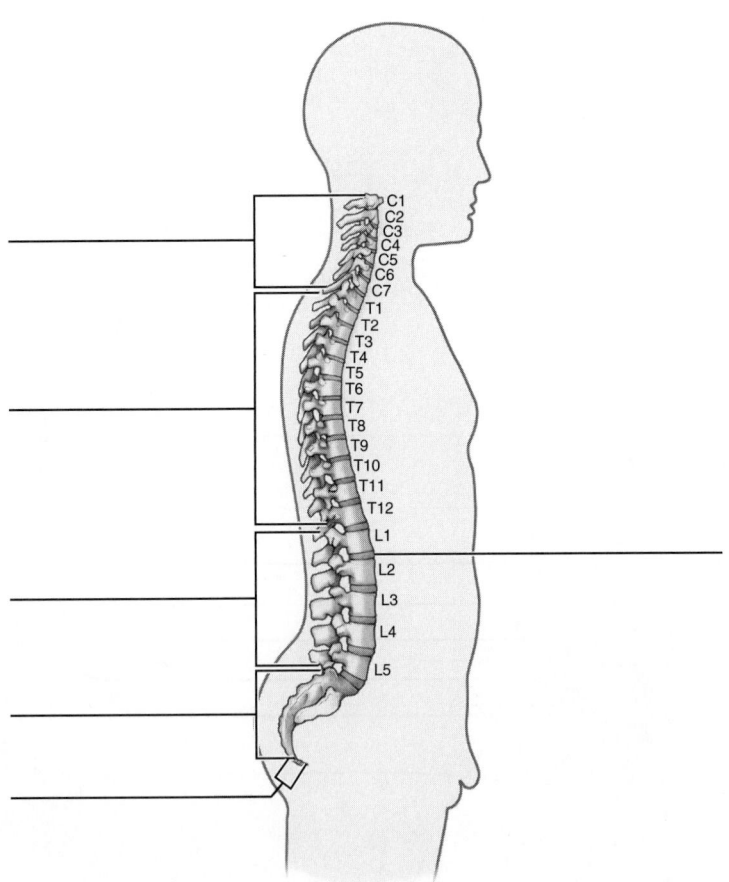

Basic Anatomy and Physiology CHAPTER 11 123

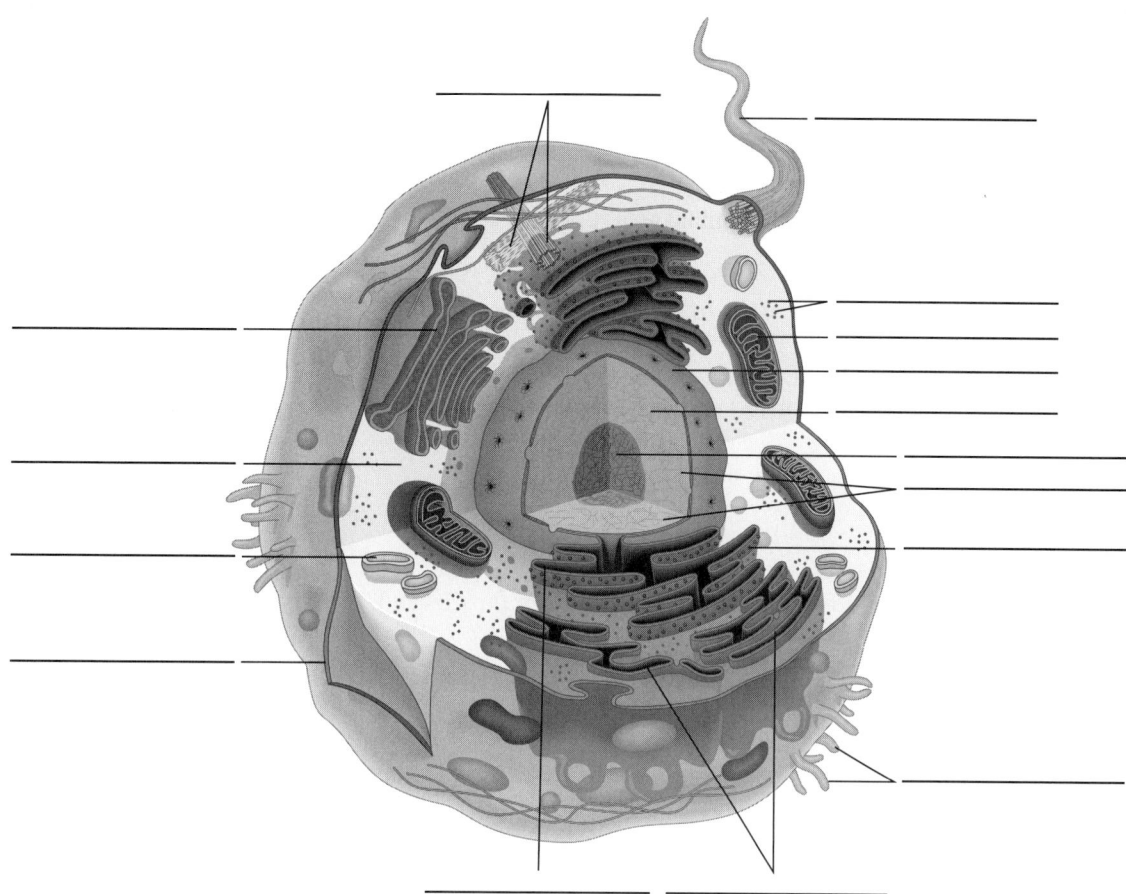

CHAPTER QUIZ

Multiple Choice

Identify the letter of the choice that best completes the statement or answers the question.

1. _____ is a vertical cut that divides the body into right and left portions.
   A. Frontal
   B. Midsagittal
   C. Sagittal
   D. Transverse

2. The main muscle of breathing that lies between the thoracic and abdominal cavities is called the _____.
   A. pleura
   B. sternocleidomastoid
   C. diaphragm
   D. costal muscle

Copyright © 2010, 2005 by Saunders, an imprint of Elsevier, Inc. All rights reserved.

3. The _____ cavity contains the teeth and tongue.
   A. buccal
   B. orbital
   C. lacrimal
   D. periodontal

4. _____ means having to do with the spinal area in the neck.
   A. Coccygeal
   B. Cervical
   C. Thoracic
   D. Lumbar

5. The _____ is the outer layer of the heart sac.
   A. pericardial membrane
   B. epicardial membrane
   C. parietal thoracic membrane
   D. none of the above

6. _____ means having to do with the spinal area between the ribs and the ilium.
   A. Lumbar
   B. Thoracic
   C. Cervical
   D. None of the above

7. _____ is the cellular activity of breaking down complex substances into simple matter.
   A. Anabolism
   B. Catabolism
   C. Cannibalism
   D. Phagocytosis

8. A _____ is an organelle responsible for breaking down larger molecules.
   A. lysosome
   B. ribosome
   C. Golgi apparatus
   D. mitochondrion

9. A substance that carries genetic information and is considered to be the "blueprint" of the cell is called _____.
   A. RNA
   B. DNA
   C. ATP
   D. PKU

10. _____ are organelles involved in cellular division.
    A. Mitochondria
    B. Ribosomes
    C. Centrioles
    D. Nucleoli

11. _____ means "not cancerous."
    A. Benign
    B. Malignant
    C. Metastatic
    D. None of the above

12. A(n) _____ solution has more solutes than any other.
    A. isotonic
    B. hypotonic
    C. hypertonic
    D. none of the above

13. A _____ is a condition or an anomaly that an infant is born with; it is not necessarily inherited.
    A. congenital
    B. hereditary
    C. genetic
    D. all the above

14. An X-linked disorder that causes malformation of the skull is _____.
    A. hydrocephalus
    B. cleft palate
    C. Turner syndrome
    D. Klinefelter syndrome

15. _____ is an X-linked recessive muscular wasting disease.
    A. Tay-Sachs disease
    B. PKU
    C. Turner syndrome
    D. Muscular dystrophy

16. The _____ is the main muscle of the heart.
    A. pericardium
    B. epicardium
    C. endocardium
    D. myocardium

17. Muscle fibers that are divided by bands of stripes are called _____.
    A. nonstriated muscle
    B. striated muscle
    C. smooth muscle
    D. cardiac muscle

18. Tissue occurring outside the cell is called _____.
    A. dense tissue
    B. fibrous tissue
    C. extracellular
    D. intracellular tissue

19. _____ nerves carry impulses from the senses to the brain.
    A. Afferent
    B. Efferent

20. Cells that provide support for nervous tissue are called _____ cells.
    A. glitter
    B. glial
    C. astro
    D. familial

Copyright © 2010, 2005 by Saunders, an imprint of Elsevier, Inc. All rights reserved.

Matching

Match each prefix or suffix with its correct definition.

_____ 21. cephal/o   A. to secrete

_____ 22. plasia   B. nose

_____ 23. crin/o   C. vein

_____ 24. phleb/o   D. sweat glands

_____ 25. col/o   E. head

_____ 26. rhin/o   F. joint

_____ 27. myel/o   G. spinal cord

_____ 28. articul/o   H. growth, formation of tissue

_____ 29. my/o   I. large intestine

_____ 30. hidr/o   J. muscle

NAME: _____ DATE: _____

12 Cardiovascular System

VOCABULARY REVIEW

Matching: Match each term with the correct definition.

A. cardiovascular system

B. myocardium

C. atrium

D. ventricle

E. aorta

F. cardiac cycle

G. electrocardiogram

H. infarction

I. ischemia

J. cardiologist

K. vasoconstrict

L. aneurysm

M. embolus

N. apex

O. pericardium

P. chordae tendineae

Q. systole

R. thrombus

S. cyanosis

_____ 1. When the blood vessel is made more narrow

_____ 2. Lower chambers of the heart

_____ 3. Systole and diastole that produce the heartbeat

_____ 4. Twisted and swollen vein

_____ 5. Tip of the heart

_____ 6. Main muscle layer of the heart wall

_____ 7. Recording of the cardiac cycle

_____ 8. Symptoms of pain and weakness in the legs that subside with rest

_____ 9. Bluish discoloration of the nails or skin caused by lack of oxygen in the blood

_____ 10. Largest artery in the body

_____ 11. Contraction of the heart

_____ 12. Abnormal heart sound

_____ 13. Body system that consists of the heart and blood vessels

_____ 14. Death of tissue because of lack of blood to area

_____ 15. Smallest blood vessel that moves oxygen into and removes waste products from body tissues

_____ 16. Stationary clot

_____ 17. Sac that surrounds the heart

CHAPTER 12 Cardiovascular System

T. cardiomegaly

U. murmur

V. sequela

W. varix

X. capillary

Y. claudication

Z. diastole

_____ 18. Upper chamber of the heart

_____ 19. Physician who specializes in the structure, function, and diseases of the heart

_____ 20. Fibrous cords that prevent atrioventricular valves from collapsing under pressure

_____ 21. Enlargement of the heart

_____ 22. Relaxation of the heart

_____ 23. Secondary result of another disease; aftereffect

_____ 24. Clot that moves through the bloodstream

_____ 25. Deficiency of blood supply because of an obstruction

_____ 26. Weakness in the wall of an artery

THEORY RECALL

True/False

Indicate whether the statement is true or false.

_____ 1. The heart is a solid, muscular pump that averages 72 beats/minute.

_____ 2. The outermost layer of the heart wall is the epicardium.

_____ 3. When the blood leaves the left atrium, it passes through the pulmonary semilunar valve.

_____ 4. The atrioventricular node is known as the body's natural pacemaker.

_____ 5. The foramen ovale is an opening in the septum between the atria before birth.

Multiple Choice

Identify the letter of the choice that best completes the statement or answers the question.

1. The inner muscle layer of the heart is called the _____.
   A. myocardium
   B. endocardium
   C. pericardium
   D. epicardium

2. The _____ is the partition between the two sides of the heart.
   A. chamber
   B. atria
   C. ventricle
   D. septum

3. The vein that brings blood low in oxygen from the head and upper limbs is called the _____.
   A. inferior vena cava
   B. aorta
   C. superior vena cava
   D. pulmonary artery

4. Movement of blood from the heart to the lungs and back is known as _____.
   A. fetal circulation
   B. coronary circulation
   C. systemic circulation
   D. pulmonary circulation

5. Death of tissue because of lack of blood to an area is called _____.
   A. ecchymosis
   B. ischemia
   C. infarction
   D. diaphoresis

6. _____ is narrowing of aorta causing a decrease in blood flow.
   A. Atrial septal defect
   B. Patent ductus arteriosus
   C. Coarctation of the aorta
   D. Myocarditis

7. The _____ artery is used to check for blood supply to lower extremities; supplies blood to muscles of foot and toes.
   A. femoral
   B. dorsalis pedis
   C. subclavian
   D. radial

8. _____ is used to check pulse in young children for CPR.
   A. Radial
   B. Carotid
   C. Temporal
   D. Brachial

9. Small arteries are called _____.
   A. arterioles
   B. atrerioles
   C. artirioles
   D. arteroles

10. A _____ carries deoxygenated blood toward the heart.
    A. capillary
    B. lumen
    C. vein
    D. thrombus

11. Pain and numbness in the fingers, hands, and feet is a symptom of _____.
    A. phlebitis
    B. congestive heart failure
    C. Raynaud disease
    D. embolus

12. Heparin is a(n) _____.
    A. beta blocker
    B. anticoagulant
    C. diuretic
    D. statin

13. In the average man, the heart weighs _____ g.
    A. 200
    B. 300
    C. 400
    D. 500

14. The purpose of the cardiac valves is to prevent _____ of blood into the atria.
    A. regurgitation
    B. deoxygenation
    C. hypertrophy
    D. none of the above

15. An abnormal heart sound is called a(n) _____.
    A. arrhythmia
    B. regurgitation
    C. diastole
    D. murmur

16. The _____ extend(s) along the outer walls of the ventricles. When the impulse passes through, the ventricles contract.
    A. bundle of His
    B. atrioventricular nodes
    C. ventricular septum
    D. Purkinje fibers

17. The _____ is an opening located in the septum between the atria of the fetal heart, allowing blood to be pumped to fetal tissue.
    A. cardiac fontanel
    B. semipulmonary artery
    C. foramen ovale
    D. none of the above

18. An _____ is a tracing of the electrical activity of the heart.
    A. EMG
    B. ECG
    C. EKG
    D. B and C

19. The _____ supplies blood to the right atrium and right ventricle.
    A. marginal artery
    B. circumflex artery
    C. anterior descending artery
    D. popliteal artery

20. A heart rate of less than 60 beats/minute is considered _____.
    A. bradycardia
    B. asystole
    C. palpitation
    D. angina

21. Which of the following statements is correct?
    A. Each ventricle contracts on its own allowing the atria to fill with oxygen-poor blood.
    B. Systemic circulation is the movement of oxygenated blood through the heart and back out to body tissues.
    C. A normal cardiac cycle shows the P, Q, R, S, and U waves.
    D. Hypertension is considered to be a blood pressure of 130/90 mm Hg.

22. The _____ opens when the right atrium contracts.
    A. bicuspid valve
    B. mitral valve
    C. tricuspid valve
    D. pulmonary valve

23. Which one of the following is considered to be the "natural pacemaker" of the heart?
    A. Purkinje
    B. Bundle of His
    C. Atrioventricular node
    D. Sinoatrial node

24. This diagnostic test displays a visual picture of the heart while in motion.
    A. Venography
    B. Electrocardiography
    C. Echocardiography
    D. Arteriography

25. What heart condition causes fever, malaise, chest pain that increases with inspiration or heartbeat, dyspnea, and tachycardia?
    A. Myocardial infarction
    B. Pericarditis
    C. Atrial stenosis
    D. Patent ductus arteriosus

Copyright © 2010, 2005 by Saunders, an imprint of Elsevier, Inc. All rights reserved.

CHAPTER 12 Cardiovascular System

Sentence Completion

Complete each sentence or statement.

ACE inhibitor	constrict	occlusion
heart block	prehypertension	patent
atherosclerosis	Tetralogy of Fallot	prophylactic
aorta	pericarditis	hypoxia
congestive heart failure	hypertension	
dilate	syncope	

1. _____ occurs when the heart muscle is unable to pump blood efficiently, causing the heart to enlarge, and the lungs to fill with blood.

2. _____ is caused by abnormal embryonic development and includes four defects.

3. _____ is a condition of low oxygen levels.

4. _____ is a measure taken to prevent disease.

5. _____ is an obstruction.

6. _____ is another name for fainting.

7. _____ is a blood pressure between 120/80 and 140/90 mm Hg.

8. _____ means to decrease in size.

9. _____ is a progressive thickening of inner walls of arteries.

10. The drug classification for captopril is _____.

Short Answers

1. Discuss the disorders of the conduction system.

   _____

   _____

   _____

Copyright © 2010, 2005 by Saunders, an imprint of Elsevier, Inc. All rights reserved.

2. List three noninvasive procedures for evaluating heart function to include the internal structures, motions of the heart, and major blood vessels.

3. Explain the cardiac cycle.

4. List the two modifications in the fetal heart that allow blood to bypass the fetal lungs and return blood from the placenta to the vena cava.

5. Explain the importance of the hepatic portal circulation.

CRITICAL THINKING

1. One of your patients has recently received a diagnosis of CAD and is scheduled to have a stress test done. Create a dialogue between you, as the medical assistant, and the patient regarding his recent diagnosis. If you are unfamiliar with this diagnosis, research it. If you were the patient, what questions would you ask? What would you want to know?

_____

_____

_____

_____

_____

_____

_____

_____

_____

_____

_____

_____

_____

_____

_____

PRACTICAL APPLICATIONS

If you have accomplished the objectives in this chapter, you will be able to make better choices as a medical assistant. Take a look at this situation and decide what you would do.

Dr. Kim Kea will examine Mr. Stan Baleaut later today as a routine follow-up for high blood pressure and possible coronary artery disease. Mr. Baleaut tells Erin, the medical assistant, that he has some left arm pain and has been having some heart palpitations and wants Dr. Kea to check this. As Erin takes Mr. Baleaut's blood pressure, she obtains a reading of 150/88 mm Hg and a pulse rate of 92 beats/minute. Dr. Kea examines Mr. Baleaut and orders a stat ECG to rule out a diagnosis of MI. As Erin is completing the ECG Mr. Baleaut has several questions about vital signs and ECGs. Erin needs to educate him in several areas.

Cardiovascular System CHAPTER 12

1. What causes systolic blood pressure, and what is happening when this is measured? What causes diastolic pressure?

2. What is the pulse rate measuring?

3. What is the route of the conduction system through the heart?

4. In the past, Mr. Baleaut has worn a Holter monitor, and now wants to know why this was necessary when he had an ECG.

5. What is a myocardial infarction, and what are the symptoms that Mr. Baleaut needs to know?

CHAPTER 12 Cardiovascular System

6. What is congestive heart failure, and what are the symptoms that Mr. Baleaut needs to know?

_____
_____
_____
_____

APPLICATION OF SKILLS

1. Label the word parts of the following terms. Use *P* to indicate a prefix, *CF* to indicate a combining form, *R* to indicate a root, *S* to indicate a suffix. (Example: abnormal—ab *P* norm *R* al *S*)
   A. cardiologist _____
   B. cyanosis _____
   C. endocardium _____
   D. ischemia _____
   E. tricuspid _____

2. Change the following from singular to plural or vice versa.
   A. lumen _____
   B. septum _____
   C. artery _____
   D. varices _____
   E. atria _____

3. Write out the meaning of each the following abbreviations.
   A. MVP _____
   B. CAD _____
   C. MI _____
   D. ASD _____
   E. AV _____

4. Label the diagrams.

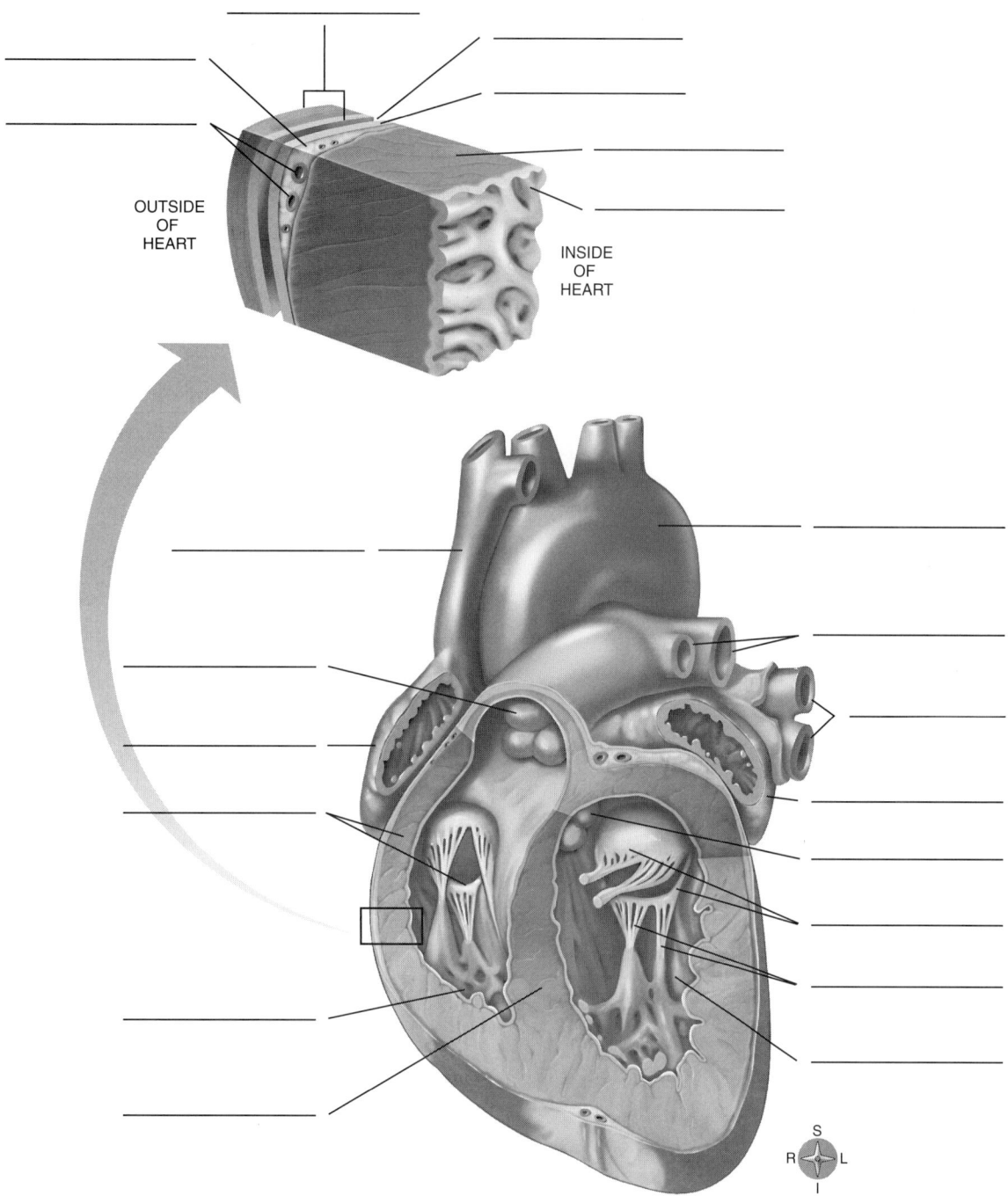

CHAPTER 12 Cardiovascular System

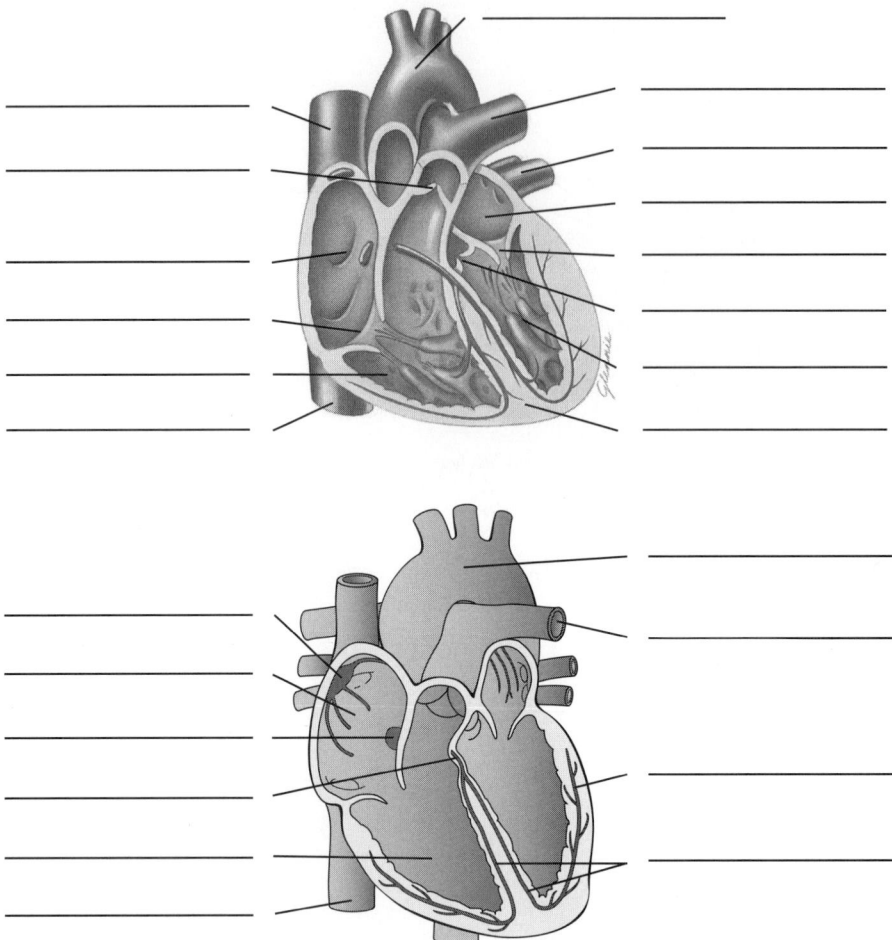

5. Trace the systemic flow of blood from the right atrium back to the right atrium.

CHAPTER QUIZ

Multiple Choice

Identify the letter of the choice that best completes the statement or answers the question.

1. The outermost layer of the heart wall is called the _____.
   A. myocardium
   B. epicardium
   C. pericardium
   D. endocardium

2. The combining form for "blood vessel" is _____.
   A. cardi/o
   B. atri/o
   C. angi/o
   D. varic/o

Copyright © 2010, 2005 by Saunders, an imprint of Elsevier, Inc. All rights reserved.

3. The upper chambers of the heart are called _____.
   A. arterioles
   B. ventricles
   C. venules
   D. atria

4. The space between the lungs where the heart, esophagus, and trachea lie is called the _____.
   A. mediastinum
   B. diaphragm
   C. apex
   D. septum

5. The _____ are the tricuspid and bicuspid valves, which prevent the blood in the ventricles from backing up into the atria when the ventricles contract.
   A. chorea tendineae
   B. cardiac valves
   C. pulmonary valves
   D. none of the above

6. A specialized group of cardiac cells that function as the heart's natural pacemaker are called the _____.
   A. SA node
   B. AV node
   C. bundle of His
   D. Purkinje fibers

7. _____ is the movement of blood through the heart.
   A. Systemic circulation
   B. Pulmonary circulation
   C. Coronary circulation
   D. Fetal circulation

8. The _____ is the heart valve that prevents backflow of blood into the right ventricle.
   A. mitral valve
   B. pulmonary semilunar valve
   C. tricuspid valve
   D. aortic semilunar valve

9. _____ is enlargement of the heart.
   A. Cardiomegaly
   B. Hypertrophy
   C. Sequel
   D. Hypoxia

10. A(n) _____ is a weakness in the wall of an artery.
    A. thrombus
    B. ischemia
    C. infraction
    D. aneurysm

Copyright © 2010, 2005 by Saunders, an imprint of Elsevier, Inc. All rights reserved.

11. These drugs relax blood vessels and improve cardiac output.
    A. Beta blockers
    B. Antiarrhythmic
    C. Antianginal
    D. Angiotensin

12. Atenolol is an example of a(n) _____.
    A. antiarrhythmic
    B. angiotensin
    C. beta blocker
    D. statin

13. The _____ is the space between the lungs where the heart, esophagus, and trachea are located.
    A. sternum
    B. pericardium
    C. atrium
    D. mediastinum

14. The _____ artery is on the thumb side of the wrist.
    A. ulnar
    B. radial
    C. popliteal
    D. brachial

15. _____ is death of the tissue of the heart muscle caused by lack of oxygen to the tissues.
    A. Myocardial infarction
    B. Angina pectoris
    C. Congestive heart failure
    D. Pericarditis

16. _____ is progressive thickening of the inner walls of a vessel leading to an occlusion.
    A. Congestive heart failure
    B. Atherosclerosis
    C. Arteriosclerosis
    D. Pericarditis

17. _____ is(are) an abnormal occurrence of swollen and twisted veins to the legs and anus.
    A. Embolus
    B. Occlusion
    C. Varicosities
    D. Phlebitis

18. _____ occurs when valves do not close properly.
    A. ABE
    B. MVP
    C. CAD
    D. EKG

19. These drugs reduce the level of low-density lipoprotein.
    A. Statins
    B. Beta blockers
    C. Vitamins
    D. Antianginal

20. Ischemia can cause a(n) _____.
    A. pericarditis
    B. valve prolapse
    C. myocardial infarction
    D. ABE or SBE

Matching

Match each prefix or suffix with its correct definition.

_____ 21. -ole   A. vein

_____ 22. ox/o   B. to view

_____ 23. phleb/o   C. carbon dioxide

_____ 24. scop/o   D. small

_____ 25. -capnia   E. oxygen

13 Blood, Lymphatic, and Immune Systems

VOCABULARY REVIEW

Matching: Match each term with the correct definition.

A. hematopoiesis

B. erythropoiesis

C. macrophage

D. hemolysis

E. type and crossmatch

F. ecchymosis

G. stem cell

H. interstitial fluid

I. lymph nodes

J. thymus gland

K. attenuated

L. petechiae

M. interferons

N. pathogens

O. vaccination

_____ 1. Altered, weakened

_____ 2. Production of blood cells

_____ 3. Disease-producing bacteria

_____ 4. Bruised or bluish area of skin caused by trauma to a blood vessel

_____ 5. Breakup of red blood cells

_____ 6. Small, oval-shaped bodies of lymphoid tissue

_____ 7. Proteins produced by T cells and cells infected with viruses that block the ability of a virus to reproduce

_____ 8. Process of determining a person's blood type

_____ 9. Process of red blood cell formation

_____ 10. Cells responsible for destroying worn-out red blood cells

_____ 11. Fluid between the cells of the tissue

_____ 12. Process of giving a small sample of the disease into the body

_____ 13. Lymphatic organ located in the mediastinum and a primary site for T-cell formation

_____ 14. Cells from which all cells develop

_____ 15. Spots appearing on the skin as a result of hemorrhages within the dermis

THEORY RECALL

True/False

Indicate whether the statement is true or false.

_____ 1. An individual with type O blood is considered a universal donor, and crossmatching is not needed.

_____ 2. Plasma is a pale yellow fluid that accounts for more than half the blood volume.

_____ 3. Lymph from the entire body drains eventually into the thoracic duct.

_____ 4. Lymph contains platelets, which allow clots to form in lymphatic vessels.

_____ 5. Antigens induce the immune system to take certain actions.

Multiple Choice

Identify the letter of the choice that best completes the statement or answers the question.

1. This mature blood cell has no nucleus.
   A. Erythrocyte
   B. Leukocyte
   C. Platelet
   D. Neutrophil

2. A normal adult red blood cell count ranges from _____.
   A. 4.5 to 5.5 million/mm^3
   B. 5.5 to 6.5 million/mm^3
   C. 6.5 to 7.5 million/mm^3
   D. 7.5 to 8.5 million/mm^3

3. Which of the following can carry oxygen?
   A. Leukocyte
   B. Thrombocyte
   C. Platelet
   D. Erythrocyte

4. Heme is broken down into this pigment, which is excreted in bile.
   A. Amino acids
   B. Iron
   C. Bilirubin
   D. Glucose

5. Which type of white blood cells plays a major role in immunity to infectious diseases?
   A. Monocytes
   B. Eosinophils
   C. Lymphocytes
   D. Basophils

6. _____ are white blood cells that react to the release of histamine in the body.
   A. Eosinophils
   B. Lymphocytes
   C. Basophils
   D. Neutrophils

7. _____ is a blood test that determines the percentage of each type of white blood cell present in a blood sample.
   A. Gram stain
   B. Differential count
   C. Platelet count
   D. Erythrocyte sedimentation rate

8. _____ is a hormone that is secreted by the thymus that helps to develop the T cells.
   A. Trinomial 3
   B. Terexel
   C. Testosterone
   D. Thymosin

9. A _____ is a person with neither A nor B antigens in his or her blood.
   A. universal donor
   B. universal recipient

10. A _____ is a cell fragment responsible for clotting.
    A. protozoan
    B. petechiae
    C. platelet
    D. fibrin

11. Inborn immunity or natural immunity is called _____.
    A. acquired immunity
    B. active immunity
    C. genetic immunity
    D. nonspecific immunity

12. The blood carries _____ to target organs, and removes excess fluids from body tissues.
    A. interferons
    B. hormones
    C. prothrombin
    D. stem cells

13. Erythropoiesis is the formation of _____.
    A. platelets
    B. red blood cells
    C. white blood cells
    D. all of the above

14. Many types of blood cells are produced in the _____.
    A. liver
    B. red bone marrow
    C. spleen
    D. pancreas

15. Erythropoietin is a hormone _____.
    A. released by the kidney to stimulate red blood cell formation
    B. released by the liver to stimulate red blood cell formation
    C. released by the kidney to stimulate red and white blood cell formation
    D. that causes the recycling of iron for production of red blood cells

16. Which of the following Rh factor combinations could cause agglutination of an infant's red blood cells?
    A. Mother −, father +, infant +
    B. Mother −, father +, infant −
    C. Mother +, father −, infant +
    D. Mother +, father +, infant −

17. In stage II of clot formation, prothrombin is converted to _____.
    A. fibrin
    B. fibrinogen
    C. thrombin
    D. thromboplastin

18. Which blood type would an individual with antibody B in their plasma be?
    A. Type A
    B. Type B
    C. Type AB
    D. Type O

19. _____, a pale yellow fluid, is approximately 90% water.
    A. Plasma
    B. Antibodies
    C. Antigens
    D. Whole blood

20. The human body has more _____ than _____.
    A. red blood cells; white blood cells
    B. white blood cells; red blood cells

21. Which of the following is correct?
    A. Granulocytes = neutrophils, lymphocytes, basophils
    B. Granulocytes = neutrophils, basophils, eosinophils
    C. Granulocytes = lymphocytes, monocytes, neutrocytes
    D. Granulocytes = lymphocytes, eosinophils, monocytes

22. Platelet factors combine with _____ and calcium to form thrombin, which cause(s) platelets to become sticky and form a plug.
    A. fibrinogen
    B. fibrin
    C. prothrombin
    D. coagulants

23. Which one of the following situations could cause hemolytic disease of the newborn?
    A. Rh-positive mother + Rh-positive father
    B. Rh-negative mother + Rh-negative father
    C. Rh-positive mother + Rh-negative father
    D. Rh-negative mother + Rh-positive father

CHAPTER 13 Blood, Lymphatic, and Immune Systems

24. Which one of the following is *not* a component of the lymphatic system?
    A. Lymphatic fluid
    B. Lymph node
    C. Gallbladder
    D. Tonsils

25. Which of the following is not a lymph organ?
    A. Thymus
    B. Spleen
    C. Pancreas
    D. Tonsils

Sentence Completion

Complete each sentence or statement.

erythroblastosis fetalis	lymphocytes
lymph nodes	eosinophils
pernicious anemia	neutrophils
AIDS	waste
leukemia	malaria
inguinal	polycythemia
hemophilia	

1. Urea, uric acid, and amino acids are examples of _____ substances carried in the blood.

2. _____ are a type of blood cell that is the first responder to an infection or damaged site. It is phagocytic in nature.

3. _____ are the smallest type of white blood cell.

4. _____ is a megaloblastic anemia resulting in a decrease of hydrochloric acid.

5. _____ is caused by the protozoan *Plasmodium*.

6. _____ is the medical term for "hemolytic disease of the newborn."

7. _____ is a syndrome that is caused by a virus that attacks an individual's entire immune system.

8. _____ is an inherited disorder characterized by a failure to form blood-clotting factor VIII.

9. _____ produce lymphocytes and monocytes.

10. _____ lymph nodes are located in the groin.

Short Answers

1. What are the two main types of immunity?

   _____

   _____

2. List three diseases of the immune system, and describe the etiology, signs and symptoms, diagnosis, therapy, and interventions for each.

   _____

   _____

   _____

   _____

   _____

   _____

   _____

   _____

   _____

3. Describe the considerations associated with the testing of AIDS patients.

   _____

   _____

   _____

   _____

   _____

4. List the three types of blood cells, and describe the functions of each.

___

CRITICAL THINKING

1. One of your patients has recently received a diagnosis of HIV. Create a dialogue between you, as the medical assistant, and the patient regarding his recent diagnosis. If you are unfamiliar with this diagnosis, research it. If you were the patient, what questions would you ask? What would you want to know?

___

PRACTICAL APPLICATIONS

If you have accomplished the objectives in this chapter, you will be able to make better choices as a medical assistant. Take a look at this situation and decide what you would do.

Pierce Fisher has come to the health clinic today to see Dr. Giffin for a routine physical examination. Pierce tells Lisa, the medical assistant, that he has been having episodes of dizziness and has some pain in his RLQ. Lisa notices that although Pierce's blood pressure is WNL, his temperature and pulse are elevated. Dr. Giffin examines Pierce and orders a stat CBC with a differential count to rule out a diagnosis of appendicitis. As Lisa is completing the blood draw, Pierce has several questions about his blood work and what it can tell the physician about his condition.

When Pierce's blood results come back, would you be able to tell what the results indicate? The blood tests return with the following results:

Hgb 14.6
Hct 46.1
WBCs 20,000
RBCs 5.3
Segs 75
Bands 1%
Eos 0%
Basos 0%
Mono 2%
Lymphs 22%
Platelets 350,000

1. What does the CBC measure, and why did the physician order a differential count?

_____
_____
_____

2. Which of these results are abnormal, and which indicate a possible acute infection?

_____
_____
_____

APPLICATION OF SKILLS

1. Label the word parts of the following terms. Use *P* to indicate a prefix, *CF* to indicate a combining form, *R* to indicate a root, *S* to indicate a suffix. (Example: abnormal—ab *P* norm *R* al *S*)
    A. agglutination _____
    B. basophil _____
    C. polycythemia _____
    D. reticulocyte _____
    E. hemoglobin _____

2. Change the following from singular to plural or vice versa.
    A. thrombus _____
    B. ecchymosis _____
    C. antibody _____
    D. immunity _____
    E. fungi _____

Copyright © 2010, 2005 by Saunders, an imprint of Elsevier, Inc. All rights reserved.

3. Write out the meaning of each the following abbreviations.
   A. HD _____
   B. HSV _____
   C. HIV _____
   D. KS _____
   E. HISTO _____

4. Label the diagram.

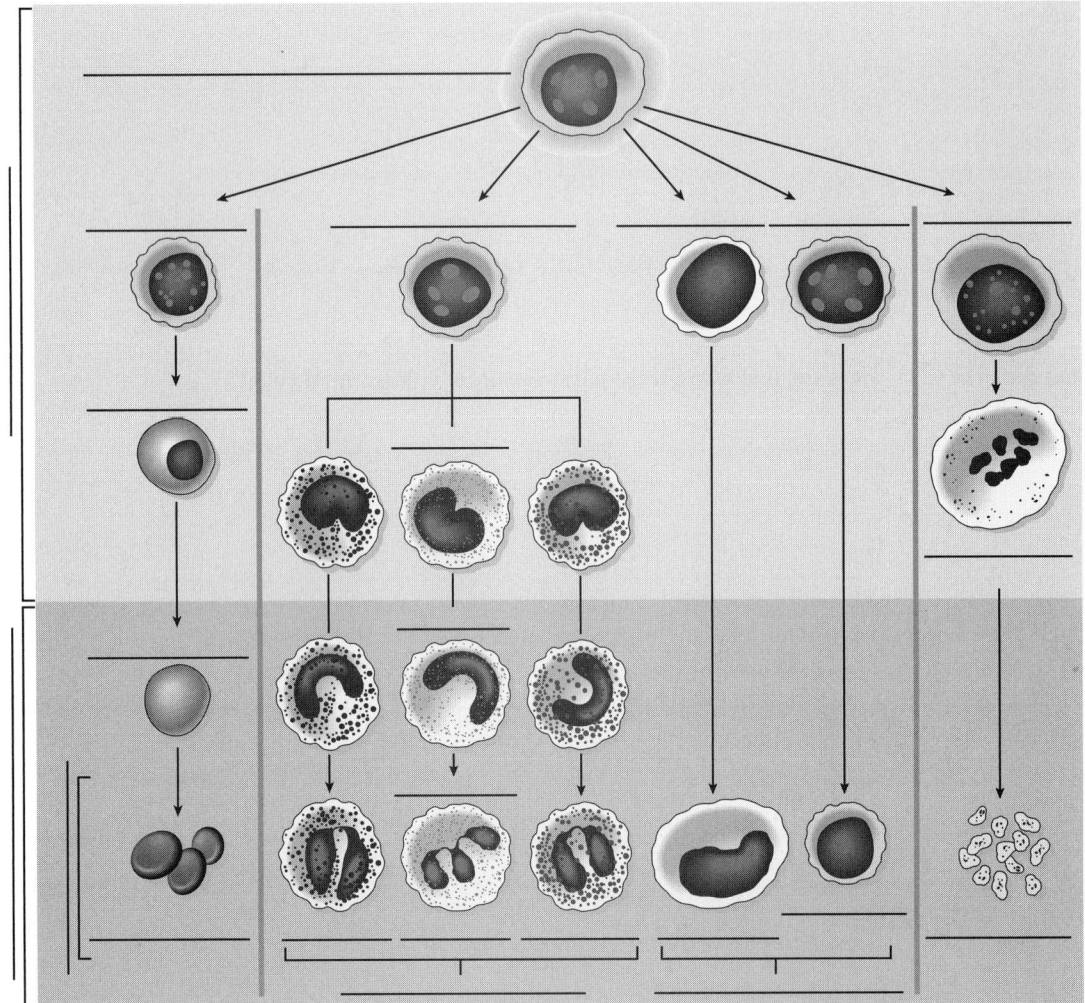

CHAPTER QUIZ

Multiple Choice

Identify the letter of the choice that best completes the statement or answers the question.

1. A hematocrit of 40% means that in every 100 mL of whole blood, there are _____.
   A. 40 red blood cells, and the remainder is plasma
   B. 40 mL of plasma and 60 mL of red blood cells
   C. 40 mL of red blood cells and 60 mL of plasma
   D. 40 mL of red blood cells and 60 mL of serum

2. Under the microscope, erythrocytes appear as _____.
   A. biconcave disks, without nuclei
   B. biconcave disks, with nuclei
   C. disks that are thick on the edges with nuclei
   D. Erythrocytes can be seen only with an electron microscope

3. Which of the following is *not* a leukocyte?
   A. Basophil
   B. Reticulocyte
   C. Neutrophil
   D. Monocyte

4. Type AB blood is considered to be the universal recipient because _____.
   A. it does not contain an Rh antigen
   B. it does not contain either anti-A or anti-B antibodies
   C. both the A and B antigens are missing
   D. A and C

5. Calcium is used in the clotting process during _____.
   A. stage I
   B. stage II
   C. stage I and II
   D. Calcium is not used in the clotting process

6. A type of blood cell produced by lymph nodes is _____.
   A. eosinophils
   B. erythrocytes
   C. neutrophils
   D. monocytes

7. The thymus is located in the _____.
   A. right upper quadrant
   B. epigastric region
   C. mediastinum
   D. neck

8. The tonsils located near the base of the tongue are called the _____.
   A. palatine tonsils
   B. pharyngeal tonsils
   C. lingual tonsils
   D. laryngeal tonsils

9. Which of the following is *not* true of the spleen?
   A. It forms red blood cells.
   B. It destroys red blood cells.
   C. It holds blood.
   D. It produces granular and agranular leukocytes.

10. Most of the body's lymph is drained by the _____.
    A. right lymphatic duct
    B. left lymphatic duct
    C. thoracic duct
    D. abdominal duct

Copyright © 2010, 2005 by Saunders, an imprint of Elsevier, Inc. All rights reserved.

11. The body's first line of defense is (are) _____.
    A. the skin
    B. lymphocytes
    C. basophils
    D. B and C

12. The most numerous type of phagocyte is the _____.
    A. neutrophil
    B. T cell
    C. stem cell
    D. basal cell

13. Which of the following is an autoimmune disease?
    A. AIDS
    B. Emphysema
    C. Hodgkin disease
    D. Measles

14. HIV invades and kills _____ first.
    A. B cells
    B. leukocytes
    C. T cells
    D. macrophages

15. Examples of lymphocytes are _____.
    A. B cells
    B. T cells
    C. A and B
    D. macrophages

Matching

Match each prefix, abbreviation, or suffix with its correct definition.

_____ 16. -lytic   A. hematocrit

_____ 17. ana-   B. antibody

_____ 18. -crit   C. again

_____ 19. Ab   D. pertaining to destruction

_____ 20. Ag   E. antigen

NAME: _____   DATE: _____

14 Respiratory System

VOCABULARY REVIEW

Matching: Match each term with the correct definition.

A. respiration

B. expiration

C. inspiration

D. cilia

E. sinuses

F. adenoids

G. nasopharynx

H. pharynx

I. epiglottis

J. trachea

K. bronchi

L. alveoli

M. pleura

N. phrenic nerve

O. pons

P. cardiopulmonary resuscitation

Q. spirometer

R. asphyxia

S. pulmonary edema

_____ 1. Nosebleed

_____ 2. Occurs when there is an increase in carbon dioxide in tissues, and hence oxygen deficiency

_____ 3. Tiny air sacs at the end of the bronchioles through which gases are exchanged

_____ 4. Process of taking air into the lungs

_____ 5. Lymph tissues located in the nasopharynx

_____ 6. Cavities in the skull connected with the nasal cavities

_____ 7. Passageway that conducts air to and from the lungs

_____ 8. Instrument used to measure breathing volumes

_____ 9. Process of inhaling oxygen to the lungs and exhaling carbon dioxide

_____ 10. Passageway of oxygen to the bronchioles

_____ 11. Passageway that transports air into the lungs and food and liquids into the esophagus

_____ 12. Incomplete lung expansion; lung collapse

_____ 13. Results in abnormal distention and destruction of the alveoli

_____ 14. Top of the pharynx; extends from the posterior nares to the soft palate

_____ 15. Part of the brainstem responsible for automatic control of respiration

T. pulmonary function tests

U. epistaxis

V. atelectasis

W. bronchodilators

X. emphysema

Y. pulmonary embolism

Z. tuberculosis

_____ 16. Process of air leaving the lungs

_____ 17. Serous membrane that provides moisture to prevent friction during movement

_____ 18. Collection of fluid in the lungs

_____ 19. Respiratory drugs that relax the bronchi

_____ 20. Hairlike projections derived from epithelial cells

_____ 21. Bacterial infection of the lungs, although this bacterium can affect other areas of the body

_____ 22. Emergency measure used when a person stops breathing and heart rate ceases

_____ 23. Flap that prevents food from entering the larynx and trachea

_____ 24. Nerve responsible for stimulating the diaphragm in breathing

_____ 25. Tests that measure how well the lungs inhale and exhale air, and how efficiently they transfer oxygen into the blood

_____ 26. Occurs when a clot dislodges and obstructs the pulmonary artery branch partially or completely

THEORY RECALL

True/False

Indicate whether the statement is true or false.

_____ 1. The lower respiratory tract warms, moisturizes, and cleans the air that is taken in during expiration.

_____ 2. Ventilation is the cyclic process of moving air into and out of the lungs.

_____ 3. Bronchoscopy is an endoscopic procedure used to examine the bronchial tubes visually.

_____ 4. COPD is an acronym for coronary obstruction pulse deficient.

_____ 5. The heart is responsible for the process of respiration.

Multiple Choice

Identify the letter of the choice that best completes the statement or answers the question.

1. The upper respiratory tract includes all of the following *except* _____.
   A. sinuses
   B. lungs
   C. pharynx
   D. larynx

2. _____ is a substance that decreases surface tension within the alveoli.
   A. Phlegm
   B. Pleura fluid
   C. Surfactant
   D. Interstitial fluid

3. The _____ is a muscular tube that is a passageway for food between the pharynx and the stomach.
   A. esophagus
   B. trachea
   C. bronchioles
   D. larynx

4. The medical term for the "voice box" is _____.
   A. nasopharynx
   B. pharynx
   C. larynx
   D. laryngopharynx

5. The area of the brain that controls conscious respiration is the _____.
   A. cerebellum
   B. cerebral cortex
   C. medulla oblongata
   D. pons

6. The medical term for "difficulty speaking" is _____.
   A. aphonia
   B. dysphonia
   C. dyspnea
   D. apnea

7. Radiographic method used to visualize the lungs is called a(n) _____.
   A. x-ray
   B. CT scan
   C. MRI
   D. PFT

8. A(n) _____ is a test that measures how well the lungs inhale and exhale air.
   A. x-ray
   B. CT scan
   C. MRI
   D. PFT

9. _____ is an acute respiratory disorder in children.
   A. Croup
   B. Epistaxis
   C. Laryngitis
   D. Sinusitis

10. The medical term for the "common cold" is _____.
    A. croup
    B. laryngitis
    C. pertussis
    D. rhinitis

11. Which one of the following is *not* a sinus of the respiratory system?
    A. frontal
    B. ethmoidal
    C. temporal
    D. sphenoidal

12. _____ are lymphatic tissues that filter out bacteria and viruses, preventing their entry into the respiratory tract.
    A. Lymph nodes
    B. Tonsils
    C. Lymphatic vessels
    D. Cilia

13. The epiglottis is attached to the base of the _____.
    A. palatine tonsils
    B. nasal septum
    C. tongue
    D. oropharynx

14. The right lung has _____ lobes.
    A. two
    B. three
    C. four
    D. none of the above

15. When atmospheric pressure is _____ than the pressure within the lungs, inspiration occurs.
    A. greater
    B. less

16. Air is inspired when the diaphragm is stimulated by _____.
    A. hormones
    B. carbon dioxide
    C. glucose
    D. phrenic nerve

17. Jim has been a heavy smoker for 25 years and has a decreased expiratory reserve volume and exhibits a barrel-shaped chest cavity. His probable diagnosis is _____.
    A. emphysema
    B. asthma
    C. bronchitis
    D. pneumonia

18. The combining form for "lung" is _____.
    A. bronch/o
    B. lung/o
    C. rhin/o
    D. pneum/o

19. The suffix for "breathing" is _____.
    A. -phonia
    B. -pnea
    C. -oxia
    D. none of the above

20. An antitussive _____.
    A. promotes expulsion of mucus from the respiratory tract
    B. blocks histamine production
    C. suppresses the cough reflex
    D. reduces congestion

21. Robitussin is an example of a(n) _____.
    A. antihistamine
    B. antitussive
    C. decongestant
    D. expectorant

22. Clubbing occurs at the ends of the fingers because of:
    A. Incomplete lung expansion
    B. Blood in the pleural cavity
    C. Low blood oxygen levels
    D. Birth defect

23. The pulmonary function test that measures the amount of air taken into and out of the lungs during respiration is called _____.
    A. TV
    B. ERV
    C. TLC
    D. IRV

24. A high-pitched breathing associated with obstructed airway heard during inspiration is called _____.
    A. rales
    B. wheezes
    C. stridor
    D. rhonchi

25. _____ is a viral infection of the upper respiratory tract.
    A. Pharyngitis
    B. Rhinitis
    C. Influenza
    D. Pneumonia

Sentence Completion

Complete each sentence or statement.

PFT	epistaxis	tuberculosis
pertussis	influenza	sinusitis
RV (residual volume)	ARDS	surfactant
pneumonia	emphysema	pneumothorax
inhalation	croup	
exhalation	pertussis	

1. _____ is caused by a virus and usually follows an upper respiratory infection.

2. The intervention for _____ is to receive an immunization at 2, 4, and 6 months of age.

3. _____ results in abnormal distention and destruction of the alveoli.

4. _____ starts out as an URI, but progresses with chills, dyspnea, and purulent sputum.

5. _____ measures the amount of air that remains in the lungs after a maximal expiration.

6. _____ is a bacterial infection of the lungs, requiring mandatory reporting to the county public health office.

7. _____ is the abbreviation for adult respiratory distress syndrome.

8. Respiratory distress syndrome is caused by an inadequate amount of _____ at birth.

9. Vital capacity is the amount of air that can be _____ after maximum _____.

10. _____ occurs when air enters the spaces between the pleural spaces.

Short Answers

1. List the four main structures in the lower respiratory tract, and describe the function of each.

   _____
   _____
   _____
   _____

2. Explain the purpose (the function) of the respiratory system.

   _____
   _____
   _____

3. Explain the importance of pulmonary function tests such as spirometry in the diagnosis of respiratory problems.

   _____
   _____
   _____
   _____

4. List 10 common signs and symptoms of respiratory diseases and disorders.

   _____
   _____
   _____
   _____

CRITICAL THINKING

1. Bill Johnson is a 52-year-old man who smokes two packs of cigarettes a day. Mr. Johnson has been diagnosed with emphysema, and the physician has asked you, the medical assistant, to discuss the alternatives with him to quit smoking. Describe at least three alternatives, listing their advantages and disadvantages.

   _____
   _____
   _____
   _____

Copyright © 2010, 2005 by Saunders, an imprint of Elsevier, Inc. All rights reserved.

2. Write one sentence appropriately using at least 10 of the respiratory abbreviations listed in the textbook.

___

PRACTICAL APPLICATIONS

If you have accomplished the objectives in this chapter, you will be able to make better choices as a medical assistant. Take a look at this situation and decide what you would do.

Mr. Chazara, with a long history of smoking cigarettes and cigars, has been diagnosed with chronic obstructive pulmonary disease (COPD) with constriction of the bronchi. He is dyspneic with stridor and wheezing. When he is seen by the physician, an order is written for spirometry testing. The testing is positive for a mild loss of vital capacity and for moderately decreased forced expiratory volume. Because of the decreases in lung capacity, an order is also written for arterial blood gas measurements (ABGs). In addition, Mr. Chazara has sinus congestion and a productive cough, but has no fever; he needs medications for the congestion and the loss of lung function.

1. What is the cause and effect of long-term cigarette and cigar smoking on the lungs?

___

2. What does the diagnosis of chronic obstructive pulmonary disease mean?

___

3. What effect does the upper respiratory infection of sinus congestion and the productive cough have on COPD?

___

4. Why would you expect Mr. Chazara to be dyspneic with stridor and wheezing? Explain what each of these medical terms means.

5. What is spirometry testing?

6. What do increased residual volume and decreased vital capacity indicate?

7. Why would a bronchodilator be prescribed?

8. Why would an expectorant rather than an antitussive be prescribed?

9. Why would an arterial blood gas measurement be ordered?

APPLICATION OF SKILLS

1. Label the word parts of the following terms. Use *P* to indicate a prefix, *CF* to indicate a combining form, *R* to indicate a root, *S* to indicate a suffix. (Example: abnormal—ab *P* norm *R* al *S*)
   A. apnea _____
   B. atelectasis _____
   C. dysphonia _____
   D. pneumothorax _____
   E. spirometer _____

2. Change the following from singular to plural or vice versa.
   A. alveoli _____
   B. thorax _____
   C. thrombus _____
   D. adenoid _____
   E. bronchiole _____

3. Write out the meaning of each the following abbreviations.
   A. COPD _____
   B. SOB _____
   C. URI _____
   D. PFT _____
   E. ABGs _____

4. Label the diagrams.

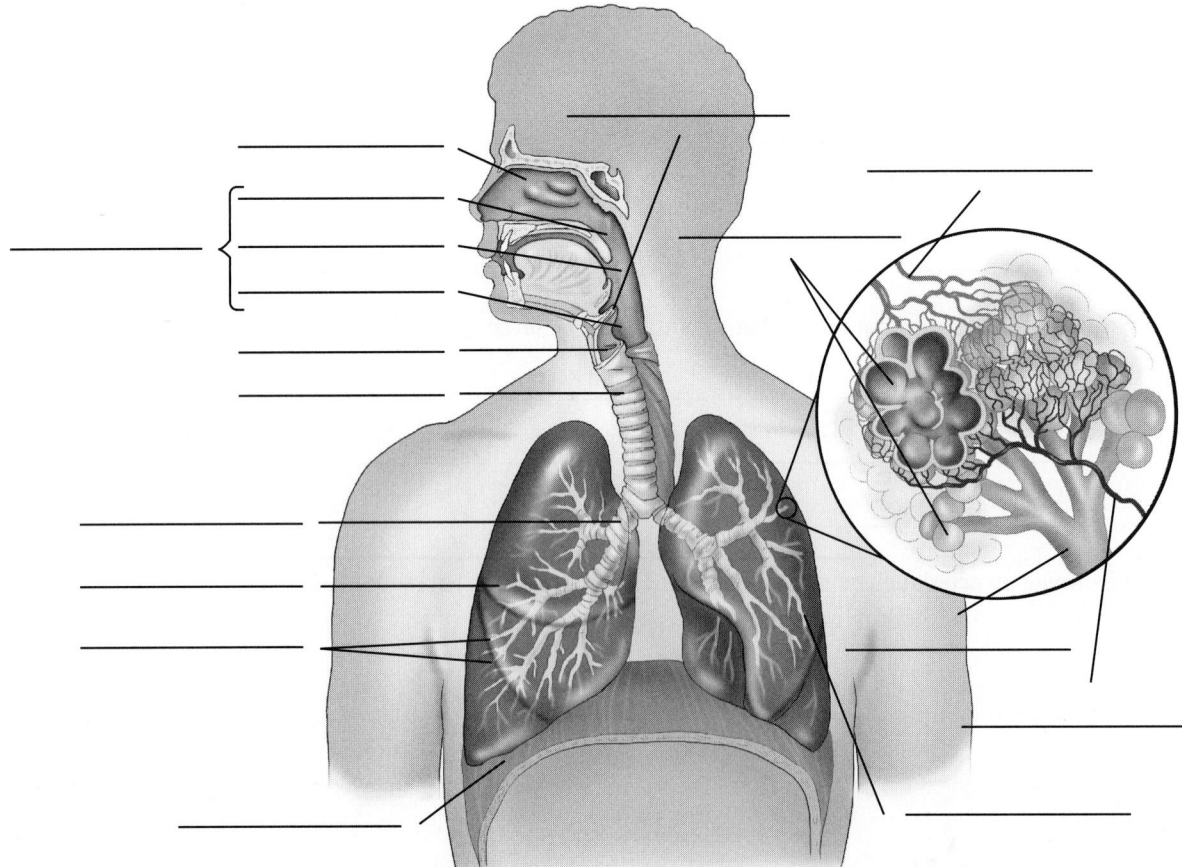

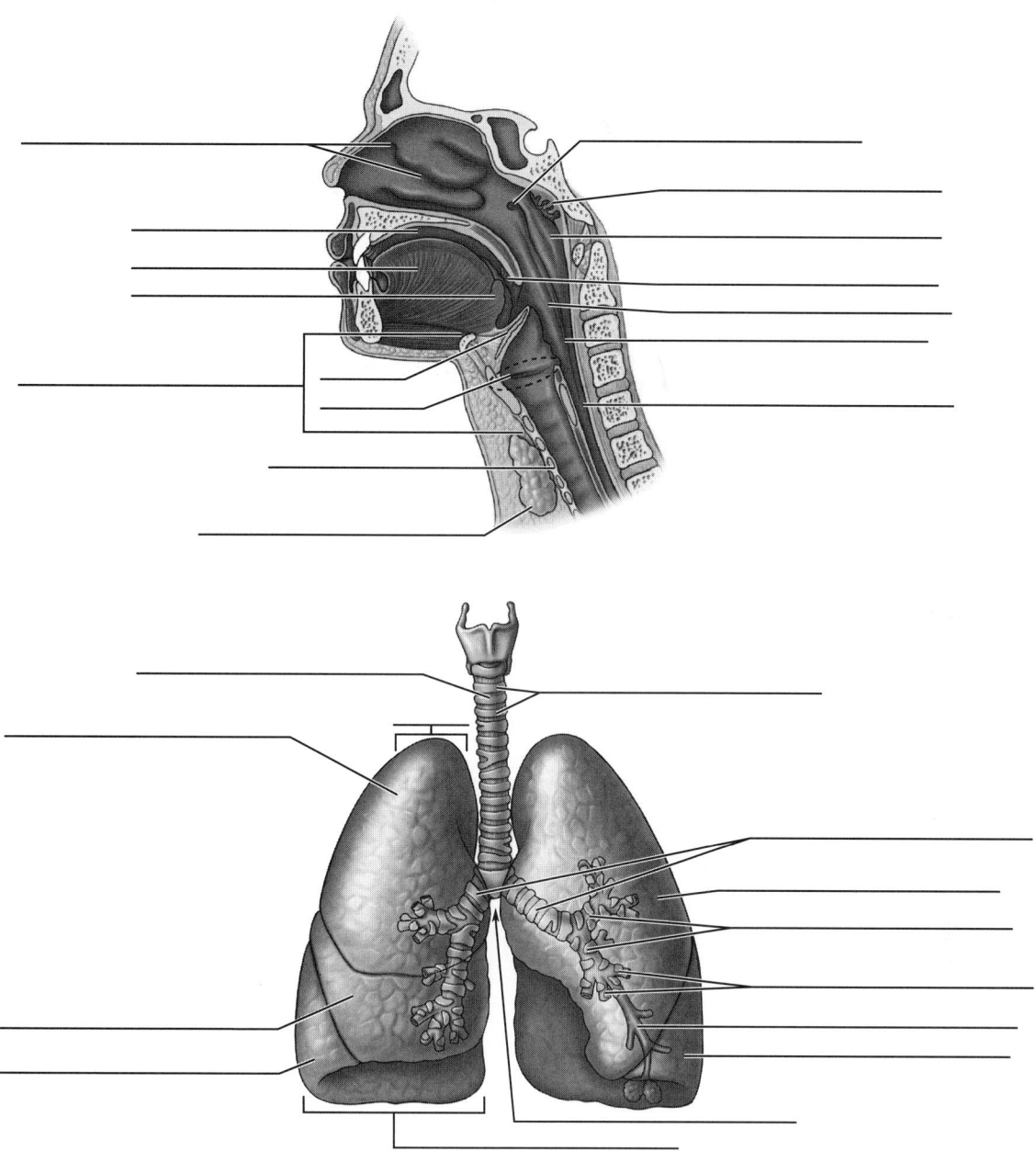

CHAPTER QUIZ

Multiple Choice

Identify the letter of the choice that best completes the statement or answers the question.

1. The external openings of the nose are called _____.
    A. nostrils
    B. sinuses
    C. septum
    D. cilia

Copyright © 2010, 2005 by Saunders, an imprint of Elsevier, Inc. All rights reserved.

2. The passageway that conducts air to and from the lungs is called the _____.
   A. esophagus
   B. trachea
   C. bronchioles
   D. laryngopharynx

3. The combining form for "diaphragm" is _____.
   A. spir/o
   B. phren/o
   C. adenoid/o
   D. diaphragm/o

4. The pressure of outside air is called _____.
   A. external respiration
   B. internal respiration
   C. osmotic pressure
   D. atmospheric pressure

5. The flap that prevents food from entering the larynx and trachea is called the _____.
   A. alveoli
   B. surfactant
   C. epiglottis
   D. epistaxis

6. The area of the brain responsible for automatic control of respiration is the _____.
   A. medulla
   B. midbrain
   C. cerebral cortex
   D. cerebellum

7. _____ is a series of x-ray pictures taken at different angles creating cross-sectional pictures of the organ.
   A. Chest x-ray
   B. Computed tomography
   C. Magnetic resonance imaging
   D. Pulmonary function tests

8. _____ is an abnormal enlargement of the ends of the fingers caused by low oxygen levels in the blood.
   A. Hemoptysis
   B. Dysphonia
   C. Asphyxia
   D. Clubbing

9. The medical term for "difficulty breathing" is _____.
   A. dysphonia
   B. apnea
   C. dyspnea
   D. aphonia

10. The medical term for "inadequate oxygen in tissues" is _____.
    A. asphyxia
    B. hypoxia
    C. hemoptysis
    D. pneumothorax

11. _____ are the crackling sounds heard during inspiration using auscultation.
    A. Rales
    B. Rhonchi
    C. Wheezes
    D. Stridor

12. The medical term for "inflammation of the throat" is _____.
    A. croupitis
    B. laryngitis
    C. pharyngitis
    D. rhinitis

13. A combination of respiratory diseases including chronic bronchitis, asthma, and emphysema is called _____.
    A. CPR
    B. PET
    C. CBAE
    D. COPD

14. A bacterial infection of the lungs that can also affect other areas of the body is _____.
    A. pleurisy
    B. pulmonary embolism
    C. SIDS
    D. tuberculosis

15. _____ measures the amount of air that can be exhaled after maximum inhalation.
    A. Tidal volume
    B. Residual volume
    C. Vital capacity
    D. Total lung capacity

16. _____ measures the amount of air that remains in the lungs after a maximal expiration.
    A. Tidal volume
    B. Residual volume
    C. Vital capacity
    D. Total lung capacity

17. _____ is the term for "incomplete lung expansion; lung collapse."
    A. Asphyxia
    B. Atelectasis
    C. Hemoptysis
    D. Hypoxia

18. The medical term for "blood in the pleural cavity" is _____.
    A. hemothorax
    B. pneumothorax
    C. hemoptysis
    D. hemostasis

19. The medical term for "whooping cough" is _____.
    A. croup
    B. bronchitis
    C. pertussis
    D. influenza

Copyright © 2010, 2005 by Saunders, an imprint of Elsevier, Inc. All rights reserved.

20. A(n) _____ is the medication given to patients with asthma.
    A. antibiotic
    B. antitussive
    C. immunization
    D. bronchodilator

Matching

Match each prefix or suffix with its correct definition.

_____ 21. rhin/o   A. breathing

_____ 22. alveol/o   B. level of oxygen

_____ 23. -pnea   C. nose

_____ 24. -oxia   D. process

_____ 25. -ation   E. alveoli

15 Digestive System

VOCABULARY REVIEW

Matching: Match each term with the correct definition.

A. digestion

B. alimentary canal

C. bolus

D. uvula

E. mastication

F. enzyme

G. peristalsis

H. chyme

I. gastroenteritis

J. mesentery

K. peritoneum

L. stomach

M. vagus nerve

N. villi

O. vermiform appendix

P. defecation

Q. liver

R. hepatic duct

S. insulin

_____ 1. Duct from the liver to the gallbladder

_____ 2. Serous membrane that lines the walls of the abdominal cavity and folds over and protects the intestines

_____ 3. Reflux into the esophagus of stomach acids and food

_____ 4. Digestive tract; extends from the mouth to the anus

_____ 5. Wavelike motions that propel food through the digestive tract

_____ 6. Enlarged, saclike portion of the alimentary canal; one of the main organs of digestion

_____ 7. Small mass of tissue hanging from the soft palate at the back of the mouth

_____ 8. Organ that secretes bile; active in the formation of certain blood proteins and the metabolism of carbohydrates, fats, and proteins

_____ 9. Inflammation of the liver caused by a viral infection

_____ 10. Food broken down by chewing and mixed with saliva

_____ 11. Protein produced by living organisms that causes biochemical changes

_____ 12. Vascular projections of the small intestine for absorption of nutrients

_____ 13. Membrane that attaches itself to the small and large intestines and holds them in place

_____ 14. Difficulty in defecation caused by hard, compacted stool; lack of water absorption in the large intestine

T. metabolism

U. constipation

V. flatulence

W. jaundice

X. regurgitation

Y. hepatitis

Z. volvulus

_____ 15. Colon twisting on itself

_____ 16. Chewing

_____ 17. Physical and chemical breakdown of food

_____ 18. Attached to the cecum

_____ 19. Digestive gas

_____ 20. Inflammation of the stomach and intestines

_____ 21. Energy production after the absorption of nutrients

_____ 22. Elimination of feces

_____ 23. Hormone functions to regulate the metabolism of carbohydrates and fats, especially the conversion of glucose to glycogen, which lowers the blood glucose level

_____ 24. Semiliquid contents of the stomach after it has been mixed with stomach acid

_____ 25. Controls secretions of hydrochloric acid, in addition to many other responsibilities

_____ 26. Yellowish discoloration of the skin caused by a breakdown of bilirubin

THEORY RECALL

True/False

Indicate whether the statement is true or false.

_____ 1. The alimentary canal is a muscular tube that extends from the mouth to the anus and is approximately 30 feet long.

_____ 2. The liver is the largest organ in the digestive system.

_____ 3. The trachea carries the bolus to the stomach via the process of peristalsis.

_____ 4. The duodenum is where the final breakdown of nutrients occurs.

_____ 5. The LES allows chyme to exit into the small intestine.

Multiple Choice

Identify the letter of the choice that best completes the statement or answers the question.

1. _____ is the process of taking nutrition into the body.
   A. Absorption
   B. Elimination
   C. Ingestion
   D. None of the above

2. Which one of the following is *not* one of the four areas of the taste buds of the tongue?
   A. Sweet
   B. Metallic
   C. Salty
   D. Sour

3. The top portion of the stomach is called the _____.
   A. fundus
   B. rugae
   C. body
   D. frenulum

4. The combining form for "mouth" is _____.
   A. cheil/o
   B. enter/o
   C. pylor/o
   D. stomat/o

5. A large pouch forming the first part of the large intestine is called the _____.
   A. cecum
   B. appendix
   C. colon
   D. jejunum

6. The suffix for "digestions" is _____.
   A. -emesis
   B. -pepsia
   C. -stalsis
   D. -phage

7. _____ is fluid that is secreted by the liver, stored in the gallbladder, and discharged into the duodenum.
   A. Chyme
   B. Bolus
   C. Feces
   D. Bile

8. The suffix for "hernia" is _____.
   A. -cele
   B. -clysis
   C. -pexy
   D. -ose

9. The medical abbreviation that means "before meals" is _____.
   A. BE
   B. BM
   C. AC
   D. NPO

10. The second part of the small intestine, responsible for absorption, is the _____.
    A. duodenum
    B. jejunum
    C. vermiform appendix
    D. cecum

11. The _____ is an organ that has endocrine and exocrine functions.
    A. liver
    B. spleen
    C. pancreas
    D. appendix

12. The medical term for "forceful expulsion of the stomach contents" is _____.
    A. emesis
    B. dyspepsia
    C. flatulence
    D. ascites

13. The process of converting smaller molecules into larger molecules is called _____.
    A. cannibalism
    B. metabolism
    C. catabolism
    D. anabolism

14. Frequent bowel movements of loose, watery stools is _____.
    A. flatulence
    B. ascites
    C. emesis
    D. none of the above

15. Dilated veins in the rectum and anus are called _____.
    A. caries
    B. hemorrhoids
    C. varicose veins
    D. glossitis

16. The medical term for "gallstones" is _____.
    A. cholelithiasis
    B. choledocolithotomy
    C. cholecystitis
    D. diverticulitis

17. _____ are usually benign growths that can be attached to the mucosal lining of the colon.
    A. Hemorrhoids
    B. Polyps
    C. Caries
    D. None of the above

18. Telescoping of one part of the intestine into another is called _____.
    A. diverticulitis
    B. gastroenteritis
    C. intussusception
    D. celiac sprue

19. A(n) _____ is a lesion of the mucosal lining of the stomach or intestine.
    A. pyloric stenosis
    B. volvulus
    C. ulcer
    D. celiac sprue

20. The medical term for "vomiting blood" is _____.
    A. gastritis
    B. intussusception
    C. ascites
    D. hematemesis

21. _____ is a viral infection of the parotid glands.
    A. Melena
    B. Mumps
    C. Measles
    D. Ulcers

22. Which one of the following is *not* a stage of digestion?
    A. Ingestion
    B. Respiration
    C. Absorption
    D. Elimination

23. When food is chewed and mixed with saliva, it becomes known as _____.
    A. bolus
    B. chyme
    C. feces
    D. phlegm

24. The oral ingestion of a suspension for imaging of the esophagus is what type of diagnostic test?
    A. Cholecystography
    B. Barium enema
    C. Barium swallow
    D. Endoscopy

25. When permanent teeth replace baby teeth, there are four _____.
    A. canines
    B. molars
    C. bicuspids
    D. none of the above

CHAPTER 15   Digestive System

Sentence Completion

Complete each sentence or statement.

lipase	lactose intolerance	gallbladder
deciduous	descending colon	laxatives
permanent	ascending colon	NPO
hepatic duct	rectum	polyps
cystic duct	anus	celiac sprue
pepsin	liver	

1. The _____ leads from the liver into the gallbladder.

2. The first set of teeth is called _____.

3. Gastric juices contain the enzyme _____.

4. _____ is the inability for the body to process dairy products.

5. The _____ is the part of the intestinal tract that moves up the right side of the body toward the lower part of the liver.

6. The _____ is continuous with the sigmoid colon and measures about 5 inches in length.

7. The liver, _____, and pancreas all empty their secretions into the duodenum.

8. _____ cause the evacuation of the bowel by increasing bulk of the feces, softening the stool, or lubricating the intestinal wall.

9. Bile leaves the gallbladder through the _____.

10. _____ is the abbreviation for "nothing by mouth."

Short Answers

1. Explain the purpose of the digestive system.

2. List the four stages of the digestive process.

Copyright © 2010, 2005 by Saunders, an imprint of Elsevier, Inc. All rights reserved.

3. Trace the pathway of food through the gastrointestinal tract.

4. Explain the role of the mouth in digestion.

5. Explain the role of the stomach in digestion.

6. What causes jaundice?

CRITICAL THINKING

1. Using Boxes 15-1 and 15-2 in the textbook, create a patient history using a minimum of 10 of the terms on the list.

2. Clarence Johansen is 67 years old and has been encouraged by his wife to have a colon check-up. The physician ordered a standard cleansing diet and is going to perform a sigmoidoscopy this afternoon. Explain to Mr. Johansen the purpose of a sigmoidoscopy, why it is necessary, and how the procedure is performed.

PRACTICAL APPLICATIONS

If you have accomplished the objectives in this chapter, you will be able to make better choices as a medical assistant. Take a look at this situation and decide what you would do.

Saril Paratel, age 69, was brought to the physician's office with fever and pain in the right lower quadrant of her abdomen. The pain has lasted for 3 days and has become progressively worse over the past 36 hours. The pain originally started in the umbilical area, but over time moved to McBurney's point. Last night she had nausea and vomiting. She has not had a bowel movement for 4 days. Saril had dyspepsia for several days before this episode of pain. She has also noticed that fatty foods tend to cause flatulence with some pain in her right upper quadrant, radiating into her back at the right shoulder. No history of hematemesis is given, but malaise has been present for several weeks. When asked about diarrhea, Saril answers that her stools 5 days ago were soft, formed, and frequent, so yes, she had diarrhea. The white blood cell count ordered by the physician is reported as WBC 15,600 with a differential of 76% neutrophils, 6% bands, 25% lymphs, 0% basos, 1% monos, and 10% eos. The physician refers Saril to a surgeon because he wants her to be evaluated for possible appendicitis and to rule out the cause of the right upper quadrant pain. (*Hint*: Use Appendix C.)

1. **What gastrointestinal organs are found in the right lower quadrant?**

2. **Where is McBurney's point?**

3. **What is appendicitis?**

4. What is hematemesis, and why would this be important in this case study?

5. What is the difference between emesis and regurgitation?

6. Did Saril really have diarrhea? Explain your answer.

7. What did the white blood cell count indicate?

8. How did the white blood cell differential confirm that Saril might have appendicitis?

9. What organs of digestion are found in the right upper quadrant?

CHAPTER 15 Digestive System

10. What disease processes might be seen with right upper quadrant pain that radiates into the right back at the shoulder with associated flatulence?

___

___

___

___

APPLICATION OF SKILLS

1. Label the word parts of the following terms. Use *P* to indicate a prefix, *CF* to indicate a combining form, *R* to indicate a root, *S* to indicate a suffix. (Example: abnormal—ab *P* norm *R* al *S*)
   A. amylase ___
   B. cholecystectomy ___
   C. catabolism ___
   D. hematemesis ___
   E. sublingual ___

2. Change the following from singular to plural or vice versa.
   A. appendix ___
   B. diverticula ___
   C. diagnoses ___
   D. lumina ___
   E. viscus ___

3. Write out the meaning of each the following abbreviations.
   A. ac ___
   B. BE, BaE ___
   C. IVC ___
   D. IC ___
   E. GA ___

4. Label the diagrams.

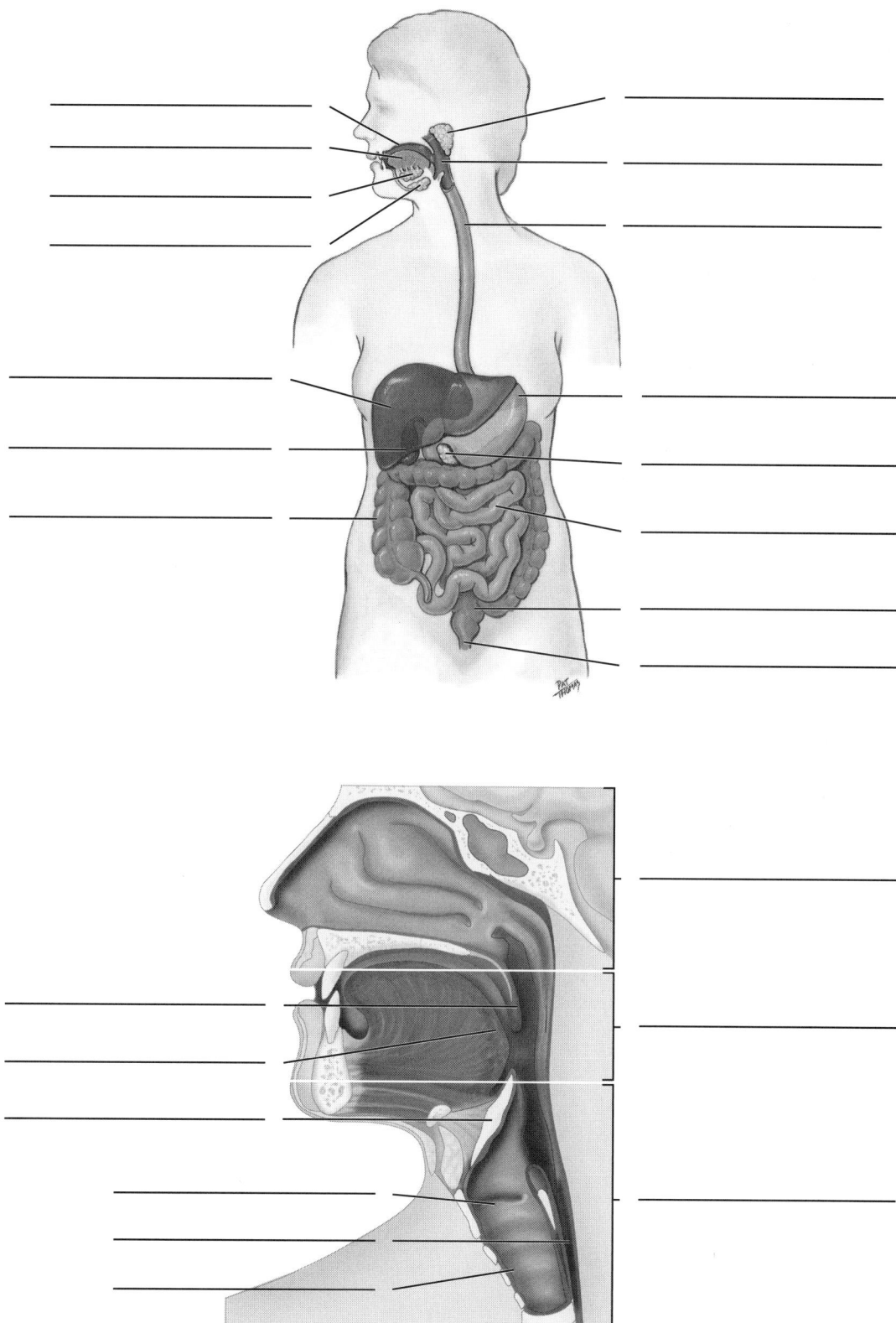

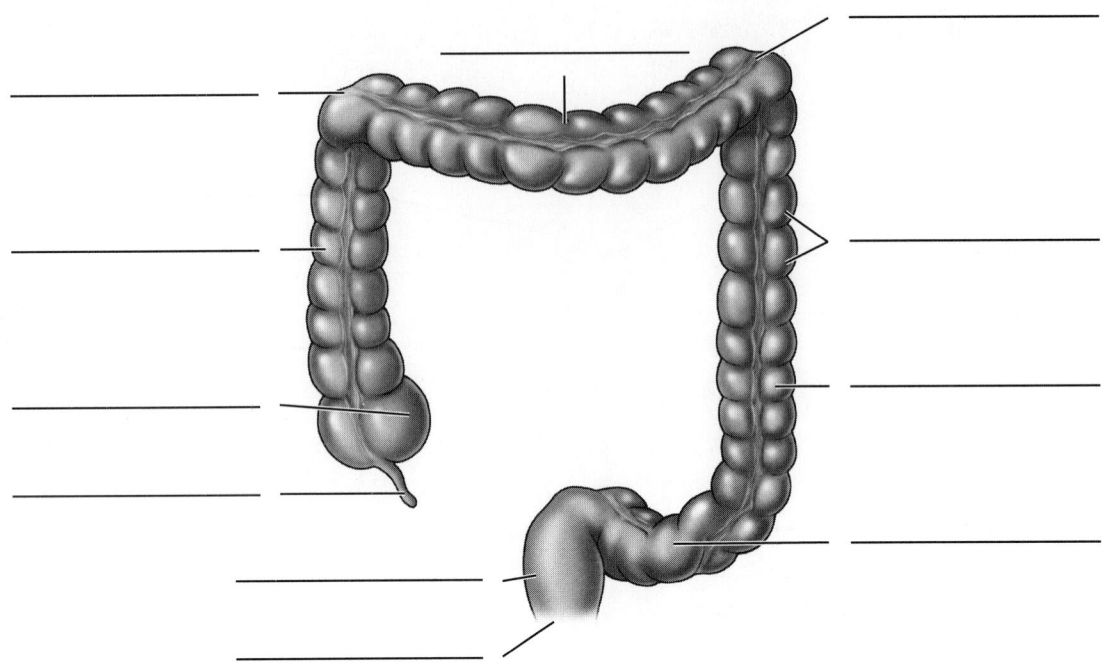

CHAPTER QUIZ

Multiple Choice

Identify the letter of the choice that best completes the statement or answers the question.

1. A toothache is a symptom of _____.
   A. glossitis
   B. caries
   C. gingivitis
   D. thrush

2. The therapy for GERD is _____.
   A. to elevate the head of the bed 4 to 6 inches
   B. the removal of plaque and antibiotic therapy
   C. a bland diet to reduce acid
   D. a gluten-free diet

3. _____ is the narrowing of the pyloric sphincter.
   A. Intussusception
   B. Pyloric stenosis
   C. Endoscopy
   D. Pyloricectomy

4. _____ is an inflammation of small outpouches in the colon.
   A. Gastritis
   B. Colitis
   C. Diverticulitis
   D. Hepatitis

5. _____ is an inflammation of the liver caused by a viral infection and contracted by coming in contact with an infected person's blood or body fluids.
   A. HIV
   B. Hepatitis C
   C. Crohn disease
   D. Hepatitis B

6. _____ is a loss of appetite.
   A. Anorexia
   B. Dyspepsia
   C. Colic
   D. Ascites

7. _____ is a yellowish discoloration of skin caused by the lack of breakdown of bilirubin in the blood.
   A. Hematemesis
   B. Melena
   C. Jaundice
   D. Cirrhosis

8. _____ cause evacuation of the bowel by stimulating nerves in the intestines, resulting in increased peristalsis.
   A. Antacids
   B. Antiemetics
   C. Cathartics
   D. Laxatives

9. _____ is the physical and chemical change nutrients undergo after absorption.
   A. Metabolism
   B. Anabolism
   C. Catabolism
   D. Hemabolism

10. The _____ is (are) the largest organ of the body.
    A. heart
    B. liver
    C. lungs
    D. stomach

11. Which one of the following vitamins is *not* stored in the liver?
    A. A
    B. B_{12}
    C. C
    D. E

12. Which one of the following is *not* an accessory organ of the digestive system?
    A. Appendix
    B. Pancreas
    C. Gallbladder
    D. Liver

Copyright © 2010, 2005 by Saunders, an imprint of Elsevier, Inc. All rights reserved.

13. _____ occurs when the stomach protrudes through the diaphragm into the chest cavity.
    A. An ulcer
    B. Spastic colon
    C. Appendicitis
    D. A hiatal hernia

14. Which one of the following is the correct spelling for the medical term meaning "inflammation of the gallbladder"?
    A. Koleecystitis
    B. Cholesisitis
    C. Cholecystitis
    D. Coaleesystitis

15. _____ are usually benign growths that can be attached to the mucosal lining of the colon.
    A. Hemorrhoids
    B. Polyps
    C. Varices
    D. Ulcers

16. The _____ is the portion of the digestive tract that extends from the sigmoid colon to the anal canal
    A. descending colon
    B. duodenum
    C. ascending colon
    D. rectum

17. The medical term for "difficulty swallowing" is _____.
    A. dysphonia
    B. dysphagia
    C. dyspepsia
    D. dysuria

18. The second part of the small intestine responsible for absorption is the _____.
    A. jejunum
    B. rectum
    C. duodenum
    D. ileum

19. The _____ are the teeth located in the front of the mouth.
    A. molars
    B. canines
    C. incisors
    D. bicuspids

20. Absorption of nutrients occurs in the _____.
    A. stomach
    B. pancreas
    C. small intestine
    D. large intestine

Complete the following table:

Digestive Juices	Site of Action	Enzyme(s)	Changes in Foods
Saliva	_____	**Amylase**	_____
Gastric juice and HCl	_____	**Pepsin**	Begins _____ digestion
_____	Small intestine	Lipase	Acts on _____
Intestinal juice	Small intestine	Lactase, maltase, sucrase	Breaks down _____
Bile	Small intestine	*None*	_____

Matching

Match each prefix or suffix with its correct definition.

_____ 1. hepato/o A. bile

_____ 2. chol/e B. barium enema

_____ 3. ac C. after meals

_____ 4. BaE D. digestion

_____ 5. glyc/o E. sugar

_____ 6. -ase F. anus

_____ 7. pc G. liver

_____ 8. -pepsia H. bladder or sac

_____ 9. cyst/o I. enzyme

_____ 10. proct/o J. before meals

16 Nervous System

VOCABULARY REVIEW

Matching: Match each term with the correct definition.

A. nerve

B. neurons

C. dendrites

D. myelin sheath

E. dermatome

F. synapse

G. brain

H. hypothalamus

I. meninges

J. oxytocin

K. thalamus

L. spinal column

M. reflex

N. gait

O. psychiatry

_____ 1. Manner of walking

_____ 2. Functional unit of a nerve that transmits impulses; located within the CNS

_____ 3. Bone structure that surrounds and protects the spinal cord

_____ 4. Medical science that deals with the origin, diagnosis, prevention, and treatment of developmental and emotional components of physical disorders

_____ 5. Protective covering of the brain and spinal cord

_____ 6. Surface area of the body where the afferent fibers travel from a spinal root

_____ 7. Covering of an axon

_____ 8. Involuntary reaction that occurs because of a stimulus

_____ 9. Located in the skull; main functioning unit of the CNS that contains many neurons

_____ 10. Bundle of fibers containing neurons and blood vessels

_____ 11. Space from the end of one neuron to the beginning of the next neuron

_____ 12. Hormone that is stored in the posterior pituitary gland and needed for uterine contractions

_____ 13. Responsible for relaying messages from parts of the body; monitors sensory stimuli

_____ 14. Receive nerve impulses

_____ 15. Controls activities of the pituitary gland; secretes oxytocin and ADH; regulates the autonomic nervous system

THEORY RECALL

True/False

Indicate whether the statement is true or false.

_____ 1. The endocrine system is the main communication and control system of the body.

_____ 2. There are 16 pairs of cranial nerves.

_____ 3. A general increase in nerve conduction occurs with age.

_____ 4. The ANS consists of the parasympathetic and sympathetic nervous systems.

_____ 5. The largest and most numerous of neuroglia are astrocytes.

Multiple Choice

Identify the letter of the choice that best completes the statement or answers the question.

1. Phagocytic cells that do not transmit impulses and are located within the CNS are called _____.
   A. glial cells
   B. astrocytes
   C. ganglia
   D. none of the above

2. _____ are nerve cells that engulf cellular waste and destroy microorganisms in nerve tissue.
   A. Astrocytes
   B. Ependymal cells
   C. Microglial cells
   D. Oligodendroglial cells

3. The _____ is known as the "little brain."
   A. brainstem
   B. cerebellum
   C. diencephalon
   D. cerebrum

4. The middle layer of the meninges is called the _____.
   A. dura mater
   B. pia mater
   C. arachnoid
   D. none of the above

Copyright © 2010, 2005 by Saunders, an imprint of Elsevier, Inc. All rights reserved.

5. _____ are(is) (a) chemical substance(s) that cause(s) a nerve impulse.
   A. Neurotransmitters
   B. Aqueous humor
   C. Oxytocin
   D. Cerebrospinal fluid

6. The combining form for "brain" is _____.
   A. neur/o
   B. dur/o
   C. rhiz/o
   D. encephal/o

7. _____ are used to produce sleep.
   A. Analgesics
   B. Hypnotics
   C. Sedatives
   D. Anesthetics

8. Paxil is an example of an _____.
   A. antimanic
   B. antipsychotic
   C. anxiolytic
   D. antidepressant

9. What roman numeral is the trigeminal nerve?
   A. III
   B. IV
   C. V
   D. X

10. A _____ headache occurs unilaterally and involves an eye, temple, cheek, and forehead. These headaches start during sleep and can last for several weeks.
    A. tension
    B. cluster
    C. migraine
    D. none of the above

11. A(n) _____ is the surgical puncture performed to remove CSF for examination.
    A. spinal tap
    B. angiography
    C. myelography
    D. electroneuromyography

12. A test that measures muscle activity and aids in diagnosing neuromuscular problems is called a(n) _____.
    A. electroencephalogram
    B. angiogram
    C. electromyogram
    D. nerve conduction study

13. A(n) _____ seizure begins with an outcry and movements that are first tonic and then clonic.
    A. petit mal
    B. myoclonic
    C. partial
    D. grand mal

14. _____ occurs when a blood vessel ruptures or a blood clot occludes a blood vessel, which decreases blood flow to the brain.
    A. ALS
    B. CVA
    C. MS
    D. TIA

15. _____ is inflammation of the brain and spinal cord coverings.
    A. Meningitis
    B. Parkinson's disease
    C. Multiple sclerosis
    D. Alzheimer's disease

16. Neuralgia of the fifth cranial nerve is called _____.
    A. Alzheimer's disease
    B. tic douloureux
    C. transient ischemic attack
    D. shingles

Sentence Completion

Complete each sentence or statement.

neuron	antisocial	depression
narcissistic	post-traumatic stress	psychosis
MMPI	neurilemma	paranoid
autism	dementia	bipolar
OCD	Rorschach	

1. The functional unit of the nervous system is the _____.

2. _____ measures personality characteristics through forced-choice questions.

3. _____ is an impaired perception of reality.

4. A(n) _____ test measures a patient's ability to integrate intellectual and emotional fears.

5. _____ is an irreversible impairment of intellectual activities.

6. _____ is a disorder marked by severe mood swings from hyperactivity to sadness.

7. _____ behavior demonstrates a lack of empathy and sensitivity to the needs of others.

8. _____ is a severe anxiety following trauma. Impairment affects daily living.

9. _____ is a disorder characterized by preoccupation with inner thoughts.

10. _____ is a continuous sheath around the myelin.

Short Answers

1. Describe the organization of the nervous system and identify its two main divisions.

   _____
   _____
   _____
   _____

2. List the main divisions of the central nervous system.

   _____
   _____
   _____

3. Describe the functions of the sympathetic and parasympathetic nervous system.

   _____
   _____
   _____
   _____
   _____
   _____
   _____

CRITICAL THINKING

1. Describe a past event that caused your sympathetic and parasympathetic nervous system to respond.

2. Clara Evanston is an 83-year-old patient who has been gradually exhibiting signs of Alzheimer's disease. Her husband is her primary caregiver and is finding it increasingly difficult to manage her care. On Clara's recent office visit, Mr. Evanston asked you to explain the progression of Clara's symptoms and what suggestions you have for her care. Explain to Mr. Evanston the progression of symptoms and what suggestions you would give him. Research Alzheimer's disease as needed.

PRACTICAL APPLICATIONS

If you have accomplished the objectives in this chapter, you will be able to make better choices as a medical assistant. Take a look at this situation and decide what you would do.

Sally Jones, age 72, complained of dizziness with a loss of sensation on the left side that lasted only for a few minutes over the past few weeks. She also had a headache that lasted only during the paresthesia. She has a long history of moderately controlled hypertension for which she has taken antihypertensives, "When I thought about them." Dr. Smith was concerned that she might be having TIAs. He prescribed a vasodilator and a mild analgesic for the headache when he saw her last week. Today she was brought to the emergency department with sudden left-side hemiplegia and a headache, but no aphasia. Except for the hypertension, Sally has been in relatively good health for her age. On admission, her blood pressure was 210/120 mm Hg, and she was semialert. Dr. Smith ordered a CT scan, and it showed an infarct to the right frontotemporal lobes. Sally was admitted to the hospital for observation and possible treatment.

Copyright © 2010, 2005 by Saunders, an imprint of Elsevier, Inc. All rights reserved.

CHAPTER 16 Nervous System

1. What is a TIA? Why was that a precursor to the condition for which Sally was admitted to the hospital?

2. Why were the dizziness, loss of sensation, and the headache over the past few weeks important in making a diagnosis of TIA?

3. Why did Dr. Smith give Sally vasodilators?

4. Define paresthesia, aphasia, and hemiplegia.

5. Why was the control of blood pressure important in the prevention of illness?

6. Why is the paralysis on the left side of the body when the right side of the brain is involved? Why does Sally not have aphasia?

7. Why did Dr. Smith order a CT scan rather than an MRI?

___

8. What is a common name for the disease process for which Dr. Smith is treating Sally?

___

9. What type of problems would you expect Sally to have because the infarct is in the frontal and temporal lobes?

___

APPLICATION OF SKILLS

1. Label the word parts of the following terms. Use *P* to indicate a prefix, *CF* to indicate a combining form, *R* to indicate a root, *S* to indicate a suffix. (Example: abnormal—ab *P* norm *R* al *S*)
   A. dysphasia ___
   B. epidural ___
   C. meningitis ___
   D. neurilemma ___
   E. poliomyelitis ___

2. Change the following from singular to plural or vice versa.
   A. vertebra ___
   B. foramen ___
   C. meninx ___
   D. axons ___
   E. amebae ___

3. Write out the meaning of each the following abbreviations.
   A. ALS ___
   B. CVA ___
   C. TIA ___
   D. MS ___
   E. EEG ___

4. Label the diagrams.

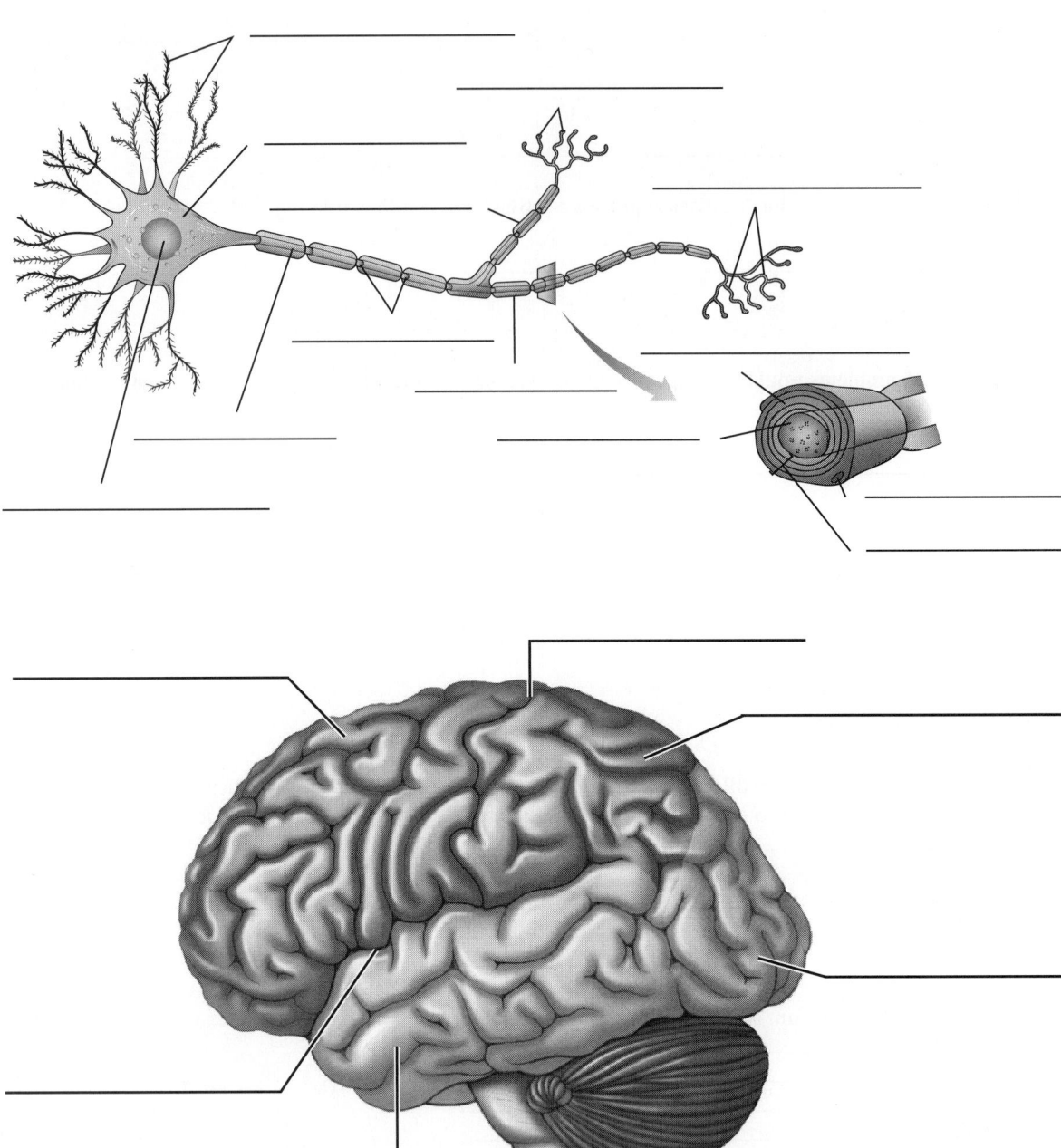

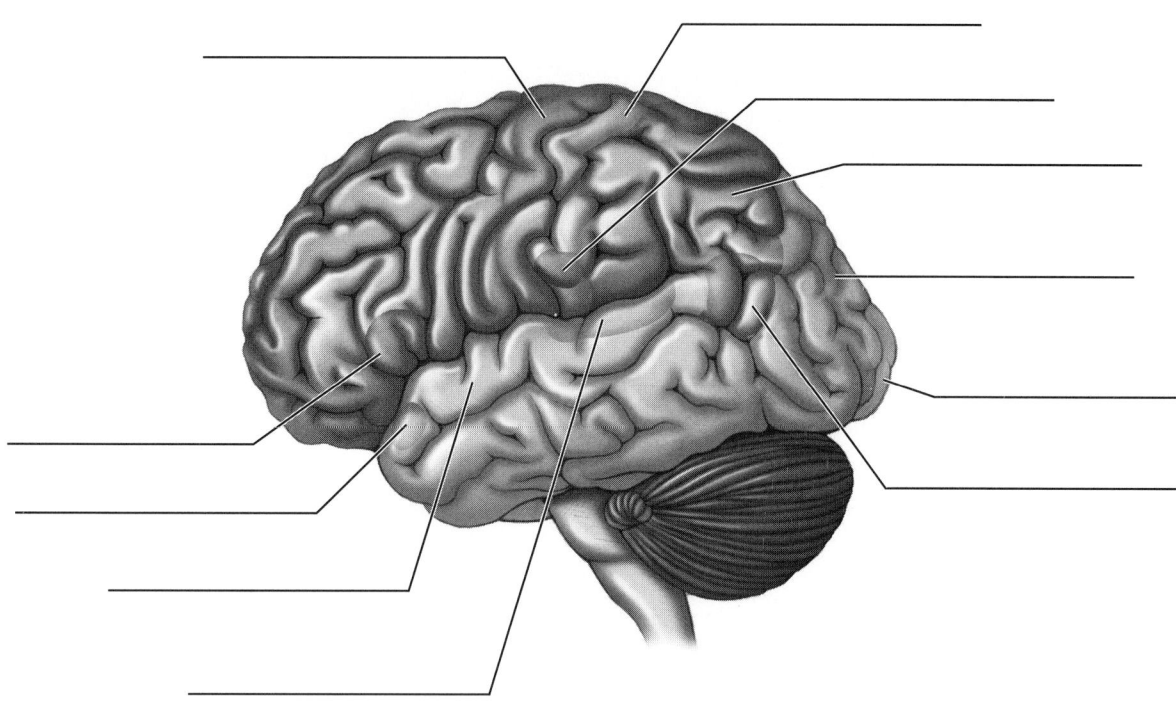

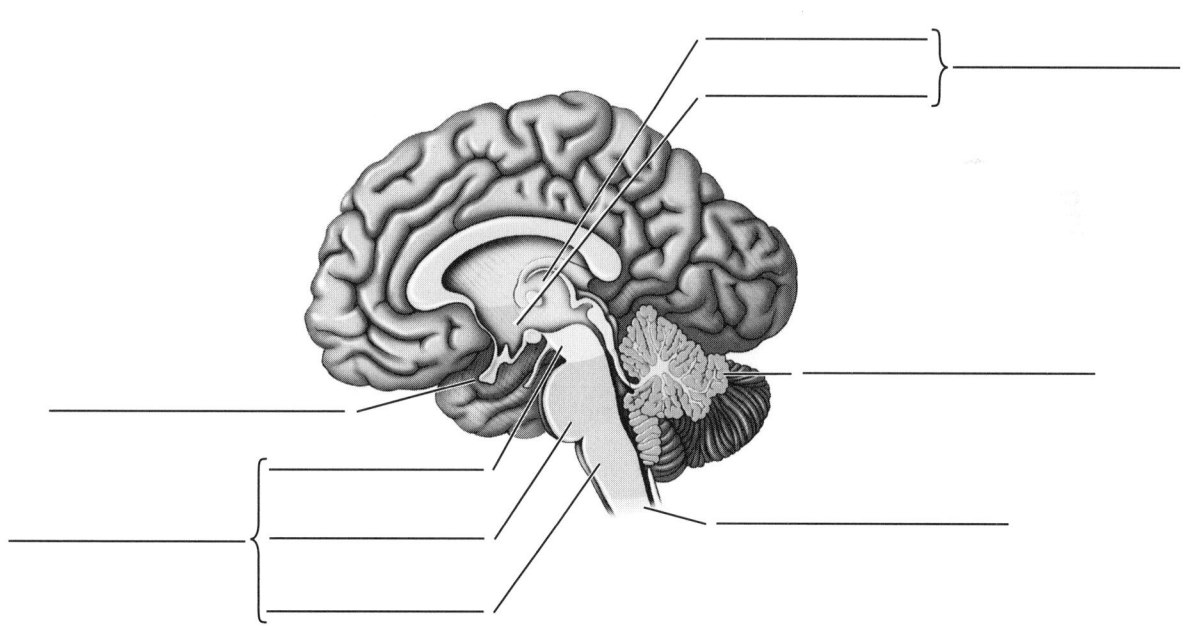

CHAPTER QUIZ

Multiple Choice

Identify the letter of the choice that best completes the statement or answers the question.

1. The _____ of a nerve cell carries impulses to other neurons and body tissue.
   A. nodes of Ranvier
   B. dendrites
   C. synapse
   D. axon

2. _____ neurons transmit nerve impulses from the CNS to muscles and glands.
   A. Efferent
   B. Integrative
   C. Afferent
   D. None of the above

3. Star-shaped nerve cells that hold blood vessels, closer to nerve cells, and transport water and salts between nerve cells are called _____.
   A. microglial cells
   B. oligodendroglial cells
   C. astrocytes
   D. ependymal cells

4. A sterile watery fluid formed within the ventricles of the brain is _____.
   A. CNS
   B. CSF
   C. PNS
   D. PSF

5. A(n) _____ reflex extends the foot when the tendon at the heel is tapped.
   A. abdominal
   B. Achilles
   C. Babinski
   D. plantar

6. _____ is the inability to focus one's attention for short periods or for engaging in quiet activities, or both.
   A. ADHD
   B. COPD
   C. Colic
   D. Kernig sign

7. _____ occurs when a blood vessel ruptures or a blood clot occludes a blood vessel that decreases blood flow to the brain.
   A. TIA
   B. ALS
   C. CVA
   D. OCD

8. _____ is an acute inflammation of the dorsal root ganglia of a dermatome.
   A. Meningitis
   B. Shingles
   C. Tic douloureux
   D. Encephalitis

9. _____ is a feeling of persistent sadness.
   A. Depression
   B. Anxiety
   C. Narcissism
   D. Paranoia

10. A(n) _____ is a test that records neuromuscular activity by electrical stimulation.
    A. CT scan
    B. MRI
    C. EEG
    D. EMG

11. _____ is a disorder characterized by a preoccupation with inner thoughts and marked unresponsiveness to social contact.
    A. Delusional disorder
    B. Autism
    C. Obsessive-compulsive disorder
    D. Munchausen syndrome

12. There are _____ pairs of spinal nerves.
    A. 12
    B. 31
    C. 36
    D. 42

13. The ANS consists of _____.
    A. the peripheral and afferent nervous systems
    B. the sympathetic and parasympathetic nervous systems
    C. the sympathetic and efferent nervous systems
    D. the parasympathetic and somatic nervous system

14. Along a neuron, the correct pathway for impulse conduction is _____.
    A. dendrite, axon, cell body, receptor
    B. dendrite, cell body, axon
    C. axon, cell body, dendrite
    D. receptor, axon, cell body

15. The white matter of the nervous system is composed of _____.
    A. myelinated fibers
    B. nuclei
    C. nonmyelinated fibers
    D. ganglia

16. When an impulse reaches a synapse, _____.
    A. two nerve fibers come in direct contact
    B. impulses pass in either direction
    C. an electrical spark jumps the gap
    D. chemical transmitters are released

Copyright © 2010, 2005 by Saunders, an imprint of Elsevier, Inc. All rights reserved.

17. Meningitis is an _____.
    A. inflammation of the brain
    B. inflammation of the meninges
    C. inflammation of the spinal cord
    D. inflammation of third ventricle

18. The brainstem does not include _____.
    A. the pons
    B. the medulla
    C. the midbrain
    D. the cerebellum

19. Tic douloureux is a painful neuralgia of the _____ nerve.
    A. trigeminal
    B. vagus
    C. abducens
    D. olfactory

20. Which of the following cranial nerves is responsible for movements of the tongue?
    A. Vagus
    B. Trigeminal
    C. Trochlear
    D. Hypoglossal

17 Sensory System

VOCABULARY REVIEW

Matching: Match each term with the correct definition.

A. equilibrium

B. vertigo

C. tactile

D. accommodation

E. ophthalmoscope

F. cerumen

G. eustachian tube

H. ossicles

I. decibels

J. otolaryngologist

K. semicircular canals

L. instillation

M. irrigation

N. conduction

O. hearing acuity tests

_____ 1. Pertains to the sense of touch

_____ 2. Loud/soft measurement of sound

_____ 3. Hand-held instrument used for viewing the internal structure of the eye

_____ 4. Small bones of the middle ear

_____ 5. Controls equilibrium

_____ 6. Adjustment that allows for vision at various distances

_____ 7. Yellow-brown substance produced by the sweat glands in the external ear

_____ 8. Dizziness

_____ 9. Specialist in the treatment of ear, nose, and throat diseases

_____ 10. Tube that connects the middle ear with the nasopharynx and acts to equalize pressure between the outer and middle ear

_____ 11. Balance

_____ 12. Process of placing medication into an area as prescribed by a physician

_____ 13. Washing or rinsing out an area to remove foreign matter

_____ 14. Tests used to check for hearing loss

_____ 15. Ability to move from one area to another, as in hearing with transmission of sound through nervous tissue

CHAPTER 17 Sensory System

THEORY RECALL

True/False

Indicate whether the statement is true or false.

_____ 1. An ophthalmologist treats disorders of the eye.

_____ 2. Antiseptics are used to reduce growth of bacteria in the eye.

_____ 3. The middle ear functions to maintain balance, equilibrium, and awareness of position.

_____ 4. Eyelashes protrude from sweat glands on the edge of the lid.

_____ 5. Lysozyme is an enzyme present in tears that acts as an antiseptic.

Multiple Choice

Identify the letter of the choice that best completes the statement or answers the question.

1. The suffix for "hearing" is _____.
   A. -acusis
   B. -geusia
   C. -kinesia
   D. -otia

2. _____ soften and break down ear wax.
   A. Anti-infectives
   B. Vasodilators
   C. Ceruminolytics
   D. Anxiolytics

3. The _____ nerve controls salivation, swallowing, and taste.
   A. olfactory
   B. trochlear
   C. glossopharyngeal
   D. hypoglossal

4. Which one of the following is *not* an extrinsic eye muscle?
   A. Superior rectus
   B. Lateral rectus
   C. Superior oblique
   D. Ciliary

5. Which eye muscle elevates or rolls the eyeball upward?
   A. Inferior rectus
   B. Medial rectus
   C. Superior oblique
   D. Inferior oblique

6. _____ is used to measure intraocular pressure.
   A. Amsler grid
   B. Gonioscopy
   C. Tonometry
   D. All of the above

7. _____ occurs when the aqueous humor does not drain properly, and the intraocular pressure increases and compresses the choroid layer, diminishing blood supply to the retina.
   A. Cataract
   B. Glaucoma
   C. Strabismus
   D. Myopia

8. _____ is a refraction error caused by the abnormal curvature of the cornea and lens.
   A. Astigmatism
   B. Ptosis
   C. Strabismus
   D. Hyperopia

9. _____ is a buildup of excess fluid in the semicircular canals, which places excess pressure on the canals, vestibule, and cochlea.
   A. Otosclerosis
   B. Mastoiditis
   C. Meniere disease
   D. None of the above

10. An _____ is a record produced by an audiometer.
    A. audiogram
    B. audiologist
    C. audiometry
    D. none of the above

11. Rinne and Weber tests are types of _____.
    A. blood tests
    B. hearing tests
    C. postpartum tests
    D. prenatal tests

12. Impulses are transmitted from the inner ear to the acoustic nerve via the _____.
    A. vestibular nerve
    B. cochlear nerve
    C. oculomotor nerve
    D. none of the above

13. Blood vessels are found in which of the following parts of the eye?
    A. Cornea
    B. Lens
    C. Choroid
    D. Aqueous humor

Copyright © 2010, 2005 by Saunders, an imprint of Elsevier, Inc. All rights reserved.

14. The white of the eye is referred to as the _____.
    A. sclera
    B. choroid
    C. cornea
    D. pupil

15. All of the following are taste sensations *except* _____.
    A. sweet
    B. spicy
    C. sour
    D. bitter

16. The sense of smell is accomplished by the _____ nerve.
    A. olfactory
    B. auditory
    C. optic
    D. vagus

17. The opening in the center of the iris in the eye is called the _____.
    A. sclera
    B. pupil
    C. lens
    D. retina

18. Accessory organs of the eye contain all of the following *except* _____.
    A. eyebrows
    B. eyelashes
    C. rods and cones
    D. lacrimal apparatus

19. Myopia is _____.
    A. nearsightedness
    B. "old eyes"
    C. farsightedness
    D. abnormal curvature of the cornea

20. Another term for "cross-eyed" is _____.
    A. myopia
    B. strabismus
    C. amblyopia
    D. diplopia

Sentence Completion

Complete each sentence or statement.

presbycusis	sebum
astigmatism	cerumen
glaucoma	Meniere
cataract	Weber
Rinne	

1. _____ is the progressive hearing loss occurring in old age.

2. A(n) _____ test compares bone conduction and air conduction of sound using a tuning fork.

3. The _____ test assesses the hearing in both ears at once.

4. _____ is the medical name for "ear wax."

5. _____ is a condition that occurs when aqueous humor does not drain properly.

Short Answers

1. Explain the purpose of the sensory system.

2. Discuss the changes that occur in the ear during the aging process. What effect do these changes have on communication?

CRITICAL THINKING

1. Jason Ball is a 56-year-old patient that comes to the clinic today with a complaint of gradual hearing loss. The physician wants you to get Jason ready for the hearing acuity tests. What tests does the physician want to perform, and how are they performed?

_____

_____

_____

_____

_____

_____

PRACTICAL APPLICATIONS

If you have accomplished the objectives in this chapter, you will be able to make better choices as a medical assistant. Take a look at this situation and decide what you would do.

Bob DeMarce, age 42, complained of vertigo, tinnitus, and a sensation of fullness of the right ear for the last month. He states that each episode did not follow a certain event. He denies any ear pain, fever, headache, or nausea.

Past medical history includes a recent ear infection that was treated with amoxicillin for 10 days. On examination, Dr. Bailey finds that the tympanic membrane is dull and inflamed. It is decided that Bob has had otitis media that failed to resolve.

Do you understand what otitis media is, and how Bob's earlier treatment relates to it? The symptoms of Meniere's disease, a disorder of the inner ear, mimic some of the symptoms present with otitis media.

1. **How are otitis media and Meniere's disease similar? How are they different?**

_____

_____

_____

_____

_____

_____

2. Why were the symptoms of vertigo, tinnitus, and a sensation of fullness over the past month important in making a diagnosis of otitis media?

3. What is Meniere's disease, and what other symptoms does it have?

4. What type of diagnostic tests would be done to confirm a diagnosis of Meniere's disease?

5. What would be the recommended lifestyle changes for Bob?

APPLICATION OF SKILLS

1. Label the word parts of the following terms. Use *P* to indicate a prefix, *CF* to indicate a combining form, *R* to indicate a root, *S* to indicate a suffix. (Example: abnormal—ab *P* norm *R* al *S*)
   A. audiologist _____
   B. aural _____
   C. otopyorrhea _____
   D. intraocular _____
   E. myopia _____

Copyright © 2010, 2005 by Saunders, an imprint of Elsevier, Inc. All rights reserved.

2. Change the following from singular to plural or vice versa.
   A. cornea _____
   B. stapes _____
   C. iris _____
   D. conjunctiva _____
   E. pinna _____

3. Write out the meaning of each the following abbreviations.
   A. Acc _____
   B. ENT _____
   C. HEENT _____
   D. PERRLA _____
   E. VA _____

4. Label the diagrams.

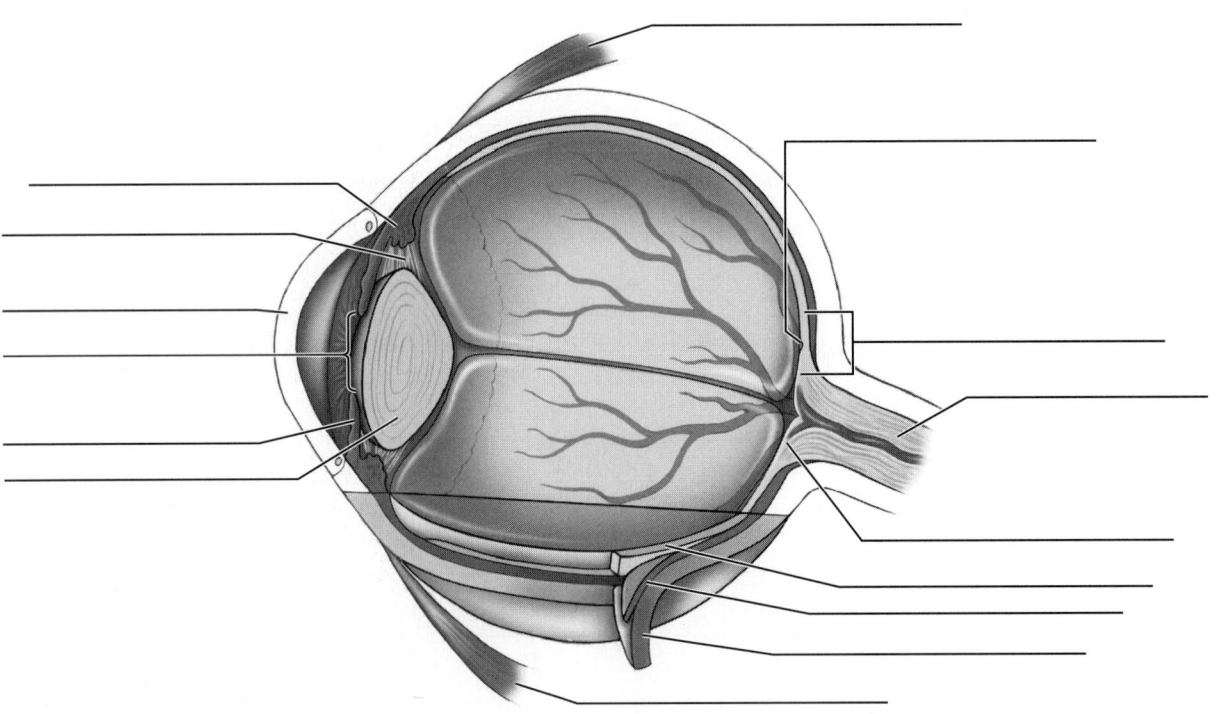

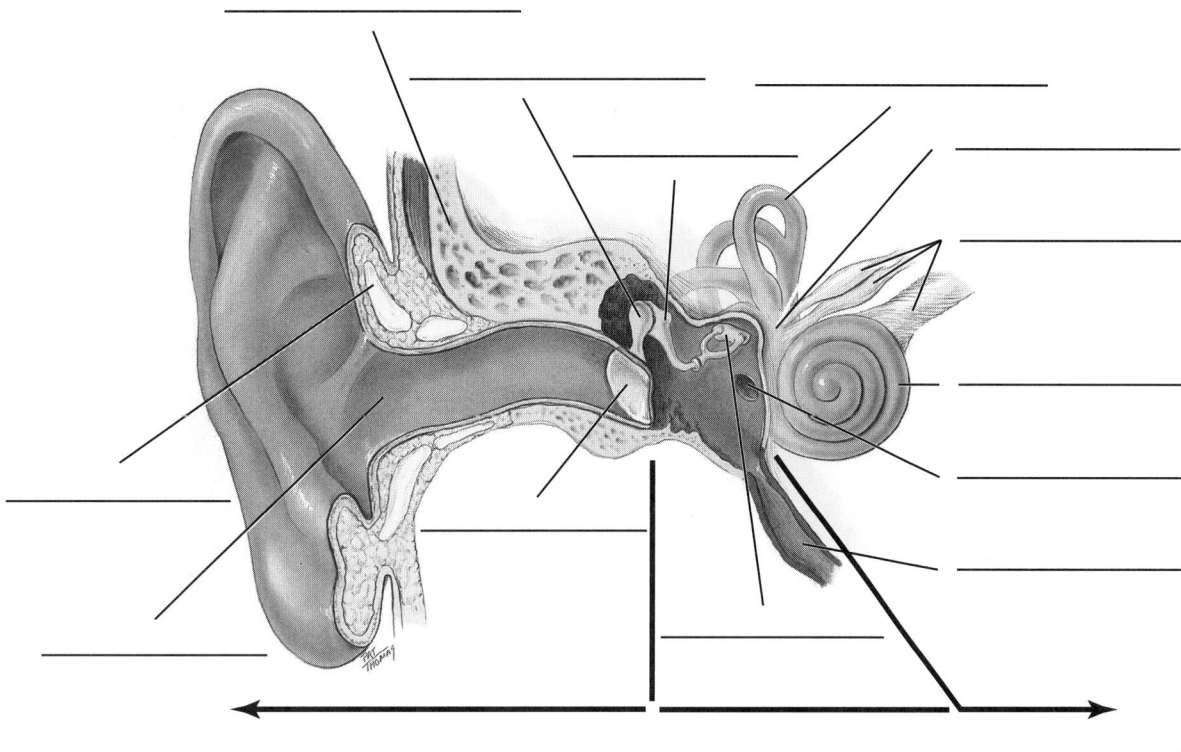

5. Wear a blindfold for 1 hour to block your vision completely. Participate in all of your regular activities—get dressed, brush your teeth, do household chores. Write one paragraph describing your experience. Identify the points that you could share with a recently blind patient or a patient who is losing his or her eyesight.

CHAPTER QUIZ

Multiple Choice

Identify the letter of the choice that best completes the statement or answers the question.

1. _____ is the anterior portion of the sclera; also means "transparent—allows light through."
   A. Iris
   B. Chorioid
   C. Lens
   D. Cornea

2. Which one of the following is *not* a muscle of the eye?
   A. Oblique
   B. Canthus
   C. Rectus
   D. All of the above are muscles of the eye

3. _____ occurs when the lens loses its ability to change shape during accommodation for close objects.
   A. Presbycusis
   B. Strabismus
   C. Presbyopia
   D. Hyperopia

4. The _____ is the external flap of the ear.
   A. pinna
   B. auricle
   C. A and B
   D. none of the above

5. The medical term for "pinkeye" is _____.
   A. chalazion
   B. conjunctivitis
   C. strabismus
   D. hordeolum

6. _____ is a buildup of excess fluid in the semicircular canals, which places excess pressure on the canals, vestibule, and cochlea.
   A. Meniere disease
   B. Vertigo
   C. Otosclerosis
   D. Presbycusis

7. Which one of the following is *not* an ossicle?
   A. Malleus
   B. Incus
   C. Stapes
   D. All of the above are ossicles

8. The _____ of the ear lies below the vestibule and is shaped like a snail shell.
   A. labyrinth
   B. eustachian tube
   C. organ of Corti
   D. cochlea

9. All of the following are taste buds *except* _____.
   A. sweet
   B. sour
   C. acid
   D. bitter

10. The auditory ossicles include all of the following *except* _____.
    A. malleus
    B. incus
    C. pinna
    D. stapes

11. Which of the following is *not* a structure of the middle ear?
    A. Incus
    B. Stapes
    C. Eustachian tube
    D. Vestibule

12. Which of the following structures is *not* a part of the external ear?
    A. Auricle
    B. Tympanic membrane
    C. Eustachian tube
    D. External auditory canal

13. Blood vessels are found in which part of the eye?
    A. Sclera
    B. Lens
    C. Choroid
    D. Rods

14. What part of the eye consists of nervous tissue?
    A. Sclera
    B. Choroid
    C. Iris
    D. Retina

15. The vitreous humor maintains the shape of the eye and _____.
    A. refracts light
    B. provides support to the retina
    C. secretes tears
    D. allows for near and far vision

Matching

Match each prefix or suffix with its correct definition.

_____ 16. -geusia   A. eye

_____ 17. ocul/o   B. sound

_____ 18. acous   C. ear condition

_____ 19. opt/o   D. sense of taste

_____ 20. -otia   E. vision

18 Skeletal System

VOCABULARY REVIEW

Matching: Match each term with the correct definition.

A. cartilage

B. epiphyseal plate

C. ossification

D. foramen

E. periosteum

F. cranium

G. fontanels

H. paranasal sinuses

I. sella turcica

J. sutures

K. nasal conchae

L. vomer

M. spinous process

N. vertebra

O. sternum

P. process

Q. amphiarthroses

R. orthopedic

S. bone scan

_____ 1. Joint with slight movement

_____ 2. Pertaining to treatment of the bones and joints

_____ 3. Outer covering of the bone that provides nourishment to the bone

_____ 4. Immovable joints

_____ 5. Area of each end of a long bone responsible for bone growth

_____ 6. Air-filled spaces within the skull

_____ 7. Caused when more bone cells are destroyed than are made; a decrease in bone density

_____ 8. Extend out from vertebral bone to serve as attachments for the ribs

_____ 9. Repair of a fracture when the skin has been surgically opened

_____ 10. Elastic substance attached to the end of some bones

_____ 11. Use of nuclear medicine to detect pathologies of bone

_____ 12. Pertaining to the study and analysis of human work devices that affect the anatomy

_____ 13. Breastbone

_____ 14. Skull; fusion of 8 cranial bones with 14 facial bones that protect the brain

_____ 15. Cancer that has spread from its original site to a new site

_____ 16. Calcification of bone

T. open reduction

U. subluxation

V. osteomyelitis

W. osteoporosis

X. metastasized

Y. crepitation

Z. ergonomic

_____ 17. Hole or opening for passage of nerves, blood vessels, and ligaments

_____ 18. Partial dislocation of a joint

_____ 19. Joints rubbing against each other

_____ 20. Forms the lower wall between the nostrils; nasal septum

_____ 21. Soft spots; located between the cranial bones

_____ 22. Projection on a bone

_____ 23. Facial bones above the roof of the mouth and the walls of the nasal cavities

_____ 24. Infection of the bone marrow and bone

_____ 25. Bony projection in the sphenoid bone that holds the pituitary gland

_____ 26. Protects the spinal cord

THEORY RECALL

True/False

Indicate whether the statement is true or false.

_____ 1. The skeletal system is the bony framework of the body and is made up of 206 bones.

_____ 2. Proper levels of calcium in the bloodstream are maintained in the blood by the pituitary hormone.

_____ 3. Long bones are located only in the upper and lower extremities.

_____ 4. The largest bone in the face is the maxilla.

_____ 5. Articulations are joints where two or more bones come together.

Multiple Choice

Identify the letter of the choice that best completes the statement or answers the question.

1. The combining form for "bone" is _____.
   A. chondr/o
   B. bon/o
   C. oste/o
   D. none of the above

2. Naproxen is an _____ prescribed to relieve and control inflammation.
   A. anti-inflammatory
   B. antibiotic
   C. antiarthritic
   D. analgesic

3. _____ is the visual examination of a joint with the use of a scope.
   A. Arthrography
   B. Myeloscopy
   C. Bone scan
   D. Arthroscopy

4. _____ is a disease of adults in which deficiency of calcium and vitamin D occurs.
   A. Rickets
   B. Osteomyelitis
   C. Osteomalacia
   D. Scurvy

5. _____ is a lateral curvature of the spine.
   A. Scoliosis
   B. Lordosis
   C. Kyphosis
   D. None of the above

6. The suffix meaning "to break" is _____.
   A. -cyto
   B. -clast
   C. -blast
   D. -malacia

7. Which one of the following is *not* a type of joint?
   A. Amphiarthroses
   B. Diarthroses
   C. Synarthroses
   D. Articulothroses

8. _____ are the long bones of the foot.
   A. Metatarsals
   B. Tarsals
   C. Metacarpals
   D. Carpals

9. The _____ is the longest and strongest bone in the body.
   A. ulnar
   B. tibia
   C. femur
   D. humerus

10. The _____ and the _____ are located behind the nose and eye sockets.
    A. xiphoid; manubrium bones
    B. incus; stapes bones
    C. sphenoid; ethmoid bones
    D. mandible; maxilla bones

11. Which of the following is *not* a distinct region of a long bone?
    A. Metaphysis
    B. Paraphysis
    C. Diaphysis
    D. Epiphysis

12. An example of _____ cartilage can be found in the outer ear.
    A. fibrous
    B. hyaline
    C. elastic
    D. retractable

13. A(n) _____ is a bone-reabsorbing cell.
    A. osteoblast
    B. osteoclast
    C. osteocyte
    D. none of the above

14. _____ is made of connective tissue and blood vessels.
    A. Bone marrow
    B. Periosteum
    C. Lamellae
    D. Compact bone

15. The bone that extends from the top of the eye orbits to the top of the head forming the forehead is called the _____.
    A. temporal bone
    B. parietal
    C. occipital
    D. frontal

16. The main shaft of a bone is called the _____.
    A. diaphysis
    B. epiphysis
    C. metaphysis
    D. paraphysis

17. The _____ bones are located within the eye orbits and along the side of the nose.
    A. palatine
    B. zygomatic
    C. lacrimal
    D. vomer

Copyright © 2010, 2005 by Saunders, an imprint of Elsevier, Inc. All rights reserved.

18. The first vertebra is called the _____ and supports the head.
    A. axis
    B. atlas
    C. sphenoid
    D. coccyx

19. Adults have _____ vertebrae.
    A. 12
    B. 26
    C. 33
    D. 42

20. The part of the sternum that is used as a landmark for CPR is the _____.
    A. manubrium
    B. body
    C. xiphoid process
    D. none of the above

21. The medical term for "shoulder blades" is _____.
    A. scapulae
    B. clavicles
    C. humerus
    D. ulna

22. The wrist has eight small bones called _____.
    A. metatarsals
    B. tarsals
    C. metacarpals
    D. carpals

23. Which one of the following is *not* a pelvic bone?
    A. Acetabulum
    B. Ilium
    C. Ischium
    D. Pubis

24. Which one of the following is the "heel" bone?
    A. Talus
    B. Calcaneus
    C. Navicular
    D. Cuboid

25. _____ is (are) a capsule made up of tough, fibrous connective tissue and filled with synovial fluid.
    A. Vertebrae
    B. Meniscus
    C. Bursae
    D. Tendons

Sentence Completion

Complete each sentence or statement.

red	phalanges	irregular
cartilage	zygomatic bone	periosteum
occipital	haversian system	saddle
axial skeleton	pivot	
appendicular skeleton	parietal	
yellow	mandible	

1. The _____ is a structural unit of the bone that receives nutrition and removes wastes.

2. The _____ contains the bones of the central section of the skeleton, which includes the bones of the head and trunk.

3. The bones of the spinal column; sphenoid; and ethmoid bones of the skull, sacrum, coccyx, and mandible are _____ [type] bones.

4. _____ is connective tissue attached to bone and does not contain mineral salts.

5. _____ bone marrow is responsible for the manufacture of red and white blood cells.

6. The _____ is the covering on the outer surface of a bone.

7. The _____ bone forms the back part of the cranial floor and is the covering for the back portion of the brain.

8. The medical term for "cheek bones" is _____.

9. The medical term for the fingers and toes is _____.

10. _____ joints allow for rotation.

Short Answers

1. List the four types of bone shapes and give an example of each.

_____

_____

_____

_____

Copyright © 2010, 2005 by Saunders, an imprint of Elsevier, Inc. All rights reserved.

2. List the five major functions of the skeletal system.

3. List three types of joints.

4. Describe the four main types of movement.

5. At birth, an infant has more bones than an adult. Explain the difference.

CRITICAL THINKING

1. One of your patients, Felicia Robinson, has been diagnosed with osteoporosis. She is 78 years old. Provide Felicia with information regarding this condition.

2. How would you explain to a patient the purpose of a goniometer?

PRACTICAL APPLICATIONS

If you have accomplished the objectives in this chapter, you will be able to make better choices as a medical assistant. Take a look at this situation and decide what you would do.

At age 14, Celia was injured in a skiing accident. She had a simple fracture of the end of the tibia and into the tarsals in her left leg. The fracture was located at the epiphyseal line. She also subluxated her knee in the same accident. The fracture was repaired with a closed reduction. After she wore a long leg cast for 8 weeks, an arthroscopy was performed on the knee to verify the tendons and ligaments had not been torn or stretched because weight bearing was difficult. Before the arthroscopy, an arthrogram was performed on the knee; this was negative. The arthroscopy was also negative. Over time, Celia seemed to recover from the fracture and had no problems until lately.

Celia is now 52 and has pain in the ankle attributed to arthritis. She has also been diagnosed with early osteoporosis as a result of a bone density scan. The physician ordered analgesics for arthralgia and vitamin D and calcium supplements for osteoporosis. Celia expresses concern while talking with Steve, the medical assistant, that the osteoporosis and arthritis will progress as she ages. She also has questions about some of the terms the physician used in talking with her.

1. What is a simple fracture?

2. What is a closed reduction?

Copyright © 2010, 2005 by Saunders, an imprint of Elsevier, Inc. All rights reserved.

3. What is subluxation of a joint?

4. Where is the tibia? Where are the tarsals?

5. What type of bone is the tibia? What type of bones are the tarsals?

6. Why would a fracture at the epiphysis be important in a child or young adult?

7. What is an arthrogram? What is arthroscopy?

8. Why would a bone scan be used in diagnosing osteoporosis?

9. Why would analgesics be ordered for arthritis?

10. What is arthralgia?

11. Why would vitamin D and calcium supplements be ordered for a patient with osteoporosis?

12. What are the dangers for Celia if the osteoporosis progresses?

CHAPTER 18 Skeletal System

APPLICATION OF SKILLS

1. Label the word parts of the following terms. Use *P* to indicate a prefix, *CF* to indicate a combining form, *R* to indicate a root, *S* to indicate a suffix. (Example: abnormal—ab *P* norm *R* al *S*)
   A. osteoarthropathy _____
   B. patellar _____
   C. periosteoedema _____
   D. arthritis _____
   E. xiphoid _____

2. Change the following from singular to plural or vice versa.
   A. bursa _____
   B. phalanx _____
   C. ilium _____
   D. arthroscopy _____
   E. sulcus _____

3. Write out the meaning of each the following abbreviations.
   A. BK _____
   B. DJD _____
   C. OA _____
   D. ROM _____
   E. Tx _____

4. Label the diagrams.

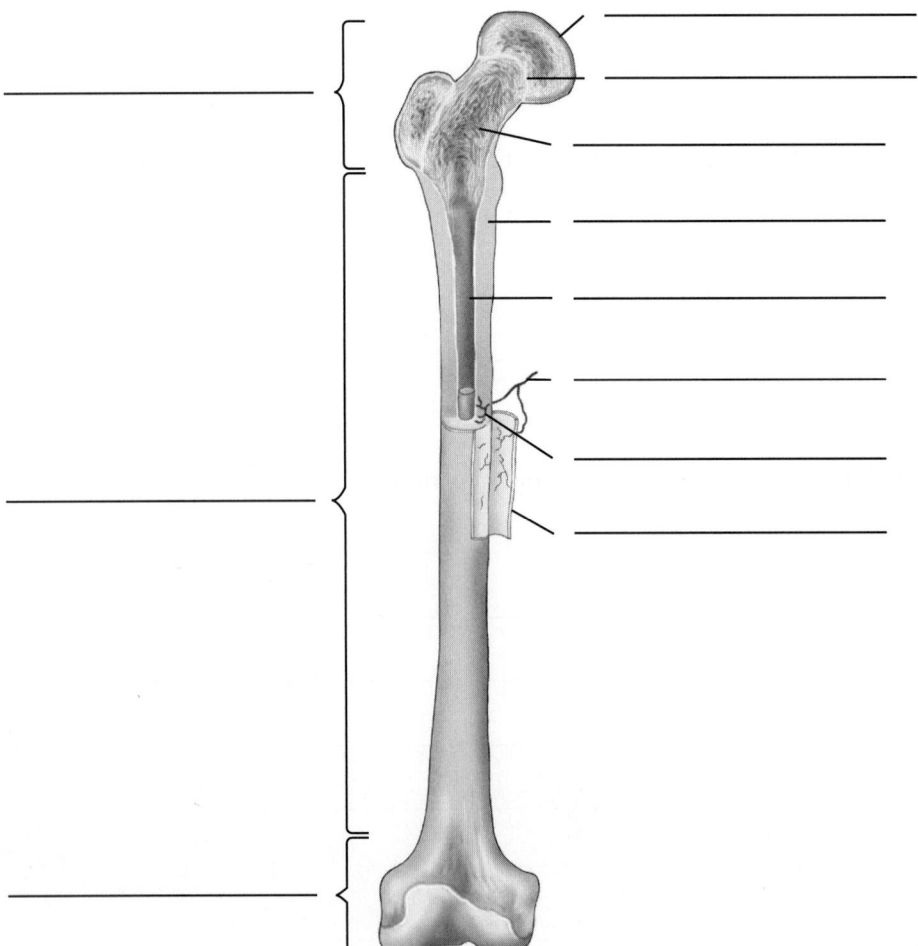

Skeletal System **CHAPTER** 18 **217**

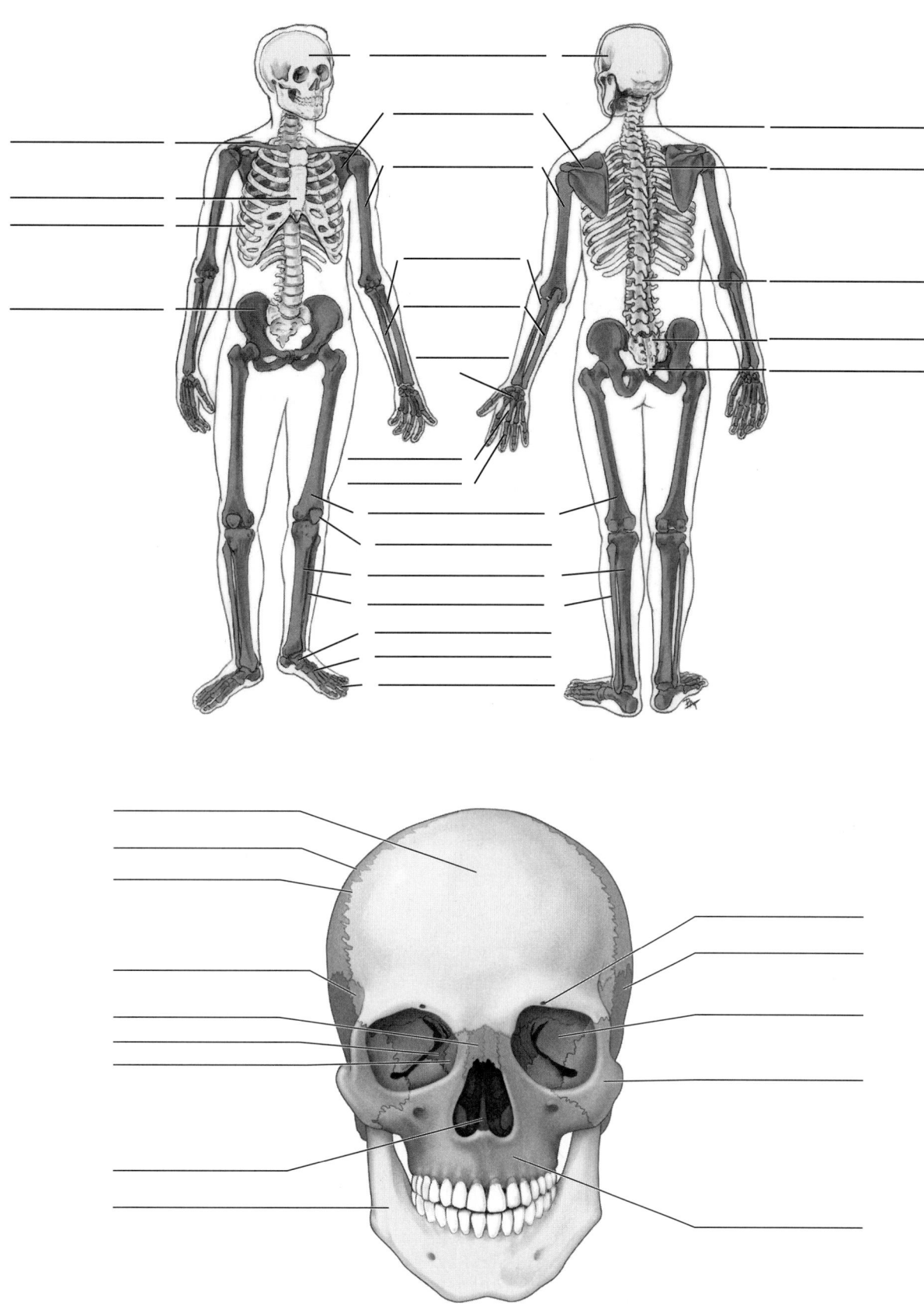

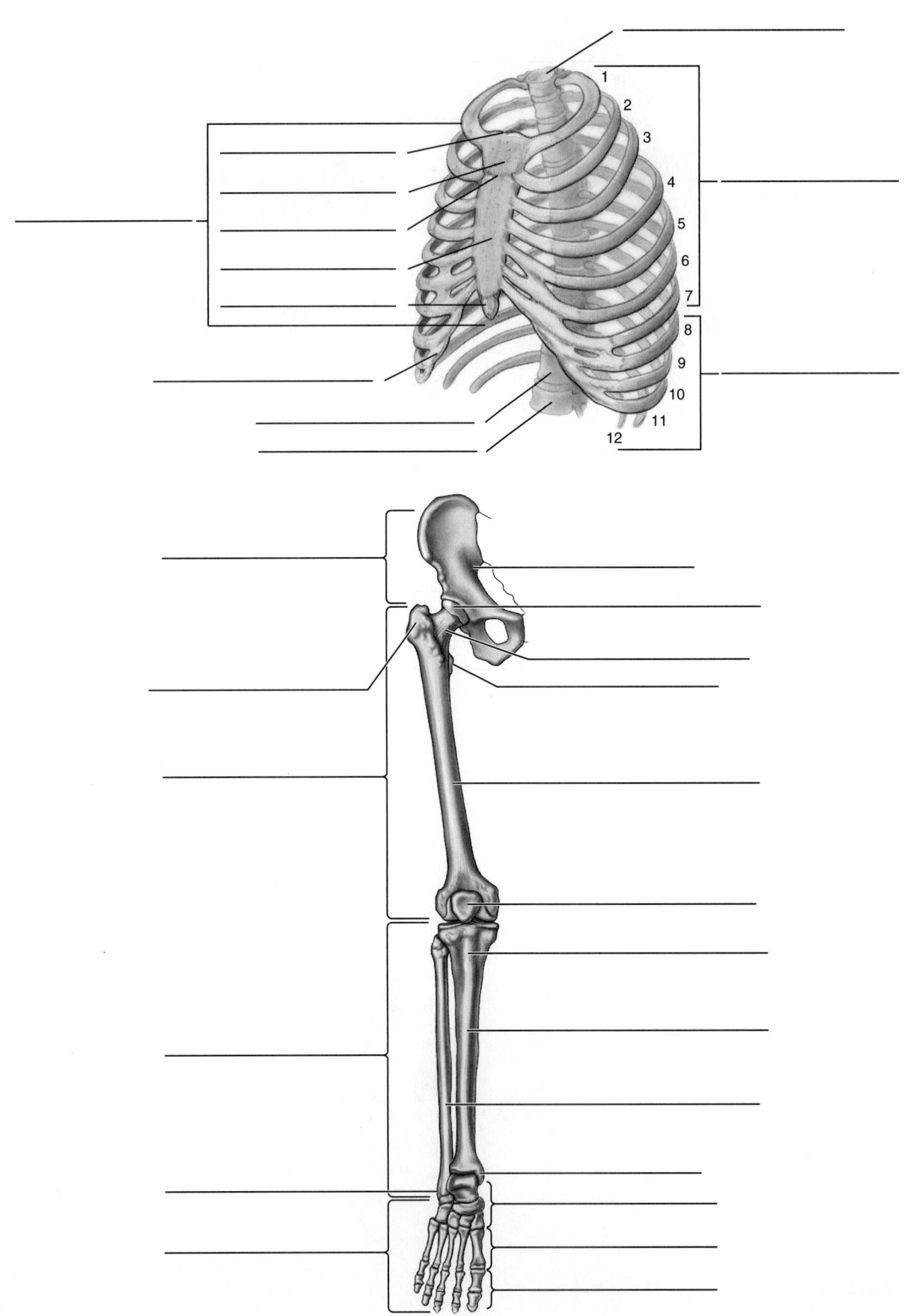

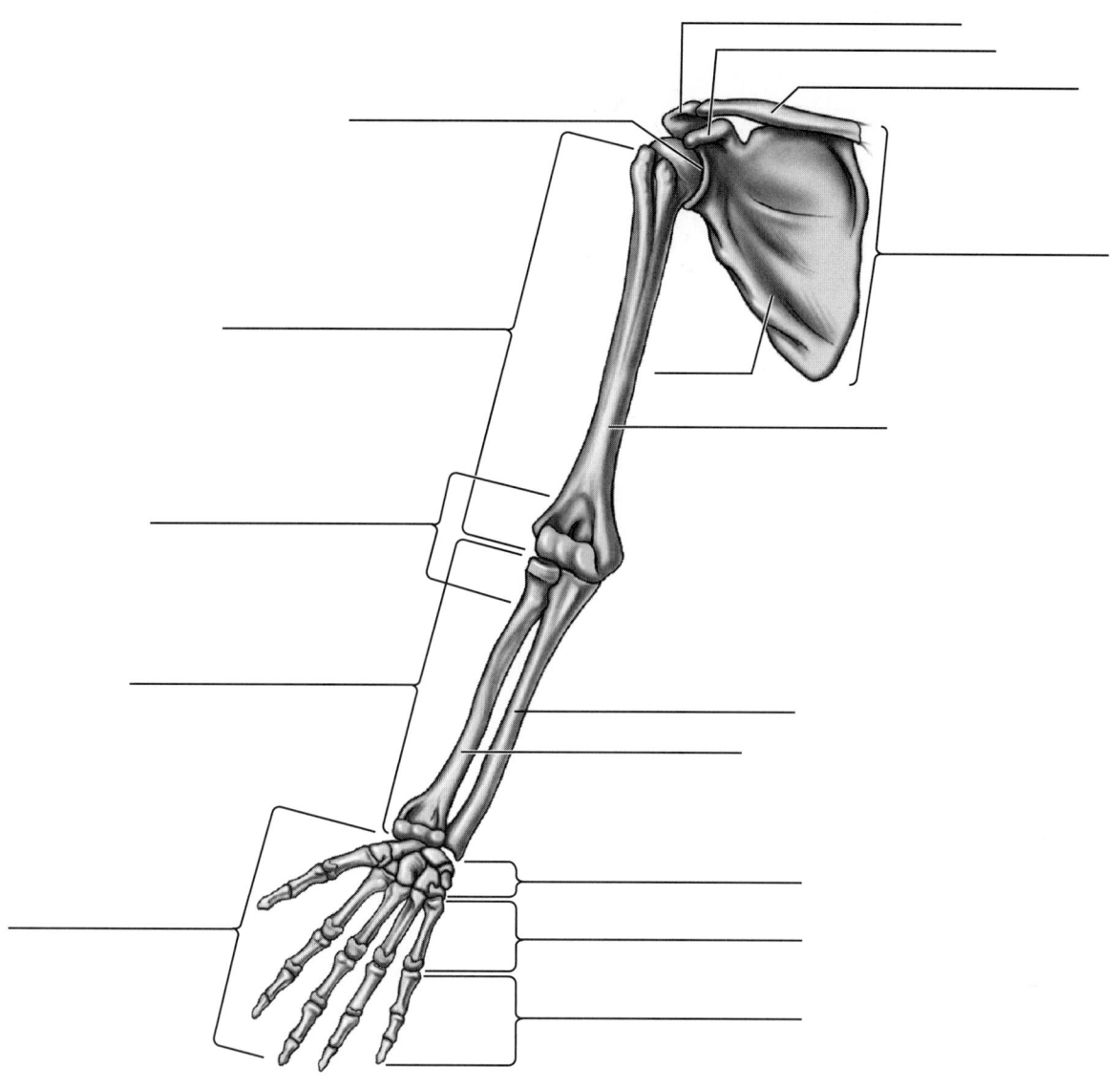

5. Using the classroom model of a human skeleton, identify each bone by sight.

CHAPTER QUIZ

Multiple Choice

Identify the letter of the choice that best completes the statement or answers the question.

1. _____ are bone-building cells.
   A. Osteoblasts
   B. Osteoclasts
   C. Osteocytes
   D. None of the above

2. The hormone that helps to maintain a proper level of calcium in the blood is _____.
   A. ADH
   B. LDH
   C. PTH
   D. none of the above

3. The _____ is the growth line for long bones in children.
   A. diaphysis
   B. epiphysis
   C. metaphysis
   D. paraphysis

4. The _____ vertebrae are the lower five vertebrae.
   A. cervical
   B. thoracic
   C. lumbar
   D. sacral

5. The bone of the upper arm is called the _____.
   A. humerus
   B. radius
   C. femur
   D. ulna

6. The eight small bones of the wrist are called _____.
   A. tarsals
   B. metatarsals
   C. carpals
   D. metacarpals

7. A joint that allows flat surfaces to move across each other is a _____.
   A. hinge joint
   B. ball-and-socket joint
   C. condyloid joint
   D. gliding joint

8. _____ is motion that occurs when the extremity is moved away from the body.
   A. Abduction
   B. Adduction
   C. Flexion
   D. Circumduction

9. A fracture in which the bone protrudes through the skin is a(n) _____.
   A. oblique fracture
   B. closed fracture
   C. open fracture
   D. greenstick fracture

10. When a bone breaks because of a twisting motion, it is called a _____.
    A. greenstick fracture
    B. spiral fracture
    C. compound fracture
    D. simple fracture

11. _____ is caused when more bone cells are destroyed than are made.
    A. Paget's disease
    B. Sarcoma
    C. Osteoarthritis
    D. Osteoporosis

12. _____ is the result of uric acid not being metabolized.
    A. Carpal tunnel syndrome
    B. Gouty arthritis
    C. Rheumatoid arthritis
    D. Ankylosis

13. A _____ is a depression or hollow space in a bone for attachments.
    A. foramen
    B. condyle
    C. fontanel
    D. fossa

14. A _____ is a narrow opening between parts of a bone that allows blood vessels or nerves to pass.
    A. fissure
    B. tuberosity
    C. foramen
    D. fossa

15. The medical term for "death of bone tissue" is _____.
    A. ostealgia
    B. osteonecrosis
    C. A and B
    D. neither A nor B

16. The medical term for "swayback" is _____.
    A. lordosis
    B. kyphosis
    C. scoliosis
    D. necrophysis

17. _____ occurs when the spinal column in the lumbar and sacral area does not close properly.
    A. Paget's disease
    B. Gouty arthritis
    C. Rheumatoid arthritis
    D. Spina bifida

18. The combining form for "vertebrae" is _____.
    A. clavicul/o
    B. spin/o
    C. spondyl/o
    D. rachi/o

Copyright © 2010, 2005 by Saunders, an imprint of Elsevier, Inc. All rights reserved.

19. Antiarthritics relieve symptoms of _____.
    A. pain
    B. arthritis
    C. gout
    D. inflammation

20. A large, rounded knuckle-like prominence that joins with another bone is called a _____.
    A. foramen
    B. fissure
    C. tuberosity
    D. condyle

Matching

Match each prefix or suffix with its correct definition.

_____ 21. -clast   A. wrist

_____ 22. rachi/o   B. softening

_____ 23. carp/o   C. ribs

_____ 24. -malacia   D. to break

_____ 25. cost/o   E. spine

19 Muscular System

VOCABULARY REVIEW

Matching: Match each term with the correct definition.

A. adenosine triphosphate (ATP)

B. antagonistic

C. lactic acid

D. synergistic

E. tonus

F. fascia

G. Achilles tendon

H. aponeurosis

I. tendon

J. isometric

K. tetany

L. contractility

M. elasticity

N. insertion

O. origin

P. prime mover

Q. atrophy

R. cramps

S. electromyography

T. fibromyalgia

_____ 1. Enzyme in skeletal muscle that produces energy

_____ 2. Muscle anchored to a moving bone

_____ 3. Muscle tension increases, but the muscle does not shorten

_____ 4. Progressive weakness and atrophy of muscles

_____ 5. Fibrous sheath that covers, supports, and separates muscles

_____ 6. Twitching and cramping of a muscle because of low blood calcium

_____ 7. Painful muscle spasms

_____ 8. Strongest tendon in the body; attaches the calf muscle to the heel

_____ 9. Muscle that is responsible for movement when a group of muscles is contracting at the same time

_____ 10. Syndrome that causes chronic pain in the muscles and soft tissue surrounding the joints

_____ 11. Exerting an opposite action to that of another

_____ 12. Ability to shorten and thicken when stimulated

_____ 13. Acting or working together

_____ 14. White, cordlike structure that serves to connect muscle to bone

_____ 15. Ability of a muscle to return to its original length after stretching

_____ 16. Involuntary muscle twitches

U. hernia

V. myalgia

W. myasthenia gravis

X. spasms

Y. sprain

Z. torticollis

_____ 17. When the intestines bulge through a weakness in a muscle wall

_____ 18. Slight tension in the muscle, which is always present, even at rest

_____ 19. Result of a shortened sternocleidomastoid muscle, causing the head and neck to tilt to one side

_____ 20. Wide, flat tendon that connects muscle to bone

_____ 21. Muscles anchored to nonmoving bones

_____ 22. Overstretching or tearing a ligament or joint

_____ 23. Waste product of muscle metabolism

_____ 24. Procedure that records the electrical activity of muscles

_____ 25. Wasting away of muscle tissues caused by nonuse over long periods

_____ 26. Muscle pain

THEORY RECALL

True/False

Indicate whether the statement is true or false.

_____ 1. The three main functions of muscles are to cause movement, provide support, and produce heat and energy.

_____ 2. When muscles are arranged in synergistic pairs, one muscle moves in one direction, and the antagonist causes movement in the opposite direction.

_____ 3. Chemical energy is used to make muscles contract.

_____ 4. Muscles are red because they contain myoglobin, and they have a rich blood supply.

_____ 5. The fixator is the muscle that is responsible for movement when a group of muscles are contracting at the same time.

Multiple Choice

Identify the letter of the choice that best completes the statement or answers the question.

1. The gluteus maximus is named for _____.
   A. origin/insertion
   B. size
   C. shape
   D. fiber direction

2. _____ move a bone away from the midline.
   A. Abductors
   B. Adductors
   C. Levators
   D. Flexors

3. _____ are ringlike muscles that close an opening.
   A. Abductors
   B. Flexors
   C. Sphincters
   D. Rotators

4. The muscles of mastication control the _____.
   A. eyelids
   B. mandible
   C. atlas
   D. vertebrae

5. Which one of the following is *not* an abdominal muscle?
   A. Lateral oblique
   B. External oblique
   C. Internal oblique
   D. Rectus abdominis

6. Stress-induced muscle tension can result in _____ and stiffness in the neck.
   A. sprain
   B. torticollis
   C. hernia
   D. myalgia

7. _____ is caused by a bacterium that enters the body through a deep open wound.
   A. Trichinosis
   B. Tetanus
   C. Torticollis
   D. Myalgia

8. The suffix that means "weakness" is _____.
   A. -trophy
   B. -stenosis
   C. -asthenia
   D. -osis

Copyright © 2010, 2005 by Saunders, an imprint of Elsevier, Inc. All rights reserved.

9. The combining form for "muscle" is _____.
   A. fasci/o
   B. kines
   C. kinesi/o
   D. my/o

10. The abbreviation for nonsteroidal anti-inflammatory drugs is _____.
    A. NSAIDs
    B. NADSs
    C. NSAIFs
    D. none of the above

11. The _____ is the smallest and deepest muscle of the buttocks.
    A. pectoralis minimus
    B. gluteus minimus
    C. adductor muscle
    D. internal oblique

12. The _____ is a fan-shaped muscle over the temporal bone.
    A. orbicularis oris
    B. zygomaticus
    C. masseter
    D. temporalis

13. The large muscle of the posterior neck and shoulder is the _____.
    A. sternocleidomastoid
    B. frontalis
    C. trapezius
    D. external intercostals

14. The point of origin to insertion for the buccinator muscle is _____.
    A. temporal bone to mandible
    B. mandible and maxilla to skin around mouth
    C. cranial aponeurosis to eyebrows
    D. none of the above

15. The muscle that flexes the neck and rotates the head is called the _____.
    A. trapezius
    B. zygomaticus
    C. sternocleidomastoid
    D. internal intercostals

16. The point of origin to insertions for the biceps brachii is _____.
    A. clavicle and scapula to humerus
    B. ilium and lower vertebrae to femur
    C. vertebrae to humerus
    D. scapula to radius

17. The _____ forms muscle mass at the medial side of each thigh.
    A. rotator cuff
    B. gluteus maximus
    C. adductor muscles
    D. latissimus dorsi

18. The _____ dorsiflexes the foot.
    A. sartorius
    B. soleus
    C. iliopsoas
    D. tibialis anterior

19. A group of four muscles that form the fleshy mass of the anterior thigh is called _____.
    A. quadriceps femoris
    B. triceps brachii
    C. biceps femoris
    D. rectus femoris

20. The muscle that originates in the ischial tuberosity and inserts at the proximal tibia is called _____.
    A. sartorius
    B. hamstrings
    C. trapezius
    D. none of the above

21. _____ is a skeletal muscle relaxant.
    A. Mytelase
    B. Vicodin
    C. Flexeril
    D. Lodine

22. The medical term for "muscle pain" is _____.
    A. contusion
    B. myalgia
    C. myosis
    D. none of the above

23. _____ is a progressive weakening and atrophy of muscles.
    A. Myasthenia gravis
    B. Fibromyalgia
    C. Muscular dystrophy
    D. Tetany

24. Muscle _____ is an injury that involves overstretching or tearing of muscle fibers.
    A. strain
    B. sprain
    C. fracture
    D. all of the above

25. Which muscle is known as "swimmer's muscle"?
    A. Achilles tendon
    B. sartorius
    C. gastrocnemius
    D. latissimus dorsi

Copyright © 2010, 2005 by Saunders, an imprint of Elsevier, Inc. All rights reserved.

Sentence Completion

Complete each sentence or statement.

ligaments	tendons	synergists
cardiac	biceps	triceps
skeletal	sarcopenia	diaphragm
orbicularis oris	rotators	
antagonist	sternocleidomastoid	

1. _____ connect muscles to bone.

2. _____ is the skeletal muscle loss experienced by the aging population.

3. The _____ is known as the "praying muscle."

4. The medical term for the "kissing muscle" is _____.

5. _____ move a joint on its axis. The serratus anterior is an example.

6. The subclavius is an example of a(n) _____ muscle.

7. The _____ is the muscle of respiration.

8. The _____ are examples of muscle with three attachments.

9. _____ are muscles that help prime movers by stabilizing the movement.

10. _____ muscle is striated and involuntary.

Short Answers

1. State the three functions of muscles, and explain the importance of each.

   _____
   _____
   _____
   _____
   _____
   _____

2. Explain the basic structure of muscle.

3. Explain how a muscle contracts.

4. List seven ways muscles can be named.

CRITICAL THINKING

1. Mrs. Greenbaum was given a prescription for an anti-inflammatory for muscle pain in her back 6 months ago. Her back is inflamed again, and she would like the prescription refilled, but she cannot remember the name of the medication. What are five anti-inflammatory medications that could have been Mrs. Greenbaum's prescription? (Reference the *Physicians' Desk Reference* as needed.)

2. Timothy injured his ankle playing hockey. The physician ordered a radiograph and determined the ankle was sprained. He applied a figure-eight bandage and provided Timothy with a pair of crutches, instructing him to remain non–weight bearing for 7 days. What other instructions would be given to a patient with a sprained ankle?

CHAPTER 19   Muscular System

PRACTICAL APPLICATIONS

If you have accomplished the objectives in this chapter, you will be able to make better choices as a medical assistant. Take a look at this situation and decide what you would do.

Tommy has been playing sports for many years, since his childhood. He has used weights to increase and strengthen the muscles of his body. Tommy has often wondered just how the muscles of his body work to make him move and what happens when one muscle contracts. He knows that some muscles are involuntary and some are voluntary.

This morning, Tommy was skiing and fell and twisted his ankle. The emergency physician told him that he had strained and sprained his ankle. In explanation, the physician also said that the extensors in the ankle had the greatest injury, and the contusion was going to become worse if Tommy did not keep ice on the ankle overnight. Because of the severity of the injury, Tommy is to see an orthopedist in the morning. The orthopedist ordered anti-inflammatory drugs and muscle relaxants.

Tommy has some questions for the medical assistant about muscles, about what the anti-inflammatory drugs will do, and about what this might have done to his muscles had he been older.

1. How do muscles work to make the body move?

   _____
   _____
   _____

2. What are synergistic muscles?

   _____
   _____
   _____

3. What are antagonistic muscles?

   _____
   _____
   _____

4. What do voluntary muscles do in the body?

   _____
   _____
   _____

5. Define "involuntary muscles."

   _____
   _____
   _____

Copyright © 2010, 2005 by Saunders, an imprint of Elsevier, Inc. All rights reserved.

6. What is the difference between a sprain and a strain?

7. What are the signs of a sprain?

8. Why would anti-inflammatory drugs and muscle relaxants be prescribed?

9. If Tommy were older, what would the physician expect the aging process to have done to his skeletal muscles?

10. What are isotonic and isometric movements?

APPLICATION OF SKILLS

1. Label the word parts of the following terms. Use *P* to indicate a prefix, *CF* to indicate a combining form, *R* to indicate a root, *S* to indicate a suffix. (Example: abnormal—ab *P* norm *R* al *S*)
   A. tenomyoplasty   _____
   B. myelogram   _____
   C. myorrhaphy   _____
   D. rhabdomyoma   _____
   E. electromyography _____

Copyright © 2010, 2005 by Saunders, an imprint of Elsevier, Inc. All rights reserved.

2. Change the following from singular to plural or vice versa.
    A. sarcoma _____
    B. datum _____
    C. deformity _____
    D. analysis _____
    E. basis _____

3. Write out the meaning of each the following abbreviations.
    A. PT _____
    B. OT _____
    C. NSAID _____
    D. EMG _____
    E. DTR _____

4. Label the diagrams.

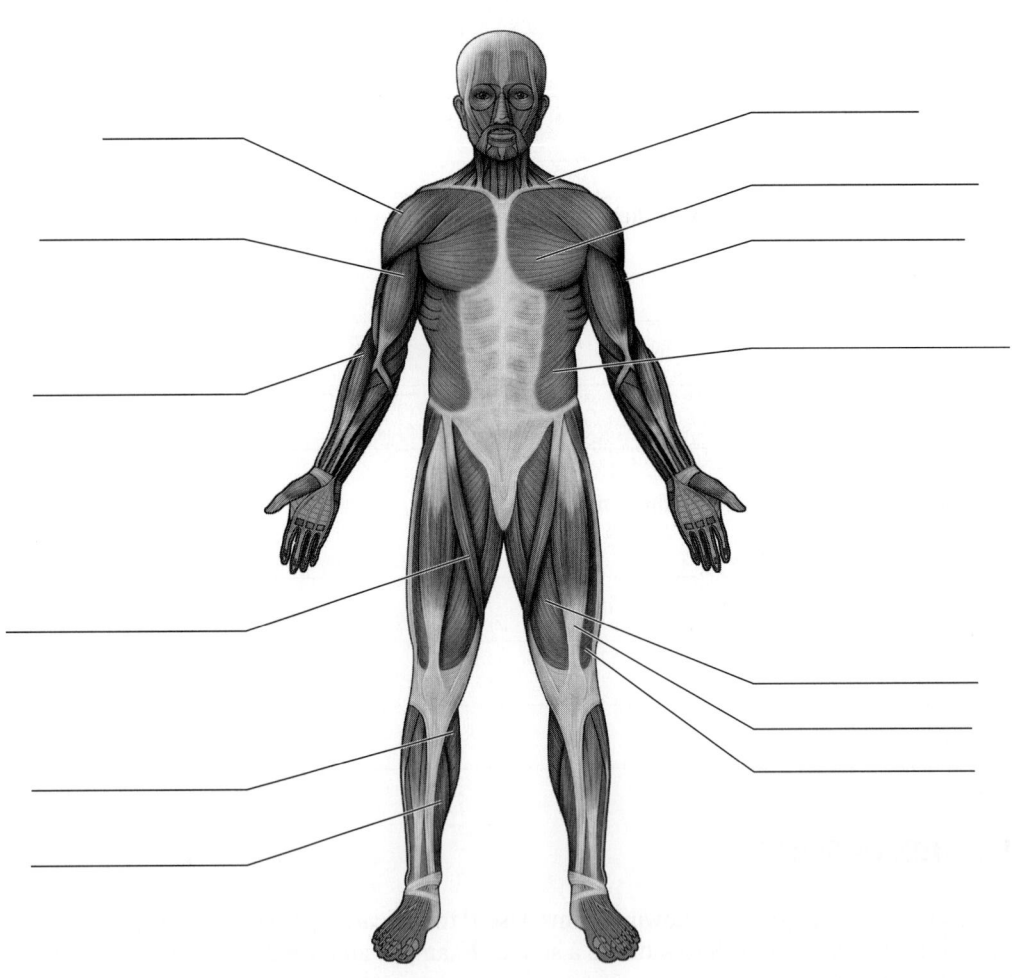

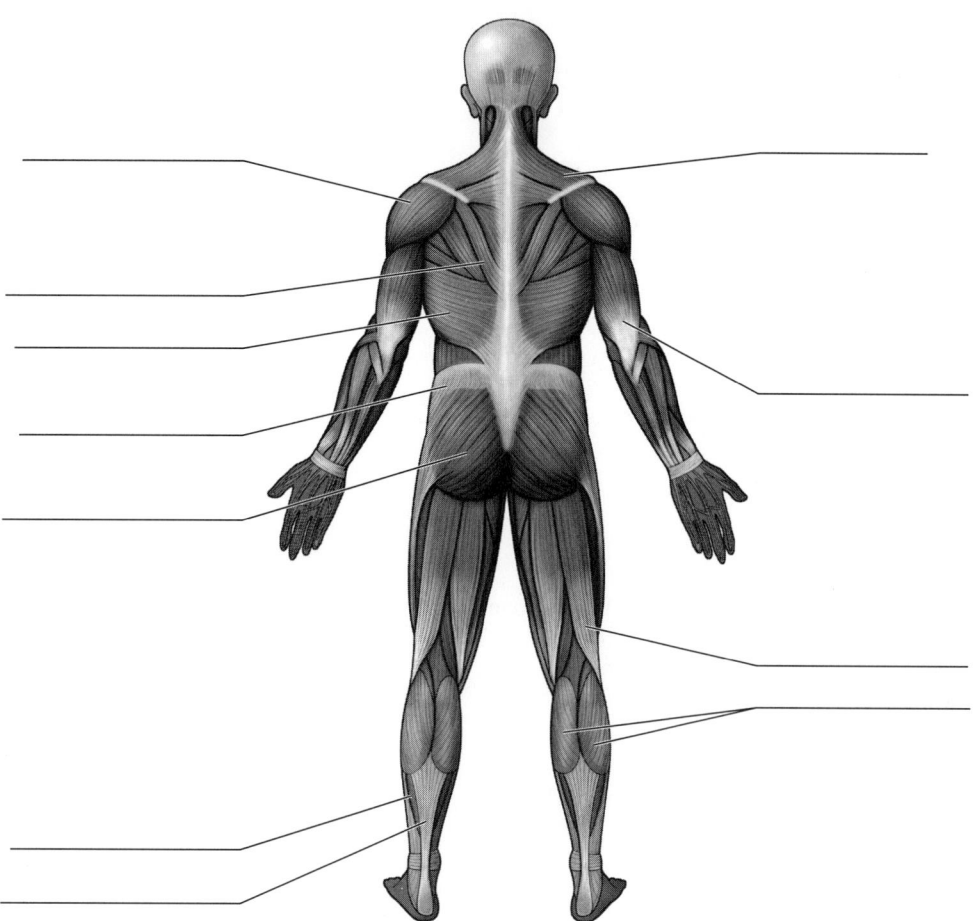

CHAPTER QUIZ

Multiple Choice

Identify the letter of the choice that best completes the statement or answers the question.

1. The enzyme in skeletal muscles that produce energy is _____.
   A. GH
   B. ATP
   C. ADH
   D. PTH

2. The strongest tendon in the body is the _____.
   A. Achilles tendon
   B. aponeurosis
   C. hamstrings
   D. none of the above

3. The medical term for "lacking muscle tone" is _____.
   A. atonic
   B. rigidity
   C. dystonic
   D. flaccid

Copyright © 2010, 2005 by Saunders, an imprint of Elsevier, Inc. All rights reserved.

4. Muscles that lower a bone are called _____.
   A. flexors
   B. depressors
   C. extensors
   D. fixators

5. Muscles that move a joint on its axis are called _____.
   A. extensors
   B. adductors
   C. rotators
   D. sphincters

6. The muscle of the shoulder shaped like an upside-down Greek letter "D" is _____.
   A. biceps
   B. iliopsoas
   C. deltoid
   D. pectoralis major

7. The wasting away of muscles caused by nonuse over long periods is called _____.
   A. atrophy
   B. dystrophy
   C. dystonic
   D. atonus

8. The medical term for "muscle and tendon inflammation" is _____.
   A. myalgia
   B. myosis
   C. atrophy
   D. fibromyositis

9. Overstretching or tearing a ligament or joint is called _____.
   A. strain
   B. sprain
   C. myalgia
   D. dystrophy

10. The medical term for "wryneck" is _____.
    A. spasms
    B. cramps
    C. torticollis
    D. hernia

11. The _____ is a muscle located in the groin.
    A. latissimus dorsi
    B. quadriceps femoris
    C. semitendinosus
    D. iliopsoas

12. The _____ forms the curved calf of the leg.
    A. trapezius
    B. gastrocnemius
    C. buccinator
    D. masseter

13. The muscle that originates in the zygomatic arch and inserts to the mandible is the _____.
    A. frontalis
    B. sternocleidomastoid
    C. masseter
    D. orbicularis oculi

14. The muscle that closes the jaw is the _____.
    A. external intercostals
    B. temporalis
    C. zygomaticus
    D. frontalis

15. Muscle _____ cause involuntary muscle twitches.
    A. spasms
    B. cramps
    C. isotonic contractions
    D. none of the above

16. _____ is the procedure that records the electrical activity of muscles.
    A. EEG
    B. ECG
    C. EMG
    D. MRI

17. Skeletal muscles are described best by which of the following?
    A. Striated and involuntary
    B. Smooth and involuntary
    C. Striated and voluntary
    D. Smooth and voluntary

18. _____ is the ability of a muscle to shorten and thicken when given proper stimulation.
    A. Irritability
    B. Contractility
    C. Elasticity
    D. Extensibility

19. _____ are specialized synergists that stabilize the origin of a prime mover.
    A. Rotators
    B. Extensors
    C. Levators
    D. Fixators

20. Triceps brachii are an example of _____ muscles.
    A. abductor
    B. levator
    C. extensor
    D. depressor

20 Urinary System

VOCABULARY REVIEW

Matching: Match each term with the correct definition.

A. erythropoietin

B. uremia

C. antidiuretic hormone

D. filtration

E. kidney

F. nephron

G. retroperitoneal

H. urine

I. ureters

J. micturition

K. urinary bladder

L. urethral meatus

M. urethra

N. albuminuria

O. bacteriuria

P. incontinence

Q. blood urea nitrogen (BUN)

R. cystoscopy

S. intravenous pyelography

_____ 1. Inability to retain urine or feces

_____ 2. Hollow muscular sac that holds urine before it is excreted from the body

_____ 3. Process where substances are filtered out

_____ 4. Occurs when toxins accumulate in the blood

_____ 5. Progressive loss of nephrons, resulting in loss of renal function

_____ 6. Urethral opening to the outside of the body

_____ 7. Main functioning unit of the kidney

_____ 8. Measures the amount of nitrogenous waste in the circulatory system

_____ 9. Artificial kidney machine filters the patient's blood and returns the filtered blood back to the patient

_____ 10. Hormone responsible for reducing urine production

_____ 11. Bacteria in urine

_____ 12. Main organ of the urinary system

_____ 13. Medication that causes increased urine excretion

_____ 14. Hormone responsible for red blood cell production

_____ 15. Transports urine from the bladder to the outside of the body

T. KUB (kidney, ureters, and bladder)

U. urinalysis

V. acute renal failure (ARF)

W. dialysis

X. diuretics

Y. hemodialysis

Z. renal failure

_____ 16. Visual examination of the urinary bladder using a cystoscope

_____ 17. Located behind the peritoneum

_____ 18. Pair of muscular tubes that carry urine from the kidneys to the bladders

_____ 19. Renal failure occurring suddenly because of trauma

_____ 20. Presence of large amounts of protein in urine; usually a sign of renal disease or heart failure

_____ 21. Process used to clean the blood of toxins

_____ 22. Imaging of the kidneys, ureters, and bladder without a contrast medium

_____ 23. Liquid and dissolved substances excreted by the kidneys

_____ 24. Physical, chemical, or microscopic examination of the urine

_____ 25. Urination

_____ 26. Imaging of the kidneys, ureters, and bladder with a contrast medium

THEORY RECALL

True/False

Indicate whether the statement is true or false.

_____ 1. Reabsorption retains essential elements the body needs to maintain pH and homeostasis.

_____ 2. The ureters extend from the bladder to the outside of the body.

_____ 3. The adrenal glands release the hormone aldosterone.

_____ 4. The cortex is the inner layer of the kidney.

_____ 5. The glomerulus is a group of capillaries responsible for filtering the blood.

Multiple Choice

Identify the letter of the choice that best completes the statement or answers the question.

1. The hormone responsible for blood pressure control is called _____.
   A. azotemia
   B. erythropoietin
   C. renin
   D. ADH

2. Cuplike edges of the renal pelvis that collect urine are called _____.
   A. Bowman's capsule
   B. calyces
   C. nephrons
   D. rugae

3. _____ is the backflow of urine from the bladder up into the ureters.
   A. Urinary reflux
   B. Micturition reflex
   C. Urination
   D. Filtration

4. _____ is a condition of having no urine production or output.
   A. Micturition
   B. Enuresis
   C. Anuresis
   D. Dysuria

5. _____ is the medical term for "excessive urination at night."
   A. Oliguria
   B. Polydipsia
   C. Ketonuria
   D. Nocturia

6. _____ occurs when a donor kidney is surgically placed in patients to function as their own.
   A. Incontinence
   B. Kidney transplant
   C. Peritoneal dialysis
   D. Hemodialysis

7. The combining form for "bladder" is _____.
   A. ureter/o
   B. olig/o
   C. glomerul/o
   D. cyst/o

8. _____ are used as a genitourinary muscle relaxant.
   A. Diuretics
   B. Antispasmodics
   C. Analgesics
   D. Antihypertensives

9. _____ is a diuretic that increases urination.
   A. Lasix
   B. Macrobid
   C. Gantrisin
   D. Pyridium

10. In the process of urine formation, _____ is the step where wastes are eliminated into the collection duct in the form of urine.
    A. filtration
    B. reabsorption
    C. secretion of toxins
    D. excretion

11. _____ is increased urine production.
    A. Anuresis
    B. Dysuria
    C. Diuresis
    D. Oliguria

12. _____ is the medical term for "pus in the urine."
    A. Dysuria
    B. Pyuria
    C. Enuresis
    D. Polyuria

13. _____ is an abnormal presence of glucose in the urine.
    A. Albuminuria
    B. Oliguria
    C. Anuresis
    D. Glycosuria

14. Which of the following laboratory tests measures the amount of nitrogenous waste in the circulatory system?
    A. BUN
    B. KUB
    C. UA
    D. IVP

15. A(n) _____ is an imaging study of the kidneys, ureters, and bladder with contrast media.
    A. KUB
    B. IVP
    C. BUN
    D. UA

16. The normal value for specific gravity of urine is which one of the following?
    A. 0.10 to 0.12
    B. 0.00 to 0.10
    C. 1.10 to 1.25
    D. 0.05 to 1.10

17. The medical term for "kidney stones" is _____.
    A. cholelithiasis
    B. cystolithiasis
    C. pelvic calculi
    D. renal calculi

Copyright © 2010, 2005 by Saunders, an imprint of Elsevier, Inc. All rights reserved.

18. Inflammation of the renal pelvis to include the connective tissue of the kidneys is called _____.
    A. glomerulonephritis
    B. pyelonephritis
    C. renalonephritis
    D. cystonephritis

19. _____ is an analgesic that produces an anesthetic effect on the lining of the urinary tract.
    A. Pyridium
    B. Lasix
    C. Macrobid
    D. Gantrisin

20. The combining form for "urea; nitrogen" is _____.
    A. vesic/o
    B. ure/o
    C. azot/o
    D. none of the above

21. Which one of the following is *not* a function of the kidneys?
    A. Filtration
    B. Reabsorption
    C. Excretion
    D. To produce leukocytes and secrete nitrites

22. Your blood passes through your kidneys approximately _____ times a day.
    A. 100
    B. 200
    C. 300
    D. 400

23. Because of the _____ in urine, some people tend to form kidney stones.
    A. solutes
    B. crystals
    C. leukocytes
    D. water

24. The part of the collection system where sodium is mainly reabsorbed is the _____.
    A. Bowman's capsule
    B. loop of Henle
    C. calyces
    D. distal convoluted tubule

25. Each kidney consists of approximately _____ nephrons.
    A. 1 million
    B. 100,000
    C. 3 million
    D. 300,000

Sentence Completion

Complete each sentence or statement.

Bowman's capsule	retroperitoneally (1½	ureters
nephrons	to 2 inches)	medulla
hilum	glomerulonephritis	renal artery
loop of Henle	lithotripsy	pyramids
peritoneal dialysis	urethral meatus	

1. The C-shaped structure that surrounds the glomerulus is the called the _____.

2. _____ can be performed with minimal equipment and in the patient's home. The procedure takes approximately 30 minutes and is done four times a day, 7 days a week.

3. _____ is an inflammation of the glomeruli.

4. _____ can be performed to remove calculi.

5. Blood enters the kidney through the _____.

6. _____ force urine into the bladder with the movements of their muscular walls.

7. The two kidneys are located _____ in the lumbar area of the spine.

8. The _____ is the urethral opening to the outside of the body.

9. The depression on the medial side of each kidney where the blood vessels, ureters, and nerves enter and exit the kidney is called the _____.

10. The main functioning units of the kidney are the _____.

Short Answers

1. State the five major functions of the urinary system.

2. Explain the purpose of urine, and describe urine formation.

3. Common signs and symptoms of urinary system disorders are:

4. Explain the purpose of dialysis and list two types.

5. What would happen if there were no loop of Henle in the nephron?

CRITICAL THINKING

1. Samuel, a 27-year-old male patient, is complaining that it is painful to urinate, that he has to "go" all the time, and he cannot seem to control it; even during the night, he wakes up to go to the bathroom three or four times a night. He also has pain directly above the pubic bone. The physician orders a complete UA, and a culture and sensitivity. You have the patient collect a urine sample and take it to the laboratory to perform the UA. Samuel's urine is cloudy, and on dipstick examination, you find the leukocytes and nitrites are increased. The microscopic examination confirmed the increase.

    A. What do you think the physician's diagnosis will be?

    _____
    _____

    B. What is the medical term for "having to go all the time, painful urination, and excessive urination at night"?

    _____
    _____

    C. What will be the most likely course of therapy?

    _____
    _____

    D. What should you, as the medical assistant, encourage the patient to do?

    _____
    _____

2. Obtain brochures from the kidney center or dialysis center in your area. (You may research on the Internet or the school's resource library if a center is unavailable in your area.) Determine the services provided by the center, hours of operation, and location. This information will be beneficial when you are required to provide patients with the same or similar information.

PRACTICAL APPLICATIONS

If you have accomplished the objectives in this chapter, you will be able to make better choices as a medical assistant. Take a look at this situation and decide what you would do.

Juanita is a regular patient in the medical office and has been in good health most of her life. At her office visit, she is complaining of pain in the flanks, in her thighs, in her lower abdomen, and in her back under her ribs. She also says that she has had burning and frequency of urination that has become progressively worse for about 2 weeks. She says when she has to go to the bathroom, she has to hurry or she will not make it. The burning is not on the perineum, but occurs as she starts the flow of urine. These symptoms have only made her incontinence worse, and she now has nocturia. When asked if she can pinpoint anything new in her routine hygiene, she states that she has recently been using a perfumed soap on a regular basis to take her bath. On obtaining a urinalysis, hematuria is present. In addition, white blood cells are found on microscopic examination. The physician has prescribed medications for treating what he has diagnosed as urinary cystitis. Juanita would like to talk to the medical assistant to ask some questions.

Copyright © 2010, 2005 by Saunders, an imprint of Elsevier, Inc. All rights reserved.

CHAPTER 20 Urinary System

1. Why do women have inflammation of the urinary tract more often than men?

2. What is hematuria? What is pyuria?

3. Would you expect Juanita to have pyuria because she has hematuria?

4. What is incontinence?

5. What is the difference between incontinence and enuresis?

6. What is the name of the symptom that is used to describe feeling the need to urinate immediately?

7. Why are urinary antiseptics used in treating urinary cystitis after anti-infective drugs have been prescribed?

8. What is urinary frequency?

_____

_____

9. What is nocturia?

_____

_____

APPLICATION OF SKILLS

1. Label the word parts of the following terms. Use *P* to indicate a prefix, *CF* to indicate a combining form, *R* to indicate a root, *S* to indicate a suffix. (Example: abnormal—ab *P* norm *R* al *S*)
   A. antidiuretic _____
   B. nephrosclerosis _____
   C. renal _____
   D. urinalysis _____
   E. urologist _____

2. Change the following from singular to plural or vice versa.
   A. glomerulus _____
   B. calyx _____
   C. calculus _____
   D. nephrosis _____
   E. urinalysis _____

3. Write out the meaning of each the following abbreviations.
   A. ADH _____
   B. BUN _____
   C. C & S _____
   D. IVP _____
   E. UTI _____

4. Label the diagrams.

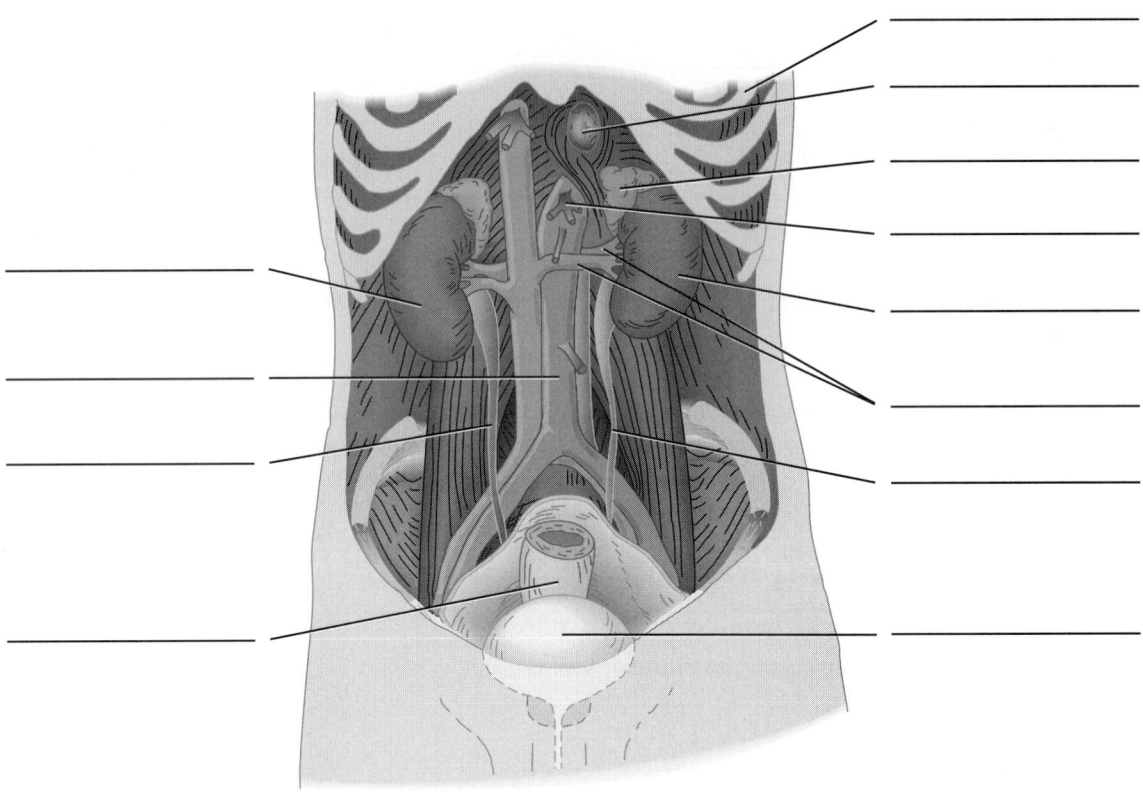

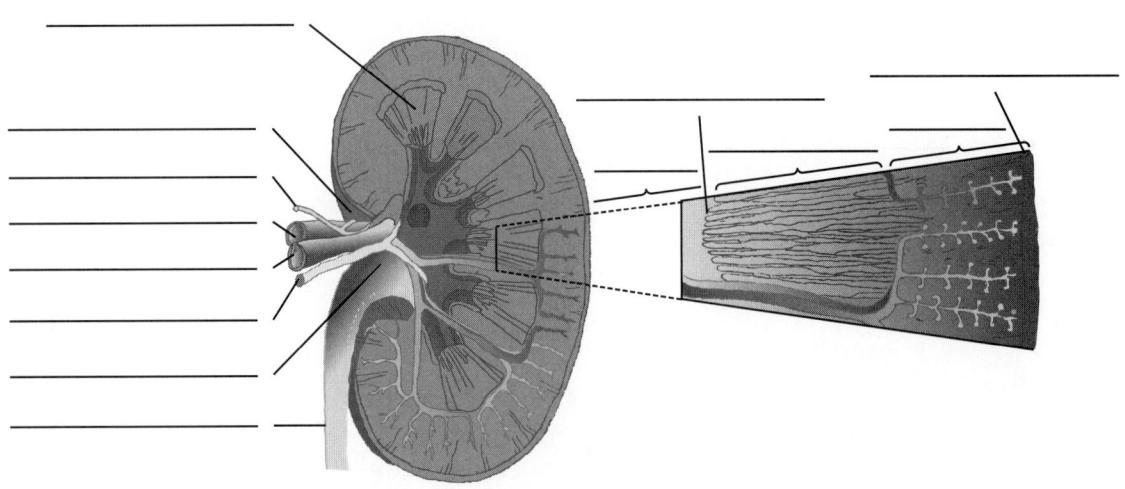

Urinary System **CHAPTER** 20 247

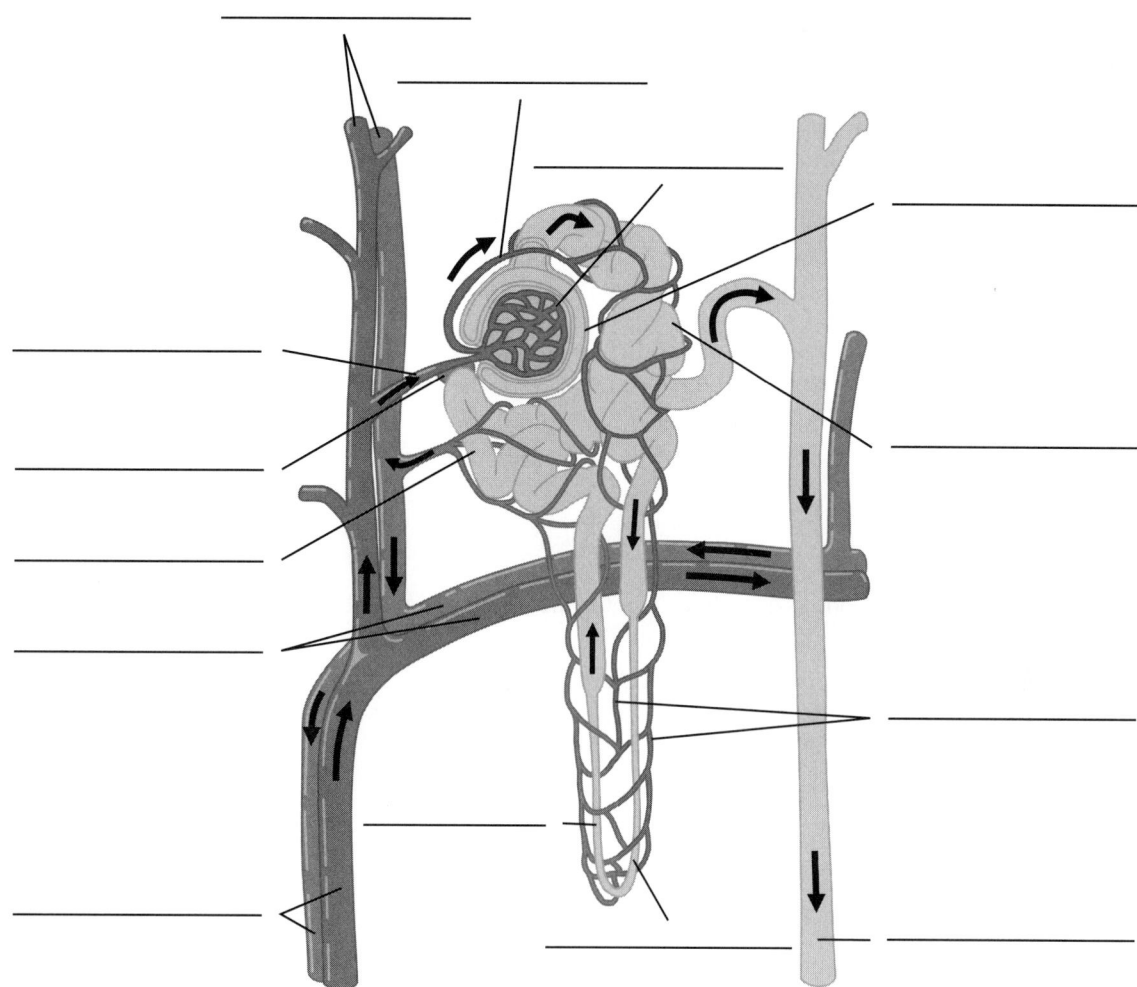

CHAPTER QUIZ

Multiple Choice

Identify the letter of the choice that best completes the statement or answers the question.

1. The medical term for "kidney stones" is _____.
   A. peritoneal calculi
   B. cystolithiasis
   C. renal calculi
   D. renolithiasis

2. The main functioning units of the kidneys are _____.
   A. ureters
   B. Bowman's capsules
   C. pyramids
   D. none of the above

Copyright © 2010, 2005 by Saunders, an imprint of Elsevier, Inc. All rights reserved.

3. The outer layer of the kidneys is called the _____.
   A. pyramid
   B. cortex
   C. medulla
   D. calyces

4. _____ is the hormone responsible for increased sodium reabsorption.
   A. Erythropoietin
   B. Aldosterone
   C. Antidiuretic hormone
   D. Renin

5. _____ occurs when toxins accumulate in the blood.
   A. Erythropoietin
   B. Bacteriuria
   C. Uremia
   D. Anuresis

6. The depression where blood vessels, nerves, and the ureters enter and exit the kidney is called the _____.
   A. hilum
   B. loop of Henle
   C. Bowman's capsule
   D. medulla

7. _____ are muscular folds that allow the bladder to expand.
   A. Calyces
   B. Rugae
   C. Pyramids
   D. Trigone

8. The _____ transports urine from the bladder to the outside of the body.
   A. ureters
   B. nephrons
   C. urethra
   D. glomeruli

9. _____ is painful or difficult urination.
   A. Anuresis
   B. Oliguria
   C. Enuresis
   D. Dysuria

10. An increase in the number of times urination occurs over a short time is called _____.
    A. urgency
    B. frequency
    C. immediacy
    D. none of the above

11. _____ are medications that increase urine excretion.
    A. Antispasmodics
    B. Analgesics
    C. Diuretics
    D. Pyuretics

12. _____ is the progressive loss of nephrons, resulting in loss of renal function.
    A. Renal failure
    B. Glomerulonephritis
    C. Cystitis
    D. Hematuria

13. The normal pH of urine is _____.
    A. 4.5
    B. 5.0
    C. 6.5
    D. 7.0

14. The main function of the kidneys is to filter _____ and other waste products from the blood.
    A. sodium
    B. urea
    C. glucose
    D. nutrients

15. The average daily production of urine is _____.
    A. 1 to 1.5 L
    B. 1.5 to 2.5 L
    C. 2 to 3 L
    D. none of the above

16. _____ is an enzyme that reacts with a blood protein to form a substance that stimulates the adrenal gland to secrete aldosterone.
    A. Lipase
    B. Glucose
    C. Vitamin C
    D. Renin

17. The _____ narrow(s) to form the ureters, which empties into the bladder.
    A. renal pelvis
    B. hilum
    C. medulla
    D. pyramids

18. When urine flows from the bladder back into the ureters, this is known as urinary _____.
    A. regurgitation
    B. incontinence
    C. micturition
    D. reflux

19. A(n) _____ treats diseases and disorders of the urinary system.
    A. gynecologist
    B. endocrinologist
    C. urologist
    D. bacteriologist

20. Inflammation of the renal pelvis including the connective tissue of the kidneys is called _____.
    A. pyelonephritis
    B. cystonephritis
    C. glomerulonephritis
    D. renalonephritis

Copyright © 2010, 2005 by Saunders, an imprint of Elsevier, Inc. All rights reserved.

21 Reproductive System

VOCABULARY REVIEW

Matching: Match each term with the correct definition.

A. gametes

B. gonads

C. circumcision

D. insemination

E. prostate gland

F. spermatozoa

G. testosterone

H. areola

I. endometrium

J. estrogen

K. infertility

L. lactiferous ducts

M. mammary glands

N. perimetrium

O. follicle-stimulating hormone

P. human chorionic gonadotropin

Q. mammogram

R. menses

_____ 1. Stage from the second week to the eighth week of gestation

_____ 2. Sperm cells

_____ 3. Radiographs of the breast

_____ 4. Reproductive cells; eggs and sperm

_____ 5. Process of expulsion of the fetus; childbirth

_____ 6. Gland that produces an alkaline fluid that neutralizes the acidity of the urethra and of the vaginal secretions

_____ 7. Joining of the egg and the sperm

_____ 8. Surgical removal of the prepuce

_____ 9. Hormone responsible for male sex characteristics

_____ 10. Surrounds the nipple; dark-colored skin

_____ 11. Cells scraped off the cervix are examined under a microscope for malignancy

_____ 12. Before birth

_____ 13. Inability to become pregnant

_____ 14. Monthly bloody discharge from the lining of the uterus

_____ 15. Sex glands; ovaries and testes

_____ 16. Toxic condition in pregnancy that produces high blood pressure and decreased kidney function

S. Papanicolaou (Pap) smear

T. embryo

U. fertilization

V. parturition

W. prenatal

X. zygote

Y. gestational diabetes

Z. toxemia

_____ 17. Introduction of semen into the female

_____ 18. Hormone produced during pregnancy; responsible for the release of progesterone and estrogen to maintain the endometrium

_____ 19. Serous layer of the uterus

_____ 20. Fertilized egg; contains all the genetic material

_____ 21. Hormone that causes the egg to ripen in the graafian follicle

_____ 22. Ducts that transport milk to each nipple

_____ 23. Inner lining of the uterus; holds the fertilized egg; vascular layer

_____ 24. Glands located within the breasts that are responsible for producing milk

_____ 25. Occurs when a pregnant woman is unable to metabolize carbohydrates; develops during the latter part of pregnancy and usually terminates with delivery

_____ 26. Hormone that prepares the uterus for the implantation of the fertilized egg and promotes female sex characteristics

THEORY RECALL

True/False

Indicate whether the statement is true or false.

_____ 1. The two main functions of the reproductive system are to produce offspring and to produce hormones.

_____ 2. Sperm mature and are stored in the epididymis.

_____ 3. Infertility is the inability to have or sustain an erection during sexual intercourse.

_____ 4. Progesterone is responsible for the development of primary and secondary sex characteristics in females.

_____ 5. A typical menstrual cycle lasts 28 days.

Multiple Choice

Identify the letter of the choice that best completes the statement or answers the question.

1. A gland that produces a fluid that acts as a lubricant is called _____.
   A. Cowper's gland
   B. epididymis
   C. glans penis
   D. graafian follicle

2. The _____ is a thick muscular layer of the uterus.
   A. endometrium
   B. myometrium
   C. perimetrium
   D. none of the above

3. The _____ is(are) where sperm are formed within the testes.
   A. prostate gland
   B. vas deferens
   C. epididymis
   D. seminiferous tubules

4. The male gonads are called (the) _____.
   A. penis
   B. scrotum
   C. spermatozoa
   D. testes

5. The female gonads are called (the) _____.
   A. uterus
   B. ovaries
   C. fallopian tubes
   D. graafian follicles

6. The area between the vagina and the anus is called the _____.
   A. cervix
   B. perimetrium
   C. perineum
   D. areola

7. A combination of physical and emotional symptoms that appear before the start of the menstrual flow and stop with its onset is _____.
   A. menopause
   B. menses
   C. toxic shock syndrome
   D. premenstrual syndrome

8. _____ is a hormone that allows for milk expulsion and the onset of labor.
   A. Oxytocin
   B. Progesterone
   C. Prolactin
   D. Testosterone

9. The muscular area located between the cervix and the vulva is called the _____.
   A. perineum
   B. vagina
   C. uterus
   D. fallopian tube

10. The _____ is a tube leading from the bladder through the penis by which semen is ejaculated.
    A. seminal vesicles
    B. seminiferous tubules
    C. ureter
    D. urethra

11. The organ that provides nourishment and oxygen to the fetus during pregnancy is called the _____.
    A. uterus
    B. placenta
    C. umbilical cord
    D. cervix

12. Sperm are produced at a rate of _____ per day.
    A. 100,000
    B. 500,000
    C. 300 million
    D. 500 million

13. Primary sex characteristics in a male include all of the following *except* _____.
    A. growth of pubic, facial, and underarm hair
    B. growth of the penis and scrotum
    C. growth and activity of internal reproductive structures
    D. all of the above are primary sex characteristics

14. The _____ produce(s) a mucus-like fluid that provides nutrition and energy for the mobile sperm. This fluid accounts for 60% of the semen volume.
    A. epididymis
    B. seminiferous tubules
    C. seminal vesicles
    D. vas deferens

15. A human gestation period is usually _____ from the time of fertilization.
    A. 266 days
    B. 40 weeks
    C. three trimesters
    D. all of the above

16. An Apgar score of less than _____ indicates a newborn needs medical attention.
    A. 2
    B. 5
    C. 7
    D. 9

17. Proscar is an example of a(n) _____.
    A. BPH medication
    B. contraceptive
    C. ovulation stimulant
    D. treatment for menopause

Copyright © 2010, 2005 by Saunders, an imprint of Elsevier, Inc. All rights reserved.

18. The name of the blood test for prostatic hypertrophy is _____.
    A. VDRL
    B. PSA
    C. FTA
    D. ABS

19. A painless lump in the testicle may indicate _____.
    A. prostatitis
    B. prostatic cancer
    C. testicular cancer
    D. epididymis

20. Which one of the following conditions can be caused by a bacterial infection?
    A. Benign prostatic hyperplasia
    B. Testicular cancer
    C. Endometriosis
    D. None of the above

21. _____ is an imaging procedure that uses contrast media to visualize the uterus and fallopian tubes.
    A. Hysterosalpingography
    B. Mammography
    C. Colposcopy
    D. Cervicography

22. An imaging procedure using high-frequency sound waves to view the pelvic area is _____.
    A. colposcopy
    B. ultrasonography
    C. mammography
    D. cervicography

23. _____ is the displacement of the uterus into the vagina.
    A. Candidiasis
    B. Fibrocystic disease of the uterus
    C. Prolapsed uterus
    D. Toxic shock syndrome

24. _____ is(are) fluid-filled sacs that form on or near the ovaries.
    A. Ovarian cysts
    B. Endometriosis
    C. Fibroids
    D. None of the above

25. _____ is the premature partial or complete separation of the placenta from the uterine wall.
    A. Toxemia
    B. Ectopic pregnancy
    C. Placenta previa
    D. Placenta abruption

Sentence Completion

Complete each sentence or statement.

epididymitis	cryptorchidism	lactiferous ducts
chlamydia	graafian follicle	Apgar score
foreskin (prepuce)	uterus	gonorrhea
cervix	seventh	ectopic pregnancy
fifth	sixth	

1. _____ occurs when one or both testes do not descend and remain in the abdomen.

2. Circumcision is a procedure that removes the fold of skin at the end of the penis called the _____.

3. At ovulation, the egg is expelled from the _____ and is swept into the fallopian tube.

4. The _____ is known as the neck of the uterus.

5. _____ transport milk to the nipple.

6. The embryo reaches the uterus around the _____ day.

7. Movement of the fetus occurs around the _____ month.

8. One minute after birth, a newborn is evaluated using a system called a(n) _____.

9. _____ occurs when the fertilized egg implants outside the uterus, usually in the fallopian tubes.

10. _____ is a sexually transmitted disease with symptoms that include purulent vaginal discharge, genital pain, and dysuria.

CHAPTER 21 Reproductive System

Short Answers

1. Trace the pathway that sperm follow through the five major structures of the male reproductive system, beginning with the testes and ending with the urethra.

2. Explain the purpose of semen.

3. List, identify, and describe the seven parts of the female reproductive system.

4. Explain the menstrual cycle including the key stages.

CRITICAL THINKING

1. A newborn at 1 minute after birth presents with a heart rate less than 100 beats/min, respiratory rate that is slow and irregular, muscle tone that is limp, reflex of grimace, and pale in color. What is the infant's Apgar score? At 3 minutes, the heart rate was greater than 100 beats/min, the respiratory rate was slow and irregular, muscle tone showed reflex of extremities, reflex withdrew foot, and torso was pink but extremities were blue. What is the infant's 3-minute score?

2. Kelly is a 22-year-old female patient. Kelly started menstruation at age 14 and has been sexually active for the past 3 years. She is being seen today with a chief complaint of vaginal itching. On examination, the physician detects a foul-smelling, green frothy discharge, and after receiving laboratory test results, he diagnoses the condition as trichomoniasis and prescribes an antibiotic. The physician asks you to talk with Kelly about her sexual partners because this condition requires that all sexual partners be treated with an antibiotic. Left untreated, this condition can lead to sterility. The physician also asks you to discuss safe sex practices and contraception with Kelly. Use your text, your institution's resource reference library, and the Internet to address this issue as needed.

PRACTICAL APPLICATIONS

If you have accomplished the objectives in this chapter, you will be able to make better choices as a medical assistant. Take a look at this situation and decide what you would do.

Valerie has called her gynecologist for her annual Pap smear. The receptionist wanted to be sure that Valerie did not make her appointment during the time of her menses. Her menarche was at age 14. She has taken oral contraceptives in the past. She is now approaching age 50 and has excessive bleeding with each menstrual period. Her LMP was 1 week ago, and she is to have the Pap smear with her physical examination today. The medical assistant asks Valerie if she performs monthly BSEs. Dr. Jones started ordering a mammogram for Valerie on a yearly basis at age 35 because of a family history of fibrocystic disease of the breasts. Valerie asks Dr. Jones about taking HRT because she seems to be approaching menopause and has PMS with each menstrual period. Dr. Jones replies that she will discuss this with Valerie after the Pap smear report has been returned. Do you understand why the various aspects of Valerie's appointment were handled the way they were?

1. Why is it important that Valerie not make her appointment for her Pap smear during the time of menses?

___

___

___

2. What are the five stages of the menstrual cycle?

___

___

___

___

3. What is menarche? Are menstrual periods regular immediately after menarche?

4. What is HRT? What classifications of medications are given for HRT? What classifications of medications are given for oral contraception?

5. What is a BSE, and why is this important to be done approximately 1 week after menses?

6. What is fibrocystic disease of the breast? Why are mammograms and BSEs important for someone with this condition?

7. What is PMS?

8. What are the signs of menopause?

APPLICATION OF SKILLS

1. Label the word parts of the following terms. Use *P* to indicate a prefix, *CF* to indicate a combining form, *R* to indicate a root, *S* to indicate a suffix. (Example: abnormal—ab *P* norm *R* al *S*)
   A. spermatogenesis _____
   B. varicocele _____
   C. oligospermia _____
   D. antenatal _____
   E. dysmenorrhea _____

2. Change the following from singular to plural or vice versa.
   A. testis _____
   B. epididymis _____
   C. spermatozoon _____
   D. cervix _____
   E. areola _____

3. Write out the meaning of each the following abbreviations.
   A. GU _____
   B. TUR _____
   C. BCP _____
   D. D&C _____
   E. LMP _____

4. Label the diagrams.

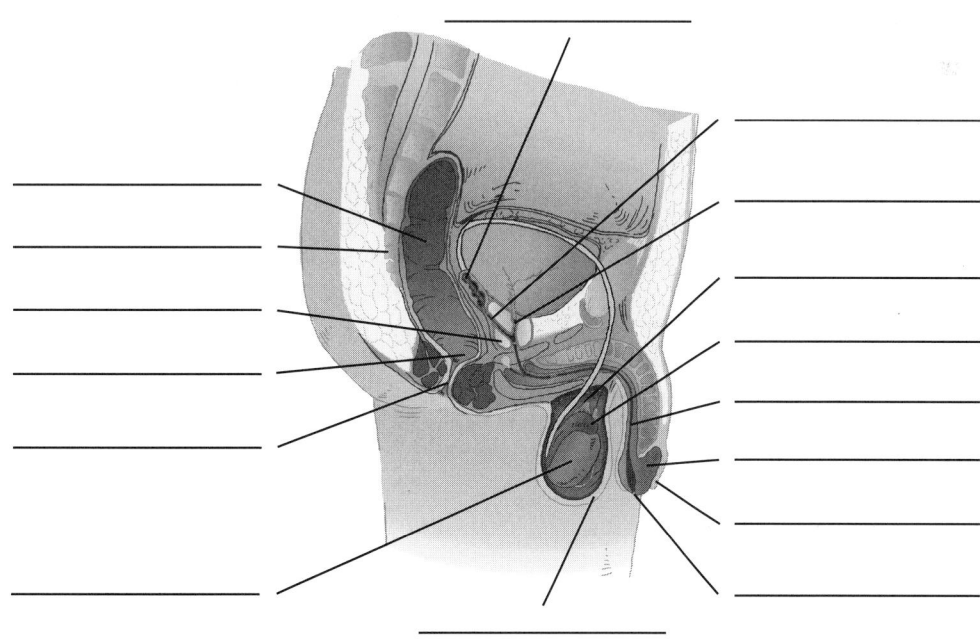

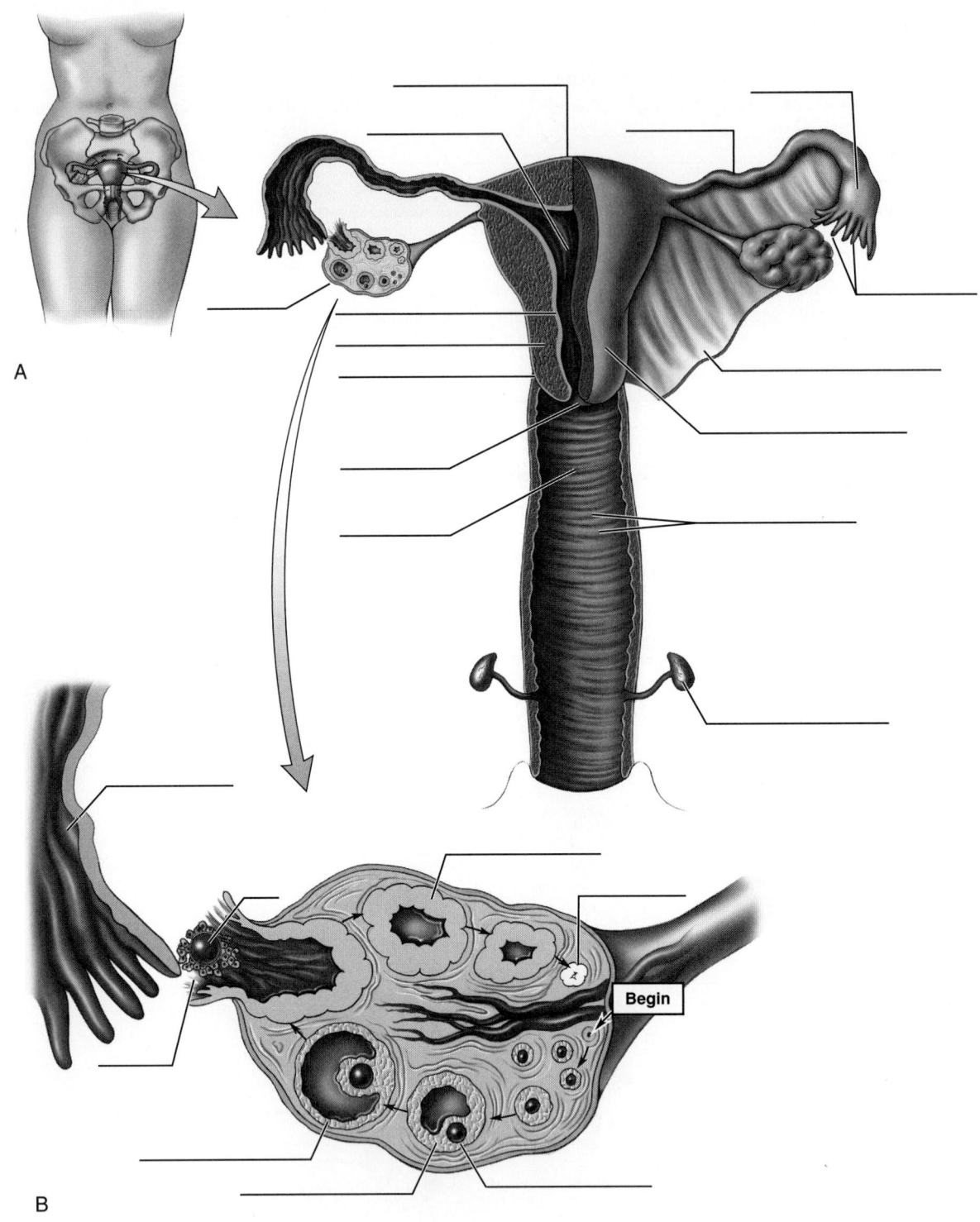

CHAPTER QUIZ

Multiple Choice

Identify the letter of the choice that best completes the statement or answers the question.

1. _____ are reproductive cells—eggs and sperm.
    A. Ovaries
    B. Testes
    C. Gonads
    D. Gametes

2. The _____ is where seminal vesicles and the vas deferens come together.
    A. seminiferous tubules
    B. bulbourethral gland
    C. ejaculatory duct
    D. urethra

3. The _____ is the organ that receives the egg.
    A. vagina
    B. uterus
    C. fallopian tube
    D. graafian follicle

4. _____ is the hormone that prepares the uterus for the implantation of the fertilized egg and promotes female sex characteristics.
    A. Estrogen
    B. Testosterone
    C. Progesterone
    D. Oxytocin

5. The _____ connect(s) the ovaries to the uterus.
    A. ureters
    B. fallopian tubes
    C. graafian follicles
    D. perineum

6. _____ occurs when the attachment of the placenta implants in the lower portion of the uterus and partially or completely covers the cervix.
    A. Ectopic pregnancy
    B. Placenta abruptio
    C. Placenta previa
    D. Endometriosis

7. The serous layer of the uterus is called the _____.
    A. perimetrium
    B. endometrium
    C. myometrium
    D. osometrium

8. _____ is a fungal yeast infection of the vagina.
   A. Trichomoniasis
   B. Syphilis
   C. Human papilloma virus
   D. Candidiasis

9. The muscular area located between the cervix and the vulva is called the _____.
   A. labia majora
   B. vagina
   C. uterus
   D. perineum

10. _____ is the medical term for "undescended or hidden testes."
    A. Epididymis
    B. Prostatitis
    C. Cryptorchidism
    D. None of the above

11. The hormone responsible for the stimulation of milk production is _____.
    A. estrogen
    B. oxytocin
    C. progesterone
    D. prolactin

12. _____ is the cessation of the menstrual cycle.
    A. Menarche
    B. Menses
    C. Menstruation
    D. Menopause

13. The hormone that increases during pregnancy and provides for pregnancy test results is _____.
    A. estrogen
    B. human chorionic gonadotropin
    C. testosterone
    D. prolactin

14. The _____ releases progesterone and estrogen to thicken the uterine wall for pregnancy.
    A. corpus luteum
    B. luteinizing hormone
    C. graafian follicle
    D. human chorionic gonadotropin

15. The _____ is where sperm is stored.
    A. vas deferens
    B. seminal vesicles
    C. scrotum
    D. epididymis

16. Gestation including the beginning day of the LMP is _____.
    A. 266 days
    B. 280 days
    C. 324 days
    D. none of the above

17. When fertilization occurs, the fusion of the sperm and egg forms a(n) _____.
    A. zygote
    B. fetus
    C. embryo
    D. infant

18. During parturition, crowning occurs and the fetus is expelled in the _____ stage.
    A. first
    B. second
    C. third
    D. fourth

19. An Apgar score of less than _____ indicates a newborn needs medical attention.
    A. 9
    B. 8.5
    C. 8
    D. 7

20. The abbreviation of an intrauterine device for contraception is _____.
    A. CVD
    B. DUI
    C. IUD
    D. PID

Matching

Match each prefix, suffix, or abbreviation with its correct definition.

_____ 21. ureth/o   A. vagina

_____ 22. orchi/o   B. human chorionic gonadotropin

_____ 23. TURP   C. ovary

_____ 24. gravida   D. urethra

_____ 25. hCG   E. testis

_____ 26. colp/o   F. pregnant woman

_____ 27. metr/o   G. fallopian tubes

_____ 28. oophor/o   H. uterus

_____ 29. salping/o   I. transurethral resection of the prostate

_____ 30. ov/o   J. egg

22 Endocrine System

VOCABULARY REVIEW

Matching: Match each term with the correct definition.

A. endocrine gland

B. exocrine gland

C. hormone

D. target organ

E. sella turcica

F. calcium tetany

G. adrenal cortex

H. steroid

I. adrenal medulla

J. islet of Langerhans

K. feedback

L. endocrinologist

M. anorexia

N. goiter

O. fasting blood sugar (FBS)

P. glucose tolerance test (GTT)

Q. hormone level test

R. radioactive iodine (RAI) uptake scan

S. thyroid function tests (TFTs)

T. acromegaly

_____ 1. Occurs when insufficient ADH is released from the posterior pituitary

_____ 2. Pancreas cells that produce the hormone insulin and cause secretion of the hormone glucagon

_____ 3. Blood test that indicates the amount of glucose present after a period of fasting

_____ 4. Main disease of the insulin-producing pancreas

_____ 5. Glands whose secretion reaches the epithelial surface, usually through a duct

_____ 6. Blood test measuring the body's ability to break down glucose

_____ 7. Specialist who treats diseases resulting from dysfunction of the endocrine system

_____ 8. Underproduction of thyroid glands in childhood causing a low metabolic rate, slow growth, and mental retardation

_____ 9. Secretes epinephrine and norepinephrine

_____ 10. Glands that secrete hormones through the bloodstream

_____ 11. Continuous muscle spasms caused by an abnormal level of calcium in the blood

_____ 12. Process that allows the body to stay in homeostasis

_____ 13. Lack of appetite

_____ 14. Organic compound derived from fats

_____ 15. Blood test measuring the amounts of ADH, cortisol, growth, and parathyroid hormones

U. diabetes insipidus

V. cretinism

W. Graves disease

X. Addison disease

Y. diabetes mellitus

_____ 16. Internal secretion by a gland or an organ that serves to regulate a body function

_____ 17. Results in adults when there is an overproduction of thyroid hormone

_____ 18. Enlargement of thyroid gland not due to a tumor

_____ 19. Outer portion of the adrenal gland that secretes steroids

_____ 20. Contains receptors that cause it to react to certain hormones

_____ 21. Results from a deficiency of adrenocortical hormones

_____ 22. Blood test assessing T_3, T_4, and calcitonin

_____ 23. Depression in the sphenoid bone in the cranial cavity; holds the pituitary gland

_____ 24. Occurs in an adult when an excessive amount of growth hormone is secreted

_____ 25. Detects the thyroid's ability to concentrate and retain iodine

THEORY RECALL

True/False

Indicate whether the statement is true or false.

_____ 1. Hormones are secreted directly into the bloodstream by glands that are referred to as ductless glands.

_____ 2. Sweat glands, sebaceous glands, and mammary glands all are part of the endocrine system.

_____ 3. The pineal gland is approximately the size of a pea and is held in the sella turcica.

_____ 4. Mineralocorticoids control sodium, potassium, and water balance, mainly through action on the kidneys.

_____ 5. The thyroid secretes five hormones.

CHAPTER 22 Endocrine System

Multiple Choice

Identify the letter of the choice that best completes the statement or answers the question.

1. The hormone responsible for contractions of the uterus during labor is _____.
   A. oxytocin
   B. ADH
   C. HCG
   D. aldosterone

2. The gland located in the neck on both sides of the trachea and larynx is _____.
   A. pituitary
   B. pineal
   C. thyroid
   D. none of the above

3. The gland located above the kidneys that helps to control the body's metabolic rate is _____.
   A. prostate gland
   B. thymus
   C. pineal
   D. adrenal

4. The hormone _____ is secreted by the thymus.
   A. norepinephrine
   B. thymosin
   C. insulin
   D. melatonin

5. _____ is an increase of potassium in the blood.
   A. Hypocalcemia
   B. Hyperkalemia
   C. Hypernatremia
   D. Exophthalmia

6. _____ is a deficiency of glucose in the blood.
   A. Hypocalcemia
   B. Hyponatremia
   C. Hyperkalemia
   D. Hypoglycemia

7. _____ is the undergrowth of bone and body tissue in children.
   A. Graves disease
   B. Dwarfism
   C. Gigantism
   D. Cushing syndrome

8. _____ results from underactive thyroid secretion in adults.
   A. Exophthalmos
   B. Goiter
   C. Myxedema
   D. Addison disease

9. _____ is the hormone that responds to natural light and plays a role in sleep.
   A. Epinephrine
   B. Aldosterone
   C. Glucocorticoid
   D. Melatonin

10. _____ is the hormone that breaks down glycogen into glucose.
    A. Prostaglandin
    B. Insulin
    C. Thymosin
    D. Glucagon

11. There are _____ parathyroid glands.
    A. three
    B. four
    C. five
    D. none of the above

12. The islets of Langerhans are scattered throughout the _____ and play a key role in the production of hormones used to regulate blood glucose.
    A. kidneys
    B. pancreas
    C. brain
    D. spleen

13. The pineal gland is a small cone-shaped organ in the brain that secretes _____.
    A. melatonin
    B. insulin
    C. prostaglandins
    D. none of the above

14. A(n) _____ feedback effect occurs when the gland is stimulated to increase hormone secretion instead of turning it off.
    A. equilateral
    B. bilateral
    C. positive
    D. negative

15. The combining form for "pituitary gland" is _____.
    A. adren/o
    B. crin/o
    C. hypophys/o
    D. natr/o

16. Which one of the following is the abbreviation for triiodothyronine?
    A. Trid
    B. T_3
    C. T_4
    D. none of the above

17. An example of a corticosteroid is _____.
    A. Amaryl
    B. Pitocin
    C. Deltasone
    D. Tapazole

18. A nondiabetic range for hemoglobin A_{1c} is _____.
    A. 4% to 6%
    B. 6% to 7%
    C. 7% to 8%
    D. 8% to 10%

19. Which one of the following is *not* a warning sign of type 1 diabetes?
    A. Weight loss
    B. Unexplained irritability
    C. Nausea and vomiting
    D. Excessive hunger

20. The _____ is responsible for water reabsorption in the kidneys.
    A. anterior lobe of the pituitary gland
    B. posterior lobe of the pituitary gland
    C. adrenal cortex
    D. adrenal medulla

21. The hormone _____ stimulates growth and hormone activity of the testes and ovaries.
    A. ACTH
    B. MSH
    C. ADH
    D. FSH

22. The hormone _____ helps in carbohydrate metabolism and is active during stress.
    A. cortisol
    B. prolactin
    C. estrogen
    D. glucagon

23. _____ increases heart rate and blood pressure and is active during times of stress.
    A. Thyroxine
    B. Epinephrine
    C. Thyroid-stimulating hormone
    D. ADH

24. The medical term for "excessive urination" is _____.
    A. polyphagia
    B. polydipsia
    C. polyphobia
    D. polyuria

25. _____ is a test used to evaluate bone density, hypoparathyroidism, and the size of the adrenal gland.
    A. CT scan
    B. MRI
    C. Radiography
    D. Ultrasonography

Sentence Completion

Complete each sentence or statement.

adrenal gland	acromegaly	exophthalmus
pheochromocytoma	pituitary gland	gigantism
myxedema	goiter	non–insulin-dependent
hirsutism	corticoids	diabetes
cretinism	glucose tolerance test	

1. The _____ is known as the master gland.

2. _____ are steroid hormones produced by the adrenal cortex.

3. _____ is abnormal hairiness, especially in women.

4. _____ is a blood test that measures the body's ability to break down a concentrated glucose solution.

5. An enlargement of the thyroid gland caused by inadequate thyroid synthesis is called a(n) _____.

6. Signs and symptoms of _____ include a swollen face, enlargement of the lips, and a swollen and protruding tongue.

7. Signs and symptoms of _____ include elevated blood levels of HGH. Radiographs may show a pituitary tumor.

8. _____ is caused by the impaired ability of the thyroid gland to produce T_4.

9. When the target cells cannot take up sufficient quantities of insulin, it is referred to as _____.

10. Overproduction of the hormone cortisol may cause _____.

CHAPTER 22   Endocrine System

Short Answers

1. Explain the two main functions of the endocrine system.
   _____
   _____

2. Compare and contrast endocrine and exocrine glands.
   _____
   _____
   _____
   _____

3. Identify and locate the seven major endocrine glands.
   _____
   _____
   _____
   _____
   _____
   _____
   _____

4. Name two organs that secrete hormones, and explain what hormone is secreted by each.
   _____
   _____
   _____
   _____

CRITICAL THINKING

1. Joanna is a 25-year-old mother of two. Joanna has recently been diagnosed with IDDM. Explain to Joanna what IDDM is, and how it is monitored and treated. (Use your text, your institution's resource reference library, and the Internet as needed.)

   _____

   _____

   _____

   _____

2. Simon is a 19-year-old man who has been treated for gigantism. Explain the etiology, signs and symptoms, therapy, and interventions. (Use your text, your institution's resource reference library, and the Internet as needed.)

   _____

   _____

   _____

   _____

PRACTICAL APPLICATIONS

If you have accomplished the objectives in this chapter, you will be able to make better choices as a medical assistant. Take another look at this situation and decide what you would do.

Juliette, age 4, cannot get enough water to drink and has to void frequently. Her mother says that Juliette eats all the time, but she is losing weight. She is also lethargic. Sometimes her mother thinks that Juliette's breath has a fruity odor, although she does not chew fruit-flavored gum or eat fruit-flavored candy. After Dr. Jay checks Juliette, she tells her mother that she is concerned that Juliette has diabetes mellitus. Dr. Jay wants to do further testing as quickly as possible. She orders a fasting blood glucose test, which comes back with an elevated value. She follows this with a glucose tolerance test. When the glucose tolerance test result is abnormally high, Dr. Jay prescribes insulin for Juliette.

1. **What type of diabetes mellitus would you expect Juliette to have at age 4?**

   _____

2. **What is the difference between IDDM and NIDDM?**

   _____

   _____

   _____

Copyright © 2010, 2005 by Saunders, an imprint of Elsevier, Inc. All rights reserved.

3. Are the symptoms listed for Juliette typical of the symptoms found for patients with diabetes?

4. What are the medical terms for "being hungry all the time," "having excessive thirst," and "having to void often"?

5. What other specific treatment would be needed to keep Juliette's blood glucose level lowered?

6. What is the term for an "elevated blood sugar level"? What is the term for "sugar in the urine"?

7. What is a fasting glucose test? What is a glucose tolerance test?

8. Diabetes insipidus has many of the same symptoms as diabetes mellitus. What symptoms are the same?

9. What glands and hormones are associated with diabetes insipidus?

10. **What is positive feedback? What is negative feedback? Why are these important in the endocrine system?**

_____
_____
_____
_____
_____
_____

APPLICATION OF SKILLS

1. Label the word parts of the following terms. Use *P* to indicate a prefix, *CF* to indicate a combining form, *R* to indicate a root, *S* to indicate a suffix. (Example: abnormal—ab *P* norm *R* al *S*)
   A. adrenopathy _____
   B. diabetes _____
   C. hyperkalemia _____
   D. myxedema _____
   E. pineal _____

2. Change the following from singular to plural or vice versa.
   A. cortex _____
   B. thyrotoxicosis _____
   C. papilla _____
   D. ovum _____
   E. ovary _____

3. Write out the meaning of each the following abbreviations.
   A. DI _____
   B. GH _____
   C. TFT _____
   D. FBS _____
   E. ADH _____

274 CHAPTER 22 Endocrine System

4. Label the diagram.

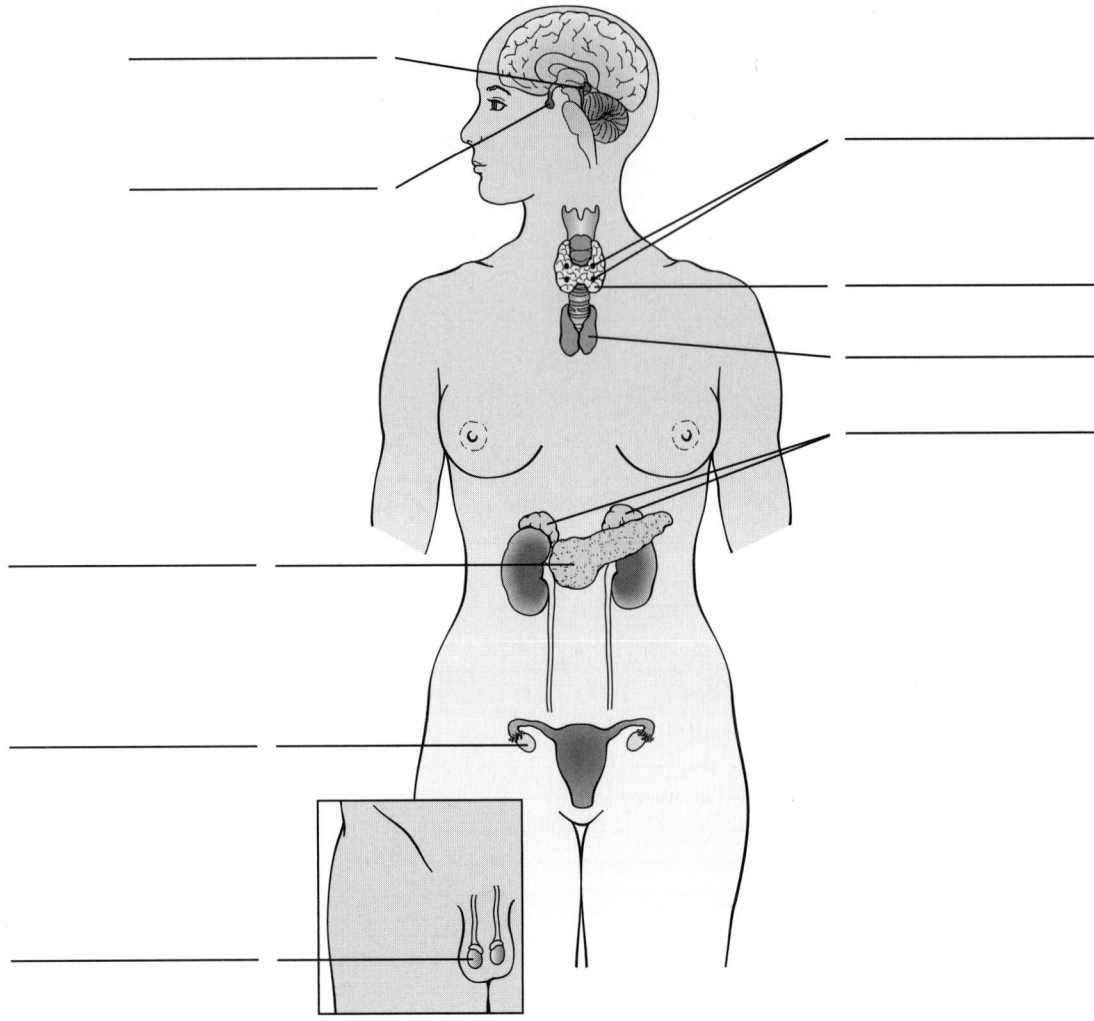

CHAPTER QUIZ

Multiple Choice

Identify the letter of the choice that best completes the statement or answers the question.

1. The _____ gland(s) is(are) known as the master gland.
   A. pineal
   B. adrenal
   C. pituitary
   D. thyroid

2. The _____ gland(s) is(are) located above the kidneys.
   A. adrenal
   B. thymus
   C. parathyroid
   D. pineal

Copyright © 2010, 2005 by Saunders, an imprint of Elsevier, Inc. All rights reserved.

3. _____ is(are) hormone(s) responsible for the regulation of blood pressure, pain threshold, inflammation, and blood clotting.
   A. Antidiuretics
   B. Corticosteroids
   C. Prostaglandins
   D. Insulin

4. _____ is an increase of glucose in the blood.
   A. Hypoglycemia
   B. Hyperglycemia
   C. Hypercalcemia
   D. Hypokalemia

5. _____ is an increase of sodium in the blood.
   A. Hypercalcemia
   B. Hyperglycemia
   C. Hypokalemia
   D. Hypernatremia

6. _____ is a blood test measuring the amounts of ADH, cortisol, and growth and parathyroid hormones.
   A. A_{1c}
   B. FBS
   C. Hormone level test
   D. Thyroid function test

7. _____ results in adults when there is an overproduction of thyroid hormone.
   A. Graves disease
   B. Cushing syndrome
   C. Diabetes mellitus
   D. Cretinism

8. _____ glands are glands whose secretion reaches the epithelial surface usually through a duct.
   A. Endocrine
   B. Exocrine
   C. Both endocrine and exocrine
   D. Neither endocrine nor exocrine

9. _____ is a type of corticosteroid.
   A. Pitocin
   B. Amaryl
   C. Deltasone
   D. Synthroid

10. _____ is a warning sign of diabetes type 1.
    A. Blurred vision
    B. Slow healing
    C. Numbness and tingling of the hands and feet
    D. None of the above

11. Which one of the following is a hormone produced by the thyroid gland?
    A. GH
    B. Calcitonin
    C. Parathormone
    D. Aldosterone

12. The adrenal medulla secretes which one of the following hormones?
    A. Testosterone
    B. Aldosterone
    C. Epinephrine
    D. Insulin

13. _____ is a lack of appetite.
    A. Exophthalmia
    B. Hirsutism
    C. Hypokalemia
    D. Anorexia

14. The medical term for "excessive thirst" is _____.
    A. polydipsia
    B. polyphagia
    C. polyuria
    D. none of the above

15. A(n) _____ is used to check for change in the size of soft tissue such as the pituitary, pancreas, and hypothalamus.
    A. CT scan
    B. MRI
    C. radiograph
    D. ultrasound

16. _____ is a blood test ordered to assess the amount of T_3, T_4, and calcitonin circulating in the blood.
    A. FBS
    B. GTT
    C. TFTs
    D. None of the above

17. _____ occurs in an adult when an excessive amount of growth hormone is secreted. The bones and soft tissue of the hands, feet, and face experience overgrowth.
    A. Dwarfism
    B. Gigantism
    C. Cretinism
    D. Acromegaly

18. The intervention for cretinism is _____.
    A. emotional support
    B. lifetime hormone replacement therapy
    C. encouraging the patient to follow diet, reduce stress, and avoid infections
    D. encouraging the patient to follow prescribed therapy for his or her lifetime

19. The clinical presentation of a "moon face," "buffalo hump," and truncal obesity is indicative of _____.
    A. diabetes mellitus
    B. Cushing syndrome
    C. diabetes insipidus
    D. Addison disease

20. _____ is described as an enlargement of the thyroid gland caused by inadequate thyroid synthesis.
    A. Goiter
    B. Acromegaly
    C. Addison disease
    D. Cushing syndrome

Matching

Match each prefix or suffix with its correct definition.

_____ 21. kal/i   A. sodium

_____ 22. natr/o   B. calcium

_____ 23. calc/o   C. secrete

_____ 24. crin/o   D. potassium

_____ 25. hypophys/o   E. pituitary gland

23 Integumentary System

VOCABULARY REVIEW

Matching: Match each term with the correct definition.

A. dermatologist

B. turgor

C. dermis

D. keratin

E. melanin

F. whorls

G. sebaceous glands

H. sudoriferous glands

I. nails

J. cyst

K. polyp

L. benign

M. malignant melanoma

N. abrasion

O. contusion

P. laceration

Q. rule of nines

R. abscess

S. cicatrix

T. decubitus ulcer

_____ 1. Black, asymmetrical lesion with uneven borders that grows faster than normal moles

_____ 2. Sweat glands; maintain body temperature

_____ 3. Contagious epithelial growths caused by a virus

_____ 4. Localized collection of pus that occurs on the skin or any body tissue

_____ 5. Specialist in the treatment of diseases and conditions of the skin

_____ 6. Abscess that occurs around a hair follicle

_____ 7. Not malignant

_____ 8. Ridges that fit snugly over the papillae on top of the dermis; coils or spirals that form fingerprints

_____ 9. Parasitic skin disorder caused by lice

_____ 10. Scar formation

_____ 11. Stalklike growth extending out from the mucous membrane

_____ 12. Pressure sore; bedsore

_____ 13. Waterproof protein that toughens the skin

_____ 14. Growths of hard keratin that protect the ends of the fingers and toes

_____ 15. Blood vessels rupture and blood seeps into the tissue

_____ 16. Viral infection of the skin characterized by "cold sores" and "fever blisters"

_____ 17. Oil glands; release oil that lubricates the skin and hair

U. furuncle

V. pruritus

W. vitiligo

X. herpes simplex

Y. pediculosis

Z. verrucae

_____ 18. Severe itching

_____ 19. Jagged cuts; tissue edges are irregular

_____ 20. Thick-walled sac that contains fluid or semisolid material

_____ 21. Normal tension in the skin

_____ 22. Loss of pigment in the skin; milk-white patches

_____ 23. Epidermis is scraped off

_____ 24. Layer of skin that lies beneath the epidermis

_____ 25. System for evaluating the burns on a patient's total body surface area

_____ 26. Dark pigment that provides color to the skin and protects against the sun's ultraviolet rays

THEORY RECALL

True/False

Indicate whether the statement is true or false.

_____ 1. The skin is composed of the dermis, epidermis, and subcutaneous layer.

_____ 2. The epidermis is the deepest layer of the skin.

_____ 3. The dermis is thicker than the epidermis and lies beneath it.

_____ 4. A macule is a split or crack in the skin.

_____ 5. An incision is a smooth cut into the skin.

Multiple Choice

Identify the letter of the choice that best completes the statement or answers the question.

1. _____ is the most common inflammation of the skin, accompanied by papules, vesicles, and crusts.
   A. Furuncle
   B. Keloid
   C. Eczema
   D. Urticaria

2. Xylocaine is an example of a(n) _____ that blocks pain at the site where it is administered.
   A. anti-inflammatory
   B. analgesic
   C. antiviral
   D. none of the above

3. Salicylic acid is a(n) _____ medication used to remove warts.
   A. keratolytic
   B. antiviral
   C. corticosteroid
   D. anti-infective

4. _____ is a microscopic examination of skin lesions to screen for herpes virus.
   A. Wood's light examination
   B. Blood antibody titer
   C. Tzanck test
   D. Skin biopsy

5. Signs and symptoms of _____ include red, itchy rash with bull's eye appearance; joint pain; and malaise.
   A. impetigo
   B. Lyme disease
   C. scleroderma
   D. scabies

6. _____ is a skin infection caused by fungus, classified according to body region.
   A. Lyme disease
   B. Scabies
   C. Tinea
   D. Pediculosis

7. A narrow band of epidermis at the base and sides of the nail is called the _____.
   A. nail bed
   B. lunula
   C. nail root
   D. cuticle

8. The medical term for "baldness" is _____.
   A. alopecia
   B. cicatrix
   C. onychomycosis
   D. none of the above

9. _____ is a parasitic skin disorder caused by lice.
   A. Onychomycosis
   B. Pediculosis
   C. Scabies
   D. Tinea

10. _____ are large abscesses that involve connecting furuncles.
    A. Cicatrix
    B. Melanoma
    C. Polyps
    D. Carbuncles

11. A sac or tube that anchors and contains an individual hair is called the _____.
    A. shaft
    B. follicle
    C. root
    D. none of the above

12. The medical term for a "precancerous growth of the skin" is _____.
    A. polyp
    B. vesicle
    C. actinic keratosis
    D. comedo

13. The skin layer that is mainly composed of adipose tissue and loose connective tissue is the _____.
    A. subcutaneous
    B. dermis
    C. epidermis
    D. B and C

14. The medical term for a "flat discolored area of the skin" is _____.
    A. papule
    B. lesion
    C. wheal
    D. macule

15. Which degree of burn is reddened blistering of the dermis and epidermis layers of the skin?
    A. first
    B. second
    C. third
    D. fourth

16. The medical term for "removal of surface epidermis by scratching, burning, or abrasion" is _____.
    A. erosion
    B. ichthyosis
    C. excoriation
    D. none of the above

17. An idiopathic hereditary dermatitis with dry, scaly, silver patches, usually on both arms, both legs, and the scalp, is called _____.
    A. psoriasis
    B. eczema
    C. urticaria
    D. scleroderma

18. The medical term for an "erosion of the skin (bedsore)" is _____.
    A. lesion
    B. pustule
    C. polyp
    D. decubitus ulcer

19. Phase 1 on the healing process is known as the _____ phase.
    A. inflammation
    B. granulation
    C. maturation
    D. none of the above

20. A(n) _____ is an overgrowth of fibrous tissue at the site of scar tissue.
    A. ulcer
    B. polyp
    C. keloid
    D. furuncle

Copyright © 2010, 2005 by Saunders, an imprint of Elsevier, Inc. All rights reserved.

21. Benadryl is an example of a(n) _____ medication.
    A. antipruritic
    B. antiviral
    C. antifungal
    D. anesthetic

22. _____ is an infection of the skin and subcutaneous tissue caused by bacteria.
    A. Psoriasis
    B. Cellulitis
    C. Pediculosis
    D. Impetigo

23. In the condition of _____, the skin hardens and becomes leathery. Organs may also be affected by decreasing in size, and joints may swell and be painful.
    A. Lyme disease
    B. psoriasis
    C. scleroderma
    D. scabies

24. The combining form for "skin" is _____.
    A. albino/o
    B. diaphor/o
    C. histi/o
    D. dermat/o

25. The maturation phase of healing is phase _____.
    A. 1
    B. 2
    C. 3
    D. 4

Sentence Completion

Complete each sentence or statement.

sebum	Bx	basal cell carcinoma
sweat	Tx	lunula
pore	Rx	vesicle
cyst	albino	ichthy/o
ung	squamous cell carcinoma	

1. A person unable to form melanin has very white skin with no pigmentation and is referred to as a(n) _____.

2. A(n) _____ is the duct opening that provides a pathway for fluid to leave the body.

3. The _____ is a white half-moon shape at the base of the nail.

4. Oil glands release _____.

5. A clear blister is called a _____.

6. A(n) _____ is a thick-walled sac that contains fluid or semisolid material.

7. _____ are skin cancers that appear as firm papules with ulcerations.

8. The abbreviation for "ointment" is _____.

9. The abbreviation for "biopsy" is _____.

10. The term for "scalelike" is _____.

Short Answers

1. List the three main functions of the skin.

_____
_____
_____

2. Identify the three layers of the skin, and describe the structure and function of each.

_____
_____
_____
_____
_____
_____
_____

3. List and briefly describe nine common skin lesions.

4. What is the rule of nines?

CRITICAL THINKING

1. Mrs. Kimerfield called the office this afternoon because her 8-year-old daughter Melanie brought a note home from school informing Mrs. Kimerfield that several of Melanie's classmates have head lice, and that there is the potential that Melanie may also have it. Explain to Mrs. Kimerfield what to look for and how to treat it. (Use your text, your institution's resource reference library, and the Internet as needed.)

2. Identify the following types of fungal infections, by stating their location and a typical treatment of each. (Use your text, your institution's resource reference library, and the Internet as needed.)

   Tinea corporis _____

   Tinea pedis _____

   Tinea unguium _____

Tinea cruris _____

Tinea faciei _____

Tinea capitis _____

PRACTICAL APPLICATIONS

If you have accomplished the objectives in this chapter, you will be able to make better choices as a medical assistant. Take another look at this situation and decide what you would do.

Marilyn was taking a shower 2 weeks ago and found a large black mole on her shoulder. At first she wanted to ignore it, but after talking with her friend, she decided that she should see her family practice physician. This physician sent her to Dr. Nelson, a dermatologist, who diagnosed her lesion as a possible malignant melanoma. Dr. Nelson asked if she had any pruritus, a fissure, or crusting of the lesion. As Dr. Nelson examined Marilyn's shoulder, he noticed petechiae, ecchymosis, and purpura. When asked about these findings, Marilyn told the physician that the mole had itched and she had scratched the area in her sleep. On her leg was a furuncle that was inflamed and hot and appeared to have a pus formation. On completing the physical examination, Dr. Nelson noticed that Marilyn had the tendency to keloid formation based on the appearance of her old appendectomy scar. Marilyn had quite a few questions for the medical assistant about the meaning of some of the terms used by Dr. Nelson. Marilyn left the dermatologist's office with surgery scheduled for removal of the melanoma 2 days later.

1. **What is the etiology of a malignant melanoma?**

   _____

   _____

2. **How do the signs of a malignant melanoma differ from those of a benign lesion?**

   _____

   _____

   _____

3. **Define pruritus, fissure, and crusting.**

   _____

   _____

   _____

   _____

Copyright © 2010, 2005 by Saunders, an imprint of Elsevier, Inc. All rights reserved.

4. What are petechiae? What is ecchymosis? What is a purpura?

5. What is the difference between a furuncle and a carbuncle?

6. Why would the physician be concerned that Marilyn had a history of keloids?

7. What are the stages of the healing process that you could expect Marilyn to have after surgery?

8. What is a closed wound? Give two examples.

9. What is an open wound? Give two examples.

_____

_____

_____

_____

APPLICATION OF SKILLS

1. Label the word parts of the following terms. Use *P* to indicate a prefix, *CF* to indicate a combining form, *R* to indicate a root, *S* to indicate a suffix. (Example: abnormal—ab *P* norm *R* al *S*)
   A. cutaneous _____
   B. excoriation _____
   C. keloid _____
   D. melanoma _____
   E. onychitis _____

2. Change the following from singular to plural or vice versa.
   A. stria _____
   B. bulla _____
   C. comedo _____
   D. stratum _____
   E. petechia _____

3. Write out the meaning of each the following abbreviations.
   A. UV _____
   B. Ung _____
   C. BSA _____
   D. I & D _____
   E. Decub _____

4. Label the diagrams.

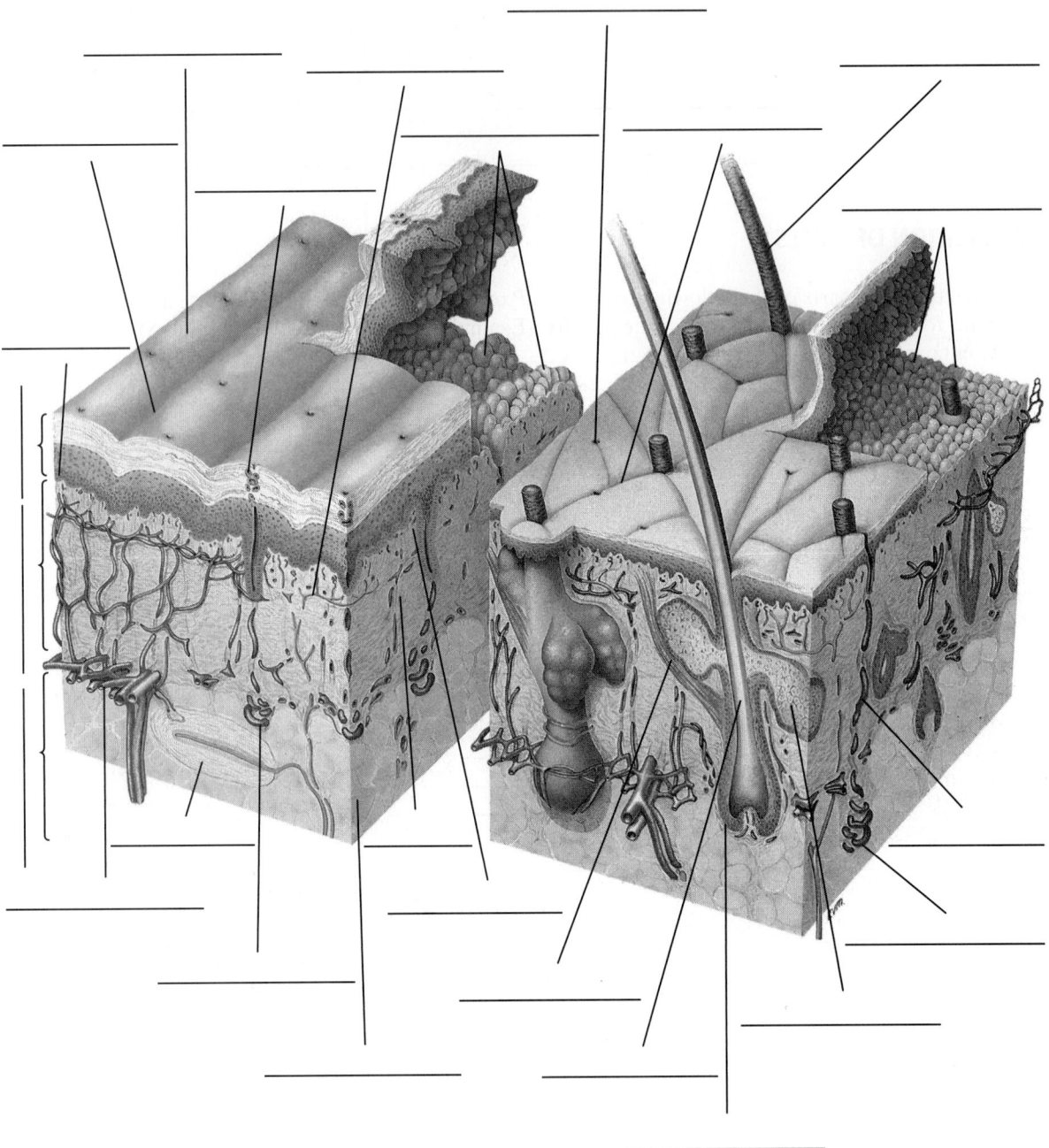

Integumentary System CHAPTER 23

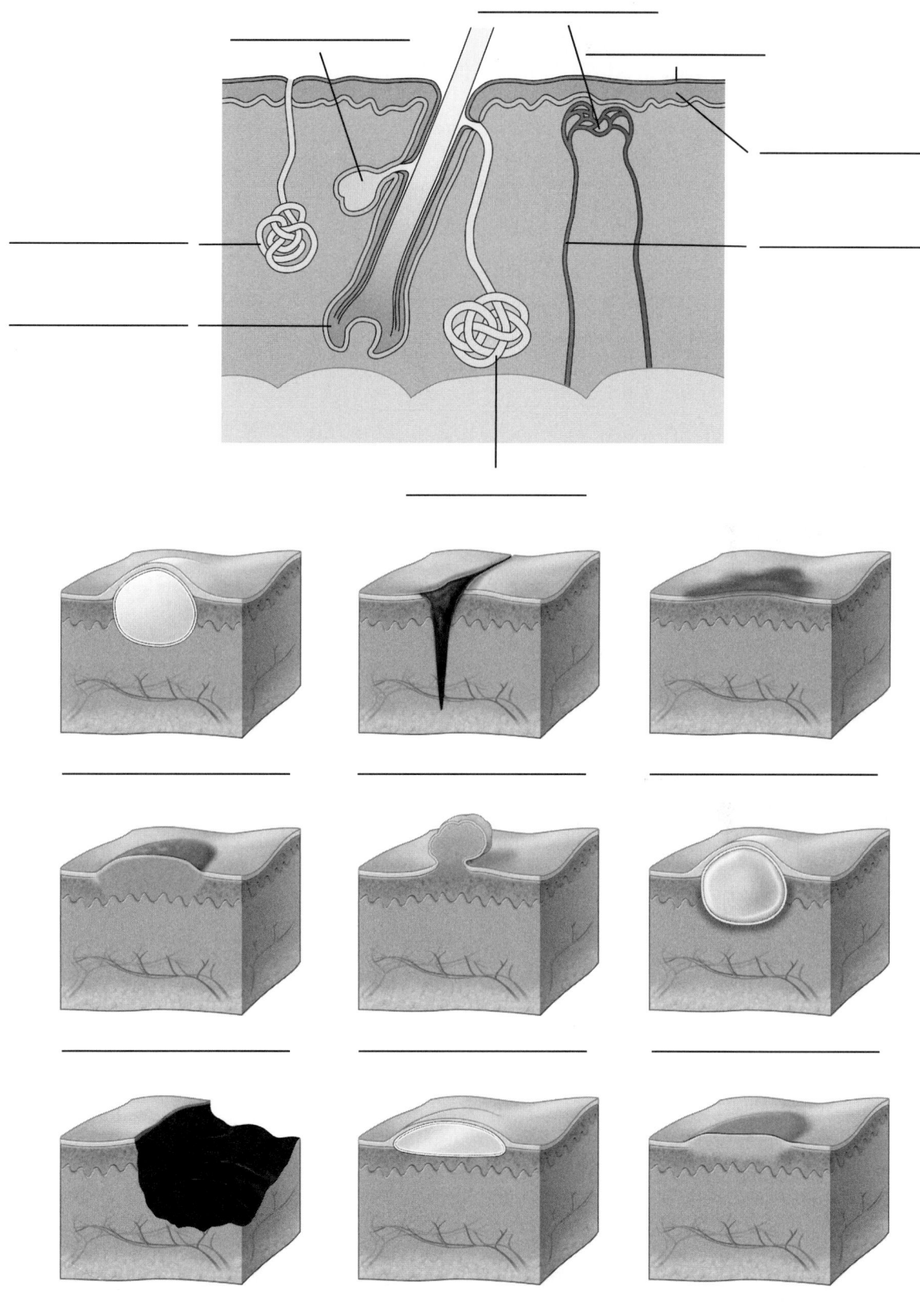

CHAPTER QUIZ

Multiple Choice

Identify the letter of the choice that best completes the statement or answers the question.

1. A(n) _____ has jagged cuts and tissue edges that are irregular.
   A. laceration
   B. incision
   C. abrasion
   D. contusion

2. _____ is an idiopathic, chronic systemic disease of the skin in which the skin hardens and becomes leathery.
   A. Impetigo
   B. Scleroderma
   C. Cellulitis
   D. Psoriasis

3. A(n) _____ is a split or crack in the skin.
   A. purpura
   B. contusion
   C. fissure
   D. onychomycosis

4. _____ are flat, pinpoint red spots.
   A. Ichthyosis
   B. Purpura
   C. Urticaria
   D. Petechiae

5. The deepest layer of skin is the _____.
   A. subcutaneous tissue
   B. epidermis
   C. dermis
   D. none of the above

6. A(n) _____ is an abscess that occurs around a hair follicle.
   A. carbuncle
   B. ulcer
   C. furuncle
   D. excoriation

7. _____ are oil glands that release oil that lubricates the skin and hair.
   A. Sudoriferous glands
   B. Sebaceous glands
   C. Lymph glands
   D. Adenoids

8. The _____ is phase 2 of the healing process; collagen forms.
   A. inflammatory phase
   B. maturation phase
   C. granulation phase
   D. none of the above

9. _____ is the normal tension of skin.
    A. Turgor
    B. Rigor
    C. Flaccidity
    D. Cicatrix

10. A(n) _____ is a malignant skin lesion that is raised, with blood vessels around the edges.
    A. squamous cell carcinoma
    B. basal cell carcinoma
    C. malignant melanoma
    D. actinic keratosis

11. _____ is a skin disorder caused by itch mites.
    A. Lyme disease
    B. Pediculosis
    C. Scabies
    D. Tinea cruris

12. A patient with _____ exhibits blisters on the lips, inside of the mouth, and occasionally the nose.
    A. pediculosis
    B. verrucae
    C. tinea corporis
    D. herpes simplex

13. The combining form for "tissue" is _____.
    A. kerat/o
    B. histi/o
    C. hidr/o
    D. onych/o

14. Ung is the abbreviation for _____.
    A. "ointment"
    B. "nail border"
    C. "urgent"
    D. none of the above

15. Tetracycline is an example of a medication used for treating _____.
    A. fungi
    B. acne
    C. lice
    D. psoriasis

16. Zovirax is an example of a medication used for treating _____.
    A. scabies
    B. herpes simplex
    C. athlete's foot
    D. burns

17. A Wood's light examination is used to detect _____.
    A. fungal skin infections
    B. reaction of the body to allergens
    C. viral infections
    D. bacterial infections

Copyright © 2010, 2005 by Saunders, an imprint of Elsevier, Inc. All rights reserved.

18. A burn patient's total body surface area is evaluated according to the _____ to determine the extent and severity of the burn.
    A. core body temperature
    B. full-thickness measurement
    C. rule of nines
    D. total body weight

19. The medical term for "ringworm" is _____.
    A. tinea capitis
    B. tinea corporis
    C. tinea faciei
    D. tinea pedis

20. The medical term for a "pore that is blocked, usually with sebum and bacteria" is _____.
    A. polyp
    B. furuncle
    C. comedo
    D. fissure

Matching

Match each prefix or suffix with its correct definition.

_____ 21. hidr/o   A. fungus

_____ 22. ichthy/   B. yellow

_____ 23. myc/o   C. sweat

_____ 24. xanth/o   D. dry

_____ 25. xer/o   E. scalelike

24 The Medical Office

VOCABULARY REVIEW

Matching: Match each term with the correct definition.

A. Americans with Disabilities Act (ADA)

B. breach of confidentiality

C. Health Insurance Portability and Accountability Act (HIPAA) of 1996

D. agenda

E. fax machine (facsimile)

F. itinerary

G. notebook computer

H. personal digital assistants (PDAs)

I. postage meter

J. preventive maintenance

K. facilities management

L. policy manual

M. procedures manual

N. back ordered

O. capital goods

P. disposable goods

Q. inventory records

R. invoice

_____ 1. Document received with an order that lists the items ordered and itemizes those sent and those to arrive at a later date

_____ 2. Status of being out of stock; items that will be shipped at a later date

_____ 3. Office equipment that scans document, translates the information to electronic impulses, and transmits an exact copy of the original document from one location to another through a telephone line

_____ 4. Pocket-sized computer used for appointments, telephone numbers, notes, and other information used on a daily basis

_____ 5. Break in a patient's right to privacy

_____ 6. Entity that sells supplies, equipment, and services

_____ 7. Expendable or consumable supplies that are used and then discarded

_____ 8. Equipment that is reusable but less expensive and durable than capital equipment

_____ 9. Travel document that describes the overall trip and indicates what is scheduled to happen each day

_____ 10. Form prepared by the vendor describing the products sold by item number, quantity, and the price; used for paying the vendor

_____ 11. Provides for accessible routes and fixtures for use by the disabled

_____ 12. Regular servicing meant to prevent the breakdown of equipment

S. lead time

T. noncapital goods

U. order quantity

V. packing slip

W. purchase order

X. reorder point

Y. safety stock

Z. vendor

AA. warranty card

_____ 13. Card that accompanies a purchased item that provides protection for the buyer against defective parts for 90 days

_____ 14. Time it takes to receive an order once placed

_____ 15. Document used to order supplies; contains the name, address, and telephone number of a vendor, and the quantity, price, and description of the items ordered

_____ 16. Document that includes the length of the meeting, topics to be covered, their order, and the person responsible for each

_____ 17. Maintaining the atmosphere and physical environment of an office

_____ 18. Optimal quantity of a supply to be ordered at one time

_____ 19. Manual containing specific instructions on how procedures are to be performed

_____ 20. Small, portable computer that can be carried easily

_____ 21. Documentation of physical assets and information that includes item description, date of purchase, price, and where purchased. Equipment serial numbers and service agreements are also recorded

_____ 22. Extra items on hand to avoid running out of stock (back-up supply)

_____ 23. Automated stamp machine

_____ 24. Mandates patient rights by providing guidelines for health care providers and insurance carriers to maintain confidentiality

_____ 25. Goods that are durable and are expected to last a few years; expensive

_____ 26. Minimum quantity of a supply to be available before a new order is placed

_____ 27. Manual that explains the day-to-day operations of the medical office and provides general information that affects all employees

THEORY RECALL

True/False

Indicate whether the statement is true or false.

_____ 1. A supply order should be paid only from a statement.

_____ 2. A postage meter provides a convenient way to print postage for all mail services, including periodicals.

_____ 3. HIPAA provides federal regulations that require all public buildings be accessible to everyone.

_____ 4. A dedicated telephone line permits documents to be sent and received 24 hours a day by fax.

_____ 5. When leasing equipment, the office owns the equipment.

Multiple Choice

Identify the letter of the choice that best completes the statement or answers the question.

1. Tongue blades, syringes, and printer paper all are examples of _____ goods.
   A. disposable
   B. special
   C. capital
   D. none of the above

2. The _____ is the optimal quantity of a supply to be ordered at one time.
   A. reorder point
   B. safety stock
   C. order quantity
   D. lead time

3. When an order is received, a(n) _____ is included in the package.
   A. purchase order
   B. packing slip
   C. invoice
   D. statement

4. Which one of the following is the first step in organizing a meeting?
   A. Prepare an agenda.
   B. Select a location and a meeting room.
   C. Send reminder notices to all participants.
   D. Assemble materials needed for the meeting.

5. Which one of the following is *not* needed to make travel arrangements for the physician?
   A. Dates of travel
   B. Number of people traveling
   C. Hotel reservations
   D. Favorite food

6. A _____ explains the day-to-day operations of the medical office.
   A. policy manual
   B. guidebook
   C. procedure manual
   D. none of the above

7. When a medical office is closed and unavailable to handle incoming calls, which one of the following is the most efficient method routinely used?
   A. Answering service
   B. Answering machine
   C. Forwarding all calls to the physician's home phone
   D. A and B are equally efficient

8. Maintenance of a procedure manual requires that _____.
   A. the physician's attorneys approve it
   B. the physician sends a memo once a year to remind everyone there is a procedure manual
   C. all employees are required to date and initial that they have read the manual
   D. none of the above

9. Which one of the following is *not* considered a medical office marketing tool?
   A. Brochure
   B. Web page
   C. Press release
   D. All of the above are marketing tools

10. Leasing is essentially _____ equipment for the office.
    A. buying
    B. renting
    C. A and B
    D. neither A nor B

11. Inventory records are used in maintaining an adequate supply for use in the office, for _____ purposes, and in case of fire or theft.
    A. depreciation
    B. capitation
    C. entrepreneurship
    D. none of the above

12. The first step in preparing a document for fax transmission after gathering supplies and equipment is to _____.
    A. copy the patient's file
    B. check the file for a release of information
    C. prepare a cover sheet
    D. photocopy the materials to be faxed on yellow paper for better transmission

13. _____ items are usually expensive and are expected to be permanent or at least last several years.
    A. Disposable
    B. Nondurable
    C. Capital
    D. None of the above

14. The best color of ink to use on a faxed document is _____.
    A. blue
    B. red
    C. black
    D. purple

15. If a fax is marked "for physician only," what should the medical assistant do?
    A. Do not accept the fax.
    B. Hand it directly to the physician.
    C. Give it to the office manager for his or her decision.
    D. Annotate it and then give to the physician.

16. When maintaining office equipment, a file should be created for _____ or type of equipment.
    A. vendor
    B. medical assistant
    C. physician
    D. none of the above

17. To meet the minimum standards of the ADA, a wheelchair ramp longer than _____ feet must have two railings.
    A. 6
    B. 8
    C. 10
    D. 12

18. Internal restrooms must be _____ inches wide to be in compliance with the ADA.
    A. 24
    B. 32
    C. 36
    D. 42

19. Which one of the following is *not* a legal concern regarding fax machines and HIPAA regulations?
    A. Confidentiality–authorization signed
    B. Amount of information being sent
    C. Location of fax machine
    D. All of the above are legal concerns

20. A(n) _____ is a document that includes the length of a meeting, topics to be covered, their order, and the person responsible for each.
    A. itinerary
    B. agenda
    C. HIPAA mandate
    D. none of the above

Sentence Completion

Complete each sentence or statement.

risk management	facilities management	personal digital
back-ordered	purchase order	assistant (PDA)
tickler file	agenda	postage meter
lead time	itinerary	
warranty card	breach of confidentiality	

CHAPTER 24 The Medical Office

1. When ordering supplies, a(n) _____ is typically initiated to keep track of what was ordered and when.

2. A(n) _____ describes an overall trip and indicates what is scheduled to happen each day.

3. You may want to create a(n) _____ to remind you that maintenance is routinely required on your office equipment.

4. A(n) _____ is a break in a patient's right to privacy.

5. A pocket-sized computer used for appointments and telephone numbers is called a(n) _____.

6. A(n) _____ is an automated stamp machine.

7. _____ is the time it takes to receive an order.

8. An item that is _____ is temporarily out of stock and will be shipped at a later date.

9. _____ is the term used for maintaining the atmosphere and physical environment of an office.

10. A(n) _____ is a card that accompanies a purchased item that provides protection for the buyer against defective parts for 90 days.

Short Answers

1. Design a plan for a medical office reception area that reflects HIPAA and ADA regulations, and incorporates the seven considerations for a reception area.

_____

_____

_____

_____

2. List six types of office equipment, and explain how each is used in the medical office.

3. Explain why inventory records are kept.

4. List three factors to be considered when establishing an inventory control system.

5. The office manager asks you to photocopy a single copy of several patient documents. After you make sure the machine is turned on and warmed up, what steps would you follow to complete the task?

6. Explain the importance of routine maintenance of office equipment.

7. As a new employee in a medical practice, you have been asked to read the Office Policy Manual and Procedures Manual. What would you expect to be included under the following headings?
   a. Purpose of Manual: _____
   b. Mission Statement: _____
   c. Hours of Operation: _____
   d. Payroll: _____
   e. Performance Evaluations: _____
   f. Benefits: _____
   g. Training: _____
   h. Appointment scheduling: _____

CRITICAL THINKING

1. The physician has requested a 10-mL syringe be available in examination room 3 for an I&D of a sebaceous cyst. When you went to the storage room to obtain the syringe, the box was empty. After searching the examination rooms, you were able to locate one 10-mL syringe, which you took into the physician. After the procedure, you check the inventory supply reorder form for 10-mL syringes. No one has requested that 10-mL syringes be ordered. The office is completely out of 10-mL syringes; what would you now do?

2. Since the above-described incident, you have been asked to take over the supply ordering. What time management principles must you put in place to make certain this task is accomplished?

3. Part of your role as a medical assistant is to be a patient advocate. What does this mean to you, and how would you go about accomplishing this goal?

PRACTICAL APPLICATIONS

If you have accomplished the objectives in this chapter, you will be able to make better choices as a medical assistant. Take a look at this situation and decide how to apply what you have learned.

Janine is a new member of the office staff. She has not had any training in the medical assisting field, but has been working as a receptionist in a loan office. On her first day at work, Janine is assigned to work at the front desk with the receptionist. As the patients for the day come in, Janine asks many personal questions about each patient and then proceeds to tell the receptionist what she knows about the patient. When told to be sure the names of the patients have been obliterated from the sign-in sheet, she uses a yellow highlighter. As she answers the telephone, everyone in the office can hear her conversations. Janine immediately moves the large plants in the reception area around so one is partially blocking the doorway. A fax from a surgeon arrives for Dr. Lopez, and Janine lays it on the front counter next to the sign-in sheet until she has a chance to give it to Dr. Lopez. When asked to move the fax, Janine replies that it would definitely be easier if the fax was just placed next to the front window rather than in the back room so she would not have to walk so far. Also, Janine does not understand why this office needs a dedicated line for the fax machine. Why not just let the fax line be connected to the multiline telephone at the front desk?

Janine was asked to leave 1 week later after she refused to maintain the equipment. As the office personnel looked for the manuals for the new equipment that had been purchased, no manuals could be found, and when she was contacted, Janine admitted discarding them.

What should Janine be told about why she was asked to leave her job at the medical office?

1. **In many ways, Janine has broken confidentiality in the medical office as required by HIPAA. Name three ways that are obvious.**

_____

_____

_____

_____

2. What is HIPAA, and how does it affect patient care?

3. Why is a multiline phone system important in a medical office?

4. What special features should be considered when deciding on a phone system for a medical office?

5. How is ADA important in the medical office? What are three of the design features that are important for patient safety?

6. How did Janine make Dr. Lopez's office dangerous for a person with a physical disability?

7. Why is it important to keep manuals that are sent with new equipment?

8. Would you want Janine to be a fellow employee in a medical office with you? Defend your answer.

APPLICATION OF SKILLS

Procedure Check-off Sheets (*) and assignments from MACC on the Evolve site at http://evolve.elsevier.com/klieger/medicalassisting (**)

1. Perform Procedure 24-1: Prepare, Send, and Receive a Fax.*

2. Perform Procedure 24-2: Maintain Office Equipment.*

3. Perform Procedure 24-3: Inventory Control: Ordering and Restocking Supplies.*
   A. MACC CD
      MACC/Professionalism/Operational functions/Establishing and maintaining a supply inventory and ordering system**

4. Perform Procedure 24-4: Develop and Maintain a Current List of Community Resources.*

5. Complete a Purchase Order (located in Chapter 24 in the Supplemental Chapter Materials section at the back of this Workbook) using the following information:

Vendor	Item	On hand	Unit price	Reorder point	ID #	Amount to reorder
XYZ SUPPLY	10 mL syringe		$15.00/bx (100/bx)	25 each	O6-82-231	1 BX

10176 Way Short Dr.
Lions, KY 67809
789-675-3434
Next Day delivery

CHAPTER QUIZ

Multiple Choice

Identify the letter of the choice that best completes the statement or answers the question.

1. _____ mandates patient rights by providing guidelines for health care providers and insurance carriers.
   A. HIPAA
   B. ADA
   C. AMA
   D. State government

2. A(n) _____ is a piece of office equipment that scans a document, translates the information, and transmits an exact copy of the original over telephone lines.
   A. e-mail
   B. postage meter
   C. fax machine
   D. personal digital assistant

3. A document that includes the length of a meeting, topics to be covered, their order, and the person responsible for each is called a(n) _____.
   A. itinerary
   B. agenda
   C. minutes
   D. memo

4. _____ goods are durable and expensive, and are expected to last a few years.
   A. Expendable
   B. Noncapital
   C. Capital
   D. None of the above

5. A(n) _____ is(are) documentation of physical assets and information that includes item description, date of purchase, and price.
   A. invoice
   B. inventory records
   C. packaging slip
   D. purchase order

6. _____ is the concept of maintaining the atmosphere of the physical environment of an office.
   A. Back ordering
   B. Safety stocking
   C. Facilities management
   D. Preventive maintenance

7. Which one of the following is the first step in organizing a meeting?
   A. Assemble materials needed for the meeting.
   B. Send reminder notices to all participants.
   C. Select a location and a meeting room.
   D. Prepare an agenda.

Copyright © 2010, 2005 by Saunders, an imprint of Elsevier, Inc. All rights reserved.

8. A(n) _____ contains specific instructions on how tasks are to be performed.
   A. policy manual
   B. procedure manual
   C. guidebook
   D. none of the above

9. Which one of the following is *not* needed to make travel arrangements for the physician?
   A. Dates of travel
   B. Mode of transportation
   C. Hotel reservations
   D. Allergies

10. _____ occurs when a sign-in sheet is used that requests the patient to identify the reason for their visit.
    A. Fraud
    B. Malfeasance
    C. Breach of contract
    D. Breach of confidentiality

11. Which one of the following is *not* a function of a medical office reception area?
    A. Provides a place to greet patients on their arrival
    B. Provides an area for patients to wait for provider
    C. Allows intake of patient information
    D. All are functions

12. To provide a comfortable reception area for patients, the temperature should not be more than _____ ° F.
    A. 64
    B. 68
    C. 70
    D. 73

13. Only artificial plants or flowers should be used in the patient waiting area.
    A. True
    B. False

14. A typical multiline telephone system has _____ buttons.
    A. three
    B. six
    C. nine
    D. none of the above

15. The _____ feature on the telephone calls the last number dialed.
    A. call forwarding
    B. conference calling
    C. privacy
    D. repeat call

16. The _____ calling feature on a telephone system allows the physician to have a three-way conversation with consulting physicians and patient's families.
    A. conference
    B. dedicated
    C. call forwarding
    D. caller ID

17. A(n) _____ is a business entity that handles patient calls during hours the medical practice is closed.
    A. voice mail
    B. answering service
    C. pager
    D. answering machine

18. _____ is the science of adjusting the work environment so that injuries will be prevented.
    A. Osteopathy
    B. Chiropractics
    C. Ergonomics
    D. None of the above

19. Mail that has been metered in the office takes longer to reach its destination.
    A. True
    B. False

20. Leased equipment cannot be sold because it is not owned by the practice.
    A. True
    B. False

25 Computers in the Medical Office

VOCABULARY REVIEW

Matching: Match each term with the correct definition.

A. boot up

B. cold boot

C. default

D. floppy disk

E. hard drive

F. host

G. ink-jet printer

H. Internet service provider

I. menus

J. motherboard

K. network

L. password

M. peripherals

N. prompt

O. read-only memory

P. search engine

Q. software

R. spreadsheet

S. touch screen

_____ 1. Productivity software that allows the computer user to work with facts and figures

_____ 2. Monitor that displays options that can be selected by touching them on the screen

_____ 3. List of commands or options, typically found on the top of the computer screen, that can be selected by the user

_____ 4. Computer system that scans and reads typewritten characters and converts them to digitized files

_____ 5. Term used to indicate that a computer system has been activated and is ready to use

_____ 6. External disk storage device that holds large amounts of data

_____ 7. Computers interconnected to exchange information

_____ 8. Main device in the computer used to store and retrieve information

_____ 9. External components attached to the computer, such as the speakers

_____ 10. Secondary storage device for computer data

_____ 11. "Intelligence" of a computer; tells the computer what to do; computer program

_____ 12. Company that provides a "host" access to the Internet

_____ 13. Uniform resource locator; Internet address

_____ 14. Starting the computer when it has been in "off" mode

_____ 15. Printer that produces characters and graphics by imprinting ink onto paper

T. tutorial

U. URL

V. warm boot

W. wizard

X. zip drive

Y. database management

Z. optical character recognition

_____ 16. Productivity software application that helps the user do calculations by entering numbers and formulas in a grid of rows and columns

_____ 17. Circuit board that contains memory chips; power supply, and vital components for processing data in the computer

_____ 18. Sequence of screens that direct the user to produce test-based documents

_____ 19. Selection or option automatically chosen by most computer programs if not directed by the user to do otherwise

_____ 20. Term used when the computer system has been on and must be restarted because it "freezes up"

_____ 21. Special set of characters known only to the user and the person who assigned the characters; designed to secure and protect unauthorized entry to a computer

_____ 22. Stored data that can be read but not changed

_____ 23. Self-guided step-by-step learning process that teaches generic skills needed to use software

_____ 24. Message displayed by the computer to request information or to help the user proceed

_____ 25. Specialized program designed to find specific information on the Internet

_____ 26. Computer that is the main computer in a system of connected terminals

THEORY RECALL

True/False

Indicate whether the statement is true or false.

_____ 1. Messages are transmitted over the Internet when a URL is entered into the browser.

_____ 2. The "motherboard" is an external component attached to the computer.

_____ 3. A 3.5-inch floppy disk holds more information than a CD-ROM.

_____ 4. Wizards are a sequence of screens that directs users through multiple steps to help them accomplish a desired task.

_____ 5. Word processing is a system of entering and editing text that requires interaction between a person and a computer.

CHAPTER 25 Computers in the Medical Office

Multiple Choice

Identify the letter of the choice that best completes the statement or answers the question.

1. A computer's function is to _____ data.
   A. input
   B. generate
   C. store
   D. all of the above

2. The OCR computer system _____ and reads typewritten data.
   A. saves
   B. scans
   C. distributes
   D. replies

3. _____ is(are) a system of entering and editing text that requires interaction between a person and a computer.
   A. PDF processing
   B. Spreadsheet
   C. Word processing
   D. Search engines

4. Hardware located outside of the computer is called _____.
   A. adjuncts
   B. peripherals
   C. accessories
   D. random memory

5. A major priority is to protect the hard drive. It is necessary to run a backup tape _____.
   A. daily
   B. weekly
   C. monthly
   D. bimonthly

6. _____ contains memory chips, power supply, and vital components for processing.
   A. Keyboard
   B. Monitor
   C. Motherboard
   D. Modems

7. _____ are rated by the size and number of dots or pixels.
   A. Scanners
   B. Monitors
   C. Laser printers
   D. None of the above

8. _____ copy is also known as a printed copy.
   A. Soft
   B. Hard
   C. Warm
   D. Cold

9. Browsers and websites contain _____ that allow a user to enter a topic or group of words into a text box to retrieve information or locate a website.
    A. Web addresses
    B. ISP numbers
    C. domain names
    D. search engines

10. _____ software aids in manipulating numerical data for financial management, such as for setting up a budget.
    A. Word processing
    B. Spreadsheet
    C. Data fields
    D. None of the above

11. A _____ is a device that transfers data from one computer to another over telephone or cable lines.
    A. motherboard
    B. scanner
    C. modem
    D. sound card

12. A _____ is a combination of letters and numbers that serves to identify the person using the computer.
    A. browser
    B. password
    C. user ID
    D. privacy code

13. _____ is the sum total of managing all of the facets of running a medical practice.
    A. Database management
    B. Practice management
    C. Employee management
    D. Financial management

14. _____ is a special set of numbers or characters or a combination of numbers and characters known only to the user.
    A. Browser
    B. Password
    C. User ID
    D. Privacy code

15. The "reports" feature of any practice management program allows the medical practice to manage all of the following *except* _____.
    A. cash flow
    B. budget
    C. patient schedules
    D. physician's personal finances

16. The _____ is the main device a computer uses to store and retrieve information.
    A. modem
    B. email
    C. hard drive
    D. soft drive

Copyright © 2010, 2005 by Saunders, an imprint of Elsevier, Inc. All rights reserved.

17. _____ contains instructions to the CPU on how to set itself up when the system is initially turned on.
    A. RAM
    B. ISP
    C. URL
    D. ROM

18. The _____ is the "brain" of the computer.
    A. URL
    B. CPU
    C. ISP
    D. RAM

19. When computers are interconnected to exchange information, it is referred to as a(n) _____.
    A. network
    B. scanner
    C. Internet
    D. wizard

20. A group of computers and other devices that are connected within the same building is called a(n) _____.
    A. WAN
    B. LAN
    C. WAR
    D. LAW

Sentence Completion

Complete each sentence or statement.

bit	wizards	CPU menu
read-only	wide area network	monitor
URL	point	
scanner	byte	
Internet service	toggle key	
provider (ISP)	random-access	

1. _____ memory is the read and write memory that a computer can use for storage, when the computer is working.

2. _____ is a group of computers and other devices that are connected between buildings, cities, and countries.

3. A(n) _____ uses a light source similar to a photocopier to copy a picture or document placed on its bed and send it through the modem or cable to the computer.

4. A(n) _____ is a company that provides a host access to the Internet.

5. In a word processing software program, font and _____ are the size and style of the typeface; number of characters per inch.

Short Answers

1. Describe the eight basic hardware parts of a computer.

   _____
   _____
   _____
   _____
   _____
   _____
   _____
   _____

2. Explain why menus were developed.

   _____
   _____
   _____
   _____

3. List three safeguards for protecting patient privacy.

   _____
   _____
   _____

4. List the four most common tasks of medical practice software.

CRITICAL THINKING

1. Explain how the central processing unit processes data.

2. Explain what the following keys represent:
   a. Esc _____
   b. function keys _____
   c. Home _____
   d. End _____
   e. toggle key _____
   f. shift _____

PRACTICAL APPLICATIONS

If you have accomplished the objectives in this chapter, you will be able to make better choices as a medical assistant. Take a look at this situation and decide what you would do.

Dr. Santos has just hired Terrell, a medical assistant, to transfer demographic and insurance data from the current paper records to the computerized patient accounting system. Terrell's assignment is to ensure that all the information on current patients is up to date in the computer, and that the latest updates and additions to the computer program are installed. As each new patient arrives at the office, Terrell has the duty of obtaining information for the data entry. He must ensure that the appointment has been scheduled into the computer so that medical notes and insurance information will be available as needed. Kate, an established patient, comes to the office and sees the new computer system in operation. Terrell explains that the office is becoming more technologically advanced, and that the computer will be used to schedule appointments, store transcription, and manage patient accounts in the future.

Would you be prepared to use the computer to perform data entry, scheduling, and other medical office tasks?

1. What functions would you expect to be accomplished by the computer?

2. What administrative tasks can be done on a computer?

3. What clinical tasks can be done on the computer?

4. How can a computer assist the health care professional who wants more information on uncommon diseases?

5. How is word processing used in a physician's office?

6. What is meant by "backing up" a computer? Why is backing up at the end of the day so important?

7. What are the three types of networks? Which would you expect to find in a small private practice? Which would you probably find in a medical practice that has multiple sites over a large area?

8. What is the importance of HIPAA in regard to computer use?

APPLICATION OF SKILLS

1. You are in charge of a local health clinic. You have been asked to submit a request for a microprocessor, related peripheral devices, and application software. The computer is to help with the clinic management duties. Itemize your request.

CHAPTER QUIZ

Multiple Choice

Identify the letter of the choice that best completes the statement or answers the question.

1. To safeguard data files of the medical practice, it is a good practice to back-up data _____.
   A. once a week
   B. monthly
   C. bimonthly
   D. daily

2. Hardware is the mechanical devices and physical components of a computer.
   A. True
   B. False

3. The _____ is the brain of the computer.
   A. CPU
   B. ROM
   C. RAM
   D. OCR

4. The _____ is a pointing device that can either be connected to the computer or be independent.
   A. mouse
   B. trackball
   C. touch pad
   D. all of the above

5. The _____ is the main device a computer uses to store and retrieve information.
   A. RAM
   B. hard drive
   C. CPU
   D. ROM

6. Floppy disks are currently about _____ inches square.
   A. 2½
   B. 3½
   C. 4½
   D. 5¼

7. _____ have high external storage capacity.
   A. Floppies
   B. CDs
   C. Zip drives
   D. ROMs

8. A printed copy is referred to as a _____.
   A. hard copy
   B. soft copy
   C. warm copy
   D. cold copy

9. Messages are transmitted over the Internet when a URL is entered into a browser.
   A. True
   B. False

10. _____ were developed to allow novice computer users to access various options without having to remember specific commands.
    A. Prompts
    B. Tutorials
    C. OCR computer systems
    D. Scanners

11. A wizard is a sequence of screens that directs the user through a multiuse software task.
    A. True
    B. False

12. A(n) _____ allow(s) computer users to enter a topic, word, or group of words into a textbox to locate information.
    A. ISP
    B. URL
    C. search engine
    D. comain name

13. _____ is a system of entering and editing text that requires interaction between a person and a computer.
    A. Spreadsheet
    B. Word processing
    C. Data
    D. None of the above

14. Practice management software can generate in-house reports of a patient's entire clinical history.
    A. True
    B. False

15. _____ protocol is the way computers exchange information over the Internet.
    A. ROM
    B. "http//:"
    C. "www."
    D. ISP address

16. Which one of the following is *not* a common Internet domain?
    A. ".edu"
    B. ".com"
    C. ".mcg"
    D. ".net"

17. Which one of the following is *not* a major consideration when purchasing practice management software?
    A. Physician's preference
    B. Office budget
    C. In-house training availability
    D. Whether it comes with built-in software games to relieve stress

18. Some practice management software programs can be purchased with fully loaded CPT codes.
    A. True
    B. False

19. Currently in medical practices, a _____ is used to back-up practice information.
    A. 3.5-inch floppy disk
    B. VHS tape
    C. CD-ROM
    D. hard drive

20. The purpose of a _____ is to store large amounts of related information, which allows multiple users to manipulate data for various purposes.
    A. word processing document
    B. spreadsheet
    C. database
    D. all of the above

NAME: _____   DATE: _____

26 Medical Office Communication

VOCABULARY REVIEW

Matching: Match each term with the correct definition.

A. autopsy report

B. certified mail

C. cluster scheduling

D. consultation report

E. discharge summary

F. double booking

G. established patient

H. full-block format

I. history and physical (H&P) report

J. matrix

K. medical practice information booklet

L. modified-block format

M. modified-wave scheduling

N. new patient

O. open-hour scheduling

P. operative report

Q. progress notes

R. registered mail

_____ 1. Appointment scheduling technique that schedules more than one patient during the same appointment time period

_____ 2. Appointment scheduling technique based on the theory that each patient visit will not require the allotted time

_____ 3. Special mail-handling method used when the contents have a declared monetary value

_____ 4. Appointment scheduling technique that groups several appointments for similar types of examination; also called categorization scheduling

_____ 5. Appointment scheduling technique that divides an hour block into average-appointment time slots

_____ 6. Booklet or brochure that provides nonmedical information for patients about standard office policies

_____ 7. Letter format in which all lines are flush with the left margin except the first line of new paragraph, date, closing, and signature (which are centered)

_____ 8. Medical report that lists a surgical procedure performed, any pathologic specimens, the findings, and the medical personnel involved

_____ 9. Appointment scheduling technique that provides a definite time period for the patient to be seen

_____ 10. Letter format that has all lines flush with the left margin

_____ 11. Medical report written by a specialist who sees a patient referred by a primary physician and then returns care to the primary physician

S. time-specified scheduling

T. wave scheduling

_____ 12. Appointment scheduling technique that allows patients to be seen without an appointment

_____ 13. Medical report that provides details about the cause of a person's illness and death through internal and external examination findings

_____ 14. Written findings of a patient's condition

_____ 15. Patient who has not received professional services from the physician or the medical office in the past 3 years

_____ 16. Medical report that provides a comprehensive review of a patient's hospital stay

_____ 17. Patient who has received professional services from the physician or the medical office in the past 3 years

_____ 18. Format used to mark off or reserve time in a schedule

_____ 19. Special mail-handling method used to prove an item was mailed and received

_____ 20. Medical report that consists of a patient's subjective and objective data

THEORY RECALL

True/False

Indicate whether the statement is true or false.

_____ 1. The HIPAA privacy rule allows for incidental disclosure of patient information as long as appropriate safeguards and rules are in place and followed.

_____ 2. Cluster scheduling is similar to wave scheduling, but instead of more than one patient being scheduled at the beginning of the hour, two patients are scheduled to see the physician at the same time.

_____ 3. A patient should be notified if they will be required to wait more than 20 minutes for the physician.

_____ 4. Mail should be arranged in order of importance and placed on the physician's desk.

_____ 5. The subject line of a business letter should be typed four lines below the salutation.

Multiple Choice

Identify the letter of the choice that best completes the statement or answers the question.

1. What is the purpose of the medical information booklet/brochure?
   A. Provides answers to nonmedical questions
   B. Outlines a treatment plan
   C. Provides the patient with a wound care instruction sheet
   D. None of the above

2. A medical assistant's/receptionist's voice should be _____ when answering the telephone.
   A. high-pitched and loud
   B. expressive but pleasant
   C. low-pitched and monotone
   D. none of the above

3. Of the following supplies, a(n) _____ is *not* necessary to answer the telephone efficiently.
   A. patient's chart
   B. message pad or notebook
   C. pen/pencil
   D. appointment book

4. Of the following, which ending of a telephone conversation is most appropriate?
   A. "Bye bye"
   B. "Talk to ya later"
   C. "Ciao"
   D. "Thank you for calling, Ms. Jones"

5. When speaking with a caller, a medical assistant should *never* _____.
   A. identify himself or herself
   B. use slang terms
   C. ask questions
   D. listen attentively

6. When placing a caller on hold, the medical assistant should _____.
   A. ask the caller if he or she minds being on hold for a moment and then wait for response
   B. say, "Just a minute," and put the caller on hold
   C. say, "I'm putting you on hold," and then push the hold button
   D. none of the above

7. Which one of the following is *not* a common type of call a medical assistant would receive on a routine basis?
   A. Emergency
   B. Payment or account balance information request
   C. Appointment
   D. Sales/telemarketing

8. Which one of the following would *not* be an acceptable outgoing telephone call a medical assistant would make as part of a routine day?
   A. Call to mother about dinner plans
   B. Call to make outpatient appointments
   C. Call to change or confirm a patient's appointment
   D. All of the above are calls a medical assistant would routinely make

9. Which medical office professional would professionally handle an incoming call regarding a patient who has been poisoned?
   A. Physician
   B. Medical assistant
   C. Medical administrative assistant
   D. Pharmaceutical sales representative

10. If another physician calls the office to speak to the physician, you should _____.
    A. take a message and send the message to the physician
    B. transfer the call to the clinical medical assistant
    C. transfer the call immediately to the physician in most circumstances
    D. none of the above

11. When an outside laboratory calls with laboratory test results, you should _____.
    A. transfer the call to the physician
    B. transfer the call to the individual requested by the laboratory
    C. transfer the call to the business office manager
    D. take a message and return the call later

12. If a patient "no-shows" an appointment, the medical assistant should _____.
    A. erase the patient's name so another patient can be scheduled
    B. write in ink next to the patient's name that the appointment was a no-show, and document the occurrence in the patient's chart
    C. do nothing
    D. never schedule the patient for another appointment

13. The appointment book is a legal document; the medical assistant must use only _____ to write in the appointment book.
    A. green ink
    B. red ink
    C. black ink
    D. pencil

14. When a new patient calls the office for an appointment, you need all of the following information except _____.
    A. name
    B. address
    C. employer's name
    D. purpose of the visit

15. _____ gives each patient an appointment for a definite period of time.
    A. Wave scheduling
    B. Open-hour scheduling
    C. Cluster scheduling
    D. None of the above

16. Practices that schedule half of their patients on the hour and the other half on the half-hour are using _____ scheduling.
    A. wave
    B. modified-wave
    C. cluster
    D. none of the above

17. _____ mail includes all sealed or unsealed letters up to and including 11 oz.
    A. First class
    B. Second class
    C. Third class
    D. Fourth class

18. Which class of mail is used to send journals and magazines?
    A. First class
    B. Second class
    C. Third class
    D. Fourth class

19. When mailing an item that has a declared monetary value and is being sent first class, it is sent as _____ mail.
    A. certified
    B. insured
    C. registered
    D. restricted

20. Which one of the following instructions describes how to fold a letter correctly for a size #10 envelope?
    A. Fold the letter in thirds face-up.
    B. Fold the letter in half and then into thirds face-down.
    C. Fold the letter in half face-up.
    D. Do not fold the letter.

21. Which one of the following instructions does *not* apply when addressing an envelope?
    A. Use single spacing and block format.
    B. Use correct punctuation.
    C. Use the two-letter abbreviation for states.
    D. Use only capital letters to start words throughout the address.

22. When using letterhead, the _____ contains the name and address with Zip code to whom the letter is written.
    A. salutation
    B. enclosure notation
    C. inside address
    D. copy notation

23. The _____ notation lists all of the people receiving the letter in addition to the addressee.
    A. enclosure
    B. copy
    C. reference
    D. salutation

24. Immediately after a surgical procedure, a(n) _____ is dictated by the surgeon about the procedure.
    A. H&P report
    B. consultation report
    C. pathology report
    D. operative report

Copyright © 2010, 2005 by Saunders, an imprint of Elsevier, Inc. All rights reserved.

CHAPTER 26 Medical Office Communication

25. A(n) _____ is a final progress note about a patient who is leaving the hospital.
    A. radiology report
    B. H&P report
    C. discharge summary
    D. pathology summary

26. A(n) _____ includes the preliminary diagnosis for a patient's cause of death.
    A. H&P report
    B. discharge summary
    C. progress note
    D. autopsy report

Sentence Completion

Complete each sentence or statement.

time zone	proofread	USPS website
telephone call	cluster	established patient
personal	matrix	appointment reminder
time specified	transcriptionist	card
abbreviations	manuscript	
business correspondence	memo	

1. Using _____ allows the medical assistant to indicate the reason for an appointment without writing out the reason using complete words and sentences.

2. A(n) _____ is any patient who has been seen in the past 3 years by the physician or provider in the practice.

3. A(n) _____ helps patients remember their next appointment and can be given to the patient at the end of their current appointment.

4. A second method of reminding a patient about their appointment is to give them a(n) _____.

5. The _____ is a great resource for familiarization of postal laws, regulations, and procedures.

6. Letters marked _____ are separated from other mail and delivered unopened to the person to whom they are addressed.

7. When you need to call a person or company in a different state, it is important to know in which _____ the person or company is located.

8. Most offices establish a _____ or develop some other format to block off time that is not to be used in patient scheduling.

9. In _____ scheduling, several appointments for similar types of examinations are grouped.

10. Before sending any written or keyed correspondence, you must _____ it to be certain the document is free of errors.

11. A(n) _____ is written for employees within the medical office setting to provide details about an upcoming event or meeting or to relay office policy decisions.

12. A(n) _____ is an article for a journal or other publication.

13. A(n) _____ is a person who listens to recorded dictation and converts it into a written document.

Short Answers

1. List the seven types of information documented when taking a telephone message.

_____

_____

_____

_____

_____

_____

_____

CHAPTER 26   Medical Office Communication

2. Why is it important to know the reason for a patient's office visit when making an appointment over the telephone?

   _____
   _____
   _____
   _____

3. Briefly describe the process of putting a caller on hold if more than one line is ringing.

   _____
   _____
   _____
   _____

4. List three pieces of information needed when scheduling an appointment for an established patient.

   _____
   _____
   _____
   _____

5. Explain how to accommodate a patient who is habitually late for appointments.

   _____
   _____
   _____
   _____

6. List and describe the steps involved in preparing outgoing mail.

   _____
   _____
   _____
   _____

Copyright © 2010, 2005 by Saunders, an imprint of Elsevier, Inc. All rights reserved.

7. List the basic guidelines for effective written correspondence.

   _____
   _____
   _____
   _____
   _____
   _____

8. You have been assigned to sort and open today's mail. List the steps you would follow.

   _____
   _____
   _____
   _____
   _____
   _____

9. List two complimentary closings in each of the following categories.

   Great respect: _____

   Formal: _____

   Less formal: _____

   Friendly: _____

CRITICAL THINKING

1. It has been an incredibly busy Monday, and the telephones have not stopped ringing. You currently have six callers on hold. Prioritize each caller by using a scale of 1 to 6, with 1 being the most important call to handle and 6 being the least important call to handle, and then write a brief summary of how each of the following callers should be handled.
   _____ a. Dr. Jacobs is on line 1 and is waiting to speak to the physician.
   _____ b. Hartley is on line 2 and would like to make an appointment for next month.
   _____ c. Sara Raphael is on line 3 and would like her prescription of Vicodin refilled as she is still in a lot of pain. This is her third refill request.
   _____ d. Porter is on line 4 and is calling to discuss his wife's pregnancy test results.
   _____ e. Caria Thopher is on line 5 with a personal call for the clinical medical assistant Grace.
   _____ f. The laboratory is on line 6 and would like to give someone test results.

2. You have been asked to explain the general office policies to a new patient. What key information would you cover?

   _____
   _____
   _____
   _____

3. Using the following information, decide how you would screen the incoming calls:

Health Care Member	Abbreviation	Responsibilities
Physician	P	Acute illness, hospital regarding current status of patient
Front Office Manager	FO	Appointments, consultation requests, pharmaceutical representatives
Back Office Manager	BO	Prescription refills, questions regarding current treatment
Insurance Specialist	IS	Billing and insurance information

_____ a. Patient has concerns about medication that the physician has prescribed.
_____ b. Insurance carrier requests information
_____ c. Pharmacy calls regarding prescription refill request
_____ d. Another physician calls and ask to speak to the physician
_____ e. Patient calls to report no relief from pain with current medication
_____ f. Patient calls for a copy of her records to be sent to another physician

PRACTICAL APPLICATIONS

If you have accomplished the objectives in this chapter, you will be able to make better choices as a medical assistant. Take a look at this situation and decide what you would do.

Tara is a new medical assistant at a physician's office. Dr. Vickers has hired her to answer the phone and to greet patients as they arrive, and to assist with making appointments as needed. On a particularly busy day, the phone is ringing with two lines already on hold, and a new patient arrives at the reception desk. Steve, the physician's assistant, asks Tara to make an appointment for another patient to see Dr. Vickers as soon as possible. Because the office makes appointments in a modified wave, Steve tells the patient to wait to be seen because Tara has found an opening in about a half hour. In all the confusion, Tara does not return to the patients who are on hold for several minutes, and one of the calls is an emergency. Tara is short-tempered with the new patient who has arrived at the office. Tara's frustration about the busy schedule she is expected to keep shows, and the new patient states that she is not sure that she has chosen the best physician's office for her medical care.

1. What effect will Tara's frustration have on this medical office? How would you have handled the situation differently?

_____

_____

2. Why is the role of the receptionist so important in putting a patient at ease?

_____

_____

3. When answering the phone, what are the voice qualities that are important in making a good impression?

_____

_____

4. What are the guidelines necessary in answering multiline calls?

5. What information should be obtained from a patient when making appointments?

6. Why is a patient information booklet important for a new patient?

7. What is modified-wave appointment scheduling? What are the problems with this type of scheduling?

8. What is double-booking scheduling? What are the dangers of double-booking?

9. How should Tara have handled the callers placed on hold?

APPLICATION OF SKILLS

Procedure Check-off Sheets (*) and assignments from MACC on the Evolve site at http://evolve.elsevier.com/klieger/medicalassisting (**)

1. Perform Procedure 26-1: Give Verbal Instructions on How to Locate the Medical Office.*
2. Perform Procedure 26-2: Create a Medical Practice Information Brochure.*
3. Perform Procedure 26-3: Answer a Multiline Telephone System.*
   A. MACC
      MACC/Administrative skills/General office duties/The telephone/Taking a telephone message**
      Practice taking two telephone messages
   B. Complete message form using information provided
4. Perform Procedure 26-4: Prepare and Maintain an Appointment Book.*
   A. MACC
      MACC/Administrative skills/General office duties/Appointments/Preparing and maintaining the appointment book
   B. Use a blank appointment page and information sheet to complete assignment
5. Perform Procedure 26-5: Schedule a New Patient.*
   A. MACC
      MACC/Administrative skills/General office duties/Appointments/Scheduling a new patient**
   B. Use a blank appointment page and information sheet to complete assignment
6. Perform Procedure 26-6: Schedule Outpatient and Inpatient Appointments.*
   A. MACC (Practice)
      MACC/Administrative skills/General office duties/Appointments/Scheduling an outpatient diagnostic test**
   B. MACC (Practice)
      MACC/Administrative skills/General office duties/Appointment/Scheduling an inpatient admission and an inpatient surgical procedure**
   C. Use surgical request forms to complete the assignments
7. Perform Procedure 26-7: Compose Business Correspondence.*
   A. MACC (Practice) MACC/Professionalism/Communication/Proofreading written correspondence**
   B. Use information sheet to complete assignment
8. Perform Procedure 26-8: Compose a Memo.*
   A. Use information sheet to complete assignment

CHAPTER QUIZ

Multiple Choice

Identify the letter of the choice that best completes the statement or answers the question.

1. A patient who has not been seen in the medical office for _____ is considered a new patient.
   A. 6 months
   B. 12 months
   C. 3 years
   D. 5 years

2. A letter that has all lines flush with the left margin except for the first line of a new paragraph and date, closing, and signature lines, is in _____ format.
   A. modified-block
   B. full-block
   C. abstract
   D. manuscript

3. A _____ is a document used for formal publication.
   A. matrix
   B. memo
   C. progress notes
   D. manuscript

4. A triage manual is important because it _____.
   A. helps the receptionist screen incoming calls and determine the level of urgency
   B. provides the receptionist with information about the practice's policies and services
   C. provides a list of routine questions to ask a patient scheduling an appointment
   D. none of the above

5. Which one of the following is *not* a piece of information you need to obtain when taking a telephone message?
   A. Caller's name
   B. Caller's telephone number
   C. Caller's date of birth
   D. Caller's message

6. In which one of the following types of schedules does every patient have an appointment for a definite time?
   A. Wave scheduling
   B. Time-specified scheduling
   C. Modified-wave scheduling
   D. Cluster scheduling

7. A _____ is used for interoffice communication.
   A. manuscript
   B. formal business letter
   C. memo
   D. journal

8. _____ help(s) the medical assistant see what needs to be corrected before sending out correspondence.
   A. Proofreader marks
   B. A dictionary
   C. Spell-check
   D. All of the above

9. _____ reports are initiated by the medical office before treatment begins.
   A. Radiology
   B. Consultation
   C. Discharge summary
   D. History and physical

10. _____ describes the surgical procedure and includes pathologic specimens, results, and personnel involved.
    A. H&P
    B. OP report
    C. Autopsy
    D. Discharge summary

11. _____ requires that someone listens to recorded information and produces the information in a written document.
    A. Dictation
    B. Proofreading
    C. Shorthand
    D. Transcription

12. _____ mail is used when it is necessary to prove that a letter was delivered.
    A. Registered
    B. Certified
    C. Express
    D. Overnight

13. _____ is(are) special services offered by the U.S. Postal Service and Western Union.
    A. Air mail
    B. Telegrams
    C. Mailgrams
    D. Express mail

14. If a patient calls the office with a question about an insurance payment, the _____ would typically handle the call.
    A. physician
    B. clinical medical assistant
    C. administrative medical assistant
    D. none of the above

15. _____ is the abbreviation used on the appointment book for a complete physical examination.
    A. CPE
    B. CPX
    C. CPR
    D. None of the above

16. The abbreviation S/R noted in the appointment book means the patient is being seen for _____.
    A. surgery
    B. superficial reattachment
    C. suture removal
    D. sinus/respiratory disorder

17. Scheduling in which more than one patient is booked for the same time slot on the schedule is called _____.
    A. cluster scheduling
    B. double booking
    C. modified-wave scheduling
    D. open-hour booking

18. Your physician just called the office; she is going to be 2 hours late to see patients this morning because of an emergency with a patient at the hospital. Which of the following is the best way to handle this situation?
    A. Call the scheduled patients, explain the situation, and offer to reschedule their appointment.
    B. Call the scheduled patients and explain the situation and that it would be best if they could arrive at their scheduled time, as it will be a first-come, first-serve basis when the physician arrives.
    C. Inform the patients of the delay, and ask them to wait patiently and offer them a beverage.
    D. None of the above

19. When scheduling a patient for a hospital admission, you must have a written order from the physician.
    A. True
    B. False

20. If the physician receives a letter marked "Personal," you should open it immediately, annotate it, and place on the physician's desk.
    A. True
    B. False

27 Medical Records and Chart Documentation

VOCABULARY REVIEW

Matching: Match each term with the correct definition.

A. acronym

B. active file

C. aging labels

D. caption

E. coding

F. conditioning

G. cross-reference

H. database

I. electronic medical record

J. filing

K. indexing

L. key unit

M. numerical filing

N. out guides

O. problem-oriented medical record

P. progress notes

Q. purge

R. SOAP

_____ 1. Patient medical records kept in a computer file; also called "paperless chart"

_____ 2. Data concerning a patient's medical care and its results

_____ 3. Method of filing that organizes records by their final digits

_____ 4. Words that describe the contents, name, or subject matter on a label

_____ 5. Method of arranging files using numbers

_____ 6. To clean out, as with excessive data in patient files

_____ 7. Type of chart format that divides each patient problem into subjective data, objective data, assessment, and plan for treatment

_____ 8. Process of removing staples and paper clips and mending a document before filing

_____ 9. Information source and storage

_____ 10. Separators that replace a file folder when it is removed from the file cabinet; contains a notation of the date and the name of who signed out the file

_____ 11. Arranging documents in a particular order for filing ease

_____ 12. Process of underlining a keyword to indicate how a document should be filed

_____ 13. Word formed from the first letter of several words

_____ 14. Chart format that is arranged according to a patient's health complaint

_____ 15. First unit to be filed

S. sorting

T. terminal-digit filing

_____ 16. Notification system showing a file stored in more than one place

_____ 17. Records of current patient

_____ 18. Process of determining how a record will be filed

_____ 19. Labels on a chart that identify the year

_____ 20. Process of putting documents in a folder

THEORY RECALL

True/False

Indicate whether the statement is true or false.

_____ 1. Medical records provide evidence of patient assessments, interventions, and communications.

_____ 2. Progress notes are a list of the current medications taken by the patient.

_____ 3. SOAP formatting is extremely advantageous when more than one physician is treating the patient because all information pertaining to a specific problem can be located in a concise format.

_____ 4. The proper method of correcting errors in a medical record is to use correction fluid and re-enter the correct information.

_____ 5. The caption on a file label is used to identify the contents of the file.

_____ 6. A patient can authorize a release of information over the telephone.

_____ 7. HIPAA is a federal law that protects the confidentiality of a patient's medical information.

_____ 8. A patient has a right to a copy of his or her medical records, including psychiatric records.

_____ 9. When a patient has a hyphenated name, it is considered two separate units.

_____ 10. Color coding of charts reduces misfiling.

Multiple Choice

Identify the letter of the choice that best completes the statement or answers the question.

1. The _____ process is the determination of how a record will be filed.
   A. indexing
   B. sorting
   C. annotating
   D. none of the above

Copyright © 2010, 2005 by Saunders, an imprint of Elsevier, Inc. All rights reserved.

2. In alphabetical filing, a _____ name is used as the key indexing unit.
   A. first
   B. middle
   C. last
   D. any of the above

3. Which of the following names would be filed before Mary Lynn Sommers?
   A. Mary Anne Winters
   B. M. Sorenson
   C. Mary Samuels
   D. Miriam Sommers

4. Which of the following names would be filed first?
   A. John Johnston
   B. Johnny Johnsten
   C. J. Jackson
   D. Jeremiah Jacobson

5. Which one of the following would be filed first?
   A. Professor Elijah Carlson
   B. President Eldon Anderson
   C. Congressman Elliason
   D. General George Franklin

6. _____ filing organizes a number by the final digits of the number.
   A. End-numeric
   B. Alpha-numeric
   C. First-digit
   D. None of the above

7. A file is "_____" when a checkmark is placed on the document indicating it should be filed.
   A. conditioned
   B. indexed
   C. sorted
   D. released

8. Inactive files are the files of a patient who has not visited the practice in _____.
   A. a time span set by the practice
   B. 1 year
   C. 3 years
   D. 7 years

9. A _____ is a reminder aid that organizes events by date.
   A. database file
   B. tickler file
   C. giggle file
   D. reminder file

10. Which one of the following files is *not* a standard form included in a patient record?
    A. Health history
    B. Consent to treatment
    C. Birth certificate
    D. Consent to disclose health information

11. If an established patient sees the physician for a _____, a new file must be made because the patient's complete health information would not be made available to an employer.
    A. pregnancy
    B. home-related injury
    C. work-related injury
    D. natural disaster

12. _____ regulations require providers to issue a written statement to each patient telling them about how the patient's health information may be used.
    A. HIPAA
    B. OSHA
    C. CLIA
    D. State

13. When initiating a file for a new patient, the first step in the procedure is to _____.
    A. create a file label
    B. attach alphabetical, color-coded labels
    C. attach an encounter form
    D. obtain and review a patient information form

14. If two patients have the exact same name, which of the following would determine which patient's file is filed first?
    A. Address
    B. Date of birth
    C. Social Security number
    D. The patient who has seen the physician more frequently

15. A _____ medical record is arranged according to the patient's health complaint.
    A. CCPH
    B. POMR
    C. SOAP
    D. none of the above

16. "My ankle hurts" is which one of the following types of information?
    A. Subjective
    B. Objective
    C. Assessment
    D. Plan

17. Which one of the following is "objective information"?
    A. There is swelling and bruising of the ankle and foot.
    B. The foot is hot to the touch.
    C. When the patient is walking to the examination room, you notice it is painful for the patient to put weight on the foot.
    D. All of the above is objective information.

18. All entries in a patient's record should begin with the _____.
    A. patient's name
    B. date of the encounter
    C. physician's signature
    D. none of the above

19. When choosing a filing system, the practice needs to consider all of the following *except* _____.
    A. available space
    B. potential volume of patients
    C. available budget
    D. what is esthetically pleasing

20. _____ has established rules to assist in efficient alphabetical filing.
    A. ARMA
    B. AAMA
    C. AHIMA
    D. None of the above

21. Which one of the following is a disadvantage to numerical filing?
    A. Expansion is unlimited.
    B. It is more confidential.
    C. It is easy to misfile.
    D. It is easy to remove inactive files.

22. The filing system that has stationary shelves and a door cover that slides up and back into a cabinet and can hold approximately 1000 records is a _____ file cabinet.
    A. vertical
    B. drawer
    C. lateral, open-shelf
    D. lateral, drawer

23. As computerization becomes increasingly sophisticated in medical offices, the use of electronic medical records is growing in popularity and will soon become the industry standard. Which one of the following is *not* an advantage of this type of system?
    A. All entries are legible.
    B. The record can be accessed by multiple practitioners at the same time.
    C. There is an inability to secure all records and maintain confidentiality.
    D. Printouts are easily retrieved.

24. _____ are dividers of a different size and color than a file folder. They should always be used when a file is removed from the storage system.
    A. Manila envelopes
    B. Out guides
    C. Book markers
    D. File labels

25. The _____ filing method uses letters of the alphabet to determine how files are arranged.
    A. Mendoza
    B. alphabetical
    C. numerical
    D. indexing

Sentence Completion

Complete each sentence or statement.

first	last	subjective
numerical	Social Security	Arabic
straight-number	number	numeric
tickler file	objective	
conditioning	prepositions	

1. _____ information is factual information and can be measured.

2. Professional titles, general titles, and professional numerical and seniority suffixes are always indexed _____.

3. _____, articles, conjunctions, and symbols are considered separate indexing units.

4. In the _____ filing method, patient files are given numbers and arranged in numerical sequence.

5. Because patient addresses may change frequently, most medical offices use the patient's date of birth or _____ rather than the address when two patient names are identical.

6. Numbers expressed in digit form are indexed before alphabetical letters or words and _____ are filed before Roman numerals.

7. Files that are filed using the _____ filing method are more likely to be misfiled, and a file list must be constantly updated and maintained.

8. _____ filing is the most common form of numerical filing.

9. _____ a file before being filed ensures the file is in good condition because all staples and paper clips are removed, and any torn edges are mended.

10. If the medical office does not have a computerized reminder system, it is an excellent idea for the medical assistant to create a(n) _____ about upcoming events such as license renewal, payments, and call-backs.

Copyright © 2010, 2005 by Saunders, an imprint of Elsevier, Inc. All rights reserved.

Short Answers

1. List the three steps for correcting an entry error in the patient's medical record.

2. State the three considerations for selecting a filing system.

3. Discuss the advantages and disadvantages of numerical filing.

4. Discuss the advantages and disadvantages of alphabetical filing.

5. List six supplies typically used with a filing system.

6. Explain the need to purge files regularly in a medical practice.

CRITICAL THINKING

1. Mr. Meredith called the office this morning inquiring about the status of laboratory results for his wife, Sharon. Sharon was seen last Friday in the office, and the laboratory results came in this morning. The laboratory reports have been filed in her patient file and are in a stack of files on Dr. Henry's desk for review. Describe how you would handle this call.

PRACTICAL APPLICATIONS

If you have accomplished the objectives in this chapter, you will be able to make better choices as a medical assistant. Take a look at this situation and decide what you would do.

Deanna is a new administrative medical assisting extern at Dr. Juanea's office. Shirley, the office manager, asks Deanna to prepare a file for a new patient who will be seen tomorrow in the office. Shirley tells Deanna to be sure that she has color-coded the file folder, and that the necessary forms have been included inside. In this office, the medical records are problem-oriented, and all records are SOAP format; both are new concepts to Deanna, who was taught to prepare source-oriented records. After Deanna has prepared the new patient's file, Shirley asks her to pull the necessary records for tomorrow's appointments from the lateral open-shelf file cabinet containing patient records filed in alphabetical order. As she pulls the records, Deanna is to annotate the patient list for tomorrow's schedule. With Shirley's assistance, Deanna will also purge the inactive patient records.

Would you be able to perform these tasks?

1. **Why is the medical record necessary? What are its uses?**

   _____
   _____
   _____
   _____

2. **What is meant by "color-coding" a patient file?**

   _____
   _____

3. **What forms should Deanna be sure are in the new record?**

   _____
   _____
   _____

4. **What is meant by problem-oriented medical records?**

   _____
   _____

Copyright © 2010, 2005 by Saunders, an imprint of Elsevier, Inc. All rights reserved.

5. What does SOAP mean?

6. What is a source-oriented patient record?

7. What are the advantages and disadvantages of open-shelf filing?

8. Why is alphabetical filing advantageous? What are the disadvantages?

9. What will Deanna do to annotate a patient list?

10. What is purging a file or a record? Why should patient records be purged on a regular basis?

APPLICATION OF SKILLS

1. Arrange the following patient names in the correct order based on the type of filing system mentioned:
   - Linda Fulmour 231232
   - Jon Ruger 626084
   - Cindy Kettle 312443
   - Reggie Clark 372764
   - Steve Marrow 545972

   A. File names alphabetically:

   _____
   _____
   _____
   _____
   _____

   B. File names using the straight digit filing method:

   _____
   _____
   _____
   _____
   _____

   C. File names using the terminal two digit filing method:

   _____
   _____
   _____
   _____
   _____

2. Identify whether the following is subjective (S) or objective (O) information.
   a. x-ray results _____
   b. complaints of dizziness and nausea _____
   c. weight loss of 5 lb since the patient's last visit _____
   d. patient's personal information (e.g., date of birth, address) _____
   e. clinical information about the patient (e.g., treatments, vital signs) _____

Copyright © 2010, 2005 by Saunders, an imprint of Elsevier, Inc. All rights reserved.

3. Use Box 27-4 for reference and practice charting the following information:
   a. Date: 9/7/20xx
      Vitals: T, 99° F; P, 90; R, 18; BP, 210/110 LA sitting, LA 190/100 standing
      Patient tells you he has had several nosebleeds over the last 2 days and a headache that will not go away even after he has taken multiple aspirin tablets.

      _____

      _____

      _____

      _____

   b. Date: 10/8/20xx
      Vitals: T, 98.2° F; P, 72; R, 18; BP, 150/90 LA sitting, 146/86 standing
      Patient is returning to see the physician for BP medication follow-up. Patient states he is feeling better since he has started taking the medication.

      _____

      _____

      _____

      _____

APPLICATION OF SKILLS

Procedure Check-off Sheets (*) and assignments from MACC on the Evolve site at http://evolve.elsevier.com/klieger/medicalassisting (**)

1. Perform Procedure 27-1: Pull Patient Records for a Manual Record System.*

2. Perform Procedure 27-2: Register a New Patient.*

3. Perform Procedure 27-3: Initiate a Patient File for a New Patient Using Color-Coded Tabs.*
   A. MACC/Administrative skills/General office duties/The medical record/Initiating a medical file for a new patient**(Practice)
      Set up and organize a medical file for a new patient that contains the personal data necessary for a complete record and any other information required by the medical office
   B. MACC (Practice)
      MACC/General office duties/The medical record/Color coding patient charts**

4. Perform Procedure 27-4: Add Supplementary Items to an Established Patient File.*
   A. MACC (Practice)
      MACC/Administrative skills/General office duties/The medical record/Adding supplementary items to established patient file**
      Add supplemental documents and progress notes to patient files, observing standard steps in filing, while creating an orderly file that facilitates ready reference to any item of information

Copyright © 2010, 2005 by Saunders, an imprint of Elsevier, Inc. All rights reserved.

5. Perform Procedure 27-5: Maintain Confidentiality of Patients and Their Medical Records.*
   A. MACC (Practice)
      MACC/Administrative skills/General office duties/The medical record/Preparing a record release form**

6. Perform Procedure 27-6: File Medical Records Using the Alphabetical System.*
   A. MACC (Practice)
      MACC/Administrative skills/General office duties/The medical record/Filing medical records using the alphabetical system**
      Correctly file a set of patient charts, using an established alphabetical filing system

7. Perform Procedure 27-7: File Medical Records Using the Numerical System.*
   A. MACC (Practice)
      MACC/Administrative skills/General office duties/The medical record/Filing medical charts using the numerical system**
      Correctly file a set of patient charts, using an established numerical filing system

CHAPTER QUIZ

Multiple Choice

Identify the letter of the choice that best completes the statement or answers the question.

1. _____ is a method of arranging files using straight numbers.
   A. Alphabetical filing
   B. Numerical filing
   C. Terminal digit filing
   D. Problem-oriented filing

2. _____ is the process of determining how a record will be filed.
   A. Conditioning
   B. Indexing
   C. Coding
   D. Purging

3. Word(s) that describe the content's name or subject matter on a label is called _____.
   A. acronym
   B. key unit
   C. cross-reference
   D. caption

4. _____ is a chart format that uses dividers to separate the different types of patient information.
   A. Problem-oriented medical record format
   B. Electronic medical record format
   C. Source-oriented format
   D. None of the above

5. A type of chart format that divides each patient problem into subjective data, objective data, assessment, and plan for treatment is _____.
   A. SOAP
   B. POMR
   C. SOBP
   D. WRI

Copyright © 2010, 2005 by Saunders, an imprint of Elsevier, Inc. All rights reserved.

6. A _____ is entered into the patient's record and is used to update the status of the patient's health. These are added to the patient's chart each time the patient visits the office.
   A. problem list
   B. tickler file
   C. progress note
   D. caption

7. The physician owns the medical record, but the patient owns the information.
   A. True
   B. False

8. When might a medical assistant use a patient's date of birth as an indexing unit for filing?
   A. Never
   B. When two patients have the same name and same address
   C. When two patients have the same name but different addresses
   D. When a patient does not have a permanent address

9. Which one of the following names would be filed first?
   A. Lolita Gonzales
   B. Edward Green III
   C. Cleo Gonzales Esq.
   D. Juanita Esperanza

10. Which one of the following names would be filed second?
    A. Lolita Gonzales
    B. Edward Green III
    C. Cleo Gonzales Esq.
    D. Juanita Esperanza

11. Which one of the following names would be filed first?
    A. Aurelia Hunter
    B. Laura Hinkleman
    C. Sister Mary Catherine
    D. Kimberly Edades

12. Which one of the following names would be filed first?
    A. Timothy O'Shea
    B. Simon Samuelson
    C. Kelly Sherwin
    D. Belinda deLarue

13. Professional titles and professional, numerical, and seniority suffixes are always indexed _____.
    A. first
    B. second
    C. last
    D. does not matter

14. Which one of the following is a charting *"don't"*?
    A. Chart anything you did not see or do.
    B. Use black ink because it is easier to photocopy.
    C. Verify the name on the file before charting.
    D. All of the above are *"don'ts"*.

15. Which one of the following is *not* part of the decision when selecting a filing system?
    A. Selection of supplies
    B. Types of storage equipment
    C. Available space
    D. All of the above would be considered when selecting a filing system.

16. In which filing system are records more protected in case of fire?
    A. Lateral-open shelf
    B. Vertical-drawer
    C. Rotary
    D. Lateral-drawer

17. _____ filing is most commonly used in small to medium-sized offices.
    A. Alphabetical
    B. Numerical
    C. Terminal-digit
    D. Geographical

18. Which one of the following is a disadvantage of direct filing?
    A. The correct spelling of the name must be known to find a folder.
    B. Alphabetical filing is the easiest system to learn.
    C. Only one sorting is required.
    D. None of the above is a disadvantage of direct filing.

19. All punctuation is disregarded when indexing personal and business names.
    A. True
    B. False

20. When filing, the first name of the patient is considered the key unit.
    A. True
    B. False

28 Financial Management

VOCABULARY REVIEW

Matching: Match each term with the correct definition.

A. accounting

B. accounts receivable

C. aging report

D. asset

E. balance sheet

F. credit

G. daysheet

H. debit

I. deposit

J. employee's withholding allowance certificate

K. endorse

L. exemption

M. financial statements

N. gross wages

O. income statement

P. liability

Q. net income

R. nonsufficient funds

_____ 1. Amount of money not able to be collected

_____ 2. Amount remaining after liabilities are subtracted from assets

_____ 3. Writing a check using a future date, so that check can be deposited only after the date on check

_____ 4. State of a checkbook and a bank statement being in balance

_____ 5. To sign or place a signature on the back of a check that transfers the rights of ownership of funds

_____ 6. Report that shows how long debt has gone unpaid

_____ 7. Reports that indicate the financial condition of a business

_____ 8. Money placed in an account of a financial institution

_____ 9. Form that each new employee fills out to declare exemption from tax withholdings for earnings

_____ 10. Recording system using a specially designed document device for the increased efficiency of recording daily transactions; also called one-write system

_____ 11. Total amount of money earned by employee before deductions are taken

_____ 12. Financial activity of a business

_____ 13. Indication that the payer did not have adequate funds in the bank to cover the amount of a check written

_____ 14. Numerical language of business that describes its activities

_____ 15. Record of patient transactions showing an amount due

_____ 16. Reports showing the results of income and expenses over time

S. one-write system

T. owner's equity

U. payable

V. payroll

W. pegboard system

X. postdated

Y. reconciled

Z. statement of owner's equity

AA. T-account

BB. third-party check

CC. transaction

DD. write-off

_____ 17. Another name for pegboard system

_____ 18. Amount owed; debt

_____ 19. Employees' salaries, wages, bonuses, net pay, and deductions

_____ 20. Amount representing a payment; recorded on the right side of an accounting sheet

_____ 21. Amount of money earned that is not taxable

_____ 22. Resulting figure when income is greater than expenditures

_____ 23. Anything of value owned by a business that can be used to acquire other items

_____ 24. Amount representing a charge or debt owed; recorded on the left side of a T-account

_____ 25. Representing liability; accounts payable are money and funds owed to someone else

_____ 26. Check signed over to another party, who is not the original payee

_____ 27. Report on the financial condition of a business on a certain date

_____ 28. Journal for recording the day's activities

_____ 29. Tool used to analyze the effect of a transaction on an account

_____ 30. Report that shows changes in the owner's financial interest over time

THEORY RECALL

True/False

Indicate whether the statement is true or false.

_____ 1. A write-off is done when a portion or the entire amount of the charges cannot be collected.

_____ 2. The statement-receipt is a charge form that lists the ICD-9 and CPT codes most frequently used in the medical practice.

_____ 3. Checks marked paid in full should not be accepted unless the amount covers the entire current balance.

_____ 4. Bookkeeping is the basic process of recording the financial activities of the business.

_____ 5. The income statement reports the changes in the owner's financial interest during a reporting period, and gives an explanation on why the investment has changed.

Copyright © 2010, 2005 by Saunders, an imprint of Elsevier, Inc. All rights reserved.

Multiple Choice

Identify the letter of the choice that best completes the statement or answers the question.

1. The legislation requiring a disclosure statement informing a patient of a procedure's total cost, including finance charges, which is required when a patient will make more than four payments, is called _____.
   A. Federal Insurance Contributions Act
   B. Federal Truth in Lending Act
   C. Federal Employees' Compensation Act
   D. Federal Unemployment Act

2. A(n) _____ is when money is prepared and sent to a financial institution to be placed in an account.
   A. deposit
   B. ABA number
   C. endorsement
   D. debit

3. _____ are sometimes given to other health care professionals and their families.
   A. Adjustments
   B. Professional discounts
   C. Write-offs
   D. Exemptions

4. Payroll is the financial record of employees' _____.
   A. salaries
   B. wages
   C. deductions
   D. all of the above

5. A(n) _____ is the amount of an individual's earnings that is exempt from income taxes based on the number of dependents.
   A. deduction
   B. exemption
   C. withholding
   D. none of the above

6. The total earnings paid to an employee after payroll taxes and other deductions have been taken is called _____.
   A. salary
   B. net pay
   C. wages
   D. all of the above

7. The legislation that provides funds to support retirement benefits, dependents of retired workers, and disability benefits is called _____.
   A. Federal Insurance Contribution Act
   B. Federal Unemployment Tax Act
   C. Federal Employees' Compensation Act
   D. none of the above

8. _____ acts as a journal for recording the day's activities.
   A. Daysheet
   B. Pegboard
   C. Ledger card
   D. Payroll register

9. _____ contains demographics about the patient and important billing information.
   A. Daysheet
   B. Pegboard
   C. Ledger card
   D. None of the above

10. _____ is a fixed fee that is paid by the patient at each office visit.
    A. Co-insurance
    B. Co-payment
    C. Restrictive endorsement
    D. None of the above

11. A(n) _____ shows the results of income and expenses over time, usually a month or year.
    A. balance sheet
    B. financial statement
    C. income statement
    D. accounts payable statement

12. A(n) _____ are reports that tell the owner the fiscal condition of the practice.
    A. balance sheet
    B. financial statement
    C. income sheet
    D. none of the above

13. A(n) _____ fund is an amount of cash kept on hand that is used for making small payments for incidental supplies.
    A. gross wages
    B. owner's equity
    C. petty cash
    D. none of the above

14. _____ is a document indicating the activity in an account.
    A. Statement-receipt
    B. Statement of ownership
    C. Statement
    D. Superbill

15. The _____ is also known as the Wage and Hour Law.
    A. Social Security law
    B. Fair Labor Standards Act
    C. Tax Payment Act
    D. Federal Unemployment Act

CHAPTER 28 Financial Management

16. The _____ requires employers not only to withhold income tax and pay it to the IRS, but also to keep accurate records of the names, addresses, and Social Security numbers of individuals employed.
    A. Social Security law
    B. Federal Labor Standards Act
    C. Tax Payment Act
    D. Federal Unemployment Act

17. Federal law requires _____ to be deducted from the employee's gross pay.
    A. Social Security tax
    B. Medicare tax
    C. federal income tax
    D. all of the above

18. _____ is(are) part of the accounting equation.
    A. Assets
    B. Liabilities
    C. Owner's equity
    D. All of the above

19. In T-accounts, the left side is also known as a(n) _____.
    A. asset
    B. credit
    C. debit
    D. equity

20. _____ is the listing of a physician's charges for service.
    A. Balance sheet
    B. Fee schedule
    C. Ledger cards
    D. None of the above

Sentence Completion

Complete each sentence or statement.

bookkeeping	owner's equity	nonsufficient
net income	accounting	funds
income statement	balance sheet	encounter form
adjustment	creditor	voucher
assets	deposit slip	
	debtor	

1. _____ is considered the "language" of business.

2. _____ reports the financial condition of a medical practice on a given date.

3. When a patient does not have enough money in his or her bank account, it will be returned for _____.

4. _____ is a person owing a debit.

5. _____ is also known as a superbill.

6. The resulting figure when income is greater than expenditures is called _____.

7. _____ is a paper showing the date, amount of transaction, what was purchased, and who purchased the item.

8. _____ is the listing of all cash and checks to be deposited to a certain account of a business's financial institution.

9. The amount remaining after the liabilities are subtracted from the assets is called _____.

10. A(n) _____ is an amount that is added or subtracted from the physician's fee, changing the patient's account balance.

Short Answers

1. List and explain the three important accounting principles.

   _____
   _____
   _____
   _____
   _____

2. Define bookkeeping.

   _____
   _____
   _____
   _____
   _____

Copyright © 2010, 2005 by Saunders, an imprint of Elsevier, Inc. All rights reserved.

3. Compare and contrast bookkeeping and accounting.

4. Explain the difference between accounts receivable and accounts payable.

5. Explain the two major purposes for using the pegboard system.

6. List the five verifications you must make to accept a check.

7. Explain in detail the four types of endorsements.

8. Explain the four types of billing cycles.

9. List and describe the various financial statements.

10. Describe the impact of the Fair Debt Collections Act and the Federal Truth in Lending Act of 1968 as they apply to collections.

11. List the different types of adjustments that can be made to a patient's account.

CRITICAL THINKING

1. You started working for Dr. Palmer 2 weeks ago as the administrative medical assistant. Dr. Palmer asked you this morning to create a list of all the patients with an outstanding balance on their account, determine which accounts are overdue, and send collection letters to all patients with an outstanding account balance more than 120 days. You determine that only one account, Marjory Kreswin, has an outstanding balance more than 120 days past due. Draft a collection letter stating that she has 10 days to bring the balance current or you will be required to send her account to a collection agency.

PRACTICAL APPLICATIONS

If you have accomplished the objectives in this chapter, you will be able to make better choices as a medical assistant. Take a look at this situation and decide what you would do.

Meredith is the office manager for a private physician. She is responsible for the financial management of the office. She is the person who tracks the assets and liabilities for the accountant and interprets "owner equity" so that the physician will know the net value of the practice. As part of her job description, Meredith also disburses petty cash. She ensures that the vouchers, with receipts attached, and the cash on hand balance at the end of each workday. As each patient leaves the office, the payments for office visits are collected. The goal is to collect whatever is necessary from patients (co-payment, co-insurance) on the day of service. If patient receivables are current, outstanding insurance claims become the main focus for accounts receivable. Another one of Meredith's duties is to approve or disapprove of professional discounts and write-offs as fee adjustments. Finally, she generates collection letters and telephone calls for overdue and delinquent accounts.

Would you be able to perform these responsibilities in the medical office?

1. What are assets? What are liabilities?

   _____
   _____
   _____
   _____

2. Why is it important for a physician to be aware of the owner equity before spending money for new equipment?

   _____
   _____
   _____
   _____

3. What is petty cash, and how is it used by the medical office?

   _____
   _____
   _____

Copyright © 2010, 2005 by Saunders, an imprint of Elsevier, Inc. All rights reserved.

4. Why is it important for Meredith to complete a petty cash voucher each time that money is removed from the petty cash fund?

5. Why is it important to keep accounts receivable at a low level?

6. What are professional discounts?

7. What is a write-off?

8. How should a collection phone call be handled?

APPLICATION OF SKILLS

Procedure Check-off Sheets (*) and assignments from MACC on the Evolve site at http://evolve.elsevier.com/klieger/medicalassisting (**)

1. Perform Procedure 28-1: Manage an Account for Petty Cash.*
    A. MACC (Practice)
       MACC/Administrative skills/Financial management/Accounts receivable and payable/Accounting for petty cash**
          Establish a petty cash fund, maintain an accurate record of expenditures, and replenish the fund as necessary

2. Perform Procedure 28-2: Post Service Charges and Payments to the Patient's Account.*
   A. MACC
      MACC/Administrative skills/Financial management/Accounts receivable and payable/Posting service charges and payments using a pegboard**
         Post service charges and payments using a daysheet

3. Perform Procedure 28-3: Record Adjustments and Credits to the Patient's Account.*
   A. MACC/Administrative skills/Financial management/Accounts receivable and payable/Posting service charges and payments using a daysheet** (continued from Procedure 28-2 screens 18-55)

4. Perform Procedure 28-4: Prepare a Bank Deposit.*
   A. MACC (Practice)
      MACC/Administrative skills/Financial management/Banking/Preparing a bank deposit**
         Correctly prepare a bank deposit for the day's receipts, and complete appropriate office records related to the deposit

5. Perform Procedure 28-5: Reconcile a Bank Statement.*
   A. MACC (Practice)
      MACC/Administrative skills/Financial management/Banking/Reconciling a bank statement**
         Correctly reconcile a bank statement with the checking account

6. Perform Procedure 28-6: Explain Professional Fees before Services Are Provided.*

7. Perform Procedure 28-7: Establish Payment Arrangements on a Patient Account.*

8. Perform Procedure 28-8: Explain a Statement of Account to a Patient.*
   A. MACC (Practice)
      MACC/Administrative skills/Financial management/Billing and collection/Explaining professional fees**
         Explain the physician's fees so that the patient understands his or her obligations

9. Perform Procedure 28-9: Prepare Billing Statements and Collecting Past-Due Accounts.*
   A. MACC (Practice)
      MACC/Administrative skills/Financial management/Billing and collections/Preparing monthly billing statements**
         Process monthly statements, and evaluate accounts for collection procedures

CHAPTER QUIZ

Multiple Choice

Identify the letter of the choice that best completes the statement or answers the question.

1. _____ is an amount owed by the medical practice.
   A. Asset
   B. Liability
   C. Owner's equity
   D. None of the above

2. _____ reports the changes in the owner's financial interest during a reporting period and why the interest has changed.
   A. Bank statement
   B. Financial statement
   C. Income statement
   D. Statement of owner's equity

3. _____ is a special device used to write the same information on several forms at one time.
   A. Daysheet
   B. Encounter form
   C. Pegboard
   D. None of the above

4. _____ is a charge form that lists the ICD-9 and CPT codes most frequently used in medical practices.
   A. Receipt-charge slip
   B. Encounter form
   C. Superbill
   D. B and C

5. _____ is collected to support the federal health insurance program for people 65 years old and older.
   A. FUTA
   B. FICA
   C. Medicare tax
   D. SUTA

6. The Wage and Hour Law is also known as the Fair Labor Standards Act.
   A. True
   B. False

7. _____ records debit and credit activity of a patient in the practice.
   A. Financial statement
   B. Income statement
   C. Ledger card
   D. None of the above

8. _____ is a numbered form used to track petty cash withdrawals.
   A. Transaction
   B. Ledger
   C. Voucher
   D. All of the above

9. The pegboard system is also known as the one-write system.
   A. True
   B. False

10. An AR report that is beneficial to the financial success of the medical practice is called the _____ report.
    A. aging
    B. financial
    C. summary
    D. none of the above

Copyright © 2010, 2005 by Saunders, an imprint of Elsevier, Inc. All rights reserved.

11. _____ is a fixed percentage of a medical cost, paid by the patient.
    A. Co-pay
    B. Co-insurance
    C. A and B
    D. Neither A nor B

12. _____ is(are) part of the accounting equation.
    A. Assets
    B. Liabilities
    C. Owner's equity
    D. All the above

13. _____ endorsement is a type of endorsement in which only a signature is listed on the back of the check.
    A. Blank
    B. Restrictive
    C. Qualified
    D. None of the above

14. The amount recorded on the right side of the T-account is called a debit.
    A. True
    B. False

15. _____ contains demographics about the patient and important billing information.
    A. Financial statement
    B. Ledger cards
    C. Encounter forms
    D. None of the above

16. When accepting a check for payment, you must verify _____.
    A. current address
    B. correct provider name
    C. affixed signature
    D. all of the above

17. The ABA number _____.
    A. helps to identify the payer's bank
    B. is located on the right corner of each check
    C. helps to identify the location of the bank
    D. all the above

18. Federal law requires _____ to be deducted from a person's gross pay.
    A. SUTA
    B. Medicare tax
    C. medical insurance premiums
    D. none of the above

19. Total earnings paid to an employee after payroll taxes and other deductions have been taken out is called gross pay.
    A. True
    B. False

20. Accounting is considered the language of business.
    A. True
    B. False

29 Medical Coding

VOCABULARY REVIEW

Matching: Match each term with the correct definition.

A. acute

B. chief complaint

C. concurrent condition

D. contributory factors

E. diagnosis

F. eponym

G. established patient

H. guidelines

I. instructional terms

J. key components

K. main term

L. medical decision making

M. medical necessity

N. morbidity rate

O. new patient

P. pertinent past, family, and social history

Q. presenting problem

R. primary diagnosis

S. referral

T. review of systems

_____ 1. Condition considered as the patient's major health problem; used in outpatient coding

_____ 2. Occurring over the long-term or recurring frequently

_____ 3. *ICD-9-CM* supplementary codes for factors influencing health status and reasons for contact with health services when a diagnosis needs further explanation, or when the patient has no disease process for coding

_____ 4. Rules that determine items necessary to interpret and report procedures and services appropriately

_____ 5. Issues that affect a decision

_____ 6. Disease, condition, noun, synonym, or eponym that helps the coder find the correct code or range of codes in an index

_____ 7. *ICD-9-CM* supplementary codes for external causes of injury and poisoning

_____ 8. Person who has not received professional services from the physician, or another physician of the same specialty, who belongs to the same group practice, within the past 3 years

_____ 9. Three main factors taken into account when selecting a level of E/M service in CPT coding

_____ 10. Transfer of a patient's care to another health care provider at the request of a member of the health care team

_____ 11. Occurring now; of short-term duration

_____ 12. Approach to managing a patient's care when a provider asks other health care providers to assist

_____ 13. That which is reasonable and necessary for the diagnosis or treatment of illness or injury, or to improve the function of a malformed body member

U. secondary condition

V. subjective findings

W. E-codes

X. V-codes

Y. chronic

Z. coordination of care

AA. history of present illness

BB. modifier

CC. greatest specificity

DD. principal diagnosis

_____ 14. Chronological description of the patient's present illness from the first sign or symptom to the present

_____ 15. Pertinent background information about a patient's family and the patient visiting a health care provider

_____ 16. Condition that occurs at the same time as the primary diagnosis and affects the patient's treatment or recovery from the primary condition

_____ 17. Rate of disease or illness or proportion of diseased individuals in a given population or location

_____ 18. Condition the patient experiences at the same time as the primary diagnosis

_____ 19. Statement in the patient's own words describing the reason for the office visit; should be documented in the patient's words

_____ 20. Information provided by the patient and generally not measurable by health care professionals

_____ 21. Determination of the nature of a disease based on signs, symptoms, and laboratory findings

_____ 22. Symptoms, disease, or condition that is currently causing a problem, and that is the reason for the patient visiting a health care provider

_____ 23. Individual who has been treated by a physician or another physician of the same specialty who belongs to the same group practice in the past 3 years

_____ 24. How the physician looks at all the information gathered on examining and testing the patient, and then factors this into a decision for a treatment plan

_____ 25. Inventory of body systems obtained through a series of questions seeking to identify signs and symptoms that the patient may be experiencing or has experienced

_____ 26. Words or phrases that have a special meaning to provide needed information

_____ 27. Person or persons for whom something has been named, or the name is so derived

_____ 28. Means by which the reporting physician can indicate a service or procedure performed has been altered by some specific circumstance, but its definition or code has not changed

_____ 29. Coding to the highest level of documentation available; not using only a 3-digit code when a 4-digit or 5-digit code exists to describe the disease or procedure better

_____ 30. Diagnosis, determined after study, that was the cause for a patient's hospital admission; used only for inpatient coding

THEORY RECALL

True/False

Indicate whether the statement is true or false.

_____ 1. "Diagnosis" is defined as determining the nature of a disease based on signs, symptoms, and laboratory findings.

_____ 2. A primary diagnosis is the condition established to be chiefly responsible for triggering the admission of the patient to the hospital for treatment.

_____ 3. CPT stands for Current Procedural Terminology.

_____ 4. The chief complaint is a statement usually made by the patient in his or her own words that describes the reason for the visit.

_____ 5. The U.S. National Center for Health Services is used to track mortality and morbidity rates.

Multiple Choice

Identify the letter of the choice that best completes the statement or answers the question.

1. Volume _____ of the *ICD-9-CM* is a numerical listing of the diseases and injury codes and consists of 17 chapters.
   A. 1
   B. 2
   C. 3
   D. 4

2. Volume _____ of the *ICD-9-CM* is included when it will be used specifically for hospital coding.
   A. 1
   B. 2
   C. 3
   D. 4

3. The first *CPT Manual* appeared in _____.
   A. 1956
   B. 1966
   C. 1976
   D. none of the above

Copyright © 2010, 2005 by Saunders, an imprint of Elsevier, Inc. All rights reserved.

4. _____ is a key component in a determination of the level of E/M service to be selected.
   A. History
   B. Examination
   C. The difficulty of medical decision making
   D. All of the above

5. Volume _____ of the *ICD-9-CM* consists of an alphabetical listing of terms and codes.
   A. 1
   B. 2
   C. 3
   D. 4

6. _____ provide a classification of environmental events, circumstances, and conditions as the cause of injury, poisoning, and other adverse effects.
   A. E-codes
   B. V-codes
   C. *ICD-9-codes*
   D. *CPT-codes*

7. _____ owns and publishes the disease classification and releases an updated version of *ICD* about every 10 years.
   A. London Bills of Mortality
   B. World Health Organization
   C. Health Insurance Portability and Accountability
   D. None of the above

8. _____ is a type of examination.
   A. Comprehensive
   B. Detailed
   C. Problem focused
   D. All of the above

9. _____ is a type of medical decision making.
   A. High complexity
   B. Straightforward
   C. Moderate complexity
   D. All of the above

10. A medical record must include _____.
    A. the nature of the problem
    B. the appropriate amount of time spent with the patient
    C. A and B
    D. neither A nor B

11. In _____, the U.S. Congress passed the Medical Catastrophic Coverage Act.
    A. 1937
    B. 1948
    C. 1988
    D. 2000

12. A _____ is a disorder that is affecting the patient at the same time as the primary diagnosis, but is not necessarily affecting the prognosis of the primary condition.
    A. concurrent condition
    B. secondary condition
    C. systemic condition
    D. none of the above

13. The _____ is used by hospitals and allows for four concurrent conditions, ranked in the order of severity.
    A. CMS 1500
    B. UB-92
    C. A and B
    D. neither A nor B

14. Volume _____ codes of the *ICD-9-CM* represent the means for the hospital to receive reimbursement for its facility overhead.
    A. 1
    B. 2
    C. 3
    D. 4

15. Effective diagnostic and procedural coding requires _____.
    A. a good knowledge of terminology
    B. familiarity with the *ICD-9* and *CPT*
    C. discipline to read all explanations from medical records
    D. all of the above

Sentence Completion

Complete each sentence or statement.

subcategories	category III	appendices
present illness	titles	new patient
chief complaint	red	CPT
guidelines	bold	counseling
mortality	history	

1. The _____ code manual lists and describes codes for services and procedures.

2. _____ codes are temporary codes used for new technology, services, and procedure.

3. _____ requires the health care provider to render a service at the request of another health care professional, such as a second opinion.

4. The _____ is whatever symptoms, illness, or injury is causing the encounter.

Copyright © 2010, 2005 by Saunders, an imprint of Elsevier, Inc. All rights reserved.

5. _____ is death from a particular disease.

6. In CPT Volume 1, all titles and codes are printed in _____.

7. _____ are groups of 4-digit code numbers listed after 3-digit categories.

8. _____ is information regarding past events.

9. _____ are additional information segments related to coding.

10. A(n) _____ is a patient who has not received any professional services from the physician, or another physician of the same specialty, who belongs to the same group practice, within the past 3 years.

Short Answers

1. List six agencies and organizations that use *ICD-9-CM* codes.

   _____

   _____

   _____

2. Explain what "main term" means, and list four items represented by main terms in *ICD-9-CM* coding.

   _____

   _____

   _____

   _____

3. Explain the purpose of the *ICD-9-CM* system.

   _____

   _____

   _____

4. Explain three factors that must be determined before the process of E/M coding begins.

5. Explain what a "special report" should include.

CRITICAL THINKING

1. Dr. Peterson has asked you to update her family practice's superbill with new diagnostic and procedure codes. She handed you the following list and would like you to have it completed by the end of the day.
    A. Locate the procedure codes for the following:
    - Office Visits—New Patient
      Problem focused/straightforward decision making
      Expanded focused/straightforward decision making
      Detailed/low complexity decision making
      Comprehensive/moderate complexity decision making
      Comprehensive/high complexity decision making
    - Office Visits—Established Patient
      Nurse visit
      Problem focused/straightforward decision making
      Expanded focus/low complexity decision making
      Detailed/moderate complexity decision making
      Comprehensive/high complexity decision making
    - Office Consultations
      Problem focused
      Expanded focused
      Detailed
      Comprehensive/moderate complexity
      Comprehensive/high complexity
    - Injections
      Trigger point/one to two muscles
      Arthrocentesis, small joint
      Arthrocentesis, large joint
    - Office Procedures
      ECG
      Cerumen removal
      Nebulizer treatment

- Radiology
  - Chest x-ray, PA and lateral _____
  - Sinuses, three views _____
  - Forearm, two views _____
  - Ankle, three views _____
- Surgery
  - Abscess, skin, simple I&D _____
  - Skin tag removal (≤15) _____
  - Skin tag removal (each additional—≥16) _____
  - Destruction of lesion, first _____
  - Destruction of lesion, 2 through 14 _____

B. Locate the diagnostic codes for the following:
   - Hypertension, benign _____
   - Edema _____
   - Urinary frequency _____
   - Gout _____
   - Anemia _____
   - Hypothyroidism _____
   - Lymphadenopathy _____
   - Dermatitis, contact _____
   - Diabetes mellitus _____
   - Fatigue and malaise _____
   - Otitis media _____
   - Sinusitis, acute _____
   - GERD _____
   - Arthritis _____
   - Back pain, lumbar _____
   - Abdominal pain, unspecified _____
   - Rectal bleeding _____
   - Dysuria _____
   - Chronic obstructive pulmonary disease (COPD) _____
   - Asthma _____
   - Upper respiratory infection (URI) _____
   - Conjunctivitis _____
   - Cerumen impaction _____
   - Syncope _____

PRACTICAL APPLICATIONS

If you have accomplished the objectives in this chapter, you will be able to make better choices as a medical assistant. Take another look at this situation and decide what you would do.

Jenny, a medical assistant, is the insurance clerk in a large medical practice. She has been with the practice for 10 years and has gradually learned how to perform coding. She uses the *ICD-9-CM* codes and the *CPT-4* codes daily. Phyllis, a long-time patient, was seen today with a chief complaint of a sore throat, influenza, and a chronic cough. Phyllis has diabetes mellitus, hypertension, and chronic obstructive pulmonary disease. The physician examined her respiratory tract and listened to her heart, and checked her other body systems. He also reviewed her symptoms and took a past history as it related to her presenting symptoms. The medical decision making was more complex for Phyllis because many medications used for cough contain sugar.

When Phyllis left the office, Jenny immediately began the process of coding her visit. Would you be able to code this visit?

Medical Coding CHAPTER 29

1. Why is coding a medical visit so important, and what is actually being accomplished by coding?

2. What part of the medical visit is coded using *ICD-9-CM* codes?

3. What part of the medical visit is coded using *CPT* codes?

4. What is a diagnosis?

5. What is the difference between Volume 1 and Volume 2 of the *ICD-9-CM* manual?

6. What is a chief complaint? Which of the listed symptoms is the chief complaint?

7. What is the primary diagnosis? What are the concurrent conditions? What are the secondary conditions?

CHAPTER 29   Medical Coding

8. Why are words such as "probable," "suspected," and "rule out" not used with outpatient diagnosis coding?

9. How would you code the *CPT* E/M code pertaining to the history? How would you use *CPT* codes for the medical decision making?

APPLICATION OF SKILLS

Procedure Check-off Sheets (*) and assignments from MACC on the Evolve site at http://evolve.elsevier.com/klieger/medicalassisting (**)

1. Perform Procedure 29-1 Diagnostic Coding.*
   A. MACC (Practice)
      MACC/Administrative skills/Health insurance activities/Assigning *ICD-9-CM* codes**
      Assign the proper *ICD-9-CM* code based on medical documentation for auditing and billing purposes

2. Perform Procedure 29-2 Procedural Coding.*
   A. MACC (Practice)
      MACC/Administrative skills/Health insurance activities/Assigning *CPT* codes**
      Assign the proper *CPT* code based on medical documentation for auditing and billing purposes

CHAPTER QUIZ

Multiple Choice

Identify the letter of the choice that best completes the statement or answers the question.

1. _____ are codes used for external causes of injury and poisoning.
   A. A
   B. E
   C. V
   D. J

2. Volume _____ is included in the *ICD-9 CM* manual only when it will be used specifically for hospital coding.
   A. 1
   B. 2
   C. 3
   D. none of the above

3. The first *CPT* book appeared in _____ as a result of an effort by the AMA to create a method of accurately and universally identifying all medical and surgical procedures and services.
   A. 1938
   B. 1945
   C. 1966
   D. 1978

4. The *ICD-9-CM* books are updated every _____.
   A. 6 months
   B. 2 years
   C. year
   D. 3 years

5. The _____ is used by hospitals and allows for four concurrent conditions, ranked in the order of severity.
   A. CMS 1500
   B. UB-92
   C. A and B
   D. neither A nor B

6. "Diagnosis" is defined as the determination of the nature of a disease based on signs, symptoms, and laboratory findings.
   A. True
   B. False

7. *ICD-9* Volume _____ consists of an alphabetical listing of terms and codes with special tables.
   A. 1
   B. 2
   C. 3
   D. 4

8. Effective diagnostic and procedural coding requires _____.
   A. a good knowledge of terminology
   B. familiarity with the *ICD-9-CM* and *CPT*
   C. discipline to read all explanations from medical records.
   D. all of the above

9. In 1948, the World Health Organization developed a publication that could be used to track morbidity rates.
   A. True
   B. False

Copyright © 2010, 2005 by Saunders, an imprint of Elsevier, Inc. All rights reserved.

10. In the *ICD-9-CM* Volume _____, all of the titles and codes are printed in bold.
    A. 1
    B. 2
    C. 3
    D. 4

11. Volume _____ of the *ICD-9-CM* is the numerical listings of disease and injury codes and consists of 17 chapters.
    A. 1
    B. 2
    C. 3
    D. 4

12. _____ is a key component in a determination of the level of E/M service to be selected.
    A. History
    B. Examination
    C. Difficulty of medical decision making
    D. All of the above

13. _____ codes are supplementary codes for factors influencing health status and reasons for contact with health services when a diagnosis needs further explanation, or when the patient has no disease process for coding.
    A. E
    B. F
    C. J
    D. V

14. A primary diagnosis is the condition considered to be the patient's major health problem.
    A. True
    B. False

15. CPT stands for Current Procedure Terminology.
    A. True
    B. False

16. A medical record must include the _____.
    A. nature of the problem
    B. appropriate amount of time spent with the patient
    C. A and B
    D. neither A nor B

17. The semicolon is critical when coding procedures.
    A. True
    B. False

18. _____ is *not* a type of examination.
    A. Comprehensive
    B. Detailed
    C. Problem focused
    D. Exhaustive

19. In *ICD-9-CM* coding, a main term represents a _____.
    A. disease
    B. condition
    C. noun
    D. all of the above

20. The chief complaint is a statement usually made by the patient in his or her own words that describes the reason for the visit.
    A. True
    B. False

30 Medical Insurance

VOCABULARY REVIEW

Matching: Match each term with the correct definition.

A. allowable charges

B. birthday rule

C. capitation

D. CHAMPVA

E. clearinghouse

F. CMS-1500

G. comprehensive plan

H. coordination of benefits

I. cost containment

J. curriculum vitae

K. explanation of benefits

L. fraud

M. gatekeeper

N. Healthcare Common Procedure Coding System

O. HIPAA

P. health maintenance organization

Q. indemnity plan

R. major medical benefits

_____ 1. Person retired from the U.S. military services

_____ 2. Medical insurance plan that covers basic and major medical costs

_____ 3. American Hospital Association 2003 update of "Patient's Bill of Rights"

_____ 4. Person or company involved in the physician-patient relationship, but not part of implied contract

_____ 5. Amount of a professional service fee that an insurance company is willing to accept

_____ 6. Type of physician's resume listing education, in-service training, hospital affiliations, professional organizations, and any publications written

_____ 7. Insurance plan in which patients pay the provider and submit a claim form for reimbursement from their insurance company

_____ 8. Form sent by the insurance carrier to the patient and the medical practice that explains the amount of reimbursement or the reason for denial of a submitted claim

_____ 9. The 10-digit lifetime identification number issued to health care providers by Medicare

_____ 10. Organization that receives electronic claim forms from medical providers and processes them for payment

_____ 11. Physician responsible for most of the ongoing care of a patient

_____ 12. Scale that uses a complex formula to determine Medicare fees based on geographical area expenses

S. managed care

T. national provider identification

U. nonparticipating provider

V. partial disability

W. patient care partnership

X. precertification

Y. preferred provider organization

Z. primary care physician

AA. release of information

BB. resource-based relative value scale

CC. third party

DD. TRICARE

EE. usual, customary, and reasonable

FF. veteran

_____ 13. Managed care plan that pays a predetermined amount to a provider over a set time regardless of the number of services rendered to their subscribers in the period

_____ 14. Civilian Health and Medical Program of the Department of Veterans Affairs; health benefits program that provides coverage to the spouse or widow(er) of a U.S. military veteran

_____ 15. Primary care physician designated by an HMO to provide ongoing care to a patient and to authorize referrals to specialists when deemed necessary

_____ 16. Insurance rule that states the policy of the parent whose birthday is first in the calendar year holds the primary insurance for any dependent

_____ 17. Health insurance claims form, also known as the "universal" claim form that can be filled with all insurance companies; formally HCFA-1500

_____ 18. Standardized coding system that uses CPT, national, and local codes to process Medicare claims; used primarily for supplies, materials, injections, and certain procedures and services not defined in CPT

_____ 19. State in which a person can perform a portion of his or her job duties

_____ 20. Organization that provides comprehensive health care services for plan participants at a fixed rate

_____ 21. Health care system that provides a list of providers who have signed a contract with the insurance carrier to provide services to the insured

_____ 22. Comprehensive federal health care program for all active duty and retired U.S. military personnel and eligible family members; formally known as CHAMPUS

_____ 23. Insurance term stating that total reimbursement from primary and secondary insurance companies will not exceed the total cost of the charges

_____ 24. Intentional misrepresentation of medical facts as they relate to a claim for health care services

_____ 25. Insurance coverage beyond basic medical benefits used for expenses incurred by lengthy illness or serious injury

_____ 26. Physician who has not signed a contract with an insurance company to participate in health care for the insured

CHAPTER 30 Medical Insurance

_____ 27. Referring to typically charged or prevailing fees for health care services in a geographical area

_____ 28. Term referring to methods used to control the increasing cost of health care

_____ 29. Method used for determining in advance how much the patient's insurance policy will reimburse for a particular service or procedure

_____ 30. Federal legislation to improve health insurance availability for individuals who lose coverage

_____ 31. Network of health care services and benefits designed for a group of individuals who pay premiums to join the insurance plan

_____ 32. Authorization signed by the patient that gives the provider permission to disclose certain health information to the insurance carrier or other health care providers or pertinent parties (e.g., attorney) as deemed appropriate

THEORY RECALL

True/False

Indicate whether the statement is true or false.

_____ 1. A preferred provider organization is a health care delivery arrangement that offers insured individuals certain incentives if they choose health care providers from a list of providers who are contracted with the PPO.

_____ 2. The Consolidated Omnibus Reconciliation Act (COBRA) was enacted in 1996, and requires employers with five or more employees to continue to offer coverage of their group health plan to employees for 18 months in the event of voluntary or involuntary termination of employment.

_____ 3. Disability income insurance is insurance that pays benefits to the policyholder if he or she becomes unable to work as a result of an illness or injury that is not related to work.

_____ 4. A medical savings account is used only for medical care with taxed dollars.

_____ 5. CMS-1500 is the name given to a universal claim form used to report outpatient services to all government programs.

Multiple Choice

Identify the letter of the choice that best completes the statement or answers the question.

1. _____ rules apply when a patient is covered by more than one insurance policy.
   A. Co-payment
   B. COB
   C. Co-insurance
   D. Managed care

2. _____ is(are) (a) reason(s) for dramatic increases in health care costs.
   A. Underpayment of premiums
   B. Overuse and misuse of medical supplies
   C. Not enough people wanting insurance
   D. Increase in the elderly population

3. _____ have policies in which major medical and basic benefits apply.
   A. Comprehensive plans
   B. Fee-for-service plans
   C. Managed care plans
   D. PPOs

4. _____ is a method of structuring fees.
   A. Usual, customary, and reasonable
   B. Capitation
   C. Relative value scale
   D. All of the above

5. _____ is a method of setting Medicare fees.
   A. RVU
   B. RBRVS
   C. RVS
   D. URC

6. The Medicare program was developed in _____, initially as a national health insurance for elderly people.
   A. 1932
   B. 1948
   C. 1959
   D. 1966

7. CHAMPVA is a health benefits program that provides coverage to the spouse or widower and to the children of veterans who _____.
   A. are rated permanently and totally disabled because of service-connected disability
   B. were rated permanently and totally disabled because of a service-connected condition at the time of death
   C. died during active duty and whose dependents are not otherwise eligible for TRICARE benefits
   D. all of the above

Copyright © 2010, 2005 by Saunders, an imprint of Elsevier, Inc. All rights reserved.

8. _____ is when an individual has loss of speech, loss of hearing in both ears, loss of sight in both eyes, or loss of the use of two limbs.
   A. Total disability
   B. Partial disability
   C. Residual disability
   D. Catastrophic disability

9. _____ is a secondary insurance policy for Medicare-eligible individuals.
   A. MediCal
   B. Medicaid
   C. MediGap
   D. Medi-Medi

10. _____ is a statement giving the health care provider permission to disclose certain health information to the patient's insurance carrier.
    A. ROI
    B. OCR
    C. FECA
    D. RVS

11. A(n) _____ has no errors or omissions, and is the best defense against delays or rejections.
    A. clean claim
    B. electronic claim
    C. paper claim
    D. quick claim

12. A(n) _____ policy is an insurance policy purchased by a company for its employees or by a group representing similar professions.
    A. Individual
    B. Private
    C. Group
    D. Public

13. CMS is responsible for the operation of the Medicare program and for the selection of the regional insurance companies, called _____.
    A. fiscal intermediaries
    B. adjusters
    C. agents
    D. none of the above

14. The patient must be _____ years of age to qualify for Medicare, unless the person is disabled.
    A. 55
    B. 60
    C. 65
    D. 70

15. _____ covers nonmilitary employees of the federal government.
    A. FICA
    B. FECA
    C. HCFA
    D. SSDI

Sentence Completion

Complete each sentence or statement.

eligible visit	total disability	episode of care
clearinghouse	precertification	gatekeeper
deductible	fiscal	benefit
goalkeeper	intermediary	individual policy
network	group policy	
premium	co-insurance	

1. _____ is a term used to describe and measure the various health care services and encounters rendered in connection with a specific injury or period of illness.

2. _____ is an insurance contract purchased by individuals who are not eligible for group policies, or who do not qualify for government-sponsored plans.

3. _____ is the method used for determining in advance how much the patient's insurance policy will reimburse or pay for a particular service or procedure.

4. _____ is an organization that receives claims from medical facilities, checks them for completeness and accuracy, and forwards them electronically to the proper carrier.

5. The primary care physician who can refer patients to specialists is also known as the _____.

6. A(n) _____ is the yearly amount the patient "must pay out of pocket" before the insurance will pay on any claims.

7. A(n) _____ is the monthly, quarterly, or annual payment for insurance coverage.

8. _____ is a state in which an individual is unable to perform the requirements of any employment.

9. _____ is an organized group of participating providers for an insurance plan; policies may have "in-network" or "out-of-network" benefits.

10. _____ is an agent or insurance company that processes Medicare claims.

Copyright © 2010, 2005 by Saunders, an imprint of Elsevier, Inc. All rights reserved.

Short Answers

1. Explain how insurance companies establish UCR fees.

2. Explain the two ways HMOs are organized.

3. Explain in detail the three parts of Medicare.

4. Explain the advantages of electronic claims over paper claims.

5. List those who are eligible for TRICARE.

6. List the steps you would take to verify a new patient's insurance coverage.

CRITICAL THINKING

1. You have a patient, Celeste, whose parents are getting divorced. Celeste's mother is the parent who typically brings Celeste to the physician's office. On this visit, however, Celeste's father brings her in. He claims that Celeste's mother is responsible for paying her medical bills. You personally know that her father is supposed to carry the insurance policy for Celeste. How would you handle this situation? Research on the Internet or using resources in your community to answer this question.

PRACTICAL APPLICATIONS

If you have accomplished the objectives in this chapter, you will be able to make better choices as a medical assistant. Take another look at this situation and decide what you would do.

Dr. Jay has hired Maria as his insurance clerk. Maria's previous experience was with household liability claims and coverage. She has not had experience with the CMS-1500 or with coding of medical conditions. She is unaware that the claim begins with the appointment and patient registration, and ends with payment by the insurer. Jude Beck, a new patient of Dr. Jay, is seen in the office for what seems to be diabetes mellitus. An ECG, urinalysis, and blood test were done during the visit without checking with Mr. Beck's insurance first. In his notes, Dr. Jay states that he must "rule out diabetes mellitus," so Maria codes this as the "primary diagnosis" and sends the claim without a final diagnosis. When the results of the laboratory work are received, Dr. Jay documents in the medical record that the final diagnoses are dehydration and hypertension with tachycardia. When the registration form was completed, Mr. Beck failed to check off which of his insurance companies is primary and which is secondary. In processing the claim, Maria sends it with a diagnosis of "diabetes mellitus" to one of the two insurance companies, which turns out to be the secondary insurer. The claim is denied because there is no EOB attached from the primary payer. Maria does not resubmit the claim to the company that is actually the primary carrier.

Could you explain to Maria what went wrong and how the claim should have been handled?

1. **Why is it important for the registration form to be completed accurately?**

2. Why would the secondary insurance not pay for the claim before payment by the primary carrier?

3. What are the guidelines for coding a "rule out" diagnosis in the outpatient setting?

4. Why is preauthorization so important when dealing with insurance?

5. What is the implication for Mr. Beck of Maria not tracking the claims?

6. What is an "EOB"?

7. Why does the EOB of primary insurance need to be sent to the secondary insurance?

8. Why is a "clean claim" so important in obtaining insurance payment?

APPLICATION OF SKILLS

Procedure Check-off Sheets (*) and assignments from MACC on the Evolve site at http://evolve.elsevier.com/klieger/medicalassisting (**)

1. Perform Procedure 30-1: Apply Managed Care Policies and Procedures.*
   A. MACC (Practice)
      MACC/Administrative skills/Health insurance activities/Obtaining a managed care precertification**
      Obtain precertification from a patient's HMO for requested services or procedures
   B. MACC
      MACC/Administrative skills/Health insurance activities/Obtaining a managed care referral**
      Obtain a referral from a patient's HMO for requested consultation or treatment

2. Perform Procedure 30-2: Complete the CMS-1500 Claim Form.*
   A. MACC (Practice)
      MACC/Administrative skills/Health insurance activities/Assigning *ICD-9-CM* codes**
      Assign the proper *ICD-9-CM* code based on medical documentation for auditing and billing purposes
   B. MACC (Practice)
      MACC/Administrative skills/Health insurance activities/Assigning *CPT* codes**
      Assign the proper *CPT* codes based on medical documentation for auditing and billing purposes
   C. MACC (Practice)
      MACC/Administrative skills/Health insurance activities/Completing and insurance claim form**
      Apply third-party guidelines to prepare an insurance claim
      Complete an insurance claim form
      Use physician's fee schedule to determine the charges

CHAPTER QUIZ

Multiple Choice

Identify the letter of the choice that best completes the statement or answers the question.

1. _____ rules apply when a patient is covered by more than one insurance policy.
   A. Co-payment
   B. COB
   C. Co-insurance
   D. Managed care

Copyright © 2010, 2005 by Saunders, an imprint of Elsevier, Inc. All rights reserved.

2. Disability income insurance is insurance that pays benefits to the policyholder if he or she becomes unable to work as a result of an illness or injury that is not related to work.
   A. True
   B. False

3. _____ program was developed in 1966, initially as a national health insurance for elderly people.
   A. Medicaid
   B. Workers' Compensation
   C. Blue Cross/Blue Shield
   D. Medicare

4. COBRA was enacted in 1985 and requires employers of _____ or more employees to continue to offer coverage in their group health care plan to former employees.
   A. 5
   B. 10
   C. 20
   D. 50

5. Medical savings accounts are used only to pay for medical care with pretax dollars.
   A. True
   B. False

6. CMS is responsible for the operation of the Medicare program, and for selection of the regional insurance companies, called _____.
   A. fiscal intermediaries
   B. adjusters
   C. agents
   D. none of the above

7. _____ is one of the methods of structuring fees.
   A. Relative value scale
   B. Capitation
   C. Usual, customary, and reasonable
   D. All the above

8. A person who is not permanently disabled must be _____ years of age to qualify for Medicare.
   A. 55
   B. 60
   C. 65
   D. 68

9. _____ is a method of setting Medicare fees.
   A. RVU
   B. RBRVS
   C. RVS
   D. URC

10. A(n) _____ is an insurance policy purchased by a company for its employees.
    A. individual policy
    B. group policy
    C. private policy
    D. public policy

11. _____ has policies in which major medical and basic benefits apply.
    A. Comprehensive plan
    B. Fee-for-service plan
    C. Managed care plan
    D. PPO

12. When an individual has loss of speech, loss of hearing in both ears, loss of sight in both eyes, or loss of the use of two limbs, it is referred to as a _____ disability.
    A. total
    B. residual
    C. catastrophic
    D. partial

13. _____ covers nonmilitary employees of the federal government.
    A. FICA
    B. FECA
    C. FEMA
    D. FAMA

14. _____ is (are) (a) reason(s) for dramatic increases in health care costs.
    A. Overuse and misuse of medical supplies
    B. Not enough people wanting insurance
    C. Increase in the elderly population
    D. None of the above

15. The CMS-1500 is the name given to a universal claim form used to report outpatient services to all government health programs.
    A. True
    B. False

16. _____ is a fixed fee that is paid by the patient at each visit.
    A. Co-payment
    B. Co-insurance
    C. Premium
    D. Allowable charge

17. _____ is a documented medical condition that is present in the patient before the insurance policy goes into effect.
    A. Precertification
    B. Preauthorization
    C. Pre-existing condition
    D. None of the above

18. _____ is a term used to describe and measure the various health care services provided for a specific injury or period of illness.
    A. Medical necessity
    B. Episode of care
    C. Guidelines
    D. Comprehensive plan

19. A proof of education, training, and experience is termed a curriculum vitae.
    A. True
    B. False

20. CHAMPUS is a health care program for members of the U.S. military.
    A. True
    B. False

31 Infection Control and Asepsis

VOCABULARY REVIEW

Matching: Match each term with the correct definition.

A. anaerobes

B. autoclave

C. bacilli

D. Centers for Disease Control and Prevention

E. cocci

F. disinfection

G. exposure incident

H. indirect contact

I. material safety data sheet

J. method of transmission

K. normal flora

L. parasite

M. protozoa

N. rickettsiae

O. Right to Know law

P. route of entry

Q. spirilla

R. sterile

S. sterilization strip

_____ 1. Way in which a microorganism enters the body

_____ 2. Microorganisms that do not require oxygen to grow

_____ 3. Bacteria that appear in chains

_____ 4. Work practices that minimize the possibility of infectious exposure to employees

_____ 5. Federal agency responsible for establishing guidelines to prevent the spread of disease-producing microorganisms

_____ 6. Infectious organism that needs a host to live or survive

_____ 7. Microorganisms that easily transfer to a host because of its location

_____ 8. Fact sheet about chemicals that includes handling precautions and first-aid procedures after a person has been exposed to a chemical

_____ 9. Free from all microorganisms, including spores

_____ 10. Destruction or inhibition of the activity of pathogens, but not of spores

_____ 11. Smallest of all microorganisms, visible only under electron microscopy

_____ 12. Way that microorganisms are passed on to other hosts or objects

_____ 13. Cleaning the hands with an antiseptic solution using a prescribed time and action to remove the most microorganisms possible

_____ 14. Equipment that sterilizes objects through the use of steam under pressure or gas

T. streptococci

U. surgical asepsis

V. susceptible host

W. transient flora

X. viruses

Y. work practice controls

Z. surgical handwash

_____ 15. Removal of all microorganisms from an object, including spores

_____ 16. Microorganisms that naturally occur within certain body systems

_____ 17. Contact with blood or other biohazardous and infectious materials that occur at work

_____ 18. Microorganisms that live in a particular species of insect and are transmitted through its bite

_____ 19. Rod-shaped bacteria

_____ 20. Person, insect, or animal that can be infected easily by a particular microorganism

_____ 21. Round or spherical bacteria

_____ 22. Chemical indicator embedded within the center of a wrapped, dense pack that shows conditions for sterilization within the pack

_____ 23. Method by which microorganisms are transmitted other than by person-to-person contact

_____ 24. Single-celled animals

_____ 25. Hazard communication standard that allows each employee to know of potential exposure problems

_____ 26. Spiral or corkscrew-shaped bacteria

THEORY RECALL

True/False

Indicate whether the statement is true or false.

_____ 1. Pathogens are not harmful and are not disease-producing microorganisms.

_____ 2. Sanitization destroys pathogens.

_____ 3. Standard Precautions must be observed at all times and for all patients regardless of age, gender, and diagnosis.

_____ 4. To be considered sterile, an item must be free from all microorganisms, including spores.

_____ 5. Steam sterilization is the primary method used to sterilize instruments in the medical office.

Multiple Choice

Identify the letter of the choice that best completes the statement or answers the question.

1. _____ are found in the air we breathe, on our skin, on everything we touch, and in our food.
   A. Bacteria
   B. Microorganisms
   C. Protozoa
   D. Pathogens

2. _____ are single-celled animals found in contaminated water and decaying material.
   A. Bacteria
   B. Microorganisms
   C. Protozoa
   D. Fungi

3. _____ is the process of making an area clean and free of infection-causing microorganisms.
   A. Medical asepsis
   B. Surgical asepsis
   C. Autoclaving
   D. Disinfection

4. The use of a(n) _____ provides the only true indication that an item is sterile.
   A. autoclave tape
   B. biological indicator
   C. chemical indicator
   D. sterilization strip

5. _____ include yeast and molds.
   A. Bacteria
   B. Fungi
   C. Rickettsiae
   D. Viruses

6. OSHA mandates that employers must provide _____.
   A. an exposure control plan
   B. implementation of engineering controls
   C. PPEs
   D. all of the above

7. The CDC recommends the use of _____-based handrubs by all health care providers during patient care.
   A. alcohol
   B. soap
   C. gel
   D. lotion

8. Antiseptic handrubs, handwashing, antiseptic handwash, and surgical handwashing are examples of _____.
   A. good hygiene
   B. hand hygiene
   C. Standard Precautions
   D. none of the above

Copyright © 2010, 2005 by Saunders, an imprint of Elsevier, Inc. All rights reserved.

9. _____ reduces the number of microorganisms on an item.
   A. Disinfection
   B. Sanitization
   C. Sterilization
   D. All of the above

10. _____ gloves are used when performing clean procedures.
    A. Nondisposable
    B. Nonsterile disposable
    C. Sterile nondisposable
    D. Sterile disposable

11. When storing autoclaved instruments, the packages with the _____ date are placed up front.
    A. earliest
    B. most recent
    C. oldest
    D. date does not affect how autoclaved instruments are stored

12. _____ are equipment and facilities that minimize the possibility of exposure to microorganisms.
    A. Autoclaves
    B. Engineering controls
    C. Work practice controls
    D. None of the above

13. _____ are microorganisms that need oxygen to live.
    A. Aerobes
    B. Anaerobes
    C. Pathogens
    D. Protozoa

14. _____ are bacteria with a hard wall capsule that is resistant to heat.
    A. Bacilli
    B. Cocci
    C. Staphylococci
    D. Diplococci

15. _____ are bacteria that appear to be corkscrew-shaped.
    A. Bacilli
    B. Streptococci
    C. Staphylococci
    D. Spirilla

16. A _____ is an infected person who has disease-causing germs, but may not have symptoms of the disease.
    A. carrier
    B. reservoir host
    C. A and B
    D. Neither A nor B

17. Non–disease-producing microorganisms are also called _____.
    A. microorganisms
    B. diplococci
    C. fungi
    D. nonpathogens

18. A device that is impregnated with a special dye that changes color when exposed to the sterilization process is a(n) _____.
    A. biological indicator
    B. chemical indicator
    C. alcohol-based handwash
    D. all of the above

19. A method by which microorganisms are transmitted other than via person-to-person contact is _____.
    A. direct contact
    B. indirect contact
    C. infection control
    D. sanitization

20. _____ is the process of making an area clean and free of infectious materials.
    A. Medical asepsis
    B. Surgical asepsis
    C. Sanitization
    D. Sterilization

Sentence Completion

Complete each sentence or statement.

sterilization	viruses	transient flora
medical asepsis	pathogens	normal flora
	nonpathogens	gloves
OSHA	rickettsiae	cocci
CDC	bacteria	

1. _____ refers to microorganisms that grow on the surface of the skin that are usually nonpathogenic.

2. _____ are parasites that need a host to survive and cannot live outside the body.

3. _____ occurs naturally on the skin and in the body, and they fight off infection when they remain in their normal location.

4. _____ reduces hand contamination by 75%.

5. _____ are nonharmful and are not disease-producing microorganisms.

6. _____ can reproduce only if they are within a living cell.

7. _____ mandates and enforces the use of Standard Precautions.

8. _____ occurs by using heat, steam under pressure, gas, UV light, or chemicals.

Short Answers

1. List the three primary conditions that must be met for steam sterilization to occur.

   _____
   _____

2. List and describe the five classifications of bacteria.

   _____
   _____
   _____
   _____

3. Describe the chain of infection.

   _____
   _____
   _____
   _____

4. Explain the four clinical situations when you would use alcohol-based handrubs.

   _____
   _____
   _____
   _____

5. List four ways to determine whether items were exposed to conditions necessary for sterilization.

   _____
   _____
   _____
   _____

Infection Control and Asepsis **CHAPTER 31**   **391**

CRITICAL THINKING

1. When you check today's schedule, you notice that Dr. Sondheim has four minor surgical procedures scheduled. The clinic has only two full minor surgery packs, one of which was used yesterday for a laceration repair. You sanitized the instruments before you went home, but you did not autoclave them. It is a good thing that the second surgery is 2 hours from now. You can use the sterilized pack for the first surgery and have the second pack ready before Dr. Sondheim needs it. In the laboratory/preparation area, you start accumulating all of the supplies you are going to need for the day. You check on the autoclaved pack to ensure the dates are good. The pack is 3 days past the 30-day expiration date.
    A. Can you use the 3-day outdated instrument pack? Explain your answer.

    _____

    _____

    _____

    B. Explain the steps involved in sterilizing an instrument pack.

    _____

    _____

    _____

    _____

    C. Develop an exposure control plan to include the following (compare what you have written with the one in your classroom):
    - Barrier protection
    - Environmental protection
    - Housekeeping controls
    - Safety training programs
    - Follow-up
    - Documentation
    - MSDS
    - Engineering controls

PRACTICAL APPLICATIONS

If you have accomplished the objectives in this chapter, you will be able to make better choices as a medical assistant. Take another look at this situation and decide what you would do.

Janine is a new medical assistant in the office of Dr. McGee, a specialist in infectious diseases. Janine did her practical experience in a pediatric practice, often caring for children with viral and bacterial infections. As she begins her new employment, Janine asks to see the MSDSs and the current Exposure Control Plan. She also wants to know where the PPEs for her use are stored.

During patient care, medical workers often come in direct contact with many microorganisms, as Janine will in an office that specializes in infectious diseases. Janine's supervisor wants to be sure she is prepared to protect patients, other staff, and herself from infection. The supervisor reviews with Janine the importance of proper handwashing in infection control. Another important task for Janine will be performing medical asepsis and surgical asepsis on a regular basis, so the supervisor assesses Janine's ability to perform these skills. The supervisor asks Janine what is done at the end of the day before leaving the office to break the

Copyright © 2010, 2005 by Saunders, an imprint of Elsevier, Inc. All rights reserved.

cycle of infection. Janine responds that all medical workers should remove any garments that have been in direct contact with pathogens and nonpathogens, and each person should carefully sanitize his or her hands.

Would you be prepared to take the necessary precautions to stop the spread of infection in the medical office?

1. What are "MSDSs"? What are "PPEs"? Why are both important to the health care worker?

2. What is "OSHA," and what are the requirements that a medical office must have to meet the OSHA standards?

3. What is included in the "Exposure Control Plan"?

4. What is the "chain of infection," and why is hand sanitization important in breaking this chain?

5. What is the difference between handwashing and hand sanitization in maintaining hand hygiene? Give two indications for the appropriate use of each.

6. What is the difference between medical asepsis and surgical asepsis?

7. What is the difference between sanitization and disinfection?

8. Is there a degree of sterilization in surgical asepsis? Defend your answer.

9. What is a nonpathogen? What is a pathogen?

10. How should Janine handle infectious waste from patients with a bacterial infection who are seen by Dr. McGee?

APPLICATION OF SKILLS

Procedure Check-off Sheets (*) and assignments from MACC on the Evolve site at http://evolve.elsevier.com/klieger/medicalassisting (**)

1. Perform Procedure 31-1: Practice Standard Precautions.*
   A. Demonstrate knowledge, by verbal or written communication as required by instructor, of the basic guidelines approved by OSHA and recommended by the CDC for a postexposure action plan as outlined in Procedure 31-1 in textbook

2. Perform Procedure 31-2: Properly Dispose of Biohazardous Materials.*

3. Perform Procedure 31-3: Perform Proper Handwashing for Medical Asepsis.*

4. Perform Procedure 31-4: Perform Alcohol-Based Hand Sanitization.*

5. Perform Procedure 31-5: Apply and Remove Clean, Disposable (Nonsterile) Gloves.*

6. Perform Procedure 31-6: Sanitize Instruments.*

7. Perform Procedure 31-7: Perform Chemical Sterilization.*

8. Perform Procedure 31-8: Wrap Instruments for the Autoclave.*

9. Perform Procedure 31-9: Sterilize Articles in the Autoclave.*

CHAPTER QUIZ

Multiple Choice

Identify the letter of the choice that best completes the statement or answers the question.

1. Spiral or corkscrew-shaped bacteria are known as _____.
   A. diplococci
   B. staphylococci
   C. spirilla
   D. spores

2. Microorganisms that naturally occur within certain body systems are known as _____.
   A. nonpathogens
   B. normal flora
   C. pathogens
   D. parasites

3. _____ is the primary method used to sterilize instruments in the medical office.
   A. Autoclaving
   B. Disinfection
   C. Sanitization
   D. Sterilization

4. _____ destroys pathogens.
   A. Autoclaving
   B. Disinfection
   C. Sanitization
   D. Sterilization

5. _____ is the removal of all pathogenic and nonpathogenic microorganisms from an object.
   A. Medical asepsis
   B. Sanitization
   C. Sterilization
   D. Surgical asepsis

6. When drawing blood, sterile gloves are used.
   A. True
   B. False

7. _____ is a primary condition that must be met for steam sterilization to occur.
   A. Appropriate time period depending on size of surgical pack or instrument
   B. Pressure of 15 pounds
   C. Temperature of 250° F to 270° F
   D. All of the above

8. _____ provides the only true indication that an item is sterile.
   A. Autoclave tape
   B. Biological indicators
   C. Chemical indicators
   D. Sterilization strips

9. Sanitization occurs by using heat, steam under pressure, gas, UV light, or chemicals.
   A. True
   B. False

10. _____ is hazard communication standard that allows each employee to know of potential exposure problems.
    A. OSHA
    B. Right to Know law
    C. Material safety data sheet
    D. Exposure control plan

11. The way microorganisms are transmitted (passed on, spread) to other hosts is known as _____.
    A. indirect contact
    B. method of transmission
    C. route of entry
    D. none of the above

12. Maintaining the hands in a clean state by using soap and water, antiseptic solution, or alcohol-based handrubs is known as _____.
    A. antiseptic handwash
    B. handwashing
    C. hand hygiene
    D. medical asepsis

13. Established policies and procedures that must be followed to minimize the risk of spreading disease-producing microorganisms are known as _____.
    A. infection control
    B. PPE
    C. Right to Know law
    D. workplace controls

14. The Centers for Disease Control and Prevention is a federal agency that enforces the use of safety measures in place under Standard Precautions.
    A. True
    B. False

15. Microorganisms that feed on organic material are known as _____.
    A. fungi
    B. parasites
    C. spirilla
    D. viruses

16. Microorganisms that do not require oxygen to grow are known as _____.
    A. aerobic
    B. anaerobic
    C. nonpathogenic
    D. sterile

17. Microorganisms are microscopic animals capable of reproducing.
    A. True
    B. False

18. Paper-wrapped or muslin-wrapped autoclaved items can be stored for _____.
    A. 15 days
    B. 30 days
    C. 6 months
    D. 1 year

19. Gloves reduce hand contamination by an average of _____%.
    A. 50
    B. 65
    C. 70
    D. 75

20. Normal flora refers to organisms that grow on the surface of the skin and are picked up easily by the hands.
    A. True
    B. False

NAME: _____   DATE: _____

32 Preparing the Examination Room

VOCABULARY REVIEW

Matching: Match each term with the correct definition.

A. audiometer

B. tuning fork

C. otoscope

D. specimen

E. percussion hammer

F. tape measure

G. ophthalmoscope

H. tongue depressor

I. lubricant

J. penlight

_____ 1. Instrument used to hold the tongue down or move it from side to side when examining the mouth

_____ 2. Agent used to reduce friction by making a surface moist; used to facilitate anal and vaginal examinations

_____ 3. Instrument used to test hearing acuity by air or bone conduction

_____ 4. Instrument used to measure tendon reflexes

_____ 5. Instrument used to examine internal structure of the eye

_____ 6. Electronic instrument used to test hearing

_____ 7. Sample of a larger part, such as body tissue or cells

_____ 8. Instrument used to examine the ear canal and eardrum

_____ 9. Device used to measure body parts and wound length

_____ 10. Instrument used to enhance examination in a cavity, and to check for pupillary response to light

THEORY RECALL

True/False

Indicate whether the statement is true or false.

_____ 1. Confidentiality is a key issue for patients.

_____ 2. It is acceptable to leave prescription pads on the counter in examination rooms because even if a patient took the pad he or she could not use it.

_____ 3. A medical assistant should be present while a patient changes into a gown.

_____ 4. An otoscope may have a short and wide speculum attached, and can be used by the physician to examine the nasal area.

_____ 5. Examination tables must be covered with nonpermeable latex as directed by OSHA.

Multiple Choice

Identify the letter of the choice that best completes the statement or answers the question.

1. An instrument used to measure tendon reflexes is a(n) _____.
   A. audiometer
   B. percussion hammer
   C. tape measure
   D. tuning fork

2. The _____ test is used when a patient states hearing is better in one ear than in the other.
   A. audiometer
   B. Rinne
   C. verbal
   D. Weber

3. Appropriate accommodations need to be made in examination rooms to ensure that the room is accessible to all patients, including patients in wheelchairs, as directed by _____.
   A. CDC
   B. OSHA
   C. ADA
   D. none of the above

4. Which one of the following is the correct spelling for the medical term for a blood pressure cuff?
   A. Syphgmomanometer
   B. Sphygmomanometer
   C. Syfigmomanometer
   D. None of the above

5. A _____ holds used needles and other sharps for disposal.
   A. biohazardous waste container
   B. puncture-resistant container
   C. sealable stainless steel canister
   D. none of the above

6. _____ requires that all contaminated work surfaces be decontaminated using appropriate disinfectant as soon as possible after a procedure or immediately if potential infectious contamination has occurred.
   A. CDC
   B. Office procedure manual
   C. OSHA
   D. Exposure control plan

7. _____ is(are) used to collect specimens and remove debris.
   A. Cotton-tipped applicator
   B. Lubricant
   C. Sterile saline
   D. Sharp/sharp operating scissors

8. _____ is an instrument used to test hearing acuity through vibration.
   A. Audiometer
   B. Otoscope
   C. Percussion hammer
   D. Tuning fork

9. _____ is an instrument used for viewing a cavity.
   A. Penlight
   B. Tongue depressor
   C. Speculum
   D. None of the above

10. The _____ test compares air conduction with bone conduction.
    A. audiometer
    B. percussion hammer
    C. Rinne
    D. Weber

11. _____ disinfects skin and equipment surfaces.
    A. Sterile saline
    B. Isopropyl alcohol 70%
    C. Johnson & Johnson Wet Wipes
    D. None of the above

12. Lubricants used in a medical office should be _____.
    A. water-soluble
    B. oil-based
    C. consistent with the ingredients of household detergent
    D. none of the above

13. Examination tables and counter surfaces must be cleaned in between patients with _____.
    A. sterile saline
    B. 70% isopropyl alcohol wipe
    C. 10% bleach solution
    D. all of the above

14. All instruments used during an examination must be removed, cleaned, and _____.
    A. sanitized
    B. disinfected
    C. sterilized
    D. all of the above

15. Which one of the following is a specialty item that would be added to an examination tray for a Pap smear?
    A. Sigmoidoscope
    B. Ophthalmoscope
    C. Tuning fork
    D. Vaginal speculum

Sentence Completion

Complete each sentence or statement.

health	otoscope	speculum
safety	ophthalmoscope	Weber
CDC	body secretions	ADA
HIPAA	percussion hammer	

1. _____ measures should be taken to ensure patients do not injure themselves in the office.

2. _____ mandates the privacy and confidentiality of patients.

3. Gloves are always worn when coming in contact with _____.

4. _____ is used for tapping the tendon in the elbow, wrist, ankle, and knee to test for reflex action.

5. _____ is used to examine the internal structures of the eye.

Short Answers

1. Describe what safety measures need to be taken in the medical office so that patients do not injure themselves.

   _____
   _____
   _____
   _____

2. List equipment for a physical examination typically found in an examination room.

   _____
   _____
   _____
   _____

Copyright © 2010, 2005 by Saunders, an imprint of Elsevier, Inc. All rights reserved.

3. List the four major areas of treatment plan preparation that the medical assistant can address.

4. List four general considerations taken when preparing an examination room for a patient.

CRITICAL THINKING

1. Today is your first day of your Practicum, and the medical assistant that you will be training with has asked you to set up Room 3 for a routine physical examination. List the items you need to have available for the physician, describe how each one is used, and describe the preparation of the examination room.

PRACTICAL APPLICATIONS

If you have accomplished the objectives in this chapter, you will be able to make better choices as a medical assistant. Take another look at this situation and decide what you would do.

Julie, a medical assistant who was not educated in a medical assisting program, has been hired by a local family physician to assist with physical examinations. Today is her second day on the job. Her mentor has called in sick, so Julie is responsible for the clinical area by herself. Another physician, Dr. Johnson, will be performing the invasive procedures, and Julie is expected to have the room and patient ready for Dr. Johnson's examinations.

Julie finds the room too warm for her comfort, and she knows that it will be too warm for the physician in a lab coat, so she lowers the thermostat to 67° F. As Mrs. Sito is undressing, Julie barges into the room and leaves the door open. A male patient walks by and sees Mrs. Sito undressed. During the examination, Dr. Johnson asks for the ophthalmoscope and otoscope. When he tries to use these, the necessary light will not work, so he asks for a penlight. Julie leaves the room to find the penlight and a tape measure. Dr. Johnson reaches for a cotton-tipped applicator and tongue depressors. Noticing that the supply is low, he asks Julie, "Would you please fill these containers?" Julie immediately departs to fill the jars, leaving Dr. Johnson alone with the patient, who needs a pelvic examination.

After Mrs. Sito leaves the room, Julie decides that the table paper does not look used. Thinking she will save the physician some money in supplies, she does not change the paper covering and brings in 5-year-old Joey Novelle, placing him on the table Mrs. Sito has just vacated. The sink still contains the dirty instruments used for the other patients. Joey's mother tells Dr. Johnson that she has never seen someone placed on dirty table paper, and she does not want her child to see dirty instruments in the sink. At the end of Joey's physical examination, Dr. Johnson takes Julie to his office and explains that if she cannot properly prepare and clean the examination room in the future, he will have to find someone to replace her.

If you worked with Julie, what are some suggestions you would make to help her perform her duties more effectively?

1. **What part did the lack of education in the medical assisting field play in Julie making mistakes?**

2. **What temperature is appropriate for the patient examination room?**

3. **Why should Julie have been very careful to keep the door closed to the examination room where a patient was placed?**

4. **What is the use of the ophthalmoscope and otoscope?**

5. Should Julie have left the room to fill the containers of cotton-tipped applicators and tongue depressors? Explain your answer.

_____

_____

_____

_____

6. Why is changing the examination table's paper covering such an important task?

_____

_____

_____

_____

7. Do you think that Joey's mother and Dr. Johnson had a right to be upset?

_____

_____

_____

_____

8. What effect did the room's lack of preparation have on the appointments for that day?

_____

_____

_____

_____

APPLICATION OF SKILLS

1. With a partner, gather the equipment and supplies required to perform a routine physical examination. Explain to your partner what each item is used for.

2. Practice the procedure using the MACC on the Evolve site *http://evolve.elsevier.com/klieger/medicalassisting,* and then practice and perform the task in the classroom: MACC/Clinical skills/Patient care/The physical exam/Assisting with a physical exam and maintaining/preparing exam room.

CHAPTER QUIZ

Multiple Choice

Identify the letter of the choice that best completes the statement or answers the question.

1. _____ is used when a patient states that the hearing is better on one side than the other.
   A. Audiometer test
   B. Tuning fork
   C. Rinne test
   D. Weber test

2. _____ is always worn when coming in contact with patient body secretions.
   A. Latex gloves
   B. Powdered gloves
   C. Disposable gloves
   D. Sterile gloves

3. A _____ should be available in the examination room for a patient to access an examination table.
   A. stepstool
   B. footrest
   C. pullout platform
   D. any of the above

4. Prescription pads should not be left on the counter in examination rooms.
   A. True
   B. False

5. The medical assistant should prepare the examination room _____ the patient arrives.
   A. after
   B. before
   C. when
   D. none of the above

6. The Americans with Disabilities Act requires that appropriate accommodations be made in examination rooms so that all patients, including patients in wheelchairs, have access.
   A. True
   B. False

7. _____ is(are) typically kept in examination rooms for physical examination.
   A. Cotton-tipped applicators
   B. Disposable gloves
   C. Tongue depressors
   D. Otoscope

8. Confidentiality is not an issue for most patients.
   A. True
   B. False

9. _____ regulates that all contaminated work surfaces must be decontaminated using an appropriate disinfectant as soon as the patient leaves.
   A. Office policy manual
   B. CDC
   C. Exposure control plan
   D. State law

10. _____ protects the patient's right to privacy.
    A. CDC
    B. OSHA
    C. HIPAA
    D. Office policy

11. Examination table paper needs to be changed _____.
    A. every morning
    B. twice a day
    C. at the end of the day
    D. after each patient

12. When the medical assistant is preparing the patient for carrying out the treatment plan, the medical assistant should _____.
    A. ensure the patient understands the instructions
    B. ensure the patient's living environment will allow for compliance
    C. ensure the patient is not hearing impaired
    D. all of the above

13. _____ is an instrument for viewing a cavity.
    A. Penlight
    B. Otoscope
    C. Speculum
    D. Tongue depressor

14. _____ is an instrument to view the internal structure of the eye.
    A. Audiometer
    B. Otoscope
    C. Ophthalmoscope
    D. Penlight

15. The medical assistant should stay in the examination room while a patient changes into a gown.
    A. True
    B. False

33 Body Measurements and Vital Signs

VOCABULARY REVIEW

Matching: Match each term with the correct definition.

A. afebrile

B. apical pulse

C. baseline

D. brachial artery

E. carotid artery

F. diastolic pressure

G. dorsalis pedis artery

H. femoral artery

I. hypotension

J. inspiration

K. popliteal artery

L. pulse rate

M. radial pulse

N. rales

O. respiratory rate

P. rhonchi

Q. sphygmomanometer

R. stridor

S. systolic pressure

T. tachycardia

_____ 1. Numerical measurement of heartbeats or respirations per minute; characteristic of measuring the pulse or respiration

_____ 2. High-pitched sounds heard when bronchial tubes are narrowed by disease

_____ 3. Without fever

_____ 4. Artery located behind the knee

_____ 5. Area of the eardrum

_____ 6. Pulse rate of less than 60 beats/min

_____ 7. Instrument used to measure blood pressure

_____ 8. Underarm area

_____ 9. First measurable sound of blood pressure when the heart contracts

_____ 10. Measurement of blood pressure that is below the expected range for the patient's age group

_____ 11. Heartbeat that is taken with a stethoscope over the apex of the heart

_____ 12. Systematic measurement of a patient's temperature, pulse rate, respiration, and blood pressure

_____ 13. Minimum ("resting") pressure of blood against arteries occurring late in ventricular resting of the heart

_____ 14. Cycle of breathing including inspiration and expiration in 1 minute

_____ 15. Measurement of a vital sign that serves as a basis to which all subsequent measurements of that vital sign are compared

U. tympanic

V. vital signs

W. wheezes

X. axillary

Y. rate

Z. bradycardia

_____ 16. Pulse rate greater than 100 beats/min

_____ 17. Act of taking a breath or breathing in; inhaling

_____ 18. Artery located in the upper arm

_____ 19. Shrill sound heard on inspiration

_____ 20. Artery located in the thigh

_____ 21. Number of heartbeats per minute

_____ 22. Artery located on both sides of the neck

_____ 23. Low-pitched sounds created as air goes through narrowed bronchi

_____ 24. Artery located in the foot

_____ 25. Breathing sounds of "tissue paper being crumpled" caused by fluid or secretions in the bronchus

_____ 26. Pulse felt at the wrist over the radius

THEORY RECALL

True/False

Indicate whether the statement is true or false.

_____ 1. Body temperature is the measurement of the amount of heat within a person's body.

_____ 2. It is okay to place a blood pressure cuff over clothing if the patient's sleeve is too tight to pull up.

_____ 3. Children should have their height recorded at each visit.

_____ 4. When recording blood pressures, the systolic number is recorded on the bottom.

_____ 5. It is better to use a smaller blood pressure cuff when in doubt.

Multiple Choice

Identify the letter of the choice that best completes the statement or answers the question.

1. Bradycardia is a pulse rate lower than _____ beats/min.
    A. 40
    B. 50
    C. 60
    D. 65

2. _____ is a low-pitched sound created as air goes through mucus or narrowed bronchi.
   A. Stridor
   B. Rales
   C. Rhonchi
   D. Wheezes

3. _____ is the most common place to measure pulse rate.
   A. Apical
   B. Brachial pulse
   C. Radial pulse
   D. Popliteal pulse

4. _____ is a measurement of the number of times the heart beats in a minute.
   A. Pulse rate
   B. Pulse
   C. Heart rate
   D. Heartbeat

5. _____ thermometers usually have digital read-outs and are hand held.
   A. Disposable
   B. Electronic
   C. Mercury-free glass
   D. Tympanic

6. The weight of an infant should _____ by 6 months compared with birth weight.
   A. double
   B. triple
   C. quadruple
   D. none of the above

7. Mercury-free glass thermometers have a _____ color-coded end.
   A. red
   B. green
   C. yellow
   D. blue

8. A _____ usually takes 1 to 2 seconds to register.
   A. disposable oral thermometer
   B. temperature-sensitive tape
   C. tympanic thermometer
   D. mercury-free thermometer

9. When taking a patient's pulse, it is best if you take it for _____.
   A. 10 seconds and multiply by 6
   B. 15 seconds and multiply by 4
   C. 30 seconds and multiply by 2
   D. 60 seconds

10. _____ pulse rate is taken over the apex of the heart.
    A. Apical
    B. Brachial
    C. Carotid
    D. Temporal

11. An adult respiratory rate is _____ breaths per minute.
    A. 10 to 15
    B. 16 to 20
    C. 20 to 40
    D. 25 to 40

12. When taking blood pressure, the normal range for adult systolic pressure is _____.
    A. 60 to 90 mm Hg
    B. 90 to 118 mm Hg
    C. 100 to 120 mm Hg
    D. 100 to 140 mm Hg

13. An older adult's height should be measured _____.
    A. every 3 years
    B. every 2 years
    C. every year
    D. every visit

14. "Bradycardia" is _____.
    A. slow breathing
    B. slow heart rate
    C. fast breathing
    D. fast heart rate

15. To take a(n) _____ pulse, a stethoscope must be used.
    A. apical
    B. femoral
    C. radial
    D. temporal

16. _____ is concerned with breathing patterns.
    A. Respiratory rate
    B. Respiratory rhythm
    C. Respiratory depth
    D. None of the above

17. _____ is(are) high-pitched sounds that occur when bronchial tubes are narrowed by disease.
    A. Stridor
    B. Rales
    C. Rhonchi
    D. Wheezing

18. _____ measure(s) body temperature by measuring the body temperature inside the ear canal or the membrane of the ear.
    A. Digital thermometers
    B. Temperature-sensitive tape
    C. Tympanic thermometers
    D. None of the above

19. The head circumference of a child is approximately _____% of an adult's circumference by 1 year of age.
    A. 70
    B. 75
    C. 80
    D. 85

20. _____ can increase or decrease a pulse rate.
    A. Alcohol
    B. Nicotine
    C. Medications
    D. All of the above

Sentence Completion

Complete each sentence or statement.

rate	oral	expiration
inspiration	aural	stethoscope
Celsius	axillary	temperature-sensitive tape
volume	growth chart	
lubb-dupp	rhythm	

1. A(n) _____ is an instrument used to listen to body sounds.

2. The heart makes a(n) _____ sound.

3. A(n) _____ temperature is taken under the arm.

4. _____ is the strength or force of each heartbeat.

5. _____ is the temperature scale that uses 0° as the freezing point and 100° as the boiling point of water.

6. _____ provides documentation of a child's progress of height and weight from infancy.

7. When taking a temperature with _____, apply it to the forehead or on the abdomen.

8. _____ is the time interval between each heartbeat.

CHAPTER 33 Body Measurements and Vital Signs

9. _____ refers to the numerical measurement of heartbeats or respirations per minute.

10. _____ is another word for "breathing in."

Short Answers

1. List the four components of vital signs.

   _____
   _____

2. Describe three examples of volume.

   _____
   _____

3. List six factors that might influence someone's blood pressure.

   _____
   _____
   _____
   _____

4. List five general guidelines for using a stethoscope.

   _____
   _____
   _____
   _____

5. List the three characteristics of the pulse that medical assistants should note in documentation.

   _____
   _____
   _____

Copyright © 2010, 2005 by Saunders, an imprint of Elsevier, Inc. All rights reserved.

CRITICAL THINKING

1. Whitney Carleton is 18 years old and the single parent of a 4-month-old girl. She has brought her daughter in for a check-up because the infant feels hot and is crying all the time. Dr. Donaldson has asked you to measure the infant's vital signs. Whitney is a very nervous new mother, and she wants you to explain everything you are going to do. You ask Whitney if she has taken the infant's temperature. She tells you she has not because she does not have a thermometer, and she does not know how to check her temperature. Explain to Whitney how to conduct a rectal examination to determine if her infant's temperature is increased.

PRACTICAL APPLICATIONS

If you have accomplished the objectives in this chapter, you will be able to make better choices as a medical assistant. Take another look at this situation and decide what you would do.

Stephanie works for a general practitioner who sees pediatric, adult, and geriatric patients. Dr. Karas wants height and weight measurements for patients at each visit, regardless of the patient's age. Dr. Karas also wants head and chest circumference measurements taken for pediatric patients up to age 3 years. Travis, a new patient, is a young teenager who does not want to have his weight and height measured because he is obese. He balks at having his temperature taken, stating that he knows he is not ill and "absolutely does not need to have that done." Stephanie tries explaining to Travis the differences in temperature, pulse, respiration, and blood pressure in different age groups. Finally, Travis agrees to have his temperature taken with a tympanic thermometer. When Stephanie starts to take Travis's blood pressure, he resists and tells her that he is scared and just knows that taking his blood pressure will hurt. Stephanie finally convinces Travis that she needs to take all his vital signs to prepare him for Dr. Karas' examination.

Would you be prepared to explain to a new patient the importance of taking body measurements and vital signs?

1. **Why would Dr. Karas want height and weight measurements on each visit for patients in all age groups?**

   _____
   _____

2. **Why are growth charts important in treating pediatric patients?**

   _____
   _____
   _____

3. **Why are head and chest circumference measurements important in pediatric patients?**

   _____
   _____
   _____

Copyright © 2010, 2005 by Saunders, an imprint of Elsevier, Inc. All rights reserved.

4. How can Stephanie convince Travis that it is important for his height and weight to be taken with each visit? How can she make the weight mensuration less upsetting to Travis?

5. What are the differences in temperature, pulse, respirations, and blood pressure in age groups?

6. How would a tympanic temperature reading differ from an oral temperature?

7. What does Stephanie need to explain to Travis about taking blood pressure?

8. Because Travis is upset, should Stephanie take his blood pressure immediately? Explain your answer.

9. What measurements are included in taking a patient's vital signs?

APPLICATION OF SKILLS

Procedure Check-off Sheets (*) and assignments from MACC on the Evolve site at http://evolve.elsevier.com/klieger/medicalassisting (**)

1. Perform Procedure 33-1: Measure Weight and Height of an Adult.*

2. Perform Procedure 33-2: Measure Weight and Length of an Infant.*

3. Perform Procedure 33-3: Measure Head and Chest Circumference of an Infant.*

4. Perform Procedure 33-4: Measure Oral Body Temperature Using a Mercury-Free Glass Thermometer.*

5. Perform Procedure 33-5: Measure Oral Body Temperature Using a Rechargeable Electronic or Digital Thermometer.*

6. Perform Procedure 33-6: Measure Rectal Body Temperature Using a Rechargeable Electronic or Digital Thermometer.*

7. Perform Procedure 33-7: Measure Axillary Body Temperature Using a Rechargeable Electronic or Digital Thermometer.*

8. Perform Procedure 33-8: Measure Body Temperature Using a Tympanic Thermometer.*

9. Perform Procedure 33-9: Measure Body Temperature Using a Disposable Oral Thermometer.*

10. Perform Procedure 33-10: Measure Radial Pulse.*

11. Perform Procedure 33-11: Measure Apical Pulse.*

12. Perform Procedure 33-12: Measure Respiratory Rate.*

13. Perform Procedure 33-13: Measure Blood Pressure.*

CHAPTER QUIZ

Multiple Choice

Identify the letter of the choice that best completes the statement or answers the question.

1. The birth weight of an infant should _____ in the first 6 months.
   A. double
   B. triple
   C. quadruple
   D. stay the same

2. Children should have their height recorded _____.
   A. each month
   B. every 6 months
   C. every visit
   D. every year

3. Growth charts provide information on the height and weight pattern of a child from infancy.
   A. True
   B. False

4. When the ventricles contract, the first measurable pressure is the _____ pressure.
   A. blood
   B. diastolic
   C. systolic
   D. none of the above

5. The mercury-free thermometer tip color, _____, signifies that it is to be used orally.
   A. blue
   B. green
   C. red
   D. yellow

6. It is better to use a larger cuff when in doubt of which size to use.
   A. True
   B. False

7. _____ is(are) a low-pitched sound created as air goes through the bronchi.
   A. Stridor
   B. Rales
   C. Rhonchi
   D. Wheezes

8. An infant's head circumference is approximately _____% of an adult's head circumference by age 1.
   A. 50
   B. 60
   C. 70
   D. 80

9. Hypotension is a blood pressure that exceeds the acceptable range for the patient's age group.
   A. True
   B. False

10. _____ is the number of times the heart beats in a minute.
    A. Pulse
    B. Pulse rate
    C. Heart rate
    D. None of the above

11. When using a(n) _____, the temperature typically registers within 60 seconds.
    A. disposable oral thermometer
    B. temperature-sensitive tape
    C. tympanic thermometer
    D. electronic thermometer

12. Adults have a respiration rate of _____.
    A. 10 to 15
    B. 16 to 20
    C. 20 to 25
    D. 22 to 28

13. Normal adult systolic range is _____ mm Hg.
    A. 80 to 100
    B. 90 to 110
    C. 100 to 120
    D. 110 to 125

14. Respiratory rate can be described as being normal, slow, or rapid.
    A. True
    B. False

15. A heart rate greater than _____ beats/min is considered to be tachycardia.
    A. 80
    B. 90
    C. 95
    D. 100

16. It is recommended to take a patient's pulse for _____.
    A. 15 seconds and multiply by 4
    B. 20 seconds and multiply by 3
    C. 30 seconds and multiply by 2
    D. 60 seconds

17. The _____ artery is the most common place for a pulse to be measured in an adult.
    A. apical
    B. brachial
    C. femoral
    D. radial

18. When listening to the heart with a stethoscope, the sound you hear is _____.
    A. lupp-dupp
    B. lubb-dubb
    C. lubb-dupp
    D. none of the above

19. Blood pressure can be measured over clothes.
    A. True
    B. False

20. The _____ pulse must be taken with a stethoscope.
    A. apical
    B. brachial
    C. popliteal
    D. radial

34 Obtaining the Medical History

VOCABULARY REVIEW

Matching: Match each term with the correct definition.

A. charting

B. demographics

C. familial

D. Health Insurance Portability and Accountability Act (HIPAA)

E. hereditary

F. objective information

G. past history

H. release of information

I. review of systems

J. social history

K. subjective information

L. symptoms

M. chief complaint

N. open-ended questions

O. signs

_____ 1. Step-by-step review of each body system

_____ 2. Biographical data; personal information

_____ 3. Subjective data reported by the patient

_____ 4. Able to be seen or measured

_____ 5. Summary of a patient's prior health

_____ 6. Found in a family member

_____ 7. Overview of a patient's lifestyle

_____ 8. Documenting what is observed or what is told by the patient

_____ 9. Not able to be seen or measured

_____ 10. Government act mandating that appropriate measures be taken to protect a patient's personal information

_____ 11. Legal form signed by a patient that indicates who can see the patient's health records

_____ 12. Acquired through genetic makeup

_____ 13. Reason why the patient wants to see the physician

_____ 14. Questions that require more than a "yes" or "no" answer

_____ 15. Observable evidence that can be seen or measured

THEORY RECALL

True/False

Indicate whether the statement is true or false.

_____ 1. The first step in interviewing any patient is to ensure the interview is private and free of interruptions.

_____ 2. Information that can be measured or observed is called "objective information."

_____ 3. Effective communication slows down the medical assistant in her or his search for necessary information.

_____ 4. It is important to be reactive to shocking details the patient tells the medical assistant.

_____ 5. The medical assistant must report what is seen, heard, felt, and smelled.

Multiple Choice

Identify the letter of the choice that best completes the statement or answers the question.

1. Charting must be _____.
   A. clear
   B. correct
   C. nonjudgmental
   D. all of the above

2. The personal data section of a medical history is completed by the _____.
   A. physician
   B. medical assistant
   C. patient
   D. insurance company
   E. either B or C

3. Symptoms that cannot be seen are referred to as _____ information.
   A. assessment
   B. objective
   C. subjective
   D. present illness

4. The medical assistant should start the charting with _____.
   A. a clean progress note sheet
   B. the date and time
   C. a pen, blue ink only
   D. a bottle of whiteout in hand to make necessary corrections

5. When interviewing the patient, the medical assistant should _____.
   A. be quick, efficient, and to the point
   B. relay personal stories to make the patient feel more at ease
   C. show genuine concern for the patient
   D. make assumptions as to the patient's answers

Copyright © 2010, 2005 by Saunders, an imprint of Elsevier, Inc. All rights reserved.

6. The _____ section contains more description about the current illness.
   A. social history
   B. present illness
   C. past history
   D. family history

7. The review of systems starts _____.
   A. as the patient walks in the door
   B. at the patient's feet and moves upward
   C. at the patient's head and moves downward
   D. none of the above

8. The medical assistant should ask _____.
   A. only the 13 standard questions of a physical examination
   B. yes or no questions
   C. open-ended questions
   D. direct questions

9. _____ is a brief statement of only one or two signs or symptoms.
   A. CC
   B. PH
   C. SH
   D. PI

10. _____ statements that pertain to the patient are key to providing a good database for the patient's physical examination.
    A. Encoding
    B. Charting
    C. Expanding on
    D. None of the above

11. The physician's treatment plan is based on _____.
    A. latest trends in technology
    B. laboratory findings only
    C. information gathered during history taking and physical examination
    D. physical examination only

12. Patients have _____ to expect that their confidential information is being protected.
    A. the right
    B. the privilege
    C. guarantees
    D. laws

Sentence Completion

Complete each sentence or statement.

diagnosis	family history	demographic
present illness	release of information	past history
familial	HIPAA	review of symptoms
social history		

1. _____ is a health inventory of a patient's immediate family.

2. _____ information includes the patient's name, address, date of birth, and telephone number.

3. _____ is an expansion of the patient's chief complaint.

4. _____ must be completed before a patient's chart can be shared with another physician.

5. _____ presents an overview of the patient's lifestyle.

Short Answers

1. List six pieces of information that need to be included when gathering the patient's past history.

   _____
   _____
   _____

2. List the four areas on which observations are based.

   _____
   _____
   _____
   _____

3. List the seven sections of the medical history form.

   _____
   _____
   _____

4. List five items the medical assistant should remember about charting.

   _____
   _____
   _____
   _____
   _____

Copyright © 2010, 2005 by Saunders, an imprint of Elsevier, Inc. All rights reserved.

CHAPTER 34   Obtaining the Medical History

CRITICAL THINKING

1. Melinda was Cindy's eighth patient after lunch. The last thing Cindy felt like doing was taking Melinda back to the examination room. Melinda always had a zillion questions and a story for everything. Trying to get to the reason Melinda was in to see the physician was always a challenge. Today, when Cindy went to retrieve Melinda from the waiting area, she was not even smiling. She was shuffling her feet and staring at the ground all the way back to the examination room. Cindy asked Melinda what was wrong and commented that Melinda did not seem to be herself today. Melinda responded, "No, dear, I'm just fine; don't you worry." But Cindy was worried that what Melinda was saying did not coincide with how she was acting.

    A. Describe what verbal and nonverbal communication is occurring between Cindy and Melinda.

    _____
    _____
    _____
    _____

    B. If you had to guess, what do you think is going on with Melinda, based just on the brief exchange given here?

    _____
    _____
    _____
    _____

PRACTICAL APPLICATIONS

If you have accomplished the objectives in this chapter, you will be able to make better choices as a medical assistant. Take another look at this situation and decide what you would do.

Dr. Walker, an obstetrician/gynecologist and internal medicine physician, has hired Jenny to assist with taking medical histories for his patients. Dr. Walker sees many patients who have high-risk pregnancies because of an infectious disease. Sarah, a new patient who is 4 months' pregnant, has been referred to Dr. Walker because she is at risk for several infectious diseases. Jenny goes to the waiting room and starts to ask Sarah questions about her pregnancy and her past medical history. Sarah tells Jenny that she does not want to discuss this with a medical assistant and would rather give the information to Dr. Walker. Jenny adamantly tells Sarah that if she does not want to cooperate, Dr. Walker will not see her as a patient. Sarah begins to cry, but starts telling her history to Jenny. Trying to impress Sarah during the interview, Jenny uses medical terminology to ask questions, and she never looks at Sarah or makes any observations about Sarah's remarks. After the history taking, Sarah is escorted to the examination room, where her vital signs are taken. After discussing her previous illnesses and family history, Dr. Walker examines Sarah and orders several laboratory tests, including tests for HIV and for syphilis. His tentative diagnosis is "possible HIV infection," and he confirms her pregnancy of 4 months. On leaving the office, Sarah makes an appointment for 2 weeks to discuss her test results and final diagnosis with Dr. Walker.

What should Jenny have done differently as a medical assistant initially taking Sarah's history?

Copyright © 2010, 2005 by Saunders, an imprint of Elsevier, Inc. All rights reserved.

1. Did Jenny handle the taking of the medical history correctly? Where should the history have been taken?

2. What actions would cause Sarah to think that Jenny is incompetent in taking a medical history?

3. Why is effective communication between the patient and the medical assistant so important when taking a medical history?

4. What is the "chief complaint," and how should it be documented?

5. What are signs? What are symptoms?

6. What is the correct name for the "tentative diagnosis"? What is the difference between this diagnosis and the "final diagnosis"?

7. Why would it be incorrect for the insurance coder to use the tentative diagnosis on the insurance claim form? What could be the repercussions if the laboratory tests are negative?

8. Why would it have been important for Jenny to observe Sarah during the taking of the medical history?

APPLICATION OF SKILLS

Procedure Check-off Sheets (*) and assignments from MACC on the Evolve site at http://evolve.elsevier.com/klieger/medicalassisting (**)

1. Perform Procedure 34-1: Complete a Medical History Form.*

2. Perform Procedure 34-2: Recognize and Respond to Verbal and Nonverbal Communication.*

CHAPTER QUIZ

Multiple Choice

Identify the letter of the choice that best completes the statement or answers the question.

1. The medical assistant must ensure _____ to obtain a good interview with a patient.
    A. confidentiality
    B. privacy
    C. an interruption-free environment
    D. all of the above

2. Symptoms that cannot be measured are known as (the) _____.
    A. chief complaint
    B. objective information
    C. present illness
    D. subjective information

3. A release-of-information form must be on file for a patient's information to be released to another physician.
    A. True
    B. False

4. _____ gives an overview of the patient's eating, drinking, smoking, and exercise habits.
    A. Family history
    B. Past history
    C. Review of systems
    D. Social history

5. _____ provide(s) observable information that can be measured.
    A. Chief complaint
    B. Signs
    C. Symptoms
    D. Past history

6. When charting, the medical assistant must be _____.
    A. clear and concise
    B. judgmental and critical
    C. selective and indecisive
    D. quick and decisive

7. _____ information includes a patient's name, address, date of birth, and gender.
    A. Familial
    B. Social
    C. Demographic
    D. Past history

8. The ROS starts with the _____.
    A. feet
    B. head
    C. when the patient walks in the door
    D. none of the above

Copyright © 2010, 2005 by Saunders, an imprint of Elsevier, Inc. All rights reserved.

9. The medical assistant has to report only what he or she hears to the physician.
   A. True
   B. False

10. Identification of a disease or condition based on review of signs and symptoms, laboratory reports, history, and procedures is known as the _____.
    A. chief complaint
    B. diagnosis
    C. objective information
    D. past history

11. _____ should be held in the strictest confidence.
    A. Family history
    B. Social history
    C. Past history
    D. All of the above

12. A medical assistant is allowed to chart his or her opinions about the patient's present history.
    A. True
    B. False

13. Information that can be measured or observed is _____.
    A. objective
    B. subjective
    C. assessment
    D. social history

14. _____ are observable evidence that can be seen or measured.
    A. Signs
    B. Symptoms

15. _____ is acquired through genetic makeup.
    A. Heredity
    B. Social history
    C. Environmental history
    D. None of the above

35 Assisting with the Physical Examination

VOCABULARY REVIEW

Matching: Match each term with the correct definition.

A. accommodation

B. auscultation

C. BSE

D. crepitus

E. diaphoresis

F. distention

G. erythema

H. gingivitis

I. goniometer

J. herpes simplex

K. jaundice

L. lithotomy position

M. macrotia

N. murmur

O. pallor

P. patent

Q. percussion

R. perforation

S. PERRLA

T. presbycusis

_____ 1. Patient's back is on the table; horizontal recumbent position

_____ 2. Crackling sound heard in the lungs or joints

_____ 3. Paleness

_____ 4. Humming or low-pitched fluttering sound of the heart heard on auscultation

_____ 5. Viral infection of the lip-skin junction; cold sore

_____ 6. Rattling sounds heard in the lungs, usually at the base

_____ 7. Ability of the eye to see objects in the distance, and then adjust to a close object

_____ 8. Ability to see at different distances

_____ 9. Patient assumes the dorsal recumbent position first; then the buttocks are moved to the end of the table and the feet are placed in stirrups

_____ 10. Decrease in hearing ability resulting from aging

_____ 11. Swollen

_____ 12. Tapping to check for reflexes or sounds of body cavities

_____ 13. Ringing in the ears

_____ 14. Listening for signs using a stethoscope

_____ 15. Open; not obstructed

_____ 16. Patient is first in the supine position, then turns onto left side with the right leg sharply bent upward

_____ 17. Skin resiliency

428 CHAPTER 35 Assisting with the Physical Examination

U. prone position

V. rhonchi

W. Sims' position

X. supine position

Y. thrill

Z. tinnitus

AA. turgor

BB. vertigo

CC. visual acuity

DD. sitting position

_____ 18. Ears larger than 10 cm

_____ 19. Yellowish appearance to the skin and eyes

_____ 20. Pupils equal, round, and reactive to light and accommodation

_____ 21. Excessive perspiration

_____ 22. Palpable vibration

_____ 23. Device used to measure joint movements and angles

_____ 24. Breast-self examination

_____ 25. Dizziness

_____ 26. Inflammation of the gums

_____ 27. Tear or hole in an organ or body part

_____ 28. Reddish discoloration of the skin

_____ 29. Patient lies on the abdomen with the head turned slightly to the side

_____ 30. Patient's body is at a 90-degree angle

THEORY RECALL

True/False

Indicate whether the statement is true or false.

_____ 1. When the medical assistant is positioning and draping the patient, he or she should always consider the patient's comfort and minimize the area of exposure.

_____ 2. When a patient is in semi-Fowler's position, the table must be at a 90-degree angle.

_____ 3. The medical assistant must assist an elderly patient with disrobing.

_____ 4. The receptionist is responsible for having the patient ready in a room for the medical assistant.

_____ 5. A patient can withdraw consent for an examination after the form has been put into the chart.

Multiple Choice

Identify the letter of the choice that best completes the statement or answers the question.

1. The _____ position helps the patient breathe easier.
   A. dorsal recumbent
   B. knee-chest
   C. Fowler's
   D. Sims'

2. _____ is the medical term for "ringing of the ears."
   A. Crepitus
   B. Tinnitus
   C. Presbycusis
   D. Vertigo

3. (A) _____ must be provided if the examination is beyond a wellness physical.
   A. chaperone
   B. gown
   C. patient's informed consent
   D. none of the above

4. Failure to secure consent for a procedure such as a colonoscopy is considered _____.
   A. assault and battery
   B. an OSHA violation
   C. dangerous
   D. consent is not required for a colonoscopy

5. The _____ position is most often used to begin a physical examination because the upper extremities are clearly accessible.
   A. horizontal recumbent
   B. sitting
   C. Sims'
   D. standing

6. When a patient is in full-Fowler's position, the table is at a _____-degree angle.
   A. 30
   B. 45
   C. 60
   D. 90

7. The _____ position can be used for rectal examination and enema administration.
   A. knee-chest
   B. prone
   C. Sims'
   D. supine

8. The physician uses a(n) _____ to examine the interior of the eye.
   A. otoscope
   B. ophthalmoscope
   C. speculum
   D. none of the above

9. The _____ chart is used to test a person's ability to read at a prescribed near distance.
   A. Jaeger
   B. Ishihara
   C. Snellen
   D. rotating E chart

10. When using the Snellen eye chart, the patient should be _____ feet from the chart.
    A. 10
    B. 15
    C. 20
    D. 25

11. The patient's type of gown will be decided by _____.
    A. patient's preference
    B. procedure to be performed
    C. the AMA
    D. all of the above

12. Patients have the right to refuse treatment.
    A. True
    B. False

13. _____ is a yellowish discoloration of the skin and eyes.
    A. Bruit
    B. Cyanosis
    C. Jaundice
    D. Erythema

14. _____ is a low-pitched fluttering sound made by the heart.
    A. Rales
    B. Thrill
    C. Turgor
    D. Murmur

15. _____ is the touching or feeling of body organs, lymph nodes, and tissue.
    A. Auscultation
    B. Palpation
    C. Percussion
    D. Turgor

16. Patient _____ must be the prime consideration for the medical assistant during positioning of the patient.
    A. safety
    B. ethnicity
    C. body size
    D. modesty

17. The _____ eye chart has rows of letters.
    A. Jaeger
    B. Ishihara
    C. Snellen
    D. none of the above

18. The _____ position is most often used for nonflexible sigmoidoscopy.
    A. Sims'
    B. Fowler's
    C. knee-chest
    D. dorsal recumbent

19. When a physician needs to determine the patient's coordination and balance through observation, the patient would be in the _____ position.
    A. dorsal recumbent
    B. sitting
    C. prone
    D. standing

20. _____ is a visual viewing of all body parts and surface areas for symmetry.
    A. Palpation
    B. Auscultation
    C. Inspection
    D. Percussion

21. _____ is when a patient has trouble focusing and vision is blurred. The shape of the cornea or lens prevents light from projecting onto the retina.
    A. Hypermetropia
    B. Myopia
    C. Presbyopia
    D. Astigmatism

22. Which method of vision testing works best for preschoolers?
    A. Jaeger
    B. Ishihara
    C. Snellen
    D. None of the above

23. Of the following, which item would *not* be used for a distance visual acuity test?
    A. Eye occluder
    B. Snellen eye chart
    C. Ophthalmoscope
    D. All would be used

24. The medical assistant's major role in preparing a patient for a _____ is to have the patient gowned, appropriately positioned, and draped for the physician.
    A. CPX
    B. BMI
    C. CXR
    D. PXR

25. Which one of the following items is *not* required for a routine physical examination?
    A. Tape measure
    B. Vaginal speculum
    C. Percussion hammer
    D. Tuning fork

CHAPTER 35 Assisting with the Physical Examination

Sentence Completion

Complete each sentence or statement.

palpation	otoscope	ophthalmoscope
turgor	dorsal recumbent	PERRLA
Weber	lithotomy	Snellen
auscultation	HEENT	

1. _____ involves the use of a stethoscope to detect sounds of the heart, respiratory system, and intestines.

2. The _____ position is the best position for the Pap smear and pelvic examination.

3. _____ involves the use by the physician of his or her hands to locate and touch major organs and lymph nodes to detect tenderness in an area.

4. The _____ chart tests for distant visual acuity.

5. The _____ aids physicians in checking the appearance of the eardrum and ear canal.

Short Answers

1. List the nine examination positions with which a medical assistant should be familiar.

   _____
   _____
   _____
   _____

2. Describe the three types of Snellen charts, and give one example of why each would be used.

   _____
   _____
   _____
   _____
   _____
   _____

3. Explain the difference between implied and informed consent.

CRITICAL THINKING

1. Magdalena Jimenez has recently moved to the United States; her mother is enrolling her in school and has made an appointment for a school physical. Magdalena does not speak English, and her mother speaks very little. You do not speak Spanish. Describe how you would proceed with Magdalena's physical examination. Which Snellen chart would you use to assess Magdalena's visual acuity?

2. In what body system would you expect to see the following terms and abbreviations used in documentation?
   a. LMP
   b. distention
   c. turgor
   d. bruit
   e. PERRLA
   f. rhonchi
   g. BPH
   h. perforation
   i. pallor
   j. thrill

PRACTICAL APPLICATIONS

If you have accomplished the objectives in this chapter, you will be able to make better choices as a medical assistant. Take a look at this situation and decide what you would do.

Beth is a medical assistant in the office of Dr. Havidiz, a family practitioner. Dr. Havidiz treats many low-income families, and many women in the community see him for gynecological visits. Holly, a new patient, comes to see Dr. Havidiz for a possible vaginal infection. Her demeanor shows her fear of the physician's

Copyright © 2010, 2005 by Saunders, an imprint of Elsevier, Inc. All rights reserved.

office, especially because this is the first time she has seen Dr. Havidiz. Dr. Havidiz was called to the hospital to see a critically ill patient earlier in the day, so appointments are delayed.

There is an available examination room when Holly arrives, so Beth takes her to the room and tells her to undress completely. Beth does not tell Holly how to put on the gown, but she stands in the room and watches Holly undress. While Holly is undressing, Beth asks the questions necessary to obtain the medical history. Beth then places Holly on the examination table in the lithotomy position and immediately leaves the room, giving the impression that she is in a great hurry. After 15 minutes, Holly has discomfort in her back but dares not move from the position because she does not want to delay the examination. After 30 minutes, Holly wonders just how much longer it will take for Dr. Havidiz to come and check her. Finally, Dr. Havidiz arrives and the examination begins.

During the examination, Beth leaves the room to answer a personal phone call, leaving Dr. Havidiz and Holly alone. As Holly leaves the office, she is in tears from back pain and appears to be very upset. Beth shows no sympathy or empathy for Holly. Two days later, Holly asks that her records be transferred to another physician and tells Dr. Havidiz that she has never been treated as rudely as she was in his office.

How might this situation have been avoided?

1. How did Beth invade Holly's privacy?

_____

_____

_____

2. Under what conditions should Beth have taken Holly's history?

_____

_____

3. Why was it important to tell Holly how to put on the gown for the examination? How should the drape have been applied?

_____

_____

_____

_____

4. What examination methods would you expect the medical assistant to use while preparing Holly for an examination?

_____

_____

_____

_____

Copyright © 2010, 2005 by Saunders, an imprint of Elsevier, Inc. All rights reserved.

5. What methods of examination would you expect the physician to use during the examination?

6. What positions should have been used for Holly while she was waiting for the pelvic examination? What positions are inappropriate for a long wait? What explanation should Beth have given when placing Holly in the position?

7. How should Beth have handled the delay?

8. Why is it unethical for Beth to leave the room during the physical examination?

9. Do you think that Holly had a legitimate complaint to Dr. Havidiz about her treatment? Explain your answer.

APPLICATION OF SKILLS

Procedure Check-off Sheets (*) and assignments from MACC on the Evolve site at http://evolve.elsevier.com/klieger/medicalassisting (**)

1. Perform Procedure 35-1: Assist with the Physical Examination.*

2. Perform Procedure 35-2: Sitting Position.*

3. Perform Procedure 35-3: Recumbent Position.*

4. Perform Procedure 35-4: Lithotomy Position.*

5. Perform Procedure 35-5: Sims' Position.*

6. Perform Procedure 35-6: Prone Position.*

7. Perform Procedure 35-7: Knee-Chest Position.*

8. Perform Procedure 35-8: Fowler's Position.*

9. Perform Procedure 35-9: Assess Distance Visual Acuity Using a Snellen Chart.*

10. Perform Procedure 35-10: Assess Color Vision Using the Ishihara Test.*

11. Perform Procedure 35-11: Assess Near Vision Using a Jaeger Card.*

CHAPTER QUIZ

Multiple Choice

Identify the letter of the choice that best completes the statement or answers the question.

1. _____ is the position that helps the patient breathe better when in respiratory distress.
    A. Dorsal recumbent
    B. Lithotomy
    C. Fowler's
    D. Sims'

2. _____ is used by the physician to check the nervous system.
    A. Auscultation
    B. Palpation
    C. Percussion
    D. Inspection

3. The medical assistant must choose the right type and size of gown for the examination being performed.
    A. True
    B. False

4. _____ is another name for "ringing in the ears."
   A. Crepitus
   B. Turgor
   C. Tinnitus
   D. Vertigo

5. Listening for body sounds, usually with a stethoscope, is called _____.
   A. auscultation
   B. inspection
   C. palpation
   D. thrill

6. Patients cannot withdraw their consent once it has been given and documented in their chart.
   A. True
   B. False

7. Bluish coloration of the skin because of lack of oxygen is called _____.
   A. bruit
   B. cyanosis
   C. jaundice
   D. gingivitis

8. _____ is(are) crackling sounds heard in the lungs, usually at the base.
   A. Bruit
   B. Crepitus
   C. Rales
   D. Rhonchi

9. Taking a patient's pulse is done by palpation.
   A. True
   B. False

10. The _____ position is most often used for a colonoscopy.
    A. dorsal recumbent
    B. knee-chest
    C. Fowler's
    D. prone

11. Color vision is tested with the _____ test.
    A. Ishihara
    B. Jaeger
    C. Snellen
    D. rotating E chart

12. A patient in the supine position whose head is at a 45-degree angle is in the _____ position.
    A. dorsal recumbent
    B. full-Fowler's
    C. semi-Fowler's
    D. supine

13. The physician uses a(n) _____ to visualize the eardrum or tympanic membrane.
    A. ophthalmoscope
    B. otoscope
    C. speculum
    D. none of the above

14. Ears smaller than 4 cm are known as macrotia.
    A. True
    B. False

15. The back and lower extremities can be examined with the patient in the _____ position.
    A. lithotomy
    B. prone
    C. sitting
    D. standing

16. Observation of the reaction of the pupils to the exposure of direct light is documented using which one of the following acronyms?
    A. PUPIL
    B. PERRLA
    C. AAOLX3
    D. none of the above

17. A device used to measure joint movements and angles is called a _____.
    A. flexible cloth tape measure
    B. yardstick
    C. goniometer
    D. pelvimeter

18. Decrease in hearing ability resulting from aging is called _____.
    A. myopia
    B. presbyopia
    C. presbycusis
    D. tinnitus

19. Medical term for "dizziness" is _____.
    A. tinnitus
    B. turgor
    C. macrotia
    D. vertigo

20. The medical term for "excessive sweating" is _____.
    A. diaphoresis
    B. crepitus
    C. gingivitis
    D. turgor

36 Electrocardiography

VOCABULARY REVIEW

Matching: Match each term with the correct definition.

A. alternating current interference

B. amplifier

C. arrhythmia

D. artifact

E. atrioventricular node

F. augmented leads

G. baseline

H. bipolar leads

I. bundle branches

J. bundle of His

K. cardiac cycle

L. electrocardiogram

M. galvanometer

N. interval

O. ischemia

P. myocardial infarction

Q. normal sinus rhythm

R. paroxysmal atrial tachycardia

S. PR interval

_____ 1. Condition in which the ventricles receive an impulse prematurely and contract early

_____ 2. Knot of specialized cells in the lower portion of the right atrium that produces the heart's electrical impulses

_____ 3. ECG pattern that represents heart-specific electrical activity

_____ 4. ECG pattern that shows the length of a wave with a segment

_____ 5. Graphic picture of the heart's electrical activity

_____ 6. Body tremors caused by voluntary or involuntary muscle movement

_____ 7. Electrical interference that appears as small, uniform spikes on ECG paper

_____ 8. Sudden onset and ending of atrial tachycardia

_____ 9. Normal, small upward curve that occasionally follows a complete ECG cycle after PQRST

_____ 10. Standard limb leads

_____ 11. Rhythm measurement that starts at the SA node; occurs within an established time frame; and follows an expected, established pattern

_____ 12. Cardiac fibers that receive impulses from the bundle branches and take them throughout the heart muscle

_____ 13. Abnormal heart rate, rhythm, and conduction system

_____ 14. Device that detects and converts the amplified electrical signal into a tracing on the ECG machine

_____ 15. Heated device that records the heart's activity on heat-sensitive graph paper

T. premature ventricular contraction

U. Purkinje fibers

V. QRS complex

W. repolarization

X. somatic tremor

Y. standardization

Z. stylus

AA. tracing

BB. U wave

CC. ventricular fibrillation

DD. wandering baseline

EE. wave

_____ 16. Small band of atypical cardiac muscle fibers that receive electrical impulses from the AV node

_____ 17. Resting phase of the ECG cycle

_____ 18. Line that separates the various cardiac waves; representative of the space between heartbeats while the heart is "resting"; also called isoelectric line

_____ 19. Time interval between atrial contraction and the beginning of ventricular contraction

_____ 20. Life-threatening condition of ventricular twitching that causes inefficient pumping action, stopping blood circulation

_____ 21. Device on the electrocardiograph that magnifies or enlarges the heart's electrical impulses so that they can be recorded

_____ 22. Poor blood supply to body tissue causing a lack of oxygen to that tissue

_____ 23. ECG pattern that shows when the impulse moves through the ventricle and reaches the Purkinje fibers, depicting contraction of both ventricles

_____ 24. Shift on the ECG tracing from the baseline or center of the paper

_____ 25. Unwanted changes in an ECG tracing caused by movement, machine malfunction, or other factors

_____ 26. Heart attack; death of the heart tissue caused by blockage of the heart's blood vessels

_____ 27. One heartbeat; one contraction/relaxation phase of the heart

_____ 28. Recording of the ECG cycle

_____ 29. Leads that measure cardiac activity from one electrode on the body at a time; recordings are augmented so that they can be read

_____ 30. Bundle of cardiac fibers that receive electrical impulses from the bundle of His

_____ 31. Process of ensuring that an ECG taken on one machine would compare with a tracing taken on another machine

THEORY RECALL

True/False

Indicate whether the statement is true or false.

_____ 1. Electrocardiography is a painless, noninvasive procedure often done as a part of a routine examination.

_____ 2. The QRS complex shows the time interval between the ventricular contraction and the beginning of ventricular relaxation.

_____ 3. Artifact occurs when a tracing shifts from the baseline, or center of the paper, and moves over the ECG paper.

_____ 4. The medical assistant must never interpret the ECG.

_____ 5. Repolarization is a discharge of electrical energy that causes contraction.

Multiple Choice

Identify the letter of the choice that best completes the statement or answers the question.

1. Leads I, II, and III are called _____ leads.
   A. augmented
   B. bipolar
   C. chest
   D. precordial

2. In standard limb leads or bipolar leads, the _____ is always negative.
   A. right arm
   B. right leg
   C. left arm
   D. left leg

3. Lead _____ is considered to be the rhythm strip.
   A. I
   B. II
   C. III
   D. IV

4. The resting phase of the heart is also known as _____.
   A. depolarization
   B. polarization
   C. relaxation
   D. repolarization

5. _____ shows how long it takes for the electrical impulse to go from the SA node to the AV node.
   A. QT interval
   B. QRS complex
   C. PR interval
   D. PR segment

Copyright © 2010, 2005 by Saunders, an imprint of Elsevier, Inc. All rights reserved.

6. _____ measure the activity of one electrode on the body surface.
   A. Bipolar leads
   B. Chest leads
   C. Standard limb leads
   D. Unipolar leads

7. _____ results from excessive electrical impulses from external sources and appears as small, uniform spikes on the ECG tracing.
   A. AC interference
   B. Artifact
   C. Arrhythmia
   D. Wandering baseline

8. Arrhythmia can mean abnormality in _____.
   A. conduction
   B. heart rate
   C. heart rhythm
   D. all of the above

9. The _____ wave is represented by a downward deflection following the P wave.
   A. Q
   B. R
   C. S
   D. T

10. _____ wave indicates the resting phase of the heart.
    A. P
    B. Q
    C. S
    D. T

11. _____ represents the time interval necessary for an electrical impulse to cause the atrial contraction and beginning the contraction of the ventricles.
    A. QT interval
    B. PR interval
    C. ST segment
    D. QRS

12. The first electrical impulse shown on an ECG is the _____ wave.
    A. T
    B. P
    C. S
    D. U

13. _____ is defined by three or more consecutive PVCs.
    A. Ventricular fibrillation
    B. Ventricular tachycardia
    C. Paroxysmal atrial tachycardia
    D. None of the above

14. _____ is the most life-threatening of all arrhythmias.
    A. Premature ventricular contraction
    B. Premature atrial contraction
    C. Ventricular tachycardia
    D. Ventricular fibrillation

15. _____ is a condition in which an electrical impulse in the atria starts before the next expected heartbeat.
    A. PAC
    B. PVC
    C. PAT
    D. NRS

16. When performing a Holter monitor ECG, the test should be conducted over a(n) _____ hour period.
    A. 8- to 12-
    B. 12- to 24-
    C. 24- to 48-
    D. 48- to 60-

17. The SA node is located in the _____.
    A. lower right atrium
    B. upper right atrium
    C. lower left atrium
    D. upper left atrium

18. Sinus bradycardia is a heartbeat of less than _____ beats/min.
    A. 50
    B. 60
    C. 80
    D. 100

19. A standardization mark is a mark made on the ECG paper that indicates the ECG can be interpreted against other ECGs.
    A. True
    B. False

20. A stylus records the motion on graph paper located in the machine by burning the impression on the heat-sensitive paper.
    A. True
    B. False

Sentence Completion

Complete each sentence or statement.

electrodes	segment	amplifier
baseline	ischemia	Q
cardiac cycle	treadmill test	Holter monitor
artifact	S	stylus
somatic tremor	standardization	interval
galvanometer	sinus bradycardia	
sinus tachycardia	U	

CHAPTER 36 Electrocardiography

1. _____ is a rhythmic cycle of a contraction and a relaxation process of the heart.

2. _____ is the process of ensuring that an ECG taken on one machine would compare with a tracing taken on another machine.

3. _____ is an abnormally rapid heartbeat.

4. _____ is an exercise ECG that is performed to determine if the heart is receiving enough blood during a time of stress.

5. The _____ wave is a small upward curve that may occasionally occur following a normal ECG tracing.

6. _____ are small devices made of a conductive material that are used to pick up the electrical activity of the heart generated by the myocardial cells.

7. _____ is a body tremor caused by voluntary or involuntary muscle movement.

8. A(n) _____ is worn and the diary is kept for a prescribed amount of time to evaluate heart activity over a period of time.

9. On an ECG tracing, the _____ indicates time and shows an entire wave with a segment.

10. The _____ magnifies the heart's electrical signal so that it can be recorded.

Short Answers

1. List and explain where precordial leads are placed.

   _____

   _____

   _____

2. List five problems an ECG can detect.

3. Explain the procedures for preparing a patient for a Holter monitor.

4. Explain the placement of the electrodes on the skin.

CRITICAL THINKING

1. Ruth Darcy is a 78-year-old patient who is in the office today for a refill check on her heart medication. She looks a little diaphoretic and pale. When you go to escort her back to the examination room, you ask, "Ruth, how are you feeling today?" Ms. Darcy answers, "Not one of my better days, dear. Definitely not one of my better days. Got a little pain in my chest; probably just indigestion from the sandwich I had at lunch. It feels awfully hot in here." You escort Ms. Darcy to the examination room, and then go notify the physician that Ms. Darcy is not doing well. Dr. Barnard asks you to do a set of vitals quickly and get her hooked up to the ECG and run a strip. Ms. Darcy's blood pressure is 220/98 mm Hg, her pulse is 112 beats/min, and her respirations are 24.

Copyright © 2010, 2005 by Saunders, an imprint of Elsevier, Inc. All rights reserved.

A. Describe your conversation and explanation of the procedure with Ms. Darcy as you are getting her ready for the ECG.

_____

_____

_____

_____

_____

B. Describe the steps of preparing Ms. Darcy for the ECG and the procedure for running the ECG.

_____

_____

_____

_____

_____

PRACTICAL APPLICATIONS

If you have accomplished the objectives in this chapter, you will be able to make better choices as a medical assistant. Take a look at this situation and decide what you would do.

Jim, a 55-year-old long-time smoker who is also overweight, has taken his grandchildren to the beach for the day. Mary, Jim's wife, notices that Jim is a little short of breath and seems to rub his chest often, so she asks if he is okay. Jim tells Mary that he thinks that he needs to get to a doctor because he has chest pain that is not subsiding. They drop off the children and immediately go to the medical office.

On arrival, Jim tells Gomez, the medical assistant, about his chest pain, which now seems to be in his left arm and left jaw. Gomez tells Jim that it is "probably just indigestion" and lets Jim sit in the waiting room. Finally, observing that Jim is very short of breath and is clasping his chest, Gomez asks the attending physician, Dr. Startz, if he can obtain an ECG.

Receiving approval for the ECG, Gomez quickly loads the paper into the electrocardiograph, not taking the necessary care to prevent markings on the ECG paper. Jim has suntan oil on his body, and his chest is hairy, so the electrodes do not attach with sufficient pressure to stay on the skin when the leads are placed on the tabs. Gomez places the electrodes in a haphazard manner, with no consideration of the way the tabs are facing. By this time, Jim is scared and experiencing a great deal of pain, which is causing diaphoresis, trembling, and twisting. Jim starts to sing and talk to relieve his tension, and the ECG has many artifacts. In a hurry to get the ECG to Dr. Startz because of Jim's declining condition, Gomez does not notice that the ECG also contains a wandering baseline. Even the rhythm strip is not readable.

On examination, Dr. Startz realizes the seriousness of Jim's condition and immediately sends him to the hospital, where another ECG and admission to the CICU are ordered. At the end of the day, Dr. Startz is upset and tells Gomez that if he cannot get a presentable ECG in an emergency situation, he might lose his job.

If you were the medical assistant in this situation, what would you have done?

1. What are Jim's risk factors for coronary artery disease?

2. What symptoms did Jim have at the beach and later in the medical office?

3. Since Jim came to the office complaining of chest pain, what would have been the appropriate action for Gomez to take?

4. Why does ECG paper need to be handled carefully?

5. How should Gomez have prepared Jim's chest for the ECG, and what effect did no preparation have on the ECG tracing?

6. What is an "artifact"? What actions by Jim caused the artifacts on the ECG?

7. What is a "wandering baseline," and what does this indicate?

8. How should the electrodes be turned when placed on the body?

9. How does a medical assistant obtain a rhythm strip on an ECG? What does the rhythm strip show?

10. What is the role of the medical assistant in obtaining an ECG tracing?

APPLICATION OF SKILLS

Label the ECG tracings.

1.
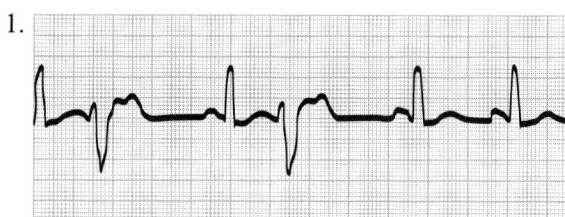
_____

2.
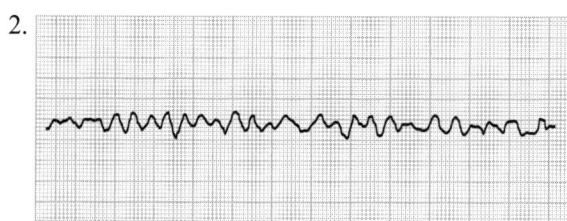
_____

3.
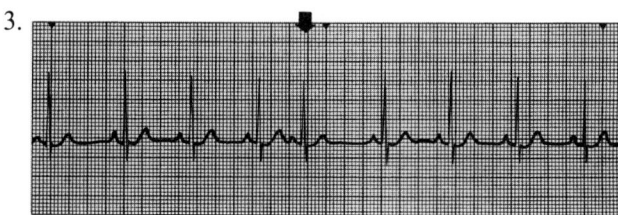
_____

(Modified from Huang S, et al: *Coronary care nursing,* Philadelphia, 1989, Saunders.)

4.
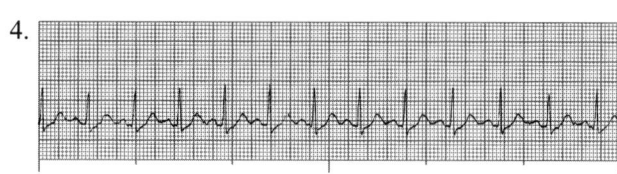
_____

(Modified from Aehlert B: *Pocket reference for ECGs made easy,* ed 3, St Louis, 2006, Mosby.)

5.
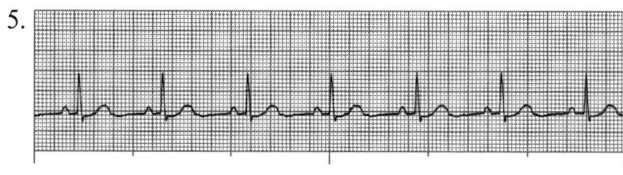
_____

(Modified from Aehlert B: *Pocket reference for ECGs made easy,* ed 3, St Louis, 2006, Mosby.)

Copyright © 2010, 2005 by Saunders, an imprint of Elsevier, Inc. All rights reserved.

6.

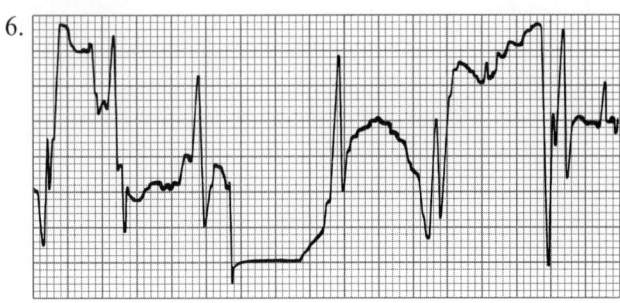

(Modified from Aehlert B: *ECGs made easy,* ed 3, St Louis, 2006, Mosby.)

7.

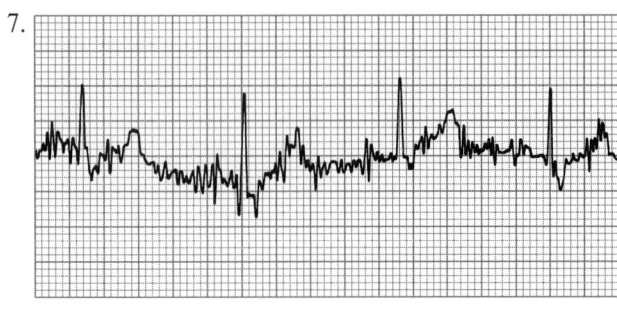

(Modified from Aehlert B: *ECGs made easy,* ed 3, St Louis, 2006, Mosby.)

8.

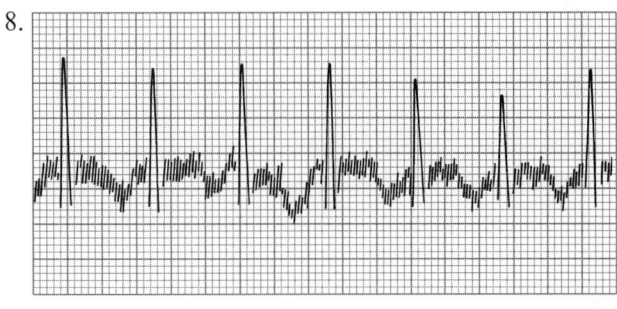

(Modified from Aehlert B: *ECGs made easy,* ed 3, St Louis, 2006, Mosby.)

Procedure Check-off Sheets (*) and assignments from MACC on the Evolve site at http://evolve.elsevier.com/klieger/medicalassisting (**)

1. Perform Procedure 36-1: Obtain a 12-Lead Electrocardiogram ECG Using a Single-Channel Electrocardiograph.*

2. Perform Procedure 36-2: Obtain a 12-Lead Electrocardiogram ECG Using a Three-Channel Electrocardiograph.*

3. Perform Procedure 36-3: Apply and Remove a Holter Monitor.*

CHAPTER QUIZ

Multiple Choice

Identify the letter of the choice that best completes the statement or answers the question.

1. It is perfectly acceptable for the medical assistant to provide the patient a clue as to the results of the ECG.
   A. True
   B. False

2. When attaching electrodes, the _____ is always positive.
   A. left leg
   B. left arm
   C. right leg
   D. right arm

3. An _____ is a wave on an ECG caused by something other than the electrical activity of the heart.
   A. artifact
   B. interference
   C. AC interference
   D. none of the above

4. A _____ occurs when an electrical impulse starts before the next expected beat.
   A. PAC
   B. PAT
   C. PVC
   D. QRS

5. _____ is a sudden onset of tachycardia measuring 150 to 250 beats/min.
   A. PAC
   B. PAT
   C. PVC
   D. QRS

6. _____ is the most deadly of all arrhythmias.
   A. V tach
   B. V fib
   C. PVC
   D. None of the above

7. _____ is the resting phase of the cardiac cycle.
   A. Contraction
   B. Depolarization
   C. Polarization
   D. Repolarization

8. The _____ wave represents the first electrical impulse.
   A. P
   B. Q
   C. R
   D. S

Copyright © 2010, 2005 by Saunders, an imprint of Elsevier, Inc. All rights reserved.

9. _____ enlarge(s) the heart's electrical signal so that it can be recorded.
   A. Leads
   B. Stylus
   C. Galvanometer
   D. Amplifier

10. The rhythm strip is lead _____.
    A. I
    B. II
    C. III
    D. IV

11. _____ results from electrolyte imbalances, caffeine, stress, cardiac disease, and emotions.
    A. PAC
    B. PVC
    C. PAT
    D. V fib

12. Leads I, II, and III are called _____ leads.
    A. augmented
    B. precordial
    C. standard
    D. chest

13. Holter monitoring is an ECG that is monitored over a(n) _____ hour period.
    A. 8- to 10-
    B. 12- to 24-
    C. 24- to 48-
    D. 48- to 60-

14. The _____ represents the time between atrial contraction and the beginning of ventricular stimulation.
    A. P wave
    B. ST interval
    C. PR interval
    D. QRS complex

15. _____ wave represents the resting phase of the cardiac cycle.
    A. S
    B. P
    C. T
    D. U

16. A device that detects and converts the amplified electrical signal into a tracing on the ECG machine is the _____.
    A. galvanometer
    B. pacemaker
    C. amplifier
    D. electrodes

17. The _____ is a rhythm measurement that starts at the SA node; occurs within an established time frame; and follows an expected, established form.
    A. PVC
    B. PAC
    C. PAT
    D. NSR

18. Unwanted changes in an ECG tracing caused by movement, machine malfunction, or other reasons are called _____.
    A. polarization
    B. ischemia
    C. artifacts
    D. arrhythmia

19. _____ are leads that measure cardiac activity from one electrode on the body at a time; recordings are augmented so that they can be read.
    A. Augmented leads
    B. Ischemic leads
    C. Laser leads
    D. Baseline leads

20. A small band of atypical cardiac muscle fibers that receive electrical impulses from the AV node is(are) the _____.
    A. SA node
    B. Purkinje fibers
    C. bundle of His
    D. myocardium

37 Radiography and Diagnostic Testing

VOCABULARY REVIEW

Matching: Match each term with the correct definition.

A. angiogram

B. caliper

C. claustrophobia

D. computer imaging

E. contrast medium

F. dosimeter

G. fluoroscopic imaging

H. intravenous pyelogram

I. lower gastrointestinal series

J. magnetic resonance imaging

K. mammography

L. nuclear medicine

M. open MRI

N. positron emission tomography

O. radiograph

P. radiopaque

Q. tomography

R. tracer

S. transducer

T. ultrasonography

_____ 1. Use of high-frequency sound waves to produce images

_____ 2. X-ray technique used to detect abnormalities of the breast

_____ 3. Diagnostic radiograph of the blood vessels using a contrast medium

_____ 4. Techniques that use radioactive material for patient diagnosis and treatment

_____ 5. Special photographic film that blackens in response to light

_____ 6. Radiographic imaging in which the view allows the radiologist to view image in motion

_____ 7. Procedure in which a sugar tracer is injected into the body and picked up by cancer cells, which send out signals that can be picked up by a camera, forming pictures of various body parts

_____ 8. Radiopaque substance that enhances an image

_____ 9. Able to be seen using an x-ray technique

_____ 10. Procedure in which strong magnetic field and radio waves are used to produce images to view body structures

_____ 11. Fear of closed places

_____ 12. Radiographic examination of the esophagus, stomach, and upper small intestine during and after the introduction of a contrast medium

_____ 13. Device that monitors the quantity of an x-ray exposure to health care workers

_____ 14. Picture or image created on film when exposed to x-rays

_____ 15. Hinged instrument that measures thickness or diameter

U. upper gastrointestinal series

V. x-ray tube

W. digital radiographic imaging

X. computed tomography

Y. x-ray film

Z. ultrasound

_____ 16. Radiographic examination of the lower intestinal tract during and after introduction of a contrast medium

_____ 17. Special radiographic medium that tags body cells, such as cancer cells

_____ 18. Vacuum tube that creates x-radiation

_____ 19. Radiography using computer imaging instead of conventional film or screen imaging

_____ 20. Imaging of soft tissue and internal organs using high-frequency sound waves

_____ 21. Radiographic view of the kidneys using contrast dye injected intravenously

_____ 22. Techniques that display images with the use of contrast media

_____ 23. Imaging table with more space used for MRI versus the enclosed narrow magnet tube

_____ 24. Device that is moved over the skin to record sound waves

_____ 25. Computerized procedure that views the target organ or body area from different angles in a three-dimensional view

_____ 26. Radiography that views the body or organ as a whole in a cross-sectional view

THEORY RECALL

True/False

Indicate whether the statement is true or false.

_____ 1. There is no advance preparation required for a patient to have a standard x-ray procedure.

_____ 2. It is acceptable for a patient to move during an x-ray procedure because the exposure time is of short duration.

_____ 3. Typical contrast media are barium and iodine.

_____ 4. A sugar tracer is used when performing a CT scan.

_____ 5. All states allow medical assistants to perform x-ray procedures.

Multiple Choice

Identify the letter of the choice that best completes the statement or answers the question.

1. _____ is the use of radiography to see the body or an organ as a whole in a cross-sectional or "slice" view.
   A. MRI
   B. PET
   C. Tomography
   D. Ultrasonography

2. When a patient is scheduled for a head and chest CT examination with contrast, the patient instructions should include _____.
   A. a normal diet
   B. no food or fluids for 8 hours
   C. no food or water 24 hours before examination
   D. fast for 6 hours

3. The PET scan can be used to help in the diagnosis of _____.
   A. Alzheimer's disease
   B. oncological conditions
   C. neurological conditions
   D. all of the above

4. _____ is a radiograph of the gallbladder.
   A. Cholecystogram
   B. Upper GI series
   C. Mammogram
   D. All of the above

5. _____ is a branch of medicine dealing with radiation.
   A. Radiograph
   B. Radiology
   C. Nuclear medicine
   D. Ultrasonography

6. Which one of the following is *not* a typical route for administration of a contrast medium?
   A. Enema
   B. Injection
   C. Swallowed (oral)
   D. Inhalation

7. A(n) _____ x-ray provides an image of the lungs, heart, and large blood vessels.
   A. chest
   B. nuclear
   C. MRI
   D. fluoroscopy

8. _____ uses high-frequency sound waves to create an image.
   A. Fluoroscopic imaging
   B. Mammography
   C. Ultrasonography
   D. Tomography

9. A(n) _____ chest x-ray has the patient facing the tube and the film holder at the back of the patient.
   A. AP
   B. PA
   C. lateral
   D. oblique

10. Before performing an MRI, it is important for the medical assistant to ask the patient about _____.
    A. pregnancy
    B. metal medical devices that the patient may have on or in them
    C. whether they can lay still for 30 minutes
    D. all of the above

11. The medical assistant should _____ when performing an x-ray.
    A. stand in the room with the patient for support
    B. stand in front of a lead barrier for better visualization
    C. stand behind a lead barrier for personal safety
    D. any of the above are acceptable depending on office policy

12. When preparing for a PET scan, the patient must fast _____ hours before the procedure.
    A. 6
    B. 12
    C. 24
    D. 48

13. If a report from the radiologist is not received within _____, the medical assistant must make a follow-up call.
    A. 1 day
    B. 3 days
    C. 5 days
    D. 1 week

14. _____ allows the physician to see in detail the inside of the body without the use of x-rays.
    A. CT
    B. PET
    C. MRI
    D. Lower GI series

15. In a(n) _____ chest x-ray, the x-ray beam is directed at an angle through the body part.
    A. PA
    B. AP
    C. lateral
    D. oblique

Sentence Completion

Complete each sentence or statement.

contrast	shellfish/iodine	digital radiographic imaging
medium	when was the last	claustrophobia
dosimeter	menstrual cycle	radiopaque
transducer	positron emission	lower GI
diagnostic imaging	tomography	
muscle	mammogram	

1. _____ is a problem for some patients who are uncomfortable in enclosed areas.

2. All employees working in the area of x-ray must wear a(n) _____ to monitor the amount of x-ray exposure.

3. When a patient is having a procedure requiring contrast medium, the medical assistant must ask the patient about _____ allergies.

4. An instrument that is moved over the skin to record sound waves during an ultrasound procedure is called a(n) _____.

5. _____ is used in ultrasonography, magnetic resonance imaging, computed tomography, and nuclear medicine.

6. If the patient is of childbearing age, it is important for the medical assistant to ask _____.

7. _____ is(are) techniques used to produce a picture image that does not involve radiation.

8. _____ tissue does not absorb electromagnetic energy, so it does not appear on an x-ray film.

9. _____ an imaging method that can evaluate the entire body with a single procedure.

10. _____ is an x-ray of breast tissue.

Short Answers

1. Explain the patient preparation for a mammogram.

_____

_____

_____

_____

2. Explain the two items the medical assistant must inform the patient of before the procedure.

CRITICAL THINKING

1. Dr. Goldberg has ordered an MRI on Mrs. Frankle. What instructions would you give Mrs. Frankle for preparing for the procedure? Your instructor may require that you verbally answer this question in a role-play format, providing you with the opportunity to practice your patient education skills.

PRACTICAL APPLICATIONS

If you have accomplished the objectives in this chapter, you will be able to make better choices as a medical assistant. Take a look at this situation and decide what you would do.

Suzanne is a medical assistant who works for Dr. Sahara. Dr. Sahara has a medical office with the equipment for basic radiography. She sends her patients to specialized radiographic offices when more extensive testing is necessary. Dr. Sahara informs Suzanne that she has ordered these diagnostic imaging tests: (1) gallbladder ultrasound for middle-aged Mr. Donnolly; (2) baseline mammography for 40-year-old Mrs. Martens; (3) MRI for Mrs. Smith because of a possible brain lesion; and (4) chest radiograph for Mr. Charles, a patient with parkinsonism, because of possible pneumonia. Mr. Charles' chest x-ray film is inconclusive, so Dr. Sahara sends him back for a CT scan. When the CT scan is suspicious, Dr. Sahara orders a PET scan for Mr. Charles 2 days later, and the results come back positive for cancer.

Would you be able to prepare patients for these procedures? Could you answer patient questions concerning the procedures?

1. What protective equipment and safety features should Suzanne use when she is taking x-ray films in Dr. Sahara's office?

2. If Suzanne were asked to perform "AP, PA, oblique, and lat" views of a forearm, in what positions would she place the arm?

3. What preparation would be needed for Mr. Donnolly's ultrasound of the gallbladder? Why would contrast media be used when the original x-ray films of the gallbladder were taken?

Copyright © 2010, 2005 by Saunders, an imprint of Elsevier, Inc. All rights reserved.

4. What does the white area on an x-ray film indicate? What does the gray area indicate? What does the black area indicate?

5. What preparation is necessary for Mrs. Martens' mammogram? What would happen if she were not prepared for the test?

6. Why was MRI used for diagnosing a possible brain lesion?

7. What patient preparation is necessary for a chest radiograph?

8. Why did Dr. Sahara order a CT scan when the chest x-ray was inconclusive?

9. What does the PET scan show that is not in evidence with MRI? What is used as the tracer for cancer cells?

10. How would Mr. Charles' parkinsonism affect his x-ray films and MR images?

11. What role does the medical assistant play in scheduling patients for imaging tests?

   _____

   _____

12. What should Suzanne do if the x-ray report on the PET scan does not arrive within the week?

   _____

   _____

CHAPTER QUIZ

Multiple Choice

Identify the letter of the choice that best completes the statement or answers the question.

1. _____ is a branch of medicine dealing with radioactive substances.
   A. Radiograph
   B. Radiography
   C. Radiology
   D. None of the above

2. Muscle tissue can absorb as much electromagnetic energy as bones.
   A. True
   B. False

3. _____ is an imaging method that can evaluate the entire body through the use of a sugar tracer.
   A. CT
   B. MRI
   C. PET
   D. X-ray

4. A(n) _____ provides an image of the lungs, heart, and large blood vessels.
   A. chest x-ray
   B. mammogram
   C. MRI
   D. CAT scan

5. The medical assistant should stand _____ a lead screen when taking an x-ray.
   A. beside
   B. behind
   C. in front of
   D. between the patient and

6. The Medical Practice Policy and state laws determine if the medical assistant is allowed to take x-rays.
   A. True
   B. False

Copyright © 2010, 2005 by Saunders, an imprint of Elsevier, Inc. All rights reserved.

7. Before instilling a contrast medium, the medical assistant should _____.
   A. establish the patient is not pregnant.
   B. ask about allergies to shellfish
   C. ask the patient if they have a ride with them
   D. none of the above

8. In patient preparation of a PET scan, the patient should _____.
   A. fast for at least 6 hours
   B. avoid food and fluids for at least 8 hours before the procedure
   C. advise and remove all metal medical devices
   D. avoid caffeine for several days before the procedure

9. _____ is an image created through the use of high-frequency sound waves.
   A. CT
   B. Mammogram
   C. MRI
   D. Ultrasound

10. When a patient is scheduled for a chest x-ray, the preparation should include _____.
    A. fasting minimally for 6 hours
    B. no drink or food for 8 hours
    C. *not* emptying the bladder before the procedure
    D. no advance preparation is required

11. _____ is used to see the body or a whole organ in a cross-sectional view.
    A. PET
    B. MRI
    C. Tomography
    D. X-ray

12. The radiology report should be received no later than _____ from the time the procedure was performed.
    A. 2 hours
    B. 8 hours
    C. 2 days
    D. 1 week

13. A transducer is a device moved over the skin to record sound waves.
    A. True
    B. False

14. When taking a(n) _____ chest view x-ray, the patient is facing the film holder, and the x-ray tube is to the back.
    A. AP
    B. PA
    C. lateral
    D. oblique

15. _____ allows for the introduction of contrast media, and may include movement of that contrast media through the body.
    A. Fluoroscopy
    B. MRI
    C. Mammography
    D. X-ray

38 Therapeutic Procedures

VOCABULARY REVIEW

Matching: Match each term with the correct definition.

A. ambulation device

B. bandage turns

C. cast

D. cerumen

E. cold therapy

F. compress

G. coupling agent

H. elastic bandage

I. figure-eight turn

J. gait patterns

K. goniometer

L. heating pad

M. immobilization

N. instillation

O. irrigation

P. orthopedist

Q. patent

R. pressure ulcer

S. recurrent turn

T. soak

_____ 1. Limb immobilizer made of fiberglass used for simple fractures and sprains

_____ 2. Physician whose specialty is to correct musculoskeletal disorders

_____ 3. Bandage containing elastic that stretches and molds to the body part to which it is applied

_____ 4. Plaster or fiberglass mold applied to immobilize a body part

_____ 5. Process of placing medication into an area as prescribed by a physician

_____ 6. Bandage turn used for a stump or the head that begins with a circular turn and progresses back and forth, overlapping each turn until the area is covered

_____ 7. Procedure that requires a body part to be immersed in water warm enough to increase blood flow to an area or cold enough to slow blood flow to the area

_____ 8. Any device that assists a patient to walk

_____ 9. Patterns of walking used with crutches

_____ 10. Lightweight mobility device providing a stable platform that is used when a patient needs optimal stability and support

_____ 11. Therapy using ice or cold application to reduce or prevent swelling by decreasing circulatory flow to the injured body part

_____ 12. Water-soluble lotion or gel used to transmit energy provided by an ultrasound wand

_____ 13. Gauze bandage made in a tubular shape that can be used to cover rounded body parts

_____ 14. Earwax

U. stockinette

V. synthetic cast

W. therapeutic procedures

X. tubular gauze

Y. ultrasound therapy

Z. walker

AA. Kling-type bandage

BB. forearm crutches

_____ 15. Bandage turn that is applied on a slant and progresses upward and then downward to support a dressing or joint

_____ 16. Ulcer created when the skin over a bony area has contact and pressure with an irritating source for long periods

_____ 17. Electrical device that delivers a set temperature of heat for heat therapy

_____ 18. Knitted cotton material used over extremities to cover an area before application of cast material

_____ 19. Method of arranging a bandage on a body part

_____ 20. Prevention of movement; inability to move

_____ 21. Open; not obstructed

_____ 22. Instrument used to measure angles

_____ 23. Therapy that uses high-frequency sound waves to produce heat and vibrations to aid in the healing of inflammation in soft tissue

_____ 24. Folded pad of soft absorbent material used for hot or cold therapy

_____ 25. Washing of or rinsing out an area to remove foreign matter

_____ 26. Procedures done to enhance the body's healing processes and assist in patient mobility

_____ 27. Gauze bandaging material that stretches and molds to irregular-shaped areas

_____ 28. Devices that provide contact with the hand and forearm

THEORY RECALL

True/False

Indicate whether the statement is true or false.

_____ 1. Of all ambulatory devices, a cane provides the most support for the patient.

_____ 2. Ear treatments are never performed as part of an ear examination.

_____ 3. All irrigation solutions must be sterile.

_____ 4. An air cast is used primarily for immobilization.

_____ 5. It is acceptable for the patient to scratch an itch underneath the cast if the patient is very careful.

Multiple Choice

Identify the letter of the choice that best completes the statement or answers the question.

1. There are _____ basic bandage turns used either for support or to secure a dressing.
   A. two
   B. four
   C. five
   D. eight

2. _____ is an application to the skin used to treat an infectious condition or to treat a traumatized body part and promote circulation.
   A. Cold therapy
   B. Heat therapy
   C. Ultrasound
   D. None of the above

3. [A] _____ is(are) prescribed when the patient needs optimal stability and support while remaining mobile.
   A. cane
   B. crutches
   C. walker
   D. all of the above

4. A _____ bandage is used on areas that are uniform in width, such as fingers and wrists.
   A. circular
   B. figure eight
   C. recurrent
   D. spiral turn

5. When performing ultrasound to an affected area, [a(n)] _____ must be used.
   A. ambulatory device
   B. coupling agent
   C. increased wattage
   D. pressure

6. _____ crutch(es) is(are) used by patients with poor arm strength.
   A. Forearm
   B. One
   C. Platform
   D. Would not be able to use crutches

7. _____ finger(s) width should fit between the crutch pads and the axilla.
   A. One
   B. Two
   C. Three
   D. Four

8. The _____-point gait is less stable than the four-point gait but much quicker for the patient.
   A. one
   B. two
   C. three
   D. none of the above

9. Usually a(n) _____ applies a cast.
   A. orthopedist
   B. medical assistant
   C. surgeon
   D. specially trained nurse

10. The advantage of applying a fiberglass cast versus a plaster cast is that _____.
    A. it is easier to put on
    B. it is lighter in weight
    C. it is more supportive
    D. a plaster cast comes in only one color

11. When fitting a patient with crutches, the elbow flex should be _____ degrees.
    A. 5 to 10
    B. 10 to 15
    C. 15 to 25
    D. 25 to 30

12. When performing eye irrigation, the medical assistant should rinse _____.
    A. toward the center of the eye
    B. toward the inner corner of the eye
    C. toward the outer corner of the eye
    D. with patient's head tilted forward

13. A _____ turn bandage is used when the area to be bandaged is of varying widths, such as the forearm and the lower calf of the leg.
    A. figure eight
    B. recurrent
    C. spiral
    D. spiral reverse turn

14. _____ are devices used when full weight cannot be placed on an injured area.
    A. Canes
    B. Crutches
    C. Walkers
    D. None of the above

15. When instilling eardrops, it is important to remember to instill the drops toward the _____ of the canal.
    A. bottom
    B. center
    C. roof
    D. it does not matter which way the drops are instilled

16. A chemical hot or cold pack has an active life of _____ minutes.
    A. 15
    B. 10 to 15
    C. 30 to 45
    D. 30 to 60

17. Heat compresses promote _____.
    A. increased circulation
    B. faster removal of waste products
    C. new cell growth
    D. all of the above

18. A plaster cast completely dries in approximately _____ hours.
    A. 12
    B. 24
    C. 48
    D. 72

19. When irrigating an ear of an adult patient, the medical assistant should straighten the ear canal by gently pulling the ear _____.
    A. upward and backward
    B. downward and forward
    C. upward and forward
    D. downward and backward

20. An ear irrigation is performed to _____.
    A. introduce medication into the ear canal
    B. dislodge materials such as insects and earwax
    C. chill the tympanic membrane
    D. all of the above

Sentence Completion

Complete each sentence or statement.

cane	walker	figure-eight
cast spreader	cast padding	cold therapy
compress	recurrent turn	circular
ice bag	capillary refill	ultrasound
instillation	cerumen	

1. _____ is the medical name for "earwax."

2. The application of _____ reduces or prevents swelling.

3. _____ uses high-frequency waves.

4. A(n) _____ is used to open up a cast.

5. _____ bandage is most frequently used for a stump area or for the head.

6. A(n) _____ is a hand-held device that provides minimal support for walking.

7. A(n) _____ bandage application is when each turn overlaps the previous turn.

8. After a bandage or cast has been applied, it is very important that the medical assistant check for _____ below the bandaged area.

9. _____ is cotton material applied over the stockinette to protect the skin and to prevent pressure sores over bony areas.

10. A(n) _____ turn bandage is most often used to hold a dressing in place or support a joint area.

Short Answers

1. Explain and describe the five stages involved in the application of a cast.

   _____
   _____
   _____

2. List three uses for bandages.

   _____
   _____
   _____

3. List and explain the three types of bandages most commonly used in a medical office.

   _____
   _____
   _____
   _____

4. List and explain the four different gait patterns.

   _____
   _____
   _____
   _____
   _____

CRITICAL THINKING

1. Samuel Olsen is a 10-year-old patient who has fallen at the school playground and injured his left arm. His mother brings him to the clinic, and the physician orders AP and lateral radiographs of the left forearm, proximal and distal views. You take the x-rays, and the physician diagnoses a fractured ulna and would like for you to set up for a fiberglass cast. List the materials you need to assemble for the cast, and briefly describe your role as a medical assistant in casting.

_____
_____
_____
_____
_____
_____

PRACTICAL APPLICATIONS

If you have accomplished the objectives in this chapter, you will be able to make better choices as a medical assistant. Take a look at this situation and decide what you would do.

A multispecialty practice has medical assistants who work with each of the specialists. Allene, a medical assistant who has not had the benefit of training, works with Dr. Sumar, an ophthalmologist. Gerald, a graduate of a medical assisting program, works with Dr. Herzog, an orthopedist. The ophthalmologist and the otolaryngologist share the same examination room, but they use it on different days. Allene is not very busy one day, so she decides to clean the medicine cabinet and rearrange the drugs. She moves the ophthalmic medications to the spot where the otic medications are usually stored, and vice versa. When Dr. Sumar treats a patient with conjunctivitis the next day, Allene hands him an otic preparation for the eye instillation. Luckily, Dr. Sumar reads the label on the medication before instilling the drops into the patient's eye. Later in the day, Dr. Sumar reprimands Allene for handing him the otic drops.

Gerald is the person who communicates to the orthopedic patients the necessity of correct application of the bandaging and the care of a cast after its application. For patients who need cold or heat therapy, Gerald is responsible for the applications as ordered by Dr. Herzog, and Gerald performs the ultrasound treatments as indicated. During ultrasound treatments, Gerald is very careful to have sufficient coupling agent and to keep the head of the machine moving at all times.

Would you be able to step into the role of Allene or Gerald and perform their duties successfully?

1. Why is it important for ophthalmic and otic preparations to remain in the same storage places?

_____
_____
_____

Copyright © 2010, 2005 by Saunders, an imprint of Elsevier, Inc. All rights reserved.

CHAPTER 38 Therapeutic Procedures

2. **What is the danger of placing otic medications into the patient's eye?**

3. **Would the ear patient have a problem if the ophthalmic preparation had been used for the ear instillation?**

4. **What reasons do you believe led to Allene's reprimand? What actions during the cleaning process could have caused the medication error?**

5. **Why is it important for Gerald to teach patients to apply bandages from distal to proximal?**

6. **What does Gerald need to teach a patient about caring for a plaster cast?**

7. **Why is it important for Gerald to keep the head of the ultrasound machine moving at all times?**

8. Why should Gerald be concerned if the patient complains of heat during an ultrasound treatment?

___

___

___

APPLICATION OF SKILLS

1. Perform Procedure 38-1: Perform an Ear Irrigation.

2. Perform Procedure 38-2: Perform an Ear Instillation.

3. Perform Procedure 38-3: Perform an Eye Irrigation.

4. Perform Procedure 38-4: Perform an Eye Instillation.

5. Perform Procedure 38-5: Apply a Tubular Gauze Bandage.

6. Perform Procedure 38-6: Apply an Ice Bag.

7. Perform Procedure 38-7: Apply a Cold Compress.

8. Perform Procedure 38-8: Apply a Chemical Cold Pack.

9. Perform Procedure 38-9: Apply a Hot Water Bag.

10. Perform Procedure 38-10: Apply a Heating Pad.

11. Perform Procedure 38-11: Apply a Hot Compress.

12. Perform Procedure 38-12: Apply a Hot Soak.

13. Perform Procedure 38-13: Administer an Ultrasound Treatment.

14. Perform Procedure 38-14: Measure for Axillary Crutches.

15. Perform Procedure 38-15: Instruct the Patient in Crutch Gaits.

16. Perform Procedure 38-16: Instruct the Patient in the Use of a Walker.

17. Perform Procedure 38-17: Instruct the Patient in the Use of a Cane.

18. Perform Procedure 38-18: Assist in Plaster-of-Paris or Fiberglass Cast Application.

Copyright © 2010, 2005 by Saunders, an imprint of Elsevier, Inc. All rights reserved.

CHAPTER QUIZ

Multiple Choice

Identify the letter of the choice that best completes the statement or answers the question.

1. The _____ bandage application is most commonly used to hold dressings in place or support a joint area.
   A. circular turn
   B. figure eight turn
   C. spiral reverse
   D. recurrent turn

2. Heat therapy is used when trying to reduce or prevent swelling.
   A. True
   B. False

3. Heat therapy cannot be used when _____ exists.
   A. damaged skin areas
   B. pregnancy
   C. major circulatory problems
   D. all of the above

4. The top of the crutch pads should be _____ inch(es) from the axillary areas.
   A. 1
   B. 2
   C. 3
   D. 4

5. _____ bandages are used to mold around irregular areas, and are most often used to support dressings.
   A. Elastic
   B. Fabric
   C. Kling
   D. Tubular

6. Overuse of hot or cold therapies can cause the opposite of the desired effect.
   A. True
   B. False

7. _____ are used when more mobility and support are needed than a cane can provide.
   A. Axillary crutches
   B. Lofstrand crutches
   C. Platform crutches
   D. None of the above

8. _____ is a typical sign of circulation impairment.
   A. Lack of pain sensation
   B. Tingling
   C. Red coloration
   D. Feeling warm to the touch

9. A hot soak requires a body part to be totally immersed in a water bath.
   A. True
   B. False

10. A chemical hot/cold pack lasts with desired effect for about _____.
    A. 10 minutes
    B. 20 to 30 minutes
    C. 30 to 45 minutes
    D. 30 to 60 minutes

11. The _____ bandage is most often used for a stump area.
    A. figure eight
    B. recurrent
    C. spiral
    D. spiral reverse

12. When performing an eye irrigation, the medical assistant _____.
    A. irrigates from the back of the patient with the patient's head tilted back toward the medical assistant
    B. has the patient tilt head away from affected eye
    C. has the patient tilt head away from the unaffected eye
    D. uses slightly warm tap water for irrigation

13. A(n) _____ is normally used for more complicated fractures.
    A. air cast
    B. plaster cast
    C. splint
    D. synthetic cast

14. A cast usually dries within _____ hours.
    A. 8
    B. 12
    C. 48
    D. 72

15. When applying heat to an area, you are _____.
    A. promoting growth of new cells
    B. removing waste from the area
    C. increasing nutrients to the area
    D. all of the above

Copyright © 2010, 2005 by Saunders, an imprint of Elsevier, Inc. All rights reserved.

39 Specialty Diagnostic Testing

VOCABULARY REVIEW

Matching: Match each term with the correct definition.

A. abstinence

B. Apgar score

C. barrier method

D. Bethesda System

E. blood chemistry

F. candidiasis

G. colposcopy

H. conduction

I. corpus luteum

J. culture and sensitivity

K. dysplasia

L. endocervical curettage

M. estimated date of delivery

N. forced vital capacity

O. *Gardnerella*

P. guaiac test

Q. hearing acuity tests

R. human chorionic gonadotropin

S. morning-after pill

T. Nägele's rule

_____ 1. Slide preparation used to observe for fungal or bacterial growth

_____ 2. Process or action of giving birth

_____ 3. Laboratory test that reveals the levels of chemicals in the blood

_____ 4. Measurement of the maximum volume of air that can be expired when the patient exhales forcefully

_____ 5. Instrument used to view the sigmoid region of the colon

_____ 6. Hormone found during pregnancy that maintains the corpus luteum during pregnancy

_____ 7. Laboratory test ordered to identify a microorganism and its susceptibility to antibiotics

_____ 8. Small endocrine tissue located on the surface of the ovary after the release of an egg; secretes the progesterone required to maintain the endometrium during implantation and pregnancy

_____ 9. Contraceptive method that prohibits sexual contact between partners

_____ 10. Tests used to check for hearing loss

_____ 11. Tests done to assess lung function

_____ 12. Infection with *Trichomonas* protozoa spread through sexual contact, making it an STD

_____ 13. Birth control method that places a physical barrier between the egg and the sperm

_____ 14. Removal of endocervical tissue by scraping

_____ 15. Method used to calculate a pregnant woman's due date by adding 7 days to the first day of the LMP, subtracting 3 months, and adding 1 year

U. oximetry sensor
V. parturition
W. photodetector
X. protozoa
Y. puerperium
Z. pulmonary function tests
AA. pulse oximetry
BB. serum pregnancy test
CC. sigmoidoscope
DD. specimen adequacy
EE. spirometry
FF. titer
GG. trichomoniasis
HH. vaginal irrigation
II. vital capacity
JJ. wet mount

_____ 16. Term that refers to the condition of a specimen

_____ 17. Device that records the percentage of oxygen in the blood after a light source passes through arterial blood

_____ 18. Examination of vaginal and cervical tissue with a colposcope

_____ 19. Test for hidden (occult) blood in the stool or other body secretions

_____ 20. Oral contraceptive that uses large doses of hormones to prevent conception after sexual intercourse

_____ 21. Method to measure the amount of oxygen in a patient's blood

_____ 22. System of measurement used to evaluate an infant at birth

_____ 23. Abnormal development of tissue

_____ 24. Single-celled parasitic organisms that have the ability to move

_____ 25. Measurement of the volume of air that can be expired when the patient exhales completely

_____ 26. Fungal infection affecting vaginal mucosa, skin, and other areas

_____ 27. A pregnant woman's probable due date for birth based on her last menstrual period

_____ 28. Device attached to a patient's finger that detects oxygen content in arterial blood

_____ 29. Type of test that measures lung volume and capacity over time

_____ 30. Ability to move from one area to another, as in hearing with transmission of sound through nervous tissue

_____ 31. Genus of bacteria that exists in the vagina and can cause infection if pH is not balanced

_____ 32. Blood test to detect the presence of human chorionic gonadotropin

_____ 33. Time period after childbirth; postpartum

_____ 34. Measurement of the amount of a substance in a specimen

_____ 35. Grading system used for a Pap smear

_____ 36. Instillation of large amounts of solution into the vagina as a method of cleansing

THEORY RECALL

True/False

Indicate whether the statement is true or false.

_____ 1. The American Cancer Society strongly recommends that at age 30, besides performing monthly BSE, you should have a clinical breast examination performed by a physician.

_____ 2. A cytology laboratory requisition must accompany all specimens to the laboratory for microscopic examination and evaluation.

_____ 3. A fecal occult test can identify the cause of rectal bleeding.

_____ 4. Bacteria are single-celled parasitic organisms that have the ability to move.

_____ 5. It is highly recommended that another woman be present when a male physician performs a pelvic examination.

Multiple Choice

Identify the letter of the choice that best completes the statement or answers the question.

1. Trichomoniasis is an infection caused by _____.
   A. bacteria
   B. fungi
   C. protozoa
   D. yeast

2. A(n) _____ is a procedure performed to examine and treat a portion of the digestive system.
   A. endoscope
   B. proctology
   C. sigmoidoscopy
   D. none of the above

3. An initial prenatal examination consists of _____.
   A. blood chemistry panel
   B. glucose testing
   C. measurement of fetal heart tones
   D. ultrasound

4. _____ is a screening to measure the volume of air that can be expired when the patient exhales completely.
   A. Forced vital capacity
   B. Vital capacity
   C. Pulse oximetry
   D. PFT

5. An _____ is a record produced by an audiometer.
   A. audiogram
   B. audiologist
   C. audiometry
   D. none of the above

6. _____ care is the care a pregnant woman receives before the birth of a child.
   A. Postpartum
   B. Prenatal
   C. Puerperium
   D. Obstetrics

7. A BSE should be performed _____.
   A. every time you shower
   B. at least once a week
   C. at least once a month
   D. twice a year

8. A patient should be instructed to not douche or insert any medications for at least _____ hours before a Pap test.
   A. 2
   B. 8
   C. 12
   D. 24

9. _____ is performed to detect the presence of lung dysfunction.
   A. Vital capacity
   B. Forced vital capacity
   C. Spirometry
   D. All of the above

10. Rinne and Weber tests are types of _____.
    A. blood tests
    B. hearing tests
    C. postpartum tests
    D. prenatal tests

11. A(n) _____ is an examination performed to establish the location of internal reproductive organs.
    A. colorectal examination
    B. obstetric examination
    C. pelvic examination
    D. Pap examination

12. _____ has symptoms of frothy discharge, dysuria, and itching.
    A. Candidiasis
    B. Trichomoniasis
    C. *Gardnerella*
    D. Vaginal infection

13. Contraceptive barrier methods include _____.
    A. condoms
    B. hormones
    C. IUD
    D. morning-after pill

14. Candidiasis may result from _____.
    A. antibiotic use
    B. chemicals
    C. fungus
    D. sexual activity

15. The Bethesda System has _____ main categories of reporting.
    A. two
    B. three
    C. four
    D. five

16. _____ is a condition that can occur during pregnancy when the effects of insulin are blocked by hormones produced in the placenta.
    A. Type 2 diabetes
    B. Type 1 diabetes
    C. Gestational diabetes
    D. All of the above

17. The _____ is a small endocrine gland located on the surface of the ovary after the release of an egg.
    A. corpus christi
    B. corpus luteum
    C. pineal corpus
    D. chorionic gonadotropin

18. _____ rule is a method used to calculate a woman's due date by adding 7 days to the first day of the LMP, subtracting 3 months, and adding 1 year (as necessary).
    A. Robert's
    B. Nägele's
    C. Frost's
    D. Weber's

19. A _____ is a slide preparation used to observe for fungal or bacterial growth.
    A. wet mount
    B. dry mount
    C. covered mount
    D. stained mount

20. _____ is the time period after childbirth.
    A. Prenatal
    B. Parturition
    C. Obstetrics
    D. Puerperium

Sentence Completion

Complete each sentence or statement.

lithotomy	Rinne	pulse oximetry
Papanicolaou test	"fishy"	sterilization
STD	placenta	vital capacity
vaginitis	spirometry	vaginal speculum
Weber	intrauterine device	

1. _____ is a screening tool that evaluates the squamous epithelial tissue covering the visible part of the cervix.

2. _____ is an inflammation of the vaginal tissue caused by fungi, bacteria, protozoa, or irritation from chemicals or foreign objects.

3. The most frequent complaint of a patient with *Gardnerella* is _____ odor.

4. The _____ test assesses the hearing in both ears at once.

5. _____ is a noninvasive procedure used to measure the oxygen level of a patient's blood.

6. _____ is a birth control device that prevents a fertilized egg from implanting in the uterine wall.

7. _____ is a contraceptive method that does not allow the egg or sperm to travel the normal pathway in the body.

8. When undergoing a pelvic examination, the patient is in the _____ position.

9. The _____ is special tissue that attaches to the uterus during pregnancy and provides nutrients and oxygen to the fetus.

10. An instrument used in a pelvic examination to view the cervix is called a(n) _____.

Short Answers

1. List the five items found in a postpartum visit.

_____

_____

_____

_____

Copyright © 2010, 2005 by Saunders, an imprint of Elsevier, Inc. All rights reserved.

480 CHAPTER 39 Specialty Diagnostic Testing

2. List the four parts of a gynecologic examination.

3. Explain the patient preparation for a sigmoidoscopy.

4. Explain the method called "liquid prep."

5. Each slide prepared from each specimen must be labeled with the location from which the sample was taken. List the three labels that are placed on the slides.

CRITICAL THINKING

1. Breast cancer is the most prevalent form of cancer in American women. Analysis is a means of looking for genetic indicators for breast cancer to determine a woman's risk of developing breast cancer. Dr. Schanze is seeing Mrs. Pettre today, and because of her family history of breast cancer will recommend she have a BRCA analysis done. What are some other factors that would be considered before recommending this analysis? How is the test done? What type of information is available to the physician and the patient that would help to decide further treatment?

2. Early detection of testicular cancer is possible when a man does regular self-examinations. Today you will be providing, Joe Vali, a patient, with information about testicular cancer and instructing him how to perform the testicular examination. List facts that are important for Joe to understand and steps for him to follow when doing the self-examination.

PRACTICAL APPLICATIONS

If you have accomplished the objectives in this chapter, you will be able to make better choices as a medical assistant. Take a look at this situation and decide what you would do.

Kari, age 20, is a new patient in the office of Dr. Berg, a gynecologist. Francine is the medical assistant for Dr. Berg and has been on the job for only about 2 weeks. Arriving for her appointment, Kari is given the history and physical paperwork to fill out because she is a new patient. When Francine calls Kari to the back to question her further on some specifics regarding her menstrual periods and sexual activity, four other patients are sitting close to Kari in the laboratory/workup area. Later, Francine is overheard discussing Kari's history with coworkers by more patients in the waiting room.

After taking Kari to the examination room, Francine tells her to get undressed without providing instructions for putting on the gown and drape. When Francine returns to see if Kari is undressed, she then places her into the lithotomy position for what turns out to be a 30-minute wait.

When Dr. Berg starts to examine Kari, Francine leaves the room and tells Dr. Berg to call her when he is ready to do the pelvic examination. During the breast examination, Kari asks Dr. Berg about birth control and tells him that she has been sexually active with a partner who has been diagnosed with a sexually transmitted disease (STD). Dr. Berg completes the pelvic examination, obtaining a Pap smear and cultures for STD and a wet prep. Dr. Berg takes the wet mount to the microscope for observation. He sees Francine in the hallway chatting with some coworkers and asks where she was when he needed her during the pelvic examination. She explains she never heard him call for assistance.

Dr. Berg returns to the examination room and begins discussing forms of birth control with Kari, asking if she would rather have a barrier method, an intrauterine device, or a hormonal method such as birth control pills. He also explains to her that she has trichomoniasis, an STD, as seen on the wet prep. Dr. Berg gives Kari a prescription to treat the trichomoniasis for herself and her sexual partner.

Would you be prepared to handle this situation better than Francine did?

Copyright © 2010, 2005 by Saunders, an imprint of Elsevier, Inc. All rights reserved.

1. What was unethical about the way Francine took Kari's history? What HIPAA regulations did Francine not follow?

2. What are the issues concerning the privacy of Kari's medical record when Francine discussed the symptoms and patient history with coworkers?

3. How did Francine mishandle the preparation of the patient and the assistance with the physical examination?

4. Why do you think that Kari did not tell Francine about the sexual partner with an STD? Would you have told Francine if you had been in Kari's situation? Why?

5. What are the elements of a pelvic examination, and how should the medical assistant help with these?

6. Why would Dr. Berg do a gonorrhea and chlamydia culture? What other methods did Dr. Berg use to diagnose trichomoniasis?

7. What medication would you expect Dr. Berg to prescribe for both sexual partners, and why do both partners need to be treated?

8. What is included in barrier methods of birth control? What is included in hormonal methods? How is an IUD effective?

APPLICATION OF SKILLS

1. Claudia Pearsonn, a 24-year-old white woman, came to the clinic on April 10, 20xx, and stated she thought she was pregnant. Her LMP was February 2, 20xx. Her vitals were BP 120/80, pulse 72 beats/min, respirations 16, and temperature 98° F. Her weight was 115 lb. Her urinalysis was negative for glucose and protein. Pregnancy test was positive. Pap smear was done. Blood was drawn for blood type, CBC, and rubella titer. Medical history was unremarkable. Begin a Pregnancy Flow Sheet on the patient. Calculate her EDD.

    May 15, 20xx, Claudia returns for her next visit. Her vitals remain the same, but her weight now is 120 lb. Urine is still negative for protein and glucose. Patient complains of fatigue. Her laboratory results are as follows:

    Hb 14 g/dL
    Hct 46%
    RBC 4.2 million/mm^3
    WBC 9333/mm^3
    Platelets 250,000/mm^3
    Titer for rubella positive
    Blood type is O Rh−
    Father's blood type A Rh+ (verified through military paperwork)
    Pap results without abnormalities

    Continue updating the flow chart for a pregnancy that progresses normally and concludes 3 days post her due date.

    When would you most likely record fetal heart tones? Fundal height would progress at what rate? When does edema of the extremities occur?

PREGNANCY FLOW SHEET

LMP. _____ MO. ___ DAY ___ YEAR ___
☐ NORMAL ☐ ABNORMAL
EDC. _____
PRE. PREG. WT. _____
QUICKENING DATE _____

LAST NAME _____ FIRST _____ MIDDLE _____
PAT. HOSP. # _____
PRENATAL CLINIC / PHYSICIAN _____
PAT. CLINIC # _____

DATE	WEIGHT THIS VISIT	BLOOD PRESSURE	URINE PROTEIN	URINE SUGAR	EST. WEEKS GEST. AGE (DATES/SIZE)	FUNDAL HEIGHT (CMS)	FETAL HEART TONES FHT	PRESENTATION	FETAL MOVEMENTS	EDEMA	COMMENTS / COMPLAINTS / TREATMENT	NEXT VISIT	CHECK IF ADDT. NOTES	INITIALS OF DR.

TELEPHONE CALLS

DATE / PERSON	QUEST.	ADVICE	DATE / PERSON	QUEST.	ADVICE

INITIAL LABORATORY RESULTS   DATE: _____
BLOOD TYPE / RH: PATIENT: ___ / ___ FATHER: ___ / ___
HEMOGLOBIN: _____ HEMATOCRIT: _____ WBC: _____
URINE: GLUCOSE: _____ PROTEIN: _____ MICRO: _____ CULTURE: _____
ANTIBODY SCREEN: _____ SICKLE CELL: _____
SEROLOGY: _____ RUBELLA TITER: _____
PAP TEST: _____ CERVICAL CULTURE: _____
TAY SACHS: _____ GC: _____
CHLAMYDIA: _____ ALPHA FETOPROTEIN: _____
ULTRASOUND: DATE: _____ RESULTS: _____
ULTRASOUND: DATE: _____ RESULTS: _____
GENETIC STUDY
___ AMNIOCENTESIS   DATE: _____ RESULTS: _____
___ CHORIONIC VILLI BIOPSY DATE: _____ RESULTS: _____

POSTTERM (42 Wks.) MANAGEMENT
___ NST (date) _____
___ CST (date) _____

RhoGAM (28 - 32 Weeks)
☐ Indicated ☐ Given DATE: _____

GLUCOSE SCREEN (27 - 32 WEEKS)
DATE: _____ RESULT: _____

HERPES CULTURE	HEPATITIS
DATE / RESULT	DATE / TEST / RESULT
/	/ /
/	/ /
/	/ /
/	/ /

M.D. SIGNATURE _____ DATE _____

(Sku #19-773 courtesy of Bibbero Systems, Inc., Petaluma, CA; (800) 242-2376; Fax (800) 242-9330; www.bibbero.com.)

Procedure Check-off Sheets (*) and assignments from MACC on the Evolve site at http://evolve.elsevier.com/klieger/medicalassisting (**)

1. Perform Procedure 39-1: Teach Breast Self-Examination.*
2. Perform Procedure 39-2: Assist with a Gynecological Examination.*
3. Perform Procedure 39-3: Assist with a Follow-up Prenatal Examination.*
4. Perform Procedure 39-4: Instruct the Patient in Obtaining a Fecal Specimen.*
5. Perform Procedure 39-5: Test for Occult Blood.*
6. Perform Procedure 39-6: Assist with Sigmoidoscopy.*
7. Perform Procedure 39-7: Perform Spirometry Testing (Pulmonary Function Testing).*
8. Perform Procedure 39-8: Instruct a Patient in the Use of a Peak Flow Meter.
9. Perform Procedure 39-9: Perform Pulse Oximetry.*

CHAPTER QUIZ

Multiple Choice

Identify the letter of the choice that best completes the statement or answers the question.

1. According to the American Cancer Society, at age _____, in addition to the BSE and clinical breast examination, an annual mammogram is recommended.
   A. 20
   B. 30
   C. 40
   D. 50

2. Patient preparation for a sigmoidoscopy should include _____.
   A. an enema
   B. a high-fiber diet
   C. 16 oz of water
   D. a mild sedative

3. Spirometry is performed when _____.
   A. lung assessment before major surgery is advised
   B. assessment of a patient's response to treatment is required
   C. it is desired to screen a patient at risk because of smoking or the environment
   D. all of the above

4. A(n) _____ examination is an internal examination to evaluate the size and location of reproductive organs.
   A. pelvic
   B. prenatal
   C. Pap
   D. obstetric

5. Candidiasis is an inflammation of the vaginal tissue caused by fungi, bacteria, protozoa, or chemical irritation.
   A. True
   B. False

6. The _____ secretes the progesterone required to maintain the endometrium during implantation and pregnancy.
   A. uterus
   B. vaginal walls
   C. corpus luteum
   D. placenta

7. _____ is a noninvasive test that measures the oxygen levels of the body.
   A. Forced vital capacity
   B. Pulse oximetry
   C. Vital capacity
   D. PFT

8. Pap smear results are recorded according to _____.
   A. Bethesda System
   B. office policy
   C. laboratory policy
   D. state policy

9. Gynecologic examinations should include not only a bimanual examination, but also a rectal examination.
   A. True
   B. False

10. _____ is an instrument used to visualize and inspect the internal genitalia.
    A. Gooseneck lamp
    B. Spatula
    C. Speculum
    D. None of the above

11. BSE should be performed _____.
    A. every day
    B. once a week
    C. once a month
    D. once every 2 months

12. Barrier devices include _____.
    A. diaphragms
    B. hormones
    C. IUDs
    D. morning-after pills

13. _____ has symptoms of yellowish green discharge, itching, and vaginal irritation.
    A. Candidiasis
    B. *Gardnerella*
    C. Trichomoniasis
    D. Pelvic infection

14. The first postpartum examination after a cesarean birth should occur _____ after birth.
    A. 12 hours
    B. 1 week
    C. 2 weeks
    D. 1 month

15. When testing for occult blood, a test card impregnated with guaiac reagent is used.
    A. True
    B. False

40 Introduction to the Physician's Office Laboratory

VOCABULARY REVIEW

Matching: Match each term with the correct definition.

A. 24-hour urine specimen

B. exudate

C. blood bank

D. centrifuge

E. Center for Medicare and Medicaid Services

F. certificate of provider-performed microscopy procedures

G. certificate of waiver

H. chain of evidence

I. Clinical Laboratory Improvement Amendments of 1988

J. coagulation studies

K. compound

L. crossmatching

M. drug screening

N. eyepiece

O. forensics

P. first morning specimen

Q. heparin

R. laboratory requisition

_____ 1. Urine or blood specimen collected at specified intervals

_____ 2. Fluid with cellular debris

_____ 3. Tests performed to study microorganisms

_____ 4. Solutions used when testing specimens in the laboratory

_____ 5. Having two sets of lenses on a microscope

_____ 6. Part of the microscope that holds the objectives

_____ 7. Mechanism just below microscope stage that adjusts light

_____ 8. Urine or blood specimen taken after a meal

_____ 9. Laboratory equipment that separates solids or semisolids from a liquid by gravity

_____ 10. Laboratory form showing the identification of a specimen and the laboratory test to be performed

_____ 11. Certificate that allows a physician office laboratory to perform low-complexity testing

_____ 12. Materials suspended in liquid that are not dissolvable

_____ 13. Part of a microscope through which the viewer looks to see an object

_____ 14. Urine or blood collection to determine the presence or absence of specific substances

_____ 15. Liquid portion of the blood

_____ 16. Process designed to monitor and evaluate the quality and accuracy of test results

_____ 17. Federal agency that oversees financial regulations of Medicare and Medicaid

S. microbiology

T. midstream clean-catch urine specimen

U. nosepiece

V. iris diaphragm

W. phlebotomy

X. plasma

Y. postprandial specimens

Z. reagents

AA. solutes

BB. sputum

CC. timed specimen

DD. urinalysis

EE. quality assurance

FF. quality control

_____ 18. Urine specimen that requires a strict cleaning procedure and collection during the middle of voiding

_____ 19. Collection of urine over a 24-hour period to test kidney function, checking for high levels of creatinine, uric acid, hormones, electrolytes, and medications

_____ 20. Lung secretions produced by the bronchi

_____ 21. Urine specimen taken when the patient first awakens; most concentrated specimen

_____ 22. Process of identifying blood compatibility by determining proteins on the red blood cells of the donor and recipient

_____ 23. Analysis of urine including physical, chemical, and microscopic properties

_____ 24. Organization that conducts studies for ABO blood grouping and Rh typing

_____ 25. Process of drawing blood from a vein; venipuncture

_____ 26. Collection of evidence

_____ 27. Studies that evaluate the clotting process of blood

_____ 28. Natural substance that prevents clotting; a vacuum tube additive that prevents the clotting of blood in the tube

_____ 29. Collection routine for a specimen used as evidence

_____ 30. Certificate that allows a physician in the office laboratory to conduct low-complexity and moderate-complexity tests

_____ 31. Legislation enacted to ensure the quality of laboratory results by setting performance standards

_____ 32. Process that provides for accuracy of laboratory tests performed by using a known value for a precheck.

THEORY RECALL

True/False

Indicate whether the statement is true or false.

_____ 1. The "coarse" focus adjustment knob on a microscope is used to bring the specimen into sharper focus.

_____ 2. Quality assurance and quality control mean the same thing.

_____ 3. A clean-catch urine specimen is used for a culture and sensitivity test.

_____ 4. There are five levels of CLIA tests.

_____ 5. All medical offices have a POL.

Multiple Choice

Identify the letter of the choice that best completes the statement or answers the question.

1. The oil-immersion lens on a microscope is _____ power.
   A. ×4
   B. ×10
   C. ×40
   D. ×100

2. _____ tests are performed to study bacteria, fungi, viruses, and parasites in body fluids.
   A. Chemistry
   B. Hematology
   C. Microbiology
   D. Serology

3. _____ specimen is the most frequently collected urine specimen from a patient.
   A. Clean-catch
   B. Midstream
   C. Timed
   D. Random

4. To ensure the reliability of test results, quality assurance requires the medical office to have _____.
   A. written policies
   B. patient education on collection requirements
   C. written procedures
   D. all of the above

5. Quality control requires all the following actions *except* _____.
   A. use of control samples
   B. using outdated reagents
   C. instrument calibration
   D. proper documentation

6. Medical laboratories are regulated by _____.
   A. the laboratory director
   B. state law and federal laws
   C. federal laws only
   D. state laws only

7. Urine collected must be processed within _____, or it must be refrigerated until the tests can be performed.
   A. 30 minutes
   B. 1 hour
   C. 6 hours
   D. 1 day

8. Laboratory safety guidelines include all of the following *except* _____.
   A. wearing laboratory coats
   B. wearing clogs
   C. placing broken glass in a sharps container
   D. cleaning of work area before and after a procedure

9. _____ is the part of the microscope that connects the objectives and ocular lenses to the base.
   A. Arm
   B. Condenser
   C. Eyepieces
   D. Iris diaphragm

10. _____ tests require proficient testing, test management, and specialized training.
    A. CLIA-waived
    B. Minimal-complexity
    C. Moderate-complexity
    D. High-complexity

11. The _____ of the microscope is the platform that holds the slide for viewing.
    A. condenser
    B. nosepiece
    C. objective
    D. stage

12. An oil-immersion lens has a magnification of _____.
    A. 40×
    B. 400×
    C. 1000×
    D. 100×

13. When using the oil-immersion lens to identify a specimen, the total magnification would be _____.
    A. 1000×
    B. 100×
    C. 400×
    D. 40×

14. Processing blood or urine in a centrifuge can leave _____ depending on the specimen used.
    A. solutes
    B. serum
    C. plasma
    D. all of the above

15. A urine specimen must be processed within _____ of collection.
    A. 30 minutes
    B. 45 minutes
    C. 1 hour
    D. 2 hours

16. The _____ knob is used to bring the specimen into focus when a lower power objective is used.
    A. coarse focus
    B. medium focus
    C. fine focus
    D. nonfocus

17. _____ is the secretion from the lungs produced in the bronchi and throat.
    A. Saliva
    B. Sputum
    C. Spit
    D. All of the above

18. A _____ is the most concentrated specimen, and is the best for studying cells.
    A. first morning specimen
    B. random specimen
    C. midstream clean catch
    D. 24-hour specimen

19. _____ tests are performed to study the body's immune response by detecting antibodies in the serum.
    A. Chemistry
    B. Hematology
    C. Microbiology
    D. Serology

20. A culture swab in transport media must be processed within _____.
    A. 8 hours
    B. 12 hours
    C. 24 hours
    D. 48 hours

Sentence Completion

Complete each sentence or statement.

CDC	quality control	waived
POL	CLIA 88	OSHA
coagulation studies	timed	rapid screening test
stool	random	binocular/compound
sputum	24-hour	quality assurance

1. A(n) _____ is a program for laboratory testing, and is designed to monitor and evaluate the quality and accuracy of the test results.

2. _____ is monitored through the CMS.

3. _____ tests do not require personnel to have a high level of specific training.

4. A(n) _____ microscope has two eyepieces.

5. A(n) _____ urine specimen is testing for kidney function over a full day's collection, rather than a random specimen.

Copyright © 2010, 2005 by Saunders, an imprint of Elsevier, Inc. All rights reserved.

6. The GTT is an example of a(n) _____ specimen.

7. _____ can be used to detect group A beta-hemolytic streptococci.

8. _____ is the end product of the digestive process.

9. The amount of regulation in which a _____ is subjected depends on the complexity of tests performed.

10. _____ is the study that evaluates the clotting process of blood.

Short Answers

1. Explain the three different laboratory methods of obtaining a specimen.

   _____
   _____
   _____
   _____

2. Explain five quality control actions as they relate to the required accuracy of tests.

   _____
   _____
   _____
   _____

3. List six categories and types of tests performed in the POL.

   _____
   _____
   _____
   _____
   _____
   _____

CRITICAL THINKING

1. You have just started working at a community clinic, where your patients have a variety of ethnicity and ages. This afternoon you have a patient who speaks very little English, and you need to provide him with instructions on how to collect a urine sample. An interpreter is unavailable. Describe how you would handle this situation.

_____
_____
_____
_____
_____
_____

PRACTICAL APPLICATIONS

If you have accomplished the objectives in this chapter, you will be able to make better choices as a medical assistant. Take a look at this situation and decide what you would do.

The full-time laboratory technician at Dr. Macinto's office is on sick leave for a week. Dr. Macinto asks Sherri, a medical assistant, to fill in for the sick technician. Sherri has just been hired from another office, where she was trained by the physician. She has not done laboratory tests, and has not prepared patients for laboratory work.

On the first day, Dr. Macinto asks Sherri to collect a midstream urine sample on a patient for a culture and sensitivity, and to send some of the urine to an outside laboratory for a drug screen. Sherri hands the urine collection container to the patient without any instructions and allows the patient to go to the bathroom alone to collect the specimen. When the specimen is collected, Sherri leaves the drug screen on the counter to await the arrival of the laboratory courier for transport to the outside laboratory. Neither Sherri nor the courier signs for the specimen. The laboratory form is incomplete, and no documentation was made of the collection of the specimen.

1. **What instructions should Sherri have given the patient for preparation for a midstream urine specimen?**

_____
_____
_____
_____

Copyright © 2010, 2005 by Saunders, an imprint of Elsevier, Inc. All rights reserved.

2. How should urine for a drug screen be collected? What was the problem with leaving the specimen on the counter for the laboratory courier to collect?

3. Would the results of the test have been acceptable in a court case or to an employer who desired this information before hiring the person?

4. What is the difference between quality control and quality assurance? Is Dr. Macinto's office practicing quality assurance when Sherri is working in the laboratory?

5. Why is quality control so important when performing laboratory tests?

6. What is Dr. Macinto's responsibility in regard to Sherri's actions?

APPLICATION OF SKILLS

Procedure Check-off Sheets (*) and assignments from MACC on the Evolve site at http://evolve.elsevier.com/klieger/medicalassisting (**)

1. Perform Procedure 40-1: Use Methods of Quality Control (QC).*
   A. MACC
      Clinical skills/Diagnostic testing/Specimen collection and testing/Instructing how to obtain a urine specimen and performing urinalysis**

2. Perform Procedure 40-2: Focus the Microscope.*
   A. MACC
      Clinical skills/Diagnostic testing/Specimen collection and testing/Preparing a urine sediment and using a microscope**

3. Perform Procedure 40-3: Complete a Laboratory Requisition.*
   A. MACC
      Clinical skills/Patient care/The physical examination/Assisting with a gynecologic examination**
   B. MACC
      Clinical skills/Diagnostic testing/Specimen collection and testing/Obtaining a wound specimen and preparing for transport to an outside laboratory**
   C. MACC
      Clinical skills/Diagnostic testing/Specimen collection and testing/Performing a venipuncture using the evacuated tube method**
   D. MACC
      Clinical skills/Diagnostic testing/Specimen collection and testing/Performing a venipuncture using the butterfly and syringe method**

4. Perform Procedure 40-4: Collect a Specimen for Transport to an Outside Laboratory.*
   A. MACC
      Clinical skills/Diagnostic testing/Specimen collection and testing/Obtaining a wound specimen and preparing for transport to an outside laboratory**

5. Perform Procedure 40-5: Screen and Follow-up on Patient Test Results.*
   A. MACC
      Clinical skills/Diagnostic testing/Specimen collection and testing/Obtaining a wound specimen and performing a rapid strep test**

6. Perform Procedure 40-6: Collect a Specimen for CLIA-Waived Throat Culture and Strep A Test.*
   A. MACC
      Clinical skills/Diagnostic testing/Specimen collection and testing/Obtaining a wound specimen and performing a rapid strep test**

7. Perform Procedure 40-7: Obtain a Urine Specimen from an Infant Using a Pediatric Urine Collector.*

8. Perform Procedure 40-8: Instruct Patient in the Collection of a Midstream Clean-Catch Urine Specimen.*
   A. MACC
      Clinical skills/Diagnostic testing/Specimen collection and testing/Instructing how to obtain a urine specimen and performing urinalysis

9. Perform Procedure 40-9: Instruct Patient in Collection of a 24-Hour Urine Specimen.*

Copyright © 2010, 2005 by Saunders, an imprint of Elsevier, Inc. All rights reserved.

CHAPTER QUIZ

Multiple Choice

Identify the letter of the choice that best completes the statement or answers the question.

1. _____ is the most common urine specimen collected.
   A. Clean catch
   B. A 24-hour
   C. Midstream
   D. Random

2. _____ tests are performed on serum.
   A. Hematology
   B. Chemistry
   C. Serology
   D. Microbiology

3. A level of CLIA tests is _____.
   A. low complexity
   B. medium complexity
   C. middle complexity
   D. waived

4. _____ evaluate(s) the clotting process of blood.
   A. Blood banks
   B. Serology
   C. Coagulation studies
   D. Microbiology

5. The scanning lens on a binocular microscope is _____ power.
   A. ×4
   B. ×10
   C. ×40
   D. ×100

6. The centrifuge is a piece of equipment that separates solid material from liquid through centrifugal force.
   A. True
   B. False

7. Urine must be processed _____, or refrigeration is required to maintain a quality specimen.
   A. immediately
   B. within 30 minutes
   C. within 1 hour
   D. within 2 hours

8. _____ tests assess the formed elements of whole blood.
   A. Chemistry
   B. Hematology
   C. Microbiology
   D. Serology

9. Cultures being transported in a swab-transport media system should be processed within _____ hours.
   A. 8
   B. 10
   C. 12
   D. 24

10. If a wound is deep, an aerobic culture kit may be used.
    A. True
    B. False

11. A _____ requires the patient to follow a strict cleaning procedure.
    A. first-morning specimen
    B. midstream clean-catch specimen
    C. random specimen
    D. timed specimen

12. A 24-hour urine specimen _____.
    A. tests for glucose
    B. tests for drugs
    C. tests kidney function
    D. all of the above

13. _____ tests are performed to study the body's immune responses.
    A. Hematology
    B. Serology
    C. Chemistry
    D. Microbiology

14. Fasting requires the patient refrain from _____.
    A. eating
    B. drinking
    C. eating and drinking
    D. consuming carbohydrates 12 hours before the test

15. When completing a laboratory requisition, it is unnecessary to include the _____.
    A. diagnosis
    B. date and time of specimen of collection
    C. anticipated treatment
    D. patient's insurance information

16. A glucose tolerance test (GTT) requires a specimen be collected _____.
    A. every hour
    B. every ½ hour
    C. every 20 minutes
    D. before ingestion of a special glucose solution

17. The _____ method of blood drawing is the most comfortable for the patient.
    A. butterfly
    B. capillary
    C. venipuncture
    D. syringe

18. The purpose of engineering controls is to _____.
    A. promote safety in the laboratory
    B. instruct patients on how procedures are to be performed
    C. help the laboratory workers to get organized
    D. publish the "Right-to-know directives"

19. The mechanical stage control knob _____.
    A. allows the slide to be moved up and down
    B. allows the slide to be moved from right to left and front to back
    C. adjusts the amount of light reaching the objective
    D. None of the above

20. A certificate of waiver is issued to a physician office laboratory qualified to perform only medium-complexity tests.
    A. True
    B. False

NAME: _____   DATE: _____

41 Phlebotomy

VOCABULARY REVIEW

Matching: Match each term with the correct definition.

A. bacteremia

B. butterfly method

C. evacuated tube

D. filter paper

E. order of draw

F. quantity not sufficient

G. syringe method

H. venipuncture

I. pipette

_____ 1. Blood collection method using a syringe and sterile needle

_____ 2. Bacteria in the blood; sepsis

_____ 3. Order or manner in which blood collection tubes are to be drawn

_____ 4. Blood collection method using a winged infusion set

_____ 5. Insufficient amount of a specimen for performing the desired test

_____ 6. Blood collection tube in which the internal atmosphere is a vacuum allowing blood to flow into the tube

_____ 7. Puncture of a vein to obtain a venous blood sample

_____ 8. Special paper used to pass a liquid through or to collect a blood specimen

_____ 9. Narrow tube used for transferring liquids by suction

THEORY RECALL

True/False

Indicate whether the statement is true or false.

_____ 1. Sodium citrate inhibits thrombin formation to preventing clotting.

_____ 2. It is imperative that previously used lancets be bleached and reused.

_____ 3. The medical assistant should always listen to the patients when they suggest where successful blood draws have been taken in the past.

_____ 4. Chemistry tests include RBC, WBC, and platelet counts.

_____ 5. The arch of the foot can be used for a capillary puncture site.

Multiple Choice

Identify the letter of the choice that best completes the statement or answers the question.

1. What is the first step to accurate laboratory tests results?
   A. Specimen collection
   B. Specimen labeling
   C. Specimen processing and transport
   D. Patient identification

2. The best way to identify a patient accurately is to _____.
   A. ask the patient for his or her Social Security number
   B. ask the patient his or her date of birth
   C. ask the patient to spell his or her last name
   D. B and C

3. A Hemogard is _____.
   A. the plastic top that fits over an evacuated tube
   B. currently only on a blood culture tube
   C. an extra piece of equipment required for syringe draws
   D. needed only if the patient has small veins

4. The syringe method of venipuncture is used when the patient _____.
   A. has a fear of needles
   B. has small, fragile veins
   C. is a young adult
   D. none of the above

5. A _____ gauge needle is used to draw a large sample of blood directly from a vein.
   A. 16- to 18-
   B. 18- to 22-
   C. 22- to 25-
   D. 25- to 27-

6. The order of draw was established by _____.
   A. OSHA
   B. CLSI
   C. CLIA
   D. CDC

7. When performing a capillary puncture, the finger must not be squeezed because _____.
   A. the platelets would break up
   B. the red blood cells might hemolyze
   C. the white blood cells may be damaged
   D. it is okay to squeeze to get an adequate specimen

8. _____ is used when only a small amount of blood is needed.
   A. Butterfly draw
   B. Capillary puncture
   C. Syringe draw
   D. Venipuncture

9. When drawing blood, _____ areas should be avoided.
   A. bruised
   B. scarred
   C. tattooed
   D. all are correct

10. Warming a site before collecting blood _____.
    A. inhibits blood flow
    B. softens the skin to make it easier to puncture
    C. increases blood flow
    D. none of the above

11. A specimen required for a PKU screening can be obtained by _____.
    A. throat culture
    B. arterial puncture
    C. venipuncture
    D. capillary puncture

12. The butterfly method of blood collection is used for _____.
    A. difficult-to-find veins
    B. infants
    C. small children
    D. all of the above

13. No more than ____ venipuncture attempts by the same medical assistant should be done on a patient.
    A. two
    B. three
    C. four
    D. five

14. When collecting a blood sample for serum, the specimen must sit for a minimum of _____ to allow a clot to form.
    A. 10 minutes
    B. 15 minutes
    C. 20 to 30 minutes
    D. 1 hour

15. A _____-top tube is used to collect specimens for plasma or whole blood for blood counts.
    A. blue
    B. gold
    C. lavender
    D. red

16. Microhematocrit centrifuge is used to _____.
    A. process blood in a capillary tube
    B. process blood in a venipuncture tube
    C. process urine in a conical bottom tube
    D. process urine in a round bottom tube

Copyright © 2010, 2005 by Saunders, an imprint of Elsevier, Inc. All rights reserved.

Sentence Completion

Complete each sentence or statement.

red	plasma	lancet
lavender	EDTA	clot activator
gray	green	heparin
sodium citrate	blue	serum
CLIA	CLSI	

1. _____ is an additive in the lavender tube that removes calcium to prevent blood from clotting.

2. A(n) _____ is a small, sterile, needle-like piece of metal used to make a small puncture in the skin.

3. The additive contained in evacuated tubes used for coagulation studies is a(n) _____.

4. A _____ contains silica particles to enhance clot formation.

5. The additive that inhibits thrombin formation to prevent clotting is _____.

6. A _____ stopper tube is used for chemistry tests.

7. Blood for hematology testing is drawn in a _____ stopper tube.

8. _____ is the liquid portion of blood minus the clotting factors.

9. _____ is the agency that established the order of draw for blood specimens.

10. Potassium oxalate is the additive in the _____ tube.

Short Answers

1. Describe four poor capillary collection techniques that could render the results useless.

   _____
   _____
   _____
   _____
   _____

2. Explain the difference between multisample and single-sample needles.

   _____
   _____
   _____
   _____
   _____

CRITICAL THINKING

1. This morning you are assigned to draw blood on all patients scheduled. Your first draw is on a 6-year-old boy who looks very frightened. Describe how you would approach this situation.

   _____
   _____
   _____
   _____
   _____
   _____
   _____

PRACTICAL APPLICATIONS

If you have accomplished the objectives in this chapter, you will be able to make better choices as a medical assistant. Take a look at this situation and decide what you would do.

The full-time laboratory technician at Dr. Macinto's office is on sick leave for another week. Dr. Macinto asks Sherri, a medical assistant, to continue to fill in for the sick technician. Remember Sherri had just been hired from another office, where she was trained by the physician. She has not done laboratory tests and has not prepared patients for laboratory work.

Mrs. Gorchetzki, a postmastectomy patient, is seen next. Dr. Macinto has ordered a fasting blood glucose and a fasting blood chemistry test. Without talking to Mrs. Gorchetzki about the preparation she has made for the test, Sherri gathers the supplies for the testing. Mrs. Gorchetzki mentions that she had bacon and eggs for breakfast. Sherri draws the blood glucose using a capillary puncture. Sherri performs the testing before doing quality control for the day. When the specimen is drawn for the blood chemistry, the laboratory request form asks for serum. Sherri starts the process of drawing the venipuncture specimen from the side of the mastectomy in a heparinized tube. Mrs. Gorchetzki tries to tell Sherri to collect the specimen from the other arm because it is easier to draw blood from that arm, but Sherri does not listen.

When Sherri places the specimen in the centrifuge, she spins only one tube. She pipettes off the liquid and sends it to the laboratory. As it turns out, the liquid sent to the laboratory is plasma, but the laboratory had requested serum.

What things would you have done differently in this situation?

1. **What color tube should have been used for the blood chemistry? What is the common tube used for whole blood and plasma?**

   _____

   _____

   _____

2. **Why shouldn't Sherri have used the arm on the side of the mastectomy? What should she have done when Mrs. Gorchetzki told her that there was a vein that was usually used for venipuncture?**

   _____

   _____

   _____

3. **Why is it important to close the cover of a centrifuge when it is operating?**

   _____

   _____

   _____

4. **After Mrs. Gorchetzki stated that she had eaten breakfast, what should Sherri have done rather than collecting the blood specimens? What part of quality assurance was broken by Mrs. Gorchetzki's action of eating?**

   _____

   _____

   _____

5. What is Dr. Macinto's responsibility in regard to Sherri's actions?

APPLICATION OF SKILLS

1. Label the veins in the arm.

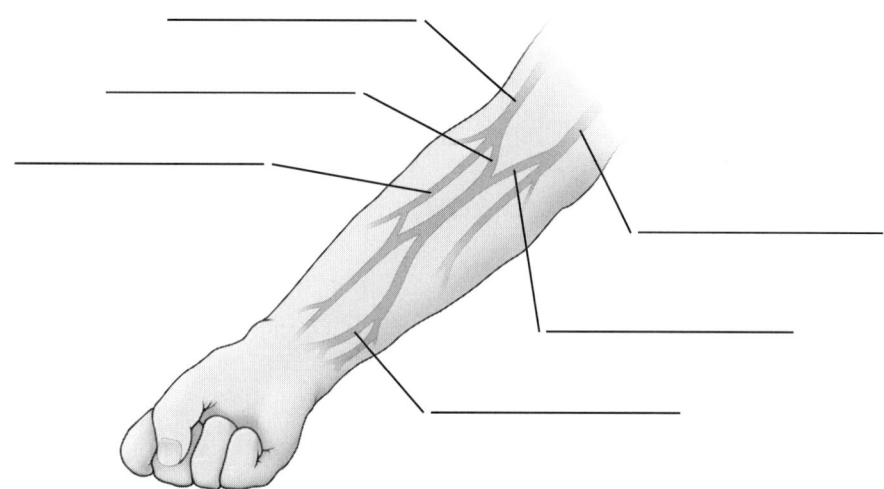

Procedure Check-off Sheets (*) and assignments from MACC on the Evolve site at http://evolve.elsevier.com/ klieger/medicalassisting (**)

1. Perform Procedure 41-1: Use a Sterile Disposable Microlancet for Skin Puncture.*
   A. MACC
      Clinical skills/Diagnostic testing/Specimen collection and testing/Performing a capillary puncture and spun microhematocrit**

2. Perform Procedure 41-2: Collect a Blood Specimen for a Phenylketonuria (PKU) Screening Test.*

3. Perform Procedure 41-3: Perform Venipuncture Using the Evacuated Tube Method (Collection of Multiple Tubes).*
   A. MACC
      Clinical skills/Diagnostic testing/Specimen collection and testing/Performing a venipuncture using the evacuated tube method**

4. Perform Procedure 41-4: Perform Venipuncture Using the Syringe Method.*
   A. MACC
      Clinical skills/Diagnostic testing/Specimen collection and testing/Performing a venipuncture using the butterfly and syringe method**

5. Perform Procedure 41-5: Perform Venipuncture Using the Butterfly Method (Collection of Multiple Evacuated Tubes)*

Copyright © 2010, 2005 by Saunders, an imprint of Elsevier, Inc. All rights reserved.

A. MACC
Clinical skills/Diagnostic testing/Specimen collection and testing/Performing a venipuncture using the butterfly and syringe method**

6. Perform Procedure 41-6: Separate Serum from Whole Blood.*

CHAPTER QUIZ

Multiple Choice

Identify the letter of the choice that best completes the statement or answers the question.

1. _____ is a small, sterile, needle-like piece of metal used to make a small puncture.
   A. Butterfly
   B. Lancet
   C. Syringe
   D. Vacutainer

2. Venipuncture is performed with a sterile _____ gauge needle to obtain a large venous specimen for diagnostic testing.
   A. 15- to 20-
   B. 18- to 20-
   C. 18- to 22-
   D. 20- to 25-

3. _____ is used when a small amount of blood is needed.
   A. Butterfly
   B. Capillary
   C. Syringe
   D. Venipuncture

4. When doing a venipuncture, the needle should be _____ gauge.
   A. 15 to 18
   B. 18 to 22
   C. 22 to 24
   D. 24 to 26

5. A _____-top tube is used for a CBC.
   A. red
   B. green
   C. lavender
   D. gold

6. The _____ method is used on small, fragile veins.
   A. butterfly
   B. lancet
   C. venipuncture
   D. syringe

7. The _____ method of blood drawing is the most comfortable for the patient.
   A. butterfly
   B. capillary
   C. venipuncture
   D. syringe

Copyright © 2010, 2005 by Saunders, an imprint of Elsevier, Inc. All rights reserved.

8. If serum is required for a test, it should be drawn in a _____-top tube
   A. red/gray marbled
   B. purple
   C. green
   D. light blue

9. Errors that affect specimen quality include _____.
   A. leaving the tourniquet on longer than 1 minute.
   B. using too small a needle
   C. having the patient pump their fist
   D. all of the above

10. Substances that prevent blood from clotting are called _____.
    A. clot activators
    B. anticoagulant
    C. fixatives
    D. electrolytes

42 Laboratory Testing in the Physician's Office

VOCABULARY REVIEW

Matching: Match each term with the correct definition.

A. 2-hour postprandial test

B. acetone

C. agar

D. automated urine analyzer

E. bilirubin

F. bilirubinuria

G. C&S

H. casts

I. chemistry profile

J. complete blood count

K. crenated

L. culture plate

M. diaphoresis

N. EDTA

O. enzyme immunoassay

P. fatty cast

Q. galactosemia

R. glucose reagent strip

S. glycosylated hemoglobin

T. Gram stain

_____ 1. To inoculate or put specimen onto a culture plate in an established pattern

_____ 2. Hyaline cast with fatty cells

_____ 3. Chemical formed when fats are metabolized rather than glucose

_____ 4. Excessive sweating

_____ 5. Fat deposits on the inside wall of an artery

_____ 6. Opening in a vessel, intestines, or tube

_____ 7. By-product of hemoglobin breakdown; orange-yellow pigment of bile

_____ 8. Pregnancy test that uses a color change reaction

_____ 9. Hemoglobin A_{1c}; test that measures the amount of glucose attached to hemoglobin over a 3-month period

_____ 10. Amount of a substance able to be measured; actual amounts

_____ 11. Hardened protein material shaped like the lumen of the kidney tubule and washed out by urine

_____ 12. Shrunken; formation of notches on the edges of red blood cells

_____ 13. High-density lipoprotein; "good" cholesterol

_____ 14. Epithelial cells released by the kidney indicating disease

_____ 15. Blood test that details the chemical composition of the blood

_____ 16. Method to measure ESR using a self-zeroing tube calibrated from 0 to 200

_____ 17. Damaged, burst cells; hemolyzed red blood cells are colorless and cannot be seen under magnification

U. HDL

V. hemoglobin

W. hemolyzed

X. hyaline cast

Y. ketonuria

Z. lumen

AA. myoglobinuria

BB. plaque

CC. precipitates

DD. quantitative

EE. reagent tablet

FF. renal epithelial cells

GG. serum cholesterol

HH. streak

II. total cholesterol

JJ. turbid

KK. urochrome

LL. Westergren method

_____ 18. Test measuring a patient's ability to metabolize food 2 hours after a meal

_____ 19. Globin from damaged muscle cells in the urine

_____ 20. Yellow pigment derived from urobilin that is left over when hemoglobin breaks down during red blood cell destruction

_____ 21. Equipment that uses light photometry to analyze a reagent test strip

_____ 22. Chemical pad on a dipstick that tests for the presence of sugar

_____ 23. White, fatlike substance made in the liver

_____ 24. Seaweed extract used to make media solid for bacterial cultures

_____ 25. Total count of each blood element

_____ 26. Common casts found in urine that are pale and transparent; appear in unchecked hypertension

_____ 27. Combined measurement of LDL and HDL cholesterol

_____ 28. Culture and sensitivity; test to determine which antibiotic is most effective against cultured organisms

_____ 29. Tablet that reacts to a specific substance, confirming its presence

_____ 30. Presence of ketones in the urine

_____ 31. Covered container with nutritional substances that support growth of bacteria

_____ 32. Red blood cell component that carries oxygen and gives blood its color

_____ 33. Not clear or transparent; particles floating within; cloudy

_____ 34. Appearance of bilirubin in the urine

_____ 35. Staining method used to identify the shape and pattern of microorganisms

_____ 36. Particles in a solution brought on by a chemical reaction

_____ 37. Galactose in the blood

_____ 38. Anticoagulant used for preserving blood for hematology studies

CHAPTER 42 Laboratory Testing in the Physician's Office

THEORY RECALL

True/False

Indicate whether the statement is true or false.

_____ 1. Cholesterol is metabolized only from foods that are eaten and is not produced by the body.

_____ 2. RBCs are larger than WBCs.

_____ 3. A hematocrit reading can be performed with venous or capillary blood.

_____ 4. LDL is considered "good" cholesterol.

_____ 5. Finding casts in urine is not of any importance.

Multiple Choice

Identify the letter of the choice that best completes the statement or answers the question.

1. A patient must fast at least _____ hours to perform a fasting blood glucose test.
   A. 2
   B. 8
   C. 12
   D. 24

2. Gram staining separates bacteria into _____ groups.
   A. two
   B. three
   C. four
   D. five

3. Throat cultures are usually cultured on _____.
   A. blood agar
   B. seaweed broth
   C. chocolate agar
   D. None of the above

4. A color that describes normal urine is _____.
   A. brown
   B. red
   C. light straw
   D. green

5. _____ is(are) a waste product of fat metabolism.
   A. Bilirubin
   B. Ketones
   C. Glucose
   D. Nitrates

6. hCG levels are detectable _____ days after fertilization.
   A. 2
   B. 5
   C. 10
   D. 14

7. _____ carry oxygen to the body.
   A. Leukocytes
   B. Platelets
   C. RBCs
   D. WBCs

8. When performing a Wintrobe ESR, the sample must sit in the sedimentation rack for _____ to obtain a valid reading.
   A. 30 minutes
   B. 45 minutes
   C. 1 hour
   D. 1½ hours

9. The chemical pad for blood on the reagent strip reacts to _____.
   A. intact RBCs
   B. hemoglobin
   C. myoglobin
   D. all of the above

10. Bilirubin appearing in urine is a clear sign of liver and biliary tract dysfunction.
    A. True
    B. False

11. Normal 24-hour adult urine volume output is _____ mL.
    A. 500 to 750
    B. 750 to 2000
    C. 1000 to 2000
    D. 1500 to 2500

12. Proteinuria is an indication of all of the following *except* _____.
    A. congestive heart failure
    B. heavy exercising
    C. UTI
    D. stroke

13. You would count _____ white blood cells when performing a differential blood cell count.
    A. 50
    B. 100
    C. 125
    D. 150

14. Normal range for urine specific gravity is _____.
    A. 1.00 to 1.125
    B. 1.01 to 1.020
    C. 1.01 to 1.025
    D. 1.01 to 1.015

15. The life of an RBC is _____ days.
    A. 80
    B. 100
    C. 110
    D. 120

16. Examination of a urine slide first takes place under _____ power.
    A. ×10
    B. ×20
    C. ×40
    D. ×100

17. _____ casts have a saw-toothed edge.
    A. Fatty
    B. Granular
    C. Hyaline
    D. Waxy

18. Emotional stress may manifest as _____ in the urine.
    A. fat
    B. glucose
    C. protein
    D. nitrates

19. _____ is the study of microorganisms, especially pathogenic organisms.
    A. Bacteriology
    B. Cytology
    C. Microbiology
    D. Pathology

20. _____ is(are) the end product of nitrate metabolism.
    A. Acetone
    B. Bacteria
    C. Nitrites
    D. Squamous epithelial cells

Sentence Completion

Complete each sentence or statement.

yeast	24	WBCs
2-hour postprandial test	hemoglobinuria	renal or transitional epithelial cells
fasting	ketones	bacteria
RBCs	lysis	point-of-care tests
	artifacts	

1. A(n) _____ is used to screen for diabetes mellitus, and to monitor the effects of a patient's insulin regimen

2. Cultured microorganisms must grow in an incubator for _____ hours.

3. _____ is the presence of intact RBCs in the urine.

4. _____ found in large numbers is an indication of kidney problems.

5. Rod-shaped organisms found in urine are known as _____.

6. Powder, fibers, and hair are known as _____ in urine.

7. _____ is(are) formed in bone marrow and in lymphoid tissue.

8. _____ involve(s) a test done in the physician's office for immediate feedback.

9. _____ is the destruction of RBCs caused by an antibody-antigen response.

10. _____ are oval-shaped, vary in size, and have small buds.

Short Answers

1. List five factors that can affect the quality of blood smear.

_____
_____
_____
_____

2. List 10 tests routinely done during a urinalysis.

3. Explain the purpose of a hemoglobin measurement.

4. Explain the purpose and procedure of a glucose tolerance test.

CRITICAL THINKING

1. Ann is a new employee at Dr Paul's practice. In observing her trainer, she discovers that this office does not perform all of the diagnostic tests that her last employer did. What might cause this difference, and how is it determined which office performs what tests?

PRACTICAL APPLICATIONS

If you have accomplished the objectives in this chapter, you will be able to make better choices as a medical assistant. Take a look at this situation and decide what you would do.

Dr. Carlson does not have a medical laboratory technician. Instead, she depends on the medical assistant to provide the test results of laboratory specimens that are ordered. Because of his training in a medical assisting program, Jerry, Dr. Carlson's medical assistant, is aware of the importance of quality control and quality assurance, and that both should be done on a daily basis.

As part of the daily routine, Jerry is expected to perform physical and chemical testing of urine using reagent strips. Dr. Carlson also allows Jerry to examine specimens using a microscope to identify the urine sediment. Jerry completes hemoglobin testing using HemoCue and uses a centrifuge to spin hematocrits. As Jerry reads the hematocrit, he finds that the anticoagulated blood has separated into three layers, each of which has a specific characteristic. Because CLIA-waived tests are often performed in a physician's office, Jerry and other medical assistants must be able to perform these tests on a daily basis.

Would you be capable of performing these tasks?

1. What is meant by a "CLIA-waived" test?

_____

_____

_____

_____

2. What do reagent strips show? Are all reagent strips the same?

_____

_____

_____

_____

3. Why is it important for Jerry to wait for the designated amount of time before reading the results of a reagent strip?

_____

_____

_____

_____

Copyright © 2010, 2005 by Saunders, an imprint of Elsevier, Inc. All rights reserved.

4. When checking a urine specimen for physical properties, what is Jerry looking for?

5. What influences the physical properties of urine?

6. Can Jerry perform a microscopic examination of urine under CLIA standards? If not, what part of the microscopic examination can he perform?

7. What type of pregnancy tests can Jerry perform in the physician's office? What are the indications of a positive pregnancy test in each test?

8. When should a urine specimen be collected for a pregnancy test?

9. Can Jerry perform hemoglobin and hematocrit measurements? Why or why not?

10. What are the three layers found in centrifuged whole blood? How are these used to measure a microhematocrit?

APPLICATION OF SKILLS

Procedure Check-off Sheets (*) and assignments from MACC on the Evolve site at http://evolve.elsevier.com/klieger/medicalassisting (**)

1. Perform Procedure 42-1: Urinalysis Using Reagent Strips.*

2. Perform Procedure 42-2: Prepare a Urine Specimen for Microscopic Examination.*

3. Perform Procedure 42-3: Perform a Urine Pregnancy Test.*

4. Perform Procedure 42-4: Determine a Hemoglobin Measurement Using a HemoCue.*

5. Perform Procedure 42-5: Perform a Microhematocrit Test.*

6. Perform Procedure 42-6: Determine Erythrocyte Sedimentation Rate (ESR, Nonautomated) Using the Westergren Method.*

7. Perform Procedure 42-7: Prepare a Blood Smear.*

8. Perform Procedure 42-8: Perform Cholesterol Testing.*

9. Perform Procedure 42-9: Perform Glucose Testing.*

10. Perform Procedure 42-10: Obtain a Bacterial Smear from a Wound Specimen.*

Copyright © 2010, 2005 by Saunders, an imprint of Elsevier, Inc. All rights reserved.

CHAPTER QUIZ

Multiple Choice

Identify the letter of the choice that best completes the statement or answers the question.

1. _____ are produced in the red bone marrow.
   A. Leukocytes
   B. Platelets
   C. RBCs
   D. WBCs

2. Glucose in the urine may indicate _____.
   A. heavy meal
   B. emotional stress
   C. high doses of vitamin C
   D. all of the above

3. Normal range for specific gravity is _____.
   A. 1.00 to 1.010
   B. 1.01 to 1.015
   C. 1.01 to 1.025
   D. 1.01 to 1.125

4. _____ casts are commonly found in urine and are pale and transparent.
   A. Fatty
   B. Granular
   C. Hyaline
   D. Waxy

5. Myoglobinuria is the result of severe muscle injury caused by trauma.
   A. True
   B. False

6. _____ is the chemical formed when fats are metabolized.
   A. Hemoglobin
   B. Ketone
   C. Glucose
   D. Yeast

7. When bilirubin is broken down by the intestinal bacteria, it is known as _____.
   A. nitrates
   B. nitrites
   C. urobilinogen
   D. urochrome

8. _____ is the measurement of the percentage of packed RBCs in a volume of whole blood.
   A. CBC
   B. ESR
   C. Hematocrit
   D. Hemoglobin

9. The Westergren method of ESR requires that the tube sit upright for _____.
   A. 30 minutes
   B. 1 hour
   C. 1½ hours
   D. 2 hours

10. _____ cholesterol is known as the "good cholesterol."
    A. Low-density lipoprotein
    B. High-density lipoprotein
    C. Total cholesterol
    D. All of the above

11. _____ is the most sensitive test of the patient's ability to metabolize glucose.
    A. Fasting blood glucose
    B. The 2-hour postprandial test
    C. Glucose tolerance test
    D. Multistik 10 reagent strip test

12. _____ carry oxygen to the body.
    A. Leukocytes
    B. Platelets
    C. RBCs
    D. WBCs

13. Sediment is the top, liquid portion of a specimen that has been centrifuged to remove solid particles.
    A. True
    B. False

14. Increased WBCs in urine are an indication of _____.
    A. arthritis
    B. kidney disease
    C. transplant rejection
    D. all of the above

15. The appearance of particles in urine can be described as _____.
    A. dark
    B. light
    C. turbid
    D. transparent

16. The normal volume of urine an adult can excrete is _____ mL in a 24-hour period.
    A. 500 to 1000
    B. 750 to 1000
    C. 750 to 1500
    D. 750 to 2000

17. Hemoglobin is the component that gives WBCs their color.
    A. True
    B. False

18. _____ is a culture medium used to support growth of microorganisms.
    A. Agar
    B. Broth
    C. Semisolid medium
    D. All of the above

19. Petri dishes need to be placed in an incubator for _____ hours to promote microorganism growth.
    A. 12
    B. 24
    C. 48
    D. 72

20. The life span of an RBC is _____ days.
    A. 30
    B. 60
    C. 100
    D. 120

NAME: DATE:

43 Understanding Medications

VOCABULARY REVIEW

Matching: Match each term with the correct definition.

A. adverse reaction

B. booster dose

C. caplet

D. contraindications

E. controlled substances

F. cumulative dose

G. curative dose

H. diagnostic drug

I. divided dose

J. elixirs

K. emulsion

L. enteric-coated tablet

M. initial dose

N. inscription

O. layered tablet

P. lethal dose

Q. maintenance dose

R. nomogram

S. ointment

T. parenteral

_____ 1. Capsule that contains time-released beads of medication

_____ 2. Rod-shaped, compressed powdered drug form

_____ 3. Amount of medication that proves deadly to a patient

_____ 4. Lozenges

_____ 5. Undesirable and unexpected effects of medications that may be harmful

_____ 6. Total amount of medication that is administered in separate doses

_____ 7. Semisolid mixture of medications that has an oil base for external use

_____ 8. Solution that has undissolved particles and must be shaken to distribute evenly before administration

_____ 9. Route for medication given under the skin or other than the digestive system

_____ 10. Drugs that have a potential for abuse, misuse, and addiction

_____ 11. Tablet with a special coating that dissolves in the small intestine

_____ 12. Liquid medications mixed with an alcohol base

_____ 13. Medication that lessens or prevents the effect of a disease

_____ 14. Drug that heals disease or cures infection

_____ 15. First dose of medication administered

_____ 16. Guidelines for drug administration: right patient, drug, dose, route, time, technique, and documentation

_____ 17. Solutions containing alcohol, water, sugar, and a drug or combination of drugs

Copyright © 2010, 2005 by Saunders, an imprint of Elsevier, Inc. All rights reserved.

U. percutaneous
V. prophylactic drug
W. scored tablet
X. seven rights
Y. spansule
Z. suspension
AA. therapeutic drug
BB. tinctures
CC. toxicity
DD. troches

_____ 18. Harmful effects of drugs on body

_____ 19. Route for medication given through the skin

_____ 20. Medication given to increase chances for long-term immunity, as with immunizations

_____ 21. Chart that shows the relationship of body surface area to height and weight in calculating drug dosage, usually for a child or an infant, but may be used with adults

_____ 22. Tablet with indentations across the middle that allows it to be broken in half

_____ 23. Substance in an oil-based liquid that must be shaken before use

_____ 24. Factors that indicate a medication should not be prescribed because potential risks outweigh potential benefits

_____ 25. Amount of medication needed by the body to maintain its desired effect

_____ 26. Medication that restores the body to its presymptomatic state

_____ 27. Total amount of medication in the body after repeated doses; medication that accumulates in the body one time

_____ 28. Drug that assists with diagnosing a disease during a procedure, such as radiopaque dye with x-rays

_____ 29. Section of a prescription where the name of the medication is entered

_____ 30. Tablet containing two or more ingredients layered to dissolve and be absorbed at different times

THEORY RECALL

True/False

Indicate whether the statement is true or false.

_____ 1. Prescriptions are legal documents.

_____ 2. Pharmacokinetics is the study of the biochemical and physiological effects of a drug within the body.

_____ 3. When documenting an immunization injection, the serum manufacturer's name must be noted in the patient's medical record.

_____ 4. Drug samples need to be documented in the patient's chart.

_____ 5. The physician's DEA number does not need to be written on a prescription for controlled substances.

Multiple Choice

Identify the letter of the choice that best completes the statement or answers the question.

1. Most drugs can be identified by _____.
   A. chemical name
   B. generic name
   C. trade name
   D. all of the above

2. The recommended adult dose is based on an age range from _____ years.
   A. 20 to 40
   B. 20 to 30
   C. 20 to 50
   D. 20 to 60

3. The _____ is the agency responsible for enforcing the Controlled Substance Act.
   A. AAMA
   B. AMA
   C. DEA
   D. FDA

4. Medication exists in _____ forms.
   A. two
   B. three
   C. four
   D. five

5. Schedule _____ drugs have no acceptable medical use.
   A. I
   B. II
   C. III
   D. IV

6. Which one of the following is not a solid form of medications?
   A. Spansules
   B. Powders
   C. Sublingual tablets
   D. Elixirs

7. _____ can be an oil-based, water-based, alcohol-based, or soap-based medication intended to be rubbed into the skin.
   A. Cream
   B. Liniment
   C. Lotion
   D. Ointment

8. _____ is a liquid with dissolved particles.
   A. Solute
   B. Solution
   C. Solvent
   D. Tincture

9. _____ is a drug used to lessen or prevent the effects of a disease.
   A. Curative
   B. Prophylactic
   C. Replacement
   D. Therapeutic

10. Section 2 of the PDR _____.
    A. includes all participating drug companies
    B. lists each product alphabetically
    C. provides generic and brand name products by page number
    D. provides photographs of various drug forms and products

11. Medication dosage is prescribed for a patient based on _____.
    A. height
    B. nationality
    C. weight
    D. past history

12. Records concerning the dispensing of drugs must be kept for a minimum of _____ year(s).
    A. 1
    B. 2
    C. 5
    D. 10

13. The *Physicians' Desk Reference* is published _____ in conjunction with the pharmaceutical companies whose products are represented.
    A. annually
    B. biannually
    C. every 2 years
    D. only as changes occur

14. Package inserts are included with samples and prescription drugs from the pharmacy.
    A. True
    B. False

15. The United States Pharmacopeia/National Formulary is published _____ by the Council on Pharmacology of the American Medical Association.
    A. annually
    B. every 2 years
    C. every 5 years
    D. every 10 years

16. Dosages for _____ are most frequently calculated according to body weight.
    A. children
    B. elderly individuals
    C. young adults
    D. middle-aged adults

17. Solutions consist of one or more medications dissolved in _____.
    A. alcohol
    B. normal saline
    C. water
    D. any of the above

18. _____ are solutions of sugar and water that contain drugs.
    A. Aerosols
    B. Suspension
    C. Syrups
    D. Tincture

19. A _____ is the amount of medication that proves deadly to a patient.
    A. curative dose
    B. lethal dose
    C. maintenance dose
    D. all of the above

20. A(n) _____ is a hard candy-like tablet that dissolves in the mouth and releases medication.
    A. elixir
    B. suppository
    C. lozenge
    D. none of the above

Sentence Completion

Complete each sentence or statement.

elixir	emulsion	capsule
subscription	pharmacokinetics	Controlled Substances
drug	inscription	Act
pharmacology	buccal tablet	controlled substances
III	replacement drug	II

1. _____ is the study of drugs and how they affect the body.

2. The _____ is legislation whose purpose is to control the manufacture, free offering, and selling of drugs that have potential for abuse.

3. Schedule _____ drugs do not have to be ordered on a special form, but records must be kept.

4. _____ is a substance suspended in an oil-based liquid into which it does not mix.

5. The _____ is the line on a prescription that provides for the name of the medication ordered, its strength, and the drug's form.

6. _____ is the study of what happens to a drug from the time it enters the body until it leaves.

7. _____ is medication that replaces substances normally found in the body.

8. _____ is a tablet that dissolves when placed between cheek and gum.

9. A(n) _____ or medicine is any substance that produces a chemical change in the body.

10. _____ must be locked, separate from other drugs, in a locked cabinet.

Short Answers

1. List the seven rights, and give the reason for each.

   _____
   _____
   _____
   _____
   _____
   _____
   _____

2. Explain the three rules for discarding a controlled substance.

   _____
   _____
   _____
   _____
   _____

3. List the three basic considerations when administrating an immunization.

___

4. What is the purpose of the vaccine information statement (VIS)? Why is it handed out whenever certain vaccinations are given?

___

5. List the current VIS dates for the following vaccinations (www.immunize.org/vis):
    a. Chickenpox   _____
    b. DTaP/DT/DTP   _____
    c. Hepatitis A   _____
    d. Hepatitis B   _____
    e. Hib   _____
    f. HPV   _____
    g. Influenza (LAIV) _____
    h. Influenza   _____
    i. MMR   _____
    j. PCV   _____
    k. PPV   _____
    l. Polio   _____
    m. Rotavirus   _____
    n. Shingles   _____
    o. Tdap   _____

6. Vaccines HAVRIX and VAQTA are given for prevention of what disease? (*Hint*: Use the Internet to research this question.)

___

CRITICAL THINKING

1. Calculate the following drug orders, and make the necessary conversions.
    a. The physician orders 30 mg of Lasix IM. You have Lasix 40 mg/mL on hand. How many mL would you give to an adult patient?

b. The physician orders 3 mg of Ativan IM. You have a 10-mL vial of Ativan 2 mg/mL on hand. How many mL would you give to an adult patient?
c. The physician orders 7.5 mg of Compazine IM q3-4h for nausea and vomiting. You have a 10-mL vial of Compazine 5 mg/mL on hand. How many mL would you give to an adult patient?
d. The physician orders 60 mg of Demerol IM q4h. You have Demerol 75 mg/1.5 mL on hand. How many mL would you give to an adult patient?
e. The physician orders ¼ gr of codeine SQ q4h PRN for pain. You have a 20-mL vial of codeine 30 mg/mL on hand. How many mL would you give to an adult patient?
f. The physician orders digoxin 600 mcg IM stat. You have digoxin 0.5 mg/2 mL on hand. How many mL would you give to an adult patient?
g. The physician orders Bicillin 2,400,000 U, IM stat. You have a 10-mL vial of Bicillin containing 600,000 U/mL on hand. How many mL would you give to an adult patient?
h. The physician orders Lanoxin 200 mcg IM. You have 250 mcg/mL of Lanoxin on hand. How many mL would you give to an adult patient?
i. The physician orders hydrochlorothiazide 12.5 mg PO. You have 25-mg tablets available. How many tablets would you give to an adult patient?

2. Convert the following measurements:
   a. 1 mg is _____ g.
   b. There are _____ mL in a liter.
   c. 10 mL = _____ cc.
   d. Which is largest: kilogram, gram, or milligram? _____
   e. Which is smallest: kilogram, gram, or milligram? _____
   f. 1 liter = _____ cc.
   g. 1000 mcg = _____ mg.
   h. 1 kg = _____ lb.
   i. 1 cm = _____ mm.

3. Select the correct notation:
   a. .3 g, 0.3 gm, 0.3 g, .3 gm, 0.30 g _____
   b. 1⅓ ml, 1.33 mL, 1.33 ML, 1⅓ ML, 1.330 mL _____
   c. 5 Kg, 5.0 kg, kg 05, 5 kg, 5 kG _____
   d. 1.5 mm, 1½ mm, 1.5 Mm, 1.50 MM, 1½ MM _____
   e. mg 10, 10 mG, 10.0 mg, 10 mg, 10 MG _____

4. Spell out these metric abbreviations:
   a. mcg _____
   b. mm _____
   c. mL _____
   d. kg _____
   e. cc _____
   f. cm _____
   g. g _____

5. Convert the following:
   a. 100 mg = _____ g
   b. 150 mcg = _____ mg
   c. 30 mg = _____ g
   d. 0.9 mg = _____ mcg
   e. 1500 mg = _____ g
   f. 250 mcg = _____ mg
   g. 4 mg = _____ g
   h. 450 mcg = _____ mg

i. 0.065 gm = _____ mg
j. 800 mcg = _____ mg
k. 3.62 g = _____ mg
l. 1000 mcg = _____ mg

6. Convert the following (round off):
   a. .030 g = _____ mg
   b. 45 oz = _____ cc
   c. ¼ gr = _____ mg
   d. 15 gr = _____ g
   e. ⅙ gr = _____ g
   f. 0.3 g = _____ gr
   g. 1/150 gr = _____ mg
   h. 60 mg = _____ gr
   i. 15 mg = _____ gr
   j. 5 mg = _____ gr

PRACTICAL APPLICATIONS

If you have accomplished the objectives in this chapter, you will be able to make better choices as a medical assistant. Take a look at this situation and decide what you would do.

Glenn is a medical assistant in an office of a family physician. His employer, Dr. Carbello, sees patients of all ages. Because Glenn lives in a state where medical assistants are allowed to call in prescriptions to the pharmacy, one of his regular duties is to call in prescriptions. Glenn is also responsible for performing the inventory on scheduled medications. Today, Dr. Carbello has asked Glenn to call a pharmacy with a prescription for meperidine for a patient who has a severe pain in her back.

After examining another patient, Mrs. Vouch, Dr. Carbello orders an antihistamine for itching, to be given by injection, and an antipyretic. Dr. Carbello tells Glenn to be sure that he tells Mrs. Vouch the side effects of the medications. Mrs. Vouch is also given a prescription for the antihistamine and antipyretic to take at home. The antihistamine is a capsule and the antipyretic is a tablet. Both these medications have systemic effects, and both can have indications of a toxic effect. As Mrs. Vouch leaves the office, Glenn asks her to call in the next week to tell him how the medications are helping with the itching.

If you were Glenn, would you be able to explain the side effects of the medications to Mrs. Vouch?

1. What is the importance of doing an inventory of Schedule II medications in the medical office?

_____
_____
_____

2. Can Glenn call in a Schedule II medication? Why or why not?

_____
_____
_____

Copyright © 2010, 2005 by Saunders, an imprint of Elsevier, Inc. All rights reserved.

CHAPTER 43 Understanding Medications

3. What type of illness would you expect to be treated with an antihistamine?

4. What is the purpose of an antipyretic? List some common antipyretics?

5. What are the "seven rights" that Glenn must follow when giving medications?

6. If Glenn does not know the interactions and the side effects of the antihistamine, what resource can he use to obtain this information?

7. What is the difference between a side effect and an adverse reaction?

8. What is the difference between a capsule and a tablet?

9. What is the difference between a systemic effect and a local effect? Give an example of each.

10. Why is it important for Glenn to explain "toxic effect" when the patient will be taking the medication at home on a regular basis?

11. What should Glenn document in the medical record at the office visit? What should he document when Mrs. Vouch calls in the next week?

12. Why is it important for Glenn to understand a drug's actions before giving the drug?

13. How are administering, prescribing, and dispensing a medication different?

14. How are the chemical name, generic name, and trade name of a medication different?

APPLICATION OF SKILLS

1. You work at a pediatric clinic, and today the office manager has asked you to develop a fact sheet that can be handed out to parents or guardians concerning follow-up instructions dealing with care of the child and reactions that often occur after vaccinations.

2. Write prescriptions for the following:
    a. Dr. Smith wants Mary Dole to have Cipro 250 mg, q12h for 7 days for a UTI. No refills.
    b. Dr. Smith wants to start Bill Durham on Capoten 12.5 mg, PO bid for his newly diagnosed hypertension for 30 days. Dr. Perez also wants Mr. Durham to take Lasix 20 mg PO every morning for 30 days.
    Mary Dole: DOB 9/23/52; address 675 Lake Terrace Rd., Right City, USA 00021
    Bill Durham: DOB 2/14/56; address 892 South Lake Dr., Right City, USA 00023

```
            Joan Smith, M.D.
            456 Anywhere Lane
            Right City USA 00020
            Office (555-123-4567)
            Fax (555-321-7654)
```

Patient Name _____ DOB _____ Date _____
Address _____

R } Superscription

Inscription { _____

Subscription { _____

Signature { _____

☐ Dispense as written
☐ May substitute generic
Refill   None   1   2   3   4   5

Signature: *Joan Smith MD*
DEA#: _____

Joan Smith, M.D.
456 Anywhere Lane
Right City USA 00020
Office (555-123-4567)
Fax (555-321-7654)

Patient Name _____ DOB _____ Date _____
Address _____

R } Superscription

Inscription {
Subscription {
Signature   {

☐ Dispense as written
☐ May substitute generic

Refill None 1 2 3 4 5   Signature: *Joan Smith MD* _____
                                     DEA#: _____

Joan Smith, M.D.
456 Anywhere Lane
Right City USA 00020
Office (555-123-4567)
Fax (555-321-7654)

Patient Name _____ DOB _____ Date _____
Address _____

R } Superscription

Inscription {
Subscription {
Signature   {

☐ Dispense as written
☐ May substitute generic

Refill None 1 2 3 4 5   Signature: *Joan Smith MD* _____
                                     DEA#: _____

Copyright © 2010, 2005 by Saunders, an imprint of Elsevier, Inc. All rights reserved.

3. You are to administer 0.25 mg of a medication IM from a vial labeled 0.125 mg/2 mL. How many mL would you administer? _____

4. You are to administer 250,000 units of a medication. The label on the vial shows there at 1,000,000 units/5 mL. How many mL would you administer? _____

5. The physician orders 0.75 g of medication. On hand you have a vial labeled 1000 mg/2 mL. How many mL would you administer? _____

6. Create a Fact Sheet that identifies the following for the listed medications:
   - Trade name, generic name, and drug classification
   - Indications for its use
   - Contraindications
   - Form and recommended dosage and administration
   - Side effects

   Medications:
   Ativan
   Antivert
   Ditropan
   Flexeril
   Lortab
   Zovirax
   Flagyl

7. Perform Procedure 43-1: Prepare and File an Immunization Record.

CHAPTER QUIZ

Multiple Choice

Identify the letter of the choice that best completes the statement or answers the question.

1. _____ is the study of drugs and how they affect the body.
   A. Pharmacology
   B. Pharmacodynamics
   C. Pharmacokinetics
   D. None of the above

2. _____ is a drug used to lessen or prevent the effects of a disease.
   A. Curative
   B. Prophylactic
   C. Replacement
   D. Therapeutic

3. The recommended adult dose is based on an age range of _____ years.
   A. 20 to 40
   B. 20 to 50
   C. 20 to 60
   D. 20 to 70

4. _____ is the nonproprietary name of a drug.
   A. Chemical name
   B. Generic name
   C. Trade name
   D. Over-the-counter

5. DEA tests and approves food, drug, and cosmetic products for the marketplace.
   A. True
   B. False

6. Schedule _____ drugs have a use, but severe restrictions apply.
   A. I
   B. II
   C. III
   D. IV

7. The *Physicians' Desk Reference* is published _____.
   A. annually
   B. biannually
   C. every 2 years
   D. every 3 years

8. Medication is prescribed for a patient based on _____.
   A. age
   B. body weight
   C. gender
   D. all of the above

9. Documentation should be done _____.
   A. immediately after the procedure
   B. just before the procedure
   C. at the end of the day
   D. when you have the time

10. _____ is a medication that is evenly distributed within the solution after shaking but not dissolved.
    A. Emulsion
    B. Elixir
    C. Solution
    D. Suspension

11. The combination vaccine Comvax provides protection against _____.
    A. Hib and HepB
    B. PCV and IPV
    C. MMR and MCV4
    D. DTaP and HepB

12. _____ is the section of a prescription with instructions to the patient about how to take the medication.
    A. Inscription
    B. Signature
    C. Subscription
    D. Superscription

13. When dispensing drugs, the records must be kept for _____.
    A. 30 days
    B. 6 months
    C. 1 year
    D. 2 years

14. When a patient is given samples of drugs, the samples must be logged into the patient's chart.
    A. True
    B. False

15. _____ is a semisolid, cone-shaped medication that dissolves within a body cavity.
    A. Buccal tablet
    B. Sublingual tablet
    C. Spansule capsule
    D. Suppository

16. Most drugs are identified by _____.
    A. chemical name
    B. generic name
    C. trade name
    D. all of the above

17. The _____ is responsible for enforcing the Controlled Substance Act.
    A. DEA
    B. FDA
    C. AMA
    D. none of the above

18. The United States Pharmacopeia/National Formulary is published every _____ year(s).
    A. 1
    B. 2
    C. 4
    D. 5

19. Package inserts are included only in prescription drugs received from a pharmacy.
    A. True
    B. False

20. The physician's DEA number must be on the prescription.
    A. True
    B. False

21. Convert the following:
    A. 10 cc = _____ oz
    B. 10 gr = _____ g
    C. 0.75 cc = _____ m
    D. m 25 = _____ mL
    E. 0.5 g = _____ mg
    F. 30 gr = _____ g
    G. gr iii = _____ mg
    H. oz i = _____ cc
    I. 0.5 mL = _____ m
    J. $1/100$ gr = _____ mg

K. 0.05 g = _____ mg
L. 0.05 mg = _____ mcg
M. 0.1 g = _____ mg
N. 0.375 mg = _____ mcg
O. 0.2 g = _____ mg
P. 0.1 mg = _____ mcg

22. Spell out the following metric abbreviations:
    A. kg: _____
    B. g: _____
    C. cc: _____
    D. mL: _____
    E. cm: _____
    F. mcg: _____
    G. mm: _____

23. Calculate the amount you will prepare for each dose.
    A. Order: Vit. B12 0.5 mg IM once/wk
       Supply: Vit. B12 1 mg/mL 10-mL vial

       _____

    B. Order: Slow-K 16 mEq PO stat
       Supply: Slow-K 8 mEq tablets

       _____

    C. Order: Duricef 1 g PO QID AC
       Supply: Duricef 500-mg capsules

       _____

    D. Order: Lanoxin 0.125 mg PO QD
       Supply: Lanoxin 0.25-mg tablets

       _____

    E. Order: Motrin 600 mg PO BID
       Supply: Motrin 300-mg tablets

       _____

NAME: _____ DATE: _____

44 Administering Medications

VOCABULARY REVIEW

Matching: Match each term with the correct definition.

A. ampule

B. antipyretics

C. aspiration

D. beveled

E. bleb

F. dorsogluteal

G. enteral

H. hub

I. induration

J. isotonic solutions

K. lumen

L. Mantoux test

M. meniscus

N. nebulizer

O. parenteral

P. shaft

Q. spacer

R. subcutaneous

S. syringe

T. transdermal patch

_____ 1. Hollow tube made of glass or plastic marked with specific measurements and with a tip that attaches to a needle

_____ 2. Fluid-filled raised area under the skin

_____ 3. Tuberculin test

_____ 4. Opening of a needle

_____ 5. Part of a needle that determines its length

_____ 6. Specially shaped single-dose glass container that contains a dose of medication and has been hermetically sealed

_____ 7. Intramuscular technique for administering medication that requires the pulling back or displacement of tissue using the injection to prevent discoloration of the skin

_____ 8. Area of hardened tissue that occurs as a result of sensitivity to an allergen

_____ 9. Air compressor unit that forces medication into the lungs

_____ 10. Taken through the digestive system

_____ 11. Vacuum-sealed bottle that contains a sterile solution with or without medication or a sterile oil-based substance

_____ 12. Pulling back, as in using suction to draw up blood in a syringe

_____ 13. Taken into the body through the skin by way of a needle

_____ 14. Solutions that contain the same salt concentration as a person's body fluids

_____ 15. Medications that reduce fever

_____ 16. Injection given into fatty layers of the skin beneath the dermis

Copyright © 2010, 2005 by Saunders, an imprint of Elsevier, Inc. All rights reserved.

U. vastus lateralis muscle

V. ventrogluteal

W. vial

X. wheal

Y. winged infusion set

Z. Z-track method

_____ 17. Muscle area formed by the gluteus medius and gluteus minimus

_____ 18. Part of the needle that fits or locks onto a syringe

_____ 19. "Butterfly needles"; special needles with tabs that resemble butterfly wings used to grasp during insertion

_____ 20. Slanted; the slant of a needle that makes piercing the skin easier

_____ 21. Attachment added to a metered-dose inhaler that acts as a reservoir and changes the characteristics of the medication

_____ 22. Area of gluteus muscle in upper outer portion of the buttocks

_____ 23. Adhesive-backed patch that contains a premeasured dose of medication that is absorbed through the skin

_____ 24. Thigh muscle located between the greater trochanter of the femur and the knee

_____ 25. Fluid-filled bump; raised hivelike bump on the surface of skin seen after a properly placed intradermal injection

_____ 26. Concave level where air and a liquid come together; the surface of fluid when placed in a column or container

THEORY RECALL

True/False

Indicate whether the statement is true or false.

_____ 1. Vaginal medication usually works within 15 to 30 minutes of application.

_____ 2. Aspiration is performed on all injections.

_____ 3. The advantage of parenteral administration of a drug is that it has slow absorption.

_____ 4. Oral medications come in either solid or liquid.

_____ 5. A medical assistant must be very careful not to allow medication to spill out when inverting an ampule.

Multiple Choice

Identify the letter of the choice that best completes the statement or answers the question.

1. _____ is the most frequently used route of administration.
   A. Inhalation
   B. Oral
   C. Parenteral
   D. Topical

2. When administering an intradermal injection, usually _____ mL of medication is given.
   A. 0.01 or less
   B. 0.1 or less
   C. 1.0 or less
   D. 2.0 or less

3. _____ is a solution used to maintain adequate fluids in the body or to prevent dehydration.
   A. Hydrating solution
   B. Hypertonic solution
   C. Isotonic solution
   D. Maintenance solution

4. The _____ syringe is the most commonly used, and is calibrated in tenths and millimeter and minims.
   A. 0.5-mL
   B. 1-mL
   C. 3-mL
   D. 5-mL

5. A(n) _____ injection is placed 1 to 2 inches below the acromion process and across from the axilla.
   A. intradermal
   B. deltoid
   C. subcutaneous
   D. ventrogluteal

6. As a medical assistant, you should have a patient who has just received an injection wait for _____ minutes for observation of any adverse reactions.
   A. 5 to 10
   B. 10 to 15
   C. 15 to 30
   D. 30 to 60

7. Typically, the action of an oral medication takes _____ to take effect.
   A. 15 to 30 minutes
   B. 30 to 60 minutes
   C. 1 to 1½ hours
   D. 1 to 2 hours

8. A(n) _____ gauge needle is used when administering a subcutaneous injection.
   A. 18- to 23-
   B. 23- to 25-
   C. 25- to 28-
   D. 28- to 30-

9. _____ is the fastest route of absorption when administering medication.
   A. Oral
   B. Intradermal
   C. Intravenous
   D. Subcutaneous

10. The preferred site for the administration of an intradermal injection is _____.
    A. forearm
    B. calf
    C. lower abdomen
    D. all of the above

11. When pouring liquid into a cup, always _____.
    A. pour with cup on the table
    B. read amount from the highest point of curvature
    C. rinse cup with water before pouring
    D. pour liquid at eye level

12. Which one of the following is the best method for administering medication to a patient with nausea and vomiting when the chance for further gastrointestinal upset is possible?
    A. Liquids
    B. Vaginal suppositories
    C. Rectal suppositories
    D. Tablets

13. When performing an intradermal injection, a _____ angle is used.
    A. 0- to 10-degree
    B. 5- to 10-degree
    C. 10- to 15-degree
    D. 15- to 20-degree

14. The most common IM injection site is the _____.
    A. deltoid muscle
    B. fatty area on the back of the arm
    C. forearm
    D. stomach

15. Topical drug reactions occur within _____ after being administered.
    A. 10 minutes
    B. 30 minutes
    C. 45 minutes
    D. 1 hour

16. The _____ injection area is free of nerves and major blood vessels.
    A. mid-deltoid
    B. dorsogluteal
    C. vastus lateralis
    D. ventrogluteal

17. An intramuscular injection is administered at a _____ angle.
    A. 10- to 15-degree
    B. 45-degree
    C. 90-degree
    D. none of the above

18. Winged butterfly infusion sets are most commonly used when a _____.
    A. patient is receiving multiple therapies
    B. patient has small veins
    C. patient is undergoing long-term therapies
    D. patient has good veins

19. When withdrawing medications from an ampule, a _____ needle should be used.
    A. filtered
    B. big-bore (hole)
    C. short-length
    D. small-bore

20. Topical medications include _____.
    A. creams
    B. lotions
    C. transdermal patches
    D. all of the above

Sentence Completion

Complete each sentence or statement.

prefilled cartridge	22	deltoid
unit	gauge	vastus lateralis
vial	bore	Z-track
needles	hub	inhalation drugs
ampule	hilt	18
subcutaneous	nebulizer	

1. _____ is a single-dose glass container that has been hermetically sealed.

2. The _____ of the needle describes the lumen of the needle.

3. A(n) _____ injection is placed into the fatty layer beneath the dermis.

4. _____ are absorbed into the bloodstream through capillary action.

5. _____ is the muscle of choice when giving an infant or a child an injection.

6. _____ injection prevents leakage of irritating medication to the skin level.

7. A(n) _____ provides a mist of medication.

8. _____ are sterile metal objects constructed to fit on the tip of a syringe.

9. Needles used most frequently range from _____ (thickest) to 30 (thinnest) and are color-coded for easier identification.

10. A(n) _____ contains a single dose of medication for injection.

Short Answers

1. Give four guidelines for preparing and administering oral medications.

   _____
   _____
   _____
   _____

2. Give four functions performed by body fluids.

   _____
   _____
   _____
   _____

3. List and explain the four categories of IV solutions.

   _____
   _____
   _____
   _____

4. As a result of the Needlestick Safety and Prevention Act, OSHA requires (*hint*: use the Internet):

   _____
   _____
   _____
   _____

CRITICAL THINKING

1. Edith, the medical assistant for Dr Wade, is asked to administer a tuberculin test and an antibiotic injection to a patient. When drawing the medications up, she placed them in 3-cc syringes with 25-gauge needles. While taking them to the patient, she forgets which medications were which. Because she is in a hurry, she chooses to give them both via an IM route. Was Edith correct in giving both injections IM? Explain why or why not.

_____

_____

_____

_____

2. Jason is a 6-year-old boy with asthma. Today Dr. Spence decides that Jason must have nebulizer treatments available at home. He asks you to teach Jason and his mother how to use a nebulizer. Create a Fact Sheet that will assist them to follow your instructions at home. Include supplies they will need, how to measure the prescribed medications, and how to assemble the nebulizer cup and mouthpiece. Also include how to begin the treatment, the length of time the treatment should be given, and what to do if Jason becomes dizzy or jittery. Demonstrate proper cleaning and storage of the equipment.

PRACTICAL APPLICATIONS

If you have accomplished the objectives in this chapter, you will be able to make better choices as a medical assistant. Take a look at this situation and decide what you would do.

Sue, a medical assistant with no formal training, has been asked by her employer, Dr. Kenyon, to give Dylan, age 3 years, a single dose of acetaminophen 250 mg. Dylan's record shows that he is allergic to penicillin and has had a severe rash in the past. Sue goes to the medicine cabinet and removes amoxicillin, 250-mg tablets, and takes a single tablet to Dylan. Sue does not bother to read the label except when taking the medication from the shelf. Dylan's mother tells Sue that her child is unable to swallow the tablet, but Sue continues to give the tablet, telling the mother that at age 3, Dylan should be able to swallow a tablet.

Sue leaves Dylan and his mother with the tablet. Margie, the other medical assistant in the office, asks Sue to prepare a medication for Mrs. Abbott, who needs a 1-mL estrogen injection. Margie tells Sue that this aqueous medication will be given intramuscularly, and that she will be back to give the medication. In preparing the estrogen medication from a vial, Sue shakes the medicine and then draws it into a 5-mL syringe with a 25-gauge, ⁵⁄₈-inch needle. Margie returns and gives the medication that Sue prepared.

In the meantime, Dylan has choked on the tablet and is having difficulty breathing. Because Sue left the room, she is unaware of the situation. When Dr. Kenyon arrives in the room, he immediately recognizes a problem and calls in both Sue and Margie to help remove the tablet from Dylan's throat.

What would you have done differently as a medical assistant?

1. When should Sue have checked the medication to be sure she had the correct medication?

_____

_____

Copyright © 2010, 2005 by Saunders, an imprint of Elsevier, Inc. All rights reserved.

CHAPTER 44 Administering Medications

2. Does it make any difference that the medication ordered was acetaminophen and the medication given was amoxicillin? What are the specific dangers in this case?

3. Was the ordered dosage of the acetaminophen correct for a 3-year-old child? What should Sue have done to be sure the dosage was correct?

4. Why is it important for Sue to know the correct dosage of a medication rather than assuming that the physician is correct?

5. Why is oral administration of acetaminophen the correct route for a 3-year-old child?

6. If Dylan was unable to swallow a tablet, what form of medication could Sue have given him?

7. What are the dangers of giving a tablet to a child who is unable to swallow that form of solid medication?

8. If Dr. Kenyon had prescribed an injection of antibiotic for Dylan, where would the appropriate site have been for administration?

9. What mistake did Sue make while removing the medication from the vial? What mistake did she make in the selection of the syringe and the needle?

10. Because Sue prepared the medication for administration and Margie administered the injection and documented the procedure, who is responsible if a mistake is made? Explain your answer.

APPLICATION OF SKILLS

Procedure Check-off Sheets (*) and assignments from MACC on the Evolve site at http://evolve.elsevier.com/klieger/medicalassisting (**)

1. Perform Procedure 44-1: Administer Oral Medication.*

2. Perform Procedure 44-2: Apply a Transdermal Patch.*

3. Perform Procedure 44-3: Instruct the Patient in Administering Medication Using a Metered-Dose Inhaler with the Closed Mouth Technique.*

4. Perform Procedure 44-4: Reconstitute a Powdered Drug.*

5. Perform Procedure 44-5: Prepare a Parenteral Medication from a Vial.*

6. Perform Procedure 44-6: Prepare a Parenteral Medication from an Ampule.*

7. Perform Procedure 44-7: Administer an Intradermal Injection.*

8. Perform Procedure 44-8: Administer a Subcutaneous Injection.*

9. Perform Procedure 44-9: Administer an Intramuscular Injection to a Pediatric Patient.*

10. Perform Procedure 44-10: Administer an Intramuscular Injection to an Adult.*

11. Perform Procedure 44-11: Administer an Intramuscular Injection Using the Z-Track Technique.*

CHAPTER QUIZ

Multiple Choice

Identify the letter of the choice that best completes the statement or answers the question.

1. The _____-mL syringe is the syringe most often used.
   A. 0.5
   B. 1
   C. 3
   D. 5

Copyright © 2010, 2005 by Saunders, an imprint of Elsevier, Inc. All rights reserved.

2. When administering an intradermal, the angle of insertion should be _____ degrees.
   A. 10 to 15
   B. 20
   C. 45
   D. 90

3. A(n) _____ injection is given in the fatty layer beneath the dermis.
   A. deltoid
   B. intradermal
   C. intramuscular
   D. subcutaneous

4. A mid-deltoid injection should be given in the upper outer quadrant of the hip.
   A. True
   B. False

5. The most common area to give an IM injection is _____.
   A. deltoid
   B. vastus lateralis
   C. gluteus muscles
   D. all of the above

6. The goal of IV fluid administration is to correct or replace fluid volume and restore electrolyte balance.
   A. True
   B. False

7. A dorsogluteal injection should be administered at a _____ degree angle.
   A. 10- to 15-
   B. 20- to 30-
   C. 45-
   D. 90-

8. The most frequently used route of medication administration is _____.
   A. oral
   B. parenteral
   C. injection
   D. topical

9. Administration of IV fluids allows for rapid absorption.
   A. True
   B. False

10. _____ are administered to replace electrolytes in severe cases of diarrhea and vomiting.
    A. Hydrating fluids
    B. Isotonic solutions
    C. Maintenance solutions
    D. Hypertonic solutions

11. _____ is an injection site used from infancy to adulthood because it lacks major nerves and blood vessels.
    A. Deltoid
    B. Forearm
    C. Vastus lateralis
    D. Ventrogluteal

12. _____ is a liquid preparation in a water base that is applied to the skin.
    A. Cream
    B. Lotion
    C. Ointment
    D. All of the above

13. _____ is a hand-held device that dispenses medication into the airway.
    A. Nebulizer
    B. Metered-dose inhaler
    C. Prefilled cartridge unit
    D. Spacer

14. Another name for the Mantoux test is the tuberculin test.
    A. True
    B. False

15. A(n) _____ gauge needle is used to administer a subcutaneous injection.
    A. 18- to 21-
    B. 21- to 23-
    C. 23- to 25-
    D. 25- to 28-

16. Oral medication action usually takes _____ minutes.
    A. 10 to 15
    B. 20 to 30
    C. 30 to 60
    D. 40 to 60

17. When pouring liquid medications, you should _____.
    A. read the highest curvature of the liquid
    B. pour medication at eye level
    C. pour it on a level surface
    D. none of the above

18. Topical medication drug actions usually occur within _____.
    A. 10 minutes
    B. 20 minutes
    C. 30 minutes
    D. 1 hour

19. Rectal medications may be used because they cause less gastrointestinal upset.
    A. True
    B. False

20. The medical assistant should check the medication against the physician's order _____.
    A. once
    B. twice
    C. three times
    D. four times

Copyright © 2010, 2005 by Saunders, an imprint of Elsevier, Inc. All rights reserved.

45 Minor Office Surgery

VOCABULARY REVIEW

Matching: Match each term with the correct definition.

A. ambulatory surgery setting

B. approximate

C. box lock

D. cicatrix

E. closed wound

F. curette

G. debridement

H. dilating

I. dissecting

J. exudates

K. general anesthetic

L. hemostatic forceps

M. jaws

N. ligate

O. open technique

P. pick-ups

Q. purulent

R. retracting

S. sanguineous

T. serous

_____ 1. Wound drainage that consists of serum or clear fluid

_____ 2. Instrument with serrated tips, ratchets, and a box lock used to clamp off blood vessels or to grasp materials

_____ 3. Area where an instrument is hinged

_____ 4. Sterile technique; used to prevent the spread of microorganisms when skin or mucous membranes have been broken

_____ 5. Long-handled instrument with a metal loop on one end that is used to scrape inside a cavity

_____ 6. Wound drainage that consists of pus

_____ 7. Break in the skin or soft tissue

_____ 8. Wound drainage such as oozing pus or serum

_____ 9. Application of only sterile gloves for performing a sterile procedure

_____ 10. Sterile material, such as gauze, used to cover a wound

_____ 11. Making wider or larger, as in a dilating instrument used to increase the diameter of an opening

_____ 12. Holding part of a clamp

_____ 13. Special handwashing technique that decreases the total number of pathogens present; surgical scrub

_____ 14. Nonhospital setting where surgery is performed and the patient is not hospitalized

_____ 15. Pulling back tissue, as in a retracting instrument used to hold tissue away from a surgical area

_____ 16. Scar tissue

U. skin lesion removal

V. sterile dressing

W. surgical asepsis

X. surgical handwashing

Y. towel clamps

Z. wound

_____ 17. Common name for thumb forceps; also used by some physicians as another name for transfer forceps or sponge forceps

_____ 18. Removal of warts or other skin lesions through the use of a freezing agent or surgery

_____ 19. Instrument with sharp points used to hold the edges of a sterile towel together, usually to form a drape

_____ 20. To bring together skin edges

_____ 21. Removal of foreign or dead material from a wound

_____ 22. To tie off

_____ 23. Wound drainage that consists of blood

_____ 24. Tissues that are injured, such as a bruise, but the skin is not broken

_____ 25. Medication that produces unconsciousness by depressing the central nervous system

_____ 26. Cutting apart or separating tissue, as in dissecting instrument used to cut between tissue

THEORY RECALL

True/False

Indicate whether the sentence or statement is true or false.

_____ 1. Catgut sutures are used in areas that heal slower, and when absorption of suture material needs to stay in place longer.

_____ 2. When sterile dressing is applied to a wound, sterile technique must be used.

_____ 3. Surgical asepsis is the highest level of protection for patients.

_____ 4. The medical assistant should always wash a wound from the center outward.

_____ 5. Local anesthesia produces unconsciousness by depressing the central nervous system.

Multiple Choice

Identify the letter of the choice that best completes the statement or answers the question.

1. Scalpel blades range in size from _____.
   A. 5 to 10
   B. 10 to 15
   C. 5 to 25
   D. 10 to 30

2. _____ scalpels are used for growth removal.
   A. Concave
   B. Convex
   C. Straight
   D. Pointed

3. _____ is a break in the soft tissue of the body that does not extend beyond the subcutaneous tissue.
   A. Closed wound
   B. Open wound
   C. Deep wound
   D. Superficial wound

4. When charting the condition of a wound, the _____ must be charted in the patient's chart.
   A. amount of drainage
   B. appearance of drainage
   C. consistency of drainage
   D. all of the above

5. _____ have blunt ends with serrated tips used for removing or applying dressing materials.
   A. Dressing forceps
   B. Sponge forceps
   C. Tissue forceps
   D. Towel clamps

6. Scar tissue is made up of all of the following *except* _____.
   A. connective tissue
   B. epithelial cells
   C. muscle tissue
   D. fibrous tissue

7. Before surgery, a patient must have _____.
   A. a second opinion
   B. given informed consent
   C. received a reimbursement check from the insurance company
   D. completed a living will

8. _____ have a sharp, pointed, slender tip and a spring mechanism used to grasp fine objects or particles.
   A. Hemostats
   B. Splinter forceps
   C. Thumb forceps
   D. Towel clamps

9. Scalpels and curettes are examples of _____ instruments.
   A. cutting
   B. dilating
   C. probing
   D. retracting

10. _____ drainage consists of blood from broken capillaries.
    A. Serous
    B. Sanguineous
    C. Serosanguineous
    D. Purulent

11. Patients who have had minor surgery usually return to the physician's office in approximately _____ to have their dressing changed.
    A. 2 to 4 days
    B. 6 to 8 days
    C. 5 to 10 days
    D. 2 weeks

12. Sebaceous cysts commonly occur on all of the following *except* the _____.
    A. back
    B. ears
    C. face
    D. feet

13. _____ anesthesia is accomplished when an anesthetic is injected into and around a set of nerves.
    A. Local
    B. Topical
    C. Regional
    D. General

14. A(n) _____ for gloving ensures that the nonsterile hands never touch the outside of the gown or glove.
    A. closed technique
    B. open technique
    C. lateral technique
    D. all of the above

15. _____ have thick blades with a fine cutting edge used to dissect and cut muscle tissue.
    A. Dissecting scissors
    B. Operating scissors
    C. Suture scissors
    D. Littauer scissors

Sentence Completion

Complete each sentence or statement.

curette	serous	surgical scrub
forceps	closed wound	surgical asepsis
scissors	thumb forceps	purulent
tissue forceps	sanguineous	retractor
laceration repair	anesthesia	

CHAPTER 45 Minor Office Surgery

1. _____ is used when the skin surface is broken.

2. _____ are two-pronged instruments for grasping or holding body tissue.

3. _____ is the lack of feeling or absence of normal feeling caused by a substance, hypnosis, or traumatic injury.

4. _____ have serrated tips and a spring mechanism used to pick up or hold tissue.

5. _____ is a surgical procedure that cleans and debrides a wound with a suture closure.

6. A(n) _____ wound does not show a break in the skin.

7. _____ drainage consists of pus.

8. _____ are instruments used to hold back the edges of a wound.

9. _____ is a long-handled instrument with a metal loop on one end.

10. The _____ removes dead skin, oils, dirt, and pathogenic microorganisms.

Short Answers

1. List five guidelines that medical assistants should follow when handling and maintaining instruments.

   _____
   _____
   _____
   _____
   _____

2. List the three classifications of wound healing.

   _____
   _____
   _____
   _____

3. Explain the four factors that help in the healing process.

CRITICAL THINKING

1. Dr. Taylor has three minor office surgeries scheduled back-to-back today. He has asked for you to assist him in each procedure. Describe the general procedure guidelines that you will use for each procedure.

PRACTICAL APPLICATIONS

If you have accomplished the objectives in this chapter, you will be able to make better choices as a medical assistant. Take a look at this situation and decide what you would do.

Shirley, a patient of Dr. Jones, has arrived at the office for removal of a cyst on her face that has been present for about 2 months. Anna is the medical assistant at the front desk, and Lori is the clinical medical assistant for Dr. Jones. Shirley has been asked to cleanse the area around the lesion with an antiseptic wash for the past 2 days. Shirley wants to know exactly what will be done and if she has to sign papers. Anna tells her that these papers can be signed at any time before the actual opening of the wound. Anna also tells Shirley that Lori will explain what will be done after Shirley is taken to the room where minor surgery is done.

As Lori sets up the surgical tray, she uses surgical asepsis. She uses a sterile tray and peel-back wrappers to set up the needed instruments. On the tray are a scalpel, several hemostat forceps, a probe, a needle holder, scissors, and two retractors.

After the surgery, Lori is in a hurry and piles the instruments in the basin before sanitizing them. When she documents the procedure for Dr. Jones, she documents only the date and the type of surgery.

Would you be prepared to step into Anna's or Lori's shoes and perform the needed tasks correctly?

1. What questions should Anna ask Shirley as she arrives at the office for the surgery?

2. Because Shirley is to receive a tranquilizer intravenously, what preparation should have been made for Shirley's safe return home?

3. Can Shirley wait to sign informed consent until after the incision has been made? Explain your answer.

4. Explain what role Lori can take in obtaining informed consent.

5. What is surgical asepsis? How does it differ from medical asepsis?

6. What is the difference between a sterile tray and peel-wrapped instruments? What is the indication of the use of each of these?

7. Explain the use of a scalpel, forceps, probe, needle holder, and retractors.

8. What did Lori miss in the correct documentation of the surgical procedure?

9. How did Lori mishandle the instruments after the procedure?

10. What instructions would you expect Lori to give to Shirley after the surgical procedure?

11. How would the lack of correct documentation affect the coding of this surgical procedure for insurance reimbursement?

Copyright © 2010, 2005 by Saunders, an imprint of Elsevier, Inc. All rights reserved.

APPLICATION OF SKILLS

Procedure Check-off Sheets (*) and assignments from MACC on the Evolve site at http://evolve.elsevier.com/klieger/medicalassisting (**)

1. Perform Procedure 45-1: Perform Handwashing for Surgical Asepsis.*

2. Perform Procedure 45-2: Apply a Sterile Gown and Gloves.*

3. Perform Procedure 45-3: Apply Sterile Gloves.*

4. Perform Procedure 45-4: Remove Contaminated Gloves.*

5. Perform Procedure 45-5: Open a Sterile Package.*

6. Perform Procedure 45-6: Pour a Sterile Solution.*

7. Perform Procedure 45-7: Assist with Minor Office Surgery.*

8. Perform Procedure 45-8: Remove Sutures or Staples and Change a Wound Dressing Using a Spiral Bandage.*

9. Perform Procedure 45-9: Apply and Remove Adhesive Skin Closures.*

CHAPTER QUIZ

Multiple Choice

Identify the letter of the choice that best completes the statement or answers the question.

1. Scissors, biopsy punches, and curettes are _____ instruments.
   A. clamping
   B. dissecting
   C. probing
   D. retracting

2. Scalpel blades range in size from _____.
   A. 5 to 10
   B. 10 to 15
   C. 10 to 25
   D. 10 to 35

3. _____ are two-pronged instruments used for grasping or holding body tissue.
   A. Forceps
   B. Curettes
   C. Retractors
   D. Scissors

4. _____ have delicate, straight blades for cutting through tissue.
   A. Bandage scissors
   B. Dissecting scissors
   C. Operating scissors
   D. Suture scissors

5. A _____ does not show a break in the skin.
   A. closed wound
   B. open wound
   C. deep wound
   D. superficial wound

6. Local anesthetics produce unconsciousness.
   A. True
   B. False

7. _____ occurs when a large wound is not closely approximated and may heal from the base of the wound upward.
   A. Primary intention healing
   B. Secondary intention healing
   C. Tertiary intention healing
   D. None of the above

8. A _____ scalpel blade is used for incision and drainage.
   A. concave
   B. convex
   C. curved
   D. pointed

9. Probes are instruments used to feel inside a body cavity.
   A. True
   B. False

10. _____ drainage consists of serum.
    A. Purulent
    B. Sanguineous
    C. Serous
    D. Serosanguineous

11. Patients must return to the physician's office in approximately _____ days for a dressing change.
    A. 1 to 3
    B. 3 to 5
    C. 5 to 10
    D. 10 to 14

12. _____ is accomplished when a local anesthetic is injected into and around a set of nerves.
    A. Topical anesthesia
    B. Regional anesthesia
    C. General anesthesia
    D. Local anesthesia

Copyright © 2010, 2005 by Saunders, an imprint of Elsevier, Inc. All rights reserved.

13. _____ is a wound that does not extend beyond the subcutaneous layer.
    A. Open
    B. Superficial
    C. Closed
    D. Deep wound

14. The surgical scrub removes dead skin, dirt, and pathogenic microorganisms.
    A. True
    B. False

15. _____ may be used to close wounds.
    A. Band-Aids
    B. Staples
    C. Superglue
    D. All of the above

16. _____ are instruments with serrated rings at the tips used to hold gauze sponges.
    A. Hemostats
    B. Thumb forceps
    C. Sponge forceps
    D. Dressing forceps

17. _____ is used when nonsterile hands never touch the outside of the gown or glove.
    A. Aseptic technique
    B. Closed technique
    C. Open technique
    D. Sterile technique

18. _____ have a sharp, pointed, slender tip used to grasp fine objects.
    A. Hemostats
    B. Thumb forceps
    C. Splinter forceps
    D. Sponge forceps

19. Curettes are instruments used to hold back the edges of a wound.
    A. True
    B. False

20. Surgical asepsis is the highest level of protection for patients.
    A. True
    B. False

46 Basic First Aid and Medical Office Emergencies

VOCABULARY REVIEW

Matching: Match each term with the correct definition.

A. anaphylactic shock

B. automated external defibrillator

C. burn

D. cardiac arrest

E. cerebrovascular accident

F. defibrillation

G. direct pressure

H. epistaxis

I. fracture

J. full-thickness burn

K. Heimlich maneuver

L. hemorrhagic shock

M. hypothermia

N. insulin shock

O. Kussmaul breathing

P. metabolic shock

Q. neurogenic shock

R. "Rule of nines"

S. seizure

T. splint

_____ 1. Severe infection with toxins that prevent blood vessels from constricting, causing blood to pool away from vital organs

_____ 2. Sudden cessation of breathing and heart activity

_____ 3. Not responding to stimuli

_____ 4. Break or crack in a bone caused by trauma or disease

_____ 5. Breathing pattern that begins with very deep, gasping respirations that become rapid and are associated with severe diabetic acidosis and coma

_____ 6. Cerebrovascular accident; condition caused by narrowing cerebral vessels; hemorrhage into the brain; and formation of an embolus or thrombus resulting in a lack of blood supply to the brain

_____ 7. Form of hyperthermia caused by dehydration causing a loss of consciousness

_____ 8. Chronic brain disorder in which an individual has seizures

_____ 9. Severe allergic reaction caused by hypersensitivity to a substance

_____ 10. Methods of evaluating a surface area of a burn; the surface is divided into regions with percentage assigned

_____ 11. Fainting

_____ 12. Firm material used to immobilize above and below a fracture to prevent further damage

_____ 13. Electrical shock to the heart to maintain heart rhythm

_____ 14. Shock caused by inadequate blood supply to tissues as a result of trauma, burns, or internal bleeding

_____ 15. Machine that analyzes a patient's cardiac rhythm and delivers an electrical shock if indicated

U. stroke

V. syncope

W. unconscious

X. septic shock

Y. heat stroke

Z. epilepsy

_____ 16. Loss of nerve control over the circulatory system causing decreased blood supply to an area

_____ 17. Burn that destroys the epidermis and dermis including the nerve endings; third-degree burn

_____ 18. Decreased body temperature

_____ 19. Injury or destruction of tissue caused by excessive physical heat, chemicals, electricity, or radiation

_____ 20. Sudden involuntary muscle activity leading to a change in level of consciousness and behavior

_____ 21. Lack of oxygen to the brain caused by narrowing or ruptured cerebral vessels

_____ 22. Abdominal thrust used in an emergency to dislodge the cause of a blockage

_____ 23. Nosebleed

_____ 24. Type of shock caused by excessive loss of body fluids and metabolites

_____ 25. Pressure applied directly over a wound

_____ 26. State that occurs when the body has too much insulin and not enough glucose to use the insulin; severe hypoglycemia

THEORY RECALL

True/False

Indicate whether the statement is true or false.

_____ 1. When a patient is having an epileptic seizure, it is important to place something between the patient's teeth.

_____ 2. Indirect pressure is applied over the wound.

_____ 3. Insulin shock occurs when a patient has taken too much insulin in relation to the amount of food eaten, causing the available glucose to be depleted.

_____ 4. Abdominal thrust is an emergency procedure used to dislodge the cause of a blockage.

_____ 5. All chemical burns should be washed with water immediately.

Multiple Choice

Identify the letter of the choice that best completes the statement or answers the question.

1. _____ occurs when the brain does not receive enough oxygen.
   A. Cerebrovascular accident
   B. Heart attack
   C. Shock
   D. Fainting

2. Epilepsy seizures can be brought on by _____.
   A. low blood sugar
   B. high fever
   C. head trauma
   D. all of the above

3. Arterial blood is _____ color.
   A. bright red
   B. dark red
   C. pale red
   D. none of the above

4. _____ occurs when the body is subjected to excessive heat.
   A. Heat exhaustion
   B. Heat stroke
   C. Sunstroke
   D. Hypothermia

5. _____ is a fracture of a bone that does not break but bends the bone.
   A. Compound
   B. Greenstick
   C. Simple
   D. Open

6. _____ can lead to ketoacidosis.
   A. Infection
   B. Glucose overload
   C. Common cold
   D. All of the above

7. To control bleeding or hemorrhage, you should initially _____.
   A. apply ice over the wound
   B. apply direct pressure
   C. apply a tourniquet above the injury
   D. immobilize the body part

8. When a patient feels lightheaded, the medical assistant needs to _____.
   A. stand the patient up
   B. have the patient lower head to knee level
   C. help patient to lithotomy position
   D. place a warm compress on the patient's forehead

Copyright © 2010, 2005 by Saunders, an imprint of Elsevier, Inc. All rights reserved.

9. _____ occurs when one end of a bone is separated from its original position in a joint.
   A. Dislocation
   B. Fracture
   C. Sprain
   D. Strain

10. A patient who is having a CVA complains of _____.
    A. lightheadedness
    B. warm tingly sensation
    C. sudden confusion
    D. difficulty concentrating

11. Epistaxis can be caused by _____.
    A. low altitude
    B. upper respiratory infection
    C. hypotension
    D. exercise

12. _____ is when the cardiac muscle can no longer pump blood throughout the body.
    A. Cardiogenic shock
    B. Hemorrhagic shock
    C. Insulin shock
    D. Septic shock

13. The body temperature of a person with heat exhaustion is _____.
    A. 100° F to 102° F
    B. 101° F to 102° F
    C. 102° F to 103° F
    D. 103° F to 104° F

14. With a sprain, the RICE treatment must begin within _____.
    A. 10 to 20 minutes
    B. 30 minutes
    C. 45 minutes
    D. 1 hour

15. Treatment for hypothermia requires the body part to be gradually warmed in water, which should not exceed _____.
    A. 99° F
    B. 100° F
    C. 105° F
    D. 108° F

Sentence Completion

Complete each sentence or statement.

bleeding	shock	burn
incident report	heat stroke	choking
first aid	splint	fainting, syncope
body mechanics	Kussmaul	
strain	CPR	

1. _____ is the temporary care given to an injured or ill person until the victim can be provided complete emergency treatment.

2. _____ is a temporary loss of consciousness caused by an inadequate blood supply to the brain.

3. _____ is a progressive circulatory collapse of the body brought on by insufficient blood flow to all parts of the body.

4. _____ is the loss of blood from a ruptured, punctured, or cut blood vessel.

5. _____ occurs when the body is subjected to high temperatures and humidity for a long time.

6. A(n) _____ immobilizes an affected body part and can be made from any available firm material.

7. Respirations that become very deep and gasping and then become rapid are known as _____ breathing.

8. _____ is an injury to or destruction of body tissue caused by excessive physical heat.

9. Using proper _____ is necessary when performing daily work activities and is essential when responding to any emergency situation.

10. A _____ describes any unusual occurrence that happens while a person is on the property of a health care facility.

Short Answers

1. Describe the symptoms of a heart attack.

   _____

   _____

   _____

2. List the four steps in wound care.

3. Explain what the acronym RICE stands for.

4. OSHA has developed many workplace standards that are directed at reducing injuries to employees. All safety programs are designed to prevent occurrences from happening. If you had to develop a safety plan for employees and patients, what would it be? (*Hint*: Review what you have learned from your initial school orientation [e.g., fire drill, tornado drill], facilities management, and laboratory safety. Read more at: www.osha.gov/Publications/osha3088.html.)
   a. personal

   b. environmental

   c. fire hazard/prevention

d. laboratory

CRITICAL THINKING

1. You and a friend are out on a lunchtime jog when she starts complaining of shortness of breath. You both write it off as being out of shape and continue. Back at the office, you notice your friend's lips are bluish in color, and her skin tone is gray. You ask her if she is feels okay. She states she is sweaty, and her chest feels a little heavy. What would you do next? Explain what the friend's statement tells you.

2. Use the following information to complete an incident report:
   Date: 9/21/20XX
   1:30 P.M.: You were in examination room #2 when you heard someone calling for help. On investigating you found Mrs. Jessie Cash, a patient of Dr. Morales, on the floor of the patient bathroom. She says that she felt a bit dizzy when she went to get up from the toilet and eased herself to the floor. Dr. Morales examines Mrs. Cash and does not observe any broken bones. Her blood pressure is 130/90 mm Hg, pulse is 90 beats/min, and respirations are 20. Dr. Morales requests that her blood glucose level be checked, and it is 100 mg/dL. She is helped to her feet and escorted to an examination room for further observation. After 30 minutes, her vital signs remain stable, and she states she is fine. She had come into the office today for a blood pressure check and a renewal of her allergy medication.
   Jessie Cash, Mrs.
   10290 Eagles Glen Ave.
   Anywhere, USA 56790
   908-765-3467
   DOB: 7/30/46

```
                        XYZ MEDICAL CENTER

    Date of Incidence: _____  Time: _____ AM/PM

    Location of Incident: _____

    Name of injured person: _____

    Address: _____
    _____

    Phone Number: _____

    Date of birth: _____  Male _____  Female _____

    Who was injured person? (circle one)   Patient   Visitor   Employer

    Description of incident: _____
    _____
    _____
    _____

    What was the nature of the injury to the person: _____
    _____

    Action taken: _____
    _____
    _____
    _____

    Injury requires hospital visit?   Yes: _____  No: _____

    Name of hospital: _____

    Address: _____

    Signature of injured party:
    _____ Date _____

    *No medical attention was desired and/or required.
    Signature of injured party:
    _____ Date _____

    Person reporting incident:
    _____ Date _____

    Signature: _____
```

3. Discuss what must be included in an emergency plan for a physician's office.

PRACTICAL APPLICATIONS

If you have accomplished the objectives in this chapter, you will be able to make better choices as a medical assistant. Take a look at this situation and decide what you would do.

Mariah has type 1 diabetes mellitus and takes insulin. Dr. Naguchi is aware that Mariah does not follow her diet as she should, and that her exercise habits are inconsistent, so her diabetes is often unstable.

Mariah lives in the southern United States, where it is currently 108° F outside and very humid. Earlier today, Mariah was in the garden gathering vegetables. Later she started canning the vegetables. Her house has minimal air-conditioning. In her haste to complete what needed to be done in the garden, Mariah did not eat her lunch as she should have, although she took her entire dose of insulin. During the afternoon Mariah began to feel weak, experiencing dizziness and sweating, and her skin felt cool and clammy. Don, her husband, drove her the three blocks to Dr. Naguchi's office because she started complaining of chest pain and difficulty breathing.

As soon as she arrives, Mariah appears to faint and falls, injuring her left ankle. As the medical assistant, Janis is the first health care professional to see what is happening to Mariah. After seeing Mariah, Dr. Naguchi orders an x-ray of her ankle to see whether she has a sprain, strain, or fracture.

If you were in Janis's place, would you know what to do in this situation?

1. What are the external factors that could have caused the symptoms that Mariah showed?

_____

_____

_____

_____

2. How should Janis handle this problem when several individuals are in the waiting room with Don and Mariah?

_____

_____

_____

_____

_____

_____

3. What questions should Janis immediately ask Don?

_____

_____

_____

_____

_____

_____

_____

Copyright © 2010, 2005 by Saunders, an imprint of Elsevier, Inc. All rights reserved.

CHAPTER 46 Basic First Aid and Medical Office Emergencies

4. What recent activities could have contributed to Mariah's problems?

5. If Mariah fainted and you were the medical assistant, what would you do for her immediately while someone was notifying the physician?

6. Knowing that Mariah has diabetes, what do you think might have happened, and what would you expect Dr. Naguchi to order for her?

7. Why would you be suspicious of hyperthermia? What should Janis do for these symptoms?

8. What symptoms does Mariah have that might indicate a heart attack?

9. How do a sprain, strain, and fracture differ, and how is each treated? What treatment is common to all three conditions?

APPLICATION OF SKILLS

For these assignments, complete on a separate piece of paper and turn in to your instructor for review.

1. You have been selected to be part of the crisis management team at your school. Your assignment is the following:
   a. List the expectations of the crisis management team in a disaster setting. For example, assign who will be "in charge." Who will be in charge of logistics?
   b. Develop tasks or competencies for the medical assistant related to the organization and management of disaster preparedness, response, and recovery.
   c. Create a list of community resources needed for an emergency situation, including names, telephone numbers, and contact persons.

2. Participate in a tabletop exercise as provided by your instructor.

CHAPTER QUIZ

Multiple Choice

Identify the letter of the choice that best completes the statement or answers the question.

1. _____ can lead to ketoacidosis.
   A. Infection
   B. Common cold
   C. Glucose overload
   D. All of the above

2. With vein damage, the color of the external bleeding is _____.
   A. bright red
   B. light red
   C. dark red
   D. pale red

3. _____ shock is when there is a loss of nerve control over the circulatory system, causing decreased blood supply to an area.
   A. Insulin
   B. Metabolic
   C. Neurogenic
   D. Psychogenic

4. Patients who are being seen for heat exhaustion will have a core temperature of _____.
   A. 99° F to 101° F
   B. 101° F to 102° F
   C. 102° F to 103° F
   D. 103° F to 104° F

5. A stroke is also called a _____.
   A. CVD
   B. CVA
   C. CHF
   D. CAD

6. A sprain is a full or partial tear of a ligament.
   A. True
   B. False

7. _____ is a form of hyperthermia marked with pale, cool, and clammy skin.
   A. Shock
   B. Heat exhaustion
   C. Heat stroke
   D. None of the above

8. _____ burn is a burn that destroys the epidermis and dermis, including the nerve endings.
   A. Full-thickness
   B. First-degree
   C. Second-degree
   D. Minor

9. Heimlich maneuver should be done only on conscious patients with an airway obstruction.
    A. True
    B. False

10. A child must be older than _____ years to feel for the carotid pulse as a part of CPR.
    A. 1
    B. 3
    C. 5
    D. 7

11. When one end of bone is separated from its original position in a joint, it is called a _____.
    A. dislocation
    B. fracture
    C. strain
    D. sprain

12. When warming an area that has frostbite, the warming solutions should be no warmer than _____.
    A. 105° F
    B. 120° F
    C. 125° F
    D. 130° F

13. A(n) _____ fracture pierces through the skin.
    A. closed
    B. open
    C. greenstick
    D. compound

14. Treatment for a sprain should begin within _____ minutes.
    A. 10 to 20
    B. 15 to 30
    C. 20 to 40
    D. 30 to 45

15. When a patient has an epileptic seizure, it is important to remember not to place anything between the patient's teeth because it could become an airway obstruction.
    A. True
    B. False

NAME: _____   DATE: _____

47 Beginning Your Job Search

VOCABULARY REVIEW

Matching: Match each term with the correct definition.

A. chronological resume

B. cover letter

C. employment agencies

D. functional resume

E. heading

F. job application

G. job interview

H. networking

I. objective

J. placement service

K. references

L. resume

_____ 1. Agencies that assist job seekers in finding employment

_____ 2. Type of resume that lists education and job experience from most recent to earliest

_____ 3. Document that provides an employer with the work history and personal information about a potential employee

_____ 4. Form that, when completed, provides information about the person applying for employment

_____ 5. Part of a resume that states the career goal(s) of the person looking for employment

_____ 6. Agencies that charge a fee to an individual for finding employment or to an employer for finding an employee

_____ 7. Verbal, face-to-face interaction that allows the employer to form an impression about the job applicant

_____ 8. Resume section that includes the demographics about the applicant

_____ 9. List of people who can vouch for the job seeker's characteristics and work habits; can be provided to a potential employer on request

_____ 10. Job tool that serves to introduce an applicant to the person in charge of screening resumes for employment opportunities

_____ 11. Interacting with people met through various professional, education, and social activities to assist in job search

_____ 12. Type of resume that relates the person's skills to the type of employment sought

THEORY RECALL

True/False

Indicate whether the statement is true or false.

_____ 1. The classifieds can list medical assistants only in the medical section of the "Help Wanted" section of the newspaper.

_____ 2. All schools have a placement service to help students find jobs.

_____ 3. Networking is only for professional office personnel.

_____ 4. Greet your interviewer with direct eye contact.

_____ 5. A resume needs to pique a potential employer's interest.

Multiple Choice

Identify the letter of the choice that best completes the statement or answers the question.

1. Answer all questions at an interview _____.
   A. honestly
   B. with what you think they want to hear
   C. with one-word answers
   D. none of the above

2. When writing your cover letter, it is okay to _____.
   A. rely on the computer to correct spelling
   B. not correct errors because the employer will not notice
   C. have two people proofread it
   D. ask the receptionist at the interview to proof it

3. The objective section of a resume should reflect _____.
   A. the demographic information of the applicant
   B. the career goal of the applicant
   C. the educational history of the applicant
   D. references available to the applicant

4. Ads describe _____ of the position.
   A. duties
   B. hours
   C. pay scale
   D. location

5. A medical assistant who practices patient-centered professionalism is _____.
   A. diligent
   B. responsible
   C. honest
   D. all of the above

Copyright © 2010, 2005 by Saunders, an imprint of Elsevier, Inc. All rights reserved.

6. The medical assistant should be _____ when an interview does not result in a job offer.
   A. disappointed
   B. angry
   C. encouraged to improve
   D. all of the above

7. A follow-up note/thank-you note should be sent to the interviewer after an interview _____.
   A. always
   B. only if you think it went well
   C. does not matter if you do or do not
   D. only when you think it went badly

8. The impression that will be remembered by the interviewer is _____.
   A. the first 10 seconds of the interview
   B. the follow-up
   C. when the applicant is leaving the interview
   D. the interaction during the interview

9. Your _____ is a major part of your overall image.
   A. communication style
   B. attire
   C. hairstyle
   D. none of the above

10. When interviewing over the telephone, make sure you have _____.
    A. a second person listening on another line
    B. a pen and paper
    C. soft music playing in the background
    D. used a cell phone so it cannot be traced

11. The medical assistant needs to revise his or her cover letter _____.
    A. once a year
    B. only when changing jobs
    C. for each job interview
    D. never if you have a well-written cover letter

12. A cover letter should be _____.
    A. accurate
    B. brief
    C. concise
    D. all of the above

13. When developing your resume, it is a good practice to _____.
    A. inform your reference names that you are interviewing, and that they may be called
    B. ask for permission to include a potential reference's name on your resume
    C. not include references on your resume; it is not required and you need to provide them only if you are hired
    D. all of the above are correct

14. A private employment agency _____.
    A. does not charge a placement fee
    B. charges only the client a placement fee
    C. charges only the employer a placement fee
    D. can charge the employer or the potential employee or both

15. Larger facilities list employment opportunities _____.
    A. with an employment agency only
    B. only in the newspaper
    C. on a telephone hotline
    D. only within the company

Sentence Completion

Complete each sentence or statement.

objective	references	do not
do	job interview	thank you note
job application	networking	cover letter
functional resume		

1. _____ is interacting with contacts or people you have met through various professional, educational, and social activities.

2. A(n) _____ accompanies a resume and basically introduces the medical assistant to the person in charge of screening job applicants.

3. _____ argue about salary when you think it is too low.

4. A(n) _____ should be a win-win situation for the employer and the applicant.

5. _____ is a type of resume that relates the person's skill to the type of employment sought.

6. _____ is(are) a list of people who can vouch for the job seeker's character and work habits.

7. _____ is a form that, when completed, provides information about the person applying for employment.

8. The _____ is the part of a resume that states the career goals of the person looking for employment.

Short Answers

1. List the five information sections of a resume.

2. List the four ways to contact an employer.

3. List the seven traits that a job interviewer will remember about an applicant.

CRITICAL THINKING

1. You are a newly graduated medical assistant and are very excited to be entering the medical workforce. After doing a job search on a medical website, you find the job of your dreams. You have a resume from last summer that is not updated to reflect your most recent accomplishments. Even so, you decide it is better to get your resume there quickly; instead of taking the time to rewrite it, you decide to fax it to the potential employer. Describe your thoughts on this approach and support your answer.

_____

_____

_____

_____

_____

_____

_____

PRACTICAL APPLICATIONS

If you have accomplished the objectives in this chapter, you will be able to make better choices as a medical assistant. Take a look at this situation and decide what you would do.

Dora has recently completed a medical assisting program and will be looking for new employment as a medical assistant in an ambulatory care setting. As she begins her search, she goes to the school placement office to see if the counselor knows of any jobs in the area. The counselor, Ms. Smith, states that she is unaware of any openings at present, but will keep Dora in mind should someone call.

Next, Dora turns to the newspaper ads. She writes her resume and cover letter quickly because she is excited about a position she saw advertised in the classifieds. She is typically good at writing, so she does not bother to ask a friend to proofread her resume and cover letter this time. (After all, it would only slow her down.) She is in such a hurry to apply for the job in the newspaper that she does not proofread or spell-check her materials. As a result, several words are misspelled, and the information that is supposed to be in chronological order is not.

Despite the errors on Dora's resume and cover letter, she obtains an interview with a potential employer. When she arrives, she is surprised that the employer expects her to complete an application before the interview. After completing the application, she answers the employer's interview questions and asks a few of her own. Overall, she has a good feeling about this interview.

After the interview, Dora returns home and waits to hear from the potential employer, taking no further action and hoping that she has been chosen for the job.

Do you think Dora would be hired for this job? What would you have done differently?

1. What are the advantages of using a newspaper ad?

_____

_____

_____

2. With whom would you network when seeking employment in your area?

3. If you were the employer, how would you feel about a resume that had misspelled words? Would you still consider hiring this person?

4. Who should proofread a resume? Why?

5. Why is the order of work experience on a resume important?

6. If an ad requests that an applicant apply "in person" and you send a fax or e-mail, do you think the employer would consider your application? Explain your answer.

7. Why is a cover letter so important?

8. Why do you think that an employer may ask applicants to complete an application at the interview? What do you need to do to make a good impression on the application?

9. Why is a thank-you letter after an interview important?

10. Do you think you would have been chosen for the job if you had made the aforementioned mistakes? Explain your answer.

APPLICATION OF SKILLS

1. Write a cover letter.

2. Write a resume.

3. Write a reference sheet.

4. Write a thank-you card.

CHAPTER QUIZ

Multiple Choice

Identify the letter of the choice that best completes the statement or answers the question.

1. A chronological resume is a type of resume that lists education and job experience from most recent to earliest.
    A. True
    B. False

2. _____ is a job tool introduces an applicant to the person in charge of screening resumes for employment opportunities.
    A. Cover letter
    B. Job application
    C. Resume
    D. Interview

3. _____ is a document given to the interviewer to provide him or her with an applicant's work history and personal information.
    A. Job application
    B. Cover letter
    C. Resume
    D. Reference sheet

4. An ad may describe the potential employee's _____, duties, and desired characteristics.
    A. hours
    B. qualifications
    C. pay scale
    D. location

5. Public employment agencies _____.
    A. charge a fee to the applicant who is looking for a job
    B. charge a fee to the employer who is hiring
    C. offer free placement service
    D. none of the above

6. Networking is interacting with people you have met through various professional, educational, and social activities.
    A. True
    B. False

7. The cover letter should be _____.
    A. updated every year
    B. updated for each job applied for
    C. updated only when changing jobs
    D. it is not necessary to update

8. When a telephone interview is done, the applicant should _____.
   A. have music in the background
   B. use a cell phone only
   C. have a pen and paper available
   D. none of the above

9. Typical information asked on a job application might be _____.
   A. age of children
   B. Social Security number
   C. references
   D. next of kin

10. The applicant should answer questions _____.
    A. with what you think the employer wants to hear
    B. completely
    C. with one-word answers
    D. with excitement

11. The cover letter is what the employer most wants to read.
    A. True
    B. False

12. When using a person as a reference, the applicant should _____.
    A. ask permission before putting the person on the list
    B. tell the person you are using him or her
    C. there is no need to tell the person about it
    D. none of the above

13. When the applicant is not offered a job, he or she should _____.
    A. be angry
    B. learn from the experience
    C. be disappointed
    D. be happy

14. To send a follow-up note is strictly the applicant's decision.
    A. True
    B. False

15. When greeting your interviewer, the applicant should _____.
    A. have a firm handshake
    B. not look them in the eyes
    C. lead the conversation
    D. have dressed in flashy clothes

Copyright © 2010, 2005 by Saunders, an imprint of Elsevier, Inc. All rights reserved.

APPENDIX A

Supplemental Chapter Materials

APPENDIX A

Supplemental Chapter Materials

Student Name: _____ DATE: _____

PROCEDURE 2-1 CHECKLIST: BEING A PROFESSIONAL

TASK: Complete a self-survey checklist to increase your awareness of areas needing improvement before entering the job market.

CONDITIONS: Using the checklist as a tool, assess your professional characteristics, abilities, and image. Discuss expectations with your instructor.

EQUIPMENT AND SUPPLIES
- Checklist and pen or pencil

STANDARDS: Complete the procedure within _____ minutes and achieve a minimum score of _____%.

Time began _____   Time ended _____

Steps	Possible Points	Student	Instructor
Professional characteristics			
1. Dependability:			
a. I am punctual.	10		
b. I am efficient.	5		
c. I am reliable	10		
2. Loyalty:			
a. I turn in quality work.	10		
b. I complete work on time.	10		
c. I display consistent work habits.	10		
d. I accept decisions.	5		
e. I display ethical behavior.	15		
3. Positive Attitude:			
a. I am enthusiastic.	10		
b. I set goals.	10		
c. I seek out learning opportunities.	10		
d. I am a team player.	10		
e. I accept constructive criticism.	5		
f. I adapt to change.	5		
g. I complete assignments on time.	10		
4. Integrity:			
a. I am trustworthy.	15		
b. I keep information confidential.	10		
c. I make ethical decisions.	15		
5. Diplomacy:			
a. I use tact when dealing with classmates.	10		
b. I display courtesy and empathy when appropriate.	10		

Steps	Possible Points	Student	Instructor
6. Confidence: a. I display leadership.	10		
b. I make decisions based on consensus.	5		
c. I prioritize assignments.	5		
Professional abilities 7. Competence: a. I complete assignments on time.	10		
b. I request assistance when unfamiliar with assignment or instructions.	15		
8. Dexterity: a. I display quality manual skills.	10		
b. I am able to assist with lifting or positioning.	10		
9. Effective communication: a. I use correct grammar.	10		
b. I spell correctly.	10		
c. I have good penmanship.	5		
10. Nonverbal Communication: a. I smile when communicating with others.	10		
Professional image 11. Personal Hygiene: a. I bathe or shower, use deodorant, and brush my teeth every morning.	20		
12. Grooming: a. My hair is neat and off my face and collar. I don't use extreme hair colors or highlights or any ornaments or decorations in my hair.	10		
b. My fingernails are clean and short. I don't use colored nail polish or artificial nails.	10		
c. If I use makeup or wear perfume/after-shave, it is minimal.	10		
d. I wear minimal jewelry, no more than a wedding ring, a wristwatch, and a single pair of nondangling earrings. I do not have any visible body piercings except perhaps for earrings.	10		

Copyright © 2010, 2005 by Saunders, an imprint of Elsevier, Inc. All rights reserved.

Steps	Possible Points	Student	Instructor
13. Dress: a. I wear a uniform that is clean, pressed, in good condition, and that fits properly over appropriate undergarments.	20		
b. I wear clean stockings without holes or tears.	10		
c. I wear clean and polished closed-toe shoes (not Crocs) with clean laces.	10		
14. Professional Appearance: a. I don't chew gum.	10		
b. I don't smell like cigarette smoke.	10		
c. I don't slouch.	5		
d. If I have tattoos, they are hidden from view.	10		
Total Points Possible	430		

Comments: Total Points Earned _____

Divided by _____

Total Possible Points = _____% Score

Instructor's Signature _____

Copyright © 2010, 2005 by Saunders, an imprint of Elsevier, Inc. All rights reserved.

CONSENT FOR SURGERY

DATE:_____

TIME:_____

I authorize the performance of the following procedure(s)_____
_____on_____
To be performed by_____, MD.

The following have been explained to me by Dr._____

    1. Nature of the procedure:_____

    2. Reason(s) for procedure:_____

    3. Possible risks:_____

    4. Possible complications:_____

I understand that no warranty or guarantee of the effectiveness of the surgery can be made.

I have been informed of possible alternative treatments including_____
_____and of the likely consequences of receiving no treatment, and I freely consent to this procedure.

I hereby authorize the above named surgeon and his/her assistants to provide additional services including administering anesthesia and / or medications, performing needed diagnostic tests including but not limited to radiology, and any other additional services deemed necessary for my well-being. I consent to have removed tissue examined by a pathologist who may then dispose of the tissue as he/she sees fit.

Signed_____ Relationship to patient_____
        Patient / Parent / Guardian

Witness_____

Copyright © 2010, 2005 by Saunders, an imprint of Elsevier, Inc. All rights reserved.

**Patient Consent to the Use and Disclosure of Health Information
for Treatment, Payment, or Health Care Operations**

I understand that as part of my health care, the practice originates and maintains paper and/or electronic records describing my health history, symptoms, examination and test results, diagnoses, treatment, and any plans for future care or treatment. I understand that this information serves as:

- A basis for planning my care and treatment,
- A means of communication among professionals who contribute to my care,
- A source of information for applying my diagnosis and treatment information to my bill,
- A means by which a third-party payer can verify that services billed were actually provided,
- A tool for routine health care operations, such as assessing quality and reviewing the competence of staff.

I have been provided the opportunity to review the *"Notice of Patient Privacy Information Practices"* **that provides a more complete description of information uses and disclosures. I understand that I have the following rights:**

- The right to review the *"Notice"* prior to acknowledging this consent,
- The right to restrict or revoke the use or disclosure of my health information for other uses or purposes, and
- The right to request restrictions as to how my health information may be used or disclosed to carry out treatment, payment, or health care operations.

Restrictions:

I request the following restrictions to the use or disclosure of my health information:

_____
_____

May discuss treatment, payment, or health care operation with the following persons:

(Please check all that apply)   Spouse [ ]   Your Children [ ]   Relatives [ ]   Others [ ]   Parents [ ]

Please list the names and relationship, if you checked "Relatives" or "Others" above

_____
_____

Messages or Appointment Reminders: (Please check all that apply)

May we leave a message on your answering machine at home [ ] or at work [ ]. **Do not leave a message** [ ]
May we leave a message with someone at your **home** using the doctor's name or the practice name: Yes [ ]   No [ ]
May we leave a message with someone at your **work** using the doctor's name or the practice name: Yes [ ]   No [ ]
Messages will be of a nonsensitive nature, such as appointment reminders.

I understand that as part of treatment, payment, or health care operations, it may become necessary to disclose health information to another entity, i.e., referrals to other health care providers, labs, and/or other individuals or agencies as permitted or required by state or federal law.

I fully understand and accept the information provided by this consent.

_____   _____   _____
Signature   Print name of person signing   Date

*If other than patient is signing, are you the parent, legal guardian, custodian, or have Power of Attorney for this patient for treatment, payment, or health care operations? Yes [ ]   No [ ]

_____

FOR OFFICE USE ONLY
[ ] Patient refused to sign the consent form.
[ ] Restrictions were added by the patient (see restrictions listed above)
[ ] "Consent form" received and reviewed by _____ on (date) _____
[ ] "Consent form" placed in the patient's medical record on (date) _____

Copyright © 2010, 2005 by Saunders, an imprint of Elsevier, Inc. All rights reserved.

GENERAL MEDICAL HEALTH CARE

AUTHORIZATION FOR RELEASE OF MEDICAL INFORMATION

I, _____ ___/___/___ _____ hereby authorize
    Print Patient's Name   Date of Birth   Social Security Number

General Medical Health Care 1234 Riverview Road, Anytown, FL 33333

to release medical, including HIV Antibody Testing, Psychiatric/Psychological, Alcohol and/or Drug Abuse information records to:

To: _____

Address _____
    (Street)   (City)   (State)   (Zip)

For the purpose of: 1. Drs. appointment on: _____

                    2. Other: _____

                                Please Specify Reason for Disclosure

I understand that if I consent to the release of any of my medical records, the results of any HIV Antibody Testing, Psychiatric/Psychological, Alcohol and/or Drug Abuse information will be released.

I understand this consent may be cancelled upon written notice to the hospital, except that action by the hospital has been taken in reliance on this authorization, and that this authorization shall remain in force for a 90-day period in order to effect the purpose for which it is given. Alcohol and drug abuse information, if present, has been disclosed from records whose confidentiality is protected by Federal Law. FEDERAL REGULATIONS (42CFR, part II) prohibit making any further disclosure of records without the specific written authorization of the undersigned, or as otherwise permitted by such regulations. The confidentiality of HIV antibody test results is protected by Florida Law [Fla. Stat.ANN. 381.609 (2) (F)], which prohibits any further disclosure by a person to whom this information has been disclosed, without specific written consent of the undersigned or as otherwise permitted by state law.

_____   From: _____ To: _____
(Date of Authorization)   (Dates to be Released)

_____
Patient's Signature

_____
Parent, Legal Guardian, or Authorized Representative Signature

_____
Relationship to Patient

_____
Witness

Copyright © 2010, 2005 by Saunders, an imprint of Elsevier, Inc. All rights reserved.

Student Name: _____   DATE: _____

PROCEDURE 24-1 CHECKLIST: PREPARE, SEND, AND RECEIVE A FAX

TASK: Correctly prepare, send, and receive information by facsimile (fax), maintaining confidentiality.

CONDITIONS: Given the proper equipment and supplies, the student will be required to prepare, send, and receive a fax.

EQUIPMENT AND SUPPLIES
- Create a cover sheet
- Document to be faxed
- Document to be received
- Release of information
- Pen
- Telephone/fax machine
- Demographic information

STANDARDS: Complete the procedure within _____ minutes and achieve a minimum score of _____%.

Time began _____   Time ended _____

Steps	Possible Points	First Attempt	Second Attempt
1. Gather equipment and supplies	5		

2. Prepare a fax to send:
  a. Create a cover sheet:
    — create the name of the practice, address, and phone number
	10		

— format the cover letter to include all needed information and a disclaimer	5		
b. Obtain document to be faxed.	5		
c. Check file for release of information	5		
d. Obtain the demographic information for the intended recipient.	5		
e. Complete the cover sheet by filling in the required information.	10		
f. Prepare the document.	5		
3. Send a fax: a. Place the cover sheet and document in the fax machine as required by the manufacturer	10		
b. Dial the telephone fax number of the recipient.	10		
c. Press start.			

Steps	Possible Points	First Attempt	Second Attempt
d. When the document is completely through the machine, press the button if required or wait to receive a transmittal report.	10		
e. Remove the document from the machine and attach the transmittal report to the document.	5		
4. Receive a fax: a. Immediately remove the document from the machine.	5		
b. Determine the intended recipient or review for action.	5		
c. Deliver the document to the intended person, perform the action, or file the document.	5		
Total Points Possible	100		

Comments: Total Points Earned _____

Divided by _____

Total Possible Points = _____% Score

Instructor's Signature _____

Copyright © 2010, 2005 by Saunders, an imprint of Elsevier, Inc. All rights reserved.

Student Name: _____ DATE: _____

PROCEDURE 24-2: MAINTAIN OFFICE EQUIPMENT

TASK: Create an office document that identifies office equipment and allows for product information and maintenance data to be recorded.

CONDITIONS: Given the proper equipment and supplies, the student will be required to create an inventory and maintenance log for standard medical office equipment.

EQUIPMENT AND SUPPLIES
- List of office equipment, including all administrative and medical equipment, such as:

Computer(s)	Electrocardiograph machine
Telephone system	Glucometer
Transcription machine	Cholesterol machine
Fax machine	Electronic thermometer(s)
Photocopy machine	Sigmoidoscope
Postage meter with labels	Ultrasound equipment
Printer	X-ray equipment

- File folder(s)
- Postage scale
- Medical equipment and office supply catalogs (used to gather information)
- Computer spreadsheet and word processing software or inventory sheet provided by instructor for completion
- Pen or pencil

STANDARDS: Complete the procedure within _____ minutes and achieve a minimum score of _____%.

Time began _____   Time ended _____

Steps	Possible Points	First Attempt	Second Attempt
1. Create an equipment inventory form for administrative and clinical equipment used in the facility. (Use classroom equipment.) (Use provided Equipment Inventory form as a model.)	20		
2. Complete required information.	10		
3. Create a file folder for administrative equipment. Also, create one for clinical equipment, and insert any product information, maintenance or service agreements into the appropriate folder.	20		
4. Create and complete a maintenance log for each piece of equipment. Attach maintenance log on left inside cover of file folder. a. Use provided Equipment Maintenance Log form as a model. b. List the manufacturer, item description, date of purchase, purchase price, item location, identification number, and whether or not a service agreement is in place.	20		

Copyright © 2010, 2005 by Saunders, an imprint of Elsevier, Inc. All rights reserved.

Steps	Possible Points	First Attempt	Second Attempt
5. Physically inspect each piece of equipment listed on the Equipment Inventory. a. Ensure that each piece of equipment is in proper working order and is calibrated as mandated by the manufacturer. b. Look for frayed cords, broken parts, and improper functioning. Note in the last column the date and status of the equipment.	20		
Total Points Possible	90		

Comments: Total Points Earned _____

Divided by _____

Total Possible Points = _____ % Score

Instructor's Signature _____

Equipment Inventory—Sample   **Month:** October 2009

Manufacturer	Item Description	Date	Purchase Price	Location	Id #	Date Inspected and Status
Burdick	Atria 3100 Resting ECG	1/19/09	$3300.00	Ex Rm 3	213456UH	10/3—Needs calibration
Welch Allen	Spot Vital Sign	3/10/08	$2300.00	Tx Rm	2Z34C567	10/4—OK

Equipment Maintenance Log—Sample   **Month:** October 2009

Manufacturer	Item Description	Date	Purchase Price	Location	Id #	Service Agreement (Yes or No)	Date Last Serviced (Problem)
Burdick	Atria 3100 Resting ECG	1/19/09	$3300.00	Ex Rm 3	213456UH	Yes	10/07/09 (calibration)

Copyright © 2010, 2005 by Saunders, an imprint of Elsevier, Inc. All rights reserved.

Student Name: _____   DATE: _____

PROCEDURE 24-3 CHECKLIST: INVENTORY CONTROL: ORDERING AND RESTOCKING SUPPLIES

TASK: Create an inventory system for expendable supplies used in the physician's office or clinic.

CONDITIONS: Given the proper equipment and supplies, role-play with a student or instructor the proper method of performing inventory control and ordering supplies.

EQUIPMENT AND SUPPLIES
- MACC/computer
- Supply list
- File box
- Supply inventory order cards—3 × 5 or 5 × 7 index cards
- Blank file box divider cards
- Pen or pencil

STANDARDS: Complete the procedure within _____ minutes and achieve a minimum score of _____%.

Time began _____   Time ended _____

Steps	Possible Points	First Attempt	Second Attempt
1. Create a list of all disposable supplies used in the facility. (Use provided Inventory Supply List form as a model.)	10		
a. Separate list into administrative and clinical supplies.	10		
b. Identify the vendor for each item.	10		
2. Create a divider card for each vendor.	5		
3. File the completed vendor divider cards.	5		
4. Create an inventory card for each disposable supply item on the supply list.	10		
5. Enter the unit price.	5		
6. Establish the reorder point.	5		
7. Inventory all items on the inventory list.	10		
8. Write the current number on hand next to the item on the supply list.	10		
9. Compare the quantity on hand with the reorder point on the inventory control card.	10		
10. Locate the inventory control card for each item that is highlighted.	5		
11. Order supplies. a. When an order has been placed, indicate the date ordered on the inventory card, amount ordered, and unit price.	5		

Copyright © 2010, 2005 by Saunders, an imprint of Elsevier, Inc. All rights reserved.

Steps	Possible Points	First Attempt	Second Attempt
12. When order is received, indicate the date and quantity received.	5		
13. Re-file the cards when the complete order has been received and the information is recorded.	5		
14. Restock the items. a. Place new items on the shelf behind the currently stocked supplies.	5		
Total Points Possible	115		

Comments: Total Points Earned _____

Divided by _____

Total Possible Points = _____% Score

Instructor's Signature _____

Inventory Supply List—Sample   Date:

Vendor	Item	On Hand	Unit Price	Reorder Point	ID #	Amount to Reorder
XYZ SUPPLY	Hand sanitizer 1200 mL		6.99 each	2	03-45-611	6
MED SUPPLY	Antimicrobial soap gallon		14.50 each	1	04-72-807	3

Copyright © 2010, 2005 by Saunders, an imprint of Elsevier, Inc. All rights reserved.

Student Name: _____   DATE: _____

PROCEDURE 24-4 CHECKLIST: DEVELOP AND MAINTAIN A CURRENT LIST OF COMMUNITY RESOURCES

TASK: Gather information from your local phone book, library, and newspaper or search the Internet, and create a reference document/brochure to increase a medical practice's visibility in the community and provide information to patients.

CONDITIONS: Given the proper equipment and supplies, the student will be required to gather community marketing information within his or her community and create a marketing tool/brochure to increase a medical practice's visibility in the community and provide information to patients.

EQUIPMENT AND SUPPLIES
- Local telephone book
- Local/state newspaper
- Internet access
- Computer spreadsheet and word processing software
- Pen or pencil

STANDARDS: Complete the procedure within _____ minutes and achieve a minimum score of _____%.

Time began _____   Time ended _____

Steps	Possible Points	First Attempt	Second Attempt
1. Research the resources available in your area using the local phone book, local/state newspaper, local library, or Internet. A minimum of five resources must be contacted. Also include three resources for emergency preparedness. (Use provided Sample as a model.) Total: eight resources	40		
2. Create a list for each resource available that includes agency name, a telephone number, address, contact person, hours of operation, and what types of services each agency provides.	10		

PROCEDURE 24-4

Steps	Possible Points	First Attempt	Second Attempt
3. Key the information gathered into a document using a word processing software program or a spreadsheet software program. Double-check your information for accuracy. Print a hard copy, and save an electronic file on the computer.	15		
Total Points Possible	65		

Comments: Total Points Earned _____

Divided by _____

Total Possible Points = _____% Score

Instructor's Signature _____

Agency Resource List

Agency (Hours)	Address	Phone/Contact	Notes
Hospice patient care program (24 hours/day 7 days/week)	6798 Crosswinds Upton GA 33746	777-867-9860/Mary Clark	Support services to terminally ill patients
CASA (24 hours/day 7 days/week)	1011 1st Ave Artview GA 33745	777-464-6765/crisis line	24-hour crisis for domestic violence

PURCHASE ORDER

No._____

Bill to:

XYZ Medical Center
901 South Street
Anytown, USA 33322

Ship to:

XYZ Medical Center
901 South Street
Anytown, USA 33322

Vendor: _____
_____
_____

Terms: _____

ORDER #	DESCRIPTION	QTY.	COLOR	SIZE	UNIT PRICE	TOTAL PRICE
					SUBTOTAL	
					TAX	
					SHIPPING	
					TOTAL	

(Modified from Hunt SA: *Fundamentals of medical assisting student mastery manual,* Philadelphia, 2002, Saunders.)

Copyright © 2010, 2005 by Saunders, an imprint of Elsevier, Inc. All rights reserved.

PURCHASE ORDER No._____

Bill to:

XYZ Medical Center
901 South Street
Anytown, USA 33322

Ship to:

XYZ Medical Center
901 South Street
Anytown, USA 33322

Vendor: _____
_____
_____

Terms: _____

ORDER #	DESCRIPTION	QTY.	COLOR	SIZE	UNIT PRICE	TOTAL PRICE
					SUBTOTAL	
					TAX	
					SHIPPING	
					TOTAL	

(Modified from Hunt SA: *Fundamentals of medical assisting student mastery manual,* Philadelphia, 2002, Saunders.)

Student Name: _____ DATE: _____

PROCEDURE 26-1 CHECKLIST: GIVE VERBAL INSTRUCTIONS ON HOW TO LOCATE THE MEDICAL OFFICE

TASK: Provide verbal instructions to a caller on how to locate the medical office using role-play.

CONDITIONS: Given the proper equipment and supplies, the student will be required to give verbal instructions to a patient on how to locate the medical office. (Instructor will provide address for medical office and patient address. For example, the school's address can be used for the medical office, and the student's home address can be used for the patient's address.)

EQUIPMENT AND SUPPLIES
- Telephone or telephone training system
- City map
- Pen or pencil
- Telephone/fax machine

STANDARDS: Complete the procedure within _____ minutes and achieve a minimum score of _____%.

Time began _____   Time ended _____

Steps	Possible Points	First Attempt	Second Attempt
1. Gather equipment and supplies.	5		
2. Address the patient or caller in a polite and professional manner.	20		
3. Determine the place of origin for the patient.	10		
4. Determine the most direct route to the medical office, with alternate routes if possible. Provide the caller with major cross streets or landmarks.	25		
5. Allow the caller sufficient time to write the directions.	10		
6. Provide the caller with the office's telephone number.	10		
7. Ask the caller if he or she has any questions.	10		
8. Politely end the call after answering any questions.	10		
Total Points Possible	100		

Comments: Total Points Earned _____

Divided by _____

Total Possible Points = _____% Score

Instructor's Signature _____

Student Name: _____ DATE: _____

PROCEDURE 26-2 CHECKLIST: CREATE A MEDICAL PRACTICE INFORMATION BROCHURE

TASK: Create a patient information booklet for a "mock" medical practice that explains general office policies.

CONDITIONS: Given the proper equipment and supplies, the student will be required to create an informational brochure for his or her "mock" practice.

EQUIPMENT AND SUPPLIES
- Computer
- Software program that allows for brochure layouts
- Examples of local medical practice brochures and local medical office policies
- Pen or pencil

STANDARDS: Complete the procedure within _____ minutes and achieve a minimum score of _____ %.

Time began _____   Time ended _____

Steps	Possible Points	First Attempt	Second Attempt
1. Write and key a short paragraph describing each of the following topics and other information as needed. a. Description of the practice	10		
b. Physical location of facility	10		
c. Parking options	10		
d. Telephone numbers, e-mail addresses, and web pages	10		
e. Office hours	10		
f. Names and credentials of staff members	10		
g. Types of services	10		
h. Appointment scheduling and cancellation policies	10		
i. Payment options	10		
j. Prescription refill policy	10		
k. Types of accepted insurance	10		
l. Referral policy	10		
m. Release or records policy	10		
n. Emergency protocols	10		
o. Name of contact person in the event the physician is unavailable	10		
p. Frequently asked questions	10		
q. Any special considerations	10		

Copyright © 2010, 2005 by Saunders, an imprint of Elsevier, Inc. All rights reserved.

Steps	Possible Points	First Attempt	Second Attempt
2. Proofread keyed paragraphs.	15		
3. Determine the layout of the brochure to provide ready access of information to patient. Including the following considerations: a. Visually pleasing	5		
b. Placement of logo	5		
c. Name, address, and telephone number of practice prominently placed	5		
4. Print the final version of the brochure. Submit to instructor for approval.	5		
5. Using your brochure as a source reference, explain the general office policies to your patient (instructor).	25		
Total Points Possible	230		

Comments: Total Points Earned _____

Divided by _____

Total Possible Points = _____% Score

Instructor's Signature _____

Student Name: _____   DATE: _____

PROCEDURE 26-3 CHECKLIST: ANSWER A MULTILINE TELEPHONE SYSTEM

TASK: Answer a multiline telephone system in a professional manner, by responding to a request for action, placing a call on hold, transferring a call to another party, and accurately recording a message for action by another staff member or in a patient's medical record; either role-play or actual procedure.

CONDITIONS: Given the proper equipment and supplies, role-play with a student or instructor how to respond to a telephone request for action, place a call on hold, transfer a call to another party, and accurately record a message for action by another staff member or in a patient's medical record.

EQUIPMENT AND SUPPLIES
- MACC/computer (Practice)
- Telephone
- Appointment book
- Message form/pad
- Telephone triage reference guide (use Table 26-1)
- Physician referral sheet
- Pen or pencil
- Headset (optional)
- Information sheet

STANDARDS: Complete the procedure within _____ minutes and achieve a minimum score of _____%.

Time began _____   Time ended _____

Steps	Possible Points	First Attempt	Second Attempt
1. Answer the telephone by third ring using good telephone techniques: a. Pleasant tone b. Moderate rate c. Sufficient volume	20		
2. Greet with: a. Appropriate time of day b. Identify the office and yourself c. Verify the identity of the caller d. Request the caller's telephone number	20		
3. Provide the caller with the requested information or service, if possible (i.e., appointment; referral). Your instructor will provide the situation.	10		
4. If you are unable to assist the caller, transfer the caller to the person who can assist him or her, using office protocol. Ask permission to put the caller on hold, and wait for an affirmative response. Transfer the call according to the telephone system in use. If the caller does not want to hold, take a message.	20		

Copyright © 2010, 2005 by Saunders, an imprint of Elsevier, Inc. All rights reserved.

Steps	Possible Points	First Attempt	Second Attempt
5. If multiple lines are ringing, use correct techniques for two ringing lines. a. Answer the first line and ask permission to place the first caller on hold. b. Answer the second line and ask permission to place this caller on hold. c. Return to the first line and provide the requested information, service, or action (take a message). d. Return to the second line and thank the caller for holding. Provide the caller with the requested information, service, or action.	20		
6. Take a message by collecting required information for return of the call. Confirm the information with the caller and, if possible, provide an expected call back time.	30		
7. End the call in an appropriate manner, and forward the message on to the physician.	10		
Total Points Possible	130		

Comments: Total Points Earned _____

Divided by _____

Total Possible Points = _____% Score

Instructor's Signature _____

Information for Procedure 26-3

Patient Cathy Chaps called at 8:30 a.m. to report that she has been feeling poorly the last couple of days and wants to see Dr. Chase today. She describes her condition as being feverish, severe headache, and chest congestion. She has no known allergies to medication. You inform her that there are not any openings today, but she could be seen tomorrow at 1:00 p.m. Ms. Chaps requests that Dr. Chase return her call at 777-125-5412. You confirm her pharmacy's name and phone number, and tell her you will give the message to Dr. Chase.

Pharmacy: MedRite 272-4132

Use today's date and your initials

MESSAGE FROM										
For Dr.	Name of Caller		Rel. to pt.	Patient		Pt. Age	Pt. Temp.	Message Date	Message Time PM	Urgent ☐YES ☐NO
Message:								Allergies		
Respond to Phone #				Best Time To Call AM PM	Pharmacy Name/#		Patient's Chart Attached ☐YES ☐NO	Patient's Chart #		Initials
DOCTOR–STAFF RESPONSE										
Doctor's/Staff Orders/Follow-up Action										
				Call Back ☐YES ☐NO		Chart Mes. ☐YES ☐NO	Follow-up Date	Follow-up Completed–Date/Time PM		Response By:

(From Potter BA: *Instructor's manual and curriculum guide for medical office administration,* Philadelphia, 2003, Saunders.)

Student Name: _____ DATE: _____

PROCEDURE 26-4 CHECKLIST: PREPARE AND MAINTAIN AN APPOINTMENT BOOK

TASK: Establish the matrix of an appointment book page, and schedule a patient appointment.

CONDITIONS: Given the proper equipment and supplies, the student will be required to matrix an appointment book and schedule appointments.

EQUIPMENT AND SUPPLIES
- MACC/computer (Practice)
- Appointment book page
- Office policy for office hours, procedure times, and list of physician's availability (information sheet)
- Pencil

STANDARDS: Complete the procedure within _____ minutes and achieve a minimum score of _____%.

Time began _____   Time ended _____

Steps	Possible Points	First Attempt	Second Attempt
1. Identify and mark the matrix according to office policy.	25		
2. Allow appointment times for emergency visits and unexpected needs.	10		
3. Schedule appointment providing the needed information for appropriate patient care, for canceling appointment, and for efficient time management.	15		
Total Points Possible	50		

Comments: Total Points Earned _____

Divided by _____

Total Possible Points = _____% Score

Instructor's Signature _____

PROCEDURE 26-4

Information for Procedure 26-4

> **OFFICE HOURS**
> Monday-Thursday: 8:30 a.m.-5:00 p.m.
> Lunch: M-Th: Noon-1:30 p.m.
> Friday: 8:30 a.m.-Noon
>
> **PHYSICIANS' AVAILABILITY**
> Dr. Bert makes hospital rounds every day from 4:30-6:00 p.m.
> Dr. Ernie makes hospital rounds every day from 7:30-9:30 a.m.
> (Both physicians set aside 1:30-2:00 for call backs)
> (This month Dr. Ernie is seeing all new patients)

Office Hours

	Monday	Tuesday	Wednesday	Thursday	Friday
Dr. Bert	8:30-noon	8:30-noon	8:30-noon	8:30-noon	8:30-noon
	2:00-4:15	2:00-4:15	2:00-4:15	2:00-4:15	
Dr. Ernie	10:00-noon	10:00-noon	10:00-noon	10:00-noon	10:00-noon
	2:00-5:00	2:00-5:00	2:00-5:00	2:00-5:00	

Scheduling Guidelines

15 Minutes	30 Minutes	45 Minutes	60 Minutes
UTI	**Physical** (afternoon appt only)	Eye injury	**New patient**
URI	Sports (SpPX)	Suspected fracture/bad sprain	Initial visit (NP)
HTN	School (ScPX)	Ear wash	Consultation (C)
Pain/infection:	Preop		Referral (R)
Ear/eye/throat	Postop visit		**Minor office surgery:**
Sinus	Asthma		Lesion removal (2)
Abdominal	Muscle strain/pain		I&D
Flu symptoms/fever	Diabetes		Ingrown toenail
Rechecks/follow-up:	Migraine		**Wellness visit** (morning appt only):
Wound			Female: PAP
BP			Male: Prostate
Allergies			ECG
Rash/hives			Blood work

Use the following information to complete the appointment schedule for Wednesday May 15, 20xx.

Patient/Phone #	Reason	Provider	Preferred Time
Bird, Jay 555-2756	Wellness visit	Bert	Morning
Warren, Lyle 727-5421	Ear wash	Ernie	Afternoon
Wells, Lucy 899-6543	New patient; history of diabetes		Anytime
Davis, Blake (minor) 437-7890	Sports physical	Ernie	After 2:45
Davis, Byron (minor) 437-7890	Sports physical	Ernie	After 2:45
Ricks, Darin 627-4414	Burning on urination	Bert	Morning
Jackson, Hue 876-6767	Hurt his back while playing baseball	Bert	Afternoon
Lee, Cindy 789-5543	Sinus pressure	Bert	Morning
Rademaker, Pete 987-9876	Consult	Bert	Morning
Wilson, Joan 765-9642	Referral	Ernie	Afternoon
Reese, Floyd 765-4321	BP/medication check	Ernie	Anytime
Kirwan, Paul 567-4343	Chest congestion	Bert	Anytime
Brown, Mary 756-6576	Migraine headaches for the past 2 days	Ernie	Anytime
James, Scott 765-1212	Sore throat	Bert	Morning
Mann, Grace 789-1441	Preop physical	Bert	Morning
Jones, LeRoy 876-4680	Fell yesterday and right wrist and forearm swollen	Bert	Anytime
White, Chester 555-7876	Postop	Bert	Anytime
Scullard, Lynelle 234-6867	Blood sugar is out of range	Ernie	Anytime
Deed, Joe 987-3579	Asthma	Bert	Late afternoon

Copyright © 2010, 2005 by Saunders, an imprint of Elsevier, Inc. All rights reserved.

			DAY / DATE				
			8	00			
				15			
				30			
				45			
			9	00			
				15			
				30			
				45			
			10	00			
				15			
				30			
				45			
			11	00			
				15			
				30			
				45			
			12	00			
				15			
				30			
				45			
			1	00			
				15			
				30			
				45			
			2	00			
				15			
				30			
				45			
			3	00			
				15			
				30			
				45			
			4	00			
				15			
				30			
				45			
			5	00			
				15			
				30			
				45			

Copyright © 2010, 2005 by Saunders, an imprint of Elsevier, Inc. All rights reserved.

Student Name: DATE:

PROCEDURE 26-5 CHECKLIST: SCHEDULE A NEW PATIENT

TASK: Schedule a new patient for an office visit.

CONDITIONS: Given the proper equipment and supplies, the student will be required to schedule a new patient appointment.

EQUIPMENT AND SUPPLIES
- MACC/computer (Practice)
- Appointment book page
- Office policy for office hours, procedure times, and list of physician's availability (information sheet)
- Telephone
- Pencil

STANDARDS: Complete the procedure within _____ minutes and achieve a minimum score of _____%.

Time began _____   Time ended _____

Steps	Possible Points	First Attempt	Second Attempt
1. Identify and mark the matrix according to office policy.	5		
2. Obtain preliminary information necessary for scheduling an appropriate appointment.	10		
3. Obtain the patient's demographic information and chief complaint.	10		
4. Determine whether the patient was referred by another physician.	10		
5. Enter the appointment in the appointment book using information and alternatives for maintenance of appointment book.	10		
6. Obtain additional information at the time the appointment is made as per office policies or patient needs.	10		
Total Points Possible	**55**		

Comments: Total Points Earned _____

Divided by _____

Total Possible Points = _____% Score

Instructor's Signature _____

PROCEDURE 26-5

Copyright © 2010, 2005 by Saunders, an imprint of Elsevier, Inc. All rights reserved.

Information for Procedure 26-5

> **OFFICE HOURS**
> Monday-Thursday: 8:30 a.m.-5:00 p.m.
> Lunch: M-Th: Noon-1:30 p.m.
> Friday: 8:30 a.m.-Noon
>
> **PHYSICIANS' AVAILABILITY**
> Dr. Bert makes hospital rounds everyday from 4:30-6:00 p.m.
> Dr. Ernie makes hospital rounds everyday from 7:30-9:30 a.m.
> (Both physicians set aside 1:30-2:00 p.m. for call backs)
> (This month both physicians are seeing new patients)

Office Hours

	Monday	Tuesday	Wednesday	Thursday	Friday
Dr. Bert	8:30-noon	8:30-noon	8:30-noon	8:30-noon	8:30-noon
	2:00-4:15	2:00-4:15	2:00-4:15	2:00-4:15	
Dr. Ernie	10:00-noon	10:00-noon	10:00-noon	10:00-noon	10:00-noon
	2:00-5:00	2:00-5:00	2:00-5:00	2:00-5:00	

All new patients are scheduled for a 60-minute visit.

1. Prepare appointment page using the above-listed data.

2. Today's date is October 28, 200xx, a Friday.

3. June Abbott, a new patient, called to make an appointment for October 28. She requests an early morning appointment. She is new to the area and does not have a preference to which physician she sees. Her address is 7890 Wild Wind Trail, Anytown, KY. Her phone number is 965-3456. She has Aetna HMO Basic Insurance. Schedule her appointment.

4. Charles Royal called last week to make an appointment with Dr. Ernie. He was referred by his physician because of a chronic skin condition. His address is 876 #4B, Anytown, USA. His phone number is 876-2121. He has Blue Cross/Blue Shield insurance. His appointment is for 10:00 a.m.

Copyright © 2010, 2005 by Saunders, an imprint of Elsevier, Inc. All rights reserved.

Supplemental Chapter Materials APPENDIX A 629

			DAY				
			DATE				
				00			
			8	15			
				30			
				45			
				00			
			9	15			
				30			
				45			
				00			
			10	15			
				30			
				45			
				00			
			11	15			
				30			
				45			
				00			
			12	15			
				30			
				45			
				00			
			1	15			
				30			
				45			
				00			
			2	15			
				30			
				45			
				00			
			3	15			
				30			
				45			
				00			
			4	15			
				30			
				45			
				00			
			5	15			
				30			
				45			

FORM NO. 56-7315 © 1974 BIBBERO SYSTEMS, INC. • PETALUMA, CA • TO REORDER CALL TOLL FREE: (800) BIBBERO (800 242-2376) OR FAX: (800) 242-9330 MFG. IN U.S.A. (REV. 7/94)

PROCEDURE 26-5

Copyright © 2010, 2005 by Saunders, an imprint of Elsevier, Inc. All rights reserved.

Student Name: _____   DATE: _____

PROCEDURE 26-6 CHECKLIST: SCHEDULE OUTPATIENT AND INPATIENT APPOINTMENTS

TASK: Schedule a patient for a physician-ordered test or procedure and admission in an outpatient or an inpatient setting or inpatient admission with the time frame requested by the physician, confirm the appointment with the patient, and issue all required instructions.

CONDITIONS: Given the proper equipment and supplies, the student will be required to schedule outpatient and inpatient appointments.

EQUIPMENT AND SUPPLIES
- MACC/computer (Practice)
- Physician's order for an outpatient or an inpatient diagnostic test procedure or inpatient admission
- Patient chart
- Surgical request forms (2)
- Test preparation or preadmission instructions
- Telephone
- Information sheet

STANDARDS: Complete the procedure within _____ minutes and achieve a minimum score of _____ %.

Time began _____   Time ended _____

Steps	Possible Points	First Attempt	Second Attempt
Outpatient (Complete Surgical Request Form)			
1. Schedule appointment using an order for an outpatient diagnostic test or procedure and the expected time frame for results.	15		
2. Precertify the procedure or test with the patient's insurance company.	10		
3. Determine patient availability.	10		
4. Contact the facility and schedule the procedure or test.	10		
5. Notify the patient of the arrangements.	10		
6. Conduct follow-up.	10		
Inpatient			
1. Schedule hospital admission.	15		
2. Precertify the admission with the patient's insurance company.	10		
3. Determine patient availability.	10		
4. Contact the facility and schedule the procedure or test.	10		

Copyright © 2010, 2005 by Saunders, an imprint of Elsevier, Inc. All rights reserved.

Steps	Possible Points	First Attempt	Second Attempt
5. Notify the patient of the arrangements.	10		
6. Conduct follow-up.	10		
Total Points Possible	130		

Comments: Total Points Earned _____

Divided by _____

Total Possible Points = _____ % Score

Instructor's Signature _____

Information for Procedure 26-6

Requesting Information

Outpatient:

Thomas Black, MD Surgeon   Date: 6/8/20xx

Need is immediate

Date needed: 6/9/20xx

(Patient is available 6/9/20xx to 6/11/20xx)

Time requested: 9:00 a.m.

Patient Name: Barbara Leaper

Procedure: Needle biopsy left breast

Procedure Code: 19102

Diagnosis: Breast Neoplasm

Diagnostic Code: 239.3

Estimated surgery time: 1 hour

Barbara Leaper is to report to XYZ Medical Center for a needle biopsy of a left breast mass on Thursday, June 10, 20xx, at 6:00 a.m. She should be NPO after midnight the evening before her surgery. Her biopsy is scheduled for 10:00 a.m. Her insurance carrier is Aetna and has approved the procedure.

All laboratory work is to be completed on Monday, June 7, 20xx, at XYZ Medical Centers laboratory.

Inpatient:
Clint Sellick, MD Date: 10/18/20xx
Need is urgent
Date needed: 10/19/20xx
(Patient is available 10/19/20xx to 10/21/20xx)
Time requested: 8:00 a.m.
Patient Name: Carolyn Moss
Procedure: Small bowel resection
Procedure Code: 44120
Diagnosis: Partial bowel obstruction
Diagnostic Code: 560.9
Estimated surgery time: 3 hours
Carolyn Moss is to report to XYZ Medical Center for a bowel resection on Wednesday, 10/19/20xx, at 5:00 a.m. She should be NPO after midnight the evening before her surgery. Her surgery is scheduled for 11:00 a.m. Her insurance carrier is Cigna and has approved the procedure.
All laboratory work is to be completed on Monday, October 17, 20xx, at XYZ Medical Centers' laboratory.

Copyright © 2010, 2005 by Saunders, an imprint of Elsevier, Inc. All rights reserved.

XYZ Medical Center

SURGICAL REQUEST AND INFORMATION

This portion is to be completed by requesting surgeon.

Surgeon: ❏ Thomas Black
❏ Clint Sellick
❏ Lynn Johnson

Schedule: ❏ URGENT ❏ IMMEDIATE ❏ PATIENT CONVENIENCE

Date Requested: _____ Time Requested: _____

Patient Name: _____

Procedure: _____

Procedure Code(s): _____

Diagnosis(es): _____

Diagnosis(es) Code(s): _____

Estimated Surgery Time: _____

Surgical Assistant Requested: _____

Additional Information: _____

This portion is to be completed by scheduling personnel.

Surgery Date: _____ Time: _____
                Day   Date

Authorization Obtained: ❏ YES ❏ NO ❏ REQUESTED

If authorization has been requested and response is pending, list date and contact information from the initial request.

Requested From: _____ Date: _____
               (Carrier and person)

Telephone: _____ Ext: _____

Completed By: _____

Date Completed: _____

(Modified from Buck CJ: *Student manual with daily tasks for practice kit for medical front office skills,* St Louis, 2009, Saunders.)

Copyright © 2010, 2005 by Saunders, an imprint of Elsevier, Inc. All rights reserved.

XYZ Medical Center

SURGICAL REQUEST AND INFORMATION

This portion is to be completed by requesting surgeon.

Surgeon: ❑ Thomas Black
❑ Clint Sellick
❑ Lynn Johnson

Schedule: ❑ URGENT ❑ IMMEDIATE ❑ PATIENT CONVENIENCE

Date Requested: _____ Time Requested: _____

Patient Name: _____

Procedure: _____

Procedure Code(s): _____

Diagnosis(es): _____

Diagnosis(es) Code(s): _____

Estimated Surgery Time: _____

Surgical Assistant Requested: _____

Additional Information: _____

This portion is to be completed by scheduling personnel.

Surgery Date: _____ Time: _____
             Day   Date

Authorization Obtained: ❑ YES ❑ NO ❑ REQUESTED

If authorization has been requested and response is pending, list date and contact information from the initial request.

Requested From: _____ Date: _____
          (Carrier and person)

Telephone: _____ Ext: _____

Completed By: _____

Date Completed: _____

(Modified from Buck CJ: *Student manual with daily tasks for practice kit for medical front office skills,* St Louis, 2009, Saunders.)

Student Name: _____ DATE: _____

PROCEDURE 26-7 CHECKLIST: COMPOSE BUSINESS CORRESPONDENCE

TASK: Compose, key, and proofread a business letter ready for mailing referring a patient to a specialist, using the guidelines of a common style.

CONDITIONS: Given the proper equipment and supplies, the student will be required to compose, key, and proofread a business letter.

EQUIPMENT AND SUPPLIES
- MACC/computer (practice)
- Computer with a word processing software
- Printer, or typewriter
- Paper
- Letterhead stationery
- Pen or pencil
- Information sheet
- # 10 business envelope
- Reference material (dictionary)

STANDARDS: Complete the procedure within _____ minutes and achieve a minimum score of _____%.

Time began _____   Time ended _____

Steps	Possible Points	First Attempt	Second Attempt
1. Assemble all needed equipment and supplies.	5		
2. Prepare a rough draft of the letter.	25		
3. Proofread the letter and correct errors.	10		
4. Prepare the final draft of the letter and proofread for errors.	10		
5. Print a copy on letterhead and prepare document for signature by appropriate person.	10		
6. Prepare the correspondence for mailing (fold).	20		
7. Address envelope for mailing.	5		
8. Calculate correct postage.	5		
9. Place in the outgoing tray for mail.	10		
Total Points Possible	100		

Comments: Total Points Earned _____

Divided by _____

Total Possible Points = _____% Score

Instructor's Signature _____

Copyright © 2010, 2005 by Saunders, an imprint of Elsevier, Inc. All rights reserved.

Information for Procedure 26-7

- Use the letterhead stationery supplied or create one using a template from your word processing package

- Create a letter from your physician, Lloyd Fisher, MD, referring his patient (John Silver) to Jane Main, MD, a dermatologist. Use good grammatical style and proofreading techniques.

- Use the following demographics:

  - John Silver, 2120 Trailer Way, Anytown, USA, 33342

  - Jane Main, MD, 6767 Folder Way, Anytown, USA, 33340, phone: 789-9876

  - Date: March 15, 20xx

- Prepare letter using full block format

XYZ Medical Center

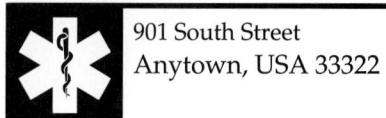

901 South Street
Anytown, USA 33322

(Modified from Buck CJ: *Student manual with daily tasks for practice kit for medical front office skills,* St Louis, 2009, Saunders.)

Copyright © 2010, 2005 by Saunders, an imprint of Elsevier, Inc. All rights reserved.

Student Name: _____   DATE: _____

PROCEDURE 26-8 CHECKLIST: COMPOSE A MEMO

TASK: Compose, key, and proofread a memo.

CONDITIONS: Given the proper equipment and supplies, the student will be required to compose, key, and proofread a memo.

EQUIPMENT AND SUPPLIES
- Computer
- Paper or memo form
- Pen or pencil
- Information sheet

STANDARDS: Complete the procedure within _____ minutes and achieve a minimum score of _____%.

Time began _____   Time ended _____

Steps	Possible Points	First Attempt	Second Attempt
1. Assemble all needed equipment and supplies.	5		
2. Create a memo form, using the guidelines presented in the chapter, or use one supplied.	15		
3. Fill in the required data.	10		
4. Ensure the format is correct.	10		
5. Distribute the memo to the proper recipients.	10		
Total Points Possible	50		

Comments: Total Points Earned _____

Divided by _____

Total Possible Points = _____% Score

Instructor's Signature _____

Information for Procedure 26-8

- Use the memo form supplied or create one using a template from your word processing package.

- Create a memo to all employees from Lloyd Fisher, MD, announcing a meeting to be held May 15, 20xx, in the conference room to discuss employee benefits. Be concise and include all the required elements of a memo.

- Date the memo May 2, 20xx.

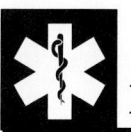 **XYZ Medical Center**

Memo

To:
From:
CC:
Date:
Re:

(Modified from Buck CJ: *Student manual with daily tasks for practice kit for medical front office skills,* St Louis, 2009, Saunders.)

Copyright © 2010, 2005 by Saunders, an imprint of Elsevier, Inc. All rights reserved.

Student Name: _____   DATE: _____

PROCEDURE 27-1 CHECKLIST: PULL PATIENT RECORDS FOR A MANUAL RECORD SYSTEM

TASK: Before the start of the business day, pull patient charts for daily appointment schedule.

CONDITIONS: Given the proper equipment and supplies, the student will be required to role-play with another student or an instructor the proper method for pulling patient records based on a full day's appointment schedule (10 to 12 patient files requested of 30 to 50 files).

EQUIPMENT AND SUPPLIES
- Computer
- Appointment book, appointment list
- Pen or pencil
- Tape
- Out guide
- Two-hole punch
- Patient files

STANDARDS: Complete the procedure within _____ minutes and achieve a minimum score of _____%.

Time began _____   Time ended _____

Steps	Possible Points	First Attempt	Second Attempt
1. Assemble all equipment and supplies.	5		
2. Locate and review the day's schedule.	5		
3. Generate the daily appointment list (type, photocopy, or print from the computer).	5		
4. Identify the full name of each scheduled patient.	5		
5. Obtain the patient's records from the filing system; place a check mark next to each patient's name on the appointment book as each record is obtained.	10		
6. Review each record for completeness.	5		
7. Annotate the appointment list with any special considerations.	5		

PROCEDURE 27-1

Steps	Possible Points	First Attempt	Second Attempt
8. Arrange all records sequentially by appointment time.	5		
9. Place the records in a specified location that is out of view from unauthorized individuals.	5		
Total Points Possible	50		

Comments: Total Points Earned _____

Divided by _____

Total Possible Points = _____% Score

Instructor's Signature _____

Student Name: _____   DATE: _____

PROCEDURE 27-2 CHECKLIST: REGISTER A NEW PATIENT

TASK: Complete a registration form for a new patient, obtaining all required information for credit and insurance claims.

CONDITIONS: Given the proper equipment and supplies, the student will be required to complete a new patient registration form by role-playing with another student or an instructor.

EQUIPMENT AND SUPPLIES
- Computer
- Registration form
- Pen
- Clipboard
- Private conference area

STANDARDS: Complete the procedure within _____ minutes and achieve a minimum score of _____%.

Time began _____   Time ended _____

Steps	Possible Points	First Attempt	Second Attempt
1. Assemble all equipment and supplies.	5		
2. Establish a new patient status.	5		
3. Obtain and document the required information. (When role-playing this procedure, information obtained can be fictitious.)	25		
4. Review the entire form for completeness; make corrections as required.	15		
Total Points Possible	50		

Comments: Total Points Earned _____

Divided by _____

Total Possible Points = _____% Score

Instructor's Signature _____

Copyright © 2010, 2005 by Saunders, an imprint of Elsevier, Inc. All rights reserved.

REGISTRATION
(PLEASE PRINT)

Home Phone: _____ Today's Date: _____

PATIENT INFORMATION

Name _____ Soc. Sec.# _____
        Last Name   First Name   Initial

Address _____

City _____ State _____ Zip _____

Cell Phone _____ E-mail: _____ Fax #: _____

Single ____ Married ____ Widowed ____ Separated ____ Divorced ____ Sex M ____ F ____ Age ____ Birthdate _____

Patient Employed by _____ Occupation _____

Business Address _____ Business Phone _____

By whom were you referred? _____

In case of emergency who should be notified? _____ Phone _____
                                               Name   Relation to Patient

PRIMARY INSURANCE

Person Responsible for Account _____
                                Last Name   First Name   Initial

Relation to Patient _____ Birthdate _____ Soc. Sec.# _____

Address (if different from patient's) _____ Phone _____

City _____ State _____ Zip _____

Person Responsible Employed by _____ Occupation _____

Business Address _____ Business Phone _____

Insurance Company _____

Contract # _____ Group # _____ Subscriber # _____

Name of other dependents covered under this plan _____

ADDITIONAL INSURANCE

Is patient covered by additional insurance? ____ Yes ____ No

Subscriber Name _____ Relation to Patient _____ Birthdate _____

Address (if different from patient's) _____ Phone _____

City _____ State _____ Zip _____

Subscriber Employed by _____ Business Phone _____

Insurance Company _____ Soc. Sec.# _____

Contract # _____ Group # _____ Subscriber # _____

Name of other dependents covered under this plan _____

ASSIGNMENT AND RELEASE

I, the undersigned, certify that I (or my dependent) have insurance coverage with _____
                                                                                                 Name of Insurance Company(ies)

and assign directly to Dr. _____ insurance benefits, if any, otherwise payable to me for services rendered. I understand that I am financially responsible for all charges whether or not paid by insurance. I hereby authorize the doctor to release all information necessary to secure the payment of benefits. I authorize the use of this signature on all insurance submissions.

_____ _____ _____
Responsible Party Signature   Relationship   Date

ORDER # 58-8425 • © 1996 BIBBERO SYSTEMS, INC. • PETALUMA, CALIFORNIA • TO REORDER CALL TOLL FREE: (800) 242-2376 OR FAX: (800) 242-9330   (REV. 12/06)

(Form # 58-8425-P; courtesy of Bibbero Systems, Inc., Petaluma, CA; (800) 242-2376; fax (800) 242-9330; www.bibbero.com.)

Student Name: _____   DATE: _____

PROCEDURE 27-3 CHECKLIST: INITIATE A PATIENT FILE FOR A NEW PATIENT USING COLOR-CODED TABS

TASK: Set up and organize a file that contains the personal data necessary for a complete record and other information required by the medical office for a new patient. This should be completed using a color-coded filing system.

CONDITIONS: Given the proper equipment and supplies, the student will be required to initiate a patient file for a new patient using color-coded tabs.

EQUIPMENT AND SUPPLIES
- MACC/computer
- End-cut file
- A-Z color-coded tabs (self-adhesive)
- Blank file label (self-adhesive)
- Color-coded year label (annual age dating label)
- Medical alert or other label types as appropriate
- Forms:
  - Patient information
  - Assignment of benefits
  - Waiver
  - Treatment authorizations
  - Referral slips
  - Health history
  - Hospital discharge summaries
  - Surgery reports
  - Progress notes
  - Visit log
  - Prescription flow sheet
  - Laboratory reports
  - Diagnostic reports
  - Consultation reports
  - Miscellaneous correspondence

STANDARDS: Complete the procedure within _____ minutes and achieve a minimum score of _____%.

Time began _____   Time ended _____

Steps	Possible Points	First Attempt	Second Attempt
1. Assemble all equipment and supplies.	5		
2. Obtain and review a completed patient information form.	10		
3. Place the completed and reviewed form on the left inside cover of the file, using the method preferred by the medical facility.	10		
4. Place progress note form and prescription flow sheet on the inside right cover of the file with the progress note form on top. File additional forms in reverse chronological order, meaning the most recent on top.	10		
5. Create a file label.	10		

Copyright © 2010, 2005 by Saunders, an imprint of Elsevier, Inc. All rights reserved.

Steps	Possible Points	First Attempt	Second Attempt
6. Attach the file label in the center of the file tab.	10		
7. Attach alphabetical, color-coded labels.	10		
8. Attach the current year "aging" label above the first-name initial tab.	5		
9. Compile the file. Place the appropriate patient information, healthy history, and other forms in the patient file.	10		
10. Attach a "Medical Alert" label on the front of the file.	5		
11. Prepare a ledger card or enter the patient information into a computerized management program.	10		
12. Attach an encounter form (super bill) to the outside of the patient's file.	5		
Total Points Possible	100		

Comments: Total Points Earned _____

Divided by _____

Total Possible Points = _____% Score

Instructor's Signature _____

XYZ Medical Center

Patient Health History

Today's Date: _____

Name: _____ Date of Birth: _____

Marital Status:　　S　　M　　D　　W

Reason for today's visit: _____

Nutrition and Activity

Diet (check one):　❏ Good　❏ Poor

Level of Physical Activity (check one):
　❏ Very Active　　❏ Active　　❏ Sedentary　　❏ Inactive

Medical History (Please list any you currently have or have had in the past)

Allergies: _____

Significant illnesses or conditions: _____

_____

Current medications: _____

Hospitalizations or Surgery: _____

Injuries requiring medical treatment: _____

Family History

Have any members of your family had any of the following (check one):

❏ Asthma　　　　　　　　❏ Diabetes　　　　　　　　❏ Bleeding Disorder
❏ Glaucoma　　　　　　　❏ Heart Disease　　　　　　❏ Drug/Alcohol Addiction
❏ Hypertension　　　　　❏ Mental Illness　　　　　　❏ Strokes
❏ Cancer (list) _____　❏ Other (list) _____

Family relationship for any of the above condition(s) checked: _____

_____

Social History

Occupation: _____

Are you sexually active?　❏ Yes　　❏ No

Have you ever had a sexually transmitted infection (STI)?　❏ Yes　　❏ No

If yes, please list the STI type(s) and treatment(s) used _____

Do you consume alcohol?　❏ Yes　　❏ No

Do you smoke?　❏ Yes　　❏ No

If yes, average weekly consumption and drink of choice _____

If yes, check all that apply:　❏ Cigarettes　❏ Pipe tobacco　❏ Cigars

Do you chew tobacco?　❏ Yes　　❏ No

How much tobacco do you consume on average per day? _____

How long have you used tobacco? _____

Do you or have you used illegal substance(s)?　❏ Yes　　❏ No

If yes, please list _____

(Modified from Buck CJ: *Student manual with daily tasks for practice kit for medical front office skills,* St Louis, 2009, Saunders.)

Copyright © 2010, 2005 by Saunders, an imprint of Elsevier, Inc. All rights reserved.

**Patient Consent to the Use and Disclosure of Health Information
for Treatment, Payment, or Health Care Operations**

I understand that as part of my health care, the practice originates and maintains paper and/or electronic records describing my health history, symptoms, examination and test results, diagnoses, treatment, and any plans for future care or treatment. I understand that this information serves as:

- A basis for planning my care and treatment,
- A means of communication among professionals who contribute to my care,
- A source of information for applying my diagnosis and treatment information to my bill,
- A means by which a third-party payer can verify that services billed were actually provided,
- A tool for routine health care operations, such as assessing quality and reviewing the competence of staff.

I have been provided the opportunity to review the *"Notice of Patient Privacy Information Practices"* **that provides a more complete description of information uses and disclosures. I understand that I have the following rights:**

- The right to review the *"Notice"* prior to acknowledging this consent,
- The right to restrict or revoke the use or disclosure of my health information for other uses or purposes, and
- The right to request restrictions as to how my health information may be used or disclosed to carry out treatment, payment, or health care operations.

Restrictions:

I request the following restrictions to the use or disclosure of my health information:
_____
_____

May discuss treatment, payment, or health care operation with the following persons:

(Please check all that apply)   Spouse [ ]   Your Children [ ]   Relatives [ ]   Others [ ]   Parents [ ]

Please list the names and relationship, if you checked "Relatives" or "Others" above
_____
_____

Messages or Appointment Reminders: (Please check all that apply)

May we leave a message on your answering machine at home [ ] or at work [ ]. **Do not leave a message** [ ]
May we leave a message with someone at your **home** using the doctor's name or the practice name: Yes [ ]   No [ ]
May we leave a message with someone at your **work** using the doctor's name or the practice name: Yes [ ]   No [ ]
Messages will be of a nonsensitive nature, such as appointment reminders.

I understand that as part of treatment, payment, or health care operations, it may become necessary to disclose health information to another entity, i.e., referrals to other health care providers, labs, and/or other individuals or agencies as permitted or required by state or federal law.

I fully understand and accept the information provided by this consent.

_____   _____   _____
Signature   Print name of person signing   Date

*If other than patient is signing, are you the parent, legal guardian, custodian, or have Power of Attorney for this patient for treatment, payment, or health care operations?   Yes [ ]   No [ ]

FOR OFFICE USE ONLY
[ ] Patient refused to sign the consent form.
[ ] Restrictions were added by the patient (see restrictions listed above)
[ ] "Consent form" received and reviewed by _____ on (date) _____
[ ] "Consent form" placed in the patient's medical record on (date) _____

PROCEDURE 27-3

GENERAL MEDICAL HEALTH CARE

AUTHORIZATION FOR RELEASE OF MEDICAL INFORMATION

I, _____ ____/____/____ _____ hereby authorize
     Print Patient's Name   Date of Birth   Social Security Number

General Medical Health Care 1234 Riverview Road, Anytown, FL 33333

to release medical, including HIV Antibody Testing, Psychiatric/Psychological, Alcohol and/or Drug Abuse information records to:

To: _____

Address _____
        (Street)   (City)   (State)   (Zip)

For the purpose of: 1. Drs. appointment on: _____

                         2. Other: _____

                                     Please Specify Reason for Disclosure

I understand that if I consent to the release of any of my medical records, the results of any HIV Antibody Testing, Psychiatric/Psychological, Alcohol and/or Drug Abuse information will be released.

I understand this consent may be cancelled upon written notice to the hospital, except that action by the hospital has been taken in reliance on this authorization, and that this authorization shall remain in force for a 90-day period in order to effect the purpose for which it is given. Alcohol and drug abuse information, if present, has been disclosed from records whose confidentiality is protected by Federal Law. FEDERAL REGULATIONS (42CFR, part II) prohibit making any further disclosure of records without the specific written authorization of the undersigned, or as otherwise permitted by such regulations.
The confidentiality of HIV antibody test results is protected by Florida Law [Fla. Stat.ANN. 381.609 (2) (F)], which prohibits any further disclosure by a person to whom this information has been disclosed, without specific written consent of the undersigned or as otherwise permitted by state law.

_____   From: _____ To: _____
     (Date of Authorization)   (Dates to be Released)

_____
       Patient's Signature

_____
Parent, Legal Guardian, or Authorized
    Representative Signature

_____
    Relationship to Patient

_____
         Witness

CONSENT FOR SURGERY

DATE:_____

TIME:_____

I authorize the performance of the following procedure(s)_____
_____on_____
To be performed by_____, MD.

The following have been explained to me by Dr._____

    1. Nature of the procedure:_____

    2. Reason(s) for procedure:_____

    3. Possible risks:_____

    4. Possible complications:_____

I understand that no warranty or guarantee of the effectiveness of the surgery can be made.

I have been informed of possible alternative treatments including_____
_____and of the likely consequences of receiving no treatment, and I freely consent to this procedure.

I hereby authorize the above named surgeon and his/her assistants to provide additional services including administering anesthesia and / or medications, performing needed diagnostic tests including but not limited to radiology, and any other additional services deemed necessary for my well-being. I consent to have removed tissue examined by a pathologist who may then dispose of the tissue as he/she sees fit.

Signed_____ Relationship to patient_____
        Patient / Parent / Guardian

Witness_____

PROCEDURE 27-3

Copyright © 2010, 2005 by Saunders, an imprint of Elsevier, Inc. All rights reserved.

XYZ Medical Center – Progress Notes	
Patient Name:	Chart Number:

REGISTRATION
(PLEASE PRINT)

Home Phone: _____   Today's Date: _____

PATIENT INFORMATION

Name _____ Soc. Sec.# _____
       Last Name   First Name   Initial

Address _____

City _____ State _____ Zip _____

Cell Phone _____ E-mail: _____ Fax #: _____

Single ___ Married ___ Widowed ___ Separated ___ Divorced ___ Sex M ___ F ___ Age ___ Birthdate _____

Patient Employed by _____ Occupation _____

Business Address _____ Business Phone _____

By whom were you referred? _____

In case of emergency who should be notified? _____ Phone _____
                                                Name   Relation to Patient

PRIMARY INSURANCE

Person Responsible for Account _____
                                  Last Name   First Name   Initial

Relation to Patient _____ Birthdate _____ Soc. Sec.# _____

Address (if different from patient's) _____ Phone _____

City _____ State _____ Zip _____

Person Responsible Employed by _____ Occupation _____

Business Address _____ Business Phone _____

Insurance Company _____

Contract # _____ Group # _____ Subscriber # _____

Name of other dependents covered under this plan _____

ADDITIONAL INSURANCE

Is patient covered by additional insurance? ___ Yes ___ No

Subscriber Name _____ Relation to Patient _____ Birthdate _____

Address (if different from patient's) _____ Phone _____

City _____ State _____ Zip _____

Subscriber Employed by _____ Business Phone _____

Insurance Company _____ Soc. Sec.# _____

Contract # _____ Group # _____ Subscriber # _____

Name of other dependents covered under this plan _____

ASSIGNMENT AND RELEASE

I, the undersigned, certify that I (or my dependent) have insurance coverage with _____
                                                                                           Name of Insurance Company(ies)

and assign directly to Dr. _____ insurance benefits, if any, otherwise payable to me for services rendered. I understand that I am financially responsible for all charges whether or not paid by insurance. I hereby authorize the doctor to release all information necessary to secure the payment of benefits. I authorize the use of this signature on all insurance submissions.

_____   _____   _____
     Responsible Party Signature   Relationship   Date

ORDER # 58-8425 • © 1996 BIBBERO SYSTEMS, INC. • PETALUMA, CALIFORNIA • TO REORDER CALL TOLL FREE: (800) 242-2376 OR FAX: (800) 242-9330   (REV. 12/06)

(Form # 58-8425-P; courtesy of Bibbero Systems, Inc., Petaluma, CA; (800) 242-2376; fax (800) 242-9330; www.bibbero.com.)

Copyright © 2010, 2005 by Saunders, an imprint of Elsevier, Inc. All rights reserved.

Visit Log

Date	Physician	Reason	Action

Copyright © 2010, 2005 by Saunders, an imprint of Elsevier, Inc. All rights reserved.

Prescription Flow Sheet

Date	Medication	Dosage	Refill

Copyright © 2010, 2005 by Saunders, an imprint of Elsevier, Inc. All rights reserved.

Student Name: _____ DATE: _____

PROCEDURE 27-4 CHECKLIST: ADD SUPPLEMENTARY ITEMS TO AN ESTABLISHED PATIENT FILE

TASK: Add supplemental documents and progress notes to patient files, observing standard steps in filing while creating an orderly file that facilitates ready reference to any information.

CONDITIONS: Given the proper equipment and supplies, the student will be required to add supplementary items to an established patient file.

EQUIPMENT AND SUPPLIES
- MACC/computer
- Patient file
- Assorted documents (provided by instructor)
- Stapler
- Clear tape
- Two-hole punch
- Alphanumeric sorter

STANDARDS: Complete the procedure within _____ minutes and achieve a minimum score of _____%.

Time began _____   Time ended _____

Steps	Possible Points	First Attempt	Second Attempt
1. Assemble all equipment and supplies.	5		
2. Retrieve the appropriate file from the file storage area.	5		
3. Condition the document.	5		
4. Release the document.	5		
5. Index and code the document.	10		
6. Sort for filing.	5		
7. File each document according to categories into the established patient's file, with the most recent document on top.	10		
8. Return file to storage area.	5		
Total Points Possible	50		

Comments: Total Points Earned _____

Divided by _____

Total Possible Points = _____ % Score

Instructor's Signature _____

Copyright © 2010, 2005 by Saunders, an imprint of Elsevier, Inc. All rights reserved.

Student Name: _____ DATE: _____

PROCEDURE 27-5 CHECKLIST: MAINTAIN CONFIDENTIALITY OF PATIENTS AND THEIR MEDICAL RECORDS

TASK: Explain through role-playing how to maintain confidentiality of patient information and their medical records.

CONDITIONS: Given the proper equipment and supplies, the student will be required to explain how to maintain confidentiality of patient information and their medical records.

EQUIPMENT AND SUPPLIES
- MACC/computer
- Authorization form for "Release of Medical Records"
- HIPAA release form

STANDARDS: Complete the procedure within _____ minutes and achieve a minimum score of _____ %.

Time began _____   Time ended _____

Steps	Possible Points	First Attempt	Second Attempt
1. Assemble all supplies and equipment.	5		
2. Select a partner to be a patient as you assume the role of the administrative medical assistant.	5		
3. Explain to the "patient" through role-playing how the integrity of confidences shared in the office is maintained regarding the following medical office types:	15		
a. Attorney is calling the office to gain information about a patient	5		
b. Release of information about a minor	5		
c. Advertising and media	5		
d. Computerized medical records	5		
4. Explain to the "patient" through role-playing how confidences shared in the office are maintained regarding the following specialty topics:	15		
a. Child abuse	5		
b. Sexually transmitted diseases	5		
c. Sexual assault	5		
d. Mental health	5		
e. AIDS and HIV	5		
f. Substance abuse	5		

Copyright © 2010, 2005 by Saunders, an imprint of Elsevier, Inc. All rights reserved.

Steps	Possible Points	First Attempt	Second Attempt
5. Explain to the "patient" through role-playing how the following situations regarding confidentiality issues are handled in the medical office:	15		
a. Subpoenaed medical records	5		
b. HIPAA guidelines	5		
c. Areas of mandated disclosure by state and federal regulations	5		
6. Explain to the "patient" through role-playing the "Patient's Bill of Rights."	15		
7. Explain to the "patient" through role-playing how to complete an authorization form for release of medical records.	15		
Total Points Possible	150		

Comments: Total Points Earned _____

Divided by _____

Total Possible Points = _____% Score

Instructor's Signature _____

**Patient Consent to the Use and Disclosure of Health Information
for Treatment, Payment, or Health Care Operations**

I understand that as part of my health care, the practice originates and maintains paper and/or electronic records describing my health history, symptoms, examination and test results, diagnoses, treatment, and any plans for future care or treatment. I understand that this information serves as:

- A basis for planning my care and treatment,
- A means of communication among professionals who contribute to my care,
- A source of information for applying my diagnosis and treatment information to my bill,
- A means by which a third-party payer can verify that services billed were actually provided,
- A tool for routine health care operations, such as assessing quality and reviewing the competence of staff.

I have been provided the opportunity to review the *"Notice of Patient Privacy Information Practices"* **that provides a more complete description of information uses and disclosures. I understand that I have the following rights:**

- The right to review the *"Notice"* prior to acknowledging this consent,
- The right to restrict or revoke the use or disclosure of my health information for other uses or purposes, and
- The right to request restrictions as to how my health information may be used or disclosed to carry out treatment, payment, or health care operations.

Restrictions:

I request the following restrictions to the use or disclosure of my health information:
_____
_____

May discuss treatment, payment, or health care operation with the following persons:

(Please check all that apply)   Spouse [ ]   Your Children [ ]   Relatives [ ]   Others [ ]   Parents [ ]

Please list the names and relationship, if you checked "Relatives" or "Others" above
_____
_____

Messages or Appointment Reminders: (Please check all that apply)

May we leave a message on your answering machine at home [ ] or at work [ ]. **Do not leave a message** [ ]
May we leave a message with someone at your **home** using the doctor's name or the practice name: Yes [ ]   No [ ]
May we leave a message with someone at your **work** using the doctor's name or the practice name: Yes [ ]   No [ ]
Messages will be of a nonsensitive nature, such as appointment reminders.

I understand that as part of treatment, payment, or health care operations, it may become necessary to disclose health information to another entity, i.e., referrals to other health care providers, labs, and/or other individuals or agencies as permitted or required by state or federal law.

I fully understand and accept the information provided by this consent.

_____   _____   _____
Signature   Print name of person signing   Date

*If other than patient is signing, are you the parent, legal guardian, custodian, or have Power of Attorney for this patient for treatment, payment, or health care operations?   Yes [ ]   No [ ]

FOR OFFICE USE ONLY
[ ] Patient refused to sign the consent form.
[ ] Restrictions were added by the patient (see restrictions listed above)
[ ] "Consent form" received and reviewed by _____ on (date) _____
[ ] "Consent form" placed in the patient's medical record on (date) _____

Copyright © 2010, 2005 by Saunders, an imprint of Elsevier, Inc. All rights reserved.

GENERAL MEDICAL HEALTH CARE

AUTHORIZATION FOR RELEASE OF MEDICAL INFORMATION

I, _____ ____/____/____ _____ hereby authorize
    Print Patient's Name   Date of Birth   Social Security Number

General Medical Health Care 1234 Riverview Road, Anytown, FL 33333

to release medical, including HIV Antibody Testing, Psychiatric/Psychological, Alcohol and/or Drug Abuse information records to:

To: _____

Address _____
       (Street)   (City)   (State)   (Zip)

For the purpose of: 1. Drs. appointment on: _____

                          2. Other: _____

                             Please Specify Reason for Disclosure

I understand that if I consent to the release of any of my medical records, the results of any HIV Antibody Testing, Psychiatric/Psychological, Alcohol and/or Drug Abuse information will be released.

I understand this consent may be cancelled upon written notice to the hospital, except that action by the hospital has been taken in reliance on this authorization, and that this authorization shall remain in force for a 90-day period in order to effect the purpose for which it is given. Alcohol and drug abuse information, if present, has been disclosed from records whose confidentiality is protected by Federal Law. FEDERAL REGULATIONS (42CFR, part II) prohibit making any further disclosure of records without the specific written authorization of the undersigned, or as otherwise permitted by such regulations. The confidentiality of HIV antibody test results is protected by Florida Law [Fla. Stat.ANN. 381.609 (2) (F)], which prohibits any further disclosure by a person to whom this information has been disclosed, without specific written consent of the undersigned or as otherwise permitted by state law.

_____   From: _____ To: _____
(Date of Authorization)   (Dates to be Released)

_____
Patient's Signature

_____
Parent, Legal Guardian, or Authorized
Representative Signature

_____
Relationship to Patient

_____
Witness

Copyright © 2010, 2005 by Saunders, an imprint of Elsevier, Inc. All rights reserved.

Student Name: _____   DATE: _____

PROCEDURE 27-6 CHECKLIST: FILE MEDICAL RECORDS USING THE ALPHABETICAL SYSTEM

TASK: Correctly file a set of patient records using an established alphabetical filing system.

CONDITIONS: Given the proper equipment and supplies, the student will be required to file medical charts using the alphabetical system.

EQUIPMENT AND SUPPLIES
- MACC/computer
- Patient files
- Alphanumeric sorter

STANDARDS: Complete the procedure within _____ minutes and achieve a minimum score of _____%.

Time began _____   Time ended _____

Steps	Possible Points	First Attempt	Second Attempt
1. Assemble all supplies and equipment.	5		
2. Retrieve the appropriate patient files from the file storage area.	15		
3. Use an out guide.	10		
4. Complete documentation as appropriate.	15		
5. Add any supplemental forms or records generated according to office procedures.	15		
6. Sort the files alphabetically, using a "desktop sorter" if possible.	15		
7. Remove the files from the sorter and return the files to the storage area, correctly filing them.	15		
8. Remove out guide.	10		
Total Points Possible	100		

Comments: Total Points Earned _____

Divided by _____

Total Possible Points = _____% Score

Instructor's Signature _____

PROCEDURE 27-6

Student Name: _____ DATE: _____

PROCEDURE 27-7 CHECKLIST: FILE MEDICAL RECORDS USING THE NUMERICAL SYSTEM

TASK: Correctly file a set of patient charts, using an established numerical filing system.

CONDITIONS: Given the proper equipment and supplies, the student will be required to file medical charts using a numerical system.

EQUIPMENT AND SUPPLIES
- MACC/computer
- Patient files
- Numerical sorter

STANDARDS: Complete the procedure within _____ minutes and achieve a minimum score of _____%.

Time began _____   Time ended _____

Steps	Possible Points	First Attempt	Second Attempt
1. Assemble all supplies and equipment.	5		
2. Retrieve the proper numerical code from the appropriate system file.	15		
3. Use an out guide.	10		
4. Complete documentation as appropriate.	15		
5. Add any supplemental forms or records generated according to office procedures.	15		
6. Sort the files numerically, using a "desktop sorter" if possible.	15		
7. Remove the files from the sorter and return the files to the storage area, correctly filing them into the appropriate numerical sequence.	15		
8. Remove out guide.	10		
Total Points Possible	100		

Comments: Total Points Earned _____

Divided by _____

Total Possible Points = _____% Score

Instructor's Signature _____

PROCEDURE 27-7

Copyright © 2010, 2005 by Saunders, an imprint of Elsevier, Inc. All rights reserved.

Student Name: _____ DATE: _____

PROCEDURE 28-1 CHECKLIST: MANAGE AN ACCOUNT FOR PETTY CASH

TASK: Establish a petty cash fund, maintain an accurate record of expenditures, and replenish the fund as necessary.

CONDITIONS: Given the proper equipment and supplies, the student will be required to establish a petty cash fund, maintain an accurate record of expenditures, and replenish the fund as necessary.

EQUIPMENT AND SUPPLIES
- MACC/computer (practice)
- Petty cash box or envelope
- Petty cash expense record
- List of petty cash expenditures
- Two blank checks
- Petty cash vouchers
- Calculator
- Pen or pencil
- Information sheet

STANDARDS: Complete the procedure within _____ minutes and achieve a minimum score of _____%.

Time began _____   Time ended _____

Steps	Possible Points	First Attempt	Second Attempt
1. Assemble all supplies and equipment.	5		
2. Establish the amount needed in the petty cash fund.	5		
3. Write a check for the determined amount, and put the cash in the petty cash box or envelope.	10		
4. Record the beginning balance to the petty cash record.	5		
5. Prepare a petty cash voucher for each amount withdrawn from the fund, and attach a sales receipt or an explanation of the payment.	10		
6. Enter each expense in the petty cash expense record, allocating the expenses to the correct disbursement categories. Calculate the new balance in the fund.	10		
7. When the fund balance has reached the established minimum, count the remaining currency in the petty cash box.	10		
8. Total all vouchers in the petty cash box.	10		

PROCEDURE 28-1

Copyright © 2010, 2005 by Saunders, an imprint of Elsevier, Inc. All rights reserved.

Steps	Possible Points	First Attempt	Second Attempt
9. Add the voucher total to the amount in the petty cash fund. This should equal the original amount of the petty cash fund.	5		
10. Prepare a check for "cash" for the amount that was used from the fund for incidental expenses. Enter the check number on the petty cash expense record.	10		
11. Cash the check, and add the replacement cash to the cash box.	5		
12. Record the amount added to the fund on the expense record.	5		
13. Bring the balance forward.	10		
Total Points Possible	100		

Comments: Total Points Earned _____

Divided by _____

Total Possible Points = _____ % Score

Instructor's Signature _____

Information for Procedure 28-1

It is August 1, 20XX, and you have been placed in charge of the "Petty Cash Fund" in your medical office. It has been determined that the fund will begin with a balance of $100.00. The office manager has you write the check and secures the physician's signature. She requests that you cash the check at the nearby bank. The following transactions occur during the month of August:

1. August 2: Amanda is sent on an errand to get miscellaneous office supplies (copier paper, staple, and batteries). The total amount is $15.50.

2. August 2: Postage due amounts to $3.20.

3. August 5: The office is sponsoring an open house to introduce a new physician joining the staff and sends Thalia to the local store to get paper products, coffee, and pastries for the event. She returns with a receipt for $37.47. She informs you that she bought a soda and chips for herself for $1.75, and it is included on the receipt.

4. August 10: Dr. Zee turns in his parking receipts for $20.00.

5. August 15: Inesha is sent to the drug store to purchase 2 × 2 NS gauze dressings, bandages, and trash bags. The receipt totals $12.50.

6. August 22: Postage due amounts to $2.23.

7. August 31: Reconcile petty cash fund.

Copyright © 2010, 2005 by Saunders, an imprint of Elsevier, Inc. All rights reserved.

Amount $ _____	No. _____
Date _____ **RECEIVED OF PETTY CASH**	
For _____	
Charge to _____	
_____	
Approved by	Received by
_____	_____

Amount $ _____	No. _____
Date _____ **RECEIVED OF PETTY CASH**	
For _____	
Charge to _____	
_____	
Approved by	Received by
_____	_____

Amount $ _____	No. _____
Date _____ **RECEIVED OF PETTY CASH**	
For _____	
Charge to _____	
_____	
Approved by	Received by
_____	_____

(Modified from Kinn ME, Woods MA: *The medical assistant,* ed 8, Philadelphia, 1999, Saunders.)

Copyright © 2010, 2005 by Saunders, an imprint of Elsevier, Inc. All rights reserved.

| Amount $ _____   No. _____ |
| Date _____ **RECEIVED OF PETTY CASH** |
| For _____ |
| Charge to _____ |
| _____ |
| Approved by   Received by |
| _____   _____ |

| Amount $ _____   No. _____ |
| Date _____ **RECEIVED OF PETTY CASH** |
| For _____ |
| Charge to _____ |
| _____ |
| Approved by   Received by |
| _____   _____ |

| Amount $ _____   No. _____ |
| Date _____ **RECEIVED OF PETTY CASH** |
| For _____ |
| Charge to _____ |
| _____ |
| Approved by   Received by |
| _____   _____ |

(Modified from Kinn ME, Woods MA: *The medical assistant,* ed 8, Philadelphia, 1999, Saunders.)

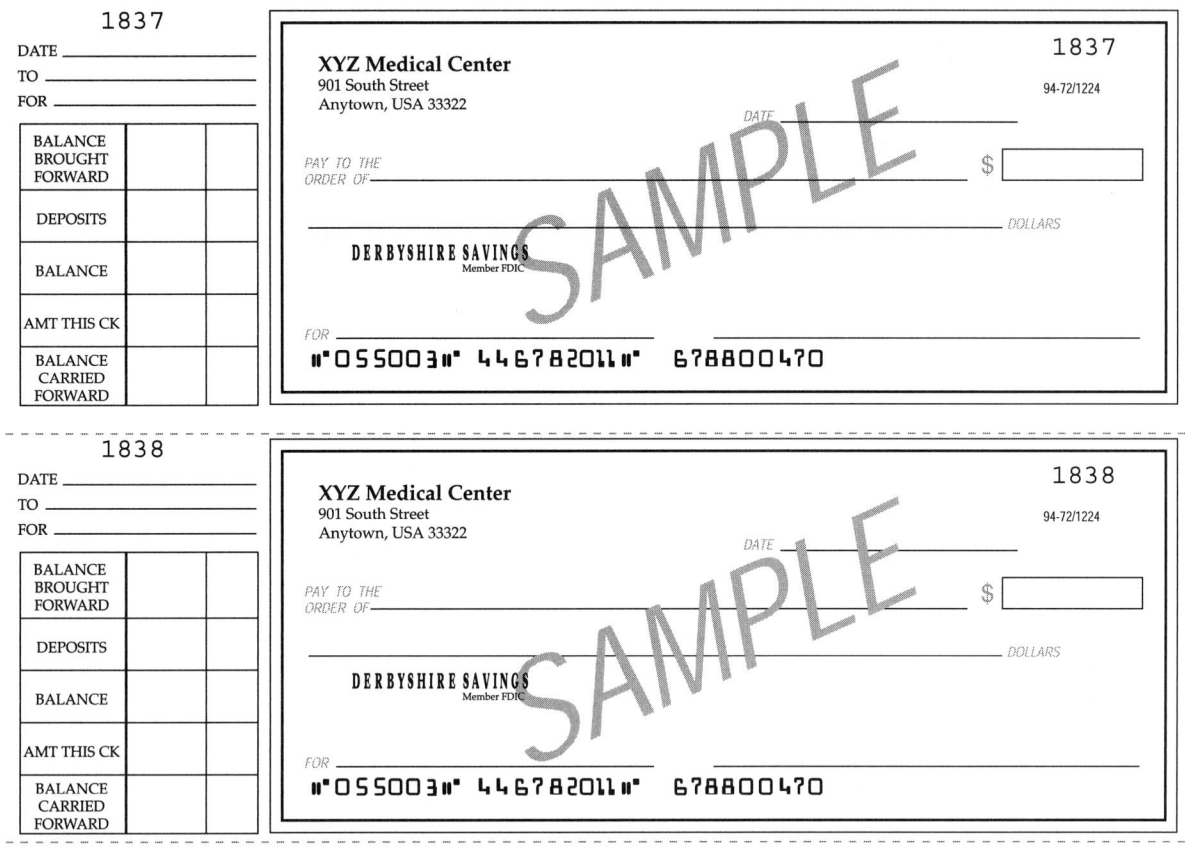

(Modified from Hunt SA: *Fundamentals of medical assisting student mastery manual,* Philadelphia, 2002, Saunders.)

Use the expense record, checks, and petty cash vouchers to complete the exercise.

Voucher #	Date	Description	Amount	Office	Auto	Misc	Balance
	8/1/XX	Fund established					

PROCEDURE 28-1

Copyright © 2010, 2005 by Saunders, an imprint of Elsevier, Inc. All rights reserved.

Student Name: _____ DATE: _____

PROCEDURE CHECKLIST 28-2: POST SERVICE CHARGES AND PAYMENTS TO THE PATIENT'S ACCOUNT

TASK: Post service charges and payments to a daysheet and ledger card, and prepare receipt.

CONDITIONS: Given the proper equipment and supplies, the student will be required to post service charges and payments.

EQUIPMENT AND SUPPLIES
- MACC/computer (practice)
- Calculator
- Daysheet (daily journal)
- Ledger cards
- Previous day's balance
- List of patients and services
- Fee schedule
- Receipt
- Encounter form
- Information sheet
- Pen or pencil

STANDARDS: Complete the procedure within _____ minutes and achieve a minimum score of _____%.

Time began _____   Time ended _____

Steps	Possible Points	First Attempt	Second Attempt
1. Assemble all supplies and equipment.	5		
2. Prepare the daysheet for today's activities.	15		
3. Date the daysheet and carry forward appropriate previous page balances. a. "A" $1220 b. "B1" $2015 c. "B2" $105 d. "C" $902 e. "D" $1802	10		
4. Complete the ledger cards for patients scheduled for appointments including demographics. (See information sheet.)	10		
5. Prepare the ledger card and the charge slip for today's visit. (If preparing just the ledger card, move to Step 8.)	10		
6. Attach the charge slip to patient's chart, and store ledger card as appropriate.	10		

PROCEDURE 28-2

685

Copyright © 2010, 2005 by Saunders, an imprint of Elsevier, Inc. All rights reserved.

Steps	Possible Points	First Attempt	Second Attempt
7. Locate, on the pegboard, the receipt with the number that matched the number on the patient's charge slip.	10		
8. After professional visit, reinsert receipt-charge slip and the patient's ledger card to the daysheet, and complete encounter form.	10		
9. Obtain payment, and record the payment amount and the new balance.	10		
10. Remove the completed receipt from the pegboard and give the patient the receipt.	10		
11. Refile the ledger card.	10		
12. Check all columns of the daysheet using a pencil to verify totals are accurately recorded.	10		
13. At the end of the day, total the figures in each column, and add to prove sheet balances.	10		
14. Add previous page totals and today's totals and prove balances of columns.	10		
15. Write, in ink, the proof totals on the bottom of the daysheet, and add the total number of pages in the Sheet Number space at the top of the daysheet pages.	10		
Total Points Possible (Using Pegboard)	150		
Total Points Possible (Not Using Pegboard)	130		

Comments: Total Points Earned _____

Divided by _____

Total Possible Points = _____ % Score

Instructor's Signature _____

Information for Procedure 28-2

For each patient you will complete the following:
- Ledger card
- Encounter form for the day's activities
- Enter transaction on the daysheet
- Complete a receipt

Ledger Cards: Previous Balance (PB)

Linda Martinez	Kathleen Peavy	Henry Nadkarni
678 Main St	3214 Trailway Dr	9087 Oneway
Lindale, WI 87645	Largo, WI 87654	Brentlawn, WI 87625
Home: 657-543-8897	Home: 657-987-3232	Home: 432-987-3218
(PB: -0-)	(PB: $515.00)	(PB: $57)

James Muno	Katie Curley	David Stern
633 Pinecone Rd	2656 Cerlew	967 45th St
Lawton, WI 87624	Busk, WI 87653	Ridgewood, WI 87654
Home: 657-678-9806	Home: 657-358-3452	Home: 432-953-1246
(PB: -0-)	(PB: -0-)	(PB: $65)

Date: 7/31/XX for Daysheet Activities
The physicians offer a 30% discount for self-pay patients and accept assignment (taking the payment that the insurance company provides) from most insurance companies.

Transactions:

1. Linda Martinez is a new patient. She just moved to the area and wants to establish herself with a physician because there is a history of diabetes in the family. Dr. Lopez has an opening at 8:30 a.m. Besides the office visit (99201) charge, Dr. Lopez orders an ECG (93000) and a urinalysis (81002). Her total for today is $112.00, and because she has no insurance she writes a check (#907) for $78.40. Dr. Lopez would like to see her again in 3 months.

2. Kathleen Peavy is seeing Dr. Lawler today at 9:00 a.m. for a follow-up visit after her surgery 10 days ago. There is no charge for today's visit (99212). Her insurance company (Blue Cross/Blue Shield) has been billed $515.00 for her surgery. Dr. Lawler wants to see her again in 1 month.

3. Henry Nadkarni is seeing Dr. Hughes today at 9:15 a.m. to have a stress test (93015). His total charges for today are $343.00, which includes his office visit (99212) and stress test. Dx: 786.50. Dr. Hughes is referring him to a cardiologist. When leaving, Mr. Nadkarni pays his $20.00 co-payment with cash. Aetna will be billed for today's services.

4. James Muno has an appointment at 9:15 a.m. with Dr. Lopez. His chief complaint today is he is having trouble hearing. After examination, Dr. Lopez orders ear irrigation for the removal of impacted cerumen. His insurance company (Ciega) will be billed for the office visit (99212) and cerumen removal. No follow-up is necessary unless symptoms reoccur.

5. Katie Curley, a long-time patient of Dr. Hughes, sees him today for recurring respiratory problems (SOB) and chest pain. An ECG was done followed by spirometry testing. Dx: COPD. Her office visit (99213) plus the ECG and spirometry testing totaled $160.00. Her insurance company (ABC) will be billed. Dr Hughes wants to see her in 1 month to evaluate her new medication.

6. David Stern sees Dr. Lawler today for a sigmoidoscopy. His office visit (99212) and procedure total $193.00 He writes a check (#207) for $65.00 to cover an outstanding balance. Dr. Lawler would like to see him in 3 months unless he has another episode of rectal bleeding. Dx: Rectal bleeding.

PATIENT LEDGER

XYZ Medical Center
901 South Street
Anytown, USA 33322
(123) 456-7890

STATEMENT TO:

DATE	PROFESSIONAL SERVICE	CHARGE	PAYMENT	ADJUST-MENT	NEW BALANCE
			PREVIOUS BALANCE		

(Modified from Hunt SA: *Fundamentals of medical assisting student mastery manual,* Philadelphia, 2002, Saunders.)

Copyright © 2010, 2005 by Saunders, an imprint of Elsevier, Inc. All rights reserved.

PATIENT LEDGER

XYZ Medical Center
901 South Street
Anytown, USA 33322
(123) 456-7890

STATEMENT TO:

DATE	PROFESSIONAL SERVICE	CHARGE	PAYMENT	ADJUST-MENT	PREVIOUS BALANCE
					NEW BALANCE

(Modified from Hunt SA: *Fundamentals of medical assisting student mastery manual,* Philadelphia, 2002, Saunders.)

PATIENT LEDGER

XYZ Medical Center
901 South Street
Anytown, USA 33322
(123) 456-7890

STATEMENT TO:

DATE	PROFESSIONAL SERVICE	CHARGE	PAYMENT	ADJUST-MENT	PREVIOUS BALANCE
					NEW BALANCE

(Modified from Hunt SA: *Fundamentals of medical assisting student mastery manual,* Philadelphia, 2002, Saunders.)

Copyright © 2010, 2005 by Saunders, an imprint of Elsevier, Inc. All rights reserved.

PATIENT LEDGER

XYZ Medical Center
901 South Street
Anytown, USA 33322
(123) 456-7890

STATEMENT TO:

DATE	PROFESSIONAL SERVICE	CHARGE	PAYMENT	ADJUST-MENT	PREVIOUS BALANCE
					NEW BALANCE

(Modified from Hunt SA: *Fundamentals of medical assisting student mastery manual,* Philadelphia, 2002, Saunders.)

Copyright © 2010, 2005 by Saunders, an imprint of Elsevier, Inc. All rights reserved.

PATIENT LEDGER

XYZ Medical Center
901 South Street
Anytown, USA 33322
(123) 456-7890

STATEMENT TO:

				PREVIOUS BALANCE	
DATE	PROFESSIONAL SERVICE	CHARGE	PAYMENT	ADJUST-MENT	NEW BALANCE

(Modified from Hunt SA: *Fundamentals of medical assisting student mastery manual,* Philadelphia, 2002, Saunders.)

Copyright © 2010, 2005 by Saunders, an imprint of Elsevier, Inc. All rights reserved.

PATIENT LEDGER

XYZ Medical Center
901 South Street
Anytown, USA 33322
(123) 456-7890

STATEMENT TO:

DATE	PROFESSIONAL SERVICE	CHARGE	PAYMENT	ADJUST-MENT	PREVIOUS BALANCE	
					NEW BALANCE	

(Modified from Hunt SA: *Fundamentals of medical assisting student mastery manual,* Philadelphia, 2002, Saunders.)

PROCEDURE 28-2

Date: _____ Sheet #: _____ Day sheet

| Date | Reference | Description | Charge | Credits | | Current balance | Previous balance | | Name | Receipt | ABA | Cash | Checks |
				Payment	Adjustment								

	Column A	Column B-1	Column B-2	Column C	Column D				Cash	Checks

Proof of posting

This page	
Previous page	
Month-to-date	

Column D total	
Plus column A total	
Subtotal	
Less total cols. B-1 and B-2	
Must equal column C	

Accounts receivable control

Previous day total	
Plus total charges	
Subtotal	
Less payments/adjustments	
Total accounts receivable	$0.00

Accounts receivable proof

Accounts receivable first of the month	
Plus column A month-to-date	
Subtotal	
Less columns B-1 and B2 month-to-date	
Total accounts receivable	$0.00

Total deposit $0.00

Copyright © 2010, 2005 by Saunders, an imprint of Elsevier, Inc. All rights reserved.

JOURNAL OF DAILY CHARGES & PAYMENTS

	DATE	PROFESSIONAL SERVICE	FEE	PAYMENT	ADJUST-MENT	NEW BALANCE	OLD BALANCE	PATIENT'S NAME	
1									1
2									2
3									3
4									4
5									5
6									6
7									7
8									8
9									9
10									10
11									11
12									12
13									13
14									14
15									15
16									16
17									17
18									18
19									19
20									20
21									21
22									22
23									23
24									24
25									25
26									26
27									27
28									28
29									29
30									30
31								TOTALS THIS PAGE	31
32								TOTAL PREVIOUS PAGE	32
33								TOTALS MONTH TO DATE	33
			COLUMN A	COLUMN B	COLUMN C	COLUMN D	COLUMN E		

MEMO _____

DAILY - FROM LINE 31
ARITHMETIC POSTING PROOF

Column E	$
Plus Column A	
Sub-Total	
Minus Column B	
Sub-Total	
Minus Column C	
Equals Column D	

MONTH - FROM LINE 31
ACCOUNTS RECEIVABLE PROOF

Accts. Receivable Previous Day	$
Plus Column A	
Sub-Total	
Minus Column B	
Sub-Total	
Minus Column C	
Accts. receivable End of Day	

YEAR TO DATE - FROM LINE 33
ACCOUNTS RECEIVABLE PROOF

Accts. Receivable beginning of Month	$
Plus Column A MONTH TO DATE	
Sub-Totaln C	
Minus Column B MONTH TO DATE	
Sub-Total	
Minus Column C MONTH TO DATE	
Accts. receivable End of Day MONTH TO DATE	

(From Buck CJ: *Student manual with daily tasks for practice kit for medical front office skills,* St Louis, 2009, Saunders.)

Copyright © 2010, 2005 by Saunders, an imprint of Elsevier, Inc. All rights reserved.

FEE SCHEDULE

XYZ Medical Center
901 South Street
Anytown, USA 33322
(123) 456-7890

Federal Tax ID Number: 00-0000000

BCBS Group Number: 14982
Medicare Group Number: 14982

OFFICE VISIT, NEW PATIENT

Focused, 99201	$45.00
Expanded, 99202	$55.00
Intermediate, 99203	$60.00
Extended, 99204	$95.00
Comprehensive, 99205	$195.00
Consultation, 99245	$250.00

OFFICE VISIT, ESTABLISHED PATIENT

Minimal, 99211	$40.00
Focused, 99212	$48.00
Intermediate, 99213	$55.00
Extended, 99214	$65.00
Comprehensive, 99215	$195.00

OFFICE PROCEDURES

EKG, 12 lead, 93000	$55.00
Stress EKG, Treadmill, 93015	$295.00
Sigmoidoscopy, Flex; 45330	$145.00
Spirometry, 94010	$50.00
Cerumen Removal, 69210	$40.00
Collection & Handling	
Lab Specimen, 99000	$9.00
Venipuncture, 35415	$9.00
Urinalysis, 81000	$20.00
Urinalysis, 81002 (Dip Only)	$12.00
Influenza Injection, 90724	$20.00
Pneumococcal Injection, 90732	$20.00
Oral Polio, 90712	$15.00
DTaP, 90700	$20.00
Tetanus Toxoid, 90703	$15.00
MMR, 90707	$25.00
HIB, 90737	$20.00
Hepatitis B, newborn to age 11 years, 90744	$60.00
Hepatitis B, 11-19 years, 90745	$60.00
Hepatitis B, 20 years and above 90746	$60.00
Intramuscular Injection, 90788	
Penicillin	$30.00
Cephtriaxone	$25.00
Solu-Medrol	$23.00
Vitamin B-12	$13.00
Subcutaneous Injection, 90782	
Epinephrine	$18.00
Susphrine	$25.00
Insulin, U-100	$15.00

COMMON DIAGNOSTIC CODES

Ischemic Heart Disease	414.9
w/o myocardial infarction	411.89
w/coronary occlusion	411.81
Hypertension, Malignant	401.0
Benign	401.1
Unspecified	401.9
w/congest. heart failure	402.91
Asthma, Bronchial	493.9
w/ COPD	493.2
allergic, w/ S.A.	493.91
allergic, w/o S.A.	493.90
Kyphosis	737.10
w/osteoporosis	733.0
Osteoporosis	733.00
Otitis Media, Acute	382.9
Chronic	382.9

(Modified from Hunt SA: *Fundamentals of medical assisting student mastery manual,* Philadelphia, 2002, Saunders.)

XYZ Medical Center
901 South Street
Anytown, USA 33322
(123) 456-7890

GUARANTOR NAME AND ADDRESS	PATIENT NO.	PATIENT NAME		DOCTOR NO.	DATE
	DATE OF BIRTH	TELEPHONE NO.	INSURANCE		
			CODE	DESCRIPTION	CERTIFICATE NO.

OFFICE - NEW

X	CPT	SERVICE	FEE
	99201	Prob Foc/Straight	
	99202	Exp Prob/Straight	
	99203	Detailed/Low	
	99204	Compre/Moderate	
	99205	Compre/High	

OFFICE - ESTABLISHED

X	CPT	SERVICE	FEE
	99211	Nurse/Minimal	
	99212	Prob Foc/Straight	
	99213	Exp Prob/Low	
	99214	Detailed/Moderate	
	99215	Compre/High	

OFFICE - CONSULT

X	CPT	SERVICE	FEE
	99241	Prob/Foc/Straight	
	99242	Exp Prob/Straight	
	99243	Detailed/Low	
	99244	Compre/Moderate	
	99245	Compre/High	

PREVENTIVE CARE - ADULT

X	CPT	SERVICE	FEE
	99385	18-39 Initial	
	99386	40-64 Initial	
	99387	65+ Initial	
	99395	18-39 Periodic	
	99396	40-64 Periodic	
	99397	65+ Periodic	

GASTROENEROLOGY

X	CPT	SERVICE	FEE
	45300	Sigmoidoscopy Rig	
	45305	Sigmoid Rig w/bx	
	45330	Sigmoidoscopy Flex	
	45331	Sigmoid Flex w/bx	
	45378	Colonoscopy Diag	
	45380	Colonoscopy w/bx	
	46600	Anoscopy	

CARDIOLOGY & HEARING

X	CPT	SERVICE	FEE
	93000	EKG (Global)	
	93015	Stress Test (Global)	
	93224	Holter (Global)	
	93225	Holter Hook Up	
	93227	Holter Interpretation	
	94010	Pulm Function Test	
	92551	Audiometry Screen	

INJECTIONS & IMMUNIZATION

X	CPT	SERVICE	FEE
	86585	TB Skin Test	
	90716	Varicella Vaccine	
	90724	Flu Vaccine	
	90732	Pneumovax	
	90718	TD Immunization	
	90782	Injection IM*	
	90788	Injection IM Antibiot*	
		Injection joint*	
SM	MED	MAJOR	
(circle one)			
FOR ALL INJECTIONS, SUPPLY DRUG INFORMATION			

REPAIR & DERMATOLOGY

X	CPT	SERVICE	FEE
	17110	Warts: #	
		Tags: #	
		Lesion Excis	
		Lesion Destruct	
	SIZE CM:	SITE:	
	MALIG:	PREMAL/BEN:	
	(Check One Above)		
		Simple Closure	
		Intermed Closure	
	SIZE CM:	SITE:	
	10060	I&D Abscess	
	10080	I&D Cyst	

OTHER

SUPPLIES/DRUGS*
DRUG NAME:
UNIT/MEASURE:
QUANTITY

DIAGNOSTIC CODES: ICD-9-CM

- ☐ 789.0 Abdominal Pain
- ☐ 795.0 Abnormal Pap Smear
- ☐ 706.1 Acne Vulgaris
- ☐ 477.0 Allergic Rhinitis
- ☐ 285.9 Anemia, NOS
- ☐ 281.0 Pernicious
- ☐ 411.1 Angina, Unstable
- ☐ 427.9 Arythmia, NOS
- ☐ 440.9 Arteriosclerosis
- ☐ 714.0 Arthritis, Rheumatoid
- ☐ 414.0 ASHD
- ☐ 493.90 Asthma, Bronchial W/O Status Ast.
- ☐ 493.91 Asthma, Bronchial W/Status Ast.
- ☐ 466.1 Bronchiolitis, Acute
- ☐ 466.0 Bronchitis, Acute
- ☐ 727.3 Bursitis
- ☐ 786.50 Chest Pain
- ☐ 574.20 Cholelithiasis
- ☐ 372.30 Conjunctivitis, Unspecified
- ☐ 564.0 Constipation
- ☐ 496 COPD
- ☐ 692.9 Dermatitis, Allergic
- ☐ 250.01 Diabetes Mellitus, ID
- ☐ 250.00 Diabetes Mellitus, NID
- ☐ 558.9 Diarrhea
- ☐ 562.11 Diverticulitis
- ☐ 562.10 Diverticulosis

- ☐ 782.3 Edema
- ☐ 492.8 Emphysema
- ☐ V16.0 Family History Of Diabetes
- ☐ 780.6 Fever of Undetermined Origin
- ☐ 578.9 G.I. Bleeding, Unspecified
- ☐ 727.41 Ganglion of Joint
- ☐ 535.0 Gastritis, Acute
- ☐ V72.3 Arythmia, NOS
- ☐ 748.0 Headache
- ☐ 550.90 Hernia, Inguinal, NOS
- ☐ 054.9 Herpes Simplex
- ☐ 053.9 Herpes Zoster
- ☐ 708.9 Hives/Urticaria
- ☐ 401.1 Hypertension, Benign
- ☐ 401.0 Hypertension, Malignant
- ☐ 402.90 Hypertension, W/O CHF
- ☐ 244.9 Hypothyroidism, Primary
- ☐ 380.4 Impacted Cerumen
- ☐ 487.1 Influenza
- ☐ 564.1 Irritable Bowel Syndrome
- ☐ 464.0 Laryngitis, Acute
- ☐ 454.9 Leg Varicose Veins
- ☐ 424.0 Mitral Valve Prolapse
- ☐ 412 Myocardial Infarction, Old
- ☐ 715.90 Osteoarthritis, Unspec. Site
- ☐ 620.2 Ovarian Cyst

- ☐ 614.9 Pelvic Inflammatory Disease
- ☐ 685.1 Pilonidal Cyst
- ☐ 462 Pharyngitis, Acute
- ☐ 627.1 Postmenopausal Bleeding
- ☐ 625.4 Premenstrual Tension
- ☐ 782.1 Rash
- ☐ 569.3 Rectal Bleeding
- ☐ 398.90 Rheumatic Heart Disease, NOS
- ☐ 431.9 Sinusitis, Acute, NOS
- ☐ 782.1 Skin Eruption, Rash
- ☐ 845.00 Sprain, Ankle
- ☐ 848.9 Sprain, Muscle, Unspec. Site
- ☐ 785.6 Swollen Glands
- ☐ 246.9 Thyroid Disease, Unspecified
- ☐ 463 Tonsillitis, Acute

- ☐ 474.0 Tonsillitis, Chronic
- ☐ 465.9 Upper Respiratory Infection, Acute
- ☐ 599.0 Urinary Tract Infection
- ☐ V03.9 Vaccination/Bacterial Dis.
- ☐ V06.8 Vaccination/Combination
- ☐ V04.8 Vaccination, Influenza
- ☐ 616.10 Vaginitis, Vulvitis, NOS
- ☐ 780.4 Vertigo
- ☐ 787.0 Vomiting, Nausea
- ☐ _____
- ☐ _____
- ☐ _____
- ☐ _____
- ☐ _____

RETURN APPOINTMENT

_____ Days
_____ Weeks
_____ Months

Authorization Number:
▶ _____

BALANCE DUE

DATE OF SERVICE	CPT CODE	DIAGNOSIS CODE(S)	CHARGE

Place of Service:
( ) Office
( ) Emergency Room
( ) Inpatient Hospital
( ) Outpatient Hospital
( ) Nursing Home

TOTAL CHARGE	$
AMOUNT PAID	$
PREVIOUS BAL	$
BALANCE DUE	$

Check #: _____
(Circle Method of Payment)
CASH CHECK MC VISA

Physician's Signature
▶ _____

PROCEDURE 28-2

XYZ Medical Center
901 South Street
Anytown, USA 33322
(123) 456-7890

GUARANTOR NAME AND ADDRESS	PATIENT NO.	PATIENT NAME	DOCTOR NO.	DATE
	DATE OF BIRTH	TELEPHONE NO.	INSURANCE	
			CODE / DESCRIPTION	CERTIFICATE NO.

OFFICE - NEW
X	CPT	SERVICE	FEE
	99201	Prob Foc/Straight	
	99202	Exp Prob/Straight	
	99203	Detailed/Low	
	99204	Compre/Moderate	
	99205	Compre/High	

OFFICE - ESTABLISHED
X	CPT	SERVICE	FEE
	99211	Nurse/Minimal	
	99212	Prob Foc/Straight	
	99213	Exp Prob/Low	
	99214	Detailed/Moderate	
	99215	Compre/High	

OFFICE - CONSULT
X	CPT	SERVICE	FEE
	99241	Prob/Foc/Straight	
	99242	Exp Prob/Straight	
	99243	Detailed/Low	
	99244	Compre/Moderate	
	99245	Compre/High	

PREVENTIVE CARE - ADULT
X	CPT	SERVICE	FEE
	99385	18-39 Initial	
	99386	40-64 Initial	
	99387	65+ Initial	
	99395	18-39 Periodic	
	99396	40-64 Periodic	
	99397	65+ Periodic	

GASTROENEROLOGY
X	CPT	SERVICE	FEE
	45300	Sigmoidoscopy Rig	
	45305	Sigmoid Rig w/bx	
	45330	Sigmoidoscopy Flex	
	45331	Sigmoid Flex w/bx	
	45378	Colonoscopy Diag	
	45380	Colonoscopy w/bx	
	46600	Anoscopy	

CARDIOLOGY & HEARING
X	CPT	SERVICE	FEE
	93000	EKG (Global)	
	93015	Stress Test (Global)	
	93224	Holter (Global)	
	93225	Holter Hook Up	
	93227	Holter Interpretation	
	94010	Pulm Function Test	
	92551	Audiometry Screen	

INJECTIONS & IMMUNIZATION
X	CPT	SERVICE	FEE
	86585	TB Skin Test	
	90716	Varicella Vaccine	
	90724	Flu Vaccine	
	90732	Pneumovax	
	90718	TD Immunization	
	90782	Injection IM*	
	90788	Injection IM Antibiot*	
		Injection joint*	
SM	MED	MAJOR (circle one)	
FOR ALL INJECTIONS, SUPPLY DRUG INFORMATION			

REPAIR & DERMATOLOGY
X	CPT	SERVICE	FEE
	17110	Warts: #	
		Tags: #	
		Lesion Excis	
		Lesion Destruct	
	SIZE CM:	SITE:	
	MALIG:	PREMAL/BEN:	
		(Check One Above)	
		Simple Closure	
		Intermed Closure	
	SIZE CM:	SITE:	
	10060	I&D Abscess	
	10080	I&D Cyst	

OTHER

SUPPLIES/DRUGS*
DRUG NAME:
UNIT/MEASURE:
QUANTITY

DIAGNOSTIC CODES: ICD-9-CM

- [ ] 789.0 Abdominal Pain
- [ ] 795.0 Abnormal Pap Smear
- [ ] 706.1 Acne Vulgaris
- [ ] 477.0 Allergic Rhinitis
- [ ] 285.9 Anemia, NOS
- [ ] 281.0 Pernicious
- [ ] 411.1 Angina, Unstable
- [ ] 427.9 Arythmia, NOS
- [ ] 440.9 Arteriosclerosis
- [ ] 714.0 Arthritis, Rheumatoid
- [ ] 414.0 ASHD
- [ ] 493.90 Asthma, Bronchial W/O Status Ast.
- [ ] 493.91 Asthma, Bronchial W/Status Ast.
- [ ] 466.1 Bronchiolitis, Acute
- [ ] 466.0 Bronchitis, Acute
- [ ] 727.3 Bursitis
- [ ] 786.50 Chest Pain
- [ ] 574.20 Cholelithiasis
- [ ] 372.30 Conjunctivitis, Unspecified
- [ ] 564.0 Constipation
- [ ] 496 COPD
- [ ] 692.9 Dermatitis, Allergic
- [ ] 250.01 Diabetes Mellitus, ID
- [ ] 250.00 Diabetes Mellitus, NID
- [ ] 558.9 Diarrhea
- [ ] 562.11 Diverticulitis
- [ ] 562.10 Diverticulosis

- [ ] 782.3 Edema
- [ ] 492.8 Emphysema
- [ ] V16.0 Family History Of Diabetes
- [ ] 780.6 Fever of Undetermined Origin
- [ ] 578.9 G.I. Bleeding, Unspecified
- [ ] 727.41 Ganglion of Joint
- [ ] 535.0 Gastritis, Acute
- [ ] V72.3 Arythmia, NOS
- [ ] 748.0 Headache
- [ ] 550.90 Hernia, Inguinal, NOS
- [ ] 054.9 Herpes Simplex
- [ ] 053.9 Herpes Zoster
- [ ] 708.9 Hives/Urticaria
- [ ] 401.1 Hypertension, Benign
- [ ] 401.0 Hypertension, Malignant
- [ ] 402.90 Hypertension, W/O CHF
- [ ] 244.9 Hypothyroidism, Primary
- [ ] 380.4 Impacted Cerumen
- [ ] 487.1 Influenza
- [ ] 564.1 Irritable Bowel Syndrome
- [ ] 464.0 Laryngitis, Acute
- [ ] 454.9 Leg Varicose Veins
- [ ] 424.0 Mitral Valve Prolapse
- [ ] 412 Myocardial Infarction, Old
- [ ] 715.90 Osteoarthritis, Unspec. Site
- [ ] 620.2 Ovarian Cyst

- [ ] 614.9 Pelvic Inflammatory Disease
- [ ] 685.1 Pilonidal Cyst
- [ ] 462 Pharyngitis, Acute
- [ ] 627.1 Postmenopausal Bleeding
- [ ] 625.4 Premenstrual Tension
- [ ] 782.1 Rash
- [ ] 569.3 Rectal Bleeding
- [ ] 398.90 Rheumatic Heart Disease, NOS
- [ ] 431.9 Sinusitis, Acute, NOS
- [ ] 782.1 Skin Eruption, Rash
- [ ] 845.00 Sprain, Ankle
- [ ] 848.9 Sprain, Muscle, Unspec. Site
- [ ] 785.6 Swollen Glands
- [ ] 246.9 Thyroid Disease, Unspecified
- [ ] 463 Tonsillitis, Acute

- [ ] 474.0 Tonsillitis, Chronic
- [ ] 465.9 Upper Respiratory Infection, Acute
- [ ] 599.0 Urinary Tract Infection
- [ ] V03.9 Vaccination/Bacterial Dis.
- [ ] V06.8 Vaccination/Combination
- [ ] V04.8 Vaccination, Influenza
- [ ] 616.10 Vaginitis, Vulvitis, NOS
- [ ] 780.4 Vertigo
- [ ] 787.0 Vomiting, Nausea

RETURN APPOINTMENT
_____ Days
_____ Weeks
_____ Months

Authorization Number:
▶ _____

BALANCE DUE

DATE OF SERVICE	CPT CODE	DIAGNOSIS CODE(S)	CHARGE

Place of Service:
( ) Office
( ) Emergency Room
( ) Inpatient Hospital
( ) Outpatient Hospital
( ) Nursing Home

TOTAL CHARGE	$
AMOUNT PAID	$
PREVIOUS BAL	$
BALANCE DUE	$

Check #: _____
(Circle Method of Payment)
CASH   CHECK   MC   VISA

Physician's Signature
▶ _____

XYZ Medical Center
901 South Street
Anytown, USA 33322
(123) 456-7890

GUARANTOR NAME AND ADDRESS	PATIENT NO.	PATIENT NAME	DOCTOR NO.	DATE
	DATE OF BIRTH	TELEPHONE NO.	INSURANCE	
			CODE / DESCRIPTION	CERTIFICATE NO.

OFFICE - NEW
X	CPT	SERVICE	FEE
	99201	Prob Foc/Straight	
	99202	Exp Prob/Straight	
	99203	Detailed/Low	
	99204	Compre/Moderate	
	99205	Compre/High	

OFFICE - ESTABLISHED
X	CPT	SERVICE	FEE
	99211	Nurse/Minimal	
	99212	Prob Foc/Straight	
	99213	Exp Prob/Low	
	99214	Detailed/Moderate	
	99215	Compre/High	

OFFICE - CONSULT
X	CPT	SERVICE	FEE
	99241	Prob/Foc/Straight	
	99242	Exp Prob/Straight	
	99243	Detailed/Low	
	99244	Compre/Moderate	
	99245	Compre/High	

PREVENTIVE CARE - ADULT
X	CPT	SERVICE	FEE
	99385	18-39 Initial	
	99386	40-64 Initial	
	99387	65+ Initial	
	99395	18-39 Periodic	
	99396	40-64 Periodic	
	99397	65+ Periodic	

GASTROENEROLOGY
X	CPT	SERVICE	FEE
	45300	Sigmoidoscopy Rig	
	45305	Sigmoid Rig w/bx	
	45330	Sigmoidoscopy Flex	
	45331	Sigmoid Flex w/bx	
	45378	Colonoscopy Diag	
	45380	Colonoscopy w/bx	
	46600	Anoscopy	

CARDIOLOGY & HEARING
X	CPT	SERVICE	FEE
	93000	EKG (Global)	
	93015	Stress Test (Global)	
	93224	Holter (Global)	
	93225	Holter Hook Up	
	93227	Holter Interpretation	
	94010	Pulm Function Test	
	92551	Audiometry Screen	

INJECTIONS & IMMUNIZATION
X	CPT	SERVICE	FEE
	86585	TB Skin Test	
	90716	Varicella Vaccine	
	90724	Flu Vaccine	
	90732	Pneumovax	
	90718	TD Immunization	
	90782	Injection IM*	
	90788	Injection IM Antibiot*	
		Injection joint*	
SM	MED	MAJOR (circle one)	
FOR ALL INJECTIONS, SUPPLY DRUG INFORMATION			

REPAIR & DERMATOLOGY
X	CPT	SERVICE	FEE
	17110	Warts: #	
		Tags: #	
		Lesion Excis	
		Lesion Destruct	
	SIZE CM:	SITE:	
	MALIG:	PREMAL/BEN:	
	(Check One Above)		
		Simple Closure	
		Intermed Closure	
	SIZE CM:	SITE:	
	10060	I&D Abscess	
	10080	I&D Cyst	

OTHER

SUPPLIES/DRUGS*
DRUG NAME:
UNIT/MEASURE:
QUANTITY

DIAGNOSTIC CODES: ICD-9-CM

- ☐ 789.0 Abdominal Pain
- ☐ 795.0 Abnormal Pap Smear
- ☐ 706.1 Acne Vulgaris
- ☐ 477.0 Allergic Rhinitis
- ☐ 285.9 Anemia, NOS
- ☐ 281.0 Pernicious
- ☐ 411.1 Angina, Unstable
- ☐ 427.9 Arythmia, NOS
- ☐ 440.9 Arteriosclerosis
- ☐ 714.0 Arthritis, Rheumatoid
- ☐ 414.0 ASHD
- ☐ 493.90 Asthma, Bronchial W/O Status Ast.
- ☐ 493.91 Asthma, Bronchial W/Status Ast.
- ☐ 466.1 Bronchiolitis, Acute
- ☐ 466.0 Bronchitis, Acute
- ☐ 727.3 Bursitis
- ☐ 786.50 Chest Pain
- ☐ 574.20 Cholelithiasis
- ☐ 372.30 Conjunctivitis, Unspecified
- ☐ 564.0 Constipation
- ☐ 496   COPD
- ☐ 692.9 Dermatitis, Allergic
- ☐ 250.01 Diabetes Mellitus, ID
- ☐ 250.00 Diabetes Mellitus, NID
- ☐ 558.9 Diarrhea
- ☐ 562.11 Diverticulitis
- ☐ 562.10 Diverticulosis

- ☐ 782.3 Edema
- ☐ 492.8 Emphysema
- ☐ V16.0 Family History Of Diabetes
- ☐ 780.6 Fever of Undetermined Origin
- ☐ 578.9 G.I. Bleeding, Unspecified
- ☐ 727.41 Ganglion of Joint
- ☐ 535.0 Gastritis, Acute
- ☐ V72.3 Arythmia, NOS
- ☐ 748.0 Headache
- ☐ 550.90 Hernia, Inguinal, NOS
- ☐ 054.9 Herpes Simplex
- ☐ 053.9 Herpes Zoster
- ☐ 708.9 Hives/Urticaria
- ☐ 401.1 Hypertension, Benign
- ☐ 401.0 Hypertension, Malignant
- ☐ 402.90 Hypertension, W/O CHF
- ☐ 244.9 Hypothyroidism, Primary
- ☐ 380.4 Impacted Cerumen
- ☐ 487.1 Influenza
- ☐ 564.1 Irritable Bowel Syndrome
- ☐ 464.0 Laryngitis, Acute
- ☐ 454.9 Leg Varicose Veins
- ☐ 424.0 Mitral Valve Prolapse
- ☐ 412   Myocardial Infarction, Old
- ☐ 715.90 Osteoarthritis, Unspec. Site
- ☐ 620.2 Ovarian Cyst

- ☐ 614.9 Pelvic Inflammatory Disease
- ☐ 685.1 Pilonidal Cyst
- ☐ 462   Pharyngitis, Acute
- ☐ 627.1 Postmenopausal Bleeding
- ☐ 625.4 Premenstrual Tension
- ☐ 782.1 Rash
- ☐ 569.3 Rectal Bleeding
- ☐ 398.90 Rheumatic Heart Disease, NOS
- ☐ 431.9 Sinusitis, Acute, NOS
- ☐ 782.1 Skin Eruption, Rash
- ☐ 845.00 Sprain, Ankle
- ☐ 848.9 Sprain, Muscle, Unspec. Site
- ☐ 785.6 Swollen Glands
- ☐ 246.9 Thyroid Disease, Unspecified
- ☐ 463   Tonsillitis, Acute

- ☐ 474.0 Tonsillitis, Chronic
- ☐ 465.9 Upper Respiratory Infection, Acute
- ☐ 599.0 Urinary Tract Infection
- ☐ V03.9 Vaccination/Bacterial Dis.
- ☐ V06.8 Vaccination/Combination
- ☐ V04.8 Vaccination, Influenza
- ☐ 616.10 Vaginitis, Vulvitis, NOS
- ☐ 780.4 Vertigo
- ☐ 787.0 Vomiting, Nausea
- ☐ _____ _____
- ☐ _____ _____
- ☐ _____ _____
- ☐ _____ _____

RETURN APPOINTMENT
_____ Days
_____ Weeks
_____ Months

Authorization Number:
▶ _____

BALANCE DUE

DATE OF SERVICE	CPT CODE	DIAGNOSIS CODE(S)	CHARGE

Place of Service:
( ) Office
( ) Emergency Room
( ) Inpatient Hospital
( ) Outpatient Hospital
( ) Nursing Home

TOTAL CHARGE	$
AMOUNT PAID	$
PREVIOUS BAL	$
BALANCE DUE	$

Check #: _____
(Circle Method of Payment)
CASH   CHECK   MC   VISA

Physician's Signature
▶ _____

PROCEDURE 28-2

XYZ Medical Center
901 South Street
Anytown, USA 33322
(123) 456-7890

GUARANTOR NAME AND ADDRESS	PATIENT NO.	PATIENT NAME	DOCTOR NO.	DATE
	DATE OF BIRTH	TELEPHONE NO.	INSURANCE	CERTIFICATE NO.
			CODE / DESCRIPTION	

OFFICE - NEW
X	CPT	SERVICE	FEE
	99201	Prob Foc/Straight	
	99202	Exp Prob/Straight	
	99203	Detailed/Low	
	99204	Compre/Moderate	
	99205	Compre/High	

OFFICE - ESTABLISHED
X	CPT	SERVICE	FEE
	99211	Nurse/Minimal	
	99212	Prob Foc/Straight	
	99213	Exp Prob/Low	
	99214	Detailed/Moderate	
	99215	Compre/High	

OFFICE - CONSULT
X	CPT	SERVICE	FEE
	99241	Prob/Foc/Straight	
	99242	Exp Prob/Straight	
	99243	Detailed/Low	
	99244	Compre/Moderate	
	99245	Compre/High	

PREVENTIVE CARE - ADULT
X	CPT	SERVICE	FEE
	99385	18-39 Initial	
	99386	40-64 Initial	
	99387	65+ Initial	
	99395	18-39 Periodic	
	99396	40-64 Periodic	
	99397	65+ Periodic	

GASTROENEROLOGY
X	CPT	SERVICE	FEE
	45300	Sigmoidoscopy Rig	
	45305	Sigmoid Rig w/bx	
	45330	Sigmoidoscopy Flex	
	45331	Sigmoid Flex w/bx	
	45378	Colonoscopy Diag	
	45380	Colonoscopy w/bx	
	46600	Anoscopy	

CARDIOLOGY & HEARING
X	CPT	SERVICE	FEE
	93000	EKG (Global)	
	93015	Stress Test (Global)	
	93224	Holter (Global)	
	93225	Holter Hook Up	
	93227	Holter Interpretation	
	94010	Pulm Function Test	
	92551	Audiometry Screen	

INJECTIONS & IMMUNIZATION
X	CPT	SERVICE	FEE
	86585	TB Skin Test	
	90716	Varicella Vaccine	
	90724	Flu Vaccine	
	90732	Pneumovax	
	90718	TD Immunization	
	90782	Injection IM*	
	90788	Injection IM Antibiot*	
		Injection joint*	

SM   MED   MAJOR   (circle one)
FOR ALL INJECTIONS, SUPPLY DRUG INFORMATION

REPAIR & DERMATOLOGY
X	CPT	SERVICE	FEE
	17110	Warts: #	
		Tags: #	
		Lesion Excis	
		Lesion Destruct	
		SIZE CM: SITE: MALIG: PREMAL/BEN: (Check One Above)	
		Simple Closure	
		Intermed Closure	
		SIZE CM: SITE:	
	10060	I&D Abscess	
	10080	I&D Cyst	

OTHER
(blank)

SUPPLIES/DRUGS*
DRUG NAME:
UNIT/MEASURE:
QUANTITY

DIAGNOSTIC CODES: ICD-9-CM

- 789.0 Abdominal Pain
- 795.0 Abnormal Pap Smear
- 706.1 Acne Vulgaris
- 477.0 Allergic Rhinitis
- 285.9 Anemia, NOS
- 281.0 Pernicious
- 411.1 Angina, Unstable
- 427.9 Arythmia, NOS
- 440.9 Arteriosclerosis
- 714.0 Arthritis, Rheumatoid
- 414.0 ASHD
- 493.90 Asthma, Bronchial W/O Status Ast.
- 493.91 Asthma, Bronchial W/Status Ast.
- 466.1 Bronchiolitis, Acute
- 466.0 Bronchitis, Acute
- 727.3 Bursitis
- 786.50 Chest Pain
- 574.20 Cholelithiasis
- 372.30 Conjunctivitis, Unspecified
- 564.0 Constipation
- 496 COPD
- 692.9 Dermatitis, Allergic
- 250.01 Diabetes Mellitus, ID
- 250.00 Diabetes Mellitus, NID
- 558.9 Diarrhea
- 562.11 Diverticulitis
- 562.10 Diverticulosis

- 782.3 Edema
- 492.8 Emphysema
- V16.0 Family History Of Diabetes
- 780.6 Fever of Undetermined Origin
- 578.9 G.I. Bleeding, Unspecified
- 727.41 Ganglion of Joint
- 535.0 Gastritis, Acute
- V72.3 Arythmia, NOS
- 748.8 Headache
- 550.90 Hernia, Inguinal, NOS
- 054.9 Herpes Simplex
- 053.9 Herpes Zoster
- 708.9 Hives/Urticaria
- 401.1 Hypertension, Benign
- 401.0 Hypertension, Malignant
- 402.90 Hypertension, W/O CHF
- 244.9 Hypothyroidism, Primary
- 380.4 Impacted Cerumen
- 487.1 Influenza
- 564.1 Irritable Bowel Syndrome
- 464.0 Laryngitis, Acute
- 454.0 Leg Varicose Veins
- 424.0 Mitral Valve Prolapse
- 412 Myocardial Infarction, Old
- 715.90 Osteoarthritis, Unspec. Site
- 620.2 Ovarian Cyst

- 614.9 Pelvic Inflammatory Disease
- 685.1 Pilonidal Cyst
- 462 Pharyngitis, Acute
- 627.1 Postmenopausal Bleeding
- 625.4 Premenstrual Tension
- 782.1 Rash
- 569.3 Rectal Bleeding
- 398.90 Rheumatic Heart Disease, NOS
- 431.9 Sinusitis, Acute, NOS
- 782.1 Skin Eruption, Rash
- 845.00 Sprain, Ankle
- 848.9 Sprain, Muscle, Unspec. Site
- 785.6 Swollen Glands
- 246.9 Thyroid Disease, Unspecified
- 463 Tonsillitis, Acute

- 474.0 Tonsillitis, Chronic
- 465.9 Upper Respiratory Infection, Acute
- 599.0 Urinary Tract Infection
- V03.9 Vaccination/Bacterial Dis.
- V06.8 Vaccination/Combination
- V04.8 Vaccination, Influenza
- 616.10 Vaginitis, Vulvitis, NOS
- 780.4 Vertigo
- 787.0 Vomiting, Nausea

RETURN APPOINTMENT
_____ Days
_____ Weeks
_____ Months

Authorization Number: _____

BALANCE DUE
DATE OF SERVICE	CPT CODE	DIAGNOSIS CODE(S)	CHARGE

Place of Service:
( ) Office
( ) Emergency Room
( ) Inpatient Hospital
( ) Outpatient Hospital
( ) Nursing Home

TOTAL CHARGE	$
AMOUNT PAID	$
PREVIOUS BAL	$
BALANCE DUE	$

Check #: _____
(Circle Method of Payment)
CASH   CHECK   MC   VISA

Physician's Signature
▶ _____

XYZ Medical Center
901 South Street
Anytown, USA 33322
(123) 456-7890

GUARANTOR NAME AND ADDRESS	PATIENT NO.	PATIENT NAME		DOCTOR NO.	DATE
	DATE OF BIRTH	TELEPHONE NO.	INSURANCE		
			CODE / DESCRIPTION	CERTIFICATE NO.	

OFFICE - NEW

X	CPT	SERVICE	FEE
	99201	Prob Foc/Straight	
	99202	Exp Prob/Straight	
	99203	Detailed/Low	
	99204	Compre/Moderate	
	99205	Compre/High	

OFFICE - ESTABLISHED

X	CPT	SERVICE	FEE
	99211	Nurse/Minimal	
	99212	Prob Foc/Straight	
	99213	Exp Prob/Low	
	99214	Detailed/Moderate	
	99215	Compre/High	

OFFICE - CONSULT

X	CPT	SERVICE	FEE
	99241	Prob/Foc/Straight	
	99242	Exp Prob/Straight	
	99243	Detailed/Low	
	99244	Compre/Moderate	
	99245	Compre/High	

PREVENTIVE CARE - ADULT

X	CPT	SERVICE	FEE
	99385	18-39 Initial	
	99386	40-64 Initial	
	99387	65+ Initial	
	99395	18-39 Periodic	
	99396	40-64 Periodic	
	99397	65+ Periodic	

GASTROENEROLOGY

X	CPT	SERVICE	FEE
	45300	Sigmoidoscopy Rig	
	45305	Sigmoid Rig w/bx	
	45330	Sigmoidoscopy Flex	
	45331	Sigmoid Flex w/bx	
	45378	Colonoscopy Diag	
	45380	Colonoscopy w/bx	
	46600	Anoscopy	

CARDIOLOGY & HEARING

X	CPT	SERVICE	FEE
	93000	EKG (Global)	
	93015	Stress Test (Global)	
	93224	Holter (Global)	
	93225	Holter Hook Up	
	93227	Holter Interpretation	
	94010	Pulm Function Test	
	92551	Audiometry Screen	

INJECTIONS & IMMUNIZATION

X	CPT	SERVICE	FEE
	86585	TB Skin Test	
	90716	Varicella Vaccine	
	90724	Flu Vaccine	
	90732	Pneumovax	
	90718	TD Immunization	
	90782	Injection IM*	
	90788	Injection IM Antibiot*	
		Injection joint*	

SM MED MAJOR
(circle one)
FOR ALL INJECTIONS, SUPPLY DRUG INFORMATION

REPAIR & DERMATOLOGY

X	CPT	SERVICE	FEE
	17110	Warts: #	
		Tags: #	
		Lesion Excis	
		Lesion Destruct	

SIZE CM: SITE:
MALIG: PREMAL/BEN:
(Check One Above)

| | | Simple Closure | |
| | | Intermed Closure | |

SIZE CM: SITE:

| | 10060 | I&D Abscess | |
| | 10080 | I&D Cyst | |

OTHER

SUPPLIES/DRUGS*

DRUG NAME:
UNIT/MEASURE:
QUANTITY

DIAGNOSTIC CODES: ICD-9-CM

- [ ] 789.0 Abdominal Pain
- [ ] 795.0 Abnormal Pap Smear
- [ ] 706.1 Acne Vulgaris
- [ ] 477.0 Allergic Rhinitis
- [ ] 285.9 Anemia, NOS
- [ ] 281.0 Pernicious
- [ ] 411.1 Angina, Unstable
- [ ] 427.9 Arythmia, NOS
- [ ] 440.9 Arteriosclerosis
- [ ] 714.0 Arthritis, Rheumatoid
- [ ] 414.0 ASHD
- [ ] 493.90 Asthma, Bronchial W/O Status Ast.
- [ ] 493.91 Asthma, Bronchial W/Status Ast.
- [ ] 466.1 Bronchiolitis, Acute
- [ ] 466.0 Bronchitis, Acute
- [ ] 727.3 Bursitis
- [ ] 786.50 Chest Pain
- [ ] 574.20 Cholelithiasis
- [ ] 372.30 Conjunctivitis, Unspecified
- [ ] 564.0 Constipation
- [ ] 496 COPD
- [ ] 692.9 Dermatitis, Allergic
- [ ] 250.01 Diabetes Mellitus, ID
- [ ] 250.00 Diabetes Mellitus, NID
- [ ] 558.9 Diarrhea
- [ ] 562.11 Diverticulitis
- [ ] 562.10 Diverticulosis

- [ ] 782.3 Edema
- [ ] 492.8 Emphysema
- [ ] V16.0 Family History Of Diabetes
- [ ] 780.6 Fever of Undetermined Origin
- [ ] 578.9 G.I. Bleeding, Unspecified
- [ ] 727.41 Ganglion of Joint
- [ ] 535.0 Gastritis, Acute
- [ ] V72.3 Arythmia, NOS
- [ ] 748.0 Headache
- [ ] 550.90 Hernia, Inguinal, NOS
- [ ] 054.9 Herpes Simplex
- [ ] 053.9 Herpes Zoster
- [ ] 708.9 Hives/Urticaria
- [ ] 401.1 Hypertension, Benign
- [ ] 401.0 Hypertension, Malignant
- [ ] 402.90 Hypertension, W/O CHF
- [ ] 244.9 Hypothyroidism, Primary
- [ ] 380.4 Impacted Cerumen
- [ ] 487.1 Influenza
- [ ] 564.1 Irritable Bowel Syndrome
- [ ] 464.0 Laryngitis, Acute
- [ ] 454.9 Leg Varicose Veins
- [ ] 424.0 Mitral Valve Prolapse
- [ ] 412 Myocardial Infarction, Old
- [ ] 715.90 Osteoarthritis, Unspec. Site
- [ ] 620.2 Ovarian Cyst

- [ ] 614.9 Pelvic Inflammatory Disease
- [ ] 685.1 Pilonidal Cyst
- [ ] 462 Pharyngitis, Acute
- [ ] 627.1 Postmenopausal Bleeding
- [ ] 625.4 Premenstrual Tension
- [ ] 782.1 Rash
- [ ] 569.3 Rectal Bleeding
- [ ] 398.90 Rheumatic Heart Disease, NOS
- [ ] 431.9 Sinusitis, Acute, NOS
- [ ] 782.1 Skin Eruption, Rash
- [ ] 845.00 Sprain, Ankle
- [ ] 848.9 Sprain, Muscle, Unspec. Site
- [ ] 785.6 Swollen Glands
- [ ] 246.9 Thyroid Disease, Unspecified
- [ ] 463 Tonsillitis, Acute

- [ ] 474.0 Tonsillitis, Chronic
- [ ] 465.9 Upper Respiratory Infection, Acute
- [ ] 599.0 Urinary Tract Infection
- [ ] V03.9 Vaccination/Bacterial Dis.
- [ ] V06.8 Vaccination/Combination
- [ ] V04.8 Vaccination, Influenza
- [ ] 616.10 Vaginitis, Vulvitis, NOS
- [ ] 780.4 Vertigo
- [ ] 787.0 Vomiting, Nausea
- [ ] _____
- [ ] _____
- [ ] _____
- [ ] _____

RETURN APPOINTMENT

_____ Days
_____ Weeks
_____ Months

Authorization Number:
▶ _____

BALANCE DUE

DATE OF SERVICE	CPT CODE	DIAGNOSIS CODE(S)	CHARGE

Place of Service:
( ) Office
( ) Emergency Room
( ) Inpatient Hospital
( ) Outpatient Hospital
( ) Nursing Home

TOTAL CHARGE	$
AMOUNT PAID	$
PREVIOUS BAL	$
BALANCE DUE	$

Check #: _____
(Circle Method of Payment)
CASH CHECK MC VISA

Physician's Signature
▶ _____

PROCEDURE 28-2

APPENDIX A Supplemental Chapter Materials

XYZ Medical Center
901 South Street
Anytown, USA 33322
(123) 456-7890

GUARANTOR NAME AND ADDRESS	PATIENT NO.	PATIENT NAME	DOCTOR NO.	DATE
	DATE OF BIRTH	TELEPHONE NO.	INSURANCE: CODE / DESCRIPTION	CERTIFICATE NO.

OFFICE - NEW
X	CPT	SERVICE	FEE
	99201	Prob Foc/Straight	
	99202	Exp Prob/Straight	
	99203	Detailed/Low	
	99204	Compre/Moderate	
	99205	Compre/High	

OFFICE - ESTABLISHED
X	CPT	SERVICE	FEE
	99211	Nurse/Minimal	
	99212	Prob Foc/Straight	
	99213	Exp Prob/Low	
	99214	Detailed/Moderate	
	99215	Compre/High	

OFFICE - CONSULT
X	CPT	SERVICE	FEE
	99241	Prob Foc/Straight	
	99242	Exp Prob/Straight	
	99243	Detailed/Low	
	99244	Compre/Moderate	
	99245	Compre/High	

PREVENTIVE CARE - ADULT
X	CPT	SERVICE	FEE
	99385	18-39 Initial	
	99386	40-64 Initial	
	99387	65+ Initial	
	99395	18-39 Periodic	
	99396	40-64 Periodic	
	99397	65+ Periodic	

GASTROENEROLOGY
X	CPT	SERVICE	FEE
	45300	Sigmoidoscopy Rig	
	45305	Sigmoid Rig w/bx	
	45330	Sigmoidoscopy Flex	
	45331	Sigmoid Flex w/bx	
	45378	Colonoscopy Diag	
	45380	Colonoscopy w/bx	
	46600	Anoscopy	

CARDIOLOGY & HEARING
X	CPT	SERVICE	FEE
	93000	EKG (Global)	
	93015	Stress Test (Global)	
	93224	Holter (Global)	
	93225	Holter Hook Up	
	93227	Holter Interpretation	
	94010	Pulm Function Test	
	92551	Audiometry Screen	

INJECTIONS & IMMUNIZATION
X	CPT	SERVICE	FEE
	86585	TB Skin Test	
	90716	Varicella Vaccine	
	90724	Flu Vaccine	
	90732	Pneumovax	
	90718	TD Immunization	
	90782	Injection IM*	
	90788	Injection IM Antibiot*	
		Injection joint*	

SM   MED   MAJOR
(circle one)

FOR ALL INJECTIONS, SUPPLY DRUG INFORMATION

REPAIR & DERMATOLOGY
X	CPT	SERVICE	FEE
	17110	Warts: #	
		Tags: #	
		Lesion Excis	
		Lesion Destruct	
		SIZE CM: SITE:	
		MALIG: PREMAL/BEN:	
		(Check One Above)	
		Simple Closure	
		Intermed Closure	
		SIZE CM: SITE:	
	10060	I&D Abscess	
	10080	I&D Cyst	

OTHER
(blank rows)

SUPPLIES/DRUGS*
DRUG NAME:
UNIT/MEASURE:
QUANTITY

DIAGNOSTIC CODES: ICD-9-CM

- ☐ 789.0 Abdominal Pain
- ☐ 795.0 Abnormal Pap Smear
- ☐ 706.1 Acne Vulgaris
- ☐ 477.0 Allergic Rhinitis
- ☐ 285.9 Anemia, NOS
- ☐ 281.0 Pernicious
- ☐ 411.1 Angina, Unstable
- ☐ 427.9 Arythmia, NOS
- ☐ 440.9 Arteriosclerosis
- ☐ 714.0 Arthritis, Rheumatoid
- ☐ 414.0 ASHD
- ☐ 493.90 Asthma, Bronchial W/O Status Ast.
- ☐ 493.91 Asthma, Bronchial W/Status Ast.
- ☐ 466.1 Bronchiolitis, Acute
- ☐ 466.0 Bronchitis, Acute
- ☐ 727.3 Bursitis
- ☐ 786.50 Chest Pain
- ☐ 574.20 Cholelithiasis
- ☐ 372.30 Conjunctivitis, Unspecified
- ☐ 564.0 Constipation
- ☐ 496 COPD
- ☐ 692.9 Dermatitis, Allergic
- ☐ 250.01 Diabetes Mellitus, ID
- ☐ 250.00 Diabetes Mellitus, NID
- ☐ 558.9 Diarrhea
- ☐ 562.11 Diverticulitis
- ☐ 562.10 Diverticulosis

- ☐ 782.3 Edema
- ☐ 492.8 Emphysema
- ☐ V16.0 Family History Of Diabetes
- ☐ 780.6 Fever of Undetermined Origin
- ☐ 578.9 G.I. Bleeding, Unspecified
- ☐ 727.41 Ganglion of Joint
- ☐ 535.0 Gastritis, Acute
- ☐ V72.3 Arythmia, NOS
- ☐ 748.0 Headache
- ☐ 550.90 Hernia, Inguinal, NOS
- ☐ 054.9 Herpes Simplex
- ☐ 053.9 Herpes Zoster
- ☐ 708.9 Hives/Urticaria
- ☐ 401.1 Hypertension, Benign
- ☐ 401.0 Hypertension, Malignant
- ☐ 402.90 Hypertension, W/O CHF
- ☐ 244.9 Hypothyroidism, Primary
- ☐ 380.4 Impacted Cerumen
- ☐ 487.1 Influenza
- ☐ 564.1 Irritable Bowel Syndrome
- ☐ 464.9 Laryngitis, Acute
- ☐ 454.9 Leg Varicose Veins
- ☐ 424.0 Mitral Valve Prolapse
- ☐ 412 Myocardial Infarction, Old
- ☐ 715.90 Osteoarthritis, Unspec. Site
- ☐ 620.2 Ovarian Cyst

- ☐ 614.9 Pelvic Inflammatory Disease
- ☐ 685.1 Pilonidal Cyst
- ☐ 462 Pharyngitis, Acute
- ☐ 627.1 Postmenopausal Bleeding
- ☐ 625.4 Premenstrual Tension
- ☐ 782.1 Rash
- ☐ 569.3 Rectal Bleeding
- ☐ 398.90 Rheumatic Heart Disease, NOS
- ☐ 431.9 Sinusitis, Acute, NOS
- ☐ 782.1 Skin Eruption, Rash
- ☐ 845.00 Sprain, Ankle
- ☐ 848.9 Sprain, Muscle, Unspec. Site
- ☐ 785.6 Swollen Glands
- ☐ 246.9 Thyroid Disease, Unspecified
- ☐ 463 Tonsillitis, Acute

- ☐ 474.0 Tonsillitis, Chronic
- ☐ 465.9 Upper Respiratory Infection, Acute
- ☐ 599.0 Urinary Tract Infection
- ☐ V03.9 Vaccination/Bacterial Dis.
- ☐ V06.8 Vaccination/Combination
- ☐ V04.8 Vaccination, Influenza
- ☐ 616.10 Vaginitis, Vulvitis, NOS
- ☐ 780.4 Vertigo
- ☐ 787.0 Vomiting, Nausea
- ☐ _____ _____
- ☐ _____ _____
- ☐ _____ _____
- ☐ _____ _____

RETURN APPOINTMENT
_____ Days
_____ Weeks
_____ Months

Authorization Number:
▶ _____

BALANCE DUE

DATE OF SERVICE	CPT CODE	DIAGNOSIS CODE(S)	CHARGE

Place of Service:
( ) Office
( ) Emergency Room
( ) Inpatient Hospital
( ) Outpatient Hospital
( ) Nursing Home

TOTAL CHARGE	$
AMOUNT PAID	$
PREVIOUS BAL	$
BALANCE DUE	$

Check #: _____
(Circle Method of Payment)
CASH   CHECK   MC   VISA

Physician's Signature
▶ _____

(Modified from Hunt SA: *Fundamentals of medical assisting student mastery manual,* Philadelphia, 2002, Saunders.)

Copyright © 2010, 2005 by Saunders, an imprint of Elsevier, Inc. All rights reserved.

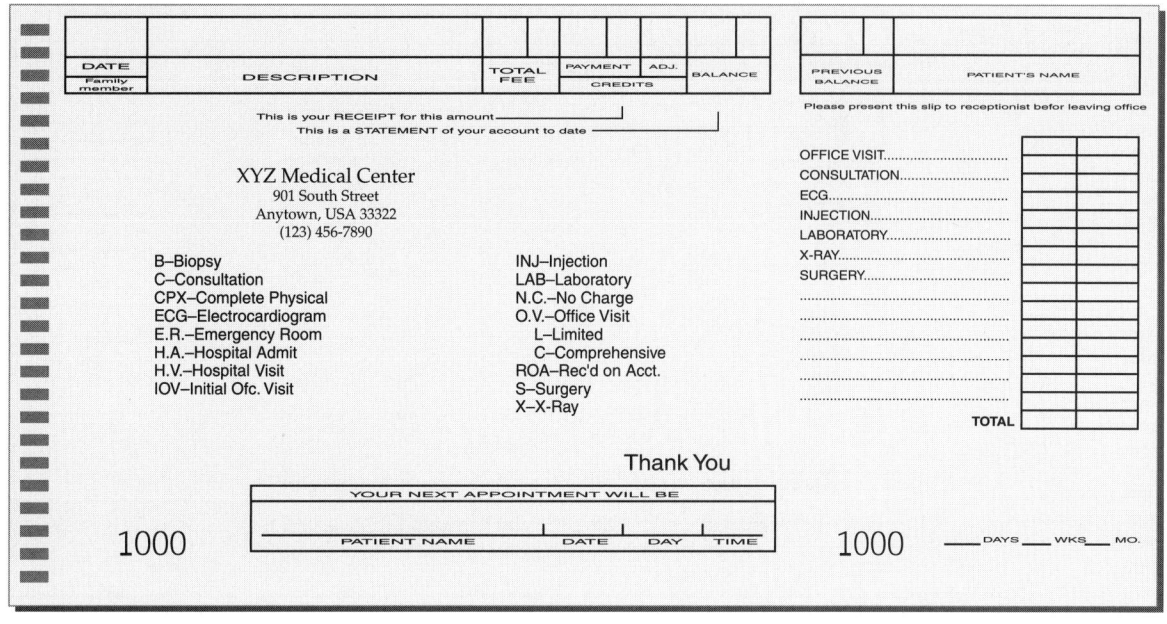

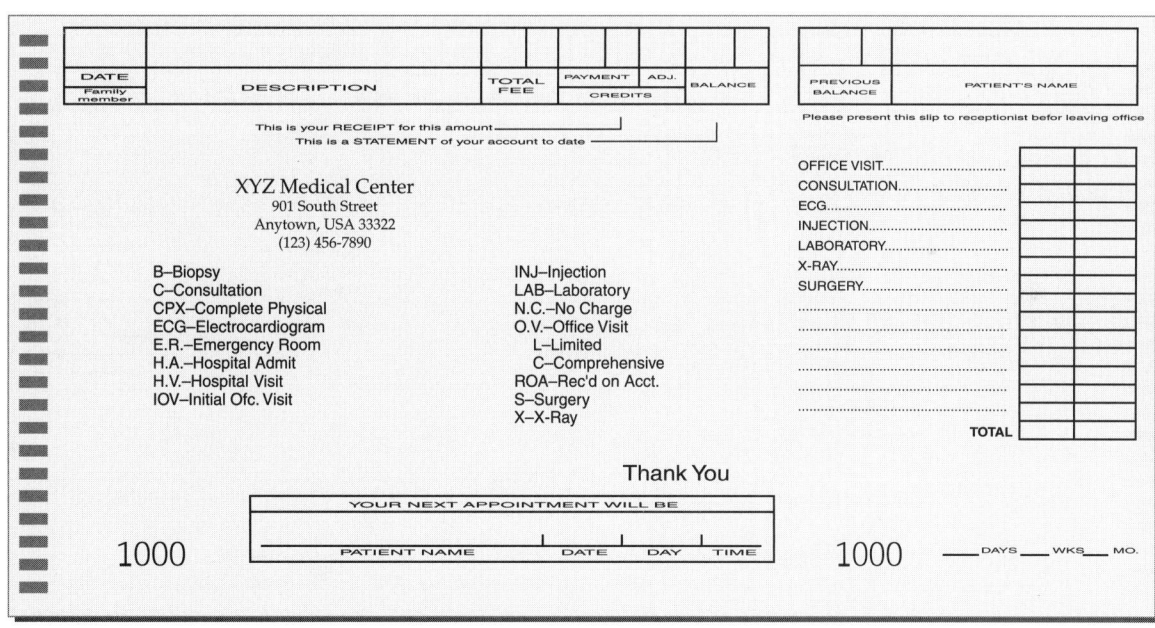

(Modified from Hunt SA: *Fundamentals of medical assisting student mastery manual,* Philadelphia, 2002, Saunders.)

APPENDIX A Supplemental Chapter Materials

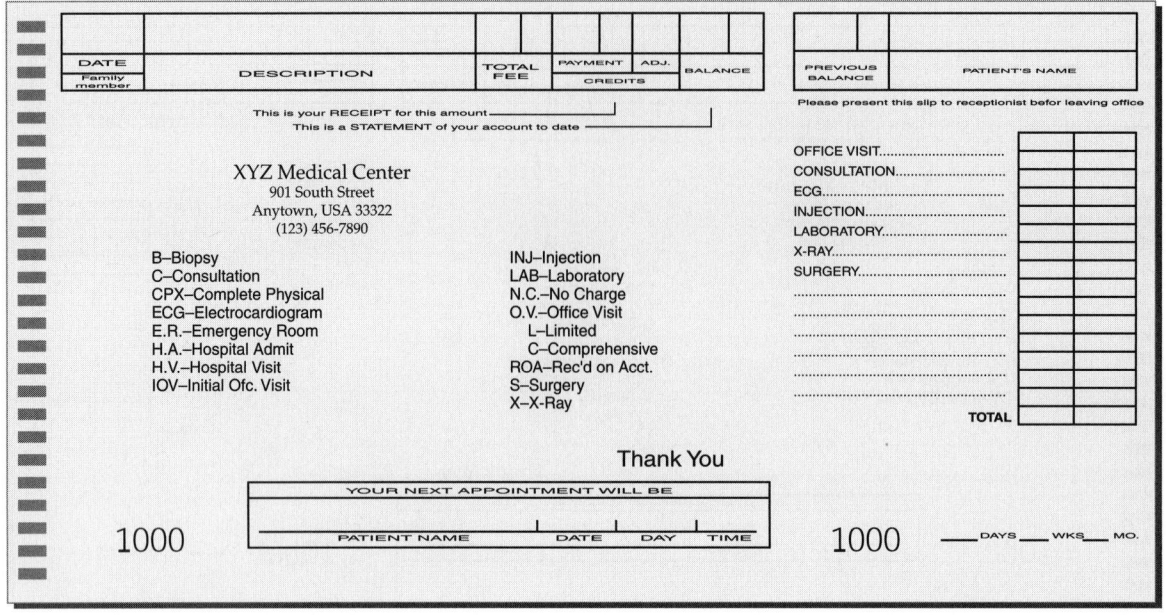

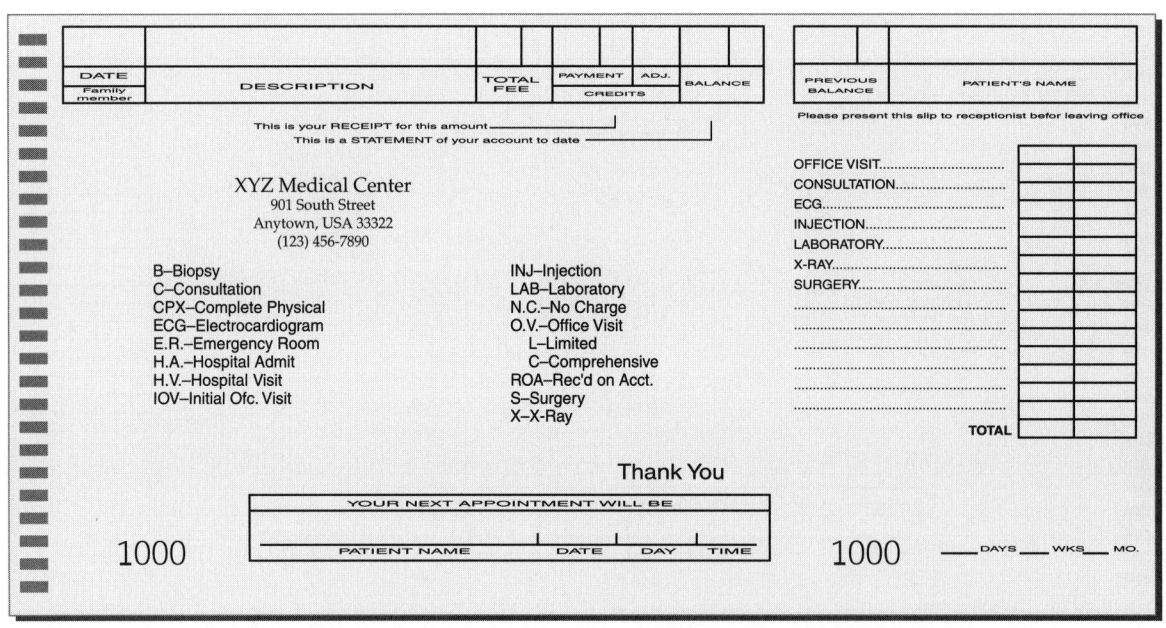

(Modified from Hunt SA: *Fundamentals of medical assisting student mastery manual,* Philadelphia, 2002, Saunders.)

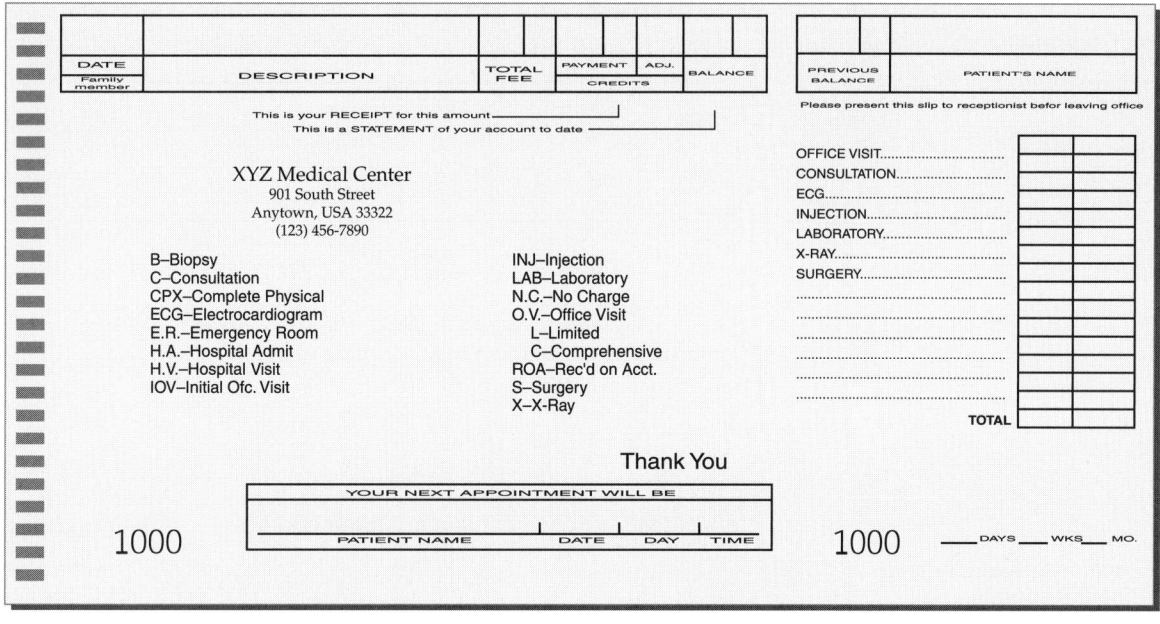

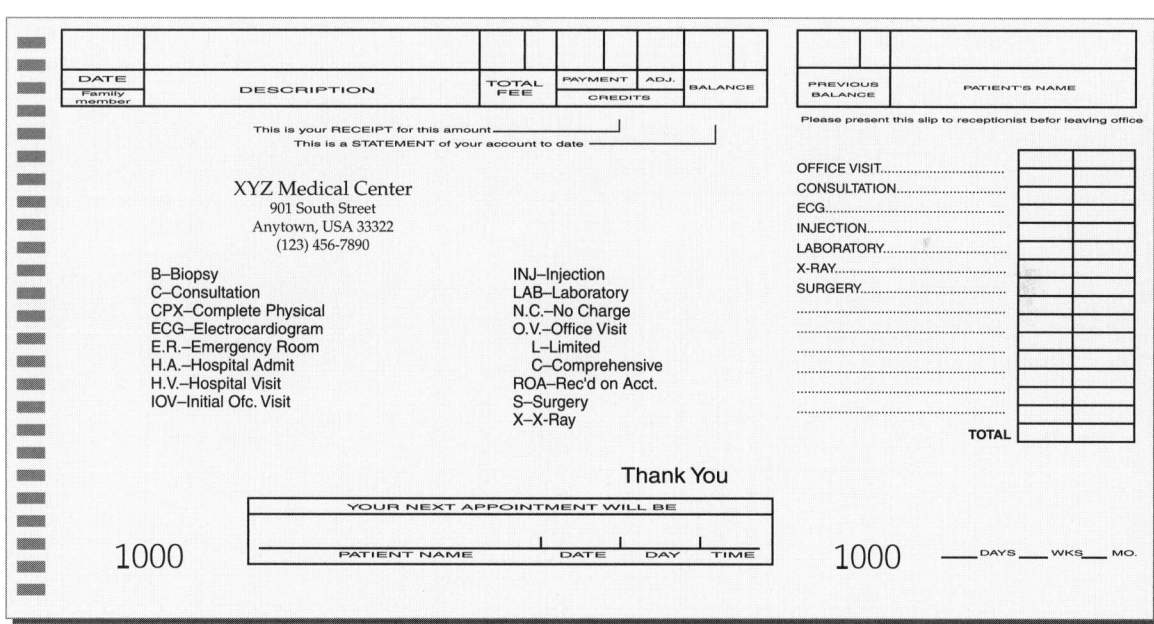

(Modified from Hunt SA: *Fundamentals of medical assisting student mastery manual,* Philadelphia, 2002, Saunders.)

Student Name: _____ DATE: _____

PROCEDURE 28-3 CHECKLIST: RECORD ADJUSTMENTS AND CREDITS TO THE PATIENT'S ACCOUNT

TASK: Record adjustments such as insurance payments, write-offs, professional discounts, and nonsufficient funds (NSF) using a daysheet.

CONDITIONS: Given the proper equipment and supplies, the student will be required to file record adjustments such as insurance payments, write-offs, professional discounts, and nonsufficient funds.

EQUIPMENT AND SUPPLIES
- MACC/computer (practice)
- Calculator
- Daysheet (daily journal)
- Ledger cards (use those from Procedure 28-2)
- Previous day's balance
- List of patients and services (information sheet)
- Sample checks
- Pen or pencil

STANDARDS: Complete the procedure within _____ minutes and achieve a minimum score of _____%.

Time began _____   Time ended _____

Steps	Possible Points	First Attempt	Second Attempt
Preparation: 1. Assemble all supplies and equipment.	5		
2. Information sheet: a. Record all transactions to the daysheet	25		
b. Post check from collection agency	5		
c. Post NSF	5		
d. Make necessary adjustments	10		
e. Process credit balance	5		
f. Process refunds	5		
g. Complete proof of posting	10		
Recording adjustments: 1. Use ledger cards (from Procedure 28-2). If using the pegboard, align it with the first available empty row on the daysheet. Otherwise, proceed to Step 2.	10		
2. Complete each ledger card as appropriate for a payment on account.	10		
3. Re-file the ledger card.	5		

Steps	Possible Points	First Attempt	Second Attempt
4. Provide information for a refund if the patient's account has a credit balance showing the adjustment for the refund on the ledger card using the appropriate information. Prepare check for signing.	10		
Recording nonsufficient funds: 1. Use ledger cards from Procedure 28-2. If using the pegboard, align it with the first available empty row on the daysheet. Otherwise, proceed to Step 2.	5		
2. Complete the ledger card as appropriate for recording an NSF check.	10		
3. Re-file the ledger card and prepare necessary documents for notification to patient.	5		
Total Points Possible	125		

Comments: Total Points Earned _____

Divided by _____

Total Possible Points = _____ % Score

Instructor's Signature _____

Information for Procedure 28-3

DATE: 8/03/XX For Day Sheet activities
The physicians offer a 30% discount for self-pay patients and accept assignment (taking the payment that the insurance company provides) from most insurance companies. Buzz Collections has an agreement in place that states the collection agency is entitled to 60% of all money collected from outstanding accounts. A $30.00 service fee is assessed on all returned checks for NSF.

Note: Previous day balances and the patients' current balances have been entered on the day sheet.

Transactions: Record the following on the day sheet:

1. Kimmith Jones is a new patient of Dr. Hughes. He travels a lot and wants to get the flu shot. He has made an appointment to receive a full physical next month. Dr. Hughes reviews his health history, does an assessment of his current health status, and has the medical assistant give him the flu shot. The office visit is $45, and the flu shot is $25. On leaving, he pays his co-pay with check #679. His insurance company will be billed.

2. Robin Briggs comes to the office today for a well woman's visit. Her office visit is $65.00, and the Pap smear is $50.00. She pays her co-pay of $10.00, and the remainder is billed to her insurance company.

3. Mick Dixon sees Dr. Lawler today for a follow-up on his new BP medication. The office visit is $48. When checking out, his pays $50.00 on his outstanding balance.

4. Steve Rossi is a new patient of Dr. Lopez. He has a history of heart disease. The office visit charge is $195.00 and $55.00 for the ECG. On check-out, he pays his co-pay of $25.00 with check #1010.

5. Janice Powers sees Dr. Lawler for an upper respiratory infection. Her office visit charge is $48.00. Her insurance company will be billed.

Mary Sunshine, the office manager, brings you the payments and other related items from today's mail. Correctly post and make adjustments on the daysheet. Process refunds accordingly using the checks supplied.

1. Buzz Collection Agency sends check #4376 in the amount of $320.00. Patient Ruppert Harrison had an outstanding balance of $1500.00 and his account was sent to the agency after being 120 days outstanding. The agency arranged to have Mr. Ruppert pay $800.00 to settle the account.

2. Jon Johnson sends check #420 for $100.00 to go toward his outstanding balance. His outstanding balance is $80.00. How do you handle this?

3. Linda Martinez's check for $78.40 has been returned for NSF.

4. BCBS sends check #7125 for $283.25 for Kathleen Peavy's procedure. The physicians accept assignment from Blue Cross/Blue Shield.

5. Make the correct entry to indicate a refund will be made. Correctly complete a refund check.

Copyright © 2010, 2005 by Saunders, an imprint of Elsevier, Inc. All rights reserved.

PROCEDURE 28-3

Date: _____ Sheet #: _____ Day sheet

Date	Reference	Description	Charge	Credits Payment	Credits Adjustment	Current balance	Previous balance		Name	Receipt	ABA	Cash	Checks

	Column A	Column B-1	Column B-2	Column C	Column D

Proof of posting		Accounts receivable control	
This page		Previous day total	
Previous page		Plus total charges	
Month-to-date		Subtotal	
Column D total		Less payments/adjustments	
Plus column A total		**Total accounts receivable**	$0.00
Subtotal			
Less total cols. B-1 and B-2			
Must equal column C			

	Cash	Checks
Total deposit		

Accounts receivable proof	
Accounts receivable first of the month	
Plus column A month-to-date	
Subtotal	
Less columns B-1 and B2 month-to-date	
Total accounts receivable	$0.00

JOURNAL OF DAILY CHARGES & PAYMENTS

	DATE	PROFESSIONAL SERVICE	FEE	PAYMENT	ADJUST-MENT	NEW BALANCE	OLD BALANCE	PATIENT'S NAME	
1									1
2									2
3									3
4									4
5									5
6									6
7									7
8									8
9									9
10									10
11									11
12									12
13									13
14									14
15									15
16									16
17									17
18									18
19									19
20									20
21									21
22									22
23									23
24									24
25									25
26									26
27									27
28									28
29									29
30									30
31								TOTALS THIS PAGE	31
32								TOTAL PREVIOUS PAGE	32
33								TOTALS MONTH TO DATE	33
			COLUMN A	COLUMN B	COLUMN C	COLUMN D	COLUMN E		

MEMO _____

DAILY - FROM LINE 31
ARITHMETIC POSTING PROOF

Column E	$
Plus Column A	
Sub-Total	
Minus Column B	
Sub-Total	
Minus Column C	
Equals Column D	

MONTH - FROM LINE 31
ACCOUNTS RECEIVABLE PROOF

Accts. Receivable Previous Day	$
Plus Column A	
Sub-Total	
Minus Column B	
Sub-Total	
Minus Column C	
Accts. receivable End of Day	

YEAR TO DATE - FROM LINE 33
ACCOUNTS RECEIVABLE PROOF

Accts. Receivable beginning of Month	$
Plus Column A MONTH TO DATE	
Sub-Totaln C	
Minus Column B MONTH TO DATE	
Sub-Total	
Minus Column C MONTH TO DATE	
Accts. receivable End of Day MONTH TO DATE	

(From Buck CJ: *Student manual with daily tasks for practice kit for medical front office skills,* St Louis, 2009, Saunders.)

Copyright © 2010, 2005 by Saunders, an imprint of Elsevier, Inc. All rights reserved.

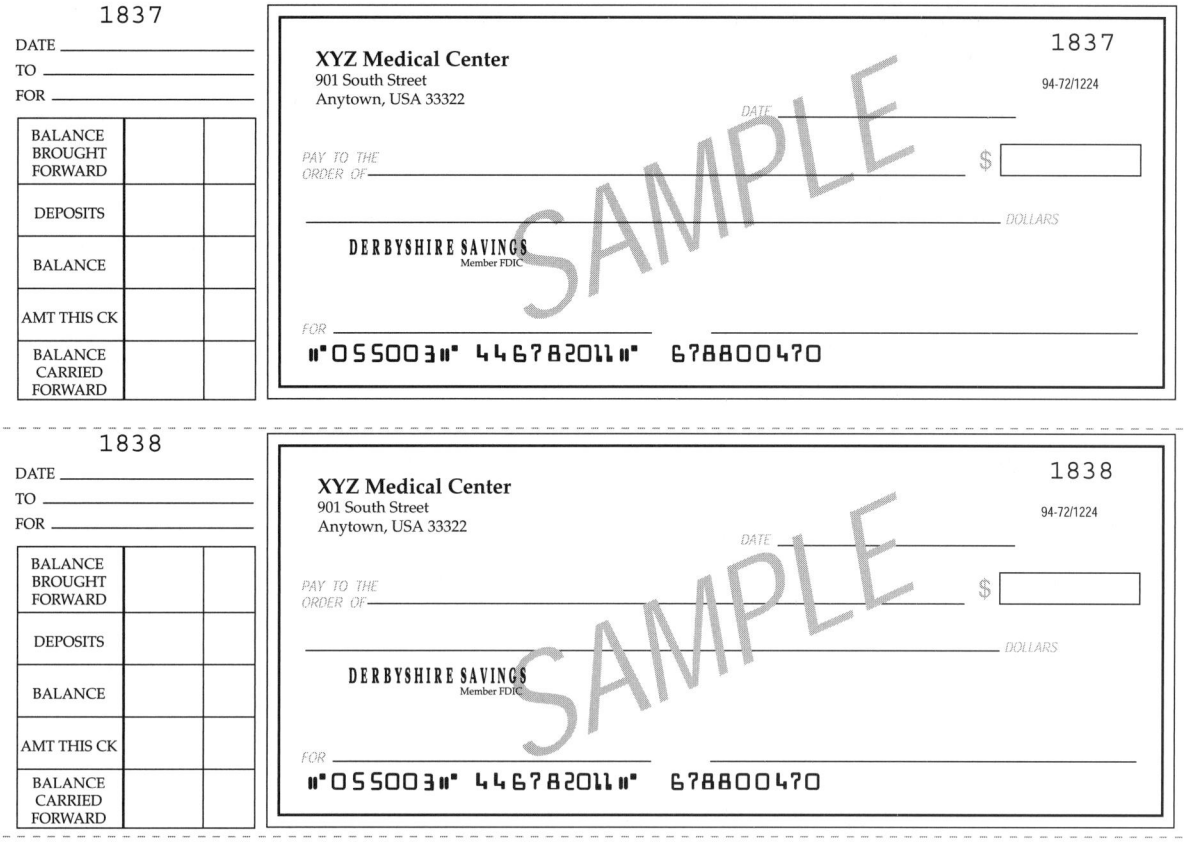

(Modified from Hunt SA: *Fundamentals of medical assisting student mastery manual,* Philadelphia, 2002, Saunders.)

PROCEDURE 28-3

Date:
Sheet #:
Day sheet

Date	Reference	Description	Charge	Credits Payment	Credits Adjustment	Current balance	Previous balance	Name	Receipt	ABA	Cash	Checks

	Column A	Column B-1	Column B-2	Column C	Column D
	$876.00	$567.00	$0.00	$2,188.97	$680.00

	Cash	Checks

Proof of posting

		Accounts receivable control	
This page		Previous day total	
Previous page		Plus total charges	
Month-to-date		Subtotal	
		Less payments/adjustments	
Column D total		**Total accounts receivable**	**$0.00**
Plus column A total			
Subtotal		Total deposit	
Less total cols. B-1 and B-2			
Must equal column C			

Accounts receivable proof

Accounts receivable first of the month	
Plus column A month-to-date	
Subtotal	
Less columns B-1 and B2 month-to-date	
Total accounts receivable	**$0.00**

Student Name: _____ DATE: _____

PROCEDURE 28-4 CHECKLIST: PREPARE A BANK DEPOSIT

TASK: Correctly prepare a bank deposit for the day's receipts, and complete appropriate office records related to the deposit.

CONDITIONS: Given the proper equipment and supplies, the student will be required to prepare a bank deposit.

EQUIPMENT AND SUPPLIES
- MACC/computer (practice)
- Deposit slip
- Endorsement stamp (optional)
- Pen or pencil
- Calculator
- Check register

STANDARDS: Complete the procedure within _____ minutes and achieve a minimum score of _____%.

Time began _____   Time ended _____

Steps	Possible Points	First Attempt	Second Attempt
1. Assemble all supplies and equipment.	5		
2. Use daysheet 2 total.	5		
3. Separate cash and check totals.	5		
4. Simulate preparing the checks for deposit.	5		
5. Complete the deposit slip, documenting each check appropriately (use daysheet 2).	10		
6. Total the amount of deposit, entering the total as appropriate.	5		
7. Record the appropriate amount of the deposit in the office checkbook (check register).	10		
8. Photocopy the front and back of the deposit slip if duplicate deposit slip is unavailable.	5		
9. Place the currency, checks, and completed deposit slip in appropriate place for deposit.	5		
Total Points Possible	55		

Comments: Total Points Earned _____

Divided by _____

Total Possible Points = _____% Score

Instructor's Signature _____

Copyright © 2010, 2005 by Saunders, an imprint of Elsevier, Inc. All rights reserved.

Information for Procedure 28-4

Check Register

Check #	Date	Description	Payment	Ref	Deposit	Balance
	7/27	Balance brought forward				8234.68
	7/27	ABC Printing	125.45			8109.23
	7/27	Deposit			563.00	8672.23
	7/30	Office supply	67.89			8604.34
	7/30	Deposit			325.00	8929.34
3663	7/31	Payroll account	3765.00			5164.34
	7/31	Deposit			163.40	5327.74
	8/1	Woodburn Mortgage	1789.00			3538.74
		Deposit			345.00	3883.74
	8/2	U.S. Postmaster	220.00			3663.74
		Deposit			258.60	3922.34
	8/3	Jon Johnson	20.00			3902.34
	8/3					

DEPOSIT TICKET

FOR CLEAR COPY, PRESS FIRMLY WITH BALL POINT PEN.

State Bank
500 Main Ave.
Anytown, USA 33322

DATE _____

	DOLLARS	CENTS
CURRENCY		
COIN		
LIST EACH CHECK		
1.		
2.		
3.		
4.		
5.		
6.		
7.		
8.		
9.		
10.		
11.		
12.		
13.		
14.		
15.		
16.		
17.		
18.		
19.		
20.		

PLEASE ENTER TOTAL

TOTAL DEPOSIT

DEPOSITS MAY NOT BE AVAILABLE FOR IMMEDIATE WITHDRAWAL

PLEASE BE SURE ALL ITEMS ARE PROPERLY ENDORSED

TOTAL ITEMS

50-17/223-0107

CHECKS AND OTHER ITEMS ARE RECEIVED FOR DEPOSIT SUBJECT TO THE PROVISIONS OF THE UNIFORM COMMERCIAL CODE OR ANY APPLICABLE COLLECTION AGREEMENT

1: 45890277": 6334792445 08" 6221

(Modified from Potter BA: *Medical office administration: a worktext,* Philadelphia, 2003, Saunders.)

Student Name: _____ DATE: _____

PROCEDURE 28-5 CHECKLIST: RECONCILE A BANK STATEMENT

TASK: Reconcile a bank statement.

CONDITIONS: Given the proper equipment and supplies, the student will be required to reconcile a bank statement.

EQUIPMENT AND SUPPLIES
- MACC/computer (practice)
- Information sheet:
  Ending (closing) balance of previous statement
  Beginning balance of current statement
  Other information in current bank statement
  List of canceled checks for current month
  Deposits in transit
  Checkbook balance
- Calculator
- Pen or pencil

STANDARDS: Complete the procedure within _____ minutes and achieve a minimum score of _____%.

Time began _____   Time ended _____

Steps	Possible Points	First Attempt	Second Attempt
1. Assemble all supplies and equipment.	5		
2. Compare the closing balance of the previous statement with the beginning balance of the current statement.	10		
3. Compare the checks written with the items on the statement using appropriate means to verify checks have cleared the bank.	20		
4. List and total the outstanding checks.	10		
5. Complete the bank statement reconciliation worksheet on the back of the bank statement.	10		
6. Reconcile deposits, including any positive adjustments made by bank.	10		
7. Add outstanding deposits to the bank statement reconciliation formula.	10		
8. Calculate the corrected bank statement balance.	10		

Copyright © 2010, 2005 by Saunders, an imprint of Elsevier, Inc. All rights reserved.

Steps	Possible Points	First Attempt	Second Attempt
9. Adjust the checkbook balance by subtracting any bank charges that appear on the bank statement.	10		
10. If the checkbook balance and the statement balance do not agree, check the appropriate figures and make adjustments as necessary.	5		
Total Points Possible	100		

Comments: Total Points Earned _____

Divided by _____

Total Possible Points = _____% Score

Instructor's Signature _____

Information for Procedure 28-5

Bank Statement:	
Ending Balance: Prior Statement	$7627.10
Ending Balance: New Statement	$8232.71
Service Charge	$6.25
Beginning Balance: Current Statement	$7627.10
Checkbook Balance	$8285.90
Adj Checkbook Balance	$_____

Other Information:

Outstanding checks:	
#705	$18.45
#712	$247.94
#724	$82.71
#735	$27.23
Deposits in transit:	$423.27

THIS WORKSHEET IS PROVIDED TO HELP YOU BALANCE YOUR ACCOUNT

1. Go through your register and mark each check, withdrawal, Express ATM transaction, payment, deposit, or other credit listed on this statement. Be sure that your register shows any interest paid into your account, and any service charges, automatic payments, or Express Transfers withdrawn from your account during this statement period.

2. Using the chart below, list any outstanding checks, Express ATM withdrawals, payments, or any other withdrawals (including any from previous months) that are listed in your register but are not shown on this statement.

3. Balance your account by filling in the spaces below.

ITEMS OUTSTANDING	
NUMBER	AMOUNT
TOTAL	$

ENTER

The NEW BALANCE shown on
this statement_____$

ADD

Any deposits listed in your register $
or transfers into your account $
which are not shown on this $
statement.   +$ _____

TOTAL

CALCULATE THE SUBTOTAL_____$

SUBTRACT

The total outstanding checks and
withdrawals from the chart at left_____-$

CALCULATE THE ENDING BALANCE

This amount should be the same
as the current balance shown in
your check register_____$

(Modified from Hunt SA: *Fundamentals of medical assisting student mastery manual,* Philadelphia, 2002, Saunders.)

Student Name: _____ DATE: _____

PROCEDURE 28-6 CHECKLIST: EXPLAIN PROFESSIONAL FEES BEFORE SERVICES ARE PROVIDED

TASK: Explain professional fees to the patient to establish understanding of his or her obligations before receiving services.

CONDITIONS: Given the proper equipment and supplies, the student will role-play with another student or an instructor how to explain professional fees to the patient.

EQUIPMENT AND SUPPLIES
- Information sheet
- Physician's fee schedule
- Surgical cost estimate
- Estimate of medical expenses form
- Private area for discussion

STANDARDS: Complete the procedure within _____ minutes and achieve a minimum score of _____%.

Time began _____   Time ended _____

Steps	Possible Points	First Attempt	Second Attempt
1. Assemble all supplies and equipment.	5		
2. Provide privacy for discussion.	5		
3. Display a professional attitude.	10		
4. Provide an estimate of anticipated fees before services are provided.	10		
5. Determine whether the patient has specific concerns that may hinder payment.	10		
6. Make appropriate arrangements for further discussion between the physician (instructor) and patient (student) if further explanation is necessary.	10		
Total Points Possible	50		

Comments: Total Points Earned _____

Divided by _____

Total Possible Points = _____% Score

Instructor's Signature _____

731

Copyright © 2010, 2005 by Saunders, an imprint of Elsevier, Inc. All rights reserved.

Information for Procedure 28-6

Fee Schedule

Facial Contouring	Price Range
Face lift	$6000-6500
Face lift, neck lift	$6600-7500
Deep midface lift with lower eyelid surgery	$3600-4000
Submental lipectomy with neck muscle tightening	$1950-2300
Surgery of the forehead	$3000-3550
Forehead lift coronal	$3600-4000
Browlift	$2500-3200
Surgery of the Eyelid	
Upper eyelid surgery	$1975-2450
Lower eyelid surgery	$2225-2700
Surgery of the Nose	
Primary rhinoplasty	$5200-5500
Secondary rhinoplasty	$1600-6500

Estimate of Medical Expenses

All estimates include the surgical fee along with the hospital, which includes anesthesia, operating room, and recovery room. Although insurance generally does not cover the cost of cosmetic surgery, flexible financing is available.

Situation

The patient, Mrs. Smith, wants to have some cosmetic surgery done on her eyelids. She knows her insurance will not cover the procedure. She has asked the office to provide an estimate of the cost. Today she is coming into the office and you have been asked to explain to her the financial impact of having this surgery.

Surgical Fee:

Upper eyelids	$2000	_____
Lower eyelids	$2000	_____
Upper and lower eyelids	$3800	_____

Hospital Fee:

Anesthesia	$1000
Operating room	$1500
Recovery room	$500
Subtotal	**$3000**
Total	_____

Student Name: _____ DATE: _____

PROCEDURE 28-7 CHECKLIST: ESTABLISH PAYMENT ARRANGEMENTS ON A PATIENT ACCOUNT

TASK: Establish a payment plan for paying for services on a large ("high-dollar") or overdue account.

CONDITIONS: Given the proper equipment and supplies, the student will role-play with another student or an instructor making payment arrangements on a patient account.

EQUIPMENT AND SUPPLIES
- Patient's billing statement (ledger card and account information)
- Calendar
- "Truth in Lending" form
- Paper
- Pen
- Private area for discussion
- Information sheet

STANDARDS: Complete the procedure within _____ minutes and achieve a minimum score of _____%.

Time began _____   Time ended _____

Steps	Possible Points	First Attempt	Second Attempt
1. Assemble all supplies and equipment.	5		
2. Determine that all information on the billing statement is correct.	10		
3. Discuss payment arrangements accepted by the practice.	20		
4. Explain any finance charges that will accrue on the account (for the purposes of this activity, use a 2% finance charge).	10		
5. Determine date of first payment.	5		
6. Prepare "Truth in Lending" statement.	15		
7. Have the person responsible for the account sign the form if the agreement requires more than four installments.	10		
8. Document the agreement by making notes to the ledger card in the appropriate place in the patient chart.	15		
9. Copy the statement and provide copy to patient. Place original in patient record or other place as appropriate under office policy.	10		
Total Points Possible	100		

Comments: Total Points Earned _____

Divided by _____

Total Possible Points = _____% Score

Instructor's Signature _____

Information for Procedure 28-7

Mr. Jefferson is coming to the office today to discuss his account balance. Currently his account is 90 days overdue—$1500.00. He had been out of work for 6 months, and last week he returned to work. He wants to avoid having his outstanding account balance sent to a collection agency. You have been assigned to discuss the situation with Mr. Jefferson.

Federal Truth in Lending Statement

Patient: James Jefferson

Address: _____

_____

1.	Cash price (service fee)	$_____
2.	Cash down payment	$_____
3.	Unpaid balance	$_____
4.	Amount financed	$_____
5.	Finance charge	$_____
6.	Annual percentage rate	$_____
7.	Total of payments (4 + 5)	$_____
8.	Deferred payment (1 + 5)	$_____

Copyright © 2010, 2005 by Saunders, an imprint of Elsevier, Inc. All rights reserved.

Student Name: _____   DATE: _____

PROCEDURE 28-8 CHECKLIST: EXPLAIN A STATEMENT OF ACCOUNT TO A PATIENT

TASK: Explain a statement of account to a patient to establish understanding of his or her obligations.

CONDITIONS: Given the proper equipment and supplies, the student will role-play with another student or an instructor the explanation of a statement of account to a patient.

EQUIPMENT AND SUPPLIES
- MACC/computer (practice)
- Patient statement
- Physician's fee schedule
- Private area for discussion

STANDARDS: Complete the procedure within _____ minutes and achieve a minimum score of _____%.

Time began _____   Time ended _____

Steps	Possible Points	First Attempt	Second Attempt
1. Assemble all supplies and equipment.	5		
2. Determine that the patient has the correct statement, and discover what seems to be the problem.	5		
3. Examine the statement for any possible errors.	10		
4. Review with the patient each of the items that appears on the statement.	15		
5. If an error is located, correct it immediately, and apologize to the patient.	5		
6. Address patient concerns hindering payment arrangements.	5		
7. If there was no error and your discussion does not resolve the patient's concerns, make arrangements for a discussion between the physician and patient to resolve the problem.	5		
Total Points Possible	50		

Comments: Total Points Earned _____

Divided by _____

Total Possible Points = _____ % Score

Instructor's Signature _____

Copyright © 2010, 2005 by Saunders, an imprint of Elsevier, Inc. All rights reserved.

Information for Procedure 28-8

Patient Jay Newton calls the office today and is upset because he received a statement in the mail saying he owes the office $36.00. He cannot understand how that can be because he has insurance. He wants to come in and see the person responsible for this mistake. You have been assigned to see Mr. Newton when he comes to the office tomorrow morning at 9:00 a.m.

STATEMENT

XYZ Medical Centers
901 South St.
Anytown, USA 33322

Responsible Party:

Jay Newton
7658 Juiceway
Anytown, USA 76567

Account: 10394876

Billing Date: 9/23/20xx

Service date	Patient	Description	Charge	Insurance paid	Adj	Patient paid	Balance due
8/17/20xx	Jay	OV 99214 Asthma 493.92	282.00				282.00
8/17/20xx	Jay	Aerosol 94640 Asthma 493.92	43.00				325.00
9/01/20xx		Payment insurance		157.00 (99214)	100.00		68.00
9/01/20xx		Payment insurance		22.00 (94640)	10.00		36.00

Please pay ➤ $36.00

Student Name: _____   DATE: _____

PROCEDURE 28-9 CHECKLIST: PREPARE BILLING STATEMENTS AND COLLECT PAST-DUE ACCOUNTS

TASK: Process monthly statements and evaluate accounts for collection procedures.

CONDITIONS: Given the proper equipment and supplies, the student will prepare statements for billing and process collection letters for past due accounts.

EQUIPMENT AND SUPPLIES
- MACC/computer (practice)
- Patient ledger cards (use from Procedure 28-2)
- Patient information form
- Collection form letters
- Stationery and envelopes
- Collection agency commission requirements
- Pen or pencil

STANDARDS: Complete the procedure within _____ minutes and achieve a minimum score of _____%.

Time began _____   Time ended _____

Steps	Possible Points	First Attempt	Second Attempt
Preparing billing statements:			
1. Assemble all supplies and equipment.	5		
2. Determine the billing schedule for the medical practice (provided by instructor).	5		
3. Determine the accounts with outstanding balances. (Use information sheet.)	20		
4. Separate the accounts for routine billing and for past due actions.	20		
Performing routine billing:			
5. Prepare ledger cards for billing statements	25		
6. Print out computer-generated statements as applicable or photocopy ledger cards.	25		
7. Prepare statements for mailing.	15		
Collecting past due accounts:			
8. Obtain all patient ledger cards with past due balances.	15		

PROCEDURE 28-9

Copyright © 2010, 2005 by Saunders, an imprint of Elsevier, Inc. All rights reserved.

Steps	Possible Points	First Attempt	Second Attempt
9. Separate accounts according to the action required, according to length of aging of account.	15		
10. Create the appropriate form letter for each account using company stationery, "mail" (turn in to the instructor) to the patient, or turn accounts over to collection agency (instructor) as appropriate.	55		
Total Points Possible	200		

Comments: Total Points Earned _____

Divided by _____

Total Possible Points = _____% Score

Instructor's Signature _____

Information for Procedure 28-9

You have been instructed by the physician to prepare monthly statements and to provide the physician with information concerning past due accounts and documentation regarding actions that have been taken to recover money owed to the practice. You review the aging report and select accounts that are at least 60 days past due. You look through prior correspondence and record the information in the comments column.

Today's date: September 30, 20xx

Patient Name	1-30	30-60	60-90	90-120	Comments
Dey, Judith			1500	2500	$4000— Her insurance was billed and the claims denied. The office has filed an appeal and yesterday was informed that a check for $3200 will be going in the mail this week. The office does not accept assignment with this insurance company.
Huey, Alfonso		360	700	1500	$2560—His insurance company was billed for all office visits and procedures. The amount remaining is the 20% still owed by the patient. He has been called twice. The first time he stated he would look into it, and the second time a message was left on his answering machine to call the office without response.

Corseni, Albert	150	300	500		$950—The patient was notified on his last visit the need to collect on his account. Patient stated that he lost his job and is looking for work. He is doing odd jobs and will try and set something up.
Schultz, Madeline		50	100	150	$300—After reviewing her account, it was found that the person entering the checks failed to recognize that the physician accepts assignment from her insurance.
Plotner, Howard				3500	$3500—Two phone calls were placed, and when the last was placed the receptionist received a message that the phone number was no longer in service. The last letter was returned stamped "Moved No Forwarding Address."
Totals	150	710	2800	7650	**$11,310**

1. After reviewing the accounts, the physician asks you to figure out what percentage of the money owed is 90-120 days overdue. _____

2. The physician then provided the following actions:
   Dey—Call and set up a payment plan. Document the plan agreed on.
   Huey—Send a collection letter. Create a letter appropriate for this situation.
   Corseni—Send a letter asking him to come into the office to establish a payment plan.
   Schultz—No action. Adjustments to be made to patient's account to bring the balance to $0.
   Plotner—Send to collections with all information.

Student Name: _____ DATE: _____

PROCEDURE 29-1 CHECKLIST: DIAGNOSTIC CODING

TASK: Assign the proper *International Classification of Diseases (ICD-9-CM)* code based on medical documentation to the highest degree of specificity.

CONDITIONS: Given the proper equipment and supplies, the student will assign the proper *ICD-9-CM* code based on medical documentation to the highest degree of specificity.

EQUIPMENT AND SUPPLIES
- MACC/computer (practice)
- Current *ICD-9-CM* codebook
- Medical dictionary
- Patient's medical records or information sheet
- Pen or pencil

STANDARDS: Complete the procedure within _____ minutes and achieve a minimum score of _____%.

Time began _____   Time ended _____

Steps	Possible Points	First Attempt	Second Attempt
1. Assemble all supplies and equipment.	5		
2. Identify the key term in the diagnostic statement.	10		
3. Locate the diagnosis in the Alphabetic Index (Volume 2, Section 1) of the *ICD-9-CM* codebook.	20		
4. Read and use footnotes, symbols, or instructions.	15		
5. Locate the diagnosis in the Tabular List (Volume 1).	10		
6. Read and use the inclusions and exclusions noted in the Tabular List.	10		
7. Assign the code to the highest degree of specificity appropriate.	20		
8. Document in the medical record.	10		

Copyright © 2010, 2005 by Saunders, an imprint of Elsevier, Inc. All rights reserved.

744 APPENDIX A Supplemental Chapter Materials

Steps	Possible Points	First Attempt	Second Attempt
9. Ask yourself these final questions (*no* points awarded for this section): a. Have you coded to the highest degree of specificity?	0		
b. When you transferred the code to the patient form and to subsequent records and forms, did you record the code accurately?			
c. Are there any secondary diagnoses or conditions addressed during the encounter that need to be coded?			
Total Points Possible	100		

Comments: Total Points Earned _____

Divided by _____

Total Possible Points = _____% Score

Instructor's Signature _____

Information for Procedure 29-1

Use Volumes 1 and 2 of the *ICD-9* coding book and write the correct code(s) in the space provided.
1. Fibrocystic disease of breast _____
2. Concussion syndrome _____
3. Bleeding duodenal ulcer _____
4. Insulin-dependent diabetes mellitus with gangrene _____
5. Fitting of hearing aid _____
6. Family history of malignant neoplasm of breast _____
7. Open fracture of maxilla resulting from fall from horse _____
8. Hypertensive cardiovascular disease with congestive heart failure _____
9. Adenocarcinoma of lower-outer quadrant of left breast _____
10. Malignant neoplasm of the prostate with metastasis to vertebral column _____

Copyright © 2010, 2005 by Saunders, an imprint of Elsevier, Inc. All rights reserved.

Student Name: _____ DATE: _____

PROCEDURE 29-2 CHECKLIST: PROCEDURAL CODING

TASK: Assign the proper *Current Procedural Terminology (CPT)* code to the highest degree of specificity based on medical documentation for auditing and billing purposes.

CONDITIONS: Given the proper equipment and supplies, the student will assign the proper *(CPT)* code to the highest degree of specificity based on medical documentation for auditing and billing purposes.

EQUIPMENT AND SUPPLIES
- MACC/computer (practice)
- Current *CPT* code book
- Medical dictionary
- Patient's medical records or information sheet
- Pen or pencil

STANDARDS: Complete the procedure within _____ minutes and achieve a minimum score of _____%.

Time began _____   Time ended _____

Steps	Possible Points	First Attempt	Second Attempt
1. Assemble all supplies and equipment.	5		
2. Read the introduction, guidelines, and notes of a current *CPT* code book.	10		
3. Review all service and procedures performed on the day of the encounter. Include all medications administered, and trays and equipment used.	20		
4. Identify the main term in the procedure.	15		
5. Locate the main term in the alphabetical index. Review any subterms listed alphabetically under the main term.	10		
6. Verify the code sets in the tabular (numerical) list. Select the code with the greatest specificity.	10		
7. Determine if a modifier is required.	20		
8. Assign the code using all necessary steps for proper code determination.	10		

Copyright © 2010, 2005 by Saunders, an imprint of Elsevier, Inc. All rights reserved.

Steps	Possible Points	First Attempt	Second Attempt
9. Ask yourself these final questions (*no* points awarded for this section): a. Have you coded to the highest degree of specificity?	0		
b. When you transferred the code to the patient form and to subsequent records and forms, did you record the code accurately?			
c. Are there any secondary diagnoses or conditions addressed during the encounter that need to be coded?			
Total Points Possible	100		

Comments: Total Points Earned _____

Divided by _____

Total Possible Points = _____% Score

Instructor's Signature _____

Information for Procedure 29-2

Use *CPT* coding book and write the correct code(s) in the space provided. Use modifiers if needed.

1. E&M new patient, detailed examination _____
2. Excision malignant lesion, 1.5 cm trunk _____
3. Control nasal hemorrhage, simple _____
4. Pericardiocentesis, initial _____
5. Double coronary venous bypass grafts _____
6. Incision and drainage of a hematoma, epididymis _____
7. Removal of corneal foreign body _____
8. Hemodialysis, single physician evaluation _____
9. 24-Hour Holter monitor (continuous ECG report) _____
10. The patient was seen in the emergency department after reinjuring her forearm and wrist. A reduction of closed Colles' fracture had been performed a week earlier, and a new set of x-rays (complete) revealed a nonalignment of the fracture site. A reduction was performed again with manipulation by the same on-call orthopaedist who performed the first reduction. _____

Student Name: _____   DATE: _____

PROCEDURE 30-1 CHECKLIST: APPLY MANAGED CARE POLICIES AND PROCEDURES

TASK: Obtain precertification and preauthorization/referral from a patient's HMO for requested services or procedures.

CONDITIONS: Given the proper equipment and supplies, the student will role-play with another student or an instructor applying managed care policies and procedures.

EQUIPMENT AND SUPPLIES
- MACC/computer (practice)
- Photocopy of patient's insurance identification card
- Patient's information form
- Patient's progress notes
- Precertification form
- Preauthorization form
- Pen or pencil
- *ICD-9* and *CPT* books

STANDARDS: Complete the procedure within _____ minutes and achieve a minimum score of _____%.

Time began _____   Time ended _____

Steps	Possible Points	First Attempt	Second Attempt
Precertification: 1. Assemble all supplies and equipment.	5		
2. Gather documents and information necessary to obtain a managed care precertification.	5		
3. Review the records to ensure all information is available.	5		
4. Complete the precertification/referral form.	5		
5. Proofread the entire form to ensure that it is accurate.	10		
6. Send the form to the insurance carrier for review and action (submit to the instructor).	5		
7. Wait for a response from the managed care organization (instructor returns paper).	5		
8. Process and place a copy of the completed form in the patient's file. Give the original to the patient (student).	5		

PROCEDURE 30-1

Copyright © 2010, 2005 by Saunders, an imprint of Elsevier, Inc. All rights reserved.

Steps	Possible Points	First Attempt	Second Attempt
Preauthorization: 9. Complete the preauthorization form.	5		
10. Proofread the form to ensure accuracy.	10		
11. Send the form to the insurance carrier for review and action (submit to the instructor).	5		
12. Repeat Steps 7 and 8.	10		
Total Points Possible	75		

Comments: Total Points Earned _____

Divided by _____

Total Possible Points = _____ % Score

Instructor's Signature _____

Information for Procedure 30-1

You are the medical assistant assigned to call a patient's insurance company for precertification of diagnostic procedures or hospitalization. Use the following information to complete the form. Before calling the insurance company, look up the *ICD-9* and *CPT* codes. Dr. Sherber is a participating provider of ABC HMO.

DATE: 2/23/20xx
PATIENT NAME: Thomas Kovach
Address: 19794 Westwood Blvd, Anytown, USA, 33324
DOB: 9/28/1952
SS #: 344-88-8765

Physician: Steven Fildo, MD (321876)
XYZ MEDICAL CENTER
901 South St
Anytown, USA 333222
Phone: 676-767-5432
Fax: 676-767-4523

Progress Note:
Patient presents today with complaints of severe heartburn. He currently is on Nexium 40 mg once daily for treatment of GERD. Will request an UGI series be performed at SunCoast Outpatient Clinic by John Sperber, MD, this week.

Using the same patient, insurance, and physician information, complete a preauthorization form for a sleep study to be done at SunCoast Outpatient Clinic. The patient has had problems with snoring and feeling tired all the time, and he is awakened at night with severe headaches that go away after he has gotten up. Dx: sleep apnea. Procedure: sleep study. Use coding books to look up *ICD-9* and *CPT* codes.

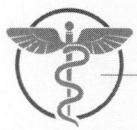

STANDARD HEALTHCARE HMO

PRE-CERTIFICATION REQUEST

Fill out form completely
Current clinical information, indicating medical necessity, must be faxed with authorization request form. Lack of this information will result in a delay in the authorization process.

Date: _____ Contact Person: _____

Office Phone Number: _____ Office Fax Number: _____

PATIENT DEMOGRAPHICS

Patient Name: _____ ID #: _____ PCP #: _____

SPECIALIST REFERRAL Referral Status: (Check One) In-Network _____ Out-of-Network _____

Specialist Physician: _____ Referring Physician: _____

Diagnosis: _____ Reason for Referral: _____

Auth Number: _____ Expiration Date: _____

REQUEST FOR PROCEDURES, TESTING, AND ADMISSIONS
(In-Network and Out-of-Network)

Facility: _____ Physician: _____

Diagnosis: _____ Diagnosis Code(s): _____

Procedure Code(s): _____

Scheduled Date: _____ **Mark One:** __Inpatient __Outpatient __Ambulatory Surgery

Prior authorization is not required for referrals to chiropractors, podiatrists, and dermatologists, but they must be contracted providers for Standard Healthcare HMO plans. Diagnostic testing must be performed at a contracted facility.

Please forward completed form to: Standard Healthcare HMO   Fax: 555-912-4415

Auth Number: _____ # of Visits: _____ Expiration Date: _____

SHHMO APPROVAL COMPLETED BY: _____ **Phone #:** _____
(Authorized SHHMO Signature)

Use of this form does not guarantee eligibility of coverage and does not supersede any member benefit plan limitations or the provider's contractual limitations.

Confidentiality Note:
The information contained in this facsimile message may be legally privileged and confidential information intended only for the use of the individual or entity named above. If the reader of this message is not the intended recipient, you are hereby notified that any dissemination, distribution, or copying of this fax is strictly prohibited. If you have received this fax in error, please immediately notify the sender above and return the original message to us at the address below by the U.S. Postal Service. Thank you for your cooperation.

Customer Service:
Standard Healthcare HMO
1500 Summitt Avenue
Western, NY 99992
(555) 800-6000

XYZ Medical Center

PREAUTHORIZATION REQUEST FORM

PATIENT INFORMATION

Last Name: _____ First Name: _____

DOB: _____ Member #: _____ Group #: _____

PREAUTHORIZATION REQUEST INFORMATION

Please list *both* procedure/product code *and* narrative description:

CPT / HCPCS Code(s): _____ Durable Medical Equipment: ☐ Rental ☐
Purchase _____
Description: _____

Date of Service: _____ Length of Stay (if applicable): _____
Place of Service or Vendor Name: _____
Assistant Surgeon Requested? ☐ Yes ☐ No   **Please list *both* diagnosis(es) code *and* narrative description:** _____

1. ICD-9 Code: _____
   Description: _____
2. ICD-9 Code: _____

Ordering Physician/Provider: _____ Office Location: _____
                            FIRST <u>AND</u> LAST NAMES PLEASE
Referring Physician/Provider: _____
                            FIRST <u>AND</u> LAST NAMES PLEASE; REQUIRED FOR PRIME PLANS
Date: _____ Contact Person: _____ Phone: _____

> *Please Note: Incomplete forms will delay the preauthorization process.*
> *Requests received after 3:00 PM are processed the next working day.*
> PacificSource responds to preauthorization requests within 2 working days.
> A determination notice will be mailed to the requesting provider, facility, and patient.
> *Please attach pertinent chart notes as appropriate.*

FOR INTERNAL OFFICE USE ONLY:
STATUS: APPROVED / DENIED / PENDING / EXPLANATION
DATE: _____ ACUITY: _____ INITIALS: _____
Reason/Status _____
_____

Field 11 Notes _____ LOS Approved _____
☐ Chart notes filed with preauthorization
Notes _____
Field 10 Facility Copy _____

901 South Street • Anytown, USA 33322 • (123) 456-7890
MEDICAL AFFAIRS DEPARTMENT CONFIDENTIAL FAX: (123) 555-2051

9/8/2003

PROCEDURE 30-1

(Modified from Beik JI: *Health insurance today,* ed 2, St Louis, 2009, Saunders.)

Student Name: _____ DATE: _____

PROCEDURE 30-2 CHECKLIST: COMPLETE THE CMS-1500 CLAIM FORM

TASK: Apply third-party guidelines and use a physician's fee schedule to complete an insurance claim form.

CONDITIONS: Given the proper equipment and supplies, the student will role-play with another student or an instructor completing a CMS-1500 claim form.

EQUIPMENT AND SUPPLIES
- MACC/computer (practice)
- Photocopy of patient's insurance identification card
- Patient information form
- Patent encounter form
- Patient medical record
- Physician's fee schedule
- CMS-1500 insurance claim form (2)
- Pen or pencil

STANDARDS: Complete the procedure within _____ minutes and achieve a minimum score of _____%.

Time began _____   Time ended _____

Steps	Possible Points	First Attempt	Second Attempt
1. Assemble all supplies and equipment.	5		
2. Identify the patient's primary third-party payer, or the company or agency to which the claim will be submitted.	15		
3. Enter the name and address of the third-party payer in the top right corner of the insurance form using all-capital letters and no punctuation.	15		
4. Complete blocks 1-13 of the form.	50		
5. Complete the Physician/Supplier Section, blocks 14-33 of the CMS-1500 form.	100		
6. Review the claim for completion and corrections.	15		
7. Submit the claim (to instructor).	0		
Total Points Possible	200		

Comments: Total Points Earned _____

Divided by _____

Total Possible Points = _____ % Score

Instructor's Signature _____

PROCEDURE 30-2

Copyright © 2010, 2005 by Saunders, an imprint of Elsevier, Inc. All rights reserved.

Information for Procedure 30-2

Physician: Steven Fildo, MD (321876)
XYZ MEDICAL CENTER
901 South St
Anytown, USA 333222
Phone: 676-767-5432
Fax: 676-767-4523
NPI 5670984324
EIN# 65-5670984

Office Fees		Place-of-Service Codes	
99212	$60	Office	11
99213	$90	Inpatient	21
99214	$115	Outpatient	22
99215	$130	Emergency—hospital	23
Procedures			
93000 ECG	$60		
71020 chest x-ray	$75		

1. Mary Pickering has been a patient of Dr. Fildo for several years. She has been having headaches for the last few days. After examining her, Dr. Fildo is sending her for sinus x-rays. Complete a CMS-1500 for today's visit. Code the visit (focused) and the chief complaint.

PATIENT INFORMATION

Name: Mary Pickering

SS#: 999-08-7654

Address: 6754 Circle Way

City: Linn

State: USA

Zip Code: 33376

Home phone: 676-987-4343

DOB: 7/15/1976

Gender: Female

Patient status: Single

Occupation: Teacher

Copyright © 2010, 2005 by Saunders, an imprint of Elsevier, Inc. All rights reserved.

Employer: Morgan County School System

Employer phone: 676-964-5342

Spouse:

Spouse's SS#:

Spouse's DOB:

Spouse's employer:

Sample Insurance Card

BLUE CROSS AND BLUE SHIELD
Insured: Mary Pickering
I.D. 98654364323   DR: S. Fildo
Group #: 234769
MEMBER SERVICES: 800-987-8234   DR: $20   ER: $200
PROVIDERS CALL: 800-675-9087   SP: 35   HO: 700/A
BEHAVIORAL HEALTH: 800-243-5674   AS: 300   UC: 50 MH: 30

2. Beverly J. Pourch has a history of coronary artery disease and asthma. She presents today with complaints of mild chest discomfort and difficulty breathing, and has had episodes of wheezing during the week. After an extensive examination, Dr. Fildo orders a chest x-ray and an ECG. Complete a CMS-1500 form for today's visit. Code the visit (comprehensive) and the chief complaint.

PATIENT INFORMATION

Name: Beverly J. Pourch

SS#: 247-97-4565

Address: 987 Bridgeway

City: Sun City

State: USA

Zip Code: 33354

Home phone: 676-876-4567

DOB: 4/25/1946

Gender: Female

Patient status: Married

Occupation: Retired

Employer:

Copyright © 2010, 2005 by Saunders, an imprint of Elsevier, Inc. All rights reserved.

Employer phone:

Spouse: George T. Pourch

Spouse's SS#: 234-23-5543

Spouse's DOB: 2/23/1943

Spouse's employer: Retired

Spouse's employer:

Sample Insurance Card

MEDICARE HEALTH INSURANCE
1-800-MEDICARE (1-800-633-4227)

Name of Beneficiary:
Beverly J. Pourch

Medicare Claim Number	Sex
986-54-2364-A	Female
Is Entitled to:	**Effective Date:**
Hospital (Part A)	4/01/20XX
Medical (Part B)	4/01/20XX

HEALTH INSURANCE CLAIM FORM

1500

APPROVED BY NATIONAL UNIFORM CLAIM COMMITTEE 08/05

PICA

CARRIER

1. MEDICARE MEDICAID TRICARE CHAMPUS CHAMPVA GROUP HEALTH PLAN FECA BLK LUNG OTHER
   (Medicare #) (Medicaid #) (Sponsor's SSN) (Member ID#) (SSN or ID) (SSN) (ID)

1a. INSURED'S I.D. NUMBER (For Program in Item 1)

2. PATIENT'S NAME (Last Name, First Name, Middle Initial)

3. PATIENT'S BIRTH DATE MM DD YY SEX M F

4. INSURED'S NAME (Last Name, First Name, Middle Initial)

5. PATIENT'S ADDRESS (No., Street)

6. PATIENT RELATIONSHIP TO INSURED
   Self Spouse Child Other

7. INSURED'S ADDRESS (No., Street)

CITY STATE

8. PATIENT STATUS
   Single Married Other
   Employed Full-Time Student Part-Time Student

CITY STATE

ZIP CODE TELEPHONE (Include Area Code) ( )

ZIP CODE TELEPHONE (Include Area Code) ( )

9. OTHER INSURED'S NAME (Last Name, First Name, Middle Initial)

10. IS PATIENT'S CONDITION RELATED TO:

11. INSURED'S POLICY GROUP OR FECA NUMBER

a. OTHER INSURED'S POLICY OR GROUP NUMBER

a. EMPLOYMENT? (Current or Previous) YES NO

a. INSURED'S DATE OF BIRTH MM DD YY SEX M F

b. OTHER INSURED'S DATE OF BIRTH MM DD YY SEX M F

b. AUTO ACCIDENT? YES NO PLACE (State)

b. EMPLOYER'S NAME OR SCHOOL NAME

c. EMPLOYER'S NAME OR SCHOOL NAME

c. OTHER ACCIDENT? YES NO

c. INSURANCE PLAN NAME OR PROGRAM NAME

d. INSURANCE PLAN NAME OR PROGRAM NAME

10d. RESERVED FOR LOCAL USE

d. IS THERE ANOTHER HEALTH BENEFIT PLAN? YES NO *If yes*, return to and complete item 9 a-d.

READ BACK OF FORM BEFORE COMPLETING & SIGNING THIS FORM.

12. PATIENT'S OR AUTHORIZED PERSON'S SIGNATURE I authorize the release of any medical or other information necessary to process this claim. I also request payment of government benefits either to myself or to the party who accepts assignment below.

SIGNED _____ DATE _____

13. INSURED'S OR AUTHORIZED PERSON'S SIGNATURE I authorize payment of medical benefits to the undersigned physician or supplier for services described below.

SIGNED _____

PATIENT AND INSURED INFORMATION

14. DATE OF CURRENT: MM DD YY ILLNESS (First symptom) OR INJURY (Accident) OR PREGNANCY(LMP)

15. IF PATIENT HAS HAD SAME OR SIMILAR ILLNESS. GIVE FIRST DATE MM DD YY

16. DATES PATIENT UNABLE TO WORK IN CURRENT OCCUPATION FROM MM DD YY TO MM DD YY

17. NAME OF REFERRING PROVIDER OR OTHER SOURCE

17a.
17b. NPI

18. HOSPITALIZATION DATES RELATED TO CURRENT SERVICES FROM MM DD YY TO MM DD YY

19. RESERVED FOR LOCAL USE

20. OUTSIDE LAB? YES NO $ CHARGES

21. DIAGNOSIS OR NATURE OF ILLNESS OR INJURY (Relate Items 1, 2, 3 or 4 to Item 24E by Line)
   1. _____ . _____   3. _____ . _____
   2. _____ . _____   4. _____ . _____

22. MEDICAID RESUBMISSION CODE ORIGINAL REF. NO.

23. PRIOR AUTHORIZATION NUMBER

24. A. DATE(S) OF SERVICE From MM DD YY To MM DD YY	B. PLACE OF SERVICE	C. EMG	D. PROCEDURES, SERVICES, OR SUPPLIES (Explain Unusual Circumstances) CPT/HCPCS MODIFIER	E. DIAGNOSIS POINTER	F. $ CHARGES	G. DAYS OR UNITS	H. EPSDT Family Plan	I. ID. QUAL.	J. RENDERING PROVIDER ID. #
1									NPI
2									NPI
3									NPI
4									NPI
5									NPI
6									NPI

25. FEDERAL TAX I.D. NUMBER SSN EIN

26. PATIENT'S ACCOUNT NO.

27. ACCEPT ASSIGNMENT? (For govt. claims, see back) YES NO

28. TOTAL CHARGE $

29. AMOUNT PAID $

30. BALANCE DUE $

31. SIGNATURE OF PHYSICIAN OR SUPPLIER INCLUDING DEGREES OR CREDENTIALS (I certify that the statements on the reverse apply to this bill and are made a part thereof.)

SIGNED _____ DATE _____

32. SERVICE FACILITY LOCATION INFORMATION

a. NPI b.

33. BILLING PROVIDER INFO & PH # ( )

a. NPI b.

PHYSICIAN OR SUPPLIER INFORMATION

NUCC Instruction Manual available at: www.nucc.org

APPROVED OMB-0938-0999 FORM CMS-1500 (08/05)

PROCEDURE 30-2

1500

HEALTH INSURANCE CLAIM FORM

APPROVED BY NATIONAL UNIFORM CLAIM COMMITTEE 08/05

PICA PICA

CARRIER

1. MEDICARE (Medicare #) MEDICAID (Medicaid #) TRICARE CHAMPUS (Sponsor's SSN) CHAMPVA (Member ID#) GROUP HEALTH PLAN (SSN or ID) FECA BLK LUNG (SSN) OTHER (ID)

1a. INSURED'S I.D. NUMBER (For Program in Item 1)

2. PATIENT'S NAME (Last Name, First Name, Middle Initial)

3. PATIENT'S BIRTH DATE MM DD YY SEX M F

4. INSURED'S NAME (Last Name, First Name, Middle Initial)

5. PATIENT'S ADDRESS (No., Street)

6. PATIENT RELATIONSHIP TO INSURED Self Spouse Child Other

7. INSURED'S ADDRESS (No., Street)

CITY STATE

8. PATIENT STATUS Single Married Other

CITY STATE

ZIP CODE TELEPHONE (Include Area Code) ( )

Employed Full-Time Student Part-Time Student

ZIP CODE TELEPHONE (Include Area Code) ( )

9. OTHER INSURED'S NAME (Last Name, First Name, Middle Initial)

10. IS PATIENT'S CONDITION RELATED TO:

11. INSURED'S POLICY GROUP OR FECA NUMBER

a. OTHER INSURED'S POLICY OR GROUP NUMBER

a. EMPLOYMENT? (Current or Previous) YES NO

a. INSURED'S DATE OF BIRTH MM DD YY SEX M F

b. OTHER INSURED'S DATE OF BIRTH MM DD YY SEX M F

b. AUTO ACCIDENT? YES NO PLACE (State)

b. EMPLOYER'S NAME OR SCHOOL NAME

c. EMPLOYER'S NAME OR SCHOOL NAME

c. OTHER ACCIDENT? YES NO

c. INSURANCE PLAN NAME OR PROGRAM NAME

d. INSURANCE PLAN NAME OR PROGRAM NAME

10d. RESERVED FOR LOCAL USE

d. IS THERE ANOTHER HEALTH BENEFIT PLAN? YES NO *If yes*, return to and complete item 9 a-d.

READ BACK OF FORM BEFORE COMPLETING & SIGNING THIS FORM.

12. PATIENT'S OR AUTHORIZED PERSON'S SIGNATURE I authorize the release of any medical or other information necessary to process this claim. I also request payment of government benefits either to myself or to the party who accepts assignment below.

SIGNED ____ DATE ____

13. INSURED'S OR AUTHORIZED PERSON'S SIGNATURE I authorize payment of medical benefits to the undersigned physician or supplier for services described below.

SIGNED ____

PATIENT AND INSURED INFORMATION

14. DATE OF CURRENT: MM DD YY ILLNESS (First symptom) OR INJURY (Accident) OR PREGNANCY(LMP)

15. IF PATIENT HAS HAD SAME OR SIMILAR ILLNESS. GIVE FIRST DATE MM DD YY

16. DATES PATIENT UNABLE TO WORK IN CURRENT OCCUPATION MM DD YY FROM TO

17. NAME OF REFERRING PROVIDER OR OTHER SOURCE

17a.

17b. NPI

18. HOSPITALIZATION DATES RELATED TO CURRENT SERVICES MM DD YY FROM TO

19. RESERVED FOR LOCAL USE

20. OUTSIDE LAB? YES NO $ CHARGES

21. DIAGNOSIS OR NATURE OF ILLNESS OR INJURY (Relate Items 1, 2, 3 or 4 to Item 24E by Line)

1. ____ . ____

2. ____ . ____

3. ____ . ____

4. ____ . ____

22. MEDICAID RESUBMISSION CODE ORIGINAL REF. NO.

23. PRIOR AUTHORIZATION NUMBER

24. A. DATE(S) OF SERVICE From MM DD YY To MM DD YY	B. PLACE OF SERVICE	C. EMG	D. PROCEDURES, SERVICES, OR SUPPLIES (Explain Unusual Circumstances) CPT/HCPCS MODIFIER	E. DIAGNOSIS POINTER	F. $ CHARGES	G. DAYS OR UNITS	H. EPSDT Family Plan	I. ID. QUAL.	J. RENDERING PROVIDER ID. #
1								NPI	
2								NPI	
3								NPI	
4								NPI	
5								NPI	
6								NPI	

25. FEDERAL TAX I.D. NUMBER SSN EIN

26. PATIENT'S ACCOUNT NO.

27. ACCEPT ASSIGNMENT? (For govt. claims, see back) YES NO

28. TOTAL CHARGE $

29. AMOUNT PAID $

30. BALANCE DUE $

31. SIGNATURE OF PHYSICIAN OR SUPPLIER INCLUDING DEGREES OR CREDENTIALS (I certify that the statements on the reverse apply to this bill and are made a part thereof.)

SIGNED DATE

32. SERVICE FACILITY LOCATION INFORMATION

a. NPI b.

33. BILLING PROVIDER INFO & PH # ( )

a. NPI b.

PHYSICIAN OR SUPPLIER INFORMATION

NUCC Instruction Manual available at: www.nucc.org

APPROVED OMB-0938-0999 FORM CMS-1500 (08/05)

PROCEDURE 30-2

Student Name: _____ DATE: _____

PROCEDURE 31-1 CHECKLIST: PRACTICE STANDARD PRECAUTIONS

TASK: Identify and demonstrate the application of standard precautions, as assigned by the instructor.

CONDITIONS: Given the proper equipment and supplies, the student will be required to role-play the proper method for practicing standard precautions.

NOTE: The student should practice the procedure using the MACC located on the Evolve site at http://evolve.elsevier.com/klieger/medicalassisting, and then practice and perform the task in the classroom: MACC/Clinical skills/Infection control/Practicing Standard Precautions.

EQUIPMENT AND SUPPLIES
- MACC/computer (practice)
- Personal protective equipment (PPE)—eyewear, gown, boots (shoe covers), mask, gloves
- Current Standard Precautions
- Biohazardous waste container
- Puncture-resistant sharps container
- Pen or pencil
- Classroom Exposure Control Plan/Post exposure plan

STANDARDS: Complete the procedure within _____ minutes and achieve a minimum score of _____%.

Time began _____   Time ended _____

Steps	Possible Points	First Attempt	Second Attempt
1. Assemble all supplies and equipment.	5		
2. Select the appropriate PPE for the assigned procedure (given by your instructor).	10		
3. Identify the body substance isolation (BSI) procedures (verbal or written).	10		
4. Apply transmission-based precautions as they apply to the assigned procedure (as given by your instructor).	10		
5. Explain Standard Precautions as they apply to all body fluids, secretions, and excretions; blood; nonintact skin; and mucous membranes (verbal).	10		
6. Explain the importance of continuing education as it relates to practices using Standard Precautions (verbal).	20		

Steps	Possible Points	First Attempt	Second Attempt
7. Demonstrate the proper use of the following exposure control devices: Sharps container Eyewash stations Fire extinguishers Biohazardous waste containers	20		
8. Demonstrate proper documentation of Standard Precautions training including the time requirement for the training or retraining record.	10		
9. Review the classroom's Exposure Control Plan. Date and initial.	5		
Total Points Possible	100		

Comments: Total Points Earned _____

Divided by _____

Total Possible Points = _____ % Score

Instructor's Signature _____

Student Name: _____   DATE: _____

PROCEDURE 31-2 CHECKLIST: PROPERLY DISPOSE OF BIOHAZARDOUS MATERIALS

TASK: Identify waste classified as biohazardous, and select appropriate containers for proper disposal. Assemble all equipment and demonstrate disposal of actual or simulated waste, following exposure control guidelines.

CONDITIONS: Given the proper equipment and supplies, the student will be required to role-play the proper method for properly disposing of biohazardous materials. The instructor will provide specific instruction on what to dispose of.

NOTE: The student should practice the procedure using the MACC located on the Evolve site at http://evolve.elsevier.com/klieger/medicalassisting: MACC/Clinical skills/Infection control/Practicing Standard Precautions.

EQUIPMENT AND SUPPLIES
- Personal protective equipment (PPE)—eyewear, gown, boots (shoe covers), mask, gloves
- Current Standard Precautions
- Biohazardous waste container
- Puncture-resistant sharps container

STANDARDS: Complete the procedure within _____ minutes and achieve a minimum score of _____%.

Time began _____   Time ended _____

Steps	Possible Points	First Attempt	Second Attempt
1. Assemble all supplies and equipment.	5		
2. Select the appropriate PPE.	5		
3. Verbally communicate a list identifying waste classified as biohazardous.	10		
4. Identify the universal biohazardous symbol, and describe the proper use of the biohazardous spill cleanup kits.	10		
5. Explain housekeeping safety controls.	20		
6. Identify and review material safety data sheets (MSDS). List the various pieces of information included on MSDS.	20		

Copyright © 2010, 2005 by Saunders, an imprint of Elsevier, Inc. All rights reserved.

Steps	Possible Points	First Attempt	Second Attempt
7. Document the decontamination of equipment procedures. Create a decontamination action log.	20		
8. Describe the importance of ongoing safety training.	10		
Total Points Possible	100		

Comments: Total Points Earned _____

Divided by _____

Total Possible Points = _____% Score

Instructor's Signature _____

Student Name: _____   DATE: _____

PROCEDURE 31-3 CHECKLIST: PERFORM PROPER HANDWASHING FOR MEDICAL ASEPSIS

TASK: Prevent the spread of pathogens by aseptically washing hands, following Standard Precautions.

CONDITIONS: Given the proper equipment and supplies, the student will be required to demonstrate the proper method of performing handwashing for medical asepsis.

NOTE: The student should practice the procedure using the MACC located on the Evolve site at http://evolve.elsevier.com/klieger/medicalassisting: MACC/Clinical skills/Infection control/Sanitizing hands.

EQUIPMENT AND SUPPLIES
- MACC/computer
- Liquid antibacterial soap
- Nailbrush or orange stick
- Paper towels
- Warm running water
- Regular waste container

STANDARDS: Complete the procedure within _____ minutes and achieve a minimum score of _____%.

Time began _____   Time ended _____

Steps	Possible Points	First Attempt	Second Attempt
1. Assemble all supplies and equipment.	5		
2. Remove rings and watch, or push watch up on forearm.	5		
3. Stand close to the sink, without allowing clothing to touch the sink.	5		
4. Turn on the faucets, using a paper towel.	5		
5. Adjust the water temperature to warm—not hot or cold. Explain why proper water temperature is important.	10		
6. Discard the paper towel in the proper waste container.	5		
7. Wet hands and wrists under running water, and apply liquid antibacterial soap. Hands must be held lower than the elbows at all times. Hands must not touch the inside of the sink.	10		
8. Work soap into a lather by rubbing the palms together using a circular motion.	10		
9. Clean the fingernails with a nail brush or an orange stick.	5		

Copyright © 2010, 2005 by Saunders, an imprint of Elsevier, Inc. All rights reserved.

Steps	Possible Points	First Attempt	Second Attempt
10. Rinse hands thoroughly under running water, holding them in a downward position and allowing soap and water to run off the fingertips.	10		
11. Repeat procedure if hands are grossly contaminated.	10		
12. Dry hands gently and thoroughly using a clean paper towel. Discard paper towel in proper waste container.	10		
13. Using a dry paper towel, turn the faucets off, clean the area around the sink, and discard towel in regular waste container.	10		
Total Points Possible	100		

Comments: Total Points Earned _____

Divided by _____

Total Possible Points = _____% Score

Instructor's Signature _____

Student Name: _____ DATE: _____

PROCEDURE 31-4 CHECKLIST: PERFORM ALCOHOL-BASED HAND SANITIZATON

TASK: Apply an alcohol-based hand rub to prevent the spread of pathogens.

CONDITIONS: Given the proper equipment and supplies, the student will be required to demonstrate the proper method of performing alcohol-based hand sanitization for medical asepsis.

NOTE: The student should practice the procedure using the MACC located on the Evolve site at http://evolve.elsevier.com/klieger/medicalassisting: MACC/Clinical skills/Infection control/Sanitizing hands.

EQUIPMENT AND SUPPLIES
- MACC/computer
- Alcohol-based hand rub containing 60% to 95% ethanol or isopropanol (gel, foam, lotion)

STANDARDS: Complete the procedure within _____ minutes and achieve a minimum score of _____%.

Time began _____   Time ended _____

Steps	Possible Points	First Attempt	Second Attempt
1. Assemble all supplies and equipment.	5		
2. Visibly inspect hands for obvious contaminants or debris.	5		
3. Remove rings.	5		
4. Open container and apply product to the palm of one hand, following manufacturer's recommendations regarding the amount of product to use.	10		
5. Close container and replace in specified location.	5		
6. Spread gel evenly, covering all surfaces of hands and fingers, 1 to 1½ inches above the wrist.	10		
7. Rub hands together until hands are dry (approximately 15 to 30 seconds).	10		
Total Points Possible	50		

Comments: Total Points Earned _____

Divided by _____

Total Possible Points = _____% Score

Instructor's Signature _____

Copyright © 2010, 2005 by Saunders, an imprint of Elsevier, Inc. All rights reserved.

Student Name: _____ DATE: _____

PROCEDURE 31-5 CHECKLIST: APPLY AND REMOVE CLEAN, DISPOSABLE (NONSTERILE) GLOVES

TASK: Apply and remove disposable (nonsterile) gloves properly.

CONDITIONS: Given the proper equipment and supplies, the student will be required to apply and remove nonsterile disposable gloves.

NOTE: The student should practice the procedure using the MACC located on the Evolve site at http://evolve.elsevier.com/klieger/medicalassisting: MACC/Clinical skills/Infection control/Practicing Standard Precautions.

EQUIPMENT AND SUPPLIES
- MACC/computer
- Alcohol-based hand rub
- Nonsterile disposable gloves
- Biohazardous waste container

STANDARDS: Complete the procedure within _____ minutes and achieve a minimum score of _____%.

Time began _____   Time ended _____

Steps	Possible Points	First Attempt	Second Attempt
Applying gloves: 1. Assemble all supplies and equipment.	5		
2. Select the correct size and style of gloves according to office policy.	5		
3. Sanitize hands as described in Procedure 31-3 or 31-4.	10		
4. Apply gloves and adjust them to ensure a proper fit.	5		
5. Inspect the gloves carefully for tears, holes, or punctures before and after application.	5		
Removing gloves: 1. Grasp the outside of one glove with the first three fingers of the other hand (approximately 1 to 2 inches below the cuff).	10		
2. Stretch the soiled glove by pulling it away from the hand, and slowly pull the glove downward off the hand. Usually the dominant hand is ungloved first.	10		

Copyright © 2010, 2005 by Saunders, an imprint of Elsevier, Inc. All rights reserved.

Steps	Possible Points	First Attempt	Second Attempt
3. After the glove is pulled free from the hand, ball it in the palm of the gloved hand.	10		
4. Remove the other glove by placing the index and middle fingers of the ungloved hand inside the glove of the gloved hand; turn the cuff downward. Be careful not to touch the outside of the soiled glove.	10		
5. Stretch the glove away from the hand and pull the cuff downward over the hand and over the balled-up glove, turning it inside out and with the balled glove inside.	10		
6. Carefully dispose of the gloves in a marked biohazardous waste container.	10		
7. Sanitize hands.	10		
Total Points Possible	100		

Comments: Total Points Earned _____

Divided by _____

Total Possible Points = _____ % Score

Instructor's Signature _____

Student Name: _____   DATE: _____

PROCEDURE 31-6 CHECKLIST: SANITIZE INSTRUMENTS

TASK: Properly sanitize contaminated instruments by cleansing with detergent and water to reduce the number of microorganisms or by using an ultrasound cleaner.

CONDITIONS: Given the proper equipment and supplies, the student will be required to demonstrate the proper method of sanitizing instruments in preparation for autoclaving. The instructor may select the method of sanitization—manual or ultrasonic cleaner or both.

NOTE: The student should practice the procedure using the MACC located on the Evolve site at http://evolve.elsevier.com/klieger/medicalassisting: MACC/Clinical skills/Infection control/Sanitizing and wrapping instruments for the autoclave.

EQUIPMENT AND SUPPLIES
- MACC/computer
- Disposable gloves
- Rubber (utility) gloves
- Fluid-resistant laboratory apron
- Laboratory safety goggles
- Stiff nylon brush
- Container to hold instruments
- Instrument cleaning solution, stain remover, and lubricant
- Ultrasonic cleaner, if applicable
- Material safety data sheet (MSDS) for cleaning solutions
- Towel

STANDARDS: Complete the procedure within _____ minutes and achieve a minimum score of _____%.

Time began _____   Time ended _____

Steps	Possible Points	First Attempt	Second Attempt
Manual method: 1. Assemble all supplies and equipment.	5		
2. Review MSDS for the chemical agent being used.	5		
3. Apply appropriate personal protective equipment (PPE).	5		
4. Apply utility gloves over the disposable gloves.	10		
5. Mix cleaning solution for the instruments, following manufacturer's directions on the label. Alternatively, prepare the ultrasound cleaning device, following manufacturer's directions.	10		
6. Remove contaminated instruments from area of use, and place them in a covered container, separating the instruments as appropriate.	10		
7. Rinse all instruments under cool running water to remove organic material.	10		

Steps	Possible Points	First Attempt	Second Attempt
8. Using a scrub brush and cleaning solution, loosen any debris on the instruments.	10		
9. Check instruments for stain or rust or both, and treat appropriately.	10		
10. Rinse all instruments.	10		
11. Dry each instrument with a paper towel.	10		
12. Dispose of cleaning solution, drying material, or remaining contaminated material as appropriate.	10		
13. Lubricate hinged instruments as appropriate.	10		
14. Remove and dispose of PPE as appropriate.	5		
15. Sanitize hands.	5		
Ultrasonic method: 1. Assemble all supplies and equipment.	5		
2. Review MSDS for the chemical agent being used.	5		
3. Apply appropriate PPE.	5		
4. Prepare ultrasonic cleaning solution according to manufacturer's recommendations.	10		
5. Separate sanitized instruments into different types of metals and by delicate and sharp instruments.	10		
6. Open hinged instruments and place them in the ultrasonic cleaner, completely submerging them.	10		
7. Turn on the ultrasonic machine and set the timer for the recommended period of time for type of instrument.	10		
8. Remove the instruments at the end of the cycle and dry.	10		
9. Change the ultrasonic cleaner according to manufacturer's instructions as appropriate.	5		
10. Cover container between uses.	5		
Total Points Possible	200		

Comments: Total Points Earned _____

Divided by _____

Total Possible Points = _____% Score

Instructor's Signature _____

Copyright © 2010, 2005 by Saunders, an imprint of Elsevier, Inc. All rights reserved.

Student Name: _____   DATE: _____

PROCEDURE 31-7 CHECKLIST: PERFORM CHEMICAL STERILIZATION

TASK: Properly sterilize items using a chemical agent.

CONDITIONS: Given the proper equipment and supplies, the student will be required to demonstrate the proper method of performing chemical sterilization of instruments.

EQUIPMENT AND SUPPLIES
- Chemical agent, disinfectant
- Material safety data sheet (MSDS)
- Disposable gloves
- Stainless steel or glass container with cover
- Towels
- Articles to be sterilized

STANDARDS: Complete the procedure within _____ minutes and achieve a minimum score of _____%.

Time began _____   Time ended _____

Steps	Possible Points	First Attempt	Second Attempt
1. Assemble all supplies and equipment.	5		
2. Review MSDS for the chemical agent being used.	5		
3. Apply appropriate personal protective equipment (PPE).	5		
4. Place the sanitized items in the chemical solution for sterilization. Instruments must be completely covered in the chemical agent.	10		
5. Place the airtight lid on the container.	5		
6. Treat the items for the required time.	10		
7. Before using the instruments, remove the items from the chemical and rinse completely. Lift out the stainless steel tray and rinse in a sterile distilled water bath.	10		
8. Using sterile transfer forceps, remove the items from the tray for use.	10		
9. Dry items before use with a sterile towel.	10		
10. Remove gloves and sanitize hands.	5		
Total Points Possible	75		

Comments: Total Points Earned _____

Divided by _____

Total Possible Points = _____% Score

Instructor's Signature _____

Student Name: _____ DATE: _____

PROCEDURE 31-8 CHECKLIST: WRAP INSTRUMENTS FOR THE AUTOCLAVE

TASK: Wrap sanitized instruments for autoclaving.

CONDITIONS: Given the proper equipment and supplies, the student will be required to demonstrate the proper method of wrapping instruments in preparation for autoclaving.

NOTE: The student should practice the procedure using the MACC located on the Evolve site at http://evolve.elsevier.com/klieger/medicalassisting: MACC/Clinical skills/Infection control/Sanitizing & wrapping instruments for the autoclave.

EQUIPMENT AND SUPPLIES
- MACC/computer
- Autoclave wrapping material
- Autoclave tape
- Sterilization indicator strip
- Sterilization pouch
- Waterproof pen
- 10 4- × 4-inch gauze squares
- One forceps
- One Kelly hemostat
- One S/S operating scissors
- Other items as designated
- One instrument to be wrapped separately

STANDARDS: Complete the procedure within _____ minutes and achieve a minimum score of _____%.

Time began _____   Time ended _____

Steps	Possible Points	First Attempt	Second Attempt
1. Assemble all supplies and equipment.	5		
2. Sanitize hands.	5		
3. Place instruments on appropriate size wrapper.	10		
4. Place a sterilization strip in the center of the pack.	10		
5. Wrap instruments in proper manner.	10		
6. Repeat the wrapping process for the outside wrap, if applicable.	10		
7. Secure the package with autoclave tape.	10		
8. Label the autoclave tape with a waterproof pen.	10		
9. Set the package aside until it is time to autoclave.	5		

PROCEDURE 31-8

Copyright © 2010, 2005 by Saunders, an imprint of Elsevier, Inc. All rights reserved.

Steps	Possible Points	First Attempt	Second Attempt
Individual instrument: 10. Label the pouch.	5		
11. Place the instrument carefully into the sterilization pack in the correct position for appropriate removal.	10		
12. Seal the pouch.	5		
13. Set aside the package until it is time to autoclave.	5		
Total Points Possible	100		

Comments: Total Points Earned _____

Divided by _____

Total Possible Points = _____% Score

Instructor's Signature _____

Copyright © 2010, 2005 by Saunders, an imprint of Elsevier, Inc. All rights reserved.

Student Name: _____ DATE: _____

PROCEDURE 31-9 CHECKLIST: STERILIZE ARTICLES IN THE AUTOCLAVE

TASK: Properly sterilize supplies and medical equipment using an autoclave.

CONDITIONS: Given the proper equipment and supplies, the student will be required to demonstrate sterilization of articles in the autoclave.

NOTE: The student should practice the procedure using the MACC located on the Evolve site at http://evolve.elsevier.com/klieger/medicalassisting: MACC/Clinical skills/Infection control/Sterilizing articles in the autoclave.

EQUIPMENT AND SUPPLIES
- MACC/computer
- Distilled water
- Heat-resistant gloves
- Wrapped packs
- Other autoclavable items as required
- Autoclave with instruction manual
- Autoclave log
- Pen

STANDARDS: Complete the procedure within _____ minutes and achieve a minimum score of _____%.

Time began _____   Time ended _____

Steps	Possible Points	First Attempt	Second Attempt
1. Assemble previously wrapped autoclave packs, other items to sterilize, and all other supplies and equipment.	5		
2. Fill the autoclave reservoir with distilled water.	5		
3. Properly load the autoclave chamber with previously prepared items.	10		
4. Fill chamber with distilled water to fill line.	5		
5. Close the door tightly.	5		
6. Turn the control knob to the "on" or "autoclave" setting to start the autoclave.	10		
7. Check the pressure gauge for appropriate pounds of pressure and proper temperature.	10		
8. Set the timer for the required time.	10		
9. After sterilization is complete, turn the control knob to "vent."	5		

Copyright © 2010, 2005 by Saunders, an imprint of Elsevier, Inc. All rights reserved.

Steps	Possible Points	First Attempt	Second Attempt
10. Open the door ½ to 1 inch when appropriate.	5		
11. Allow items to dry.	5		
12. Use heat-resistant gloves to remove items from the chamber.	5		
13. Turn the autoclave control knob to the "off" position.	5		
14. Inspect each pack for any breaks in sterilization technique.	5		
15. Appropriately store autoclaved articles.	5		
16. Maintain the autoclave log with all required information.	5		
Total Possible Points	100		

Comments: Total Points Earned _____

Divided by _____

Total Possible Points = _____% Score

Instructor's Signature _____

Student Name: _____   DATE: _____

PROCEDURE 33-1 CHECKLIST: MEASURE WEIGHT AND HEIGHT OF AN ADULT

TASK: Correctly obtain accurate height and weight measurements on an adult patient.

CONDITIONS: Given the proper equipment and supplies, the student will be required to role-play with another student or an instructor the proper method for measuring the height and weight of an adult patient.

NOTE: The student should practice the procedure using the MACC located on the Evolve site at http://evolve.elsevier.com/klieger/medicalassisting: MACC/Clinical skills/Patient care/Patient preparation/Obtaining height and weight.

EQUIPMENT AND SUPPLIES
- MACC/computer (practice)
- Paper towel
- Balance scale with bar measure for height
- Patient's medical record
- Pen

STANDARDS: Complete the procedure within _____ minutes and achieve a minimum score of _____%.

Time began _____   Time ended _____

Steps	Possible Points	First Attempt	Second Attempt
Weight: 1. Assemble all supplies and equipment.	5		
2. Sanitize hands.	5		
3. Check the scale to ensure it is properly balanced.	10		
4. Greet and identify the patient.	5		
5. Explain the procedure to the patient.	5		
6. Instruct the patient to remove shoes and empty items from pockets.	10		
7. Assist the patient on to the scale facing forward as necessary.	10		
8. Instruct the patient to stand still and not to hold on to objects for support.	10		
9. Balance the scale by moving the large weight (50-lb increment) first, and then the small (1-lb increment) weight until the scale is balanced.	5		

PROCEDURE 33-1

779

Copyright © 2010, 2005 by Saunders, an imprint of Elsevier, Inc. All rights reserved.

Steps	Possible Points	First Attempt	Second Attempt
10. Read the results.	5		
11. Return the balance weights to the resting position of "0."	5		
12. Record the weight in the patient's medical record.	5		
Height: 1. Instruct the patient to stand erect and look straight ahead, with his or her back to the scale. (The patient must turn around on scale from being weighed.)	10		
2. Raise the height bar above the person's head.	5		
3. Open the bar, taking care not to hit the patient's head.	5		
4. Move the bar down gently until it rests level on top of the patient's head.	10		
5. Assist the patient in stepping off the scale as appropriate.	5		
6. Read and record the measurement in the patient's medical record; convert from inches to feet and inches as per office policy.	20		
7. Assist the patient as needed in putting his or her shoes back on.	5		
8. Return the bar to the resting position.	5		
9. Sanitize hands.	5		
Total Points Possible	150		

Comments: Total Points Earned _____

Divided by _____

Total Possible Points = _____% Score

Instructor's Signature _____

Student Name: _____   DATE: _____

PROCEDURE 33-2 CHECKLIST: MEASURE WEIGHT AND LENGTH OF AN INFANT

TASK: Correctly measure the weight and length of an infant to monitor development.

CONDITIONS: Given the proper equipment and supplies, the student will be required to role-play the proper method for measuring the weight and length of an infant, using a mannequin.

NOTE: The student should practice the procedure using the MACC located on the Evolve site at http://evolve.elsevier.com/klieger/medicalassisting: MACC/Clinical skills/Patient care/The physical exam/Taking pediatric measurements and plotting on a growth chart.

EQUIPMENT AND SUPPLIES
- MACC/computer (patient)
- Infant scale with disposable plastic-lined drape or pad cover
- Flexible tape measure
- Infant growth charts, male or female, as appropriate
- Patient's medical record
- Pen
- Ruler

STANDARDS: Complete the procedure within _____ minutes and achieve a minimum score of _____%.

Time began _____   Time ended _____

Steps	Possible Points	First Attempt	Second Attempt
Weight:			
1. Assemble all supplies and equipment.	5		
2. Sanitize hands.	5		
3. Unlock the pediatric scale and balance as necessary.	10		
4. Greet the parent or guardian, and identify the patient.	10		
5. Explain the procedure to the parent or guardian.	10		
6. Place the plastic-lined disposable drape or pad cover on the scale.	10		
7. Undress the infant, including the diaper.	10		
8. Gently place the infant on his or her back on the scale.	10		
9. Weigh the infant by first moving the pound weight and then the ounce weight until the scale balances.	10		
10. Read the results.	10		

781

Copyright © 2010, 2005 by Saunders, an imprint of Elsevier, Inc. All rights reserved.

Steps	Possible Points	First Attempt	Second Attempt
11. Record the infant's weight in the medical record.	10		
12. Return the balance weights to the resting position.	10		
13. Remove the infant from the scale. (If you are measuring the length of the infant on a scale that has length measurement included, do not perform Steps 13 and 14 at this time.)	10		
14. Discard the scale drape or pad.	10		
Length (measured on the infant scale): 1. Position the infant in the scale by placing the vertex of the infant head against the headboard at the zero mark, asking the parent or guardian to hold the infant in place.	10		
2. Read the length in inches to the nearest fraction of an inch.	10		
3. Record the results.	10		
4. Remove the infant from the scale.	10		
5. Discard the scale drape or pad.	10		
6. Read and record the measurement in the patient's medical record.	10		
Length (measured using the examination table): 7. Position the infant on his or her back in the center of the examination table.	10		
8. Ask the parent or guardian to hold the infant in place.	5		
9. With a pen, mark a line on the table paper level with the patient's head.	10		
10. Holding the infant, stretch the leg and foot down and place a mark at the heel.	10		
11. Gently remove the infant from the table.	10		

Steps	Possible Points	First Attempt	Second Attempt
12. Measure the length between the two pen marks using the tape measure.	10		
13. Inform the parent or guardian of the measurements and have the parent or guardian replace the diaper.	10		
14. Discard the protective paper on the examination table in the appropriate container.	10		
15. Sanitize hands.	5		
16. Plot the infant's weight and length on the growth charts and in the patient's medical record.	20		
Total Points Possible	290		

Comments: Total Points Earned _____

Divided by _____

Total Possible Points = _____ % Score

Instructor's Signature _____

Copyright © 2010, 2005 by Saunders, an imprint of Elsevier, Inc. All rights reserved.

Student Name: _____ DATE: _____

PROCEDURE 33-3 CHECKLIST: MEASURE HEAD AND CHEST CIRCUMFERENCE OF AN INFANT

TASK: Accurately measure the head circumference and chest circumference of an infant.

CONDITIONS: Given the proper equipment and supplies, the student will be required to role-play the proper method for measuring the weight and length of an infant, using a mannequin.

NOTE: The student should practice the procedure using the MACC located on the Evolve site at http://evolve.elsevier.com/klieger/medicalassisting: MACC/Clinical skills/Patient care/The physical exam/Taking pediatric measurements & plotting on a growth chart.

EQUIPMENT AND SUPPLIES
- MACC/computer (practice)
- Flexible tape measure
- Infant growth charts, male or female, as appropriate
- Patient's medical record
- Pen
- Ruler

STANDARDS: Complete the procedure within _____ minutes and achieve a minimum score of _____%.

Time began _____   Time ended _____

Steps	Possible Points	First Attempt	Second Attempt
Head circumference: 1. Assemble all supplies and equipment.	5		
2. Sanitize hands.	5		
3. Greet the parent or guardian, and identify the patient.	5		
4. Explain the procedure to the parent or guardian.	5		
5. Position the infant.	5		
6. Position the tape measure around the infant's head above the ears and just over the eyebrows.	10		
7. Read the tape measure to the nearest ¼ inch.	10		
8. Write the results on the examination paper.	5		
Chest circumference: 1. Place the tape around the infant's chest at the nipple line.	5		
2. Read the tape measure to the nearest ¼ inch.	5		

Copyright © 2010, 2005 by Saunders, an imprint of Elsevier, Inc. All rights reserved.

Steps	Possible Points	Frist Attempt	Second Attempt
3. Write the results on the examination paper.	5		
4. Hand the infant back to the parent or guardian.	5		
5. Inform the parent or guardian of the measurements, and record the results in the patient's medical record.	10		
6. Discard the protective paper on the examination table in the appropriate container if the examination will not be done on the same table.	5		
7. Sanitize hands.	5		
8. Plot points on the growth chart and connect the dots using a ruler.	10		
Total Points Possible	100		

Comments: Total Points Earned _____

Divided by _____

Total Possible Points = _____% Score

Instructor's Signature _____

Copyright © 2010, 2005 by Saunders, an imprint of Elsevier, Inc. All rights reserved.

Information for Procedures 33-2 and 33-3

Record the following data on the appropriate growth chart for Susan Rivers, and calculate the percentiles:

	Weight	Percentile	Length	Percentile
Birth	8 lb.		18 inches	
3 mo	12 lb.		19¾ inches	
6 mo	14 lb.		20½ inches	
9 mo	19 lb., 7 oz.		22 inches	
12 mo	22 lb.		24¼ inches	
15 mo	23 lb., 10 oz.		25 inches	
18 mo	25 lb.		26¼ inches	

Record the following data on the appropriate growth chart for Joseph Craine, and calculate the percentiles:

	Weight	Percentile	Length	Percentile
Birth	7 lb., 2 oz.		20 inches	
3 mo	11 lb., 6 oz.		22½ inches	
6 mo	15 lb., 1 oz.		25¾ inches	
9 mo	18 lb., 5 oz.		27¼ inches	
12 mo	21 lb., 10 oz.		30 inches	
15 mo	23 lb., 5 oz.		32¼ inches	
18 mo	27 lb.		33 inches	

Copyright © 2010, 2005 by Saunders, an imprint of Elsevier, Inc. All rights reserved.

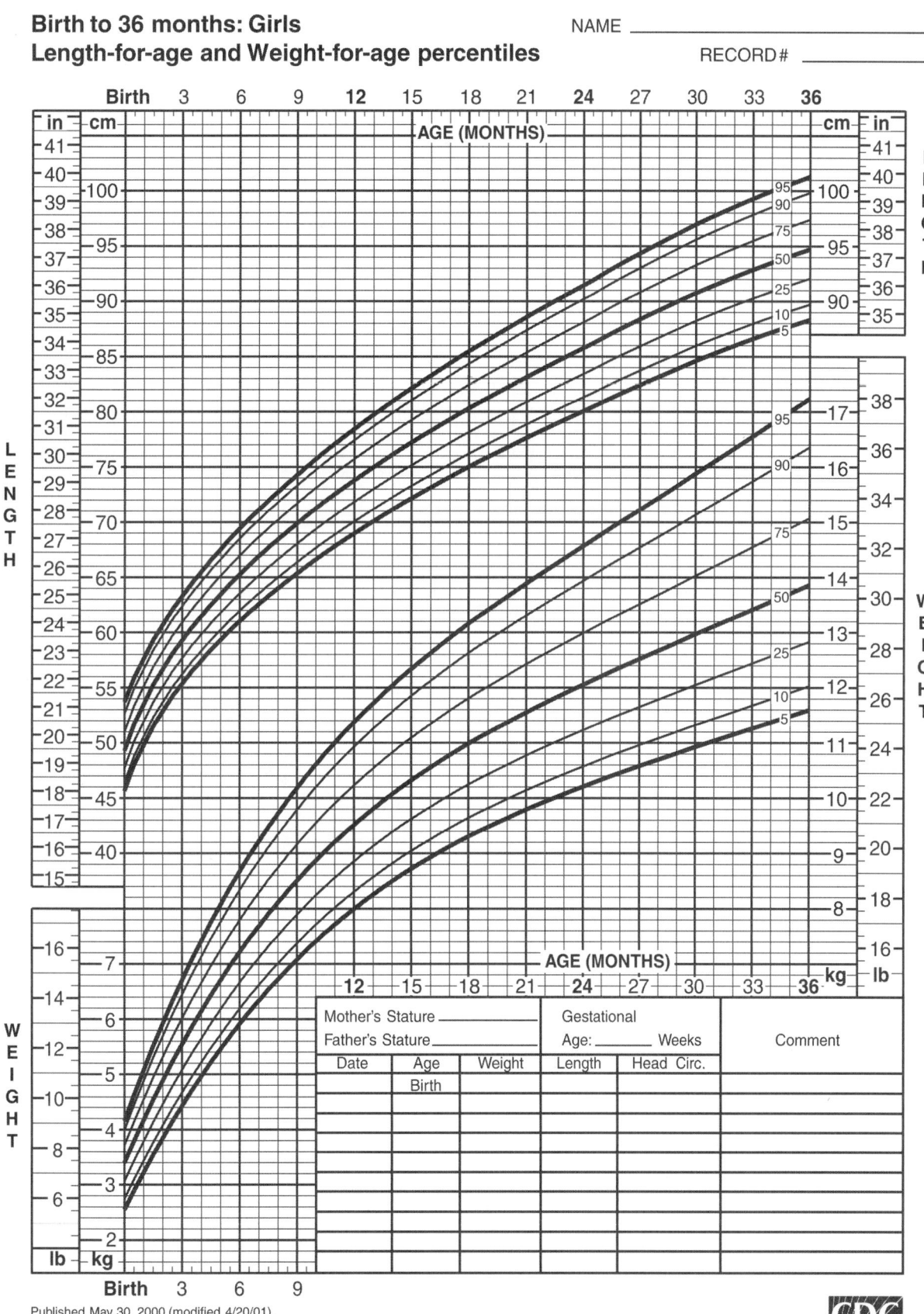

APPENDIX A Supplemental Chapter Materials

Birth to 36 months: Boys
Head circumference-for-age and
Weight-for-length percentiles

NAME _____

RECORD # _____

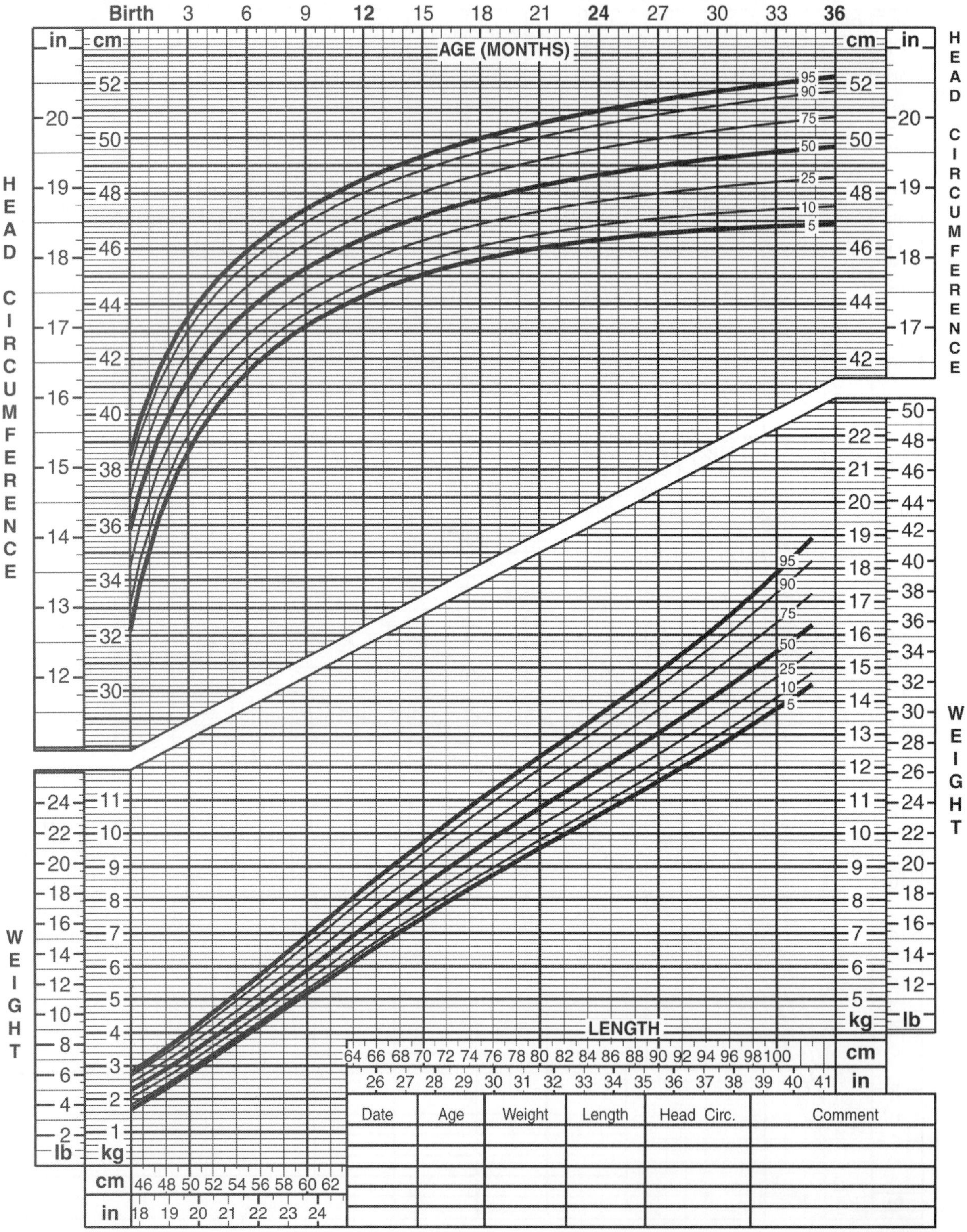

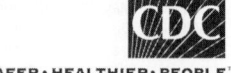

Published May 30, 2000 (modified 10/16/00).
SOURCE: Developed by the National Center for Health Statistics in collaboration with
the National Center for Chronic Disease Prevention and Health Promotion (2000).
http://www.cdc.gov/growthcharts

SAFER · HEALTHIER · PEOPLE™

Copyright © 2010, 2005 by Saunders, an imprint of Elsevier, Inc. All rights reserved.

Student Name: _____   DATE: _____

PROCEDURE 33-4 CHECKLIST: MEASURE ORAL BODY TEMPERATURE USING A MERCURY-FREE GLASS THERMOMETER

TASK: Accurately measure and record a patient's oral temperature.

CONDITIONS: Given the proper equipment and supplies, the student will be required to role-play with another student or an instructor the proper method for measuring an oral body temperature using a mercury-free glass thermometer.

EQUIPMENT AND SUPPLIES
- Mercury-free glass oral thermometer
- Thermometer sheath
- Disposable gloves
- Biohazardous waste container
- Pen
- Patient's medical record

STANDARDS: Complete the procedure within _____ minutes and achieve a minimum score of _____%.

Time began _____   Time ended _____

Steps	Possible Points	First Attempt	Second Attempt
1. Assemble all supplies and equipment.	5		
2. Sanitize hands.	5		
3. Greet and identify the patient.	5		
4. Explain the procedure to the patient.	5		
5. Determine if the patient has recently had a hot or cold beverage to drink, or if he or she has smoked.	5		
6. Put on gloves and remove the thermometer from its holder, without touching the bulb end with your fingers.	5		
7. Inspect the thermometer for chips or cracks.	5		
8. Read the thermometer to ensure that the temperature is well below 96.0°F. Shake down thermometer as necessary.	5		
9. Cover the thermometer with a protective thermometer sheath.	5		
10. Ask the patient to open his or her mouth and place the probe tip under the tongue.	5		
11. Ask the patient to hold, not clasp, the thermometer between the teeth and to close the lips snugly around it to form an airtight seal.	5		

Copyright © 2010, 2005 by Saunders, an imprint of Elsevier, Inc. All rights reserved.

Steps	Possible Points	First Attempt	Second Attempt
12. Leave the thermometer in place for a minimum of 3 minutes.	5		
13. Remove the thermometer and read the results.	10		
14. Holding the thermometer by the stem, remove the protective sheath and discard in a biohazardous waste container.	5		
15. Sanitize the thermometer following the manufacturer's recommendations.	5		
16. Remove gloves and discard in biohazardous waste container.	5		
17. Return the thermometer to its storage container.	5		
18. Sanitize hands.	5		
19. Document the results in the patient's medical record.	5		
Total Points Possible	100		

Comments: Total Points Earned _____

Divided by _____

Total Possible Points = _____% Score

Instructor's Signature _____

Student Name: _____ DATE: _____

PROCEDURE 33-5 CHECKLIST: MEASURE ORAL BODY TEMPERATURE USING A RECHARGEABLE ELECTRONIC OR DIGITAL THERMOMETER

TASK: Accurately measure and record a patient's oral temperature.

CONDITIONS: Given the proper equipment and supplies, the student will be required to role-play with another student or an instructor the proper method for measuring an oral body temperature using a rechargeable electronic or digital thermometer.

NOTE: The student should practice the procedure using the MACC located on the Evolve site at http://evolve.elsevier.com/klieger/medicalassisting: MACC/Clinical skills/Patient care/The physical exam/Obtaining digital oral, digital rectal & tympanic body temperatures.

EQUIPMENT AND SUPPLIES
- MACC/computer
- Rechargeable electronic or digital thermometer
- Probe cover
- Waste container
- Pen
- Patient's medical record

STANDARDS: Complete the procedure within _____ minutes and achieve a minimum score of _____%.

Time began _____   Time ended _____

Steps	Possible Points	First Attempt	Second Attempt
1. Assemble all supplies and equipment.	5		
2. Sanitize hands.	5		
3. Greet and identify the patient.	5		
4. Explain the procedure to the patient.	5		
5. Remove the thermometer unit from its rechargeable base, and attach the blue collar probe for measuring oral temperature.	10		
6. Remove the thermometer probe cover from the probe holder, and attach to thermometer probe.	5		
7. Ask the patient to open his or her mouth. Place the probe tip under the tongue.	10		
8. Ask the patient to close his or her mouth.	5		
9. When the alert signal is seen or heard, remove the probe from the patient's mouth.	10		

Copyright © 2010, 2005 by Saunders, an imprint of Elsevier, Inc. All rights reserved.

Steps	Possible Points	First Attempt	Second Attempt
10. Read the result in the LED window of the unit.	10		
11. Dispose of the thermometer tip.	5		
12. Return the probe to the stored position on the thermometer.	5		
13. Place the thermometer unit back on the rechargeable base.	5		
14. Sanitize hands.	5		
15. Document results in the patient's medical record.	10		
Total Points Possible	100		

Comments: Total Points Earned _____

Divided by _____

Total Possible Points = _____% Score

Instructor's Signature _____

Student Name: _____ DATE: _____

PROCEDURE 33-6 CHECKLIST: MEASURE RECTAL BODY TEMPERATURE USING A RECHARGEABLE ELECTRONIC OR DIGITAL THERMOMETER

TASK: Accurately measure and record a patient's rectal temperature.

CONDITIONS: Given the proper equipment and supplies, the student will be required to role-play with a mannequin the proper method for measuring the rectal temperature using a rechargeable electronic or digital thermometer.

NOTE: The student should practice the procedure using the MACC located on the Evolve site at http://evolve.elsevier.com/klieger/medicalassisting: MACC/Clinical skills/Patient care/Patient preparation/Obtaining digital oral, digital rectal, & tympanic body temperature.

EQUIPMENT AND SUPPLIES
- MACC/computer
- Rechargeable electronic or digital thermometer
- Probe cover
- Disposable gloves
- Lubricant
- Biohazardous waste container
- Pen
- Patient's medical record
- Soft tissue
- Gauze squares

STANDARDS: Complete the procedure within _____ minutes and achieve a minimum score of _____ %.

Time began _____   Time ended _____

Steps	Possible Points	First Attempt	Second Attempt
1. Assemble all supplies and equipment.	5		
2. Sanitize hands.	5		
3. Greet and identify the patient.	5		
4. Explain the procedure to the patient.	5		
5. Remove the thermometer unit from its rechargeable base, and attach the red collar probe for measuring rectal temperature.	5		
6. Remove the thermometer probe cover from the probe holder and attach to thermometer probe.	5		
7. Place a plastic-lined disposable drape or pad cover on the table.	5		
8. Put on disposable gloves.	5		

Copyright © 2010, 2005 by Saunders, an imprint of Elsevier, Inc. All rights reserved.

Steps	Possible Points	First Attempt	Second Attempt
9. Undress the child, including the diaper. (Position an adult patient in the Sims' position and properly drape. Expose the rectal area of an adult patient.)	5		
10. Squeeze approximately 1 inch of lubricant onto a gauze square; lubricate the first 2 inches of the probe cover for an adult and 1 inch for a child.	5		
11. If patient is a child, have the parent or guardian (classmate) hold the child firmly but comfortably so that the child lies still, to avoid injury to the rectal wall.	5		
12. Insert the tip about 1 to 2 inches for an adult or ½ inch for a child.	5		
13. When the alert signal is seen or heard, read the results in the LED window of the unit.	5		
14. Remove the probe cover.	5		
15. Return the probe to the stored position on the thermometer.	5		
16. Place the thermometer unit back on the rechargeable base.	5		
17. Wipe the patient's anal area with tissue.	5		
18. Remove soiled gloves and discard in a biohazardous waste container.	5		
19. Sanitize hands.	5		
20. Document results in the patient's medical record using ® to indicate rectal temperature was obtained.	5		
Total Points Possible	100		

Comments: Total Points Earned _____

Divided by _____

Total Possible Points = _____% Score

Instructor's Signature _____

Student Name: _____ DATE: _____

PROCEDURE 33-7 CHECKLIST: MEASURE AXILLARY BODY TEMPERATURE USING A RECHARGEABLE ELECTRONIC OR DIGITAL THERMOMETER

TASK: Accurately measure and record a patient's axillary temperature.

CONDITIONS: Given the proper equipment and supplies, the student will be required to role-play with another student or an instructor the proper method for measuring the axillary temperature using a rechargeable electronic or digital thermometer.

EQUIPMENT AND SUPPLIES
- Rechargeable electronic or digital thermometer
- Probe cover
- Waste container
- Pen
- Patient's medical record

STANDARDS: Complete the procedure within _____ minutes and achieve a minimum score of _____%.

Time began _____   Time ended _____

Steps	Possible Points	First Attempt	Second Attempt
1. Assemble all supplies and equipment.	5		
2. Sanitize hands.	5		
3. Greet and identify the patient.	5		
4. Explain the procedure to the patient.	5		
5. Remove the thermometer unit from its rechargeable base, and attach the probe with the blue collar for measuring axillary temperature.	10		
6. Remove the thermometer probe from the probe holder and attach thermometer cover.	5		
7. Remove the patient's clothing as needed to access the axillary region.	5		
8. Pat the axilla and axillary area dry as needed.	5		
9. Place the probe into the center of the patient's armpit.	5		
10. Instruct the patient to hold the arm snugly across the chest until the thermometer sends the alert signal that the temperature has been taken.	5		

Steps	Possible Points	First Attempt	Second Attempt
11. When the alert signal is seen or heard, remove the probe from the patient's armpit.	5		
12. Read the results in the LED window of the unit.	10		
13. Dispose of the probe cover.	5		
14. Return the probe to the stored position on the thermometer.	5		
15. Place the thermometer unit back on the rechargeable base.	5		
16. Sanitize hands.	5		
17. Document results in the patient's medical record.	10		
Total Points Possible	100		

Comments: Total Points Earned _____

Divided by _____

Total Possible Points = _____ % Score

Instructor's Signature _____

Student Name: DATE:

PROCEDURE 33-8 CHECKLIST: MEASURE BODY TEMPERATURE USING A TYMPANIC THERMOMETER

TASK: Accurately measure and record a patient's temperature using a tympanic thermometer.

CONDITIONS: Given the proper equipment and supplies, the student will be required to role-play with another student the proper method for measuring the tympanic temperature using a tympanic thermometer.

NOTE: The student should practice the procedure using the MACC located on the Evolve site at http://evolve.elsevier.com/klieger/medicalassisting: MACC/Clinical skills/Patient care/Patient preparation/Obtaining digital oral, digital rectal, & tympanic body temperature.

EQUIPMENT AND SUPPLIES
- MACC/computer
- Tympanic thermometer
- Disposable probe cover
- Pen
- Patient's medical record
- Biohazardous waste container

STANDARDS: Complete the procedure within _____ minutes and achieve a minimum score of _____%.

Time began _____   Time ended _____

Steps	Possible Points	First Attempt	Second Attempt
1. Assemble all supplies and equipment.	5		
2. Sanitize hands.	5		
3. Greet and identify the patient.	5		
4. Explain the procedure to the patient.	5		
5. Remove the thermometer from the charger.	5		
6. Check to ensure the mode for interpretation of temperature is set to "oral" mode.	10		
7. Check the lens probe to ensure it is clean and not scratched.	5		
8. Turn on the thermometer.	5		
9. Insert the probe firmly into a disposable plastic probe cover.	5		
10. Wait for a digital "READY" display.	5		

Copyright © 2010, 2005 by Saunders, an imprint of Elsevier, Inc. All rights reserved.

Steps	Possible Points	First Attempt	Second Attempt
11. With the hand that is not holding the probe, pull adult patient's ear up and back to straighten the ear canal. For a small child, pull the patient's ear down and back to straighten the ear canal.	10		
12. Insert the probe into the patient's ear and tightly seal the ear canal opening.	10		
13. Position the probe.	5		
14. Depress the activation button.	5		
15. Release the activation button and wait 2 seconds.	5		
16. Remove the probe from the ear and read the temperature.	5		
17. Note the reading, making sure that the screen displays "oral" as the mode of interpretation.	5		
18. Discard the probe cover in a biohazardous waste container.	5		
19. Replace the thermometer on the charger base.	5		
20. Sanitize hands.	5		
21. Document results in the patient's medical record using Ⓣ to indicate a tympanic temperature was obtained.	10		
Total Points Possible	125		

Comments: Total Points Earned _____

Divided by _____

Total Possible Points = _____% Score

Instructor's Signature _____

Student Name: _____ DATE: _____

PROCEDURE 33-9 CHECKLIST: MEASURE BODY TEMPERATURE USING A DISPOSABLE ORAL THERMOMETER

TASK: Accurately measure and record a patient's oral temperature using a disposable thermometer.

CONDITIONS: Given the proper equipment and supplies, the student will be required to perform the proper method for measuring an oral temperature using a disposable oral thermometer.

EQUIPMENT AND SUPPLIES
- Disposable thermometer
- Disposable gloves
- Biohazardous waste container
- Pen
- Patient's medical record

STANDARDS: Complete the procedure within _____ minutes and achieve a minimum score of _____ %.

Time began _____   Time ended _____

Steps	Possible Points	First Attempt	Second Attempt
1. Assemble all supplies and equipment.	5		
2. Sanitize hands.	5		
3. Greet and identify the patient.	5		
4. Explain the procedure to the patient.	5		
5. Put on disposable gloves.	5		
6. Open the thermometer packaging.	5		
7. Place the thermometer under the patient's tongue and wait 60 seconds.	5		
8. Remove the thermometer and read the results by looking at the colored dots.	5		
9. Discard the thermometer and gloves in a biohazardous waste container.	5		
10. Sanitize hands.	5		
11. Document results in the patient's medical record.	10		
Total Points Possible	60		

Comments: Total Points Earned _____

Divided by _____

Total Possible Points = _____ % Score

Instructor's Signature _____

Student Name: DATE:

PROCEDURE 33-10 CHECKLIST: MEASURE RADIAL PULSE

TASK: Accurately measure and record the rate, rhythm, and quality of a patient's pulse.

CONDITIONS: Given the proper equipment and supplies, the student will be required to role-play with another student or an instructor the proper method for measuring a patient's radial pulse.

NOTE: The student should practice the procedure using the MACC located on the Evolve site at http://evolve.elsevier.com/klieger/medicalassisting: MACC/Clinical skills/Patient care/Patient preparation/Obtaining pulse & respiration.

EQUIPMENT AND SUPPLIES
- MACC/computer (practice)
- Watch with a second hand
- Patient's medical record
- Pen

STANDARDS: Complete the procedure within _____ minutes and achieve a minimum score of _____ %.

Time began _____   Time ended _____

Steps	Possible Points	First Attempt	Second Attempt
1. Assemble all supplies and equipment.	5		
2. Sanitize hands.	5		
3. Greet and identify the patient.	5		
4. Explain the procedure to the patient.	5		
5. Observe the patient for any signs that may indicate an increase or decrease in the pulse rate because of external conditions.	5		
6. Position the patient.	5		
7. Place the index and middle fingertips over the radial artery while resting the thumb on the back of the patient's wrist.	10		
8. Apply moderate, gentle pressure directly over the site until the pulse can be felt.	10		
9. Count the pulse for 60 seconds.	10		
10. Sanitize hands.	5		
11. Document the results in the patient's chart; include the pulse rate, rhythm, and volume.	10		
Total Points Possible	75		

Comments: Total Points Earned _____

Divided by _____

Total Possible Points = _____ % Score

Instructor's Signature _____

Copyright © 2010, 2005 by Saunders, an imprint of Elsevier, Inc. All rights reserved.

Student Name: _____ DATE: _____

PROCEDURE 33-11 CHECKLIST: MEASURE APICAL PULSE

TASK: Accurately measure and record the rate, rhythm, and quality of a patient's pulse.

CONDITIONS: Given the proper equipment and supplies, the student will be required to role-play with another student or an instructor the proper method for measuring a patient's apical pulse.

EQUIPMENT AND SUPPLIES
- Watch with a second hand
- Stethoscope
- Alcohol wipe
- Patient's medical record
- Pen

STANDARDS: Complete the procedure within _____ minutes and achieve a minimum score of _____%.

Time began _____   Time ended _____

Steps	Possible Points	First Attempt	Second Attempt
1. Assemble all supplies and equipment.	5		
2. Sanitize hands.	5		
3. Greet and identify the patient.	5		
4. Explain the procedure to the patient.	5		
5. Clean the earpieces of the stethoscope with an alcohol wipe.	5		
6. Position the patient in a supine or sitting position.	10		
7. Position the stethoscope over apex of heart.	10		
8. Count the number of beats for 1 full minute.	10		
9. Clean the stethoscope earpieces and diaphragm with an alcohol wipe.	5		
10. Sanitize hands.	5		
11. Document the results in the patient's chart; include the pulse rate, rhythm, and volume.	10		
Total Points Possible	75		

Comments: Total Points Earned _____

Divided by _____

Total Possible Points = _____% Score

Instructor's Signature _____

Copyright © 2010, 2005 by Saunders, an imprint of Elsevier, Inc. All rights reserved.

Student Name: _____ DATE: _____

PROCEDURE 33-12 CHECKLIST: MEASURE RESPIRATORY RATE

TASK: Accurately measure and record a patient's respiratory rate.

CONDITIONS: Given the proper equipment and supplies, the student will be required to role-play with another student the proper method for measuring a patient's respiratory rate.

NOTE: The student should practice the procedure using the MACC located on the Evolve site at http://evolve.elsevier.com/klieger/medicalassisting: MACC/Clinical skills/Patient care/Patient preparation/Obtaining pulse & respiration.

EQUIPMENT AND SUPPLIES
- MACC/computer (practice)
- Watch with a second hand
- Patient's medical record
- Pen

STANDARDS: Complete the procedure within _____ minutes and achieve a minimum score of _____%.

Time began _____   Time ended _____

Steps	Possible Points	First Attempt	Second Attempt
1. Assemble all supplies and equipment.	5		
2. Sanitize hands.	5		
3. Greet and identify the patient.	5		
4. Explain the procedure to the patient.	5		
5. Count each respiration for 30 seconds and multiply by 2. (If breathing pattern is inaccurate, count for 1 full minute.)	15		
6. Sanitize hands.	5		
7. Document the results in the patient's chart; include the respiratory rate, rhythm, and depth. Document any irregularities found.	10		
Total Points Possible	50		

Comments: Total Points Earned _____

Divided by _____

Total Possible Points = _____% Score

Instructor's Signature _____

Copyright © 2010, 2005 by Saunders, an imprint of Elsevier, Inc. All rights reserved.

Student Name: _____   DATE: _____

PROCEDURE 33-13 CHECKLIST: MEASURE BLOOD PRESSURE

TASK: Accurately measure and record a patient's blood pressure by palpation and auscultation.

CONDITIONS: Given the proper equipment and supplies, the student will be required to role-play with another student the proper method for measuring a patient's blood pressure.

NOTE: *The student should practice the procedure using the MACC located on the Evolve site at http://evolve.elsevier.com/klieger/medicalassisting: MACC/Clinical skills/Patient care/Patient preparation/Obtaining blood pressure.*

EQUIPMENT AND SUPPLIES
- MACC/computer (practice)
- Stethoscope
- Aneroid sphygmomanometer in proper size for patient
- Alcohol wipe
- Patient's medical record
- Pen

STANDARDS: Complete the procedure within _____ minutes and achieve a minimum score of _____%.

Time began _____   Time ended _____

Steps	Possible Points	First Attempt	Second Attempt
1. Assemble all supplies and equipment.	5		
2. Sanitize hands.	5		
3. Greet and identify the patient.	5		
4. Explain the procedure to the patient.	5		
5. Position the patient comfortably in a sitting or supine position.	5		
6. Palpate the brachial artery.	10		
7. Position the blood pressure cuff, wrap the cuff snugly and evenly around the patient's arm, and secure the end.	10		
8. Position the aneroid gauge for direct viewing at a distance of no more than 3 feet.	10		
9. Measure the systolic pressure by palpation.	15		
10. Deflate the cuff completely, and wait at least 60 seconds before reinflating.	10		
11. Clean the stethoscope.	5		
12. Place the earpieces of the stethoscope in your ears, with the earpieces directed slightly forward.	5		

Copyright © 2010, 2005 by Saunders, an imprint of Elsevier, Inc. All rights reserved.

Steps	Possible Points	First Attempt	Second Attempt
13. Position the head of the stethoscope over the brachial artery of the arm.	5		
14. Close the valve to the manometer.	5		
15. Pump the cuff at a smooth rate to approximately 20 to 30 mm Hg above the palpated systolic pressure.	10		
16. Loosen the thumbscrew slightly to open the valve and release the pressure on the cuff, slowly and steadily.	10		
17. Obtain the systolic reading.	10		
18. Continue to release the air from the cuff at a moderately slow rate.	5		
19. Listen for the disappearance of the Korotkoff sounds; obtain diastolic pressure.	10		
20. Release the air remaining in the cuff quickly by loosening the thumbscrew to open the valve completely.	5		
21. Remove the earpieces of the stethoscope from your ears, and remove the cuff from the patient's arm.	5		
22. Sanitize hands.	5		
23. Document the results in the patient's chart.	10		
24. Clean the earpieces and diaphragm with an alcohol wipe, and properly store the equipment.	5		
Total Points Possible	175		

Comments: Total Points Earned _____

Divided by _____

Total Possible Points = _____ % Score

Instructor's Signature _____

Charting for Procedures 33-1 through 33-13

Date	Chart

Date	Chart

Date	Chart

Date	Chart

Copyright © 2010, 2005 by Saunders, an imprint of Elsevier, Inc. All rights reserved.

	Chart
Date	

	Chart
Date	

	Chart
Date	

	Chart
Date	

	Chart
Date	

	Chart
Date	

	Chart
Date	

	Chart
Date	

	Chart
Date	

	Chart
Date	

	Chart
Date	

	Chart
Date	

Student Name: _____ DATE: _____

PROCEDURE 34-1 CHECKLIST: COMPLETE A MEDICAL HISTORY FORM

TASK: Obtain and record a patient's medical history using verbal and nonverbal communication skills and applying the principles of accurate documentation in the patient's medical record.

CONDITIONS: Given the proper equipment and supplies, the student will be required to role-play with another student or an instructor the proper method for obtaining and recording a patient's medical history.

NOTE: The student should practice the procedure using the MACC located on the Evolve site at http://evolve.elsevier.com/klieger/medicalassisting: MACC/Clinical skills/Patient care/Patient preparation/Obtaining & recording a medical history.

EQUIPMENT AND SUPPLIES
- MACC/computer (practice)
- Medical history form
- Patient's medical record
- Pen (red and black ink)
- Clipboard
- Quiet private area

STANDARDS: Complete the procedure within _____ minutes and achieve a minimum score of _____%.

Time began _____   Time ended _____

Steps	Possible Points	First Attempt	Second Attempt
1. Assemble all supplies and equipment.	5		
2. Greet and identify the patient.	5		
3. Escort the patient to a quiet, comfortable room that is well lit and affords privacy.	5		
4. Explain why information is needed, and reassure the patient that the information will be kept confidential.	10		
5. Seat the patient, and then sit near the patient at eye level.	5		
6. Review the completed portion of the medical history form, looking for omissions or incomplete answers. Verify information as needed.	15		
7. Speak clearly and distinctly; maintain eye contact as appropriate with the patient.	10		
8. Remember to record all information legibly in black ink.	5		
9. Ask the patient to state the reason for today's visit.	10		

Copyright © 2010, 2005 by Saunders, an imprint of Elsevier, Inc. All rights reserved.

Steps	Possible Points	First Attempt	Second Attempt
10. Record the information briefly and concisely, using the patient's own words as much as possible.	20		
11. Ask the patient about prescription, over-the-counter, and herbal medications or treatments; record all medications the patient is taking.	10		
12. Inquire about allergies to medications, food, and other substances; record any allergies in red ink on every page of the history form. Record no allergies as appropriate.	10		
13. Review and record information in all sections of the family history form.	10		
14. Thank the patient for providing the information.	10		
15. Review the record for errors before giving to the physician.	10		
16. Use the information to complete the patient's record as directed.	10		
Total Points Possible	150		

Comments: Total Points Earned _____

Divided by _____

Total Possible Points = _____ % Score

Instructor's Signature _____

Identification Information   Today's Date _____

Name_____ Date of Birth_____

Occupation _____ Marital Status _____

PART A – PRESENT HEALTH HISTORY

I. CURRENT MEDICAL PROBLEMS
Please list the medical problems for which you came to see the doctor. About when did they begin?

Problems   Date Began
_____   _____
_____   _____
_____   _____

What concerns you most about these problems?
_____
_____

If you are being treated for any other illness or medical problems by another physician, please describe the problems and write the name of the physician or medical facility treating you.

Illness or Medical Problem   Physician or Medical Facility   City
_____   _____   _____
_____   _____   _____

II. MEDICATIONS
Please list all medications you are now taking, including those you buy without a doctor's prescription (such as aspirin, cold tablets or vitamin supplements).

_____   _____   _____
_____   _____   _____

III. ALLERGIES AND SENSITIVITIES
List anything that you are allergic to such as certain foods, medications, dust, chemicals or soaps, household items, pollens, bee stings, etc., and indicate how each affects you.

Allergic To: Effect   Allergic To: Effect
_____   _____   _____   _____
_____   _____   _____   _____

IV. GENERAL HEALTH, ATTITUDE AND HABITS

How is your overall health now?	Health now:	Poor ____ Fair ____ Good ____ Excellent ____
How has it been most of your life?	Health has been:	Poor ____ Fair ____ Good ____ Excellent ____

In the past year:
- Has your appetite changed? .... Appetite: Decreased ____ Increased ____ Stayed same ____
- Has your weight changed? .... Weight: Lost ____ lbs. Gained ____ lbs. No change ____
- Are you thirsty much of the time? .... Thirsty: No ____ Yes ____
- Has your overall 'pep' changed? ..... Pep: Decreased ____ Increased ____ Stayed same ____

Do you usually have trouble sleeping? ..... Trouble sleeping: No ____ Yes ____
How much do you exercise? .... Exercise: Little or none ____ Less than I need ____ All I need ____
Do you smoke? .... Smokes: No ____ Yes ____ If yes, how many years? ____
How many each day? .... ____ Cigarettes ____ Cigars ____ Pipesfull
Have you ever smoked? .... Smoked: No ____ Yes ____ If yes, how many years? ____
How many each day? .... ____ Cigarettes ____ Cigars ____ Pipesfull
Do you drink alcoholic beverages? ...... Alcohol: No ____ Yes ____ I drink ____ Beers ____ Glasses of wine
                                                ____ Drinks of hard liquor - per day
Have you ever had a problem with alcohol? ... Prior problem: No ____ Yes ____
How much coffee or tea do you usually drink? ... Coffee/Tea: ____ cups of coffee or tea a day
Do you regularly wear seatbelts? .... Seatbelts: No ____ Yes ____

DO YOU:	Rarely/Never	Occasionally	Frequently	DO YOU:	Rarely/Never	Occasionally	Frequently
Feel nervous?	____	____	____	Ever feel like committing suicide?	____	____	____
Feel depressed?	____	____	____	Feel bored with your life?	____	____	____
Find it hard to make decisions?	____	____	____	Use marijuana?	____	____	____
Lose your temper?	____	____	____	Use "hard drugs"?	____	____	____
Worry a lot?	____	____	____	Do you want to talk to the doctor about a personal matter? No ____ Yes ____			
Tire easily?	____	____	____				
Have trouble relaxing?	____	____	____				
Have any sexual problems?	____	____	____				

Created and Developed by "Medical Economics" Professional Systems
Copyright © 1979, 1983 Bibbero Systems International, Inc.   STOCK NO. 19-742-4   8/95   Page 1

Copyright © 2010, 2005 by Saunders, an imprint of Elsevier, Inc. All rights reserved.

PART A – PRESENT HEALTH HISTORY (continued)

IV. GENERAL HEALTH, ATTITUDE AND HABITS (continued)

Have you recently had any changes in your: If yes, please explain:

Marital status?	No____ Yes____	_____
Job or work?	No____ Yes____	_____
Residence?	No____ Yes____	_____
Financial status?	No____ Yes____	_____
Are you having any legal problems or trouble with the law?	No____ Yes____	_____

PART B – PAST HISTORY

I. FAMILY HEALTH

Please give the following information about your immediate family:

Relationship	Age, if Living	Age At Death	State of Health Or Cause of Death
Father	_____	_____	_____
Mother	_____	_____	_____
Brothers and Sisters	_____	_____	_____
	_____	_____	_____
	_____	_____	_____
Spouse	_____	_____	_____
Children	_____	_____	_____
	_____	_____	_____
	_____	_____	_____

Have any **blood relatives** had any of the following illnesses? If so, indicate relationship (mother, brother, etc.)

Illness	Family Members
Asthma	_____
Diabetes	_____
Cancer	_____
Blood Disease	_____
Glaucoma	_____
Epilepsy	_____
Rheumatoid Arthritis	_____
Tuberculosis	_____
Gout	_____
High Blood Pressure	_____
Heart Disease	_____
Mental Problems	_____
Suicide	_____
Stroke	_____
Alcoholism	_____
Rheumatic Fever	_____

II. HOSPITALIZATIONS, SURGERIES, INJURIES

Please list all times you have been hospitalized, operated on, or seriously injured.

Year	Operation, Illness, Injury	Hospital and City
_____	_____	_____
_____	_____	_____
_____	_____	_____

III. ILLNESS AND MEDICAL PROBLEMS

Please mark with an (X) any of the following illnesses and medical problems you have or have had and indicate the year when each started. If you are not certain when an illness started, write down an approximate year.

Illness	(x)	(Year)	Illness	(x)	(Year)
Eye or eye lid infection	___	___	Hernia	___	___
Glaucoma	___	___	Hemorrhoids	___	___
Other eye problems	___	___	Kidney or bladder disease	___	___
Ear trouble	___	___	Prostate problem (male only)	___	___
Deafness or decreased hearing	___	___	Mental problems	___	___
Thyroid trouble	___	___	Headaches	___	___
Strep throat	___	___	Head injury	___	___
Bronchitis	___	___	Stroke	___	___
Emphysema	___	___	Convulsions, seizures	___	___
Pneumonia	___	___	Arthritis	___	___
Allergies, asthma or hay fever	___	___	Gout	___	___
Tuberculosis	___	___	Cancer or tumor	___	___
Other lung problems	___	___	Bleeding tendency	___	___
High blood pressure	___	___	Diabetes	___	___
Heart attack	___	___	Measles/Rubeola	___	___
High cholesterol	___	___	German measles/Rubella	___	___
Arteriosclerosis (Hardening of arteries)	___	___	Polio	___	___
			Mumps	___	___
Heart murmur	___	___	Scarlet fever	___	___
Other heart condition	___	___	Chicken pox	___	___
Stomach/duodenal ulcer	___	___	Mononucleosis	___	___
Diverticulosis	___	___	Eczema	___	___
Colitis	___	___	Psoriasis	___	___
Other bowel problems	___	___	Venereal disease	___	___
Hepatitis	___	___	Genital herpes	___	___
Liver trouble	___	___	HIV test	___	___
Gallbladder trouble	___	___	AIDS	___	___

CONFIDENTIAL

© 1979, 1983 Bibbero Systems International, Inc. (REV. 6/92)   To Order Call: 800-BIBBERO (800 242-2376) Or Fax: (800 242-9330)   STOCK NO. 19-742-4   8/95

PART C – BODY SYSTEMS REVIEW

MEN: Please answer questions 1 through 12, then skip to question 18.
WOMEN: Please start on question 6.

MEN ONLY

1. Have you had or do you have prostate trouble? .... No _____ . Yes _____
2. Do you have any sexual problems or a problem with impotency? .... No _____ . Yes _____
3. Have you ever had sores or lesions on your penis? .... No _____ . Yes _____
4. Have you ever had any discharge from your penis? .... No _____ . Yes _____
5. Do you ever have pain, lumps or swelling in your testicles? .... No _____ . Yes _____

Check here if you wish to discuss any special problems with the doctor .... ☐

	Rarely/Never	Occasionally	Frequently

MEN & WOMEN

6. Is it sometimes hard to start your urine flow? .... _____ _____ _____
7. Is urination ever painful? .... _____ _____ _____
8. Do you have to urinate more than 5 times a day? .... _____ _____ _____
9. Do you get up at night to urinate? .... _____ _____ _____
10. Has your urine ever been bloody or dark colored? .... _____ _____ _____
11. Do you ever lose urine when you strain, laugh, cough or sneeze? .... _____ _____ _____
12. Do you ever lose urine during sleep? .... _____ _____ _____

WOMEN ONLY

Do you:

	Rarely/Never	Occasionally	Frequently

13.
 a. Have any menstrual problems? .... _____ _____ _____
 b. Feel rather tense just before your period? .... _____ _____ _____
 c. Have heavy menstrual bleeding? .... _____ _____ _____
 d. Have painful menstrual periods? .... _____ _____ _____
 e. Have any bleeding between periods? .... _____ _____ _____
 f. Have any unusual vaginal discharge or itching? .... _____ _____ _____
 g. Ever have tender breasts? .... _____ _____ _____
 h. Have any discharge from your nipples? .... _____ _____ _____
 i. Have any hot flashes? .... _____ _____ _____
14. How many times, if any, have you been pregnant? .... _____
15. How many children born alive? .... _____
16. Are you taking birth control pills? .... No _____ Yes _____
17. Do you examine your breasts monthly for lumps? .... No _____ Yes _____
17a. What was the date of your last menstrual period? .... Date _____

Check here if you wish to discuss any special problem with the doctor .... ☐

	Rarely/Never	Occasionally	Frequently

MEN & WOMEN

18. In the past year have you had any:
 a. Severe shoulder pain? .... _____ _____ _____
 b. Severe back pain? .... _____ _____ _____
 c. Muscle or joint stiffness or pain due to sports, exercise or injury? .... _____ _____ _____
 d. Pain or swelling in any joints not due to sports, exercise or injury? .... _____ _____ _____

19. Do you have dry skin or brittle fingernails? .... No _____ Yes _____
20. Do you bruise easily? .... No _____ Yes _____
21. Do you have any moles that have changed in color or in size? .... No _____ Yes _____
22. Do you have any other skin problems? .... No _____ Yes _____

23. In the last 3 months have you had:
 a. A fever that lasted more than one day? .... No _____ Yes _____
 b. Sores or cuts that were hard to heal? .... No _____ Yes _____
 c. Any cold sores (fever blisters)? .... No _____ Yes _____
 d. Any lumps in your neck, armpits or groin? .... No _____ Yes _____
 e. Do you ever have chills or sweat at night? .... No _____ Yes _____

24. Have you traveled out of the country in the last 2 years? .... No _____ Yes, Traveled in: _____

25. Write in the dates for the shots you have had: ....
 { Measles _____ Smallpox _____
   Mumps _____ Tetanus _____
   Polio _____ Typhoid _____ }

26. Have you had a tuberculin (TB) skin test? .... No _____ Yes _____ Date _____
 If so, was it negative or positive? .... Neg _____ Pos _____

27. Have you had an HIV test for AIDS? .... No _____ Yes _____ Date _____
 If so, was it negative or positive? .... Neg _____ Pos _____

CONFIDENTIAL

PROCEDURE 34-1

29.	Do you wear contact lenses?	No_____	Yes_____	
30.	Has your vision changed in the last year?	No_____	Yes_____	

		Rarely/Never	Occasionally	Frequently
31.	How often do you have:			
	a. Double vision?	_____	_____	_____
	b. Blurry vision?	_____	_____	_____
	c. Watery or itchy eyes?	_____	_____	_____
32.	Do you ever see colored rings around lights?	_____	_____	_____
33.	Do others tell you you have a hearing problem?	_____	_____	_____
34.	Do you have trouble keeping your balance?	_____	_____	_____
35.	Do you have any discharge from your ears?	_____	_____	_____
36.	Do you ever feel dizzy or have motion sickness?	_____	_____	_____

37.	Do you have any problems with your hearing?	No_____	Yes_____	Hearing Problems
38.	Do you ever have ringing in your ears?	No_____	Yes_____	Ringing in ears

		Rarely/Never	Occasionally	Frequently
39.	How often do you have:			
	a. Head colds?	_____	_____	_____
	b. Chest colds?	_____	_____	_____
	c. Runny nose?	_____	_____	_____
	d. Stuffed up nose?	_____	_____	_____
	e. Sore/hoarse throat?	_____	_____	_____
	f. Bad coughing spells?	_____	_____	_____
	g. Sneezing spells?	_____	_____	_____
	h. Trouble breathing?	_____	_____	_____
	i. Nose bleeds?	_____	_____	_____
	j. Cough blood?	_____	_____	_____

40.	Have you ever worked or spent time:		
	a. On a farm?	No_____	Yes_____
	b. In a mine?	No_____	Yes_____
	c. In a laundry or mill?	No_____	Yes_____
	d. In very dusty places?	No_____	Yes_____
	e. With or near toxic chemicals?	No_____	Yes_____
	f. With or near radioactive materials?	No_____	Yes_____
	g. With or near asbestos?	No_____	Yes_____

		Rarely/Never	Occasionally	Frequently
41.	Do you get out of breath easily when you are active (like climbing stairs)?	_____	_____	_____
42.	Do you ever feel light-headed or dizzy?	_____	_____	_____
43.	Have you ever fainted or passed out?	_____	_____	_____
44.	Do you sometimes feel your heart is racing or beating too fast?	_____	_____	_____
45.	When you exercise do you ever get pains in your chest or shoulders?	_____	_____	_____
46.	Do you have any leg cramps or pain in your thighs or legs when walking?	_____	_____	_____
47.	Do you ever have to sit up at night to breathe easier?	_____	_____	_____
48.	Do you use two pillows at night to help you breathe easier?	_____	_____	_____
49.	Would you say you are a restless sleeper?	_____	_____	_____
50.	Are you bothered by leg cramps at night?	_____	_____	_____
51.	Do you sometimes have swollen ankles or feet?	_____	_____	_____

		Rarely/Never	Occasionally	Frequently
52.	How often, if ever:			
	a. Are you nauseated (sick to your stomach)?	_____	_____	_____
	b. Do you have stomach pains?	_____	_____	_____
	c. Do you burp a lot after eating?	_____	_____	_____
	d. Do you have heartburn?	_____	_____	_____
	e. Do you have trouble swallowing your food?	_____	_____	_____
	f. Have you vomited blood?	_____	_____	_____
	g. Are you constipated?	_____	_____	_____
	h. Do you have diarrhea (watery stools)?	_____	_____	_____
	i. Are your bowel movements painful?	_____	_____	_____
	j. Are your bowel movements bloody?	_____	_____	_____
	k. Are your bowel movements dark or black?	_____	_____	_____
53.	Have you ever had a sigmoidoscopy?	No_____	Yes_____	Date_____

(Form # 19-742-4; courtesy of Bibbero Systems, Inc., Petaluma, CA; (800) 242-2376; fax (800) 242-9330; www.bibbero.com.)

Copyright © 2010, 2005 by Saunders, an imprint of Elsevier, Inc. All rights reserved.

Student Name: _____   DATE: _____

PROCEDURE 34-2 CHECKLIST: RECOGNIZE AND RESPOND TO VERBAL AND NONVERBAL COMMUNICATION

TASK: Recognize and respond to basic verbal and nonverbal communication.

CONDITIONS: Given the proper equipment and supplies, the student will be required to role-play with another student the proper method for recognizing and responding to basic verbal and nonverbal communication.

NOTE: The student should practice the procedure using the MACC located on the Evolve site at http://evolve.elsevier.com/klieger/medicalassisting: MACC/ Professionalism/Communication/Recognizing & responding to verbal/nonverbal communication.

EQUIPMENT AND SUPPLIES
No equipment or supplies are required; instructor can supply different scenarios to direct the communication process.

STANDARDS: Complete the procedure within _____ minutes and achieve a minimum score of _____%.

Time began _____   Time ended _____

Steps	Possible Points	First Attempt	Second Attempt
1. Greet the patient, smile to welcome the patient, and introduce yourself.	5		
2. Verify the patient's name, and use it with a courtesy title, unless instructed otherwise by the patient.	5		
3. Establish a comfortable physical environment, while respecting individual ethnic and cultural differences.	5		
4. Verify the patient feels comfortable.	5		
5. Establish the topic of discussion as directed.	5		
6. Observe the patient for nonverbal communication cues.	10		
7. Ask open-ended questions. Verify that the patient understands the questions.	10		
8. Practice active listening; provide feedback.	10		

Copyright © 2010, 2005 by Saunders, an imprint of Elsevier, Inc. All rights reserved.

Steps	Possible Points	First Attempt	Second Attempt
9. Near the end of the discussion, provide the patient the opportunity to ask questions or provide further clarifications.	10		
10. Thank the patient for his or her comments, and signal the end of the discussion.	10		
Total Points Possible	75		

Comments: Total Points Earned _____

Divided by _____

Total Possible Points = _____% Score

Instructor's Signature _____

Charting for Procedures 34-1 and 34-2

Date	Chart

Date	Chart

Date	Chart

Date	Chart

Student Name: _____ DATE: _____

PROCEDURE 35-1 CHECKLIST: ASSIST WITH THE PHYSICAL EXAMINATION

The instructor may choose to do this procedure last or incorporate the other procedures into this procedure (i.e., positions and eye tests).

TASK: Prepare a patient and assist the physician or health care practitioner with a basic physical examination.

CONDITIONS: Given the proper equipment and supplies, the student will be required to role-play with another student or an instructor the proper method for assisting with a basic physical examination.

NOTE: The student should practice the procedure using the MACC located on the Evolve site at http://evolve.elsevier.com/klieger/medicalassisting: MACC/Clinical skills/Patient care/The physical exam/Assisting with a physical exam & maintaining and preparing exam room.

EQUIPMENT AND SUPPLIES
- MACC/computer (practice)
- Examination table
- Table paper
- Patient gown
- Drape
- Urine specimen container
- Snellen chart
- Patient's medical record
- Balance scale
- Tongue depressor
- Plastic-backed paper towel
- Stethoscope
- Sphygmomanometer
- Otoscope
- Ophthalmoscope
- Pen (black ink)
- Disposable gloves

STANDARDS: Complete the procedure within _____ minutes and achieve a minimum score of _____%.

Time began _____   Time ended _____

Steps	Possible Points	First Attempt	Second Attempt
1. Sanitize hands.	5		
2. Assemble equipment and supplies.	5		
3. Obtain the patient's medical record.	5		
4. Greet and identify the patient.	5		
5. Explain the procedure to the patient.	5		
6. Measure weight and height, and document the results.	10		
7. Measure visual acuity and document the results.	10		

Steps	Possible Points	First Attempt	Second Attempt
8. Have the patient obtain a urine sample (if office policy).	5		
9. Escort the patient to the examination room.	5		
10. Measure the patient's vital signs, and document the results.	10		
11. Provide a gown and drape to the patient and allow the patient to change into the gown. Inform the physician when the patient is ready, and make the patient's medical record available to the physician.	10		
12. Assist physician with eye exam.	10		
13. Assist physician with ear exam.	10		
14. Assist physician with nasal exam.	10		
15. Assist physician with throat exam.	10		
16. Assist physician with heart and lung exam.	10		
17. Assist physician with testing and examination of the upper extremity reflexes.	10		
18. Position the patient as required.	10		
19. Assist the patient from the examination table as appropriate.	10		
20. Allow the patient time to change from gown to street clothes.	10		
21. Allow time for further discussion between the physician and patient regarding prescriptions, medications, and a return visit. Ask the patient if he or she has any questions.	10		
22. Document any instructions given to the patient in the medical record.	10		

Copyright © 2010, 2005 by Saunders, an imprint of Elsevier, Inc. All rights reserved.

Steps	Possible Points	First Attempt	Second Attempt
23. Clean the examination room according to Standard Precautions, and take used equipment to appropriate place for sanitization.	10		
24. Sanitize hands.	5		
Total Points Possible	200		

Comments: Total Points Earned _____

Divided by _____

Total Possible Points = _____% Score

Instructor's Signature _____

Copyright © 2010, 2005 by Saunders, an imprint of Elsevier, Inc. All rights reserved.

Student Name: _____ DATE: _____

PROCEDURE 35-2 CHECKLIST: SITTING POSITION

TASK: Properly position and drape the patient for examination of the head, neck, chest, and upper extremities, and measurement of vital signs.

CONDITIONS: Given the proper equipment and supplies, the student will be required to role-play with another student or an instructor the proper method for positioning the patient in the sitting position.

NOTE: The student should practice the procedure using the MACC located on the Evolve site at http://evolve.elsevier.com/klieger/medicalassisting: MACC/Clinical skills/Patient care/The physical exam/Assisting with a physical exam & maintaining and preparing exam room.

EQUIPMENT AND SUPPLIES
- MACC/computer (practice)
- Examination table
- Table paper
- Patient gown
- Drape

STANDARDS: Complete the procedure within _____ minutes and achieve a minimum score of _____%.

Time began _____   Time ended _____

Steps	Possible Points	First Attempt	Second Attempt
1. Sanitize hands.	5		
2. Assemble equipment and supplies.	5		
3. Greet and identify the patient.	5		
4. Explain the procedure to the patient.	5		
5. Provide a gown for the patient, and instruct the patient to change into the gown with opening in the front or back depending on type of assessment to be done.	5		
6. Pull out the footrest of the table, and assist the patient to a sitting position.	5		
7. Drape the patient for modesty.	5		
8. When the examination is complete, assist the patient from the table.	5		
9. Clean the examination room according to Standard Precautions.	5		
10. Sanitize hands.	5		
Total Points Possible	50		

Comments: Total Points Earned _____

Divided by _____

Total Possible Points = _____% Score

Instructor's Signature _____

Copyright © 2010, 2005 by Saunders, an imprint of Elsevier, Inc. All rights reserved.

Student Name: _____ DATE: _____

PROCEDURE 35-3 CHECKLIST: RECUMBENT POSITION

TASK: Properly position and drape the patient for catheter insertion, examinations of the abdomen, and general examination procedures.

CONDITIONS: Given the proper equipment and supplies, the student will be required to role-play with another student or an instructor the proper method for positioning the patient in the recumbent position.

NOTE: The student should practice the procedure using the MACC located on the Evolve site at http://evolve.elsevier.com/klieger/medicalassisting: MACC/Clinical skills/Patient care/The physical exam/Assisting with a physical exam & maintaining and preparing exam room.

EQUIPMENT AND SUPPLIES
- MACC/computer (practice)
- Examination table
- Table paper
- Patient gown
- Drape

STANDARDS: Complete the procedure within _____ minutes and achieve a minimum score of _____%.

Time began _____   Time ended _____

Steps	Possible Points	First Attempt	Second Attempt
1. Sanitize hands.	5		
2. Assemble equipment and supplies.	5		
3. Greet and identify the patient.	5		
4. Explain the procedure to the patient.	5		
5. Provide a gown for the patient, and instruct the patient to change into the gown with opening in the front or back depending on type of assessment to be done.	5		
6. Pull out the footrest of the table, and assist the patient to a sitting position.	10		
7. Place the patient in the recumbent position.	10		
8. Drape the patient as appropriate.	10		
9. When the examination is complete, assist the patient from the recumbent position and into a sitting position. Assist the patient from the table.	5		

Copyright © 2010, 2005 by Saunders, an imprint of Elsevier, Inc. All rights reserved.

Steps	Possible Points	First Attempt	Second Attempt
10. Clean the examination room according to Standard Precautions.	10		
11. Sanitize hands.	5		
Total Points Possible	75		

Comments: Total Points Earned _____

Divided by _____

Total Possible Points = _____% Score

Instructor's Signature _____

Student Name: _____   DATE: _____

PROCEDURE 35-4 CHECKLIST: LITHOTOMY POSITION

TASK: Properly position and drape the patient in the lithotomy position for a vaginal, pelvic, or rectal examination.

CONDITIONS: Given the proper equipment and supplies, the student will be required to role-play with another student or an instructor the proper method for positioning the patient in the lithotomy position.

NOTE: The student should practice the procedure using the MACC located on the Evolve site at http://evolve. elsevier.com/klieger/medicalassisting: MACC/Clinical skills/Patient care/The physical exam/Assisting with a physical exam & maintaining and preparing exam room.

EQUIPMENT AND SUPPLIES
- MACC/computer (practice)
- Examination table
- Table paper
- Patient gown
- Drape

STANDARDS: Complete the procedure within _____ minutes and achieve a minimum score of _____%.

Time began _____   Time ended _____

Steps	Possible Points	First Attempt	Second Attempt
1. Sanitize hands.	5		
2. Assemble equipment and supplies.	5		
3. Greet and identify the patient.	5		
4. Explain the procedure to the patient.	5		
5. Provide a gown for the patient, and instruct the patient to change into the gown with opening in the back.	5		
6. Pull out the footrest of the table, and assist the patient to a sitting position.	10		
7. Place the patient in the supine position.	10		
8. Drape the patient as appropriate.	10		
9. Pull out the stirrups and place the patient in the lithotomy position. Place both legs in the stirrups at the same time.	10		
10. Have the patient slide the buttocks to the edge of the table.	10		

Copyright © 2010, 2005 by Saunders, an imprint of Elsevier, Inc. All rights reserved.

Steps	Possible Points	First Attempt	Second Attempt
11. When the examination is complete, assist the patient from the lithotomy position and into the supine position and into a sitting position. Support both legs and remove from stirrups at the same time. Assist the patient from the table.	10		
12. Clean the examination room according to Standard Precautions.	10		
13. Sanitize hands.	5		
Total Points Possible	100		

Comments: Total Points Earned _____

Divided by _____

Total Possible Points = _____% Score

Instructor's Signature _____

Copyright © 2010, 2005 by Saunders, an imprint of Elsevier, Inc. All rights reserved.

Student Name: _____   DATE: _____

PROCEDURE 35-5 CHECKLIST: SIMS' POSITION

TASK: Properly position and drape the patient for a vaginal or rectal examination.

CONDITIONS: Given the proper equipment and supplies, the student will be required to role-play with another student or an instructor the proper method for positioning the patient in the Sims' position.

NOTE: The student should practice the procedure using the MACC located on the Evolve site at http://evolve.elsevier.com/klieger/medicalassisting: MACC/Clinical skills/Patient care/The physical exam/Assisting with a physical exam & maintaining and preparing exam room.

EQUIPMENT AND SUPPLIES
- MACC/computer (practice)
- Examination table
- Table paper
- Patient gown
- Drape

STANDARDS: Complete the procedure within _____ minutes and achieve a minimum score of _____%.

Time began _____   Time ended _____

Steps	Possible Points	First Attempt	Second Attempt
1. Sanitize hands.	5		
2. Assemble equipment and supplies.	5		
3. Greet and identify the patient.	5		
4. Explain the procedure to the patient.	5		
5. Provide a gown for the patient, and instruct the patient to change into the gown with opening in the back.	5		
6. Pull out the footrest of the table, and assist the patient to a sitting position.	10		
7. Place the patient in the supine position.	10		
8. Drape the patient as appropriate so rectal area can be viewed while providing patient modesty.	10		
9. Place the patient in Sims' position.	10		
10. Adjust the drape as the physician examines the anal area.	10		
11. When the examination is complete, assist the patient from the Sims' position and into the supine position and into a sitting position. Assist the patient from the examination table.	10		

Copyright © 2010, 2005 by Saunders, an imprint of Elsevier, Inc. All rights reserved.

Steps	Possible Points	First Attempt	Second Attempt
12. Clean the examination room according to Standard Precautions.	10		
13. Sanitize hands.	5		
Total Points Possible	100		

Comments: Total Points Earned _____

Divided by _____

Total Possible Points = _____% Score

Instructor's Signature _____

Student Name: _____ DATE: _____

PROCEDURE 35-6 CHECKLIST: PRONE POSITION

TASK: Properly position and drape the patient for examination of the back.

CONDITIONS: Given the proper equipment and supplies, the student will be required to role-play with another student or an instructor the proper method for positioning the patient.

NOTE: The student should practice the procedure using the MACC located on the Evolve site at http://evolve.elsevier.com/klieger/medicalassisting: MACC/Clinical skills/Patient care/The physical exam/Assisting with a physical exam & maintaining and preparing exam room.

EQUIPMENT AND SUPPLIES
- MACC/computer (practice)
- Examination table
- Table paper
- Patient gown
- Drape

STANDARDS: Complete the procedure within _____ minutes and achieve a minimum score of _____%.

Time began _____   Time ended _____

Steps	Possible Points	First Attempt	Second Attempt
1. Sanitize hands.	5		
2. Assemble equipment and supplies.	5		
3. Greet and identify the patient.	5		
4. Explain the procedure to the patient.	5		
5. Provide a gown for the patient, and instruct the patient to change into the gown with opening in the back.	5		
6. Pull out the footrest of the table, and assist the patient to a sitting position.	10		
7. Place the patient in the supine position.	10		
8. Drape the patient as appropriate for patient modesty.	10		
9. Place the patient in the prone position.	10		
10. Adjust the drape as necessary.	10		
11. When the examination is complete, assist the patient from the prone position and into the supine position and into a sitting position. Assist the patient from the examination table.	10		

Copyright © 2010, 2005 by Saunders, an imprint of Elsevier, Inc. All rights reserved.

Steps	Possible Points	First Attempt	Second Attempt
12. Clean the examination room according to Standard Precautions.	10		
13. Sanitize hands.	5		
Total Points Possible	100		

Comments: Total Points Earned _____

Divided by _____

Total Possible Points = _____% Score

Instructor's Signature _____

Copyright © 2010, 2005 by Saunders, an imprint of Elsevier, Inc. All rights reserved.

Student Name: DATE:

PROCEDURE 35-7 CHECKLIST: KNEE-CHEST POSITION

TASK: Properly position and drape the patient for a proctologic examination.

CONDITIONS: Given the proper equipment and supplies, the student will be required to role-play with another student or an instructor the proper method for positioning the patient in the knee-chest position.

NOTE: The student should practice the procedure using the MACC located on the Evolve site at http://evolve.elsevier.com/klieger/medicalassisting: MACC/Clinical skills/Patient care/The physical exam/Assisting with a physical exam & maintaining and preparing exam room.

EQUIPMENT AND SUPPLIES
- MACC/computer (practice)
- Examination table
- Table paper
- Patient gown
- Drape
- Tissue

STANDARDS: Complete the procedure within _____ minutes and achieve a minimum score of _____%.

Time began _____   Time ended _____

Steps	Possible Points	First Attempt	Second Attempt
1. Sanitize hands.	5		
2. Assemble equipment and supplies.	5		
3. Greet and identify the patient.	5		
4. Explain the procedure to the patient.	5		
5. Provide a gown for the patient, and instruct the patient to change into the gown with opening in the back.	5		
6. Pull out the footrest of the table, and assist the patient to a sitting position.	10		
7. Place the patient in the supine position.	10		
8. Drape the patient as appropriate for patient modesty.	10		
9. Place the patient in the prone position.	10		
10. Have the patient bend the arms at the elbows and rest them alongside the head.	10		
11. Place the patient in the knee-chest position.	10		
12. Adjust the drape as the physician examines the rectal area.	10		

Copyright © 2010, 2005 by Saunders, an imprint of Elsevier, Inc. All rights reserved.

Steps	Possible Points	First Attempt	Second Attempt
13. Wipe the rectal area with tissue as appropriate after the exam to remove excess lubricant.	10		
14. When the examination is complete, assist the patient from the knee-chest position and into the prone position, into a supine position, and into a sitting position. Assist the patient from the examination table.	10		
15. Clean the examination room according to Standard Precautions.	10		
16. Sanitize hands.	5		
Total Points Possible	130		

Comments: Total Points Earned _____

Divided by _____

Total Possible Points = _____ % Score

Instructor's Signature _____

Student Name: _____ DATE: _____

PROCEDURE 35-8 CHECKLIST: FOWLER'S POSITION

TASK: Properly position and drape the patient for examination of the head, chest, abdomen, and extremities.

CONDITIONS: Given the proper equipment and supplies, the student will be required to role-play with another student or an instructor the proper method for positioning the patient in Fowler's position.

NOTE: The student should practice the procedure using the MACC located on the Evolve site at http://evolve.elsevier.com/klieger/medicalassisting: MACC/Clinical skills/Patient care/The physical exam/Assisting with a physical exam & maintaining and preparing exam room.

EQUIPMENT AND SUPPLIES
- MACC/computer (practice)
- Examination table
- Table paper
- Patient gown
- Drape

STANDARDS: Complete the procedure within _____ minutes and achieve a minimum score of _____%.

Time began _____   Time ended _____

Steps	Possible Points	First Attempt	Second Attempt
1. Sanitize hands.	5		
2. Assemble equipment and supplies.	5		
3. Greet and identify the patient.	5		
4. Explain the procedure to the patient.	5		
5. Provide a gown for the patient, and instruct the patient to change into the gown with opening in the back.	5		
6. Pull out the footrest of the table, and assist the patient to a sitting position.	10		
7. Place the patient in Fowler's position or semi-Fowler's position, supporting head with pillow as appropriate.	10		
8. Drape the patient as appropriate for patient modesty and exam being performed.	10		

Copyright © 2010, 2005 by Saunders, an imprint of Elsevier, Inc. All rights reserved.

Steps	Possible Points	First Attempt	Second Attempt
9. When the examination is complete, assist the patient from the examination table. Raise head off table as appropriate.	10		
10. Clean the examination room according to Standard Precautions.	10		
11. Sanitize hands.	5		
Total Points Possible	80		

Comments: Total Points Earned _____

Divided by _____

Total Possible Points = _____% Score

Instructor's Signature _____

Student Name: _____   DATE: _____

PROCEDURE 35-9 CHECKLIST: ASSESS DISTANCE VISUAL ACUITY USING A SNELLEN CHART

TASK: Accurately measure visual acuity using a Snellen eye chart, and document the procedure in the patient's medical record.

CONDITIONS: Given the proper equipment and supplies, the student will be required to measure visual acuity using a Snellen chart.

NOTE: The student should practice the procedure using the MACC located on the Evolve site at http://evolve.elsevier.com/klieger/medicalassisting: MACC/Clinical skills/ Patient care/The physical exam/Measuring visual acuity.

EQUIPMENT AND SUPPLIES
- MACC/computer (practice)
- Snellen eye chart
- Eye occluder
- Well-lit examination room
- Floor mark (20 ft from chart)
- Patient's medical record
- Pen

STANDARDS: Complete the procedure within _____ minutes and achieve a minimum score of _____%.

Time began _____   Time ended _____

Steps	Possible Points	First Attempt	Second Attempt
1. Sanitize hands.	5		
2. Assemble equipment and supplies.	5		
3. Greet and identify the patient.	5		
4. Explain the procedure to the patient.	5		
5. Ask the patient if he or she is wearing contact lenses, and observe for eyeglasses.	10		
6. Place the patient in a comfortable position 20 ft from the chart.	10		
7. Select the appropriate Snellen chart for the patient, and position the center of the chart at the patient's eye level. Stand next to the chart during the test to indicate to the patient the line to be identified.	10		
8. Ask the patient to cover the left eye with the eye occluder, keeping the eye open.	10		

Copyright © 2010, 2005 by Saunders, an imprint of Elsevier, Inc. All rights reserved.

Steps	Possible Points	First Attempt	Second Attempt
9. Measure the visual acuity of the right eye by asking the patient to identify verbally each letter (or picture or rotating "E" direction) in the row on the Snellen chart, starting with the 20/70 line.	10		
10. Proceed up or down the chart as necessary.	10		
11. Observe the patient for any unusual symptoms while he or she is reading the letters, such as squinting, tilting the head, or watering eyes.	10		
12. Repeat the procedure to test the left eye by covering the right eye.	10		
13. Record the results appropriately, indicating the errors for each eye.	10		
14. Repeat the procedure without covering the eye.	10		
15. If appropriate, repeat the procedure without corrective lenses.	10		
16. Chart the procedure.	10		
17. Sanitize or discard the occluder as appropriate.	5		
18. Sanitize hands.	5		
Total Points Possible	150		

Comments: Total Points Earned _____

Divided by _____

Total Possible Points = _____% Score

Instructor's Signature _____

Student Name: _____ DATE: _____

PROCEDURE 35-10 CHECKLIST: ASSESS COLOR VISION USING THE ISHIHARA TEST

TASK: Measure color visual acuity accurately using the Ishihara color-blindness test.

CONDITIONS: Given the proper equipment and supplies, the student will be required to role-play with another student or an instructor the proper method for measuring color visual acuity using the Ishihara color-blindness test.

EQUIPMENT AND SUPPLIES
- Ishihara color plate book
- Cotton swab
- Well-lit examination room (natural light preferred)
- Watch with second hand
- Patient's medical record
- Pen or pencil

STANDARDS: Complete the procedure within _____ minutes and achieve a minimum score of _____%.

Time began _____   Time ended _____

Steps	Possible Points	First Attempt	Second Attempt
1. Sanitize hands.	5		
2. Assemble equipment and supplies.	5		
3. Greet and identify the patient.	5		
4. Explain the procedure to the patient.	5		
5. In a well-lit room, use the first plate in the book as an example, and instruct the patient on how the examination will be conducted using the plate.	10		
6. Hold the color plates 30 inches from the patient.	10		
7. Ask the patient to identify the number on the plate or, using a cotton-tipped swab, to trace the winding path.	10		
8. Record the results for each plate, and continue until the patient has viewed and responded to all 11 plates.	10		
9. Appropriately record the results in the patient's medical record.	10		
10. Return the Isihara book to its proper place.	10		

PROCEDURE 35-10

Copyright © 2010, 2005 by Saunders, an imprint of Elsevier, Inc. All rights reserved.

Steps	Possible Points	First Attempt	Second Attempt
11. Discard cotton-tipped swab as appropriate.	5		
12. Sanitize hands.	5		
Total Points Possible	90		

Comments: Total Points Earned _____

Divided by _____

Total Possible Points = _____% Score

Instructor's Signature _____

Student Name: _____ DATE: _____

PROCEDURE 35-11 CHECKLIST: ASSESS NEAR VISION USING A JAEGER CARD

TASK: Measure near visual acuity accurately using a Jaeger near-vision acuity card, and document the procedure in the patient's medical record.

CONDITIONS: Given the proper equipment and supplies, the student will be required to role-play with another student or an instructor the proper method for assessing near vision using a Jaeger card.

EQUIPMENT AND SUPPLIES
- Jaeger card
- Occluder
- Well-lit examination room
- Patient's medical record
- Pen

STANDARDS: Complete the procedure within _____ minutes and achieve a minimum score of _____%.

Time began _____   Time ended _____

Steps	Possible Points	First Attempt	Second Attempt
1. Sanitize hands.	5		
2. Assemble equipment and supplies.	5		
3. Greet and identify the patient.	5		
4. Explain the procedure to the patient.	5		
5. In a well-lit room, seat the patient in a comfortable position.	10		
6. Provide the patient with the Jaeger card and instruct the patient to hold the card 14 to 16 inches away from the eyes. Measure the distance for accuracy.	15		
7. Ask the patient to read out loud the paragraphs on the card; cover the left eye and then the right eye with the occluder.	15		
8. Document the number at which the patient stopped reading for each eye.	10		
9. Return the Jaeger card to its proper storage place.	10		

Copyright © 2010, 2005 by Saunders, an imprint of Elsevier, Inc. All rights reserved.

Steps	Possible Points	First Attempt	Second Attempt
10. Sanitize or discard the occluder as appropriate.	10		
11. Sanitize hands.	10		
Total Points Possible	100		

Comments: Total Points Earned _____

Divided by _____

Total Possible Points = _____ % Score

Instructor's Signature _____

Copyright © 2010, 2005 by Saunders, an imprint of Elsevier, Inc. All rights reserved.

Charting for Procedures 35-1 through 35-11

Date	Chart

Date	Chart

Date	Chart

Date	Chart

	Chart
Date	

	Chart
Date	

	Chart
Date	

	Chart
Date	

	Chart
Date	

	Chart
Date	

	Chart
Date	

	Chart
Date	

Student Name: _____   DATE: _____

PROCEDURE 36-1 CHECKLIST: OBTAIN A 12-LEAD ECG USING A SINGLE-CHANNEL ELECTROCARDIOGRAPH

TASK: Obtain an accurate 12-lead ECG tracing by running a single-channel electrocardiograph with manual capacity.

CONDITIONS: Given the proper equipment and supplies, the student will be required to obtain an accurate 12-lead ECG tracing.

NOTE: The student should practice the procedure using the MACC located on the Evolve site at http://evolve.elsevier.com/klieger/medicalassisting: MACC/Clinical skills/Diagnostic testing/Patient testing/Performing an electrocardiogram.

EQUIPMENT AND SUPPLIES
- MACC/computer (practice)
- Single-channel electrocardiograph with lead wires
- ECG paper
- Disposable electrodes (self-adhesive)
- ECG mounting form and mounting supplies such as an ECG paper cutter, if applicable
- Examination table with footstool or step
- Alcohol wipes (70% isopropyl)
- 4- × 4-inch gauze squares
- Disposable razor
- Patient gown
- Drape
- Blanket (optional)
- Small pillow

STANDARDS: Complete the procedure within _____ minutes and achieve a minimum score of _____%.

Time began _____   Time ended _____

Steps	Possible Points	First Attempt	Second Attempt
1. Sanitize hands.	5		
2. Assemble equipment and supplies.	5		
3. Greet and identify the patient.	5		
4. Explain the procedure to the patient.	5		
5. Ask the patient to remove all possible sources of electrical interference.	5		
6. Prepare the patient by removing clothes as appropriate; drape and gown the patient.	5		
7. Position the patient in a relaxed position, being sure to prevent stress from the position. Ask the patient to remain still and not talk.	10		

Steps	Possible Points	First Attempt	Second Attempt
8. Prepare the patient's skin for electrode placement; remove hair and oil as appropriate.	10		
9. Position the ECG machine, and turn it on.	5		
10. Label the beginning of the ECG paper with the patient's name, date, time, and current cardiovascular medications, or input the information directly into the machine.	5		
11. Properly apply the limb electrodes.	10		
12. Properly apply the chest electrodes.	10		
13. Connect the lead wires to the electrodes.	5		
14. Standardize the ECG machine.	10		
15. Record ECG as appropriate for machine.	10		
16. Ask the patient to lie as still as possible during the tracing; correct artifacts as necessary. If the ECG reading is inaccurate, run the lead again.	10		
17. If an arrhythmia or abnormal tracing occurs during the procedure, notify the nurse or physician immediately.	5		
18. When an accurate ECG has been obtained, disconnect the patient from the electrocardiograph by removing all of the lead wires and electrodes.	5		
19. Discard electrodes and any other waste material in the appropriate waste container.	5		
20. Thank the patient and allow the patient to dress.	5		
21. Sanitize hands.	5		
22. Document any special information on the ECG tracing.	10		
23. Cut and mount the ECG as appropriate.	5		

Steps	Possible Points	First Attempt	Second Attempt
24. Handle the recording carefully, and place the mounted recording in the appropriate place to be reviewed by the physician.	5		
25. Document the procedure.	10		
26. Clean and return all equipment to its proper place.	5		
Total Points Possible	175		

Comments: Total Points Earned _____

Divided by _____

Total Possible Points = _____% Score

Instructor's Signature _____

Student Name: _____ DATE: _____

PROCEDURE 36-2 CHECKLIST: OBTAIN A 12-LEAD ECG USING A THREE-CHANNEL (MULTICHANNEL) ELECTROCARDIOGRAPH

TASK: Obtain an accurate 12-lead ECG tracing by running a three-channel electrocardiograph.

CONDITIONS: Given the proper equipment and supplies, the student will be required to obtain an accurate 12-lead ECG tracing.

EQUIPMENT AND SUPPLIES
- Three-channel electrocardiograph with lead wires
- ECG paper
- Disposable electrodes (self-adhesive)
- ECG mounting form and mounting supplies such as an ECG paper cutter, if applicable
- Examination table with footstool or step
- Alcohol wipes (70% isopropyl)
- 4- × 4-inch gauze squares
- Disposable razor
- Patient gown
- Drape
- Blanket (optional)
- Small pillow

STANDARDS: Complete the procedure within _____ minutes and achieve a minimum score of _____%.

Time began _____   Time ended _____

Steps	Possible Points	First Attempt	Second Attempt
1. Sanitize hands.	5		
2. Assemble equipment and supplies.	5		
3. Greet and identify the patient.	5		
4. Explain the procedure to the patient.	5		
5. Ask the patient to remove all possible sources of electrical interference.	5		
6. Prepare the patient by removing clothes as appropriate; drape and gown the patient.	5		
7. Position the patient in a relaxed position, being sure to prevent stress from the position.	5		
8. Prepare the patient's skin for electrode placement; remove hair and oil as appropriate.	10		
9. Position the ECG machine and turn it on.	5		

Copyright © 2010, 2005 by Saunders, an imprint of Elsevier, Inc. All rights reserved.

Steps	Possible Points	First Attempt	Second Attempt
10. Turn on the electrocardiograph, and enter the patient data using the soft-touch keypad. Label the beginning of the ECG paper with the patient's name, date, time, and current cardiovascular medications.	5		
11. Properly apply the limb electrodes.	10		
12. Properly apply the chest electrodes.	10		
13. Connect the lead wires to the electrodes.	5		
14. Press the "Start" or "Auto" button on the machine and run the ECG tracing.	10		
15. Record ECG as appropriate for machine.	10		
16. Ask the patient to lie as still as possible during the tracing; correct artifacts as necessary. If the ECG reading is inaccurate, run the lead again.	10		
17. If an arrhythmia or abnormal tracing occurs during the procedure, notify the nurse or physician immediately.	5		
18. When an accurate ECG has been obtained, disconnect the patient from the electrocardiograph by removing all of the lead wires and electrodes.	5		
19. Discard electrodes and any other waste material in the appropriate waste container.	5		
20. Thank the patient and allow the patient to dress.	5		
21. Sanitize hands.	5		
22. Document any special information on the ECG tracing.	10		
23. Cut and mount the ECG as appropriate.	10		
24. Handle the recording carefully, and place the mounted recording in the appropriate place to be reviewed by the physician.	5		

Steps	Possible Points	First Attempt	Second Attempt
25. Document the procedure.	10		
26. Clean and return all equipment to its proper place.	5		
Total Points Possible	175		

Comments: Total Points Earned _____

Divided by _____

Total Possible Points = _____% Score

Instructor's Signature _____

Copyright © 2010, 2005 by Saunders, an imprint of Elsevier, Inc. All rights reserved.

Student Name: _____   DATE: _____

PROCEDURE 36-3 CHECKLIST: APPLY AND REMOVE A HOLTER MONITOR

TASK: Demonstrate the correct procedure for applying and removing a Holter monitor.

CONDITIONS: Given the proper equipment and supplies, the student will be required to role-play with another student or an instructor the proper method for applying and removing a Holter monitor for patient instruction.

EQUIPMENT AND SUPPLIES
- Holter monitor with battery
- Blank magnetic tape
- Patient activity diary
- Carrying case
- Disposable razor
- Belt or shoulder strap
- Disposable electrodes (self-adhesive)
- Nonallergenic tape
- Electrode cable with lead wires
- Gauze squares
- Alcohol wipes (70% isopropyl)

STANDARDS: Complete the procedure within _____ minutes and achieve a minimum score of _____%.

Time began _____   Time ended _____

Steps	Possible Points	First Attempt	Second Attempt
Applying the monitor: 1. Sanitize hands.	5		
2. Assemble equipment and supplies.	5		
3. Greet and identify the patient.	5		
4. Explain the procedure to the patient.	5		
5. Prepare the equipment, ensuring that all batteries are charged adequately, and a blank tape is in the machine.	10		
6. Place the patient in either a sitting position or a supine position on the examination table.	5		
7. Locate and prepare the skin at electrode placement sites.	5		
8. Prepare and apply the electrodes.	5		
9. Repeat Step 8 until all electrodes are firmly applied.	5		
10. Attach lead wires to the electrodes, and place a strip of adhesive nonallergenic tape over the wires just below each electrode.	5		

Copyright © 2010, 2005 by Saunders, an imprint of Elsevier, Inc. All rights reserved.

Steps	Possible Points	First Attempt	Second Attempt
11. Connect the lead wires to the electrode cable, and tape the cable to the patient's chest.	5		
12. Check the recorder's effectiveness by using the start-up procedure recommended by the manufacturer.	10		
13. Instruct the patient to redress while being careful not to pull on the lead wires.	5		
14. Insert the recorder into its carrying case and strap it over the patient's clothing using a waist belt or shoulder strap.	5		
15. Set the Holter monitor, and record the start time.	10		
16. Complete the patient identification section of the patient's activity diary.	10		
17. Give the diary to the patient and provide verbal and written instructions on the use of the monitor and proper documentation. Ensure that the date and time of application are recorded.	10		
18. Ask the patient if he or she has any questions or would like clarification of any instructions.	5		
19. Instruct the patient on when to return for removal of the monitor.	5		
20. Sanitize hands.	5		
21. Remind the patient not to forget the diary.	5		
22. Document the procedure.	10		
Removing the monitor: 23. Sanitize hands.	5		
24. Assist the patient with removing clothing from the waist up.	5		
25. Turn off the monitor, remove the monitor strap, and detach it from the lead wires.	5		
26. Remove the lead wires and electrodes from the patient.	5		
27. Clean the skin at the electrode sites.	5		

Steps	Possible Points	First Attempt	Second Attempt
28. Allow the patient to redress and assist the patient as necessary.	5		
29. Obtain the activity diary from the patient.	5		
30. Sanitize hands.	5		
31. Place the cassette in the computerized analyzer for recording.	10		
32. Attach the patient activity diary printout to the patient's medical record, chart the time that the monitor was returned, and give the results of diary to the physician.	10		
Total Points Possible	200		

Comments: Total Points Earned _____

Divided by _____

Total Possible Points = _____ % Score

Instructor's Signature _____

Copyright © 2010, 2005 by Saunders, an imprint of Elsevier, Inc. All rights reserved.

Charting for Procedures 36-1 through 36-3

Date	Chart

Date	Chart

Date	Chart

Date	Chart

Copyright © 2010, 2005 by Saunders, an imprint of Elsevier, Inc. All rights reserved.

Student Name: _____ DATE: _____

PROCEDURE 38-1 CHECKLIST: PERFORM AN EAR IRRIGATION

TASK: Simulate irrigation of the external ear canal to remove cerumen.

CONDITIONS: Given the proper equipment and supplies, the student will be required to perform proper irrigation of an external ear to remove cerumen.

EQUIPMENT AND SUPPLIES
- Irrigating solution (may use warm tap water)
- Container to hold irrigating solution (sterile)
- Disposable gloves
- Irrigating syringe or Reiner's ear syringe
- Ear basin for drainage
- Disposable barrier drape
- Cotton balls or gauze squares
- Otoscope with probe cover
- Biohazardous waste container
- Towel
- Patient's medical record

STANDARDS: Complete the procedure within _____ minutes and achieve a minimum score of _____%.

Time began _____   Time ended _____

Steps	Possible Points	First Attempt	Second Attempt
1. Sanitize hands.	5		
2. Assemble equipment and supplies.	5		
3. Obtain the patient's medical record, and verify the physician's order, the solution to use, and the ear to be treated.	10		
4. Greet and identify the patient. Escort the patient to the examination room and seat the patient on the end of the examination table.	5		
5. Explain the procedure to the patient.	10		
6. Warm the irrigating solution to body temperature by running the container under warm tap water.	5		
7. Put on disposable gloves (latex-free if patient as an allergy).	5		
8. Examine the ear with the otoscope.	15		
9. Position the patient by tilting the head slightly forward and toward the affected ear.	15		

867

Copyright © 2010, 2005 by Saunders, an imprint of Elsevier, Inc. All rights reserved.

Steps	Possible Points	First Attempt	Second Attempt
10. Place a water-resistant disposable barrier on the patient's shoulder on the affected side. Provide an ear basin, and ask the patient to hold the basin snugly against the head underneath the affected ear.	10		
11. Using the solution ordered to perform the irrigation, moisten cotton balls or 2- × 2-inch gauze squares and clean the outer ear.	10		
12. Pour the warmed solution into the sterile basin.	5		
13. Fill the ear-irrigating syringe with the ordered solution, being sure to expel air bubbles from the syringe.	10		
14. Straighten the ear canal as appropriate for age.	10		
15. Irrigate the ear by inserting the tip of the irrigating syringe into the ear and injecting the irrigating solution toward the roof of the canal.	15		
16. Irrigate until the solution has been used, or until the desired results have been achieved. Save solution for physician to observe if appropriate.	10		
17. Examine the ear canal with the otoscope at the end of the procedure. Gently dry the outside of the ear with a cotton ball or 2- × 2-inch gauze squares.	10		
18. Explain to the patient that the ear may feel sensitive for a few hours. Have the patient lie on the examination table with the affected ear down for approximately 15 minutes.	10		
19. Remove gloves, and sanitize the hands.	5		
20. Inform the physician that procedure is complete. Provide otoscope for inspection as appropriate.	5		

Copyright © 2010, 2005 by Saunders, an imprint of Elsevier, Inc. All rights reserved.

Steps	Possible Points	First Attempt	Second Attempt
21. Provide clarification of questions as appropriate.	5		
22. Escort the patient to the reception area.	5		
23. Document the procedure.	10		
24. Clean the equipment and examination room.	5		
Total Points Possible	200		

Comments: Total Points Earned _____

Divided by _____

Total Possible Points = _____% Score

Instructor's Signature _____

Student Name: _____ DATE: _____

PROCEDURE 38-2 CHECKLIST: PERFORM AN EAR INSTILLATION

TASK: Simulate ear instillation with prescribed medication in the affected ear.

CONDITIONS: Given the proper equipment and supplies, the student will be required to demonstrate the proper method for instilling prescribed medication into an affected ear.

EQUIPMENT AND SUPPLIES
- Otic drops with sterile dropper
- Cotton balls or gauze squares
- Disposable gloves (nonlatex)
- Patient's medical record

STANDARDS: Complete the procedure within _____ minutes and achieve a minimum score of _____%.

Time began _____   Time ended _____

Steps	Possible Points	First Attempt	Second Attempt
1. Sanitize hands.	5		
2. Assemble equipment and supplies.	5		
3. Obtain the patient's medical record.	5		
4. Verify the physician's order, otic drops to be instilled, and correct ear.	5		
5. Greet and identify the patient. Escort the patient to the examination room and seat the patient on the end of the examination table.	5		
6. Explain the procedure to the patient.	5		
7. Put on disposable gloves.	5		
8. Warm the medication, if necessary, and draw the medication into a dropper.	10		
9. Position the ear.	5		
10. Instill the medication in the ear as ordered (discard unused medication left in dropper).	10		
11. Instruct the patient to rest on the unaffected side for approximately 5 minutes.	5		
12. If appropriate, place cotton ball in ear canal.	5		
13. Remove gloves, and sanitize hands.	5		
14. Provide the patient with verbal and written follow-up instructions. Allow for questions.	5		

Copyright © 2010, 2005 by Saunders, an imprint of Elsevier, Inc. All rights reserved.

Steps	Possible Points	First Attempt	Second Attempt
15. Escort the patient to the reception area.	5		
16. Document the procedure.	10		
17. Clean the equipment and examination room.	5		
Total Points Possible	100		

Comments: Total Points Earned _____

Divided by _____

Total Possible Points = _____% Score

Instructor's Signature _____

Copyright © 2010, 2005 by Saunders, an imprint of Elsevier, Inc. All rights reserved.

Student Name: _____ DATE: _____

PROCEDURE 38-3 CHECKLIST: PERFORM AN EYE IRRIGATION

TASK: Simulate irrigation of the patient's eye to remove foreign particles and to soothe irritated tissue.

CONDITIONS: Given the proper equipment and supplies, the student will be required to demonstrate the proper method for irrigating the patient's eye.

EQUIPMENT AND SUPPLIES
- Sterile irrigating solution (as ordered)
- Sterile container for solution
- Sterile bottled solution with syringe tip, eye wash cup, or appropriate equipment for eye irrigation
- Disposable gloves (latex-free)
- Basin for the returned solution
- Sterile gauze squares
- Disposable moisture-resistant towel
- Biohazardous waste container
- Patient's medical record
- Tissues

STANDARDS: Complete the procedure within _____ minutes and achieve a minimum score of _____%.

Time began _____   Time ended _____

Steps	Possible Points	First Attempt	Second Attempt
1. Sanitize hands.	5		
2. Assemble equipment and supplies.	5		
3. Obtain the patient's medical record and verify order.	5		
4. Obtain the correct solution ordered by the physician.	5		
5. Greet and identify the patient. Escort the patient to the examination room and seat the patient on the end of the examination table.	5		
6. Explain procedure to patient.	5		
7. Warm the irrigating solution to body temperature by running the container under warm running tap water (98.6° to 100° F).	5		
8. Position the patient, and apply moisture-resistant barrier to shoulder of affected side.	5		
9. Put on disposable gloves.	5		

Steps	Possible Points	First Attempt	Second Attempt
10. Remove any debris or discharge from the patient's eyelid using moisturized cotton balls. Wipe from inner to outer canthus.	10		
11. Prepare the irrigating solution.	10		
12. Expose the lower conjunctiva by separating the eyelids with the gloved index finger and thumb, and ask the patient to stare at a fixed spot.	10		
13. Irrigate the affected eye(s) from inner to outer canthus.	10		
14. Continue with the irrigation until the correct amount of solution has been used or as ordered by the physician.	10		
15. Dry the eyelids from the inner to the outer canthus using dry cotton balls or dry gauze squares.	10		
16. Wipe the face and neck as needed.	10		
17. Remove gloves, and sanitize hands.	5		
18. Provide any further follow-up instructions. (Inform the patient that the eye may be red and irritated. If it lasts 2 days or longer, report it to the office.) Allow for questions.	10		
19. Escort the patient to the reception area.	5		
20. Document the procedure.	10		
21. Clean the equipment and examination room.	5		
Total Points Possible	150		

Comments: Total Points Earned _____

Divided by _____

Total Possible Points = _____ % Score

Instructor's Signature _____

Student Name: _____ DATE: _____

PROCEDURE 38-4 CHECKLIST: PERFORM AN EYE INSTILLATION

TASK: Simulate instillation as prescribed medication in the affected eye.

CONDITIONS: Given the proper equipment and supplies, the student will be required to perform a proper instillation of eye medication.

EQUIPMENT AND SUPPLIES
- Ophthalmic drops with sterile eyedropper, or ophthalmic ointment as ordered by physician
- Sterile gauze squares
- Tissues
- Disposable gloves (nonlatex)
- Patient's medical record

STANDARDS: Complete the procedure within _____ minutes and achieve a minimum score of _____%.

Time began _____   Time ended _____

Steps	Possible Points	First Attempt	Second Attempt
1. Sanitize hands.	5		
2. Assemble equipment and supplies.	5		
3. Obtain the patient's medical record and verify order.	5		
4. Obtain correct "ophthalmic" medication.	5		
5. Greet and identify the patient. Escort the patient to the examination room and seat the patient on the end of the examination table.	10		
6. Explain the procedure to the patient.	10		
7. Place the patient in a sitting or supine position.	5		
8. Put on disposable powder-free gloves, and prepare the medication.	5		
9. Prepare the eye for instillation (ask the patient to stare at a fixed spot during the instillation).	10		
10. Expose the lower conjunctival sac of the eye to be treated.	5		

Copyright © 2010, 2005 by Saunders, an imprint of Elsevier, Inc. All rights reserved.

Steps	Possible Points	First Attempt	Second Attempt
11. Instill the medication according to physician's order. Instill drops in the center of the lower conjunctival sac of the affected eye, or place a thin ribbon of ointment along the length of the lower conjunctival sac from inner to outer canthus, holding the tip of the dropper or ointment tube approximately ½ inch above the eye sac, never allowing the applicator to touch the eye.	15		
12. Discard any unused solution from the eye dropper, and replace the dropper into the bottle.	10		
13. Ask the patient to close the eyes gently, and rotate the eye. Ask patient not to squeeze the eyelids.	15		
14. Blot-dry the eyelids from the inner to the outer canthus with a dry gauze square to remove any excess medication. Use a separate tissue for each eye.	10		
15. Remove gloves, and sanitize the hands.	5		
16. Provide verbal and written follow-up instructions.	5		
17. Document the procedure.	15		
18. Clean the equipment and examination room.	10		
Total Points Possible	150		

Comments: Total Points Earned _____

Divided by _____

Total Possible Points = _____% Score

Instructor's Signature _____

Student Name: DATE:

PROCEDURE 38-5 CHECKLIST: APPLY A TUBULAR GAUZE BANDAGE

TASK: Properly apply a gauze bandage to the affected area.

CONDITIONS: Given the proper equipment and supplies, the student will be required to demonstrate the proper method for applying a tubular gauze bandage.

EQUIPMENT AND SUPPLIES
- Tube gauze applicator
- Roll of tubular gauze
- Adhesive tape
- Patient's medical record

STANDARDS: Complete the procedure within _____ minutes and achieve a minimum score of _____%.

Time began _____   Time ended _____

Steps	Possible Points	First Attempt	Second Attempt
1. Sanitize hands.	5		
2. Assemble equipment and supplies.	5		
3. Obtain the patient's medical record.	5		
4. Greet and identify the patient. Escort the patient to the examination room and seat the patient on the end of the examination table.	5		
5. Explain the procedure to the patient.	5		
6. Prepare the bandage according to the manufacturer's directions and the necessary length for the needed bandage.	10		
7. Gently slide the applicator over the proximal end of the appendage.	5		
8. Anchor the bandage at the proximal end of the appendage, pulling the applicator away from the proximal end toward the distal portion.	10		
9. Pull the applicator approximately 1 inch past the distal end of the patient's appendage.	5		
10. Rotate the applicator one full turn to anchor the bandage.	5		
11. Push the applicator toward the proximal end.	5		
12. Repeat Steps 8 through 11 until desired layers of gauze has been applied.	20		
13. Remove the applicator, and trim the excess gauze as needed.	5		

Copyright © 2010, 2005 by Saunders, an imprint of Elsevier, Inc. All rights reserved.

Steps	Possible Points	First Attempt	Second Attempt
14. Secure the bandage with adhesive tape or by securing the length of tube gauze remaining on the applicator around the patient's wrist or ankle.	10		
15. Provide instructions on care of bandage.	10		
16. Document the procedure.	10		
17. Clean the equipment and examination room.	5		
Total Possible Points	125		

Comments: Total Points Earned _____

Divided by _____

Total Possible Points = _____% Score

Instructor's Signature _____

Copyright © 2010, 2005 by Saunders, an imprint of Elsevier, Inc. All rights reserved.

Student Name: _____   DATE: _____

PROCEDURE 38-6 CHECKLIST: APPLY AN ICE BAG

TASK: Properly apply an ice bag to a swollen area.

CONDITIONS: Given the proper equipment and supplies, the student will be required to apply an ice bag properly.

EQUIPMENT AND SUPPLIES
- Ice bag with protective covering
- Small pieces of ice (ice chips or crushed ice)
- Patient's medical record
- Towel or protective covering

STANDARDS: Complete the procedure within _____ minutes and achieve a minimum score of _____%.

Time began _____   Time ended _____

Steps	Possible Points	First Attempt	Second Attempt
1. Sanitize hands.	5		
2. Assemble equipment and supplies.	5		
3. Obtain the patient's medical record.	5		
4. Greet and identify the patient. Escort the patient to the examination room and seat the patient on the end of the examination table.	5		
5. Explain the procedure to the patient.	10		
6. Properly fill the bag ½ to ⅔ full with ice chips or crushed ice.	5		
7. Remove air from bag and replace cap.	5		
8. Dry the outside of the bag and place in protective covering.	5		
9. Apply ice bag to the affected area, asking patient if the temperature is tolerable. Check patient after approximately 5 minutes.	15		
10. Leave bag in place for 20 to 30 minutes or as ordered by physician.	10		
11. Refill the bag with ice and change protective covering as needed.	5		
12. Sanitize hands.	5		

Steps	Possile Points	First Attempt	Second Attempt
13. Provide written and verbal follow-up instructions to the patient.	5		
14. Document the procedure.	10		
15. Properly sanitize and store ice bag covering.	5		
Total Points Possible	100		

Comments: Total Points Earned _____

Divided by _____

Total Possible Points = _____% Score

Instructor's Signature _____

Student Name: DATE:

PROCEDURE 38-7 CHECKLIST: APPLY A COLD COMPRESS

TASK: Properly apply a cold compress to an affected area.

CONDITIONS: Given the proper equipment and supplies, the student will be required to apply a cold compress.

EQUIPMENT AND SUPPLIES
- Ice cubes
- Washcloths or gauze squares (compress)
- Basin
- Towel
- Ice bag
- Patient's medical record

STANDARDS: Complete the procedure within _____ minutes and achieve a minimum score of _____%.

Time began _____   Time ended _____

Steps	Possible Points	First Attempt	Second Attempt
1. Sanitize hands.	5		
2. Assemble equipment and supplies.	5		
3. Obtain the patient's medical record.	5		
4. Greet and identify the patient. Escort the patient to the examination room and seat the patient on the end of the examination table.	5		
5. Prepare the cold water by adding ice for the compress.	5		
6. Prepare an ice bag.	5		
7. Prepare and apply the cold compress.	5		
8. Cover the compress with an ice bag in accordance with office policy.	5		
9. Ask the patient if the temperature is tolerable.	5		
10. Prepare compress and repeat application for prescribed duration.	10		
11. Periodically check the patient's skin for signs of blueness or numbness. Check for increased pain at site. Notify physician as necessary. Ask the patient if the site is painful.	10		

Copyright © 2010, 2005 by Saunders, an imprint of Elsevier, Inc. All rights reserved.

Steps	Possible Points	First Attempt	Second Attempt
12. Add ice as needed to keep water cold.	5		
13. At end of prescribed time, dry the affected area.	5		
14. Sanitize hands.	5		
15. Provide written and verbal follow-up instructions. Allow for questions from patient.	5		
16. Document the procedure.	10		
17. Properly care for the equipment and return to storage. Clean the equipment and examination room.	5		
Total Points Possible	100		

Comments: Total Points Earned _____

Divided by _____

Total Possible Points = _____% Score

Instructor's Signature _____

Student Name: _____ DATE: _____

PROCEDURE 38-8 CHECKLIST: APPLY A CHEMICAL COLD PACK

TASK: Properly activate and apply a chemical cold pack.

CONDITIONS: Given the proper equipment and supplies, the student will be required to activate and apply a chemical cold pack.

EQUIPMENT AND SUPPLIES
- Chemical cold pack
- Protective covering
- Patient's medical record

STANDARDS: Complete the procedure within _____ minutes and achieve a minimum score of _____%.

Time began _____   Time ended _____

Steps	Possible Points	First Attempt	Second Attempt
1. Sanitize hands.	5		
2. Assemble equipment and supplies.	5		
3. Obtain the patient's medical record.	5		
4. Greet and identify the patient. Escort the patient to the examination room and seat the patient on the end of the examination table.	5		
5. Explain the procedure to the patient.	10		
6. Follow manufacturer's instructions to activate the cold pack.	10		
7. Apply a cover to the pack and apply to the proper area.	15		
8. Administer cold therapy for the prescribed time.	10		
9. Discard the bag in the appropriate waste receptacle.	10		
10. Sanitize the hands.	5		
11. Provide verbal and written follow-up instructions.	10		
12. Document the procedure.	10		
Total Points Possible	100		

Comments: Total Points Earned _____

Divided by _____

Total Possible Points = _____% Score

Instructor's Signature _____

Copyright © 2010, 2005 by Saunders, an imprint of Elsevier, Inc. All rights reserved.

Student Name: _____   DATE: _____

PROCEDURE 38-9 CHECKLIST: APPLY A HOT WATER BAG

TASK: Fill and apply a hot water bag to an affected area.

CONDITIONS: Given the proper equipment and supplies, the student will be required to apply a hot water bag.

EQUIPMENT AND SUPPLIES
- Hot water bag with protective covering
- Pitcher to hold water
- Bath thermometer
- Patient's medical record

STANDARDS: Complete the procedure within _____ minutes and achieve a minimum score of _____%.

Time began _____   Time ended _____

Steps	Possible Points	First Attempt	Second Attempt
1. Sanitize hands.	5		
2. Assemble equipment and supplies.	5		
3. Obtain the patient's medical record.	5		
4. Greet and identify the patient. Escort the patient to the examination room.	5		
5. Explain the procedure to the patient.	10		
6. Prepare the water to be used in the hot water bag.	10		
7. Fill the hot water bag ⅓ to ½ full.	5		
8. Expel excess air.	5		
9. Dry the outside of the bag, and test for leakage.	5		
10. Cover with protective covering, and place the hot water bag on the affected area. Ensure that the patient is in a comfortable position.	10		
11. Apply the water bag for the prescribed time, refilling the bag with hot water as needed to maintain proper temperature, and checking patient.	10		

Copyright © 2010, 2005 by Saunders, an imprint of Elsevier, Inc. All rights reserved.

Steps	Possible Points	First Attempt	Second Attempt
12. Sanitize the hands.	5		
13. Provide verbal and written follow-up instructions.	5		
14. Document the procedure.	10		
15. Care for the hot water bag and store properly.	5		
Total Points Possible	100		

Comments: Total Points Earned _____

Divided by _____

Total Possible Points = _____% Score

Instructor's Signature _____

Student Name: _____ DATE: _____

PROCEDURE 38-10 CHECKLIST: APPLY A HEATING PAD

TASK: Apply a heating pad to an affected area.

CONDITIONS: Given the proper equipment and supplies, the student will be required to apply a heating pad to prescribed area.

EQUIPMENT AND SUPPLIES
- Heating pad
- Protective covering
- Patient's medical record

STANDARDS: Complete the procedure within _____ minutes and achieve a minimum score of _____%.

Time began _____   Time ended _____

Steps	Possible Points	First Attempt	Second Attempt
1. Sanitize hands.	5		
2. Assemble equipment and supplies. Inspect the heating pad to ensure it is in proper working order. Place the heating pad in the protective covering.	15		
3. Obtain the patient's medical record.	5		
4. Greet and identify the patient. Escort the patient to the examination room, and explain the procedure to the patient.	10		
5. Connect the heating pad to the electrical outlet, and set controls to proper setting as prescribed by physician.	5		
6. Place the patient in a position of comfort. Apply the heating pad to the affected area and check on patient during the prescribed time.	10		
7. Sanitize the hands.	5		
8. Provide verbal and written follow-up instructions. Allow for questions.	5		
9. Document the procedure.	10		
10. Store the equipment appropriately.	5		
Total Points Possible	75		

Comments: Total Points Earned _____

Divided by _____

Total Possible Points = _____% Score

Instructor's Signature _____

Copyright © 2010, 2005 by Saunders, an imprint of Elsevier, Inc. All rights reserved.

Student Name: _____   DATE: _____

PROCEDURE 38-11 CHECKLIST: APPLY A HOT COMPRESS

TASK: Apply a hot compress to an affected area according to physician's order.

CONDITIONS: Given the proper equipment and supplies, the student will be required to apply a hot compress to an affected area to increase circulation.

EQUIPMENT AND SUPPLIES
- Solution ordered by physician or commercially prepared hot, moist heat packs.
- Bath thermometer
- Washcloths or gauze squares
- Basin
- Towel
- Patient's medical record

STANDARDS: Complete the procedure within _____ minutes and achieve a minimum score of _____%.

Time began _____   Time ended _____

Steps	Possible Points	First Attempt	Second Attempt
1. Sanitize hands.	5		
2. Assemble equipment and supplies.	5		
3. Obtain the patient's medical record.	5		
4. Greet and identify the patient. Escort the patient to the examination room, and explain the procedure.	10		
5. Fill the basin with ordered solution, and check temperature.	10		
6. Place the patient in a comfortable position, cover the compress with a waterproof cover, and apply the compress to the affected area.	15		
7. Ask the patient if the temperature is tolerable.	10		
8. Prepare additional compresses as needed and reapply the compress; periodically check the patient's comfort, and replace the cooled water if necessary.	10		
9. After the prescribed time has elapsed, gently dry the area.	5		
10. Sanitize the hands.	5		

Copyright © 2010, 2005 by Saunders, an imprint of Elsevier, Inc. All rights reserved.

Steps	Possible Points	First Attempt	Second Attempt
11. Provide verbal and written follow-up instructions.	5		
12. Document the procedure.	10		
13. Care for the equipment and return it to its storage place.	5		
Total Points Possible	100		

Comments: Total Points Earned _____

Divided by _____

Total Possible Points = _____% Score

Instructor's Signature _____

Student Name: _____   DATE: _____

PROCEDURE 38-12 CHECKLIST: APPLY A HOT SOAK

TASK: Apply a hot soak to an affected area as prescribed by physician.

CONDITIONS: Given the proper equipment and supplies, the student will be required to apply a hot soak to an affected area.

EQUIPMENT AND SUPPLIES
- Soaking solution ordered by physician
- Bath thermometer
- Basin
- Towels
- Patient's medical record

STANDARDS: Complete the procedure within _____ minutes and achieve a minimum score of _____%.

Time began _____   Time ended _____

Steps	Possible Points	First Attempt	Second Attempt
1. Sanitize hands.	5		
2. Assemble equipment and supplies.	5		
3. Obtain the patient's medical record.	5		
4. Greet and identify the patient. Escort the patient to the examination room, and explain the procedure.	10		
5. Fill the basin with ordered solution and check temperature.	5		
6. Place the patient in a comfortable position, and gently and slowly immerse the patient's affected body part into the solution.	15		
7. Ask the patient if the temperature is tolerable.	5		
8. Apply the soak for the appropriate amount of time as ordered. Periodically check the patient and temperature of the water, replacing the cooled water with hot water as appropriate.	15		
9. After the prescribed time has elapsed, gently dry the area.	10		
10. Sanitize the hands.	5		

Steps	Possible Points	First Attempt	Second Attempt
11. Provide verbal and written follow-up instructions. Allow for questions.	5		
12. Document the procedure.	10		
13. Properly care for the equipment and return it to storage place.	5		
Total Points Possible	100		

Comments: Total Points Earned _____

Divided by _____

Total Possible Points = _____% Score

Instructor's Signature _____

Student Name: _____ DATE: _____

PROCEDURE 38-13 CHECKLIST: ADMINISTER AN ULTRASOUND TREATMENT

TASK: Administer an ultrasound treatment according to physician's order.

CONDITIONS: Given the proper equipment and supplies, the student will be required to administer an ultrasound treatment.

EQUIPMENT AND SUPPLIES
- Ultrasound machine
- Coupling agent
- Paper towels or tissues
- Patient's medical record

STANDARDS: Complete the procedure within _____ minutes and achieve a minimum score of _____%.

Time began _____   Time ended _____

Steps	Possible Points	First Attempt	Second Attempt
1. Sanitize hands.	5		
2. Assemble equipment and supplies.	5		
3. Obtain the patient's medical record.	5		
4. Greet and identify the patient. Escort the patient to the examination room, and explain the procedure.	10		
5. Prepare the patient and place the patient in a comfortable position to allow access for the type of ultrasound treatment ordered by the physician.	5		
6. Apply coupling gel to cover the treatment area completely.	10		
7. Use the ultrasound applicator head to spread the coupling agent evenly over the treatment area before turning on machine.	10		
8. Set ultrasound machine to "on," and place to the intensity level and time ordered by physician.	10		
9. Increase the intensity level to the level ordered.	10		
10. Place the applicator head at a right angle into the coupling agent on the patient's skin.	10		
11. Depending on the area of the body being treated, move the applicator in either a continuous back-and-forth motion or a circular motion.	10		

Copyright © 2010, 2005 by Saunders, an imprint of Elsevier, Inc. All rights reserved.

Steps	Possible Points	First Attempt	Second Attempt
12. If the patient complains of any pain, burning, or discomfort, stop the procedure immediately, and notify the physician.	10		
13. Continue ultrasound treatment until the prescribed time has expired.	5		
14. Remove the applicator head from the patient's skin, and turn the intensity control to the minimum position.	10		
15. Wipe excessive coupling agent from the patient's skin and applicator head.	5		
16. Instruct the patient to dress; assist as needed.	5		
17. Sanitize the hands.	5		
18. Document the procedure.	10		
19. Properly care for the equipment and return it to its appropriate storage place.	10		
Total Points Possible	150		

Comments: Total Points Earned _____

Divided by _____

Total Possible Points = _____% Score

Instructor's Signature _____

Student Name: _____ DATE: _____

PROCEDURE 38-14 CHECKLIST: MEASURE FOR AXILLARY CRUTCHES

TASK: Measure a patient for axillary crutches.

CONDITIONS: Given the proper equipment and supplies, the student will be required to measure a patient properly for crutches.

EQUIPMENT AND SUPPLIES
- Crutches
- Goniometer
- Patient's medical record

STANDARDS: Complete the procedure within _____ minutes and achieve a minimum score of _____%.

Time began _____   Time ended _____

Steps	Possible Points	First Attempt	Second Attempt
1. Sanitize hands.	5		
2. Assemble equipment and supplies.	5		
3. Obtain the patient's medical record.	5		
4. Greet and identify the patient. Escort the patient to the examination room, and explain the procedure.	10		
5. Position the patient in the standing position. Place crutch in axillary area, and position the crutch tips to create an appropriate triangle.	15		
6. Ask the patient to stand erect with a crutch beneath each axilla and to support his or her weight on the hand grips.	5		
7. To avoid pressure on axillary area, adjust the crutches.	5		
8. Adjust the handgrip so that elbows are at a 15-degree angle.	10		
9. Perform a final check of the crutch measurement so that no damage to body will occur.	15		
Total Points Possible	75		

Comments: Total Points Earned _____

Divided by _____

Total Possible Points = _____% Score

Instructor's Signature _____

Copyright © 2010, 2005 by Saunders, an imprint of Elsevier, Inc. All rights reserved.

Student Name: _____ DATE: _____

PROCEDURE 38-15 CHECKLIST: INSTRUCT THE PATIENT IN CRUTCH GAITS

TASK: Provide proper instructions for the appropriate crutch gait, depending on the injury or condition.

CONDITIONS: Given the proper equipment and supplies, the student will be required to instruct a patient on the proper crutch gait.

EQUIPMENT AND SUPPLIES
- Properly adjusted crutches
- Patient's medical record

STANDARDS: Complete the procedure within _____ minutes and achieve a minimum score of _____%.

Time began _____   Time ended _____

Steps	Possible Points	First Attempt	Second Attempt
1. Sanitize hands.	5		
2. Assemble equipment and supplies.	5		
3. Obtain the patient's medical record.	5		
4. Greet and identify the patient.	5		
5. Explain the procedure to the patient.	10		
6. Ask the patient to stand erect and face straight ahead.	5		
7. Position the crutches.	5		
8. Instruct the patient in the four-point gait, and obtain verbal and practical feedback.	10		
9. Instruct the patient in the three-point gait, and obtain verbal and practical feedback.	10		
10. Instruct the patient in the two-point gait, and obtain verbal and practical feedback.	10		
11. Instruct the patient in the swing gaits, and obtain verbal and practical feedback.	10		
12. Provide patient with appropriate written instruction.	5		
13. Sanitize the hands.	5		
14. Document the instructions.	10		
Total Points Possible	100		

Comments: Total Points Earned _____

Divided by _____

Total Possible Points = _____ % Score

Instructor's Signature _____

Student Name: _____ DATE: _____

PROCEDURE 38-16 CHECKLIST: INSTRUCT THE PATIENT IN THE USE OF A WALKER

TASK: Accurately measure and provide patient instructions for proper use of a walker.

CONDITIONS: Given the proper equipment and supplies, the student will be required to measure and provide instructions for proper use of a walker.

EQUIPMENT AND SUPPLIES
- Walker
- Patient's medical record

STANDARDS: Complete the procedure within _____ minutes and achieve a minimum score of _____%.

Time began _____   Time ended _____

Steps	Possible Points	First Attempt	Second Attempt
1. Sanitize hands.	5		
2. Provide a walker for instructional purposes.	5		
3. Obtain the patient's medical record.	5		
4. Greet and identify the patient, and explain the procedure to the patient.	5		
5. Adjust the walker to the proper height.	5		
6. Instruct the patient to pick up the walker and move it 6 inches forward.	5		
7. Have the patient move the dominant foot and then the nondominant foot into the "cage" of the walker.	10		
8. Caution the patient to be sure he or she has good balance before moving the walker ahead again.	10		
9. Repeat Steps 7 and 8 as appropriate.	5		
10. Observe the patient for several repetitions until the patient understands instructions and can safely have mobility with the walker.	10		
11. If the walker folds for storage or transport, instruct the patient on the appropriate method of folding the walker. Demonstrate and practice as needed.	10		

Copyright © 2010, 2005 by Saunders, an imprint of Elsevier, Inc. All rights reserved.

Steps	Possible Points	First Attempt	Second Attempt
12. Provide written instructions for use of the walker.	5		
13. Sanitize the hands.	5		
14. Document the instructions.	10		
15. If using facility's equipment, return to proper storage.	5		
Total Points Possible	100		

Comments: Total Points Earned _____

Divided by _____

Total Possible Points = _____% Score

Instructor's Signature _____

Student Name: _____ DATE: _____

PROCEDURE 38-17 CHECKLIST: INSTRUCT THE PATIENT IN THE USE OF A CANE

TASK: Measure and provide instructions for proper use of cane.

CONDITIONS: Given the proper equipment and supplies, the student will be required to measure and provide instruction on cane use.

EQUIPMENT AND SUPPLIES
- Cane
- Patient's medical record

STANDARDS: Complete the procedure within _____ minutes and achieve a minimum score of _____%.

Time began _____   Time ended _____

Steps	Possible Points	First Attempt	Second Attempt
1. Sanitize hands.	5		
2. Obtain cane if applicable.	5		
3. Obtain the patient's medical record.	5		
4. Greet and identify the patient, and explain the procedure.	10		
5. Measure cane to correct height on the unaffected side.	10		
6. Position the cane.	5		
7. Instruct the patient to move the cane and the affected leg forward at the same time.	10		
8. Repeat steps to ensure the patient understands the use of and can manage the cane.	5		
9. Sanitize the hands.	5		
10. Provide written instructions for use at home.	5		
11. Document the instructions.	10		
12. As appropriate, return equipment to proper storage.	5		
Total Points Possible	80		

Comments: Total Points Earned _____

Divided by _____

Total Possible Points = _____% Score

Instructor's Signature _____

901

Copyright © 2010, 2005 by Saunders, an imprint of Elsevier, Inc. All rights reserved.

Student Name: _____   DATE: _____

PROCEDURE 38-18 CHECKLIST: ASSIST IN PLASTER-OF-PARIS OR FIBERGLASS CAST APPLICATION

TASK: Provide supplies and assistance during cast application, and instruct the patient in cast care.

CONDITIONS: Given the proper equipment and supplies, the student will be required to assist with the application of a plaster-of-Paris or fiberglass cast.

EQUIPMENT AND SUPPLIES
- Cast material
- Stockinette to fit extremity
- Sheet wadding (cast padding)
- Basin or bucket to hold warm water
- Scissors
- Disposable glove
- Hand cream
- Patient's medical record

STANDARDS: Complete the procedure within _____ minutes and achieve a minimum score of _____%.

Time began _____   Time ended _____

Steps	Possible Points	First Attempt	Second Attempt
1. Sanitize hands.	5		
2. Assemble equipment and supplies.	5		
3. Obtain the patient's medical record.	5		
4. Greet and identify the patient, and explain the procedure.	10		
5. Place the patient in a comfortable position to allow access for the type of cast being applied.	5		
6. Clean and dry the area to be cast. Observe the area for any broken skin, redness, and bruising.	10		
7. Prepare the area by appropriately applying stockinette.	10		
8. Prepare the area by wrapping area in cast padding.	10		
9. Apply disposable gloves at proper time to assist with case application.	10		
10. Prepare the plaster-of-Paris or fiberglass roll.	10		
11. Assist as needed by holding the body part in the position requested by the physician. Reassure the patient as needed.	15		

Copyright © 2010, 2005 by Saunders, an imprint of Elsevier, Inc. All rights reserved.

Steps	Possible Points	First Attempt	Second Attempt
12. Repeat Steps 10 and 11 as needed.	10		
13. Assist with folding the stockinette down over the edge of casting material as appropriate.	5		
14. Provide scissors or a plastic knife to the physician to trim areas around thumb, fingers, or toes as necessary.	10		
15. Provide appropriate verbal and written instructions and isometric exercise instructions as prescribed by the physician.	5		
16. Clean the equipment and examination room. Return unused supplies to proper storage.	5		
17. Remove glove and sanitize the hands.	5		
18. Provide patient with written instructions for possible danger signs and symptoms.	5		
19. Document the procedure.	10		
Total Points Possible	150		

Comments: Total Points Earned _____

Divided by _____

Total Possible Points = _____% Score

Instructor's Signature _____

Charting for Procedures 38-1 through 38-18

Date	Chart

Date	Chart

Date	Chart

Date	Chart

Copyright © 2010, 2005 by Saunders, an imprint of Elsevier, Inc. All rights reserved.

	Chart
Date	

	Chart
Date	

	Chart
Date	

	Chart
Date	

	Chart
Date	

	Chart
Date	

	Chart
Date	

	Chart
Date	

Copyright © 2010, 2005 by Saunders, an imprint of Elsevier, Inc. All rights reserved.

	Chart
Date	

	Chart
Date	

	Chart
Date	

	Chart
Date	

	Chart
Date	

	Chart
Date	

	Chart
Date	

	Chart
Date	

Copyright © 2010, 2005 by Saunders, an imprint of Elsevier, Inc. All rights reserved.

Student Name: _____ DATE: _____

PROCEDURE 39-1 CHECKLIST: TEACH BREAST SELF-EXAMINATION

TASK: Instruct the patient to perform breast self-examination (BSE).

CONDITIONS: Given the proper equipment and supplies, the student will be required to provide instructions for performing a breast self-examination.

NOTE: The student should practice the procedure using the MACC located on the Evolve site at http://evolve.elsevier.com/klieger/medicalassisting: MACC/Clinical skills/Patient care/Teaching breast self-examination.

EQUIPMENT AND SUPPLIES
- Small pillow or rolled towel
- Model of breast with known irregularities
- BSE instruction sheet
- Patient's medical record

STANDARDS: Complete the procedure within _____ minutes and achieve a minimum score of _____%.

Time began _____   Time ended _____

Steps	Possible Points	First Attempt	Second Attempt
1. Sanitize hands.	5		
2. Assemble equipment and supplies.	5		
3. Obtain the patient's medical record.	5		
4. Greet and identify the patient. Escort the patient to the examination room, and ask her to have a seat on the end of the examination table.	10		
5. Explain the importance of performing the monthly BSE.	10		
6. Provide an instruction card, and explain the steps for BSE.	5		
7. Instruct patient to inspect both breasts visually in a mirror for color, texture, and symmetry.	5		
8. Instruct patient to raise both arms at the same time and to check both breasts and nipples for reaction to movement.	5		
9. Instruct patient to rest palms on hips and press down firmly, and then to flex the chest and tighten the chest muscles while observing breast.	5		

Copyright © 2010, 2005 by Saunders, an imprint of Elsevier, Inc. All rights reserved.

Steps	Possible Points	First Attempt	Second Attempt
10. Instruct patient to bend forward at the waist with hands on hips and to check for dimpling of the skin or nipples.	5		
11. Instruct patient to stand up and gently squeeze the nipple of each breast with the fingertips for any discharge.	5		
12. Instruct patient to use the pads of her index, middle, and ring fingers to palpate the model to determine abnormalities.	5		
13. Using the model, instruct patient to use a small circular motion, in a systematic pattern, over all areas of the breast (about the size of a dime) and to apply continuous pressure while palpating both breasts for lumps or thickening of breast tissue.	15		
14. Palpate toward the nipple, keeping fingers on the breast to avoid missing a spot.	5		
15. Check the entire breast, from the armpit to breastbone and from the collarbone to the bra line.	10		
16. Position the patient for inspection of her own breasts, and instruct her to follow a pattern while palpating her own breasts in a standing position.	10		
17. Instruct patient to place her right hand on her right shoulder and palpate her right breast with her left hand, checking for lumps, thickening, or hard knots.	10		
18. Instruct patient to repeat the process and to examine her left breast.	5		
19. After having adequately completed the return demonstration, assist patient with dressing as necessary.	5		

Steps	Possible Points	First Attempt	Second Attempt
20. Provide the patient with an instruction card, and ask if there are any questions.	5		
21. Remind the patient that the health care provider will answer any questions she may have about any abnormalities found.	5		
22. Document the instructions in the patient's medical record.	10		
Total Points Possible	150		

Comments: Total Points Earned _____

Divided by _____

Total Possible Points = _____% Score

Instructor's Signature _____

Copyright © 2010, 2005 by Saunders, an imprint of Elsevier, Inc. All rights reserved.

Student Name: _____   DATE: _____

PROCEDURE 39-2 CHECKLIST: ASSIST WITH A GYNECOLOGICAL EXAMINATION

TASK: Prepare a patient for and assist the health care provider with a gynecological examination, including Pap smear (direct smear method and "liquid prep" method).

CONDITIONS: Given the proper equipment and supplies, the student will be required to prepare a patient for and assist with a gynecological examination, including a Pap smear.

NOTE: The student should practice the procedure using the MACC located on the Evolve site at http://evolve.elsevier.com/klieger/medicalassisting: MACC/Clinical skills/Patient care/Assisting with a gynecologic exam.

EQUIPMENT AND SUPPLIES
- Patient gown and drape
- Nonsterile disposable gloves
- Gauze squares
- Disposable vaginal speculum or sterilized stainless steel speculum
- Light source
- Lubricant (water-based)
- Tissues
- Cytology requisition
- Transport media
- Urine specimen container
- Biohazardous waste container
- Patient's medical record

"Dry Prep" (Direct Smear) Method

- Wooden spatula
- Endocervical brush; cotton-tipped applicator
- Microscope slides with frosted edge
- Slide holder
- Cytology fixative

"Liquid Prep" Method

- Cervical broom
- Plastic spatula
- Transport medium vial

STANDARDS: Complete the procedure within _____ minutes and achieve a minimum score of _____%.

Time began _____   Time ended _____

Steps	Possible Points	First Attempt	Second Attempt
1. Sanitize hands.	5		
2. Assemble equipment and supplies.	5		
3. Obtain the patient's medical record.	5		
4. Greet and identify the patient.	5		

Copyright © 2010, 2005 by Saunders, an imprint of Elsevier, Inc. All rights reserved.

Steps	Possible Points	First Attempt	Second Attempt
5. Ask the patient if she needs to empty her bladder before the exam.	5		
6. Escort the patient to the examination room, and ask the patient to have a seat on the end of the examination table.	5		
7. Obtain and record the following preliminary patient information: a. Vital signs	5		
b. Height and weight	5		
c. Menstrual and obstetric history	5		
d. Any particular patient concerns or complaints	5		
8. Complete the cytology requisition form.	10		
9. Ask the patient to undress completely and put on the gown with opening on the back, and to sit at the end of the examination table with the drape across her lap. Assistant leaves the room and knocks on door before entering.	5		
10. Position and drape the patient for a breast examination, and assist physician as needed.	5		
11. Adjust the drape for the abdominal examination in the supine position, and assist physician as needed.	10		
12. Position and drape the patient into the lithotomy position for the pelvic examination.	10		
13. Apply disposable gloves.	5		
14. Fold back the corner of the drape to expose the perineal area; adjust and focus the light on the perineum for the physician.	5		
15. Warm the vaginal speculum using warm water.	5		
16. Assist the physician with the pelvic examination by encouraging the patient to breathe deeply and evenly.	5		

Steps	Possible Points	First Attempt	Second Attempt
17. Prepare slides for the specimens with labeling as required by laboratory. Pass instruments and equipment as needed.	10		
18. Pass spatula for cervical specimen. Hold the glass slide marked "C" for the physician to apply the specimen. Discard the applicator in biohazardous waste container.	10		
19. Pass the endocervical brush. Hold out the slide with an "E" to receive the next specimen. Discard the endocervical brush in biohazardous waste container.	10		
20. Hand the physician a cotton-tipped applicator to collect a vaginal specimen. Hold out the slide marked with a "V." Discard the applicator in biohazardous waste container.	10		
21. Spray the Pap slides immediately with fixative (within 10 seconds).	10		
22. If performing "liquid prep" method, label the liquid-prep vial or slides as required by the laboratory and place the liquid-prep vial or slides in a biohazardous transport bag.	10		
23. Assist the physician with the bimanual pelvic examination, including passing speculum and encouraging deep breathing. Assist with occult blood test, including the developing of guaiac slide.	10		
24. Dispose of disposable speculum, guaiac slide, and gloves in a biohazardous waste container.	5		
25. Assist the patient from the lithotomy position and down from the examination table.	5		
26. Instruct the patient to dress.	5		
27. Leave the room and complete the cytology requisition form.	5		

Copyright © 2010, 2005 by Saunders, an imprint of Elsevier, Inc. All rights reserved.

Steps	Possible Points	First Attempt	Second Attempt
28. Attach the completed cytology form to either the microscope slide holder or the transport medium vial, and chart the transport to the laboratory.	5		
29. Clean the examination room in preparation for the next patient.	5		
30. Sanitize the hands.	5		
31. Document the procedure in the patient's medical record.	10		
Total Points Possible	225		

Comments: Total Points Earned _____

Divided by _____

Total Possible Points = _____% Score

Instructor's Signature _____

Student Name: _____ DATE: _____

PROCEDURE 39-3 CHECKLIST: ASSIST WITH A FOLLOW-UP PRENATAL EXAMINATION

TASK: Assist the physician during a follow-up prenatal visit.

CONDITIONS: Given the proper equipment and supplies, the student will be required to assist the physician during a follow-up prenatal examination.

EQUIPMENT AND SUPPLIES
- Flexible, nonstretchable centimeter tape measure
- Nonsterile disposable gloves
- Doppler fetal pulse detector
- Lubricant (water-based)
- Ultrasound coupling agent
- Vaginal speculum
- Examining gown and drape
- Biohazardous waste container
- Patient's medical record

STANDARDS: Complete the procedure within _____ minutes and achieve a minimum score of _____%.

Time began _____   Time ended _____

Steps	Possible Points	First Attempt	Second Attempt
1. Sanitize hands.	5		
2. Assemble equipment and supplies.	5		
3. Obtain the patient's medical record.	5		
4. Greet and identify the patient.	5		
5. Collect the first morning urine specimen that the patient has brought from home.	5		
6. Weigh and document the results in the patient's medical record.	10		
7. Escort patient to the examination room, and explain the procedure.	5		
8. Document problems, concerns, or complaints.	5		
9. Measure the patient's vital signs, and document the results in the patient's medical record.	10		
10. Prepare the patient for the examination by applying drape and gown.	10		
11. Test the urine specimen using a reagent strip, and document the results in the patient's medical record.	10		

919

Copyright © 2010, 2005 by Saunders, an imprint of Elsevier, Inc. All rights reserved.

Steps	Possible Points	First Attempt	Second Attempt
12. Inform the physician that the patient is ready to be examined, and provide the physician with the medical record for review.	5		
13. Position and drape the patient, just before the physician is ready to start the examination.	10		
14. Assist the physician as required for the prenatal examination, passing instruments and equipment as needed. Collect and prepare specimens as requested. Apply gloves as appropriate.	10		
15. After the examination, assist the patient from the examination table.	10		
16. Remove gloves and dispose of disposable equipment in correct container as appropriate.	5		
17. Allow patient time to redress.	5		
18. Provide the patient education, and clarify any of the physician's instructions as appropriate.	10		
19. Apply gloves to clean the examination room in preparation for the next patient. Discard gloves in appropriate waste container.	10		
20. Sanitize hands.	5		
21. Document appropriate information in the patient's medical record.	5		
Total Points Possible	150		

Comments: Total Points Earned _____

Divided by _____

Total Possible Points = _____% Score

Instructor's Signature _____

Copyright © 2010, 2005 by Saunders, an imprint of Elsevier, Inc. All rights reserved.

Student Name: _____ DATE: _____

PROCEDURE 39-4 CHECKLIST: INSTRUCT THE PATIENT IN OBTAINING A FECAL SPECIMEN

TASK: Provide the patient with accurate and complete instructions on the preparation and collection of a stool sample for testing.

CONDITIONS: Given the proper equipment and supplies, the student will be required to provide the patient with instructions on the preparation and collection of a stool sample.

NOTE: The student should practice the procedure using the MACC located on the Evolve site at http://evolve.elsevier.com/klieger/medicalassisting: MACC/Clinical skills/Diagnostic testing/Instructing how to obtain a fecal specimen and testing for occult blood.

EQUIPMENT AND SUPPLIES
- Hemoccult slide testing kit
- 3 occult blood slides
- 3 applicator sticks
- Diet and collection instruction sheet
- Patient's medical record

STANDARDS: Complete the procedure within _____ minutes and achieve a minimum score of _____%.

Time began _____   Time ended _____

Steps	Possible Points	First Attempt	Second Attempt
1. Sanitize hands.	5		
2. Assemble equipment and supplies.	5		
3. Greet and identify the patient.	5		
4. Explain the procedure to the patient. Escort the patient to the examination room.	10		
5. Provide the patient with verbal and written instructions including diet modification and other conditions that might affect the test results, such as menses.	10		
6. Provide the patient with the Hemoccult slide test kit.	5		
7. Instruct the patient to use a ballpoint pen to complete the required information on the front of the card.	5		
8. Inform the patient of the requirements for proper care and storage of the slides.	5		
9. Instruct patient to collect a stool specimen in the toilet from the first bowel movement after the 48-hour preparation period.	5		

PROCEDURE 39-4

Copyright © 2010, 2005 by Saunders, an imprint of Elsevier, Inc. All rights reserved.

Steps	Possible Points	First Attempt	Second Attempt
10. Explain the stool collection procedure to the patient; include the matter of obtaining specimen and the means of placing specimen on slide.	10		
11. Instruct the patient to allow the slides to air dry minimally overnight.	5		
12. Instruct the patient to repeat the process on the next two bowel movements, repeating the collection steps.	5		
13. When all three specimens have been collected and allowed to air dry, instruct the patient to place the cardboard slides in the envelope, carefully seal, and return it as soon as possible to the medical office.	5		
14. Ensure that patient understands the instructions required for patient preparation, collection, and processing of the stool specimens, and for storage of the slides.	5		
15. Document that instructions have been provided in the patient's medical record.	10		
16. Sanitize the hands.	5		
Total Points Possible	100		

Comments: Total Points Earned _____

Divided by _____

Total Possible Points = _____ % Score

Instructor's Signature _____

Student Name: _____ DATE: _____

PROCEDURE 39-5 CHECKLIST: TEST FOR OCCULT BLOOD

TASK: Accurately develop the occult blood slide test, and document the results.

CONDITIONS: Given the proper equipment and supplies, the student will be required to demonstrate competency in developing an occult blood slide test and document the results.

NOTE: The student should practice the procedure using the MACC located on the Evolve site at http://evolve.elsevier.com/klieger/medicalassisting: MACC/Clinical skills/Diagnostic testing/Instructing how to obtain a fecal specimen & testing for occult blood.

EQUIPMENT AND SUPPLIES
- Prepared cardboard slides
- Reference card
- Developing solution
- Nonsterile disposable gloves
- Biohazardous waste container
- Patient's medical record

STANDARDS: Complete the procedure within _____ minutes and achieve a minimum score of _____%.

Time began _____   Time ended _____

Steps	Possible Points	First Attempt	Second Attempt
1. Sanitize hands.	5		
2. Assemble supplies, including test kit reference card.	5		
3. Check the expiration date on the developing solution bottle.	10		
4. Obtain the patient's medical record.	5		
5. Apply nonsterile disposable gloves.	5		
6. Prepare the patient by removing clothes as appropriate; drape and gown the patient.	5		
7. Prepare the slides.	10		
8. Develop slides according to manufacturer's instructions.	10		
9. Read the results within 60 seconds.	10		
10. Perform quality control procedure on slide, and document the results in the quality control laboratory log book.	10		
11. Properly dispose of the Hemoccult slides in a biohazardous waste container.	10		

Copyright © 2010, 2005 by Saunders, an imprint of Elsevier, Inc. All rights reserved.

Steps	Possible Point	First Attempt	Second Attempt
12. Remove gloves and sanitize hands.	5		
13. Document the results.	10		
Total Points Possible	100		

Comments: Total Points Earned _____

Divided by _____

Total Possible Points = _____% Score

Instructor's Signature _____

Student Name: _____   DATE: _____

PROCEDURE 39-6 CHECKLIST: ASSIST WITH SIGMOIDOSCOPY

TASK: Assist the physician and the patient during sigmoidoscopy.

CONDITIONS: Given the proper equipment and supplies, the student will be required to assist the physician and patient during sigmoidoscopy.

EQUIPMENT AND SUPPLIES
- Nonsterile disposable gloves
- Sterile specimen container with preservative
- Flexible sigmoidoscope
- 4- × 4-inch gauze squares
- Water-soluble lubricant
- Tissue wipes
- Drape
- Biopsy forceps
- Biohazardous waste container
- Patient's medical record

STANDARDS: Complete the procedure within _____ minutes and achieve a minimum score of _____%.

Time began _____   Time ended _____

Steps	Possible Points	First Attempt	Second Attempt
1. Sanitize hands.	5		
2. Assemble equipment and supplies.	5		
3. Obtain the patient's medical record.	5		
4. Greet and identify the patient. Escort the patient to the examination room, and explain the procedure to the patient.	5		
5. Ask the patient if he or she needs to empty his or her bladder before the examination.	5		
6. Assist patient in preparing for exam by gowning, positioning, and draping the patient.	5		
7. Assist physician in application of disposable gloves. Lubricate the physician's gloved index finger.	10		
8. Lubricate the distal end of the sigmoidoscope for insertion into anus.	10		
9. Assist the physician with the suction equipment as required.	5		

PROCEDURE 39-6

925

Copyright © 2010, 2005 by Saunders, an imprint of Elsevier, Inc. All rights reserved.

Steps	Possible Points	First Attempt	Second Attempt
10. On completion of the examination, apply clean gloves, and clean the patient's anal area with tissues to remove excess lubricant.	5		
11. Remove gloves and sanitize hands.	5		
12. Assist the patient from the examination table; instruct the patient to dress.	5		
13. Provide the patient with a restroom to expel any air that was used to inflate the colon during the procedure.	5		
14. Prepare the laboratory requisition form and accompanying specimens.	10		
15. Clean the examination room and clean equipment in preparation for the next patient.	5		
16. Document the procedure in the patient's medical record.	10		
Total Points Possible	100		

Comments: Total Points Earned _____

Divided by _____

Total Possible Points = _____% Score

Instructor's Signature _____

Student Name: _____ DATE: _____

PROCEDURE 39-7 CHECKLIST: PERFORM SPIROMETRY (PULMONARY FUNCTION TESTING)

TASK: Prepare and operate a simple spirometer to measure lung volume.

CONDITIONS: Given the proper equipment and supplies, the student will be required to demonstrate competency in performing spirometry.

NOTE: The student should practice the procedure using the MACC located on the Evolve site at http://evolve.elsevier.com/klieger/medicalassisting: MACC/Clinical skills/Diagnostic testing/Performing a spirometry test.

EQUIPMENT AND SUPPLIES
- Spirometry machine
- Disposable mouthpiece
- Disposable tubing
- Nose clips
- Biohazardous waste container
- Patient's medical record

STANDARDS: Complete the procedure within _____ minutes and achieve a minimum score of _____%.

Time began _____   Time ended _____

Steps	Possible Points	First Attempt	Second Attempt
1. Sanitize hands.	5		
2. Assemble equipment and supplies.	5		
3. Obtain the patient's medical record.	5		
4. Greet and identify the patient. Escort the patient to the examination room, and explain the procedure to the patient.	10		
5. Measure the patient's height and weight.	5		
6. Enter the patient's information into the spirometer.	5		
7. Perform the spirometry test.	15		
8. Instruct the patient in breathing.	15		
9. Coach the patient into performing the task to the best of his or her ability.	10		
10. Allow rest periods for the patient, if needed.	5		
11. Ensure that the physician reviews the spirometry results.	10		
12. Before documenting the procedure, make the patient comfortable, and put the equipment away.	10		

PROCEDURE 39-7

Copyright © 2010, 2005 by Saunders, an imprint of Elsevier, Inc. All rights reserved.

Steps	Possible Points	First Attempt	Second Attempt
13. Discard the disposable components of the spirometry test in a biohazardous waste container.	10		
14. Sanitize the hands.	5		
15. Document the test results.	10		
Total Points Possible	125		

Comments: Total Points Earned _____

Divided by _____

Total Possible Points = _____ % Score

Instructor's Signature _____

Student Name: _____ DATE: _____

PROCEDURE 39-8 CHECKLIST: INSTRUCT THE PATIENT IN THE USE OF A PEAK FLOW METER

TASK: Properly provide instructions to a patient in the use of a peak flow meter.

CONDITIONS: Given procedure, proper equipment, and supplies, the student will be required to role play with another student and provide accurate and complete instructions on the proper way to use a peak flow meter.

EQUIPMENT AND SUPPLIES
- Peak flow meter
- Patient's medical record

STANDARDS: Complete the procedure within _____ minutes and achieve a minimum score of _____ %.

Time began _____   Time ended _____

Steps	Possible Points	First Attempt	Second Attempt
1. Sanitize hands.	5		
2. Assemble equipment and supplies.	5		
3. Obtain the patient's medical record.	5		
4. Greet the patient, introduce yourself, and confirm the patient's identity.	10		
5. Escort the patient to the examination room, and explain the procedure to the patient.	10		
6. Instruct the patient to stand up straight and how to hold the meter, and set indicator to zero.	15		
7. Instruct the patient to take a deep breath and to place the mouthpiece in his or her mouth with the lips around the mouthpiece.	15		
8. Instruct the patient to blow out hard (fast hard puff).	15		
9. Write down the number, reset the indicator to zero, and have the patient repeat the procedure two more times and write down the numbers.	15		
10. Determine the highest number.	5		
11. Provide the patient with a booklet to record daily readings.	5		
12. Sanitize the hands.	5		
13. Document the test results and patient education in the medical record.	15		
Total Points Possible	125		

Comments: Total Points Earned _____

Divided by _____

Total Possible Points = _____ % Score

Instructor's Signature _____

Copyright © 2010, 2005 by Saunders, an imprint of Elsevier, Inc. All rights reserved.

Student Name: _____   DATE: _____

PROCEDURE 39-9 CHECKLIST: PERFORM PULSE OXIMETRY

TASK: Accurately determine a patient's blood oxygen saturation using pulse oximetry.

CONDITIONS: Given the proper equipment and supplies, the student will be required to demonstrate the competency of performing pulse oximetry.

EQUIPMENT AND SUPPLIES
- Pulse oximeter
- Probe
- Alcohol prep pads
- Patient's medical record

STANDARDS: Complete the procedure within _____ minutes and achieve a minimum score of _____%.

Time began _____   Time ended _____

Steps	Possible Points	First Attempt	Second Attempt
1. Sanitize hands.	5		
2. Assemble equipment and supplies.	5		
3. Obtain the patient's medical record.	5		
4. Greet and identify the patient. Escort the patient to the examination room.	5		
5. Explain the procedure to the patient.	5		
6. Ask the patient to have a seat in a comfortable position with arms well supported.	5		
7. Connect the oximeter finger probe to the monitor.	10		
8. Turn on the power switch.	5		
9. Wipe the probe clean with the alcohol prep pad and let dry.	10		
10. Apply the oximeter probe to the patient's finger.	10		
11. Wait while the system stabilizes.	5		
12. Read the pulse rate and the arterial blood saturation on the digital display.	10		

Copyright © 2010, 2005 by Saunders, an imprint of Elsevier, Inc. All rights reserved.

Steps	Possible Points	First Attempt	Second Attempt
13. Remove the sensor from the patient's finger.	5		
14. Sanitize hands.	5		
15. Document the pulse oximetry results in the patient's medical record.	10		
Total Points Possible	100		

Comments: Total Points Earned _____

Divided by _____

Total Possible Points = _____% Score

Instructor's Signature _____

Charting for Procedures 39-1 through 39-9

Date	Chart

Date	Chart

Date	Chart

Date	Chart

Copyright © 2010, 2005 by Saunders, an imprint of Elsevier, Inc. All rights reserved.

	Chart
Date	

	Chart
Date	

	Chart
Date	

	Chart
Date	

	Chart
Date	

	Chart
Date	

	Chart
Date	

Student Name: _____ DATE: _____

PROCEDURE 40-1 CHECKLIST: USE METHODS OF QUALITY CONTROL (QC)

TASK: Practice quality control procedures in the medical laboratory to ensure accuracy of test results through detection and elimination of errors.

CONDITIONS: Given the proper equipment and supplies, the student will demonstrate the proper methods of quality control.

EQUIPMENT AND SUPPLIES
- Quality control log book/log sheets on a clip board
- Quality control samples (as provided in CLIA-waived prepackaged test kits)
- hCG pregnancy test
- Patient's sample
- Patient's medical record
- Copy of CLIA 88 guidelines (Internet)
- Copy of state regulation and guidelines (Internet search for your state)

STANDARDS: Complete the procedure within _____ minutes and achieve a minimum score of _____%.

Time began _____   Time ended _____

Steps	Possible Points	First Attempt	Second Attempt
1. Sanitize hands.	5		
2. Assemble equipment and supplies.	5		
3. Obtain the quality control (QC) sample provided in a CLIA-waived prepackaged kit.	5		
4. Check the expiration date on the prepackaged test kit and on each QC specimen.	10		
5. Perform QC using the test kit supplied.	5		
6. Obtain the specimen from the patient, and identify the specimen as belonging to the patient.	15		
7. Perform testing of the specimen following the specific protocols outlined for the sample by the manufacturer.	20		
8. Perform QC testing as outlined by the manufacturer's protocols for the specimen being tested.	10		
9. Determine the results for the patient's specimen and the QC sample.	10		

Copyright © 2010, 2005 by Saunders, an imprint of Elsevier, Inc. All rights reserved.

Steps	Possible Points	First Attempt	Second Attempt
10. Sanitize the hands.	5		
11. Document the results in the QC log book and the patient's medical record.	10		
Total Points Possible	100		

Comments: Total Points Earned _____

Divided by _____

Total Possible Points = _____% Score

Instructor's Signature _____

hCG Control Log

Manufacturer/Kit Name: _____

Lot # _____

Expire Date: _____

Date	Specimen: Control/Patient	Result: +/−	Control Within Limits (Y/N)	Doc PT Chart	Initials

Copyright © 2010, 2005 by Saunders, an imprint of Elsevier, Inc. All rights reserved.

Student Name: _____ DATE: _____

PROCEDURE 40-2 CHECKLIST: FOCUS THE MICROSCOPE

TASK: Focus the microscope on a prepared slide from low power to high power and oil immersion.

CONDITIONS: Given the proper equipment and supplies, the student will be required to demonstrate the proper method for focusing a microscope.

EQUIPMENT AND SUPPLIES
- Microscope with cover
- Lens paper
- Lens cleaner
- Specimen slide (supplied by instructor)
- Soft cloth
- Tissue or gauze

STANDARDS: Complete the procedure within _____ minutes and achieve a minimum score of _____%.

Time began _____   Time ended _____

Steps	Possible Points	First Attempt	Second Attempt
1. Sanitize hands.	5		
2. Assemble equipment and supplies.	5		
3. Clean the ocular and objective lenses of the microscope with lens paper and lens cleaner.	10		
4. Turn on the light source, and adjust the ocular lenses to fit your eye span.	5		
5. Place the slide on the stage, and secure it in the slide clip.	10		
6. Rotate the nosepiece to the scanning objective (×4) or to the low-power objective (×10) if the scanning objective is not attached to your microscope.	10		
7. Adjust the coarse focus adjustment knob.	5		
8. Open the diaphragm to allow in the maximum amount of light.	10		
9. Focus the specimen.	5		
10. Focus the specimen further into finest detail by using the fine focus adjustment knob.	10		

Copyright © 2010, 2005 by Saunders, an imprint of Elsevier, Inc. All rights reserved.

Steps	Possible Points	First Attempt	Second Attempt
11. Adjust the diaphragm and condenser to regulate and adjust the amount of light focused on the specimen to obtain the sharpest image.	10		
12. Rotate the nosepiece to high power, and use fine adjustment as needed to bring specimen in focus.	10		
13. Examine the specimen by scanning the slide using the stage movement knob to move it in four directions.	10		
14. Examine the specimen as required for the procedure or test, and report the results.	10		
15. On completion of the examination of the specimen, lower the stage or raise the objective, turn off the light, and remove the slide from the stage.	10		
16. Return objectives to highest placement and turn objective to lowest power.	10		
17. Clean the stage with lens paper or gauze.	5		
18. When clean, cover the microscope with a dust cloth and return it to storage.	5		
19. Sanitize the hands.	5		
Total Points Possible	150		

Comments: Total Points Earned _____

Divided by _____

Total Possible Points = _____% Score

Instructor's Signature _____

Copyright © 2010, 2005 by Saunders, an imprint of Elsevier, Inc. All rights reserved.

Student Name: DATE:

PROCEDURE 40-3 CHECKLIST: COMPLETE A LABORATORY REQUISITION

TASK: Complete a laboratory requisition form accurately for specimen testing.

CONDITIONS: Given the proper equipment and supplies, the student will be required to complete a laboratory requisition form.

EQUIPMENT AND SUPPLIES
- Physician's written order for laboratory tests
- Laboratory requisition form (supplied by instructor)
- Patient's medical record
- Pen

STANDARDS: Complete the procedure within _____ minutes and achieve a minimum score of _____%.

Time began _____   Time ended _____

Steps	Possible Points	First Attempt	Second Attempt
1. Obtain the patient's medical record, and confirm the physician's orders for laboratory testing.	5		
2. Obtain the laboratory requisition form for the laboratory where the test will be performed; ensure that the laboratory is acceptable for patient's insurance policy.	10		
3. Complete the section of the requisition requiring the physician's name and address.	5		
4. Complete the patient's demographic information.	5		
5. Complete the section of the requisition requiring the patient's insurance and billing information.	10		
6. Complete the desired laboratory testing information.	10		
7. Complete the section of the requisition requiring date and time of specimen collection.	10		
8. Enter the patient's diagnosis code on the requisition as required.	10		
9. Enter the type and amount of medication the patient is taking if appropriate for test to be performed.	10		
10. Complete the patient authorization to release and assign the benefits portion as applicable.	10		

Copyright © 2010, 2005 by Saunders, an imprint of Elsevier, Inc. All rights reserved.

Steps	Possible Points	First Attempt	Second Attempt
11. Attach copy of insurance identification cards if required by laboratory.	5		
12. Attach the laboratory requisition securely to the specimen before sending it to the laboratory.	5		
13. Document in the patient's medical record and in the laboratory log book showing the laboratory where specimen was sent for testing.	5		
Total Points Possible	100		

Comments: Total Points Earned _____

Divided by _____

Total Possible Points = _____% Score

Instructor's Signature _____

Patient Information for Procedure 40-3

John Doe is a 25-year-old patient of Dr. Heal. Today Dr. Heal orders a chemistry panel to be drawn on John Doe.

Dx: Hyperlipidemia
Medications: Crestor

John Heal, MD
United Health Center
1925 Oregon Ave
Our Town, USA 65432

Insurance: ABC Medical Insurance
4567 Darnway Blvd
West Town, USA 67890
ID # 67890BF34

John Doe
1234 West End St
Our Town, USA 65411
(678) 456-3487

Patient Laboratory Log Sheet for Procedure 40-3

Date	Patient	Specimen	Result	Sent to Lab	Initials

Copyright © 2010, 2005 by Saunders, an imprint of Elsevier, Inc. All rights reserved.

Student Name: _____   DATE: _____

PROCEDURE 40-4 CHECKLIST: COLLECT A SPECIMEN FOR TRANSPORT TO AN OUTSIDE LABORATORY

TASK: Collect a specimen to be sent to an outside laboratory.

CONDITIONS: Given the proper equipment and supplies, the student will be required to demonstrate the proper method of collecting a specimen for transport to an outside laboratory.

EQUIPMENT AND SUPPLIES
- Specimen and container (throat culture)
- Disposable gloves
- Label
- Laboratory request form (instructor will provide)
- Patient's medical record
- Laboratory log book/log sheet
- Pen

STANDARDS: Complete the procedure within _____ minutes and achieve a minimum score of _____%.

Time began _____   Time ended _____

Steps	Possible Points	First Attempt	Second Attempt
1. Ensure that the patient has followed any advance preparation or special instructions necessary for test accuracy.	5		
2. Review the requirements in the laboratory directory for collection and handling of the specimen ordered by the physician.	5		
3. Complete the laboratory requisition form.	10		
4. Sanitize hands.	5		
5. Assemble equipment and supplies.	5		
6. Greet and identify the patient, and escort the patient to the examination room.	5		
7. Collect the specimen using OSHA standards. Ensure that specimen has been collected according to laboratory specifications.	10		
8. Process the specimen further as required by the outside laboratory.	5		
9. Clearly label the tubes and specimen containers, and prepare for transport to outside laboratory.	10		

Copyright © 2010, 2005 by Saunders, an imprint of Elsevier, Inc. All rights reserved.

Steps	Possible Points	First Attempt	Second Attempt
10. Record information about the collection in the patient's medical record and laboratory log book.	10		
11. Properly handle and store the specimen, according to the laboratory's specifications.	10		
12. Remove gloves and sanitize the hands.	5		
Total Points Possible	85		

Comments: Total Points Earned _____

Divided by _____

Total Possible Points = _____ % Score

Instructor's Signature _____

Patient Information for Procedure 40-4

Jasmine Dole is a 46-year-old patient of Dr. Heal. Her complaint today is a sore throat and ear pain. Dr. Heal orders a throat culture to be done for C&S.

Dx: Sore throat with ear pain
Medications: None

John Heal, MD
United Health Center
1925 Oregon Ave
Our Town, USA 65432

Insurance: TRUE Medical Insurance
1234 Barn Blvd
East Town, USA 67822
ID # 76543HF1234

Jasmine Dole
4321 South End St
Our Town, USA 65466
(678) 654-0987

Patient Laboratory Log Sheet for Procedure 40-4

Date	Patient	Specimen	Result	Sent to Lab	Initials

Copyright © 2010, 2005 by Saunders, an imprint of Elsevier, Inc. All rights reserved.

Student Name: _____ DATE: _____

PROCEDURE 40-5 CHECKLIST: SCREEN AND FOLLOW-UP ON PATIENT TEST RESULTS

TASK: Follow-up with a patient who has abnormal test results.

CONDITIONS: Given the proper equipment and supplies, the student will screen and follow-up with a patient's test results.

EQUIPMENT AND SUPPLIES
- Laboratory test results (see Fig. 40-7)
- Tickler file (3- × 5-inch cards or computer software program) or laboratory log of patient results
- Pen
- Patient's medical record

STANDARDS: Complete the procedure within _____ minutes and achieve a minimum score of _____%.

Time began _____   Time ended _____

Steps	Possible Points	First Attempt	Second Attempt
1. Review the test results as returned from the laboratory.	5		
2. Attach the laboratory report to the patient's medical record, and submit it to the physician for review.	5		
3. If the physician requests that you schedule the patient for a follow-up appointment, determine the most appropriate method of contact, using HIPAA guidelines.	10		
4. Contact the patient and schedule an appointment.	10		
Total Points Possible	30		

Comments: Total Points Earned _____

Divided by _____

Total Possible Points = _____% Score

Instructor's Signature _____

Patient Information

Use the information from Procedure 40-3. Use results from Figure 40-7. Physician requests that patient is scheduled for follow-up. Chart appropriately on charting boxes provided after Procedure 40-9.

Student Name: _____ DATE: _____

PROCEDURE 40-6 CHECKLIST: COLLECT A SPECIMEN FOR CLIA-WAIVED THROAT CULTURE AND STREP A TEST

TASK: Collect an uncontaminated throat specimen to test for group A beta-hemolytic streptococci, and perform a rapid strep test.

CONDITIONS: Given the proper equipment and supplies, the student will collect a specimen to perform a CLIA-waived throat culture and rapid strep.

EQUIPMENT AND SUPPLIES
- Nonsterile disposable gloves
- Sterile polyester (Dacron) swab
- Facemask
- Culture transport system
- Test tube rack
- Tongue depressor
- Gooseneck lamp
- Timer
- Biohazardous waste container
- Patient's medical record

STANDARDS: Complete the procedure within _____ minutes and achieve a minimum score of _____%.

Time began _____   Time ended _____

Steps	Possible Points	First Attempt	Second Attempt
Specimen collection for throat culture: 1. Sanitize hands.	5		
2. Assemble equipment and supplies.	5		
3. Obtain the patient's medical record.	5		
4. Greet and identify the patient, and escort the patient to the examination room.	5		
5. Instruct the patient to sit on the end of the examination table, and explain the procedure to the patient.	5		
6. Put on gloves and facemask.	5		
7. Prepare the culture transport system.	5		
8. Prepare the polyester (Dacron) swab.	5		
9. Visually inspect the patient's throat.	5		

Steps	Possible Points	First Attempt	Second Attempt
10. Remove the culture transport system from the peel-apart package, being careful to prevent contamination caused by touching tip to any extraneous objects.	5		
11. Remove the Dacron swab from the paper wrapper, again being careful not to contaminate it by touching the tip.	5		
12. Place both swabs in your right hand with the tips close together, almost like one swab.	5		
13. Ask the patient to tilt the head back and open the mouth.	5		
14. Use a tongue depressor to hold the tongue away from testing materials.	5		
15. Carefully insert the swabs into the patient's mouth without touching the inside of the mouth, tongue, or teeth.	10		
16. Ask the patient to say "Ahh."	5		
17. Firmly swab the back of the throat (posterior pharynx) with a figure-eight motion between the tonsillar areas.	10		
18. Continue to hold down the tongue with the depressor, and carefully remove the swabs from the patient's mouth without touching the tongue, teeth, or inside of the cheeks.	10		
19. Discard the tongue depressor in a biohazardous waste container.	5		
20. Remove and discard the cap from the tube, and place the swab from the transport system firmly into the bottom of the tube so that it is dampened with the transport medium, and secure tightly. Return the Dacron swab to the original wrapper.	10		
21. Label the transport tube and swab with the patient's name.	10		

Steps	Possible Points	First Attempt	Second Attempt
22. When the specimens have been returned to their individual packaging, remove personal protective equipment (PPE) and sanitize the hands.	5		
Rapid strep test (Quickvue): 23. Sanitize the hands.	5		
24. Put on PPE (if not already applied).	5		
25. Assemble equipment and supplies, being sure to have sufficient supplies for quality control.	5		
26. Unwrap each of the three cassettes that are wrapped in foil pouches.	5		
27. Record the lot number and expiration date of the kit on the log sheets.	10		
28. Label each cassette for the controls and the patient.	10		
29. Insert the swab into the swab chamber of the cassette.	5		
30. Ensure that a glass ampule is inside. Break ampule.	5		
31. Shake the bottle vigorously five times to mix the solution.	5		
32. Fill the swab chamber to the rim with the extraction solution and remove the required amount.	10		
33. Set the time for the required time, and do not move the cassette during that time.	5		
34. Examine the results window at the end of required minutes. Check for positive or negative test results (according to manufacturer's directions).	10		
35. Sanitize hands.	5		
36. Record the known controls on the quality control log sheet.	10		

Steps	Possible Points	First Attempt	Second Attempt
37. Record the results from the patient's cassette, including the internal quality assurance.	10		
38. Document the test results.	10		
Total Points Possible	250		

Comments: Total Points Earned _____

Divided by _____

Total Possible Points = _____% Score

Instructor's Signature _____

Patient Laboratory Log Sheet for Procedure 40-6

Date	Patient	Specimen	Result	Sent to Lab	Initials

Copyright © 2010, 2005 by Saunders, an imprint of Elsevier, Inc. All rights reserved.

Quickvue Control Log

Manufacturer/Kit Name: _____

Lot # _____

Expire Date: _____

Date	Specimen: Control/Patient	Result: +/−	Control Within Limits (Y/N)	Doc PT Chart	Initials

Copyright © 2010, 2005 by Saunders, an imprint of Elsevier, Inc. All rights reserved.

Student Name: _____   DATE: _____

PROCEDURE 40-7 CHECKLIST: OBTAIN A URINE SPECIMEN FROM AN INFANT USING A PEDIATRIC URINE COLLECTOR

TASK: Collect an uncontaminated urine specimen from an infant.

CONDITIONS: Given the proper equipment and supplies, the student will role-play obtaining a urine specimen from an infant using a pediatric urine collector.

EQUIPMENT AND SUPPLIES
- Nonsterile disposable gloves
- Antiseptic wipes or gauze squares and antiseptic solution
- Sterile water and sterile gauze squares
- Pediatric urine collector bag
- Sterile urine specimen container and label
- Patient's medical record

STANDARDS: Complete the procedure within _____ minutes and achieve a minimum score of _____%.

Time began _____   Time ended _____

Steps	Possible Points	First Attempt	Second Attempt
1. Sanitize hands.	5		
2. Assemble equipment and supplies.	5		
3. Obtain the patient's medical record.	5		
4. Greet the infant's parent or guardian and identify the patient, and escort them to the examination room.	5		
5. Explain the procedure to the parent or guardian.	5		
6. Don disposable gloves.	5		
7. Position the infant in a supine position, and remove diaper, asking parent or guardian to help spread the legs.	10		
8. Clean the infant's genitalia thoroughly as with a clean-catch procedure.	10		
9. Prepare the urine collection bag by removing peel-off tab.	10		
10. Firmly attach the urine collection bag to the perineum of a girl or base of penis of a boy.	10		

PROCEDURE 40-7

Copyright © 2010, 2005 by Saunders, an imprint of Elsevier, Inc. All rights reserved.

Steps	Possible Points	First Attempt	Second Attempt
11. Loosely diaper the infant, and, having the parent or guardian remain with the infant, check the urine collection bag every 15 minutes until a urine specimen is obtained, or provide instructions to parent or guardian to check for specimen and bring bag to office.	10		
12. Remove gloves and sanitize hands.	5		
13. When a sufficient volume of urine has been collected, apply new gloves and gently remove the urine collection bag.	10		
14. Clean the genital area and re-diaper the infant.	10		
15. Transfer the urine specimen into a sterile urine container, and tightly secure the lid.	10		
16. Label the specimen.	10		
17. Process the specimen based on the laboratory protocol.	10		
18. Remove gloves and sanitize the hands.	5		
19. Document the procedure.	10		
Total Points Possible	150		

Comments: Total Points Earned _____

Divided by _____

Total Possible Points = _____% Score

Instructor's Signature _____

Patient Information

Urine specimen was processed in-house. The specimen was positive ++ for leukocytes and positive for nitrites. Prescription for:

Cefotaxime 150 mg/kg IM divided q6-8h   Safe to use in infants <6 wk of age; used with ampicillin in infants aged 2-8 wk

Patient Laboratory Log Sheet for Procedure 40-7

Date	Patient	Specimen	Result	Sent to Lab	Initials

Copyright © 2010, 2005 by Saunders, an imprint of Elsevier, Inc. All rights reserved.

Patient Laboratory Log Sheet for Procedure #

Student Name: _____ DATE: _____

PROCEDURE 40-8 CHECKLIST: INSTRUCT A PATIENT IN THE COLLECTION OF A MIDSTREAM CLEAN-CATCH URINE SPECIMEN

TASK: Instruct a patient in the correct method for obtaining a midstream clean-catch urine specimen.

CONDITIONS: Given the proper equipment and supplies, the student will be required to demonstrate the proper method for instructing a patient in the collection of a midstream clean-catch urine specimen.

EQUIPMENT AND SUPPLIES
- Midstream urine collection kit *or*
- Sterile specimen container with lid and 3 antiseptic towelettes

STANDARDS: Complete the procedure within _____ minutes and achieve a minimum score of _____%.

Time began _____   Time ended _____

Steps	Possible Points	First Attempt	Second Attempt
1. Sanitize hands.	5		
2. Assemble equipment and supplies, and verify the order.	5		
3. Greet and identify the patient, and escort the patient to the examination room.	5		
4. Label the container with the patient's name and clinic identification number.	10		
5. Instruct the patient to wash and dry his or her hands.	10		
6. Instruct the patient to loosen the top of the collection container and not to touch the inside of the container.	10		
7. Provide the patient with instructions.	5		
Total Points Possible	50		

Comments: Total Points Earned _____

Divided by _____

Total Possible Points = _____% Score

Instructor's Signature _____

PROCEDURE 40-8

Student Name: _____ DATE: _____

PROCEDURE 40-9 CHECKLIST: INSTRUCT A PATIENT IN THE COLLECTION OF A 24-HOUR URINE SPECIMEN

TASK: Instruct a patient in the correct method for obtaining a 24-hour urine specimen, and process the urine specimen.

CONDITIONS: Given the proper equipment and supplies, the student will be required to provide instructions to a patient in the collection of a 24-hour urine specimen.

EQUIPMENT AND SUPPLIES
- Large urine collection container
- Written instruction sheet
- Laboratory requisition
- Patient's medical record

STANDARDS: Complete the procedure within _____ minutes and achieve a minimum score of _____%.

Time began _____   Time ended _____

Steps	Possible Points	First Attempt	Second Attempt
1. Sanitize hands.	5		
2. Assemble equipment and supplies.	5		
3. Greet and identify the patient, and escort the patient to the examination room.	5		
4. Explain the procedure to the patient, ensuring that patient drinks normal amounts of fluids and does not consume alcoholic beverages.	10		
5. Provide the patient with the collection container.	5		
6. Instruct the patient to empty bladder as usual on the first morning of the procedure and to collect the next specimen in a collection hat or other suitable container. Continue collecting all specimens, including the first morning specimen the second day.	30		
7. Keep the container refrigerated with lid on.	10		
8. When the patient returns the specimen, ask the patient whether he or she encountered any difficulties during the 24-hour collection process.	10		

Copyright © 2010, 2005 by Saunders, an imprint of Elsevier, Inc. All rights reserved.

Steps	Possible Points	First Attempt	Second Attempt
9. Prepare the specimen for transport to the laboratory.	10		
10. Document the results.	10		
Total Points Possible	100		

Comments: Total Points Earned _____

Divided by _____

Total Possible Points = _____ % Score

Instructor's Signature _____

Charting for Procedures 40-1 through 40-9

Date	Chart

Date	Chart

Date	Chart

Date	Chart

Copyright © 2010, 2005 by Saunders, an imprint of Elsevier, Inc. All rights reserved.

	Chart
Date	

	Chart
Date	

	Chart
Date	

	Chart
Date	

Copyright © 2010, 2005 by Saunders, an imprint of Elsevier, Inc. All rights reserved.

	Chart
Date	

	Chart
Date	

	Chart
Date	

	Chart
Date	

Copyright © 2010, 2005 by Saunders, an imprint of Elsevier, Inc. All rights reserved.

Student Name: _____ DATE: _____

PROCEDURE 41-1 CHECKLIST: USE A STERILE DISPOSABLE MICROLANCET FOR SKIN PUNCTURE

TASK: Obtain a capillary blood specimen acceptable for testing using the index or middle finger.

CONDITIONS: Given the proper equipment and supplies, the student will be required to use a sterile disposable microlancet for puncturing the skin to obtain a capillary sample.

EQUIPMENT AND SUPPLIES
- MACC/computer
- Nonsterile disposable gloves
- Alcohol wipes
- Sterile disposable microlancet with semiautomated lancet device or semiautomatic, single-use lancet system
- Sterile 2- × 2-inch gauze pads
- Sharps container
- Bandage and adhesive
- Patient's medical record

Supplies for Ordered Test

- Microhematocrit capillary tubes
- Microcontainers
- Glass slides
- Glucometer or cholesterol device
- Clay sealant tray

STANDARDS: Complete the procedure within _____ minutes and achieve a minimum score of _____%.

Time began _____ Time ended _____

Steps	Possible Points	First Attempt	Second Attempt
1. Sanitize hands.	5		
2. Assemble equipment and supplies, and verify order.	5		
3. Greet and identify the patient, and escort the patient to the examination room.	5		
4. Explain the procedure to the patient.	5		
5. Open the sterile gauze packet, and place the gauze pad on the inside of its wrapper.	5		
6. Open the sterile lancet system.	5		
7. Position the patient comfortably either sitting or lying down with the palmar surface of the hand facing up and the arm supported.	10		
8. Select the appropriate puncture site.	10		

Copyright © 2010, 2005 by Saunders, an imprint of Elsevier, Inc. All rights reserved.

Steps	Possible Points	First Attempt	Second Attempt
9. Warm the site to increase blood flow.	5		
10. Apply gloves.	5		
11. Clean the puncture site with an alcohol wipe, and allow to air dry.	5		
12. Prepare the lancet as appropriate to perform the puncture.	5		
13. Dispose of the lancet in biohazardous sharps container.	5		
14. Wipe away the first drop of blood with dry gauze.	10		
15. If necessary, massage the finger by applying gentle, continuous pressure from the knuckles to the puncture site to increase the blood flow.	15		
16. Allow a second well-rounded drop of blood to form, and collect the specimen in the correct manner for the test ordered.	10		
17. Provide clean gauze square, and apply pressure directly over the site on completion of collection.	10		
18. Bandage the puncture site as appropriate.	10		
19. Remove the gloves and sanitize the hands before transporting the specimen to the laboratory for processing.	10		
20. Document the procedure (for test performed).	10		
Total Points Possible	150		

Comments: Total Points Earned _____

Divided by _____

Total Possible Points = _____ % Score

Instructor's Signature _____

Student Name: _____ DATE: _____

PROCEDURE 41-2 CHECKLIST: COLLECT A BLOOD SPECIMEN FOR A PHENYLKETONURIA (PKU) SCREENING TEST

TASK: Collect a capillary specimen for PKU screening.

CONDITIONS: Given the proper equipment and supplies, the student will be required to role-play the collection of a capillary blood specimen for PKU screening.

EQUIPMENT AND SUPPLIES
- Nonsterile disposable gloves
- Personal protective equipment (PPE)
- Sterile disposable microlancet with semiautomated lancet device or semiautomatic, single-use lancet system (lancet must be 2.4 mm in length)
- PKU test card and mailing envelope
- Alcohol wipe
- Sharps container
- Sterile 2- × 2-inch gauze pads
- Laboratory requisition form
- Patient's medical record

STANDARDS: Complete the procedure within _____ minutes and achieve a minimum score of _____%.

Time began _____   Time ended _____

Steps	Possible Points	First Attempt	Second Attempt
1. Sanitize hands.	5		
2. Verify the order, and assemble equipment and supplies.	5		
3. Greet and identify the infant's parent or guardian, identify the infant, and escort them to the examination room.	5		
4. Explain the procedure to the parent or guardian.	5		
5. Open the sterile gauze packet, and place the gauze pad on the inside of its wrapper.	5		
6. Open the sterile lancet system and assemble as needed.	5		
7. Position the infant in a supine position or lying across the parent's or guardian's lap, or positioned in the parent's or guardian's arms with the foot exposed.	10		
8. Apply gloves.	5		
9. Select an appropriate puncture site, and warm the puncture site.	10		

Steps	Possible Points	First Attempt	Second Attempt
10. Clean the puncture site with an alcohol wipe, and allow it to air dry.	10		
11. Position the lancet and perform the puncture on the medial or lateral surface of heel.	10		
12. Dispose of the lancet in biohazardous sharps container.	5		
13. Wipe away the first drop of blood with the dry gauze.	10		
14. Allow a second well-rounded drop of blood to form, and collect the specimen using a microcollection container or filter paper test cards.	10		
15. After sample is collected, apply pressure with a clean gauze square directly over the puncture site. Do not place a bandage on an infant.	10		
16. Discard contaminated materials in the appropriate biohazardous waste container.	10		
17. If a PKU test card is used, complete the information section.	10		
18. Remove gloves and sanitize hands before transporting the specimen to the laboratory for processing.	5		
19. Process the specimen for transport to laboratory.	5		
20. Document the procedure.	10		
Total Points Possible	150		

Comments: Total Points Earned _____

Divided by _____

Total Possible Points = _____% Score

Instructor's Signature _____

Student Name: _____   DATE: _____

PROCEDURE 41-3 CHECKLIST: PERFORM VENIPUNCTURE USING THE EVACUATED-TUBE METHOD (COLLECTION OF MULTIPLE TUBES)

TASK: Obtain a venous blood specimen acceptable for testing using the evacuated-tube system.

CONDITIONS: Given the proper equipment and supplies, the student will be required to perform a venipuncture using the evacuated-tube system method of collection.

EQUIPMENT AND SUPPLIES
- MACC/computer
- Nonsterile disposable gloves
- Personal protective equipment (PPE) as required
- Tourniquet (nonlatex)
- Evacuated tube holder
- Evacuated tube multidraw needle (21 or 22 gauge, 1 or 1½ inch) with safety guards
- Evacuated blood tubes for requested tests with labels (correct evacuated tube required for designated test ordered) (additive or nonadditive)
- Alcohol wipe
- Sterile 2- × 2-inch gauze pads
- Bandage (nonlatex) or nonallergenic tape
- Sharps container
- Biohazardous waste container
- Laboratory requisition form
- Patient's medical record

STANDARDS: Complete the procedure within _____ minutes and achieve a minimum score of _____%.

Time began _____   Time ended _____

Steps	Possible Points	First Attempt	Second Attempt
1. Sanitize hands.	5		
2. Verify the order, and assemble equipment and supplies.	5		
3. Greet and identify the patient, and escort the patient to the proper room. Ask patient to sit in phlebotomy chair.	5		
4. Confirm that the patient has followed the needed preparation.	5		
5. Explain the procedure to the patient.	5		
6. Prepare the evacuated-tube system.	5		
7. Open the sterile gauze packet, and place the gauze pad on the inside of its wrapper, or obtain sterile gauze pads from a bulk package.	10		
8. Position the remaining needed supplies for ease of reaching with nondominant hand. Place tube loosely in holder with label facing downward.	10		

Copyright © 2010, 2005 by Saunders, an imprint of Elsevier, Inc. All rights reserved.

Steps	Possible Points	First Attempt	Second Attempt
9. Position and examine the arm to be used in the venipuncture.	10		
10. Apply the tourniquet.	10		
11. Apply gloves and PPE.	5		
12. Thoroughly palpate the selected vein.	5		
13. Release the tourniquet.	5		
14. Prepare the puncture site using alcohol swabs.	10		
15. Reapply the tourniquet.	10		
16. Position the holder while keeping the needle covered, being certain to have control of holder. Uncover the needle.	10		
17. Position the needle so that it follows the line of the vein.	5		
18. Perform the venipuncture.	10		
19. Secure the holder and push the bottom of the tube with the thumb of your nondominant hand so that the needle inside the holder pierces the rubber stopper of the tube. (Follow the direction of the vein.)	10		
20. Change tubes (minimum of two tubes) as required by test orders.	10		
21. Gently invert tubes that contain additives to be mixed with the specimen.	10		
22. While the blood is filling the last tube, release the tourniquet and withdraw the needle. Cover the needle with the safety shield.	10		
23. Apply direct pressure on the venipuncture site, and instruct the patient to raise the arm straight above the head and maintain pressure on the site for 1 to 2 minutes.	10		
24. Discard the contaminated needle and holder into the sharps container.	10		
25. Label the tubes as appropriate for laboratory.	10		
26. Place the tube into the biohazard transport bag.	5		

Copyright © 2010, 2005 by Saunders, an imprint of Elsevier, Inc. All rights reserved.

Steps	Possible Points	First Attempt	Second Attempt
27. Check for bleeding at puncture site and apply a pressure dressing.	5		
28. Remove and discard the alcohol wipe and gloves.	5		
29. Sanitize the hands.	5		
30. Record the collection date and time on the laboratory requisition form, and place the requisition in the proper place in the biohazard transport bag.	10		
31. Ask and observe how the patient feels. Escort patient to front office.	5		
32. Clean the work area using Standard Precautions.	5		
33. Document the procedure, indicating tests for which blood was drawn and the laboratory to which blood will be sent.	10		
Total Points Possible	250		

Comments: Total Points Earned _____

Divided by _____

Total Possible Points = _____ % Score

Instructor's Signature _____

Student Name: _____ DATE: _____

PROCEDURE 41-4 CHECKLIST: PERFORM VENIPUNCTURE USING THE SYRINGE METHOD

TASK: Obtain a venous blood specimen acceptable for testing using the syringe method.

CONDITIONS: Given the proper equipment and supplies, the student will be required to perform a venipuncture using the syringe method of collection.

EQUIPMENT AND SUPPLIES
- MACC/computer
- Nonsterile disposable gloves
- Personal protective equipment (PPE)
- Tourniquet (nonlatex)
- Test tube rack
- 10-mL syringe with 21- or 22-gauge needle and safety guards
- Proper evacuated blood tubes for tests ordered
- Alcohol wipe
- Sterile 2- × 2-inch gauze pads
- Bandage (nonlatex) or nonallergenic tape
- Sharps container
- Biohazardous container
- Laboratory requisition form
- Patient's medical record

STANDARDS: Complete the procedure within _____ minutes and achieve a minimum score of _____%.

Time began _____   Time ended _____

Steps	Possible Points	First Attempt	Second Attempt
1. Sanitize hands.	5		
2. Verify the order. Assemble equipment and supplies.	5		
3. Greet and identify the patient, and escort the patient to the room for the blood draw. Position patient in phlebotomy chair or on exam table.	5		
4. Explain the procedure to the patient. Confirm that any necessary preparation has been accomplished.	5		
5. Prepare the needle and syringe, maintaining syringe sterility. Break the seal on the syringe by moving the plunger back and forth several times. Loosen the cap on the needle, and check to ensure that the hub is screwed tightly onto the syringe.	15		
6. Place the evacuated tubes to be filled in a test tube rack on a work surface in order of fill.	15		

Copyright © 2010, 2005 by Saunders, an imprint of Elsevier, Inc. All rights reserved.

Steps	Possible Points	First Attempt	Second Attempt
7. Open the sterile gauze packet, and place the gauze pad on the inside of its wrapper, or obtain sterile gauze pads from a bulk package.	5		
8. Position and examine the arm to be used in the venipuncture.	10		
9. Apply gloves and PPE.	5		
10. Thoroughly palpate the selected vein.	10		
11. Release the tourniquet.	10		
12. Prepare the puncture site and reapply tourniquet.	10		
13. If drawing from the hand, ask the patient to make a fist or bend the fingers downward. Pull the skin taut with your thumb over the top of the patient's knuckles.	15		
14. Position the syringe, and grasp the syringe firmly between the thumb and the underlying fingers.	10		
15. Follow the direction of the vein and insert the needle in one quick motion at about a 45-degree angle.	10		
16. If drawing from AC vein, with your nondominant hand, pull the skin taut beneath the intended puncture site to anchor the vein. Thumb should be 1 to 2 inches below and to the side of the vein.	15		
17. Position the syringe, and grasp the syringe firmly between the thumb and the underlying fingers.	10		
18. Follow the direction of the vein and insert the needle in one quick motion at about a 15-degree angle.	10		
19. Perform the venipuncture. If flash does not occur, gently pull back on the plunger. Do not move the needle. If blood still does not enter the syringe, slowly withdraw the needle, secure new supplies, and retry the draw.	10		
20. Anchor the syringe, and gently continue pulling back on the plunger until the required amount of blood is in the syringe.	10		

Copyright © 2010, 2005 by Saunders, an imprint of Elsevier, Inc. All rights reserved.

Steps	Possible Points	First Attempt	Second Attempt
21. Release the tourniquet.	5		
22. Remove the needle, and cover the needle with safety shield.	10		
23. Apply direct pressure on the venipuncture site, and instruct the patient to raise the arm straight above the head. Instruct the patient to maintain pressure on the site for 1 to 2 minutes.	5		
24. Transfer the blood to the evacuated tubes as soon as possible.	10		
25. Properly dispose of the syringe and needle.	10		
26. Label the tubes and place into biohazard transport bag.	10		
27. Check for bleeding at venipuncture site, and place a pressure dressing.	10		
28. Remove and discard the alcohol wipes and gloves.	5		
29. Sanitize the hands.	5		
30. Record the collection date and time on the laboratory requisition form, and place the requisition in the biohazard transport bag.	10		
31. Ask and observe how the patient feels. Escort patient to the front desk.	5		
32. Clean the work area using Standard Precautions.	5		
33. Document the procedure.	10		
Total Points Possible	255		

NOTE: Awards points for Steps 13-14-15 or 16-17-18, not both.

Comments: Total Points Earned _____

Divided by _____

Total Possible Points = _____% Score

Instructor's Signature _____

Copyright © 2010, 2005 by Saunders, an imprint of Elsevier, Inc. All rights reserved.

Student Name: _____ DATE: _____

PROCEDURE 41-5 CHECKLIST: PERFORM VENIPUNCTURE USING THE BUTTERFLY METHOD (COLLECTION OF MULTIPLE EVACUATED TUBES)

TASK: Obtain a venous blood specimen acceptable for testing using the butterfly method.

CONDITIONS: Given the proper equipment and supplies, the student will perform a venipuncture using the butterfly method of collection.

EQUIPMENT AND SUPPLIES
- MACC/computer
- Nonsterile disposable gloves
- Personal protective equipment (PPE)
- Tourniquet (nonlatex)
- Test tube rack
- Winged-infusion set with Luer adapter and safety guard
- Multidraw needle (22 to 25 gauge) and tube holder, or 10-mL syringe
- Evacuated blood tubes for requested tests with labels (correct evacuated tube required for designated test ordered)
- Alcohol wipe
- Sterile 2- × 2-inch gauze pads
- Bandage (nonlatex) or nonallergenic tape
- Sharps container
- Biohazardous container
- Laboratory requisition form
- Patient's medical record

STANDARDS: Complete the procedure within _____ minutes and achieve a minimum score of _____%.

Time began _____   Time ended _____

Steps	Possible Points	First Attempt	Second Attempt
1. Sanitize hands.	5		
2. Verify the order. Assemble equipment and supplies.	5		
3. Greet and identify the patient, and escort the patient to the proper room for venipuncture.	5		
4. Ask the patient to sit in the phlebotomy chair or on exam table.	5		
5. Explain the procedure to the patient. Verify that any preparation has been followed.	10		
6. Prepare the winged infusion set. Attached the winged infusion set to either a syringe or an evacuated tube holder.	15		
7. Open the sterile gauze packet, and place the gauze pad on the inside of its wrapper, or obtain sterile gauze pads from a bulk package.	5		

Copyright © 2010, 2005 by Saunders, an imprint of Elsevier, Inc. All rights reserved.

Steps	Possible Points	First Attempt	Second Attempt
8. Position and examine the arm to be used in the venipuncture.	10		
9. Apply the tourniquet.	10		
10. Put on gloves and PPE.	5		
11. Thoroughly palpate the selected vein.	10		
12. Release the tourniquet.	10		
13. Prepare the punctures site, and reapply the tourniquet.	5		
14. If drawing from the hand, ask the patient to make a fist or bend the fingers downward. Pull the skin taut with your thumb over the top of the patient's knuckles.	10		
15. Remove the protective shield from the needle of the infusion set, being sure the bevel is facing up. Position needle over vein to be punctured.	10		
16. Perform the venipuncture. With your nondominant hand, pull the skin taut beneath the intended puncture site to anchor the vein. Thumb should be 1 to 2 inches below and to the side of the vein. Follow the direction of the vein, and insert the needle in one quick motion at about a 15-degree angle.	20		
17. After penetrating the vein, decrease the angle of the needle to 5 degrees until a "flash" of blood appears in the tubing.	5		
18. Secure the needle for blood collection.	10		
19. Insert the evacuated tube into the tube holder or gently pull back on the plunger of the syringe. Change tubes as required by the test ordered.	10		
20. Release the tourniquet, and remove the needle.	10		
21. Apply direct pressure on the venipuncture site, and instruct the patient to raise the arm straight above the head. Maintain pressure on the site for 1 to 2 minutes, with the arm raised straight above the head.	10		
22. If a syringe was used, transfer the blood to the evacuated tubes as soon as possible.	10		

Copyright © 2010, 2005 by Saunders, an imprint of Elsevier, Inc. All rights reserved.

Steps	Possible Points	First Attempt	Second Attempt
23. Dispose of the winged infusion set.	5		
24. Label the tubes, and place the tubes into the biohazard transport bag.	5		
25. Check for bleeding and place a bandage over the gauze to create a pressure dressing.	5		
26. Remove and discard the alcohol wipe and gloves.	5		
27. Sanitize the hands.	5		
28. Record the collection date and time on the laboratory requisition form, and place the requisition in the biohazard transport bag.	10		
29. Ask and observe how the patient feels.	5		
30. Clean the work area using Standard Precautions.	5		
31. Document the procedure.	10		
Total Points Possible	250		

Comments: Total Points Earned _____

Divided by _____

Total Possible Points = _____% Score

Instructor's Signature _____

Copyright © 2010, 2005 by Saunders, an imprint of Elsevier, Inc. All rights reserved.

Student Name: _____   DATE: _____

PROCEDURE 41-6 CHECKLIST: SEPARATE SERUM FROM A BLOOD SPECIMEN

TASK: Transfer serum separated from whole blood through the process of centrifugation into a transfer tube.

CONDITIONS: Given the proper equipment and supplies, the student will transfer serum separated from whole blood through the process of centrifugation into a transfer tube.

EQUIPMENT AND SUPPLIES
- Nonsterile disposable gloves
- Personal protective equipment (PPE)
- Clotted blood specimen
- Laboratory requisition form

STANDARDS: Complete the procedure within _____ minutes and achieve a minimum score of _____%.

Time began _____   Time ended _____

Steps	Possible Points	First Attempt	Second Attempt
1. Sanitize hands.	5		
2. Assemble equipment and supplies, and verify order.	5		
3. Put on gloves and other appropriate PPE.	5		
4. Verify orders against the laboratory requisition form and the specimen tube.	5		
5. Place two stoppered red-top tubes in the centrifuge to balance the centrifuge, and close and latch the centrifuge lid securely.	10		
6. Set timer for 15 minutes.	10		
7. When the time has elapsed, allow the centrifuge to come to a complete stop before opening lid and removing the tube.	10		
8. Properly remove the stopper or apply a transfer device.	10		
9. Separate the serum from the top of the tube into a transfer tube using the transfer device or a disposable pipette. If a red/gray (marbled), speckled, or Hemogard gold tube is used, the serum may be poured into a transfer tube.	10		
10. Label the tubes, and attach the laboratory requisition form.	10		

PROCEDURE 41-6

Steps	Possible Points	First Attempt	Second Attempt
11. Properly dispose of all waste material in the appropriate waste receptacle.	5		
12. Package the specimen for transport to the laboratory.	10		
13. Remove gloves and sanitize the hands.	5		
Total Points Possible	100		

Comments: Total Points Earned _____

Divided by _____

Total Possible Points = _____ % Score

Instructor's Signature _____

Charting for Procedures 41-1 through 41-6

Date	Chart

Date	Chart

Date	Chart

Date	Chart

	Chart
Date	

	Chart
Date	

	Chart
Date	

	Chart
Date	

Student Name: _____ DATE: _____

PROCEDURE 42-1 CHECKLIST: URINALYSIS USING REAGENT STRIPS

TASK: Observe, record, and report the physical and chemical properties of a urine sample using Multistix 10-SG.

CONDITIONS: Given the proper equipment and supplies, the student will perform a urinalysis using reagent strips.

NOTE: The student should practice the procedure using the MACC located on the Evolve site at http://evolve.elsevier.com/klieger/medicalassisting, and then practice and perform the task in the classroom: MACC/Clinical skills/Diagnostic testing/Specimen collection & testing/Instructing how to obtain a urine specimen & performing urinalysis.

EQUIPMENT AND SUPPLIES
- MACC/computer
- Nonsterile disposable gloves
- Personal protective equipment (PPE)
- Multistix 10-SG reagent strips
- Normal and abnormal quality control reagent strips
- Laboratory report form
- Quality control log sheet
- Urine specimen container
- Conical urine centrifuge tubes
- Digital timer or watch with second hand
- Paper towel
- 10% Bleach solution
- Biohazardous waste container
- Patient's medical record
- Laboratory log/log sheet

STANDARDS: Complete the procedure within _____ minutes and achieve a minimum score of _____%.

Time began _____   Time ended _____

Steps	Possible Points	First Attempt	Second Attempt
1. Sanitize hands.	5		
2. Verify the order. Assemble equipment and supplies.	5		
3. Greet and identify the patient, and escort the patient to the examination room or laboratory area. Explain the procedure to patient.	5		
4. Ask patient to collect a midstream clean-catch urine specimen.	10		
5. Apply gloves and other PPE as indicated.	5		
6. While waiting for patient to collect the specimen, record the lot number and expiration date of Multistix 10-SG on the laboratory quality control log sheet.	5		

993

Copyright © 2010, 2005 by Saunders, an imprint of Elsevier, Inc. All rights reserved.

Steps	Possible Points	First Attempt	Second Attempt
7. Place controls from the manufacturer's container into the urine centrifuge tubes, and record the lot number and expiration date on the tubes if the first samples of the day.	10		
8. Observe and record the physical properties of the control samples as appropriate.	10		
9. Remove one strip from container. Recap the bottle immediately.	5		
10. Dip the strip in the abnormal control specimen and draw it out, pulling along the edge of the tube top to remove excess urine.	5		
11. Read each test on the strip after the manufacturer's recommended time has elapsed.	5		
12. Check the second hand on a watch to read the results after the recommended time has elapsed.	5		
13. After the reagent strip has been interpreted and documented on the log sheet, discard the reagent strip in the biohazardous waste container.	5		
14. Repeat the process for the normal control specimen.	10		
15. Check controls to ensure recommended ranges have been achieved.	10		
16. After the reagent strip has been read, interpreted, and documented on the log sheet, discard the reagent strip in the biohazardous waste container.	10		
17. Prepare the patient specimen for testing.	5		
18. Perform steps 9 through 16 on the patient sample, and record the result on the laboratory report form.	10		
19. Clean and disinfect the work area with a 10% bleach solution.	5		
20. Remove gloves and dispose of in a biohazardous waste container.	10		
21. Sanitize the hands.	10		

Steps	Possible Points	First Attempt	Second Attempt
22. Document the results and provide to the physician.	10		
23. Document the procedure.	10		
24. After the physician has reviewed the results, place the laboratory report form if applicable in the patient's medical record.	5		
Total Points Possible	175		

Comments: Total Points Earned _____

Divided by _____

Total Possible Points = _____ % Score

Instructor's Signature _____

Copyright © 2010, 2005 by Saunders, an imprint of Elsevier, Inc. All rights reserved.

Urine Strip/Analyzer Control Log

Manufacturer/Kit Name: _____

Lot # _____

Expire Date: _____

Date	Specimen: Control/Patient	Result: +/−	Control Within Limits (Y/N)	Doc PT Chart	Initials

Copyright © 2010, 2005 by Saunders, an imprint of Elsevier, Inc. All rights reserved.

Patient Laboratory Log Sheet for Procedure 42-1

Date	Patient	Specimen	Result	Sent to Lab	Initials

Copyright © 2010, 2005 by Saunders, an imprint of Elsevier, Inc. All rights reserved.

Urinalysis Results:

Leukocytes: _____
Nitrite: _____
Urobilinogen: _____
Protein: _____
pH: _____
Blood: _____
Specific gravity: _____
Ketones: _____
Bilirubin: _____
Glucose: _____

Leukocytes: _____
Nitrite: _____
Urobilinogen: _____
Protein: _____
pH: _____
Blood: _____
Specific gravity: _____
Ketones: _____
Bilirubin: _____
Glucose: _____

Leukocytes: _____
Nitrite: _____
Urobilinogen: _____
Protein: _____
pH: _____
Blood: _____
Specific gravity: _____
Ketones: _____
Bilirubin: _____
Glucose: _____

Leukocytes: _____
Nitrite: _____
Urobilinogen: _____
Protein: _____
pH: _____
Blood: _____
Specific gravity: _____
Ketones: _____
Bilirubin: _____
Glucose: _____

Student Name: _____ DATE: _____

PROCEDURE 42-2 CHECKLIST: PREPARE A URINE SPECIMEN FOR MICROSCOPIC EXAMINATION

TASK: Prepare a urine sample for examination using a microscope.

CONDITIONS: Given the proper equipment and supplies, the student will prepare a urine specimen for microscopic examination.

NOTE: The student should practice the procedure using the MACC located on the Evolve site at http://evolve.elsevier.com/klieger/medicalassisting, and then practice and perform the task in the classroom: MACC/Clinical skills/Diagnostic testing/Specimen collection & testing/Preparing urine sediment & using the microscope.

EQUIPMENT AND SUPPLIES
- MACC/computer
- Nonsterile disposable gloves
- Personal protective equipment (PPE)
- Urine specimen container
- Conical urine centrifuge tubes with caps
- Disposable pipette
- Microscope slide and coverslip
- Centrifuge
- Paper towel
- Biohazardous waste container
- Laboratory log book/log sheet

NOTE: Perform Procedure 42-8 and then Procedure 42-1 in preparation for a microscopic urinalysis.

STANDARDS: Complete the procedure within _____ minutes and achieve a minimum score of _____%.

Time began _____   Time ended _____

Steps	Possible Points	First Attempt	Second Attempt
1. Sanitize hands.	5		
2. Assemble equipment and supplies, and verify the order.	5		
3. Put on gloves and other PPE as indicated.	5		
4. Prepare a urine sediment sample by centrifuging. Properly fill tube and centrifuge before starting centrifuge.	10		
5. When the centrifuge stops, remove the cap from the specimen and discard it in the biohazardous waste container. Decant the supernatant fluid.	10		
6. Mix sediment with remaining urine in the bottom of the tube.	10		
7. Place microscope slide on a paper towel, and pipette a drop of the mixed urine sediment in the center of the slide. Place coverslip on slide.	10		

PROCEDURE 42-2

Copyright © 2010, 2005 by Saunders, an imprint of Elsevier, Inc. All rights reserved.

Steps	Possible Points	First Attempt	Second Attempt
8. Mount the slide on the microscope stage and adjust the coarse focus.	10		
9. Remove gloves and dispose of in a biohazardous waste container.	5		
10. Sanitize the hands.	5		
11. Inform the physician that the slide is ready for viewing.	10		
12. Record the results in the laboratory log book and medical record as reported by the physician and as office policy.	15		
Total Points Possible	100		

Comments: Total Points Earned _____

Divided by _____

Total Possible Points = _____% Score

Instructor's Signature _____

Copyright © 2010, 2005 by Saunders, an imprint of Elsevier, Inc. All rights reserved.

Patient Laboratory Log Sheet for Procedure 42-2

Date	Patient	Specimen	Result	Sent to Lab	Initials

Copyright © 2010, 2005 by Saunders, an imprint of Elsevier, Inc. All rights reserved.

Student Name: _____   DATE: _____

PROCEDURE 42-3 CHECKLIST: PERFORM A URINE PREGNANCY TEST

TASK: Perform a urine pregnancy test using a commercially prepared CLIA-waived test (Quick Vue).

CONDITIONS: Given the proper equipment and supplies, the student will be required to perform a urine pregnancy test properly.

EQUIPMENT AND SUPPLIES
- Nonsterile disposable gloves
- Personal protective equipment (PPE)
- Urine specimen (preferably first morning specimen)
- Urine pregnancy testing kit (Quick Vue)
- Biohazardous waste container
- Laboratory log book/log sheet
- Patient's medical record

STANDARDS: Complete the procedure within _____ minutes and achieve a minimum score of _____%.

Time began _____   Time ended _____

Steps	Possible Points	First Attempt	Second Attempt
1. Sanitize hands.	5		
2. Verify the order. Assemble equipment and supplies.	5		
3. Perform the quality control test as recommended by the manufacturer, and document results in the laboratory log book.	10		
4. Greet and identify the patient, and escort the patient to the examination room.	5		
5. If a urine specimen is to be collected in the office, explain the procedure to the patient.	10		
6. Provide the patient with the collection container and instructions as needed.	5		
7. Put on gloves and other PPE as indicated.	5		
8. Obtain a pregnancy test, and prepare for testing according to manufacturer's directions.	5		
9. Time the test according to manufacturer's direction.	15		
10. Interpret the test results, and dispose of the test cassette in a biohazardous waste container.	10		

Copyright © 2010, 2005 by Saunders, an imprint of Elsevier, Inc. All rights reserved.

Steps	Possible Points	First Attempt	Second Attempt
11. Remove gloves and dispose of in a biohazardous waste container.	10		
12. Sanitize the hands.	5		
13. Document the results in the patient's medical record and the laboratory log book.	10		
Total Points Possible	100		

Comments: Total Points Earned _____

Divided by _____

Total Possible Points = _____% Score

Instructor's Signature _____

Pregnancy Control Log

Manufacturer/Kit Name: _____
Lot # _____
Expire Date: _____

Date	Specimen: Control/Patient	Result: +/−	Control Within Limits (Y/N)	Doc PT Chart	Initials

Copyright © 2010, 2005 by Saunders, an imprint of Elsevier, Inc. All rights reserved.

Patient Laboratory Log Sheet for Procedure 42-3

Date	Patient	Specimen	Result	Sent to Lab	Initials

Copyright © 2010, 2005 by Saunders, an imprint of Elsevier, Inc. All rights reserved.

APPENDIX A

Patient Laboratory Log Sheet for Exercises 4.3–4.5

Student Name: _____ DATE: _____

PROCEDURE 42-4 CHECKLIST: DETERMINE A HEMOGLOBIN MEASUREMENT USING A HEMOCUE

TASK: Accurately measure the hemoglobin using a HemoCue analyzer.

CONDITIONS: Given the proper equipment and supplies, the student will determine a hemoglobin measurement using a HemoCue analyzer.

EQUIPMENT AND SUPPLIES
- Nonsterile disposable gloves
- Personal protective equipment (PPE)
- Alcohol wipes
- Sterile disposable microlancet
- Sterile 2- × 2-inch gauze squares
- HemoCue Analyzer
- Control cuvette—normal and abnormal
- Microcurette
- 10% bleach solution
- Sharps container
- Biohazardous waste container
- Patient's medical record
- Laboratory quality control log sheet

STANDARDS: Complete the procedure within _____ minutes and achieve a minimum score of _____%.

Time began _____   Time ended _____

Steps	Possible Points	First Attempt	Second Attempt
1. Sanitize hands.	5		
2. Verify the order, and assemble equipment and supplies.	5		
3. Perform the quality control test as recommended by the manufacturer, and document on the laboratory quality control log sheet if first test of the day or new container of microcassettes.	10		
4. Prepare the HemoCue analyzers for testing.	5		
5. Place the control cuvette into the holder and push into the photometer to validate the control values. Perform testing using controls and read and record results.	10		
6. Greet and identify the patient, and escort the patient to the examination room.	10		
7. Explain the procedure to the patient.	5		

Copyright © 2010, 2005 by Saunders, an imprint of Elsevier, Inc. All rights reserved.

Steps	Possible Points	First Attempt	Second Attempt
8. Sanitize the hands, and apply gloves and PPE as indicated.	10		
9. Perform capillary puncture, and dispose of the lancet in a sharps container. Wipe away the first drop of blood with a gauze pad.	10		
10. Collect the specimen.	15		
11. Wipe away excess blood from the tip of the cuvette.	10		
12. Place the cuvette in its holder and push into the photometer.	10		
13. Read and record the hemoglobin value from LED screen.	10		
14. Discard the cuvette into the rigid biohazardous container.	5		
15. Turn the equipment "off" as appropriate. Clean the equipment with a mild soap and water.	10		
16. Disinfect the work area with 10% bleach solution.	10		
17. Remove gloves and sanitize the hands.	5		
18. Document the results in the patient's medical record and the laboratory log book.	5		
Total Points Possible	150		

Comments: Total Points Earned _____

Divided by _____

Total Possible Points = _____% Score

Instructor's Signature _____

Copyright © 2010, 2005 by Saunders, an imprint of Elsevier, Inc. All rights reserved.

Patient Laboratory Log Sheet for Procedure 42-4

Date	Patient	Specimen	Result	Sent to Lab	Initials

Copyright © 2010, 2005 by Saunders, an imprint of Elsevier, Inc. All rights reserved.

HemoCue Control Log

Manufacturer/Kit Name: _____
Lot # _____
Expire Date: _____

Date	Specimen: Control/Patient	Result: +/−	Control Within Limits (Y/N)	Doc PT Chart	Initials

Copyright © 2010, 2005 by Saunders, an imprint of Elsevier, Inc. All rights reserved.

Student Name: _____ DATE: _____

PROCEDURE 42-5 CHECKLIST: PERFORM A MICROHEMATOCRIT TEST

TASK: Collect a capillary blood sample for performing a microhematocrit.

CONDITIONS: Given the proper equipment and supplies, the student will perform a microhematocrit.

NOTE: The student should practice the procedure using the MACC located on the Evolve site at http://evolve.elsevier.com/klieger/medicalassisting, and then practice and perform the task in the classroom: MACC/Clinical skills/Diagnostic testing/Specimen collection & testing/Performing a capillary puncture & spun microhematocrit.

EQUIPMENT AND SUPPLIES
- MACC/computer
- Nonsterile disposable gloves
- Personal protective equipment (PPE), as indicated
- Microhematocrit capillary tubes (heparinized)
- Sealing compound
- Alcohol wipe
- Sterile disposable microlancet
- Sterile 2- × 2-inch gauze squares
- 10% bleach solution
- Microhematocrit centrifuge or centrifuge with microhematocrit reading
- Microhematocrit reader
- Rigid biohazardous container
- Patient's medical record
- Laboratory log book

STANDARDS: Complete the procedure within _____ minutes and achieve a minimum score of _____%.

Time began _____   Time ended _____

Steps	Possible Points	First Attempt	Second Attempt
1. Sanitize hands.	5		
2. Verify the order, and assemble equipment and supplies.	5		
3. Greet and identify the patient. Escort the patient to the examination room or laboratory, and explain the procedure to the patient.	5		
4. Put on gloves and PPE as indicated.	5		
Collecting the specimen: 5. Perform a capillary puncture, and dispose of the lancet in a ridged biohazardous container.	10		
6. Wipe away the first drop of blood with a gauze pad.	5		
7. After the samples have been collected, instruct the patient to press a clean gauze square to provide direct pressure to the puncture site.	5		

Copyright © 2010, 2005 by Saunders, an imprint of Elsevier, Inc. All rights reserved.

Steps	Possible Points	First Attempt	Second Attempt
8. Seal the dry end of the capillary tubes with sealing clay.	10		
9. Leave the capillary tubes embedded in the sealing clay to prevent damage.	10		
10. Check the puncture site.	5		
11. Remove gloves and sanitize hands.	10		
Testing the specimen: 12. Place the specimen in the centrifuge after donning gloves. Be sure to keep centrifuge balanced. The sealed end should be placed toward the outer edge. Record placement to prevent errors in identifying specimens.	10		
13. Secure the locking top by placing it over the threaded bolt on the centrifuge head and turning the fastener until tight.	5		
14. Spin for 5 minutes at 2500 rpm or use the high setting. If required by centrifuge being used, lock the high speed.	10		
15. When the centrifuge comes to a complete stop, unlatch the lid, and remove the locking top if appropriate.	10		
16. Position one of the tubes in the microhematocrit reader and adjust as necessary for reading the results.	10		
17. Determine the results of spun microhematocrit.	15		
18. Record the microhematocrit results.	10		
19. Discard the capillary tube in a rigid biohazardous container.	5		
20. Repeat the reading for the second capillary tube.	10		
21. Average the two results, and record the average value as the reading for the patient.	15		
22. Disinfect the work area with 10% bleach solution.	10		

Steps	Possible Points	First Attempt	Second Attempt
23. Remove gloves and sanitize hands.	5		
24. Document the results in the patient's medical record.	10		
Total Points Possible	**200**		

Comments: Total Points Earned _____

Divided by _____

Total Possible Points = _____% Score

Instructor's Signature _____

Copyright © 2010, 2005 by Saunders, an imprint of Elsevier, Inc. All rights reserved.

Patient Laboratory Log Sheet for Procedure 42-5

Date	Patient	Specimen	Result	Sent to Lab	Initials

Copyright © 2010, 2005 by Saunders, an imprint of Elsevier, Inc. All rights reserved.

Student Name: _____ DATE: _____

PROCEDURE 42-6 CHECKLIST: DETERMINE ERYTHROCYTE SEDIMENTATION RATE (ESR, NONAUTOMATED) USING THE WESTERGREN METHOD

TASK: Properly fill a Westergren tube, and observe and report ESR results accurately.

CONDITIONS: Given the proper equipment and supplies, the student will be required to fill a Westergren tube and accurately report the results of a Westergren ESR.

EQUIPMENT AND SUPPLIES
- Nonsterile disposable gloves
- Personal protection equipment (PPE) as indicated
- Supplies to perform venipuncture
- EDTA-anticoagulated blood specimen (lavender-top tube)
- Sed-Pac ESR system (reservoir, diluents, Dispette tube) with rack
- Transfer pipette
- Timer
- 10% bleach solution
- Biohazardous waste container
- Patient's medical record
- Laboratory log book

STANDARDS: Complete the procedure within _____ minutes and achieve a minimum score of _____%.

Time began _____   Time ended _____

Steps	Possible Points	First Attempt	Second Attempt
1. Sanitize hands.	5		
2. Verify the order, and assemble equipment and supplies.	5		
3. Greet and identify the patient. Escort the patient to the examination room or laboratory, and explain the procedure to the patient.	5		
4. Put on gloves and PPE as indicated.	5		
5. Perform a venipuncture.	10		
6. Transport the specimen to laboratory.	5		
7. Transfer the specimen.	5		
8. Insert the Dispette tube into the reservoir, and push down until the tube touches the bottom of the reservoir. The Dispette tube will autozero the blood, and any excess will flow into the closed reservoir compartment.	10		
9. Place ESR tube in a rack, ensuring it remains vertical.	10		

Copyright © 2010, 2005 by Saunders, an imprint of Elsevier, Inc. All rights reserved.

Steps	Possible Points	First Attempt	Second Attempt
10. Set the timer for 1 hour.	10		
11. Read the results.	10		
12. Dispose of the ESR tube properly in a rigid biohazardous container.	10		
13. Disinfect the work area with 10% bleach solution.	5		
14. Remove gloves and sanitize the hands.	5		
15. Document the results in the patient's medical record and the laboratory log book.	10		
Total Points Possible	110		

Comments: Total Points Earned _____

Divided by _____

Total Possible Points = _____% Score

Instructor's Signature _____

Patient Laboratory Log Sheet for Procedure 42-6

Date	Patient	Specimen	Result	Sent to Lab	Initials

Copyright © 2010, 2005 by Saunders, an imprint of Elsevier, Inc. All rights reserved.

Student Name: _____   DATE: _____

PROCEDURE 42-7 CHECKLIST: PREPARE A BLOOD SMEAR

TASK: Prepare a blood smear.

CONDITIONS: Given the proper equipment and supplies, the student will prepare a blood smear.

EQUIPMENT AND SUPPLIES
- Nonsterile disposable gloves
- Personal protective equipment (PPE)
- Supplies to perform capillary puncture or venipuncture
- Glass slides (frosted end)
- Pipette or Diff-Safe
- Slide holder
- Pencil
- Sharps container

STANDARDS: Complete the procedure within _____ minutes and achieve a minimum score of _____%.

Time began _____   Time ended _____

Steps	Possible Points	First Attempt	Second Attempt
1. Sanitize hands.	5		
2. Verify the order, and assemble equipment and supplies.	5		
3. Greet and identify the patient. Escort the patient to the examination room or laboratory, and explain the procedure to the patient.	5		
4. Put on gloves and PPE as indicated.	5		
5. Label two slides on the frosted end, using a pencil, with the patient's name and the date.	10		
6. Perform a venipuncture or capillary puncture.	10		
7. Place a well-rounded, medium-sized drop (1 to 2mm) of fresh whole blood on each slide.	10		
8. Pull back the drop of blood.	10		
9. Spread forward the drop of blood.	10		
10. Evaluate the slide.	10		
11. Repeat Steps 9 and 10 for the second glass slide.	10		
12. Allow both slides to air-dry standing at an angle, with the frosted end of the slide or blood end down.	10		

Copyright © 2010, 2005 by Saunders, an imprint of Elsevier, Inc. All rights reserved.

Steps	Possible Points	First Attempt	Second Attempt
13. Dispose of the spreader slide in a sharps container; dispose of all other contaminated or regular waste appropriately.	5		
14. When the slides are completely dry (a minimum of 20 minutes), both slides can be placed in slide holders and transported to the laboratory.	5		
15. Disinfect the work area using 10% bleach solution.	5		
16. Remove gloves and sanitize the hands.	5		
Total Points Possible	120		

Comments: Total Points Earned _____

Divided by _____

Total Possible Points = _____% Score

Instructor's Signature _____

Copyright © 2010, 2005 by Saunders, an imprint of Elsevier, Inc. All rights reserved.

Student Name: _____ DATE: _____

PROCEDURE 42-8 CHECKLIST: PERFORM CHOLESTEROL TESTING

TASK: Collect and process a blood specimen accurately for cholesterol testing using a CLIA-waived test such as Cholestech LDX.

CONDITIONS: Given the proper equipment and supplies, the student will perform a cholesterol test.

EQUIPMENT AND SUPPLIES
- Nonsterile disposable gloves
- Personal protective equipment (PPE) as indicated
- Capillary puncture supplies
- Cholesterol testing device (Cholestech LDX)
- Cholesterol testing kit (capillary tube with plunger, test cassette)
- 10% bleach solution
- Sharps container
- Biohazardous waste container
- Quality control log sheet
- Patient's medical record
- Laboratory log book/log sheet

STANDARDS: Complete the procedure within _____ minutes and achieve a minimum score of _____%.

Time began _____   Time ended _____

Steps	Possible Points	First Attempt	Second Attempt
1. Sanitize hands.	5		
2. Verify the order, and assemble equipment and supplies.	5		
3. Prepare the test supplies and analyzer.	5		
4. Perform a quality control test as recommended by the manufacturer, and document on the laboratory quality control log sheet.	10		
5. Greet and identify the patient. Escort the patient to the examination room or laboratory, and explain the procedure to the patient.	5		
6. Put on gloves and PPE as indicated.	5		
7. Perform the capillary puncture.	10		
8. Put on disposable gloves. Wipe away the first drop of blood.	5		
9. Collect blood specimen in a capillary tube.	10		
10. Prepare the specimen as necessary for testing.	5		
11. Insert the cassette into the Cholestech LDX analyzer and activate the timer.	10		

PROCEDURE 42-8

Copyright © 2010, 2005 by Saunders, an imprint of Elsevier, Inc. All rights reserved.

Steps	Possible Points	First Attempt	Second Attempt
12. When the timer stops, read the results.	10		
13. Discard the cassette, capillary tube, and plunger in a rigid biohazardous container.	5		
14. Turn off the analyzer, and wipe with a damp cloth.	5		
15. Disinfect the work area using 10% bleach solution.	10		
16. Remove gloves and sanitize hands.	5		
17. Document results.	10		
Total Points Possible	120		

Comments: Total Points Earned _____

Divided by _____

Total Possible Points = _____% Score

Instructor's Signature _____

Cholesterol Control Log for Procedure 42-8

Manufacturer/Kit Name: _____
Lot # _____
Expire Date: _____

Date	Specimen: Control/Patient	Result: +/–	Control Within Limits (Y/N)	Doc PT Chart	Initials

Copyright © 2010, 2005 by Saunders, an imprint of Elsevier, Inc. All rights reserved.

Patient Laboratory Log Sheet for Procedure 42-8

Date	Patient	Specimen	Result	Sent to Lab	Initials

Copyright © 2010, 2005 by Saunders, an imprint of Elsevier, Inc. All rights reserved.

Student Name: DATE:

PROCEDURE 42-9 CHECKLIST: PERFORM GLUCOSE TESTING

TASK: Collect and process a blood specimen for glucose testing using AccuCheck.

CONDITIONS: Given the proper equipment and supplies, the student will perform a glucose test.

NOTE: The student should practice the procedure using the MACC located on the Evolve site at http://evolve.elsevier.com/klieger/medicalassisting, and then practice and perform the task in the classroom: MACC/Clinical skills/Diagnostic testing/Specimen collection & testing/Performing glucose testing using AccuCheck.

EQUIPMENT AND SUPPLIES
- MACC/computer
- Nonsterile disposable gloves
- Personal protection equipment (PPE), as indicated
- Supplies for capillary puncture
- Glucose testing equipment (AccuCheck)
- AccuCheck supplies
- Control test solution
- 10% bleach solution
- Sharps container
- Biohazardous waste container
- Patient's medical record
- Laboratory quality control log sheet
- Laboratory log book/log sheet

STANDARDS: Complete the procedure within _____ minutes and achieve a minimum score of _____%.

Time began _____   Time ended _____

Steps	Possible Points	First Attempt	Second Attempt
1. Sanitize hands.	5		
2. Verify the order, and assemble equipment and supplies.	5		
3. Prepare the analyzer according to the manufacturer's instructions.	5		
4. Perform a quality control test as recommended by the manufacturer, and document on the laboratory quality control log sheet.	10		
5. Greet and identify the patient, and escort the patient to the examination room or laboratory. Explain the procedure to patient. Determine when last food was ingested.	10		
6. Perform a capillary puncture.	10		
7. Insert a test strip into the test strip slot.	10		
8. Apply a rounded drop of blood from the capillary puncture to the test strip. Start the timer for testing.	10		

Copyright © 2010, 2005 by Saunders, an imprint of Elsevier, Inc. All rights reserved.

Steps	Possible Points	First Attempt	Second Attempt
9. Discard the test strip into the biohazardous container.	5		
10. Turn off the glucometer, and wipe it with a damp cloth.	10		
11. Disinfect the work area using 10% bleach solution.	5		
12. Remove gloves and sanitize the hands.	5		
13. Document the results in the patient's medical record and laboratory log book.	10		
Total Points Possible	100		

Comments: Total Points Earned _____

Divided by _____

Total Possible Points = _____% Score

Instructor's Signature _____

Glucometer Control Log for Procedure 42-9

Manufacturer/Kit Name: _____
Lot # _____
Expire Date: _____

Date	Specimen: Control/Patient	Result: +/−	Control Within Limits (Y/N)	Doc PT Chart	Initials

Copyright © 2010, 2005 by Saunders, an imprint of Elsevier, Inc. All rights reserved.

Patient Laboratory Log Sheet for Procedure 42-9

Date	Patient	Specimen	Result	Sent to Lab	Initials

Copyright © 2010, 2005 by Saunders, an imprint of Elsevier, Inc. All rights reserved.

Student Name: _____   DATE: _____

PROCEDURE 42-10 CHECKLIST: OBTAIN A BACTERIAL SMEAR FROM A WOUND SPECIMEN

TASK: Collect a sample of wound exudates, using sterile collection supplies, and prepare the specimen for transport to laboratory.

CONDITIONS: Given the proper equipment and supplies, the student will role-play obtaining a bacterial smear from a wound specimen.

NOTE: The student should practice the procedure using the MACC located on the Evolve site at http://evolve.elsevier.com/klieger/medicalassisting, and then practice and perform the task in the classroom: MACC/Clinical skills/Diagnostic testing/Specimen collection & testing/Obtaining a wound specimen & preparing for transport to an outside lab.

EQUIPMENT AND SUPPLIES
- MACC/computer
- Nonsterile disposable gloves
- Personal protective equipment (PPE), as indicated
- Laboratory requisition form
- Plastic-backed small drape
- Sterile gauze (4- × 4-inch)
- 10% antiseptic solution
- Surgical tape
- Bandage roll
- Marking pen
- Agar-gel transport system (sterile tube with sterile swab and semisolid solution in the bottom)
- 10% bleach solution
- Biohazardous waste container
- Patient's medical record

STANDARDS: Complete the procedure within _____ minutes and achieve a minimum score of _____%.

Time began _____   Time ended _____

Steps	Possible Points	First Attempt	Second Attempt
1. Sanitize hands.	5		
2. Verify the order, and assemble equipment and supplies.	5		
3. Prepare a laboratory requisition form for microbiology department.	5		
4. Greet and identify the patient, and escort the patient to the examination room.	5		
5. Explain the procedure to patient.	5		
6. Apply gloves and PPE as indicated.	5		
7. Position patient for easy access to the area for specimen collection.	5		

Steps	Possible Points	First Attempt	Second Attempt
8. Remove dressing and dispose in a biohazardous waste container. Inspect wound for odor, color, amount of drainage, and depth.	15		
9. Open transport system and obtain sterile swab, being careful to prevent contamination when removing from kit.	10		
10. Change gloves.	5		
11. Obtain specimen from area with greatest amount of exudates by moving the swab from side to side.	10		
12. Carefully return the swab to the tube, taking care to prevent contamination by extraneous microorganisms.	10		
13. Label the specimen.	10		
14. Place the agar-gel transport tube in a biohazard transport bag and seal the bag.	10		
15. Clean the wound using medical aseptic technique.	10		
16. Apply a clean bandage to the wound site using sterile technique.	5		
17. Dispose of all waste material appropriately, and disinfect the work area using 10% bleach solution.	5		
18. Remove gloves, and sanitize the hands.	5		
19. Complete the laboratory requisition form, and transport the specimen to laboratory as soon as possible.	10		
20. Document the procedure.	10		
Total Points Possible	150		

Comments: Total Points Earned _____

Divided by _____

Total Possible Points = _____% Score

Instructor's Signature _____

Charting for Procedures 42-1 through 42-10

Date	Chart

Date	Chart

Date	Chart

Date	Chart

	Chart
Date	

	Chart
Date	

	Chart
Date	

	Chart
Date	

Date	Chart

Date	Chart

Date	Chart

Date	Chart

Copyright © 2010, 2005 by Saunders, an imprint of Elsevier, Inc. All rights reserved.

Student Name: _____   DATE: _____

PROCEDURE 43-1 CHECKLIST: PREPARE AND FILE AN IMMUNIZATION RECORD

TASK: Prepare and file and immunization record

CONDITIONS: Given the proper equipment and supplies, the student will prepare and document an immunization in the medical record and then file the medical record.

EQUIPMENT AND SUPPLIES
- Vaccine administration record
- Patient immunization record
- Physician's orders for immunization
- Patient's medical record

STANDARDS: Complete the procedure within _____ minutes and achieve a minimum score of _____%.

Time began _____   Time ended _____

Steps	Possible Points	First Attempt	Second Attempt
1. Obtain the patient's medical record.	5		
2. Confirm the date the previous immunizations were ordered and administered.	10		
3. Verify that the immunization will be given within the required time frame.	5		
4. Enter the correct date into the patient's medical vaccine administration record and on the patient's immunization record.	10		
5. Enter the required information into the patient's immunization record.	50		
6. Document in the patient's chart and sign the entry.	10		
7. Return the patient's record to the filing system.	5		
Total Points Possible	95		

Comments: Total Points Earned _____

Divided by _____

Total Possible Points = _____% Score

Instructor's Signature _____

APPENDIX A Supplemental Chapter Materials

Information for Procedure 43-1

Today's Date: 2/24/xx.

Tyler Olson, 6 months old, is brought to the clinic today for his next series of vaccinations. Complete his vaccination record for today's visit and prior visits assuming he was brought to the clinic according to the recommended schedule (see Figure 43-11). The clinic uses the following vaccines:

Comvax	(MRK)	#1865M
Pediarix	(GSK)	#642B3
Trihibit	(SPI)	#8172AA
ProQuad	(MRK)	#0964M
PCV	(WYE)	#645-835
Rotarix	(GSK)	#908B7

Source:	F (Federally supported)	S (State supported)	P (Private insurance)

DOB: 9/21/xx

Birth: HepB	Given: 9/21	Source: S	Site: RT	Vaccine: Lot # 0976M	Mfr: MRK	VIS: 7/11/01	Given: 9/21

Copyright © 2010, 2005 by Saunders, an imprint of Elsevier, Inc. All rights reserved.

VACCINE ADMINISTRATION RECORD FOR CHILDREN AND TEENS

Patient Name: _____
Birthdate: _____
Chart number: _____

Vaccine	Type of Vaccine[1] (generic abbreviation)	Date given (mo/day/yr)	Source (F,S,P)[2]	Site[3]	Vaccine Lot #	Vaccine Mfr.	Vaccine Information Statement Date or VIS[4]	Vaccine Information Statement Date given[4]	Signature/ initials of vaccinator
Hepatitis B[5] (e.g., HepB, Hib-HepB, DTaP-HepB-IPV) Give IM.									
Diphtheria, Tetanus, Pertussis[5] (e.g., DTaP, DTaP-Hib DTaP-HepB-IPV, DT Tdap, Td) Give IM.									
Haemophilus influenzae **type b**[5] (e.g., Hib, Hib-HepB, DTaP-Hib) Give IM.									
Polio[5] (e.g., IPV, DTaP-HepB-IPV) Give IPV SC or IM. Give DTaP-HepB-IPV IM.									
Pneumococcal (e.g., PCV, conjugate; PPV, polysaccharide) Give PCV IM. Give PPV SC or IM.									
Rotavirus (Rv) Give oral (po).									
Measles, Mumps, Rubella[5] (e.g., MMR, MMRV) Give SC.									
Varicella[5] (e.g., Var, MMRV) Give SC.									
Hepatitis A (HepA) Give IM.									
Meningococcal (e.e., MCVS4; MPSV4) Give MCV4 IM and MPSV4 SC.									
Human papillomavirus (e.g., HPV) Give IM.									
Influenza[5] (e.g., TIV, inactivated; LAIV, live attenuated) Give TIV IM. Give LAIV IN.									
Other									

1. Record the generic abbreviation for the type of vaccine given (e.g., DTaP-Hib, PCV), *not* the trade name.
2. Record the source of the vaccine given as either F (Federally-supported), S (State-supported) or P (supported by Private insurance or other Private funds)
3. Record the site where vaccine was administered as either RA (Right Arm), LA (Left Arm), RT (Right Thigh), IN (Intranasal), or O (Oral).
4. Record the publication date of each VIS as well as the date it is given to the patient.
5. For combination vaccines, fill in a row for each seperate antigen in the combination.

From: Immunization Action Coalition • 1573 Selby Ave.• St. Paul, MN 55104 • (651) 647-9009 • www.immunize.org • www.vaccineinformation.org

IMMUNIZATION RECORD					
Name					
Birthdate					

Immunization	DATE	DATE	DATE	DATE	DATE
Hep B (Hepatitis B)					
DTaP (Diphtheria, Tetanus, and Pertussis)					
Hib (Haemophilus influenzae Type b)					
IPV (Inactivated Polio Vaccine)					
PCV (Pneumococcal Conjugate Vaccine)					
Rv (Rotavirus)					
MMR (Measles, Mumps, and Rubella)					
Varicella (Chickenpox)					
Hep A (Hepatitis A)					
MPSV4 (Meningococcal)					
HPV (Human papillomavirus)					
Influenza (TIV or LAIV)					
Tetanus Booster					
Other					

PROCEDURE 43-1

Copyright © 2010, 2005 by Saunders, an imprint of Elsevier, Inc. All rights reserved.

Charting for Procedure 43-1

Date	Chart

Date	Chart

Student Name: _____   DATE: _____

PROCEDURE 44-1 CHECKLIST: ADMINISTER ORAL MEDICATION

TASK:
- Interpret the physician's orders for administering oral medication.
- Calculate the required dose of the prescribed medication.
- Pour and measure an accurate dose of the prescribed medication.
- Document the medication administration in the patient's medical chart.

CONDITIONS: Given the proper equipment and supplies, the student will be required to demonstrate the proper method of interrupting a physician's order and of preparing and administering an oral medication.

*Students may be required to pour both a solid or liquid medication.

NOTE: The student should practice the procedure using the MACC located on the Evolve site at http://evolve.elsevier.com/klieger/medicalassisting, and then practice and perform the task in the classroom: MACC/Clinical skills/Patient care/Medications/Pouring an oral liquid medication.

EQUIPMENT AND SUPPLIES
- MACC /computer
- Medication ordered by physician (liquid or solid)
- Medication cup (calibrated)
- Water, as appropriate
- Patient's medical record

STANDARDS: Complete the procedure within _____ minutes and achieve a minimum score of _____%.

Time began _____   Time ended _____

Steps	Possible Points	First Attempt	Second Attempt
Solid Medication: 1. Sanitize hands.	5		
2. Verify the order, and assemble equipment and supplies.	5		
3. Follow the "seven rights" of medication administration.	5		
4. Select the right drug.	10		
5. Perform the first of the three checks of medication. Verify that the medication name on the label matched the medication name in the written orders.	15		
6. Check the expiration date of the medication.	5		
7. Read the dosage information on the label and compare it with the physician's order. Calculate the right dose using the conversion formula as needed.	15		
8. Perform the second check of the medication against the written order.	10		
9. Prepare the right dose for a solid medication and perform the third check before returning the medication to the storage.	10		

1055

Copyright © 2010, 2005 by Saunders, an imprint of Elsevier, Inc. All rights reserved.

Steps	Possible Points	First Attempt	Second Attempt
Liquid Medication: 10. Repeat steps 2 through 8	5		
11. Correctly open container, palm label, and pour medication to correct level by placing thumb at line to be administered.	15		
12. Place the cup on a flat surface, and recheck the meniscus.	10		
13. Before returning the bottle to the cabinet, perform the third check against the written order.	10		
14. Carry medicine cup(s) carefully to avoid spilling, and administer the medication(s).	10		
15. Offer water to the patient if appropriate.	5		
16. Remain with the patient until the medication has been swallowed.	5		
17. Sanitize hands.	5		
18. Document the administration of the medication, completing the seven rights.	10		
Total Points Possible	155		

Comments: Total Points Earned _____

Divided by _____

Total Possible Points = _____% Score

Instructor's Signature _____

Student Name: _____   DATE: _____

PROCEDURE 44-2 CHECKLIST: APPLY A TRANSDERMAL PATCH

TASK: Apply a transdermal patch, and provide the patient with instructions for accurate application and safe removal.

CONDITIONS: Given the proper equipment and supplies, the student will role-play the preparation and application of a transdermal patch.

EQUIPMENT AND SUPPLIES
- Medicated transdermal patch, as ordered by the physician
- Nonsterile disposable gloves
- Patient instruction sheet
- Patient's medical record

STANDARDS: Complete the procedure within _____ minutes and achieve a minimum score of _____%.

Time began _____   Time ended _____

Steps	Possible Points	First Attempt	Second Attempt
1. Sanitize hands.	5		
2. Verify the order, and assemble the equipment and supplies.	5		
3. Follow the "seven rights" of medication administration.	10		
4. Select the right drug.	5		
5. Perform the first of the three checks of the medication.	10		
6. Check the expiration date of the medication.	10		
7. Read the dosage information on the label and compare it with the physician's order.	10		
8. Perform the second check of the medication against the written order.	10		
9. Return the package to storage, checking the medication for the third time.	10		
10. Identify the patient, and explain the procedure to the patient.	10		
11. Instruct the patient that the location of the patch should be rotated to different sites at each application.	10		
12. Apply the transdermal patch, dispose of all waste materials appropriately, and disinfect the work area.	15		
13. Remove gloves. Sanitize hands.	5		

Copyright © 2010, 2005 by Saunders, an imprint of Elsevier, Inc. All rights reserved.

Steps	Possible Points	First Attempt	Second Attempt
14. Instruct the patient on safe removal of the patch, its proper disposal, and the application of a new patch at the same time as per physician's orders.	10		
15. Provide written instructions to the patient.	10		
16. Document the procedure.	15		
Total Points Possible	150		

Comments: Total Points Earned _____

Divided by _____

Total Possible Points = _____% Score

Instructor's Signature _____

Student Name: _____ DATE: _____

PROCEDURE 44-3 CHECKLIST: INSTRUCT A PATIENT IN ADMINISTERING MEDICATION USING A METERED-DOSE INHALER WITH THE CLOSED-MOUTH TECHNIQUE

TASK: Provide patient instruction for the use of a metered-dose inhaler.

CONDITIONS: Given the proper equipment and supplies, the student will provide patient instruction for the use of a metered-dose inhaler.

EQUIPMENT AND SUPPLIES
- Medication ordered by the physician
- Metered-dose inhaler (MDI)
- Spacer, if required
- Patient's medical record

STANDARDS: Complete the procedure within _____ minutes and achieve a minimum score of _____%.

Time began _____   Time ended _____

Steps	Possible Points	First Attempt	Second Attempt
1. Sanitize hands.	5		
2. Verify the order, and assemble the equipment and supplies.	5		
3. Follow the "seven rights" of medication administration.	5		
4. Select the right dose.	10		
5. Check the expiration date of the medication.	5		
6. Read the dosage information on the label and compare it with the physician's order.	10		
7. Read the dosage information on the label and compare it with the physician's order.	10		
8. Perform the second check of the medication against the written order.	10		
9. Return the package to storage, checking the medication for the third time.	10		
10. Identify the patient.	10		
11. Prepare the medication as ordered by physician.	10		
12. Instruct the patient to inhale deeply and then gently expel as much air as he or she can comfortably do so.	10		
13. Instruct the patient to place the mouthpiece in the mouth, holding the inhaler upright and closing the lips around it.	10		

Steps	Possible Points	First Attempt	Second Attempt
14. Instruct the patient to inhale slowly through the mouth, depress the medication canister fully while breathing in, and then hold breath for 10 seconds.	10		
15. Instruct the patient to exhale slowly.	10		
16. Repeat steps 12 through 15 as appropriate.	10		
17. Instruct the patient to clean the mouthpiece after each use.	10		
18. Instruct the patient to wash and dry the hands.	5		
19. Document the procedure.	5		
Total Points Possible	160		

Comments: Total Points Earned _____

Divided by _____

Total Possible Points = _____% Score

Instructor's Signature _____

Student Name: _____   DATE: _____

PROCEDURE 44-4 CHECKLIST: RECONSTITUTE A POWDERED DRUG

TASK: Reconstitute a powdered medication to its liquid dosage form.

CONDITIONS: Given the proper equipment and supplies, the student will reconstitute a powdered drug.

EQUIPMENT AND SUPPLIES
- Vial of powdered medication as ordered by physician
- 70% isopropyl alcohol wipes
- Reconstituting liquid, as indicated by manufacturer
- Appropriate needle and syringe
- Rigid biohazardous container

STANDARDS: Complete the procedure within _____ minutes and achieve a minimum score of _____%.

Time began _____   Time ended _____

Steps	Possible Points	First Attempt	Second Attempt
1. Sanitize hands.	5		
2. Verify the order, and assemble the equipment and supplies.	5		
3. Follow the "seven rights" of medication administration.	5		
4. Check the medication against the physician's order three times before administration.	5		
5. Check the patient's medical record for drug allergies or conditions that may contraindicate the injection. Check expiration date of the medication.	10		
6. Select the correct medication powder and diluent from cabinet.	10		
7. Check expiration date of the medication.	10		
8. Follow the manufacturer's instructions for reconstituting the powder to correct strength.	10		
9. Prepare the needle and syringe.	5		
10. Fill the syringe and remove the needle from the vial stopper by pulling both hands away from each other.	10		
11. Insert diluent into the medication vial. Remove needle after filling vial.	5		

Copyright © 2010, 2005 by Saunders, an imprint of Elsevier, Inc. All rights reserved.

Steps	Possile Points	First Attempt	Second Attempt
12. Mix the powder and diluent thoroughly by rolling the vial between the flattened palms until all powder has been dissolved. Label the vial with the date and time of reconstitution and your initials.	10		
13. Sanitize hands.	10		
Total Points Possible	100		

Comments: Total Points Earned _____

Divided by _____

Total Possible Points = _____ % Score

Instructor's Signature _____

Student Name: _____ DATE: _____

PROCEDURE 44-5 CHECKLIST: PREPARE A PARENTERAL MEDICATION FROM A VIAL

TASK: From a vial, measure the ordered medication dosage into a 3-mL hypodermic syringe for injection.

CONDITIONS: Given the proper equipment and supplies, the student will prepare a parenteral medication from a vial in a 3-mL syringe.

NOTE: *The student should practice the procedure using the MACC located on the Evolve site at http://evolve.elsevier.com/klieger/medicalassisting, and then practice and perform the task in the classroom: MACC/Clinical skills/Patient care/Medications/Preparing parenteral medications from a vial & ampule.*

EQUIPMENT AND SUPPLIES
- MACC/computer
- Vial of medication as ordered by physician
- 70% isopropyl alcohol wipes
- 3-mL syringe for ordered dose
- Needle with safety device appropriate for site of injection
- 2- × 2-inch gauze squares
- Sharps container

STANDARDS: Complete the procedure within _____ minutes and achieve a minimum score of _____%.

Time began _____   Time ended _____

Steps	Possible Points	First Attempt	Second Attempt
1. Sanitize hands.	5		
2. Verify the order, and assemble the equipment and supplies.	5		
3. Follow the "seven rights" of medication administration.	10		
4. Check the medication against the physician's order three times before administration.	10		
5. Check expiration date of the medication.	10		
6. Check the patient's medical record for drug allergies or conditions that may contraindicate the injection.	10		
7. Calculate the correct dose to be given, as necessary.	10		
8. Prepare the vial, needle, and syringe.	5		
9. Draw the amount of air into the syringe for the amount of medication to be administered.	5		
10. Remove the cover from the needle and insert the needle into the vial.	10		

Copyright © 2010, 2005 by Saunders, an imprint of Elsevier, Inc. All rights reserved.

Steps	Possible Points	First Attempt	Second Attempt
11. Inject the air into vial and fill the syringe with the medication.	10		
12. Remove any air bubbles and recap the needle as necessary.	10		
13. Compare the medication to the vial label, and return the medication to its proper storage.	5		
14. Sanitize hands.	10		
Total Points Possible	115		

Comments: Total Points Earned _____

Divided by _____

Total Possible Points = _____% Score

Instructor's Signature _____

PROCEDURE 44-6 CHECKLIST: PREPARE A PARENTERAL MEDICATION FROM AN AMPULE

TASK: From an ampule, measure the correct medication dosage in a 1-mL hypodermic syringe for injection.

CONDITIONS: Given the proper equipment and supplies, the student will prepare a parenteral medication from an ampule.

NOTE: The student should practice the procedure using the MACC located on the Evolve site at http://evolve.elsevier.com/klieger/medicalassisting, and then practice and perform the task in the classroom: MACC/Clinical skills/Patient care/Medications/Preparing parenteral medications from a vial & ampule.

EQUIPMENT AND SUPPLIES
- MACC/computer
- Ampule of medication ordered by physician
- Ampule breaker or 2- × 2-inch gauze squares
- 70% isopropyl alcohol wipes
- Appropriate syringe for ordered dose
- Needle with safety device
- Filter needle (used for ampule only)
- Rigid biohazardous container

STANDARDS: Complete the procedure within _____ minutes and achieve a minimum score of _____%.

Time began _____   Time ended _____

Steps	Possible Points	First Attempt	Second Attempt
1. Sanitize hands.	5		
2. Verify the order, and assemble the equipment and supplies.	5		
3. Follow the "seven rights" of medication administration.	10		
4. Check the medication against the physician's order three times before administration.	10		
5. Check expiration date of the medication.	10		
6. Check the patient's medical record for drug allergies or conditions that may contraindicate the injection.	10		
7. Calculate the correct dose to be given, as ordered by the physician.	10		
8. Clean neck of ampule.	5		
9. Prepare the syringe with a filter needle.	5		

Copyright © 2010, 2005 by Saunders, an imprint of Elsevier, Inc. All rights reserved.

Steps	Possible Points	First Attempt	Second Attempt
10. Ensure that liquid from the top of the ampule is in hollow reservoir and break the ampule.	10		
11. Remove the cover from the filter needle, and insert filter needle into the ampule. Fill syringe.	15		
12. Remove filter needle and recap.	5		
13. Remove any air bubbles and check medication.	10		
14. Check the medication label. Keep the medication ampule and syringe together until ready to administer.	10		
15. Sanitize hands.	5		
Total Points Possible	125		

Comments: Total Points Earned _____

Divided by _____

Total Possible Points = _____% Score

Instructor's Signature _____

Student Name: _____   DATE: _____

PROCEDURE 44-7 CHECKLIST: ADMINISTER AN INTRADERMAL INJECTION

TASK:
- Identify the correct syringe, needle gauge, and length for an intradermal injection.
- Select and prepare an appropriate site for an intradermal injection.
- Demonstrate the correct technique to administer an intradermal injection.
- Document an intradermal injection correctly in the medical record.

CONDITIONS: Given the proper equipment and supplies, the student will prepare and administer an intradermal injection.

NOTE: The student should practice the procedure using the MACC located on the Evolve site at http://evolve.elsevier.com/klieger/medicalassisting, and then practice and perform the task in the classroom: MACC/Clinical skills/Patient care/Medications/Performing intradermal injections.

EQUIPMENT AND SUPPLIES
- MACC/computer
- Nonsterile disposable gloves
- Medication as ordered by physician
- Tuberculin syringe for ordered dose
- Needle with safety device (26 or 27 gauge, ⅜ inch to ½ inch)
- 2- × 2-inch sterile gauze
- 70% isopropyl alcohol wipes
- Written patient instructions for post-testing as appropriate
- Rigid biohazardous container
- Patient's medical record

STANDARDS: Complete the procedure within _____ minutes and achieve a minimum score of _____%.

Time began _____   Time ended _____

Steps	Possible Points	First Attempt	Second Attempt
1. Sanitize hands.	5		
2. Verify the order, and assemble the equipment and supplies.	5		
3. Check the patient's medical record for drug allergies or conditions that may contraindicate the injection.	10		
4. Follow the "seven rights" of medication administration.	10		
5. Check the medication against the physician's order three times before administration.	10		
6. Check expiration date of the medication.	10		
7. Calculate the correct dose to be given, if necessary.	15		

PROCEDURE 44-7

1067

Copyright © 2010, 2005 by Saunders, an imprint of Elsevier, Inc. All rights reserved.

Steps	Possible Points	First Attempt	Second Attempt
8. Follow the correct procedure for drawing the medication into syringe.	10		
9. Greet and identify the patient, and explain the procedure to the patient.	10		
10. Select an appropriate injection site and properly position the patient as necessary to expose the site adequately.	10		
11. Apply gloves.	5		
12. Prepare the injection site.	10		
13. While the prepared site is drying, remove the cover from the needle.	10		
14. Pull the skin taut at the injection site.	10		
15. Inject the medication between the dermis and epidermis. Create a wheal.	10		
16. Withdraw the needle from the injection site at the same angle as it was inserted, and activate the safety device immediately.	10		
17. Dab the area with the gauze. Do not rub.	5		
18. Remove gloves and discard in a biohazardous container.	5		
19. Sanitize the hands.	5		
20. Check the patient.	5		
21. Read or discuss with the patient the test results.	10		
22. Sanitize hands.	5		
23. Document the procedure.	10		
Mantoux test: 24. Check to ensure test was given 48 to 72 hours earlier.	10		
25. After sanitizing the hands and applying nonsterile gloves, gently rub the test site with a finger and lightly palpate for induration.	10		

Steps	Possible Points	First Attempt	Second Attempt
26. Using the tape that comes with the medication, measure the diameter of the area of induration from edge to edge.	10		
27. Record the area of induration, and notify the health care provider of the measurement if not within the negative range.	10		
28. Record the reading in the medical record.	10		
Total Points Possible	245		

Comments: Total Points Earned _____

Divided by _____

Total Possible Points = _____% Score

Instructor's Signature _____

Student Name: _____ DATE: _____

PROCEDURE 44-8 CHECKLIST: ADMINISTER A SUBCUTANEOUS INJECTION

TASK:
- Identify the correct syringe, needle gauge, and length for a subcutaneous injection.
- Select and prepare an appropriate site for a subcutaneous injection.
- Demonstrate the correct technique to administer a subcutaneous injection.
- Document a subcutaneous injection correctly in the medical record.

CONDITIONS: Given the proper equipment and supplies, the student will prepare and administer a subcutaneous injection.

NOTE: The student should practice the procedure using the MACC located on the Evolve site at http://evolve.elsevier.com/klieger/medicalassisting, and then practice and perform the task in the classroom: MACC/Clinical skills/Patient care/Medications/Performing subcutaneous injections.

EQUIPMENT AND SUPPLIES
- MACC/computer
- Nonsterile disposable gloves
- Medication as ordered by physician
- Appropriate syringe for ordered dose of medication
- Appropriate needle with safety device
- 2- × 2-inch sterile gauze
- 70% isopropyl alcohol wipes
- Sharps container
- Rigid biohazardous container
- Patient's medical record

STANDARDS: Complete the procedure within _____ minutes and achieve a minimum score of _____%.

Time began _____   Time ended _____

Steps	Possible Points	First Attempt	Second Attempt
1. Sanitize hands.	5		
2. Verify the order, and assemble the equipment and supplies.	5		
3. Follow the "seven rights" of medication administration.	10		
4. Check the medication against the physician's order three times before administration.	10		
5. Check the patient's medical record for drug allergies or conditions that may contraindicate the injection.	10		
6. Check expiration date of the medication.	10		
7. Calculate correct dose to be given, if necessary.	15		
8. Follow the procedure for drawing the medication into the syringe.	5		

Steps	Possible Points	First Attempt	Second Attempt
9. Greet and identify the patient, and explain the procedure.	10		
10. Select an appropriate injection site, and properly position the patient as necessary to expose the site.	10		
11. Apply gloves.	5		
12. Prepare the injection site.	10		
13. While the prepared site is drying, remove the cover from the needle.	5		
14. Pinch the skin at the injection site and puncture the skin quickly and smoothly, ensuring that the needle is kept at a 45-degree angle.	10		
15. Aspirate the syringe to check for blood. If no blood is present, inject the medication.	10		
16. Place a gauze pad over the injection site and quickly withdraw the needle from the injection site at the same angle at which it was inserted.	10		
17. Massage the injection site, if appropriate.	5		
18. Discard the syringe and needle in a rigid biohazardous container.	5		
19. Remove gloves and discard in a biohazardous waste container.	5		
20. Sanitize the hands.	5		
21. Check on the patient.	5		
22. Document procedure.	10		
Total Points possible	175		

Comments: Total Points Earned _____

Divided by _____

Total Possible Points = _____% Score

Instructor's Signature _____

Student Name: _____ DATE: _____

PROCEDURE 44-9 CHECKLIST: ADMINISTER AN INTRAMUSCULAR INJECTION TO A PEDIATRIC PATIENT

TASK:
- Identify the correct syringe, needle gauge, and length for a pediatric intramuscular injection.
- Select and prepare an appropriate site for a pediatric intramuscular injection.
- Demonstrate the correct technique to administer an intramuscular injection to a pediatric patient.
- Document an intramuscular injection correctly in the medical record.

CONDITIONS: Given the proper equipment and supplies, the student will be required to demonstrate competency (through use of a pediatric mannequin) in the proper method of preparing and administering an intramuscular injection for a pediatric patient.

NOTE: The student should practice the procedure using the MACC located on the Evolve site at http://evolve.elsevier.com/klieger/medicalassisting, and then practice and perform the task in the classroom: MACC/Clinical skills/Patient Care/Medications/Administering intramuscular injections & recording immunizations.

EQUIPMENT AND SUPPLIES
- MACC/computer
- Nonsterile disposable gloves
- Medication order by physician
- Appropriate syringe for ordered dose
- Appropriate needle with safety device (25 or 27 gauge, $5/8$ inch to 1 inch)
- 2- × 2-inch sterile gauze
- 70% isopropyl alcohol wipes
- Rigid biohazardous container
- Biohazardous waste container
- Patient's medical record

STANDARDS: Complete the procedure within _____ minutes and achieve a minimum score of _____%.

Time began _____   Time ended _____

Steps	Possible Points	First Attempt	Second Attempt
1. Sanitize hands.	5		
2. Verify the order, and assemble the equipment and supplies.	5		
3. Follow the "seven rights" of medication administration.	10		
4. Check the medication against the physician's order three times before administration.	10		
5. Check the patient's medical record for drug allergies or conditions that may contraindicate the injection.	10		
6. Check expiration date of the medication.	10		
7. Calculate the correct dose to be given.	20		

Copyright © 2010, 2005 by Saunders, an imprint of Elsevier, Inc. All rights reserved.

Steps	Possible Points	First Attempt	Second Attempt
8. Follow the procedure for drawing the medication into syringe.	10		
9. Greet and identify the patient and the patient's parent or guardian, and explain the procedure to the patient or guardian, as appropriate.	15		
10. Select an appropriate injection site, and properly position the patient as necessary.	10		
11. Apply disposable gloves.	10		
12. Secure the patient, asking help from parent or guardian as needed.	10		
13. Prepare the injection site.	10		
14. While the prepared site is drying, remove the cover from the needle.	10		
15. Secure the skin at the injection site.	10		
16. Puncture the skin quickly and smoothly, ensuring that the needle is kept at a 90-degree angle.	15		
17. Aspirate the syringe.	10		
18. Inject the medication appropriately for base of medication (e.g., oil, water).	10		
19. Place a gauze pad over the injection site, and quickly withdraw the needle from the injection site at the same angle as insertion. Activate safety sheath over needle.	10		
20. Massage the injection site if appropriate.	5		
21. Dispose of the syringe and needle in a rigid biohazardous container.	5		
22. Remove gloves, and discard in a biohazardous waste container.	5		
23. Sanitize the hands.	5		

Steps	Possible Points	First Attempt	Second Attempt
24. Check on the patient.	5		
25. Document procedure.	10		
Total Points Possible	235		

Comments: Total Points Earned _____

Divided by _____

Total Possible Points = _____ % Score

Instructor's Signature _____

Copyright © 2010, 2005 by Saunders, an imprint of Elsevier, Inc. All rights reserved.

Student Name: _____   DATE: _____

PROCEDURE 44-10 CHECKLIST: ADMINISTER AN INTRAMUSCULAR INJECTION TO AN ADULT

TASK:
- Identify the correct syringe, needle gauge, and length for an adult intramuscular injection.
- Select and prepare an appropriate site for an adult intramuscular injection.
- Demonstrate the correct technique to administer an intramuscular injection.
- Document an intramuscular injection correctly in the medical record.

CONDITIONS: Given the proper equipment and supplies, the student will prepare and administer an intramuscular injection to an adult patient.

NOTE: The student should practice the procedure using the MACC located on the Evolve site at http://evolve.elsevier.com/klieger/medicalassisting, and then practice and perform the task in the classroom: MACC/Clinical skills/Patient care/Medications/Administering intramuscular injections & recording immunizations.

EQUIPMENT AND SUPPLIES
- MACC/computer
- Nonsterile disposable gloves
- Medication as ordered by physician
- Appropriate syringe for ordered medication dose
- Appropriate needle with safety device (21 or 25 gauge, 1 to 1½ inch)
- 2- × 2-inch sterile gauze
- 70% isopropyl alcohol wipes
- Sharps container
- Biohazardous waste container
- Patient's medical record

STANDARDS: Complete the procedure within _____ minutes and achieve a minimum score of _____%.

Time began _____   Time ended _____

Steps	Possible Points	First Attempt	Second Attempt
1. Sanitize hands.	5		
2. Verify the order, and assemble the equipment and supplies.	5		
3. Follow the "seven rights" of medication administration.	10		
4. Check the medication against the physician's order three times before administration.	10		
5. Check the patient's medical record for drug allergies or conditions that may contraindicate the injection.	10		
6. Check expiration date of the medication.	10		
7. Calculate the correct dose to be given.	20		
8. Greet and identify the patient, and explain the procedure.	10		

Copyright © 2010, 2005 by Saunders, an imprint of Elsevier, Inc. All rights reserved.

Steps	Possible Points	First Attempt	Second Attempt
9. Select an appropriate injection site by amount and density of medication. Properly position the patient as necessary to expose the site adequately.	10		
10. Apply gloves.	5		
11. Prepare the injection site.	10		
12. While the prepared site is drying, remove the cover from the needle.	10		
13. Secure the skin at the injection site.	10		
14. Puncture the skin quickly and smoothly, ensuring that the needle is kept at a 90-degree angle.	10		
15. Aspirate the syringe.	10		
16. Inject medication using proper technique for density of medication.	10		
17. Place a gauze pad over the injection site, and quickly withdraw the needle from the injection site at the same angle at which it was inserted. Activate the safety shield over the needle.	10		
18. Massage the injection site if appropriate for medication.	10		
19. Discard the syringe and needle in a sharps container.	5		
20. Remove gloves and discard in a biohazardous waste container.	5		
21. Sanitize the hands.	5		
22. Check on the patient.	10		
23. Document procedure.	10		
Total Points Possible	210		

Comments: Total Points Earned _____

Divided by _____

Total Possible Points = _____% Score

Instructor's Signature _____

Copyright © 2010, 2005 by Saunders, an imprint of Elsevier, Inc. All rights reserved.

Student Name: _____ DATE: _____

PROCEDURE 44-11 CHECKLIST: ADMINISTER AN INTRAMUSCULAR INJECTION USING THE Z-TRACK TECHNIQUE

TASK: Demonstrate the correct technique to administer an intramuscular injection using the Z-track technique.

CONDITIONS: Given the proper equipment and supplies, the student will prepare and administer an intramuscular injection using the Z-track technique.

EQUIPMENT AND SUPPLIES
- Nonsterile disposable gloves
- Medication order by physician
- Appropriate syringe for ordered dose
- Appropriate needle with safety device
- 2- × 2-inch sterile gauze
- 70% isopropyl alcohol wipes
- Rigid biohazardous container
- Biohazardous waste container
- Patient's medical record

STANDARDS: Complete the procedure within _____ minutes and achieve a minimum score of _____%.

Time began _____   Time ended _____

Steps	Possible Points	First Attempt	Second Attempt
1. Sanitize hands.	5		
2. Verify the order, and assemble the equipment and supplies.	5		
3. Follow the "seven rights" of medication administration.	10		
4. Check the medication against the physician's order three times before administration.	10		
5. Check the patient's medical record for drug allergies or conditions that may contraindicate the injection.	10		
6. Check expiration date of the medication.	10		
7. Calculate the correct dose to be given.	20		
8. Follow the correct procedure for drawing the medication into syringe.	10		
9. Greet and identify the patient, and explain the procedure to the patient.	15		

PROCEDURE 44-11

Copyright © 2010, 2005 by Saunders, an imprint of Elsevier, Inc. All rights reserved.

Steps	Possible Points	First Attempt	Second Attempt
10. Select an appropriate injection site, and properly position the patient.	5		
11. Apply disposable gloves.	5		
12. Prepare the injection site.	5		
13. While the prepared site is drying, remove the cover from the needle.	5		
14. Secure the skin at the injection site by pushing the skin away from the injection site.	10		
15. Puncture the skin quickly and smoothly, ensuring that the needle is kept at a 90-degree angle.	10		
16. Continue to hold the tissue in place while aspirating and injecting the medication.	15		
17. Inject the medication.	10		
18. Withdraw the needle.	10		
19. Release the traction on the skin to seal the track as the needle is being removed. Activate safety shield over needle.	10		
20. Discard the syringe and needle in a rigid biohazardous container.	5		
21. Remove gloves and discard in a biohazardous waste container.	5		
22. Sanitize the hands.	5		
23. Check on the patient.	5		
24. Document the procedure.	5		
25. Clean the equipment and examination room.	10		
Total Points Possible	215		

Comments: Total Points Earned _____

Divided by _____

Total Possible Points = _____% Score

Instructor's Signature _____

Copyright © 2010, 2005 by Saunders, an imprint of Elsevier, Inc. All rights reserved.

Charting for Procedures 44-1 through 44-11

Date	Chart

Date	Chart

Date	Chart

Date	Chart

Copyright © 2010, 2005 by Saunders, an imprint of Elsevier, Inc. All rights reserved.

Date	Chart

Date	Chart

Date	Chart

Date	Chart

Copyright © 2010, 2005 by Saunders, an imprint of Elsevier, Inc. All rights reserved.

	Chart
Date	

	Chart
Date	

	Chart
Date	

	Chart
Date	

Copyright © 2010, 2005 by Saunders, an imprint of Elsevier, Inc. All rights reserved.

Student Name: DATE:

PROCEDURE 45-1 CHECKLIST: PERFORM HANDWASHING FOR SURGICAL ASEPSIS

TASK: Performing a surgical handwashing (surgical scrub) following Standard Precautions.

CONDITIONS: Given the proper equipment and supplies, the student will perform a handwashing for surgical asepsis.

EQUIPMENT AND SUPPLIES
- Liquid antibacterial soap and nailbrush with orange stick, or prepackaged sterile scrub brush with antibacterial soap and orange stick
- Paper towels
- Warm running water
- Sterile towel pack
- Regular waste container and cloth hamper

STANDARDS: Complete the procedure within _____ minutes and achieve a minimum score of _____%.

Time began _____   Time ended _____

Steps	Possible Points	First Attempt	Second Attempt
1. Remove jewelry.	5		
2. Open the sterile pack containing a scrub brush with an orange stick and sterile towel.	10		
3. Load the brush with liquid antibacterial soap or use prepackaged scrub.	5		
4. Turn on the faucets using correct method for facility.	10		
5. Use a paper towel to adjust the water temperature.	10		
6. Wet hands, wrists, and forearms.	10		
7. Clean nails with a nail brush or orange stick.	5		
8. Scrub hands, wrists, and forearms.	15		
9. Rinse hands, wrists, and forearms.	10		
10. Turn off the faucets using correct method for facility.	5		
11. Dry the hands and arms with sterile towel.	10		
12. Discard used towels in a regular waste container or soiled-linen container.	5		
Total Points Possible	100		

Comments: Total Points Earned _____

Divided by _____

Total Possible Points = _____ % Score

Instructor's Signature _____

Student Name: _____   DATE: _____

PROCEDURE 45-2 CHECKLIST: APPLY A STERILE GOWN AND GLOVES

TASK: Apply a sterile gown and gloves to maintain sterile technique.

CONDITIONS: Given the proper equipment and supplies, the student will apply a sterile gown and gloves to maintain sterile technique.

EQUIPMENT AND SUPPLIES
- Supplies for surgical handwashing
- Sterile gown
- Sterile gloves
- Hair cover
- Mask
- Goggles (as needed for standard precautions)
- Regular waste container

STANDARDS: Complete the procedure within _____ minutes and achieve a minimum score of _____%.

Time began _____   Time ended _____

Steps	Possible Points	First Attempt	Second Attempt
1. Remove jewelry (rings and watch).	5		
2. Sanitize hands.	5		
3. Open sterile package's outer wrappings for sterile gloves, sterile towels, and sterile gown.	10		
4. Open the inner packages.	10		
5. Apply hair cover, mask, and goggles.	10		
6. Unfold and apply sterile gown and secure.	10		
7. Apply a sterile glove to the nondominant hand.	15		
8. Apply a sterile glove to the dominant hand.	15		
9. Adjust gloves and gown.	10		
10. Maintain sterile technique.	10		
Total Points Possible	100		

Comments: Total Points Earned _____

Divided by _____

Total Possible Points = _____ % Score

Instructor's Signature _____

Student Name: _____ DATE: _____

PROCEDURE 45-3 CHECKLIST: APPLY STERILE GLOVES

TASK: Apply sterile gloves to maintain sterile technique.

CONDITIONS: Given the proper equipment and supplies, the student will apply sterile gloves to maintain sterile technique.

NOTE: The student should practice the procedure using the MACC located on the Evolve site at http://evolve. elsevier.com/klieger/medicalassisting, and then practice and perform the task in the classroom: MACC/Clinical skills/Patient care/Minor office surgery/Donning sterile gloves.

EQUIPMENT AND SUPPLIES
- Supplies for surgical handwashing
- Sterile gloves
- Regular waste container

STANDARDS: Complete the procedure within _____ minutes and achieve a minimum score of _____%.

Time began _____   Time ended _____

Steps	Possible Points	First Attempt	Second Attempt
1. Remove jewelry (rings and watch).	5		
2. Sanitize hands.	5		
3. Open the sterile glove package's outer wrapping.	10		
4. Open the inner package.	10		
5. Aseptically sanitize the hands.	15		
6. Pick up the sterile glove for the nondominant hand by the cuff.	10		
7. Lift the entire glove from the paper and pull it onto the nondominant hand.	10		
8. Adjust the glove for the nondominant hand, being careful not to contaminate the gloved hand.	10		
9. Pick up the sterile glove for the dominant hand, being careful not to touch the fingers and palm of glove.	10		
10. Adjust the glove for the dominant hand.	5		
11. Inspect the gloves for tears.	10		
Total Points Possible	100		

Comments: Total Points Earned _____

Divided by _____

Total Possible Points = _____ % Score

Instructor's Signature _____

Copyright © 2010, 2005 by Saunders, an imprint of Elsevier, Inc. All rights reserved.

Student Name: _____   DATE: _____

PROCEDURE 45-4 CHECKLIST: REMOVE CONTAMINATED GLOVES

TASK: Remove contaminated gloves to avoid spreading contaminants.

CONDITIONS: Given the proper equipment and supplies, the student will remove contaminated gloves properly.

EQUIPMENT AND SUPPLIES
- Gloves used in procedure
- Regular waste container
- Biohazardous waste container if gloves are contaminated with blood or body fluid

STANDARDS: Complete the procedure within _____ minutes and achieve a minimum score of _____%.

Time began _____   Time ended _____

Steps	Possible Points	First Attempt	Second Attempt
1. Grasp the outside of dominant hand glove with the first three fingers of the nondominant hand 1 to 2 inches below the cuff.	10		
2. Remove the glove by pulling up to loosen glove.	5		
3. As the glove is pulled free from the hand, ball it in the palm of the gloved hand.	10		
4. Remove the second glove of nondominant hand by placing forefingers of dominant hand under the cuff and turning the glove as it is removed.	10		
5. Carefully dispose of the gloves in a regular or marked biohazardous waste container if the gloves are contaminated with blood or body fluids.	5		
6. Sanitize hands.	10		
Total Points Possible	50		

Comments: Total Points Earned _____

Divided by _____

Total Possible Points = _____ % Score

Instructor's Signature _____

Copyright © 2010, 2005 by Saunders, an imprint of Elsevier, Inc. All rights reserved.

Student Name: _____   DATE: _____

PROCEDURE 45-5 CHECKLIST: OPEN A STERILE PACKAGE

TASK: Open a sterile package, and establish a sterile field.

CONDITIONS: Given the proper equipment and supplies, the student will open a sterile package and create a sterile field.

NOTE: The student should practice the procedure using the MACC located on the Evolve site at http://evolve.elsevier.com/klieger/medicalassisting, and then practice and perform the task in the classroom: MACC/Clinical skills/Patient care/Minor office surgery/Establishing sterile field & assisting with minor office surgery.

EQUIPMENT AND SUPPLIES
- MACC/computer
- Sterile package
- Mayo stand or other sturdy surface
- Regular waste container

STANDARDS: Complete the procedure within _____ minutes and achieve a minimum score of _____%.

Time began _____   Time ended _____

Steps	Possible Points	First Attempt	Second Attempt
1. Sanitize hands.	5		
2. Verify orders, and assemble equipment and supplies.	10		
3. Check the integrity of the sterile package.	10		
4. Position the sterile package.	10		
5. Remove the tape on the sterile package.	10		
6. Open the top flap.	10		
7. Open the side flaps.	10		
8. Do not contaminate the field by touching anything with ungloved or nonsterile hands.	10		
9. Maintain sterility of the inside of the pack and the supplies within the package.	10		
Total Points Possible	85		

Comments: Total Points Earned _____

Divided by _____

Total Possible Points = _____ % Score

Instructor's Signature _____

Student Name: _____   DATE: _____

PROCEDURE 45-6 CHECKLIST: POUR A STERILE SOLUTION

TASK: Add a sterile solution to a sterile field.

CONDITIONS: Given the proper equipment and supplies, the student will add a sterile solution to a sterile field without contaminating the field.

NOTE: The student should practice the procedure using the MACC located on the Evolve site at http://evolve.elsevier.com/klieger/medicalassisting, and then practice and perform the task in the classroom: MACC/Clinical skills/Patient care/Minor office surgery/Establishing a sterile field & assisting with minor office surgery.

EQUIPMENT AND SUPPLIES
- MACC/computer
- Sterile solution
- Sterile container
- Sterile towel
- Regular waste container

STANDARDS: Complete the procedure within _____ minutes and achieve a minimum score of _____%.

Time began _____   Time ended _____

Steps	Possible Points	First Attempt	Second Attempt
1. Sanitize hands.	5		
2. Verify orders, and assemble equipment and supplies.	5		
3. Read the label three times to ensure you have the correct solution, as with any medication.	10		
4. Palm the label of the bottle.	10		
5. Remove the cap. Set the cap with the opening facing up.	15		
6. Pour a small amount of solution over the lip of the bottle into a waste receptacle for discarding, to wash away possible contaminants on the lip.	15		
7. Pour the solution from a height of 2 to 6 inches above the sterile container.	10		
8. Replace the cap on the bottle.	5		
Total Points Possible	75		

Comments: Total Points Earned _____

Divided by _____

Total Possible Points = _____% Score

Instructor's Signature _____

Copyright © 2010, 2005 by Saunders, an imprint of Elsevier, Inc. All rights reserved.

Student Name: DATE:

PROCEDURE 45-7 CHECKLIST: ASSIST WITH MINOR OFFICE SURGERY

TASK: Provide all equipment, supplies, and materials needed to perform a minor office surgery (I&D), and assist with the procedure.

CONDITIONS: Given the proper equipment and supplies, the student will assist with preparing and performing in a minor office surgical procedure.

NOTE: The student should practice the procedure using the MACC located on the Evolve site at http://evolve.elsevier.com/klieger/medicalassisting, and then practice and perform the task in the classroom: MACC/Clinical skills/Patient care/Minor office surgery/Establishing a sterile field & assisting with minor office surgery.

EQUIPMENT AND SUPPLIES
- MACC/computer
- Sterile packs

Sterile Skin Prep Pack
- 1 stainless steel bowl
- Stack of 20 sterile 4- × 4-inch gauze squares
- 2 sterile towels

Typical Sterile Pack for I&D
- Tissue forceps (Adson)
- Kelly hemostats
- Dressing forceps
- Sharp/sharp operating scissors
- Mayo dissecting scissors

Individual Sterile Items (as Indicated)
- Fenestrated drape
- Scalpel with blade appropriate for type of surgery
- Fork retractor
- 3-mL syringe 25-gauge, ⅝- to 1-inch needle, or size appropriate for type of surgery
- Sterile dressing
- 4- ×-4 sterile gauze squares

Additional Supplies—Side Table
- Bottled sterile water
- Bottle chlorhexidine gluconate (Hibiclens)
- Povidone-iodine (Betadine) swabs or other skin cleanser as preferred by physician
- Anesthesia as ordered by physician
- Roll of surgical tape
- Lister bandage scissors
- Conforming bandages
- Package of proper-sized sterile gloves
- Package of sterile towels
- 2 plastic-backed underdrapes
- Alcohol wipes
- Masks

Copyright © 2010, 2005 by Saunders, an imprint of Elsevier, Inc. All rights reserved.

- Goggles (optional)
- Biohazardous waste container
- Sharps container
- Mayo stand
- Sterile gown
- Disposable gloves
- Waterproof waste bag
- Signed consent form
- Wound culture
- Laboratory requisition
- Biohazardous transport bag
- Patient's medical record

STANDARDS: Complete the procedure within _____ minutes and achieve a minimum score of _____%.

Time began _____   Time ended _____

Steps	Possible Points	First Attempt	Second Attempt
1. Sanitize hands.	5		
2. Verify orders, and assemble equipment and supplies.	5		
3. Greet and identify the patient, and escort the patient to the examination room.	5		
4. Explain the procedure to patient.	5		
5. Obtain written and informed consent for the procedure if not already obtained.	10		
6. Verify compliance of preoperative diet and medication instructions.	5		
7. Position the Mayo stand so that it is within easy reach of the procedure site.	5		
8. Create a sterile field, using a prepackaged sterile drape, and attach a temporary disposal bag to the edge of the Mayo stand.	10		
9. Open sterile packs for surgical hand scrubs and sterile towels in the staging area (not in the examination room).	10		
10. Open a scrub pack in the examination room.	10		
11. Position the patient for the procedure.	5		
12. Perform a surgical scrub of the incision site.	10		

Steps	Possible Points	First Attempt	Second Attempt
13. Drape the area with the fenestrated drape.	10		
14. Remove the contaminated supplies from the room after completing the scrub.	10		
15. Open the sterile packs including physician's gown and set up tray.	10		
16. Assist the physician with surgical gown and gloves.	10		
17. Prepare the anesthetic as ordered by the physician.	10		
18. Hand the physician the antiseptic skin cleanser (povidone-iodine swab) in preparation of the incision site. Ask the patient if he or she has an allergy to shellfish.	10		
19. Assist with sterile items as indicated.	10		
20. Collect the surgical specimen, as required and complete laboratory requisition form.	10		
21. Monitor the patient during the procedure.	10		
22. Clean the surgical site and apply a sterile dressing.	10		
23. Monitor the patient for the next 30 minutes.	10		
24. Clean the examination room by collecting surgical instruments and taking to the utility area to rinse and place in soaking solution. Discard solutions as necessary.	15		
25. Discard any nonsharp disposable items in the biohazardous waste container.	15		
26. After the patient leaves, sanitize the room.	5		
27. Follow-up with the patient.	10		
28. Document the procedure.	10		
Total Points Possible	250		

Comments: Total Points Earned _____

Divided by _____

Total Possible Points = _____% Score

Instructor's Signature _____

Copyright © 2010, 2005 by Saunders, an imprint of Elsevier, Inc. All rights reserved.

CONSENT FOR SURGERY

DATE:_____

TIME:_____

I authorize the performance of the following procedure(s)_____
_____on_____
To be performed by_____, MD.

The following have been explained to me by Dr._____

    1. Nature of the procedure:_____

    2. Reason(s) for procedure:_____

    3. Possible risks:_____

    4. Possible complications:_____

I understand that no warranty or guarantee of the effectiveness of the surgery can be made.

I have been informed of possible alternative treatments including_____
_____and of the likely consequences of receiving no treatment, and I freely consent to this procedure.

I hereby authorize the above named surgeon and his/her assistants to provide additional services including administering anesthesia and / or medications, performing needed diagnostic tests including but not limited to radiology, and any other additional services deemed necessary for my well-being. I consent to have removed tissue examined by a pathologist who may then dispose of the tissue as he/she sees fit.

Signed_____ Relationship to patient_____
       Patient / Parent / Guardian

Witness_____

PROCEDURE 45-7

Copyright © 2010, 2005 by Saunders, an imprint of Elsevier, Inc. All rights reserved.

Student Name: _____ DATE: _____

PROCEDURE 45-8 CHECKLIST: REMOVE SUTURES OR STAPLES AND CHANGE A WOUND DRESSING USING A SPIRAL BANDAGE

TASK: Remove sutures from a healed wound as ordered by the physician, apply a sterile dressing to a wound, and apply a bandage using a spiral turn.

CONDITIONS: Given the proper equipment and supplies, the student will role-play removing sutures from a healed wound, apply a sterile dressing to a wound, and apply a spiral turn bandage over a sterile dressing

NOTE: The student should practice the procedure using the MACC located on the Evolve site at http://evolve.elsevier.com/klieger/medicalassisting, and then practice and perform the task in the classroom: MACC/Clinical skills/Patient care/Minor office surgery/Removing sutures & changing a wound dressing using a spiral bandage.

EQUIPMENT AND SUPPLIES
- MACC/computer
- Nonsterile disposable gloves
- Sterile suture removal kit or staple removal kit
- Sterile gauze pads in appropriate size for size of wound
- Antiseptic or sterile swabs
- Sterile gloves
- Waterproof waste bag
- Surgical tape
- Scissors
- Biohazardous waste container
- Patient's medical record

STANDARDS: Complete the procedure within _____ minutes and achieve a minimum score of _____%.

Time began _____   Time ended _____

Steps	Possible Points	First Attempt	Second Attempt
1. Sanitize hands.	5		
2. Verify orders, and assemble equipment and supplies. Obtain the patient's medical record.	5		
3. Greet and identify the patient, escort the patient to the examination room, and explain the procedure to the patient.	10		
4. Position patient on examination table, and expose area to be treated.	5		
5. Position the Mayo stand so that it is within easy reach of the procedure site.	5		
6. Create a sterile field, using a prepackaged sterile drape; attach a temporary disposal bag (waterproof waste bag) to the edge of the Mayo stand.	5		
7. Apply nonsterile gloves.	5		

Steps	Possible Points	First Attempt	Second Attempt
8. Remove the soiled dressing.	10		
9. Check the incision line.	10		
10. Discard the contaminated dressing, and gloves. Sanitize the hands again, and put on sterile gloves to remove the sutures or staples.	10		
11. Clean the incision line.	5		
12. Grasp the first suture to be removed. Cut the suture at the skin level away from the suture line.	10		
13. Use the dressing forceps to lift the suture at the knot straight upward, away from the suture line, and out of the skin.	10		
14. Place each suture on the gauze square after being removed. Inspect and count the sutures on the gauze square before discarding them. (Check to ensure the number of sutures applied and the number of sutures removed are the same.)	15		
To remove staples: 15. Carefully place the jaws of the staple remover under the staple to be removed.	10		
16. Firmly squeeze the staple remover handles until they are fully closed.	10		
17. Gently lift the staple remover upward to remove the staple from the incision line.	10		
18. Place the staple on a gauze square.	10		
19. Continue in this manner until all the staples have been removed.	5		
20. Inspect and count the staples on the gauze square before discarding.	10		
Cleansing and dressing a wound: 21. Clean the wound with an appropriate solution.	10		
22. Use the sterile gauze squares to absorb excess antiseptic.	10		
23. Apply a sterile dressing to cover and protect the wound and any remaining sutures.	10		

Copyright © 2010, 2005 by Saunders, an imprint of Elsevier, Inc. All rights reserved.

Steps	Possible Points	First Attempt	Second Attempt
24. After the wound is covered, remove your gloves and discard in the water-resistant waste container.	10		
25. Sanitize the hands before bandaging the dressing.	5		
26. Bandage the dressing.	10		
27. Use a spiral turn to apply the bandage to the suture site by anchoring the bandage with a circular turn. Then begin the spiral turns, being sure to cover the previous turn by one third to one half of the distance. Ensure that the turn does not stop on a pressure site.	20		
28. Check the patient's fingers and hand or toes and foot for adequate circulation.	10		
29. Assist the patient to a comfortable position.	5		
30. Instruct the patient when to return for removal of the remaining sutures if applicable.	10		
31. Disinfect the work area.	10		
32. Remove gloves and sanitize the hands.	5		
33. Provide the patient with verbal and written wound care instructions.	10		
34. Document the procedure.	10		
Total Points Possible	300		

Comments: Total Points Earned _____

Divided by _____

Total Possible Points = _____% Score

Instructor's Signature _____

Student Name: _____   DATE: _____

PROCEDURE 45-9 CHECKLIST: APPLY AND REMOVE ADHESIVE SKIN CLOSURES

TASK: Apply and remove a skin closure using a sterile technique.

CONDITIONS: Given the proper equipment and supplies, the student will apply and remove a skin closure using a sterile technique.

EQUIPMENT AND SUPPLIES
- Nonsterile disposable gloves
- Sterile cotton-tipped applicator
- Sterile gloves
- Adhesive skin closure strips
- Antiseptic solution
- Sterile 4- × 4-inch gauze squares
- Sterile dressing forceps
- Surgical tape
- Antiseptic swabs (povidone-iodine [Betadine])
- Tincture of benzoin
- Biohazardous waster container
- Patient's medical record

STANDARDS: Complete the procedure within _____ minutes and achieve a minimum score of _____%.

Time began _____   Time ended _____

Steps	Possible Points	First Attempt	Second Attempt
1. Sanitize hands.	5		
2. Verify orders, and assemble equipment and supplies.	5		
3. Obtain the patient's medical record.	5		
4. Greet and identify the patient, and escort the patient to the examination room.	5		
5. Explain the procedure to patient.	5		
6. Position patient as required, and inspect the wound.	5		
7. Position the Mayo stand so that it is within easy reach of the procedure site.	5		
8. Put on disposable gloves.	5		
9. Clean the wound thoroughly using an antiseptic solution and working from the center of the wound outward.	10		
10. Apply tincture of benzoin.	10		
11. Open the sterile adhesive strips.	5		
12. Apply sterile gloves.	5		

PROCEDURE 45-9

Copyright © 2010, 2005 by Saunders, an imprint of Elsevier, Inc. All rights reserved.

Steps	Possible Points	First Attempt	Second Attempt
13. Verify that the skin surface is dry, and position the first strip over the center of the wound.	10		
14. Continue applying adhesive strips from center outward, pulling the wound in the same direction with each strip applied.	10		
15. Apply a dry sterile dressing over the strips, as indicated by the physician.	5		
16. Remove gloves and sanitize the hands.	5		
17. Provide the patient with verbal and written wound care instructions as ordered by the physician.	10		
18. Document the procedure.	10		
Removal of skin closures: 19. Sanitize hands.	5		
20. Verify orders, and assemble equipment and supplies.	5		
21. Obtain the patient's medical record.	5		
22. Greet and identify the patient, and escort the patient to the examination room.	5		
23. Explain the procedure to the patient.	5		
24. Position the patient as required and remove the soiled dressing.	5		
25. Check the incision line.	5		
26. Place a 4- × 4-inch gauze square in close approximation with the wound. Apply clean gloves.	5		
27. Clean the site with antiseptic swab, and apply a dry sterile dressing as indicated by the physician.	5		
28. Properly dispose of all contaminated supplies.	5		
29. Disinfect the work area.	5		

Steps	Possible Points	First Attempt	Second Attempt
30. Remove gloves and sanitize hands.	5		
31. Provide the patient with verbal and written wound care instructions.	10		
32. Document the procedure.	10		
Total Points Possible	200		

Comments: Total Points Earned _____

Divided by _____

Total Possible Points = _____% Score

Instructor's Signature _____

PROCEDURE 45-9

Charting for Procedures 45-1 through 45-9

Date	Chart

Date	Chart

Date	Chart

Date	Chart

Copyright © 2010, 2005 by Saunders, an imprint of Elsevier, Inc. All rights reserved.

	Chart
Date	

	Chart
Date	

	Chart
Date	

	Chart
Date	

Copyright © 2010, 2005 by Saunders, an imprint of Elsevier, Inc. All rights reserved.

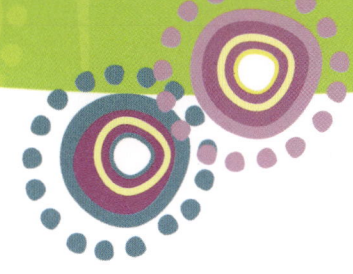

SECTION FIVE **CLINICAL MEDICAL ASSISTING**

31 Infection Control and Asepsis, 636
32 Preparing the Examination Room, 670
33 Body Measurements and Vital Signs, 679
34 Obtaining the Medical History, 715
35 Assisting with the Physical Examination, 731
36 Electrocardiography, 761
37 Radiography and Diagnostic Imaging, 793
38 Therapeutic Procedures, 808
39 Specialty Diagnostic Testing, 855
40 Introduction to the Physician's Office Laboratory, 895
41 Phlebotomy, 926
42 Laboratory Testing in the Physician's Office, 956
43 Understanding Medications, 1002
44 Administering Medications, 1036
45 Minor Office Surgery, 1085
46 Basic First Aid and Medical Office Emergencies, 1130

SECTION SIX **EMPLOYMENT AND BEYOND**

47 Beginning Your Job Search, 1151

APPENDICES

A Common Abbreviations, Acronyms, and Symbols, 1167
B Common Prefixes and Suffixes, 1173
C Common Laboratory Test Values, 1179
D English-to-Spanish Guide, 1181

Glossary, 1183

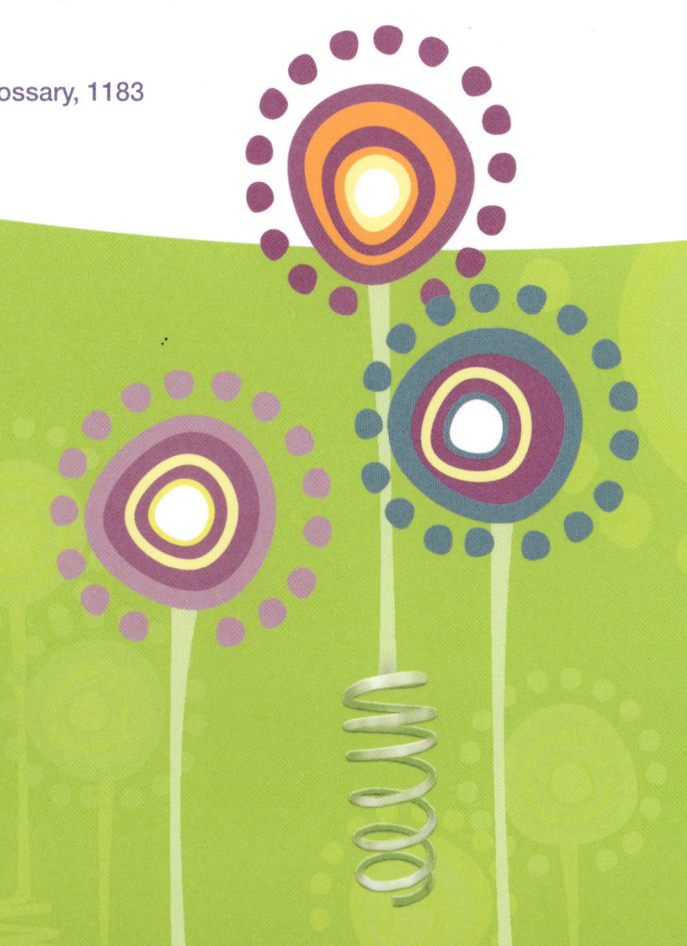
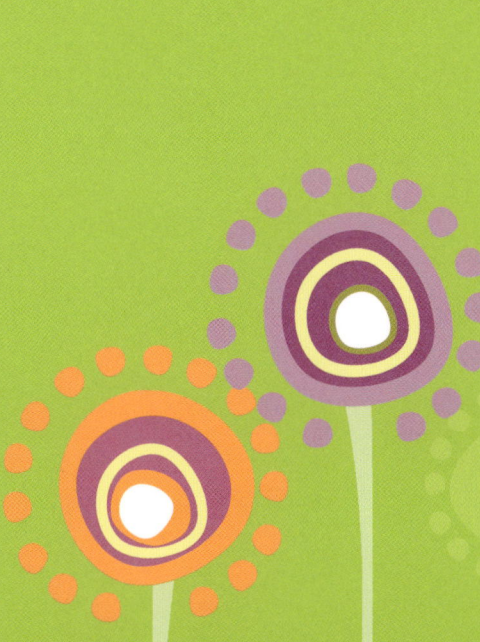

Saunders

ESSENTIALS OF
MEDICAL ASSISTING

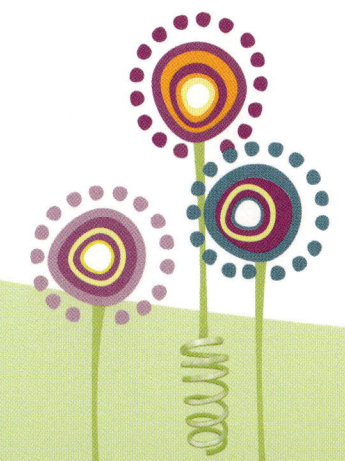

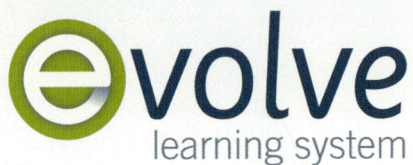
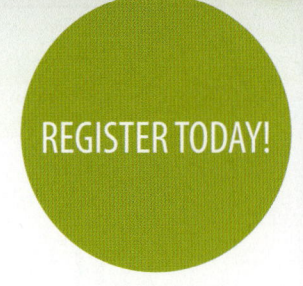

REGISTER TODAY!

To access your Student Resources, visit:

http://evolve.elsevier.com/klieger/medicalassisting

Evolve® Student Learning Resources for Klieger: Saunders Essentials of Medical Assisting, *Second Edition, offer the following features:*

- **Medical Assisting Competency Challenge**
  Interactive guided practice and application activities that allow you to experience real-world scenarios

- **Chapter Quizzes**
  Scored quizzes can serve as a valuable study tool

- **Archie Animations**
  Detailed anatomy and physiology videos

- **Body Spectrum**
  Fun and interactive coloring book that helps you study anatomy and physiology

- **Spanish-English Pronunciation Glossary**
  A pronunciation glossary to prepare you for medical office situations

- **CMA and RMA Review Questions**
  Practice questions to help you prepare for your examinations

- **Medisoft Exercises**
  Software exercises can prepare you for realistic office scenarios

- **Math Review**
  Various interactive quizzes refresh simple math knowledge, to aid you in your future career

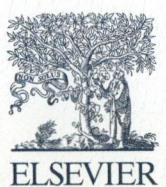
ELSEVIER

Saunders

ESSENTIALS OF MEDICAL ASSISTING

SECOND EDITION

Diane M. Klieger
RN, MBA, CMA (AAMA)

Retired Program Director, Medical Assisting
Adjunct Medical Assisting Instructor
Pinellas Technical Education Centers (PTEC)
St. Petersburg, Florida

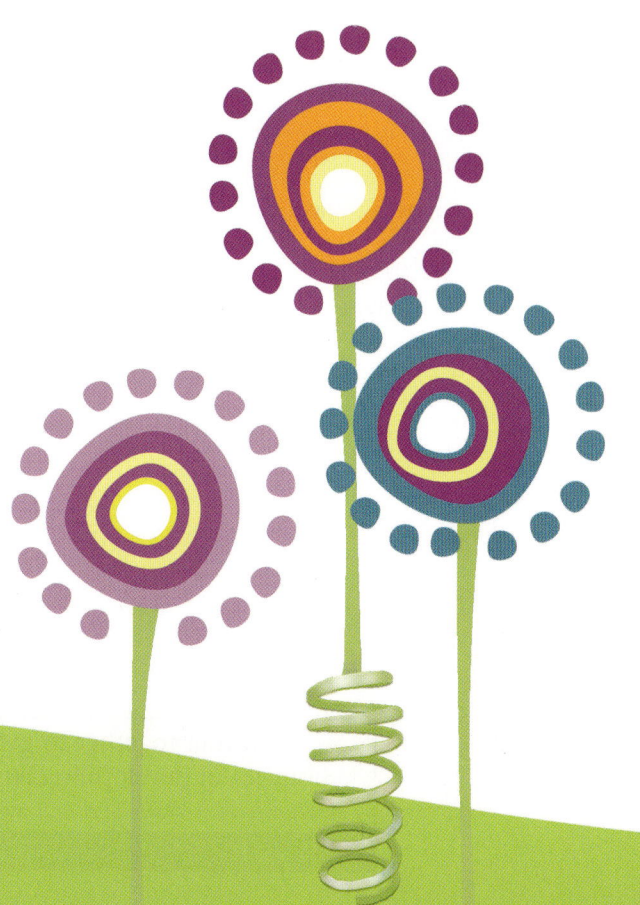

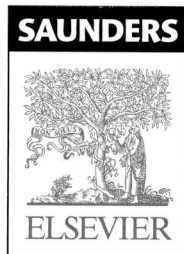
SAUNDERS
ELSEVIER

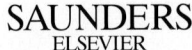

3251 Riverport Lane
Maryland Heights, Missouri 63043

SAUNDERS ESSENTIALS OF MEDICAL ASSISTING   ISBN: 978-1-4160-5674-4
Copyright © 2010, 2005 by Saunders, an imprint of Elsevier Inc.

All rights reserved. No part of this publication may be reproduced or transmitted in any form or by any means, electronic or mechanical, including photocopying, recording, or any information storage and retrieval system, without permission in writing from the publisher. Permissions may be sought directly from Elsevier's Rights Department: phone: (+1) 215 239 3804 (US) or (+44) 1865 843830 (UK); fax: (+44) 1865 853333; e-mail: healthpermissions@elsevier.com. You may also complete your request on-line via the Elsevier website at http://www.elsevier.com/permissions.

Notice

Knowledge and best practice in this field are constantly changing. As new research and experience broaden our knowledge, changes in practice, treatment and drug therapy may become necessary or appropriate. Readers are advised to check the most current information provided (i) on procedures featured or (ii) by the manufacturer of each product to be administered, to verify the recommended dose or formula, the method and duration of administration, and contraindications. It is the responsibility of the practitioner, relying on their own experience and knowledge of the patient, to make diagnoses, to determine dosages and the best treatment for each individual patient, and to take all appropriate safety precautions. To the fullest extent of the law, neither the Publisher nor the Editor/Author assumes any liability for any injury and/or damage to persons or property arising out of or related to any use of the material contained in this book.

The Publisher

Library of Congress Cataloging-in-Publication Data

Klieger, Diane M.
  Saunders essentials of medical assisting / Diane M. Klieger.—2nd ed.
      p. ; cm.
  Rev. ed. of: Saunders textbook of medical assisting / Diane M. Klieger. c2005.
  Includes index.
  ISBN 978-1-4160-5674-4 (hardcover : alk. paper) 1. Medical assistants.   2. Physicians' assistants.   3. Allied health personnel.   I. Klieger, Diane M. Saunders textbook of medical assisting.   II. Title.   III. Title: Essentials of medical assisting.
    [DNLM: 1. Physician Assistants.   2. Allied Health Personnel.   3. Office Management.   W 21.5 K646sa 2010]
  R728.8.K55 2010
  610.73′7069–dc22

2009013834

Publisher: Michael S. Ledbetter
Developmental Editor: Jennifer Bertucci
Publishing Services Manager: Catherine Jackson
Project Manager: David Stein
Design Direction: Teresa McBryan

Printed in China.

Last digit is the print number: 9   8   7   6   5   4   3   2

Working together to grow libraries in developing countries

www.elsevier.com | www.bookaid.org | www.sabre.org

ELSEVIER   BOOK AID International   Sabre Foundation

Reviewers

Lynn Augenstern, MA, CMA (AAMA)
Retired Medical Assistant Program Director
Ridley-Lowell Business and Technical Institute
Binghamton, New York

Kristi Bertrand, MPH, CMA (AAMA), CPC, PBT (ASCP)
Allied Health Department Chair
Spencerian College
Lexington, Kentucky

Norma Bird, MEd, BS, CMA (AAMA)
Medical Assisting Program Director and Master Instructor
Idaho State University College of Technology
Pocatello, Idaho

Patricia Bucho, CMA (AAMA), HT (ASCP), CPT1
Allied Health Instructor
Long Beach City College
Long Beach, California

Lou Brown, MT (ASCP), CMA (AAMA)
Program Director, Medical Assisting and Phlebotomy
Wayne Community College
Goldsboro, North Carolina

Kathy Cline, RN, ASN
Medical Assisting Program Instructor
Blue Cliff College
Alexandria, Louisiana

Joyce Combs, MS, CMA (AAMA)
Medical Assisting Program Coordinator
Bluegrass Community and Technical College
Lexington, Kentucky

Cydney Kay Condit, BS, AAS, CMA (AAMA), RPT
Allied Health Instructor
Midstate College
Peoria, Illinois

Janie Corbitt, RN, BSLA, MLS
Instructor, Health Technology Core
Central Georgia Technical College
Milledgeville, Georgia

Tracie Fuqua, BS, CMA (AAMA)
Director, Medical Assistant Program
Wallace State Community College
Hanceville, Alabama

Candace Gioia, RN, BSN, CNOR
Program Director, Surgical Technology
Pinellas Technical Education Centers
St. Petersburg, Florida

Jen Gouge, AA, RT
Coordinator, Medical Assistant Program
Peninsula College
Port Angeles, Washington

Susanna M. Hancock, AAS-MOM, RMA, CMA (AAMA), RPT, COLT/CMLA
Retired Medical Assistant Program Director/Instructor
American Institute of Health Technology
Boise, Idaho

Carolyn Helms, BS, RMA
Program Director, Medical Assisting
Atlanta Technical College
Atlanta, Georgia

Lynn Johnson, RN, MSN
Continuing Education Instructor
Pinellas Technical Education Centers
St. Petersburg, Florida

Geri Kale-Smith, MS, CMA (AAMA)
Associate Professor, Medical Office Administration Program
Harper College
Palatine, Illinois

Terrance Morton, MD
Medical Coordinator and Instructor
Tidewater Community College
Virginia Beach, Virginia

Lisa Nagle, BSed, CMA (AAMA)
Program Director, Medical Assisting
Augusta Technical College
Augusta, Georgia

Diana Reeder, AAS, CMA (AAMA)
Medical Assisting Program Coordinator
Maysville Community and Technical College
Morehead, Kentucky

Theresa A. Rieger, CMA (AAMA), CPC
Manager
Mercy Health Network Northwest Family Clinic
Oklahoma City, Oklahoma

Lisa Stephens, CMA (AAMA), AAS
Assistant Director of Education
Kaplan College
Indianapolis, Indiana

Deb Stockberger, MSN, RN
Medical Assistant Program Leader
North Iowa Area Community College
Mason City, Iowa

Karen Stone, RN
Registered Nurse; Clinical Medical Assisting Instructor
Northampton Community College
Bethlehem, Pennsylvania

Shannon Ydoyaga, MS, BBA
Program Administrator, Health Professions
Richland College
Dallas, Texas

To my grandsons,
Calvin *and* Pierce

To all students,
who provide inspiration

To my family, extended family, and friends,
who provide support

Preface

Spring into your new career with the second edition of *Saunders Essentials of Medical Assisting*! With this textbook in hand, you are about to take the first step toward a career with many fulfilling opportunities and rewards. As a medical assistant, you will be able to make a difference in the lives of others and be a part of the ever-changing world of health care. The U.S. Department of Labor's Bureau of Labor Statistics *Occupational Outlook Handbook* (2008-2009) projects that medical assisting employment will increase *at least 35%* between 2006 and 2016, which is much faster than the average for all occupations. This is largely the result of increases in the number of outpatient health care facilities. In addition, rapid advances in medical techniques and procedures have created a need for more highly skilled health care professionals.

What does this mean for you? Armed with the solid foundation of administrative and clinical knowledge and skills provided in this textbook, you will be prepared to take advantage of the tremendous opportunities that await you in the medical assisting field.

To provide high-quality care to patients, all physicians, nurses, medical assistants, and other allied health care professionals must be thoroughly educated in every aspect of their scope of practice. This textbook is a comprehensive source of the fundamental knowledge and skills you need to achieve a successful medical assisting career. It covers all content and competencies of both the Commission on Accreditation of Allied Health Education Programs (CAAHEP) and the American Medical Technologists (AMT) national curricula for medical assisting, so you can be certain that everything you will learn in this textbook reflects best practices in the field. Furthermore, you can count on this textbook to prepare you properly for either the AAMA's or the AMT's certification examination. The text content has been revised to meet current trends, and many new photographs appear throughout this edition. In addition, all lessons have been updated to reflect changes in the CAAHEP and the Accrediting Bureau of Health Education Schools (ABHES) curricula. Also, in order to more effectively organize your learning, two very comprehensive chapters in the previous edition (Circulatory and Nervous Systems) have been split, and Phlebotomy has been made a stand-alone chapter.

In addition to providing you with the basics you need to succeed, this book demonstrates the importance of your actions and words. You will learn how everything you say and do has a ripple effect on both the practice and the patient. A medical assistant's actions and words can have ethical, legal, or even lethal consequences. In every chapter, you are asked to analyze the legal and ethical consequences of a medical assistant's actions and words, including the impact on the patient, on the practice, and even on the community and beyond.

The innovative presentation of up-to-date concepts and information in this book, along with learning about the consequences of your actions, will equip you to perform your duties effectively and make the right decisions as you work with other members of the health care team to provide patients with the best care possible.

ORGANIZATIONAL STRUCTURE

Saunders Essentials of Medical Assisting is written specifically for medical assisting students. The reader-friendly writing style, authoritative content, and clear organization enable students to gain a solid understanding of the concepts and skills. The text is divided into six sections:

Section One: Strategies for Success

Section One advises students on how to get the most out of their learning experience. Highlights include the importance of applying effective study methods, strategies for managing time and accomplishing goals, proven methods for learning more effective, and tips for successful test taking.

Section Two: Foundational Concepts

Section Two provides important foundational knowledge that medical assistants need to function within the medical practice, including legal and ethical boundaries, professionalism, understanding the behavior of others, and effective communication skills. Chapter 10 is dedicated to helping students understand medical terminology.

Section Three: Anatomy and Physiology

This section is a comprehensive look at the major systems of the body, and their structure and function. Detailed illustrations provide students with valuable comprehensive knowledge of anatomy and serve as a great study resource. In addition, students are introduced to diseases and disorders that affect each body system.

Section Four: Administrative Medical Assisting

Section Four walks students through all the front-office duties that medical assistants need to understand and must be able to perform to be successful in their careers. Illustrated administrative procedures demonstrate the proper performance and explain each step of the procedure. Students are reminded of the legal and ethical consequences of their words and actions as they relate to administrative medical assisting responsibilities. Electronic medical records, which are quickly becoming central to the function of today's medical office, are also addressed in this section.

Section Five: Clinical Medical Assisting

This section provides the knowledge and skills necessary to perform clinical medical assisting duties. Illustrated step-by-step procedures show the proper performance of each procedure and break down the reasons behind each step and the need for accuracy in both performing the skill and documenting it in the medical record. As in the other sections, the importance of legal and ethical behavior is emphasized. Also, Chapter 46 addresses disaster preparedness, which is an essential topic in the current medical assisting field.

Section Six: Employment and Beyond

Section Six helps coach students in how to find a job and succeed in their career. Chapter 47 provides real solutions for finding job opportunities, developing effective self-promoting materials (resumés, cover letters), and making the most of interviews.

DISTINCTIVE FEATURES

This textbook has been designed to incorporate student-centered pedagogical (educational) features that support the intended learning objectives while actively engaging students in the content. These pedagogical features include Learning Objectives, Key Terms, Practical Application case studies, illustrated step-by-step procedures, Patient-Centered Professionalism boxes, For Your Information boxes, Web Search boxes, Chapter Summaries, detailed and helpful tables, and lists of word parts and abbreviations.

SUPPLEMENTAL STUDENT RESOURCES

Keeping in mind the diversity of medical assisting students, instructors, programs, institutions, and teaching environments, an innovative and flexible package of supplemental resources has been developed to complement *Saunders Essentials of Medical Assisting*. Each of these comprehensive supplements has been specifically designed to enrich the learning and teaching experience while supporting the ultimate goal of producing students who are well prepared for certification examinations and for thriving careers as medical assistants. These enriching supplements and unique features include an updated and helpful student workbook, the comprehensive Evolve site, and the instructor resources, which include a combination TEACH and Instructor Resource Manual, Evolve Instructor Resources, a Test Bank, and Power Point slides.

Workbook

This valuable and practical student resource matches material in the book chapter-by-chapter to help students apply and master key concepts and skills. It offers a variety of exercises to reinforce chapter material, including:
- Comprehensive reviews of terminology, anatomy, and content, reinforced by a variety of recall exercises, such as sentence completion, multiple choice, or short answer
- Skills application exercises that encourage students to put concepts into practice
- Critical thinking exercises that take information to the next level and prepare students for the real world through patient care scenarios
- Chapter quizzes that help students reinforce learning
- Skills competency checklists, which enable students and instructors to evaluate performance for each completed skill

NEW to the workbook for this edition is an appendix that contains essential and effective work papers and forms, as well as the procedure checklists for each chapter. These new forms and work papers will provide students with important practice for their future career, and will help in making the students the best possible medical assistants. Because this new appendix is logically separated by chapter and procedure, it is easily navigated.

Evolve Site

Evolve is an interactive learning environment that reinforces and expands on the concepts learned in the classroom. The resources on the Evolve site bridge information in the text with real-world practice and allow you to apply the key content and skills you've learned throughout the chapters in the textbook. On the Evolve site, whose URL is http://evolve.elsevier.com/Klieger/medicalassisting, students will find valuable resources, including:

- The **Medical Assisting Competency Challenge**, which provides realistic scenarios that cover core administrative and clinical competencies and are in line with the most current CAAHEP and ABHES content and competencies. The application activities let students try the skills on their own, as well as let them receive feedback for errors. The guided practice uses a step-by-step approach on how to perform each skill, and clinical skills show animation of how to perform key steps
- Scored, interactive **Chapter quizzes**, which serve as a great study tool
- **Archie Animations**, which provide students with detailed anatomy and physiology videos
- **Body Spectrum**, a fun and interactive coloring book that also helps students master anatomy and physiology

In addition, there are four **NEW** and exciting features to the Evolve site for this new edition. These fun and beneficial updates include:

- A **Spanish-English Pronunciation Glossary**, which helps students prepare for a diverse work environment
- Practice **CMA and RMA exam review questions**, which help students prepare for these vital examinations
- **Medisoft® activities and exercises**, which provide students with software practice
- An extensive, interactive **math review**, which provides students with invaluable mathematical knowledge both to assist them with passing their CMA/RMA examinations and to prepare them for situations in their careers where

knowledge of simple math is necessary, such as prescriptions and dosages

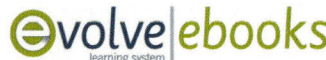
Spend less time searching and more time learning with electronic access to *Saunders Essentials of Medical Assisting, Second edition!* With easy access from your computer or any internet browser, you can easily search and navigate the book, make notes, highlight, and more. Please check with your instructor or go to http://www.elsevierhealth.com for more information.

SUPPLEMENTAL INSTRUCTOR RESOURCES

TEACH Instructor's Resource Manual

This all-encompassing manual gives instructors everything they need to teach students as effectively as possible. This combination of the TEACH Lesson Plan Manual (which provides instructors with customizable lesson plans and lecture outlines based on learning objectives) and Instructor's Manual (which provides instructors with teaching outlines and vital information about adhering to CAAHEP and ABHES competencies) gives instructors a comprehensive resource that will help them prepare their students for success in the real world. With this indispensable resource, instructors will save valuable preparation time and create a learning environment that fully engages students in classroom preparation. The lesson plans are linked to each chapter and are divided into 50-minute units, in a three column format, that map learning objectives to course content. Instructors will also have lecture outlines in Power Point with talking points and thought-provoking questions for their lectures.

Evolve Site

Evolve is an interactive learning environment that reinforces and expands on the concepts learned in the classroom. The resources on the Evolve site bridge information in the text with real-world practice and allow students to apply the key content and skills they've learned throughout the chapters in the textbook. On the Evolve site, students will find many resources (listed above) to help them succeed in the classroom and the real world. In addition to the Evolve Learning Resources available to students, an entire suite of tools exists for instructors that allows for communication between instructors and students, including discussion boards, chat rooms, e-mail, and more. Other valuable resources for instructors include:
- Two **Accreditation Correlation Grids** (one for ABHES Competencies, and one for the newly formatted CAAHEP competencies), which map out the competencies to exactly where they are covered in the text
- The **Answer Keys** to all Workbook questions, so that instructors can check the work of their students
- **Patient-Centered Professionalism Discussion Points**, which give instructors valuable discussion topics for their classroom
- A **Test Bank**, consisting of over 1,500 questions, so instructors can customize and format their exams

- An electronic version of the **TEACH Instructor's Resource Manual** chapters
- Interactive **Procedure Checklists**, which allow instructors to electronically score, print out, and track their students' progress of the procedures
- **Power Point Slides**, which contain talking points for instructors, so instructors can engage their students in classroom discussion

Test Bank

The Test Bank provides an accurate and in-depth foundation of test items for a wide variety of examination styles. Sample test questions include Matching, True/False, and Multiple Choice. Instructors have the ability to build their own exams using these Test Banks (found on the instructor's Evolve site at www.evolve.elsevier.com/klieger/medicalassisting). The Test Bank consists of over 1,500 questions and is available in both printed and electronic format so that instructors can easily prepare quizzes and exams, tailored to their classroom format.

Power Point Presentation Slides

On the Evolve® site, over 2,100 Power Point Slides are available for instructor use. These slides include a summary of key chapter material, as well as important chapter figures and images, and can easily be customized to support lectures and enhance classroom presentations. Also, these slides can be easily formatted within the Power Point program for student note-taking, or as overhead transparencies.

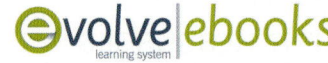
Spend less time searching and more time learning with electronic access to *Saunders Essentials of Medical Assisting, Second edition.* With easy access from your computer or any internet browser, you can search across all of your Elsevier e-textbooks; paste important text and images from multiple sources into a focused, custom document; make notes; highlight; and more. Please contact your Elsevier sales representative for more information or visit http://evolve.elsevier.com/ebooks.

DEVELOPMENT OF THIS TEXTBOOK

To ensure the accuracy of the material presented throughout this textbook, an extensive review and development process was used. This included several phases of evaluation by a variety of medical assisting instructors and experts in administrative medical assisting, anatomy and physiology, and clinical medical assisting. Many people shared their comments and suggestions. Reviewing a book or supplement takes an incredible amount of energy and attention, and many colleagues were able to take time out of their busy schedules to help ensure the validity and appropriateness of content in this textbook. The reviewers provided additional viewpoints and opinions that combine to make this text a practical, real-world learning tool.

Diane M. Klieger
RN, MBA, CMA (AAMA)

Special Features

Learning Objectives are stated at the beginning of each chapter and correspond to the organization of the chapter content.

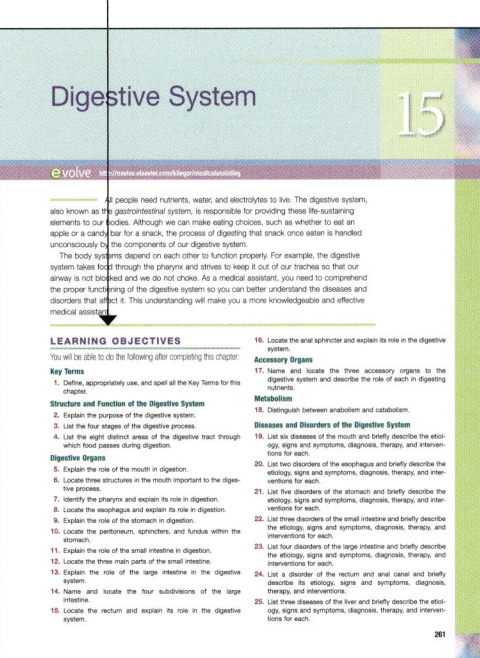

Each chapter contains a list of **Key Terms**, whose definitions can be found in the Glossary.

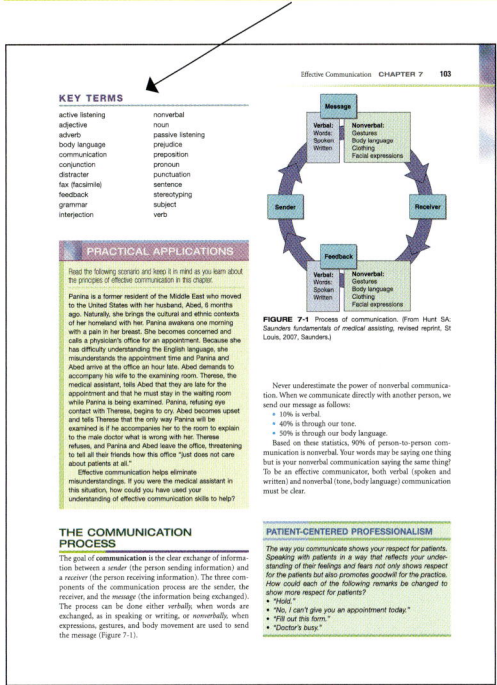

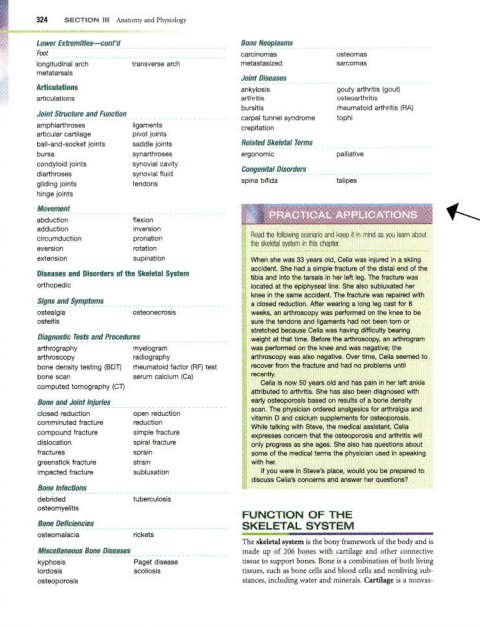

Practical Applications case studies are at the beginning of each chapter, and place chapter content into context to create interest in real-world scenarios.

Practical Applications case studies are revisited at the end of each chapter, accompanied by questions that help students apply what they've learned, as well as understand the consequences of the practical situations presented.

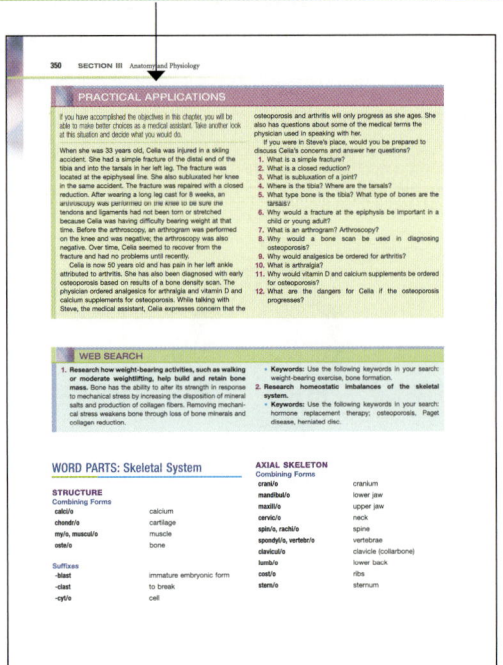

Patient-Centered Professionalism boxes at the end of major sections prompt students to think about the patient's perspective and encourage empathy.

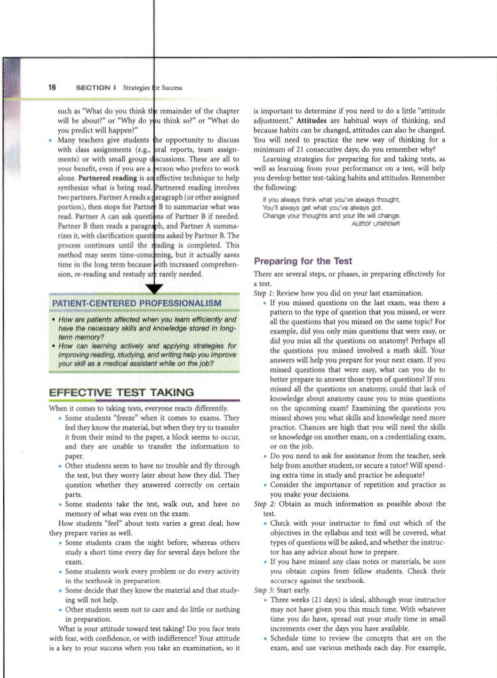

Illustrated step-by-step procedures, with charting examples and rationales, show how to perform and document administrative and clinical procedures.

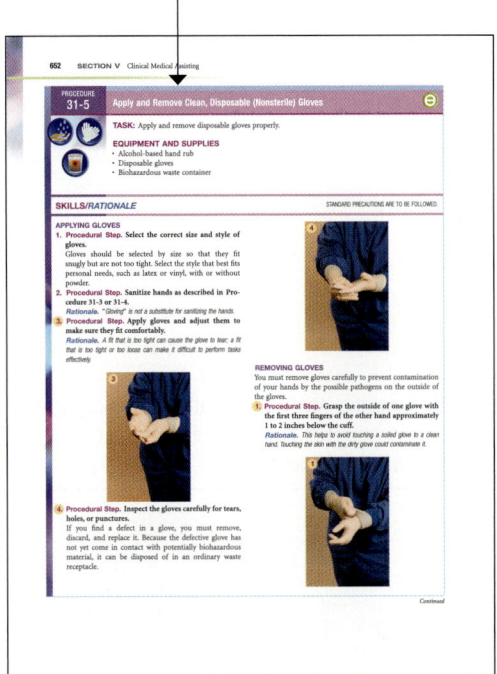

For Your Information boxes, interspersed throughout each chapter, provide pertinent additional information that allows students to further expand their knowledge of up-to-date information in the real world.

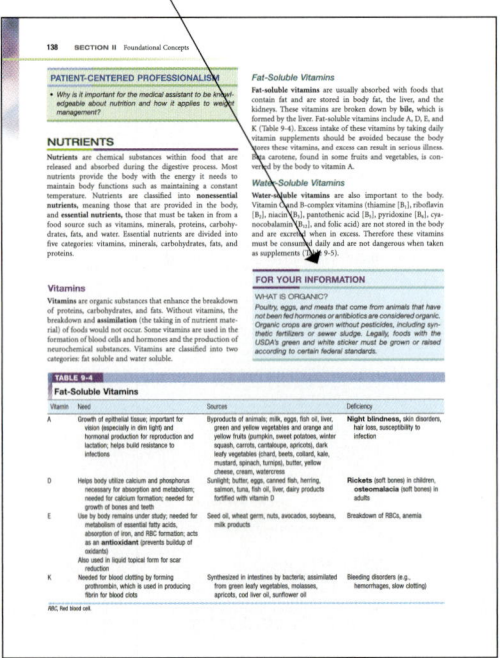

Special Features **xiii**

Web Search boxes, at the end of every chapter, suggest topics for further Internet research that expands students' comprehension of concepts and inspires them to learn beyond the text.

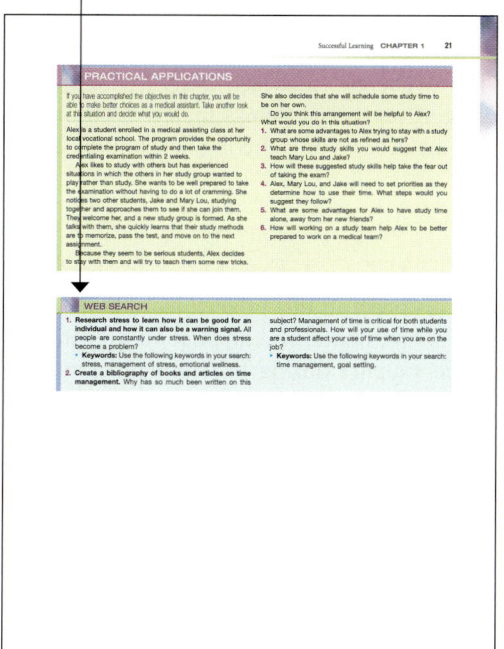

At the end of every chapter, a **Chapter Summary** of the learning objectives provides an outcome-based review of important points for each learning objective, reinforcing content the student must master. These objectives are designed to tie the chapter together, and include revisiting Patient-Centered Professionalism boxes.

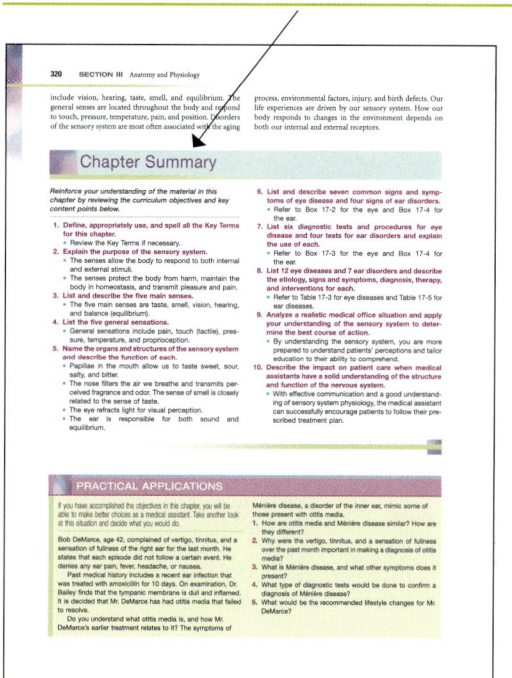

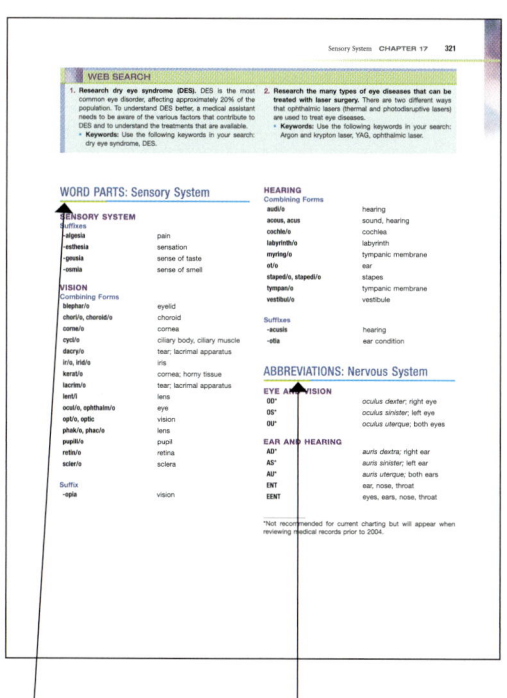

Lists of **Word Parts** and **Abbreviations**, found at the end of each chapter in the Anatomy and Physiology section, reinforce student understanding of medical terminology.

Acknowledgments

I extend a special acknowledgment to the people who brought their expertise to bear by contributing content and valuable editorial input, with particular thanks to Theresa A. Rieger, CMA (AAMA), who provided the subject matter for coding and insurance billing. Also, special thanks to Terry Allison, the photographer and friend whose patience and expertise made the process of gathering new photos in this second edition a wonderful experience.

A project of this magnitude is accomplished only with hard work and a dedicated team of editors and supporters. I wish to thank Michael Ledbetter, Publisher, for his belief in this project; Jennifer Bertucci, Developmental Editor, who worked closely with me in manuscript, figure, and illustration preparation; and Jamie Mabb, Editorial Assistant, who provided valuable support during this sometimes tedious process. Also, I was blessed to have Senior Project Manager, David Stein, assigned to this project because he guided it with great skill and experience.

Contents

SECTION ONE STRATEGIES FOR SUCCESS

1 Successful Learning, 1
  Am I Responsible for My Own Learning? 2
  Accomplishing Your Goals, 3
  Successful Study Strategies, 9
  Effective Test Taking, 16
  Conclusion, 19

2 Becoming a Professional, 22
  Professional Qualities, 23
  The Professional Medical Assistant, 25
  Professional Training, 29
  Conclusion, 34

SECTION TWO FOUNDATIONAL CONCEPTS

3 Diversity in Health Care Delivery, 36
  Medical Practice Settings, 37
  Medical Specialties, 37
  The Professional Health Care Team, 39
  Health Care Delivery Settings, 42
  Conclusion, 42

4 Law and Ethics in Health Care, 45
  Law and Licensure in Medical Practice, 46
  Law and Liability, 48
  Health Care Legislation, 54
  Ethics in Health Care, 61
  Conclusion, 68

5 Understanding Human Behavior, 72
  Psychology and Personality, 73
  Human Needs, 74
  Mental and Physical Health, 75
  Coping, 80
  Conclusion, 83

6 Understanding Patient Behavior, 85
  Development, 86
  Cultural Diversity, 95
  Response to Illness, 98
  Conclusion, 99

7 Effective Communication, 102
  The Communication Process, 103
  Effective Verbal Communication, 104
  Effective Nonverbal Communication, 105
  Effective Listening, 107
  Effective Written Communication, 109
  Effective Communication Using Electronic Technology, 112
  Conclusion, 115

8 Communicating with Patients, 118
  Role of the Medical Assistant, 119
  Different Cultures, 122
  Patients with Special Needs, 123
  Patient Education, 125
  Conclusion, 126

9 Nutrition, 130
  Dietary Guidelines, 131
  Food Guide Pyramid, 132
  Principles of Nutrition, 134
  Nutrients, 138
  Nutrition Through the Life Span, 142
  Nutrition and Chronic Disease, 144
  Diet Therapy, 145
  Conclusion, 147

10 Understanding Medical Terminology, 151
  Word Origins and Meanings, 152
  Word Parts, 153
  Guidelines for Medical Terminology, 156
  Conclusion, 163

SECTION THREE ANATOMY AND PHYSIOLOGY

11 Basic Anatomy and Physiology, 166
  Describing the Human Body, 168
  Organizational Levels of the Body, 174
  Conclusion, 193

12 Cardiovascular System, 198
  Functions of the Circulatory System, 199
  Heart, 200
  Brain and Hepatic Portal Circulation, 205
  Blood Vessels, 211
  Conclusion, 215

13 Blood, Lymphatic, and Immune Systems, 221
Functions of the Blood, 222
Composition of the Blood, 222
Lymphatic System, 229
Immune System, 236
Conclusion, 239

14 Respiratory System, 243
Structure and Function of the Respiratory System, 244
Upper Respiratory Tract, 245
Lower Respiratory Tract, 247
Breathing, 248
Respiratory Diseases and Disorders, 252
Conclusion, 258

15 Digestive System, 261
Structure and Function of the Digestive System, 263
Digestive Organs, 264
Accessory Organs, 268
Metabolism, 271
Diseases and Disorders of the Digestive System, 271
Conclusion, 276

16 Nervous System, 281
Nervous System Structure and Function, 283
Diseases and Disorders of the Nervous System, 294
Mental Health, 302
Conclusion, 303

17 Sensory System, 308
Sensory System, 309
Conclusion, 318

18 Skeletal System, 322
Function of the Skeletal System, 324
Bone and Cartilage, 325
Axial and Appendicular Skeleton, 328
Articulations, 335
Diseases and Disorders of the Skeletal System, 338
Conclusion, 345

19 Muscular System, 352
Function and Structure of Muscles, 353
Muscle Contraction, 354
Types of Muscle and Muscle Tissue, 355
Principal Skeletal Muscles, 356
Diseases and Disorders of the Muscular System, 362
Conclusion, 363

20 Urinary System, 367
Major Functions of the Urinary System, 368
Structure of the Urinary System, 369
Diseases and Disorders of the Urinary System, 373
Conclusion, 378

21 Reproductive System, 381
Function and Structure of the Reproductive System, 383
Male Reproductive System, 383
Female Reproductive System, 386
Human Development, 391
Sexually Transmitted Diseases, 396
Conclusion, 396

22 Endocrine System, 402
Endocrine System Function, 403
Major Endocrine Glands, 404
Endocrine Activity in Cells and Organs, 408
Regulation of Hormones, 410
Diseases and Disorders of the Endocrine System, 410
Conclusion, 411

23 Integumentary System, 419
Function and Structure of the Integumentary System, 420
Damage to the Skin, 423
Diseases and Disorders of the Integumentary System, 430
Conclusion, 431

SECTION FOUR ADMINISTRATIVE MEDICAL ASSISTING

24 The Medical Office, 438
Facilities Management, 439
Office Equipment, 442
Supplies, 450
Office Management, 451
Policy and Procedures Manuals, 454
Community Resources, 455
Conclusion, 456

25 Computers in the Medical Office, 460
Functions of the Computer, 461
Components of the Computer, 462
Basics of Computer Use, 465
Computer Systems in Medical Practice Management, 468
Conclusion, 471

26 Medical Office Communication, 474
Greeting Patients, 475
Managing the Telephone, 479
Scheduling Appointments, 485
Handling Mail, 493
Managing Written Correspondence, 498
Conclusion, 510

27 Medical Records and Chart Documentation, 514
   Purpose and Contents of Medical Records, 515
   Charting in the Patient's Record, 527
   Selecting a Filing System, 528
   Filing Methods, 533
   Tickler File, 537
   Review of Basic Filing Procedures, 537
   Conclusion, 539

28 Financial Management, 543
   Accounting Principles, 544
   Bookkeeping Procedures, 549
   Banking Procedures, 557
   Billing and Collections, 566
   Payroll Processing, 571
   Conclusion, 577

29 Medical Coding, 582
   Diagnostic Coding, 583
   Procedural Coding, 591
   Conclusion, 598

30 Medical Insurance, 601
   Overview of Health Insurance, 603
   Patient and Provider Roles in Medical Insurance, 604
   Medical Insurance Policies and Plans, 606
   Third-Party Medical Insurance, 610
   Medical Insurance Claim Cycle, 620
   Submitting Claims, 620
   Preventing Rejections and Delays, 629
   Claims Follow-Up, 630
   Conclusion, 630

SECTION FIVE CLINICAL MEDICAL ASSISTING

31 Infection Control and Asepsis, 636
   Infection Control, 637
   Medical Asepsis, 643
   Surgical Asepsis, 654
   Autoclave Maintenance, 657
   Conclusion, 661

32 Preparing the Examination Room, 670
   Room Preparation, 671
   Room Maintenance, 675
   Patient Preparation, 675
   Conclusion, 676

33 Body Measurements and Vital Signs, 679
   Body Measurements, 680
   Vital Signs, 690
   Conclusion, 709

34 Obtaining the Medical History, 715
   Sections of the Medical History, 716
   Interviewing Skills, 723
   Charting, 725
   Conclusion, 728

35 Assisting with the Physical Examination, 731
   Preparing the Patient, 732
   Body Mechanics, 736
   Positioning and Draping the Patient, 737
   Examination Methods, 747
   Vision Testing, 749
   Ear Examination, 755
   Conclusion, 755

36 Electrocardiography, 761
   Purpose of Electrocardiography, 762
   Electrical Impulses and ECG Patterns, 763
   Equipment and Supplies, 765
   Obtaining an Electrocardiogram, 769
   Artifacts, 779
   Cardiac Arrhythmias, 780
   Holter Monitor, 782
   Event Monitor, 784
   Cardiac Stress Testing, 784
   Conclusion, 789

37 Radiography and Diagnostic Imaging, 793
   Basics of Radiography, 794
   Film-Screen Radiography, 795
   Fluoroscopic Imaging, 798
   Computer Imaging, 799
   Employee Safety, 803
   Medical Assistant's Role, 803
   Conclusion, 804

38 Therapeutic Procedures, 808
   Ear Treatments, 809
   Eye Treatments, 812
   Bandaging, 817
   Cold and Heat Therapy, 822
   Ultrasound Therapy, 831
   Laser Therapy, 838
   Ambulatory Devices, 838
   Casts, 844
   Conclusion, 851

39 Specialty Diagnostic Testing, 855

Gynecological Examination and Testing, 856
Obstetrical Examination and Testing, 870
Colon Tests, 877
Pulmonary Function Tests, 883
Pulse Oximetry, 888
Hearing Acuity Tests, 889
Conclusion, 891

40 Introduction to the Physician's Office Laboratory, 895

Laboratory Regulations and Safety, 896
Basic Laboratory Equipment, 898
Laboratory Tests, 904
Culture Collection, 911
Urine Collection, 912
Stool Collection, 918
Sputum Collection, 922
Conclusion, 922

41 Phlebotomy, 926

Blood Collection, 927
Conclusion, 954

42 Laboratory Testing in the Physician's Office, 956

Urinalysis, 958
Blood Tests, 972
Conclusion, 998

43 Understanding Medications, 1002

Pharmacology, 1003
Drug Legislation, 1006
Drug Administration, 1011
Drug Forms, 1024
Drug Classifications, 1025
Prescriptions, 1028
Electronic Prescribing, 1030
Medication Record, 1031
Conclusion, 1031

44 Administering Medications, 1036

Oral Administration, 1037
Topical Administration, 1041
Vaginal and Rectal Administration, 1042
Inhalation, 1042
Parenteral Administration, 1045
Conclusion, 1082

45 Minor Office Surgery, 1085

Before Surgery, 1086
Surgical Asepsis, 1088
Surgical Instruments, 1089
Assisting with Minor Office Surgery, 1105
Wound Care, 1114
Conclusion, 1127

46 Basic First Aid and Medical Office Emergencies, 1130

Situations Requiring First Aid, 1131
Incident Reporting, 1132
Office Emergencies, 1133
Basic Life Support, 1145
Disaster Preparedness, 1146
Conclusion, 1148

SECTION SIX EMPLOYMENT AND BEYOND

47 Beginning Your Job Search, 1151

Organizing Your Resources, 1152
Developing Your Materials, 1153
Contacting Potential Employers, 1157
The Job Application, 1158
The Job Interview, 1160
Conclusion, 1163

APPENDICES

A. Common Abbreviations, Acronyms, and Symbols, 1167

B. Common Prefixes and Suffixes, 1173

C. Common Laboratory Test Values, 1179

D. English-to-Spanish Guide, 1181

Glossary, 1183

List of Procedures

Clinical Procedure Icons

Icons have been incorporated throughout the step-by-step procedures in this text. An illustration of each icon along with its description is outlined below.

HANDWASHING plays a crucial role in preventing the transmission of pathogens in the medical office. The medical assistant should frequently sanitize his/her hands. Also, when performing clinical procedures, the hands need to be sanitized before and after patient contact, before the application of gloves and after the removal of gloves, and after coming in contact with blood or other potentially infectious materials.

CLEAN DISPOSABLE GLOVES should be worn when a medical assistant will have hand contact with the following: blood and other potentially infectious materials, mucous membranes, nonintact skin, and contaminated articles or surfaces.

SHARPS CONTAINERS are used to contain medical needles (and other sharp medical instruments). Needles are discarded into a sharps container after a single use and are dropped into the container without touching the side of it.

BIOHAZARD CONTAINERS are closable, leakproof, and suitably constructed to contain the biohazardous contents during handling, storage, transport, or shipping. The containers must be labeled or color coded and closed before removal to prevent the contents from spilling.

PROTECTIVE EYEWEAR WITH MASKS OR FACE SHIELDS must be worn whenever it is possible that drops of blood, spray, splashes, or other possibly infectious materials may be produced, each of which creates a risk when it comes into contact with the eyes, nose, or mouth.

Chapter 24
- 24-1 Prepare, Send, and Receive a Fax, 444
- 24-2 Maintain Office Equipment, 449
- 24-3 Inventory Control: Ordering and Restocking Supplies, 452
- 24-4 Develop and Maintain a Current List of Community Resources, 457

Chapter 26
- 26-1 Give Verbal Instructions on How to Locate the Medical Office, 477
- 26-2 Create a Medical Practice Information Brochure, 478
- 26-3 Answer a Multiline Telephone System, 481
- 26-4 Prepare and Maintain an Appointment Book, 486
- 26-5 Schedule a New Patient, 490
- 26-6 Schedule Outpatient and Inpatient Appointments, 494
- 26-7 Compose Business Correspondence, 503
- 26-8 Compose a Memo, 505

Chapter 27
- 27-1 Pull Patient Records for a Manual Record System, 517
- 27-2 Register a New Patient, 518
- 27-3 Initiate a Patient File for a New Patient Using Color-Coded Tabs, 521
- 27-4 Add Supplementary Items to an Established Patient File, 523
- 27-5 Maintain Confidentiality of Patients and Their Medical Records, 525
- 27-6 File Medical Records Using the Alphabetical System, 538
- 27-7 File Medical Records Using the Numerical System, 539

Chapter 28
- 28-1 Manage an Account for Petty Cash, 547
- 28-2 Post Service Charges and Payments to the Patient's Account, 554
- 28-3 Record Adjustments and Credits to the Patient's Account, 556
- 28-4 Prepare a Bank Deposit, 561
- 28-5 Reconcile a Bank Statement, 565
- 28-6 Explain Professional Fees Before Services Are Provided, 567
- 28-7 Establish Payment Arrangements on a Patient Account, 570
- 28-8 Explain a Statement of Account to a Patient, 571
- 28-9 Prepare Billing Statements and Collect Past-Due Accounts, 573

Chapter 29
- 29-1 Diagnostic Coding, 590
- 29-2 Procedural Coding, 595

Chapter 30
- 30-1 Apply Managed Care Policies and Procedures, 618
- 30-2 Complete the CMS-1500 Claim Form, 626

Chapter 31
- 31-1 Practice Standard Precautions, 642
- 31-2 Properly Dispose of Biohazardous Materials, 644
- 31-3 Perform Proper Handwashing for Medical Asepsis, 649
- 31-4 Perform Alcohol-Based Hand Sanitization, 651
- 31-5 Apply and Remove Clean, Disposable (Nonsterile) Gloves, 652
- 31-6 Sanitize Instruments, 655
- 31-7 Perform Chemical Sterilization, 658
- 31-8 Wrap Instruments for the Autoclave, 662
- 31-9 Sterilize Articles in the Autoclave, 665

Chapter 33
- 33-1 Measure Weight and Height of an Adult, 682
- 33-2 Measure Weight and Length of an Infant, 685
- 33-3 Measure Head and Chest Circumference of an Infant, 687
- 33-4 Measure Oral Body Temperature Using a Mercury-Free Glass Thermometer, 692
- 33-5 Measure Oral Body Temperature Using a Rechargeable Electronic or Digital Thermometer, 694
- 33-6 Measure Rectal Body Temperature Using a Rechargeable Electronic or Digital Thermometer, 696
- 33-7 Measure Axillary Body Temperature Using a Rechargeable Electronic or Digital Thermometer, 698
- 33-8 Measure Body Temperature Using a Tympanic Thermometer, 699
- 33-9 Measure Body Temperature Using a Disposable Oral Thermometer, 701
- 33-10 Measure Radial Pulse, 704
- 33-11 Measure Apical Pulse, 706
- 33-12 Measure Respiratory Rate, 708
- 33-13 Measure Blood Pressure, 710

Chapter 34
- 34-1 Complete a Medical History Form, 719
- 34-2 Recognize and Respond to Verbal and Nonverbal Communication, 726

Chapter 35
- 35-1 Assist with the Physical Examination, 733
- 35-2 Sitting Position, 739
- 35-3 Recumbent Position, 740
- 35-4 Lithotomy Position, 741
- 35-5 Sims' Position, 742
- 35-6 Prone Position, 744
- 35-7 Knee-Chest Position, 745
- 35-8 Fowler's Position, 746
- 35-9 Assess Distance Visual Acuity Using a Snellen Chart, 751
- 35-10 Assess Color Vision Using the Ishihara Test, 752
- 35-11 Assess Near Vision Using a Jaeger Card, 754

Chapter 36
- 36-1 Obtain a 12-Lead ECG Using a Single-Channel Electrocardiograph, 771
- 36-2 Obtain a 12-Lead ECG Using a Three-Channel (Multichannel) Electrocardiograph, 775
- 36-3 Apply and Remove a Holter Monitor, 785

Chapter 38
- 38-1 Perform an Ear Irrigation, 810
- 38-2 Perform an Ear Instillation, 813
- 38-3 Perform an Eye Irrigation, 815
- 38-4 Perform an Eye Instillation, 818
- 38-5 Apply a Tubular Gauze Bandage, 820
- 38-6 Apply an Ice Bag, 826
- 38-7 Apply a Cold Compress, 827
- 38-8 Apply a Chemical Cold Pack, 829
- 38-9 Apply a Hot Water Bag, 830
- 38-10 Apply a Heating Pad, 832
- 38-11 Apply a Hot Compress, 833
- 38-12 Apply a Hot Soak, 835
- 38-13 Administer an Ultrasound Treatment, 836
- 38-14 Measure for Axillary Crutches, 839
- 38-15 Instruct the Patient in Crutch Gaits, 840
- 38-16 Instruct the Patient in the Use of a Walker, 845
- 38-17 Instruct the Patient in the Use of a Cane, 846
- 38-18 Assist in Plaster-of-Paris or Fiberglass Cast Application, 849

Chapter 39
- 39-1 Teach Breast Self-Examination, 858
- 39-2 Assist with a Gynecological Examination, 863
- 39-3 Assist with a Follow-up Prenatal Examination, 875
- 39-4 Instruct the Patient in Obtaining a Fecal Specimen, 879
- 39-5 Test for Occult Blood, 881
- 39-6 Assist with Sigmoidoscopy, 884
- 39-7 Perform Spirometry (Pulmonary Function Testing), 885
- 39-8 Instruct the Patient in the Use of a Peak Flow Meter, 887
- 39-9 Perform Pulse Oximetry, 890

Chapter 40
- 40-1 Use Methods of Quality Control (QC), 899
- 40-2 Focus the Microscope, 903
- 40-3 Complete a Laboratory Requisition, 906
- 40-4 Collect a Specimen for Transport to an Outside Laboratory, 908
- 40-5 Screen and Follow-up on Patient Test Results, 911

40-6	Collect a Specimen for CLIA-Waived Throat Culture and Strep A Test, 913		

- 40-6 Collect a Specimen for CLIA-Waived Throat Culture and Strep A Test, 913
- 40-7 Obtain a Urine Specimen from an Infant Using a Pediatric Urine Collector, 916
- 40-8 Instruct a Patient in the Collection of a Midstream Clean-Catch Urine Specimen, 919
- 40-9 Instruct a Patient in the Collection of a 24-Hour Urine Specimen, 920

Chapter 41

- 41-1 Use a Sterile Disposable Microlancet for Skin Puncture, 931
- 41-2 Collect a Blood Specimen for a Phenylketonuria (PKU) Screening Test, 933
- 41-3 Perform Venipuncture Using the Evacuated-Tube Method (Collection of Multiple Tubes), 935
- 41-4 Perform Venipuncture Using the Syringe Method, 944
- 41-5 Perform Venipuncture Using the Butterfly Method (Collection of Multiple Evacuated Tubes), 947
- 41-6 Separate Serum from a Blood Specimen, 953

Chapter 42

- 42-1 Urinalysis Using Reagent Strips, 963
- 42-2 Prepare a Urine Specimen for Microscopic Examination, 970
- 42-3 Perform a Urine Pregnancy Test, 973
- 42-4 Determine a Hemoglobin Measurement Using a HemoCue, 976
- 42-5 Perform a Microhematocrit Test, 978
- 42-6 Determine Erythrocyte Sedimentation Rate (ESR, Nonautomated) Using the Westergren Method, 980
- 42-7 Prepare a Blood Smear, 984
- 42-8 Perform Cholesterol Testing, 988
- 42-9 Perform Glucose Testing, 989
- 42-10 Obtain a Bacterial Smear from a Wound Specimen, 994

Chapter 43

- 43-1 Prepare and File an Immunization Record, 1019

Chapter 44

- 44-1 Administer Oral Medication, 1038
- 44-2 Apply a Transdermal Patch, 1043
- 44-3 Instruct a Patient in Administering Medication Using a Metered-Dose Inhaler with the Closed-Mouth Technique, 1046
- 44-4 Reconstitute a Powdered Drug, 1049
- 44-5 Prepare a Parenteral Medication from a Vial, 1051
- 44-6 Prepare a Parenteral Medication from an Ampule, 1053
- 44-7 Administer an Intradermal Injection, 1062
- 44-8 Administer a Subcutaneous Injection, 1067
- 44-9 Administer an Intramuscular Injection to a Pediatric Patient, 1071
- 44-10 Administer an Intramuscular Injection to an Adult, 1075
- 44-11 Administer an Intramuscular Injection Using the Z-Track Technique, 1078

Chapter 45

- 45-1 Perform Handwashing for Surgical Asepsis, 1090
- 45-2 Apply a Sterile Gown and Gloves, 1093
- 45-3 Apply Sterile Gloves, 1095
- 45-4 Remove Contaminated Gloves, 1098
- 45-5 Open a Sterile Package, 1099
- 45-6 Pour a Sterile Solution, 1106
- 45-7 Assist with Minor Office Surgery, 1109
- 45-8 Remove Sutures or Staples and Change a Wound Dressing Using a Spiral Bandage, 1119
- 45-9 Apply and Remove Adhesive Skin Closures, 1124

Successful Learning

1

evolve http://evolve.elsevier.com/klieger/medicalassisting

Have you ever read a section of a book and suddenly realized that you had no idea what you had just read? Have you ever re-read the section and still had no idea? Have you ever crammed for a test and passed it (maybe even made an A), but then promptly forgot all that you had learned? If you forgot the material that quickly, you probably memorized it for the test. Will you need that knowledge when you arrive at the workplace? If so, you will likely regret not learning it permanently when you have to waste valuable time relearning it later.

If you are reading this, you probably are interested in learning how to become a successful student. The concepts and techniques in this chapter show you how to become a better student. You will notice that many of these concepts and techniques apply to life in general, as follows:

- Effectively managing your daily schedule enables you to block off time to study. It also allows you to arrive at work on time, run errands, and accomplish everything you need to do in a day.
- Setting goals helps you prioritize your study time. It also helps you decide what is important in your life.
- Managing your stress and staying healthy allow you to perform at your best on tests. They also help you improve the quality of your life.

This chapter helps you understand the importance of good study and organizational skills and teaches you specific strategies and methods to help you accomplish your goals successfully.

LEARNING OBJECTIVES

You will be able to do the following after completing this chapter:

Key Terms
1. Define, appropriately use, and spell all the Key Terms for this chapter.

Am I Responsible for My Own Learning?
2. Distinguish between short-term and long-term memory.
3. List three benefits of good study habits.
4. Explain the role of the student and the teacher in the learning process.

Accomplishing Your Goals
5. Explain the importance of setting goals and managing your time effectively.
6. Explain how to-do lists and day planners can help you balance your studies and your life.
7. Describe how learning or studying habits can be changed.
8. Describe the negative and positive effects of stress.

Successful Study Strategies
9. State four methods for improving your understanding of what you are reading and briefly describe each.
10. State five methods of organizing and reorganizing the information you are learning and briefly describe each.
11. Explain what it means to "learn actively" and why this is important.

Effective Test Taking
12. Describe the four stages of preparing for a test.
13. List nine tips for successful test taking.
14. Explain how you can learn from feedback.
15. Explain the importance of using knowledge gained from a test to prepare for your next test.

Patient-Centered Professionalism

16. Analyze a realistic situation and apply your understanding of effective goal-setting and study strategies to determine the best course of action.
17. Describe the impact on patient care when medical assistants understand and practice strategies for successful study and time management.

KEY TERMS

acronym
anticipation guide
attitude
background knowledge
concept map
day planner
defined purpose
discussion
feedback
flashcards
goals
habit
KWL
learning log
long-term memory

matrix
mind map
mnemonic device
organize
partnered reading
personal mission statement
power notes
prioritize
reorganization
short-term memory
SQ3R
time management
to-do list
Venn diagram
word map

PRACTICAL APPLICATIONS

Read the following scenario and keep it in mind as you learn about the importance of developing effective goal-setting and study strategies in this chapter.

Alex is a student enrolled in a medical assisting class at her local vocational school. The program provides the opportunity to complete the program of study and then take the credentialing examination within 2 weeks.

Alex likes to study with others but has experienced situations in which the others in her study group wanted to play rather than study. She wants to be well prepared to take the examination without having to do a lot of cramming. She notices two other students, Jake and Mary Lou, studying together and approaches them to see if she can join them. They welcome her, and a new study group is formed. As she talks with them, she quickly learns that their study methods are to memorize, pass the test, and move on to the next assignment.

Because they seem to be serious students, Alex decides to stay with them and will try to teach them some new tricks. She also decides that she will schedule some study time to be on her own.

Do you think this arrangement will be helpful to Alex? What would you do in this situation?

AM I RESPONSIBLE FOR MY OWN LEARNING?

Are good study habits really needed to succeed in this class and in your new career? Do you already have good study habits? Could you improve on them? Will there be any benefit for you to take the time to learn additional study skills? The answers to these questions are important because they will help you develop the right attitudes and habits as you learn new information. The answers will also help you develop more confidence and greater self-esteem. Understanding the importance of developing good organization and study habits, as well as some specific strategies for academic success, are steps that will put you on the road to success.

What Is Learning?

Just what is "learning," and how do we do it? We learn when we acquire new knowledge and store it in our **long-term memory.** When we first encounter a new concept or piece of information, it goes into our **short-term memory.** The short-term memory can hold up to seven items or "chunks" of information for just under a minute (the average is only 15 to 20 seconds). After that, the information is either sent to the long-term memory for storage or forgotten. Our long-term memory is similar to a computer; information and skills stored there are saved and can be retrieved for use throughout our lifetime.

There are several ways to learn, including the following:
- *Through study.* We can read to learn new information or to help recall information.
- *Through instruction.* Instruction, or teaching, is used to help introduce us to new information or skills and provide educational experience.
- *Through experience, practice, or repetition.* Most learning occurs as a result of practice or repetition.

Studying and receiving instruction are both important parts of the learning process, but alone they are unlikely to help you move new information into your long-term memory.

Some learning happens, however, when a "light bulb goes on," or when you have what is often called an "aha moment." Those "aha moments" usually are the result of experiences, but they may be accelerated by hearing another person's comment, reading something, or meditating on or thinking about a topic. Have you ever observed a child when he or she realized that a dime was worth more than a nickel or a penny? That is an "aha moment." Experience alone may not produce long-term learning, but when it is followed with much practice and repetition, experience can "kick-start" true learning. Practice and repetition need to be done often to become a part of your long-term memory. Once the concept is ingrained into your memory, however, you will be able to recall it and use it again and again, as you have with the basic addition and subtraction facts and multiplication tables you learned in grade school.

> **FOR YOUR INFORMATION**
>
> EDUCATION
> *Education is a lifelong process. You will need to continue learning and studying long after you complete this program of study. Your employer will expect you to be involved in continuing education. The skills and habits you develop now can help you throughout your lifetime.*

Why Learn Additional Study Habits?

Study skills are the tools you use to put knowledge into your long-term memory. Memorization works well for short-term memory and occasionally for long-term memory, but it is not a dependable tool for most people who need to apply what they have learned in the workplace setting.

Developing good study habits provides the following benefits:
- Developing additional study skills will help you be more efficient with your time.
- You will be able to learn more in less time.
- These skills may also help you quickly learn new information and skills in the future, while on the job, and in your life.

Good study habits are like riding a bicycle. You will never forget them, and you will find them useful every time you pick up a technical book, just as your bicycle riding skills are useful each time you get on a bike. If you are a parent, you may find that you use these skills to help your children in their quest to learn and be successful in school.

Do I Have to Change?

Do you have to change your way of study? No, but you may choose to change because you may find that the idea of saving time by learning more quickly appeals to you. You may also be motivated to put more information needed for your career into your long-term memory to save time spent relearning later. Your motivation may come from your desire to be a good role model for your children and family. It could come from your desire to do well in school and on the job. Change is a choice; you control your decisions.

Am I Really Responsible for My Own Learning?

Who is responsible for your learning? Can you be successful on the job or in life without learning? The only person who can learn for you is *you*. Think of the most successful people you know, whether a homemaker, CEO, sales representative, minister, or president of a nation. These people are constantly learning. Think about some of the things they are learning: new and better ways to run a household, a company, a congregation, or a country. Are they learning by studying, learning from experience, learning from practice, or being taught? Often it is a combination of all these processes. Would they continue to be successful if they were not continuing to learn? Do they accept responsibility for learning, or try to put the responsibility on others? Most likely, no matter whom you chose as your examples of success, they are still learning, especially from their experiences and by studying to stay current in their fields of interest and need.

As with these successful people, you are responsible for your learning. Your teachers are responsible for providing you with experiences and resources from which you can learn. Think of your teacher as an old-fashioned shepherd tending a flock of sheep. The shepherd cannot make the sheep graze, but he can lead them to green pastures where food is abundant. The sheep must take the initiative to actually eat and satisfy their hunger. As a student in the class, you must "graze on the grass" provided by your shepherd, the teacher, to satisfy your "hunger" to prepare for a new career.

Getting Your Money's Worth

Since you are responsible for your own learning, you most likely will also want to "get your money's worth" for the time you spend in school. This means that you will need to use your time wisely. A decision to skip school or classes or to watch TV instead of studying may actually cost you money. Your class content is set up like the foundation of a building, brick by brick. If you take one day off or one brick out of this foundation, the structure falls. Staying away from class causes students to miss big chunks of their foundation, and these chunks cannot be replaced. Everything that you do that does not align with your goal of completing your training or degree can mean that you have to pay for extra time in school and that you will not be employed as quickly, thus losing money in two ways. Wasted time is costly to students, both now and in the future.

> **PATIENT-CENTERED PROFESSIONALISM**
>
> - *What are some ramifications of forgetting content, such as professional standards, ethics, and law?*

ACCOMPLISHING YOUR GOALS

When you made the decision to study medical assisting, you set a **goal** for yourself. Maybe you are just exploring medical assisting as a career option, or maybe you have decided to become a medical assistant. Either way, because you are reading this text, you have committed yourself to study medical assisting.

We set many goals in our lives; some are specific, and some are more general. One point is certain, however: if you do not have a goal, you will *not* achieve it.

Setting Goals

One way to start setting your goals is to develop a **personal mission statement.** A personal mission statement is a statement of your overall life goal or purpose. The mission statement can then be broken down into short-term goals that serve as "steps" to achieving your main life goal (Box 1-1).

Take some time to think about what it is that you want to accomplish. Do you want to "take" a course, do you want to "pass" a course, or do you want to achieve a certain grade in a course (e.g., A, B)? Set specific goals for yourself based on where you are now, where you want to be, and what you can reasonably accomplish in the given time. Box 1-2 shows a technique that can help you choose your goals.

Tips for effectively setting goals include the following:
- You are most likely to achieve goals that are realistic and challenging, yet attainable. Know your limitations and your possibilities.
- You need a way to identify if you have reached your goals successfully. Examples of clear outcomes include attending 100% of your classes, exercising at least 30 minutes every day over a set period, and obtaining a medical assisting certificate.
- You must have enough time and help to succeed.

Although it is an extremely important task, creating a list of goals is easy; the challenging part is to develop a plan and manage your time effectively to achieve these goals.

Managing Time

Once you have decided what you want to do, you need to plan what actions you will take to accomplish your goals. Planning allows you to identify the required resources and time needed to accomplish your goals. Your plan must fit your lifestyle.

BOX 1-1
Developing a Personal Mission Statement

To develop your own personal mission statement, you must answer four questions:
1. *Whose* mission?
2. *What* will I do?
3. *How* will I do it?
4. *Why* will I do it?

The following example describes a student who wants to do well in school and is forming a personal mission statement.

LIFE MISSION

Gracie is a student at a vocational school and wants to use her time and energy to accomplish all her goals. She is starting by forming her mission for her life, then breaking it down to her mission and goals for the months she will be in school.

Gracie decided that her life mission is "to assist people in having a more comfortable life by being a mom and a medical assistant to make the world a better place." Breaking it down, her personal mission statement would look like this:
1. *Who?* Gracie decided.
2. *What?* Her life mission is to assist people in having a more comfortable life.
3. *How?* By serving as a mom and medical assistant.
4. *Why?* To make the world a better place.

SCHOOL MISSION (WORKING TOWARD LIFE MISSION)

Once her mission statement was developed, Gracie went further and stated the mission for her months in school: "My *(who)* mission is to *(what)* successfully complete my studies for medical assisting by *(how)* setting aside time each day to study *(why)* so that I set a good example for my children and get good training so that I am an effective worker."

SHORT-TERM GOALS (WORKING TOWARD SCHOOL MISSION)

Gracie then used the same process to break her mission into goals. One goal was to get good grades during the first grading period by setting aside time each day so that she could learn the material. Another goal was to develop new study skills so that she could use less time studying, yet learn more and still have time to spend with her children.

BOX 1-2
The SMART Way to Choose Your Goals

Goals should make you a more efficient person by allowing you to improve on your weaknesses. One method for choosing goals is by being "SMART":

S Be *specific;* write down each goal.
M Make your goal *measurable.*
A Make your goal *attainable.*
R Make your goal *result oriented.*
T Make your goals *trackable* (i.e., you should be able to follow the steps you have taken to reach your goal).

Goals must be challenging, yet attainable. You must have a way to identify if you have reached your goals successfully. You must have enough time and help to succeed. Goals should be balanced (Figure 1-1) and stated positively. Identify what it is you really want to achieve, not what you want to avoid. Goals change as you grow and as you meet your short-term goals.

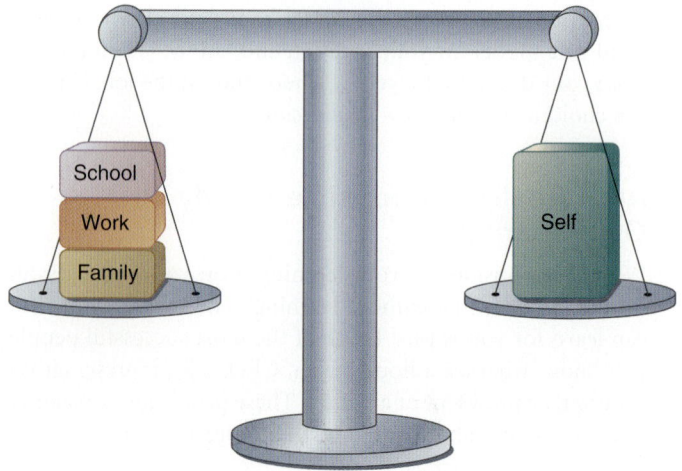

FIGURE 1-1 Goals must be balanced.

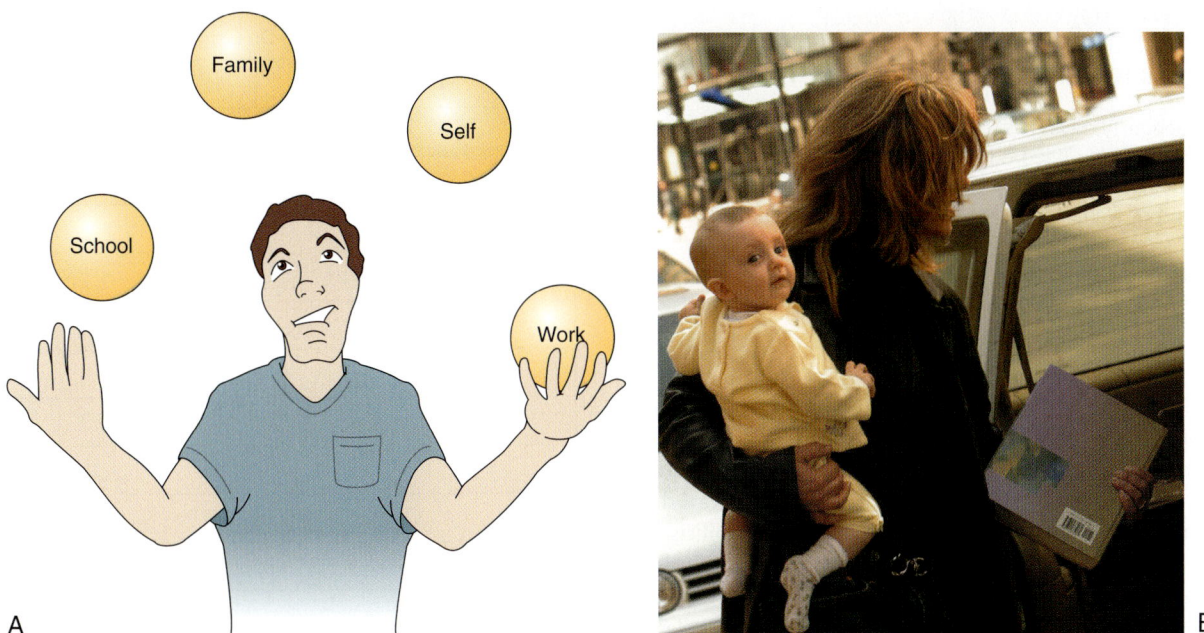

FIGURE 1-2 Learning to juggle your schedule will be a challenge.

Learning how to manage your time helps you continue your job, raise your family, and have time for yourself (Figure 1-2).

Time is often the greatest issue for students. While many students are single with few responsibilities, others have multiple responsibilities as parents, spouses, caretakers, employees, church or synagogue members, and community volunteers. Finding the time to study is a challenge. Fortunately, there are proven ways of organizing your time so that you will be able to accomplish your goals. Setting priorities and making a plan are strategies for effectively managing time.

Priorities

In our lives, some things are important to us and some things are not. The things that are important to us are considered priorities. Because we only have so much time, we must set priorities. **Prioritizing** is deciding which situations require the most attention and then listing each in descending order according to their importance to the situation. This is a learned skill and will improve with experience and practice. On a day when you have only 30 minutes to spare, do you pay bills or watch your favorite TV show? Do you run errands or study? It all depends on your priorities. Priorities can change from day to day and minute to minute. For instance, taking a nap might not be a priority on most days, but if you are recovering from illness or injury, rest may become more of a priority.

To set priorities, a decision must be made as to the importance of each task you need or want to do. We can categorize our tasks to decide which should be done first to accomplish our goals, as follows:

- "Must do," or "Priority A" (or "Priority 1"), tasks are critical to your success. Since they usually have deadlines, they almost always go on this list.
- "Should do," or "Priority B" (or "Priority 2"), tasks can be done after the "A" items are completed. The deadlines are usually a few days off.
- "Want to do," or "Priority C" (or "Priority 3"), tasks have no definite time frame. These are the "if you have time" items.

When you are feeling overwhelmed and trying to find a way to cut back, consider the following consequences:
1. If I do not do the task or activity today, what are the immediate consequences?
2. If I do not accomplish this task today, which of my goals (long term and short term) suffer?

> ### Priorities and Consequences
> Sue's ultimate goal is to make the dean's list this grading period. She has a term paper to finish. It is due tomorrow, and now she has been offered free tickets to a concert she wants to see tonight. If she does not turn her paper in on time, it will result in a lower grade. Her goal is to get on the dean's list, and the lower grade will have a definite negative impact on her ability to make the list. What should she do? Are there other options?

Setting Limits. Everyone starts the day with 86,400 seconds. How you use this time will determine your success with your goals. Effective planning requires choosing the right goals for what you want to accomplish each day. You cannot do more in one day than time permits. When you find that you often do not have enough time in the day to get everything done, take a close look at your situation and see if you can lighten your load by delegating tasks or by saying "no."

BOX 1-3

Why Is It Hard to Say "No"?

- I feel guilty saying "no."
- What if I ever need a favor?
- I want to be liked.
- I do not want to hurt the other person's feelings.
- Others will think I am self-centered.
- I do not want to look like I cannot handle a challenge.
- I do not want to be selfish.

Delegate. Managing your time efficiently sometimes requires delegating tasks to others or simply asking for help. Opting to do everything yourself rather than delegating tasks can be counterproductive in the long run. Remember, you can delegate authority, but you cannot delegate responsibility. For example, you can ask someone to do the laundry, but if he or she does not know how to operate the machine, it probably will not be done correctly. The person to whom you delegate must have the time, capabilities, and resources necessary to complete the task. When you delegate, set completion deadlines and give explicit instructions.

Learn to Say "No." The inability to say "no" can create **time management** problems. When you are asked to take on a new task or participate in an activity, think carefully about whether that activity is really necessary. Will it move you toward your goals? Is it consistent with your life mission? If the answer is "no," you should be cautious of agreeing to do the activity or task. When you say "no," you are free to do other things that meet your personal goals and mission. It is much better to say "no" than to commit to something you cannot or do not have time to do (Box 1-3).

Making a Plan

If you have a plan, you have a road map for accomplishing your goals. It is helpful to have long-term plans as well as short-term plans. A long-term plan might map out your overall goals for a month or even a year. Short-term plans can be developed for a week or even a day. Planning your time to meet your established goals is a skill that takes patience and practice.

To-Do Lists. Successful people usually have a daily plan or **to-do list** to help them accomplish their tasks (Figure 1-3). All the items on the list are prioritized into categories A, B, or C, as described previously. "A" tasks should be completed first (or when they are scheduled, such as attending a class at a specific time; here, "first" means they have priority over "B" tasks), then "B" tasks, and so on (Figure 1-4). When their schedule is interrupted, successful people set a new time to accomplish their tasks. They check or cross off their tasks as they complete them to make sure the tasks get done.

As you are organizing your tasks on the to-do list, make certain they align with your identified goals. Review your goals daily to see what you have accomplished and to make certain everything is listed. Being organized is no accident. At the end of each day, write down tomorrow's list.

FIGURE 1-3 Example of a to-do list.

FIGURE 1-4 Example of prioritized to-do list.

Day Planners and Organizers. The use of a **day planner** or organizer is critical for the success of most students. These can be purchased in most school bookstores as well as in office supply stores. Figure 1-5 shows an example of how one student used a day planner to block off time for study.

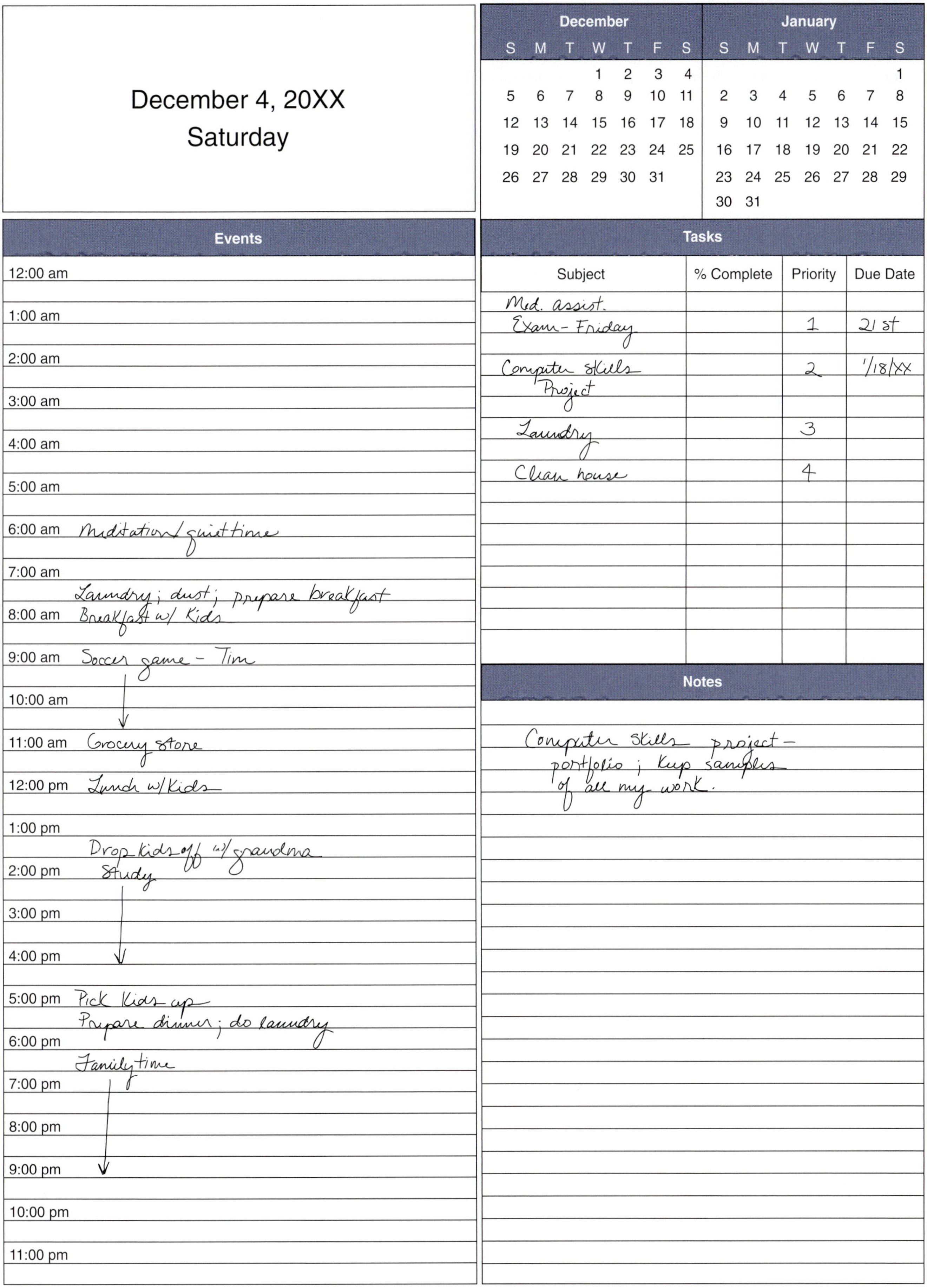

Successful Learning **CHAPTER 1** 7

	December		January
	S M T W T F S		S M T W T F S
	1 2 3 4		1
	5 6 7 8 9 10 11		2 3 4 5 6 7 8
	12 13 14 15 16 17 18		9 10 11 12 13 14 15
	19 20 21 22 23 24 25		16 17 18 19 20 21 22
	26 27 28 29 30 31		23 24 25 26 27 28 29
			30 31

December 4, 20XX
Saturday

Events

12:00 am	
1:00 am	
2:00 am	
3:00 am	
4:00 am	
5:00 am	
6:00 am	Meditation / quiet time
7:00 am	Laundry; dust; prepare breakfast
8:00 am	Breakfast w/ kids
9:00 am	Soccer game – Tim
10:00 am	
11:00 am	Grocery store
12:00 pm	Lunch w/ kids
1:00 pm	
2:00 pm	Drop kids off w/ grandma — Study
3:00 pm	
4:00 pm	
5:00 pm	Pick kids up
6:00 pm	Prepare dinner; do laundry
7:00 pm	Family time
8:00 pm	
9:00 pm	
10:00 pm	
11:00 pm	

Tasks

Subject	% Complete	Priority	Due Date
Med. assist. Exam – Friday		1	21st
Computer Skills Project		2	1/18/XX
Laundry		3	
Clean house		4	

Notes

Computer skills project – portfolio; keep samples of all my work.

FIGURE 1-5 Example of day-planner page.

Planning to Study. Studying is a choice. If you make it a priority, you must set aside time to do it. If you have children or other distractions at home, you may take an extra hour or two to stay at school or go to the library to study. The development of good study habits will reduce the amount of time you use in study, providing you more time for other pursuits.

Students also need to build breaks into their study time. Most educators recommend approximately 2 hours of study in one sitting. A 20-minute break after 2 hours will help refresh you and will prepare your mind to retain more information. Many people like to build into their study schedule a 5-minute walk after an hour to oxygenate the brain better. Breaks should include the following:
- Exercise (usually walking or stretching)
- Water
- Fresh air
- Natural light, if possible

Each of these increases the brain's retention of information and makes your study time more efficient.

Establishing Good Habits

What are some of the habits you have? Do you get up in the morning and brush your teeth? Do you have a habit of eating slow or fast? Do you have habits in your exercise program, or is your way of walking a habit? Which shoe do you put on first? Do you always put certain items, such as keys, in the same place? Understanding how habits develop can help you break bad habits and establish new ones. Doing this will bring down your stress levels and improve your health.

How Habits Develop

When you were young and learning to put on your shoes, did you always put the same shoe on first? Probably not; most likely after a few tries, however, your dominant hand led you to put your shoe comfortably on your dominant foot first. Soon you had done it this way consistently many times over a 21-day period. Finally, it became a **habit**, or a pattern or belief fixed in the brain.

Psychologists state that habits cannot be eliminated; they can only be replaced. To replace a habit, the new habit must be done consistently for 21 to 28 days, and it must be done more than once on most of these days (Box 1-4). After this, the new habit replaces the former pattern or belief.

21-Day Habit

If you want to develop a habit of asking yourself, "What do I already know about the subject of this new chapter in the text?" before you begin to read an assignment, you will first need to identify how you have started reading assignments in the past. If you just picked up the book or article and started to read, skipping the objectives or any other information at the beginning of the assignment, you need to set a goal of replacing that habit with the question, "What do I already know about the subject of this new chapter?" and take time to answer it.

21-Day Habit—cont'd

You may need to "tie a string around your finger" to remind you to start this way. A sticky note with the question written on it can be transferred from chapter to chapter as you work through the book, serving as your reminder until it becomes a habit. After you have done this consistently for 21 to 28 days, it will be a habit, and you will think of the question as you begin to read other resources.

As a student, you should make it a habit to start at the beginning of every chapter. The objectives, introductions, and vocabulary prepare your way for learning.

Stress

Stress can create bad habits. If you repeatedly stay up late at night studying and do not receive enough sleep, you will become fatigued. If your schedule is too full of unnecessary tasks, you may fall into the habit of being late everywhere you go. You will experience stress in both your personal and your professional life, with each stress impacting the others. A bad day at work or school can affect your mood at home, and vice versa. Stress can never be eliminated, but it can often be

BOX 1-4

Forming Good Learning Habits

According to research, students can best put new knowledge into their long-term memory by using it a minimum of 28 times in a 21-day time frame. This means that you will need to use your new knowledge many times in the 3-week time frame after your introduction to the information.

You may want to make a habit of reviewing daily what you have learned in the past few weeks. Instead of learning something, passing the test, and then forgetting it, make a habit of reviewing it daily. You will find that this will save you hours of preparation time for the credentialing examination and that you will go into the examination with more confidence.

It is best if you select a different way of reviewing each day; otherwise it becomes boring, and soon you are just letting the words pass through your mind instead of focusing on them. You can vary your studies in the following ways:
- On one day you might draw a web or map outlining the information you have studied.
- On another day you might use word associations and an anagram.
- The next day you could create "finger plays" or hand signals to help you recall the information.
- You can also change *where* you study. If you like nature, take advantage of good weather and sit outside occasionally to study. Most people like to have their materials in one location (free from distractions such as family or television) and use this as their main location for study, but sometimes moving to the library or outside can bring needed variety.
- Finally, you can change the *background*. Soft music or background noise helps some people learn, but it may distract others. You will need to make your own choice regarding this.

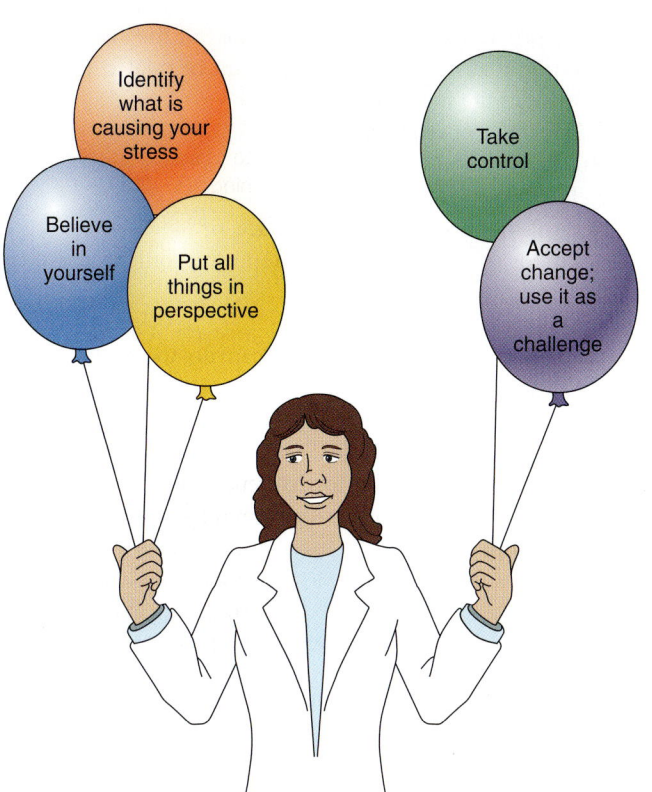

FIGURE 1-6 Managing your stress.

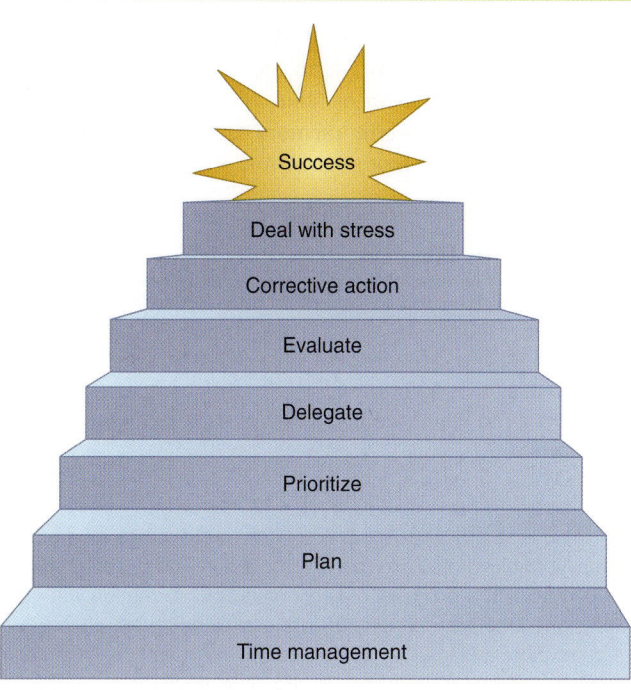

FIGURE 1-7 Steps to success.

reduced or at least managed. Some types of stress can be healthy, whereas other types are unhealthy.

No one is perfect, and trying to be perfect is not healthy. Developing the habit of controlling your situation and your schedule will help you enjoy your constantly changing environment. Relieve stress with activities you enjoy when possible. Just taking a brisk walk, sitting for 5 minutes without interruptions, or taking deep breaths can help. No matter how good you are at time management, however, the human element that makes each day unique can upset the best of plans. You achieve success by managing your time and coping with stressful situations by adjusting to what happens (Figure 1-6). Planning assists you to overcome roadblocks in your way and thus reduces stress (Figure 1-7).

Health

It is important to have healthy habits for living. Eating a well-balanced diet, getting enough sleep, exercising, and avoiding alcohol and recreational drugs not only will keep you healthy, but also will help you in stressful times. Everyone reacts to stress differently. *Positive stress* allows an individual to focus, perform well, and be at peak efficiency. *Negative stress* can have long-lasting adverse effects on physical, emotional, and behavioral health. You will learn more about the negative effects of stress in Chapter 5. If you are experiencing too much stress, you may need to make changes in your lifestyle or daily schedule so that you can be healthy.

Realize that you cannot always change unpleasant situations, but you *can* manage how they affect you. Choose to think positively, to be proactive, and to focus on the present, not the past. Doing these things will help you manage stress and stay healthy.

> **PATIENT-CENTERED PROFESSIONALISM**
>
> - How will goal setting and prioritizing affect your on-the-job performance?
> - How is the care you provide to patients affected when you are less stressed, healthier, and better organized?
> - Why is it important to make effective time management a habit, not just something you do "every once in a while"?

SUCCESSFUL STUDY STRATEGIES

Never before have students had the opportunity to know as much about their learning styles and patterns of learning as they do today. This gives you the opportunity to learn more quickly, more efficiently, and better than students in the past. Today, more is known about long-term memory. This knowledge allows students to do better on credentialing examinations and then recall more when they are on the job. It is an exciting time to be a student. With all this knowledge available, it makes sense to learn more about successful studying and test-taking techniques.

Successful studying means studying and then learning what you have studied, not just memorizing and forgetting. When you first encounter new information or a new idea, your mind stores it in your short-term memory for temporary holding.

Short-term memory can only hold material for about a minute. In addition, short-term memory typically can only hold seven or fewer items or "chunks" of information. Information in the short-term memory is either transferred to long-term memory for storage or forgotten.

> **Short-Term Memory**
>
> Try to memorize each of these lists of seven or fewer random numbers:
> List A: 4, 6, 4, 9, 2
> List B: 8, 3, 1, 7, 0, 2, 8
>   Now try to memorize these lists of eight or more random numbers:
> List C: 7, 2, 4, 3, 6, 9, 1, 2, 5
> List D: 6, 4, 9, 8, 1, 2, 4, 3, 7, 9, 5, 3
>   You probably find lists C and D more difficult to memorize than A and B. If you group the numbers in lists C and D (e.g., 72-436-9125), you have three "chunks" of information instead of eight. Use this "chunking" strategy to help you when you must learn a large number of items. For instance, you can more easily learn the bones of the body if you "chunk" them (e.g., bones of the arm, bones of the skull, bones of the leg).

Long-term memory holds information until it is needed and then retrieves it for use. Storing information into the long-term memory instead of the short-term memory can lead to greater success in your education and in the workplace. The following sections provide practical methods of (1) reading for understanding, (2) organizing to remember, and (3) learning actively.

Reading for Understanding

Many of you have probably experienced this situation since the beginning of this chapter: reading a passage and not remembering what you just read. As you study to become a medical assistant and once you are on the job, you will read a large amount of technical material, and you will need to retain it.

Having a **defined purpose** for reading or studying is important. Each time you pick up a book, you should ask yourself *why* you are reading it and *what* you expect to learn from it. This will help you focus on what you are reading. If the text or article has objectives, read those first to find the focus. If it does not, you can find it yourself by looking at the headings or boldface print in the reading. Your instructor may also give you questions to ask as you are reading. Successful students add their own questions to these to have a strong sense of purpose when reading.

It will be helpful to you now and later to learn strategies for effectively and efficiently reading and understanding what you have read. These strategies will help you move what you have read from your short-term to your long-term memory.

Format of Text

Before you begin reading a section or chapter, you should pay attention to the format of the text. The organization of the material provides clues to the importance of the information. Formatting that may indicate important or related information includes the following:

- Information found in charts
- Definitions
- Text boxes
- Print that is underlined, boldface, or italicized
- Photos or drawings that relate to the content and their descriptions
- Objectives or goals
- Suggestions of activities you can do to enhance your learning
- Use of color or white space
- Use of columns or tables

Paying attention to the format of the text can give you important clues about the main points and concepts you need to understand.

SQ3R

SQ3R is a method used to increase reading comprehension. It is an acronym that spells out the following steps of the technique:

- **Survey:** Begin by looking over the chapter, noting how it is set up. How are the headings set up? Are they centered, or "flush left"? What does this signify?
- **Question:** Next, write questions based on the headings, charts, graphs, and other elements, and place them on the left side of your notebook paper.
- **Read:** Read the text, following the headings and looking for the answers to your questions. Write your answers on the right-hand side of your paper next to your questions.
- **Recite:** Next, recite the information to a partner in your study group, or recite it aloud to yourself. (It is best to do this with another person.)
- **Review:** Finally, review all you have read. Your review may be done in many ways, such as writing one-sentence summaries of each section, creating a **mind map,** or developing an outline.

KWL

KWL (*k*now, *w*ant to know, *l*earned) is another reading strategy that can help bring focus to your reading. To use KWL, answer the following three questions in three columns (Figure 1-8):

Column 1: What do I already *know* about the subject? Brainstorm answers to this question and write them in the first column. Consider what you know and what you need to know.

Column 2: What do I *want to know* about the subject? Think about the gap between what you know and what you want or need to know, and write down your answers.

Column 3: What have I *learned* about the subject? After reading, list what you have learned. If you did not have all your questions from Column 2 answered, you will need to see other sources such as books, videos, the Internet, or your instructor.

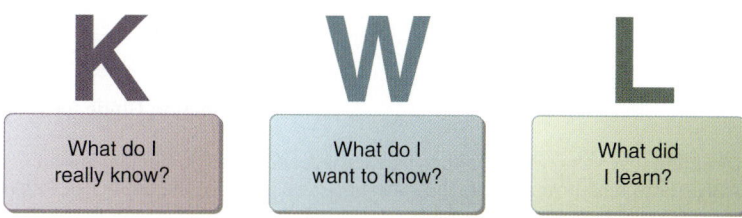

FIGURE 1-8 "KWL" strategy.

Knowing that you have some **background knowledge** of the subject is a confidence builder. Other ways you can use to determine your background knowledge include the following:
- Look at the objectives (found at the beginning of many textbook chapters, including this one) and see how many you know or are able to do.
- Take a "pretest" (either from your teacher or the author, or make your own using chapter headings).
- Use an **anticipation guide**, sometimes provided by your teacher or found in your student manual (Figure 1-9). An anticipation guide allows you to anticipate the answers to challenging questions. You can guess with no penalties and see what you know.

Once you know how much background knowledge you have and whether you can already accomplish any of the objectives, you can adjust your study time to focus on the content you do not know as well. This is investing your time wisely.

Be Active

To improve reading comprehension, you need to *read actively*. Ways you can read actively include taking notes, making outlines, reading out loud or re-reading passages, summarizing passages, writing about what you have read, telling someone else about what you have read, and asking questions. More ideas for active learning are presented in the *Learning Actively* section.

Organizing to Remember

One of the factors that determine whether information will be sent from short-term memory to long-term memory for storage or will be discarded is how the information is organized. Information that is unorganized or is organized in a way that you do not understand will be discarded, whereas information you have organized to understand will be stored.

Organizing

Before you begin to read or study new information, ask yourself how you can **organize** as you study and read to better understand the material. Organizing is putting the information into a form you understand and are likely to remember. Ways to organize information as you read or study include the following:
- Take notes. Do you want your notes to be in question-answer form, mapping form, or do you want to write out summaries of the material in sentences and paragraphs? You can even create "raps" or poems to help you remember.
- Write out questions.
- Use sticky notes to emphasize certain information.
- "Chunk" or group the information into classifications (remember, aim for seven or fewer groups or chunks).
- Use **mnemonic devices.** Mnemonic devices are memory "tricks" that help you organize information before you attempt to store it in your memory. A mnemonic device may be a story, song, poem, or word (an **acronym** made up of the first letter of each word to be remembered). A mnemonic used to remember the atrioventricular valves is LAB RAT—*l*eft *a*trium: *b*icuspid; *r*ight *a*trium: *t*ricuspid. Another example to help you remember the order of the cardiac valves in the circuit is "TRI before you BI"—*Tri*cuspid valve is located in the right side of the heart, and *bi*cuspid valve is located in the left side of the heart. "Blood flows through the *tri*cuspid *before* *bi*cuspid."
- Do selective underlining or highlighting of your notes (or your text if this is allowed).
- Create a chart.
- Do a word or **concept map** (Figure 1-10). To begin a concept map, write the concept in the center. Then draw an arm out from the concept, draw or write out a subconcept, and surround the subconcept with relevant information. You can continue several layers into the information you are mapping.
- Make a **Venn diagram** (Figures 1-11 and 1-12). A Venn diagram allows you to compare and contrast information. Circles are used for the topics being compared. The circles are arranged so that they overlap. The overlapping areas are where similarities are listed, and the other areas are used to list the differences.
- Develop a hypothesis (theory), then read the material to prove it right or wrong.
- Use a **matrix.** A matrix, sometimes called a *semantic feature analysis,* allows you to chart features of a topic. Figure 1-13 is an example of nutrients in foods in the form of a matrix.
- Use **flashcards.** Write a question or term on the front of an index card. On the back of the card, write an answer. Continue until all required material is on an index card. Shuffle the index cards and look at the card on top. Try to answer the question or explain the term. If you can answer the question or explain the term, put the card off to the side. If unable to answer, look at the answer on the back of

Name_____

Anticipation Guide for Chapter 1

Directions: Working with a partner, take turns reading each statement in Part I. If you believe the statement is true, put a check in the AGREE column. If you believe the statement is false, check the DISAGREE column. Be ready to explain your answer to each other and the class. Do not look at notes or at a book. You will have a chance later to check these resources and see how many questions you knew or guessed right.

Part I

AGREE	DISAGREE		
_____	_____	1.	Learning is the acquisition of new knowledge into short-term memory to quote back to the teacher on a test.
_____	_____	2.	Teachers are responsible for students' learning.
_____	_____	3.	In order to establish a new habit, it needs to be repeated consistently over a 21-day period of time.
_____	_____	4.	It is a waste of time to look over a book or chapter before starting to read.
_____	_____	5.	By reorganizing the content of a chapter into notes, concept maps, pictures of concepts, etc., you are helping to place new information into your long-term memory.
_____	_____	6.	A matrix or semantic feature analysis allows you to reorganize information into a quick and easily remembered format.
_____	_____	7.	SQ3R is a good way to create a defined purpose and to help remember what you have read.
_____	_____	8.	People learn best by teaching a concept to another person.
_____	_____	9.	Metacognition refers to the confidence that you have in knowing the content that you are studying.
_____	_____	10.	It is wise to go through a test and answer the easiest questions first. This creates self-confidence and helps you approach harder questions with more confidence.

Directions: You may use your textbook to find support for your answers. If the information supports your previous choice, put a check in the SUPPORT column. Use the IN YOUR OWN WORDS column to add any additional details from the resources. If the information does not support your choice, put a check in the NO SUPPORT column. Write a true statement in your own words.

Part II

SUPPORT	NO SUPPORT		IN YOUR OWN WORDS
_____	_____	1.	_____
_____	_____	2.	_____
_____	_____	3.	_____
_____	_____	4.	_____
_____	_____	5.	_____
_____	_____	6.	_____

FIGURE 1-9 Example of anticipation guide.

Successful Learning **CHAPTER 1** 13

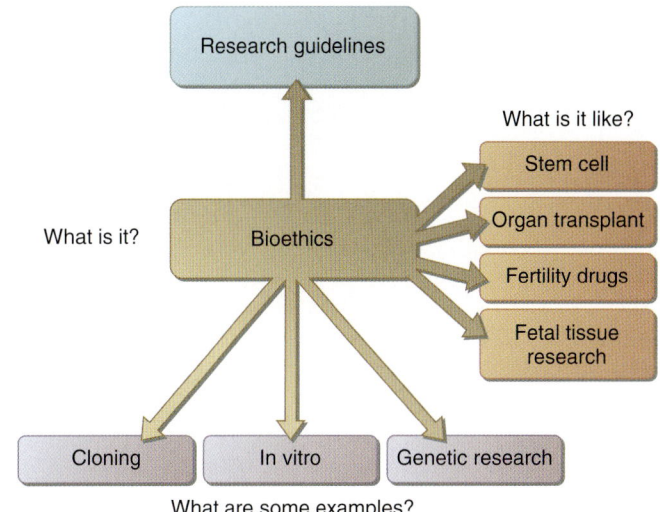

FIGURE 1-10 Concept map.

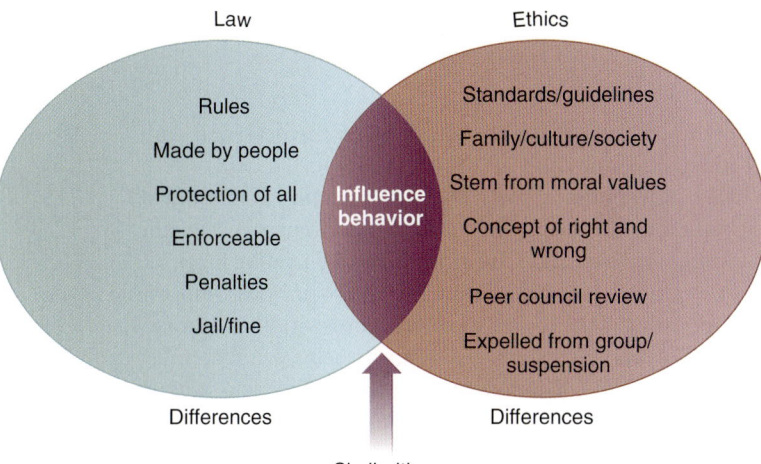

FIGURE 1-11 Example of a Venn diagram: law versus ethics.

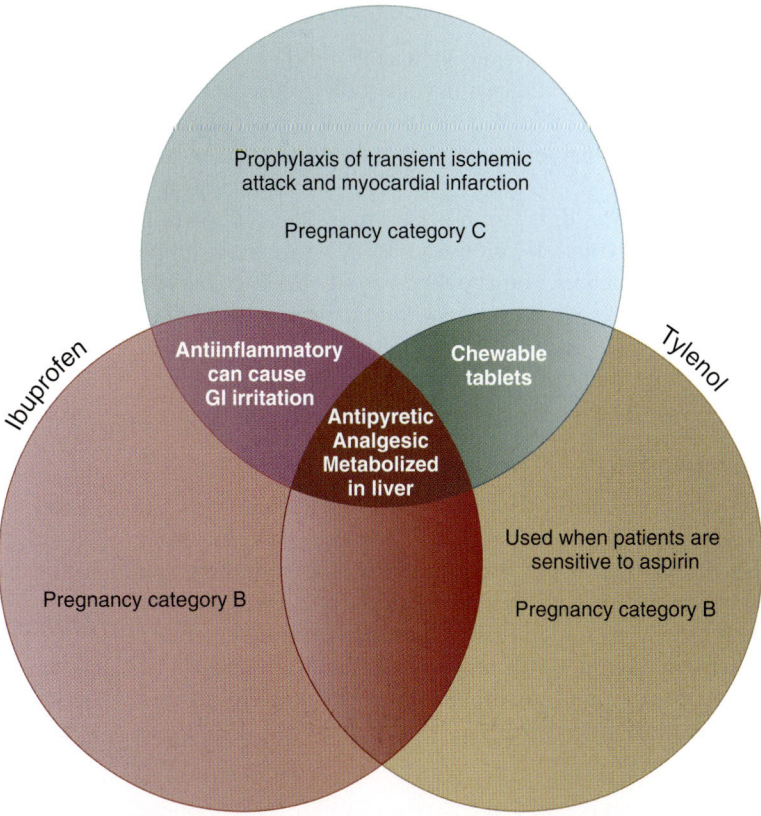

FIGURE 1-12 Example of a Venn diagram: aspirin.

Nutrients/Foods	Apples	Broccoli	Bananas	Iceberg lettuce	Cantaloupe	Carrots	Corn	Mustard greens
Vitamin A	~	x	~	~	x	x	x	x
Vitamin C	~	x	~	~	x	~	~	x
Thiamin	x	x	x	x	x	x	x	x
Riboflavin	x	x	x	x	x	x	x	x
Niacin	x	x	x	x	x	x	x	x
Carbohydrates	x	x	x	~	x	x	x	x
Fat	~	~	~	~	~	~	~	~
Protein	~	~	~	~	~	~	~	~
Calcium	~	x	~	~	~	~	~	x
Iron	~	x	~	~	~	~	~	x
Water	x	x	x	x	x	x	x	x

x = Some value
~ = Trace or none

FIGURE 1-13 Example of a matrix: nutrients/foods.

the index card. Place the card back in the deck and continue until you know all the information.
- Take **power notes.** Power notes are a simplified method of outlining that helps you make connections between the concepts presented in the lecture or in the reading material. Power notes help you determine the main ideas and the supporting details. You may use words or short phrases and occasionally sentences. *Simplicity* helps you remember the main ideas. The following outline shows you how to begin developing power notes (compare to example in Figure 1-14):
    Power 1: Main idea.
        Power 2: Detail or support for main idea.
            Power 3: Detail or support for power 2.

Sharing your notes, concept maps, or other organizing activities with other students in your study group allows you to learn from each other. You may have seen things differently than others or may have grasped concepts that others did not.

Learning styles differ from person to person, and there is no one best method. If you learn best by writing everything out in full sentences, you should do so. If you learn best by remembering key words, you may want to develop the skill of power notes. If you tend to remember things in groups of three or four items, you may want to create groupings. The bottom line is to use the method that works best for you.

Reorganizing
Sometimes organizing the information to study is not enough to help you understand it. At times you may need to rearrange the information or put it into a different form to help you comprehend the concepts. **Reorganization** in a variety of ways helps your mind to use multiple senses and remember better. For example, you may organize into groupings that make sense to you because they are numerically alike, because they begin with the same letter, or because they are in the same

```
            Power notes

    Power 1: Drug classifications
        Power 2: Analgesics
            Power 3: Tylenol
                     Aspirin
                     Ibuprofen
```
FIGURE 1-14 Example of power notes.

classification. Then, you may reorganize it in one of the other ways to reinforce your understanding. If you used an outline to take notes, reorganize your notes into a concept map, Venn diagram, or some other form. Doing this forces you to look at the concepts in a different light and helps you understand them more completely.

Learning Actively
Making sense of what you read, of the lecture you attend, and of the audiovisual supplements you see and hear is essential for long-term memory. When students cannot make sense out of what they are expected to learn, frustration results, and some quit trying, perhaps dropping out of the program of study. To make sense of what you are expected to learn, you need to be actively involved in it. Since you are involved in a job preparatory program, you likely will be encouraged to become actively involved in applying the content, as well as using some of the study strategies presented in this chapter, to activate your learning. There are ways you can learn actively while reading, writing, and studying with other students.

Reading Actively
When you are reading, you can make it an active process by doing any of the note-taking, organizing, reorganizing, or reading comprehension (e.g., SQ3R, KWL) techniques. It also

helps to ask yourself questions as you go, checking to see if you know the answers. Think about how what you are reading applies to your own life or job. If you do not know the answer to a question, research it or ask your instructor for help.

Writing Actively

If you are taking notes, writing a summary, or developing a concept map, you are writing. However, this may not be adequate to learn all the concepts you will need to complete this program of study. You will have specific assignments with this text that will encourage you to write. Just as organizing and reorganizing helps move concepts into your long-term memory, so does writing. However, simply copying is not an acceptable form of writing for learning. Copying does not engage your mind and does not have a defined purpose. You may be able to memorize what you have copied, but it will not transfer to long-term memory for use in the future on your credentialing examination or on the job. Learning logs are methods of using writing to help transfer knowledge into your long-term memory.

Learning Logs. **Learning logs** are very informal and do not require fancy penmanship; they are "for your eyes only." After a lecture, video, reading assignment, or other learning activity, sit down and write everything that you can remember that was in the activity. Do not worry about whether your form is correct; just write everything you can recall. If you have questions that need clarification, add them into your learning log. You can even include your emotions and reactions to what you learn. To enhance your learning further, you can read and share your learning log with a partner. This allows you to give and receive a response using your discussion skills and helps clarify ideas and information. You may learn from reading or hearing your partner's ideas. Figure 1-15 provides an example of a learning log.

Learning logs can also be written in creative forms, such as a letter to your partner or a friend. Another idea is to begin your learning log before you listen to the lecture or read the chapter by writing out what you already know, what you anticipate learning about, and later concluding with what you have learned (another form of a KWL). In general, learning logs should be kept simple; they are not for a grade, but for learning. Use a style that is comfortable so you can focus on the *purpose,* not perfection.

Classroom Activities and Discussion

You can learn actively whether you are reading, studying, or writing at home or sitting in class. One of the most common methods of active involvement is simply asking questions, especially thought-provoking questions. Your instructor may provide opportunities in class for experiments, interviews, and role playing. Take advantage of such activities by participating to maximize your learning. In addition, participation in groups that make decisions about issues of interest to medical assisting students will help you think through topics in your program of study and will guide you in your growth toward becoming a credentialed medical assistant.

Classroom Activities. Students who are effective at gathering information from the lectures and reading material interact with the information and reorganize it into a format that is easy for them to understand. As they listen and read, they jot down questions, make predictions as to what will happen, reorganize the content, compare and contrast ideas, and visualize outcomes. These are all activities that help transfer information into the long-term memory.

Discussion. **Discussion** is when you talk about what you have studied or read. Many teachers provide class time for discussion in small groups or with the whole class. It is important that every student have the opportunity to talk; however, if you do not have this chance in class, you will need to find another way. For example, you and some fellow students may form a study group in which you each have equal opportunity to discuss what you have read, seek clarification from each other, or explain concepts to each other. People learn best by teaching a concept to another person, so this is very important. Saying the concepts out loud and explaining them to someone else is a critical aspect of transferring information from short-term to long-term memory. You can use the following techniques when discussing concepts you are learning:

- If you are working in a study group or cooperative learning group, the use of *prediction questions* can help you learn and prove to be beneficial discussion time. Participants in the group question each other about what they predict will be covered in the next section of reading material, or about what could happen in the medical office if the scenario offered in the text occurred. Examples include questions

FIGURE 1-15 Learning log sample.

A professional = somebody who acts right to the customers. They are loyal. They go beyond the call of duty. They are honest. They show up to work on time, and don't miss a lot of days. They let the boss know when they will be late, which is rare. You can depend on them - they do what they say they will do.

Professionals act like they like their job. It is not just a matter of having a snobbish attitude - they may not even dress fancy. They come to work to do their job, and do it well. They talk to people nicely. They use "we" instead of "I" when they talk about the business - don't act like they own the whole thing when we all know they don't. They are friendly, but have boundaries, and are not overly talkative.

such as "What do you think the remainder of the chapter will be about?" or "Why do you think so?" or "What do you predict will happen?"
- Many teachers give students the opportunity to discuss with class assignments (e.g., oral reports, team assignments) or with small group discussions. These are all to your benefit, even if you are a person who prefers to work alone. **Partnered reading** is an effective technique to help synthesize what is being read. Partnered reading involves two partners. Partner A reads a paragraph (or other assigned portion), then stops for Partner B to summarize what was read. Partner A can ask questions of Partner B if needed. Partner B then reads a paragraph, and Partner A summarizes it, with clarification questions asked by Partner B. The process continues until the reading is completed. This method may seem time-consuming, but it actually saves time in the long term because with increased comprehension, re-reading and restudy are rarely needed.

> **PATIENT-CENTERED PROFESSIONALISM**
>
> - *How are patients affected when you learn efficiently and have the necessary skills and knowledge stored in long-term memory?*
> - *How can learning actively and applying strategies for improving reading, studying, and writing help you improve your skill as a medical assistant while on the job?*

EFFECTIVE TEST TAKING

When it comes to taking tests, everyone reacts differently.
- Some students "freeze" when it comes to exams. They feel they know the material, but when they try to transfer it from their mind to the paper, a block seems to occur, and they are unable to transfer the information to paper.
- Other students seem to have no trouble and fly through the test, but they worry later about how they did. They question whether they answered correctly on certain parts.
- Some students take the test, walk out, and have no memory of what was even on the exam.

How students "feel" about tests varies a great deal; how they prepare varies as well.
- Some students cram the night before, whereas others study a short time every day for several days before the exam.
- Some students work every problem or do every activity in the textbook in preparation.
- Some decide that they know the material and that studying will not help.
- Other students seem not to care and do little or nothing in preparation.

What is your attitude toward test taking? Do you face tests with fear, with confidence, or with indifference? Your attitude is a key to your success when you take an examination, so it is important to determine if you need to do a little "attitude adjustment." **Attitudes** are habitual ways of thinking, and because habits can be changed, attitudes can also be changed. You will need to practice the new way of thinking for a minimum of 21 consecutive days; do you remember why?

Learning strategies for preparing for and taking tests, as well as learning from your performance on a test, will help you develop better test-taking habits and attitudes. Remember the following:

> If you always think what you've always thought,
> You'll always get what you've always got.
> Change your thoughts and your life will change.
> *Author Unknown*

Preparing for the Test

There are several steps, or phases, in preparing effectively for a test.

Step 1: Review how you did on your last examination.
- If you missed questions on the last exam, was there a pattern to the type of question that you missed, or were all the questions that you missed on the same topic? For example, did you only miss questions that were easy, or did you miss all the questions on anatomy? Perhaps all the questions you missed involved a math skill. Your answers will help you prepare for your next exam. If you missed questions that were easy, what can you do to better prepare to answer those types of questions? If you missed all the questions on anatomy, could that lack of knowledge about anatomy cause you to miss questions on the upcoming exam? Examining the questions you missed shows you what skills and knowledge need more practice. Chances are high that you will need the skills or knowledge on another exam, on a credentialing exam, or on the job.
- Do you need to ask for assistance from the teacher, seek help from another student, or secure a tutor? Will spending extra time in study and practice be adequate?
- Consider the importance of repetition and practice as you make your decisions.

Step 2: Obtain as much information as possible about the test.
- Check with your instructor to find out which of the objectives in the syllabus and text will be covered, what types of questions will be asked, and whether the instructor has any advice about how to prepare.
- If you have missed any class notes or materials, be sure you obtain copies from fellow students. Check their accuracy against the textbook.

Step 3: Start early.
- Three weeks (21 days) is ideal, although your instructor may not have given you this much time. With whatever time you do have, spread out your study time in small increments over the days you have available.
- Schedule time to review the concepts that are on the exam, and use various methods each day. For example,

on the first day you may choose simply to read the concept or make notes about the concepts you already know well. On the second day you might make notes and create a concept map or web with them. On the third day you might take the vocabulary words and do a **word map.** On the fourth day you might take the vocabulary words and phrases and complete concept maps. On the fifth day you might create a chart of major concepts, followed by a matrix on the sixth day.

- Make a list of questions that you need to have clarified, and work with your study group or teacher to clarify them.
- On one day, write the questions that you would put on the examination if you were the teacher.
- Create flash cards by transferring them to 3 × 5 or 4 × 6 cards, and write the answers on the back. When you have a few minutes, read the questions and answer them to yourself or to a friend. Check to make sure you were correct. Soon the information will become second nature to you. These cards can go with you anywhere and can help you make good use of waiting time (e.g., physician's office).
- Study with others only after you have confidence that you know most of the material. Teaching is the best method of learning, so assist students who missed class by teaching them, and you will benefit in the process.

Step 4: Get adequate sleep and rest the night before the exam.

- Gather and organize all the resources you need, including pencils, paper, your uniform, and tools for any skills test.
- Eating a light breakfast that includes some protein helps prepare your mind for mental work.
- Exercise will help oxygenate your brain, so you might park a little farther from the building and walk briskly to the examination site.
- Deep breathing also helps supply your brain with oxygen. This helps you think more clearly and relax.
- Water is essential to a well-functioning brain, so bring a bottle of water to the examination site, if allowed. Otherwise, be sure you drink plenty of water.
- If you still feel uncomfortable with a concept, review it just before the exam.
- Gather your materials and report to the room a little early, making sure your pencils are sharp or your ink pen is full.
- If the test includes a skills section for which you will need your uniform and some medical tools, make sure you have them organized and ready.

Taking the Test

You can follow several steps to help increase your performance when taking a test.

Step 1: Take a deep breath and relax.

- Most likely, you will have instructions to be quiet. This is because most students do their best concentrating in a quiet room, or one in which classical music is playing.
- Relax, and let yourself enjoy the environment.

Step 2: Listen carefully to instructions (or read them carefully).

- The instructions are very important, so listen carefully, or read them before you begin to take the exam.
- If you are allowed to mark on the test, underline or highlight any special instructions. Have you ever taken an examination where the instructions stated that you were only to answer the last question, and turn in your paper? If you skip the instructions on such an exam, you will work much too hard!

Step 3: Skim the test.

- Make sure you know what to do in each section.
- Plan your time, especially if it is a timed exam.

Step 4: Begin answering questions immediately.

- Start by answering the easy questions. This will help build your confidence and ensure that you answer these questions correctly. Also, if you run out of time, you will have completed the easy questions, which will help your final score.
- If there are multiple-choice questions, make sure you read all the choices, even if an answer seems obvious. The question may have an option of "all of the above" or some key word that may make it more difficult than a first glance would indicate (Box 1-5).

BOX 1-5

Tips for Answering Multiple-Choice Questions

- Questions that contain the word "not" need to be studied more carefully because they may be confusing.
- Do not look for hidden meaning or read extra meaning into the questions.
- Concentrate on the *stem* (question that is being asked). Make certain you understand what is being asked.
- Think about the *context* of the question. On a chapter test the question relates to the context of the chapter, not another topic.
- Before you read the options (a, b, c, d), think through what you believe to be the correct answer. If that answer is not provided, re-read the question. Did you understand the question correctly?
- Think about which option is the best answer. Sometimes possible options can distract you from the correct answer. Use your critical thinking skills to evaluate each option and then select the answer that is the best, even if more than one answer could be correct.
- If some choices are obviously wrong, eliminate them.
- Look for similarities in the choices. If three are similar and one is different, the different one may be the correct answer.
- Look for answers that are comprehensive.

- If you are unsure about some questions, make educated guesses. Use the process of elimination to guess difficult multiple-choice or matching questions. After you eliminate answers that are not right, you can select the best answer from the remaining options. If there are words you do not know, use context clues to help you define them, or use your skills at breaking words into suffixes, prefixes, and root words. Use material on the test itself to help you answer the more difficult questions.
- To answer essay questions, make a quick outline or power notes of what you want to include. Then write out your answer. Proofread it to be sure you have answered the question. Bluffing your way through an essay question will not give you points from most instructors.
- If the test is long and has questions you are unsure of, you may use a coding system. Write a "3" next to a very difficult question, a "2" next to a difficult question, and a "1" next to those you feel confident about. Answer the 1s first, then the 2s, then the 3s. (Only use this method if your instructor allows you to write on the test.)

Step 5: Proofread what you have done.
- Check your answers to make sure you have not made any errors.
- Check your math, and be sure that short answers and essays really answer the question.

Step 6: Take a deep breath, relax, and turn in your paper.
- Have confidence that you have done your best.

Learning from Feedback

As a student taking responsibility for your own learning, it is important that you use the feedback provided to you, as well as the feedback you produce yourself, to help you grow and do better in achieving your objectives and goals. **Feedback** is the evidence of your growth, progress, or mastery provided to you by instructors. Feedback also shows you where you can make improvements. Feedback on homework, tests, and other assignments can help you focus your energy into areas that will most benefit you.

Feedback comes from your instructors in many forms, including grades, written or oral comments, and facial expressions. Grades are the most common type of feedback. Whether represented by numbers, percentages, or letters, grades give you a sense of how you are doing in comparison to the standards established by your teacher.

Analyzing Tests for Feedback

Successful students often analyze their tests, including pretests, when the tests are returned to them. After a test is graded, look over it carefully so that you know what you missed and can study more on those topics. You can spend less time on the topics you already know.

Successful students look for patterns in the questions missed, and they check to be sure they did not miss questions because of carelessness or rushing. For example, did you miss only questions about the heart, answering all other questions about organs correctly? Did you miss only questions about suffixes and prefixes? Were there vocabulary words that confused you? Looking for patterns and identifying them can help you know what you need to restudy. Failure to learn what you missed on an examination can hinder you on future exams because the remainder of your program content is likely based on the knowledge needed for this exam.

If questions were missed because of carelessness or rushing, it is important for you to develop the habit of reviewing your test before turning it in. You may also want to slow down, mark answers more carefully, or even use a ruler to be sure your questions and answers are aligned correctly.

Other Types of Feedback

You can also receive valuable feedback from your instructors and by tracking your own progress.

Instructor Feedback. The most beneficial feedback to you as a student is coaching feedback. *Coaching feedback* identifies what you are doing well but also gives directions on areas where you need to improve. The instructor may even suggest methods for improvement in weak areas. For example, if a medical assisting student is having difficulty locating the proper position for placement of the electrodes on a patient for an electrocardiogram (ECG), the instructor may suggest that the student find each location on himself or herself.

Written comments by your instructors can be extremely valuable; you should read them carefully to help you set your study and work plans for the next unit or for additional work on the existing unit. If you keep a learning log in which you identify how you are doing on each objective for your program of study, you can compare your instructor's comments to your own learning log.

Feedback from your instructor may occasionally hurt. Be mature and realize it is for your own good and is designed to help you grow, not to destroy you. The teacher is not "out to get you." Use the comments and feedback to help you improve. Your future bosses will appreciate you more.

Self-Monitoring. You can also take responsibility for your feedback. One method is to chart your progress, creating a run chart or bar graph indicating how you are doing on your assignments or tests. This would be similar to a chart maintained by a sports enthusiast preparing for a race. Just as runners or racewalkers would track number of calories, time spent in exercise, and their weight loss, you can track time spent on completing assignments and doing homework with your grades on assignments and tests. This will help you learn to track yourself and may assist you in seeing the connection between your effort and your grades. For example, if you do not get a good night's sleep and do poorly on a test, this can become evident to you on your grade-tracking system and you will be able to make better decisions in the future. You can also track the number of objectives you have accomplished for the program of study, the time frame required to accomplish each, and the evidence that you have retained the knowledge that you have gained.

Keeping track of your grades also allows you to compare your grades with the instructor's grade book.

Preparing for Your Next Examination

After you take an examination and receive feedback, you can begin to prepare for your next examination by analyzing your performance, using the following questions:
- What did you learn from taking your last examination?
- Did you learn that you were careless and made mistakes that cost you points?
- Did you learn that you consistently missed true-false questions?
- Did you learn that you did not know enough about how the organs of the body function, for example, or the procedures for submitting an insurance claim?

In preparing for your next exam, it is important to take the results of your analysis and use them to assist you in doing better. Your study plan may need to include an additional question each day on the topic you do not feel confident about, or you may need to talk with your teacher about your need to understand how a particular type of question (e.g., true-false) is written.

PATIENT-CENTERED PROFESSIONALISM

- What might happen if you crammed and passed a test about a concept such as location of the bones in the body, but then forgot the information when you were on the job because you had only memorized, not learned?
- How can good test-taking skills help you even after you have completed your credentialing examination?

CONCLUSION

Effective study and organizational habits are very important skills as you prepare for your career as a medical assistant. By continuing your good habits and replacing any bad habits with better ones, you can gain more time to spend with family and friends. You can also feel more confident about your knowledge and skills, and later you will be able to review for your credentialing examination without feeling the need to cram. You can go into your clinical duties and your first job with the confidence that you have learned the material well.

These skills will also serve you well in your future life. You may be able to teach these skills to your children and grandchildren, for example, thus helping them to be more successful in their school careers. Good study and organizational habits are keys to success in your program of study; effective learning and time-management habits are keys to success in life.

Your behavior, time-management skills, achievement of goals, and ability to work under pressure are all used by patients to measure your level of professionalism. Being organized assists in reducing stress in the workplace and ultimately benefits the patient.

Chapter Summary

Reinforce your understanding of the material in this chapter by reviewing the curriculum objectives and key content points below.

1. **Define, appropriately use, and spell all the Key Terms for this chapter.**
   - Review the Key Terms if necessary.
2. **Distinguish between short-term and long-term memory.**
   - Long-term memory is similar to a computer. It stores information and skills so that you can retrieve them when necessary throughout your life.
   - Short-term memory holds small amounts of information for short periods and then either sends the information to long-term memory to be stored or discards it.
3. **List three benefits of good study habits.**
   - Good study habits help you become more efficient with your time.
   - They help you learn more effectively in less time.
   - They prepare you for learning the rest of your life.
4. **Explain the role of the student and the teacher in the learning process.**
   - As a student, you are responsible for your own learning.
   - Your teacher is responsible for providing you with resources and opportunities to learn.
   - Your role is to make use of these resources and opportunities and make the most of your learning.
   - Good study habits are a choice.
5. **Explain the importance of setting goals and managing your time effectively.**
   - A life mission provides focus and allows you to set yearly, monthly, weekly, and even daily short-term goals.
   - Setting goals allows you to prioritize your daily tasks.
   - Effective time management helps you accomplish what you need to do and plan time for what you want to do.
6. **Explain how to-do lists and day planners can help you balance your studies and your life.**
   - To-do lists and day planners can help you determine goals for each day (what you plan to accomplish).
   - These tools help you keep track of the tasks you need to do to accomplish your goals.

- Time can be blocked off for study and for everyday tasks.
- Activities can be prioritized so that the most important ones are accomplished before the least important ones.

7. **Describe how learning or studying habits can be changed.**
   - Habits need to be replaced, not eliminated.
   - The new behavior must be consistently repeated for 21 to 28 days until it becomes a habit.

8. **Describe the negative and positive effects of stress.**
   - Positive stress allows an individual to focus, perform well, and be at peak efficiency.
   - Negative stress can have long-lasting adverse effects on physical, emotional, and behavioral health.

9. **State four methods for improving your understanding of what you are reading and briefly describe each.**
   - Understanding how the author has constructed the article or book will guide you to a quicker understanding of the content.
   - Using various methods to reorganize the content of the chapter will help you assimilate the information more quickly.
   - Thinking through what you already know about a topic provides background information, to which you can add new information, and gives you self-confidence.
   - Having a purpose for reading is more productive than just reading because it is an assignment.
   - Recognizing what you know and realizing what you do not know is an important part of the learning process.

10. **State five methods of organizing and reorganizing the information you are learning and briefly describe each.**
    Organizing information helps transfer it to long-term memory for storage.
    - Take notes: be concise, underline, and highlight.
    - "Chunk" information into blocks or groups.
    - Use mnemonic devices ("memory tricks" or acronyms), using the first letter of each word to be remembered (e.g., LAB RAT).
    - Create charts (columns and rows) to sort information.
    - Develop a hypothesis (theory), then read to prove it right or wrong.
    - Reorganizing information helps you see it in a different light and understand it more completely.
    - Learn actively: engage yourself in the material and make it your own.
    - Read actively: question the material, apply it, and research it.
    - Write actively: do not copy material, but rework it so that you remember it.
    - Use learning logs to recall the material.

11. **Explain what it means to "learn actively" and why it is important.**
    - Learning actively requires your participation, not just your attention. Knowledge gained this way will become long-term memory.
    - Discussing and writing what you have read helps solidify it in your mind.

12. **Describe the four stages of preparing for a test.**
    - Review your last exam, and learn from your previous mistakes.
    - Ask your instructor for guidelines; know what to study.
    - Start early; cramming creates stress.
    - Eat and sleep adequately the night before; feed your body and your brain.

13. **List nine tips for successful test taking.**
    - Plan to arrive early and come equipped with needed materials.
    - Make sure you understand the instructions for the test clearly, whether oral or written.
    - Carefully analyze the test questions, and budget your time.
    - Answer the easiest questions first.
    - Know the strategies for picking multiple-choice answers.
    - Answer all the questions even if you have to guess.
    - Look for context clues to confirm your answers.
    - Briefly outline essay questions; this will save you time in the long term.
    - Stop periodically; stretch, refocus your eyes, and take a deep breath.

14. **Explain how you can learn from feedback.**
    - Feedback on a test will help you prepare for the next exam, as well as for learning the next block of material.
    - Feedback helps you adjust what you are doing to correct errors and to make you more efficient.

15. **Explain the importance of using knowledge gained from a test to prepare for your next test.**
    - Consistent study habits will prevent you from feeling the need to cram and store information into your short-term memory, soon to be forgotten.
    - Learning from your mistakes can help you budget your test preparation time wisely.
    - Looking for patterns on questions that were missed on previous tests can help you improve your performance on future tests by giving you clues on what and how to study.

16. **Analyze a realistic situation and apply your understanding of effective goal-setting and study strategies to determine the best course of action.**
    - Understand your own preferences, strengths, and weaknesses, and develop a study plan that fits your life.
    - Effective study will help you store knowledge in your long-term memory so that you can use it in the future.

17. **Describe the impact on patient care when medical assistants understand and practice strategies for successful study and time management.**
    - When medical assistants have mastered the knowledge and skills they need to perform their duties, they will be prepared to provide quality care to patients.

PRACTICAL APPLICATIONS

If you have accomplished the objectives in this chapter, you will be able to make better choices as a medical assistant. Take another look at this situation and decide what you would do.

Alex is a student enrolled in a medical assisting class at her local vocational school. The program provides the opportunity to complete the program of study and then take the credentialing examination within 2 weeks.

Alex likes to study with others but has experienced situations in which the others in her study group wanted to play rather than study. She wants to be well prepared to take the examination without having to do a lot of cramming. She notices two other students, Jake and Mary Lou, studying together and approaches them to see if she can join them. They welcome her, and a new study group is formed. As she talks with them, she quickly learns that their study methods are to memorize, pass the test, and move on to the next assignment.

Because they seem to be serious students, Alex decides to stay with them and will try to teach them some new tricks. She also decides that she will schedule some study time to be on her own.

Do you think this arrangement will be helpful to Alex? What would you do in this situation?

1. What are some advantages to Alex trying to stay with a study group whose skills are not as refined as hers?
2. What are three study skills you would suggest that Alex teach Mary Lou and Jake?
3. How will these suggested study skills help take the fear out of taking the exam?
4. Alex, Mary Lou, and Jake will need to set priorities as they determine how to use their time. What steps would you suggest they follow?
5. What are some advantages for Alex to have study time alone, away from her new friends?
6. How will working on a study team help Alex to be better prepared to work on a medical team?

WEB SEARCH

1. **Research stress to learn how it can be good for an individual and how it can also be a warning signal.** All people are constantly under stress. When does stress become a problem?
   - **Keywords:** Use the following keywords in your search: stress, management of stress, emotional wellness.
2. **Create a bibliography of books and articles on time management.** Why has so much been written on this subject? Management of time is critical for both students and professionals. How will your use of time while you are a student affect your use of time when you are on the job?
   - **Keywords:** Use the following keywords in your search: time management, goal setting.

2 Becoming a Professional

evolve   http://evolve.elsevier.com/klieger/medicalassisting

Have you ever gone into a medical office and had to wait until the receptionist finished a personal phone call before acknowledging you standing there? How did it make you feel? Did you have the feeling that this person was not very concerned about you as a patient? Some may think all it takes to be a professional are the technical skills to do the job, but this is not the case. Professionalism not only includes technical skills, but also requires that you learn and apply professional social skills when dealing with patients. A medical assistant who is respectful and courteous and shows concern for a patient's well-being demonstrates a professional approach to patient care. The medical receptionist in the above example was neither respectful nor courteous and showed more concern for the personal phone call than for your well-being as a patient at the medical office.

With practice and dedication to the principles of the medical assisting profession, you can become a true professional. This chapter provides guidelines that will help you understand what it means to be a professional.

LEARNING OBJECTIVES

You will be able to do the following after completing this chapter:

Key Terms
1. Define, appropriately use, and spell all the Key Terms for this chapter.

Professional Qualities
2. List six characteristics of a professional medical assistant and briefly describe the importance of each.
3. List three abilities needed by a professional medical assistant and explain the significance of each.
4. Give an example that shows the importance of a professional personal appearance.
5. State 10 steps you can take to project a professional personal appearance on the job.

The Professional Medical Assistant
6. List eight administrative duties a medical assistant may perform regularly.
7. List eight clinical duties a medical assistant may perform regularly.

Professional Training
8. Explain the purpose of accreditation.
9. Explain the significance of becoming credentialed in medical assisting.

10. Explain the importance of maintaining professional competence through continuing education.

Patient-Centered Professionalism
11. Analyze a realistic medical office situation and apply your understanding of professional qualities and characteristics to determine the best course of action.
12. Describe the impact on patient care when medical assistants appear and behave professionally.

KEY TERMS

AAMA	diplomacy
ABHES	efficiency
administrative	empathy
ambulatory	ethical standards
AMT	ethically
CAAHEP	integrity
clinical	professional
CMA	punctuality
compassion	reliability
competence	resume
compromise	revalidation
confidential	RMA
consensus	tactful
dexterity	

PRACTICAL APPLICATIONS

Read the following scenario and keep it in mind as you learn about becoming a professional in this chapter.

Robert is a medical assistant in a medical office. His responsibility is to draw blood samples at 8 AM, but he often does not show up until 8:15 AM or later. The scheduled patients must wait and be late for work or must reschedule their appointment. When Robert does arrive, often his uniform is blood stained and wrinkled and he has not shaved or bathed before coming to work. Even if another staff member has started drawing blood, the daily operation of the office is already behind schedule. Robert also has a habit of taking a break between patients.

As the office slips even further behind with more patients waiting, Robert draws the blood but does not take time to label the tubes with the patient's name or complete the laboratory request forms. When Robert makes mistakes, the office staff must make the corrections, resulting in even more delays and confusion about which tube of blood belongs to which patient.

One day Robert is sick and stays home but does not call the office. By 8:30 AM, patients have filled the waiting room, and patients coming to see the physicians have no place to sit. The office has insufficient staff, and the patients and the office personnel are stressed.

Robert's lack of professionalism is affecting both patients and staff. What would you do differently from Robert?

PROFESSIONAL QUALITIES

What is a professional? How can you tell if others think of you as a professional medical assistant? A person who displays certain positive characteristics and demonstrates **competence** when performing tasks is thought of as a **professional.** Professionals are expected to behave according to the **ethical standards** of their chosen profession. Your personal characteristics, your professional abilities, and your personal appearance all contribute to your professionalism.

Professional Characteristics

When physician-employers are asked to identify personal qualities expected of their employees, dependability, loyalty, a positive attitude, integrity, diplomacy, and confidence top the list. These qualities are important because they have a positive impact on everyone in the workplace.

Dependability

Dependability is one of the most important qualities for medical assistants to have. If you are dependable your co-workers and the patients you care for can trust you to do your job well. Being dependable means being punctual, efficient, and reliable.

- **Punctuality** (being on time) is necessary for the office to run smoothly. If you are late, the regular routines of the office are delayed.
- **Efficiency** also helps the office run smoothly. You are efficient when you perform your tasks on time and accurately to the best of your ability.
- **Reliability** means that you do your job well and others can count (rely) on you. Patients and co-workers alike are relying on your presence; they trust you to be there.

Call to report an absence on those few occasions when you are unable to be at work. Poor attendance also affects the proper functioning of the office. When you are absent, someone else has to perform your duties. This places stress on the other employees.

You will not be considered dependable if you are late too often or take too many days off. Although you may not be a medical assistant yet, think about how dependable you are as a student. Are you punctual? Are you efficient about doing schoolwork? Can you be relied on to attend class? If not, these are all areas you can work on right now. Many employers will not hire a person who has a reputation for not being dependable. When a potential physician-employer asks your instructor about your attendance and work habits, how will your instructor be able to respond?

Loyalty

A medical assistant displays loyalty to a physician-employer in several ways, including, but not limited to, the following:
- Producing quality work all the time.
- Giving that extra push to finish the job in any situation.
- Showing good work habits consistently.
- Supporting team leaders and members by accepting decisions.
- Behaving according to the ethics of the profession.

When you begin a new job as a medical assistant, your physician-employer may not know you very well. Over time, as you prove you are dependable, competent, and trustworthy, the employer will become more loyal to you as an employee. In the same way, you will become more loyal over time to a physician-employer who shows dependability, competence, and trustworthiness.

Positive Attitude

Can you think of someone you know who has a "positive attitude"? People with positive attitudes are easy to recognize by their behavior. A positive attitude is often reflected in the tone of voice (pleasant, confident) or body language (smiling, walking with confidence, holding the head high).

You may see the following qualities in professionals with a positive attitude:
- Enthusiastic about work.
- Goal oriented.
- Seek new learning opportunities for growth.

> **BOX 2-1**
>
> **Guidelines to Effective Teamwork**
>
> 1. *All team members must share responsibility for success.* Quality patient care is achieved when all members of the team work toward a common goal.
> 2. *The team must agree to support decisions made.* If the goal of the team is to provide quality patient care, each team member must have a voice in how the goal will be achieved. The physician-employer, however, is the final decision maker. If the physician's staff does not agree with the decisions made, patient care will not be a team effort.
> 3. *Each team member needs to be flexible as changes occur.* Changes in health care techniques and laws present new challenges. The new Health Insurance Portability and Accountability Act (HIPAA) regulations, for example, may require medical office teams to alter policy or develop new policies to comply with confidentiality requirements.
> 4. *All team members must frequently evaluate progress toward goals.* Staff meetings allow goal evaluation to take place on a regular basis.
> 5. *Each team member must understand the importance of his or her role in providing quality patient care.* When individual team members do their part, the goal is fully accomplished.

- Have a good working relationship with others; are "easy to work with."
- Accept criticism and use it to improve.
- Are team players working toward common goals.
- Use "we," not "I"; they understand that quality patient care cannot be provided by only one person.
- Flexible; adjust to change easily.
- Take initiative to see all work completed.
- Look at the "big picture"; understand how one decision impacts the entire office.
- Want what is best for the medical practice.

A positive attitude is contagious in the workplace. One positive attitude can change the tone of the whole team over time. The team approach allows all members of the medical practice to contribute to the care, health, and well-being of the patient (Box 2-1).

Integrity

A person who has **integrity** is honest and straightforward. A strong emphasis is placed on this quality in the medical office. A health professional must be regarded as being trustworthy and having high moral character. As a medical assistant you will handle **confidential** (private) information and materials. Your physician-employer also needs to be able to trust you to handle money. Integrity is **ethically** doing the right thing, even when it is difficult. It means choosing to do what is right for all people, even though it may not always be what you personally want to do.

Diplomacy

Diplomacy (tact) helps build good relationships between people. Building a good relationship with patients and co-workers is based on the ability to be **tactful** (considerate and thoughtful). Patients who are ill, have been injured, or have had to sit in the waiting room for a long time may be anxious or upset. Showing courtesy, **compassion** (providing a sensitive emotional support), and **empathy** (understanding how people feel by putting yourself in their place) shows your respect for the patients. The medical assistant must have an inward desire to reduce the emotional suffering of another by showing a special kindness to those in need. You may not always agree with a patient's concerns, but you must always be tactful and show understanding. Likewise, stressful situations may arise in the medical office between co-workers. Be thoughtful and considerate of your co-workers to help the whole team work more effectively together.

Confidence

Confidence is an important quality for a health professional. If you are confident in your abilities as a medical assistant, you will be able to make decisions and provide leadership. Confident medical assistants can provide leadership by giving direction, communicating well, and offering encouragement to others. They address problems immediately, offer options, and will **compromise** (make a decision based on mutual agreement) or move toward **consensus** (majority opinion) of the group when possible. They have the ability to prioritize and handle unexpected situations by using a decision-making process (a series of steps to find an answer to a problem). You can develop leadership skills by frequently using common sense and learning from past experiences.

Professional Abilities

In addition to these personal qualities, a medical assistant must also have strong technical abilities. Competence, dexterity, and the ability to communicate effectively are needed to perform everyday duties.

Competence

Competence is the ability to get things done on time and correctly. A competent health professional can perform his or her duties well. Being a competent medical assistant does not mean you have to know everything. However, it does mean that you understand the implications of your actions. It also means you know when to ask for help and where to find it when needed.

Dexterity

Dexterity is the ability to move with skill or ease. Medical assistants must be able to lift, assist patients with movement when necessary, and operate multiple pieces of automated equipment (e.g., urine analyzer, HemoCue). These machines process valuable information in a short time, and mastery is needed to use the equipment's full potential. Medical assistants also need manual dexterity, which is the ability to move the hands with skill or ease. You will use your hands for office duties such as keyboarding, as well as for medical procedures such as taking blood pressure or drawing blood.

Effective Communication

Health professionals must have the ability to communicate effectively with patients and co-workers. You need good English skills when writing and speaking to communicate effectively. You also need to be aware of what your facial expression communicates to patients.

English Skills. Having a good vocabulary, being able to spell, and knowing the rules of English grammar are required in the workplace. Clear, understandable speech and proper use of grammar often make good first impressions. Since you may be the first member of the medical staff who speaks to a new patient calling to make an appointment, you need to create a good first impression of the medical staff. Communication is covered in more detail in Chapters 7 and 8.

Facial Expression. Can you tell how someone is feeling by the expression on his or her face? Absolutely; when you smile, for example, the patient understands that you care. Smiling is the appropriate way to greet both patients and co-workers; it says that you are pleased to see them. Also, the person at the other end of the phone line can usually feel your smile while you are talking on the phone. Would you want to walk into a medical office for an appointment and be greeted with a frown or an "I don't care" expression? It certainly would not make you feel welcome or confident about those caring for you.

Professional Image

Even though you may have all the desirable personal qualities and abilities of a medical assistant, if your image is not professional, patients and co-workers may think you are incapable of doing a good job. All health professionals, including medical assistants, need to be concerned with the image their personal appearance creates.

Personal Appearance

People need only a few seconds to form a first impression. Whether it is "fair" or "right," most of this impression is based on the person's appearance, with some based on the person's ability to communicate. First impressions are crucial. You have to make a good first impression during your interview to be hired. Once hired, you need to make a good impression on patients and co-workers. You can make a good professional impression on others by being in good health, being well groomed, and dressing appropriately for the workplace (Table 2-1). When people see that you take pride in yourself, they will have more confidence in your abilities. Your professional appearance can influence a person's final opinion of you as a medical assistant (Figure 2-1).

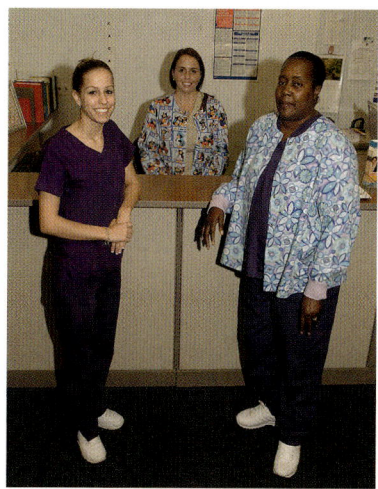

FIGURE 2-1 The properly dressed medical assistant presents a professional and positive image to patients.

PATIENT-CENTERED PROFESSIONALISM

- Why do the medical assistant's professional characteristics, professional abilities, and professional image sometimes make a difference in whether a patient will sue for an error in treatment?
- How do arriving on time, performing duties efficiently, and being dependable affect patients? How can a medical assistant help the office schedule stay on track?
- How does a medical assistant's appearance affect patients?
- What professional qualities and abilities do you currently possess? How can you improve in weaker areas?

THE PROFESSIONAL MEDICAL ASSISTANT

Medical assisting is a profession. To understand the profession and become a professional, you need to know about the professional duties of medical assistants, as well as the types of professional training available.

Professional Duties

Medical assistants perform a variety of duties depending on the type of **ambulatory** (walk-in) health care setting in which they are employed. Remember that a medical assistant works under the direct supervision of the physician and on his or her license. Medical assistants use **administrative** (office protocols and finances), **clinical** (patient care), and general *(core)* skills to assist in running the office smoothly (Boxes 2-2 and 2-3). The duties a medical assistant may perform clinically vary from state to state based on state law, policies, and procedures. You will learn more about administrative duties in Section 4 and about clinical duties in Section 5.

TABLE 2-1
Professional Appearance*

What to Do		Reasons
PERSONAL HYGIENE		
Body	Bathe or shower daily	Removes bacteria that could be harmful to patients.
	Use deodorant	Helps keep you healthy.
		Removes odors that can make others uncomfortable.
Teeth	Brush and floss teeth and use mouthwash	Helps keep you healthy.
		Removes odors that can make others uncomfortable.
GROOMING		
Hair	Away from face and off the shoulders or collar	Keeps hair from blocking your vision or falling on patients.
	Styled neatly	Does not distract co-workers or patients.
	Clean	
	No extreme colors	
	No ornaments or decorations	
Fingernails	Clean	Long or sharp fingernails can injure patients.
	Nail polish (clear)	Colored nail polish is inappropriate.
	Practical length (just over top of fingers)	Long fingernails can harbor bacteria.
Makeup	Minimal	Does not distract co-workers or patients.
Perfume, aftershave	Very little, if any	Many people are allergic to these fragrances.
Jewelry	As little as possible	Can injure patients.
	Rings: wedding ring only	Can harbor bacteria.
	Wrists: simple wristwatch only	
	Earrings: one pair only; lower lobe of ears; small studs—no dangle earrings	
	No body piercing except earrings	
DRESS		
Uniform	Clean and pressed	Dirty uniform can harbor bacteria.
	Fits properly	Improper fit or untucked shirt can interfere with your work.
	In good condition (no tears or stains)	
	Stain-resistant material	
	Neat, with shirt tucked in	
	Meets office dress code	
	Worn with undergarments (should not be visible beneath uniform)	
Stockings	Clean	Stockings or white socks help to present a professional image.
	No holes or tears	
	White socks acceptable	
Shoes	Comfortable and supportive	Supportive shoes keep your feet comfortable when standing and walking all day.
	Fit properly	
	Clean and polished	Exposed feet or toes can become injured or contaminated by splashes or spills and can spread bacteria.
	Laces clean	
	No open-toe shoes or sandals	Canvas shoes stain easily, can harbor bacteria, and are not supportive.
	No canvas shoes	
OTHER		
	No gum or candy	Good posture helps you avoid injury and strain.
	No tobacco odors	Anything that can distract patients or co-workers should be avoided.
	Maintain good posture	
	Cover visible tattoos	

*A professional appearance puts patients at ease, inspires confidence, and makes a good impression.

BOX 2-2

Occupational Analysis of the CMA (AAMA)

Competency in all areas (administrative, clinical, and general) should be presented utilizing manual and state-of-the-art methods. All skills require decision making based on critical thinking concepts.

Invasive procedures must be taught to clinical competency.

Patient care **instructions** should encompass all phases of the life cycle: pediatric, adult, and geriatric.

Adaptations for special needs patients should be addressed.

ADMINISTRATIVE SKILLS
Administrative Procedures
- Schedule, coordinate, and monitor appointments
- Schedule inpatient/outpatient admissions and procedures
- Apply third-party and managed care policies, procedures, and guidelines
- Establish, organize, and maintain patient medical record
- File medical records appropriately

Practice Finances
- Perform procedural and diagnostic coding for reimbursement
- Perform billing and collection procedures
- Perform administrative functions, including bookkeeping and financial procedures
- Prepare submittable ("clean") insurance forms

CLINICAL SKILLS
Fundamental Principles
- Identify the roles and responsibilities of the medical assistant in the clinical setting
- Identify the roles and responsibilities of other team members in the medical office
- Apply principles of aseptic technique and infection control
- Practice Standard Precautions, including hand washing and disposal of biohazardous materials
- Perform sterilization techniques
- Comply with quality assurance practices

Diagnostic Procedures
- Collect and process specimens
- Perform CLIA-waived tests
- Perform electrocardiography and respiratory testing
- Perform phlebotomy, including venipuncture and capillary puncture
- Utilize knowledge of principles of radiology

Patient Care
- Perform initial-response screening following protocols approved by supervising physician
- Obtain, evaluate, and record patient history employing critical thinking
- Obtain vital signs
- Prepare and maintain examination and treatment areas
- Prepare patient for examinations, procedures, and treatments
- Assist with examinations, procedures, and treatments
- Maintain examination/treatment rooms, including inventory of supplies and equipment
- Prepare and administer oral and parenteral (excluding intravenous [IV]) medications and immunizations (as directed by supervising physician and as permitted by state law)
- Utilize knowledge of principles of IV therapy
- Maintain medication and immunization records
- Screen and follow-up test results
- Recognize and respond to emergencies

GENERAL SKILLS
Communication
- Recognize and respect cultural diversity
- Adapt communications to individual's understanding
- Employ professional telephone and interpersonal techniques
- Recognize and respond effectively to verbal, nonverbal, and written communications
- Utilize and apply medical terminology appropriately
- Receive, organize, prioritize, store, and maintain transmittable information utilizing electronic technology
- Serve as "communication liaison" between the physician and patient

Legal Concepts
- Perform within legal (including federal and state statutes, regulations, opinions, and rulings) and ethical boundaries
- Document patient communications and clinical treatments accurately and appropriately
- Maintain medical records
- Follow employer's established policies dealing with the health care contract
- Comply with established risk management and safety procedures
- Recognize professional credentialing criteria
- Identify and respond to issues of confidentiality

Instruction
- Function as a health care advocate to meet individual patient needs
- Educate individuals in office policies and procedures
- Educate the patient within the scope of practice and as directed by supervising physician in health maintenance, disease prevention, and compliance with the patient's treatment plan
- Identify community resources for health maintenance and disease prevention to meet individual patient needs
- Maintain current list of community resources, including those for emergency preparedness and other patient care needs
- Collaborate with local community resources for emergency preparedness
- Educate patients in their responsibilities relating to third-party reimbursements

Operational Functions
- Perform an inventory of supplies and equipment
- Perform routine maintenance of administrative and clinical equipment
- Apply computer and other electronic equipment techniques to support office operations
- Perform methods of quality control

Courtesy American Association of Medical Assistants, Chicago, IL.

BOX 2-3

American Medical Technologists Registered Medical Assistant Task Listing

I. **GENERAL MEDICAL ASSISTING KNOWLEDGE**
   A. **Anatomy and Physiology**
      1. Body systems
      2. Disorders and diseases of the body
   B. **Medical Terminology**
      1. Word parts
      2. Medical terms
      3. Common abbreviations and symbols
      4. Spelling
   C. **Medical Law**
      1. Medical law
      2. Licensure, certification, and registration
   D. **Medical Ethics**
      1. Principles of medical ethics
      2. Ethical conduct
      3. Professional development
   E. **Human Relations**
      1. Patient relations
      2. Interpersonal relations
      3. Cultural diversity
   F. **Patient Education**
      1. Identify and apply proper communication methods in patient instruction
      2. Develop, assemble, and maintain patient resource materials

II. **ADMINISTRATIVE MEDICAL ASSISTING**
   A. **Insurance**
      1. Medical insurance terminology
      2. Various insurance plans
      3. Claim forms
      4. Electronic insurance claims
      5. ICD-9/CPT coding applications
      6. HIPAA-mandated coding systems
      7. Financial applications of medical insurance
   B. **Financial Bookkeeping**
      1. Medical finance terminology
      2. Patient billing procedures
      3. Collections procedures
      4. Fundamental medical office accounting procedures
      5. Office banking procedures
      6. Employee payroll
      7. Financial calculations and accounting procedures mathematics
   C. **Medical Secretary-Receptionist**
      1. Medical terminology associated with receptionist duties
      2. General reception of patients and visitors
      3. Appointment scheduling systems
      4. Oral and written communications
      5. Medical records management
      6. Charting guidelines and regulations
      7. Protect, store, and retain medical records according to HIPAA regulations
      8. Release of protected health information adhering to HIPAA regulations
      9. Transcription of dictation
      10. Supplies and equipment management
      11. Medical office computer applications
      12. Compliance with OSHA guidelines and regulations of office safety

III. **CLINICAL MEDICAL ASSISTING**
   A. **Asepsis**
      1. Medical terminology
      2. State/federal universal blood-borne pathogen/body fluid precautions
      3. Medical asepsis/surgical asepsis procedure
   B. **Sterilization**
      1. Medical terminology associated with sterilization
      2. Sanitization, disinfection, and sterilization procedures
      3. Record-keeping procedures
   C. **Instruments**
      1. Specialty instruments and parts
      2. Usage of common instruments
      3. Care and handling of disposable and reusable instruments
   D. **Vital Signs/Mensurations**
      1. Blood pressure, pulse, and respiration measurements
      2. Height, weight, and circumference measurements
      3. Various temperature measurements
      4. Recognize normal and abnormal measurement results
   E. **Physical Examinations**
      1. Patient history information
      2. Proper charting procedures
      3. Patient positions for examinations
      4. Methods of examinations
      5. Specialty examinations
      6. Visual acuity/Ishihara (color blindness) measurements
      7. Allergy testing procedures
      8. Normal/abnormal results
   F. **Clinical Pharmacology**
      1. Medical terminology associated with pharmacology
      2. Commonly used drugs and their categories
      3. Various routes of medication administration
      4. Parenteral administration of medications (subcutaneous, intramuscular, intradermal, Z-tract)
      5. Classes or drug schedules and legal prescription requirements for each
      6. Drug Enforcement Agency regulations for ordering, dispensing, storage, and documentation of medication use

BOX 2-3

American Medical Technologists Registered Medical Assistant Task Listing—cont'd

    7. Drug reference books (*PDR, Pharmacopeia, Facts and Comparisons, Nurses Handbook*)

G. Minor Surgery
1. Surgical supplies and instruments
2. Asepsis in surgical procedures
3. Surgical tray preparation and sterile field respect
4. Prevention of pathogen transmission
5. Patient surgical preparation procedures
6. Assisting physician with minor surgery, including set-up
7. Dressing and bandaging techniques
8. Suture and staple removal
9. Biohazard waste disposal procedures
10. Instruct patient in presurgical and postsurgical care

H. Therapeutic modalities
1. Various standard therapeutic modalities
2. Alternative/complementary therapies
3. Instruct patient in assistive devices, body mechanics, and home care

I. Laboratory Procedures
1. Medical laboratory terminology
2. OSHA safety guidelines
3. Quality control and assessment regulations
4. Operate and maintain laboratory equipment
5. CLIA-waived laboratory testing procedures

    6. Capillary, dermal, and venipuncture procedures
    7. Office specimen collection such as urine, throat, vaginal, wound cultures, stool, sputum, etc.
    8. Specimen handling and preparation
    9. Laboratory recording according to state and federal guidelines
    10. Adhere to the medical assistant scope of practice in the laboratory

J. Electrocardiography
1. Standard, 12-lead ECG testing
2. Mounting techniques for permanent record
3. Rhythm strip ECG monitoring on lead II

K. First Aid
1. Emergencies and first aid procedures
2. Emergency crash cart supplies
3. Legal responsibilities as a first responder

TASK INVENTORY NOTE

The tasks included in this inventory are considered by American Medical Technologists (AMT) to be *representative* of the medical assisting job role. This document should be considered dynamic to reflect the medical assistant's current role with respect to contemporary healthcare. Therefore tasks may be added, removed, or modified on an ongoing basis. Medical assistants that meet AMT's qualifications and pass a certification examination are certified as a Registered Medical Assistant (RMA).

Courtesy American Medical Technologists, Rosemont, Ill.

One advantage of a career in medical assisting is the cross-training in both administrative support functions and clinical duties. If you should decide to seek training in another health profession, such as nursing or physical therapy, your administrative and clinical knowledge and skills would be great assets in your further training.

PATIENT-CENTERED PROFESSIONALISM

- Why is it important for medical assistants to only perform those duties within their scope of training?
- What would you do if a patient or another health professional asked you to do something for which you were not trained?
- How do the transdisciplinary skills of a medical assistant affect the care patients receive?

PROFESSIONAL TRAINING

As you can see, medical assistants must master many administrative and clinical skills. Completing training programs, seeking credentials, and continuing your education are ways you can learn the knowledge and skills you need to be a successful medical assistant.

Training Programs

There are many types of training programs for medical assistants, and they vary in length. Some training programs have gone through the process of *accreditation*, which involves a review of the program by an agency that establishes standards and guidelines for training. The purpose of this voluntary process is to help training programs set, achieve, and maintain educational goals. The following nationally recognized accrediting agencies for medical-assisting programs are:

- Commission on Accreditation of Allied Health Education Programs (**CAAHEP**)
- Accrediting Bureau of Health Education Schools (**ABHES**)

Although formal training is not a requirement for employment as a medical assistant, it is encouraged in many states because of the multiple skills involved in the profession. Another reason to graduate from an accredited program is that you then become eligible for professional credentialing (e.g., CMA or RMA).

FOR YOUR INFORMATION

MEDICAL ASSISTANT TRAINING AND THE LAW

- Each state may have a statute, which lists the tasks that may be performed in that state by a medical assistant. A medical assistant must inquire into and understand the laws of the state where he or she lives.
- Some states require that medical assistants register with their state for a small fee.
- After taking and passing either the AMT or the AAMA national certification examination, a medical assistant will receive a credential. All medical assistants nationwide practice under a physician's direct supervision whether they have or have not received a credential.

BOX 2-4

Why Seek a Credential?

A *credential* is a title that signifies a person has attained certain competency standards. Passing a national exam tells employers and patients you have successfully achieved a standardized body of knowledge.

A credential allows an employer to make a hiring decision using an applicant's educational qualifications. Education, as well as other factors, sets this applicant apart from an individual who only has on-the-job training. Remember, a graduate of medical school must be licensed to begin practicing medicine. This requires not only the schooling, but also passing rigorous examinations.

Why is it not enough for a medical assistant to go through extensive education with hands-on training? Why bother to obtain a credential? Both questions can be answered if you review why you went to school. Did you go to school just to learn some skills or to get a job, or did you go to school to achieve your full potential? "Being the best you can be" requires that you take the time to tackle a national certification examination.

Credentials

One way to promote professionalism is by joining your professional organization and becoming credentialed after taking an examination (Box 2-4). Both the American Association of Medical Assistants (**AAMA**) and the American Medical Technologists (**AMT**) are nationally recognized associations for credentialing opportunities. The AAMA offers certified medical assistant (**CMA** [**AAMA**]) certification, and the AMT offers registered medical assistant (**RMA**) certification. Both the CMA (AAMA) and the RMA credentials are types of national certification (Figure 2-2).

As a professional medical assistant, being a member of a professional organization allows you to have a voice in public policy concerning the practice of medical assisting. It also provides opportunities for continuing education and networking with other medical assistants, both of which are ways to stay current in the profession. It is important to be involved in an organization that will continue to support you as a medical assistant.

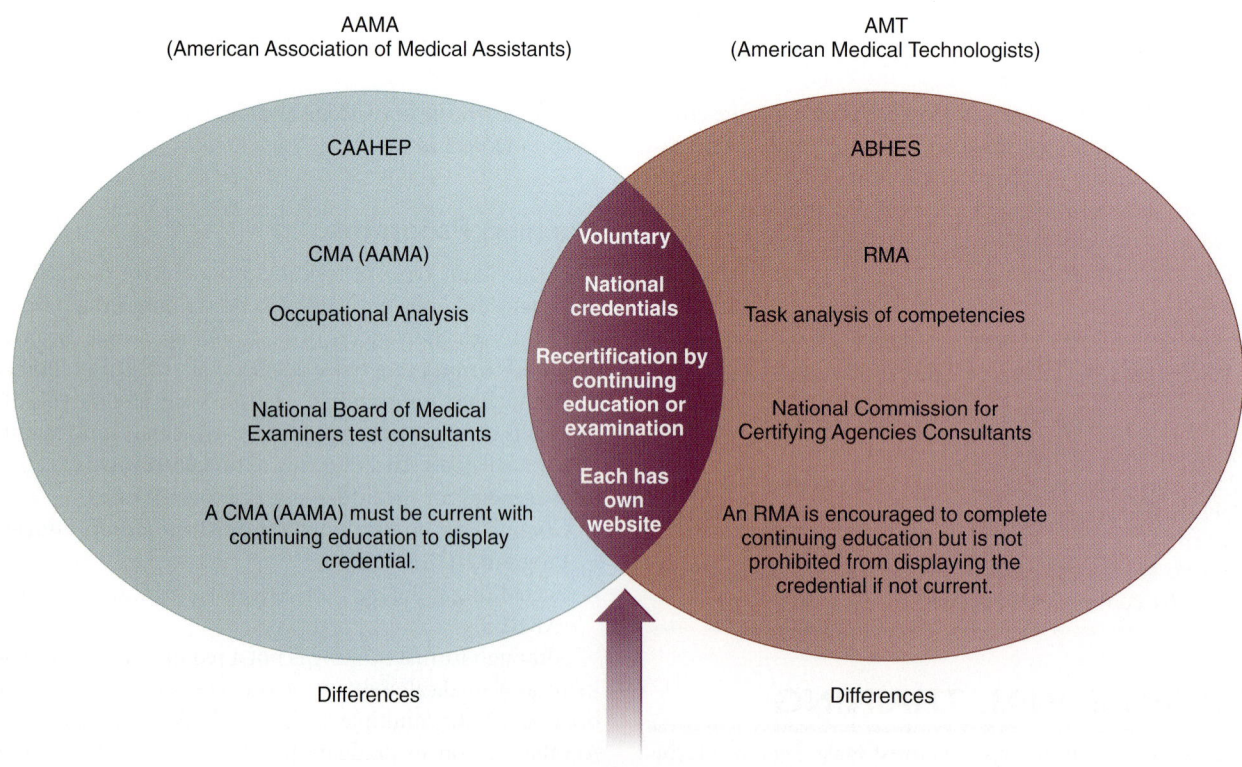

FIGURE 2-2 Venn diagram comparing the AAMA and the AMT.

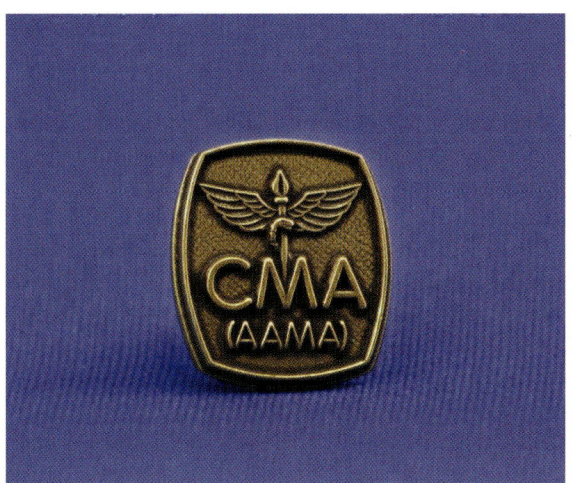

FIGURE 2-3 Pin worn by the certified medical assistant (CMA [AAMA]). (Courtesy American Association of Medical Assistants, Chicago.)

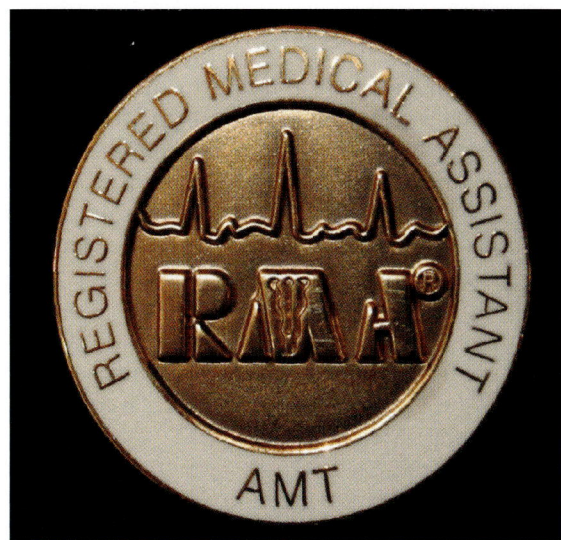

FIGURE 2-4 Pin worn by the registered medical assistant (RMA). (Courtesy American Medical Technologists, Rosemont, IL.)

BOX 2-5

American Association of Medical Assistants (AAMA) Recertification

AAMA RECERTIFICATION BY CEUs
- Acquire 60 recertification points, 30 of which must be AAMA approved CEUs
  - 10 Administrative
  - 10 Clinical
  - 10 General
  - 30 any combination of the three categories
- Current Provider Level CPR certification

CEUs, Continuing education units.

BOX 2-6

American Medical Technologists Recertification

AMT RECERTIFICATION BY CEUs
- Earn 30 points every 3 years (compliance interval as of 1/1/2006)
  - One hour is equal to one point
- Earn points through one or all of the following:
  - Formal education in field of practice
  - Field-related continuing education programs
  - Ongoing employment in field of practice
  - Authorship of written works
  - Instructional presentations
  - Professional organizational participation
  - Professional development

CEUs, Continuing education units.

CMA Credential

The CMA (AAMA) credential is awarded by the Certifying Board of AAMA (Figure 2-3). The CMA examination consists of 200 multiple-choice questions. Examinees are allowed to complete the questions in any order they choose. The examination is scored according to the number of correct responses, with no penalty for guessing. Each question receives equal scoring weight. The final score is based on a curve formed from examinees' past and present scores. Note that the AAMA requires recertification of the CMA (AAMA) credential every 5 years by either examination or continuing education units (CEUs) (Box 2-5). Failure to keep current with CEUs results in forfeiture of the right to use the CMA (AAMA) credential.

RMA Credential

The RMA credential is awarded by the AMT (Figure 2-4). The RMA examination currently has more than 200 questions; about 41% cover general subject areas, 35% clinical areas, and 24% administrative areas. Tests are administered both on computer and in paper-and-pencil modes at numerous testing centers and academic institutions almost weekly throughout the United States. Testing is available on demand as candidates complete their academic programs and fulfill application requirements. The examination is criterion-referenced in design. The questions are weighted according to difficulty, and the scores are not based on a curve, but a scale. The minimum passing score is 70.

Medical assistants certified after January 1, 2006 are required to renew their certificates every 3 years by demonstrating compliance with AMT's Certification Program (CCP). The program presents certificants with alternative means of demonstrating continued competence, including continuing education, professional activities, and ongoing employment. Certificants failing to comply with the Program are not entitled to use the RMA designation on certificate expiration (Box 2-6).

Credentialing Examinations

Medical assistant credentialing examinations are comprehensive tests of knowledge in all areas, including law and ethics, anatomy and physiology, nutrition, psychology, and administrative and clinical areas. The AAMA and the AMT administer these examinations. Table 2-2 compares eligibility requirements for the CMA (AAMA) and RMA examinations. These national examinations are taken on a voluntary basis and allow you to demonstrate your knowledge of current entry-level competencies. By taking and passing a national certification test, you become more of an asset to the physician. Showing your commitment to professionalism provides credibility to what you do.

Certification Test-Taking Skills. Preparing for the national examination requires that you refine your test-taking skills. To do this you must examine your strengths and weaknesses when taking a test. You should do the following when taking a credentialing exam:

- **Identify key words in the sentence.** Key words will direct your focus and assist with selecting the correct answer.
- **Select answers that are patient centered.** By understanding the basic principles of communication and interpersonal relationships, correct answers can be selected.
- **Understand how to approach "all of the above" and "none of the above" options.** If one answer is eliminated as *incorrect*, "all of the above" is also eliminated. If one answer can be eliminated as *correct*, "none of the above" is also eliminated.

Refer to Chapter 1 for more information on studying, preparing for an examination, and test-taking strategies. Remember, do not spend too much time on one question. If a question is causing you to feel frustrated, skip it and return to it later after you have answered the ones you know; this allows you to concentrate on what you do know. If you still do not know the answer, guess; there is no penalty for guessing.

TABLE 2-2

Comparison of Certified Medical Assistant (CMA [AAMA]) and Registered Medical Assistant (RMA) Certification

CMA	RMA
MANDATE	
Credential is voluntary in most states, not required by the federal government.	Credential is voluntary in most states, not required by the federal government.
ADDRESS	
American Association of Medical Assistants 20 N. Wacker Drive, Suite 1575 Chicago, IL 60606-2903 (800) ACT-AAMA www.aama-ntl.org	Registered Medical Assistants of American Medical Technologists 10700 Higgins Road Suite 150 Rosemont, IL 60018 (847) 823-5169 or (800) 275-1268 www.amt1.com
CREDENTIAL AWARDED BY	
Certifying Board of the American Association of Medical Assistants (AAMA)	American Medical Technologists (AMT)*
REQUIREMENTS	

The qualifications for taking the AAMA Certification Examination require only graduates of medical assisting programs accredited by the Commission on Accreditation of Allied Health Education Programs (CAAHEP) or the Accrediting Bureau of Health Education Schools (ABHES) to be eligible to take the test for initial certification and become a CMA (AAMA).†
If a student graduates from a medical assistant program that is not CAAHEP accredited at the time of graduation, but becomes CAAHEP accredited within 36 months of the date of graduation, the individual is considered to be a graduate of a CAAHEP-accredited medical assisting program and is thus eligible to take the certification examination.
Any CMA who is not a graduate of a CAAHEP-accredited medical assisting program continues to be eligible to recertify either through the continuing education method or by taking and passing the certification examination.
	The applicant must have the following qualifications:
	1. Good moral character.
	2. Graduate of an accredited high school or acceptable equivalent.
	3. One of the following requirements:
	  a. Graduate of:
	    1. Medical assistant program or institution accredited by ABHES or CAAHEP.
	    2. Medical assistant program accredited by a Regional Accrediting Commission or by a nationally accredited organization approved by the U.S. Department of Education.
	    3. Formal medical services training of the U.S. Armed Forces.
	  b. Employed in the profession of medical assisting for a minimum of 5 years, no more than 2 years of which may have been as an instructor in a post-secondary medical assisting program.
	  c. Completed a medical assistant course in a school holding national accreditation recognized by the Council on Postsecondary Accreditation (COPA) and acceptable for the AMT Board of Directors and has been employed as a medical assistant for a minimum of 1 year.

TABLE 2-2
Comparison of Certified Medical Assistant (CMA [AAMA]) and Registered Medical Assistant (RMA) Certification—cont'd

CMA	RMA
TEST SITES More than 120 test centers throughout the United States.	Approximately 200 test sites throughout the United States.
TEST DATES Beginning April 2009 testing is available at select locations on a continuous basis throughout the year as candidates complete their coursework to include a practicum. The CMA (AAMA) test will be available prior to graduation. Preliminary immediate pass/fail results will be provided. Official scores will be mailed within five to six weeks to candidates who have satisfied all examination requirements.	Testing is available upon demand as candidates complete their academic programs and fulfill application requirements. Three examination administration options are available: 1. Computer-based administration at an AMT-approved site. 2. Paper-and-pencil administration at various sites under the direction of an AMT proctor. 3. Computer-based administration at an AMT-approved school site (option available to candidates with an approved application on file and at selected school sites pre-arranged with AMT). Available to those who have been approved and a certification application is on file, and the exam has been set up prior to administration through AMT.
TEST DEVELOPMENT The AAMA Certifying Board prepares, administers, and evaluates examinations for certification and recertification and certifies successful candidates. The board includes CMAs (AAMA) currently practicing in the field and CMA (AAMA) educators.	Test questions are developed by the AMT Registered Medical Assistant Education, Qualifications, and Standards Committee. All committee members are certificants of AMT. Seven RMAs and one RMA consultant serve on the committee and are appointed by the AMT Board of Directors annually.
TESTING AGENCY The National Board of Medical Examiners (NBME) assists the AAMA as a test consultant in the development of the examination. Prometric test centers provide the test administration services.	All RMA certification examinations are conducted under the auspices of American Medical Technologists.
TEST QUESTIONS The Certification/Recertification Examination is developed from a broad range of categories.	Test questions are developed from the Registered Medical Assistant Certification Examination Construction Parameters which reflect competencies required for safe and successful practice in the field.

*Two organizations award the credential RMA, which can be confusing to graduates seeking a credential. The Registered Medical Assistant by the American Medical Technologists, Rosemont, Illinois, awards the credential by examination. The Registered Medical Assistant by the American Registry of Medical Assistants, Westfield, Massachusetts, offers registration only and does not have a certification examination requirement.
†Call AAMA for qualifications.
AMT and AAMA are two different organizations offering a choice of certification to medical assistants seeking a credential.

Continuing Education

You will have worked hard to complete school and pass the examination to be credentialed. The next step is to continue with your professional development in order to maintain your credential. *Continuing education* is a term used to describe education once the credential is received. Obtaining a license to perform certain tasks within a profession is also continuing education. Continuing education has many benefits, including the following:
- Keeping up with new knowledge.
- Reinforcing areas related to your individual job responsibilities.
- Networking with other professionals.

Continuing education is also required for recertification, or **revalidation.** Both the AAMA and the AMT require CMAs (AAMA) and RMAs to recertify to retain active status.

PATIENT-CENTERED PROFESSIONALISM

- *How can continuing education improve the care a medical assistant provides to patients?*
- *How can obtaining credentials as a medical assistant impact patients? How can it impact health care in general?*
- *What is the value in continuing to improve yourself and your skills even after you are a medical assistant?*

Career Planning

This chapter is the first of many that will prepare you for a career in medical assisting. The physician-employer is expecting more than basic skills (e.g., reading, writing, and arithmetic). Thinking skills or the ability to problem solve, make a decision, and be a creative thinker are all workplace foundation skills expected of the entry level medical assistant. Professional qualities, such as professional characteristics, abilities, and image, are added to this foundational inventory.

Improving your chances of a successful career in medical assisting is a legitimate concern that needs to be addressed early on in the educational process. Chapter 47 will bring your career planning full circle. In preparation, begin to put together a **resume**. A resume is a document that outlines your skills and experiences to let a physician-employer see at a glance how you can contribute to his or her practice. The information presented in this chapter and subsequent chapters can help you build a career profile that lists not only your professional skills (e.g., superior verbal and written communication skills) but also your technical skills (e.g., software such as Medisoft or Microsoft Word/Excel).

Never underestimate your personal professional qualities (e.g., dependability, loyalty, and integrity) since these are also necessary for career success. Two persons with the same educational background and employment history will be evaluated on many of these skills, so pay close attention to them. As you progress through this textbook, continue to modify and update your resume with additional workplace competencies you have mastered.

CONCLUSION

Medical assisting, the profession you have chosen, requires certain personal qualities and abilities, professional duties, and adequate preparation and training. It takes time and practice to develop the personal and physical qualities, skills, and knowledge needed. Time must be spent learning from others, as well as from your own experiences. When you begin a new career, you must remember the following:

1. Small improvements become significant accomplishments.
2. Determine what you do well and what needs improvement.
3. Take advantage of educational opportunities.
4. Never give up. Setbacks will occur; learn from them and use them for growth.
5. Accept responsibility for your own actions.

With hard work, patience, and dedication, you can become a true professional.

Chapter Summary

Reinforce your understanding of the material in this chapter by reviewing the curriculum objectives and key content points below:

1. **Define, appropriately use, and spell all the Key Terms for this chapter.**
   - Review the Key Terms if necessary.
2. **List six characteristics of a professional medical assistant and briefly describe the importance of each.**
   - Employers expect dependability, loyalty, a positive attitude, integrity, diplomacy, and confidence from their employees.
   - Dependability is being consistently reliable in job performance.
   - Loyalty forms when trust and respect develop between employee and employer.
   - A positive attitude is a "can do" attitude.
   - Integrity is adherence to personal moral and ethical standards.
   - Diplomacy is being able to be courteous and understanding during tense situations.
   - Confidence is being aware of your abilities and projecting this awareness.
3. **List three abilities needed by a professional medical assistant and explain the significance of each.**
   - Competence in clinical and administrative skills projects professionalism.
   - Technical skill and dexterity when using office equipment are important in providing efficient and accurate care.
   - Using proper English skills ensures effective communication and makes a good impression.
4. **Give an example that shows the importance of a professional personal appearance.**
   - Dressing for success is important since you only get one chance to make a first impression.
5. **State 10 steps you can take to project a professional personal appearance on the job.**
   - Medical assistants should consider their hygiene, dress, and overall appearance and how these things affect co-workers and patients.
   - Refer to Table 2-1.
6. **List eight administrative duties a medical assistant may perform regularly.**
   - Administrative duties of a medical assistant involve front office (appointment and procedure scheduling, inventory, ordering supplies, insurance and billing), record keeping (filing patient records), computer related (entering electronic patient records), and financial tasks (bank deposits, receiving patient co-payments).
7. **List eight clinical duties a medical assistant may perform regularly.**
   - Clinical duties of a medical assistant involve assisting with the care of the patient in areas such as taking patient histories, providing patient education, taking vital signs, dressing wounds, helping with office procedures, sterilizing instruments, drawing blood, and recording electrocardiograms (ECGs).
8. **Explain the purpose of accreditation.**

- Accreditation is an attempt to standardize the body of knowledge and skills taught in various types of medical assistant programs.
- National program accreditation can be accomplished through ABHES and CAAHEP.

9. **Explain the significance of becoming credentialed in medical assisting.**
   - It is important to obtain credentialing through either the AAMA or AMT after graduation.
   - Commitment to the profession is a good employment tool.
   - Passing a national certification examination demonstrates your knowledge and skills to employers.

10. **Explain the importance of maintaining professional competence through continuing education.**
    - Continuing education is encouraged to remain current with professional issues.

11. **Analyze a realistic medical office situation and apply your understanding of professional qualities and characteristics to determine the best course of action.**
    - A professional appearance, demeanor, and feeling of competence in performing duties are necessary for medical assistants.

12. **Describe the impact on patient care when medical assistants appear and behave professionally.**
    - Patients are more likely to follow prescribed treatment plans when they have confidence in the ability of the medical office staff and the staff projects a professional appearance.

PRACTICAL APPLICATIONS

If you have accomplished the objectives in this chapter, you will be able to make better choices as a medical assistant. Take another look at this situation and decide what you would do.

Robert is a medical assistant in a medical office. His responsibility is to draw blood samples at 8:00 AM, but he often does not show up until 8:15 AM or later. The scheduled patients must wait and be late for work or must reschedule their appointment. When Robert does arrive, often his uniform is blood stained and wrinkled and he has not shaved or bathed before coming to work. Even if another staff member has started drawing blood, the daily operation of the office is already behind schedule. Robert also has a habit of taking a break between patients.

As the office slips even further behind with more patients waiting, Robert draws the blood but does not take time to label the tubes with the patient's name or complete the laboratory request forms. When Robert makes mistakes, the office staff must make the corrections, resulting in even more delays and confusion about which tube of blood belongs to which patient.

One day Robert is sick and stays home but does not call the office. By 8:30 AM, patients have filled the waiting room, and patients coming to see the physicians have no place to sit. The office has insufficient staff, and the patients and the office personnel are stressed.

Robert's lack of professionalism is affecting both patients and staff. What would you do differently from Robert?

1. Medical assistants who are respected for their professionalism have certain personality characteristics. Which of these characteristics is Robert lacking? How is Robert's lack of professionalism affecting patients? Co-workers? The office as a whole?
2. If you were a patient in this office, how would you feel if Robert was going to draw your blood?
3. How could Robert be liable for mislabeling blood samples?
4. What actions have shown that Robert does not meet the ethical standards of a medical assistant?
5. How does the daily schedule fall behind in a medical office? Who is affected by this? What other potential problems and mistakes can you think of that might occur as a result of Robert being late?
6. If you were Robert's immediate supervisor, what would you say to Robert? How would you help him meet the professional and ethical standards expected of a medical assistant? What are some things he can do to arrive at work on time?

WEB SEARCH

1. **Research medical assisting as a career.** It is important to learn as much as you can about medical assisting, including the duties of medical assistants, the training necessary to become a medical assistant, ways to improve your skills once you become a medical assistant, and the organizations that exist to provide support to medical assistants.
   - **Keywords:** Use the following keywords in your search: medical assistant, medical assisting, AAMA, AMT.

2. **Research professionalism in other fields.** Positive professional qualities, appropriate professional abilities, and a professional image are important to other professions as well as the medical assisting profession. Are the same skills that make you a professional in medical assisting needed in other professions?
   - **Keywords:** Use the following keywords in your search: professionalism, being professional.

3 Diversity in Health Care Delivery

evolve http://evolve.elsevier.com/klieger/medicalassisting

Diversity means "having variety." People are diverse in many ways. There is variety in people's size, shape, gender, age, race, and culture. Because of these differences, health care must be diverse as well. Health care must meet the needs of both the people seeking health care and the individuals delivering health care services. Examples of the diversity of health care delivery include the different types of medical settings, practice specialties, and the health care professionals and even the settings in which health care is provided. It is important for you to learn about the various ways health care is delivered so that you can understand how the whole system works.

LEARNING OBJECTIVES

You will be able to do the following after completing this chapter:

Key Terms
1. Define, appropriately use, and spell all the Key Terms for this chapter.

Medical Practice Settings
2. List four different types of medical practice settings.

Medical Specialties
3. Explain the difference between a family practitioner and a specialist.
4. Explain what it means to be "board certified."

The Professional Health Care Team
5. List the members of the professional health care team and explain their training and duties.
6. List five types of medical organizations in which a medical assistant can find employment.

Health Care Delivery Settings
7. Explain the importance of being knowledgeable about the various health care delivery settings in your community.
8. List seven health care delivery settings other than the medical office.

Patient-Centered Professionalism
9. Analyze a realistic medical office situation and apply your understanding of the diversity in health care delivery to determine the best course of action.
10. Describe the impact on patient care when medical assistants have a solid understanding of the various settings in which health care is provided and the various roles of health care professionals.

KEY TERMS

ambulatory	JCAHO
corporation	management service organization (MSO)
diversity	partnership
entity	sole proprietorship
group practice	specialization

PRACTICAL APPLICATIONS

Read the following scenario and keep it in mind as you learn about the diversity in health care delivery in this chapter.

Jade is a recent graduate of a medical assisting program. She is looking for a job that will fit her credentials. She has not taken the credentialing examinations for medical assisting and has not had any experience in the medical field except her externship in a pediatric clinic.

Jade finds two ads in the local paper for a medical assistant. One ad specifically asks for a certified medical assistant for a group practice in a management service organization. The other ad asks for a medical assistant for a solo practice for an internist; no medical assisting credentials are specified, but applicants should have experience appropriate to the internal medicine setting. In the solo practice, Jade would be the only clinical employee for the practice. Jade decides to apply for both positions. Jade thinks that the job of a medical assistant is the same in each setting and that she is prepared for both employment opportunities.

While reading the same paper, Jade also sees an ad for a nurse for a physician partnership in obstetrics-gynecology. She decides to apply for this position as well.

What advice would you give Jade if she asked for your input?

MEDICAL PRACTICE SETTINGS

A medical practice is a business **entity.** A business entity is a particular type of business that possesses a separate existence for tax purposes such as a medical practice. Some types of business entities include corporations and limited liability companies. There are three major types of medical practices: private practice (**sole proprietorship**), **partnership** practice, and **group practice** (Table 3-1). A solo practice, or sole proprietorship, and a group practice may be a practice that has "incorporated," or become a **corporation** (e.g., Professional Service Corporation [PSA]). Often group and corporate practices have their patient billing and payment services handled by a **management service organization (MSO).** In this situation the physician is considered an employee of the MSO. Fees that a physician can charge are limited by the agreement signed by the MSO and the practice.

Medical practice settings are considered **ambulatory** care facilities. The patient comes to the office for health care and then goes home. This textbook will address this type of setting.

PATIENT-CENTERED PROFESSIONALISM

Take a moment to consider the impact of different events on various medical practice settings.
- *How are the physicians in a corporate practice setting affected by a lawsuit as compared with a physician in a private practice setting?*
- *Why do you think most practices today are group and corporate practices?*
- *How might a patient's experience differ in each of the four types of medical practice settings?*
- *How might your experience as a medical assistant differ in each of the four types of medical practice settings? Which setting do you think you would prefer?*

MEDICAL SPECIALTIES

Advances in technology have required physicians to seek additional training to keep their skills up to date. More and more physicians have decided to specialize to focus on the advances in one area. It is important for you to know about the various specialties so that you can make decisions about the type of practice in which you want to work. This knowledge will also help you when dealing with patients who are referred to different types of specialists for treatment.

Specialty Fields

Many physicians are family or general practitioners. *Family practitioners* are medical doctors that treat all ages from the newborn to the elderly. They diagnose and treat a variety of diseases and disorders, and they are patients' long-term health care providers or primary care physicians. When patients need more specialized care for specific conditions, they are referred to specialists. A *specialist* is a physician who has completed additional training and educational requirements to become more knowledgeable about specific conditions or medical areas. Table 3-2 provides an overview of some of the areas of **specialization** available. Table 3-3 lists other specialists not recognized as medical physicians who treat patients for certain disorders.

Specialty Boards and Certification

The additional training a physician can complete to become a specialist often involves a 3- to 7-year residency in the specialty area and a national board examination. There are many individual boards, each governed by the American Board of Medical Specialists (ABMS) (Figure 3-1). Continued training and education is an ongoing requirement even after board

TABLE 3-1

Differences among Medical Practice Settings

	Private Practice (Sole Proprietorship)	Partnership Practice	Group Practice
Ownership	One owner. May be incorporated.	Two owners sharing the same specialty or different specialties.	Three or more owners sharing the same specialty or multiple specialties.
Life of the business	Ends when owner dies or closes practice.	Ends when one partner dies or leaves, or when the practice closes.	Ends when a predetermined number of owners die or leave, when the practice closes, or shareholders vote to close; the physician can be replaced and the group continues.
Liability	Owner is responsible for all debt of the practice.	Each partner is responsible for debt of the practice and is liable for the other partner's actions; personal assets can be used for liabilities.	The practice is responsible for the debt incurred (owners have "incorporated," or formed a corporation).
Advantages	Owner is sole decision-maker.	More potential for profit; shared decision making.	More potential for profit; shared decision making; shared facilities, equipment, and employees; many tax advantages.
Disadvantages	Sole physician is responsible for patient care 24 hours a day.	Partners may not have similar values; each partner is held responsible for the other's actions.	Owners may not have similar values; each owner is held responsible for the actions of the other owners; individuals have less control over business decisions.

TABLE 3-2

Medical Practice Specialties

Specialty	Specialist	Scope of Practice
Aerospace medicine	Aerospace medical specialist	Researches the effect of space environment on people.
Allergy and immunology	Allergist-immunologist	Treats allergies and the immune system's response to contagious disease, transplantation, and immunizations.
Anesthesiology	Anesthesiologist	Administers and maintains anesthesia during surgery; oversees pain management.
Cardiology	Cardiologist	Provides noninvasive treatment for heart and vascular disease.
Dermatology	Dermatologist	Treats diseases of the skin.
Emergency medicine	Emergency physician, trauma physician	Treats acutely ill patients and trauma victims in emergency departments.
Endocrinology	Endocrinologist	Treats diseases of the endocrine system.
Gastroenterology	Gastroenterologist	Treats diseases of the digestive system.
Gerontology	Gerontologist	Treats diseases of elderly persons.
Gynecology	Gynecologist	Treats disorders of the female reproductive system.
Hematology	Hematologist	Treats disorders of the blood.
Infertility	Infertility specialist	Treats problems of conception and maintaining pregnancy.
Internal medicine	Internist	Provides nonsurgical treatment of internal organs.
Nephrology	Nephrologist	Treats diseases of the kidneys.
Neurology	Neurologist	Provides nonsurgical treatment of the nervous system.
Nuclear medicine	Nuclear medicine physician	Treats diseases with radionuclides.
Obstetrics	Obstetrician	Provides care during pregnancy, delivery, and aftercare of women.
Oncology	Oncologist	Treats all forms of cancer.
Ophthalmology	Ophthalmologist	Treats disorders of the eye.
Orthopedics	Orthopedist	Treats disorders of the musculoskeletal system.
Otorhinolaryngology	ENT specialist, otorhinolaryngologist	Treats disorders of the ear, nose, and throat (ENT).
Pathology	Pathologist	Examines tissue samples for signs of disease.
Pediatrics	Pediatrician	Treats both well and sick children.
Plastic surgery	Surgeon	Performs restorative (e.g., cancer, burns) and cosmetic (e.g., "facelift") surgery.
Psychiatry	Psychiatrist	Treats mental, behavioral, and emotional disorders.
Radiology	Radiologist	Uses x-ray films to diagnose and treat disease.
Surgery	Surgeon	Treats disease and trauma by surgical procedures.
Urology	Urologist	Treats male and female urological conditions and the reproductive disorders of the male.

TABLE 3-3

Additional Medical Specialties

Specialty	Specialist	Degree	Scope of Practice
Chiropractic medicine	Chiropractor	DC	Treats the patient by manipulation of the spine to relieve musculoskeletal disorders.
Dentistry	Dentist	DDS	Treats diseases and disorders of the teeth and gums.
Naprapathy	Naprapath	DN	Specialist in treatment of myofascial disorders.
Naturopathy	Naturopath	ND	Holistic treatment focusing on disease prevention and treatments using physical methods.
Optometry	Optometrist	OD	Tests vision and prepares lenses to correct refractive problems.
Oral surgery	Oral surgeon	DMD	Treats dental disorders requiring surgery.
Podiatry	Podiatrist	DPM	Treats disorders of the feet.
Psychology	Psychologist	MA and/or PhD	Counsels patients with stress- or emotion-related disorders.

certification. The following three organizations offer recognition for additional training:

American College of Surgeons: Fellow of the American College of Surgeons (FACS)

American College of Physicians: Fellow of the American College of Physicians (FACP)

American College of Family Physicians: Fellow of the American College of Family Physicians (FACFP)

PATIENT-CENTERED PROFESSIONALISM

Take a moment to consider the advantages of specialization.
- How does the existence of medical specialties improve the care provided to all patients?
- How does specialization improve the care that a single physician can provide to patients?
- How does specialization improve the entire health care system?

THE PROFESSIONAL HEALTH CARE TEAM

The physician and all other allied professionals in a medical setting make up a team. The team works together to provide health care services to a community. From the time the patient schedules an appointment, many members of the health care team are involved in providing quality care (Figure 3-2). As a medical assistant, you need to know the role of each member of the team so that you can help the team care for patients.

American Board of Allergy and Immunology
American Board of Anesthesiology
American Board of Colon and Rectal Surgery
American Board of Dermatology
American Board of Emergency Medicine
American Board of Family Practice
American Board of Internal Medicine
American Board of Medical Genetics
American Board of Neurological Surgery
American Board of Nuclear Medicine
American Board of Obstetrics and Gynecology
American Board of Ophthalmology
American Board of Otolaryngology
American Board of Pathology
American Board of Pediatrics
American Board of Physical Medicine and Rehabilitation
American Board of Plastic Surgery
American Board of Preventive Medicine
American Board of Psychiatry and Neurology
American Board of Radiology
American Board of Surgery
American Board of Thoracic Surgery
American Board of Urology

FIGURE 3-1 American medical boards.

Physician

Hippocrates, known as the "Father of Medicine," was the first to document the disease process. Today, the physician is the health care team member solely responsible for diagnosing and treating patients. Each state establishes licensing requirements through its medical board. Two often-confused types of licensed physicians are the Doctor of Medicine (MD) and the Doctor of Osteopathy (DO) (Table 3-4). The main difference between the two types of physicians is that DOs have been specially trained to perform osteopathic manipulations on patients. They view the patient as a "total person," focus on preventive care, and treat the whole body rather than a specific illness or symptoms.

Physician Assistant

The physician assistant (PA) can perform certain procedures under the physician's supervision. As a member of the health care team, the PA can perform the following duties:
1. Take medical histories.
2. Examine and treat patients.
3. Order and interpret laboratory tests and x-rays.
4. Make diagnoses.
5. Prescribe medications.

In some rural areas and inner city clinics, PAs may function as the principal provider and confer with other medical professionals as needed or as required by law. The PA should not be confused with the medical assistant. PA training requires completing a formalized program of college credit and clinical experience.

Nurse

Nursing is a profession in health care that provides for a patient's well-being. Nurses have a wide range of responsibilities depending on their educational background and skills. At one time, they worked solely in the hospital and nursing home

TABLE 3-4
Doctor of Medicine (MD) Compared with Doctor of Osteopathy (DO)

	Type of Doctor	Emphasis	Training	Licensing
MD	Medical	Treats specific symptoms of disease and injury. Family practitioner, internist, or specialty area.	Graduation from 4-year college with emphasis on scientific courses. Completion of 4 years of medical school. Completion of a residency (intensive hospital-based training). Option to practice in a specialty area with additional 2 to 6 years of training (e.g., surgery, psychiatry).	Must pass series of examinations in the state where MD will practice. Must meet the established criteria set by the medical board in that state.
DO	Medical	Uses the "whole person" approach to medicine. Assesses overall health of patient to include home and work environment, focusing on the musculoskeletal system. Primary care physicians.	Same as for MD.	Same as for MD.

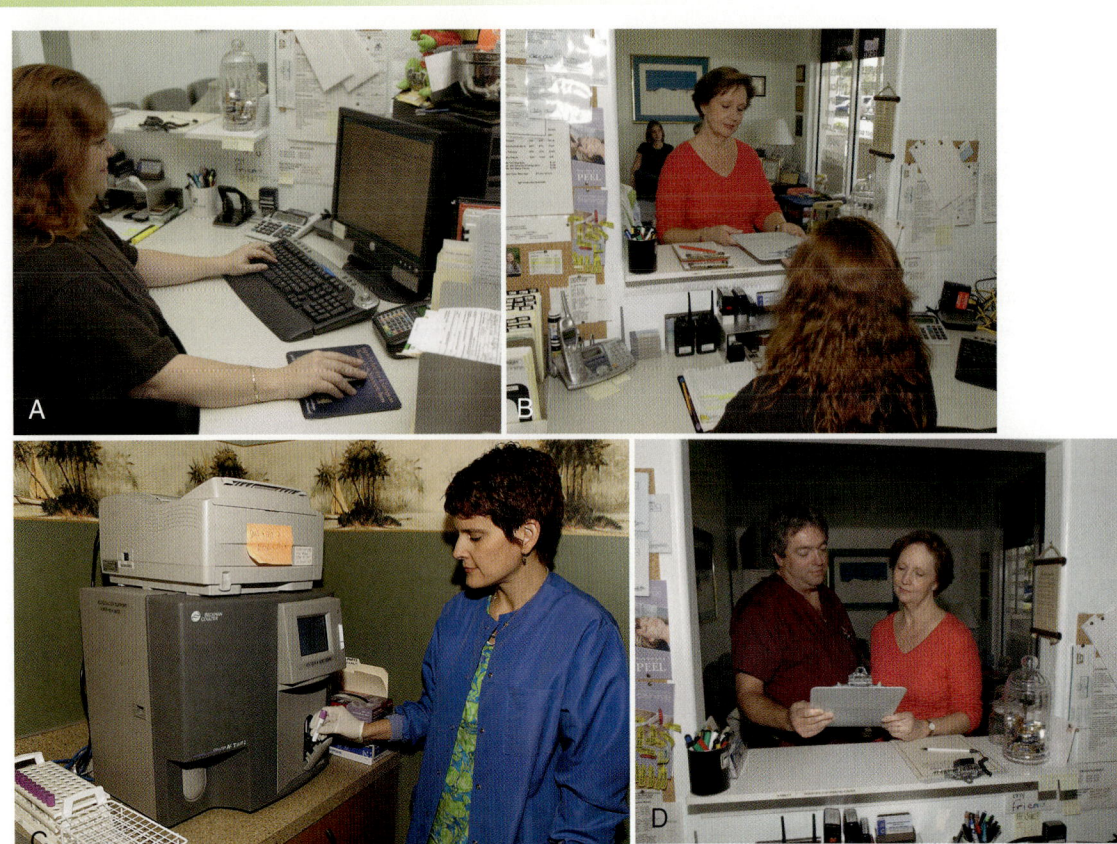

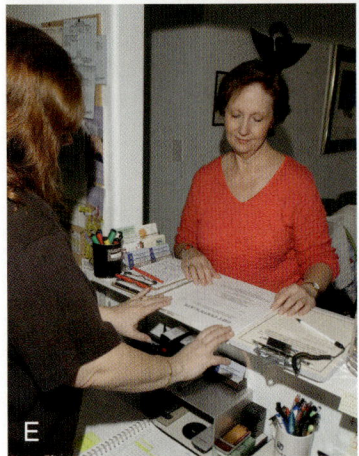

FIGURE 3-2 Patients depend on many professionals to assist with their health care treatment. **A,** Medical assistant makes an appointment for a patient. **B,** Medical assistant greets a patient arriving for her appointment. **C,** Medical technologist processes a patient's laboratory specimen to assist the physician with a diagnosis. **D,** Physician interacts with a patient. **E,** Medical assistant discusses the office visit charges with the patient.

settings, but they now work in many settings, including medical clinics, home health care agencies, hospices, and schools. All nurses are licensed by their state after passing an examination.

Nurse Practitioner

The nurse practitioner (NP) is schooled in the typical duties of a nurse but has additional training and education for diagnosis and treatment in a specialized field (e.g., family nurse practitioner [FNP], American registered nurse practitioner [ARNP]). The NP receives a Master's of Science in Nursing (MSN). Often, the NP is the first professional a patient sees for common illnesses and injuries (Figure 3-3). In some states the NP can prescribe medications.

Registered Nurse

The registered nurse (RN) has the typical bedside care duties but can also perform administrative tasks and may have supervisory responsibilities. RNs must have 2 to 4 years of college and pass the National Council Licensure Examination (NCLEX-RN).

Licensed Practical Nurse and Licensed Vocational Nurse

The licensed practical nurse (LPN) or licensed vocational nurse (LVN) is trained in basic nursing duties and works under the supervision of an RN or physician. The LPN has passed the NCLEX-PN. LPN and LVN duties are usually limited under state law. This credential can be upgraded to RN with additional educational credits and clinical training.

Certified Nursing Assistant

The certified nursing assistant (CNA) completes a state-approved course that includes a skills examination. The CNA provides basic patient care in a variety of settings, including hospitals, long-term care facilities, and home health care agencies. The CNA's duties include personal care (e.g., bathing, hygiene), assisting with food service, and taking vital signs.

Medical Assistant

A certified medical assistant (CMA) or a registered medical assistant (RMA) has completed an accredited medical assistant program and passed a national examination. You learned about this certification process in Chapter 2. The MA works under the direct supervision of a licensed physician. Many skills are needed to perform a wide variety of duties. MAs perform clinical duties such as drawing blood, performing basic laboratory tests, and assisting with examinations and procedures. They also perform administrative (office-related) duties, including scheduling appointments and billing. In addition, the MA provides valuable patient education and a communication pathway between the physician and the patient (Figure 3-4). MAs work not only in medical offices and clinics but also in hospitals, research centers, insurance companies, and correctional institutions.

Other Allied Health Professionals

In addition to physicians, physician assistants, nurses, and medical assistants, there are other allied health professionals involved with patient care. Figure 3-5 lists some of the many health care professionals you may encounter on a day-to-day basis.

PATIENT-CENTERED PROFESSIONALISM

Take a moment to consider the importance of clarifying your role as medical assistant to patients.
- *What would you do if a patient referred to you as a nurse?*
- *Does it really matter if a medical assistant is thought of as a nurse or if a nurse or physician assistant is thought of as a physician?*
- *Why is it important for all health care professionals to practice within their scope of training?*
- *How might a patient feel if she finds out later that the health professional she thought was a nurse was actually a medical assistant? What are some actions the patient might take?*

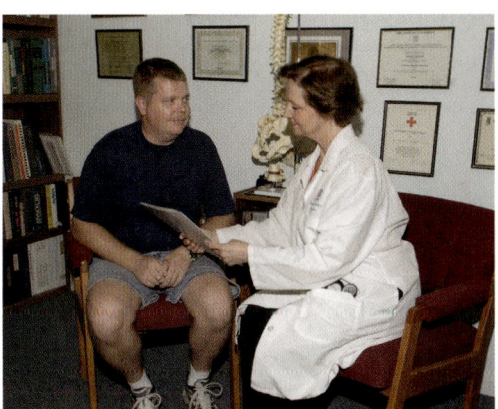

FIGURE 3-3 A nurse practitioner can diagnose and treat common acute illnesses.

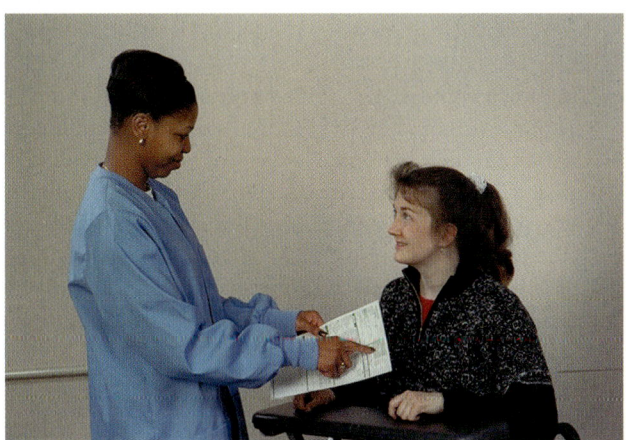

FIGURE 3-4 A medical assistant provides valuable education and information to the patient.

Medical Technologist Clinical Laboratory Technician Histologist Cytotechnologist Phlebotomist	Registered Dietitian EKG Technician Health Information Technologist Respiratory Therapist Physical Therapist Occupational Therapist Unit Secretary Radiology Technologist Medical Secretary Medical Transcriptionist Registered EMT Medical Assistant	Pharmacist Pharmacy Technician
		Surgical Technologist

FIGURE 3-5 Allied health professionals.

HEALTH CARE DELIVERY SETTINGS

The medical office is one type of health care delivery setting. As a medical assistant, one of your responsibilities will be to assist in referring patients to a variety of other health care delivery settings. For example, the primary care physician may want patients to go to an outside laboratory for blood work, a diagnostic center for x-ray films, or to a specialist, such as an endocrinologist, for further evaluation. In addition, patients may require assistance at home after a hospital stay or long-term illness. This may require the intervention of a home health care agency or hospice. You need to know about not only the various health-related services patients need but also the types of services offered in your community. Being knowledgeable about other health care delivery settings benefits patients. It allows you to interact efficiently with the health care professionals in other settings to coordinate the services patients need. The health care delivery settings most often used by patients and their families are as follows:

- **Hospital:** Provides inpatient care and treatment for acute (serious) conditions.
- **Ambulatory surgery center:** Provides outpatient services for surgery, with patients admitted and discharged on the same day.
- **Short-term care facility:** Provides a place for patients who cannot function on their own after being discharged from the hospital. Restorative care is provided so that the patient can return home.
- **Long-term care facility (skilled nursing home):** Provides 24-hour-a-day nursing services to those who are unable to function on their own on a long-term basis.
- **Assisted living facility:** Provides services and assistance to people who require minimal help, such as with cooking, laundry, and medications.
- **Home health care agency:** A contracted service that provides for the social and medical needs of patients in their homes.
- **Hospice care:** Assists and meets the needs of terminally ill patients and their families.

In 1951 a not-for-profit organization was formed to raise the level of safety and quality of care in all health care settings and referred to as the *Joint Commission on Accreditation of Healthcare Organizations* or **JCAHO.** In 2007 the name was shortened to *The Joint Commission*. Facilities volunteer to be evaluated or accredited by JCAHO because accredited organizations are deemed to have met the Medicare and Medicaid certification requirement necessary for gaining reimbursement.

PATIENT-CENTERED PROFESSIONALISM

Take a moment to consider the importance of being knowledgeable about the various types of health care delivery settings.
- *Are medical office staff qualified and prepared to deliver any type of care a patient might need?*
- *How might a terminally ill patient and his family be affected by a medical assistant who is not aware of the types of services such as hospice care? What is the difference a knowledgeable medical assistant could make to the patient and family in this situation?*
- *How can a medical assistant who knows about the health care delivery services in the community influence the entire community's opinion of the medical clinic?*

CONCLUSION

All health care professionals must perform only the duties listed under their scope of practice. If they take on the duties of professionals without the proper training, education, and licensure, they can be found guilty of practicing without a license. Physicians who allow their employees to perform duties for which they are not qualified can be found guilty for permitting this to happen. Medical boards and state legislators have established consequences for these unethical and illegal choices. Understanding your duties and training and the duties and training of other members of the health care team helps you make the right choices.

Chapter Summary

Reinforce your understanding of the material in this chapter by reviewing the curriculum objectives and key content points below.

1. **Define, appropriately use, and spell all the Key Terms for this chapter.**
   - Review the Key Terms if necessary.
2. **List three different types of medical practice settings.**
   - A private practice (sole proprietorship) is a practice owned by one person who is legally responsible for the debts and taxes of the business.
   - A partnership is a practice owned by two people who are held legally responsible for the debts and taxes of the business and whose personal assets may be used for liabilities of the practice.
   - A group practice is a practice owned by three or more people who are held legally responsible for the debts and taxes of the business. Group practices can be corporate practices or professional associations.
3. **Explain the difference between a family practitioner and a specialist.**
   - Family practitioners treat patients of all ages, from newborns to elderly persons.

- Physicians in specialty fields provide patients with current procedures and up-to-date information in their specialty.
- Specialty fields are based on a specific condition (e.g., asthma) or medical area (e.g., orthopedics).

4. **Explain what it means to be "board certified."**
   - Physicians can take additional training to gain proficiency in a specialty.
   - Physicians are considered board certified once they have completed the additional training and examination required by the national board of their specialty.

5. **List the members of the professional health care team and explain their training and duties.**
   - A medical physician can be an MD or a DO.
   - A nurse requires a license to work and includes several categories (i.e., nurse practitioner, registered nurse, licensed practical nurse, or licensed vocational nurse).
   - A physician assistant performs routine diagnostic procedures and works under the physician's supervision.
   - A medical assistant is a multiskilled professional who is knowledgeable about both administrative and clinical procedures.
   - Other allied health care professionals work with various members of the team daily.

6. **List five types of medical organizations in which a medical assistant can find employment.**
   - Medical assistants work in medical offices and clinics, hospitals, research centers, insurance companies, and correctional institutions.

7. **Explain the importance of being knowledgeable about the various health care delivery settings in your community.**
   - Medical assistants interact with health care professionals in other delivery settings to coordinate services needed by patients and their families.
   - Being aware of the various health care delivery settings in your community helps you provide better care to patients.

8. **List seven health care delivery settings other than the medical office.**
   - Hospitals, ambulatory surgery centers, short-term care facilities, long-term care facilities, assisted living facilities, home health care agencies, and hospice care are the most common types of health care delivery settings outside the medical office.

9. **Analyze a realistic medical office situation and apply your understanding of the diversity in health care delivery to determine the best course of action.**
   - Understanding the setting in which you work allows you to operate effectively within that setting.
   - Always stay within the scope of your practice.

10. **Describe the impact on patient care when medical assistants have a solid understanding of the various settings in which health care is provided and the various roles of health care professionals.**
    - Medical assistants must understand their role, as well as the role of the other health care professionals with whom they work.
    - When health care professionals work together as a team, patients benefit.

PRACTICAL APPLICATIONS

If you have accomplished the objectives in this chapter, you will be able to make better choices as a medical assistant. Take another look at this situation and decide what you would do.

Jade is a recent graduate of a medical assisting program. She is looking for a job that will fit her credentials. She has not taken the credentialing examinations for medical assisting and has not had any experience in the medical field except her externship in a pediatric clinic.

Jade finds two ads in the local paper for a medical assistant. One ad specifically asks for a certified medical assistant for a group practice in a management service organization. The other ad asks for a medical assistant for a solo practice for an internist; no medical assisting credentials are specified, but applicants should have experience appropriate to the internal medicine setting. In the solo practice Jade would be the only clinical employee for the practice. Jade decides to apply for both positions. Jade thinks that the job of a medical assistant is the same in each setting and that she is prepared for both employment opportunities.

While reading the same paper, Jade also sees an ad for a nurse for a physician partnership in obstetrics-gynecology. She decides to apply for this position as well.

What advice would you give Jade if she asked for your input?

1. Does Jade have the credentials for these employment opportunities? If so, which ones? If not, why are some or all not appropriate?
2. What advantages would a new graduate have in a group practice rather than a solo practice where he or she is the only clinical medical assistant? What experiences should Jade expect to find in each setting? What are the advantages and disadvantages of each?
3. Should Jade assume that she could take a nursing position? What are the implications of using that title? In what scope of practice does the title "nurse" place Jade?
4. What would be the legal implications for the physicians in each setting if Jade is hired?
5. What influence could Jade have on the community's perception of the physician's abilities or the scope of practice if she does not understand her own abilities and scope of training? Will her scope of practice have any effect on the physician's office? If so, how?
6. Is the physician legally responsible for Jade's actions? Explain why or why not.

WEB SEARCH

1. **Research the basics of CAM to understand the topic of integrated medicine.**
   - **Keywords:** Use the following keyword in your search: CAM
2. **Research bariatric medicine.** Although you learned about some of the different medical specialties in this chapter, many more exist. It is helpful for medical assistants to know about the various medical specialties.
   - **Keywords:** Use the following keyword in your search: bariatric medicine.

Law and Ethics in Health Care

4

evolve http://evolve.elsevier.com/klieger/medicalassisting

Law and ethics are two of the most important aspects of patient-centered professionalism. As reported in the news, the cost of health care is rising quickly. One reason is the growing number of lawsuits against physicians. Laws and ethical standards protect both the physician and the patient. A truly patient-centered health professional follows not only the law but also the ethical principles of the profession.

LEARNING OBJECTIVES

You will be able to do the following after completing this chapter:

Key Terms
1. Define, appropriately use, and spell all the Key Terms for this chapter.

Law and Licensure in Medical Practice
2. Describe the purpose of the Medical Practice Acts.
3. List the three ways health professionals can become licensed.
4. List the six licensure requirements for physicians.
5. Explain how a physician could have his or her license revoked or suspended.

Law and Liability
6. Distinguish between public law and private law.
7. Describe abandonment and give an example.
8. List the six steps in formally withdrawing from the physician-patient contract.
9. Define *expressed contract* and *implied contract* and give an example of each.
10. Explain how malpractice relates to liability.
11. Explain the difference between *intentional* negligence and *nonintentional* negligence.
12. Explain the importance of informed consent.
13. Describe the purpose of the Good Samaritan Act.
14. List three types of nonintentional negligence.
15. State the "four Ds" of negligence.
16. Explain the importance of keeping accurate medical records.
17. List 10 guidelines of risk management to avoid a lawsuit.
18. Describe the trial process.

Health Care Legislation
19. List five types of patient information that, by law, must be reported to state or local authorities.
20. Explain the purpose of a living will.
21. Explain the purpose of the Uniform Anatomical Gift Act.
22. List three laws that concern workplace issues and explain how they can protect medical assistants and other workers.

Ethics in Health Care
23. Explain the difference between ethics and law.
24. State the five parts of the American Association of Medical Assistants Code of Ethics.
25. Describe the legal and ethical importance of maintaining patient privacy and confidentiality.
26. Describe the expectations patients have for effective care.
27. List three bioethical situations and explain the considerations for each.

Patient-Centered Professionalism
28. Analyze a realistic medical office situation and apply law and ethics to determine the best course of action.
29. Describe the impact on patient care when medical assistants have a solid understanding of law and ethics.

KEY TERMS

abandonment
administrative law
age of majority
agent
assault
battery
bioethics
breach of contract
Centers for Disease Control and Prevention (CDC)
confidentiality
consideration
constitutional law
contract
criminal law
damages
emancipated minor
endorsement
ethics
euthanasia
examination
expressed contract
felony
fiduciary
genomics
Good Samaritan Act
gross negligence

Continued

KEY TERMS—cont'd

- Health Insurance Portability and Accountability Act (HIPAA)
- implied contract
- infraction
- international law
- laws
- libel
- license
- malfeasance
- malpractice
- material safety data sheet (MSDS)
- Medical Practice Acts
- misdemeanor
- misfeasance
- negligence
- noncompliance
- nonfeasance
- Occupational Safety and Health Administration (OSHA)
- Patient Care Partnership
- Patient's Bill of Rights
- private law
- public law
- *quid pro quo*
- reciprocity
- *res ipsa loquitur*
- *respondeat superior*
- risk management
- slander
- statute of limitations
- statutes
- subpoena
- subpoena *duces tecum*
- tort
- vicarious liability

PRACTICAL APPLICATIONS

Read the following scenario and keep it in mind as you learn about law and ethics in this chapter.

Jill is a medical assistant with on-the-job training in a medical office setting. She always strives to be caring, courteous, and respectful of patients and co-workers. Because of her caring attitude, the patients with whom Jill works all appreciate her attitude and her work. One of Jill's favorite patients, Shandra, a 24-year-old mother of two young children, has been diagnosed with cancer and recently was told by the physician that her condition is terminal. Shandra is at the office for an appointment and is feeling very upset about her terminal illness. She pours out her heart and fears to Jill. Wanting to comfort Shandra, Jill tells her, "Don't worry. You'll be just fine. You know the doctor will make you better."

Shandra is comforted by Jill's words and tells her how much Jill means to her. In fact, she has so much faith in Jill that she believes that she *will* be fine and tells her family what Jill has said. Sadly, a few months later, Shandra dies. Believing she would be fine, Shandra had not made any plans for her children and family. Her family is upset with the physician and with Jill. The family thinks they have been betrayed because they believed that Shandra would be fine. The family is discussing what to say to the physician about this betrayal and whether to bring a lawsuit because Shandra did not have a will.

How might this situation have been avoided? What are the possible implications for Shandra's family, Jill, the physician, and the practice?

LAW AND LICENSURE IN MEDICAL PRACTICE

In the United States, **laws** protect the physical and social well-being of the citizens. Laws, or **statutes**, are general rules and standards to regulate conduct. They must be followed or punishment occurs. During the twentieth century, a system for protecting the public from unsafe medical practitioners was mandated by law in all states. This system, spelled out in the **Medical Practice Acts**, is based on the ethical belief that practitioners should "do no harm." Medical assistants should understand this system, which involves licensure and credentialing.

Medical Practice Acts

Medical Practice Acts are statutes created by states to oversee the practice of medicine. The acts establish a medical board to review licensing requirements, guidelines for suspension and loss of licenses, and renewal requirements for physicians in the state. These acts allow the physician-employer to hire and train unlicensed health care workers, and the acts are recognized in most states. If a physician allows unlicensed health care workers to perform diagnostic or treatment procedures, the physician's license can be revoked or suspended. All 50 states have laws that protect people from unqualified persons practicing medicine.

Licensure

Many health professionals have some form of regulation of their profession to ensure competence. A **license,** the strongest form of professional regulation, is a legal document that allows a person to offer skills and knowledge to the public for pay. A license is required for persons practicing in certain professions, including doctors of medicine (MDs) and registered nurses (RNs). Rules for licensing are developed by Medical Practice Act statutes in each state. The following three ways are used to obtain a state license:

1. **Examination:** Oral and written exams for a particular state are taken and passed.
2. **Reciprocity:** A state accepts a current license from another state.
3. **Endorsement:** A state accepts the scores of a national examination.

Licenses must be renewed, and proof of continuing education must be current. A license that is not renewed by the deadline automatically becomes inactive. Practicing medicine without an active license is a **felony.**

Practicing without a License

Dr. Moore went to medical school but never took the credentialing examinations. He moved to a different location, opened an office, and began to practice family medicine without a license. The community came to respect and trust him. He

> **Practicing without a License—cont'd**
>
> had a good bedside manner and often referred patients to specialists in neighboring communities. Another physician approached him about developing a partnership, but he refused. His reluctance concerned the other physician, who did some research and found that "Dr." Moore was not truly an MD. The physician reported this to the state medical board. Dr. Moore was criminally charged for practicing without a license.

The Physician and Licensure

Box 4-1 lists the requirements physicians must meet to earn a license. Physicians are usually required to renew their license biennially (every 2 years). To renew, they are required to have 50 continuing medical education hours (CMEs) each year, including 5 hours of **risk management.** The physician must be licensed by the state to prescribe medications. To prescribe scheduled medications, such as narcotics, the physician must also obtain a license from the U.S. Drug Enforcement Agency (DEA). A physician cannot prescribe medication to anyone, including a friend or acquaintance, without first examining the person as a patient and performing the necessary tests, making a diagnosis, and properly documenting the medical record.

A physician's license can be suspended or revoked in certain situations (Box 4-2).

> **BOX 4-1**
>
> **Requirements for Physician License**
>
> - Meet individual state requirements.
> - Complete education requirements through an approved medical school.
> - Complete an approved residency program.
> - Pass all examinations required by the state board of medical examiners.
> - Be of good moral character.
> - Attain the age of majority as defined by state statute.

> **BOX 4-2**
>
> **Reasons for Revocation or Suspension of a Physician's License**
>
> 1. Conviction of a crime
>   - Felony (e.g., practicing without a license, murder, rape, larceny, or substance abuse)
>   - Fraud (e.g., billing for more treatments than given/upcoding)
> 2. Unprofessional conduct
>   - Failure to adhere to ethical standards
>   - Breach of confidence
>   - Fee splitting
>   - Addiction to drugs or alcohol
>   - Advertising falsely
>   - Incapacity to perform duties

In addition to maintaining a license to practice, the physician is responsible for hiring qualified employees. The doctrine of *respondeat superior* (RA-spon-dant su-per-e-or; Latin for "let the master answer") places the liability on the physician for an employee's actions. This means that a physician is held responsible for the actions of the employees under his or her supervision. Even though the medical assistant has a responsibility to the physician to perform all duties competently, the physician is held liable for the medical assistant's actions. This is called **vicarious liability.**

> **Vicarious Liability**
>
> Janet, a medical assistant, is driving from one office to another and stops at a bakery to pick up a cake for an office birthday party. After leaving the bakery, she speeds through a school zone, sideswiping a car and injuring three children walking home from school. Because the accident occurred while Janet was on "company business" (performing activities for her job), the physician-employer could well be named in a resulting lawsuit.

Credentialing

Credentialing is a voluntary process that health professionals can go through to earn certifications and other proof of their knowledge and skills. Credentials are earned by meeting a set of expectations. Steps in the process may include the following:

1. Graduating from an accredited program.
2. Selecting a test site.
3. Completing an application and returning it with the appropriate application fee.
4. Taking and passing the examination.
5. Renewing by completing the required continuing education units (CEUs) in a defined period.

Credentialing for physicians can also refer to the process of applying to a hospital for staff privileges. Physicians must present proof of their education and medical competency, along with peer recommendations, for approval by the hospital's board of directors.

The Medical Assistant and Credentialing

Some states have statutes that protect the medical assistant's right to practice. Other states may limit what a medical assistant can do. It is important to know the statutes of your state because you can only do what you have been trained to do and what the state law allows you to do. Credentialing is not a requirement in all states. However, it is highly recommended because it helps ensure a competency level of knowledge and training. You learned about becoming credentialed in Chapter 2.

PATIENT-CENTERED PROFESSIONALISM

- In some states a medical assistant can work without being credentialed. What do you see as the value of being credentialed?
- How might obtaining credentials as a medical assistant affect patients' views of you as a professional?
- Why do you think a medical practice would want its medical assistants to be credentialed?

LAW AND LIABILITY

Medical assistants need a good understanding of what law is and how it applies to the medical practice. Learning about the categories of law and how liability (guilt) is determined is a good place to begin. Laws can be divided into two main categories: public law and private law (also referred to as *civil law*). Each branch has its own subcategories. Both public law and private law affect the medical practice (Figures 4-1 and 4-2).

Public Law

Public law deals with offenses or crimes against the welfare or safety of the public. The main divisions are administrative, criminal, constitutional, and international law. The medical profession mainly deals with the administrative and criminal aspects of public law.

Administrative Law

Administrative law regulates business practices and is the body of law governing administrative agencies. Agencies are created by Congress or state legislatures such as the Social Security Administration or the Occupational Safety and Health Administration. The administrative agency administers law through the creation of regulations and enforcement of these regulations. The administrative branch of public law creates the state board of medical examiners for physicians.

Criminal Law

Criminal law deals with the rights and responsibilities of the government to the people and the people to the government. Box 4-3 lists the offenses considered under criminal law. This branch of public law protects the welfare and safety of the public by establishing what is legal and illegal. It also provides guidelines on how those committing crimes will be punished.

Constitutional Law

Fundamental laws of a nation or state are defined in a constitution. **Constitutional law** interprets and defends a constitution. State constitutions are subordinate to the U.S. Constitution.

International Law

International law protects and asserts the rights and privileges of a sovereign nation.

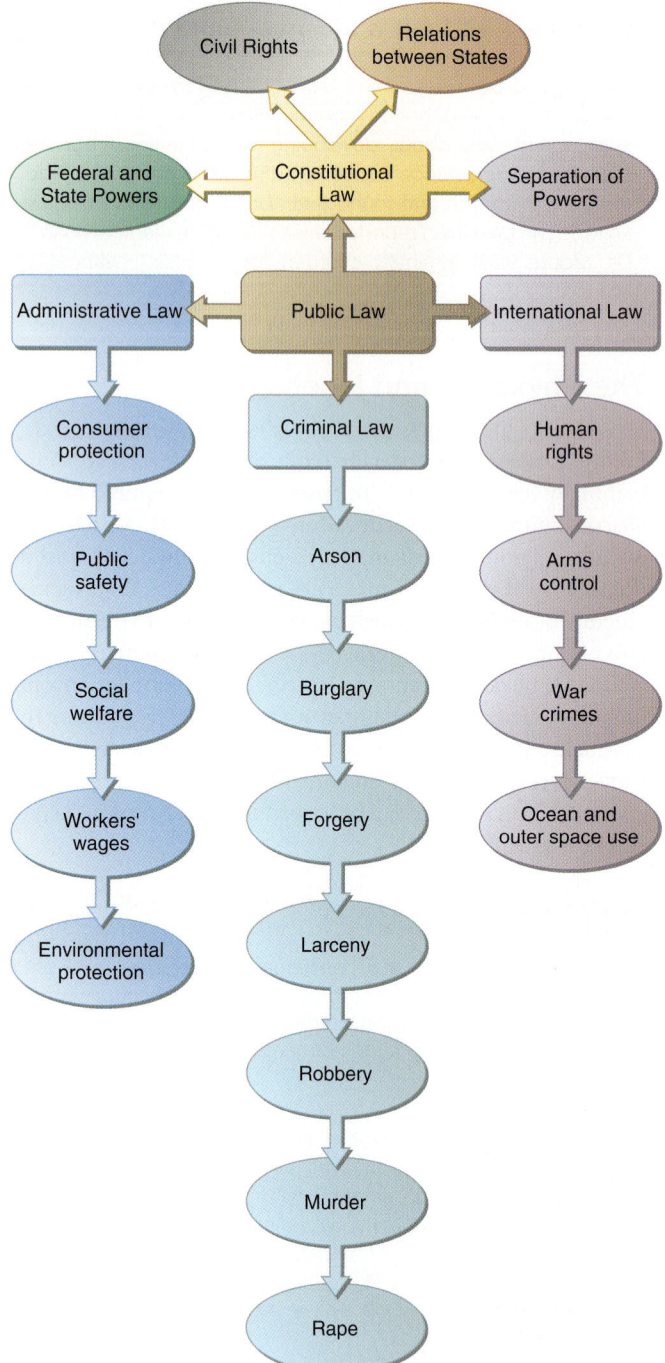

FIGURE 4-1 Public law flowchart.

Private Law

Private law, or civil law, is concerned with the enforcement of rights, the performance of duties, and other legal issues involving private individuals. Crimes considered under private law are solely against an individual person or property. The main divisions of private law are property law, family law, inheritance law, corporate law, contract law, and tort law. Contract and tort laws apply to everyday living and the medical practice more than the other divisions. Civil law reviews rules and a court judge must then apply the case as it is presented to them.

Law and Ethics in Health Care **CHAPTER 4** 49

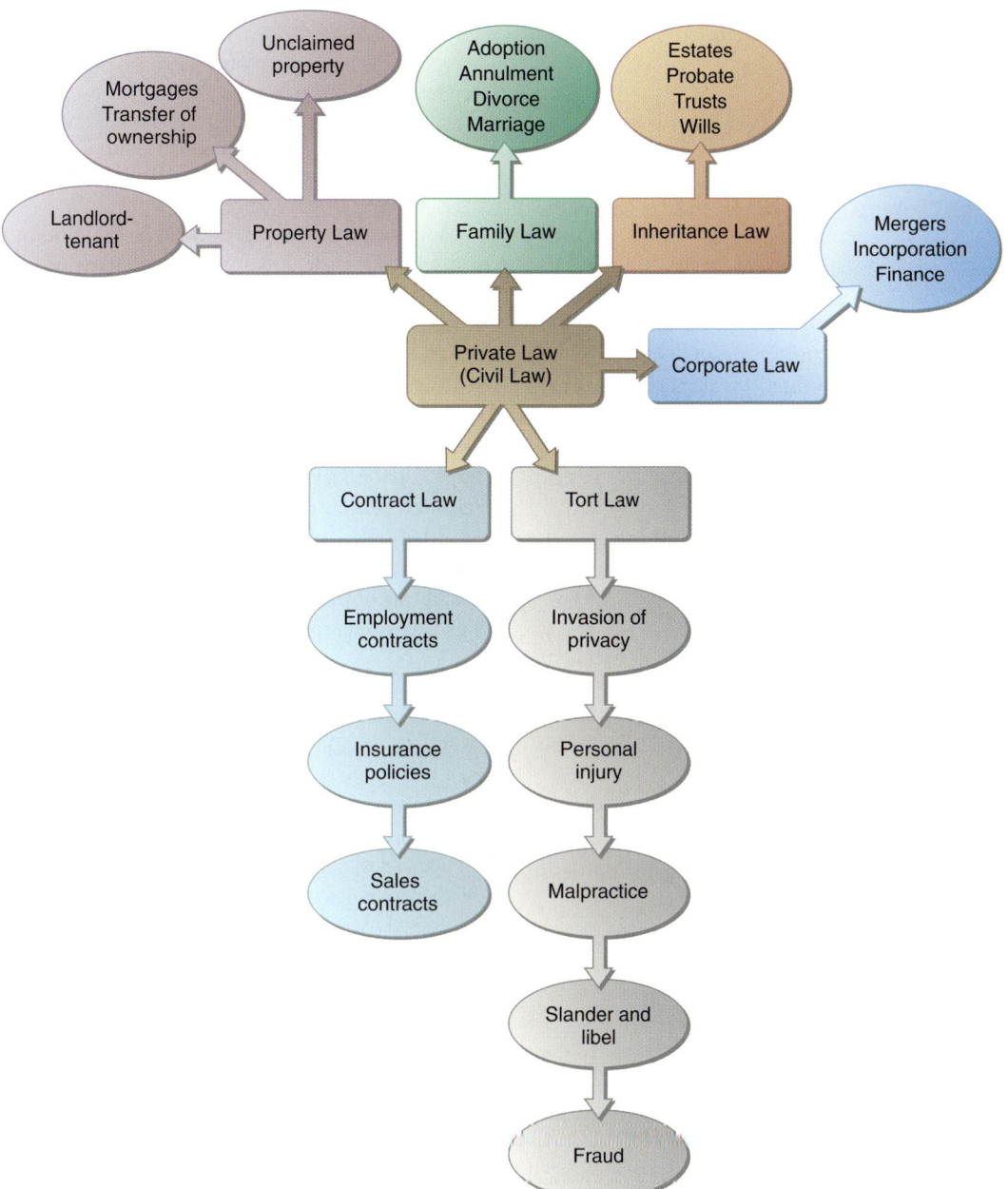

FIGURE 4-2 Private law flowchart.

BOX 4-3

Offenses Considered under Criminal Law

- **Felony:** A serious crime that is punishable, as defined in the state statute, by death or incarceration. Crimes against the public that fall into this category are murder, rape, assault, and larceny (theft of a large amount of money).
- **Misdemeanor:** A crime that is punishable in jail for less than 1 year. It is considered less serious than a felony and includes disorderly conduct and petty theft.
- **Infraction:** A violation of a law or ordinance that usually results in a fine. This is the least serious of all offenses (e.g., jaywalking).

Contract Law

Contractual agreements occur every day, both in our professional and personal lives. Health professionals must understand several aspects of contract law.

A **contract** is an agreement between two or more people promising to work toward a specific goal for adequate **consideration** (payment or benefit). The physician-patient relationship is considered a contractual agreement. The two parties in this type of contract are the physician and the patient. As with any contract, a physician-patient contract must meet certain requirements to be valid and enforceable by law, as follows:

1. **There must be an offer and acceptance among the parties. For example:**

   > Dr. Sanford is a licensed general practitioner who accepts new patients. Mr. Smith wants Dr. Sanford to become his physician. He calls Dr. Sanford's office to make an appointment. Dr. Sanford's office agrees to give Mr. Smith an appointment the next day.
   >
   > OFFER → AGREEMENT → ACCEPTANCE

   An offer must be specific and communicated in words or actions. Mr. Smith communicated his desire to become a patient by calling Dr. Sanford's office to make an appointment. Acceptance of this offer occurred when Dr. Sanford agreed to examine Mr. Smith with the understanding that Dr. Sanford would be paid for his services.

2. **There must be a valid consideration (something of value must be exchanged, such as money or services). For example:**

   > Dr. Sanford agreed to examine Mr. Smith in exchange for payment. Mr. Smith also agrees to follow Dr. Sanford's advice in exchange for being seen. The consideration in this physician-patient contract between Dr. Sanford and Mr. Smith is the money Dr. Sanford received for the examination.
   >
   > ACCEPTANCE → CONSIDERATION

   Both the patient and the physician have responsibilities in the physician-patient contract.

   The physician is expected to do the following:
   1. Diagnose and treat each patient to the best of his or her ability.
   2. Be available to the patient for care.
   3. Arrange for a substitute physician to take patient calls if unavailable (failure to do this is considered **abandonment**).

   The patient is expected to do the following:
   1. Truthfully impart past and present medical information.
   2. Follow all treatments prescribed by the physician.
   3. Take all medications.
   4. Keep all scheduled appointments.
   5. Be responsible with an appropriate (agreed-on) reimbursement plan.

3. **The agreement must have a lawful purpose. For example:**

   > Receiving medical care from a licensed physician is not illegal. Had Dr. Sanford not been licensed, however, the contract would have been invalid because Dr. Sanford would have been practicing without a license, which is a felony.

   If the service is illegal, there is no contract. State statutes govern all agreements.

4. **All parties must be competent (have the legal capacity to make a contract). For example:**

   > Both Mr. Smith and Dr. Sanford are over age 18, are considered competent (able to make sound judgments), and understand what is being agreed to, so they were able to enter into the physician-patient contract. Had Mr. Smith been underage (under 18 in most states), a parent or legal guardian would have had to form the contract with Dr. Sanford.

   A competent person is capable of making decisions for himself or herself. Anyone under the **age of majority** is considered by law to be a minor and cannot enter into a contract. An exception to this rule is the **emancipated minor,** an underage person who has legally separated from parents for various reasons (e.g., military service, marriage).

5. **The agreement must be in the form required by law.**

   Mr. Smith and Dr. Sanford's contract was verbal. Contracts may also be written, as in consent forms. Each state has a required format to be considered valid.

   When all requirements for a contract have been met, the contract is considered valid and is enforceable in a court of law. If one of the parties fails to meet the terms of the contract, this is considered **breach** (break) **of contract.** For example:

   > Dr. Sanford and Mr. Smith could breach their physician-patient contract in the following ways:
   > - Mr. Smith could fail to follow Dr. Sanford's medical advice.
   > - Dr. Sanford or his staff could promise that Mr. Smith's illness would be cured through treatment, and this promise would be in danger of being broken because of unforeseen circumstances or conditions.
   > - Dr. Sanford could promise to provide Mr. Smith with the latest treatments and then not follow through.

   Occasionally the physician may want to withdraw from the care of a patient because the patient is displaying **noncompliance** (failing to follow the treatments prescribed). To do so, the physician is required to withdraw from the physician-patient contract formally and must do the following:
   1. Notify the patient in writing.
   2. Indicate the reason(s) for the withdrawal.
   3. Give a date when this withdrawal takes effect (minimum of 30 days).
   4. Provide a list of physicians who may be willing to treat the patient.
   5. Provide for transfer of the patient's medical record.
   6. Send the letter by certified mail with return receipt requested, and retain a copy of the letter and the return receipt for legal protection.

   If a patient withdraws from a physician's care, this must be fully documented in the patient's chart. When a patient requests that his or her records be sent to another physician for transfer of care, the signed and dated records release form must be filed in the patient's chart.

   Types of Contracts. The two most common types of contracts used in a medical setting are expressed and implied contracts.

   Expressed. An **expressed contract** is one that is specifically stated aloud or written and is understood by all parties.

When a third party (e.g., not the insurance company or patient, usually a relative) agrees to pay for any medical services not covered by insurance, the expressed contract must be in writing. For example:

> Mr. Smith's adult son calls Dr. Sanford's office and says, "Send me Dad's bills and I'll pay them." This is not enforceable unless the agreement is in writing. The statute of frauds in each state indicates which contracts must be written.

Oral contracts exist when both parties agree to a specified condition with proper consideration. For example:

> During an interview between Dr. Sanford and Ms. Johnson, an applicant for a medical assisting position in his office, an agreement is reached about the job duties expected. Dr. Sanford offers Ms. Johnson a specified salary, and she accepts. A valid oral contract has been made.

Implied. An **implied contract** is one that is suggested or expected but not clearly expressed. Most of what occurs in a medical office is by implied agreement. The physician-employer places staff, including medical assistants, in a position to act as his or her **agent** (a person who is authorized to act for or in place of another). Remember that a physician is responsible for the actions of his or her employees while they are performing within their scope of training. As a medical assistant, you will encounter physician-patient contract situations. The patient will interpret your words and actions as a medical assistant to be speaking and acting for the physician and will see you in a position of trusted responsibility (**fiduciary**). For example:

> When Mr. Smith called Dr. Sanford's office for an appointment, kept the appointment, and received treatment, he was expected to pay the bill under the terms of the implied contract. Even though Dr. Sanford may not have made the appointment for Mr. Smith in person, because his staff was acting on his behalf, the physician-patient contract was still valid.

Tort Law

A **tort** is a wrongful act committed by a person against another person or property that causes harm. Tort law concerns health professionals because it deals with negligence and medical **malpractice,** or *medical professional liability,* and covers the areas where no contract exists. Malpractice is a specific type of negligence in which a professional fails to act with reasonable care. The person committing malpractice is held liable for the **damages** if the act caused harm (e.g., physical injury, damaged property, or loss of personal freedom). Remember, if the health professional does no harm, there is no tort. Torts can be classified as either intentional (willful) or nonintentional (accidental) (Figure 4-3).

Intentional Tort. Violating a person's rights or property with the intent to do harm is an *intentional tort.* **Gross negligence** is intentional negligence, or a wrongful act done (or not done) on purpose. Money is typically awarded to victims of inten-

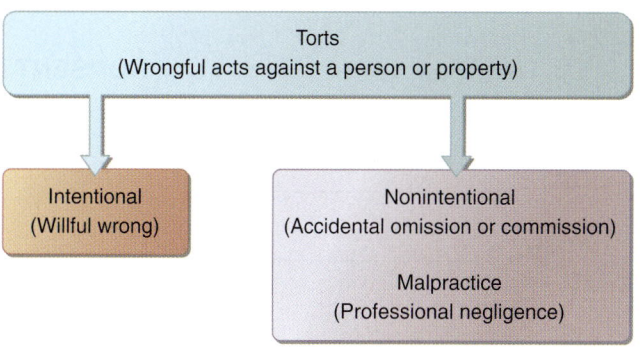

FIGURE 4-3 Classification of torts.

tional torts. Intentional torts can also result in the person being charged under criminal law. This type of tort can be broken down into the following two categories:

Assault is the threat or the perceived threat of doing bodily harm by another person.

Battery is the act of touching or doing bodily harm without consent (permission).

For example:

> Sandy Johnson, Dr. Sanford's new medical assistant, is asked to draw Mr. Smith's blood. Mr. Smith tells Sandy he doesn't want it done, but Sandy pulls Mr. Smith's arm down and draws the blood anyway. In this situation, Sandy is actually guilty of battery because she did not have Mr. Smith's consent.

You must have the patient's consent to carry out any treatment or procedure.

To avoid being accused of battery, *informed consent* must be given by the patient before a treatment or procedure. For surgical procedures the physician must explain the following, using words the patient can understand:

1. What procedure is to be done and why.
2. What is going to happen.
3. Who will be doing the procedure.
4. Whether others will or will not be involved (e.g., will there be another person assisting with the procedure).
5. What results are expected.
6. What risks are involved.
7. What the consequences are if the procedure is not done.
8. What alternative treatments are available and the risks.
9. Any other important information the patient needs to make a decision. It is best if this is in writing. See Figure 4-4, "Consent for Surgery" form. Only the physician can do the informing; a medical assistant can act as a witness.

However, what if the patient cannot give informed consent before treatment? Emergency situations in which a patient's life, health, or safety is in immediate danger are exceptions to the informed consent rule. Under the **Good Samaritan Act,** implied consent applies if no one is available to consent for the patient and if a "reasonable" person would consent under similar circumstances. The Good Samaritan Act may vary

CONSENT FOR SURGERY

DATE:_____

TIME:_____

I authorize the performance of the following procedure(s)_____
_____on_____
To be performed by_____, MD.

The following have been explained to me by Dr._____

    1. Nature of the procedure:_____

    2. Reason(s) for procedure:_____

    3. Possible risks:_____

    4. Possible complications:_____

I understand that no warranty or guarantee of the effectiveness of the surgery can be made.

I have been informed of possible alternative treatments including_____
_____and of the likely consequences of receiving no treatment, and I freely consent to this procedure.

I hereby authorize the above named surgeon and his/her assistants to provide additional services including administering anesthesia and / or medications, performing needed diagnostic tests including but not limited to radiology, and any other additional services deemed necessary for my well-being. I consent to have removed tissue examined by a pathologist who may then dispose of the tissue as he/she sees fit.

Signed_____ Relationship to patient_____
      Patient / Parent / Guardian

Witness_____

FIGURE 4-4 Consent for surgery form.

from state to state but basically provides that care given in good faith by a health professional or a non–health professional is protected from civil liability if the person provided care within their scope of training. The implied consent would end if the patient became able to answer on his or her own behalf. In this case the rescuers would let the person know what they were doing and would ask, "Is it okay to continue?"

Other examples of intentional torts follow:

1. *Defamation* of character occurs when false statements, written or spoken, are made public about another person with the intent to damage the person's reputation.

- **Libel** is defamation of character in writing.
- **Slander** is defamation of character with speech. To be considered in a court of law, a third person must be present when slander is taking place.
2. *False imprisonment* is the intentional, unlawful restraint of a patient. For example, you cannot stop a patient or employee from leaving the office.
3. *Fraud* refers to a deceitful or dishonest practice in order to induce someone to part with something of value or a legal right. Examples include not telling a patient about the risks of a procedure, performing an experimental procedure on a patient without letting the patient know it is experimental, and charging the insurance company for procedures not done.
4. *Invasion of privacy* is an unlawful intrusion into the personal life of another person without cause or disclosure of public information without the person's consent. This includes the public release of information about a person or the use of photographs of a person without the person's consent. This is a breach of confidentiality and privacy and could result in a lawsuit.

Nonintentional Tort. Ordinary **negligence** is not doing (or doing) something that a reasonable person would do (or not do). Ordinary negligence is not intentional. Forms of ordinary negligence are malfeasance, misfeasance, and nonfeasance. *Feasance* is the performance of an act.

1. **Malfeasance** is the performance of an unlawful or improper act causing or resulting in harm. An example of malfeasance is a medical assistant practicing beyond the scope of his or her training. A medical assistant cannot imply he or she is a nurse.
2. **Misfeasance** is the improper performance of an act that results in harm to the patient. Misfeasance occurs, for example, when a patient receives a burn during ultrasound therapy.
3. **Nonfeasance** is the failure to do what is expected, resulting in harm to the patient. For example, a patient comes in with an arm injury, the physician fails to order an x-ray film, and later it is found that the patient has a broken arm.

Lawsuits

More than 85% of medical lawsuits are for ordinary negligence (mistakes made in good faith). It is important for all health professionals to understand the actions that could lead to a lawsuit and the ways to avoid them (risk management). When such actions cannot be avoided, it is necessary to be familiar with the trial process so that you can be a credible witness.

Causes for Lawsuit

Four components, or "four Ds," must be present before an attorney will pursue a case for professional negligence, as follows:
1. *Duty* occurs when the physician-patient relationship is established. For example:

> A new patient sees the physician and makes a follow-up appointment for an experimental procedure.

2. *Dereliction of duty* occurs when a health care professional fails to meet accepted standards of care. **Res ipsa loquitur** (ras ep-sa lo-kwi-tur; Latin for "the thing speaks for itself") is the principle that applies when the very existence of the situation shows negligence (e.g., surgical sponge left in the abdomen after surgery). For example:

> At the follow-up appointment, the physician treats the patient with an experimental procedure, even though the physician knows he has not had adequate training to perform this procedure safely.

3. *Direct cause* or *proximate cause* must be shown between the patient's injury and the actions of the health care professional. For example:

> The patient develops a new medical problem proven to be caused by the improper performance of the procedure.

4. *Damages* (money) awarded will compensate the victim for the permanent injury (Table 4-1). For example:

> The patient is awarded money as compensation for the medical problem.

Each state has laws that limit the length of time a person has to take legal action. These **statutes of limitations** (time limits to bring forth a lawsuit) for malpractice vary in length and by situation. Medical office professionals must be aware of the statute of limitations in their state because it will impact the way medical records are kept. The dates and information recorded in the medical record can be used in a lawsuit, so the medical records must be up to date, accurate, and complete.

A patient's own negligence may impact damages awarded. In some states, if the patient has contributed to the injury, this is called *contributory negligence,* and no damages will be awarded. In some states, if the physician and the patient were both at fault, it is considered to be *comparative negligence,* and compensation will be less.

Avoiding Lawsuits or Risk Management

The best way to avoid a lawsuit for malpractice is to keep the lines of communication open between the medical staff and the patient. Establishing and maintaining a good relationship builds mutual trust and respect. Box 4-4 provides guidelines to avoid a lawsuit. Remember accurate documentation is the best form of risk management. When dealing with an angry patient the use of positive body language (e.g., smile) and a kind word can do wonders to calm the patient.

Lawsuit Process

Even when the guidelines for avoiding a lawsuit are followed, it may not always be enough. If a patient's attorney decides that the "four Ds" of negligence exist, the attorney will file a

TABLE 4-1

Damages in Lawsuits

Type of Damages	Compensation	Awarded for
GENERAL COMPENSATORY DAMAGES Payment for injuries or losses that have been demonstrated	Monetary award	Any of the following as a result from the injury: Pain Suffering Mental anguish Any physical disability
SPECIAL COMPENSATION Payment for costs incurred because of the negligent act	Monetary award	Any of the following as a result from the injury: Loss of earnings Medical bills Rehabilitation therapy
PUNITIVE DAMAGES Payment for injury or loss caused by gross negligence	Monetary award as determined by state statute	Any conduct that is considered by the court to be intentional or malicious. Award is not to compensate the plaintiff but to punish the defendant.

BOX 4-4

Guidelines to Avoid a Lawsuit (Risk Management)

NEVER:
- Promise a specific outcome, such as a cure, as a result of the procedure or treatment.
- Chart criticism or negative comments about the physician, patient, or other health care professionals. Keep your opinions to yourself.
- Verbalize negative comments about the medical staff.
- Give medical advice or diagnose, even when asked your opinion.
- Speak to the plaintiff or their attorney without the approval of the physician's attorney.
- Alter a medical record by using "white out" or correction tape.

ALWAYS:
- Listen to the patient's concerns or complaints; chart the facts or write "the patient states."
- Document accurately what you did, what you observed, and what the patient said.
- Have the physician or attorney review any patient's record before copying them.
- Perform within your scope of training.
- Practice safe work habits.
- Keep patient information confidential.
- Chart missed appointments.
- Document phone calls.
- Follow-up with test results in a timely manner by providing the patient a specific time frame in which to expect the results.
- Record when the patient has been notified of the test results and the action taken.
- Treat all patients equally and with respect.

complaint and the process begins. As a medical assistant you need to understand what happens with lawsuits in case you are involved in preparing materials for one or testifying in court. Table 4-2 shows the different phases in the lawsuit process, as well as what the medical assistant needs to know about each.

PATIENT-CENTERED PROFESSIONALISM

- *What is the benefit to patients when the medical assistant understands the contract process (and the physician-patient contract)? What is the benefit to the medical assistant and the practice?*
- *How can the lawsuit process affect patients? Medical assistants? The medical practice?*
- *Why is it better to avoid a lawsuit rather than go to trial, even in situations in which the practice would "win" the lawsuit?*
- *What should you keep in mind about your appearance, your communication, and your professionalism when testifying in court? What does it matter whether the people in the courtroom think you look and sound credible as long as you are telling the truth?*

HEALTH CARE LEGISLATION

In addition to contract law and tort law, the medical assistant needs to be aware of other national, state, and local laws and regulations. These regulations involve reporting requirements, living wills, donation of one's body or organs, debt collection, and workplace issues.

TABLE 4-2

Lawsuit Process

Phase	What Happens	What You Need to Know as a Medical Assistant
Summons	After receiving the complaint, the court issues a *summons*, and the complaint is delivered to the defendant (the physician). The defendant notifies his or her attorney and insurance carrier. A response to the summons must be filed with the court addressing the charges and making any applicable counterclaims.	You may be asked to make copies of medical records. Always check with the physician or the physician's attorney before copying them.
Collection of information	If no motions to dismiss or move the trial are approved, a period of discovery begins to uncover evidence to support charges. A *deposition* is a formal retrieval of information about the charges and is either written or given orally. An *interrogatory* is a written set of questions requiring written answers. A **subpoena** is a document requiring a person to appear in court or to be available for a deposition. A **subpoena *duces tecum*** is an order to appear in court with the original records; in this case, the patient's chart. *Testimony* is a statement given under oath about what a person knows. If the evidence is obvious (e.g., surgical instrument left inside a body cavity after surgery), testimony of an expert may not be needed. This doctrine is called *res ipsa loquitur* ("the thing speaks for itself").	You may be asked to supply information or records during this process.
Trial	A jury is selected. Each attorney makes opening statements. The plaintiff's (patient's) attorney calls witnesses, and the defendant's (physician's) attorney cross-examines. The defendant's attorney calls witnesses, and the plaintiff's attorney cross-examines. Both attorneys make closing arguments to explain why the jury should decide in their favor. The judge gives the jury instructions and asks them to reach a *verdict* based on the evidence. If the jury finds the defendant not guilty, the case is dismissed; if the jury finds the defendant guilty, a monetary settlement is awarded.	If called as a witness to testify, you need to be prepared. When you testify, your statements will be evaluated not only on what you have to say but also on how credible you appear to be. You can increase your credibility in the following ways: *Appearance* • Dress appropriately (e.g., conservative hairstyle and makeup, simple jewelry). • Do not chew gum or bite nails. • Maintain good posture. *Behavior* • Remain calm. • Make eye contact with the attorneys, judge, and jury. • Have a professional manner at all times. *Communication* • Only give answers that you know as fact. • Only give answers to what is asked. • Answer questions clearly.
Appeal	Either attorney can file an *appeal* to a higher court to reconsider the decision.	Again, you may be asked to provide more oral or written information during this phase.
Arbitration	An alternative to going to trial, in some cases, is having the dispute go before an arbitrator. Both sides present their case, and the arbitrator decides the outcome. In *binding arbitration*, the decision is final.	You may be asked to provide oral or written information for this process.

Reporting Requirements

Some issues affect the health, safety, and welfare of the general public and must be reported despite confidentiality. All states require the report of *vital statistics,* including births, deaths, and communicable diseases. Other reportable situations are injuries caused by a lethal weapon (gun or knife), bad reactions to vaccines, certain diseases in newborns (e.g., congenital syphilis), and suspected abuse (Box 4-5). Medical assistants must report all suspected child abuse, elder abuse, spousal abuse, and drug abuse. Even if abuse is only suspected, it must be reported. Every state has a statute governing the reporting of diseases that could pose potential harm to the public (e.g., *Listeriosis,* Q fever, encephalitis, etc.). Local, state, and national agencies (e.g., **Centers for Disease Control and Prevention [CDC]**) require that such diseases be reported when they are diagnosed by physicians and laboratories. Reporting allows for the collection of statistics that show how often the disease occurs, which helps to identify disease trends and track disease outbreaks. Reportable diseases are divided into the following several groups:

- Mandatory *written reporting* (e.g., gonorrhea and salmonellosis).
- Mandatory *reporting by telephone* (e.g., rubeola [measles] and pertussis [whooping cough]).
- Report of total number of cases (e.g., chickenpox and influenza).
- Mandatory reporting to the CDC (e.g., acquired immunodeficiency syndrome [AIDS], anthrax, botulism, and poliomyelitis).

The forms and reports required for each reportable incident will vary. Medical assistants must be familiar with what is required in their state.

Patient Awareness and Protection

Some health care legislation protects patients and helps make them aware of their rights. As a medical assistant, you need to understand these laws so that you will be able to follow them and explain them to patients when necessary. The Patient Self-Determination Act, the Uniform Anatomical Act, and the Fair Debt Collection Practices and Bankruptcy Acts all help protect patients' rights and wishes.

Patient Self-Determination Act

The *Patient Self-Determination Act* of 1990 requires health care institutions to give patients written information about advance directives before life-sustaining measures become necessary. *Advance directives* are documents that state people's wishes in case they become incapable of making decisions. Two forms of advance directives are the *living will* and *durable power of attorney for health care.* These documents provide written instructions and are legally binding documents.

Living Will. A living will is a statement to the family, physician, or lawyer that conveys a person's decisions about medical treatment if the person becomes unable to make the decision. The living will does not go into effect until the person becomes terminally ill (Figure 4-5).

A living will is characterized by the following:
- Must be witnessed by two persons, one of whom is neither a spouse nor a blood relative.
- Can be revoked or amended at any time by the individual who initiated it.
- Only pertains to health, *not* finances.
- Should be copied and given to the physician, family, attorney, and kept with the individual's legal papers.
- Requires a physician and the hospital staff to abide by the individual's wishes.

BOX 4-5

Characteristics of Emotional Abuse, Neglect, Child Abuse, and Elder Abuse

Emotional abuse occurs when a parent, guardian, or spouse needlessly yells, calls a person derogatory names, or tells them they are useless. An example is a parent yelling at a child, "You're stupid! You can't do anything right! What good are you?"

Neglect occurs when a safe place is not provided to live, play, and grow up. The emotional scars from neglect do not show up like bruises and burns. Forms of neglect include:
- Leaving a child alone
- Not locking up poisons (e.g., bleach, bug spray)
- Not feeding and bathing a child on a regular basis
- Not providing a child with adequate clothing for the weather
- Not providing a child with medical attention when needed

Child abuse can be physical or sexual in nature.

SIGNS OF PHYSICAL ABUSE
- Bruises on the face, lips, mouth, cheeks, buttocks, back, chest, abdomen, and inner thighs
- Welts taking the shape of an object (e.g., belt, chain, hanger, or rope) on the same areas as described for bruises
- Burns and scalds of the hands, feet, back, or buttocks
- Fractures of the nose, skull, legs, or arms
- Bite marks on any part of the body

SIGNS OF SEXUAL ABUSE
- Bruises or bleeding of genitalia, mouth, or anus
- Stains or blood on undergarments
- Difficult or painful urination
- Vaginal discharge and genital odor
- Difficulty walking
- Pregnancy

Elder abuse signs may or may not be physical in nature and include:
- Living conditions that are unclean and unsafe
- Poor personal hygiene
- Weight loss resulting from poor nutrition and fluid intake
- Frequent or recurring injuries
- New and old bruises that can be seen
- Patient who is anxious and fearful and a caregiver who is always present and does not let the patient answer questions
- Frequent trips to the emergency department
- Medications not taken or taken improperly

LIVING WILL

To my family, physician, and spiritual advisor;
To any medical facility that has been entrusted with my care;
To anyone who should have interest in my health, welfare, or affairs:

I willfully and voluntarily make this my definite expression of my desires:

If the situation arises in which I cannot participate in my own decision making regarding my health care decisions and the attending physician and another consulting physician determine I have:

☐ A Terminal Condition; meaning a condition caused by injury or illness from which there is no reasonable medical probability of recovery and which, without treatment, can be expected to cause death;

or

☐ An End-Stage Condition; meaning a condition that is caused by injury or illness which has resulted in severe and permanent deterioration, indicated by incapacity and complete physical dependency, and for which, to a reasonable degree of medical certainty, treatment of the irreversible condition would be medically ineffective;

or

☐ A Persistent Vegetative State; meaning a permanent and irreversible condition of unconsciousness in which there is (1) the absence of voluntary action or cognitive behavior of any kind and (2) an inability to communicate or interact purposefully with the environment.

Then, I request that I be allowed to die and that life-prolonging procedures not be either initiated or provided. I direct that I am not to be kept alive by ventilators, artificial means, or through "heroic measures" and that nutrition and hydration not be administered by artificial means through invasive medical procedures. I wish to be treated with dignity and do not wish to suffer the indignities of hopeless pain, loneliness, and isolation. I request that medication be administered to me to alleviate pain and suffering, acknowledging that this may hasten death but without the intention of taking my life.

Other Personal Instructions: _____

_____

I understand the full import of this declaration, and I am emotionally and mentally competent to make this declaration. These directions express my legal right to preserve my right to privacy and self-determination. Therefore, I direct my family, doctors, and all those concerned with my care to regard themselves as morally bound in accordance with my directions.

In witness whereof, I have signed this declaration this ____ Day of _____, 20____

_____   _____
Signature   Print Name

I attest that the signature or mark of the principal was knowingly and voluntarily signed in my presence. (Witnesses must be adults who are not themselves surrogates. One witness shall not be either the principal's spouse nor blood relative.)

_____   _____
Witness Signature   Witness Signature

_____   _____
Witness Name, Address, Phone Number   Witness Name, Address, Phone Number

FIGURE 4-5 Example of a living will.

Durable Power of Attorney for Health Care. The durable power of attorney for health care is a statement that gives a person's representative (including same-sex partner) clear authority and instructions about life-support decisions (Figure 4-6).

Uniform Anatomical Gift Act of 1968

Under the *Uniform Anatomical Gift Act,* competent individuals, who have reached the age of consent in their state, may donate their body or body parts after they die. The decision to donate can be stated in a will, in a written agreement, or by signing the back of the driver's license. Medical schools, research institutions, and tissue banks accept these organs, which are also used in transplant surgery or in the study of medicine.

Consumer Protection

Medical assistants should be aware of two consumer protection acts.

The *Fair Debt Collection Practices Act* provides guidelines for collecting money owed. When contacting people to collect money owed to the medical office, you may not harass them with threats or abusive language. Also, contact must only be made during reasonable hours (9 AM to 9 PM), and you can only call once a week.

The *Bankruptcy Act* protects people who have a considerable amount of debt and allows for fair payment to the people or businesses the person owes. Once a medical office has been notified of a patient's bankruptcy through the court system, no further bills or statements can be sent to the patient. The office can ask for payment for any future visits but cannot refuse to send a copy of the patient's medical record to another physician.

Miscellaneous Laws and Regulations

So far you have learned about many of the laws that protect patients' rights and wishes. Other laws protect health care professionals on the job. You need to be familiar with the laws on employment safety, work-related injuries, and disabilities. These laws exist to protect your rights as an employee. Table 4-3 lists additional laws concerning employment.

TABLE 4-3
Additional Employment Laws

National Labor Relations Act (Wagner Act) 1935	Protects the rights of workers to organize labor unions, to engage in collective bargaining, and to take part in strikes in support of their demands.
Rehabilitation Act of 1973	Recognized as civil-right statute for workers with disabilities. Paved the way for the 1990 Americans with Disabilities Act.
Age Discrimination in Employment Act 1967	Prohibits employment discrimination against persons 40 years of age or older, including hiring, promotions, wages, or firing/layoffs.
Employee Retirement Income Security Act (ERISA) 1974	Regulates employee benefit plans.

FOR YOUR INFORMATION
DOMESTIC VIOLENCE LAW

Some states (e.g., Florida) have enacted a law that requires employers to grant workers up to 3 days of leave per year for reasons related to domestic violence. This includes employees, family, or household members. To comply with the requirement, employers need to develop a policy and post it where employees will see it. Criteria must be specific as to who qualifies and must also include other conditions that apply. Guidelines include the following:

- Leave requests must be kept confidential.
- Applies to companies with at least 50 employees.
- Applies to employees who have been on the job for at least 3 months.
- Leave can be paid or unpaid.
- Employers can require employees to first exhaust their vacation days and sick days before granting domestic violence leave.
- Time off can be used to seek injunctions, obtain medical care or mental health counselors, seek help from a domestic violence shelter or similar organization, secure one's home from a perpetrator, or seek legal assistance.

Occupational Safety and Health

The *Occupational Safety and Health Act* issues and enforces rules to prevent work-related injuries, illnesses, and deaths by developing safety standards to protect employees from on-the-job exposure to chemicals, disease, and injury. Two major areas that have been addressed are the *Hazardous Chemical Standards* and the *Bloodborne Pathogens Standard.*

The Hazardous Chemical Standards focuses on exposure to chemicals. It requires that:

- All employees have a "right-to-know" within 30 days of their employment how to handle exposure to various chemicals.
- An exposure control plan must be written for the facility.
- Each chemical used on the job must have a **material safety data sheet (MSDS)** from the manufacturer on file.
- There must be a yearly inventory of all chemicals.

The Bloodborne Pathogen regulations concern exposure to blood and body fluids and tissues. Human immunodeficiency virus (HIV) and hepatitis B virus (HBV) are the two main concerns for health care workers. The Bloodborne Pathogen regulations provide the following:

- Promote the use of standard precautions established by the CDC to reduce the risk of cross-contamination. The CDC is a federal agency established to protect the health and safety of populations and people at home and abroad.
- Mandate that all employees at risk must be offered the hepatitis B vaccine within 30 days of employment at no cost to the employee. An employee can decline the vaccine by signing a *declination* (waiver). Box 4-6 lists the hepatitis B series time frame.

DURABLE POWER OF ATTORNEY FOR HEALTH CARE

Durable Power of Attorney made this _____ day of _____, 20 ___

1. I, _____, (insert name and address of principal) hereby appoint _____, (insert name and address of agent) as my attorney in fact (my agent) to act for me and in my name in any way I could act in person to make any and all decisions for me concerning my personal care, medical treatment, hospitalization, and health care and to require, withhold, or withdraw any type of medical treatment or procedure, even though my death may ensue. My agent shall have the same access to all my medical records that I have, including the right to disclose the contents to others. My agent shall also have full power to make a disposition of any part or all of my body for medical purposes, authorize an autopsy of my body, and direct the disposition of my remains.

THE ABOVE GRANT OF POWER IS INTENDED TO BE AS BROAD AS POSSIBLE SO THAT YOUR AGENT WILL HAVE AUTHORITY TO MAKE ANY DECISION YOU COULD MAKE TO OBTAIN OR TERMINATE ANY TYPE OF HEALTH CARE, INCLUDING WITHDRAWAL OF NOURISHMENT AND FLUIDS AND OTHER LIFE-SUSTAINING OR DEATH-DELAYING MEASURES, IF YOUR AGENT BELIEVES SUCH ACTION WOULD BE CONSISTENT WITH YOUR INTENT AND DESIRES. IF YOU WISH TO LIMIT THE SCOPE OF YOUR AGENT'S POWERS OR PRESCRIBE SPECIAL RULES TO LIMIT THE POWER TO MAKE AN ANATOMICAL GIFT, AUTHORIZE AUTOPSY, OR DISPOSE OF REMAINS, YOU MAY DO SO IN THE FOLLOWING PARAGRAPHS.

2. The powers granted above shall not include the following powers or shall be subject to the following rules or limitations (here you may include any specific limitations you deem appropriate, such as your own definition of when life-sustaining or death-delaying measures should be withheld; a direction to continue nourishment and fluids or other life-sustaining or death-delaying treatment in all events; or instructions to refuse any specific types of treatment that are inconsistent with your religious beliefs or unacceptable to you for any reason, such as blood transfusion, electroconvulsive therapy, or amputation):

_____
_____
_____
_____
_____
_____
_____
_____

FIGURE 4-6 Example of durable power of attorney for health care.

> **BOX 4-6**
>
> **Hepatitis B Vaccination Schedule for a New Employee**
>
> *First dose:* Must be offered within 30 days of employment at no charge to the employee.
> *Second dose:* Given 30 days after the first injection.
> *Third dose:* Given 2 months after the second dose and at least 4 months after the first dose.

- Require training for employees concerning the control and exposure plan. OSHA standards provide that job training be provided during working hours.
- Require that the labeling and the disposing of biological waste be done according to procedure.

The **Occupational Safety and Health Administration (OSHA)** is a federal agency that enforces these regulations. OSHA can inspect a workplace at any time unannounced. The sole purpose of OSHA is to ensure a safe working environment for all employees. Violations of an OSHA regulation can result in fines of $10,000 per violation.

Workers' Compensation

Even though OSHA regulates standards for safety in the workplace, work-related injuries still occur. In most states, employers with a certain number of employees (as determined by the state) must carry workers' compensation insurance. This insurance covers medical care and rehabilitation costs and offers temporary or permanent pay for the injured employee.

Title VII of the Civil Rights Act

Title VII of the Civil Rights Act of 1964 concerns hiring practices, treatment of employees, and employment of those with disabilities. Three aspects of this act that relate directly to medical assistants are protection from sexual harassment, emergency family and medical leave, and the hiring of disabled people. Complaints are filled with the Equal Employment Opportunity Commission (EEOC), which is the federal agency responsible for ending employment discrimination in the United States.

Sexual Harassment. The Equal Employment Opportunity Commission defines sexual harassment as follows:

> Unwelcome sexual advances, requests for sexual favors, and other verbal or physical conduct of a sexual nature constitute sexual harassment when (1) submission to such conduct is made either explicitly or implicitly a term or condition of an individual's employment; (2) submission to or rejection of such conduct by an individual is used as a basis for employment decisions affecting such individual; or (3) such conduct has the purpose or effect of unreasonably interfering with an individual's work performance or creating an intimidating, hostile, or offensive working environment.

This definition specifies what is not acceptable in the workplace. It protects the employee from "this for that" or the "something for something" (***quid pro quo*** [kwid pro kwo]) issues. It covers not only the acceptance or rejection of unwanted sexual conduct but also the condition of the working environment. A hostile working environment might include foul language, off-color jokes, inappropriate pictures, or other offensive actions or items that can affect another person's job performance.

Family and Medical Leave. The *Family and Medical Leave Act* (FMLA) allows an employee to take up to 12 weeks of unpaid leave per year (or within a 12-month period) for maternity leave (male or female), adoptions, and caring for ill immediate family members. It also permits extended unpaid leave for employees with serious medical conditions. To qualify, the employee must have been actively employed for 1 year. Only companies with 50 or more employees within a 75-mile radius are affected. This law protects the employee by requiring that the employee is entitled to return to their original job or one with equal pay and benefits after the leave, protection of employee benefits while on leave, and protection from retaliation by an employer for exercising rights under the Act.

Health Insurance Portability and Accountability Act. Title I of the **Health Insurance Portability and Accountability Act (HIPAA)** protects health insurance coverage for workers and their families when they change or lose their jobs. Title II, the Administrative Simplification provision, requires the establishment of national standards for electronic health care transactions and national identifiers for providers, health insurance plans and employers. The act also requires all health professionals to protect the privacy and confidentiality of patients' health information.

Hiring of Disabled People. The *Americans with Disabilities Act* (ADA) mandates equal opportunity for government services, public facilities, commercial accommodations, and transportation. It also prevents hiring discrimination against people with disabilities. If the most qualified person for the job is a person with a disability, a reasonable effort must be made to accommodate this person in the workplace. For example, a ramp or elevator could be added to accommodate an employee in a wheelchair. However, a position may be denied to a disabled individual if the accommodation creates an undue hardship (such as financial) on the company.

> **PATIENT-CENTERED PROFESSIONALISM**
>
> - How can reporting births, deaths, certain diseases, and abuse benefit patients and society?
> - Why is it important for patients to know about advance directives and living wills? If asked, could you explain these documents to a patient?
> - How do the CDC and OSHA work together to protect employees? How is patient care improved when workplace safety is practiced?
> - How does the Civil Rights Act impact you as a medical assistant? How might it impact the care that a patient receives from health professionals?

ETHICS IN HEALTH CARE

Laws are rules established by governing entities (e.g., city, state, and federal governments) that must be followed. **Ethics** are moral guidelines developed over time and influenced by family, culture, and society. Something considered unethical may not be against the law. For example:

> While shopping, Calvin finds an envelope containing $100 in the aisle of the store. The envelope has no name or any means to identify the owner. It is not against the law for him to keep it, but is it ethical? Should he turn it in to the front office, or keep it under the doctrine of "finders keepers, losers weepers"?

> If he were trying to decide whether it was ethical to keep the money he found, Calvin might answer these questions as follows:
> 1. *Is it legal?* Would it be a crime for Calvin to keep the money he found in the envelope? Keeping unidentified money found in a public place is not usually considered a crime.
> 2. *Is it well balanced?* Would keeping the envelope full of money treat everyone fairly? Calvin would benefit, but the person who lost the money would not.
> 3. *Would most people agree?* Would Calvin like it if this story were broadcast on the news? How would the people watching the news feel about Calvin's decision to keep the money? Most people would probably think Calvin should have turned the money over to the store manager or to the police.

Our personal and professional ethics influence the decisions we make and the actions we take. It is important for medical assistants to understand ethics and its importance, as well as special ethical situations that affect health care.

Ethical Standards

Your ethical standards as a health care professional are determined by many influences. Some of these influences are principles, personal integrity, professional responsibilities, confidentiality, and responsibilities to the patient.

Principles

Ethics refers to moral principles that govern a person's behavior and reflect the person's understanding of right and wrong. Throughout history there have been standards of behavior and professionalism. As times change, however, ethical standards and principles may change. Think about how standards of behavior have changed over the past several hundred years.

Personal Integrity

A person with *integrity* is seen as being honest and having high moral values. Personal integrity impacts the decisions you make. By asking yourself the following three questions, you can decide whether a solution to a problem is ethical:
1. *Is it legal?* If the solution to a problem is illegal, it is unethical.
2. *Is it well balanced?* The decision must treat everyone fairly. If one person benefits and another does not, the decision may not be ethical.
3. *Would most people agree?* Think about how you will be affected by this decision. If your decision were to be broadcast on the 6 PM news, would you still think it is the right thing to do?

If you can answer all three of these questions with a "yes," the decision is probably ethical. If not, you should think carefully and review the situation in more depth before making the decision. For example:

Professional Responsibilities

Health professionals establish a relationship with the patient, the family of the patient, their co-workers, and society in general. All have expectations about how health care professionals should behave. Sometimes a person can become torn between ethical obligations and legal obligations. For example:

> A patient at your office is HIV positive. You find out that this patient is dating your best friend's daughter. What can you do? The conflict arises from the concern for the safety of the public (best friend's daughter) and the breach of confidentiality (patient's right to privacy).

Boxes 4-7 and 4-8 illustrate expectations of the physician and the medical assistant according to their professions. Professional, patient-centered medical assistants follow their code of ethics.

FOR YOUR INFORMATION

COUNCIL ON ETHICAL AND JUDICIAL AFFAIRS
The Council on Ethical and Judicial Affairs (CEJA) develops ethics policy for the American Medical Association (AMA). The Council prepares reports that analyze and address timely ethical issues that confront physicians and the medical profession. The Council has judicial responsibilities, which include appellate jurisdiction over physician members' appeals of ethics-related decisions made by state and specialty medical societies.

Confidentiality

All health care professionals have a legal obligation to maintain the patient's privacy. A breach of **confidentiality** is not only against the law, but it is also unethical. HIPAA requires all health professionals to protect the privacy and confidentiality of patients' health information. This includes oral communication, data recorded on paper, and electronic records (see Chapter 27). Box 4-9 lists some of HIPAA's key requirements. Confidentiality breaches occur most often as a result of carelessness in elevators or hallways and when eating (e.g.,

BOX 4-7

Principles of Medical Ethics: American Medical Association

PREAMBLE

The medical profession has long subscribed to a body of ethical statements developed primarily for the benefit of the patient. As a member of this profession, a physician must recognize the responsibility not only to patients, but also to society, to other health professionals, and to self. The following Principles adopted by the American Medical Association are not laws, but standards of conduct which define the essentials of honorable behavior for the physician.

I. A physician shall be dedicated to providing competent medical services with compassion and respect for human dignity.

II. A physician shall deal honestly with patients and colleagues, and strive to expose those physicians deficient in character or competence, or who engage in fraud or deception.

III. A physician shall respect the law and also recognize a responsibility to seek changes in those requirements which are contrary to the best interests of the patient.

IV. A physician shall respect the rights of patients, of colleagues, and of other health professionals, and shall safeguard patient confidences within the constraints of the law.

V. A physician shall continue to study, apply, and advance scientific knowledge; make relevant information available to patients, colleagues, and the public; obtain consultation; and use the talents of other health professionals when indicated.

VI. A physician shall, in the provision of appropriate patient care, except in emergencies, be free to choose whom to serve, with whom to associate, and the environment in which to provide medical services.

VII. A physician shall recognize a responsibility to participate in activities contributing to an improved community.

From Code of Medical Ethics. Current Opinions of the Council on Ethical and Judicial Affairs. Copyright 1995-1999. American Medical Association.

BOX 4-8

AAMA Medical Assistant Code of Ethics

The Code of Ethics of the American Association of Medical Assistants shall set forth principles of ethical and moral conduct as they relate to the medical profession and the particular practice of medical assisting.

Members of AAMA dedicated to the conscientious pursuit of their profession, and thus desiring to merit the high regard of the entire medical profession and the respect of the general public which they serve, do pledge themselves to strive always to:

A. render service with full respect for the dignity of humanity;

B. respect confidential information obtained through employment unless legally authorized or required by responsible performance of duty to divulge such information;

C. uphold the honor and high principles of the profession and accept its disciplines;

D. seek to continually improve the knowledge and skills of medical assistants for the benefit of patients and professional colleagues;

E. participate in additional service activities aimed toward improving the health and well-being of the community.

AAMA MEDICAL ASSISTANT CREED

I believe in the principles and purposes of the profession of medical assisting.
I endeavor to be more effective.
I aspire to render greater service.
I protect the confidence entrusted to me.
I am dedicated to the care and well-being of all people.
I am loyal to my employer.
I am true to the ethics of my profession.
I am strengthened by compassion, courage and faith.

Courtesy American Association of Medical Assistants (AAMA).

"over lunch"). Even though a breach of confidentiality is not intended to be a violation of a patient's rights, it still is an invasion of the patient's privacy. Remember, HIPAA was enacted to prevent fraud and abuse in health care.

Breach of Confidentiality

A jury ordered an emergency medical technician (EMT) and her employer to pay a fine as a result of an invasion of the privacy of an overdose patient. The EMT told the patient's co-worker about the overdose, who then told others at a local hospital where both the co-worker and the overdose patient were nurses. The EMT claimed she called the co-worker out of concern for the patient. The jury decided that, regardless of her intentions, the EMT had no right to disclose confidential medical information.

Respect for the privacy of patients in your care is the law, not an option. Information about a patient may not be given out without the permission of the patient or legal guardian. Figure 4-7 provides an example of a patient consent form using HIPAA criteria. An exception to this does occur in situations where workers' compensation is an issue or instances where public safety is in question. Box 4-10 provides guidelines for releasing patient information.

Responsibilities to the Patient

Health professionals interact with people whose cultures and beliefs may not match their own. A judgmental attitude is not tolerated in health care. All health care professionals are responsible for respecting the following rights of patients:

Right to: Consideration and respect

- The patient is treated with kindness and a caring attitude.
- The patient's personal values and cultural beliefs and practices are considered when care is provided.

BOX 4-9

Patient Protections in the Health Insurance Portability and Accountability Act (HIPAA)

Following are the patient protections listed in the Department of Health and Human Services (DHHS) HIPAA Fact Sheet:

- **Access to medical records.** Patients generally should be able to see and obtain copies of their medical records and request corrections if they identify errors and mistakes. Health plans, doctors, hospitals, clinics, nursing homes, and other covered entities generally should provide access to these records within 30 days and may charge patients for the cost of copying and sending the records.
- **Notice of privacy practices.** Covered health plans, doctors, and other health care providers must provide a notice to their patients how they may use personal medical information and their rights under the new privacy regulation. Doctors, hospitals, and other direct-care providers generally will provide the notice on the patient's first visit following the April 14, 2003, compliance date and upon request. Patients generally will be asked to sign, initial, or otherwise acknowledge that they received this notice. Patients also may ask covered entities to restrict the use or disclosure of their information beyond the practices included in the notice, but the covered entities would not have to agree to the changes.
- **Limits on use of personal medical information.** The privacy rule sets limits on how health plans and covered providers may use individually identifiable health information. To promote the best quality care for patients, the rule does not restrict the ability of doctors, nurses, and other providers to share information needed to treat their patients. In other situations, though, personal health information generally may not be used for purposes not related to health care, and covered entities may use or share only the minimum amount of protected information needed for a particular purpose. In addition, patients would have to sign a specific authorization before a covered entity could release their medical information to a life insurer, a bank, a marketing firm, or another outside business for purposes not related to their health care.
- **Prohibition on marketing.** The final privacy rule sets new restrictions and limits on the use of patient information for marketing purposes. Pharmacies, health plans, and other covered entities must first obtain an individual's specific authorization before disclosing their patient information for marketing. At the same time, the rule permits doctors and other covered entities to communicate freely with patients about treatment options and other health-related information, including disease-management programs.
- **Stronger state laws.** The new federal privacy standards do not affect state laws that provide additional privacy protections for patients. The confidentiality protections are cumulative; the privacy rule will set a national "floor" of privacy standards that protect all Americans, and any state law providing additional protections would continue to apply. When a state law requires a certain disclosure—such as reporting an infectious disease outbreak to the public health authorities—the federal privacy regulations would not preempt the state law.
- **Confidential communications.** Under the privacy rule, patients can request that their doctors, health plans, and other covered entities take reasonable steps to ensure that their communications with the patient are confidential. For example, a patient could ask a doctor to call his or her office rather than home, and the doctor's office should comply with that request if it can be reasonably accommodated.
- **Complaints.** Consumers may file a formal complaint regarding the privacy practices of a covered health plan or provider. Such complaints can be made directly to the covered provider or health plan or to HHS' Office for Civil Rights (OCR), which is charged with investigating complaints and enforcing the privacy regulation. Information about filing complaints should be included in each covered entity's notice of privacy practices. Consumers can find out more information about filing a complaint at http://www.hhs.gov/ocr/hipaa or by calling (866) 627-7748.

From U.S. Department of Health and Human Services Fact Sheet: Protecting the privacy of patients' health information, April 14, 2003.

BOX 4-10

Guidelines for Release of Information

- A release of information form does not need to be signed if:
  - Information is required by law (e.g., abuse).
  - Information is court ordered.
- Provide a copy of the requested information.
- Only release information related to the request.
- Unless requested by the patient or legal guardian, never release mental health conditions or treatments for drug/alcohol conditions, unless required by law.
- Information cannot be released over the telephone.
- Never release the original medical record unless court ordered.
- Patient can rescind the authorization from the health care facility by doing the following:
  - Must be in writing.
  - Signed by the patient or patient's representative.
  - Delivered to the health care facility.
  - Takes effect when the medical facility receives it, unless the facility or others have already relied on its use (e.g., insurance company).

Patient Consent to the Use and Disclosure of Health Information for Treatment, Payment, or Health Care Operations

I understand that as part of my health care, the practice originates and maintains paper and/or electronic records describing my health history, symptoms, examination and test results, diagnoses, treatment, and any plans for future care or treatment. I understand that this information serves as:

- A basis for planning my care and treatment,
- A means of communication among professionals who contribute to my care,
- A source of information for applying my diagnosis and treatment information to my bill,
- A means by which a third-party payer can verify that services billed were actually provided,
- A tool for routine health care operations, such as assessing quality and reviewing the competence of staff.

I have been provided the opportunity to review the *"Notice of Patient Privacy Information Practices"* that provides a more complete description of information uses and disclosures. I understand that I have the following rights:

- The right to review the *"Notice"* prior to acknowledging this consent,
- The right to restrict or revoke the use or disclosure of my health information for other uses or purposes, and
- The right to request restrictions as to how my health information may be used or disclosed to carry out treatment, payment, or health care operations.

Restrictions:

I request the following restrictions to the use or disclosure of my health information:

_____

_____

May discuss treatment, payment, or health care operation with the following persons:

(Please check all that apply)   Spouse [ ]   Your Children [ ]   Relatives [ ]   Others [ ]   Parents [ ]

Please list the names and relationship, if you checked "Relatives" or "Others" above

_____

_____

Messages or Appointment Reminders: (Please check all that apply)

May we leave a message on your answering machine at home [ ] or at work [ ]. **Do not leave a message [ ]**
May we leave a message with someone at your **home** using the doctor's name or the practice name: Yes [ ]   No [ ]
May we leave a message with someone at your **work** using the doctor's name or the practice name: Yes [ ]   No [ ]
Messages will be of a nonsensitive nature, such as appointment reminders.

I understand that as part of treatment, payment, or health care operations, it may become necessary to disclose health information to another entity, i.e., referrals to other health care providers, labs, and/or other individuals or agencies as permitted or required by state or federal law.

I fully understand and accept the information provided by this consent.

_____   _____   _____
Signature   Print name of person signing   Date

*If other than patient is signing, are you the parent, legal guardian, custodian, or have Power of Attorney for this patient for treatment, payment, or health care operations? Yes [ ]   No [ ]

FOR OFFICE USE ONLY
[ ] Patient refused to sign the consent form.
[ ] Restrictions were added by the patient (see restrictions listed above)
[ ] "Consent form" received and reviewed by _____ on (date) _____
[ ] "Consent form" placed in the patient's medical record on (date) _____

FIGURE 4-7 Examples of HIPAA-compliant patient consent forms.

GENERAL MEDICAL HEALTH CARE

AUTHORIZATION FOR RELEASE OF MEDICAL INFORMATION

I, _____ ___/___/___ _____ hereby authorize
    Print Patient's Name   Date of Birth   Social Security Number

General Medical Health Care 1234 Riverview Road, Anytown, FL 33333

to release medical, including HIV Antibody Testing, Psychiatric/Psychological, Alcohol and/or Drug Abuse information records to:

To: _____

Address _____
    (Street)   (City)   (State)   (Zip)

For the purpose of: 1. Drs. appointment on: _____

                      2. Other: _____

                      Please Specify Reason for Disclosure

I understand that if I consent to the release of any of my medical records, the results of any HIV Antibody Testing, Psychiatric/Psychological, Alcohol and/or Drug Abuse information will be released.

I understand this consent may be cancelled upon written notice to the hospital, except that action by the hospital has been taken in reliance on this authorization, and that this authorization shall remain in force for a 90-day period in order to effect the purpose for which it is given. Alcohol and drug abuse information, if present, has been disclosed from records whose confidentiality is protected by Federal Law. FEDERAL REGULATIONS (42CFR, part II) prohibit making any further disclosure of records without the specific written authorization of the undersigned, or as otherwise permitted by such regulations.
The confidentiality of HIV antibody test results is protected by Florida Law [Fla. Stat.ANN. 381.609 (2) (F)], which prohibits any further disclosure by a person to whom this information has been disclosed, without specific written consent of the undersigned or as otherwise permitted by state law.

_____ From: _____ To: _____
(Date of Authorization)   (Dates to be Released)

_____
Patient's Signature

_____
Parent, Legal Guardian, or Authorized Representative Signature

_____
Relationship to Patient

_____
Witness

FIGURE 4-7, cont'd

Right to: Information
- Information is provided in terms the patient can understand.
- The physician explains the diagnosis, treatment, alternatives, and prognosis.

Right to: Refuse treatment
- The patient does not have to accept treatment.
- The patient must be informed of the health risks involved in refusing treatment.

Right to: Privacy
- The patient's records and care and the information received from the patient are kept private.
- The right to privacy is protected even after death.

Right to: Confidentiality
- Information can only be shared after the patient gives written consent.
- No information is to be shared with another health care worker unless that person is directly involved in the patient's care.

Right to: Competent care
- The patient expects all care provided to be given by a qualified person.

The American Hospital Association (AHA) has created documents to help increase awareness of a patient's rights. AHA established a **Patient's Bill of Rights** in 1998 and then created the **Patient Care Partnership** document in 2001 (Box 4-11). This brochure outlines the AHA's expectations of patients and hospitals. To enhance this resource document, the AHA created a "Blueprint for Action" to assist with the implementation of this revised plan. This document is divided into two parts, as follows:

1. An organizational checklist to assist hospitals in assessing their strengths and weaknesses.
2. Case studies highlighting action taken by hospitals to improve communication among the patients.

Special Ethical Considerations

Bioethics concerns the special ethical decisions that must be made because of advancements in medical research. The federal government has tried to anticipate and work with these advances through laws and regulations. Some special ethical considerations that relate to health care include the "right to die," fertility, abortion, genetic engineering, and resource allocation.

"Right to Die" Issues

Do people have the "right to die" if they are suffering? Dr. Jack Kevorkian brought attention to **euthanasia** by providing the means and information to terminally ill patients to allow them to commit physician-assisted suicide. Although the courts would not convict Dr. Kevorkian initially, he was found guilty of second-degree murder in 1999 and sentenced to prison. Within hours of his release in 2007, he said he still feels that people have a right to decide when they want to die and he will work to have physician-assisted suicide legalized but will not break any laws doing it. Some of the arguments for and against this issue lie in religious teachings, scientific findings, and quality-of-life issues.

Beginning-of-life issues arise when an infant is born with severe disabilities. The physicians' code implies that treatment should begin, except for those who would clearly not benefit. What if the parents do not want treatment started? Should quality-of-life issues be addressed?

End-of-life issues are more in the public eye now than ever before. People today are living longer, but is the quality of life what they expected? Do they have a right to terminate their life or ask someone to assist them in the termination? The law says "no," but some believe that in certain circumstances this is justifiable.

Some argue that we are kinder to animals with a terminal illness than we are to humans. The use of advance directives at least allows a patient some say in the matter, but are they enough? What do you think?

Fertility

Health professionals can use various ways to help women conceive or become pregnant. *In vitro fertilization* (e.g., test-tube fertilization) and *artificial insemination* are two methods. Controversy exists over whether religious and ethical principles are being violated. Fertility treatments resulting in multiple fetuses may pose a threat to the mother and babies. Physicians may recommend "selective reduction" (aborting the weakest fetuses so the others might survive), which poses an ethical dilemma for the parents.

Such types of "assisted conception" also lead to legal questions about parentage (e.g., does a surrogate mother or a sperm donor have any parental responsibilities or rights?). Some states have laws dealing with these issues, but others do not. States without laws rely on the physician to act with reasonable care. Questions regarding legal protection and parentage should be addressed to an attorney when considering these procedures.

Abortion

Roe v. Wade in 1973 was the court case that established the rights of women to control their bodies. Basically, the decision mandates that the states have no authority to regulate abortions within the first 13 weeks of pregnancy. Some states responded by denying the use of federal funds for abortions. There are many religious and scientific theories about when life begins. Does life begin at conception, at birth, or somewhere in between? Often the issue is not whether women should be able to have an abortion, but whether women should have control over their own bodies.

Genetic Engineering

Amazing progress has been made in the fields of genetics and **genomics,** which is the science of understanding the complete genetic inheritance of an organism. The same gene-splicing technology that could eliminate genetic disease in children also could be used to change how they look, how they act, or how they think. Likewise, the same genetic test that helps a physician assess disease risks and recommend preventive

BOX 4-11

The Patient Care Partnership: Understanding Expectations, Rights and Responsibilities

When you need hospital care, your doctor and the nurses and other professionals at our hospital are committed to working with you and your family to meet your health care needs. Our dedicated doctors and staff serve the community in all its ethnic, religious and economic diversity. Our goal is for you and your family to have the same care and attention we would want for our families and ourselves.

The sections explain some of the basics about how you can expect to be treated during your hospital stay. They also cover what we will need from you to care for you better. If you have questions at any time, please ask them. Unasked or unanswered questions can add to the stress of being in the hospital. Your comfort and confidence in your care are very important to us.

What to Expect During Your Hospital Stay

- **High quality hospital care.** Our first priority is to provide you the care you need, when you need it, with skill, compassion, and respect. Tell your caregivers if you have concerns about your care or if you have pain. You have the right to know the identity of doctors, nurses and others involved in your care, and you have the right to know when they are students, residents or other trainees.
- **A clean and safe environment.** Our hospital works hard to keep you safe. We use special policies and procedures to avoid mistakes in your care and keep you free from abuse or neglect. If anything unexpected and significant happens during your hospital stay, you will be told what happened, and any resulting changes in your care will be discussed with you.
- **Involvement in your care.** You and your doctor often make decisions about your care before you go to the hospital. Other times, especially in emergencies, those decisions are made during your hospital stay. When decision-making takes place, it should include:
- *Discussing your medical condition and information about medically appropriate treatment choices.* To make informed decisions with your doctor, you need to understand:
  - The benefits and risks of each treatment.
  - Whether your treatment is experimental or part of a research study.
  - What you can reasonably expect from your treatment and any long-term effects it might have on your quality of life.
  - What you and your family will need to do after you leave the hospital.
  - The financial consequences of using uncovered services or out-of-network providers.

  Please tell your caregivers if you need more information about treatment choices.
- *Discussing your treatment plan.* When you enter the hospital, you sign a general consent to treatment. In some cases, such as surgery or experimental treatment, you may be asked to confirm in writing that you understand what is planned and agree to it. This process protects your right to consent to or refuse a treatment. Your doctor will explain the medical consequences of refusing recommended treatment. It also protects your right to decide if you want to participate in a research study.
- *Getting information from you.* Your caregivers need complete and correct information about your health and coverage so that they can make good decisions about your care. That includes:
  - Past illnesses, surgeries or hospital stays.
  - Past allergic reactions.
  - Any medicines or dietary supplements (such as vitamins and herbs) that you are taking.
  - Any network or admission requirements under your health plan.
- *Understanding your health care goals and values.* You may have health care goals and values or spiritual beliefs that are important to your well-being. They will be taken into account as much as possible throughout your hospital stay. Make sure your doctor, your family and your care team know your wishes.
- *Understanding who should make decisions when you cannot.* If you have signed a health care power of attorney stating who should speak for you if you become unable to make health care decisions for yourself, or a "living will" or "advance directive" that states your wishes about end-of-life care; give copies to your doctor, your family and your care team. If you or your family need help making difficult decisions, counselors, chaplains and others are available to help.
- **Protection of your privacy.** We respect the confidentiality of your relationship with your doctor and other caregivers, and the sensitive information about your health and health care that are part of that relationship. State and federal laws and hospital operating policies protect the privacy of your medical information. You will receive a Notice of Privacy Practices that describes the ways that we use, disclose and safeguard patient information and that explains how you can obtain a copy of information from our records about your care.
- **Preparing you and your family for when you leave the hospital.** Your doctor works with hospital staff and professionals in your community. You and your family also play an important role in your care. The success of your treatment often depends on your efforts to follow medication, diet and therapy plans. Your family may need to help care for you at home.

  You can expect us to help you identify sources of follow-up care and to let you know if our hospital has a financial interest in any referrals. As long as you agree that we can share information about your care with them, we will coordinate our activities with your caregivers outside the hospital. You can also expect to receive information and, where possible, training about the self-care you will need when you go home.
- **Help with your bill and filing insurance claims.** Our staff will file claims for you with health care insurers or other programs such as Medicare and Medicaid. They also will help your doctor with needed documentation. Hospital bills and insurance coverage are often confusing. If you have questions about your bill, contact our business office. If you need help understanding your insurance coverage or health plan, start with your insurance company or health benefits manager. If you do not have health coverage, we will try to help you and your family find financial help or make other arrangements. We need your help with collecting needed information and other requirements to obtain coverage or assistance.

Reprinted with permission of the American Hospital Association, copyright 2003.

measures could also be used by health insurance carriers to deny health care coverage or by employers to withhold promotions or terminate employment.

Another issue is the ability to *clone* (duplicate). It may be possible in the future to clone humans, but is it ethical? Currently there is no federal statute outlawing embryonic stem cell research in the United States. The barriers are largely due to restrictions placed on the use of federal research dollars.

Resource Allocation

A *resource* is something of value to the public, whether a heart or liver or an appointment, or anything that has limited access. Allocation is deciding who receives the resource. Some believe that the only fair way to allocate is to use the lottery system, or "luck of the draw." Others think that a list of criteria would help with the decision process. Questions could include the following:

- Who would benefit the most?
- What would the benefit do to the quality of life?
- How long would the benefit last?
- What is the urgency of need?
- How much of the resource is needed?

Allocation of resources poses moral dilemmas. Would it be ethical to refuse a liver transplant to an alcoholic patient who declines treatment for his alcoholism? Another issue relating to resource allocation is the treatment of patients who have HIV infection or AIDS. Insurance companies create more ethical questions when they refuse insurance to individuals who have these diseases. Patients with an HIV infection or AIDS have the same rights as people with other life-threatening illnesses and should be treated with dignity and respect by health professionals.

> **PATIENT-CENTERED PROFESSIONALISM**
>
> - *What are some ways your ethics could be challenged as a medical assistant in a medical office setting?*
> - *How could releasing confidential patient information hinder a patient's chances for employment? For health or life insurance coverage? Relationships with friends and family?*
> - *You will come into contact with patients who do not share your views on bioethical issues (e.g., "right to die," cloning, or abortion). What can you do to maintain a healthy relationship with patients regardless of their ethical beliefs?*
> - *Why is it important for medical assistants to stay current on the laws associated with bioethical issues, such as the "right to die," fertility, abortion, and genetic engineering?*

CONCLUSION

To perform your duties legally and ethically, it is necessary for you to know the legal and ethical boundaries associated with medical assisting. All health professionals have a responsibility to behave legally and ethically. They respect the rights of their patients and provide competent, effective care.

Medical assistants who strive to be patient-centered professionals help their physician-employers meet patient expectations and avoid lawsuits. Always remember that one misplaced word or inappropriate action could result in legal problems not just for you, but for the whole organization in which you work. Ignorance is no excuse; it is part of your job as a patient-centered professional to *know* the laws and to follow them. While working within the law, follow the medical assistants' code of ethics to help you make choices about the "right thing" to do.

Chapter Summary

Reinforce your understanding of the material in this chapter by reviewing the curriculum objectives and key content points below.

1. **Define, appropriately use, and spell all the Key Terms for this chapter.**
   - Review the Key Terms if necessary.
2. **Describe the purpose of the Medical Practice Acts.**
   - The Medical Practice Acts were created to protect people from unqualified health care professionals.
   - The Medical Practice Acts establish a medical board to review licensing requirements, guidelines for suspension and revocation of licenses, and renewal requirements for physicians in their state.
3. **List the three ways health professionals can become licensed.**
   - The three ways to obtain a license are by examination, reciprocity, or endorsement.
4. **List the six licensure requirements for physicians.**
   - A license is a legal document that allows a person to work in a particular profession; each state will develop rules for licensing.
   - To obtain a license, physicians must (a) meet individual state requirements, (b) complete education requirements through an approved medical school, (c) complete an approved residency program, (d) pass all examinations required by the state board of medical examiners, (e) be of good moral character, and (f) attain the age of majority as defined by state statute.
5. **Explain how a physician could have his or her license revoked or suspended.**
   - A physician could have his or her license revoked or suspended because of conviction of a crime, unprofessional conduct, or incapacity to perform duties.
   - A physician-employer is ultimately responsible for the actions of his or her staff; permitting unqualified staff

to endanger patients jeopardizes the physician's right to practice.

6. **Distinguish between public law and private law.**
   - Public law is concerned with the welfare or safety of the public.
   - Private law deals with issues against private individuals.

7. **Describe abandonment and give an example.**
   - Abandonment occurs if a physician fails to provide physician coverage in his or her absence.
   - Refusal to treat in cases of noncompliance can also be considered abandonment if the patient is not formally notified and given the opportunity to transfer care to another physician.

8. **List the six steps in formally withdrawing from the physician-patient contract.**
   - The patient must be notified in writing.
   - Reasons for dismissal must be stated.
   - An effective date is given when treatment will cease.
   - A list of possible new physicians is provided.
   - A form is enclosed for transfer of the patient's records.
   - A letter is sent via certified mail, and return receipt is requested.

9. **Define *expressed contract* and *implied contract* and give an example of each.**
   - A contract requires that an offer be made by one person and accepted by another.
   - "Expressed" means spoken, stated, or written. Voluntary hospital admission requires the patient's signed forms agreeing to payment of the hospital bill.
   - "Implied" means suggested or expected. Treatment is rendered before any agreement on payment.

10. **Explain how malpractice relates to liability.**
    - Malpractice is a specific type of negligence in which a professional fails to act with reasonable care, and the person who commits malpractice is liable (held accountable for their actions).

11. **Explain the difference between *intentional* negligence and *nonintentional* negligence.**
    - Negligence is not doing something a reasonably prudent person would do in a similar situation, or doing something a reasonably prudent person would not do in a similar situation.
    - A tort is a wrongful act committed by one person against another.
    - Intentional torts include assault and battery, defamation, invasion of privacy, false imprisonment, and medical abandonment.
    - Nonintentional torts include negligence and res ipsa loquitur. The majority of U.S. malpractice suits are nonintentional torts.

12. **Explain the importance of informed consent.**
    - Informed consent must be given by the patient before treatment or procedures.
    - The physician, before treatment, must give sufficient information about the procedure (risks, alternatives) to enable the patient to make an informed decision.

13. **Describe the purpose of the Good Samaritan Act.**
    - The Good Samaritan Act allows a person to assist an injured person without fear of a lawsuit as long as they stay within their scope of training.

14. **List the three types of nonintentional negligence.**
    - Ordinary (nonintentional) negligence is the accidental commission or omission of an act.
    - Types of negligence include malfeasance, misfeasance, and nonfeasance.

15. **State the "four Ds" of negligence.**
    - The four Ds of negligence must be present before an attorney will pursue a case for professional negligence: **D**uty of care to the patient, breach of that duty (**D**ereliction of duty), **D**irect connection between breach of duty and patient injury, and **D**amage sustained by the patient.

16. **Explain the importance of keeping accurate medical records.**
    - A patient's medical record follows them for life. Accurate records ensure continuity of care for any health care team treating the patient.
    - The dates and information recorded in the medical record can be used in a lawsuit, so the medical records must be kept up to date, accurate, and complete.

17. **List 10 guidelines of risk management to avoid a lawsuit.**
    - Refer to Box 4-4.

18. **Describe the trial process.**
    - Refer to Table 4-2.

19. **List five types of patient information that, by law, must be reported to state or local authorities.**
    - Reportable events include birth, death, communicable diseases, and injuries caused by weapons or suspected abuse.

20. **Explain the purpose of a living will.**
    - A living will is a statement to the family, physician, or lawyer that conveys a person's decisions about medical treatment if the person becomes unable to make the decision.
    - The Patient Self-Determination Act provides for advanced directives concerning life-support decisions.

21. **Explain the purpose of the Uniform Anatomical Gift Act.**
    - The Uniform Anatomical Gift Act allows a person to donate his or her body or body parts after death for research or to preserve life.

22. **List three laws that concern workplace issues and explain how they can protect medical assistants and other workers.**
    - OSHA's laws and regulations protect employees from hazardous work environments. Each state has a branch of OSHA enforcement.
    - Workers' compensation laws assist employees with work-related injuries.
    - Laws enacted under the ADA prevent hiring discrimination against disabled persons.

23. **Explain the difference between ethics and law.**
    - Ethics is a moral, voluntary choice—right or wrong.
    - Law is a mandated choice—right or wrong.
    - Law you must do; ethics you should do.
    - Something that is unethical may not be illegal.

24. **State the five parts of the AAMA code of ethics.**
    - Refer to Box 4-8.

25. **Describe the legal and ethical importance of maintaining patient privacy and confidentiality.**

- Patients expect and have a right to privacy and confidentiality by law.
- The AAMA's code of ethics encourages respectful treatment of patients' privacy and confidentiality.

26. **Describe the expectations patients have for effective care.**
    - All health care workers have a responsibility to their patients to be respectful, competent, maintain a code of ethics, and to "do no harm."
    - The AHA formulated the Patient Care Partnership.

27. **List three bioethical situations and explain the considerations for each.**
    - "Right-to-die" issues, in vitro fertilization, and resource allocation are all ethical considerations.

28. **Analyze a realistic medical office situation and apply law and ethics to determine the best course of action.**
    - Always follow the law.
    - Practice the ethics established by your profession.
    - Describe the impact on patient care when medical assistants have a solid understanding of law and ethics.
    - Illegal and unethical practices can have a devastating, even lethal, impact on patients.
    - The medical practice is affected by the legal and ethical behavior of its staff.

29. **Describe the impact on patient care when medical assistants have a solid understanding of law and ethics.**
    - Illegal and unethical practices can have a devastating, even lethal, impact on patients.
    - The medical practice is affected by the legal and ethical behavior of its staff.

PRACTICAL APPLICATIONS

If you have accomplished the objectives in this chapter, you will be able to make better choices as a medical assistant. Take another look at this situation and decide what you would do.

Jill is a medical assistant with on-the-job training in a medical office setting. She always strives to be caring, courteous, and respectful of patients and co-workers. Because of her caring attitude, the patients with whom Jill works all appreciate her attitude and her work. One of Jill's favorite patients, Shandra, a 24-year-old mother of two young children, has been diagnosed with cancer and recently was told by the physician that her condition is terminal. Shandra is at the office for an appointment and feeling very upset about her terminal illness. She pours out her heart and fears to Jill. Wanting to comfort Shandra, Jill tells her, "Don't worry. You'll be just fine. You know the doctor will make you better."

Shandra is comforted by Jill's words and tells her how much Jill means to her. In fact, she has so much faith in Jill that she believes that she will be fine and tells her family what Jill has said. Sadly, a few months later, Shandra dies. Believing she would be fine, Shandra had not made any plans for her children and family. Her family is upset with the physician and with Jill. The family thinks they have been betrayed because they believed that Shandra would be fine. The family is discussing what to say to the physician about this betrayal and whether to bring a lawsuit because Shandra did not have a will.

How might this situation have been avoided? What are the possible implications for Shandra's family, Jill, the physician, and the practice?

1. Jill has been trained on the job and is uncredentialed. What are the disadvantages to Jill of not having a formal medical assisting education? Would having credentialing and an education make a difference in what Jill said to Shandra?
2. Would credentialing make a difference if Shandra's family decides to bring a lawsuit? If so, what are the benefits to the physician if the medical assistant is credentialed?
3. Why was it important for Shandra to have an advance directive?
4. What are the legal ramifications of Jill telling Shandra not to worry and that she would be fine? What ethical guidelines should be considered in this situation? Did Jill do something illegal, something unethical, neither, or both? Explain why or why not.

WEB SEARCH

1. **Research the legal history of the Terry Schiavo case.** This case focused attention on end-of-life medical ethics and the need for some type of advanced directives by individual.
   - **Keywords:** Use the following keyword in your search: Schiavo.
2. **Research OSHA laws and regulations to learn more about how they protect employees.** OSHA is concerned with protecting employees from harm while they do their jobs. OSHA also checks to see that these laws and regulations are followed and provides for punishment when they are not.
   - **Keywords:** Use the following keywords in your search: OSHA, Occupational Safety and Health Act.
3. **Research your state's statutes that require practitioners to report certain diseases/conditions to their public health department.** The Bureau of Epidemiology at the Department of Health uses data collected from each state's public health department to track incidence of disease outbreaks across the country.
   - **Keywords:** Use the following keywords in your search: public health, public health reporting, reportable diseases.

5 Understanding Human Behavior

evolve http://evolve.elsevier.com/klieger/medicalassisting

The study of human behavior helps us understand how people learn, feel emotions, and establish relationships. This knowledge can help us adjust to the instant demands of an ever-changing world. As a medical assistant, you will be required to perform a wide variety of tasks each day. Although a few of these tasks may not involve interacting with people, most of your work will depend on your ability to relate to both patients and co-workers. To relate well to others, medical assistants need to develop "USA": *understanding, sensitivity,* and *accommodation* (adjusting) to patient needs. Human relations are the key to providing professional, quality care to patients. Skill in human relations develops over time and as with other skills, must be practiced, fine-tuned, and nurtured every day.

LEARNING OBJECTIVES

You will be able to do the following after completing this chapter:

Key Terms
1. Define, appropriately use, and spell all the Key Terms for this chapter.

Psychology and Personality
2. List and briefly define the three parts that make up a person's personality according to Freud.
3. List three factors that influence personality development.

Human Needs
4. List the five types of human needs.

Mental and Physical Health
5. Explain the importance of having good self-esteem.
6. List the four types of factors that can influence perception.
7. Differentiate between experiencing fear and having a phobia.
8. List five health problems caused by anxiety or stress.
9. Explain how fear, phobia, anxiety, and stress affect a person's mental and physical health.

Coping
10. List and describe six defense mechanisms.
11. List the five stages of grief and briefly describe each in the first person.

Patient-Centered Professionalism
12. Analyze a realistic medical office situation and apply your understanding of human behavior to determine the best course of action.
13. Describe the impact on patient care when medical assistants understand human behavior.

KEY TERMS

acceptance
anger
anxiety
bargaining
compensation
defense mechanism
denial
depression
displacement
ego
empathy
fantasy
fear
fight, flight, or fright
homeostasis
hospice

id
labels
overcompensation
perception
phobias
physiological
projection
psychiatry
psychology
psychosomatic
rationalization
self-esteem
stress
subconscious
superego
sympathy

PRACTICAL APPLICATIONS

Read the following scenario and keep it in mind as you learn about human behavior in this chapter.

Sara Ann is a 22-year-old single mother and a medical assistant. She has no assistance at home with child care or with any of the chores necessary to keep up a household. Sara Ann works as many hours as she can to support herself and her two children in the best way possible. On top of all of this, going to school has added major financial problems for Sara Ann.

On many days, Sara Ann is tired and frustrated and wonders just how she will get through the day. Because of her lack of self-esteem and the lack of help, anxiety and stress are affecting the way Sara Ann deals with co-workers. Sara Ann's anxiety level often leads her to label patients. In addition, Sara Ann has difficulty adapting to any variation in the daily schedule.

Because Sara Ann feels close to some patients with whom she has spent time in the medical office, she will often discuss her personal problems with these patients. Also, Sara Ann must handle some of her personal business (banking, errands) while at work because she does not leave work early enough to do these things when the businesses are open.

Sara Ann is experiencing a lot of stress, which is having an impact on her performance at work. If you were in Sara Ann's situation, what would you do to reduce stress?

PSYCHOLOGY AND PERSONALITY

Psychology is the scientific study of the mind and the behavioral patterns of humans and animals. **Psychiatry** is a medical specialty that deals with the treatment and prevention of mental illness. Sigmund Freud, an Austrian physician, was interested in understanding the development of the mind to treat psychological problems that his patients were experiencing. He was one of the first theorists to recognize that **subconscious** memory can affect a person's health. Further studies have shown that the mind and emotions have a powerful effect on an individual's ability to stay healthy. Freud's theories attempted to explain the structure of personality and how it develops over time.

Basic Structure of Personality

Freud used a three-part organizational model to explain the structure of personality: the id, ego, and superego.

Id: The part of the brain associated with basic unconscious biological drives. The id is the main source of energy, desire, and needs gratification (the satisfying of the body's needs). For example:

> An infant cries when hungry, when the diaper is wet or soiled, and when the infant wants to be held. Gratification is received when the infant receives food, when the diaper is changed, and when the infant is held.

Ego: The part of the personality that is aware of reality and the consequences of different behaviors. Interacting with others develops the ego. For example:

> Toddlers learn that each time they use the toilet, praise is given, and when they soil their pants, praise is withheld. As they interact with their peers who are "potty-trained," toddlers want to be accepted, and praise from others (e.g., adults) is less important.

Superego: The part of the personality that acts as a conscience, or moral guide; the internalization of values and standards designed to promote proper social behavior. For example:

> It is acceptable for an infant to cry to receive gratification. As the infant grows and becomes a toddler, crying becomes unacceptable behavior and often results in negative consequences. As the superego develops, toddlers begin to behave in an acceptable way that allows them to be gratified.

Once the superego is developed, the ego acts as the gatekeeper and holds off the demands of the id until proper gratification is chosen that is acceptable to the superego. As we develop, we learn to control our impulses. For example:

> What happens when a 10-year-old boy sees a candy bar on the store counter but has no money?
> - The *id* wants to grab the candy bar and run out of the store.
> - The *ego* wants to satisfy the id but knows there will be a punishment for stealing.
> - The *superego* knows it is morally wrong to steal.
>
> Freud believes that the child's ego will repress the urges of the id because of a fear of punishment, but as the child develops, the reality of right and wrong will take over. Even though the superego uses guilt to enforce the rules, a person who does what is acceptable to the superego feels pride and self-satisfaction.

As a medical assistant, when you confront difficult decisions, listen to your superego and make the right choice.

Personality Development

As a medical assistant, you will interact with people who have all types of personalities. It is important to understand the factors that can influence the way a person's personality develops. The study of behavior indicates that the development of personality is influenced by the following factors:

- Events that take place in a person's early developmental years
- Biological (genetic) factors, such as whether a person is male or female

- Psychological (environmental) factors, such as poverty or wealth and a person's upbringing

With all the factors that impact the development of personality, it is no wonder that no two people are alike. Keep this in mind when working with patients of all personality types.

Other theorists have expanded on the ideas of Freud. Some have examined the way people gain knowledge and the way they think about things to help explain personality development.

PATIENT-CENTERED PROFESSIONALISM

- *How can understanding how personality develops help you provide better care to patients?*
- *How can understanding the components of personality help you communicate better with patients and co-workers?*
- *Why is it important to keep in mind that patients all have their own unique personalities?*
- *What is the benefit of trying to understand each patient's unique personality?*

HUMAN NEEDS

Abraham Maslow, like Freud, studied human behavior. Maslow, an American psychologist, was interested in what motivates people to do what they do. He recognized that a person's development and behavior are affected by both physical and emotional needs. He believed that all humans have needs that must be met. He placed these needs in a *hierarchy* (rank order) to show which needs take priority over others. He emphasized that all lower needs must be met before the higher needs can be satisfied.

Maslow's Hierarchy of Needs

Maslow's hierarchy of needs model has the following five categories (Figure 5-1):

1. *Physical needs.* First level: foundation of a person's motivational drive.
   - Basic needs, including air, food, water, and shelter.
   - Necessary for survival.
   - When achieved, physical needs bring about **homeostasis** (balance) to the body.
   - When *not* achieved, the person may experience illness, pain, and irritation.
2. *Safety and security needs.* Second level: a person's physical needs are already met.
   - Psychological needs, including feeling safe from harm and feeling secure about safety.
   - When achieved, safety and security needs bring a sense of stability and consistency.
   - When *not* achieved, safety is not ensured and the person must be "on guard."
3. *Social needs.* Third level: a person's physical and safety needs are already met.
   - The need to feel loved and appreciated; the need to feel a sense of belonging.

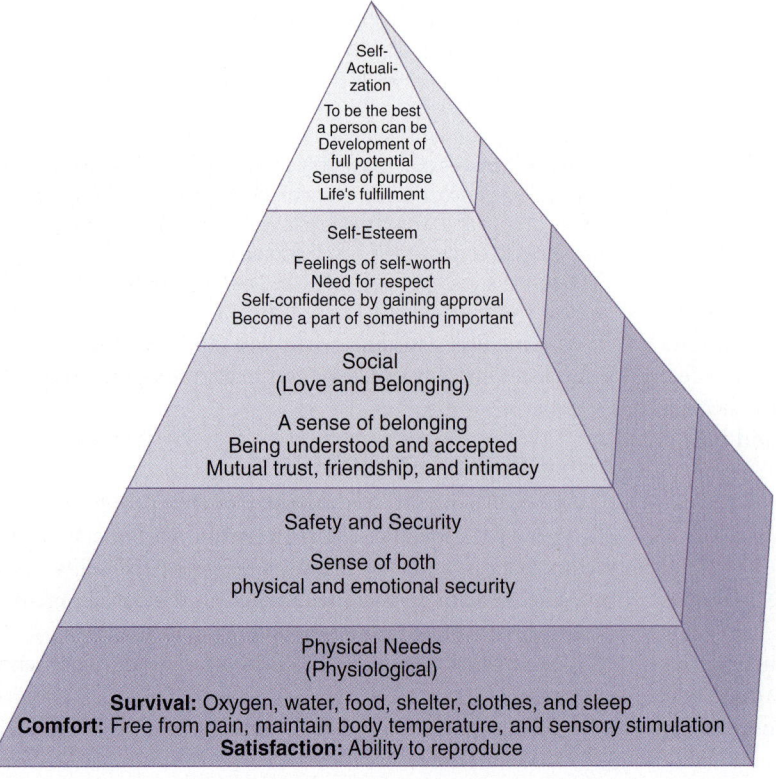

FIGURE 5-1 Maslow's hierarchy of needs pyramid.

- When achieved, social needs bring friendship and companionship.
- When *not* achieved, disappointment and loneliness may result.

4. *Self-esteem.* Fourth level: physical, safety, and social needs are already met.
   - The need to feel worthwhile and good about oneself.
   - Affected by attention and recognition from others.
   - When achieved, self-esteem creates a sense of being in control.
   - When *not* achieved, there may be a lack of appreciation for others or oneself.

5. *Self-actualization.* Fifth level: physical, safety, social, and self-esteem needs are already met.
   - The need of persons to "be all they can be" (to do their best and accomplish their goals).
   - As the most advanced level, self-actualization may never be reached because it deals with becoming the absolute best a person can be.

Box 5-1 lists Maslow's characteristics of a self-actualized person. Maslow's theories are widely used in the study of employee behavior, helping us understand what motivates people to perform well on the job. People are only motivated to reach for what they do not have, or their "unsatisfied needs." Satisfying needs is healthy, and the desire for gratification has a major influence on our actions.

Which level of Maslow's hierarchy is currently motivating you as a person? As an employee? How can you satisfy these needs and move to the next level?

PATIENT-CENTERED PROFESSIONALISM

- *Part of your job as a medical assistant is to monitor patients' compliance with the physician's treatment plan. With this in mind, how can understanding where patients are on Maslow's hierarchy of needs help you encourage them to follow their treatment plans?*
- *How can you use your understanding of a patient's needs when communicating with patients?*
- *How can understanding your own needs and the needs of your co-workers help you provide better care to patients?*

BOX 5-1

Maslow's Characteristics of a Self-Actualized Person

Effective perception of reality
Self-acceptance and acceptance of others
Having a need for privacy and solitude at times
Being problem centered rather than ego centered
Having a deep appreciation of the basic experiences of life
Having the ability for a deep interpersonal relationship
Having a good sense of humor
Having democratic attitudes
Being creative

MENTAL AND PHYSICAL HEALTH

Freud, Maslow, and many others who study human behavior agree that mental health can affect physical health. People who have a good opinion of themselves and their abilities (e.g., high self-esteem) tend to be healthier than those who think negatively about themselves. In addition, when people go through stressful situations in life, it wears down their resistance to disease. Stressful situations cause people to experience fear and anxiety, which can impact their health over time.

As a medical assistant, you need to understand the importance of a healthy self-esteem and good self-perception as well as the effect that fear and anxiety can have on health.

Self-Esteem

How people feel about themselves at any given time is referred to as their **self-esteem.** Self-esteem is the fourth level in Maslow's hierarchy. Positive or high self-esteem is having feelings of self-worth and emotional well-being. It is an "I like myself" state of mind. Individuals with negative or low self-esteem focus on mistakes and dwell on what they have not done versus what they have accomplished. Self-esteem is influenced by labels, perceptions, and the way people adapt to change.

Labels

Labels (e.g., genius, jock, stupid, nerd) placed on individuals by parents, family, and others influence how people value themselves. Research shows that labels of any type place limitations on people.

- Children described as being "shy" may never try to socialize because they are expected to be shy.
- Children labeled "special ed" students may never reach their full potential because society (the school system) has placed a label on them that says they cannot learn. Just because a student is labeled as "special ed" does not mean the student cannot learn; it only means the student learns at a different pace or by different methods. However, a child labeled as "special ed" may come to believe that he or she cannot learn at all.
- Parents brag about their child getting all "A"s and refer to the child as a "genius." If the child receives a "B" on her next report card, she may think she has lost her "genius" status.

Labels can place too much pressure on a person, especially a child. Never "label" patients or co-workers.

Self-esteem fluctuates throughout the day based on the many challenges people face. Positive self-worth is not about accomplishments but rather is an acceptance of "self" no matter what setbacks have occurred. Always remember that you must be appreciative of the "good things in life" and use your mistakes as learning experiences to improve. Take negative beliefs and change them to positive ones. As a medical assistant, it is important for you to have a healthy self-esteem. With a healthy self-esteem, you will be more confident in your ability to care for patients and more positive when interacting with both patients and co-workers.

> No one can make you feel inferior without your consent.
> *Eleanor Roosevelt*

Perception

Perception is the process of interpreting information gathered from our surroundings. How we view an event, another person, and even ourselves is influenced by our life experiences. Our first impression is often inaccurate because our subconscious mind usually focuses on existing information, and we are slow to change our original impression, even if it is wrong. It takes effort to move beyond these "old habits" or past beliefs. To some, perception matters more than reality. Many factors influence how an individual will perceive any given situation, including psychological, **physiological,** and cultural influences and social roles.

Psychological Influences. The words we use influence how we perform.

- *Past experiences.* We recall past experiences when we perform similar tasks. "I've never been very good at it" versus "With some help, I am ready to tackle this."
- *Assumptions.* We make judgments about how things will go based on how things have gone so far. If the day begins with problems, "It's going to be a bad day" versus "Up to this point, it has not been a good day, and it can only get better."
- *Expectations.* We use reports of others to form our expectations. "I heard that the test was hard, so I probably won't pass it" versus "I heard the test was hard, so I will give it my best shot."
- *Knowledge.* The facts we have will influence our approach to a problem because facts provide a place to begin. "I only know part of what I need to know to do this" versus "I know some of the facts, and I can ask for help or research the rest."
- *Personal moods.* Our mood influences our perception. When you do not want to do something, "I am not the person for this task, and I know I won't do a good job" versus "I will do a better job after I have a chance to figure out what really needs to be done."

Physiological Influences. What we sense and feel influences how we perform.

- *Senses.* It is difficult to perform if we are not comfortable. Sights, sounds, smells, things we touch or feel, and tastes can affect us. One person may feel cold in a room, whereas another may feel comfortable.
- *Age.* People of different age groups may think and use words differently. An 80-year-old and a 23-year-old will have a different meaning for the words "sweet" and "bad" because of the generation change and use of words during certain time periods
- *Number of experiences.* The amount of experience we have affects our perception. A recent graduate will approach a project differently than someone who has been in the field several years.
- *Health.* Not being healthy may take away the ability to focus. If you have a bad headache, you might not be able to type as quickly as usual.
- *Fatigue.* Proper rest is vital for peak performance. If you are tired, you could make a mistake you normally would not have made.
- *Hunger.* Satisfaction of hunger is one of the primary levels in Maslow's hierarchy. If your stomach is growling, your mind may not be on your work.
- *Biological cycles.* Different people are best at different times of the day. Some people are fresh in the morning, whereas others do not start until noon.

Cultural Influences. Our culture influences how we behave and what we believe.

- Different cultural backgrounds can lead to misunderstanding or miscommunication. A person's cultural background will determine what the person regards as caring behavior.
- Do not make assumptions regarding a patient's understanding of health maintenance, causes of disease, treatment, and prevention.
- Many cultures believe in alternative medicine, faith healers, and other approaches to health and perceive Western medicine as ineffective or wrong. Do not discount their belief system.

Social Roles. People have different beliefs about social roles.

- Different people and cultures have diverse beliefs about the roles of men and women. Some may think that women should stay home with children and that men are the heads of the household and should make all decisions. Others may think that men and women are equal partners in decision making.
- Patients who have certain beliefs about social roles may be uncomfortable, for example, with male or female physicians. Be considerate and understanding.

A person's perception of any given situation is influenced not only by physiological and psychological factors but also by personal needs and interests at the time. Medical assistants must be aware of their own perceptions versus those of patients and co-workers. Differing perceptions can cause fear and stress.

Adapting to Change

Change, whether considered to be positive or negative, can cause stress (Table 5-1). How we adapt or adjust to change has a major impact on both our physical and mental health. Adjusting or modifying our behavior depends on how we perceive the change will affect our usual routine. In early childhood, for example, infants develop feelings of security and emotional attachment by doing things the same way each time. Once these routines are established, the child will acquire new behavior or will slightly modify behavior when introduced to new situations. This is the process of adapting behavior to fit new situations. If change is introduced slowly, with full understanding and encouragement, it may be smooth and even welcomed. However, sudden changes are difficult for people to handle.

TABLE 5-1
Changes Affecting Behavior

Negative	Positive
Fired from job	Opportunity to go back to school Learn a new career
Death in family	Look at life differently Appreciate others and self
Getting a divorce	Opportunity to make new goals Go back to school
Serious accident	Learn to live with disability Become a counselor

TABLE 5-2
Common Phobias

Source	Phobia
Number 13	Triskaidekaphobia
Being alone	Monophobia
Bees	Apiphobia
Birds	Ornithophobia
Blood	Hemophobia
Confined spaces	Claustrophobia
Going to the doctor	Iatrophobia
Eating or swallowing	Phagophobia
Germs	Verminophobia
Homosexuality	Homophobia
Injections	Trypanophobia
Insects	Acarophobia
Laughter	Geliophobia
Light	Photophobia
Lightning or thunder	Brontophobia
Riding in a car	Amaxophobia
Going to school	Didaskaleinophobia
Speaking in public	Glossophobia
Spiders	Arachnophobia
Sunlight	Phengophobia
Water	Hydrophobia

As part of the life process, change occurs daily. Sometimes these changes are perceived as hassles or irritating events; these do not require a major adjustment in a person's routine. Others are seen as *minor* changes, such as moving to a middle school from an elementary school. Some changes, such as a death of a loved one, are perceived as being a *major* change, or a life changing event. Major changes challenge our ability to cope with the situation. Common situations that require an adjustment in behavior include the following:

- School-age children face changes daily in their studies, with other children, and with their teachers.
- Adolescents face issues such as appearance, feelings of self-worth, others' opinions, and their future.
- Young adults are moving from the "I" to the "we" concept concerning education, job, home, and family.
- Middle age is a change for many people because their children are independent, often leaving home, and a void is created.
- Old age may bring about the death of friends, loss of independence, and decrease in income.

As a medical assistant, it is important for you to consider the impact of a positive self-esteem, differing perceptions, and people's ability to adapt to change. Being sensitive and understanding will help you provide better care to your patients.

Fear, Anxiety, and Stress

You have learned how certain factors establish a person's self-esteem and how labels, differing perceptions, and life changes can impact a person's mental and physical health. Fear, anxiety, and stress also affect mental and physical health. As a medical assistant, you need to understand the effects of fear, anxiety, and stress so that you can be more helpful to patients in the medical office.

Fear

Fear is a *normal* reaction to a *genuine* danger. It is an emotional response that alerts the body to take appropriate action to protect itself from the danger. The emotional response causes the body to either stand up to the danger ("fight"), run away from the danger ("flight"), or freeze, "like a deer in the headlights" ("fright"). This is called the **fight, flight, or fright** response. This response is actually caused by physiological changes in the body that occur when a threat is sensed.

Examples of physiological responses to fear are sudden and can include increased heart rate, rapid breathing, and sweaty palms. Patients who are ill or injured may be experiencing fear and may display these physiological responses.

Phobias. **Phobias** are *irrational* (unreasonable) fears of objects, activities, or situations. Phobias interfere with a person's ability to function in everyday life. A person with a phobia feels powerless to do anything about the situation. When a fear is constantly on a person's mind, causing lost sleep and an inability to focus when awake, this fear is classified as a phobia. Persons with a phobia avoid situations where they might encounter the object of their fear. This is called *avoidance behavior*. In addition, the degree of physiological responses helps professionals identify phobias. People who have phobias often experience the fight, flight, or fright response when merely thinking about the fearful object or situation. For example:

> It is not abnormal to have a *fear* of poisonous snakes because of the real danger of being bitten. It is considered to be a *phobia* if a person not only fears all snakes but also avoids any situation where snakes could be present (e.g., will not go outdoors because there may be snakes).

Phobias can be classified into one of three categories: simple, social, or agoraphobia (Box 5-2).

Research has shown that phobias focus on objects and situations that people cannot predict or control such as lightning (Table 5-2). Fears tend to be very *objective* because they are very *obvious* and almost everyone would share the fear. Phobias

BOX 5-2

Types of Phobias

SIMPLE

A persistent irrational fear of a specific object or situation when in its presence.

Fears
- *Objects* (e.g., animals and reptiles such as dogs, cats, or snakes)
- *Transportation* (e.g., flying, riding in a train or car)
- *Closed spaces* (e.g., elevators, rooms with the doors closed)
- *Heights* (e.g., going up a ladder or an elevator with glass sides)

Signs and Symptoms
- Avoiding these objects or situations.
- Withdrawing from these objects or situations.

SOCIAL: ANTHROPOPHOBIA

An irrational fear of being in certain social or performing situations.

Fears
- Looking ridiculous when speaking in public.
- Interacting with authority figures.
- Being ridiculed or thought of as "strange."
- Being suspicious of or fearing harm from other people (irrationally).

Signs and Symptoms
- Avoiding or refusing to eat in public.
- Refusing invitations from others.
- Having a reclusive lifestyle.
- Trembling hands, dry throat, or lump in the throat.
- Preoccupation with some aspect of appearance (e.g., refusing to wear bathing suits in front of others, having several cosmetic surgeries to look better).

AGORAPHOBIA

An exaggerated fear of being in places where there is no escape or where embarrassment could occur.

Fears
- Being ridiculed or thought of as "strange" in public places.
- Being suspicious of others or fearing harm from other people (irrationally) in public places.

Signs and Symptoms
- Avoiding or refusing to go out (secluding oneself at home).
- Only going to stores or being in crowds if accompanied.

BOX 5-3

Medical Conditions Associated with Anxiety*

CARDIAC
Chest pain
Heart palpitations
Hypertension

RESPIRATORY
Bronchial asthma
Hyperventilation

DIGESTIVE
Duodenal ulcer
Ulcerative colitis

SENSORY
Deafness
Tinnitus
Nystagmus
Visual blurring

ENDOCRINE
Hypoglycemia
Hyperthyroidism

*Appropriate tests can help physicians determine if these anxiety-related conditions have an organic cause.

---

are fears that remain even when the person is not in any danger from the object or situation. You may encounter patients with phobias (e.g., hemophobia, the fear of blood). Always be considerate and understanding and seek help with these patients when necessary.

Anxiety

Anxiety is the feeling of apprehension, uneasiness, or uncertainty about a situation. These feelings are normal as long as the person is able to move on and function normally. We all have had periods of anxiety and worry when faced with new situations (e.g., on the first day at a new job, your heart may pound and your mouth may be dry). What makes anxiety different from a fear or phobia is that an anxiety is very *subjective*. A person may worry excessively over "bad things" that have not happened and may never happen. A person experiencing anxiety may display the following characteristics:

1. *Perception of future events is always negative.* The person may be uneasy, even for no real reason.
2. *The person almost always exhibits self-doubt.* The person may give up on something because of a lack of confidence in his or her ability.
3. *Crippling symptoms appear.* The person may be unable to sleep, may have difficulty breathing, or may have periods in which the person describes a feeling that "a tight band is around my head."
4. *Behavior and posture are different.* The person's facial expression may be tense and the voice may quiver. No eye contact is made, and the person may blush and begin to sweat and may also "fidget" and "wring" the hands.

When the biological and physical changes resulting from anxiety are long term, the body can experience physical problems and illness. These problems occur because of the added stress put on the body (e.g., ulcers, increased blood pressure). Box 5-3 lists medical conditions attributable to anxiety.

Stress

Stress is the body's response to any demand put on the body. Stress is an unavoidable fact of life. Some stress is good because it keeps a person alert and aware of what is happening (e.g., a runner may feel stress while waiting for the signal to begin the race). How well people adapt to stressful events in life is often the difference between a healthy mind and body and a life with many illnesses. For example:

Pressures of life	Raising a family	Earning a living
Conflicts	Choosing a spouse	Choosing a career
Frustrations	Renting and not owning a home	Not getting the promotion

Reactions to Stress. During periods of stress, our natural body defense systems weaken, fatigue takes over, and we become more susceptible to disease. Does stress always cause disease? Not always, but these factors influence the likelihood of illness:

1. Is the stress severe? Severe stress includes the death of a spouse or friend, a divorce, or a financial crisis.
2. Is the stress chronic (occurring every day)?
3. Does the person perceive the event as stressful?

If the answers to these questions are "yes," the probability of a stress-related illness is greater. Consider what people may do in response to stressful situations (e.g., smoke, drink, overeat, not eat). These unhealthy behaviors increase the chance of illness. Sometimes our bodies force us to take it easy when our hearts and minds refuse. Research has proved that many **psychosomatic** disorders (physical illness caused by psychological problems) are caused by the effects of stress. Our health and susceptibility to disease also depend on other factors, such as genetic makeup, environmental factors, psychological factors, and the way we cope with problems.

At the first sign of stress, our body responds. Table 5-3 shows the phases and common symptoms of stress.

Short-Term and Long-Term Stress. How you are able to cope with life's everyday challenges has both short-term and long-term effects on your body. If you allow a stressful situation to control you over a long period, it can have a great impact on your mental and physical health.

When a person does not cope with short-term stress and it becomes long-term stress, the following occurs:

Short Term	Long Term
Muscle tension	Headache, backache
Increased blood pressure	Hypertension
Heart palpitations	Heart disease
"Butterflies in stomach"	Ulcers

When a person takes steps to control the short-term stress and to prevent the effects of long-term stress, the following occurs:

TABLE 5-3

Phases and Symptoms of Stress

Type	Symptoms
AWARENESS STAGE	
Physical	Increase in blood pressure
	Heart palpitations
	Chills or heavy sweating
	Headaches
Behavioral	Constant irritability
	Inability to sleep
	Grinding the teeth (bruxism)
Psychological	Increased anxiety
	Forgetfulness
	Inability to concentrate
ENERGY-CONSERVATION	
Physical	Decreased sexual desires
	Constant tiredness
Behavioral	Constant lateness to work or school
	Missing deadlines
	Increased consumption of caffeine or alcohol
Psychological	Putting things off
	Withdrawing from friends
	Negative attitude
	Argumentative
EXHAUSTION	
Physical	Chronic stomach upsets
	Constant tiredness
	Chronic headaches
Behavioral	Withdrawal from family
Psychological	Depression (sense of hopelessness)
	Mental fatigue

Short Term	Long Term
Exercise: increased circulation	Good cardiac function
Nutrition and relaxation techniques	Improves the body's ability to resist disease

Table 5-4 lists disorders associated with long-term stress.

Managing Stress. Knowing how to manage stress in the short term provides long-term rewards. When you are able to control the stress in your everyday life, you achieve an overall feeling of satisfaction. Your life may become hectic at times because of stressful situations at home and on the job. You need to be able to manage your stress to stay healthy and provide good patient care. Follow these steps to manage stress in your life:

1. **Recognize the signs of stress.** Is it physical (e.g., fatigue, illness)? Behavioral (e.g., bad habits)? Emotional or mental (e.g., negative thoughts, worries)?
2. **Identify the cause of the stress.** Is it sickness or injury? Problems at school or work? An argument with a friend or family member?
3. **Determine the importance of the stress factor.** How important is the cause of the stress? Is it worth getting sick or upset over? What is the worst that could happen?

TABLE 5-4
Disorders Associated with Long-Term Stress

System	Disorders
Respiratory	Bronchial asthma
Digestive	Colitis
	Gastritis
	Ulcers (peptic or duodenal)
Circulatory	Hypertension
	Heart attack
	Raynaud disease
Nervous	Migraine headaches
	Cluster headaches
	Twitching
Reproductive	Sexual dysfunction
Integumentary	Eczema

BOX 5-4
Healthy Habits to Reduce Stress

1. Exercise
2. Take deep breaths and stretch several times a day
3. Get adequate sleep
4. Take time for self and family
5. Receive proper nutrition and hydrate with water
6. Laugh (Figure 5-2)

4. **Work to reduce the impact of the stress factor.** Are there workable alternatives? Can delegating some of the responsibility help the situation? Can prioritizing the duties reduce the stress? Will simple life changes and better health habits, such as those in Box 5-4, reduce your stress levels?

PATIENT-CENTERED PROFESSIONALISM

- *How might a patient be affected if a medical assistant labels him "difficult"? How will this label affect the way other health professionals interact with this patient?*
- *How can a patient's perception of your ability as a medical assistant influence her to follow a treatment plan? How can it affect the patient's confidence in coming to the medical office and the likelihood that the patient will not only come back, but also refer new patients to the office?*
- *How can understanding the differences among fear, anxiety, and stress help you provide better care to patients?*
- *How can stress interfere with your ability to care for patients?*
- *Are you experiencing anxiety or stress? What are some things you can do to reduce your anxiety or stress?*

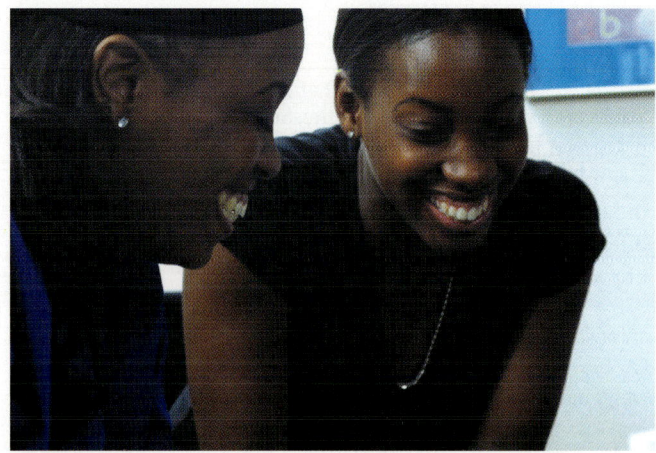

FIGURE 5-2 Laughter increases blood circulation, lowering blood pressure. Laughing not only helps you feel good about yourself but also increases the activity of your body's T cells (natural killer cells) and antibodies. Research shows that a baby begins laughing at 2 to 3 months; a 6-year-old child laughs an average of 300 times a day, and an adult only chuckles between 15 and 100 times a day. How many times have you laughed today?

COPING

You now understand the importance of managing stress in your everyday life. You also know some ways to reduce the effects of stress. You can take action when you are aware of the problem and how it can be solved, but what about other types of problems? People may have subconscious problems (problems they do not realize they have). Terminal illness is another situation that cannot be "solved" but still must be confronted. People cope with their problems and conflicts in ways that are healthy and in other ways that are not healthy. As a medical assistant, you need to know how to work with patients who are coping with conflicts or difficult situations.

Defense Mechanisms

Sometimes we have deep-seated problems that we are not aware of or that we choose to ignore. Our bodies and minds have a way of coping with these types of problems. Freud's unconscious awareness theory implies that we unconsciously avoid situations (conflicts) that could cause us feelings of anxiety (dread, uneasiness). If we cannot recognize the real problem or situation or choose not to confront it directly, we may use a **defense mechanism** to cope with the problem. Defense mechanisms are coping tools that help us deal with conflict. These behavioral responses keep our minds off of the conflict, thus preventing or decreasing anxiety and allowing us to maintain our self-image. We have all used defense mechanisms at one time or another. The key to good mental health is not using defense mechanisms too often instead of facing our real conflicts or problems.

Table 5-5 lists several types of defense mechanisms (the first seven are the most common). You may encounter patients

TABLE 5-5

Defense Mechanisms

Term	Definition	Examples
Compensation	When personal strengths in one area are emphasized to cover up a weakness in another area; can be a good thing unless the person gives up too soon on worthwhile tasks or lowers self-expectations when "the going gets tough."	A new medical assistant might brag about how well she did in school to cover up her discomfort at starting a new career. An insecure co-worker may compensate by acting tough and "bullish." A parent may give a child many material things to compensate for not being able to spend much time with the child.
Denial	Refusing to acknowledge or face the unpleasant facts of life. By denying a problem exists, the importance of the unpleasant information or situation is temporarily relieved.	A person who experiences chest pain decides that it is indigestion and buys antacids instead of going to the emergency room. A wife whose husband leaves her tells friends that they have agreed to a trial separation.
Displacement	Behaving aggressively toward someone who cannot fight back as a substitute for anger toward the source of frustration. The bottled-up feeling is taken out on something or someone less threatening (a scapegoat) than what actually caused the negative feelings.	A co-worker who is angry with the physician may take out his anger on another co-worker instead of the physician. A patient tells the physical therapist, "I hate you!" when the physical therapist is trying to help the patient recover from a painful injury.
Fantasy	Daydreaming inappropriately. People who use fantasy as a way to cope try to satisfy their desires by imagining achievements.	A trainee in a medical office daydreams about a higher position instead of working on a solution to make it happen. A student who is teased by other students imagines herself taking revenge inappropriately.
Overcompensation	Exaggerated and inappropriate behavior of a person in one area to handle inadequacy in some other area.	A co-worker who feels shy may talk too much or too loudly in an attempt to not be seen as shy. A parent who does not spend enough time with the family works overtime to provide extra money.
Projection	Projecting one's own unacceptable qualities or thoughts onto others or blaming others for these unacceptable qualities or thoughts in oneself.	A medical receptionist who cannot get promoted to office manager because of poor skills projects his failure onto another co-worker by believing the co-worker makes him look bad. A wife who has cheated on her husband may feel guilty and accuse her husband of being unfaithful.
Rationalization	Inventing excuses or reasons for one's behavior.	A medical assistant who talks about a patient's condition with a co-worker rationalizes it with the excuse that the co-worker knows the patient's family so they "need to know" about the patient's condition. A person who has paid too much for an item says, "It's a good investment and the resale value is high."
Aggression	Attacking the real or imaginary source of frustration.	A patient is upset about her medical bill and screams at the medical receptionist.
Conversion reaction	Emotional conflict causes a physical symptom.	A person loses the use of his legs after a car accident that was his fault. There is no neurological cause for the paralysis.
Intellectualization	Making emotional conflict bearable by analyzing it in a logical way.	A person diagnosed with a terminal illness dismisses it by saying, "We all have to die sometime."
Repression	Blocking out ideas, memories, and feelings that cause conflict. Repression tends to lower self-esteem.	A victim of abuse cannot remember how she got her bruises.
Regression	Behaving in an immature way when frustrated.	An older child soils his pants in reaction to the birth of a sibling.
Sublimation	Transforming an unconscious conflict into a more socially acceptable form.	An aggressive child works hard to become a star athlete instead of a bully.
Withdrawal	Physically or emotionally pulling away from people or conflict.	An office manager's reaction to office conflict is to avoid becoming involved by acting as if the conflict does not exist.

using one or more of these defense mechanisms. Keep in mind that patients can hide a variety of thoughts or feelings (e.g., anger, fear, sadness, depression, helplessness) by using defense mechanisms. It is important that you listen not only to what patients say but also to *how* they say it so that you can "read between the lines" and address the deeper issues.

Death and Dying

One of the most difficult situations that people face is death and dying. Whether they face their own death or that of a loved one, they must learn to cope with the situation. As a medical assistant you may be involved with a terminal (dying) patient. Understanding the stages of the dying process can prepare you to help patients going through this process while maintaining a good relationship with them.

Stages of Grief

Elisabeth Kübler-Ross is known for her research and theories on the dying process, which are based on many studies of terminally ill patients and their families. She believed that dying people, and often their families, go through five stages of grief when coming to terms with their impending death. These stages only establish guidelines; a person could skip a stage or even return to a stage during the dying process. How fast or slow a person moves through a stage will depend on his or her beliefs, values, inner strength, spiritual growth, and support system (family and friends). Kübler-Ross's five stages of grief are as follows:

1. **Denial** is a defense mechanism that allows the patient time to deal with the shock. It is usually a temporary phase. Reactions may include any of the following:
   - "This is not happening."
   - "It can't be true."
   - "They made a mistake at the lab."
   - Changing physicians.
   - Continuing on as if nothing is wrong.
   - Refusing to talk about the problem.
   - Refusing treatment.

   As part of the health care team, it is important that you listen to patients and not argue. Allow them to vent their frustration and remain calm. Sometimes, all that is needed is for someone to listen without interruption.

2. **Anger** is a normal reaction caused by the feeling of losing control. Emotions run high at this point, and the anger may turn to rage and resentment directed at anyone in the way. Reactions vary but usually include the following:
   - Temper tantrums.
   - "Why me?"
   - Feeling of envy toward healthy people.
   - Periods of yelling and withdrawal.

   Again, listening and allowing the person to vent help the patient deal with this phase.

3. **Bargaining** is making deals with anyone in sight, including the physician, a higher power, and the family. This phase is very goal directed and important; otherwise a person could lapse into despair. The patient may become agreeable and cooperative in an effort to buy more time. Reactions to this phase include the following:
   - "Give me just enough time to see the birth of my grandchild (or attend my child's wedding or graduation)."
   - "If I can get a second chance, I will …"

4. **Depression** can be described as an overall feeling of hopelessness. In this stage health is usually declining, pain may be increasing, symptoms are worsening, and relationships may have been severed. Reactions to depression are as follows:
   - Negative body language (e.g., no eye contact, stooped shoulders, excessive sleeping).
   - Not caring about personal appearance.
   - Relief is sought through crying.

   Listening and giving reassurance that it is normal to have these feelings benefit the dying patient more than saying the person should not feel this way. *Touch* is reported to help during this time; it is the unspoken word that often meets the need of the patient.

5. **Acceptance** is coming to terms with dying or the loss of a loved one. The patient or family can use this time together to make plans, such as finalizing a will, completing advance directives, and preparing for the funeral. If this phase is reached, the reward is the peace of mind that is achieved. Reactions to this phase are as follows:
   - Planning a trip to a place where the person has always wanted to go.
   - Giving away personal items.
   - Emptying closets of clothes.

Arriving at this stage is the most beneficial of the stages for the patient and the family. **Hospice** is a bundle of services and a team of people helping patients and their families during the end stage of a terminal illness. The hospice team (e.g., physician, nurse, social worker) works on the concept of listening to the needs of the patient and family, whether physical, psychological, or spiritual. The purpose of the team is to preserve the dignity of the dying patient. Hospice is concerned with quality of life, pain management, and offering comfort.

How to Help

Health care workers can best help during the dying process by showing more compassion and **empathy** than **sympathy**. Empathy is putting yourself in another person's situation. It means not being judgmental when anger is displayed or when the other person is vocal about the situation. Sympathy is showing concern for a person's situation. People who are dying need someone to understand their emotional state and allow them to express themselves freely. Part of this process is coming to realize that their plans for the future have changed.

Research has shown that dying patients need a good relationship with their health care team (Figure 5-3). The patient wants to be recognized as a unique and whole individual, not

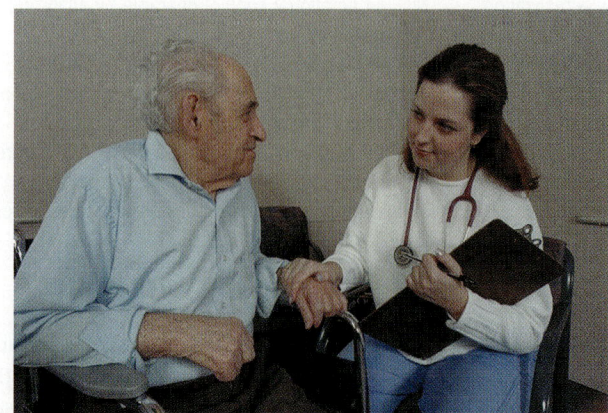

FIGURE 5-3 When dealing with terminal patients, show compassion and empathy rather than sympathy. Sometimes the best thing you can do for your patient is listen.

just a disease. The family also needs to be recognized as individual people, not just the family of a terminal patient. Studies have shown that if the family's psychological and spiritual needs are met in addition to the treatment of the patient's disease, the dying process is less distressing for all those involved.

PATIENT-CENTERED PROFESSIONALISM

- *Why do medical assistants need to understand and to be able to recognize the defense mechanisms used by patients? By co-workers? By themselves?*
- *As a medical assistant, how can understanding the stages of grief help you work with patients who are dying?*
- *How can understanding these stages benefit terminal patients' families?*
- *How does the medical practice benefit when terminal patients and their families are treated with courtesy and respect?*

CONCLUSION

As a medical assistant, you will be working with people. You will see many types of behaviors, some positive and some negative. Understanding what causes people to behave the way they do will help you to provide better care to the patients with whom you work. It will also help you to be a more effective member of the health care team. Much research and knowledge exist about human behavior. Patient-centered professionalism means studying this knowledge and applying it in your day-to-day medical assisting duties.

Chapter Summary

Reinforce your understanding of the material in this chapter by reviewing the curriculum objectives and key content points below.

1. **Define, appropriately use, and spell all the Key Terms for this chapter.**
    - Review the Key Terms if necessary.
2. **List and briefly define the three parts that make up a person's personality according to Freud.**
    - The id is concerned with basic unconscious biological drives (e.g., food, sleep).
    - The ego is aware of reality and the consequences of behavior.
    - The superego (conscience) demands that decisions be made morally and ethically.
3. **List three factors that influence personality development.**
    - Events early in life
    - Biological factors
    - Psychological factors
4. **List the five types of human needs.**
    - Abraham Maslow developed the hierarchy of needs, which deals with the stages in personal fulfillment: physical needs, safety and security needs, social needs, self-esteem, and self-actualization.
5. **Explain the importance of having good self-esteem.**
    - Self-esteem deals with feelings of self-worth. Good self-esteem permits people to fulfill their potential.
6. **List the four types of factors that can influence perception. Perception is the process of interpreting information gathered from surroundings. The four types of factors that can influence perception are as follows:**
    - Psychological influences include past experiences, assumptions, expectations, knowledge, and personal moods.
    - Physiological influences include senses, age and number of experiences, health, fatigue, hunger, and biological cycles.
    - Culture influences what we believe and how we behave; alternative medicine may be a choice.
    - Beliefs about male and female roles (social roles) also influence perception.
7. **Differentiate between experiencing fear and having a phobia.**
    - Fear is an appropriate reaction, whereas a phobia is an irrational fear causing avoidance behavior.
8. **List five health problems caused by anxiety or stress.**
    - Many health problems can be caused by anxiety or stress, including ulcers, hypertension, heart disease, headache, and backache.
9. **Explain how fear, phobia, anxiety, and stress affect a person's mental and physical health.**
    - Fear and phobias are mentally crippling and encourage avoidance behavior. Anxiety and stress are part of everyday living. Not learning to deal with these reactions exacts a physical and mental toll on the body.
10. **List and describe six defense mechanisms. Defense mechanisms are used by the unconscious mind to block out awareness of unpleasant events and help individuals deal with conflict. The most common defense mechanisms are the following:**
    - Compensation emphasizes strength to cover up a weakness.

- Denial is refusing to acknowledge that a problem exists.
- Displacement is finding a scapegoat.
- Fantasy is daydreaming inappropriately.
- Overcompensation is exaggerated behavior in one area to compensate for inadequacy in another area.
- Projection is projecting one's unacceptable qualities onto another person or blaming that person for one's shortcomings.

11. **List the five stages of grief and briefly describe each in the first person.**
    - Denial: "This can't be happening to me."
    - Anger: "I'm a good person; why is this happening to me?"
    - Bargaining: "Just let me live until the baby is born."
    - Depression: "I really am going to die, and there is nothing I can do about it."
    - Acceptance: "I have made my peace, and I am ready to go."

12. **Analyze a realistic medical office situation and apply your understanding of human behavior to determine the best course of action.**
    - Understanding why patients behave the way they do helps medical assistants interact more positively with them.

13. **Describe the impact on patient care when medical assistants understand human behavior.**
    - When patients think that the office staff understands and wants to help them, they are more likely to follow their prescribed treatment plan and be satisfied with their care.

PRACTICAL APPLICATIONS

If you have accomplished the objectives in this chapter, you will be able to make better choices as a medical assistant. Take another look at this situation and decide what you would do.

Sara Ann is a 22-year-old single mother and a medical assistant. She has no assistance at home with child care or with any of the chores necessary to keep up a household. Sara Ann works as many hours as she can to support herself and her two children in the best way possible. On top of all of this, going to school has added major financial problems for Sara Ann.

On many days, Sara Ann is tired and frustrated and wonders just how she will get through the day. Because of her lack of self-esteem and the lack of help, anxiety and stress are affecting the way Sara Ann deals with co-workers. Sara Ann's anxiety level often leads her to label patients. In addition, Sara Ann has difficulty adapting to any variation in the daily schedule.

Because Sara Ann feels close to some patients with whom she has spent time in the medical office, she will often discuss her personal problems with these patients. Also, Sara Ann must handle some of her personal business (banking, errands) while at work because she does not leave work early enough to do these things when the businesses are open.

Sara Ann is experiencing a lot of stress, which is having an impact on her performance at work. If you were in Sara Ann's situation, what would you do to reduce stress?

1. How are Sara Ann's reactions to her work understandable under the circumstances? What reactions are related to the anxiety and loss of self-esteem?
2. How are Sara Ann's reactions typical for someone who is not coping with personal or professional worlds?
3. What are some of the reactions that you would expect from Sara Ann's fellow employees about her behavior?
4. Where on Maslow's hierarchy of needs would you place Sara Ann? Why did you place her at that level?
5. Because Sara Ann has no one at home for emotional or financial support, how would you, as a patient, feel if she told you about her problems? Are her actions involving patients ethical? Why?

WEB SEARCH

1. **Research other theories about the development of personality.** Understanding the development of personality helps medical assistants provide more effective care to patients. Many theories exist that help people understand how personality develops. Learn about the personality theories of Erik Erikson, Jean Piaget, and Lawrence Kohlberg.
    - **Keywords:** Use the following keywords in your search: Erik Erikson, Jean Piaget, Lawrence Kohlberg, personality development.

2. **Research stress and its effects on humans.** Medical assistants need to understand what stress is, what causes it, how it affects people, and how it can be managed.
    - **Keywords:** Use the following keywords in your search: stress relief, stress, effects of stress, stress-related illness.

Understanding Patient Behavior

6

evolve http://evolve.elsevier.com/klieger/medicalassisting

In Chapter 5, you learned how personality, perception, motivation, self-esteem, and factors such as stress and anxiety affect human behavior. These elements, among others, also influence the way a person will *behave* as a patient in a medical setting. A patient's age not only influences the patient's behavior but also determines how the medical assistant should interact with the patient. Cultural differences can also influence patient behavior. Patients may have certain cultural beliefs that conflict with recommended treatment. There is the potential for communication problems with patients who do not speak English well. Finally, any patient can become irritated while waiting for the physician, or simply because the patient is not feeling well. This may bring on complaints or anger. Medical assistants need to understand how to work effectively with patients of all ages and stages of development as well as patients of all cultures.

LEARNING OBJECTIVES

You will be able to do the following after completing this chapter:

Key Terms
1. Define, appropriately use, and spell all the Key Terms for this chapter.

Development
2. List and describe the three areas of change during growth and development in a lifetime.
3. For each age level, list two age-appropriate ways that medical assistants can enhance interaction with patients.
4. Describe the basic developmental milestones for each developmental stage.
5. Explain why the medical assistant must understand the various body system changes involved in the aging process.

Cultural Diversity
6. List eight areas in which cultural differences exist.
7. Explain the importance of being knowledgeable about the cultural background of a patient.

Response to Illness
8. List four types of responses that patients commonly have toward illness.

9. List five things you can do when a patient becomes angry.

Patient-Centered Professionalism
10. Analyze a realistic medical office situation and apply your understanding of the patient's background and behavior to determine the best course of action.
11. Describe the impact on patient care when medical assistants understand how people react to illness and medical care and how they change at various stages of development.

KEY TERMS

adolescence
adulthood
childhood
cultural diversity
development
heredity
infancy

mental growth
physical growth
preschool
psychosocial growth
school age
toddler

PRACTICAL APPLICATIONS

Read the following scenario and keep it in mind as you learn about the importance of understanding patient behavior in this chapter.

Juan, 40 years old, has moved to the United States. His family is still in Mexico, but he hopes to find a good job soon and pay for them to come to the United States. Because Juan does not speak English very well, he has had difficulty finding employment and a place to live. Lately, he has been staying at a shelter for homeless people. His educational background is limited, and his broken English makes communicating difficult. Few Hispanic people live in the area where he has settled. Juan has lost 10 pounds, his vision is declining, and he has noticed that he is not hearing as well as he used to. Because of his constant weight loss and vision problems, Juan decided to visit the local medical office. He has heard the office provides services to those who cannot pay.

When Juan arrives at the office, his clothing is worn and torn. The new medical assistant tells Juan that he cannot be seen at the office unless he can pay for his visit before he is seen. She does not explain her statement, and because of his broken English, Juan does not ask further questions. He thinks that the physician will not see him and leaves the office very upset. He decides to start taking herbal medications and try home remedies. He now believes that seeing a physician in America just is not worth the trouble and embarrassment. Several weeks later, Juan is hospitalized with dehydration, starvation, and severe reactions to the herbal drugs.

This situation did not have to result in the hospitalization of Juan. If you were the new medical assistant, what would you have done differently?

DEVELOPMENT

Growth and change occur throughout our entire lives. Our bodies and body systems change and so does the way we think, behave, and react. We have different needs at each stage in our lives. To provide effective care for patients from all age groups, medical assistants must understand the basic changes that people go through during their lifetime. Understanding these changes allows medical assistants to meet the needs of all patients in the health care setting.

There are basically three areas or categories of change during growth and **development** that occur in the human life span, as follows:

1. **Physical growth** (physical size, motor and sensory skills)
2. **Mental growth** (cognitive development, thinking, and understanding)
3. **Psychosocial growth** (emotional and social development)

As people approach each life stage, both **heredity** (genetics) and the environment influence their development. Basic principles of growth and development include the following:

- Each person is unique from the time of conception. Standards of development are only guidelines.
- Growth is continuous; it does not occur at the same rate for everyone.
- As physical size increases, skills will increase proportionately.
- Development depends on the balance among physical, mental, and psychosocial changes.
- If basic needs are not met, an individual's growth pattern is usually altered.

The human life span can be divided into the following three major phases:

1. Infancy: infants from birth to 1 year.
2. Childhood: toddlers, preschoolers, school-age children, and adolescents.
3. Adulthood: adults in the early, middle, late, and later stages of life.

As a medical assistant, you need to understand the physical, mental, and psychosocial changes that occur in each phase so that you can interact positively with patients and their families while attending to patients' age-related needs.

Infancy (Birth to 1 Year)

Development through the **infancy** stage relies on some family structure. The family's main role is to foster security, allowing for growth and development of the personality, body, and intellect of the infant. Physical growth occurs in spurts. Research proves that normal development requires a continuous close relationship with nurturing individuals (mother, father, grandparents, guardian, caregiver).

Birth to 3 Months

PHYSICAL (SENSORY AND MOTOR)
Front fontanels (soft spot) will close
Fist to mouth
Opens and closes hand
Raises head and chest (Figure 6-1)

MENTAL (COGNITIVE)
Reacts to sound, motion, and light
Reacts to caregiver's voice
Hands and eyes coordinate
Imitates some sounds

PSYCHOSOCIAL (EMOTIONAL AND SOCIAL)
Coos when happy
Smiles at 6 weeks
Cries when tired and uncomfortable

    Medical assistants should:
- Make eye contact when speaking.
- Involve parents or guardians; when demonstrating procedures for home care, have them practice.
- Encourage repeating of cooing and happy sounds made by the infant.
- Share developmental status with caregivers and encourage bright-colored toys.
- Focus on parents' concerns.

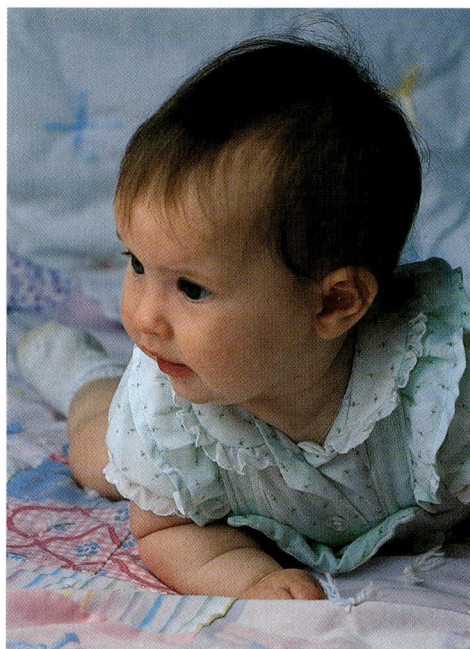

FIGURE 6-1 A 3-month-old child is able to raise the head and chest. (From Sorrentino SA: *Mosby's assisting with patient care*, ed 2, St Louis, 2004, Mosby.)

4 to 7 Months—cont'd

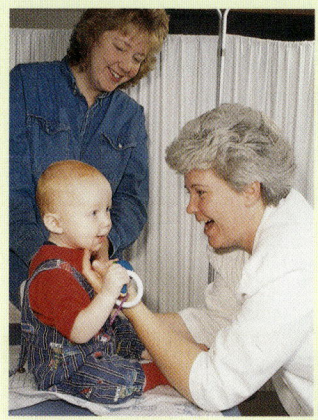

The infant responds to touch and smiling. Parental involvement increases cooperativeness.

(From Chester GA: *Modern medical assisting*, Philadelphia, 1998, Saunders.)

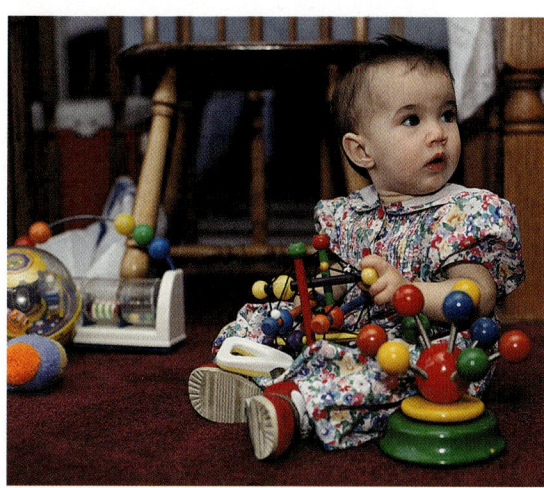

FIGURE 6-2 A 6-month-old child is able to sit and grasp objects. (From Sorrentino SA: *Mosby's assisting with patient care*, St Louis, 1999, Mosby.)

4 to 7 Months

PHYSICAL
Nose-breathes
Respirations of 60 breaths per minute
Teeth erupt
Eye coordination good
Relies on vision to explore environment
Permanent eye color
Doubles birth weight
Rolls over and sits up
Grasps objects (Figure 6-2)

MENTAL
Explores by banging, dropping, and throwing
Reaches

PSYCHOSOCIAL
Imitates inflections of voices
Shows anger or tantrums
Self-entertaining (plays with hands and feet)
  Medical assistants should:
- Make eye contact when speaking.
- Involve parents or guardians; when demonstrating procedures for home care, have them practice.
- Encourage grasping toys and toys with sound.
- Follow-up on prior health concerns.
- Share developmental status with caregivers.
- Review immunization records with caregivers.
- Focus on eating and sleeping habits.

8 to 12 Months

PHYSICAL
Crawls
Stands upright
Increased interest in exploration
Able to grasp with thumb and forefinger

MENTAL
Shakes head "no"
Waves "bye-bye"
Begins to equate sound with action (running water to bathe)

PSYCHOSOCIAL
Smiles at self in mirror (Figure 6-3)
Does not like confinement
Buries head in caregiver's shoulder (acts shy)

Continued

8 to 12 Months—cont'd

Medical assistants should:
- Make eye contact when speaking.
- Involve parents or guardians; when demonstrating procedures for home care, have them practice.
- Encourage playing with large blocks for stacking.
- Be aware of family stresses that could interfere with the child's health.

13 to 18 Months

PHYSICAL

Coordination improves Stacks objects
Feeds self (Figure 6-4) Points with index finger
Walks without support

MENTAL

Knows names and can point to body parts
Recognizes picture book upside down

PSYCHOSOCIAL

Has not grasped warnings but Has separation anxiety
  knows praise Self-loving
Tantrums more frequent

Medical assistants should:
- Make eye contact when speaking.
- Involve parents or guardians; when demonstrating procedures for home care, have them practice.
- Review immunization records with current recommended schedule.
- Review developmental status with caregivers and provide information on expectations.
- Encourage space for movement.
- Observe behavior and interaction with peers.
- Encourage identifying body parts (e.g., "Where's your nose?").

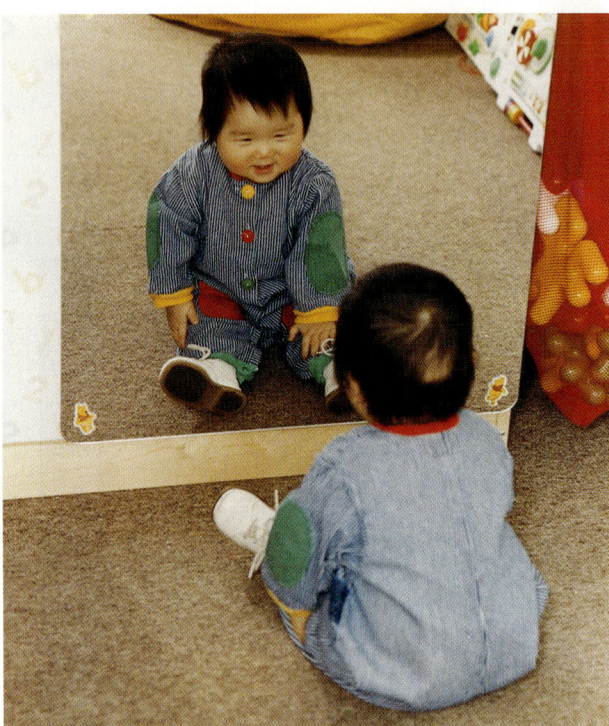

FIGURE 6-3 A 9-month-old child can enjoy his image in a mirror. (From Hockenberry MJ et al: *Wong's nursing care of infants and children*, ed 8, St Louis, 2007, Mosby.)

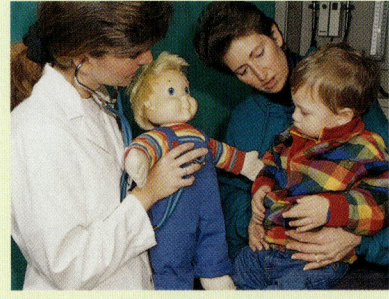

Establishing trust is important in gaining a toddler's cooperation.

(From Chester GA: *Modern medical assisting*, Philadelphia, 1998, Saunders.)

Childhood

Many changes occur during **childhood.** As a toddler becomes a preschooler, expectations about physical, mental, and psychosocial characteristics and abilities are raised. As a child becomes an adolescent, important body changes occur, and psychosocial issues are important.

Toddler (13 Months to 3 Years)

The **toddler** grows slowly, gaining only 5 to 10 pounds and growing 3 inches typically each year. Overall development speeds along as toddlers learn to walk, speak their first words, and refine their dexterity skills. They develop a unique personality, and if the environment is positive, they will explore and learn.

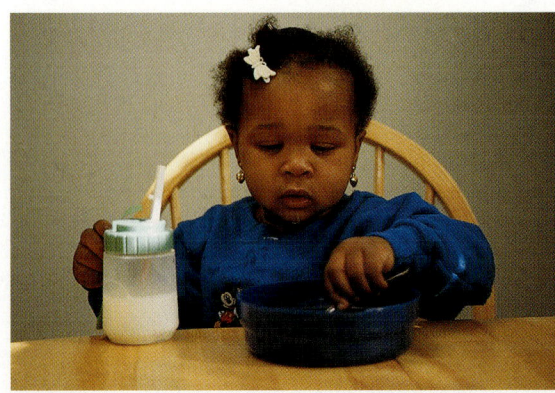

FIGURE 6-4 A toddler is able to use a spoon as coordination improves. (From Sorrentino SA: *Mosby's assisting with patient care,* ed 2, St Louis, 2004, Mosby.)

19 to 23 Months

PHYSICAL
Runs and climbs
Can kick a ball
Bladder and bowel control
Drinks from a cup (Figure 6-5)
Draws circles

MENTAL
"So big" and "all gone"
Voices frustration

PSYCHOSOCIAL
Sharing is not a concept; "mine"
Feelings are apparent
Gives hugs and kisses

   Medical assistants should:
- Make eye contact when speaking.
- Involve parents and guardians; when demonstrating procedures for home care, have them practice.
- Review schedule of immunization.
- Review developmental status with caregivers and provide information on expectations.
- Encourage action toys (e.g., pushcart, telephone).
- Focus on eating, sleeping, and elimination.
- Provide large crayons for drawing.

24 to 36 Months

PHYSICAL
Can hop
Toilet training concluded

MENTAL
Sentences and vocabulary improve
Grasps categories of animals such as cats and dogs

PSYCHOSOCIAL
Likes to help
Can play alone (Figure 6-6)
Says "no" more often

   Medical assistants should:
- Make eye contact when speaking.
- Develop rapport by explaining procedures to the child first and using words the child understands.
- Demonstrate procedures on a toy and let the child do the procedure on the toy.
- Praise expected behavior.
- Provide parents with information on accident prevention and respiratory infections because these are the main health problems of toddlers.
- Provide books or toys, blow bubbles, or pretend-play to build rapport or distract when necessary.
- Involve parents and guardians; when demonstrating procedures for home care, have them practice.

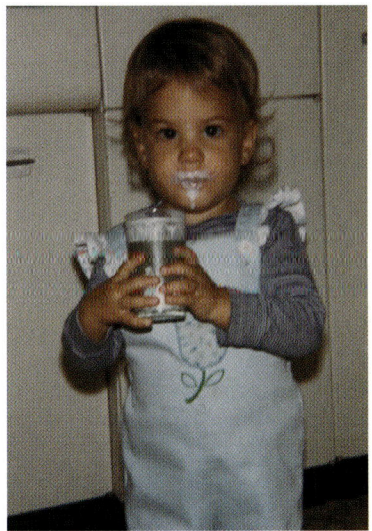

FIGURE 6-5 A toddler is able to drink from a cup. (From Mahan LK, Escott-Stump S: *Krause's food, nutrition, and diet therapy*, ed 12, St Louis, 2008, Saunders.)

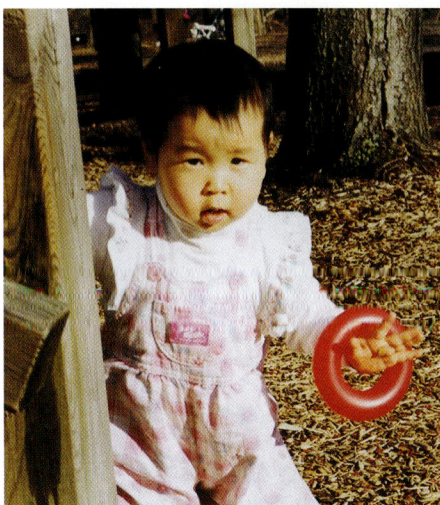

FIGURE 6-6 A toddler can self-entertain. (From Hockenberry MJ et al: *Wong's nursing care of infants and children*, ed 7, St Louis, 2005, Mosby.)

Preschool (3 to 5 Years)

By the time they reach the early **preschool** stage, children have developed attitudes, beliefs, and expectations about life. Unfavorable experiences during this phase can lead to mistrust and may hamper attempts at trying new things. Reassuring children during this phase is important.

36 to 48 Months

PHYSICAL

Can dress and undress self
Pedals and steers a tricycle
Can hold a pencil, draw, and color (Figure 6-7)
Assembles simple puzzles
Can use small scissors and small musical instruments

MENTAL

Knows the difference between same and different
Can hear and tell a story
Wants to know "why"
Can organize experiences into concepts

PSYCHOSOCIAL

Increased social awareness
Sensitive to feelings
Needs rules
Separation anxiety
Makes decisions between two possibilities

Medical assistants should:

- Make eye contact when speaking.
- Keep the caregiver in sight.
- Build rapport by letting the child help (e.g., undressing).
- Use toys, hand puppets, or nurse or doctor kits to build rapport and distract when necessary.
- Involve parents and guardians; when demonstrating procedures for home care, have them practice.

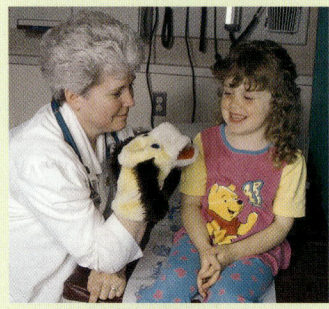

Hands-on play or puppet play helps alleviate the preschooler's fears.

(From Chester GA: *Modern medical assisting,* Philadelphia, 1998, Saunders.)

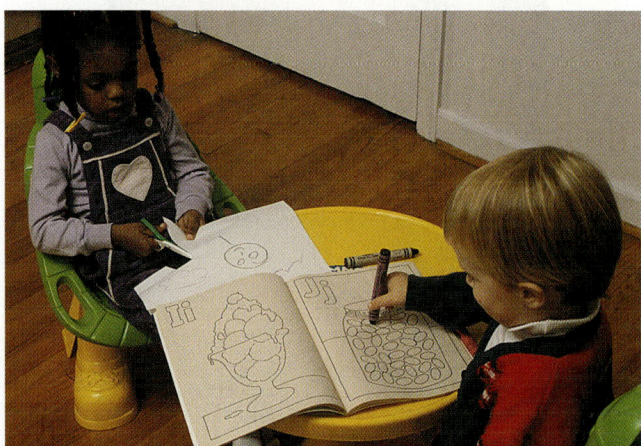

FIGURE 6-7 Three-year-old children enjoy drawing, coloring, and cut-and-paste activities. (From Sorrentino SA: *Mosby's assisting with patient care,* St Louis, 1999, Mosby.)

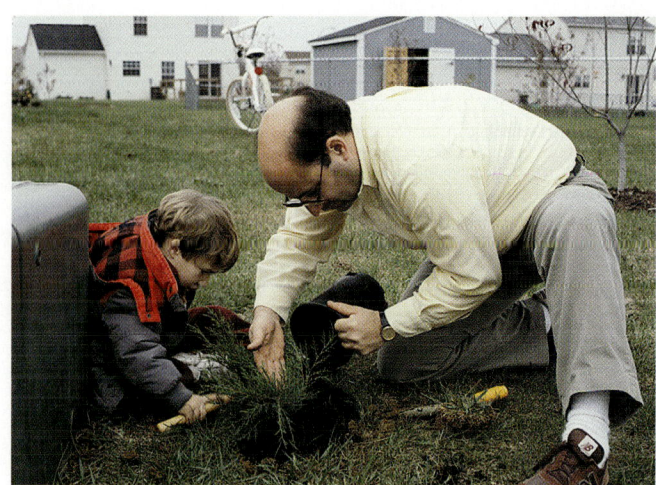

FIGURE 6-8 Five-year-old children enjoy helping a parent. (From Sorrentino SA: *Mosby's assisting with patient care,* St Louis, 1999, Mosby.)

4 to 5 Years

PHYSICAL

Grows 2 to $2\frac{1}{2}$ inches each year
Jumps rope
Can learn to print first name
Has excessive energy

MENTAL

Can count
Can learn address and telephone number
Has a short attention span
Develops self-concept and body image

PSYCHOSOCIAL

Is assertive and independent
Relates to important people, caregivers, and siblings (Figure 6-8)
Can follow rules, but will stretch them
Behavior modified by reward and punishment
Can learn manners
Makes more complex decisions among three possibilities

Medical assistants should:

- Make eye contact when speaking.
- Provide rewards for good behavior (e.g., sticker).
- Involve the child; demonstrate the procedure and let the child be involved in treatments (e.g., nebulizer).
- Let the child express feelings.
- Provide creative activities and puzzles.
- Involve parents and guardians; when demonstrating procedures for home care, have them practice.

School Age (6 to 11 Years)

If a child has progressed through other experiences with little difficulty, the **school-age** years will be a time for physical and emotional growth.

6 to 11 Years

PHYSICAL
Loses baby teeth
Growth is slow and steady
Can assume responsibility (e.g., pet care)
Likes organized sports

MENTAL
Can use logic
Will listen to other opinions
Learns to compromise
Acquires knowledge and new skills quickly

PSYCHOSOCIAL
Peers gain importance (Figure 6-9)
Family group not first
Will seek praise (Figure 6-10)
Written rules acceptable

Medical assistants should:
- Make eye contact when speaking.
- Explain procedures in correct but age-appropriate terminology.
- Respect privacy; knock before entering.
- Allow independence to make health choices.
- Tell jokes or riddles; ask if the child has any to tell.
- Praise good behavior.
- Involve parents and guardians; when demonstrating procedures for home care, have them practice.

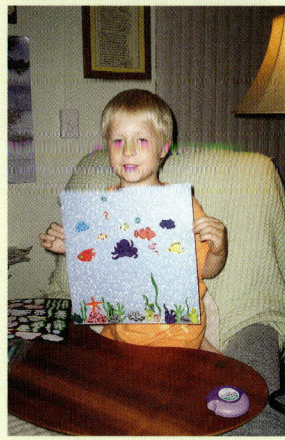

The child in early elementary school responds well to praise and recognition.

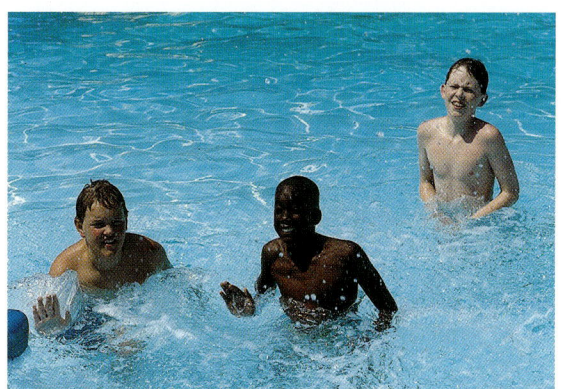

FIGURE 6-9 Belonging to a peer group is important to 6-year-old children. (From Sorrentino SA: *Mosby's assisting with patient care,* ed 2, St Louis, 2004, Mosby.)

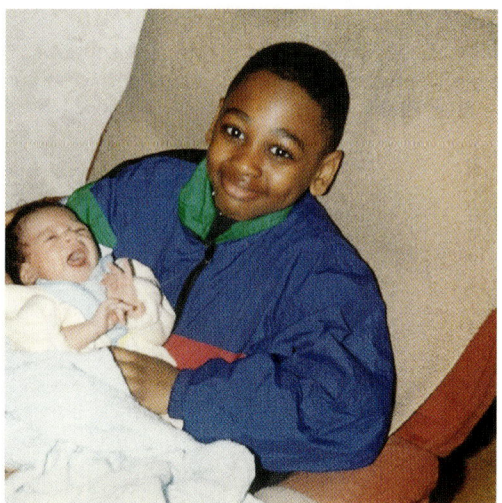

FIGURE 6-10 Being recognized as the big brother is gratifying for the school-age child. (From Jarvis C: *Physical examination and health assessment,* ed 4, Philadelphia, 2004, Saunders.)

Adolescent (12 to 18 Years)

Adolescence is the developmental stage between childhood and early adulthood. It can be the most confusing time for the adolescent and the caregiver. Peer pressure becomes an issue, and the adolescent is concerned with conforming to peers in dress, language, and goals. The caregiver does remain influential over values and long-term goals.

12 to 18 Years

PHYSICAL
Rapid growth
Some awkward movements
Increased hormones
Increased appetite
Easily fatigued
Fine motor skills improve

MENTAL
Abstract and logical thinking
Cause and effect
Self-esteem development (Figure 6-11)
Identity issues
Sets goals

12 to 18 Years—cont'd

PSYCHOSOCIAL

Confusion over growth changes
Appearance important
Self-esteem issues arise
Wants to be independent but wants some dependence
Develops relationship with the opposite gender
Peers are primary influence (Figure 6-12)

Medical assistants should:

- Make eye contact when speaking.
- Be aware that illness is a threat to self-esteem and body image.
- Allow adolescents to ask questions, and respect their opinions.
- Avoid judgments concerning appearance.
- Recognize that illness causes anxiety because the fear of always being dependent is strong.
- Let adolescents help plan care.
- Respect privacy issues.
- Be aware of possible body image problems.
- Ask about hobbies or organized physical sports.
- If appropriate, demonstrate procedures for home care and have them practice.

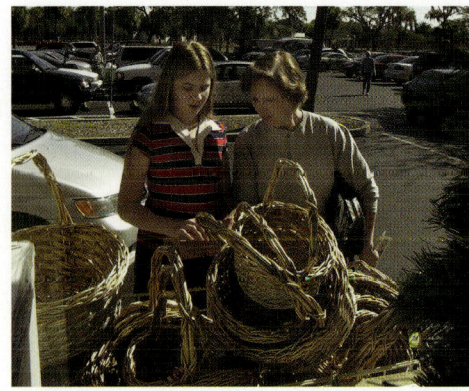

FIGURE 6-11 Every adolescent needs to be able to discuss their feelings with someone who encourages this expression of feelings and opinions.

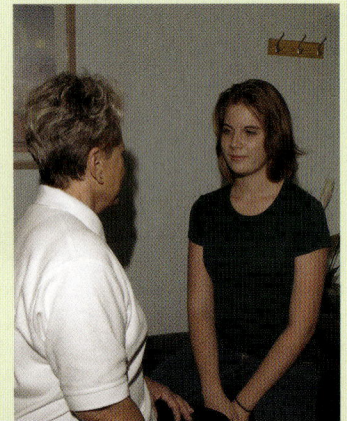

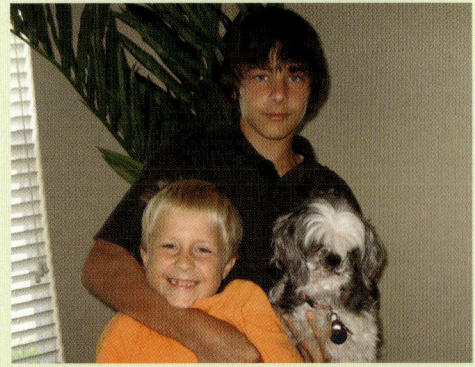

The adolescent must be treated with respect and given autonomy.

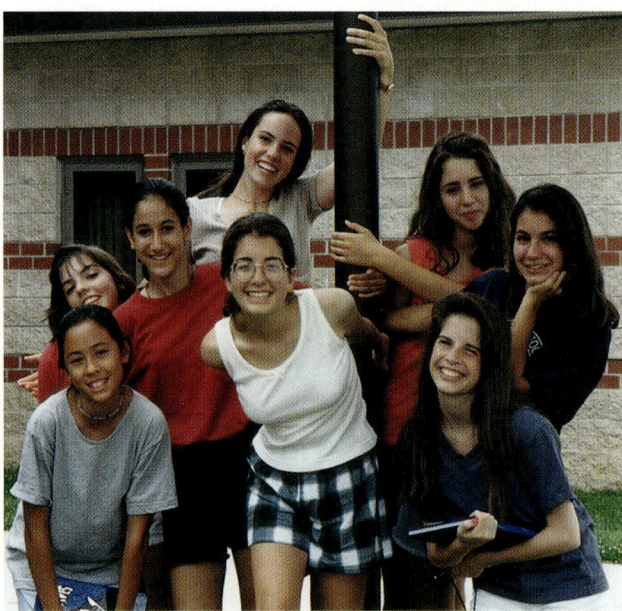

FIGURE 6-12 Peers are the primary influence for the adolescent. (From Jarvis C: *Physical examination and health assessment,* ed 4, Philadelphia, 2004, Saunders.)

Adulthood

Progression into **adulthood** is often defined by changing social roles and family expectations. This phase begins in the late teens (about age 19) and continues until the individual dies. As the body ages, changes occur in each body system.

Early Adulthood (19 to 45 Years)

PHYSICAL
Growth until age 30
Muscle efficiency peaks in late 20s
Skin tone less, with decreased moisture
Some vision changes
Decreased hearing in high tones

MENTAL
Learning easier in early years
Takes longer to focus on new things

PSYCHOSOCIAL
Ages 20 to 30: evaluates future
Looks for place in society
Ages 30 to 45: reevaluates work, family, and social issues
Plans for economic security
Sense of responsibility (Figure 6-13)
Some health care concerns

Medical assistants should:
- Make eye contact when speaking.
- Provide education for lifestyle changes.
- Explain options and offer choices.
- Understand that illness at this time may cause self-image and self-esteem issues.
- Recognize that medical treatment may be seen as a threat.
- Be aware that illness during this stage can bring on anxiety responses or depression; the patient may revert to the defense mechanism of denial, which can prevent timely recovery and treatment.
- Provide education for home health care if necessary (e.g., insulin testing).

Middle Age (45 to 59 Years)

PHYSICAL
Bone mass decreases
Muscle mass declines
Wrinkles appear
Hair decreases
Slower reflexes
Glasses may be required for reading

MENTAL
Short-term memory decreases
Looks back over life experiences
Stress response prolonged

PSYCHOSOCIAL
Begins to settle in on future goals
Concerns about health
May have to care for parents and family
May experience "empty nest" syndrome
Pursues hobbies and areas of interest (Figure 6-14)
Measures accomplishments against goals

Medical assistants should:
- Make eye contact when speaking.
- Give patients options and alternatives.
- Provide literature on optimal health.
- Provide education for home health care if necessary.

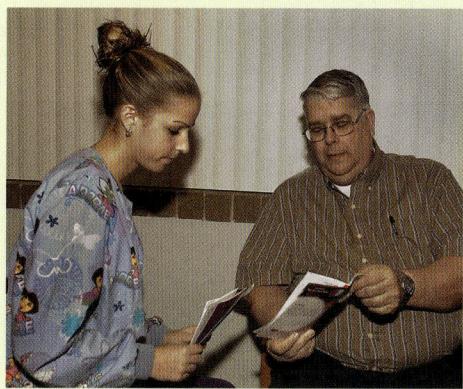

The medical assistant should use brochures to help teach patients.

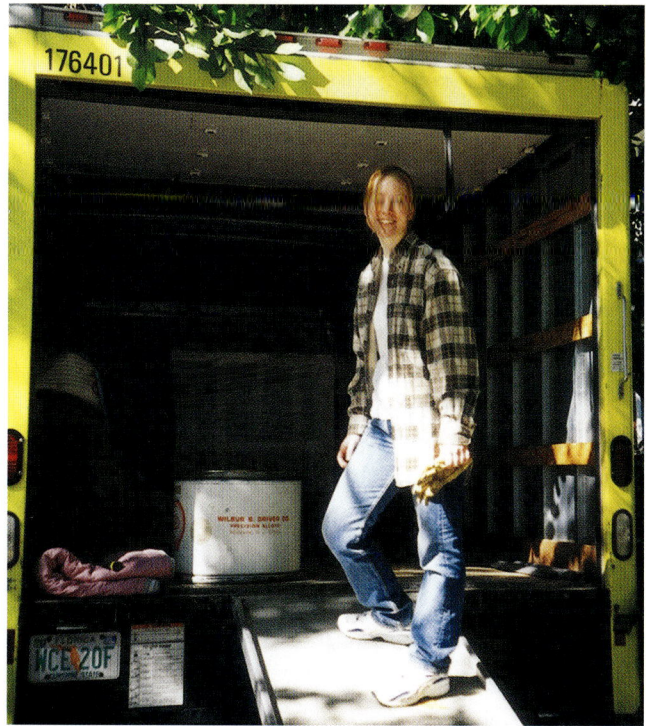

FIGURE 6-13 Young adults begin to develop a strong sense of responsibility. (From Jarvis C: *Physical examination and health assessment,* ed 4, Philadelphia, 2004, Saunders.)

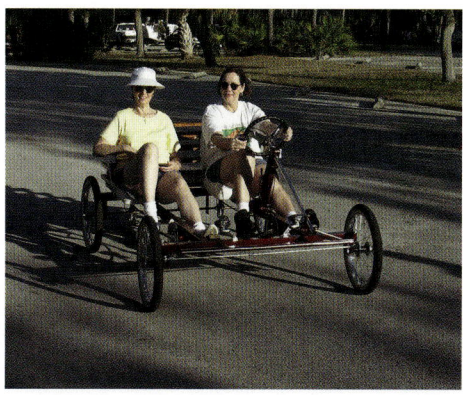

FIGURE 6-14 Middle-age adults often have more time for activities they enjoy.

Mature Adult (60 to 69 Years)

PHYSICAL
Heat and cold tolerance decreases
Circulation to extremities decreases
Skin thins and loses elasticity
Hair thins
Loss of height
Hearing loss continues
Sense of smell and taste decreases
Less saliva
Dexterity decreases

MENTAL
Life-sharing memories

PSYCHOSOCIAL
Ages 60 to 70: comfort and acceptance (Figure 6-15)
Mellowing
Privacy important
Friends important
Values high for truth and sincerity
Examines feelings of self-worth
Retirement
Changes in relationships because of death, illness, and birth of grandchildren
Comes to terms with own death

Medical assistants should:
- Make eye contact when speaking.
- Know the patient's support system.
- Know how the patient receives nutrition.
- Provide education for home health care if necessary.

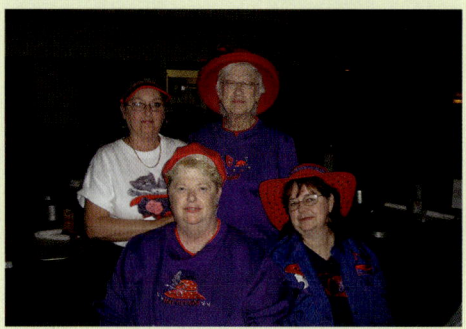
Friendship is important to mature adults.

Later Maturity (70+ Years)

PHYSICAL
Gastrointestinal system slows down
Less absorption of nutrients
Drugs processed more slowly
Fat lost, so bones protrude
Bones more porous
Skin pigment changes (Figure 6-16)
Skin sensitive and tears easily
Cardiac output slows
Hardening of blood vessels
Urinary system problems (loss of bladder muscle tone)
Balance is decreased
Sleeps less

MENTAL
Learning is possible, but slower
Short-term memory declines further

PSYCHOSOCIAL
Relationships decrease because of death
Reflective
Living arrangements may need to be adjusted (Figure 6-17)

Medical assistants should:
- Make eye contact when speaking.
- Understand how the effects of aging decrease resilience and alter lifestyle.
- Continue to assess the support system.
- Be aware that nutrition and fluid intake needs increase.
- Repeat directions as needed; mature adults may be slower to interpret sensory input.
- Provide education for home health care if necessary.

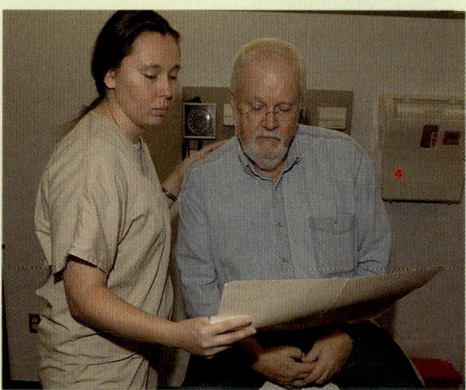
Medical assistants can help mature patients and their families accept and adjust to age-related changes.

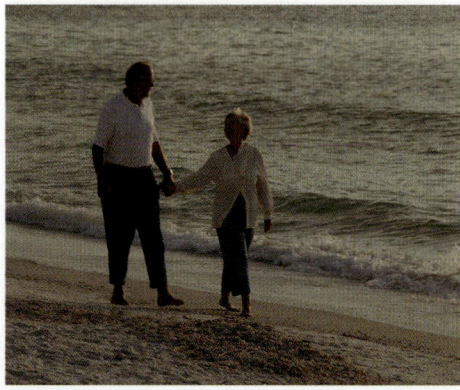

FIGURE 6-15 Love and companionship are important to the mature adult.

CULTURAL DIVERSITY

We live in a culturally diverse society. **Cultural diversity** means there is a rich mix of ethnicity, race, and religion. Within each ethnic, race, or religious group, there are a variety of individual characteristics such as gender, ability, socioeconomic status, family structure, and languages. Because our society is culturally diverse, our medical settings are also culturally diverse. As a medical assistant, you will interact with health professionals and patients of many different cultures, beliefs, and individual characteristics. You must be aware of the cultural differences of your patients. If you are not knowledgeable about different cultures, you may have unrealistic expectations about patient behavior. This will prevent effective communication between you and culturally diverse patients.

Patient behavior can vary, depending on religious, racial, ethical, economic, and social upbringing. Different cultures have different beliefs about what is acceptable and "correct" behavior in various situations. A behavior that is acceptable to someone in one culture in a certain situation may be totally unacceptable or even offensive to someone from a different culture because of differing beliefs (Box 6-1). For instance, in some cultures males are raised to be achievers while the females are expected to conform. Although this attitude is not part of most Western culture, it still is a part of other cultures and must be respected.

To understand how cultural diversity impacts medical assistants, you need to understand the importance of accepting diversity and must be knowledgeable about the cultural differences of patients.

Embracing Diversity

Medical assistants interact with people of different backgrounds daily. It is important to embrace each difference with an open mind. Do not make negative judgments concerning

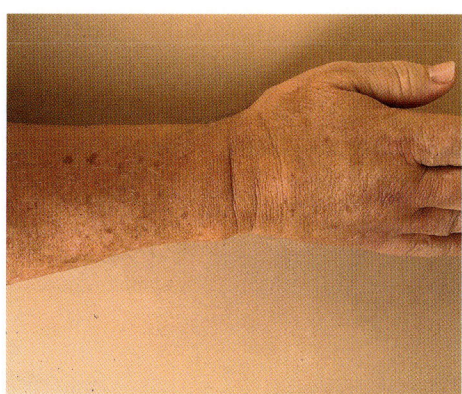

FIGURE 6-16 Skin pigment changes occur in later maturity.

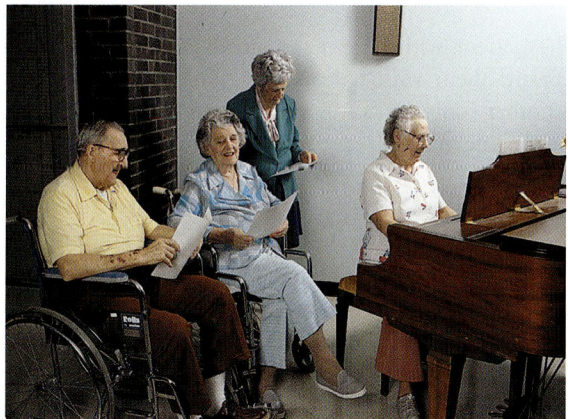

FIGURE 6-17 As a person reaches later maturity, living arrangements may need to be altered. (From Sorrentino SA: *Mosby's assisting with patient care,* St Louis, 1999, Mosby.)

PATIENT-CENTERED PROFESSIONALISM

- *An infant's physical growth occurs in spurts. Why is it important for medical assistants to know what to expect concerning an infant's cognitive and social growth at 2-month through 12-month visits? How do the infant and the family benefit from a medical assistant who understands infant physical growth?*
- *As a child progresses from a toddler to an adolescent, many psychosocial changes occur that have an impact on self-esteem. How can medical assistants use their knowledge of expected changes during this time to provide better care to an adolescent patient?*
- *As a young adult moves through the life span, what changes in physical aspects and mental focus are expected? Does a feeling of self-worth have any impact on how a person approaches these life span changes? How can medical assistants use their understanding of these changes to provide better care to adult patients?*

BOX 6-1

Different Cultures, Different Beliefs

- In the United States, the color black is a sign of mourning; to certain Asian cultures, the color white means mourning.
- Iranians (and other groups) may believe that all things are predetermined.
- Some cultures believe good health is a reward from a higher power, whereas other cultures may not believe in a higher power at all.
- Some cultures believe demons and evil spirits are the cause of illness, whereas other cultures believe illness is caused only by disease or injury.
- Many Americans believe in outward demonstrations of affection and engage in more casual touching than other cultures (e.g., slaps on the back, kissing pecks on the cheek, or handshakes). Other cultures may be more reserved about their "persona."

behavior because it differs from your own; the behavior may be the result of beliefs from a culture that has been passed down from one generation to the next.

All medical assistants have a responsibility to their profession and to patients to accept and respect the cultural beliefs of others even if they differ from their own. The goal is to be knowledgeable and sensitive to cultural attitudes and behaviors. This enables effective communication and mutual respect between the patient (and family) and the health professionals and will help establish a good relationship. To prepare yourself to work with people of many cultures and beliefs, you should research the cultural background and beliefs of the people in your community. If a classmate's ethnic background is different from your own, learn about the classmate's culture. Begin by explaining what you know or think you know about your classmate's belief system, and then ask questions about what you do not know. Gather fact-based information from reading material and compare it to your perception of the culture. In turn, you may be able to share your cultural beliefs with the classmate. Table 6-1 shows some of the health and illness beliefs of different cultures.

Understanding Cultural Differences

Knowledge of patients' cultural backgrounds and ethnic beliefs is necessary to understand their behavior. Both knowledge and understanding are valuable when assessing patients and providing care because both can help prevent misunderstandings. For example, if a culture stresses independence, illness may be considered unacceptable because it makes a person dependent on others. A patient with these beliefs may be resistant or uncooperative and may not want to be seen as being ill. Understanding this belief helps you work through the patient's resistance and provide the appropriate care.

Planning culturally appropriate and acceptable care requires medical assistants to understand the possible impact of a patient's cultural beliefs. Once a patient's beliefs are understood, health professionals can begin to integrate the cultural influences into the patient's care. Common areas in which cultural differences exist include the following:

- *Eye contact.* In some Asian cultures, direct eye contact is considered to be disrespectful and even hostile. In Western culture, however, people who do not maintain eye contact may be considered rude, defiant, or inattentive.
- *Herbal medicine.* Many Americans, including Native Americans, as well as Asian immigrants and Caribbean Islanders, believe that herbs are an important part of healing (Figure 6-18). They may be open to the idea of Western medicine if the value of their alternative form is also recognized and taken into account when prescribing medications.
- *Gestures.* Gestures can cause more misunderstandings than any other form of communication. An Asian immigrant may believe pointing a finger at someone is insulting. In some Asian (and other) countries, the pointing gesture is used to call animals. How would you feel if someone pointed at you and said, "Here, boy" or "Here, girl" as if you were a dog? It is more appropriate to gesture toward

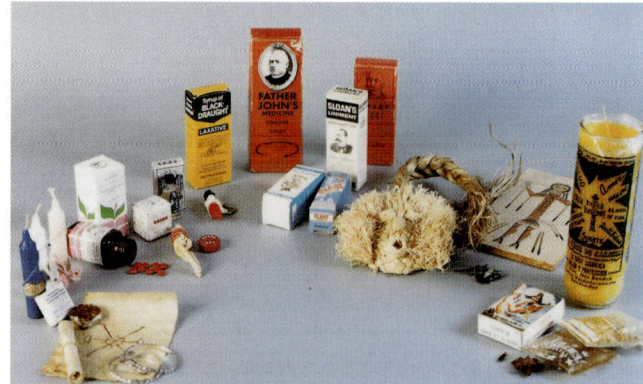

FIGURE 6-18 A variety of remedies are used by many cultural groups in the United States. (Photo by Lucy Rozier, Boston College Audio Visual Services, Boston College, Chestnut Hill, Mass. From Potter PA, Perry AG: *Fundamentals of nursing,* ed 4, St Louis, 1997, Mosby.)

the patient with your palm down, sweeping your hand toward them with the back of your hand facing down. Another common gesture in Western culture is the "okay" sign made by touching the forefinger and thumb together. In some cultures, this is seen as an obscene gesture. Shaking your head from side to side means "no" in Western culture, but to a Bulgarian or someone from Taiwan, this gesture means "yes." A simple smile seems to be universally accepted and works well when all else fails.
- *Time.* Some Latin cultures are not sensitive to time. A 1 o'clock appointment may mean "sometime around one" to them. In Western culture, being late is sometimes considered disrespectful. Be aware that the expression of time means different things to people of different cultures, and do not automatically assume the patient does not respect the medical office's time.
- *Foods.* Many Asians believe certain foods can heal or bring the body into balance, especially when an illness occurs. They believe alternating the use of hot and cold foods will achieve balance in their lives. Some cultures use hot foods for relieving a cold and use cold foods for relieving a fever.
- *Reactions.* Crying or showing any type of emotion in some cultures is seen as feminine or as a sign of weakness. Other cultures believe that saying "no" is being disrespectful; therefore a patient may say "yes" and really mean "no." Only the head of the family may make decisions and speak for the patient in some cultures. Some immigrants may not want the details of their illness to be included in the treatment plan.
- *Clothing.* Some cultures will not allow females to disrobe in the medical office unless another female member of the family is present. Religious beliefs may forbid the removal of certain garments, and the physician and medical assistant need to be sensitive to this and work around the situation.
- *Physical space.* Some cultures want to be very close during a conversation, whereas others require more personal space.

TABLE 6-1

Cross-Cultural Examples of Cultural Phenomena Affecting Health Care

Nations of Origin	Communication	Space	Time Orientation	Social Organization	Environmental Control	Biological Variations
ASIAN China Hawaii Philippines Korea Japan Southeast Asia (Laos, Cambodia, Vietnam)	National language preference Dialects, written characters Use of silence Nonverbal and contextual cuing	Noncontact people	Present	Family; hierarchical structure Devotion to tradition Many religions, including Taoism, Buddhism, Islam, Christianity	Traditional health and illness beliefs Use of traditional medicines Traditional practitioners, Chinese doctors, and herbalists	Liver cancer Stomach cancer Coccidioidomycosis Hypertension Lactose intolerance
AFRICAN West Coast (as slaves) Many African countries West Indian Islands Dominican Republic Haiti Jamaica	National languages Dialect, pidgin, Creole, Spanish, French	Close personal space	Present over future	Family, many female single parents Large, extended family networks Strong church affiliation within community Community social organization	Traditional health and illness beliefs Folk medicine tradition Traditional healer: rootworker	Sickle cell anemia Hypertension Cancer of the esophagus Stomach cancer Coccidioidomycosis Lactose intolerance
EUROPEAN Germany England Italy Ireland Spain Other European countries	National languages Many learn English immediately	Noncontact people Aloof Distant Southern countries: closer contact and touch	Future over present	Nuclear families Extended families Judeo-Christian religions Community social organizations	Primary reliance on modern health care system Traditional health and illness beliefs Some remaining folk traditions	Breast cancer Heart disease Diabetes mellitus Thalassemia
NATIVE AMERICAN 500 Native American tribes Aleuts Eskimos	Tribal languages Use of silence and body language	Space very important and has no boundaries	Present	Extremely family oriented Biological and extended families Children taught to respect traditions Community social organizations	Traditional health and illness beliefs Folk medicine tradition Traditional healer: medicine man	Accidents Heart disease Cirrhosis of the liver Diabetes mellitus
HISPANIC COUNTRIES Cuba Mexico Central and South America	Spanish or Portuguese primary language	Tactile relationships Touch Handshakes Embracing Value physical presence	Present	Nuclear family Extended families *Compadrazgo:* godparents Community social organization	Traditional health and illness beliefs Folk medicine tradition Traditional healers: *curandero, espiritista, partera, señora*	

Modified from Potter PA, Perry AG: *Basic nursing,* ed 5, St Louis, Mosby, 2003.
Compiled by Rachel Spector, RN, PhD.

Chinese people may not want to be touched by people they do not know. Some cultures will not let a female caregiver touch a male patient. Touching the head of a child is offensive to some cultures because the head is seen as sacred and can only be touched by a parent or the elder of the family.

Understanding cultural differences is important if there is to be a complete trust in the health care team. The patient interprets the workings of the medical office, the staff, and treatments from their own cultural perspective. Not everyone sees things the way you do. It will take patience and understanding to adjust to other ways of thinking, but it is worth the effort.

Although it is impossible to be familiar with all the beliefs and practices of every culture, it is necessary to understand the role that culture plays in patient behavior. Patient apathy, passiveness, or detachment concerning illness may be cultural; patients may place all their faith in the health care team and their spiritual being. Do not dismiss patients' cultural beliefs. Instead, recognize their beliefs while encouraging compliance with the treatment recommended by the physician.

PATIENT-CENTERED PROFESSIONALISM

- *Although there are many commonalities among cultures, why is it important to understand each culture's values and its beliefs about health care? How does this understanding impact a medical assistant's relationship with patients and their families?*
- *How can a person's cultural value system as it relates to lifesaving measures (e.g., transplants, feeding tubes) affect the person's treatment? What is the patient-centered, professional way for a medical assistant to work with a patient (or family) who disagrees with a prescribed medical treatment because of cultural values or beliefs?*

RESPONSE TO ILLNESS

Health care team members have expectations about how patients behave. These expectations are based on prior experience, assumptions, knowledge, and even their current moods. As you learned, a patient's behavior can be understood to some degree by taking the patient's developmental stage and cultural differences into consideration. Besides developmental stages and cultural differences, another factor that influences a patient's behavior is the patient's *response* to being ill. Some patients may exhibit behavior that is challenging or difficult to handle when they are ill. This is understandable considering people are not at their best when feeling unwell. Coping mechanisms and emotional responses can cause patients to react in a way they normally would not.

Each patient must be evaluated on his or her own merits and accepted as an individual. Illnesses and disabilities have various psychological effects on individuals. A patient who is terminally ill, for example, may react with calmness and demonstrate a strong will to get better, whereas a person with a minor illness may react as though he or she is dying. Anxiety can result if a patient sees illness as a threat to self-image. The anxiety causes the patient to react. The type of reaction depends on the person's ability to cope and the defense mechanism used. Remember that defense mechanisms allow the patient to feel in control. The health care team must assess whether the defenses used are helpful or dangerous to the eventual recovery of the patient. Reactions vary from patient to patient. However, four common patient reactions to illness are fear, talkativeness, withdrawal, and anger.

Fear

The unknown can cause fear in the patient and regression in the patient's behavior. Fear of pain and death are two very strong emotions for most people. Fear may cause one person to seek medical attention, whereas another person may avoid seeking the necessary medical help or may not follow the prescribed treatment (Figure 6-19). Fear is a natural reaction when a person is faced with a threatening situation. However, anxiety can be produced when patients worry about the "what if." This form of self-talk is pointless and destructive. To help the patient minimize the worry, you must involve the patient

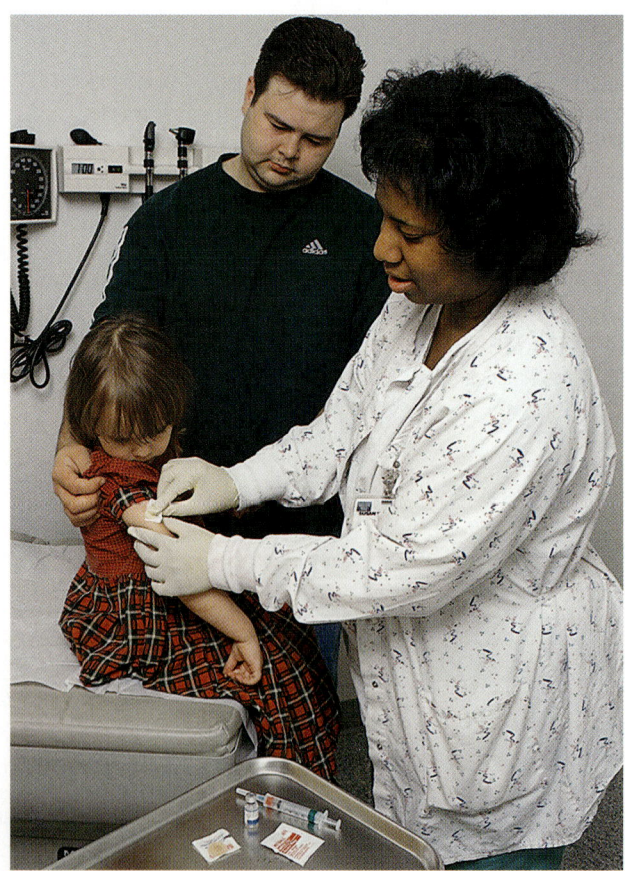

FIGURE 6-19 Fear and anxiety are strong emotions that need to be acknowledged to achieve patient cooperation, especially in children. (From deWit SC: *Fundamental concepts and skills for nursing*, ed 2, St. Louis, 2005, Saunders.)

in the treatment plan and be a good listener. Treat patients' fears with kindness and reassurance. Answer their questions honestly to provide them with information. Turning the "unknown" into the "known" by providing more information will help reduce their fears. Once fearful patients see that treatment can help them feel better, their fears are likely to decrease. For example:

> *White coat syndrome* is a situation in which a patient has an elevated blood pressure in the physician's office but not when taking it at home. The anxiety experienced by the patient appears to happen at a subconscious level during the visit. This diagnosis is confirmed after monitoring the patient's blood pressure frequently during a given period of time.

Talkativeness

The talkative patient may just be anxious, nervous, or fearful. Listen to what the patient is saying. In your own words, reflect on the feelings and ideas expressed by the patient. Make your response goal directed (e.g., "What can I do to help?"). Communication is the key with talkative patients. Try to find the core concern that is causing their talkativeness, and address this concern.

Withdrawal

Withdrawn or depressed patients do not put out the energy and involvement required to get better. They may seem very apathetic about their recovery. They lose interest in their surroundings and have a feeling of hopelessness. Their appetite is decreased, and they may have various complaints unrelated to their illness. The longer the depression continues, the less chance there will be for recovery. A withdrawn patient requires great amounts of encouragement to motivate the patient to cooperate with the treatment plan. Do not give advice; this should be done by trained professionals such as physicians, psychologists, and psychiatrists. Instead, use questions such as, "What has happened to upset you?" Focus on where you need the patient to be in the treatment plan. This type of patient will need compassion, empathy, and understanding. Encourage patients to vent without placing undue pressure on them.

Anger

The angry patient must be addressed constructively. To be effective, try to put yourself in the patient's place. You might say, "You sound upset," and "How can I help you?" Watch the patient's body language and expressions, and focus on what the patient is saying instead of worrying about what response to give. Try to find the underlying cause of the patient's anger. Helpful hints to deal with the angry patient are as follows:

1. Let the patient vent. Do not try and defend yourself or the office. Policies can be explained later, when the patient is calm and more apt to listen.
2. Make eye contact with the angry patient. Show interest in what is being said.
3. Be a good listener. Take a posture of attention (face the patient and make eye contact), and ignore putdowns. Do not allow yourself to become angry and lose control of the situation. Take notes on the patient's complaints.
4. Find some truth in the complaint; this often disarms the patient. ("You're right, we did make an error on your bill, here's what I will do to correct it" *or* "You're right, we could have handled it better. Let's start over: What is it that you need?" *or* "What would you like us to do?")
5. Never make judgmental statements. Do not become hostile or defensive. Putting patients on the defensive will cause them to lose focus, and they will shut you out.
6. Clarify what has been said (e.g., "Okay, let me see if I have all the facts").
7. The best response may be silence. With this approach, there is no argument, only the patient venting. Sometimes patients just want to be heard.
8. Avoid distractions so that the patient sees that he or she has your full attention. Take the patient out of the reception area and into a quiet place away from other patients.
9. Do not react to the patient with anger. Remain professional and courteous.

When a patient is fearful, talkative, withdrawn, or angry, always focus on objective facts and solutions. Talk about what really caused the problem and how it can be solved. Working effectively with these behaviors is not a test of power, but an opportunity to find out what a patient really needs. Avoid "why" questions because they tend to increase defensiveness. Success can only be achieved when an atmosphere of trust and cooperation is established. Use "I" statements, such as "I hear what you are saying" or "I understand," and give solutions (e.g., "Let me give you some of your options"). Never give advice; this is not within a medical assistant's scope of practice. Always maintain the integrity of the other person, and never lose your own integrity.

Box 6-2 provides additional tips for dealing with patients who react negatively to illness.

PATIENT-CENTERED PROFESSIONALISM

- *How does understanding the overall development (e.g., physical, mental, and psychosocial) of people help medical assistants respond to a patient diagnosed with a terminal illness?*
- *As a medical assistant, how would you interact with an adult patient diagnosed with cancer? What if this patient is always rude when he comes into the office?*
- *What is the benefit to terminal patients and their families when a medical assistant understands the stages of dying?*

CONCLUSION

As a medical assistant, you have no way of knowing exactly how a patient is feeling as a result of an illness, injury, or medical procedure. You can, however, understand some of the

BOX 6-2
Tips for Interacting with Patients Responding Negatively to Illness

1. Offer encouragement that is consistent with the patient's defenses, self-image, and personality needs.
2. Be aware of other problems that the patient may have such as financial or employment problems and family instability. If a patient cannot work because of an illness, the patient may be concerned about family welfare and paying the bills. This can heighten anxiety and may make the patient unresponsive to health issues.
3. Try to help patients through minor sources of irritation. This might give them the energy to focus on the real problem.

basic characteristics or typical reactions of people in different developmental stages. You can also research the backgrounds and beliefs of people of different cultures in your community so that you will have a better understanding of reactions caused by cultural differences. Finally, you can be empathetic to patients who are experiencing fear, exhibiting talkativeness, showing signs of withdrawal, or displaying anger. A patient-centered health professional is courteous and caring to all patients. It also means being knowledgeable about the different behaviors that patients exhibit and what causes these behaviors. Understanding patient behavior will help you provide effective care to patients of all ages, genders, cultures, personalities, and states of mind.

Chapter Summary

Reinforce your understanding of the material in this chapter by reviewing the curriculum objectives and key content points below.

1. **Define, appropriately use, and spell all the Key Terms for this chapter.**
   - Review the Key Terms if necessary.
2. **List and describe the three areas of change during growth and development in a lifetime.**
   - Physical growth includes an increase in physical size and the development of motor and sensory skills.
   - Mental growth includes cognitive development and increased thinking and understanding.
   - Psychosocial growth includes emotional and social development.
3. **For each age level, list two age-appropriate ways that medical assistants can enhance interaction with patients.**
   - For infants, try to involve parents or guardians in care; follow up on previous health concerns.
   - For children, explain or demonstrate procedures first, and keep the caregiver in sight.
   - For adolescents, be sure to respect their privacy; offer choices when possible.
   - For adults, provide as much patient education and information as possible; know your patient's support system.
4. **Describe the basic developmental milestones for each developmental stage.**
   - Infants develop as they discover their surroundings.
   - Toddlers discover independence and develop quickly if the environment is positive.
   - Preschoolers have perceptions about life's expectations based on their experiences.
   - School-age children experience extensive physical and emotional development.
   - Adolescents undergo physical changes and are constantly challenged by peer group pressures.
   - Adults experience role definition and body changes throughout their life span.
5. **Explain why the medical assistant must understand the various body system changes involved in the aging process.**
   - Body systems change and weaken as people age from early to late adulthood.
   - Medical assistants can help patients accept and adapt to these changes.
6. **List eight areas in which cultural differences exist.**
   - Cultural differences can be expressed in various ways, including eye contact, nontraditional medicines, gestures, concept of time, food, emotions, social roles, and physical space.
7. **Explain the importance of being knowledgeable about the cultural background of a patient.**
   - Understanding the cultural background of a patient can help you communicate more effectively with the patient and address the patient's core concerns.
8. **List four types of responses that patients commonly have toward illness.**
   - Patients may be fearful, talkative, withdrawn, or angry because of illness, injury, discomfort, or pain.
9. **List five things you can do when a patient becomes angry.**
   - Always remain calm and professional; never return a patient's anger.
   - Just listen; some patients need to vent first.
   - Agree with them; sometimes the staff is at fault.
   - Make eye contact; give patients your full attention.
   - Clarify what has been said so that you are sure you have received the message correctly.
10. **Analyze a realistic medical office situation and apply your understanding of the patient's background and behavior to determine the best course of action.**
    - Cultural behaviors, when misunderstood, can create barriers to effective communication between patients and the medical assistant.

11. **Describe the impact on patient care when medical assistants understand how people react to illness and medical care and how they change at various stages of development.**
    - Understanding how people react to illness and how they change at various stages of their development allows medical assistants to modify their approach when interacting with patients. Age-appropriate responses to the patient by the medical assistant will facilitate care.

PRACTICAL APPLICATIONS

If you have accomplished the objectives in this chapter, you will be able to make better choices as a medical assistant. Take another look at this situation and decide what you would do.

Juan, 40 years old, has moved to the United States. His family is still in Mexico, but he hopes to find a good job soon and pay for them to come to the United States. Because Juan does not speak English very well, he has had difficulty finding employment and a place to live. Lately, he has been staying at a shelter for homeless people. His educational background is limited, and his broken English makes communicating difficult. Few Hispanic people live in the area where he has settled. Juan has lost 10 pounds, his vision is declining, and he has noticed that he is not hearing as well as he used to. Because of his constant weight loss and vision problems, he decided to visit the local medical office. He has heard the office provides services to those who cannot pay.

When Juan arrives at the office his clothing is worn and torn. The new medical assistant tells Juan that he cannot be seen at the office unless he can pay for his visit before he is seen. She does not explain her statement, and because of his broken English, Juan does not ask further questions. He thinks that the physician will not see him and leaves the office very upset. He decides to start taking herbal medications and try home remedies. He now believes that seeing a physician in America just is not worth the trouble and embarrassment. Several weeks later, Juan is hospitalized with dehydration, starvation, and severe reactions to the herbal drugs.

This situation did not have to result in the hospitalization of Juan. If you were the new medical assistant, what would you have done differently?

1. What part does age play in the symptoms that Juan is experiencing? Could the symptoms be related to the illnesses as well? Explain.
2. What influence did differing cultural backgrounds have in this situation?
3. How would the situation have turned out if the new medical assistant had studied cultural differences? What activities would help the medical assistant in understanding diversity?
4. What factors led to Juan's withdrawal from medical care until he was hospitalized?
5. As the medical assistant, how would you approach Juan differently?

WEB SEARCH

1. **Research alternative medicine.** Patients of different cultural or belief systems may seek alternative medical treatments. To provide effective patient care, it is necessary for medical assistants to understand these various alternative medical practice techniques.
   Keywords: Use the following keywords in your search: alternative medicine, folk medicine, culture in medicine, ethnicity in medicine.
2. **Research various cultural beliefs about response to illness.** Every person will respond differently to illness. It is important for the medical assistant to be aware of responses based on cultural beliefs, especially if these beliefs differ from the assistant's own beliefs, to provide meaningful patient care.
   Keywords: Use the following keywords in your search: cross-cultural health care, cultural response to illness, cultural response to death and dying.

7 Effective Communication

evolve http://evolve.elsevier.com/klieger/medicalassisting

Communication is the process of sharing information, including ideas, thoughts, opinions, facts, and feelings. In order for people to satisfy their needs and help satisfy the needs of others, those needs must be known. For instance, if you need help, you have to communicate this to someone before that person will help you. Whether at home or in a medical setting, effective communication helps people build good relationships. In the same way, poor communication can cause misunderstandings that harm relationships. Effective communication helps medical assistants establish trust, obtain and provide important information, build positive relationships, and carry out their duties in an efficient, professional way.

You can become an effective communicator by learning and practicing good verbal communication skills, nonverbal communication skills, listening skills, writing skills, and communication using electronic technology.

LEARNING OBJECTIVES

You will be able to do the following after completing this chapter:

Key Terms
1. Define, appropriately use, and spell all the Key Terms for this chapter.

The Communication Process
2. State the goal of the communication process.
3. List and describe the three components of the communication process.

Effective Verbal Communication
4. List and describe the four steps in sending a message that will be understood.
5. List the three types of distracters that can prevent a message from being sent or received.
6. Explain how a verbal message can be misinterpreted.
7. Explain the process of sending a verbal message and evaluating its receipt.

Effective Nonverbal Communication
8. List and describe three ways that people communicate nonverbally.
9. Explain how a nonverbal message can be misinterpreted.

Effective Listening
10. List the three components of effective listening.
11. Compare and contrast active and passive listening and give an example of each.
12. State six steps to becoming a better listener.

Effective Written Communication
13. Recognize the parts of speech and give an example of each.
14. Demonstrate correct use of punctuation.
15. Explain the importance of choosing the correct words.
16. List six words that are frequently misspelled in the medical office.

Effective Communication Using Electronic Technology
17. Explain the importance of understanding how to communicate effectively using electronic technology.
18. List the different types of electronic technology used for communication in a medical office.
19. List six guidelines for e-mail etiquette.

Patient-Centered Professionalism
20. Analyze a realistic medical office situation and apply your understanding of effective communication to determine the best course of action.
21. Describe the impact on patient care when medical assistants consistently apply the principles of effective communication.

KEY TERMS

active listening	nonverbal
adjective	noun
adverb	passive listening
body language	prejudice
communication	preposition
conjunction	pronoun
distracter	punctuation
fax (facsimile)	sentence
feedback	stereotyping
grammar	subject
interjection	verb

PRACTICAL APPLICATIONS

Read the following scenario and keep it in mind as you learn about the principles of effective communication in this chapter.

Panina is a former resident of the Middle East who moved to the United States with her husband, Abed, 6 months ago. Naturally, she brings the cultural and ethnic contexts of her homeland with her. Panina awakens one morning with a pain in her breast. She becomes concerned and calls a physician's office for an appointment. Because she has difficulty understanding the English language, she misunderstands the appointment time and Panina and Abed arrive at the office an hour late. Abed demands to accompany his wife to the examining room. Therese, the medical assistant, tells Abed that they are late for the appointment and that he must stay in the waiting room while Panina is being examined. Panina, refusing eye contact with Therese, begins to cry. Abed becomes upset and tells Therese that the only way Panina will be examined is if he accompanies her to the room to explain to the male doctor what is wrong with her. Therese refuses, and Panina and Abed leave the office, threatening to tell all their friends how this office "just does not care about patients at all."

Effective communication helps eliminate misunderstandings. If you were the medical assistant in this situation, how could you have used your understanding of effective communication skills to help?

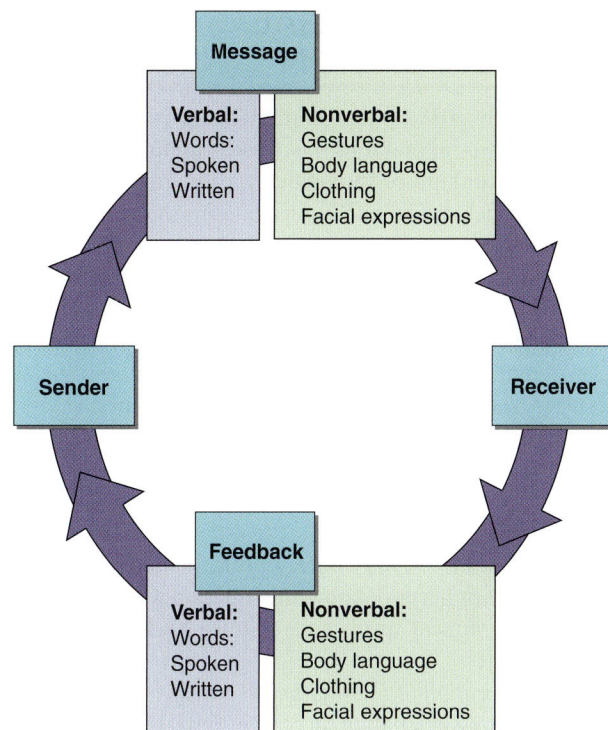

FIGURE 7-1 Process of communication. (From Hunt SA: *Saunders fundamentals of medical assisting,* revised reprint, St Louis, 2007, Saunders.)

Never underestimate the power of nonverbal communication. When we communicate directly with another person, we send our message as follows:
- 10% is verbal.
- 40% is through our tone.
- 50% is through our body language.

Based on these statistics, 90% of person-to-person communication is nonverbal. Your words may be saying one thing but is your nonverbal communication saying the same thing? To be an effective communicator, both verbal (spoken and written) and nonverbal (tone, body language) communication must be clear.

THE COMMUNICATION PROCESS

The goal of **communication** is the clear exchange of information between a *sender* (the person sending information) and a *receiver* (the person receiving information). The three components of the communication process are the sender, the receiver, and the *message* (the information being exchanged). The process can be done either *verbally,* when words are exchanged, as in speaking or writing, or *nonverbally,* when expressions, gestures, and body movement are used to send the message (Figure 7-1).

PATIENT-CENTERED PROFESSIONALISM

The way you communicate shows your respect for patients. Speaking with patients in a way that reflects your understanding of their feelings and fears not only shows respect for the patients but also promotes goodwill for the practice. How could each of the following remarks be changed to show more respect for patients?
- *"Hold."*
- *"No, I can't give you an appointment today."*
- *"Fill out this form."*
- *"Doctor's busy."*

EFFECTIVE VERBAL COMMUNICATION

Although only 10% of all communicating is done verbally, words are powerful and must be chosen carefully. We have all been hurt by unkind or thoughtless words. You have learned how using labels can impact understanding and communication. Verbal communication is an important part of every medical assistant's day. You need to be able to communicate effectively with both co-workers and patients to provide effective care. Effective verbal communication involves (1) organizing a message, (2) prioritizing information, (3) sending the message, and (4) evaluating whether the message was received.

Organize

To ensure that the message being sent is focused on what the receiver wants or needs to know, the situation must be assessed and planning done. Consider the following when organizing verbal messages:

1. *Best organization of information to convey the information.* Is a lengthy explanation necessary or a brief summary? Would an example help clarify the idea?
2. *Time frame for communicating the message.* Is it something that must be conveyed immediately, or should it wait awhile?
3. Most important, *ability of the recipient to receive the message.* Will the person understand what you mean? How can you modify your communication based on the person's characteristics, abilities, and condition?

To be understandable, the message must be clear, concise, and in words that both the sender and the receiver can understand. For example, you could ask an adult patient to "urinate in the cup," but you may have to ask a child to "pee in the cup." Both these requests communicate the same message, but the wording has been adjusted to fit the understanding of the different receivers (adult and child).

Prioritize

Information being sent must be categorized and arranged in a logical order. What do you want the listener to hear first? A disorganized message is not likely to be understood by the listener.

Transmit

The sender must choose an appropriate way to transmit (send) the message. Depending on the information to be conveyed, the sender may transmit the message over the phone, in person, or by electronic mail (Figure 7-2).

Delivery

The way a message is delivered is just as important as the message itself. Keep in mind the following about the delivery of messages:

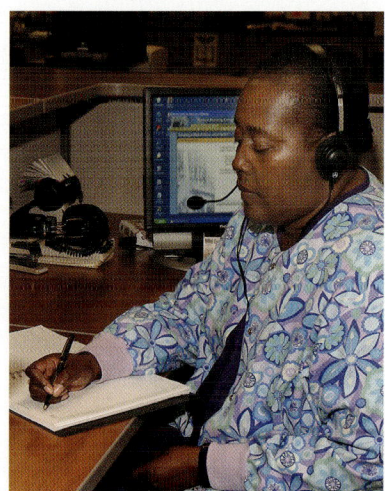

FIGURE 7-2 This medical assistant is sending a message to a patient when she confirms an appointment.

- Choose your words carefully and accurately; do not use slang terms or terminology the patient cannot understand.
- Be aware of the rate of your speech. If you talk too fast, your enunciation may become slurred, and the receiver may not be able to understand or hear all your words.
- Ensure that your message is clear and concise. Avoid a monotone voice. Vary your inflection (volume) when making points.
- Match your tone to the message you are sending. For example, use a serious tone for serious messages. Consider your volume as well; if your voice is too loud or too soft, the receiver may ignore the message.
- Give full attention to the listener. Maintain appropriate eye contact, use the listener's name, and smile if appropriate.

Distracters

A **distracter** is anything that causes the sender or receiver not to give full attention to the message. Distracters cause either the receiver to miss information provided or the sender to miscommunicate the message. For example, a person looking at her watch during an exchange of information gives the impression she wants to be someplace else. A person who constantly interrupts implies that the information being given is not important. Three major distracters you need to be aware of are the environment, your use of good grammar, and the physical well-being of the receiver.

Environment. The following environmental situations can distract a receiver and can prevent messages from being communicated:

- A noisy room with side conversations, a ringing telephone, or a TV in the background
- An uncomfortable room temperature (e.g., too warm or too cold)
- A room with either poor lighting or lights that are too bright or flickering

In each of these situations, the environment causes the receiver to pay more attention to the surroundings than to the message. When communicating, you must try to reduce the amount of *environmental interference*. For example, if you are trying to give instructions to a mother about her child and the child is misbehaving, the mother's focus is on the child and not the information being given. In this situation, you need to be patient and repeat the information when the mother is ready to listen to what you are saying. Providing written instructions to a parent or guardian for home care is also helpful.

Use of Grammar. The second major factor that distracts receivers from the information being sent is the improper use of grammar. When the sender uses improper grammar, the receiver may misunderstand the message being sent. In addition, the receiver may form a negative opinion about the sender (e.g., "this person doesn't speak properly; is she capable of performing her medical assisting duties?"). Even if the receiver believes and understands the message, he or she may not accept it because of the manner in which it is spoken. Proper use of grammar helps ensure that a message is organized well and communicated clearly. It also helps inspire confidence in the sender. Avoid using slang terms; patients may see them as unprofessional or may misinterpret their meaning altogether. Keep the medical explanations simple; do not use terminology the patient may not completely understand.

Physical Well-Being. The third major distracter is the receiver's physical well-being. If the receiver is weak from illness, in pain, or heavily medicated, he or she may not hear the message or be able to interpret or recall what is being communicated. If a family member or caregiver is not present with the patient at this time, be sure to provide written instructions for the patient to take home.

Evaluate

Even after the message is sent and received, the sender still has work to do. The message sent must be evaluated to determine how effective it was at communicating the intended information. Consider the following when evaluating a message's effectiveness:

1. Did the receiver understand the message exactly as you intended?
2. Did you obtain the expected response from the receiver?
3. Did a relationship of mutual respect and trust develop between you and the receiver?

You can answer these questions through feedback and clarification.

Assess Feedback

Receiving **feedback** (an indication that the message was received) from the receiver allows you to determine if the message was understood the way it was intended. Feedback occurs when the receiver responds to the information.

When communicating face-to-face, the feedback is immediate; you only need to observe the person's expression to decide if the message was received the way it was intended. For example, if the receiver looks confused or is silent, there usually is a problem.

When seeking feedback, you must use statements or questions that are open ended. *Open-ended questions* encourage more than a "yes" or "no" response. Open-ended questions, such as "Tell me about yourself" (rather than "How long have you lived here?"), encourage dialogue and allow patients to express more about their feelings and perceptions. These questions also give medical assistants a chance to verify that the information is accurate. *Closed-ended questions* (e.g., "yes" or "no" questions) may make patients feel rushed. If you are doing an assessment and use too many closed-ended questions, the patient may mentally tune out and provide only minimal information. Allowing the patient to ask questions and seek clarification before continuing on with the information greatly facilitates the communication process.

Seek Clarification

In some cases, you may have to repeat the information and even demonstrate what is needed from the receiver. This process, called *echoing*, helps you clarify the patient's feedback. If you discover during evaluation that the patient does not understand your message, adjust the message to fit the patient and send it again. Evaluating the effectiveness of your messages helps ensure that you are communicating clearly with patients.

PATIENT-CENTERED PROFESSIONALISM

- *What is the most effective way for the medical assistant to communicate to the patient concerning a plan of care? How does effectively communicating a plan of care to patients benefit the patient and the health care team?*
- *What are some of the ways distracters can reduce the quality of care a patient receives?*

EFFECTIVE NONVERBAL COMMUNICATION

Nonverbal communication is the exchange of messages or information without using words. Nonverbal communication can help or hinder the process of sending a message, depending on how it is used. Nonverbal communication is sometimes unintentional and unconscious, but it is still important. Understanding nonverbal communication will help you to interpret patients' nonverbal messages, as well as consider the messages you are sending as you interact with others. Your physical presentation, which includes not only your personal appearance but also your posture, movements, gestures, and facial expression, provides the patient clear signals about you. Body language, posture and movement, and personal space and distance are all forms of nonverbal communication.

Body Language

Our **body language** is as important as our words. When communicating with patients, you must observe for nonverbal signals as you listen to what they are saying (Figure 7-3). Consider how body motions, such as a nod of the head, shrug of the shoulders, or a toddler's shake of the head to indicate "no," can send a clear message. However, understand that body language can sometimes be misinterpreted. A patient may interpret a medical assistant's unsmiling facial expression as a lack of concern for the patient's well-being, when the medical assistant simply may be tired that day. Cultural differences in body language can also cause misunderstandings. Casual touching of some body parts (e.g., arms, shoulder, or face) and standing too close to a person's face may be offensive to some patients.

Always be aware of the nonverbal messages you are sending to patients. To improve communication with patients, you must understand the nonverbal messages that can be sent with the eyes, mouth, hands, and touch.

Eyes

The eyes can tell a great deal about what people are feeling. One look into a patient's eyes could reveal pain, fear, anger, or withdrawal. Our eyes send the following common nonverbal signals:

- The size of the pupil increases when looking at something of interest. The stronger the interest, the larger the pupil becomes.
- In America, looking downward or away can be interpreted as submission, giving in, or wanting to avoid a situation. When a teacher asks for a volunteer or asks a question, have you ever looked away because you didn't want to be called on?
- The eyes help create facial expressions that signal many emotions, including surprise, fear, anger, disgust, happiness, and sadness.

Mouth

The mouth can also send the following signals about what a person is feeling.

- When people are surprised, their mouths often drop open unexpectedly.
- A smile may signal acceptance, friendliness, or appreciation.
- A firm or set jaw may signal anger, impatience, or stubbornness.

Hands

The movements of the hands can send many signals such as the following:

- How would you interpret a message from someone who was pointing his or her finger at you?
- What message does a "thumbs-up" gesture send in Western culture?
- People may snap their fingers when they think of an idea, want to emphasize something, or want to get someone's attention.

Touch

Touch can send many nonverbal signals to the receiver. How touch is interpreted depends on many variables. The growth and developmental stages and experiences of a person are important. If someone comes from a family environment where hugging was an everyday expression, touch may be accepted and welcome. Someone growing up in a family who is not "touchy-feely" may be uncomfortable with touch. Common messages associated with touch follow:

- In the United States, a handshake is a social expression and can be used when meeting someone for the first time. In Europe, the handshake is an everyday greeting among women and men alike.
- Hugs are usually saved for close relationships (e.g., within families or between close friends).
- A hand on the arm, shoulder, or back can convey comfort, support, or congratulations (Figure 7-4).

In the medical field, touch can be used to express feelings of caring or concern. Touch is a basic form of communication for patients of all ages and does not require words or any

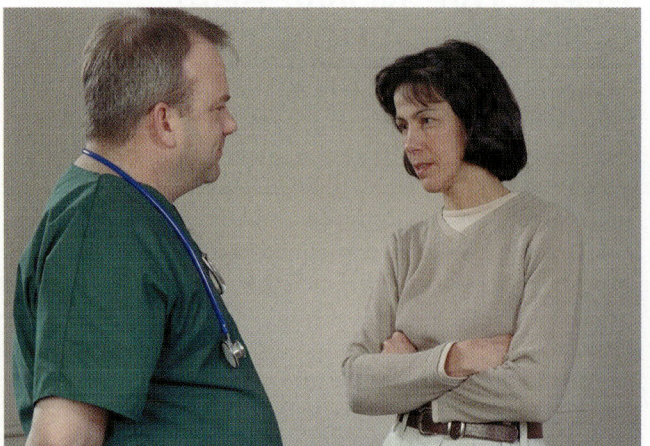

FIGURE 7-3 What is this patient trying to communicate?

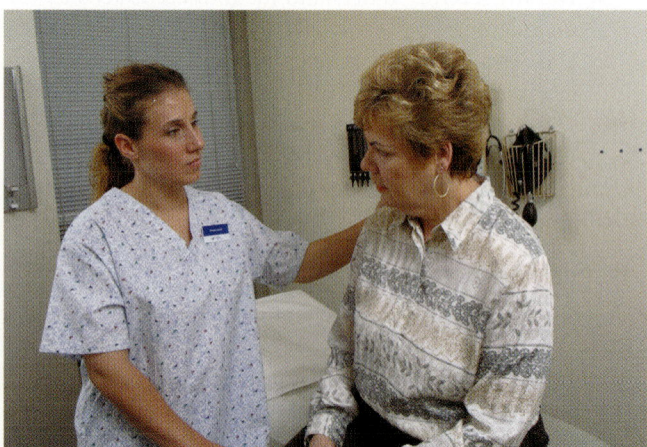

FIGURE 7-4 A medical assistant lets the patient know she cares with a simple touch.

previous experience or education to be effective. Medical assistants often use touch to offer support and to give positive reinforcement to patients. The patient's shoulders, arms, and hands are considered proper places for casual touch.

Posture and Movement

Posture and body movements are constantly sending messages. If you were speaking to a patient and his arms were folded over his chest, how would you interpret this? What might it mean if a patient turns her back to you? A patient's posture can tell you if the patient is tense or relaxed. In the same way that a patient's body movements and posture can send messages, the medical assistant's body movements and posture also send messages. For example, when questioning a patient, sitting instead of standing creates a more relaxed atmosphere and sends the message that you are taking your time.

Body movements can also imply many things. Fidgeting could signal that a patient is tired of waiting or anxious about something. Shivering could imply fear or feeling cold.

Space and Distance

When talking to another person, do you tend to stand very close to the person or farther away? The distance between people when communicating is often influenced by culture, race, gender, age, and personality. Different space considerations are as follows:

- *Public space* (12 to 25 feet apart) is generally used when people are speaking to a group, or giving lectures or presentations. An example is a teacher speaking to an entire class.
- *Social space* (2 to 4 feet apart) is mostly used in the workplace and similar situations. An example is a customer being helped by a salesperson at a store.
- *Personal space* (arm's length distance, $1\frac{1}{2}$ to $2\frac{1}{2}$ feet) is used for personal conversations in soft to moderate tones. An example is two close friends "catching up on old times."
- *Intimate space* (1 to $1\frac{1}{2}$ feet apart) is used for those times of closeness. An example is a parent comforting a small child.

The distance between people when speaking depends on their feelings, what they are doing, and the nature of their relationship.

Other Nonverbal Considerations

Other factors that influence the interpretation of nonverbal communication include the following:

- *Time.* How long it takes to send a message and how much time it takes to interpret it sends a nonverbal message.
- *Silence.* Silence can be difficult to read, whether as acceptance, nonacceptance, or not understanding.
- *Sounds.* Nonverbal communication can also be vocal. Examples include groans, sighs, or even screams when the patient is in pain.

Appearance. Just as your personal appearance as a medical assistant sends messages to patients, a patient's appearance sends messages as well. If a small child is not dressed warmly enough in cold weather, this might be interpreted as parental neglect.

Often, what you *don't* say is more important than what you do say. Make certain your actions reflect what you want sent to the receiver. By carefully observing the person, you can determine if the receiver has understood what you have said. Be careful that your facial expressions and body movements do not contradict your spoken words. Table 7-1 describes various behavioral styles of nonverbal communicators, and Box 7-1 defines some common American gestures.

PATIENT-CENTERED PROFESSIONALISM

- How can paying attention to a patient's body language improve communication between a medical assistant and the patient?
- What are some things that could happen if a patient's body language and nonverbal communication are ignored?
- Besides body language, what are some other nonverbal elements that could help you provide better care to patients?

EFFECTIVE LISTENING

Listening plays a key role in the communication process. Developing good listening skills takes practice. However, being a good listener will improve your skill in other areas of communication as well. When patients sense that you are listening to them, they become more relaxed and ready to communicate. This helps you establish rapport and prepares the patient for communicating with other members of the health care

TABLE 7-1

Behavioral Styles of Nonverbal Communicators*

	Confusion or Lack of Interest	Understanding	Anger
Gestures	Fidgeting	Reaching out	Pointing finger
Facial expressions	Blank look	Attentive	Frowning Rolling eyes
Eye contact	Downcast eyes	Direct	Glaring Staring
Posture	Slumped	Relaxed	Rigid
Tone	Weak or quiet	Appropriate volume	Loud
Rate of speech	Hesitant or slow	Matches situation	Fast Precise

*By carefully observing the nonverbal actions of the receiver, the sender of a message can decide how well it was understood and even if it has been accepted.

BOX 7-1

Common American Gestures

GREETING GESTURES
- Handshake (firm, solid grip)
- Direct eye contact (when greeting and talking)
- Arm raised with the open hand waving back and forth (signals "hello" or "goodbye"; also used in attempt to get someone's attention)

BECKONING GESTURES
- Waving to another and then scooping the hand inward (signals a person to "come over")
- Raising the index finger toward one's face, and making a "curling" motion with that finger (beckons a person to "come closer")

OTHER NONVERBAL GESTURES
- Palm facing out with the index and middle fingers in a V shape (indicates a "victory" or "peace" sign)
- Closed fist with the thumb up (indicates approval ["good job" or "way to go"] or hitchhiking)
- Whistling (indicates approval and recognition)
- Nodding or shaking the head (indicates "yes" or "no")

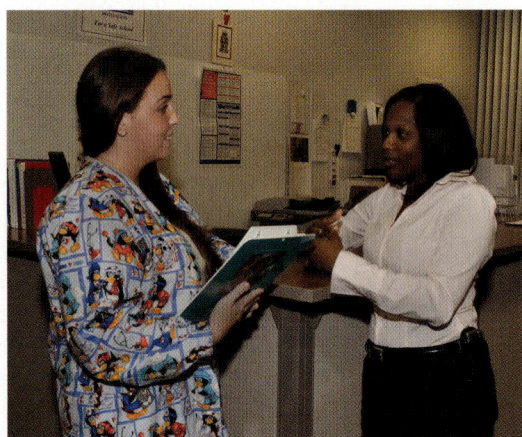

FIGURE 7-5 A medical assistant listens carefully to a patient's concerns.

team. To listen effectively, you need to concentrate on the message, analyze the message, and provide feedback.

Concentrate on the Message

As a medical assistant, your listening skills will be used daily in all your routine activities. For example, one of your typical duties may be to listen and record why patients have come to the office (Figure 7-5). You will also need to be a good listener when receiving oral instructions from the physician, coworkers, and patients. If you allow distracters to interfere with your listening, you will not obtain the information you need. This can affect the care that patients receive by causing confusion, miscommunication, and delays. Such communication mistakes can be costly in terms of time, money, goodwill, and reputation of the health care team.

Being a good listener as a medical assistant requires you to concentrate on the message being sent by the patient and its purpose. There are two types of listening: passive and active.

Passive listening involves hearing what the speaker is saying but not listening with enough effort to become personally, intensely involved in what is being said. Examples of passive listening are cooking while listening to the television, doodling on paper while the teacher is talking in class, and looking through the patient's chart while the patient chats about the weather.

Active listening requires you to demonstrate listening by maintaining eye contact and providing responses (feedback) to indicate that you are listening and really thinking about what is being said. Unless you are listening actively to the patient, you may not hear or understand part of the message.

Analyze the Message

Active listeners analyze or evaluate the speaker's words as well as the person's posture, facial expressions, tone, mannerisms, and general appearance. Analyzing the message involves thinking on the part of the listener. To analyze a message, the following two conditions must be met:

1. The listener must be *able* to understand the message. This depends on the listener's vocabulary and attitudes. If you are listening and hear words you do not understand, ask for clarification. When patients are listening to you, confirm their understanding by paraphrasing, clarifying, validating, or encouraging them to repeat the message back to you. Use the patient's nonverbal clues to help you understand the meaning of the message while you are listening.

2. The listener must be *willing* to understand the message. A listener must want to grasp the meaning of the message and be willing to understand the speaker's point of view. As a health professional, you must overcome feelings of **prejudice** (negative opinion toward an individual because of his or her affiliation with a specific group) and avoid **stereotyping** (believing that all members of a culture or group are the same). Not accepting patients as they are interferes with your ability to listen to what they are saying. When you stereotype or have feelings of prejudice toward patients, you make automatic assumptions about them that may or may not be true. If you consider a patient to be uncooperative, you may not accept the information the patient is giving you as true. This may cause you to respond incorrectly to the patient.

When listening to and responding to children, take special care to listen actively (Box 7-2). Children may not be as effective as adults at conveying their message because of their vocabulary level, or they may simply be uncomfortable or in pain.

As a medical assistant, you will need to listen in a variety of ways, both in person and on the phone. You can even apply active listening skills when reading written communication, such as mail, faxes, letters, memos, and e-mail, by "listening" between the lines to such factors as tone and perspective of

> **BOX 7-2**
>
> **Guidelines in Communicating with Children**
>
> 1. Be a good listener.
> 2. Let children speak at their own speed. Do not rush them or supply words. Let them complete their own thoughts and sentences.
> 3. Encourage self-talk.
> 4. Talk to children with words they can easily understand.
> 5. Be aware of situations that might be frightening to children, and try to reassure them.

TABLE 7-2

Six Steps to Becoming a Better Listener

L	1.	Look at the entire delivery of the message. Read facial expression, posture, and gestures.
I	2.	Interruptions should be avoided. Give your full attention to the speaker, and listen to his or her needs.
S	3.	Stay involved. Do not think about other things you have to do. Remember, not everyone is a dynamic speaker, but all speakers have something important to say.
T	4.	Transmit feedback based on your understanding of the message. Put yourself in the speaker's shoes. Ask probing questions and provide statements (without interrupting) that indicate your understanding. Listen until you have heard the entire message.
E	5.	Evaluate the information thoroughly. Use all aspects of the communication process to draw your conclusions.
N	6.	Neutralize bias and negative attitudes from your evaluation process. Treat the speaker with respect. Accept people for who they are, and do not let your attitudes interfere with listening carefully.

the writer. You can become an active listener by practicing good listening skills and by always striving to concentrate on both the verbal and nonverbal messages being sent (Table 7-2).

Provide Feedback

Feedback is incredibly important. Feedback from the listener (receiver) helps the speaker (sender) know if the message has been received. The type of feedback given by a receiver affects the sender's message. Giving a quizzical glance, having an expression of confusion, or giving the appearance of boredom sends a message back to the sender. If a patient senses that the medical assistant is distracted or preoccupied while sending the message, the patient may tune out the message altogether.

The following factors influence a receiver's feedback and may cause roadblocks to effective communication:

- *Background of the receiver.* This includes the receiver's personality, life experiences, knowledge of the subject area being covered, and interest in hearing or motivation to listen to the message being sent. If the receiver is not interested, there will be minimal or no feedback.
- *Appearance of the sender or message being sent.* This can present roadblocks if the appearance is distracting or unprofessional. If the sender looks unkempt or does not speak clearly, or if a message contains bad grammar or spelling errors, the message is either lost to the receiver or seen as unimportant.
- *Skills of the sender and receiver.* The sender of a message needs to organize the message based on the receiver's vocabulary and comprehension level. Ideally, the skills of the sender and receiver should match. A message that is "over the head" of a patient will not be understood. In the same way, using the wrong word (e.g., "Pacific" instead of "specific") changes the meaning of the intended message. A patient who understands the difference between these words may receive the impression that the medical assistant does not pay attention to detail and may even be careless about the patient's care. Even if the receiver understands the message, his or her impression of the sender is affected.

> **PATIENT-CENTERED PROFESSIONALISM**
>
> - *How are relations with patients improved when medical assistants have good listening skills?*
> - *How do poor listening skills interfere with a medical assistant's ability to provide quality patient care?*
> - *How do prejudices and stereotyping interfere with the medical assistant's ability to communicate effectively with patients?*
> - *How can effective use of feedback increase the likelihood that patients will communicate clearly and openly with the medical assistant?*

EFFECTIVE WRITTEN COMMUNICATION

People judge a medical office by how its employees look, act, think, speak, and write. If a letter with grammatical and spelling errors is sent to a patient, the patient will have a negative feeling about the medical office and may not value the contents of the letter. Good writing skills are also needed to chart properly. Chart notes must be clear, concise, and precise when recording care given to the patient. Remember that written documentation serves as a permanent, legal record of care provided to a patient. If it is not documented or if the documentation is not clear, there is no proof that a procedure took place.

Rules and principles of grammar exist to help us write clearly and effectively. It is important to know the parts of speech used to create sentences, as well as the correct way to capitalize, use numbers, and use punctuation. Further, it is helpful to study words that are frequently misused and misspelled. This section covers the major areas that often cause problems in written communication.

Grammar

Grammar is the study of words and their relationship to other words in a sentence. A **sentence** is a group of words that expresses a complete thought. The different types of words that make up sentences are referred to as the "parts of speech." There are eight parts of speech: **nouns, pronouns, verbs, adjectives, adverbs, prepositions, conjunctions,** and **interjections.**

Parts of Speech

In order to express a complete thought, a sentence must contain a **subject** (what is being discussed) and a verb (action word) (Box 7-3). A subject is usually a noun or pronoun. Understanding the purpose of each part of speech will help you write sentences that are correct, clear, and professional (Table 7-3). Numbers may be used as nouns or adjectives. Take care to express them correctly when writing (Box 7-4).

BOX 7-3

Sentence Structure

- A *sentence* is a group of words that expresses a *complete* thought.
- A *subject* is usually a noun or pronoun and indicates who is speaking or what the sentence involves. The subject often comes first in a sentence.
  Example: The patient has arrived. (*Patient* is the subject.)
- A *simple sentence* expresses only one thought.
  Example: The patient has arrived. (One thought is expressed.)
- A *compound sentence* expresses two or more thoughts, and the thoughts are joined by a conjunction.
  Example: The patient has arrived, and the physician is ready to see him. (Two thoughts are expressed: one about the patient and one about the physician.)

TABLE 7-3

Using the Parts of Speech Correctly

Part of Speech	What It Is	Examples	Function in Sentence	Sentence Examples
Noun	A word used to name things, including people, places, objects, and ideas.	Medical assistant, Calvin, phlebotomist, woman, Boston, city, store.	Often used as the subject, or the "thing" the sentence is talking about.	The *doctor* vacations in *Florida* every *year*. The *medical assistant* took his *blood pressure*.
Pronoun	A word used to take the place of a noun.	I, we, you, they, he, her, them, no one, someone, who, me, our.	Used as the subject of a sentence, to show ownership (e.g., his, hers, theirs, ours), or to talk about another person in the sentence.	Pete took *him* to the doctor's office. Give *me my* pencil.
Verb	A word or phrase used to express action, a condition, or a state of being.	Run, walk, eat, ask, is, has, was, seems, should have been.	Used to explain what is "happening" to the subject of the sentence.	The patient *came* to the office. He *is* a medical assistant. The child *seems to be* confused.
Adjective	A word used to describe a noun or pronoun.	Good, better, best, green, tall, heavy, nice, discolored, uneven, swollen.	Provides more information about a noun or pronoun (e.g., tells what kind, which one, or how many).	The *new* medical assistant started yesterday. There are *three* nurses in the office.
Adverb	A word used to describe a verb, adjective, or another adverb.	Quickly, evenly, carefully, well, too, very, soon, there, nearly.	Provides more information about how something happened or was done (e.g., tells where, when, how, why, or to what extent).	Put the chart *there*. *Carefully* remove the sutures. It is *too* late.
Preposition	A word used to begin a prepositional phrase.	*To* the left, *around* the corner, *over* the top, *before* the surgery.	Used to show the relationship between a noun and the rest of the sentence.	The request *from* the patient was *for* an afternoon appointment. The referral was received *after* lunch.
Conjunction	A word used to join words or groups of words.	And, or, but, nor, for, yet, since, if, because.	Connects related items or groups of words within a sentence; also used to join two short sentences to make one longer sentence.	The supplies *and* equipment arrived today. The patient would have been on time, *but* her car broke down.
Interjection	A word used to express strong feeling or emotion.	Wow! Yikes! Ouch! Oh,.	Often used alone and followed by an exclamation point.	*Wow!* What an improvement. *Oh,* I forgot to leave a message.

BOX 7-4

Using Numbers in Writing*

- Numbers from one through nine should be spelled out; numbers 10 and up should be written numerically.

Examples:
The speaker has two hours to give the presentation.
There are 26 pairs of nonsterile gloves left in the box.

- Numbers that begin sentences should be spelled out even if they are greater than nine. *Example:* Twenty people applied for the job.
- Fractions standing alone should be spelled out; when several fractions are being discussed, write them numerically.

Examples:
More than three fourths of the patients have medical insurance.
Between ¾ and ⅞ of all patients live within a 20-mile radius of the office.

- Ages are spelled out unless the age is being referred to as a statistic.

Examples:
Sue began working for the physician at the age of twenty-three.
All patients over the age of 50 are sent for an annual colonoscopy.

*These general guidelines may vary according to the medical specialty and subject and the publisher and textbook, as in this text (e.g., 2 hours; age 23 years).

BOX 7-5

Words Frequently Misspelled in Medical Communication

abscess	concede	physician
accommodate	definitely	physiological
agglutinate	diarrhea	pneumonia
aggressive	embarrassing	questionnaire
analysis	fluctuation	rheumatism
benefited	forty	schedule
calendar	license	sphygmomanometer
canceled	negligence	stethoscope
clientele	ophthalmoscope	surgeon
committee	patients	vacuum

BOX 7-6

Spelling Hints

WHAT DO YOU DO WHEN CHOOSING "IE" OR "EI"?

Use "i" before "e" except after "c"...

thief	chief
believe	friend
conceive	perceive

...or when it sounds like an "ay," as in "neighbor" and "weigh":

weigh	vein
eight	their

WHAT DO YOU DO WHEN ADDING ENDINGS TO WORDS?

If a word ends in a consonant, repeat the consonant if it is preceded or followed by a vowel:

ship	shipped
bag	baggage

In words ending in a silent "e," the "e" is usually dropped if the ending begins with a vowel (e.g., "ing"):

use	using
decorate	decorating

Punctuation

Punctuation helps to separate, emphasize, and clarify the different ideas within sentences and between groups of sentences (Table 7-4). Incorrect punctuation marks can change the meaning of a sentence. Carefully proofread everything you write to be sure that you have used the correct punctuation.

Word Choice

Words that sound alike, look alike, or are pronounced exactly alike can be confusing and will cause miscommunication if not correctly applied. Medical assistants must choose the word that expresses the correct meaning for the situation. Study the words in Table 7-5 so that you will be able to use them correctly.

Spelling

Spelling words incorrectly not only creates an unprofessional impression but also can cause misunderstandings and mistakes in the treatment of patients. "Ilium" and "ileum" are pronounced the same way, but *ilium* refers to the hip area, whereas *ileum* refers to the intestinal area—the difference of one letter! Surgery on the incorrect body part (ilium or ileum) could be potential malpractice. Spelling problems often occur when there are double-letter combinations (e.g., accommodate, committee) and when trying to decide if a word is one word or two (e.g., cannot, percent, all right). Box 7-5 shows other words that are frequently misspelled in medical communication. Study these words to reduce the chance of spelling them incorrectly. Box 7-6 provides hints to help you when spelling difficult words.

PATIENT-CENTERED PROFESSIONALISM

- In what ways do the written communication skills of medical assistants influence patients' attitudes, confidence, and cooperation?
- Why is the use of good grammar so important when charting? How can improper grammar in charting affect patient care?

TABLE 7-4
Using Punctuation Correctly

Punctuation	Symbol	How It Is Used	Sentence Examples
Period	.	To show where one statement or command ends and the next sentence begins.	The patient called for an appointment. Please pull the patient's records.
Question mark	?	To show where a question ends and the next sentence begins.	Will the doctor be available this afternoon? What is the fee for today's visit?
Exclamation mark	!	To add emphasis to the end of a sentence expressing strong feelings or emotion or to an interjection.	Congratulations! We are proud of you. You did it!
Comma	,	1. To separate two or more complete thoughts in a sentence joined by *and, but, or,* etc. 2. To separate items in a list or groups of words within a sentence. 3. To signal the reader to pause after an introductory word or group of words.	1. I left the patient with instructions, and I plan to follow up tomorrow. 2. The pens, pencils, and markers arrived with our order. 3. First, let me explain the procedure.
Semicolon	;	To join two or more complete thoughts in a sentence when *and, but, or,* or *nor* is not used.	The medical assistant has a new stethoscope; she prefers the other one. We have swabs; however, there may not be enough.
Colon	:	1. To introduce a list or an example or examples. 2. To add emphasis to a word.	1. We have the following: paper towels, antiseptic soap, and handrub. 2. There can be only one reason why she is late: illness.
Dash	—	To emphasize or separate something in a sentence.	This year's conference will be in Portland—be prepared for rain. He tried again—for the third time.
Apostrophe	'	1. To form contractions. 2. To show ownership.	1. It's been a great day. 2. Nate's lab coat is clean.
Parentheses	( )	To set off words that provide additional information or explanation.	The formula (see page 53) will help you make the calculation. Her aunt (the mayor) is visiting today.
Quotation marks	" "	1. To set off dialogue (conversations). 2. To signal use of the exact words of others. 3. To emphasize a term.	1. "Yes, it is," he replied. 2. The patient reports "…a bad feeling in my stomach, and a headache that has lasted for three days." 3. The term "fax" is often used to mean "facsimile."

EFFECTIVE COMMUNICATION USING ELECTRONIC TECHNOLOGY

Just 10 to 20 years ago, no one would have ever considered using electronic technology to communicate in a medical office. Today, however, medical assistants and other health professionals must use electronic technology on a daily basis. Although most patients prefer speaking to "real people" and there is no replacement for in-person communication when discussing a health problem, electronic technology provides another way for patients to receive information and contact the medical office. As with all types of communication, care must be taken to communicate effectively and with confidentiality. Many of the same principles for effective verbal, nonverbal, and written communication apply when sending and receiving messages electronically.

To function in a modern medical office, medical assistants need to understand new and evolving technologies and develop the correct skills to use them effectively. Communicating through speaking or writing typically does not require special equipment. However, electronic information systems require properly functioning software, hardware, and processing equipment to be in place before the message can be sent. Four types of electronic technology used to send and receive messages in the medical office are voice mail systems, web sites, fax machines, and electronic mail (e-mail).

Voice Mail

A *voice mail system* is an automated answering device. It allows the person calling on the phone to leave a voice message when the receiver is not available to take the call. The message is saved (stored) on a computer or an answering machine and can be retrieved later when it is convenient for the receiver to respond. In a medical office, voice mail should be retrieved at the same times each day (e.g., on arrival in the morning, after lunch hour). The voice mail system should provide callers with a time they can expect their call to be returned. The system should also provide instructions for emergency situations (e.g., "If this is an emergency, press '0,' call 911, or proceed to the emergency room"). The system is meant to help, not to

TABLE 7-5

Frequently Used Sound-Alike Words*

Word Pair	Definitions	Usage Examples
1. access 2. excess	1. To gain admission (access) to; to get at 2. Too much	1. The door was locked, so he could not **access** the papers. 2. **Excess** fat in one's diet is not good.
1. advise 2. advice	1. To recommend 2. A helpful suggestion	1. I **advise** you to hurry up. 2. I will take your **advice**.
1. affect 2. effect	1. To change or influence (verb) 2. Result; to bring out (noun)	1. Your mood **affects** your behavior. 2. The **effect** was positive.
1. already 2. all ready	1. Previously 2. Prepared	1. We have **already** finished. 2. We are **all ready** to go.
1. altogether 2. all together	1. Entirely 2. Everyone in a group	1. It is **altogether** too time consuming. 2. We were **all together** for Thanksgiving.
1. always 2. all ways	1. At all times 2. All means or methods	1. I **always** brush my teeth after meals. 2. Have you tried **all ways** possible to solve the problem?
1. anyway 2. any way	1. In any case 2. Any method	1. He decided to go **anyway**. 2. Is there **any way** you will reconsider?
1. assistance 2. assistants	1. To help 2. More than one person	1. The doctor needs your **assistance**. 2. All of the medical **assistants** were present.
1. awhile 2. a while	1. For a short time 2. A short period of time	1. They talked **awhile** on the phone. 2. In **a while**, we will close the office.
1. council 2. counsel	1. A group that advises 2. To advise	1. The national **council** meets each year. 2. The experienced medical assistant **counseled** the new assistant about a difficult situation.
1. disinterested 2. uninterested	1. Unbiased 2. Having no interest	1. He is considered a **disinterested** voter because he favors neither candidate. 2. The lecture was boring, so the listeners quickly became **uninterested**.
1. every day 2. everyday	1. Each day 2. Daily	1. Take some time for yourself **every day**. 2. Communication is an **everyday** occurrence.
1. farther 2. further	1. Physical distance (measurable) 2. Additional time or quantity	1. She walked **farther** than she had ever gone. 2. We will need **further** research to make the decision.
1. fewer 2. less	1. When items can be counted 2. When quantities cannot be counted	1. We have **fewer** patients than last year. 2. **Less** time should be wasted.
1. its 2. it's	1. Shows possession 2. Contraction for "it is"	1. The dog dropped **its** bone. 2. It looks like **it's** going to rain today.
1. patience 2. patients	1. A sense of calm; waiting 2. People seeking the care of a physician or other health care provider	1. Waiting takes **patience**. 2. There are 10 **patients** scheduled this morning.
1. principle 2. principal	1. Doctrine 2. A person who is in a leading position	1. Follow the established ethics and **principles** of your profession. 2. The **principal** called the teachers to a meeting.
1. rode 2. road	1. To have ridden 2. A path	1. We **rode** the bus to work. 2. The **road** was bumpy.
1. stationary 2. stationery	1. Not movable 2. Paper used to write letters	1. The car that ran out of gas remained **stationary**. 2. Use the office **stationery** to write the letter.
1. than 2. then	1. Used in a comparison 2. Tells when	1. We need more **than** that amount. 2. First, get the towels; **then**, place them near the sink.
1. their 2. there 3. they're	1. Belonging to them 2. A location or direction 3. Contraction for "they are"	1. **Their** car is parked in the lot. 2. You can find the records over **there**. 3. **They're** leaving the office.
1. to 2. too 3. two	1. In the direction of 2. How much or to what degree 3. How many; number	1. The patient went **to** the office. 2. The patient's mother came, **too**. 3. The **two** walked to the door together.
1. your 2. you're	1. Belonging to you 2. Contraction for "you are"	1. You dropped **your** pen. 2. **You're** going to pass the test.

*To identify the correct word or meaning, decide how the word is used in the sentence.

replace, the receptionist. All incoming calls are immediately routed to the proper location (e.g., prescription refills, scheduling or billing department). Setting up a voice mail system can be done through the telephone company or by purchasing a software package.

Advantages
- People can call all day or at any hour to leave a message.
- Messages can be retrieved from other locations.
- Length of the message is reduced because communication is only one way.

Disadvantages
- Some people want to speak to a person immediately.
- Some messages may be incoherent.

Website

A *website* usually is created to provide information about the practice to patients and the community. Items that may be on a website include but are not limited to the following:
1. Directions to the practice
2. Hours of operation
3. Practice philosophy
4. Billing and insurance information
5. Information on the medical staff
6. Answers to the most frequently asked questions (FAQs)

Advantages
- Websites can answer some types of questions (e.g., hours, location, and services) and save patients the time and effort of calling to ask.
- Websites can be quickly updated and are available 24 hours a day, 7 days a week.

Disadvantages
- All patients may not have access to the Internet.
- Providing a website may require staff members who can develop, program, and maintain the technical aspects of the website.

Fax Machine

A **facsimile,** or **fax,** machine converts written material or pictures into electronic impulses that are transmitted by telephone lines to other locations with similar equipment. Received messages are recorded magnetically and printed as a *hard copy* (on paper) by using a computer printer or fax machine. The material received is a duplicate of the original that was sent. Box 7-7 lists some important considerations for faxing materials.

Advantages
- Messages are sent and received rapidly.
- Faxing materials is often relatively inexpensive.
- Faxes are now considered forms of original and legal documents.

BOX 7-7

Fax Transmission Protocol

- Health information should only be faxed when absolutely necessary.
- For any fax using thermal paper, the fax should be photocopied before filing in the patient's record because the print on thermal paper fades over time.
- Always use a cover sheet when faxing materials. Include the sender's and the receiver's telephone numbers, fax numbers, and the name of the contact person, as well as a confidentiality disclaimer.
- Ask for the receiving office to confirm receipt of the material.
- If information is confidential, arrange for the recipient to be available when the office will fax the documents.

BOX 7-8

E-Mail Etiquette

1. Keep messages professional and to the point.
2. Do not type in "ALL CAPS." This creates the impression of shouting or yelling.
3. Use the "spell check" to create a professional document.
4. Respond to e-mail messages in a timely manner.
5. Be respectful to the receiver. Avoid sarcasm.
6. Do not forward copies of an e-mail to others unless instructed to do so by the sender.
7. Do not send confidential information.

Disadvantages
- Extra care must be taken to maintain patient confidentiality when faxing.
- Not all patients have access to a fax machine.

Electronic Mail

Written messages can be transmitted by electronic mail *(e-mail)*. Messages are sent as electronic signals from one computer to another. E-mail is faster and less expensive than mailing a letter. Office e-mail messages should be answered at least once a day. E-mail is becoming more and more common. To communicate clearly and professionally, follow established "etiquette" guidelines (proper form and manners) when e-mailing (Box 7-8).

Advantages
- Messages can be sent to groups of people at one time (e.g., all Medicare patients).
- E-mail is available 24 hours a day.
- Messages are sent and received rapidly.
- Sender can verify that messages were received.
- Staff is not making multiple phone calls or stuffing letters.

Disadvantages

- It is easy to send a message to the wrong person and thus jeopardize patient confidentiality.
- Once a message is sent, it often cannot be "unsent" or canceled.
- All patients may not have access to e-mail.

> **PATIENT-CENTERED PROFESSIONALISM**
>
> - *How are patients affected when medical assistants do not know and follow established guidelines when using electronic technology (e.g., voice mail, fax, or e-mail)?*
> - *How can you help ensure electronic technology is used in a way that provides convenience to patients but does not make them feel as if they are "just another patient"?*

CONCLUSION

A medical assistant relies on some form of communication every day to exchange information with patients. Communication must be clear, correct, and professional. The way you communicate creates an impression of you and the entire health care team. Communicating effectively and listening actively help reduce misunderstandings and mistakes in the medical office. You can improve your communication skills by understanding, applying, and practicing the principles of effective verbal, nonverbal, and written communication. Effective communication skills are an essential component of patient-centered professionalism.

Chapter Summary

Reinforce your understanding of the material in this chapter by reviewing the curriculum objectives and key content points below.

1. **Define, appropriately use, and spell all the Key Terms for this chapter.**
   - Review the Key Terms if necessary.
2. **State the goal of the communication process.**
   - Communication is the sharing of information.
3. **List and describe the three components of the communication process.**
   - The sender can be the patient or the medical assistant.
   - The receiver can be the patient or the medical assistant.
   - The message must be clearly conveyed by the sender and needs to be understood by the receiver.
4. **List and describe the four steps in sending a message that will be understood.**
   - To send a message that will be understood, the sender must organize the message, prioritize the information, transmit the message, and evaluate the effectiveness of the message.
5. **List the three types of distracters that can prevent a message from being sent or received.**
   - The environment, improper use of grammar, and physical well-being can be major distracters when sending or receiving a message.
6. **Explain how a verbal message can be misinterpreted.**
   - Improper grammar, lack of understanding on the part of the listener, and biased or negative attitudes can cause messages to be misinterpreted.
7. **Explain the process of sending a verbal message and evaluating its receipt.**
   - To be heard, the sender must organize a message logically and deliver it to the receiver in a manner that is easily understood.
   - After a message has been sent, the sender must evaluate the effectiveness of the transmission.
8. **List and describe three ways that people communicate nonverbally.**
   - Nonverbal communication includes body language, appearance, and the distance between two people when communicating.
9. **Explain how a nonverbal message can be misinterpreted.**
   - When analyzing a message being sent, the receiver must evaluate both verbal and nonverbal communications. When nonverbal communication does not match the verbal communication, conflicting messages are sent.
   - Patients of different cultures may have different beliefs and standards concerning body language.
10. **List the three components of effective listening.**
    - Effective listening requires that a listener concentrates, analyzes, and provides feedback.
11. **Compare and contrast active and passive listening and give an example of each.**
    - Active listening requires the listener to respond to the speaker's message with some type of verbal or nonverbal feedback (e.g., answer to a direct question).
    - Passive listening does not require the recipient's full attention (e.g., talking on the phone while watching TV).
12. **State six steps to becoming a better listener.**
    - Analyze or evaluate the speaker's words, posture, facial expressions, tone, mannerisms, and general appearance.
    - Refer to Table 7-2.

13. **Recognize the parts of speech and give an example of each.**
    - Every sentence must have a subject and a verb.
    - Words are classified into eight components, or parts of speech.
    - Refer to Table 7-3.
14. **Demonstrate correct use of punctuation.**
    - The way a sentence is written or spoken can alter the meaning of that sentence (e.g., "The panda eats shoots and leaves" versus "The panda eats, shoots, and leaves").
15. **Explain the importance of choosing the correct words.**
    - Some words sound alike and can cause miscommunication if not used properly (e.g., patients versus patience).
    - Miscommunication can lead to costly mistakes (e.g., ilium versus ileum).
16. **List six words that are frequently misspelled in the medical office.**
    - Refer to Box 7-5.
    - Medical terminology must be spelled correctly or errors can occur in record keeping, billing, or even treatment.
17. **Explain the importance of understanding how to communicate effectively using electronic technology.**
    - It is essential for medical assistants to be comfortable communicating with electronic technology because it is part of everyday life.
18. **List the different types of electronic technology used for communication in a medical office.**
    - Medical offices use voice mail systems, websites, fax machines, and e-mail to communicate with patients and other health professionals.
19. **List six guidelines for e-mail etiquette.**
    - Be just as courteous and professional in e-mail communication as you would on the phone, in a letter, or face-to-face. Never type in all capital letters; you will appear to be yelling at the recipient.
    - Use "spell check" before you send e-mail.
    - Be concise and professional in tone.
    - Respond to e-mails in a timely manner.
    - Do not send confidential information via e-mail.
20. **Analyze a realistic medical office situation and apply your understanding of effective communication to determine the best course of action.**
    - Cultural and ethnic barriers can cause misunderstandings and miscommunication.
    - Make every attempt to understand what patients may be communicating with their actions and expressions in addition to what they say.
21. **Describe the impact on patient care when medical assistants consistently apply the principles of effective communication.**
    - When communication is effective, confusion or even dangerous mistakes can be avoided and patient care is not adversely impacted.

PRACTICAL APPLICATIONS

If you have accomplished the objectives in this chapter, you will be able to make better choices as a medical assistant. Take another look at this situation and decide what you would do.

Panina is a former resident of the Middle East who moved to the United States with her husband, Abed, 6 months ago. Naturally, she brings the cultural and ethnic contexts of her homeland with her. Panina awakens one morning with a pain in her breast. She becomes concerned and calls a physician's office for an appointment. Because she has difficulty understanding the English language, she misunderstands the appointment time and Panina and Abed arrive at the office an hour late. Abed demands to accompany his wife to the examining room. Therese, the medical assistant, tells Abed that they are late for the appointment and that he must stay in the waiting room while Panina is being examined. Panina, refusing eye contact with Therese, begins to cry. Abed becomes upset and tells Therese that the only way Panina will be examined is if he accompanies her to the room to explain to the male doctor what is wrong with her. Therese refuses, and Panina and Abed leave the office, threatening to tell all their friends how this office "just does not care about patients at all."

Effective communication helps eliminate misunderstandings. If you were the medical assistant in this situation, how could you have used your understanding of effective communication skills to help?

1. What role did Panina and Abed's cultural and ethnic background play in the misunderstandings in the physician's office? What role did communication skills play in the misunderstandings?
2. What distracters may have caused the lack of communication between Panina and Therese?
3. What nonverbal communication between Panina and Therese could have been recognized and used to diffuse the negative situation that occurred in the physician's office?
4. Why is an understanding of ethnicity and cultural differences so important in the medical field?
5. What body parts are involved in the communication of body language?

WEB SEARCH

1. **Research the topic of communication to improve your communication skills.** Communication skills are crucial to a successful patient–medical assistant relationship. Locate information on ways you can communicate more clearly with patients and help establish good relationships.
   - **Keywords:** Use the following keywords in your search: communicating with patients, communication techniques, communication.

2. **Research techniques for interpreting nonverbal communication.** Patients provide a wealth of information nonverbally about their feelings, beliefs, and comfort. Understanding how to interpret a patient's body language is important for effective communication.
   - **Keywords:** Use the following keywords in your search: nonverbal communication, body language, patient body language.

3. **Research effective listening techniques to improve your listening skills.** Even if you are not a good listener, you can improve through learning and practice. Locate information and tips on how to be a better listener.
   - **Keywords:** Use the following keywords in your search: listening skills, listening to patients.

4. **Research effective written communication to improve your writing skills.** As with listening, writing skills can be improved through learning and practice. Locate information and tips on how you can improve your writing skills.
   - **Keywords:** Use the following keywords in your search: writing skills, writing styles, grammar, spelling.

5. **Research communication through electronic technology.** Current advances in technology allow patients or prospective patients to communicate with or gather information about the medical practice. Locate information and tips on how you can use electronic technology to communicate effectively in the medical office.
   - **Keywords:** Use the following keywords in your search: website creation, facsimile, electronic mail, voice mail, computers in medical practice.

8 Communicating with Patients

evolve   http://evolve.elsevier.com/klieger/medicalassisting

Communicating effectively with patients should be the primary goal of the medical office staff. As a medical assistant, you will be expected to listen to, understand, and even anticipate patient needs. Each patient must be treated as an individual, and the staff's actions must convey to patients that each individual is important.

This chapter helps you learn to apply the principles of effective communication discussed in Chapter 7 with patients in a medical setting and introduces you to one of the most important aspects of the medical assistant's career roles—patient education.

Patient education is the process of influencing patient behavior and causing the necessary changes in patient knowledge, attitudes, and skills that will maintain or improve the patient's health. Through patient education, medical assistants can help ensure that the prescribed treatment plan will be followed correctly. In addition, patient education is an opportunity to establish and build trusting relationships with patients.

Throughout this text, you will be introduced to many aspects of patient preparation and patient teaching necessary for performing and preparing for clinical examinations, procedures, and diagnostic tests.

LEARNING OBJECTIVES

You will be able to do the following after completing this chapter:

Key Terms
1. Define, appropriately use, and spell all the Key Terms for this chapter.

Role of the Medical Assistant
2. Understand the role of the medical assistant in patient communication.
3. Explain the concept of *holistic* care.
4. Discuss four effective communication techniques and three barriers to avoid when communicating with the patient.
5. List five ways you can improve communication with patients, and explain how better communication improves patient care and results in good service.
6. Explain the importance of handling patient complaints effectively.

Different Cultures
7. List three ways to establish trust with patients of different cultures.

Patients with Special Needs
8. List five considerations for communicating with a patient who is visually impaired.
9. List seven ways to communicate effectively with a patient who has a hearing impairment.
10. List three considerations for accommodating patients with other physical disabilities.
11. List six considerations for communicating effectively with elderly patients.
12. List six considerations for communicating effectively with children.
13. Explain the considerations for communicating with patients with a below-normal ability to reason or think, with mental impairments, or with developmental delays.
14. Explain the importance of communicating effectively with the caregivers and families of mentally impaired and developmentally delayed patients.

Patient Education
15. Explain the importance of patient education.

Patient-Centered Professionalism
16. Analyze a realistic medical office situation and apply your understanding of effective communication with patients to determine the best course of action.
17. Describe the impact on patient care when medical assistants consistently apply the principles of effective communication when interacting with patients.

KEY TERMS

affective
cognitive
holistic
litigation
maturation
patient education
psychomotor
psychosocial
rapport

PRACTICAL APPLICATIONS

Read the following scenario and keep it in mind as you learn about communicating with patients and the role of the medical assistant in this chapter.

Mr. Joplin is a spry 82-year-old and still lives in his own home. His wife died about a year ago, but Mr. Joplin has no severe medical problems and is able to care for himself. He does have visual problems caused by cataracts in his left eye, as well as joint stiffness related to his age. John, the medical assistant, approaches Mr. Joplin to escort him to the examining room. John shouts at Mr. Joplin as if he has a hearing difficulty, then walks away without assisting Mr. Joplin from the chair. When John reaches the door, he looks over his shoulder, rolls his eyes, and shouts, "Do you need some help?" Mr. Joplin looks away and refuses any assistance. Dr. Smith examines Mr. Joplin and asks John to explain the treatment so Mr. Joplin will comply. John hurriedly tells Mr. Joplin one time what is expected, then returns him to the waiting room. Several days later, Mr. Joplin calls the office to tell the receptionist to cancel his next appointment because he is going to find a new physician.

John's poor communication skills caused Dr. Smith to lose Mr. Joplin as a patient. If you were the medical assistant in this situation, what would you have done to communicate more effectively with Mr. Joplin?

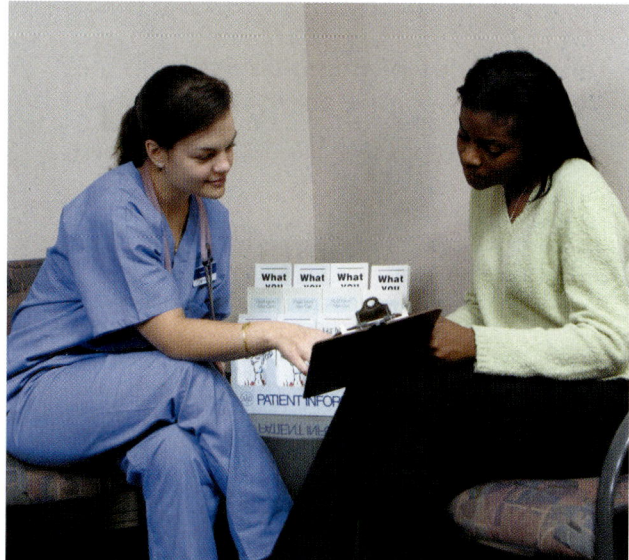

FIGURE 8-1 Through positive communication techniques, the medical assistant can meet the needs of the patient.

patient's treatment. By using positive communication techniques, medical assistants can help ensure that patient needs are met and that their experience is positive (Figure 8-1).

Keep in mind that patients' needs are not limited to their illness alone. **Holistic** health care deals with all the needs of the patient, including physical, emotional, social, economic, and spiritual needs. All of a patient's needs influence his or her behavior and compliance with treatment. This is why medical assistants must address all patient needs. A patient may not comply with treatment when he or she is nervous, angry, frightened, or confused about the illness or has financial problems. You must use what you have learned about human relations and behavior to develop a working **rapport** with patients. For example:

> A patient undergoing treatment for muscle spasms definitely has physical needs, but you must also consider the patient's emotional needs and feelings about treatment. Consider where this patient is on Maslow's Hierarchy of Needs (see Chapter 5). If the muscle spasms result in missed work, the patient may be worried about money for treatment, food, rent, and other necessities.

Box 8-1 lists ways you can apply the principles of communication to address patient needs and concerns.

ROLE OF THE MEDICAL ASSISTANT

As an employee, the medical assistant has a responsibility to the physician and the patient to provide quality care. Communicating effectively with patients is a key factor in providing quality care. The medical assistant's role in promoting effective communication is to focus on the "customers" (patients) and their needs, strive for continuous improvement, and effectively handle patient complaints.

Focusing on the Patient

Patients and their families feel respected and well taken care of when their needs are met and their concerns are addressed immediately. When patients perceive that they are important to the health care team, they tend to follow the physician's plan of care. The medical assistant is the communication link between the patient and the physician, and thus the medical assistant–patient relationship could be key to the success of a

Striving for Improvement

Finding better ways to communicate with your patients will result in quality service and patient care. Identifying the patient's understanding of the disease process, treatments involved, and tests to be performed is necessary to meet the needs of the patient. You can assess patient understanding and improve communication in the following ways:

- Communicate in simple, everyday language. Table 8-1 provides a list of positive, or therapeutic, communica-

BOX 8-1

Ten Principles of Communication in the Medical Assistant–Patient Relationship

1. Greet every patient and family member with a smile and a kind word.
2. Introduce yourself.
3. Explain all procedures before beginning the procedure and provide updates, no matter how minor.
4. Leave sufficient time for questions and answers.
5. Be available to listen when the patient has a need to complain or talk.
6. Try to resolve an issue without delay, or find someone who can resolve it.
7. Maintain a pleasant demeanor throughout the day even when stressed.
8. Dismiss the patient with a smile and a kind word.
9. Provide clear written instructions so that the patient is aware of follow-up plans.
10. Keep the patient informed with prompt phone calls (when appropriate) regarding test results. Remember that the patient is anxious and waiting.

tion techniques often used for effective communication. If overused, they become ineffective.

- Ask patients to write down questions so the issues can be explained, reinforced, and discussed to clear up misunderstandings.
- Match your approach to the patient's level of readiness and ability to learn (Figure 8-2).
- Identify any barriers to communication that may be evident, such as a history of noncompliance, a language barrier, reading ability, or physical or emotional state. Table 8-2 provides a list of communication barriers (nontherapeutic techniques) to effective communication that need to be avoided when communicating with the patient.
- Do not be afraid to say, "I don't know the answer." Remember that medical assistants do not know everything, but they do know how to find the answers.

Box 8-2 provides suggestions for improving communication during patient teaching. Effective use and working knowledge of both positive communication techniques and barriers to avoid will enhance patient care and interactions with family and patients throughout the treatment plan.

TABLE 8-1

Positive Communication Techniques

Technique and Meaning	Example	Value
CLARIFYING Seeks additional input from the patient to make clear that which is vague and to better understand the message received.	**Patient:** "When I walk I have this terrible pain in my leg." **MA:** "Tell me what you mean by terrible" or "Describe this pain."	Ensures no miscommunication and demonstrates to the patient a true interest in what the patient is saying.
FOCUSING Expands or develops a single idea or point of view.	**Patient:** "I have so many things I'm responsible for, my kids, my husband, my parents, my job." **MA:** "Of all the responsibilities you've mentioned, which is causing you the most worry?"	Directs the patient's energies to one topic.
REFLECTING Directs the patient's ideas, actions, thoughts, and feelings back to the patient.	**Patient:** "I am so upset; I thought I would be well by now!" **MA:** "You sound upset that you're not fully recovered from your stroke."	Allows the patient to hear and think about what he or she said and indicates that the patient's point of view has value.
RESTATING Paraphrasing or repeating the main thought or idea expressed by the patient.	**Patient:** "I can't sleep; I stay awake all night." **MA:** "You're having a problem sleeping?"	Lets the patient know that he or she has communicated his or her thoughts effectively.
SILENCE Periods of no verbal communication.	**Patient:** "I don't know how to explain it." **MA:** Needs to be aware of patient's nonverbal behavior. Says nothing but continues to maintain eye contact and show interest.	Can convey acceptance, support, and concern and allows the patient to organize his or her thoughts.
SUMMARIZING Organizes and sums up that which has gone on before and is a statement of main ideas expressed during an interaction.	**Patient:** Interaction has taken place between the patient and the medical assistant. **MA:** "We have discussed …"	Important process since it serves as a review of information exchanged and allows both the patient and the medical assistant to come to an agreement about what has been discussed.

Handling Patient Complaints

A patient may complain if he or she perceives the quality of the service to be unsatisfactory. Patient complaints generally fall into one of the following two categories:

1. *Administrative complaints* occur when the patient is unhappy with the performance of the support staff. Dissatisfaction may come from miscommunication or misunderstandings related to billing issues, telephone response time, waiting time, or office reception.
2. *Medical complaints* involve dissatisfaction with appointment access, poor referral follow-up, quality of service by the physician or clinical personnel, and limitation or denial of benefits.

Handling patient complaints requires the cooperation of all members of the health care team. Working together reduces the risk of a complaint not being handled promptly and can help relieve patient anxiety and hostility. Often, patients are angry and upset, as well as hostile, when voicing complaints. First, move the patient to a quiet area where they can vent their frustration out of view of the rest of the patients. Remain calm and matter of fact, and never return anger with anger. Handling patient complaints effectively can reduce the risk of **litigation** (a lawsuit). The following guidelines are useful for handling patient complaints:

- Take all complaints *seriously*. Write out all the facts of the complaint, no matter how trivial. Some complaints cannot be resolved, but they can be addressed.

> **BOX 8-2**
>
> ### Effective Communication for Patient Teaching
>
> 1. Assess the patient's readiness to learn. Ask yourself:
>   - Is the patient's appearance, behavior, and communication appropriate to the situation and age?
>   - Is the patient able to understand and participate in the treatment plan?
> 2. Include the patient's family or support group in the treatment plan, if the patient agrees.
> 3. Allow adequate time for demonstration and return demonstration by the patient. Use positive reinforcement such as, "Yes, that is correct."
> 4. Provide time for questions and concerns to be expressed by the patient. Provide honest answers only within the scope of medical assisting training.
> 5. Assist patients in fitting the new behavior or procedure into their normal activities (e.g., a patient required to exercise may need suggestions for starting a routine).
> 6. Use age-appropriate wording and learning materials for better understanding.
> 7. Chart patients' reactions and comments concerning their level of understanding.

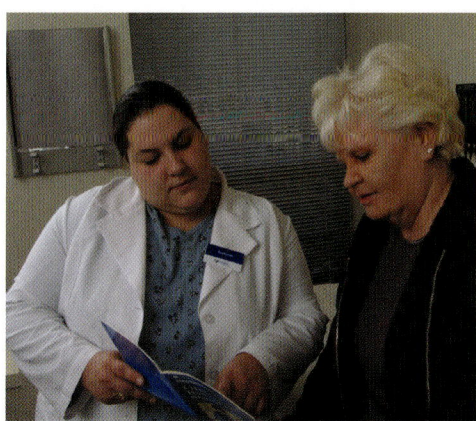

FIGURE 8-2 The medical assistant needs to individualize teaching techniques to match the patient's level of readiness.

TABLE 8-2

Barriers to Effective Communication

Technique and Meaning	Example	Threat
DEFENDING Attempting to protect someone or something from negative verbal attack.	**Patient:** "I don't like the way my doctor is handling my care." **MA:** "I'm sure your doctor has your best interests in mind."	Does not allow a patient to express an opinion; blocks further communication.
CHANGING TOPICS Introducing unrelated subjects.	**Patient:** "I'm feeling depressed." **MA:** "Have you been exercising?"	Redirects patient's concerns and implies that his or her concerns are of no value.
MAKING STEREOTYPED COMMENTS Using trite or meaningless responses.	**Patient:** "I'm too scared to have surgery." **MA:** "It's for your own good."	Implies patient's thoughts are unimportant.
REJECTING Refusing to discuss ideas or topics with the patient.	**Patient:** "I might as well just die and get it over with." **MA:** "That's silly! I don't want to hear that."	Approach closes off topic from further discussion and patient may feel rejected.

- Use *tactful* (inoffensive) language when responding to a complaint, and reassure the patient that the complaint will be investigated. Give the patient a time frame for resolution, and follow through with this plan.
- *Always* alert the physician or office manager about an unhappy patient so that he or she can defuse the situation immediately.
- *Always* inform the physician or office manager of any statements made by the patient that reflect a negative attitude. The patient's statements may reflect noncompliance with the prescribed treatment and could compromise the patient's ability to heal properly.

A large number of lawsuits result from careless actions or comments made by physicians and office staff when patients complain. A medical practice is less likely to be sued if the staff shows genuine concern for the patient's well-being by taking steps to correct problems promptly. Patients may not always remember what you did or what you said, but they will always remember *how* you made them feel. Another reason to take patient complaints seriously is because they may affect how managed care companies and state and federal agencies view the practice. Medicare has strict guidelines for handling patient complaints, and failure to follow them can lead to loss of service privileges.

PATIENT-CENTERED PROFESSIONALISM

- *How does understanding the many aspects of a patient's illness (including effects on the patient's lifestyle, work, and family) allow medical assistants to provide better patient care?*
- *What can medical assistants do to improve their communication skills with the patient? How can a medical assistant with good communication skills impact the patient's experience?*
- *Why do you think patients are less likely to sue when their complaints have been taken seriously?*

DIFFERENT CULTURES

In Chapter 6, you learned how culture and belief systems affect patient behavior. In the same way, culture and belief systems also affect the way patients perceive what the health care team says and does. It is important to understand how to communicate effectively with patients of different cultures. Providing high-quality patient care means meeting patient needs in a manner that invokes trust, shows respect for cultural beliefs, and allows patients to maintain their dignity. This can only be accomplished by understanding patients' cultural systems and standard health procedures, family interactions, and value systems. Using your understanding of patients' cultural systems in your communication approach and eliminating negative personal beliefs will help you provide quality care to patients of all cultures.

Approach

As you have learned, your actions (nonverbal communication) and words (verbal communication) should take into consideration the patient's beliefs and level of understanding. All treatment plans must allow patients to maintain their self-esteem and help establish trust in the health care team. Ways to accomplish this are as follows:

- Involve the patient and patient's family in the decision-making process when possible. Encourage them to include their cultural beliefs if appropriate.
- Ask the patient's opinion, and encourage the patient to discuss issues and potential problems.
- Do not embarrass or anger the patient by arguing about his or her beliefs.
- Be sensitive to patients' needs as individuals to help avoid cultural conflicts.
- Demonstrate active listening, or patients may feel that they are not important to you.
- Provide honest feedback to patients continuously to demonstrate respect for their feelings.

As a medical assistant, you must strive to accommodate every patient's needs. When given individualized care and shown respect, a patient is more likely to follow a treatment plan.

Personal Beliefs

All patients need to be treated with dignity and respect. You will encounter patients whose cultural beliefs differ from your own. Stereotyping and any form of discrimination are not acceptable and cannot be tolerated. You must get rid of any negative beliefs so they do not affect your communication with or care for patients.

Not listening to or refusing to understand a particular culture's point of view limits the effectiveness of the health care process. If you show resistance in accepting a patient's cultural heritage or religious beliefs, the trust necessary for effective treatment may be weakened or destroyed. The following guidelines can help you eliminate personal beliefs that are barriers to effective communication with patients:

- Do a perception check. Discuss your interpretation of the situation with the patient to see if it is correct; be specific.
- Listen to the patient's explanation and be empathetic to his or her situation.
- Answer questions within your scope of training. With the physician's guidance, explain the reasons for the needed changes and the importance of compliance.
- After the physician has explained the possible consequences of not following a treatment plan, be supportive.
- Respect the patient's decision and avoid a judgmental attitude.

Remember that the physician guides the patient care process. The medical assistant's role is an extension of the quality care process. You represent your physician, so "mirror your physician's image" to show acceptance of cultural differences.

> **PATIENT-CENTERED PROFESSIONALISM**
>
> - *How can the medical assistant know if patients of other cultures understand what is expected of them?*
> - *What nonverbal communication do you currently use that could be misinterpreted by a patient of a different culture?*

PATIENTS WITH SPECIAL NEEDS

In previous chapters, you learned how important it is to place yourself in the patient's situation. Empathy allows you to consider how a patient might feel and helps you anticipate the patient's needs. When working with patients who have special needs, this tactic is especially important. Patients with special needs may have increased anxiety because of their current illness and unfamiliar surroundings. You have a responsibility to recognize this and strive to reduce their anxiety. Do not rush these patients. Be helpful, but do not take away their dignity by automatically assuming they are not able to do something. Always ask if you can help first. If one method of communication is not working, combine it with another approach (e.g., visual aids, help from family members). Patients with special needs include those with disabilities, children and elderly persons, those with lower levels of understanding, and those with mental impairment.

Disabilities

There are many types of disabilities. In the medical office, you will work with patients who have impaired vision, impaired hearing, diminished mental capacity, and other physical disabilities. It is important to understand how to apply effective communication skills with patients having all types of disabilities.

Visual Impairment

Vision problems, such as *total blindness, presbyopia, macular degeneration, cataracts,* and *glaucoma,* all affect the ability to see. Patients may have varying degrees of sight. Unless totally blind, a patient may benefit from having written materials enlarged. A totally blind patient can benefit from instructions given on an audiocassette. Always encourage questions and obtain feedback. Guidelines for communicating with patients who have visual difficulties include the following:

- Make the patient comfortable in the unfamiliar surroundings (e.g., "Ms. Konters, the treatment room we are entering has an examination table, a chair, and a cabinet with a countertop for supplies").
- Always explain what you are going to do and alert patients before touching them (e.g., "Mr. Samuel, I am going to give you an injection in your right upper arm").
- Prevent patients from falling into or over objects by providing verbal directions (e.g., "Mrs. Jones, I will need you to move forward four steps to the chair").
- Do not increase voice volume (these patients are not hearing-impaired).

Hearing Impairment

Hearing loss is suspected when a patient speaks or responds inappropriately to a situation. Occasionally, families will comment on the patient's social withdrawal and the increased volume of the television or the radio. When you are aware of a patient's hearing loss, it is best to communicate by restating directions. Also, provide the patient with written directions. Several ways to communicate effectively with a hearing-impaired patient are as follows:

- Directly face the patient when speaking.
- When the patient is not facing you, touch the patient's arm or shoulder before speaking.
- Speak clearly in a natural tone and at a normal rate of speech; do not yell or shout.
- Use hand gestures and facial expressions as cues.
- Use visual examples and reading materials.
- Involve family or close friends and provide them with all information given to the patient.
- Minimize distractions from the environment.

Other Physical Disabilities

There are many other types of physical disabilities. Physically disabled patients require attention directly associated with their impairments. When helping physically disabled patients set goals, the medical assistant encourages realistic goals using their existing abilities to help them achieve the highest possible satisfaction and enrichment in life. Because of advances in biomedical engineering, many devices now allow disabled people to become more functional and less dependent on others.

Patients with disabilities do not expect sympathy or special considerations. They do expect that you care about them as individual patients with unique needs. Your tone of voice should reflect this caring attitude.

Age

As people age, they experience a decline in vision and hearing. This makes it difficult for the elderly patient to collect information from the surroundings. In addition, changes occur in the senses of smell, taste, and touch. Box 8-3 offers suggestions for communicating with elderly patients effectively.

At the other end of the spectrum are pediatric patients. When communicating with children, use wording and methods that are appropriate to their age, ethnicity, and level of understanding. Be familiar with the growth and developmental stages of children (see Chapter 6) so that you can communicate more effectively with them and their parents. Box 8-4 provides tips for communicating with children.

Intelligence

Some patients with special needs may have difficulty understanding or a below-normal ability to think and reason. You

BOX 8-3

Communicating with Elderly Patients

- Be an empathetic listener. This shows recognition of the aging person's hearing and visual changes, fatigue, and pain (Figure 8-3).
- If the patient wears a hearing aid, allow time for the person to adjust the volume if necessary.
- Do not shout at a hearing-impaired patient. Shouting is often associated with anger or displeasure. Speak in a low tone of voice close to the patient's good ear or directly in front of the person.
- Be careful of body language. If an elderly patient perceives you as "too busy," the patient may not report serious concerns.
- Speak clearly and slowly, using short sentences with slight pauses. Do not give lengthy explanations.
- Be patient, and wait for the elderly patient to respond. The aging process may delay the speed at which elderly patients can organize their thoughts and speech.

BOX 8-4

Communicating with Children

- Use dolls, pictures, and other models to enhance communication.
- Let children speak at their own speed. Do not rush or supply words for them; let them complete their own thoughts and sentences.
- Encourage children to talk about themselves.
- Talk to children with words they can easily understand.
- Recognize situations that might be upsetting to children and try to reassure them.
- Allow children to handle safe medical equipment (e.g., stethoscope, blood pressure cuff) (Figure 8-4).
- Sit down or bend down to talk with a child. Be at their level.

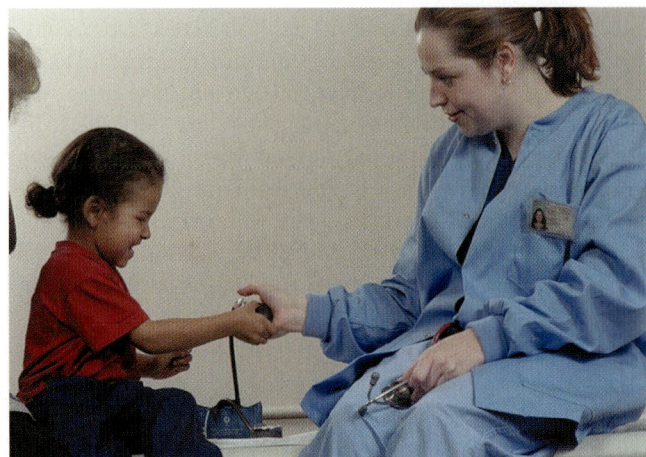

FIGURE 8-4 Children understand procedures better if they handle the equipment.

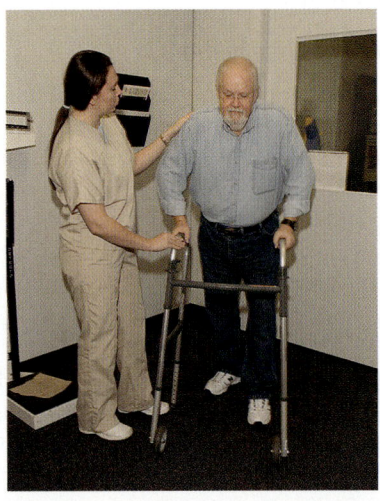

FIGURE 8-3 The medical assistant must recognize that the aging process puts limitations on the elderly patient.

must determine the patient's level of understanding and adjust your communication accordingly. You can adjust communication in these situations in the following ways:

- Use both verbal and nonverbal clues to assess both the patient's ability to read and the patient's educational and emotional background. You must adapt to the patient's ability to understand.
- Allow more time for recall because people process information at different speeds. The aging process can also delay recall.
- Do not overload the patient with information. Instead, provide small portions and evaluate feedback before moving forward with new information. Repeat or rephrase material when needed.

Finally, determine how well the information has been received. Do not mistake a patient's understanding if he or she nods and smiles when necessary information is provided. Ask questions about information that has been provided or have the patient do a return demonstration when possible.

Mental Impairment

The ability to process new information and apply it appropriately in a given setting reflects a patient's mental functioning. A person is diagnosed as mentally challenged when the person functions at a lower-than-normal intellectual level. People who are mentally challenged cannot think abstractly. They learn through repetition and habit (e.g., using the same routine daily). When communicating with mentally challenged patients, the atmosphere must be relaxed, and only one direction should be given at a time.

To communicate effectively with mentally impaired patients, you must obtain information from the caregiver about the patient's habits, routines, and personal terminology (e.g., nicknames). Rushing these individuals causes stress and may reduce their cooperation. Mentally challenged patients need to be treated with the same respect that all patients deserve.

Developmentally delayed patients are those who lag behind in **maturation.** They should not be confused with mentally impaired patients. Areas of concern with these patients include not only their mental ability but also their physical, social, and emotional functioning. To communicate effectively with developmentally delayed patients, the medical assistant needs to address their level of maturation not their chronological age. For example, an infant who is deprived of physical contact or nutrition will not progress at the same rate as an infant who receives these basic needs. The way you interact with this infant may be quite different from the way you interact with the infant who has received the basic needs.

Providing caregivers with a list of available community resources is a valuable service. Many communities have support groups and special day care centers equipped to handle mentally handicapped or developmentally delayed individuals.

> **PATIENT-CENTERED PROFESSIONALISM**
>
> - How does understanding the emotional and physical needs of a patient with special needs improve the quality of care?
> - Why is it important to understand a patient's limitations? Give an example of how understanding a patient's limitations can result in a positive patient experience.

PATIENT EDUCATION

The goal of any treatment for a disease or condition is to manage it successfully and eliminate it if possible. Successful management requires that the patient be well informed about the illness, as well as the necessary actions for controlling or correcting it. Changes in patient behavior, including dietary habits, lifestyle, and use of medications, are often important parts of the prescribed treatment plan. Understanding their illness and how it is controlled or corrected influences patients' behaviors and increases the likelihood that the treatment plan will be followed. Effective **patient education** is the key to helping patients understand the situation and the need for these changes.

A solid understanding of human behavior and effective communication techniques are necessary to perform effective patient education.

In addition to understanding human behavior and communication principles, medical assistants should know about different learning styles, as well as what takes place during the teaching process.

Learning Styles

People learn in different ways. You may have known people who learned best by doing or who learned best by watching someone else. Other people learn best by reading or listening to someone speak about how to do the task. Keeping in mind that people learn in different ways will help you find the best way to educate each individual patient. It is best to discuss expectations and goals with the patient and allow the patient to be part of developing a treatment plan. This also helps the medical assistant determine how the patient learns or processes information.

Three types of learning are cognitive, affective, and psychomotor. Learning experiences that incorporate all three types of learning are most effective because they address the whole patient.

> **FOR YOUR INFORMATION**
>
> EFFECTIVE PATIENT EDUCATION = UNDERSTANDING HUMAN BEHAVIOR + GOOD COMMUNICATION
>
> *Applying what you learned in Chapters 5 and 6 about human behavior and Chapters 7 and 8 about interpersonal communication should make the process of patient education easier.*
>
> - *Human behavior. Before a patient will be receptive to changes in behavior, the patient's basic human needs must be met. The patient must feel safe from the embarrassment that can result from lack of knowledge or differing cultural beliefs. For the patient to learn, he or she must be convinced that what is being taught is of value, is an attainable goal, and is something that can be used immediately.*
> - *Interpersonal communication. During communication, both verbal and nonverbal messages are sent and received. These messages are influenced by a variety of factors, including environment, personal space, cultural beliefs, perception, developmental stage, language mastery, and a feeling of self-worth. The patient must have the time to listen to the information. For example, if diet information is to be provided to a patient newly diagnosed with diabetes, the patient must have the time available to listen and be able to ask questions.*

Cognitive Learning

Cognitive learning is based on what a person already knows or has experienced. Memory or recall can stimulate the thought process, allowing a person to use information to analyze, plan, and evaluate a situation. Patients generally know something about a variety of health issues. When the medical assistant interviews the patient, this information can be used to create a baseline from which to start.

Learning occurs when the patient can understand information presented and when he or she places a significant meaning to its importance. This process may occur when the medical assistant demonstrates adequate knowledge about the subject area.

Affective Learning

A person's **affective** ability is concerned with the person's emotions and feelings. These, along with a person's attitudes, will cause one person to respond to a given situation or illness differently than someone else. In addition, the patient's ability to learn is affected by his or her emotions, feelings, and attitudes about health care.

The medical assistant's role is to determine how a particular patient's emotions will guide or affect the patient's ability to learn and follow through with established goals. Sincere positive feedback from the medical assistant will build a feeling of confidence in a patient.

Psychomotor Learning

Psychomotor ability relates to movement or muscular activity associated with mental processes. A patient's physical capabilities must be considered when teaching and must be treated with respect at all times throughout the patient education process. The medical assistant must be aware of the patient's ability to perform the required skill.

Teaching Process

The teaching-learning process is a critical part of the medical practice, and again, patient education is an important role of the medical assistant. To perform this role successfully, medical assistants must meet the patient's learning needs. The key to patient teaching is not to focus on how to make the patient do something, but to create a situation in which the patient will *want* to do what is needed. The process begins by assessing the patient, moving to form a plan and implementing the plan, and ends by evaluating the process.

Assess

Once the patient's learning needs have been identified, the medical assistant needs to take a quick inventory of the patient's readiness to learn by asking the following questions:

- Is the patient physically and emotionally ready for the health information to be presented? For example, does the patient have any visual or hearing difficulties? Can the patient handle the equipment? Changes associated with aging or disease process may affect the patient's ability to perform a skill.
- Will the patient be able to adapt to any **psychosocial** restrictions (e.g., alcohol)?
- Are the patient's health beliefs, behavior, and expectations in line with the treatment plan?
- What does the patient already know or understand about the illness or procedure? Checking for understanding is a critical element in patient teaching. If the patient lacks knowledge, teaching the basics (vocabulary, pathophysiology of the disease) is a good place to start. Building on prior knowledge provides a framework with which to modify or elaborate on a subject area.

The medical assistant must be willing to adapt to the patient's needs, educational level, and developmental stage.

Plan

To plan effectively, the patient's learning style must be identified and addressed. What may work for one patient may not work for another. Teaching techniques and methods must allow for the patient's learning style. A variety of tools can be used to improve a person's knowledge about a health care problem.

Provide information in ways that do not involve memorization. Plan to provide a learning experience by connecting events rather than bits and pieces. Local chapters of national organizations develop patient education materials that can serve this purpose (e.g., pamphlets, newsletters, videotapes). When using preprinted material, it is important to consider the reading ability of the patient. Also involve the patient's family and significant others if appropriate during the planning process.

Implement

The medical assistant must know the material being presented to patients well. Pretending to be knowledgeable about a subject area is not acceptable. The environment must be conducive to learning (e.g., comfortable room temperature, good lighting) because learning can take place only when the learner is focused on the material being presented. The patient must understand the language being used and should always be encouraged to ask questions.

When teaching procedures, it is helpful if the same equipment and supplies that the patient will use at home can be used to demonstrate the required action, as follows:

- The medical assistant must first demonstrate the steps when teaching a skill. *Show* patients what to do; do not tell them. It is better to demonstrate on yourself or a family member because it allows the patient to observe the entire procedure.
- Use multimedia material when possible (e.g., videotapes), and make referrals to appropriate outside resources or agencies for reinforcement of learning.
- If the patient becomes frustrated or distracted, stop the session and reschedule for a time that is more suitable for the patient and caregiver.

Evaluate

When evaluating the patient's ability to learn, use objective data. For example, ask open-ended questions to determine the patient's understanding, or ask the patient to demonstrate the procedure. Always document the date, patient education and important information provided, and the amount of time spent with the patient. (This is an important step for insurance claims.)

PATIENT-CENTERED PROFESSIONALISM

- *How would using the Internet in patient teaching benefit both the medical assistant and the patient?*

CONCLUSION

Communication may be the best tool that medical assistants have to establish a trusting relationship with patients and encourage compliance with their treatment plan. Every patient is unique. Addressing each patient's communication needs individually promotes health safety. If a patient completely understands his or her illness, the reason why a prescribed treatment is necessary, and how to properly take their medications, the treatment plan has a chance for success. A patient's culture, beliefs, background, age, intelligence, and abilities (seeing, hearing, sensing, thinking, and comprehending) all need to be analyzed to establish a communication process that best fits the patient's communication and learning style. The ability to apply the principles of effective communication to your daily interaction with patients takes much effort and practice. However, your efforts will be reflected in the positive relationships you establish with patients and the quality, professional care you provide.

An extension of the communication process is patient education. Educating patients about following through with treatment plans, improving their nutrition, and improving their overall health is one of the most important responsibilities of the medical assistant.

Chapter Summary

Reinforce your understanding of the material in this chapter by reviewing the curriculum objectives and key content points below.

1. **Define, appropriately use, and spell all the Key Terms for this chapter.**
   - Review the Key Terms if necessary.
2. **Understand the role of the medical assistant in patient communication.**
   - A medical assistant is expected to be an active listener and to understand and anticipate the patient's needs. A medical assistant also needs to communicate to patients their treatment plan, instructions for medication, and follow-up appointments.
3. **Explain the concept of holistic care.**
   - The holistic approach to health care is concerned with all the patient's needs: physical, emotional, social, economic, and spiritual.
4. **Discuss four effective communication techniques and three barriers to avoid when communicating with the patient.**
   - Refer to Table 8-1.
   - Refer to Table 8-2.
5. **List five ways you can improve communication with patients, and explain how better communication improves patient care and results in good service.**
   - Communication with patients can be improved by listening actively, involving the patient and family with decision making, being sensitive to the patient's needs, encouraging the patient to discuss issues and problems, and providing feedback to the patient.
   - Better communication improves patient care because the treatment plan (the message) has been delivered correctly by the medical assistant and has been accepted by the patient.
   - Focusing on the patient's needs and striving for improvement achieves quality care and service.
6. **Explain the importance of handling patient complaints effectively.**
   - Patients must believe that their complaints have been addressed effectively by the practice. Unhappy patients are more likely to sue or to report their dissatisfaction with the practice to others (other family members, patients, or health care workers).
   - Handling patient complaints is a skill that requires practice and the cooperation of all staff members.
   - Reducing lawsuits in the medical office starts with the patient-staff relationship.
7. **List three ways to establish trust with patients of different cultures.**
   - When dealing with cultural beliefs you do not understand, it is important to show respect.
   - You need good communication skills when interacting with patients who have cultural beliefs that are different from your own.
   - Allow the patient to maintain self-esteem at all times.
8. **List five considerations for communicating with a patient who is visually impaired.**
   Keep in mind that patients with visual impairments can have varying degrees of sight.
   - Use written materials with large print.
   - Consider using audiocassettes for patient instruction.
   - Orient the patient to unfamiliar surroundings ("There is a chair on your left in this room").
   - Give verbal visual cues when necessary ("Step down and turn around").
   - Alert the patient before touching the patient ("I'm going to wash your eye out now").
9. **List seven ways to communicate effectively with a patient who has hearing impairment.**
   Nonverbal communication is especially important to patients with hearing impairments.
   - Provide written instructions whenever possible.
   - Restate directions and instructions frequently.
   - Face patients when you are speaking to them.
   - Speak clearly and at a normal rate; do not yell or shout.
   - Involve family and caregivers.
   - Use hand gestures and facial expressions if appropriate.
   - Minimize distractions (e.g., close the door, turn down the radio).
10. **List three considerations for accommodating patients with other physical disabilities.**

- Patients with special needs (e.g., those with walkers, crutches, wheelchairs, or oxygen tanks) require multiple approaches based on their individual circumstances. Do not rush these patients.
- Be careful ushering these patients through doorways.
- These patients may need assistance in the bathroom.

11. **List six considerations for communicating effectively with elderly patients.**
    - The aging process causes many changes in the ability to process sensory information.
    - Refer to Box 8-3.
12. **List six considerations for communicating effectively with children.**
    - Adjust your communication to the level of the child.
    - Refer to Box 8-4.
13. **Explain the considerations for communicating with patients with a below-normal ability to reason or think, with mental impairments, or with developmental delays.**
    - When assessing a patient's ability to learn, acknowledge the patient's life experiences as well as formal education.
    - Review the patient's understanding of the information provided by asking questions or by having the patient perform a return demonstration of the procedure.
    - Mental impairment is diagnosed when the intellectual level is lower than the accepted range.
    - A developmentally delayed patient requires a level of communication based on maturational level, not chronological age.
14. **Explain the importance of communicating effectively with the caregivers and families of mentally impaired and developmentally delayed patients.**
    - Family members can provide information on the patient's life and experiences. This information can be used to communicate effectively with the patient.
    - Family members can assist the patient in complying with the treatment plan.
15. **Explain the importance of patient education.**
    - The purpose of patient education is to influence a patient's behavior toward a certain goal.
    - Understanding effective communication techniques and human behavior is necessary to provide optimum patient education.
16. **Analyze a realistic medical office situation and apply your understanding of effective communication with patients to determine the best course of action.**
    - Age, intelligence, special needs, and culture all impact the way medical assistants communicate with patients.
    - Communication approaches should be varied based on the needs of each patient.
17. **Describe the impact on patient care when medical assistants consistently apply the principles of effective communication when interacting with patients.**
    - When patients see the medical office staff as diligent, responsive, and caring, they are more understanding when misunderstandings occur.
    - Effectively communicating with patients of all types requires empathy, patience, effective listening, and understanding of the needs of the individual patient.

PRACTICAL APPLICATIONS

If you have accomplished the objectives in this chapter, you will be able to make better choices as a medical assistant. Take another look at this situation and decide what you would do.

Mr. Joplin is a spry 82-year-old and still lives in his own home. His wife died about a year ago, but Mr. Joplin has no severe medical problems and is able to care for himself. He does have visual problems caused by cataracts in his left eye, as well as joint stiffness related to his age. John, the medical assistant, approaches Mr. Joplin to escort him to the examining room. John shouts at Mr. Joplin as if he has a hearing difficulty, then walks away without assisting Mr. Joplin from the chair. When John reaches the door, he looks over his shoulder, rolls his eyes, and shouts, "Do you need some help?" Mr. Joplin looks away and refuses any assistance. Dr. Smith examines Mr. Joplin and asks John to explain the treatment so Mr. Joplin will comply. John hurriedly tells Mr. Joplin one time what is expected, then returns him to the waiting room. Several days later, Mr. Joplin calls the office to tell the receptionist to cancel his next appointment because he is going to find a new physician.

John's poor communication skills caused Dr. Smith to lose Mr. Joplin as a patient. If you were the medical assistant in this situation, what would you have done to communicate more effectively with Mr. Joplin?

1. Did John need to speak in a loud voice to Mr. Joplin, or did he stereotype Mr. Joplin because of his age and visual impairments?
2. Did John show professionalism? List three ways that John could have improved his interaction with Mr. Joplin.
3. What body language did John display that exhibited negative thoughts about Mr. Joplin?
4. What role did Mr. Joplin's age play in this interaction?
5. What steps could John have taken to show that he really wanted Mr. Joplin to comply with the physician's treatment plan?
6. What role did the receptionist play in this scenario? What should she have done when Mr. Joplin canceled his appointment?

WEB SEARCH

Research holistic health. It is important for the medical assistant to understand how holistic treatments can be used together with conventional medicine. Learn more about holistic treatments to enhance your own understanding.

- **Keywords:** Use the following keywords in your search: holistic, holistic medicine, holistic treatment.

9 Nutrition

http://evolve.elsevier.com/klieger/medicalassisting

Chapter 8 introduced you to the role of the medical assistant in patient communication and patient education. In this chapter, you will learn important concepts of good nutrition. Medical assistants often need to educate patients about good nutrition and provide support and encouragement for patients prescribed a special diet by their physician.

Individuals with inadequate diets and poor nutritional status are more prone to disease. Teaching patients how to make adjustments in their lifestyle (e.g., good nutrition, proper exercise, and smoking cessation) is an area in which medical assistants have the opportunity to improve patients' quality of living. To perform effective patient education in the area of nutrition, medical assistants must understand not only patient learning styles, as provided in the previous chapter, and the teaching-learning process but also dietary guidelines, principles of nutrition and nutrients, nutrition through the life span, nutrition for patients with chronic disease, and diet therapy.

LEARNING OBJECTIVES

You will be able to do the following after completing this chapter:

Key Terms
1. Define, appropriately use, and spell all the Key Terms for this chapter.

Dietary Guidelines
2. Explain the purpose of dietary guidelines.
3. List the six food groups included in the food guide pyramid and discuss the recommended daily quantities for a 2,000-calorie diet.
4. Explain the purpose of the Nutrition Labeling and Education Act (NLEA), and list the two main panels to consider when looking at a food label.

Principles of Nutrition
5. List and briefly describe five basic principles of good nutrition.
6. Demonstrate how to calculate a patient's body mass index (BMI), and indicate whether a patient is underweight, normal, overweight, or obese according to the chart.
7. List five tips for maintaining nutritional balance in the daily diet.

Nutrients
8. Differentiate between essential and nonessential nutrients.
9. Differentiate fat-soluble vitamins from water-soluble vitamins and list the major sources of each.
10. List nine major minerals and explain the sources of each and the result of deficiency.
11. List seven trace minerals and explain the sources of each and the result of deficiency.
12. Explain why the body needs carbohydrates, fats, and proteins.
13. Explain the importance of water and state the daily recommended amount.

Nutrition Through the Life Span
14. Explain dietary needs during pregnancy and lactation, infancy, toddler age, school age, adolescence, and older adulthood.

Nutrition and Chronic Disease
15. Explain the dietary needs of patients newly diagnosed with HIV and those with AIDS.
16. Explain the dietary needs for cancer patients undergoing chemotherapy.

Diet Therapy
17. List and briefly describe nine types of therapeutic diets.
18. Explain why fad diets are unhealthy and a poor choice for long-term weight loss.

Patient-Centered Professionalism
19. Analyze a realistic medical office situation and apply your understanding of patient education and nutrition to determine the best course of action.
20. Describe the impact on patient care when medical assistants have a solid understanding of nutrition and how it relates to a patient's treatment plan.

KEY TERMS

amino acids	major minerals
anorexia	malabsorption
antioxidant	malnutrition
assimilation	minerals
beriberi	monounsaturated fats
bile	night blindness
bland diet	nonessential nutrients
body mass index (BMI)	nutrients
bulimia	nutrition
caloric intake	Nutrition Labeling and Education Act (NLEA)
calories	
calorie-controlled diet	nutritional fact panel
carbohydrates	obese
cellulose	osteomalacia
cholesterol	pellagra
complex carbohydrates	pernicious anemia
complex proteins	polyunsaturated fats
Daily Value (DV)	proteins
dermatitis	recommended dietary allowances (RDAs)
diabetic diet	
display panel	regular diet
enzymes	renal failure diet
essential nutrients	rickets
fad diet	saturated fats
fat-soluble vitamins	scurvy
fatty acids	simple carbohydrates
food guide pyramid	simple proteins
glossitis	sodium-restricted diet
glycemic index	soft diet
glycerol	synthesize
goiter	therapeutic diet
high-fiber diet	trace minerals
hydrogenated	trans fatty acids
hypercholesterolemia	triglycerides
liquid diet	unsaturated fats
low-cholesterol, low-fat diet	vitamins
low-fiber diet	water-soluble vitamins

PRACTICAL APPLICATIONS

Read the following scenario and keep it in mind as you learn about patient education and nutrition.

Josephine, age 52, has just been diagnosed with type 2 diabetes mellitus related to obesity. Living in the home with Josephine are her mother, Susie, who is 80 years old; Josephine's daughter Jessie, who is 24 and pregnant; and Jessie's two very active children, ages 6 and 2. Susie has been diagnosed with a heart condition and must be on a soft diet that is low in cholesterol and sodium restricted. Josephine's concern today is how she can maintain a diet acceptable for all the medical conditions in the household while being sure the other family members will eat what is prepared. She thinks the children need sugar, but her mother needs to watch her sugar and salt intake to remain in a stable condition and not gain weight. Susie also needs her meals to be soft and easily chewable because of her decrease in intestinal motility. However, Jessie and her 2-year-old child both need a diet that allows the necessary fiber for adequate bowel activity.

If you were the medical assistant, how might you educate Josephine about nutrition and answer her questions?

DIETARY GUIDELINES

Nutrition is the scientific study of how different food groups affect the body. Improper or incomplete nutrition leads to various disorders. Proper and complete nutrition allows people to function effectively, both physically and mentally. It also helps the body resist infection and disease. Food is required for the body to grow, heal, reproduce, and maintain a healthy state. Proper nutrition influences the appearance of a person's hair, eyes, teeth, and complexion. If deprived of proper nutrition, the body is prone to illness and is not able to maintain growth and a healthy state (Table 9-1).

Many American diets have adequate **calories** (units of energy) to get through the day, but they are inadequate in the necessary nutrients to nourish the body's systems. Therefore medical assistants must be prepared to educate patients about healthy eating and explain special diets that may be prescribed by the physician.

To help patients maintain optimal health, medical assistants must understand nutritional standards and must be able to assess the recommended nutritional guidelines in foods that are eaten by the patient daily. In 1941 the National Academy of Sciences and the Food and Nutrition Board published the **recommended dietary allowances (RDAs)**. The RDAs reflected the established amounts of essential nutrients in a diet that help to decrease the risk of chronic disease and keep

TABLE 9-1

Signs and Symptoms of Poor and Good Nutrition

Tissues Involved	Poor Nutrition	Good Nutrition
Hair	Dry and brittle	Shiny
Eyes	Dull and dry	Bright and moist
Skin	Dry and scaling	Smooth, good color, and moist
MOUTH		
Lips	Lesions and cracked	Pink color
Tongue	Surface smooth, swollen, and dry	Moist and surface bumpy
Teeth	Dental caries	No caries
Gums	Inflamed and bleeding	Firm and pink

the body in homeostasis. In recent years the RDAs have been replaced on the food label with the term **Daily Value (DV)**. This term better reflects dietary standards that include a range of particular nutrients to optimize an individual's health.

FOR YOUR INFORMATION

DIETARY GUIDELINE UPDATES
The Dietary Guidelines, first published in 1980, must be reviewed every 5 years by law because the guidelines are used by federal agencies to determine the nutritional content of school lunches.

In May 2005 the U.S. Department of Health and Human Services (DHHS) and U.S. Department of Agriculture (USDA) released new guidelines that provided the American public with updated information on food and nutrition. The food guide pyramid and its accompanying dietary guidelines are not solely for public education but influence what products are manufactured and sold and set standards for federal nutrition programs, including school lunches. Dietary guidelines allow an individual to select the types and amounts of foods and adjust them to recognize factors such as age, gender, health status, pregnancy, and other conditions that would affect their daily nutritional needs. The guidelines also identify a relationship between exercise (up to 30 to 60 minutes per day to maintain proper weight) and eating. Current knowledge about weight, nutrition, and physical activity is used to offer practical advice.

FOOD GUIDE PYRAMID

The **food guide pyramid** was developed by the USDA to provide a visual picture of the six food groups common to the American diet. The updated pyramid (www.mypyramid.gov) emphasizes the consumption of fruits and vegetables and indicates more calories should come from grains rather than meat proteins and dairy products (Figure 9-1). At least 3 ounces (oz) of the recommended 6 oz of grains should be whole grains, since these are complex carbohydrates that supply the muscles and the brain with energy. These foods include bread, pasta, and cereal made from whole grains and brown rice. Limiting fats, oils, and sugars is still advised. The pyramid also emphasizes physical activity by featuring a human figure climbing up the side of the pyramid. A change was made from abstract "servings" to a more concrete measure such as cups and ounces.

The guidelines represented by the pyramid are not intended to be rigid but rather should be seen as recommendations to encourage people to eat a variety of foods from the six major food groups (Table 9-2). A diet low in fat and containing only moderate use of sugars and salt supports a healthier body. The food pyramid is a tool that provides the information needed to make good choices. Therefore the food pyramid should be used as a guide, not a strict map, for healthier eating. Certain food pyramids have been developed for specific ethnic and cultural groups (Figure 9-2). Box 9-1 provides information about the relationship between culture and nutrition.

BOX 9-1
Culture and Nutrition

People eat food not only to meet the nutritional needs of the body but also to feel pleasure, satisfaction, or even comfort in times of stress and sadness. For many, mealtime is a social event, and many joyful occasions are celebrated with food. What is considered a food will vary from one culture to another. Most cultures have their own health norms and practices. Knowing a patient's cultural traditions, ethnic background, and religion is important because these factors can influence the person's health and attitudes toward health care.

Attitudes and habits concerning food are the result of culture and society and will influence what foods are eaten most frequently. For example:
- Bread is the main staple in the diet of many countries, especially the Greek diet.
- Persons of German descent often favor pork, noodles, and sauerkraut.
- Italians relish pasta and green leafy vegetables and use large amounts of olive oil when cooking.
- The East-Asian population favors fish and rice as their main sources of food.
- Some cultures, such as Indian, use spicy seasonings when cooking.

In recent years, diabetes and gallbladder disease have been increasing among Native Americans. Changes in dietary habits, increased obesity, and genetic factors are thought to have contributed to this increase.

When a person becomes ill, he or she often must adjust their food selection based on their diet restrictions. A medical assistant must understand that a patient's diet is an important part of the patient's lifestyle and ethnicity. Offering suggestions that the patient will find appealing without compromising treatment can be a challenge.

TABLE 9-2
Recommended Daily Consumption of the Six Food Groups

Calories	Grains (Major source of energy and fiber)	Vegetables (Rich sources of fiber, potassium, and magnesium)	Fruits (Important sources of fiber, potassium, and magnesium)	Oils (Low in saturated fat)	Milk (Low-fat/fat-free major source of calcium and protein)	Protein (Lean meats, poultry, fish, beans, peas, nuts and seeds)
1,000 calories	3 oz	1 cup	1 cup	3 tsp	2 cups	2 oz
2,000 calories	6 oz	2½ cups	2 cups	6 tsp	3 cups	5½ oz
3,200 calories	10 oz	4 cups	2½ cups	11 tsp	3 cups	7 oz

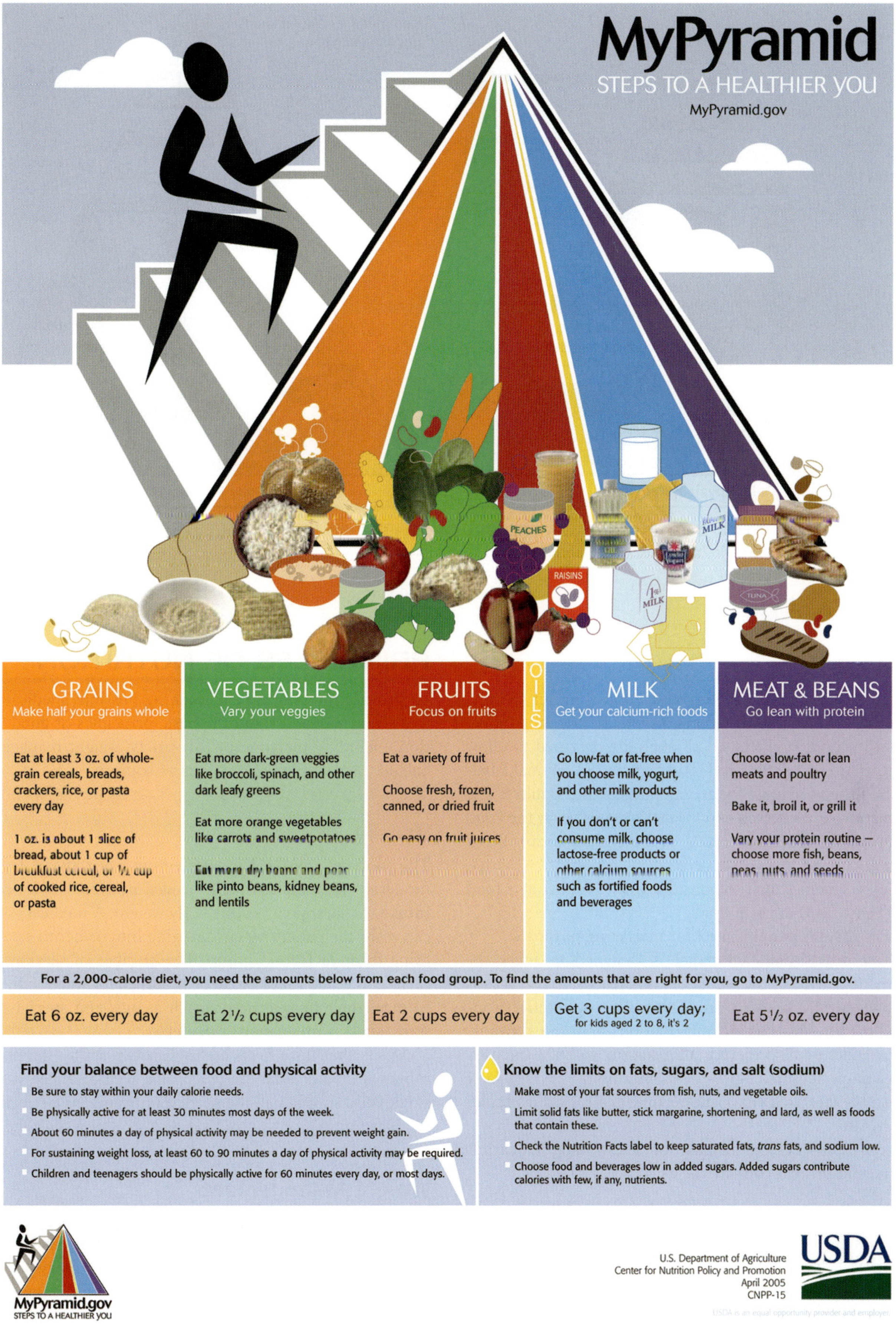

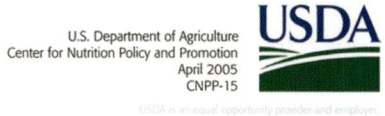

FIGURE 9-1 USDA Food Guide Pyramid. (Courtesy U.S. Department of Agriculture, Center for Nutrition Policy and Promotion, April 2005.)

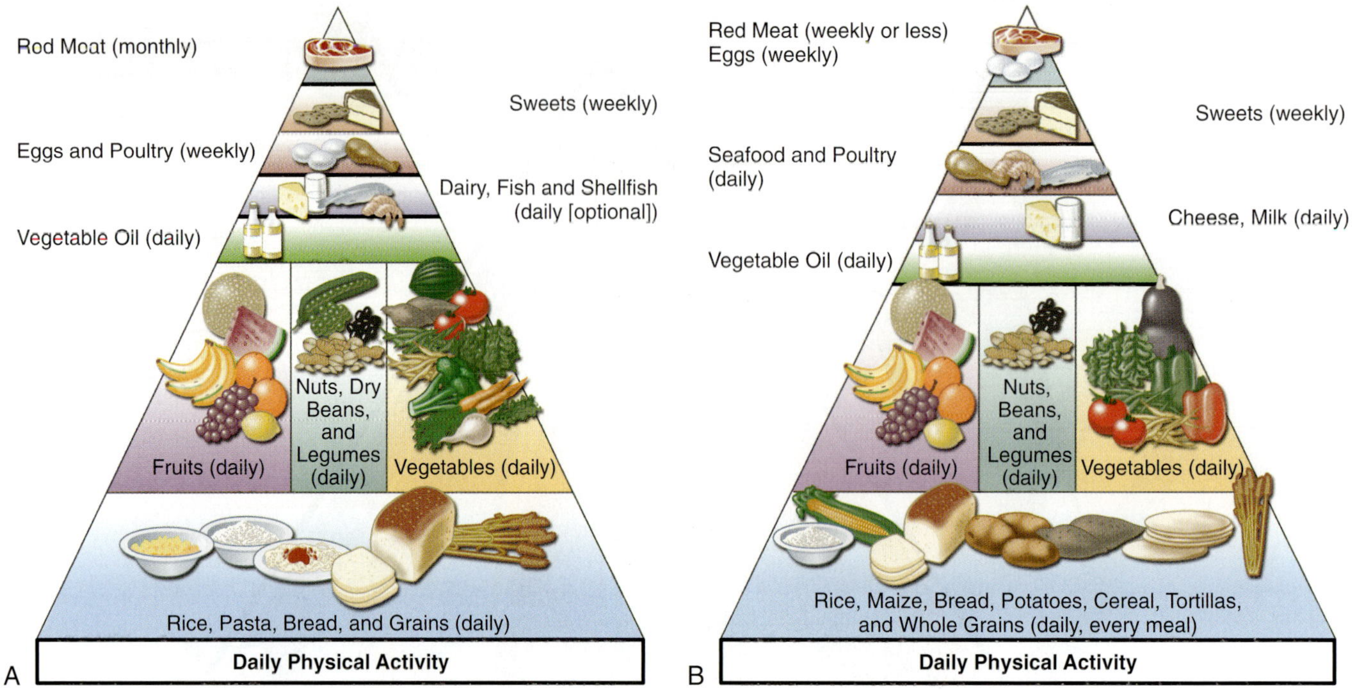

FIGURE 9-2 Ethnic Food Guide Pyramid. **A,** An Asian diet indicates that one food group is no better than another. **B,** A Latin American diet includes protein based on plants and grains.

Food Labels

In 1990 the **Nutrition Labeling and Education Act (NLEA)** was passed to assist consumers in identifying nutritional content in food products. Food labels are designed to allow consumers to make informed food choices. Nutritional labeling is required for most foods, except meat and poultry. The information contained on a food label is regulated by the Food and Drug Administration (FDA) and therefore is considered a legal document.

The two main panels to consider when looking at a food label (Figure 9-3) are as follows:
- The **display panel** is used for marketing purposes.
- The **nutritional fact panel** is designed to meet the requirements of the regulatory boards. This panel is subdivided into two sections. The main (top) section contains product-specific information, and the footnote provides general dietary information. In 2006 the government required labels to list the amount of trans-fatty acids, fats that have been linked to cardiovascular disease.

Box 9-2 provides the formula for determining fat, carbohydrate, and protein content.

PATIENT-CENTERED PROFESSIONALISM

- Why is it important for the medical assistant to understand the food guide pyramids of different cultures?

PRINCIPLES OF NUTRITION

To provide the best patient teaching possible, medical assistants need to understand the basic principles of good nutrition, including the concepts of variety, weight management, balance, and minimizing sugar and sodium.

Variety

The food pyramid encourages eating a variety of foods in moderate amounts to obtain needed nutrients and a **caloric intake** to maintain a healthy body weight. A medical assistant can assist the patient by encouraging him or her to eat something from each food group. The number of servings from each food group may have to be modified for some individuals to meet their unique needs, such as age, and special conditions, such as pregnancy or diabetes.

Foods that have been highly fortified with vitamins and minerals do not take the place of a well-balanced diet. No single food supplies all the needed nutrients, so a selection of foods from each of the six food groups is necessary daily.

Weight Management

Research shows that being overweight increases a person's risk of developing chronic diseases and conditions such as heart disease, type 2 diabetes, stroke, arthritis, respiratory problems, hypertension, osteoarthritis, and certain cancers. Being overweight causes the heart to work harder, thus increasing the risk for a heart attack.

Sample Food Label

The food label can be found on food packages in your supermarket. Reading the label tells more about the food and what you are getting. The nutrition and ingredient information is required by the government.

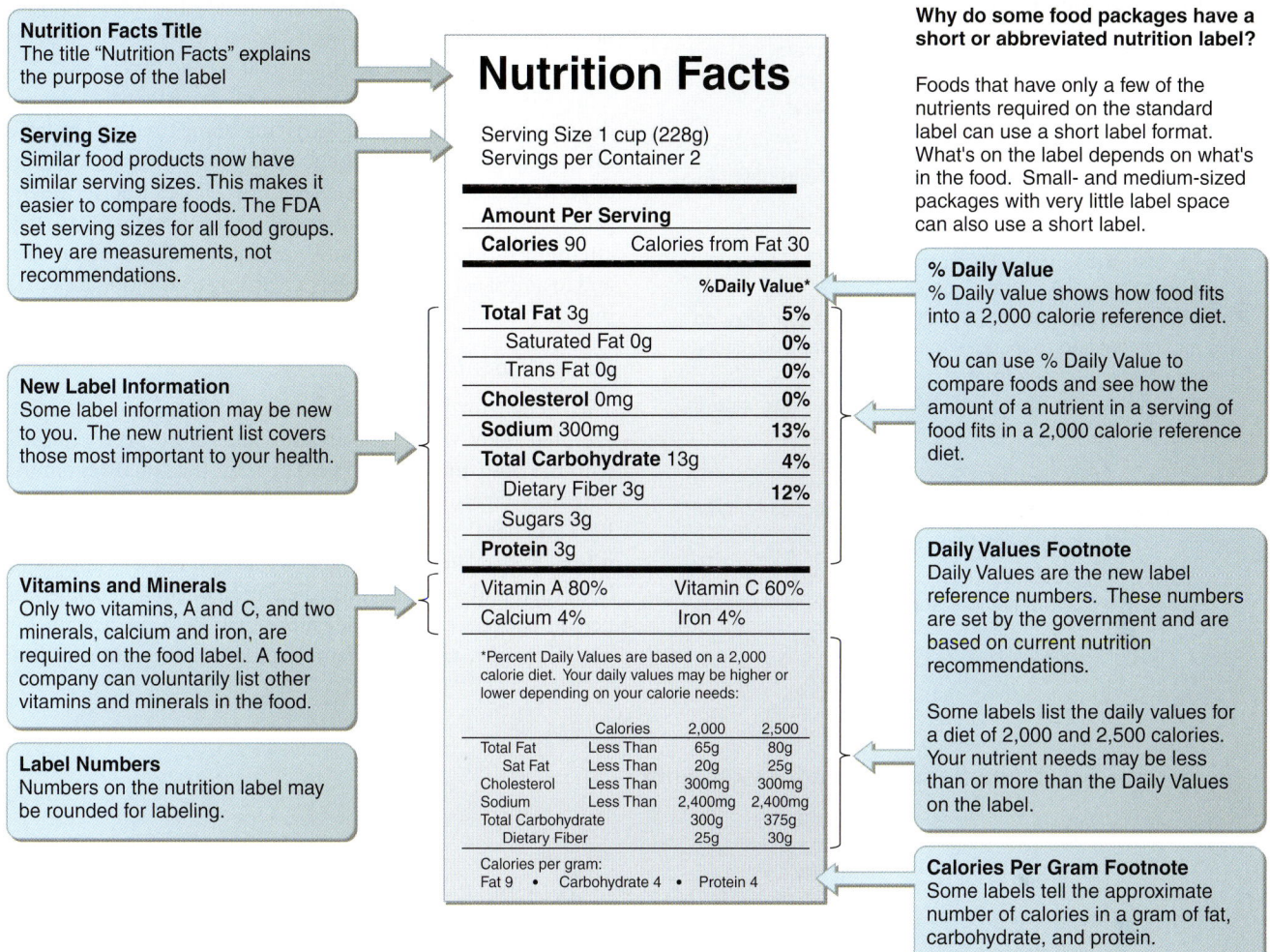

Nutrition Facts Title
The title "Nutrition Facts" explains the purpose of the label

Serving Size
Similar food products now have similar serving sizes. This makes it easier to compare foods. The FDA set serving sizes for all food groups. They are measurements, not recommendations.

New Label Information
Some label information may be new to you. The new nutrient list covers those most important to your health.

Vitamins and Minerals
Only two vitamins, A and C, and two minerals, calcium and iron, are required on the food label. A food company can voluntarily list other vitamins and minerals in the food.

Label Numbers
Numbers on the nutrition label may be rounded for labeling.

Why do some food packages have a short or abbreviated nutrition label?
Foods that have only a few of the nutrients required on the standard label can use a short label format. What's on the label depends on what's in the food. Small- and medium-sized packages with very little label space can also use a short label.

% Daily Value
% Daily value shows how food fits into a 2,000 calorie reference diet.

You can use % Daily Value to compare foods and see how the amount of a nutrient in a serving of food fits in a 2,000 calorie reference diet.

Daily Values Footnote
Daily Values are the new label reference numbers. These numbers are set by the government and are based on current nutrition recommendations.

Some labels list the daily values for a diet of 2,000 and 2,500 calories. Your nutrient needs may be less than or more than the Daily Values on the label.

Calories Per Gram Footnote
Some labels tell the approximate number of calories in a gram of fat, carbohydrate, and protein.

Key Points:

- Doubling the serving size also doubles the nutrient value and the calories.
- The calories listed provide a measure of how much energy is received from one serving and those calories derived from fat.
- Consumption of fats, cholesterol, sodium, and sugar in foods should be minimized since research shows they are responsible for chronic illness. It is recommended that these be less than 100% of their Daily Value.
- Nutrients contained in dietary fiber, protein, vitamins, and minerals improve health and assist in reducing disease. It is advised that these nutrients average to 100% daily.
- Foods containing 5% or less of dietary fiber are considered too low in dietary fiber to contribute toward the daily total.
- Foods containing 20% or higher of vitamins and minerals contribute a good amount toward the daily total as needed.

FIGURE 9-3 Sample food label.

BOX 9-2

Calorie Distribution: Fat, Carbohydrate, and Protein Content

Carbohydrates	4 calories per gram
Protein	4 calories per gram
Fat	9 calories per gram

Values from label:
Serving size: 2 tbsp = 12 g total fat, 15 g total carbohydrates, and 8 g protein
8 g protein × 4 calories = 32 calories
15 g carbohydrates × 4 = 60 calories
12 g fat × 9 calories = 108 calories
Total calories: 32 + 60 + 108 = 200 calories per serving
This means that each serving of this product has 200 calories, most of which comes from fat.
By using the values given on the food label, calculate the percentage of calories in food supplied from fat:

Grams of fat × 9 = Fat calories
(Fat calories ÷ Total calories) × 100 = % of calories from fat
Solution: 12 g × 9 = 108
(108 ÷ 200) × 100 = (10,800 ÷ 20,000)
= 5.9% of calories supplied from fat

Restriction of calories and saturated fats may be needed if reduced activity is a concern. The body only burns a certain number of calories per day during normal body functions, and calories not burned turn into fat. Take the lower number of recommended servings, and choose fewer foods high in caloric count (e.g., fats, sugars, and alcoholic beverages).

Problems with weight management can arise when people do not plan ahead for meals. Arriving home tired and hungry often leads to eating fast food (high in fat and sugar) with few or no vegetables. If this cycle continues, it can lead to weight gain. The rationale behind weight management is to pay attention to total caloric intake and not the type of calories and to adjust exercise regimens according to additional caloric intake.

Body Mass Index

The weight-for-height charts formerly used to determine accepted body weight for an individual have been replaced with the **body mass index (BMI)** chart, since the BMI simultaneously takes into account height and weight (Figure 9-4). BMI is better than the traditional height-weight tables because it is well correlated with total body fat content and applies to both men and women. BMI calculations help determine if a person is overweight, **obese** (more than 20% overweight for gender, height, and body frame), underweight, or at a healthy

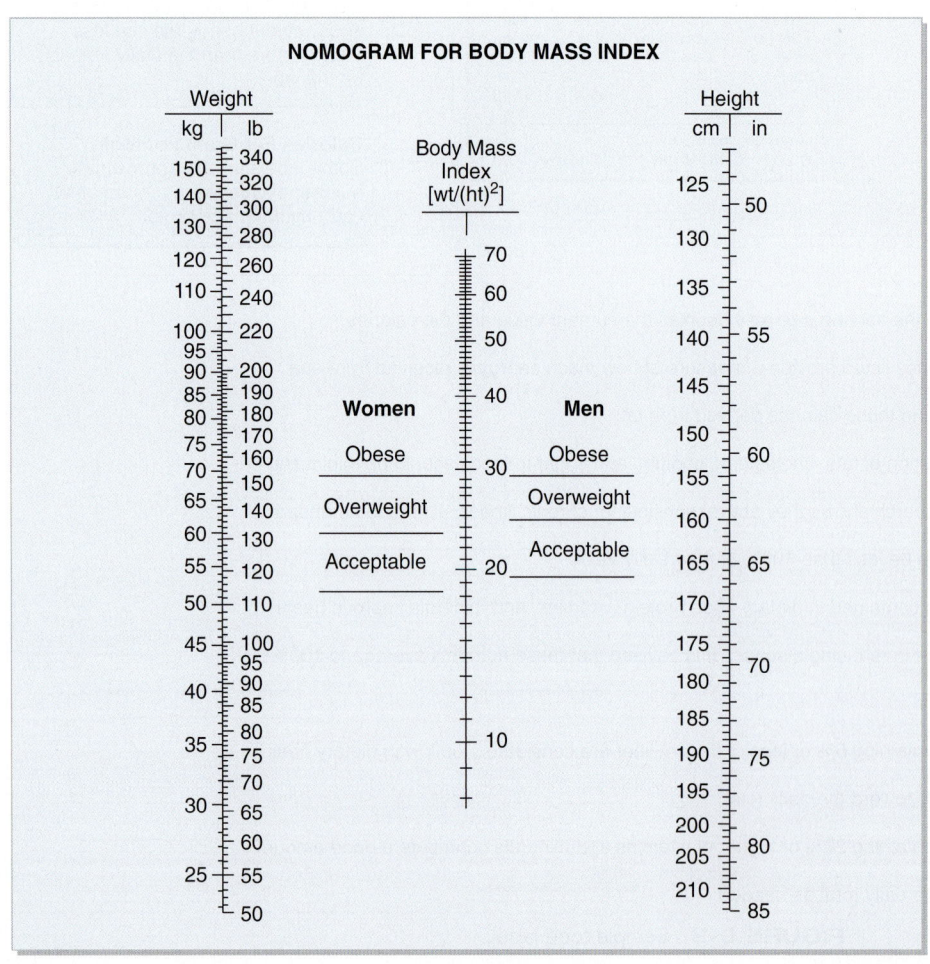

FIGURE 9-4 Nomogram for body mass index. (Modified from Young AP, Proctor DB: *Kinn's the medical assistant*, ed 10, St Louis, 2007, Saunders.)

TABLE 9-3
Body Mass Index (BMI)

Weight Status	BMI
Underweight	Less than 18.5
Normal	18.5 to 24.9
Overweight	25 to 29.9
Obese	Greater than 30

weight, as determined by the BMI range. For example, a man who weighs 246 pounds (lbs) and is 76 inches tall falls into the obese range.

Children and teens are assessed for being underweight, overweight, and at risk for becoming overweight. BMI for children is gender and age specific. For an adult, BMI is calculated by using a person's weight and height; the BMI is then compared to an established range (Table 9-3). The Mayo Clinic considers a person overweight if the person has a BMI of 25 to 29.9 and obese if the BMI is 30 or higher.

A mathematical formula is used to calculate BMI. The person's weight in kilograms is divided by the person's height in meters squared. For example:

BMI Calculation A 46-year-old woman weighs 150 lbs and is 60 inches tall. According to the following formula:

$$BMI = Weight\ (kg) \div Height\ (m^2)$$

1. Convert 150 lbs to kilograms (kg)
   (2.2 kg is equal to 1 lb)

$$150 \div 2.2 = 68\ kg$$

2. Convert 60 inches to meters (m)
   (39.37 inches = 1 m)

$$60 \div 39.37 = 1.52\ m$$

3. Square 1.52 m

$$1.52 \times 1.52 = 2.3104\ m$$

4. Substitute numbers into formula

$$BMI = kg \div m^2$$

$$68 \div 2.3104 = 29.4$$

$$BMI = 29.4$$

The BMI chart indicates that the woman is in the overweight range and is close to being obese.

Balance

A balanced diet is encouraged to provide the proper amounts of all nutrients that an individual needs for optimal health. As seen in the food pyramid, each food group has recommendations that contribute to the body's total nutritional needs for a day. Omitting any food group reduces the body's chance of homeostasis. Tips for balancing the daily diet are as follows:

1. Drink eight glasses of water daily (64 oz). This aids in proper elimination, keeps the body hydrated, and promotes clear skin.
2. Eat low-fat, lean meats (skinless chicken, fish). These supply all the essential amino acids that the body needs to build cells and repair tissue.
   - 3 oz of fish is about the size of a thick checkbook
   - 3 oz of meat or chicken is about the size of a deck of cards
3. Eat a variety of fruits and vegetables daily. These provide nutrient value and roughage (fiber), which helps with elimination.
   - A cup of fruit or vegetables is about the size of a tennis ball
4. Use low-fat or fat-free dairy products. Whole milk can cause unsaturated fatty acids to build in the bloodstream.
   - 1 oz of cheese is the size of 4 dice
5. Eat plenty of whole grains, rice, and pasta. Adequate starch and fiber provides energy and promotes elimination.

FOR YOUR INFORMATION

IMPORTANCE OF BREAKFAST

Eating a breakfast of complex carbohydrates (e.g., whole-grain cereals) and proteins starts the body off with fuel for the energy needs of the day. This is why breakfast is considered to be the most important meal of the day.

Minimize Sugar

Sugars are poor sources of vitamins and minerals; therefore, even though sugars are high in carbohydrates, their value is poor. Sugars on food labels are listed as syrups, sugars, and foods ending in "ose" such as lactose (milk sugar), fructose (fruit sugar), and sucrose (table sugar). Honey is composed of 75% sugar and contains very few nutrients. Some sugars can contribute to tooth decay, as can the lack of adequate calcium and inadequate oral hygiene.

FOR YOUR INFORMATION

THE SWEETEST SWEETENER

Blackstrap molasses contains iron, calcium, potassium, and some B vitamins and is the healthiest of all sweeteners.

Minimize Sodium

Sodium is found naturally in many foods. Therefore the addition of table salt (sodium chloride) when preparing or cooking foods, as well as eating large quantities of foods processed with salt, may contribute greatly to cardiovascular disease. In hypertension, for example, sodium in salt causes the body to accumulate fluid, causing more pressure against the blood vessel walls. The recommended intake of sodium per day is 2,400 mg. As a comparison, just 1 teaspoon of salt contains approximately 2,000 mg of sodium.

> **PATIENT-CENTERED PROFESSIONALISM**
>
> - Why is it important for the medical assistant to be knowledgeable about nutrition and how it applies to weight management?

NUTRIENTS

Nutrients are chemical substances within food that are released and absorbed during the digestive process. Most nutrients provide the body with the energy it needs to maintain body functions such as maintaining a constant temperature. Nutrients are classified into **nonessential nutrients**, meaning those that are provided in the body, and **essential nutrients**, those that must be taken in from a food source such as vitamins, minerals, proteins, carbohydrates, fats, and water. Essential nutrients are divided into five categories: vitamins, minerals, carbohydrates, fats, and proteins.

Vitamins

Vitamins are organic substances that enhance the breakdown of proteins, carbohydrates, and fats. Without vitamins, the breakdown and **assimilation** (the taking in of nutrient material) of foods would not occur. Some vitamins are used in the formation of blood cells and hormones and the production of neurochemical substances. Vitamins are classified into two categories: fat soluble and water soluble.

Fat-Soluble Vitamins

Fat-soluble vitamins are usually absorbed with foods that contain fat and are stored in body fat, the liver, and the kidneys. These vitamins are broken down by **bile**, which is formed by the liver. Fat-soluble vitamins include A, D, E, and K (Table 9-4). Excess intake of these vitamins by taking daily vitamin supplements should be avoided because the body stores these vitamins, and excess can result in serious illness. Beta carotene, found in some fruits and vegetables, is converted by the body to vitamin A.

Water-Soluble Vitamins

Water-soluble vitamins are also important to the body. Vitamin C and B-complex vitamins (thiamine [B_1], riboflavin [B_2], niacin [B_3], pantothenic acid [B_5], pyridoxine [B_6], cyanocobalamin [B_{12}], and folic acid) are not stored in the body and are excreted when in excess. Therefore these vitamins must be consumed daily and are not dangerous when taken as supplements (Table 9-5).

> **FOR YOUR INFORMATION**
>
> **WHAT IS ORGANIC?**
>
> *Poultry, eggs, and meats that come from animals that have not been fed hormones or antibiotics are considered organic. Organic crops are grown without pesticides, including synthetic fertilizers or sewer sludge. Legally, foods with the USDA's green and white sticker must be grown or raised according to certain federal standards.*

TABLE 9-4

Fat-Soluble Vitamins

Vitamin	Need	Sources	Deficiency
A	Growth of epithelial tissue; important for vision (especially in dim light) and hormonal production for reproduction and lactation; helps build resistance to infections	Byproducts of animals; milk, eggs, fish oil, liver, green and yellow vegetables and orange and yellow fruits (pumpkin, sweet potatoes, winter squash, carrots, cantaloupe, apricots), dark leafy vegetables (chard, beets, collard, kale, mustard, spinach, turnips), butter, yellow cheese, cream, watercress	**Night blindness,** skin disorders, hair loss, susceptibility to infection
D	Helps body utilize calcium and phosphorus necessary for absorption and metabolism; needed for calcium formation; needed for growth of bones and teeth	Sunlight; butter, eggs, canned fish, herring, salmon, tuna, fish oil, liver, dairy products fortified with vitamin D	**Rickets** (soft bones) in children, **osteomalacia** (soft bones) in adults
E	Use by body remains under study; needed for metabolism of essential fatty acids, absorption of iron, and RBC formation; acts as an **antioxidant** (prevents buildup of oxidants) Also used in liquid topical form for scar reduction	Seed oil, wheat germ, nuts, avocados, soybeans, milk products	Breakdown of RBCs, anemia
K	Needed for blood clotting by forming prothrombin, which is used in producing fibrin for blood clots	Synthesized in intestines by bacteria; assimilated from green leafy vegetables, molasses, apricots, cod liver oil, sunflower oil	Bleeding disorders (e.g., hemorrhages, slow clotting)

RBC, Red blood cell.

TABLE 9-5

Water-Soluble Vitamins

Vitamin	Need	Source	Deficiency
Vitamin C (ascorbic acid)	Synthesizes and maintains connective tissue; necessary for cholesterol metabolism and cortisol production in adrenal gland; maintains blood vessel strength; used in formation of hemoglobin; aids in utilization of iron in body; vital for healing and acts as an antioxidant	Citrus fruits and juices, broccoli, papayas, mangoes, potatoes, berries, cantaloupe, kiwi, Brussels sprouts, red and green peppers *Note:* Overcooking destroys most of the vitamin C in foods	**Scurvy** (affects mucous membranes, gums, and skin), slow healing
B-COMPLEX VITAMINS			
Thiamine (B_1)	Aids in nervous tissue function; co-enzyme for cellular energy; used in carbohydrate metabolism (turns complex carbohydrates into glucose or fat); helps the functioning of the brain, heart, and nervous system	Brewer's yeast, liver, pork, whole grains, nuts, beans, lentils, oatmeal	Mental confusion, **beriberi** (peripheral nerve disorder), muscle weakness
Riboflavin (B_2)	Used for normal growth; needed for protein, fat, and carbohydrate metabolism; used in formation of liver enzymes; assists adrenal glands to release hormone that stimulates production of stress-relieving hormones; helps RBC production	Milk and milk products, greens, whole grains, liver, lean meat, fish, poultry, eggs	**Dermatitis** (inflammation of skin) around mouth, lips, and nose; **glossitis** (inflamed tongue); light sensitivity
Niacin (B_3)	Aids in tissue respiration; used in cellular energy production; synthesizes fat; forms enzymes needed for carbohydrate metabolism *Note:* Formed in body from dietary amino acids	Whole grains, milk, eggs, legumes, lean meats, poultry, fish, and nuts	Dermatitis, diarrhea, mental confusion and irritability, **pellagra**
Pantothenic acid (B_5)	Used in metabolism of fats, carbohydrates, and amino acids; aids in function of adrenal gland; needed to maintain immune system	Brewer's yeast, grains, milk, green vegetables, mushrooms	Reports of burning feet syndrome, cramps, fatigue
Pyridoxine (B_6)	Used in hemoglobin synthesis; needed for formation of RBCs and neurotransmitters; used in metabolism for amino acid formation; needed for utilization of amino acids; involved in protein, sugar, and fatty acid metabolism	Meats, liver, grains, nuts, bananas, avocados, molasses, mushrooms	Anemias, low level of immunity, peripheral neuropathy, skin disorders
Cyanocobalamin (B_{12})	Needed for nerve synthesis; used in RBC development; assists in folic acid metabolism; needed for iron metabolism	Synthesized by gastrointestinal flora; meat, Brewer's yeast, eggs, milk	**Pernicious anemia** (body lacks intrinsic factor to absorb vitamin), sores in mouth, loss of coordination *Note:* Most seniors lose the ability to make stomach acid which interferes with the ability to absorb B_{12}.
Folic acid	Needed for hematopoiesis in bone marrow; needed for metabolism of sugar and amino acids; needed for fetal development for neural tube closure; needed for manufacture of antibodies	Liver, green leafy vegetables, beets, cauliflower, broccoli, citrus fruits, Brewer's yeast, eggs, nuts, sweet potatoes	Spina bifida, anencephaly, macrocytic anemia

RBC, Red blood cell.

Minerals

Minerals are inorganic substances used in the formation of hard and soft body tissues. Minerals are necessary for muscle contraction, nerve conduction, and blood clotting. Minerals are taken into the body from the foods eaten. The body uses **major minerals,** including calcium, phosphorus, magnesium, sodium, iron, iodine, and potassium, in sufficient amounts (Table 9-6). **Trace minerals,** or trace elements, are used in smaller quantities and include copper, cobalt, manganese, fluorine, and zinc. Trace minerals are found in adequate amounts in most foods (Table 9-7).

Carbohydrates

Carbohydrates produce quick body energy and are the body's primary energy source. Carbohydrates represent the most abundant food source and cost less than foods in the other food groups. **Cellulose** (chief part of the plant cell walls), which is abundant in plant carbohydrates, is important for elimination. During metabolism, carbohydrates produce energy that causes the release of water and carbon dioxide. Unabsorbed glucose increases blood sugar levels and insulin production. The glucose released by the cells is absorbed from the small intestine to be processed in the liver, then converted to glycogen to be stored for use later by the body.

Two types of carbohydrates are starches (**complex carbohydrates**) and unrefined sugars (**simple carbohydrates**). Starches are found mainly in grains, legumes, and tubers (e.g., potatoes, yams). Sugars are found in fruits and plants. Complex carbohydrates have the most nutrients. Refined sugars have a high caloric value but are basically empty in nutrient value.

TABLE 9-6

Major Minerals

Vitamin	Need	Source	Deficiency
Calcium (Ca^{++})	Needed for bone and tooth development; regulates nerve stimulation and muscle contraction, especially in heart muscle; forms intracellular cement; assists in blood-clotting process *Note:* Calcium is stored in bones and reabsorbed by blood and tissue.	Greens (beets, collards, kale, mustard, spinach, turnips); milk and milk products; canned salmon, sardines; whole-grain cereals, enriched breads; beans, peas, broccoli; cheese, eggs; nuts, seeds, soybeans	Muscle spasms, poorly formed bones and teeth, slow clotting, osteoporosis
Phosphorus (P)	Needed for energy metabolism of cells; combines with calcium in bones and teeth, allowing added strength	Milk and milk products	Fragile bones and stiff joints
Magnesium (Mg)	Needed for metabolism; important for electrical impulse in nerve and muscle cells	Most natural foods	Tremors, foot cramps, irregular heartbeat, convulsions
Sodium (Na^+)	Needed in extracellular fluid in cells; aids in normal nerve and muscle function	Most natural foods, especially vegetables and salt	Lack of muscle contractions, dehydration, weakness, cramps *Note:* Excess sodium causes edema and elevated blood pressure.
Iron (Fe)	Needed for hemoglobin production and the transport of oxygen in blood; used in cellular respiration and energy production *Note:* Iron is not easily absorbed by the digestive process and can cause GI problems such as constipation; foods high in iron need to be eaten with vitamin C–enriched foods for proper absorption.	Whole and enriched grains, dried beans and fruit, egg yolks, shellfish, lean meats and liver, dark-green vegetables, molasses, wine, nuts, soybeans, cocoa, absorbable iron supplements	Impaired behavior, fatigue, iron deficiency anemia *Note:* Women receiving hormone replacement therapy need more iron if they experience uterine bleeding; women taking oral contraceptives may need less iron.
Iodine (I)	Needed to synthesize hormone of thyroid gland that regulates metabolism and physical and mental development	Iodized salt, shellfish, garlic, cabbage, turnips, parsley	**Goiter** (enlarged thyroid) *Note:* Low iodine during pregnancy leads to birth defects and possible mental retardation.
Potassium (K^+)	Maintains normal fluid balance in body; needed for proper functioning of muscle and nervous system	Fresh fruit (apricots, bananas, cantaloupe), citrus juices, dried fruits, raw cauliflower and parsley, whole grains, soybeans, nuts, nonfat milk and tomato juice, potato skins, seafood	Poor nerve conduction, irregular heartbeat and muscle function

TABLE 9-7

Trace Minerals (Elements)

Vitamin	Need	Source	Deficiency
Copper (Cu)	Found in many enzymes and proteins in brain, blood, and liver; assists in formation of myelin sheath; assists in iron absorption and aids in proper function of vitamin C	Seafood, meat, eggs, whole-grain cereals, nuts	Anemia caused by failure of iron to assist with hemoglobin formation
Cobalt (Co)	Used in magnesium and sugar metabolism; aids in copper absorption; aids in RBC production	Brewer's yeast, fruits, vegetables, nuts, whole grains	Pernicious anemia
Manganese (Mn)	Used in energy metabolism; assists in thyroid function	Green vegetables, Brewer's yeast, eggs, fruit, whole grains, tea	Mental confusion
Fluorine (F)	Needed for tooth and bone formation; needed to minimize demineralization of bone	Water with natural or added fluorine	Dental caries, brittle bones
Zinc (Zn)	Forms enzymes; needed for release of vitamin A from liver; aids in protein metabolism and hormone production	Oysters, herring, Brewer's yeast, eggs, beef, peas, dairy, whole-grain foods, nuts, tofu, other shellfish	Impaired growth, poor wound healing, loss of appetite
Chromium (Cr)	Needed for fat and carbohydrate metabolism; aids in production of energy	Fruits, vegetables, Brewer's yeast, wheat germ, meats, molasses	Weight loss, poor glucose removal from blood (type 2 diabetes)
Selenium (Se)	Needed for normal functions of liver and connective tissue; acts as an antioxidant	Protein-rich foods	Osteoarthropathy

RBC, Red blood cell.

Sources of Carbohydrates and Cellulose

STARCHES	SUGARS	CELLULOSE
Cereals	Cane and beet sugar	Bran fruits
Breads	Carbonated beverages	Raw vegetables
Pasta	Candy	
Potatoes	Jelly	
Rice	Jams	
Grits		

Fats

Fatty acids and **glycerol** are building blocks of fat that produce oils. Fats are the most concentrated source of energy, but glycogen is the most easily stored form of energy. Glycogen is composed of carbon, hydrogen, and glycerol and is not soluble in water. The body cannot make the essential fatty acids, omega-3 oils, and omega-6 oils.

Dietary fats are broken down into fatty acids and pass into the blood to form **triglycerides** (fatty acids and glycerol), phospholipids, and sterols—namely, cholesterol (lipoprotein). Triglycerides are the most abundant lipids, and they function as the body's most concentrated source of energy.

The American diet takes in more animal fatty acids, cholesterol, and trans-fatty acids that leave the cell membrane in less-than-optimal strength. The cell wall may thus be incapable of holding water, nutrients, and electrolytes. Under current guidelines, the daily allowance of saturated fats is 20 grams. To date, no such limit has been set for trans fats.

Saturated Fats

Diets high in **saturated fats** have been linked to high cholesterol levels in the blood. Saturated fats are usually solid at room temperature and come from animal fats and tropical oils. Triglycerides are saturated fats that come from butter and lard.

Unsaturated Fats

Unsaturated fats are liquid at room temperature and are referred to as "oils." Unsaturated fats may be monounsaturated or polyunsaturated, as follows:

- **Monounsaturated fats** are liquid at room temperature and may help lower total blood cholesterol. They are thought to raise high-density lipoprotein (HDL, or "good") cholesterol and lower low-density lipoprotein (LDL, or "bad") cholesterol levels. Monounsaturated fats are found in canola, olive, and peanut oils.
- **Polyunsaturated fats** are also liquid at room temperature. They are thought to lower both HDL ("good") and LDL ("bad") cholesterol levels. Some polyunsaturated fats have a lowering effect on total blood cholesterol. Polyunsaturated fats can be found mainly in vegetable oils. **Trans-fatty acids** are formed when polyunsaturated oils are **hydrogenated,** or made solid. Foods high in hydrogenated oil are margarines, peanut butter, and baked goods.

Research indicates that the cell takes in all fatty acids, but that the omega-3 oils (found primarily in whole grains, beans and seeds, and seafood) and the omega-6 oils (found in unsaturated, nonhydrogenated vegetable oils from canola, peanuts, olive, flax, safflower, and sunflower) are the most desirable. The omega oils help maintain smoother skin, promote smoother muscle contractions, allow for better digestion, and support better cardiovascular performance.

Fatty Acid Guidelines

SATURATED FATS	UNSATURATED FATS
Animal source	Plant source
Raise cholesterol in blood	Lower cholesterol
	Monounsaturated and polyunsaturated

Cholesterol

Cholesterol is necessary for vitamin D and bile acid production. Sources of cholesterol include egg yolks and organ meats, in addition to other animal sources. Although cholesterol is important to the body, too high a level of cholesterol in the blood (**hypercholesterolemia**) is unhealthy and contributes to atherosclerosis and heart disease. As the level of blood cholesterol increases, so does the risk of developing these problems.

Sources of Fats and Cholesterol

SATURATED FATS	POLYUNSATURATED FATS	HIGH CHOLESTEROL
(Animal fats)	(Plant fats)	Organ meats
Beef	Vegetable oils (liquid)	Shrimp
Pork	Tub margarines made with safflower or corn oil	Whole milk
Eggs		Lard
Lard		Egg yolks
Solid shortening		Butter, cream
Whole milk		Baked products with butter, eggs, and whole milk

Proteins

Proteins are a group of substances composed of many **amino acids** (building blocks) linked together. Proteins are found in food sources such as whole grains, beans, nuts, and seeds (**simple proteins**). **Complex proteins** contain all the essential amino acids and are found in animal sources (e.g., eggs, meat, fish, dairy products, and poultry). The primary function of proteins is to build and repair body tissue and the formation of **enzymes**. When broken down, amino acids can be absorbed by the small intestine for nutrition. Proteins can also be converted for the body's energy. As the body uses the carbohydrates and fats, it also uses protein from the diet or protein stored in tissue.

There are 22 amino acids in proteins, and of those, the body cannot **synthesize** (make) eight of them. A diet containing these eight amino acids is essential for growth and health, thus the name "essential." Foods containing complete proteins contain all the essential amino acids. Both plants and animals provide protein, and it is important to balance the animal protein consumed with the protein from plants. For example:

Eight Essential Amino Acids The eight essential amino acids are isoleucine, leucine, lysine, methionine, phenylalanine, threonine, tryptophan, and valine. These essential amino acids can be found in animal sources of protein, milk, and eggs, as well as in peas, beans, lentils, nuts, seeds, and whole grains.

Incomplete proteins should be eaten with other protein sources. When certain amino acids are lacking, the other amino acids will convert to produce the energy needed for tissue growth, causing an excessive excretion of nitrogen from the body. When the body is exposed to increased loss of nitrogen, it responds by being deficient in energy, and **malnutrition** (inadequate nutrition) is evident.

Sources of Protein

COMPLETE PROTEINS	INCOMPLETE PROTEINS
Meat	Cereal grains
Poultry	Oatmeal
Cheese	Dried peas and beans
Fish	Peanut butter
Eggs	Nuts
Milk	Soybean products

Water

The body requires large amounts of water each day. This is because water is constantly evaporating as the body produces energy from the foods being eaten. The more protein, salt, caffeine, and alcohol consumed, the more water is needed. Water hydration is also important for removing wastes from the body. The daily recommended amount of water is 2 quarts, or more if you consume salty foods, caffeine, or alcohol.

PATIENT-CENTERED PROFESSIONALISM

- Why must the medical assistant be able to explain the difference between essential and nonessential nutrients when providing patient education?

NUTRITION THROUGH THE LIFE SPAN

For patients of all ages, an important part of the nutritional evaluation is the assessment of the ability to feed oneself, elimination, amount and content of meals, vitamin and other dietary supplements, food preferences and dislikes, food intolerances and allergies, and gastrointestinal (GI) problems. The medical assistant needs to know this information when making assessments of patients' nutritional habits.

Nutritional needs change as people age and go through different life situations.

Pregnancy and Lactation

Meeting nutritional needs during pregnancy and lactation is important to the healthy development of the child.

Nutrition during Pregnancy

Adequate nutrition during pregnancy decreases the chance of some birth defects and assists with embryonic development. Nutritional needs during pregnancy are best met by consuming the minimal number of recommended servings from the food guide pyramid, as follows:

- Foods high in folic acid are needed to prevent neural tube defects.
- To avoid constipation, diet during pregnancy should be especially high in fiber, and water intake should be increased.
- Increased calcium is essential and can be added by using skim milk, thus avoiding added fats.
- Foods high in vitamin A, such as dark-green leafy vegetables and orange vegetables and fruits, are encouraged.
- Vitamin C intake through citrus is essential.

Pregnant women need encouragement to avoid "empty-calorie" foods (e.g., sweets, junk food). Vitamin supplements are not a replacement for nutrients found in food; iron is considered the only supplement truly needed during pregnancy. Processed foods and nonessential fats and sugars should be avoided, but sodium intake should be maintained through fresh vegetables. Sodium helps increase blood volume and meets fetal requirements.

Nutrition after Childbirth

After birth, the adequacy of breast milk can be measured by the following:

- Adequate weight gain by the infant (1 to 2 lbs per month).
- Number of feedings should be between 8 and 12 in a 24-hour period.
- Diaper changes should consist of at least six wet diapers.

The diet of a lactating mother is the same as the diet during pregnancy to maintain and ensure lactation.

Infants

There are established feeding protocols for an infant's diet. Solid foods are not recommended until age 4 to 6 months for the following reasons:

- Complex carbohydrates (cereal, vegetables, and fruits) are not easily digested, and therefore nutrients are not absorbed.
- The tongue is not able to guide food at such an early age.
- Infants are not able to open and close their mouth to indicate a desire for food.

Adding solid foods as the infant grows older helps replenish depleted iron supplies. Guidelines to add foods are as follows:

- Iron-fortified rice cereal: 4 to 6 months.
- Pureed fruits and vegetables: 6 to 8 months.
  - Add one at a time.
  - Add vegetables first; fruits may be too sweet.
- Pureed meats: 6 to 8 months.
- Diluted juice from a cup: 9 months.
- Finger foods: 9 months.

Egg whites, whole milk, and orange juice are introduced after 1 year of age because these tend to cause allergies in some children.

Toddlers

Toddlers need to be given structured choices for a snack (e.g., offer carrots or sliced apples, or raisins or orange slices). Letting toddlers choose from specific options lets them demonstrate their independence and autonomy, but it still allows the caregiver to have some control. Toddlers will need smaller servings to avoid feeling overwhelmed because their growth rate slows during this period, reducing the amount of food they need.

Plan meals with the toddler's food preferences in mind (e.g., preferring apples over pears). However, foods refused should be offered again in the future to encourage variety in the diet. In addition, toddlers' feeding skills should be accepted as they are. This means caregivers must understand that hand-mouth coordination has not yet been mastered. Finger foods work well. If a child dislikes a particular food in a food group, the caregiver should be encouraged to find a suitable substitute (e.g., yogurt for milk). Providing nutritious snacks throughout the day can compensate for poor eating at mealtime. The total amount of nutrients consumed during the day is much more important than what is eaten at a single meal.

School-Age Children

School-age children need to have established, regular meal patterns. Breakfast is often earlier than they would like because of school. School-age children may eat lunch at school with other children, and they often trade food. Dietary needs for school-age children include the following:

- Calcium is needed for bone and growth development, so milk is encouraged, as is broccoli and other dark-green vegetables.
- Vitamin A foods assist with vision and healthy skin.
- Vitamin C helps maintain healthy gums and protects against infection.
- Energy is aided by the consumption of breads, pastas, rice, and cereals.
- Snacks should include milk products, fruits, and nuts; sweets and sodas should be avoided.

Adolescents

Major health problems can develop in adolescence because of inadequate nutrition, as well as from overeating or undereating. Peer pressure and food fads may have an influence on the diet of a teenager. Potato chips instead of vegetables and soft drinks instead of milk can lead to obesity, skin problems, and anemia. Teens who obtain sufficient calories from plant protein (e.g., beans, whole grains, soy products) to maintain a healthy weight may avoid protein from meat if they choose. A teenager who is a strict vegetarian may need to take a multivitamin.

The adolescent is entering a time when the body changes and adolescents have a desire to take control. The amount of body fat in girls increases before puberty, and girls also experience long bone growth. Boys develop later but catch up with increased muscle mass and long bone growth.

For many teens, the issues at hand are being accepted by their peers and having a sense of autonomy. These issues are influenced by society's emphasis on being "thin." **Anorexia** (psychological fear of gaining weight), **bulimia** (compulsive overeating followed by self-induced vomiting or laxative or diuretic abuse), and being overweight are conditions that can affect the teenager during this time.

The dietary needs of an adolescent are as follows:
- More calories and nutrients to assist with increases in bone mass, muscle density, and activity of the endocrine system.
- Foods high in zinc for energy and growth.
- Foods high in calcium, iron, and iodine.
- Increased dairy consumption.
- Include foods high in vitamin B_{12} (animal products).

Aging Individuals

As adults age, their metabolic rates often decrease. Energy levels do not increase as people age, so older adults tend to be less active. When these changes occur and eating habits do not change, older adults tend to put on weight by increasing their fat tissue. Maintaining good bone density during this time is based on physical activity and taking in the needed nutrients so that the weight gain that results is not detrimental to the person's health.

Factors that influence the older adult's dietary consumption and selection of foods include the following:

1. *Income.* Many older adults limit food choices because of cost, thus minimizing protein consumption. Carbohydrates are cheap, easy to fix, store easily, and are consumed more often.
2. *Cultural habits,* customs, race, ethnic background, and gender.
3. *Declining health.* Older adults may have trouble chewing and swallowing, so choices may be affected. The digestive system may not absorb or metabolize needed nutrients from foods as effectively as it once did.
4. *Sense of taste.* The sense of taste alters as people age because of the decreased number of taste buds. Sweets have the greatest taste for many elderly people.

Many older adults use mineral oil as a laxative. This interferes with the body's ability to absorb vital nutrients and should be discouraged.

To assist the elderly patient in nutritional selection, the medical assistant must consider all factors. Knowing the patient's home situation, income, and other demographics will help you guide the patient toward better food selections, as follows:

- The mature adult needs 6 to 8 glasses of water per day to aid in elimination.
- Calcium-rich foods for strong bones and iron-containing foods are needed to help the body use energy.
- Protecting against zinc deficiency helps the wound-healing process.
- Encouraging physical activity is important.

PATIENT-CENTERED PROFESSIONALISM

- *Why is it important for the medical assistant to understand the nutritional needs of patients at various stages in the life span?*

NUTRITION AND CHRONIC DISEASE

Patients with chronic illness have special nutritional needs. The main goal is to maintain adequate nutrition so that the immune system is at optimal strength. Patients with human immunodeficiency virus (HIV) infection, acquired immunodeficiency syndrome (AIDS), and cancer rely on their defense systems to assist them in maintaining a fight toward better health.

HIV and AIDS

Patients newly diagnosed with HIV infection are encouraged to maintain a diet high in protein, with foods adequate in the essential vitamins, minerals, vitamins A and C, vitamin B_{12}, copper, and zinc. Good nutrition is thought to prevent or delay the onset of AIDS by promoting a healthy immune system.

When HIV progresses to AIDS, the metabolic rate increases as a result of infections, stress, and GI upsets. The medications used to treat AIDS often cause nausea and diarrhea. This causes a loss of appetite and **malabsorption** of nutrients. A diet low in lactose and fat can assist in reducing these GI upsets. The addition of liquid supplements can increase caloric intake and add vitamins and proteins to the diet.

Cancer

It is important for cancer patients undergoing chemotherapy to maintain adequate nutritional intake. A diet high in protein (especially red meats), fats, carbohydrates, vitamins, and fluids is needed to keep up with the increased energy demands. Increased energy is needed because of the high metabolic rate caused by tissue breakdown. Research shows that a diet with adequate nutritional intake prevents weight loss, helps to rebuild body tissue, replaces fluid and electrolyte loss, and provides the patient with a sense of well-being.

As with any patient who has a chronic illness, the patient with cancer suffers from lack of appetite, altered taste, a feeling of fullness, chewing and swallowing difficulties, nausea, and fatigue. The patient should be encouraged to eat small but frequent meals, avoid greasy foods, and limit hot and spicy foods. Serving the patient's favorite foods often assists with taking in nourishment.

> **PATIENT-CENTERED PROFESSIONALISM**
>
> - How can the medical assistant help the patient with a chronic illness to understand the importance of nutrition?

DIET THERAPY

A **therapeutic diet** is required in many medical office situations, including preparation for special testing, increasing or decreasing caloric intake, and treating metabolic disorders. It is important for the medical assistant to understand the purpose of various diet therapies, especially in determining which foods are allowed and which should be avoided. To be successful in teaching the patient, the medical assistant must know the patient's current habits and food preferences in addition to the type of therapeutic diet needed.

Regular Diet

A **regular diet** contains all foods from the food guide pyramid and is considered to be adequate and well balanced. It provides generous amounts of all nutrients that an individual needs daily. Modifying this diet to accommodate more fiber, increased nutrients, or increased energy levels leads to a therapeutic diet prescribed to meet the special requirements of the individual patient.

Liquid Diet

A therapeutic **liquid diet** can be in the form of a clear-liquid or a full-liquid diet. Liquid diets should not be used for long periods because of inadequate protein, minerals, vitamins, and calories.

Clear-Liquid Diet

- *Purpose:* Clear liquids are generally the first type of nourishment given to a patient after surgery, in preparation for a colonoscopy, or when fluids have been lost during diarrhea or vomiting. This diet contains minimal residue and consists primarily of dissolved sugar and flavored fluids that provide calories but lack essential nutrients.
- *Recommended foods:* Water, ginger ale, plain gelatin, tea or coffee with sugar, and fat-free broth.
- *Foods to avoid:* Milk and milk products.

Full-Liquid Diet

- *Purpose:* A patient advances to a full-liquid diet after clear liquids. This diet is also prescribed when the patient has difficulty swallowing or an irritated GI tract.
- *Recommended foods:* Continue with clear liquids; custards, ice cream, sherbet, strained soup, puddings, and strained cooked cereals.
- *Foods to avoid:* Any solid food.

Soft Diet

Foods in a **soft diet** are low residue for easy digestion.
- *Purpose:* A soft diet is used to advance past a full-liquid diet, when less strain on the GI system is required, and when there is difficulty chewing.
- *Recommended foods:* Dairy products (to include soft cheese), pureed vegetables, cooked fruit, pastas, ground beef, fish, and chicken.
- *Foods to avoid:* Raw fruits and vegetables, nuts, fried foods, and gas-forming vegetables and meats.

Diabetic Diet

A **diabetic diet** may be prescribed for diabetes or hypoglycemia.
- *Purpose:* Diabetic diets are used with patients who are having difficulty with insulin secretion; this includes both hyperglycemia and hypoglycemia.

The focus is placed on having several small meals of complex-carbohydrate and protein foods. The food intake should match the type of insulin therapy used, exercise performed, and patient's age and weight.

The **glycemic index** rates carbohydrate foods on a scale from the slowest to the fastest with effects on blood glucose levels. It indicates the body's response to a particular food (after eating) compared to a standard amount of glucose. Not all carbohydrates raise the glucose level at the same rate; therefore the index allows an individual to select carbohydrates that take longer to affect blood glucose levels.

Box 9-3 provides food values in the glycemic index. Every carbohydrate is compared to glucose, which has a value of 100. Therefore carbohydrates are given a number relative to glucose in the index. Foods that are thought to be low-glycemic foods seem to have less effect on blood sugars. Foods such as instant rice and white bread have a much higher glycemic value than unprocessed foods such as whole grains and fruits (e.g., grapes, oranges).
- *Recommended foods:* A balance of protein, carbohydrate, and fat.
- *Foods to avoid:* Foods high in sugar (sweets to include baked goods, candy, and syrups).

BOX 9-3

Glycemic Index: Food Values Based on 100 (Glucose)

BEANS		BREADS		CEREALS	
baked	43	bagel	72	cornflakes	83
black	30	pita	57	oatmeal	49
chickpeas	33	rye (whole)	50	Cheerios	74
lentils	30	white	72	All Bran 7	44
COOKIES		**CRACKERS**		**DESSERTS**	
graham crackers	74	rice cakes	82	angel food cake	67
oatmeal	55	rye	63	blueberry muffin	59
shortbread	64	saltines	72	bran muffin	60
vanilla wafers	77	Wheat Thins	67	pound cake	54
FRUIT		**GRAINS**		**PASTA**	
dates (dried)	103	rice (instant)	91	spaghetti	40
banana	62	sweet corn	55	linguine	50
orange	43	brown rice	59	vermicelli	55
grapes	43	Barley	22	mac and cheese	64
JUICES		**MILK PRODUCTS**		**SWEETS**	
apple	41	yogurt	38	honey	58
grapefruit	48	milk	34	Lifesavers	70
orange	55	pudding	43	Snickers	41
pineapple	46	ice cream	50	Skittles	70

Calorie-Controlled Diet

A **calorie-controlled diet** may be a low-calorie or a high-calorie diet.

Low-Calorie Diet (1,000-1,200 Calories)

- *Purpose:* A low-calorie diet reduces calorie intake for overweight and arthritic patients.
- *Recommended foods:* Lean meats, poultry, low-carbohydrate vegetables, fruits, whole grains, and skim milk products.
- *Food to avoid:* Fatty meats, whole milk products, lima beans, corn, peas, beans, snack foods, and desserts.

High-Calorie, High-Protein Diet (>2,000 Calories)

- *Purpose:* High-calorie diets are used after surgery, with burn patients, when high fever or infection is present, when weight is below normal (e.g., hyperthyroidism, anorexia), and for patients with fractures.
- *Recommended foods:* All food groups.
- *Foods to avoid:* Fatty foods.

Low-Cholesterol, Low-Fat Diet

Research indicates that when an individual chooses a diet low in fats (**low-cholesterol, low-fat diet**), the person is able to eat a variety of foods needed for nutritional intake. Fats contain twice as many calories as an equal amount of protein or carbohydrates. A diet low in saturated fat and cholesterol helps maintain the blood cholesterol levels below 200 milligrams per deciliter (mg/dL). Total fat intake should be 30% or less of the total calories consumed. For example:

> **30% Fat Intake** Fat intake should be 30% (or less) of the total calories consumed.
>
> A diet of 1,500 calories per day would allow 450 calories to come from fat.
>
> $$1500 \times .3 (30\%) = 450$$
>
> To determine the number of grams (g) of fat, divide 450 by 9 (9 calories are provided by each gram of fat).
>
> $$450 \div 9 = 50 \text{ g}$$
>
> Therefore, in a diet of 1500 calories per day, 50 or fewer grams of fat should be consumed or 450 or fewer calories should come from fat.
>
> - *Purpose:* Low-cholesterol and low-fat diets are prescribed for patients with elevated lipids; those with liver, gallbladder, or cardiovascular disease; and patients who are obese.
> - *Recommended foods:* Skim milk products, lean fish, poultry, meats, cottage cheese, vegetables, fruits and their juices, tea and coffee, jelly, and honey.
> - *Foods to avoid:* Cheese, whole milk products, fatty meats (pork, bacon, ham, sausage, duck, goose, fatty fish), chocolate, and fried foods.

Sodium-Restricted Diet

Another type of therapeutic diet is the **sodium-restricted diet.**

- *Purpose:* Sodium-restricted diets are prescribed for patients with kidney disease, high blood pressure, or cardiovascular disease and those who have edema.
- *Recommended foods:* Natural foods without additives.
- *Foods to avoid:* Processed foods, added table salt, condiments, pickles, and olives.

Renal Failure Diet

The **renal failure diet** is ordered when a patient's kidneys are not able to get rid of all the wastes in their blood.

- *Purpose:* Controls the amount of protein and phosphorus in a patient's diet. The diet may also restrict the amount of sodium and potassium the patient consumes.
- *Recommended foods:* Per day: 1 oz of protein; ½ cup of nondairy product; 1 slice of bread (Italian, light rye); ½ cup of vegetables: alfalfa sprouts, green or wax beans, cabbage, lettuce (1 cup); fruit: canned pears, applesauce, blueberries (½ cup).
- *Foods to avoid:* Processed foods, more than 1 oz of meat, chicken, fish, eggs, dairy products, beans, peas, and nuts. Also avoid colas, beer, and cocoa.

Bland Diet

A **bland diet** may also be prescribed as a therapeutic diet.

- *Purpose:* Bland diets help avoid irritation to the GI tract (e.g., colitis, ulcers).
- *Recommended foods:* Foods low in fiber, mild seasonings, dairy, eggs, well-cooked vegetables, boiled and broiled meats, fish, poultry, and pastas.
- *Foods to avoid:* Fried foods or highly seasoned foods, alcohol or carbonated beverages, condiments, pickled products, and raw vegetables.

Low-Fiber Diet

The **low-fiber diet** is another therapeutic option.

- *Purpose:* A low-fiber diet decreases the work of the intestines (e.g., in patients with colitis, ileitis, or diverticulitis).
- *Recommended foods:* Broiled, boiled, or baked meats; fish and poultry; pastas; dairy products; well-cooked vegetables; fruit and vegetable juices; and canned fruit.
- *Foods to avoid:* Fresh fruits and vegetables, fried foods, nuts, and pickled products.

High-Fiber Diet

A **high-fiber diet** may also be needed as a therapeutic option.

- *Purpose:* To help with elimination.
- *Recommended foods:* All vegetables, raw and cooked fruits, and whole-grain foods, including breads, grains, and cereals.
- *Foods to avoid:* Fatty foods.

Fad Diets

A **fad diet** offers quick weight loss but has no long-term advantages. Research has shown that although weight loss is quick, if steps are not taken to revise eating habits, dieters regain much of the weight, if not more, by the end of the first year.

- The *Atkins diet* stresses low carbohydrates, high protein, and fats.
- The *cabbage soup diet* is a 7-day diet plan that requires a special soup to be eaten each day, with certain foods introduced each day as well.
- The *negative-calorie diet* allows only certain foods to be eaten that the body tends to burn faster.
- The *South Beach diet* is based on reducing carbohydrates initially and changing the eating habits overall for a lifetime to exclude many white flour and sugar food items.

Fad diets can result in electrolyte loss, dehydration, kidney disease, gout, and calcium depletion, which in turn can result in hospitalization. There is no substitute for eating a healthy diet, making good nutrition a habit, and ensuring adequate exercise.

> **PATIENT-CENTERED PROFESSIONALISM**
>
> - How does the medical assistant use information concerning different diet therapies?
> - How should the medical assistant answer a question about a fad diet that a patient is considering?

CONCLUSION

The medical assistant who understands basic nutritional concepts and the reasons for a particular diet therapy can assist the patient in following the prescribed dietary regimen. Unless the body receives the nutrients it requires, fat and muscle are used to supply the energy needed by the body daily. The basic life process needed to circulate the blood throughout the body, to move muscles in order to breathe, and to maintain the body temperature requires a certain amount of energy. Therefore adequate nutrition is required daily.

Nutrition is the key to the healing process, but other factors affect the body's ability to absorb or take in the required nutrients. These factors include the state of a person's digestive system, an individual's mental issues with physical appearance (e.g., "perfect" body), and economic inability to purchase nutritious foods. Dealing with the nutrition issues of patients is not only about the type of food they eat; as a medical assistant, you must also address the person as a whole. Consider what disease processes are affecting a patient's ability to eat, whether the patient is on a limited income, and whether the patient is depressed or has low self-esteem during patient teaching.

Educating patients about following through with treatment plans, improving their nutrition, and improving their overall health is one of the most important responsibilities of the medical assistant.

Chapter Summary

Reinforce your understanding of the material in this chapter by reviewing the curriculum objectives and key content points below.

1. **Define, appropriately use, and spell all the Key Terms for this chapter.**
   - Review the Key Terms if necessary.
2. **Explain the purpose of dietary guidelines.**
   - Dietary guidelines provide the public with information about the amounts of essential nutrients in a diet that assist in decreasing the risk of chronic disease.
3. **List the six food groups included in the food guide pyramid and discuss the recommended daily quantities for a 2,000-calorie diet.**
   - Review Table 9-2.
   - Grains (half should be whole grain): 6 oz.
   - Vegetables (variety): 2½ cups.
   - Fruits: 2 cups.
   - Milk: 3 cups.
   - Vegetables: 3-5 servings.
   - Fruits: 2-4 servings.
   - Meat and beans: 5½ oz.
   - Consumption of fats, sodium, and sugar in foods should be minimized. Fat sources from fish, nuts, and vegetable oils.
4. **Explain the purpose of the NLEA, and list the two main panels to consider when looking at a food label.**
   - The NLEA was enacted to assist consumers in identifying nutritional content in food products.
   - Food labels allow consumers to make better choices.
   - The display panel is used for marketing purposes, and the nutritional fact panel meets the requirements of federal regulatory boards.
   - The calories listed show how much energy is received from one serving and how many calories are derived from fat.
5. **List and briefly describe five basic principles of good nutrition.**
   - Five principles of good nutrition are variety (eating different foods in moderation), weight management (restricting calories to maintain weight), balance (eating proper amounts of foods), minimizing sugar (restricting these poor-value calories), and reducing sodium (found naturally in many foods).
   - Doubling the serving size also doubles the nutrient value and the calories.
6. **Demonstrate how to calculate a patient's BMI, and indicate whether a patient is underweight, normal, overweight, or obese according to the chart.**
   - BMI = Weight (kg) ÷ Height (m^2).
   - Review Table 9-3.
7. **List five tips for maintaining nutritional balance in the daily diet.**
   - Drinking water, eating low-fat lean meats, eating a variety of fruits and vegetables, using low-fat or fat-free dairy products, and eating plenty of whole grains, rice, and pasta are tips for maintaining balance in the daily diet.
8. **Differentiate between essential and nonessential nutrients.**
   - Essential nutrients must be taken from a food source (vitamins, minerals, proteins, carbohydrates, fats, water).
   - Nonessential nutrients are provided within the body.
   - Nutrients contained in dietary fiber, protein, vitamins, and minerals improve health and assist in reducing disease. It is advised that these nutrients average to 100% daily.
   - Foods containing 5% or more of dietary fiber are considered to be contributing toward the daily total.
   - Foods containing 20% or higher of vitamins and minerals contribute a good amount toward the daily total.
9. **Differentiate fat-soluble vitamins from water-soluble vitamins and list the major sources of each.**
   - Review Tables 9-4 and 9-5.
10. **List nine major minerals and explain the sources of each and the result of deficiency.**
    - Review Table 9-6.
11. **List seven trace minerals and explain the sources of each and the result of deficiency.**
    - Review Table 9-7.
12. **Explain why the body needs carbohydrates, fats, and proteins.**
    - Carbohydrates are the body's primary energy source.
    - Fats are the body's stored energy.
    - Proteins build and repair body tissue and break down enzymes into amino acids.
13. **Explain the importance of water and state the daily recommended amount.**
    - Water keeps the body hydrated and is important for eliminating waste.
    - The daily recommended amount of water is 2 quarts.
14. **Explain dietary needs during pregnancy and lactation, infancy, toddler age, school age, adolescence, and older adulthood.**
    - The amounts and types of nutrients vary depending on age and physical state, which determine how well the body can absorb and use the nutrients.
15. **Explain the dietary needs of patients newly diagnosed with HIV and those with AIDS.**
    - Newly diagnosed HIV patients need a diet high in protein and adequate in essential vitamins, minerals, vitamins A and C, vitamin B$_{12}$, copper, and zinc that will prevent or delay the onset of AIDS by promoting a healthy immune system.
    - Patients with AIDS may have gastrointestinal upset, stress, and infections, thus a diet low in lactose and fat should help reduce nausea and diarrhea. Increased caloric intake, vitamins, and proteins are also important.
16. **Explain the dietary needs for cancer patients undergoing chemotherapy.**
    - Patients undergoing chemotherapy need to maintain adequate nutritional intake to prevent weight loss, rebuild body tissue, replace fluid and electrolyte loss, and promote a sense of well-being. A diet high in

protein, fats, carbohydrates, vitamins, and fluids is needed to keep energy up.

17. **List and briefly describe nine types of therapeutic diets.**
    - Therapeutic diets include liquid (clear or full liquid), soft (low residue, easy to digest), diabetic (small meals with complex carbohydrates), calorie controlled (low calorie or high calorie based on losing or gaining weight), low cholesterol, low fat (restricted animal fat intake), sodium restricted (natural foods without additives), bland (non-irritating to gastrointestinal tract), low fiber (decreases work of intestines), and high fiber (increases work of intestines to help with elimination).

18. **Explain why fad diets are unhealthy and a poor choice for long-term weight loss.**
    - Fad diets can result in electrolyte loss, dehydration, kidney disease, gout, and calcium depletion.
    - Fad diets do not change a person's eating behavior for the long term and may actually increase weight gain.

19. **Analyze a realistic medical office situation and apply your understanding of patient education and nutrition to determine the best course of action.**
    - Medical assistants must understand both patient education techniques and nutrition to provide optimum education for their patients.

20. **Describe the impact on patient care when medical assistants have a solid understanding of nutrition and how it relates to the patient's treatment plan.**
    - Nutrition knowledge is a valuable tool for the promotion of health care because it helps promote actions that benefit the patient.
    - Nutritional information in the medical practice is an ongoing topic, since the effects are seen throughout the patient's life span and assist during treatment of an illness.

PRACTICAL APPLICATIONS

If you have accomplished the objectives in this chapter, you will be able to make better choices as a medical assistant. Take another look at this situation and decide what you would do.

Josephine, age 52, has just been diagnosed with type 2 diabetes mellitus related to obesity. Living in the home with Josephine are her mother, Susie, who is 80 years old; Josephine's daughter Jessie, who is 24 and pregnant; and Jessie's two very active children, ages 6 and 2. Susie has been diagnosed with a heart condition and must be on a soft diet that is low in cholesterol and sodium restricted.

Josephine's concern today is how she can maintain a diet acceptable for all the medical conditions in the household while being sure the other family members will eat what is prepared. She thinks the children need sugar, but her mother needs to watch her sugar and salt intake to remain in a stable condition and not gain weight. Susie also needs her meals to be soft and easily chewable because of her decrease in intestinal motility. However, Jessie and her 2-year-old child both need a diet that allows the necessary fiber for adequate bowel activity.

If you were the medical assistant, how might you educate Josephine about nutrition and answer her questions?

1. Why are learning styles important for the medical assistant to understand when teaching medical knowledge to the patient?
2. Why is it now so important for Josephine to read food labels? What information is found on these?
3. Why is diet so important for Josephine to follow in the treatment of type 2 diabetes mellitus? Why does she need to know the glycemic index of foods?
4. What special requirements will be needed for Susie so that she maintains a low-cholesterol diet?
5. Jessie's children want to eat pizza and french fries like their friends. How will this affect the dietary changes of Josephine, Susie, and Jessie?
6. Because Jessie has elevated blood pressure and early signs of edema in the legs and feet, what type of diet would you expect her to maintain for the remainder of her pregnancy?
7. What is found in a diabetic diet? A low-sodium diet?
8. What effect would low income have on this family?
9. What effect would culture have in planning this diet if the family were of Greek or Italian ethnicity?
10. Why is BMI a better guide for obesity than height-weight charts?
11. Why is it important that Josephine include a variety of foods in the diet for all members of the family?

WEB SEARCH

1. **Research food guide pyramids for a certain age group.** Children need nutrients that promote growth, for example, but getting a child to eat is sometimes a difficult task. Elderly persons may need fewer calories because they tend to be less active. Both groups have certain nutritional needs that must be met to promote tissue growth and maintain body function.
   - **Keywords:** Use the following keywords in your search: food guide pyramid, elderly nutrition, toddler food guide, adolescent nutritional needs.

2. **Research what policies the American Medical Association (AMA) adopted in 2007 to promote healthier food options to fight obesity in Americans.** Combating obesity by promoting healthier food options is a concern of the AMA. The AMA focused on replacing trans fats with healthier fats and oils, nutritional labeling at fast-food and chain restaurants, and tailoring items in food assistance programs to better address the health care needs of Americans.
   - **Keywords:** Use the following keywords in your search: AMA obesity, AMA healthier food, AMA trans fat.

3. **Research metabolic syndrome.** Metabolic syndrome is a combination of medical disorders that increase the risk of developing cardiovascular disease and diabetes.
   - **Keywords**: Metabolic syndrome, syndrome X, insulin resistance, or Reaven's syndrome.

Understanding Medical Terminology

10

evolve http://evolve.elsevier.com/klieger/medicalassisting

Medical terminology is the language of medicine and health care. It is used to describe and record every aspect of patient care, including medical history, diagnostic testing results, treatment, and charting progress. Medical terminology is also important in medical billing because it is used to communicate with insurance companies, providers, and other health care professionals.

By understanding the origin of medical terminology, the parts used to build medical words, and the guidelines for using medical terminology, you will be able to identify and use medical words correctly.

LEARNING OBJECTIVES

You will be able to do the following after completing this chapter:

Key Terms
1. Define, appropriately use, and spell all the Key Terms for this chapter.

Word Origins and Meanings
2. Discuss the origins of words and where the terms used in medicine often originated.
3. Explain the importance of using correct medical terminology in a medical setting.

Word Parts
4. Identify and describe the four word parts used to build medical words.
5. State the importance of understanding the function of each word part.
6. Identify three helpful tips for studying medical terminology.

Guidelines for Medical Terminology
7. Apply pronunciation guidelines to pronounce various medical terms correctly.
8. Change various medical terms from singular to plural correctly.
9. Define and give an example of an antonym, homonym, and synonym.

Patient-Centered Professionalism
10. Analyze a realistic medical office situation and apply your understanding of medical terminology to determine the best course of action.
11. Describe the impact on patient care when medical assistants have a solid grasp of the correct use of medical terminology.

KEY TERMS

antonym
combining form
combining vowel
consonant
diagnostic
diminutive
eponym
homonym

operative
plural
prefix
root word
suffix
symptomatic
synonym
vowel

PRACTICAL APPLICATIONS

Read the following scenario and keep it in mind as you learn about medical terminology in this chapter.

Dr. Smith has a medical assistant who does the medical transcription of her patient notes. The following is a note the medical assistant has transcribed on Susie Ramos:

"Seen in the office today for arteriaslcerosis and hipertension. Mrs. Ramos complained of feeling dizzy with some fertigo for three days. On questioning, Mrs. Ramos did state that she was febrile two days ago with some gastroentestinal symptoms such as darhea and nausea. She also complained of aralgia and laryngetes. On examination the toncils are red and swollen. Her blood pressure is controlled by medication. There are no complaints of chest pain or anjina, nor does she have dispnea, although she does have some orthapnea. She does have some syanosis of the hands and feet but does not complain of pain in these areas. Her sinuses are painful. Her current diagnosisses are sinisitus, athuroscleroisis, possible streptocokki infection, gastrointeritis, and faringitis."

Would you be able to point out all the mistakes this note contains to the medical assistant?

BOX 10-1

Medical Eponyms*

Specific People	Specific Places	Specific Things
McBurney point	Mayo scissors	Athlete's foot
Foley catheter	Ardmore disease	Army-navy retractor
Babinski reflex	Minnesota Multiphasic Personality Inventory (MMPI)	Housemaid knee
Crohn disease		Pinkeye
Cesarean section		Tennis elbow
	Duke staging system	
	Philadelphia chromosome	

*The possessive form ('s) is also often used with medical eponyms (e.g., McBurney's point).

WORD ORIGINS AND MEANINGS

The first steps in learning about medical terminology are to understand the origin of the words and to recognize the importance of knowing the true meaning of the words used in the medical setting.

Word Origins

The language used in the medical field comes from a combination of Greek and Latin words, eponyms, and terms that resulted from modern medical advances (e.g., pacemaker, fiberoptics). An **eponym** is the name of a specific person (or place or thing) for whom (or which) something is being named. You use eponyms every day and may not even be aware of it (e.g., the sandwich is named for the Earl of Sandwich, who asked his servant to bring him a serving of meat between two pieces of bread). In medicine, certain diagnostic and surgical procedures, diseases, instruments, and parts of the anatomy are named using eponyms (Box 10-1).

The vast majority of medical terms have Greek and Latin origins. In general, Greek words usually refer to disease and Latin words to anatomical structures.

Anatomical	Latin	Greek	Disease
kidney/renal	ren-	nephro-	nephritis
tongue/linguistic	lingua-	glossa-	glossitis

We use medical terminology because it provides one word for something that might otherwise take many words to describe. For example, you can say "arthritis" more quickly than you can say "inflammation of the joint." Understanding the origin of medical terms can help you begin to uncover their meaning.

Importance of Medical Terms

As a medical assistant, you will hear, see, and use many medical terms throughout the day. It is critical that you understand the meaning of these words in the medical setting. Consider the following situations that could result if a medical assistant used medical terminology incorrectly on the job:

- The patient could be given a treatment that is ineffective or even harmful because of an incorrect term recorded on the chart.
- The patient could be influenced by the medical assistant's incorrect use of medical terminology and lose trust in the health care team.
- The patient's health insurance company may not pay the full amount of the services (payment is based on what is recorded in the medical records).
- Lawsuits could result, word could spread, and patients could choose to leave the practice.

For these reasons, it is necessary for medical assistants to have a firm grasp of medical terminology. It is impossible to memorize all the medical words. However, by dividing words into parts, it is often possible to figure out their meaning. In the next section, you begin learning the basic root words, prefixes, and suffixes that will make it easier to understand these unfamiliar words. Box 10-2 offers helpful hints for learning and understanding medical terms.

PATIENT-CENTERED PROFESSIONALISM

- How can a medical assistant build a medical vocabulary? Why is it not necessary to memorize every medical term?
- How is patient care affected if the medical assistant is not familiar with medical terminology?
- How does a medical assistant's grasp of medical terminology affect the person's ability to communicate effectively with patients?

> **BOX 10-2**
>
> **Guidelines for Learning and Understanding Medical Terminology**
>
> 1. Pair or group words or word parts together that have an opposite meaning (antonyms).
> 2. Pair or group words or word parts together that have similar meanings (synonyms).
> 3. Look at the word and divide it into basic word parts. Decide if either an action or a condition is involved, or if the word element relates to an anatomical part.
>   If an action or condition is involved, do the following:
>   - Define the suffix.
>   - Define the root word or combining form.
>   - Define the prefix.
>   (In other words, start backward.)
>   If the word is referring to an anatomical part, do the following:
>   - Define the root word(s) or combining form.
>   - Define the suffix.
>   - Define the prefix.
> 4. Remember, there can be more than one prefix, suffix, or root word with the same meaning (synonym), so be certain you are using (or considering) the most precise, accurate word part possible.

TABLE 10-1

Parts of Three Common Medical Terms

Term and Pronunciation	Prefix	Combining Form and Root	Suffix
hematology (study of blood) he-mah-TALL-uh-jee		hemat/o (blood)	logy (study of)
cytopathology (study of cellular diseases) sye-toh-puh-THALL-uh-jee	cyto (referring to cells)	path/o (disease)	logy (study of)
chemotherapy (treatment by a chemical agent) key-mo-THAYR-uh-pee		chem/o (chemical)	therapy (treatment)

WORD PARTS

You will need to learn the meaning of many medical terms. One way you can do this is to learn about the *parts* of medical words and how they fit together. There are three word parts: root words (together with combining vowels), prefixes, and suffixes (Table 10-1).

Understanding the function of these word parts will enable you to decipher (*de* [undo the] + *cipher* [code or message]) medical terms that are unfamiliar to you.

Root Words and Combining Vowels

The **root word** is the part of the word that contains the main meaning. All medical terms have at least one root word. The root word may be used alone or combined with a vowel, usually *o* or *e*. The **combining vowel** is added to the root word before any prefixes or suffixes are added. Combining vowels do not change the meaning of a root word and are not used for all medical terms. The combining vowel makes pronunciation easier. The root word with the combining vowel is called the **combining form,** as in the following word parts of "cyto + patho + logy":

- The root word is *path*, which means "disease."
- The combining vowel is *o*.
- Therefore the combining form is *patho*.

When using combining vowels with root words, follow these guidelines:

1. Use a combining vowel before a suffix that begins with a consonant (e.g., cyt/o/pathology).
2. Use a combining vowel to join other root words (e.g., gastr/o/enteritis).
3. Do not use a combining vowel before a suffix beginning with a vowel (e.g., gastritis, not gastroitis).

It is also helpful to know some of the common root words and combining forms used in health care terminology (Table 10-2), in addition to those used to represent color (Table 10-3), chemical elements (Table 10-4), cells, and tissues (Table 10-5).

Prefixes

A **prefix** is a word part that is sometimes placed at the beginning of a root word to change its meaning by making it more specific or to create a new word. In the example "cyto + patho + logy":

- The prefix is *cyto*, which means "having to do with (pertaining to) cells."

Not all medical words have a prefix. Learning the prefixes used with number and quantity (Table 10-6), size and amount (Table 10-7), position and direction (Table 10-8), and other descriptive prefixes (Table 10-9) will help you understand medical terminology.

Suffixes

A **suffix** is a word part or series of word parts added to the end of a root word to change its meaning. By adding a suffix to a root word, the meaning changes to an *adjective, noun,* or *verb*. In the example "cyto + patho + logy":

- The suffix is *logy*, which means "the study of."
- Adding the suffix to "cytopatho" makes the term a noun.

Not all medical words have suffixes. *When analyzing medical words, begin with the* **suffix,** *then proceed to the* **root** *and* **prefix.** This may help uncover the definition or its applied

TABLE 10-2

Common Medical Roots and Combining Forms

Roots and Combining Forms	Meaning	Word Example	Definition of Example
aden/o	gland	**aden**opathy	Enlargement of glands
aer/o	air	**aer**obe	Organism requiring oxygen to live
andr/o	of man	**andr**oid	Something having human form
auto-	self	**auto**analysis	Self-evaluation
bar/o	pressure	**baro**metric	Atmospheric pressure
bi/o	life	**bio**logy	Study of life and living things
brady-	slow	**brady**cardia	Slow heart rate; below 60 beats per minute
brachy-	short (distance)	**brachy**therapy	Radiation delivered in close range to tumor site
carcin/o	cancer	**carcino**gen	Something that causes cancer
cancer/o		**cancer**ous	Pertaining to cancer
cry/o	cold	**cryo**therapy	Use of low temperatures in medical therapy
crypt/o	hidden	**crypt**orchidism	Undescended testicle
dextro-	right	**dextro**cardia	Heart located in right hemothorax, caused by disease or congenital defect
diplo-	double	**diplo**coccus	Pair of cocci bacteria; two cocci together
erg/o	work	syn**erg**ism	State of two or more parts working together
eti/o	cause of disease	**eti**ology	Study of causes or origins of disease
eu-	good, normal, healthy	**eu**genic	Good offspring or related to improving offspring
exo-,	without, outside of	**exo**biology	Study of extraterrestrial life and effects of extraterrestrial surroundings on living organisms
ecto-		**ecto**derm	Outermost layer of developing embryo
febr	fever	**febr**ile	Feverish; having a fever
gyn/o, gynec/o	female	**gyneco**logy	Study of health care for women
holo-, hol-	whole, complete	**hol**istic medicine	Something that is seen as more than the sum of its parts Treating the "whole patient"
hydr/o, hydr-	water	**hydro**cele	A swelling filled with water; accumulation of fluid in a sac-like body cavity
macro-, macr-	large, huge	**macro**scopic	Large enough to be seen with the naked eye
megalo-, mega-		**mega**dose	Dose that exceeds the amount usually given
men/o, mens	month	**meno**pause	Period marked by cessation of menstruation
meso-	middle	**meso**derm	Middle cell layer of developing embryo
micro-, micr-	small	**micro**scope	Instrument used to magnify images of small objects
morph/o	shape	**morpho**logy	Study of shape or form
narc/o	sleep	**narco**lepsy	Disorder with sudden attacks of deep sleep
nat/o	birth	neo**nat**al	Pertaining to a newborn infant
necr/o	death	**necro**sis	Death of cells or tissues through injury or disease
nyct/o	night	**nycto**phobia	Abnormal fear of night or darkness
noct/o, noct/l		**noct**urnal	Pertaining to the night
olig-, oligo-	scanty, few	**olig**uria	Producing an abnormally small amount of urine
onc/o	tumor	**onco**logy	Study and treatment of cancer
path/o	disease	**patho**physiology	Study of changes resulting from disease or injury
phot/o	light	**photo**phobia	Abnormal fear or insensitivity to light
py/o	pus	**pyo**rrhea	Inflammation of and discharge from the gums and teeth
quadri-, quadr-	four	**quadri**lateral	Having four sides
scler/o	abnormally hard	arterio**scler**osis	Hardening of the arteries
septic	poison, infection	**septic**emia	Blood poisoning
sinistro-	left	**sinistro**cerebral	Brain located toward left side of cranium
son/o	sound	**sono**gram	Image produced by ultrasonography
staphyl/o	grapelike clusters	**staphylo**coccus	Round gram-positive bacteria appearing in clusters
steno-	narrow	**steno**sis	Narrowing of a duct or passage
strept/o	twisted chains	**strepto**coccus	Round gram-positive bacteria appearing in clusters or "twisted chains"
supra-	above, superior, beyond	**supra**nasal	Superior to (above) the nose
super-		**super**acid	Excessive acid
therap	treatment	**therap**y	Treatment
therm/o	heat	**therm**al	Relating to heat

TABLE 10-3
Word Forms Representing Color

Roots and Combining Forms	Meaning	Word Example	Definition of Example
chlor/o	green	**chlor**ophane	Light-green pigment in the inner segment of the cones of the retina
chrom/o	color	**chrom**ophobic	Cell or tissue not easily stained
chromat/o		**chromat**ic	Stainable by dye
cyan/o	blue	**cyan**osis	Bluish discoloration of the skin and mucous membranes from a lack of oxygen
erythr/o	red	**erythr**oderma	Abnormal redness of the skin
rube-		**rube**lla	German measles = red rash
glauc/o	gray	**glauc**oma	Eye disease caused by obstruction of aqueous humor outflow, which gives the eye a dull-gray coating
polio-		**polio**encephalitis	Viral infection causing inflammation to gray matter of the brain
leuk/o	white	**leuk**oplakia	Condition involving white spots or patches on mucous membranes
albin/o	colorless	**albin**o	Person with a marked deficiency of pigment (color) in the hair, skin, and eyes
albumin/o		**albumin**uria	Presence of albumin in urine
melan/o	black	**melan**oma	Dark-pigmented tumor (often malignant); usually in the skin
purpur/o	purple	**purpur**a	Hemorrhages in the skin and mucous membranes resulting in the appearance of purplish spots or patches
xanthr/o, xanth/o	yellow	**xanth**oderma	Yellowish color to skin
cirrh/o		**cirrh**osis	Chronic inflammation of liver that results in yellow skin and organ tissue
lute/o		**lute**oma	Tumor cells resembling those of corpus luteum (which is yellow)

TABLE 10-4
Word Forms Representing Chemical Elements

Roots and Combining Forms	Meaning	Word Example	Definition of Example
azot/o	nitrogen (N)	**azot**emia	Nitrogenous waste in blood
calci-	calcium (Ca)	**calci**penia	Deficiency of calcium
carb-	carbon (C)	**carb**on dioxide	Colorless, odorless gas formed from carbon and oxygen
chlori-	chloride (Cl)	**chlori**duria	Excessive level of chlorides in the urine
ferr/o	iron (Fe)	**ferr**ous	Relating to or containing iron
ferr/i		**ferr**ic	Relating to or containing iron
sider/o		**sider**openia	Low iron
kali-	potassium (K)	hypo**kal**emia	Low potassium in blood
natri-	sodium (Na)	**natri**uresis	Excretion of excessive amounts of sodium in the urine
ox-	oxygen (O)	**ox**imeter	Device for measuring amount of oxygen in arterial blood

TABLE 10-5
Word Forms Representing Tissues

Roots and Combining Forms	Meaning	Word Example	Definition of Example
adip/o	fat	**adip**ose	Fat tissue
lip/o		**lip**ase	Enzyme that breaks down fats into glycerol and fatty acids
epitheli/o	epithelial	**epitheli**um	Membranous tissue covering most internal and external surfaces of body and organs
my/o	muscle	**my**ocardia	Muscular tissue of heart
neur/o	nervous	**neur**opathology	Study of diseases of the nervous system
sarc/o	connective	**sarc**olemma	Thin membrane enclosing a muscle fiber

TABLE 10-6
Prefixes Representing Number and Quantity

Prefix	Meaning	Word Example	Definition of Example
ambi-	both, both sides, around	**ambi**guous	Open to more than one interpretation; uncertain
bi-	two, twice	**bi**concave	Concave on both sides
		bifocal	Having two focal lengths (or lens types)
di-		**di**atomic	Made up of two atoms
centi-	1/100 (one hundredth)	**centi**meter	Unit of length equal to 1/100 of a meter
deca-	10	**deca**gram	Unit of mass equal to 10 grams
hemi-	half, one side, partial	**hemi**algia	Pain affecting half the body
semi-		**semi**flexion	Limb positioned midway between full flexion and full extension
		semicircular	Half of a circle in shape
kilo-	1000	**kilo**gram	Unit of mass equal to 1000 grams
micro-	1/1,000,000 (one millionth)	**micro**gram	Unit of mass equal to 1/1000 of a milligram or 1/1,000,000 of a gram
milli-	1/1000 (one thousandth)	**milli**liter	Unit of volume equal to 1/1000 of a liter
multi-, mult-	many, much	**multi**cellular	Containing multiple cells
nulli-	none	**nulli**para	Woman who has never given birth
primi-	first	**primi**tive	Simple, crude, or unsophisticated
tri-	three	**tri**angular	Shape with three angles and sides
		trifocals	Having three focal lengths (or lens types)
uni-	one	**uni**cellular	Composed of one cell
mono-		**mono**cular	Having one eye or lens

TABLE 10-7
Prefixes Representing Size and Amount

Prefix	Meaning	Word Example	Definition of Example
hetero-	unequal, different	**hetero**sexual	Sexually oriented to persons of the opposite sex
homo-	same, similar	**homo**sexual	Sexually oriented to persons of the same sex
homeo-		**homeo**pathy	Therapy based on theory that "like cures like"
iso-	equal	**iso**metric	Maintaining equal length
pan-	all	**pan**demic	Epidemic over a wide area; affecting a large population

meaning. Important types of suffixes to recognize are general suffixes (Table 10-10), common medical suffixes (Table 10-11), **symptomatic** suffixes (Table 10-12), **diagnostic** suffixes (Table 10-13), and **operative** suffixes (Table 10-14).

> **PATIENT-CENTERED PROFESSIONALISM**
>
> - *How can knowing the function and meaning of word parts help you improve your ability to communicate with patients and co-workers?*
> - *Why is it important to always use the correct prefixes, suffixes, and root words in medical settings?*
> - *What is the best way to break down a medical term to determine its meaning? Why?*

GUIDELINES FOR MEDICAL TERMINOLOGY

In addition to understanding how to determine the meaning of medical terms from the word parts, you also need to know how to correctly *use* these terms in the medical setting. Correctly using medical terminology requires an understanding of the word parts and their function. You also must know how to pronounce the words, how to make singular terms plural when needed, and how to distinguish antonyms and homonyms to be certain you are using the correct word.

Pronunciation

The pronunciation of medical words can be made easier if you keep in mind some *phonetic* (relating to sounds and speech) guidelines.

Vowels

In most cases, if a **vowel** (*a, e, i, o, u,* and sometimes *y*) is followed by another vowel, the vowel receives a long pronunciation, and a *macron* (¯) is placed over the vowel symbol. For example, "tray" is pronounced ('trā).

TABLE 10-8

Prefixes Representing Position and Direction

Prefix	Meaning	Word Example	Definition of Example
ab-	away from, away, upon	**ab**duction	Moving or drawing away from the body
ad-	toward, add, increase	**ad**duction	Moving or drawing inward toward the body
ana-	up, back against, against	**ana**bolism	Metabolic process that builds up complex materials
ante-	before, forward, in front of	**ante** cibum (a.c.)	Before meals (prescription directions)
		antecubital	Area in front of the elbow
pre-		**pre**natal	Before birth
pro-		**pro**lapse	When an organ or part of an organ slips out of place and falls forward
fore-		**fore**arm	Part of the arm between the wrist and elbow
de-	down, remove downward	**de**calcification	Process of removing calcium from bones
		deactivation	Making inactive or stopping action
cata-		**cata**bolism	Process in which complex substances are broken down in metabolism
endo-, end-	within, in, inside	**endo**scope	Instrument for examining the interior of a body cavity
intra-		**intra**bronchial	Within the bronchial area
epi-, ep-	above, on, excessive, over, beyond	**epi**dermis	Outer layer of the skin
hyper-		**hyper**tension	High blood pressure
gen-	beginning	gluconeo**gen**esis	Having to do with new formation of sugar in the blood
		genetic	Having to do with genes
inter-	between	**inter**atrial	Situated between the atria of the heart
meta-	after, beyond	**meta**carpal	Beyond the carpals (at the wrist); pertaining to the middle part of the hand
para-	around, beside, near, past	**para**nasal	Area around the nose
peri-		**peri**carditis	Inflammation of the pericardium
circum-		**circum**cision	Surgical procedure that removes the foreskin around the penis
re-	back, again	**re**verse	Turned backward in position or direction
retro-	behind, backward	**retro**peritoneal	Behind the anterior abdominal organs
post-		**post**erior	Relating to the dorsal side in humans
postero-		**postero**anterior	Direction from back to front
sub-	below, under, beneath	**sub**acute	Abnormal condition present, but the person appears well
hyp-		**hyp**notic	Inducing sleep or hypnosis
hypo-		**hypo**tension	Low blood pressure
syn-	together, joined, with	**syn**dactyly	Fusing together of the web space between fingers
		synapsis	Pairing of like chromosomes during meiosis; point of contact
con-		**con**ceive	To become pregnant with (offspring)
		conjoined twins	Siamese twins; joined together at some point of their bodies
trans-	across, through, over	**trans**hepatic	Across, through, or over the liver
		transverse	Crosswise

Vowel	Word	Phonetic Symbol
a	tray	ā
e	bean	ē
i	pie	ī
o	goat	ō
u	cue	ū
y	bye	ȳ

Vowel	Word	Phonetic Symbol
a	addict	ă
e	endless	ĕ
i	injury	ĭ
o	son	ŏ
u	umbrella	ŭ

In general, when a vowel is followed by a **consonant,** the vowel receives a short pronunciation, and a *breve* (˘) is placed over the vowel. For example, "umbrella" is pronounced (ŭm-′bre-la).

Consonants

There are some guidelines for consonants as well. Some consonants can be referred to as being "soft" or "hard" sounding.

TABLE 10-9

Descriptive Prefixes

Prefix	Meaning	Word Example	Definition of Example
a-	not, without, negate	**a**febrile	Having no fever
an-, ana-		**ana**erobic	Able to live without oxygen
un-		**un**conscious	Temporarily lacking consciousness
in-		**in**accurate	Incorrect; not accurate
im-		**im**balance	Lack of balance
non-		**non**conductor	Material that conducts little or no electricity, heat, or sound
anti-	against, opposite	**anti**body	Protein in a cell that fights bacteria and viruses
contra-		**contra**ceptive	Something that prevents conception (pregnancy)
brady-	slow	**brady**pnea	Slow breathing
		bradycardia	Slow heart rate
dis-	apart, remove, absence, free of	**dis**ability	Disadvantage or deficiency
dys-	difficult, painful	**dys**pnea	Difficulty in breathing
idio-	unknown	**idio**pathic	Having no known cause
mal-	bad	**mal**formation	Deformity; abnormal formation
neo-	new	**neo**nate	Newborn infant
ortho-	straight	**ortho**pnea	Person must be upright to breathe (sit or stand)
per-	excessive, through	**per**cutaneous	Passed or done through the skin
ultra-		**ultra**filter	Membrane that removes both large and small molecules
tachy-	fast	**tachy**cardia	Rapid heart rate

TABLE 10-10

General Suffixes

Suffix	Meaning	Word Example	Definition of Example
ADJECTIVE ENDINGS			
-ac, -iac	pertaining to, relating to	card**iac**	Relating to the heart
-ic		ischem**ic**	Relating to a decrease in blood supply to an organ or tissue
-al		inguin**al**	Relating to the groin
-ar		patell**ar**	Relating to the kneecap
-ary		axill**ary**	Relating to the axilla
-ous		tendin**ous**	Relating to the nature of a tendon
-ory		sens**ory**	Relating to the senses
-tic		necro**tic**	Relating to death of cells or tissues through injury or disease
-eal		laryng**eal**	Relating to the larynx
-ose		adip**ose**	Relating to fat
NOUN ENDINGS			
-er	one who	radiograph**er**	One who takes x-rays
-ia	condition of	pneumon**ia**	Condition caused by viruses or bacteria with inflammation of the lungs
-ism	state of being, condition	alcohol**ism**	State of having a dependence on alcohol
-um, -ium	structure or tissue	pericard**ium**	Structure or membrane surrounding the heart
-y	condition, process	aton**y**	Condition of lacking muscle tone
DIMINUTIVE ENDINGS (indicates a small version)			
-ole	small size, tiny, minute	arteri**ole**	Small terminal branch of an artery
-icle		ves**icle**	Small bladder-like cell or cavity
-ula		mac**ula**	Small spot on the cornea
-ule		pust**ule**	Small pus-filled lesion; pimple

TABLE 10-11
Common Medical Suffixes

Suffix	Meaning	Word Example	Definition of Example
-blast	not developed	myo**blast**	Undeveloped cell in an embryo
-cide	causing death	germi**cide**	Agent that kills germs; a disinfectant
-ian	specialist in a field of study	physic**ian**	Specialist in the field of medicine
-ician		pediat**rician**	Specialist who treats children and adolescents
-iatrics	treatment of, field of medicine	ped**iatrics**	Field of medicine dealing with the care of children
-iatry		psych**iatry**	Field of medicine dealing with diagnosis, treatment, and prevention of mental and emotional disorders
-logist	one who specializes	bio**logist**	One who specializes in the study of life and living things
-iatrist		pod**iatrist**	One who specializes in the treatment of nails and feet
-ist		dent**ist**	One who specializes in the care and treatment of teeth and gums
-logy	study of	hemato**logy**	Study of the blood and blood-producing organs (Figure 10-1)
-stasis	constant; standing	homeo**stasis**	State of equilibrium, or balance, in which the body is able to adapt to changes to maintain health

TABLE 10-12
Symptomatic Suffixes

Suffix	Meaning	Word Example	Definition of Example
-algia	pain	neur**algia**	Nerve pain
		ceph**algia**	Headache
-dynia		cephalo**dynia**	Pain in the head; headache
-form	resembling, similar	somato**form** disorder	A mental disorder where the mind manufactures physical symptoms to mimic a real disease
		epilepti**form**	Resembling epileptic symptoms
-oid		sarc**oid**	Resembling flesh (connective tissue)
		muc**oid**	Resembling mucus, glycoproteins similar to mucins
-genic	condition of producing	auto**genic**	Produced from within; self-generating
-gen	beginning, origin	carcino**gen**	Something that produces or causes cancer
-genesis		osteo**genesis**	Formation and development of bony tissue
-lysis	breaking down, destroying (can also stand alone as a noun)	thrombo**lysis**	Destruction of a thrombus with surgery or medication
		lysis of adhesions	Destruction of previously formed scar tissue
-mania	excessive preoccupation	ego**mania**	Excessive preoccupation with the self
-megaly	enlargement	spleno**megaly**	Enlargement of the spleen
		cardio**megaly**	Enlargement of the heart
-path	disease	psycho**path**	Person with antisocial personality disorder (psychologic disease)
-penia	decrease	leuko**penia**	Having a low number of leukocytes (white blood cells) in the circulating blood
-pnea	breathing	dys**pnea**	Difficulty in breathing; reduction or shortness of breath
-rrhea	discharge	rhino**rrhea**	Discharge from the nose (runny nose)
-spasm	involuntary contraction	chiro**spasm**	Writer's cramp
-stenosis	narrowing	tracheo**stenosis**	Narrowing of the trachea

TABLE 10-13
Diagnostic Suffixes

Suffix	Meaning	Word Example	Definition of Example
-cele	hernia	hydro**cele**	Herniated sac filled with water; accumulation of fluid in a sac-like body cavity
-coccus	round-shaped bacteria	staphylo**coccus**	Round bacteria in clusters
-ectasis	stretching; dilatation	bronchi**ectasis**	Chronic dilation of bronchial tubes (lungs)
-emia	blood condition	ur**emia**	Body waste normally excreted in the urine instead accumulates in the blood
		hyper**emia**	Increase in blood flow to a body part; engorgement
-gram	record	echocardio**gram**	Visual record produced by an echocardiograph
-graph	instrument for recording	electrocardio**graph**	Instrument used in detection and diagnosis of heart abnormalities
-graphy	process of recording	myo**graphy**	Process of recording muscular contractions
-iasis	presence of, condition of	cholelith**iasis**	Presence of gallstones
-itis	inflammation	tonsill**itis** (note spelling with two *l*'s)	Inflammation of a tonsil (note spelling with one *l*)
-lith	stone	rhino**lith**	Nose stone
-malacia	softening	osteo**malacia**	Softening of the bones
-meter	instrument for measuring	tympano**meter**	Instrument used to measure pressure in the middle ear (Figure 10-2)
-metry	process of measuring	opto**metry**	Field of practice concerned with measuring and improving vision
-oma	tumor	hemangi**oma**	Benign skin tumor; usually elevated masses of dilated blood vessels (Figure 10-3)
-opsy	to view	bi**opsy**	Removal and examination of a sample of body tissue
-osis	abnormal condition	sarcoid**osis**	Abnormal condition of developing nodules in the lungs
		neur**osis**	Mental or emotional disorder
	increase in number when referring to blood cells, of, increase of	granulocyt**osis**	Abnormal number (increase) of granulocytes in the blood
-phil	attraction for	eosino**phil**	Red granulocytes that have an attraction for allergic responses; a granular bilobed white blood cell
-philia		hemo**philia**	Disorder in which blood fails to clot normally; no attraction for blood to stick together
-poiesis	formation of	hemato**poiesis**	Formation of blood or blood cells in the body
-plasia		hyper**plasia**	Formation of excess cells in an organ or tissue
-ptosis	falling down, downward displacement	nephro**ptosis**	Downward displacement of the kidney
-rrhage	to burst forth	hemo**rrhage**	Excessive discharge of blood from the blood vessels
-rrhagia		hemo**rrhagia**	
-rrhexis	rupture	amnio**rrhexis**	Rupture of the amniotic sac
-scope	instrument	micro**scope**	Instrument used to produce magnified images of small objects
-scopy	process of examining with a scope	broncho**scopy**	Instrument; process of using an instrument for examining the interior of the bronchi
-toxic	poison	neuro**toxic**	Poisonous or toxic to nerve tissue

TABLE 10-14
Operative Suffixes

Suffix	Meaning	Word Example	Definition of Example
-centesis	surgical puncture	amnio**centesis**	Procedure in which a small sample of fluid is drawn out of the amniotic sac and uterus (Figure 10-4)
-clasia	break	osteo**clasia**	Surgical breaking of a bone
-desis	binding, fusion	arthro**desis**	Fixing a joint surgically (results in bone fusion)
-ectomy	removal, excision	tonsill**ectomy**	Removal of the tonsils
-pexy	fixing, fixation, suspension	utero**pexy**	Surgical fixation of the uterus
-plasty	surgical repair, reconstruction	septo**plasty**	Surgical reconstruction of the nasal septum
-rrhaphy	suture	hernio**rrhaphy**	Surgical repair of a hernia by suturing it back into place
-stomy	creation of a new opening	tracheo**stomy**	Surgically opening the trachea to insert a catheter or breathing tube
-tome	instrument to cut	derma**tome**	Instrument used to cut thin slices of skin
-tomy	to cut into, incision	veno**tomy**	Incision into a vein
-tripsy	crushing of	litho**tripsy**	Crushing of kidney stones or gallstones with a lithotripter (Figure 10-5)

Understanding Medical Terminology   CHAPTER 10

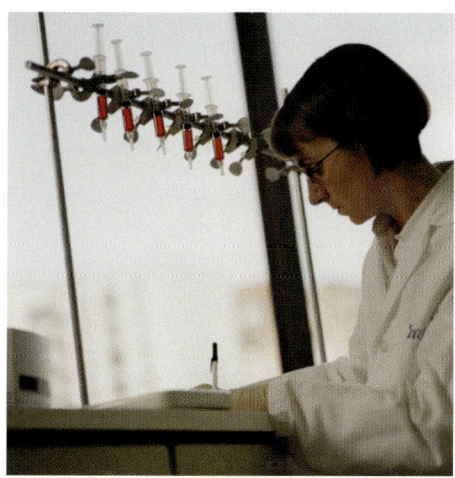

FIGURE 10-1 *Hemat/o + logy:* the study of blood. (From Shiland BJ: *Mastering healthcare terminology,* ed 2, St Louis, 2006, Saunders.)

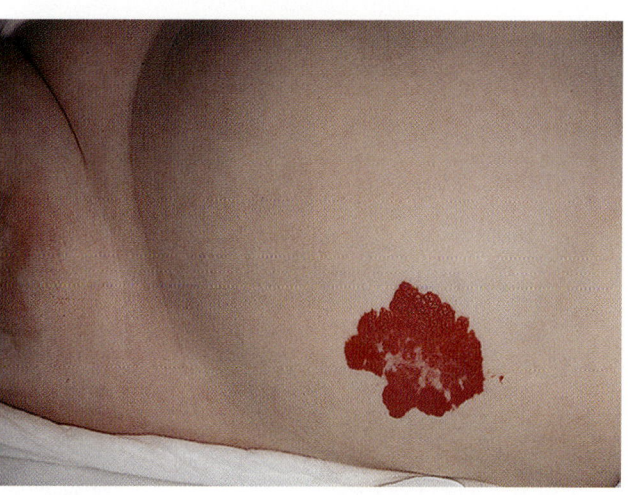

FIGURE 10-3 *Hemang/i + oma:* a benign skin tumor. (From Callen FP et al: *Color atlas of dermatology,* ed 2, Philadelphia, 2000, WB Saunders.)

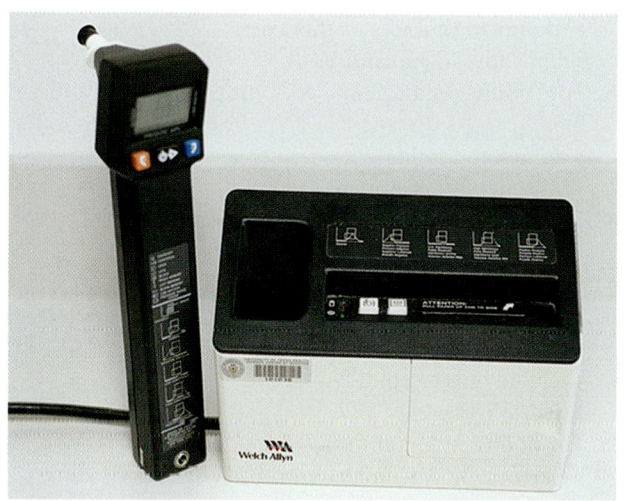

FIGURE 10-2 *Tympan/o + meter:* an instrument used to measure pressure in the middle ear. (From Seidel HM et al: *Mosby's guide to physical examination,* ed 6, St Louis, 2006, Mosby.)

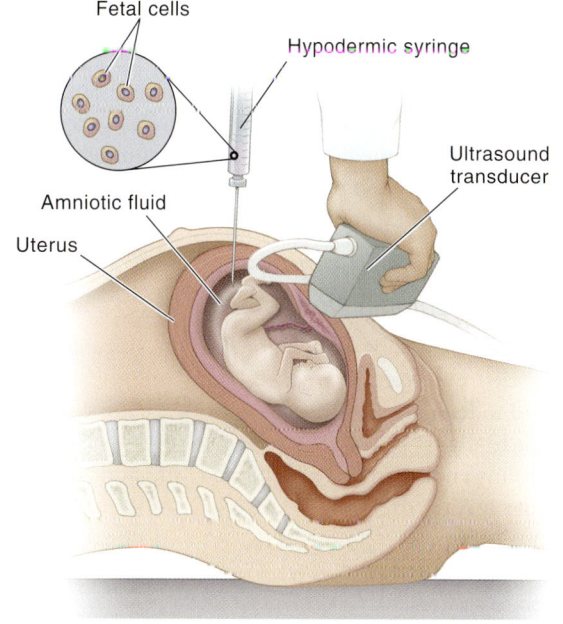

FIGURE 10-4 *Amni/o + centesis:* the removal and analysis of amniotic fluid for diagnostic purposes. (Modified from Thibodeau GA, Patton KT: *The human body in health and disease,* ed 4, St Louis, 2005, Mosby.)

Consonant	Word	Pronunciation
Soft c if before *e* or *i*	face	"s"
Soft g if before *e* or *i*	gel	"j"
Hard c if before *a, o, u*	cake	"k"
Hard g if before *a, o, u*	gate	"g"

Unusual Pronunciation

When two consonants are together, or an *x* is the first letter, the word may have an unusual pronunciation, as in the following:

Consonants	Word		Pronunciation
ch	chromosome	k	kro
ph	phalanx	f	fay
pn	pneumatic	n	noo
ps	psychology	s	sye
pt	ptosis	t	toh
eu	euthyroid	you	yoo
x	xeroderma	z	zeer
gn	gnathalgia	n	nuh

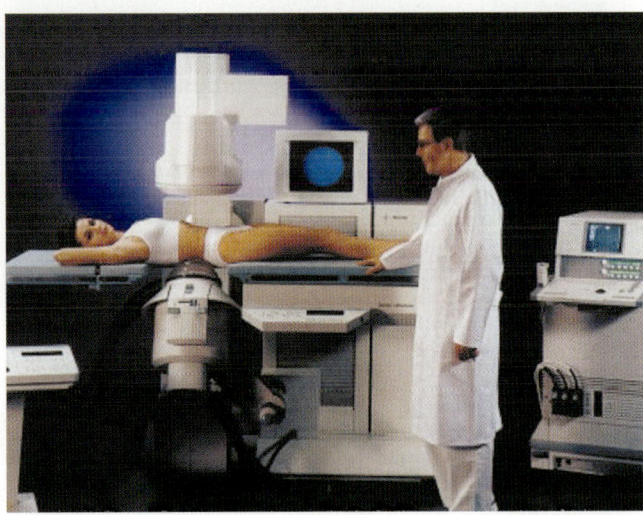
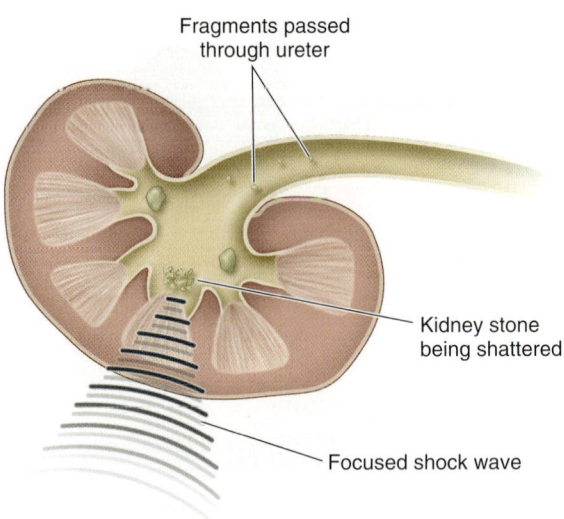

FIGURE 10-5 *Lith/o + tripsy:* the crushing of kidney stones and gallstones. (From LaFleur-Brooks M: *Exploring medical terminology: a student-directed approach,* ed 5, St Louis, 2000, Mosby.)

Plurals

A **plural** is a noun that refers to more than one. Sometimes when making a noun plural, English rules are acceptable. However, most of the medical terms that are nouns stem from Greek or Latin words and require different endings. As in any rule, there are some exceptions.

Guidelines for Forming Plural Words from English Nouns

1. A plural is formed by adding an "s" to the singular form.
   - muscle to muscles
   - hand to hands
   - digit to digits
2. For nouns ending in an "s," "ch," and "sh," add "es" to the singular form.
   - sinus to sinuses
   - church to churches
   - sash to sashes
3. For nouns ending in a "y" preceded by a consonant, change the "y" to "i" and add "es."
   - capillary to capillaries
   - ovary to ovaries
4. For nouns ending in "o," add "s" or "es."
   - tomato to tomatoes
   - auto to autos
5. For nouns ending in "f" or "fe," drop the "f" or "fe" and add "ves."
   - half to halves
   - calf to calves

Guidelines for Forming Plural Words from Latin and Greek Nouns

1. For nouns ending in "a," add an "e."
   - stria to striae
   - petechia to petechiae
2. For nouns ending in "ax" or "ix," change the "x" to "c" and add "es."
   - thorax to thoraces or thoraxes
   - appendix to appendices
3. For nouns ending in "en," drop the "en" and add "ina."
   - lumen to lumina
   - foramen to foramina
4. For nouns ending in "ex" or "ix," change to "ices."
   - cortex to cortices
   - varix to varices
5. For nouns ending in "is," change to "es" or "ides."
   - psychosis to psychoses
   - epididymis to epididymides
   - iris to irides
6. For nouns ending in "ma," change to "mata."
   - sarcoma to sarcomata (could add an "s": sarcomas)
   - carcinoma to carcinomata
7. For nouns ending in "nx," "anx," "inx," or "ynx," change to "nges."
   - phalanx to phalanges (Figure 10-6)
   - larynx to larynges
8. For nouns ending in "on," change to "a."
   - phenomenon to phenomena
   - spermatozoon to spermatozoa
9. For nouns ending in "um," change to "a."
   - diverticulum to diverticula
   - ovum to ova
10. For nouns ending in "us," change to "i."
    - bronchus to bronchi
    - alveolus to alveoli
11. For nouns ending in a "y" preceded by a consonant, change the "y" to "i" and add "es."
    - myopathy to myopathies
    - artery to arteries

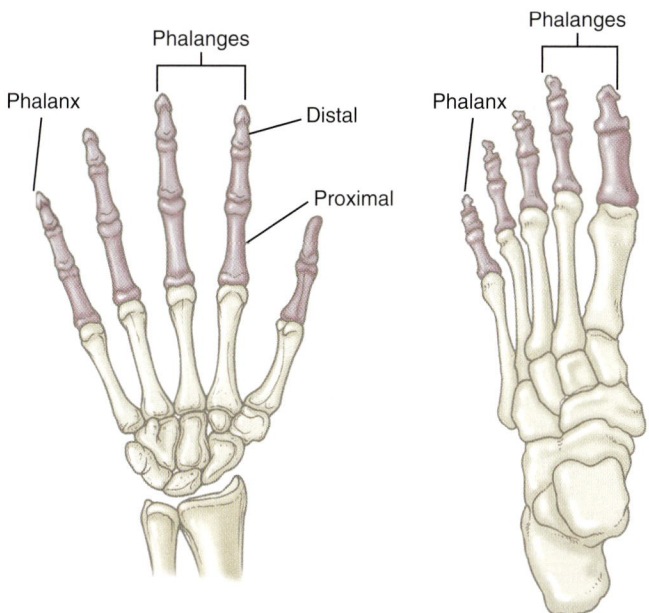

FIGURE 10-6 One phalan*x*; two or more phalan*ges*.

Antonyms

An **antonym** can be a root word, prefix, or suffix that has the *opposite* meaning of another word. If you know both a word and its antonym, you will be able to figure out words using roots, prefixes, and suffixes based on this knowledge. Examples are as follows:

good	eu	bad	mal
right	*dextro*	left	*sinistro*
toward	*ad*	away from	*ab*

Homonyms

Homonyms are words that have the same pronunciation but a different spelling and meaning. A medical example of homonyms follows:
- *ileum* (part of the small intestine)
- *ilium* (part of the hip bone)

Synonyms

Synonyms are root words, prefixes, or suffixes that have the same or almost the same meaning as another given word, prefix, or suffix. A medical example of synonyms follows:
- *pulmon/o*—lung (as in "pulmonologist")
- *pneumo*—lung (as in "pneumonia")

Both prefixes mean "lung," but they are not interchangeable. You cannot say "pneumologist" for example; "pulmonologist" is the only correct term.

PATIENT-CENTERED PROFESSIONALISM

- *How important is it to the patient that medical assistants pronounce medical terminology correctly? What about spelling words correctly and using correct plural forms? How are these skills legally and ethically important?*
- *Why do medical assistants need to be certain they are using the correct words (e.g., not confusing homonyms or antonyms) when documenting patient records?*

CONCLUSION

You will need what you have learned in this chapter as you continue through this text and the next section on anatomy and physiology. You should not continue to the next chapter until you have mastered this information. To help you become familiar with medical root words, prefixes, and suffixes, practice is essential. Effective ways to practice your medical terminology skills are to make flash cards, to practice writing the terms and their meanings, and to practice pronouncing the terms correctly. You cannot memorize all medical terms, but by learning the prefixes, combining forms, and suffixes, you can understand the meaning of most of the unfamiliar words you may encounter in a medical office. With a solid grasp of medical terminology, you will be more prepared to meet the expectations of your co-workers and patients. With practice, you will be prepared to exceed their expectations and provide high-quality care.

Chapter Summary

Reinforce your understanding of the material in this chapter by reviewing the curriculum objectives and key content points below.

1. **Define, appropriately use, and spell all the Key Terms for this chapter.**
   - Review the Key Terms if necessary.
2. **Discuss the origins of words and where the terms used in medicine often originated.**
   - The language used in medicine is a combination of Greek and Latin words, eponyms, and from modern medical advances.
   - Greek words usually refer to diseases.
   - Latin words refer to anatomical structures.
3. **Explain the importance of using correct medical terminology in a medical setting.**
   - Medical terminology is used in medical records; in communicating with the physician, the patients, and other health care workers; and for medical billing.

4. **Identify and describe the four word parts used to build medical words.**
   - The root word contains the core meaning of the term.
   - The combining vowel is added to a root word to make the combining form.
   - One or more prefixes can be added to the beginning of a root word to change the meaning of the word or to create a new word.
   - A suffix can be added to the end of a root word to change the type of word (e.g., adjective or verb to noun) or to change the meaning of the word.

5. **State the importance of understanding the function of each word part.**
   - If you understand the function of each word part, you will understand how they work together to form medical terms.
   - Understanding the function of the word parts can help you determine the meaning of unfamiliar medical terms.

6. **Identify three helpful tips for studying medical terminology.**
   - Practice makes perfect. Use flash cards, practice writing the word parts and their meanings, and look up unfamiliar parts in a medical dictionary if necessary.

7. **Apply pronunciation guidelines to pronounce various medical terms correctly.**
   - Study the pronunciation key so that you understand the pronunciation symbols.
   - Practice pronouncing difficult medical terms.

8. **Change various medical terms from singular to plural correctly.**
   - You may have to change a medical term from singular to plural to record it. Knowing the guidelines for changing English, Greek, and Latin words from singular to plural will help.

9. **Define and give an example of an antonym, homonym, and synonym.**
   - An antonym has the opposite meaning of another word (e.g., right = "dextro"; left = "sinistro").
   - A homonym has the same pronunciation as another word, but a different spelling and meaning (e.g., "ilium" = hip; "ileum" = intestine).
   - A synonym is a root word, suffix, or prefix that has the same or almost the same meaning as another root word, suffix, or prefix (e.g., "pulmon/o" = lung; "pneum/o" = lung).

10. **Analyze a realistic medical office situation and apply your understanding of medical terminology to determine the best course of action.**
    - Mistakes and misspellings in medical records can create many types of problems for both the patient and the medical office.

11. **Describe the impact on patient care when medical assistants have a solid grasp of the correct use of medical terminology.**
    - Medical assistants who use medical terminology correctly create a good impression for patients and co-workers alike. They are seen as more competent, and patient care is not compromised.

PRACTICAL APPLICATIONS

If you have accomplished the objectives in this chapter, you will be able to make better choices as a medical assistant. Take another look at this situation and decide what you would do.

Dr. Smith has a medical assistant who does the medical transcription of her patient notes. The following is a note the medical assistant has transcribed on Susie Ramos:

"Seen in the office today for arteriaslcerosis and hipertension. Mrs. Ramos complained of feeling dizzy with some fertigo for three days. On questioning, Mrs. Ramos did state that she was febrille two days ago with some gastroentestinal symptoms such as darhea and nausea. She also complained of aralgia and laryngetes. On examination the toncils are red and swollen. Her blood pressure is controlled by medication. There are no complaints of chest pain or anjina, nor does she have dispnea, although she does have some orthapnea. She does have some syanosis of the hands and feet but does not complain of pain in these areas. Her sinuses are painful. Her current diagnosisses are sinisitus, athurosclerosis, possible streptocockki infection, gastrointeritis, and faringitis."

Would you be able to point out all the mistakes this note contains to the medical assistant?

1. There are 20 mistakes in the use of medical terminology in this dictation. Find the mistakes.
2. Explain why using and spelling the correct medical term is important in the medical record.
3. Why does the medical assistant need to study medical terminology? How does a solid understanding of medical terminology benefit the care that patients receive?

WEB SEARCH

1. **Research eponyms used in medicine.** Eponyms are used often in everyday language. There are many eponyms in the field of medicine as well. It is important to understand their meaning so that you can use them correctly. For each eponym you find, identify its meaning and its origin (where it came from).
   - **Keywords:** Use the following keyword in your search: medical eponyms.
2. **Research the origin of medical language.** You know that medical language has roots in Greek and Latin. Research to learn about how medical terminology originated from Greek and Latin language and mythology, as well as from terms from other languages (e.g., French, Dutch); terms that originated from their discoverers' names; and terms originating from plants, colors, and animals.
   - **Keywords:** Use the following keywords in your search: origin of medical terms, Greek and Latin medical terminology, medical terminology language origin.

11 Basic Anatomy and Physiology

evolve http://evolve.elsevier.com/klieger/medicalassisting

The human body is fascinating, and much has been learned about how it works. The body is a *system,* almost like a machine. All the parts of the body work together to enable us to perform our daily activities. As with any machine, if a part of the body is missing or not working properly, it affects the whole system. Knowing about the *structure* (anatomy) and the *function* (physiology) of the body is crucial for health care workers, who must know what is normal in the human body and its parts before they can understand the disease process. Anatomy can be subdivided into several categories based on the method of study used and the type of information needed (Box 11-1).

Learning about human anatomy and physiology is the first step in understanding many other concepts and procedures important to your skill as a medical assistant. In this chapter, you begin to build a foundation of basic human anatomy by learning about the language used to describe the body and its parts, positions, function, structure, and organization.

LEARNING OBJECTIVES

You will be able to do the following after completing this chapter:

Key Terms
1. Define, appropriately use, and spell all the Key Terms for this chapter.

Describing the Human Body
2. List and describe the location of the three major body planes.
3. List and describe directional and positional terms and anatomical positions.
4. Identify the two main body cavities within the ventral cavity and the two main body cavities within the dorsal cavity.
5. Differentiate between abdominal quadrants and abdominal regions.

Organizational Levels of the Body
6. Describe the progression from an atom to a system.
7. Identify the main structures of a cell.
8. List and describe the transport systems used by cells.
9. List two causes for genetic disorders.
10. List five factors that can cause genes to mutate.
11. List the four main types of body tissues and describe the function of each.
12. Match major organs to their body system.
13. List the ten body systems and describe the function of each.

Patient-Centered Professionalism
14. Analyze a realistic medical office situation and apply your understanding of basic anatomy and physiology to determine the best course of action.
15. Describe the impact on patient care when medical assistants have a solid grasp of basic anatomy and physiology.

KEY TERMS

The Key Terms for this chapter have been organized into sections so that you can easily see the terminology associated with each aspect of anatomy and physiology.

anatomy	physiology

Anatomical Position and Direction

anatomical position	posterior
anterior	prone position
dorsal	superior
inferior	supine position
midline	ventral

Continued

Basic Anatomy and Physiology CHAPTER 11

Body Planes
body plane
frontal (coronal) plane
midsagittal (median) plane
sagittal (lateral) plane
transverse (cross-sectional) plane

Body Cavities
diaphragm
membrane
parietal membranes
viscera
visceral membranes

Ventral Cavity
serous membrane
ventral cavity

Abdominopelvic Cavity (Abdominal and Pelvic Cavities)
abdominal
abdominopelvic cavity
mesentery
pelvic
peritoneum
quadrants
regions
umbilicus

Thoracic Cavity
heart
lungs
mediastinum
parietal pericardial membrane
pericardial membrane
pleural cavity
thoracic cavity
visceral pleura

Dorsal Cavity
dorsal cavity
meninges

Cranial Cavity
buccal cavity
cranial cavity
lacrimal cavity
nasal cavity
orbital cavity

Spinal Cavity
cervical
coccygeal
lumbar
sacral
spinal cavity
spinal column
spinal cord
thoracic
vertebra

Additional Body Areas
appendicular area
thorax
torso

Atoms
atom
chemicals
molecules

Cells
cell
organism

Cell Structure
active transport
adenosine triphosphate (ATP)
anabolism
catabolism
cell membrane
centrioles
chromosomes
cilia
cytoplasm
deoxyribonucleic acid (DNA)
endoplasmic reticulum (ER)
extracellular
genes
Golgi apparatus
lysosomes
mitochondria
nucleolus
nucleus
organelles
ribonucleic acid (RNA)
ribosomes
semipermeable
viable

Passive Transport
crenate
diffusion
filtration
hemolyze
hypertonic
hypotonic
isotonic
osmosis
passive transport
phagocytosis
pinocytosis
plasma

Cell Division
gametes
meiosis
mitosis
somatic cells

Uncontrolled Cell Growth
benign
malignant
metastasis
neoplasm
oncology
tumor

Genetic Information in the Cell
dominant
recessive

Genetic Diseases
abnormalities
congenital
etiology
familial
genetic counseling
hereditary
insidious
mutation
predisposing factor
sign
symptom

Chromosomal Diseases/Procedure
amniocentesis
Down syndrome
Klinefelter syndrome
Turner syndrome

Single-Cell and Mutation Diseases/Signs
cleft palate, cleft lip
cystic fibrosis
dyspnea
gait
Gowers' sign
hemophilia
Huntington chorea (disease)
muscular dystrophy
palliative
pallor
phenylketonuria (PKU)
sickle cell anemia
Tay-Sachs disease
thalassemia

Tissue
connective tissue
epithelial tissue
intercellular
muscle tissue
nerve tissue
tissues

Continued

Epithelial Tissue

columnar
cuboidal
squamous

Glandular Tissue

endocrine gland
exocrine gland
glands

Muscle Tissue

cardiac muscle
fibers
involuntary
myocardium
nonstriated
skeletal muscle
smooth muscle
striated
voluntary

Connective Tissue

adipose tissue
areolar tissue
blood tissue
bone tissue
cartilage tissue
collagenous
dense tissue
elastic
elastic cartilage
fibrocartilage
fibrous tissue
hyaline cartilage
matrix
reticular
reticular tissue

Nerve Tissue

afferent nerves
efferent nerves
glial cells
neurons

BOX 11-1

Common Categories of Anatomy

Macroscopic anatomy	The study of parts of the body or organs that can be viewed with the naked eye (gross anatomy).
Microscopic anatomy	The study of the body's structure by using a microscope. *Cytology* is the study of cell formation and structure. *Histology* is the study of living tissue and structure. *Pathology* is the study of changes in tissue and cell structure and function.
Developmental anatomy	The study of growth and development from conception to birth (*embryology*).
Comparative anatomy	The study of the body and organs by comparing human anatomical features to those of other animals.
Applied anatomy	The study of the body's organ structure as it relates to diagnosis and treatment.

PRACTICAL APPLICATIONS

Read the following scenario and keep it in mind as you learn about the basic structure and function of the body in this chapter.

John Choi is a medical assistant in a primary care facility. Barb Quinn arrives and complains of pain that she thinks is in her stomach. She states that she has had vomiting with blood and also has diarrhea. She also complains of difficulty with eating; she just does not want anything to eat and says, "I have to force myself to eat." After the examination, Dr. Elory tells Ms. Quinn that based on her symptoms, he is suspicious of a cancer in her abdomen. Dr. Elory orders several diagnostic tests that will be completed the next day. Dr. Elory tells Ms. Quinn that he will call as soon as he has her test results.

John Choi needs to know enough about anatomy and physiology to understand Ms. Quinn's symptoms and Dr. Elory's observations. If you were to step into this situation, would you be prepared to assist Dr. Elory in caring for Ms. Quinn?

DESCRIBING THE HUMAN BODY

Two aspects used by medical professionals to describe the human body are anatomical directions and body planes. These directions are very important when referring to the **anatomy** and **physiology** of the human body.

Anatomical Positions and Directions

When describing the body and its structures, specific terms are used to indicate direction and position. The body is assumed to be in a correct or true **anatomical position** when the individual is *standing erect* (upright) and *facing forward,* with the *arms at the side, palms and toes facing forward, feet slightly apart,* and *legs parallel* (Figure 11-1). In the **prone position** the body is *lying on the belly* with the *face down.* The **supine position** is *lying on the back* with the *face up.* In addition, directional terms are used to describe and clarify location and position (Figure 11-2). Table 11-1 provides a list of common directional and positional terms used to describe relative positions of one body part to another.

Body Planes

In the anatomical position the body can be divided into three distinctive body planes. A **body plane** is an imaginary flat surface that divides the body into specific anatomical sections. The three major planes of the body are the frontal, sagittal (including midsagittal), and transverse planes (Figure 11-3).

- The **frontal (coronal) plane** is a vertical cut that divides the body into **anterior** (front, or **ventral**) and **posterior** (back, or **dorsal**) parts.
- The **sagittal (lateral) plane** uses a lengthwise or vertical cut that divides the body into right and left sides, whereas

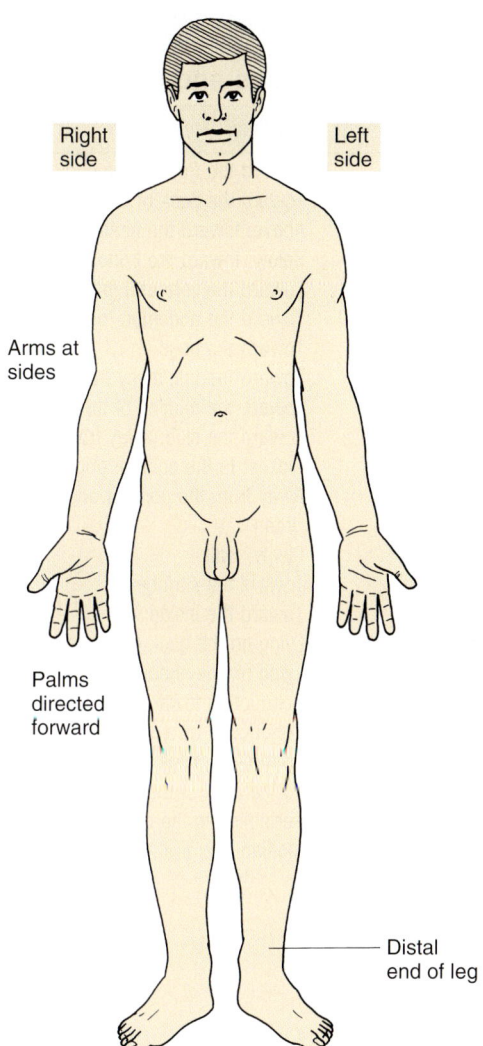

FIGURE 11-1 The body in the anatomical position. The body is standing erect (upright), face forward, arms at sides, palms and toes directed forward, and feet slightly apart. (Modified from Solomon EP: *Introduction to human anatomy and physiology*, ed 3, St Louis, 2009, Saunders.)

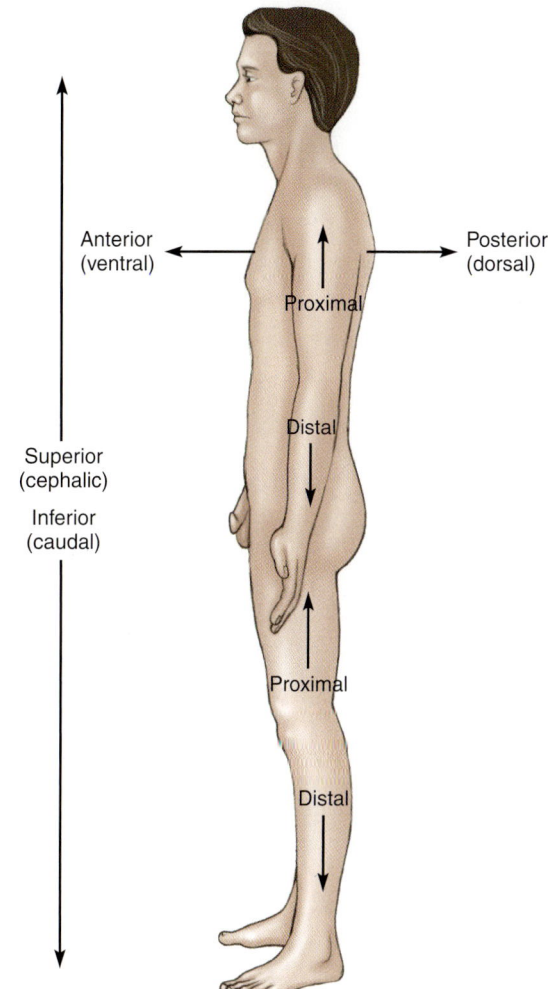

FIGURE 11-2 Positional and directional terms are used in health care to clarify location and position.

the **midsagittal (median) plane** divides the body into *equal* right and left halves by using a vertical cut down the **midline.**

- The **transverse (cross-sectional) plane** (across) is a horizontal cut that separates the body into **superior** (upper) and **inferior** (lower) portions.

Body Cavities and Membranes

A cavity is a hollow space. You are probably most familiar with the term "cavity" as it refers to a hole or hollow space in a tooth. The human body has many types of cavities that appear during embryonic development. The ventral and dorsal cavities are the two main spaces that contain the internal organs (organs of any cavity are referred to as **viscera**). Thin sheets of epithelial tissue called serous membranes line body cavities (**parietal membranes**) and cover organs (**visceral membranes**). These cavities are further subdivided into smaller cavities (Table 11-2 and Figure 11-4).

Ventral Cavity

The **ventral cavity** provides protection and allows for organ movement. It includes the thoracic (chest) cavity and the abdominopelvic (abdominal and pelvic) cavities. The ventral cavity contains organs that maintain homeostasis (balance) when the body is exposed to internal and external stimuli. For example, the beta cells of the pancreas (an organ in the ventral cavity) secrete the hormone insulin to promote the use of glucose in the cells, thus lowering blood glucose level and allowing cells to use glucose for energy. When the balance of the body is maintained, this promotes a state of good health. All organs and cavity walls are lined with a **serous membrane** that decreases friction between the layers of tissues because it produces serous fluid.

Thoracic Cavity. The **thoracic cavity** is surrounded by the rib cage that protects the **lungs** and **heart**. The lungs are situated in the **pleural cavity** and are protected from excessive friction

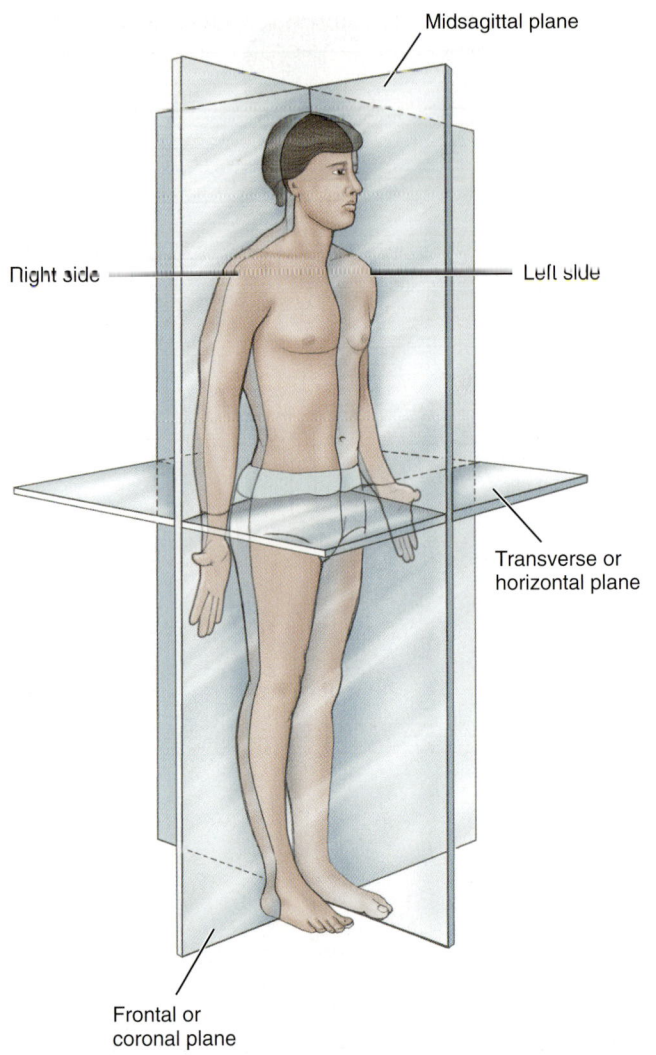

FIGURE 11-3 Body planes are imaginary cuts or sections through the body.

TABLE 11-1
Anatomical Directions and Positions

Term	Definition
Anterior	Toward the front of the body
Posterior	Toward the back of the body
Superior	Above; toward the head
Inferior	Below; toward the bottom
Dorsal	Toward the vertebral (back) surface
Ventral	Toward the abdomen (belly)
Cephalic/cranial	Toward the head
Caudal	Toward the tail; away from the head
Medial	Toward the midline of the body
Lateral	Toward the side; away from the middle
Proximal	Closest to the point of origin or attachment
Distal	Away from the point of origin or attachment
Visceral	Organ
Parietal	Cavity, wall
Superficial	Toward the surface
Deep	Toward the inside
Supine	Lying on the back (face up)
Prone	Lying on the abdomen (face down)
Afferent	Conducting toward a structure
Efferent	Conducting away from a structure
Left	To the left of the body (patient's left)
Right	To the right of the body (patient's right)
Central	Pertaining to the center
Midline	Median line; in the middle

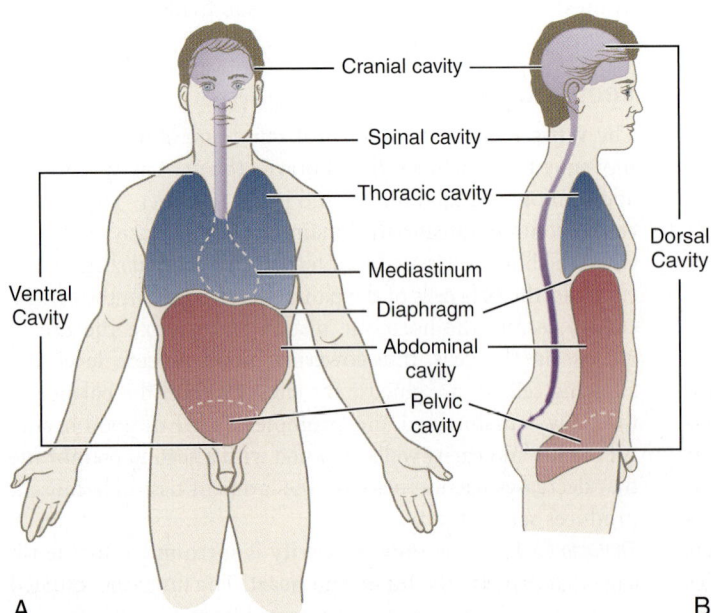

FIGURE 11-4 **A,** Frontal view showing divisions of the ventral and dorsal cavities. **B,** Lateral view of the body showing the ventral and dorsal cavities.

between these layers by a serous membrane called the **visceral pleura.** The cavity wall is also lined with a serous membrane called the *parietal pleura.*

The heart is situated in the middle of the **mediastinum** and is lined with a **parietal pericardial membrane.** A visceral sac or **pericardial membrane** protects the heart. The mediastinum also contains the trachea, esophagus, thymus gland, and major blood vessels of the heart.

The inferior border of the thoracic cavity is the **diaphragm,** the main muscle of breathing and a landmark dividing the thoracic and abdominopelvic cavities.

Abdominopelvic Cavity. The **abdominopelvic cavity** contains the **abdominal** and **pelvic** cavities. The abdominal cavity contains many digestive organs and glands. The pelvic cavity contains the internal reproductive organs, urinary bladder, and the last portion of the digestive tract. No muscular wall separates the abdominal and pelvic areas. Therefore, for purposes of description and location of pain and injury, two imaginary lines have been drawn in this area, dividing this section of the body into **quadrants** (four parts). One imaginary horizontal line is drawn between the right and left iliac crests, and a second vertical line is drawn from the end of the sternum to the pubis (Figure 11-5, *A*). The abdominal cavity is lined with a double-folded **membrane** called the parietal **peritoneum.** The abdominal organs are covered and protected by the visceral peritoneum and its folds are called the **mesentery.**

For clinical and operative purposes, the abdominal cavity can be divided into four quadrants and nine **regions.** These divisions are used to describe areas of the abdomen for purposes of location, reference, and identification.

Quadrants. The abdominal area can be divided into four clinical divisions (quadrants) by using an imaginary vertical line and a horizontal line that bisect at the center of the **umbilicus** (navel, belly button). Quadrants are used to describe location such as "pain localized in RLQ" (Figure 11-5, *B* and *C*).

- *RUQ* (right upper quadrant) of the abdomen contains the right lobe of the liver, gallbladder, the head of the pancreas, and parts of the small and large intestines.
- *LUQ* (left upper quadrant) of the abdomen contains the left lobe of the liver, the stomach, the tail of the pancreas, the spleen, and parts of the small and large intestines.
- *RLQ* (right lower quadrant) of the abdomen contains parts of the small and large intestines, the appendix, right ureter, and the right ovary and right fallopian tube in the female.

TABLE 11-2
Body Cavities

Cavity	Body System	Organs/Structures
VENTRAL		
Thoracic	Respiratory	Lungs, trachea, bronchi
	Circulatory	Heart and its major blood vessels (aorta, arteries, veins, capillaries)
	Digestive	Esophagus
	Endocrine	Thymus gland
Abdominal	Digestive	Stomach, intestines, liver, gallbladder, pancreas, appendix
	Urinary	Kidneys (retroperitoneal)
	Lymphatic	Spleen
	Circulatory	Aorta, vena cava, blood vessels
Pelvic	Urinary	Bladder, urethra, ureters
	Digestive	Rectum, intestines
	Reproductive	Internal reproductive organs
DORSAL		
Cranial	Nervous	Brain
	Endocrine	Pituitary gland, pineal gland
Spinal	Nervous	Spinal cord, peripheral nerves

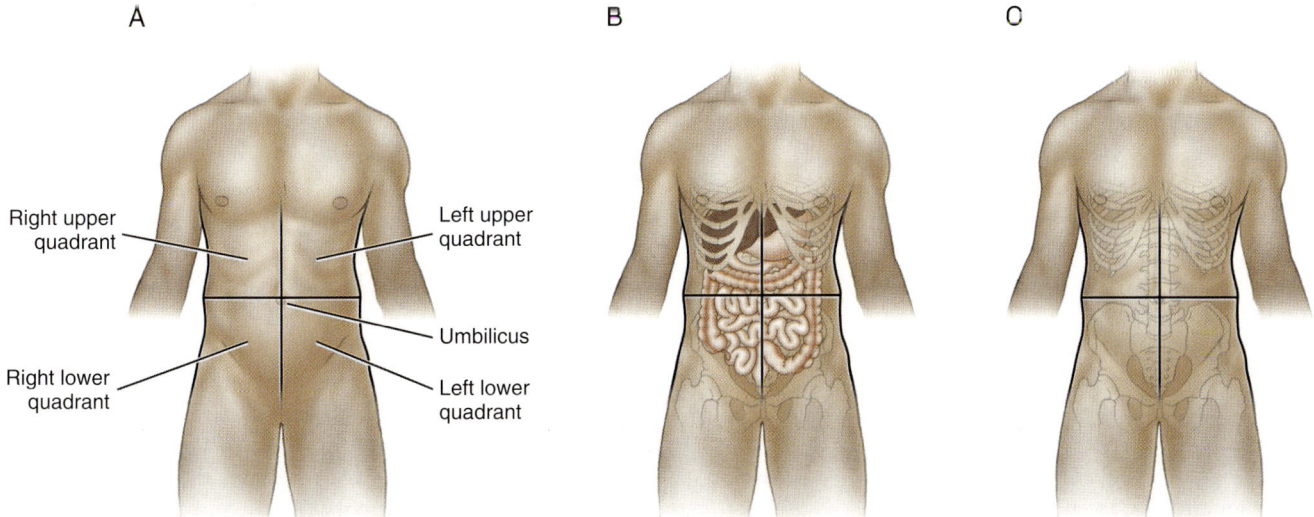

FIGURE 11-5 Quadrants. **A,** Imaginary lines showing four abdominal quadrants. **B,** Internal organs and rib cage. **C,** Skeletal view showing spinal column in midline.

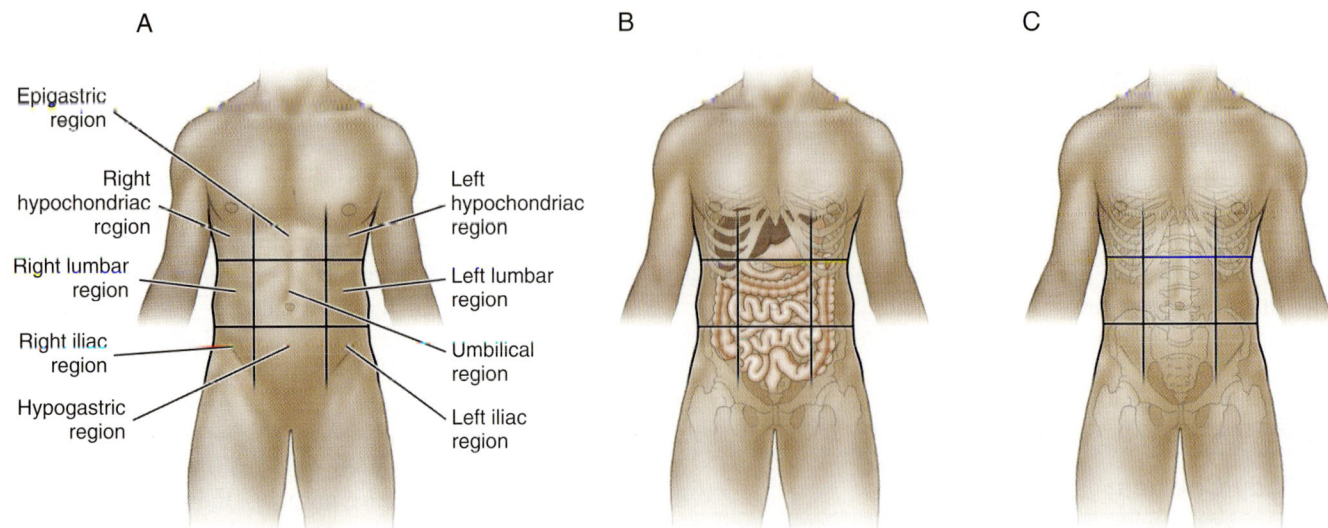

FIGURE 11-6 Regions. **A,** Tic-tac-toe lines showing nine regions of abdominopelvic area. **B,** Internal organs and rib cage. **C,** Skeletal view showing spinal column.

- LLQ (left lower quadrant) of the abdomen contains parts of the small and large intestines, left ureter, and the left ovary and left fallopian tube in the female.

Regions. A more inclusive and specific division of the abdominopelvic area includes nine sections, or regions, with the umbilicus as the center section. To help you picture it, imagine a tic-tac-toe board with the navel area as the center square. This division is used for both clinical and surgical description, location, and documentation (Figure 11-6).

Center square	Umbilical region: mesentery, transverse colon, lower part of the duodenum, jejunum, and ileum	Navel, belly button
Top middle square	Epigastric region: pyloric end of stomach, duodenum, pancreas, aorta, portion of the liver	Above navel area
Top right side square	Right hypochondriac region: right lobe of liver, gallbladder, part of duodenum, hepatic flexure of colon, part of right kidney and adrenal gland	Below ribs
Top left side square	Left hypochondriac region: stomach, spleen, tail of pancreas, splenic flexure of colon, upper portion of left kidney	Below ribs
Middle right side square	Right lumbar region: ascending colon, lower portion of right kidney, part of duodenum and jejunum	Lateral, waist, loin
Middle left side square	Left lumbar region: descending colon, lower portion of left kidney, parts of jejunum and ileum	Lateral, waist, loin
Lower center square	Hypogastric region: ileum, bladder	Below navel area
Lower right side square	Right iliac region: cecum, appendix, lower portion of ileum, right ureter, right spermatic cord in male and right ovary in female	Lower; groin, inguinal area
Lower left side square	Left iliac region: sigmoid colon, left ureter, left spermatic cord in male and left ovary in female	Lower; groin, inguinal area

Dorsal Cavity

The **dorsal cavity** cushions and protects the central nervous system (CNS) and is made up of the cranial (brain) and the spinal (spinal cord) cavities. As with the ventral cavity, membranes protect all cavity walls and organs. The brain and spinal cord are one continuous structure and covered by the **meninges.**

Cranial Cavity. The skull forms the **cranial cavity.** The skull consists of eight cranial bones and 14 facial bones and holds the brain. Additional cavities formed by the facial bones are the **orbital cavity** (eye), which contains the **lacrimal cavity,** or tear ducts; the **nasal cavity** (nose); and the **buccal cavity** (cheek) (Figure 11-7).

Spinal Cavity. The **spinal cavity** is formed by the **spinal column** (backbone). Each bone in the column is called a **ver-**

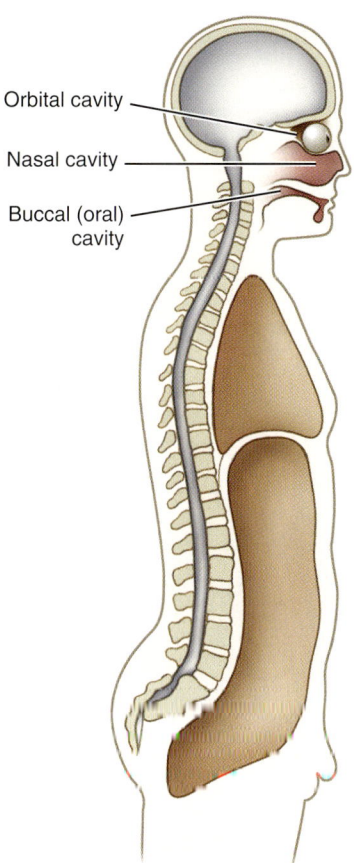

FIGURE 11-7 Additional cranial cavities.

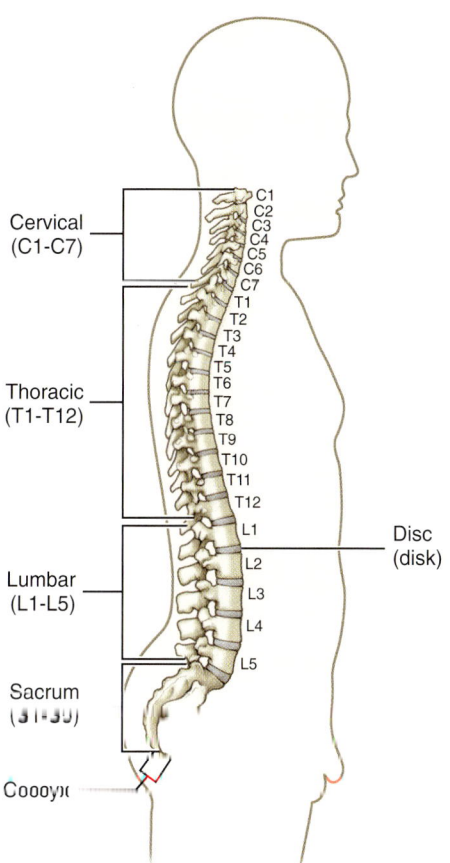

FIGURE 11-8 Divisions of the spinal column.

tebra and is named for its location along the spine. There are five divisions of the spinal column: **cervical, thoracic, lumbar, sacral,** and **coccygeal** (Figure 11-8).

Individual vertebrae are separated and cushioned by cartilaginous material called a *disc*. The **spinal cord** is not bone, as is the spinal column, but rather nerve tissue that conducts impulses to the brain *(afferent)* and back to the body *(efferent)* to cause function. Severing the spinal cord will result in paralysis.

Body Areas and Landmarks

The body can be divided into the axial and the appendicular areas (Figure 11-9).
- The *axial area* includes the head, neck, and trunk **(torso)**. The trunk includes the chest **(thorax)**, abdomen, and pelvis.
- The **appendicular area** includes the upper and lower extremities (limbs).

Figure 11-10 illustrates these and other areas and body landmarks that are important to understand as you learn about the body.

PATIENT-CENTERED PROFESSIONALISM

To communicate effectively with other health care professionals, specific terms are used to refer to anatomical directions and positions, body planes, and body cavities.
- Why is it important for medical assistants to remember that all medical terms referring to direction, position, and body planes are based on the body being in the anatomical position?
- Body planes are imaginary lines used to divide the body into various sections. It is important to know the plane or a section so the anatomical relationship of one part to another can be understood. Which field of medicine describes its finding in terms such as "sagittal" and "transverse"?
- How does having a good understanding of the words used to describe the structure and function of the human body help medical assistants improve the quality of the care they provide?

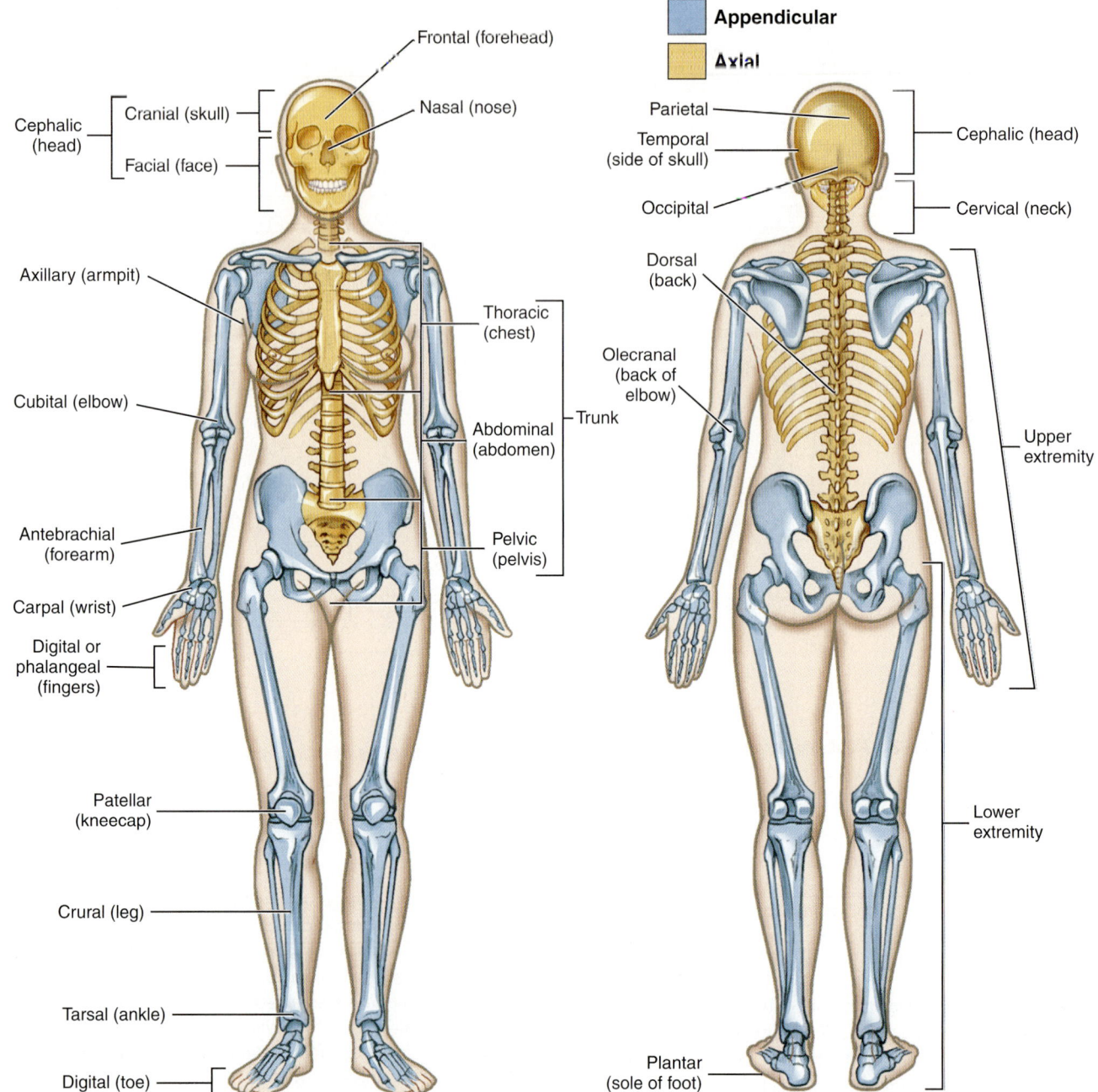

FIGURE 11-9 Axial and appendicular divisions of the body with common terms for body and anatomical regions.

ORGANIZATIONAL LEVELS OF THE BODY

Earlier in this chapter, we compared the human body to a machine with many parts working together to keep the whole running smoothly. The smallest part of the body is an atom. Groups of atoms make up a cell. A group of cells working together makes up tissue. A group of tissues working together makes up an organ. A group of organs working together makes up a system. All the systems working together to sustain life make up an **organism** (Figure 11-11). To understand how the body's parts depend on each other, it is helpful to look at the levels of organization of the body, including atoms, cells, body tissues, organs, and entire systems.

Atoms

An **atom** is the simplest part or particle of matter in both living and nonliving things. There are many types of atoms (e.g., oxygen, carbon), and when they combine with other atoms, they become **molecules** (e.g., carbon dioxide), which form **chemicals** that group together to form the components of cells.

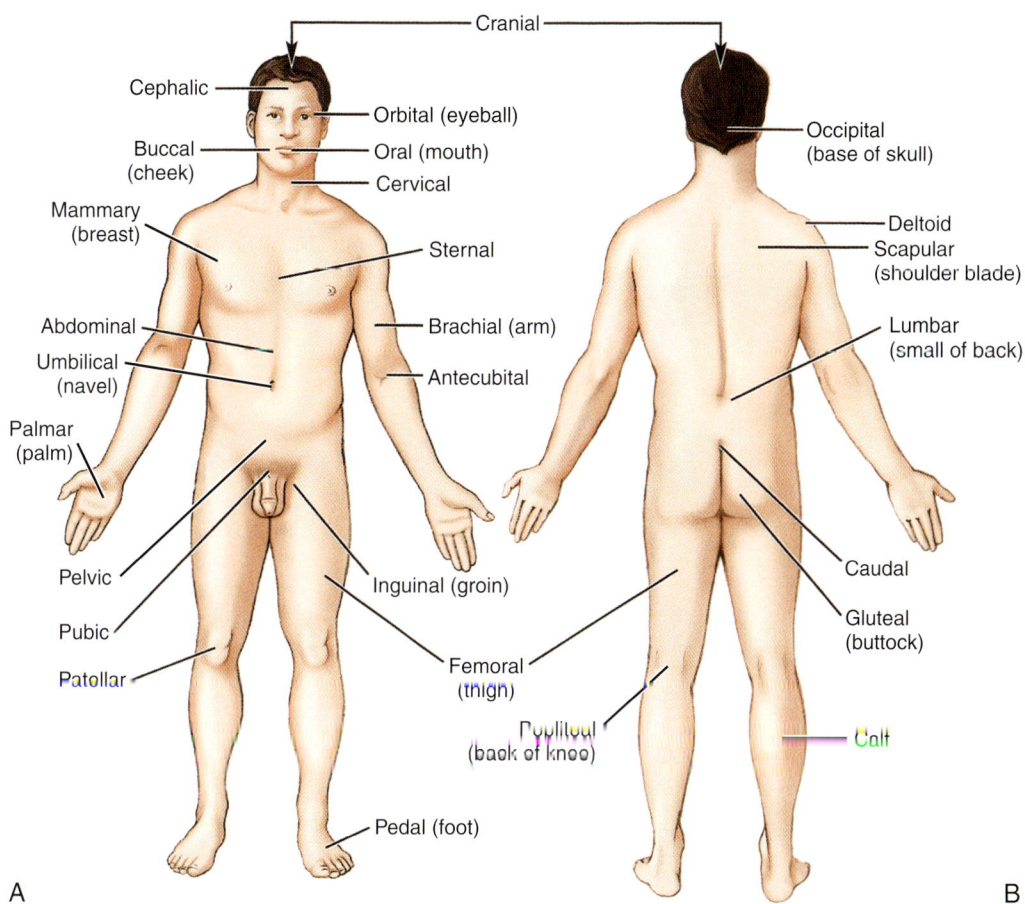

FIGURE 11-10 Anatomical landmarks: **A,** anterior view; **B,** posterior view.

Cells

The fundamental unit of all living things is the **cell**. Without the cell, there is no life. All functions of the body rely on these "building blocks," which consist of nucleic acids, proteins, lipids, carbohydrates, water, and some salts. In the human body, each cell is responsible for carrying out a *specific* function (e.g., blood cells carry oxygen to the tissues, nerve cells carry electrical impulses, and muscle cells contract). The *size* and *shape* of a cell are related to the function it will perform. For example, muscle cells are long and slender and have fibers used for contracting and relaxing. The *life span* of individual cells varies according to their function. Epithelial cells that make up the skin and mucous membrane divide frequently to replace those lost because of friction. Red blood cells live for about 120 days and white blood cells for 14 to 21 days. Blood cells are constantly being reproduced in *bone marrow*. When injured by an infection or a wound, cells will reproduce until sufficient replacement has occurred.

Medical assistants should be familiar with the structure and transportation systems of the cell. In addition, it is important to understand how cells divide and hold genetic information and how genetic diseases occur.

Cell Structure

There are three main parts of the cell: the cell membrane (wall), the cytoplasm, and the nucleus. Figure 11-12 shows a typical cell with **organelles** (structures within the cell that perform specific functions). The organelles within the cell carry out several life functions, including the following:
- Growth and reproduction
- Nourishment and waste disposal
- Reacting and adapting to change

Table 11-3 lists the basic cell structures and their functions.

Cell Membrane. Every cell is surrounded and protected by a **cell membrane,** or plasma membrane. It is made up of proteins and lipids and acts as a wall or barrier. The cell membrane encloses the contents of the cell. It is **semipermeable** and protects the inside of the cell by determining what passes in and out of the cell. The cell membrane regulates the transportation of nutrients into and wastes out of the cell.

Cytoplasm. **Cytoplasm** is the main substance of the cell. It is a fluid made of 70% water and 30% minerals, proteins, lipids, and specialized materials. It surrounds the nucleus and

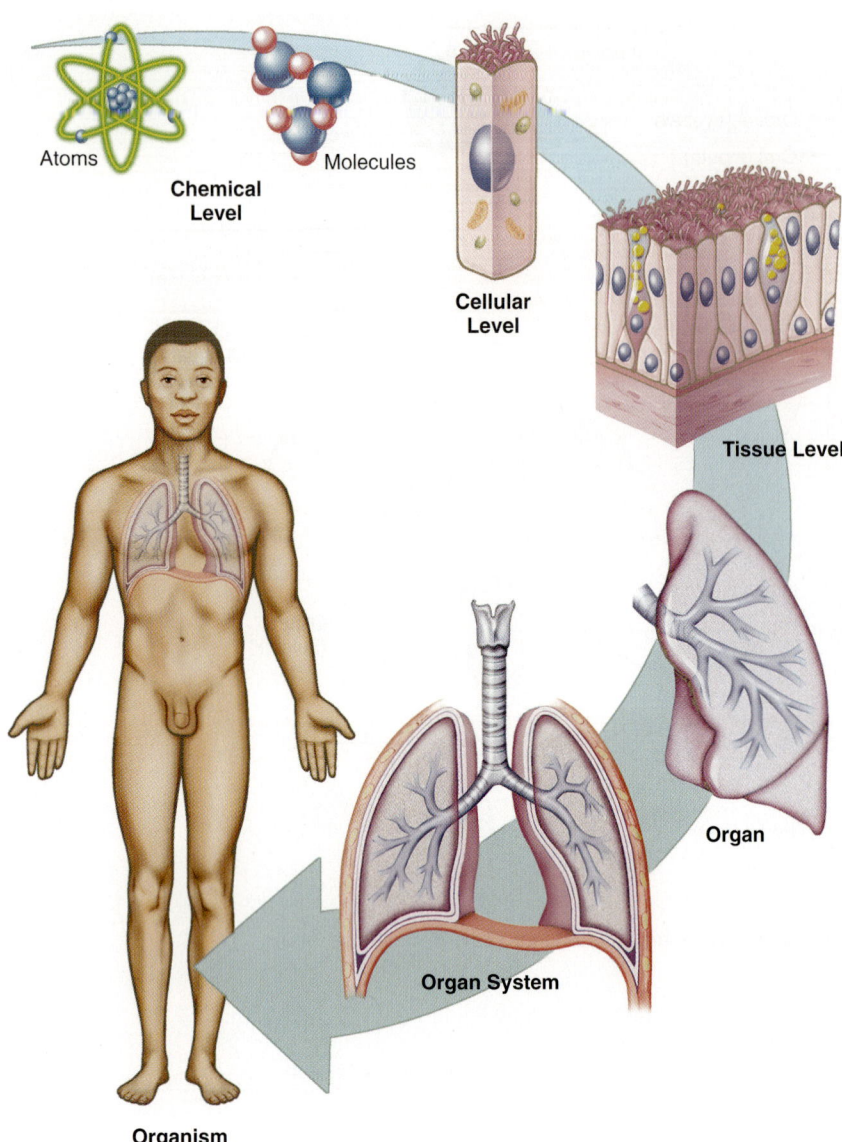

FIGURE 11-11 Organizational levels of the body, with respiratory system as an example. (From Thibodeau GA, Patton KT: *The human body in health and disease,* ed 4, St Louis, 2005, Mosby.)

holds the organelles (little organs). Cytoplasm provides the environment in which the organelles inside the cell can function.

Nucleus. The **nucleus** is the most prominent structure in the cell and is often referred to as its "command center." The nucleus controls the cell's activities such as the way it reproduces and divides. Contained within the nucleus is **deoxyribonucleic acid (DNA),** which is the cell's genetic framework that is stored within the **chromosomes.** Each chromosome contains thousands of **genes** that determine inherited characteristics and control production of certain *enzymes.* Also within the nucleus is the **nucleolus,** which is made up of **ribonucleic acid (RNA).** The function of the nucleolus is to produce RNA and combine it with protein to form **ribosomes.** RNA contains a working copy of the genetic code and carries it into the ribosomes and the cytoplasm.

Transportation Systems of the Cell

In order for all the parts of a cell, as well as the cell itself, to remain **viable** (alive), the cell must be able to receive nourishment and eliminate wastes. These tasks require the ability to transport materials into, out of, and within the cell. Several processes allow this transportation to take place. Some of these processes do not require energy to transport materials (passive transport), and some do require energy (active transport).

Passive Transport Methods. Diffusion, osmosis, and filtration are all examples of **passive transport.** These methods create their own energy for movement.

Diffusion is the random movement of dissolved particles (atoms and molecules of gases, liquids, and solids) that move from an area of higher concentration to an area of low concentration. The movement is constant and continues until both areas are equal. Have you ever been in a room in which

TABLE 11-3
Cell Structures and Functions

Cell Structure	Location	Function
Cell membrane (Plasma membrane)	Outer boundary of cell	Protects cell contents
		Regulates entry and exit of materials from cell
Nucleus	Near the center of cell	Controls cellular activity ("command center" of cell)
		Contains chromosomes composed of DNA and carrying genetic information
		Most prominent structure in cell
Nucleolus	Within the nucleus	Required for manufacture of proteins
		Made up of RNA, which is responsible for transmitting genetic information from nucleus to cytoplasm
		Forms ribosomes
Mitochondria	Scattered throughout cell	Controls release of energy from nutrients
		Forms ATP (cellular energy)
		"Power plant" of cell that produces energy as body heat
		When complex foods are taken in and combined with oxygen, energy is released (**catabolism**)
		Largest structure in cell after nucleus
Endoplasmic reticulum (ER)	Network of membranes throughout the cytoplasm	System of tubes or tunnels within cytoplasm that stores and transports proteins
		Holds ribosomes
		Joins smaller protein particles with others to form larger particles (**anabolism**)
Ribosomes	Can be attached to ER or scattered throughout cytoplasm	Manufacture (synthesize) proteins in cytoplasm
		Are small in size
Golgi apparatus	Layers of membranes near nucleus	Forms substances and produces lysosomes
		Packages proteins for export from cell
		Resembles stack of pancakes
		Secretes hormones, enzymes, and mucus from cell
Lysosomes	Small sacs throughout cytoplasm	Digest or break down materials in cell for use
		Destroy bacteria
Centrioles	Two rod-shaped bodies near nucleus	Needed during cell division to direct chromosome distribution
Cilia	Hairlike projections from cell membrane	Move substances over the cell surface
		Can be used for filtering
Flagella	Cell extension	Propel sperm cells
Cytoplasm	Within the cell membrane	Fluid that surrounds and bathes organelles in the cell

ATP, Adenosine triphosphate; *DNA*, deoxyribonucleic acid; *RNA*, ribonucleic acid.

someone enters wearing perfume or cologne? If the fragrance is strong enough, before long the entire room smells of the scent. Figure 11-13 shows how an aroma from a bottle diffuses (escapes) into the air when the top is removed. Figure 11-14 illustrates how a dye tablet placed in a liquid diffuses over time. Figure 11-15 shows how two different glucose solutions will be the same after the diffusion process.

The respiratory system uses the diffusion process to exchange the gases oxygen (O_2) and carbon dioxide (CO_2) in the lungs. When CO_2 builds up in the blood to a concentration that is higher than in the lungs, CO_2 diffuses into the lungs for expiration, and O_2 diffuses out of the lungs and into the blood for circulation to the cells.

Osmosis is the diffusion (pulling) of water molecules through a semipermeable membrane from an area of higher concentration of water to one of lower concentration (Figure 11-16). An example of this is when a patient receives intravenous (IV) fluids of normal saline (0.9%) or 5% dextrose (glucose) in water (D5W) to replace body fluids. The cell contents are equal to these two fluids and no harm comes to the patient, so the solution is considered to be an **isotonic** (same) solution. If the IV solution is **hypertonic,** say 10% glucose, the cells in the blood would shrivel up or **crenate** because the solution is higher in its glucose concentration than the cells' intracellular composition. If the solution were **hypotonic,** the cells would **hemolyze** because the cell would now pull in the lower concentration of solution, swell, and burst. Figure 11-17 shows the effects of the different types of solutions on the red blood cell.

Filtration occurs when particles are pushed through a membrane by a mechanical pressure. The particles allowed to pass depend on the size of the membrane's pores. This can be compared to the way coffee is made. Coffee grounds are placed in a filter, and water is passed through the grounds and the filter. The filter allows the small water particles through but holds back the larger particles of the coffee grounds. In the body, this is what happens with blood pressure. When the liquid portion of the blood (**plasma**) moves through the capillary walls, a pressure is exerted when the heart contracts. The pressure causes some of the blood plasma to move out of the

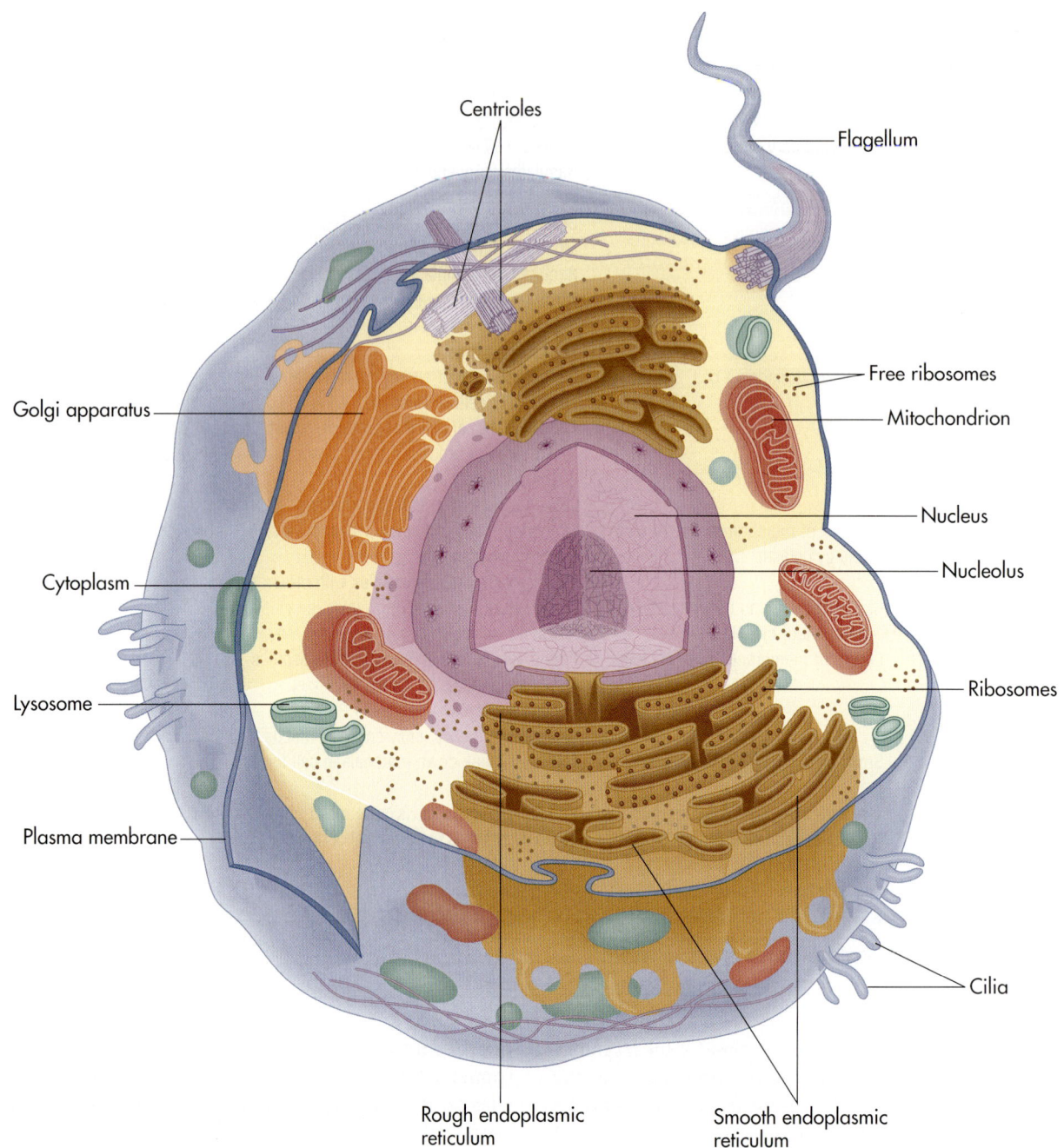

FIGURE 11-12 Basic cell structure. (From Thibodeau GA, Patton KT: *The human body in health and disease,* ed 4, St Louis, 2005, Mosby.)

capillary walls into the tissue. Normally the plasma is returned to the circulatory system by the lymphatic system. If the plasma stays inside the tissue, swelling (edema) occurs.

Active Transport Methods. **Active transport** requires cellular energy (through **adenosine triphosphate [ATP]**) and proteins within the cell membrane to carry molecules across the membrane from an area of lower concentration to one of higher concentration. This allows the cell to take what it needs from the tissue fluid. Like a salmon swimming upstream, active transport allows for movement against the natural flow.

Phagocytosis, or "cell eating," occurs when a moving cell engulfs (eats) a particle of solid material (Figure 11-18). White blood cells are "scavengers" that digest bacteria and parts of dead cells.

Pinocytosis, or "cell drinking," occurs when a stationary cell engulfs and digests droplets of a fluid.

Cell Division

Even in healthy individuals, cells die or are destroyed. In order for people to grow and for cells and tissues to be repaired when damaged or injured, single cells must divide to produce

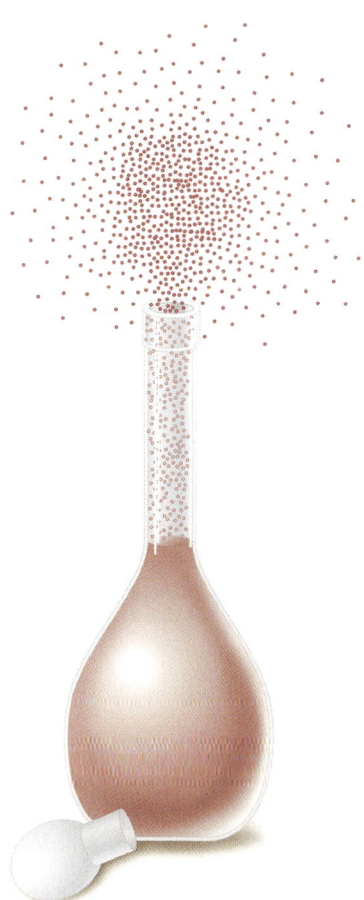

FIGURE 11-13 Diffusion of molecules into the air when a stopper is removed from a scented liquid.

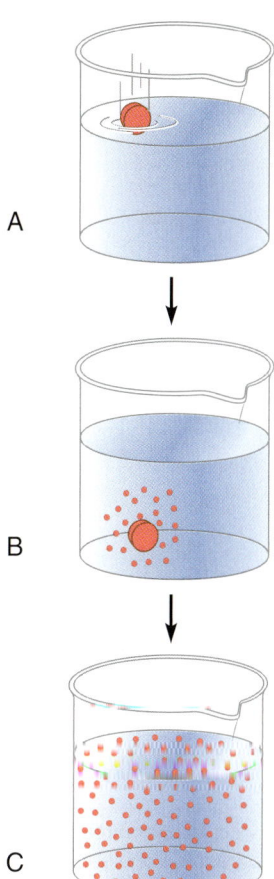

FIGURE 11-14 Diffusion. **A,** Molecules of a dye tablet are closely packed when they enter the water. **B,** Dye molecules move from an area of higher concentration toward the area of lower concentration. **C,** Dye molecules distribute evenly throughout the water. (Modified from Applegate EJ: *The anatomy and physiology learning system,* ed 3, St Louis, 2006, Saunders.)

more cells. There are two types of cell division: mitosis and meiosis. Mitosis is involved in bodily growth and repair, and meiosis occurs only in sex cells.

Mitosis. **Mitosis** is the division of body cells (**somatic cells**). This takes place when a single cell (parent cell) divides to form two identical cells (daughter cells). Before mitosis occurs, the cell actively prepares for the duplication by producing new DNA and duplicating the centrioles and mitochondria (see Table 11-3). Figure 11-19 illustrates the five stages of mitosis.

FOR YOUR INFORMATION

CELL GROWTH AND CANCER

Although cell growth and production are usually good for the body, cancer is an exception. Cancer occurs when one of a person's own cells has uncontrolled cell growth, forming a **tumor,** *or* **neoplasm,** *and the resulting cells replace the function of healthy tissue. Tumors can be* **benign** *(not cancerous) or* **malignant** *(cancerous).* **Metastasis** *occurs when these cancer cells break away from the tumor and travel to other parts of the body.* **Oncology** *is the study of cancerous tumors.*

Meiosis. In addition to mitosis, humans also undergo the process of **meiosis**. Meiosis is the division of sex cells (**gametes**). When a sperm that has 23 chromosomes (X or Y) and an ovum (egg) also with 23 chromosomes (X) join together to form a new cell called a *zygote,* this new cell then has 46 single (or 23 pairs of) chromosomes.

Genetic Information in the Cell

As you know, our genes determine our characteristics. Everything from our eye color to our height to our abilities, likes, and dislikes can be attributed directly or indirectly to our genetic makeup. Genes are either **dominant** or **recessive.** A dominant gene is prominent in the genetic makeup of an individual unless two recessive genes appear together. Genetic information is carried within the DNA in our chromosomes. A person has a total of 46 chromosomes: 23 from the mother and 23 from the father. More or less, an incorrect pairing of chromosomes will result in serious problems for a child.

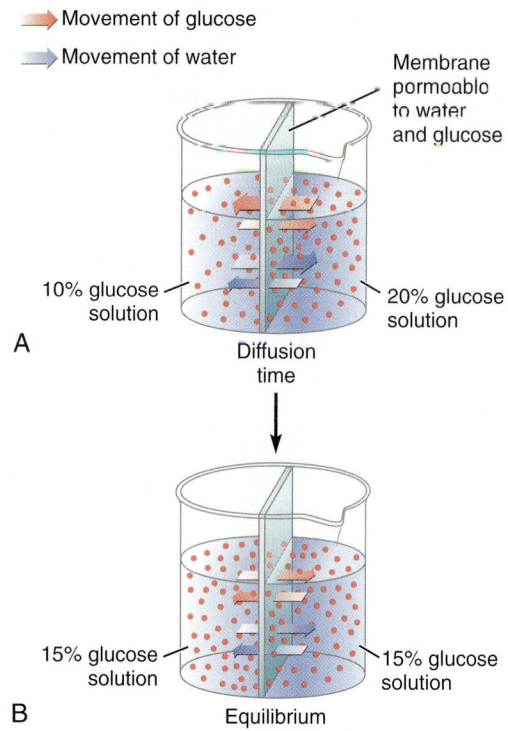

FIGURE 11-15 Diffusion through a membrane. At the start of diffusion, the membrane separates each solution. **A,** Membrane allows glucose and water to pass through it. **B,** After time, glucose solutions diffuse and become one solution.

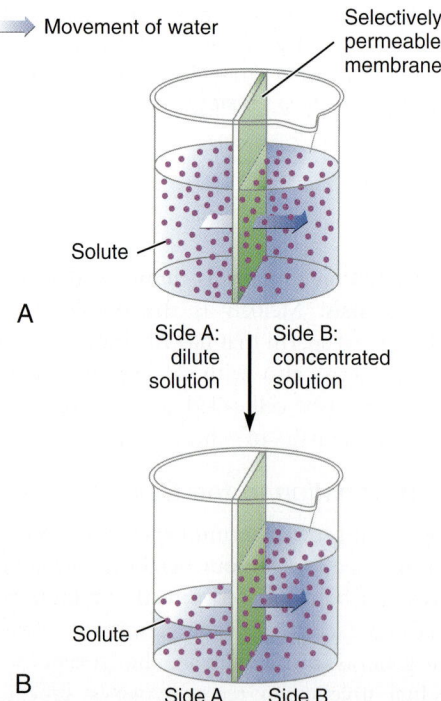

FIGURE 11-16 Osmosis. **A,** Semipermeable membrane separates two solutions. **B,** The dilute solution moves across the membrane to the concentrated solution. (Modified from Herlihy B, Maebius NK: *The human body in health and illness,* ed 3, St Louis, 2007, Saunders.)

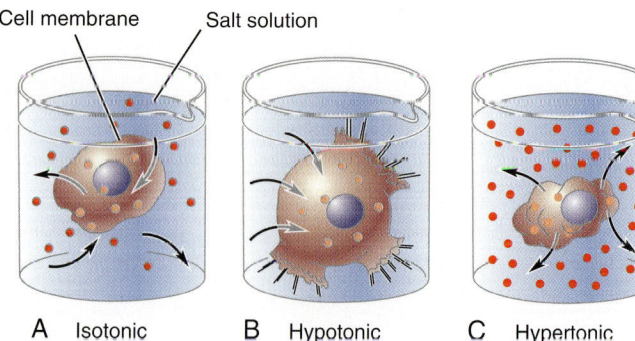

FIGURE 11-17 Osmosis in cells. **A,** Cells placed in an *isotonic* solution maintain a constant volume because the fluid within the cell and the fluid around the cell are equal. **B,** A cell placed in a *hypotonic* solution may swell because the solution surrounding the cell diffuses inward. **C,** A cell placed in a *hypertonic* solution will shrink because the solution inside the cell diffuses outward. (Modified from Herlihy B, Maebius NK: *The human body in health and illness,* ed 3, St Louis, 2007, Saunders.)

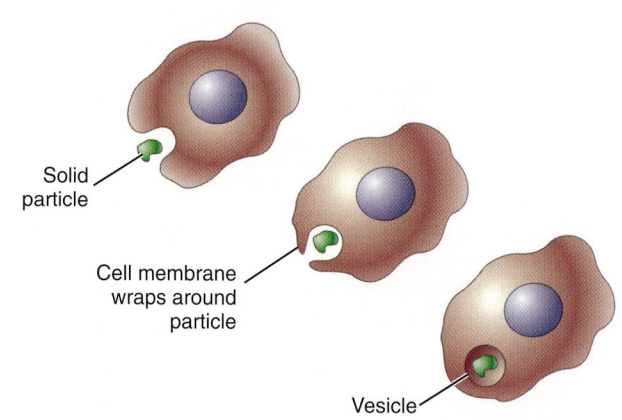

FIGURE 11-18 Phagocytosis. (Modified from Applegate EJ: *The anatomy and physiology learning system,* ed 3, St Louis, 2006, Saunders.)

Genetic Disorders

Genetic disorders occur when the structure of a gene (or genes) is altered, resulting in a *mutated* gene (**mutation**). They also occur when the number of chromosomes changes or when chromosomes are altered. Viruses, chemical toxins, drugs, the environment, and even radiation can cause alterations to the gene structure. Some disorders are inherited (**familial**), meaning that they are passed down from a family member (e.g., **hemophilia**). Heredity alone is sometimes the **predisposing factor** for a person acquiring the disease. Other genetic disorders are congenital. Not to be confused with "heredity," **congenital** refers to a condition a person is born with but not necessarily something the person has inherited (**hereditary**). For example, children born of alcoholic mothers may have *fetal alcohol syndrome* present as a congenital condition at birth.

- *Chromosomal diseases* are caused by **abnormalities** of the chromosome, either by changes in its structure or by too

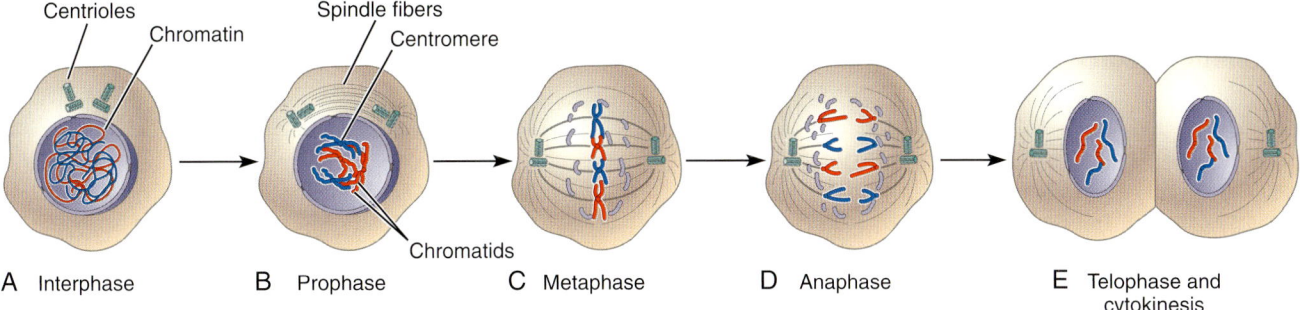

FIGURE 11-19 Mitosis. **A,** Interphase. Cell prepares for division. **B,** Prophase. Protective membrane disappears, and centrioles move to opposite ends of the cell. **C,** Metaphase. Chromosomes move to the center of the cell. **D,** Anaphase. Chromosomes separate and are pulled toward the centrioles. **E,** Telophase. Cytoplasm divides, leaving daughter cells (each with 23 pairs of chromosomes).

many or too few chromosomes. This type of disorder is not inherited (e.g., **Down syndrome, Klinefelter syndrome,** or **Turner syndrome**).
- *Single-cell diseases* or *mutated diseases* are caused by a defective gene, are usually inherited, and often affect certain cultures more than others (e.g., **Tay Sachs disease**).

Table 11-4 provides the following information on specific chromosomal and single-cell or mutated disorders:
- *Incidence:* Frequency of occurrence.
- *Etiology:* Cause or origin (**etiology**) of a disease or disorder as determined by medical diagnosis.
- *Signs and symptoms:* A **sign** is something that can be seen or measured by a medical assistant (*objective* finding), whereas a **symptom** is something that the patient can tell the medical assistant about, but that cannot be seen or measured (*subjective* finding). Both signs and symptoms are points of documentation in the patient record.
- *Diagnosis:* Identification of the nature and cause of a disease or injury through evaluation of patient history, examination, and review of laboratory data.
- *Therapy:* Treatment of an illness or disability.
- *Interventions:* Actions taken to produce a desired effect, as in therapeutic intervention, or treatment undertaken to correct a problem.

Genetic Counseling. The process of **genetic counseling** provides families with the current information about inherited diseases, whether in themselves or in their offspring. The main goal of genetic counseling is to allow individuals or couples to make informed decisions when one or both people are carriers for a genetic defect. Options may be presented, such as taking the risk, not having children at all, or terminating an existing pregnancy.

Many ethical, social, and psychological issues surround genetic counseling. Culture and religious beliefs also play an important role in the decision process. The medical assistant's role during this decision time is to remain objective and accept the patient's beliefs and wishes.

Body Tissues

We began this discussion of the body's organizational levels with an atom and then progressed to a cell. **Tissues** are formed when a group of cells with similar structure network together to carry out a specific task. They are bound together by a cement-like **intercellular** (between cells) substance that varies according to the type of tissue. Each tissue type has specific properties, and each tissue's function is related to the organ(s) of which it is a part. Based on function and appearance, there are four basic types of body tissues, as follows:
1. **Epithelial tissue** covers surfaces, lines cavities and hollow organs, and forms glands.
2. **Muscle tissue** produces movement by contracting and relaxing.
3. **Connective tissue** supports and forms the framework of the body.
4. **Nerve tissue** conducts nerve impulses.

Epithelial Tissue

Epithelial tissue offers protection by covering the body surface (skin) and lining the body cavities. The cells of epithelial tissue fit tightly together and have only small amounts of intercellular substance holding them. Epithelial cells have no blood supply of their own and rely solely on the connective tissue beneath them for oxygen and nutrients. Epithelial tissues repair quickly when injured and reproduce when worn, especially inside the mouth, intestinal tract, and the skin. The shape and the arrangement of the cells aid in identifying the different types of epithelial tissue (Table 11-5).

Epithelial tissue can also be specialized within the body to absorb and secrete. Absorption occurs when the tiny air sacs in the lungs take in oxygen, when molecules of food are pulled into the digestive tract, and when the kidneys filter blood through the capillary walls. At times, different sections of the body require protective secretions or mucus to line body cavities. For certain types of secretions, specialized epithelial cells form structures called **glands.** The two types of glands are classified by (1) what they secrete and (2) how the substance is released.

Text continued on p. 186

TABLE 11-4

Genetic Disorders

Incidence	Etiology	Signs and Symptoms	Diagnosis	Therapy	Interventions
DOWN SYNDROME (CHROMOSOMAL DISEASE)					
1:1000 births in young women; 1:300 live births when mother over age 35	Faulty meiosis of ovum; presence of extra chromosome 21 creates syndrome	Facial features abnormal at birth, short extremities (Figure 11-20); growth retardation; possible heart defects; mental retardation	**Amniocentesis** before birth; appearance at birth	Surgery to correct heart abnormalities; antibiotic and thyroid therapy as needed	Emotional support for entire family
KLINEFELTER SYNDROME (CHROMOSOMAL DISEASE)					
Affects males; 1:800 live births	Problem during gamete formation, causing an extra X chromosome XXY (47)	Abnormal development of testes, low testosterone; sterile	Physical exam and lab tests; usually not diagnosed until puberty	Psychological and hormone therapy	Emotional support for patient and family
TURNER SYNDROME (CHROMOSOMAL DISEASE)					
Affects females; 1:3000 live births	Loss of X chromosome during gamete formation XO (45)	Dwarfism, cardiac defect, absence of ovaries	Chromosomal analysis at birth	Hormone replacement and growth therapy; surgical repair for heart defects	Emotional support for family
SICKLE CELL ANEMIA (GENETIC MUTATION)					
Affects African-American population and those of northern Mediterranean ancestry; 1:600 births and when both parents have the gene	Altered shape to red blood cell (Figure 11-21)	Chronic fatigue; **dyspnea** (difficulty breathing) on exertion; joint swelling; **pallor** (pale)	Family history and lab tests; decreased hemoglobin and hematocrit, red blood cell count, and increased white blood cell and platelet count	**Palliative** (supportive) antibiotics, vaccinations, analgesics during crisis	Nutritional needs addressed: foods high in folic acid, good fluid intake, rest, daily exercise
HEMOPHILIA (X-LINKED GENETIC DISEASE)					
1.25:10,000 live male births in United States	Deficiency of clotting factors carried on genes of X chromosome	Prolonged bleeding time; joint swelling and pain	Family history and laboratory tests	Medications to improve clotting levels; supportive levels	Activity restrictions; emotional support; encouragement of good hygiene and dental care; Med-Alert tag
PHENYLKETONURIA (PKU) (METABOLIC DISORDER)					
Often affects those of Scottish and Irish descent; 1:14,000 births in United States	Autosomal recessive trait; missing enzyme that converts phenylalanine to tyrosine	Musty smell on diapers; hyperactivity; irritability	Blood screening at birth and after feeding has started; if not diagnosed soon after birth, will result in mental retardation	Special protein-restricted diet to counter lack of the enzyme responsible for breaking down an amino acid	Emotional support for family and patient as they approach school age

TABLE 11-4

Genetic Disorders—cont'd

Incidence	Etiology	Signs and Symptoms	Diagnosis	Therapy	Interventions
CYSTIC FIBROSIS (MUTATED GENE DEFECT)					
Mainly affects Caucasians of Northern European ancestry; 1:2500-3500 live births	Autosomal recessive gene	Large amounts of thick mucus in lungs; dry cough, dyspnea, tachypnea; increased salts produced by body; inability to absorb fats	Two positive sweat tests; low weight gain; family history	Supportive care for patient and family; increased salt intake, oxygen therapy, chest drainage	Increased fluid intake; be supportive and encourage support group
TAY-SACHS DISEASE (METABOLIC DISEASE CAUSED BY MUTATED GENE)					
Usually affects those of Ashkenazic Jewish ancestry; 1:3600 live births	Missing enzyme that metabolizes lipids	Delayed psychomotor development; cannot sit up and roll over; vision loss	Retinas have cherry-red spot with gray border; family history; death by age 5 years is typical	Supportive feedings and suctioning	Supportive care for family; around-the-clock care
HUNTINGTON CHOREA OR HUNTINGTON DISEASE (MUTATED GENE DEFECT)					
Each child of a parent with the disease has a 50% chance of inheriting it	Autosomal dominant trait causing the cerebral cortex and basal ganglia to degenerate	Uncontrolled involuntary movement; personality changes; dementia	Neurological assessment and imaging tests; family history, has insidious onset in early middle age	Supportive care based on symptoms	Emotional support for family and patient
THALASSEMIA (COOLEY ANEMIA) (SINGLE-CELL GENETIC BLOOD DISORDER)					
Affects persons of Mediterranean ancestry*; each child of affected parent has 50% chance of inheriting the disease	Autosomal dominant gene affecting hemoglobin production and life span of red blood cells	Progressive anemia, jaundice, pallor, lethargy, and enlarged spleen	Lab tests show decreased hemoglobin and red blood cells and increase in bilirubin in urine and feces	Folic acid replacement; supportive care	No iron supplements; need balanced diet and increased fluid intake; activity monitoring
MUSCULAR DYSTROPHY (SINGLE-GENE DEFECT)					
1:7000 live births	Inherited gene from the female X-linked decreased dystrophin (muscle protein)	Weak but well-developed muscles; slow to walk; waddling **gait** (style of walking)	**Gowers' sign** (Figure 11-22); electromyography, muscle biopsy; progressive weakening of skeletal muscles usually appears before age 5 years	Physical therapy and supportive care	Include family in all care and offer support to family and patient
CLEFT PALATE AND CLEFT LIP (POLYGENIC ERRORS)					
1:10,000 live births	Recessive X-linked gene	Hole in palate that separates mouth and nasal cavity (Figure 11-23)	Evident at birth	Surgical intervention to repair defect; ongoing process; speech therapy	Supportive care for family

*Greeks and Italians, as well as those of Southeast Asia, Southern China, and some African races.

TABLE 11-5

Classification of Epithelial Tissues

Type	Structure	Function
Simple **squamous**	Single layer of flat cells	Permits diffusion of gases in tiny air sacs of lungs (alveoli)
Stratified squamous	Many layers; surface layers flat; lower layers rounded	Covers surface area of epidermis (skin), lines vagina, mouth, and esophagus Protection
Simple **cuboidal**	Single layer of cube-shaped cells	Lines kidney tubules
Simple **columnar**	Single layer of column-shaped cells	Lines small intestines Protection Secretion Absorption
Pseudostratified columnar	Multiple incomplete layers	Respiratory tract (trachea)

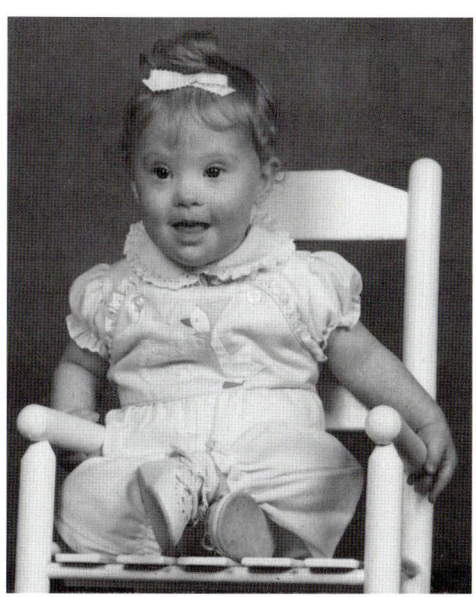

FIGURE 11-20 Infant with Down syndrome. (From Jorde LB, Carey JC, White RL, Bamshad MJ: *Medical genetics,* ed 3, St Louis, 2008, Mosby.)

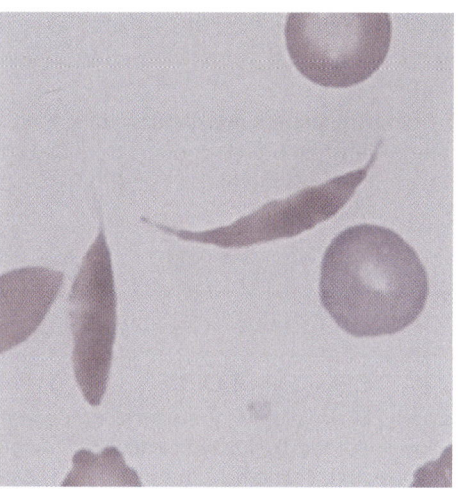

FIGURE 11-21 Appearance of sickle cells. (From Carr JH: *Clinical hematology atlas,* ed 3, St Louis, 2008, Saunders.)

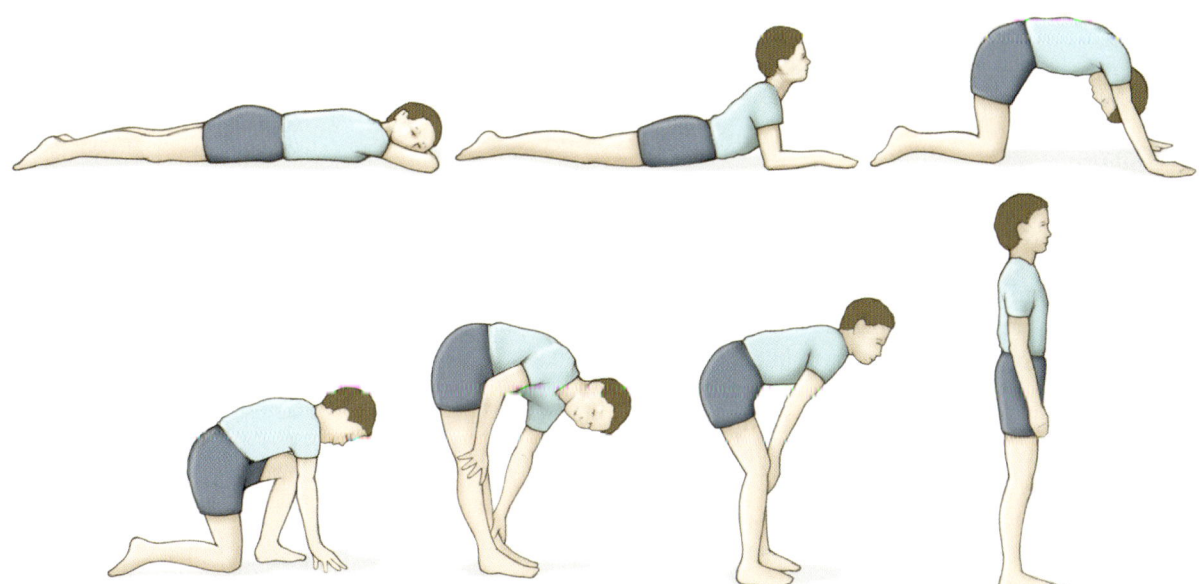

FIGURE 11-22 Child with muscular dystrophy stands up from prone position by placing hands on thighs (Gowers' sign).

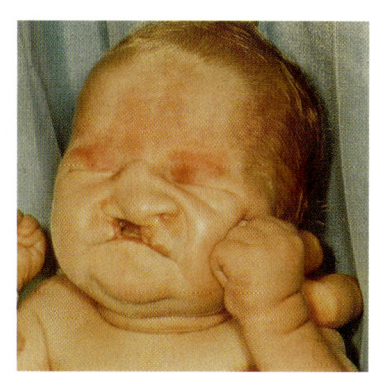

FIGURE 11-23 Infant with cleft lip. (From Ibsen OAC, Phelan JA: *Oral pathology for the dental hygienist*, ed 5, St Louis, 2009, Saunders.)

- The **exocrine glands** have ducts that take secretions to the body surface (e.g., sweat, tears, saliva, and mammary glands).
- The **endocrine glands** are ductless and discharge their hormones into the blood or tissue fluid to be absorbed by the capillaries in the body (e.g., insulin).

FOR YOUR INFORMATION

EPITHELIAL TISSUE DISORDERS
- A *carcinoma* is a malignant growth occurring in epithelial tissue and is spread by the lymphatic system.
- A *squamous cell carcinoma* can occur on the skin and in the mouth, lungs, bronchi, esophagus, or cervix (Figure 11-24).
- An *adenoma* is a benign growth of glandular epithelial tissue.
- A *papilloma* is a benign tumor of the epithelium (wart).
- An *adenocarcinoma* is a malignant growth from glandular epithelial tissue.
- An *epithelioma* is a malignant tumor derived from epithelial cells that originate in the epidermis of the skin or a mucous membrane.

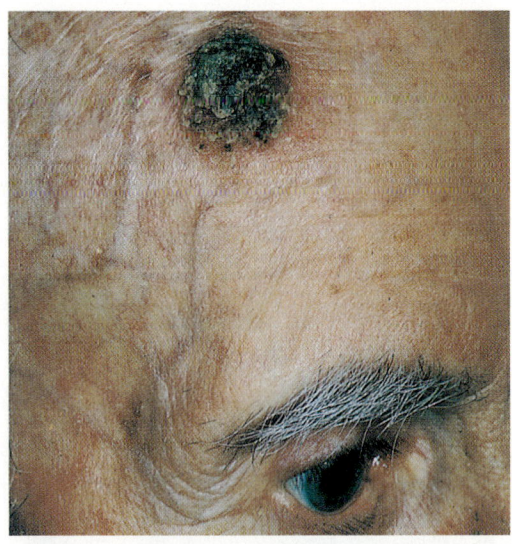

FIGURE 11-24 Example of squamous cell carcinoma. (From Habif TP: *Clinical dermatology*, ed 3, St Louis, 1996, Mosby.)

TABLE 11-6
Types of Muscle Tissue

Location	Appearance	Function	Illustration
Skeletal	Striated	Voluntary movement of skeleton Eye movements Swallowing (upper third of esophagus)	
Smooth (visceral)	Nonstriated	Involuntary movement through digestive tract Controls size of blood vessels (aids in regulation of blood pressure) Regulates size of pupils and shape of lens	
Cardiac	Striated	Involuntary contraction of heart	

Muscle Tissue

Muscle tissue contracts, or shortens, allowing movement. The muscle cells are elongated, narrow, and threadlike and are referred to as muscle **fibers**. Muscle fibers are arranged in bundles and surrounded by connective tissue. As seen in Figure 11-25, muscles can appear under the microscope to be **striated** (with stripes) or **nonstriated** (without stripes). Muscle tissue action or function is considered to be **voluntary** (made to contract by effort) or **involuntary** (contract independently regardless of effort). There are three types of muscle tissue, as follows (Table 11-6):

1. **Skeletal muscle** or striated voluntary is attached to the bones of the skeletal system by connective tissue and contracts when stimulated by a nerve impulse that produces movement. They contain many nuclei per cell.
2. **Smooth muscle** (nonstriated involuntary) or visceral muscle forms the walls of hollow organs located in the ventral cavity of the body and controls the diameter of the blood vessels. They contain only one nucleus per cell.
3. **Cardiac muscle** (striated involuntary) cells make up the heart wall (**myocardium**) and is responsible for the pumping of blood through the chambers of the heart and for the subsequent heartbeat. Cardiac muscle cells stimulate heart contraction, and nerve impulses act to speed up or slow down the heart rate. Cardiac muscle fibers have cross-striations and form unique dark bands called *intercalated disks*. These disks support the systematic contraction of the cardiac tissue.

Muscle tissues do not readily repair themselves as do epithelial tissues. Muscle tissue is often replaced with fibrous connective tissue, which affects both the structure and the function of the tissues.

Basic Anatomy and Physiology CHAPTER 11 187

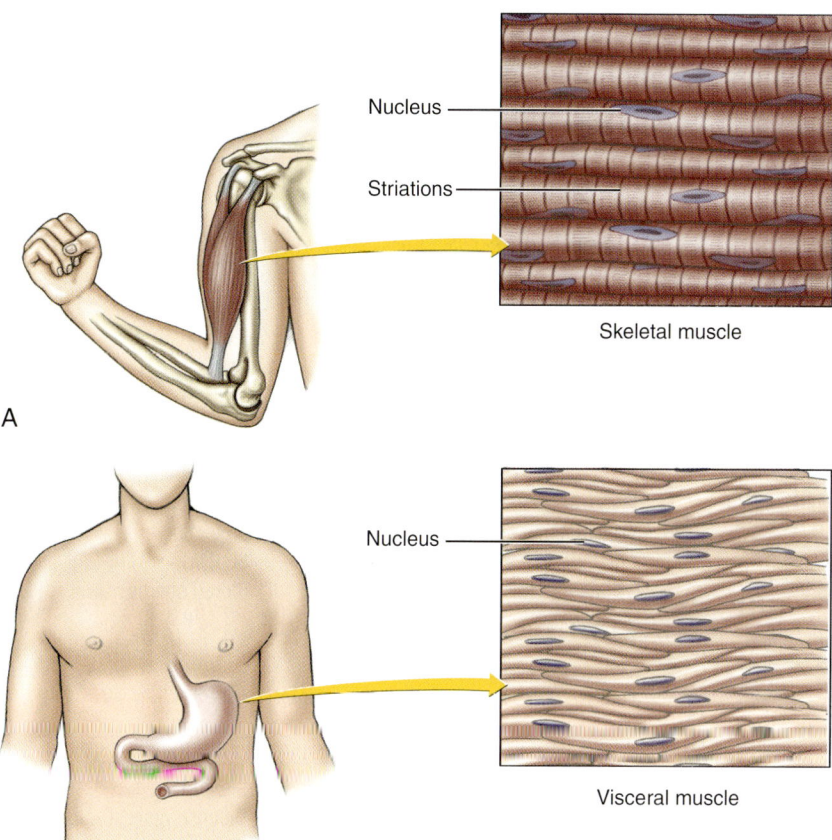

FIGURE 11-25 **A,** *Skeletal* muscle fibers are long and cylindrical with alternating light and dark bands; they are voluntary. **B,** *Visceral* muscle cells are elongated; they are involuntary. **C,** *Cardiac* muscle cells are cylindrical and striated; they are involuntary.

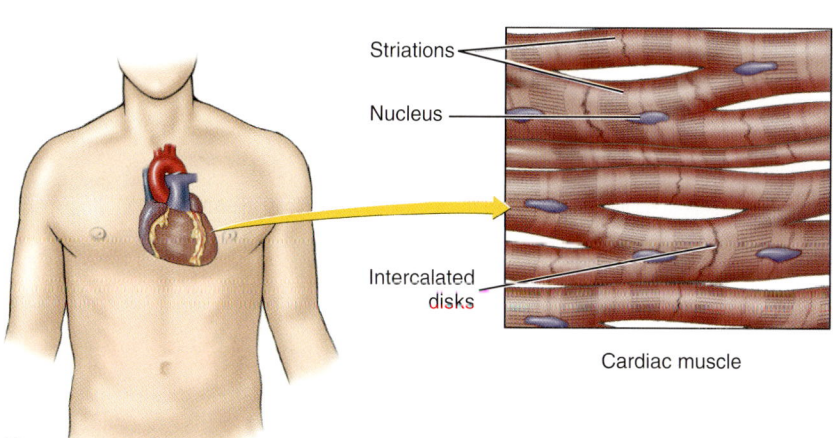

FOR YOUR INFORMATION

MUSCLE TISSUE DISORDERS
- A *rhabdomyoma* is a benign tumor of striated muscle.
- A *rhabdomyosarcoma* is a malignant tumor of striated muscle.
- A *myoma* is a tumor usually found in involuntary muscles (e.g., uterine fibroids).
- A *leiomyoma* (*leio-,* smooth) is a benign tumor of the smooth muscle.
- A *leiomyosarcoma* is a malignant tumor of the smooth muscle.

Connective Tissue

Connective tissue is the most abundant tissue in the body. It connects other tissues, provides for support of organs and other body parts, and provides protection. Connective tissue cells produce large amounts of a specialized intercellular substance called a **matrix**. The matrix can consist of a fluid, tissue fibers (either **collagenous, reticular,** or **elastic**), and a substance from which the cell was made. There are four types of connective tissue, as follows (Table 11-7):

1. **Fibrous tissue** can be classified according to its **extracellular** fibrous structure.

TABLE 11-7
Types of Connective Tissue

Type	Location	Function	Illustration
FIBROUS			
Loose (areolar)	Between organs and tissues; around blood vessels, nerves and joints	Connects skin to muscles; cushions organs Mucous membranes	Bundle of collagenous fibers / Elastic fibers
Adipose (fat)	Under the skin Around some organs and the eyes	Insulation Protection Support Stores energy	Storage area for fat
Reticular	Networks within the spleen, bone marrow, lymph nodes	Support Defense against microorganisms Filtration	Blood cell / Reticular fibers
Dense (collagenous)	Ligaments Scars Tendons Aponeuroses	Flexibility Strength	Fibroblast / Collagenous fibers
Bone (osseous)	Skeleton	Support Protection Storage of excess calcium	Osteon (Haversian system)

TABLE 11-7
Types of Connective Tissue—cont'd

Type	Location	Function	Illustration
CARTILAGE			
Hyaline	Nasal septum Covers ends of bones at joints Larynx Rings in trachea and bronchi	Flexibility Support	Matrix, Chondrocyte
Fibrocartilage	Discs between vertebrae Symphysis pubis	Support Flexibility Protection	Collagenous fibers, Cartilage cell
Elastic	Ear (external) Eustachian tube Larynx	Flexibility Support	Chondrocyte, Elastic fibers
Blood	Blood vessels	Transport Protection Regulation of body temperature Regulates body pH	Erythrocyte, Eosinophil, Neutrophil

Loose, reticular, dense, and bone illustrations from Thibodeau GA: *Anatomy and physiology*, ed 6, St Louis, 2007, Mosby.
Adipose illustration from Erlandsen SL, Magney J: *Color atlas of histology*, 1992, Mosby.

a. **Areolar** (loose) **tissue** is stretchable and is found between tissues and organs.
b. **Adipose tissue** consists of fat cells to help conserve body heat and offer a place for excess food.
c. **Reticular tissue** forms a network for the spleen, lymph nodes, and bone marrow and helps in body defenses.
d. **Dense tissue** helps anchor muscle to bone (tendon), or connects bone to bone (ligament), and forms the inner layer of the skin (dermis).

2. **Bone tissue** has fibers and a hard mineral substance that provides for protection and support of the body and allows for the attachment of muscles.

3. **Cartilage tissue** is similar to bone tissue but allows for flexibility in its support. Its collagenous fibers trap water to form a firm gel. All three types of cartilage contain these collagenous fibers, but in different amounts.
    a. **Hyaline cartilage** supports the rings of the bronchi, which aid in keeping the airway open. It also covers the ends of bones at the joints, which reduces friction during movement.
    b. **Fibrocartilage** is the strongest and most durable of the three cartilage tissues because it has large amounts of collagenous fibers. This type of cartilage serves as a shock absorber between the vertebrae and in the knee, allowing for movement.
    c. **Elastic cartilage** is the most flexible because it contains elastic fibers with the collagenous fibers. This is most evident in the tip of the nose, the external ear, and parts of the pharynx.
4. **Blood tissue** does not have fibers but has blood cells with plasma. Blood is discussed in more detail in Chapter 13.

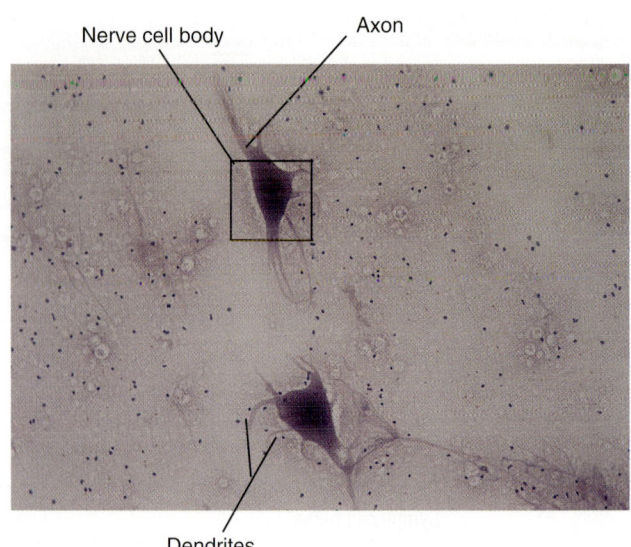

FIGURE 11-26 Nerve tissue. (From Thibodeau GA: *Anatomy and physiology,* ed 6, St Louis, 2007, Mosby.)

FOR YOUR INFORMATION

CONNECTIVE TISSUE DISORDERS

- A *lipoma* is a benign tumor containing fat.
- An *osteoma* is a benign bony tumor.
- A *sarcoma* is a malignant connective tissue tumor comprised of bone or cartilage that spreads by way of the bloodstream.

Nerve Tissue

Nerve tissue is the most highly organized tissue in the body. It is supported by connective tissue throughout the body except in the brain and spinal cord. It consists of many clusters of nerve cells called **neurons,** which carry nerve impulses (messages) throughout the body via **afferent nerves** and **efferent nerves,** and clusters of nerve cells called **glial cells,** which provide nutrition and support the activities of the neuron. Figure 11-26 shows microscopic nerve tissue. Nerve tissue and its function are discussed in more detail in Chapter 16.

FOR YOUR INFORMATION

NERVE TISSUE DISORDERS

- A *glioma* is a sarcoma composed of neuroglial cells.
- A *glioblastoma* is a malignant tumor containing immature glial cells.
- A *neurofibroma* is a connective tissue tumor involving the Schwann cells of the nerve (cells that produce myelin sheaths around neurons).

Organs

From tissue, we move to the next organizational level of the body: organs. An **organ** is composed of two or more types of tissues that allow it to perform a specific function or functions. Some organs occur in pairs (e.g., ovaries) and function independently of each other. Other organs can still function if up to 30% of the organ is damaged (e.g., kidney), and others can be removed entirely with minimal effect on the body (e.g., spleen). The skin, the largest organ in the body, is composed of all four tissue types. Individual organs are discussed in detail in subsequent chapters.

Systems

The next organizational level in the human body is the system. A body **system** is an organized grouping of structures (composed of tissues and organs) that perform a similar function. Table 11-8 lists and illustrates the body systems and their components.

The final organizational level in the human body is the entire body itself. When all the systems work together normally, they can sustain life. Starting with atoms and cells, advancing to tissues, organs, and systems, the body is an amazing machine.

PATIENT-CENTERED PROFESSIONALISM

- *The structural organization of the human body is divided into various levels: chemical (atoms and molecules), cellular, tissue, organs, and systems. What significance does each level play in the development of a person?*
- *Organs are highly organized structures with unique shapes and specialized activities. How can understanding the activities of each organ help you to understand patients' nutritional needs? Provide examples.*
- *How important is it to understand cell division and tissue types when trying to understand cancer growth and genetic disorders? How does this understanding benefit the patients you work with?*

TABLE 11-8
Body Systems

Body System	Components	Function	Illustration
CIRCULATORY Heart	Heart Arteries Veins Vessels	Responsible for transportation of blood Carries blood high in oxygen Carries blood high in carbon dioxide Carries blood (arteries, veins, or capillaries)	
Blood	Blood Red blood cells White blood cells Platelets	Carries nutrients to and wastes away from body tissues Carries oxygen to tissues Responsible for removing wastes Responsible for clotting	
Lymphatic Immune	Lymph nodes Spleen Thymus Tonsils	Defense against disease Blood reservoir Fetal immunity Filter and protect	
RESPIRATORY	Larynx Lungs Nose Pharynx Trachea	Exchanges oxygen and carbon dioxide and other waste products	
DIGESTIVE	Anus Esophagus Large intestine Liver Mouth Small intestine Stomach	Takes ingested food and provides for absorption of nutrients and elimination of solid wastes	

TABLE 11-8

Body Systems—cont'd

Body System	Components	Function	Illustration
NERVOUS	Brain Ears Eyes Nerves Spinal cord	Controls activities of body through transmission of electrical impulses; interprets sensory information	
SKELETAL	Bones Cartilage Joints Ligaments	Supports and protects internal organs; provides a framework for muscle attachment Stores minerals and is responsible for blood cell formation	
MUSCULAR	Muscles Tendons	Holds body erect and allows for movement of skeleton and internal organs; produces heat	
URINARY	Kidneys Ureters Urethra Bladder	Filters waste products from blood and forms urine	
REPRODUCTIVE	Ovaries Testes Uterus	Responsible for creation of new life	

TABLE 11-8
Body Systems—cont'd

Body System	Components	Function	Illustration
ENDOCRINE	Adrenals Ovaries Testes Pancreas Pineal Pituitary Thyroid and parathyroids Thymus	Provides for homeostasis of body and regulates body functions by means of hormone	
INTEGUMENTARY	Hair Nails Sebaceous glands Skin Sweat glands	Protects body from environment and aids in temperature regulation	

CONCLUSION

Take a moment to pull all this basic anatomy and physiology together and see why it is important to you as a medical assistant. You began this chapter learning anatomical terms that describe the human body and its structures in relation to one another (e.g., superior, RUQ, dorsal cavity). You will use these terms to communicate with other medical professionals. Next, you were introduced to the different levels of structural organization of the body (e.g., cells → tissues → organs → systems → organism). Medical assistants must understand the organizational levels of the body because of the concept of *homeostasis*, or the body being in balance. Remember that when the body is in balance, it functions normally. However, when the body is not in balance as a result of illness or injury, medical care may be needed. Two important responsibilities of medical assistants are to assist the physician and to help encourage patients to comply with their treatment plan. You need to understand the disease process to perform these responsibilities effectively.

If you do not understand cell structure, tissue formation probably will not make sense. If you do not understand tissue types, how can you understand organs? The understanding of one part leads to the understanding of another. If you do not understand how the whole body is structured and meant to function (anatomy and physiology), how can you expect to understand the disease process? The two skills you learned in this chapter (describing the human body and understanding the organizational levels of the body) serve as the foundation for the rest of the chapters in this section. With these two skills, you are prepared to learn about each of the body's systems in detail, to understand disease processes better, and ultimately, to provide the best care possible to patients.

Chapter Summary

Reinforce your understanding of the material in this chapter by reviewing the curriculum objectives and key content points below.

1. **Define, appropriately use, and spell all the Key Terms for this chapter.**
   - Review the Key Terms if necessary.
2. **List and describe the location of the three major body planes.**
   - The frontal, or coronal, plane divides the body vertically into anterior and posterior portions.
   - The sagittal plane divides the body vertically into right and left sides.
   - The transverse plane divides the body horizontally into superior and inferior portions.
3. **List and describe directional and positional terms and anatomical positions.**
   - Ventral refers to the front (anterior).

- Dorsal refers to the back (posterior).
- Superior refers to the upper region, or that which is above.
- Inferior refers to the lower region, or that which is below.
- An individual is in anatomical position when he or she is standing erect (upright), facing forward, arms at the sides, palms and toes facing forward, feet slightly apart, and legs parallel.
- The supine position is on the back with the face up.
- The prone position is on the belly with the face down.

4. **Identify the two main body cavities within the ventral cavity and the two main body cavities within the dorsal cavity.**
   - The ventral cavity contains the thoracic cavity and the abdominopelvic cavity.
   - The dorsal cavity contains the cranial cavity and the spinal cavity.

5. **Differentiate between abdominal quadrants and abdominal regions.**
   - There are four abdominal quadrants used to describe location.
   - There are nine abdominal regions used for clinical and surgical description, location, and documentation.

6. **Describe the progression from an atom to a system.**
   - Atoms make up cells, cells make up tissues, tissues make up organs, and organs make up systems.

7. **Identify the main structures of a cell.**
   - The cell membrane surrounds and protects the cell.
   - Cytoplasm is fluid that surrounds the nucleus and contains nutrients.
   - The nucleus is the "command center" of the cell, controlling a cell's activity.

8. **List and describe the transport systems used by cells.**
   - Cells must have the ability to transport materials into, out of, and within themselves.
   - Active transport requires energy; passive transport does not require energy.

9. **List two causes for genetic disorders.**
   - Chromosomal abnormalities and defective genes can cause genetic disorders.

10. **List five factors that can cause genes to mutate.**
    - Viruses, chemical toxins, drugs, the environment, and radiation can cause alterations to the gene structure.

11. **List the four main types of body tissues and describe the function of each.**
    - Epithelial tissues cover surfaces, line cavities and hollow organs, and form glands.
    - Muscle tissues produce movement by contracting and relaxing.
    - Connective tissues support and form the framework of the body.
    - Nerve tissues conduct nerve impulses.

12. **Match major organs to their body system.**
    - Refer to Table 11-8.

13. **List the ten body systems and describe the function of each.**
    - Refer to Table 11-8.

14. **Analyze a realistic medical office situation and apply your understanding of basic anatomy and physiology to determine the best course of action.**
    - To perform medical assisting duties correctly and efficiently, you must understand the basic structure and function of the body.

15. **Describe the impact on patient care when medical assistants have a solid grasp of basic anatomy and physiology.**
    - Understanding the normal structure and function of the human body helps medical assistants understand the disease process and the need for patients to follow the prescribed treatment plan.
    - This knowledge will help medical assistants communicate instructions and concepts to patients more effectively.

PRACTICAL APPLICATIONS

If you have accomplished the objectives in this chapter, you will be able to make better choices as a medical assistant. Take another look at this situation and decide what you would do.

John Choi is a medical assistant in a primary care facility. Barb Quinn arrives and complains of pain that she thinks is in her stomach. She states that she has had vomiting with blood and also has diarrhea. She also complains of difficulty with eating; she just does not want anything to eat and says, "I have to force myself to eat." After the examination, Dr. Elory tells Ms. Quinn that based on her symptoms, he is suspicious of a cancer in her abdomen. Dr. Elory orders several diagnostic tests that will be completed the next day. Dr. Elory tells Ms. Quinn that he will call as soon as he has her test results.

John Choi needs to know enough about anatomy and physiology to understand Ms. Quinn's symptoms and Dr. Elory's observations. If you were to step into this situation, would you be prepared to assist Dr. Elory in caring for Ms. Quinn?

1. John needs to chart the pain using the correct cavity for the stomach, the region of the abdominopelvic area, and the correct quadrant of the abdominal area. In what body system would John know the stomach is found?
2. How might John explain to Ms. Quinn what her symptoms mean in relation to anatomy and physiology?
3. What is cancer?
4. What does cell division have to do with cancer?
5. If Ms. Quinn had complained of pain in the left upper quadrant, what organs might have been involved?
6. If the pain was in the umbilical region, what could this mean?
7. What does pain in the right lower quadrant indicate as a possible organ involvement?
8. If Ms. Quinn had complained of shortness of breath, in what cavity would you expect the discomfort to be? What organ systems would be found in this cavity? What separates this cavity from the abdominopelvic cavity?
9. What is the difference between a sign and a symptom when discussing illness? What are the symptoms in the above scenario? What is a subjective finding and what is an objective finding in the patient's medical history?
10. What symptoms indicate a disturbance of the homeostasis of Ms. Quinn's body?

WEB SEARCH

1. **Research the various types of cancers.** Cancers are classified by their microscopic appearance and the body site from which they arise. A cancer is named from the type of tissue in which it develops. Knowing more about the types of cancer will help you interact with patients.
   - **Keywords:** Use the following keywords in your search: melanoma, sarcoma, carcinoma.
2. **Research the causes of cancer.** To better understand the diagnosis of cancer, a medical assistant needs to understand the various factors that can contribute to cancer-forming cells.
   - **Keywords:** Use the following keywords in your search: carcinogen, viruses, oncogenes, mutation.
3. **Research cancer treatments.** You may work with patients undergoing various cancer treatments. Cancer treatment can prove to be difficult because all cancer cells behave differently and sometimes a tumor has more than one type of cancer cell.
   - **Keywords:** Use the following keywords in your search: cancer treatments, metastasis, chemotherapy, radiation therapy, National Cancer Institute (NCI).

WORD PARTS: Chapter 11

ANATOMICAL POSITION

anter/o	front	later/o	side
poster/o	back	proxim/o	close
super/o	above	dist/o	far
infer/o	below	viscer/o	internal organs
dors/o	back	supra	above
ventr/o	front (belly side)	af-	toward
cephal/o	head	ef-	away
caud/o	tail	sinistr/o	left
medi/o	middle	dextr/o	right

CELLS

-cyte	cell
erythr/o	red (erythrocyte = red blood cell [RBC])
leuk/o	white (leukocyte = white blood cell [WBC])
thromb/o	clot (thrombocyte = platelet)

Cell Growth and Formation

-plasia	formation, development, and growth of tissues and cells
-aplasia	lack of development of a tissue
-anaplasia	loss of organization and structure in cell formation; characteristic of a malignant cell growth
dysplasia	abnormal growth of cells
intra	within

TISSUES
Prefixes

epi-	above
endo-	within

Combining Forms

my/o	muscle
neur/o	nerve
aden/o	gland
ex/o	out of
crin/o	to secrete
fibr/o, fibros/o	fiber
cardi/o	heart
adip/o	fat
chondr/o	cartilage

BODY SYSTEMS
Circulatory System

arter/o, arteri/o	arteries
ven/o, ven/i	veins
phleb/o	veins
vas/o, vascul/o	vessel
hem/o, hem/a	blood
hemat/o	blood

Lymphatic and Immune Systems

lymph/o	lymph
lymphaden/o	nodes
splen/o	spleen
thym/o	thymus
tonsil/lo	tonsils

Respiratory System

laryng/o	larynx
pneum/o, pneumon/o	lungs
pulmon/o	lungs
nas/o	nose
rhin/o	nose
pharyng/o	pharynx
trache/o	trachea

Digestive System

an/o	anus
proct/o	anus and rectum
esophag/o	esophagus
col/o	large intestine
hepat/o	liver
or/o	mouth
stomat/o	mouth
enter/o	small intestine
gastr/o	stomach

Nervous System

encephal/o	brain
ot/o	ears
ocul/o	eyes
ophthalm/o	eyes
myel/o	spinal cord

Skeletal System

oste/o	bones
arthr/o	joints
articul/o	joints

Muscular System

ten/o	tendons
tend/o, tendin/o	tendons
my/o	muscle

Urinary System

nephr/o	kidneys
ren/o	kidneys
ureter/o	ureters
urethr/o	urethra
cyst/o	bladder

Reproductive System

ovari/o	ovaries
oophor/o	ovaries
orchid/o, orchi/o	testes
uter/o	uterus
hyster/o	uterus
salping/o	fallopian tube

Endocrine System

adren/o	adrenals
gonad/o	gonads
pancreat/o	pancreas
pineal/o	pineal
pituit/o	pituitary
thyroid/o, thyr/o	thyroid

Integumentary System

cutane/o	skin
derm/o, dermat/o	skin
pil/o, trich/o	hair
onych/o, ungul/o	nails
seb/o	sebaceous glands
hidr/o	sweat glands

12 Cardiovascular System

evolve   http://evolve.elsevier.com/klieger/medicalassisting

As you learned in Chapter 11, the human body is made up of body systems that work together to sustain life. By understanding the normal structure and function (anatomy and physiology) of each system, medical assistants can begin to understand how disease affects each system. In this chapter on the cardiovascular system, as well as the other chapters on body systems, you are introduced to the structure and function of the system and then the types of diseases and conditions that affect the system

LEARNING OBJECTIVES

You will be able to do the following after completing this chapter:

Key Terms
1. Define, appropriately use, and spell all the Key Terms for this chapter.

Cardiovascular System
2. Name the components of the cardiovascular system.

Heart
3. Identify the four cardiac chambers and describe the function of each.
4. Locate the four cardiac valves of the heart and describe the function of each.
5. List the sequence of actions that take place in the conduction system.
6. Explain the importance of being able to recognize normal heart sounds.
7. Identify the two divisions of the autonomic nervous system that are responsible for modulating nerve conduction within the heart.
8. Trace the circulation of the blood from the heart to the lungs.
9. Trace the circulation of blood to the heart (coronary circulation).
10. Trace the movement of oxygenated blood through the heart and back out to the body tissues.
11. Trace the oxygenated blood supply to the brain.
12. Discuss the function of the hepatic portal system.
13. Explain fetal heart circulation

14. List seven forms of heart disease and describe the risk factors, etiology, signs and symptoms, diagnosis, therapy, and interventions for each.

Blood Vessels
15. List three types of blood vessels and describe the function of each.
16. List eight disorders of the blood vessels and describe the etiology, signs and symptoms, diagnosis, therapy, and interventions for each.

Patient-Centered Professionalism
17. Analyze a realistic medical office situation and apply your understanding of the cardiovascular system to determine the best course of action.
18. Describe the impact on patient care when medical assistants have a solid understanding of the structure and function of the heart and blood vessels.

KEY TERMS

The Key Terms for this chapter have been organized into sections so that you can easily see the terminology associated with each aspect of the cardiovascular system.

cardiovascular system   oxygen
  (circulatory system)

Heart
apex   sternum
diaphragm   thoracic vertebrae
mediastinum

Continued

Heart Muscle and Heart Coverings
endocardium
epicardium
myocardium
pericardium
visceral layer

Heart Chambers
atrium (plural atria)
chambers
septum (plural septa)
ventricles

Heart Valves and Related Blood Vessels
aorta
aortic semilunar valve
cardiac valves
cardiomegaly
chordae tendineae
cusps
hypertrophy
inferior vena cava
mitral (bicuspid) valve
pulmonary artery
pulmonary semilunar valve
pulmonary veins
regurgitation
superior vena cava
tricuspid valve
valve
valvular insufficiency
venae cavae

Conduction System of the Heart
conduction system

Heartbeat
cardiac cycle
diastole (S_2)
heartbeat
murmur
stethoscope
systole (S_1)

Cardiac Cycle
atrioventricular bundle
atrioventricular (AV) node
bundle of His
cardiac output
electrocardiogram (ECG)
Purkinje fibers
sinoatrial (SA) node
stroke volume

Nerve Supply of the Heart
antagonistic
arrhythmias
autonomic nervous system (ANS)
flutter
heart block
parasympathetic
sympathetic

Blood Supply
carbon dioxide (CO_2)
coronary circulation
deoxygenated blood
pulmonary circulation
systemic circulation

Coronary Circulation
anterior descending artery
circumflex artery
coronary arteries
infarction
ischemia
marginal artery
posterior descending artery

Brain and Hepatic Portal Circulation
anastomose
bifurcate
circle of Willis
external carotid arteries
internal carotid arteries
portal vein
vertebral arteries

Fetal Circulation
ductus arteriosus
ductus venosus
foramen ovale

Heart Disorders
cardiologist
cyanosis
diaphoresis
hypoxia
internist
occlusion
prophylactic
sequela
stenosis
syncope

Blood Vessels
arterioles
artery
blood vessels
capillary
diameter
varices
varix (plural varices)
vasoconstrict
vasodilate
vein
venules

Disorders of Blood Vessels
aneurysm
claudication
aneurysm
dilation
embolus
phlebitis
thrombus

PRACTICAL APPLICATIONS

Read the following scenario and keep it in mind as you learn about the cardiovascular system in this chapter.

Dr. Kim Kea will examine Mr. Stan Baleaut later today as a routine follow-up for high blood pressure and possible coronary artery disease. Mr. Baleaut tells Erin, the medical assistant, that he has some left arm pain and also has been having some heart palpitations and wants Dr. Kea to check this. As Erin takes Mr. Baleaut's blood pressure, she obtains a reading of 150/88 mm Hg and a pulse rate of 92 beats/min. Dr. Kea examines Mr. Baleaut and orders a stat ECG as a way of ruling out a diagnosis of MI. As Erin is completing the ECG, Mr. Baleaut has several questions about vital signs and ECGs. Erin needs to educate him in several areas.

FUNCTIONS OF THE CIRCULATORY SYSTEM

The **circulatory system,** also called the **cardiovascular system,** transports elements in the blood throughout the body. It also regulates body temperature and maintains homeostasis. The circulatory system does all this *systematically,* or in an organized way, as follows:

- The blood in the circulatory system delivers **oxygen** and nutrients to each cell and collects waste byproducts from cells.

- These waste products are carried to the kidneys, liver, lungs, and skin to be broken down or eliminated in urine, exhaled air, or sweat through a process called excretion.
- The blood carries hormones to target organs and removes excess fluids from body tissues.

Improper function of any part of the circulatory system can lead to the death of body tissues, organ failure, and even the death of an individual. The circulatory system consists of four separate but essential parts: (1) the heart, (2) the blood vessels, (3) the blood, and (4) the lymphatic system. Each part has its own role in transporting oxygen, eliminating wastes, and removing fluids from body tissue. The heart and the blood vessels are covered in this chapter, and the blood, lymphatic, and immune systems are discussed in Chapter 13.

> **PATIENT-CENTERED PROFESSIONALISM**
>
> - How can understanding the function and structure of the circulatory system help you communicate with patients?

HEART

Imagine working 24 hours a day, 7 days a week, with no breaks, and having your life depend on it. This is what it is like for your heart. The heart constantly pumps and circulates fluid in the circulatory system. Every day it pumps 4,000 gallons of blood at 40 miles per hour through 70,000 miles of vessels.

Medical assistants need to understand the structure of the heart, as well as how the heart beats to circulate blood, in order to comprehend the diseases that affect the heart.

Structure and Function of the Heart

The heart is a hollow, muscular pump that has four chambers. It beats an average of 72 beats per minute (beats/min or bpm) with a range of 60 to 100 beats/min, or more than 100,000 beats per day. Although heart size varies from person to person, the heart is about the size of a closed fist. In an average adult male the heart weighs approximately 300 g or about ½ lb. The heart is a dual pump system. One function of the heart is to pump enough blood to meet the needs of all body tissues and the other is to pump blood to the lungs for reoxygenation and waste removal.

It is important for medical assistants to recognize the location of the heart and its muscle, coverings, chambers, and valves.

Location

The heart is located slightly left of the center of the chest in the **mediastinum**. It is protected in the front by the **sternum** (breastbone) and the back by the **thoracic vertebrae** (backbone). The lungs are located on each side of the heart. The **apex** (tip) of the heart rests on the **diaphragm** and is pointed toward the left side of the body (Figure 12-1). The upper portion, called the *base*, lies just below the second rib.

Heart Muscle

The fibers of the heart muscle are striated, similar to skeletal muscle, but they are involuntary in action. The cardiac fibers are laced with intercalated disks that serve to join muscle fibers together, allowing for an electrical impulse to travel through both the atrial and ventricular chambers. Three different layers make up the wall of the heart: the epicardium, myocardium, and endocardium (Figure 12-2).

- The **epicardium** is the outermost of the three layers of tissues that form the heart wall. It covers the outside of the myocardium with a serous membrane known as the **visceral layer.** Together, the epicardium, lining of the blood vessels, and visceral layer form a sac, the **pericardium**, in which the heart is located.
- The **myocardium** forms the thick middle layer of the heart.
- The **endocardium** lines the heart chambers.

Heart Coverings

The outer covering of the heart is a double-layered serous membrane called the *pericardium*. This membrane secretes a pericardial fluid that lubricates the surfaces of the visceral and parietal tissues that prevents friction when the heart beats.

Heart Chambers

The heart is divided into four cavities known as **chambers:** two atria (upper chambers: left atrium and right atrium) and two ventricles (lower chambers: left ventricle and right ventricle) (Figure 12-3). Walls called **septa** (singular **septum**) divide the right and left chambers (e.g., ventricular septum, atrial septum).

- The **atria** (singular **atrium**) are the top chambers of the heart and are smaller with less muscle tissue than the ventricles because their function is to hold blood within the heart until it is moved to the ventricles.
- The **ventricles** pump blood out of the heart, first to the lungs and then to the body tissues. The left ventricle has the thickest wall because it exerts the greatest force pumping the blood throughout the body and returning it back to the heart.

Heart Valves and Related Blood Vessels

A **valve** is a structure that controls the flow of a substance by opening and closing openings so that substances can flow in only one direction. Examples of simple, everyday valves include faucets and garden hose nozzles. The purpose of the **cardiac valves** is to prevent blood from flowing back (**regurgitation**) to the atria when the ventricles contract. By looking at the flow of blood through the heart, we can see the role of the cardiac valves, as follows (Figure 12-4):

- When the right atrium receives venous blood from the **superior vena cava** and the **inferior vena cava** (together they are called the **venae cavae**), the **tricuspid valve** opens when the atrium contracts, allowing the blood to flow to the right ventricle. The tricuspid valve then closes during

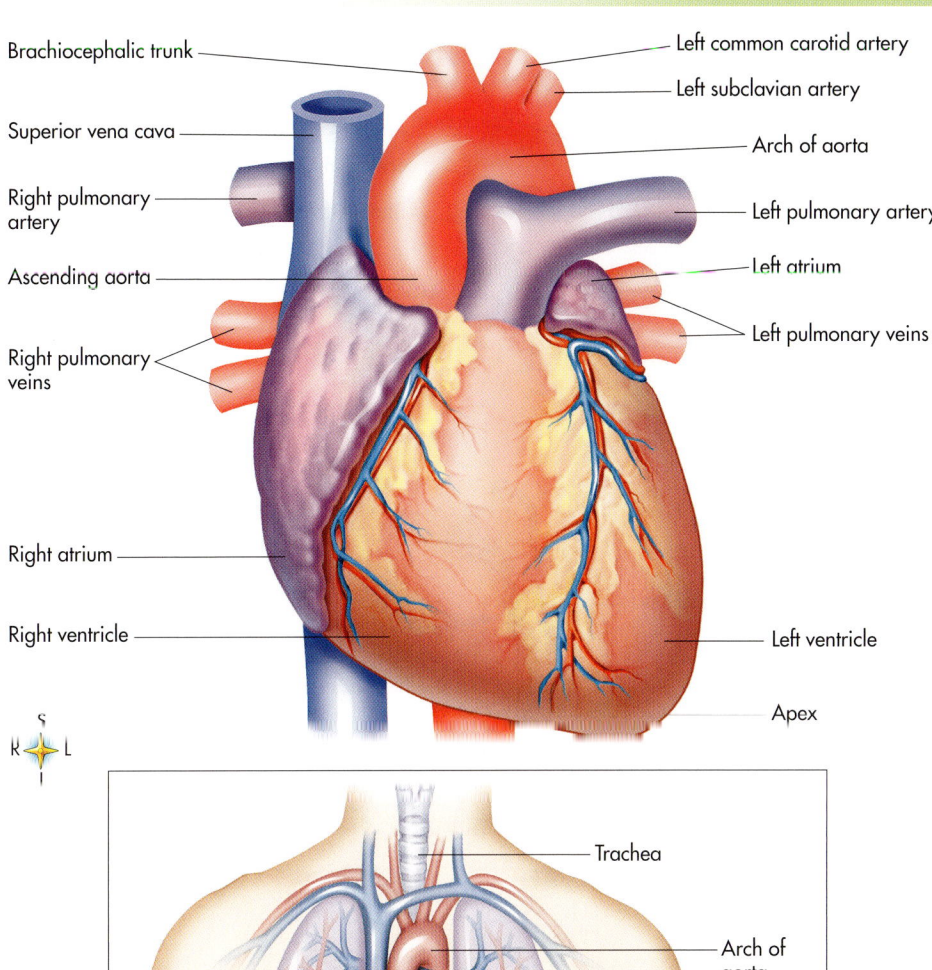

FIGURE 12-1 Location of the heart. (Modified from Thibodeau GA, Patton KT: *The human body in health and disease,* ed 4, St Louis, 2005, Mosby.)

ventricular contraction. The tricuspid is made up of three flaps (**cusps**).
- **Chordae tendineae** provide strength to the valves and prevent prolapse. These fibrous tissue cords are attached to the valve leaflets and anchored to the floor of the ventricle and prevent the valve from collapsing under pressure.
- The **pulmonary semilunar valve** prevents backflow of blood into the right ventricle. The right ventricle sends the deoxygenated blood through this semilunar valve into the **pulmonary artery** toward the lungs where the blood becomes oxygenated.
- When the oxygenated blood leaves the lungs by way of the **pulmonary veins,** it enters into the left atrium.
- When the blood leaves the left atrium, it passes through the **mitral (bicuspid) valve.** After the atrium empties into the left ventricle, the mitral valve (like the tricuspid valve) closes and prevents blood from returning to the atrium.
- When the left ventricle pumps blood to the **aorta,** the body's largest artery, the **aortic semilunar valve** prevents blood from returning to the left ventricle.

When a valve loses its ability to close tightly, it permits blood to leak back into the heart chamber through which the blood just passed. This is called **valvular insufficiency.** When this occurs, the heart chamber will **hypertrophy,** resulting in an enlarged heart (**cardiomegaly**).

Conduction System of the Heart

Your heart beats because of the heart's **conduction system.** The conduction system generates electrical signals and conducts them through the heart. These rhythmic electrical signals stimulate the heart to contract and pump blood. The system is made of two nodes (special conduction cells) and a series of conduction fibers or bundles (pathways).

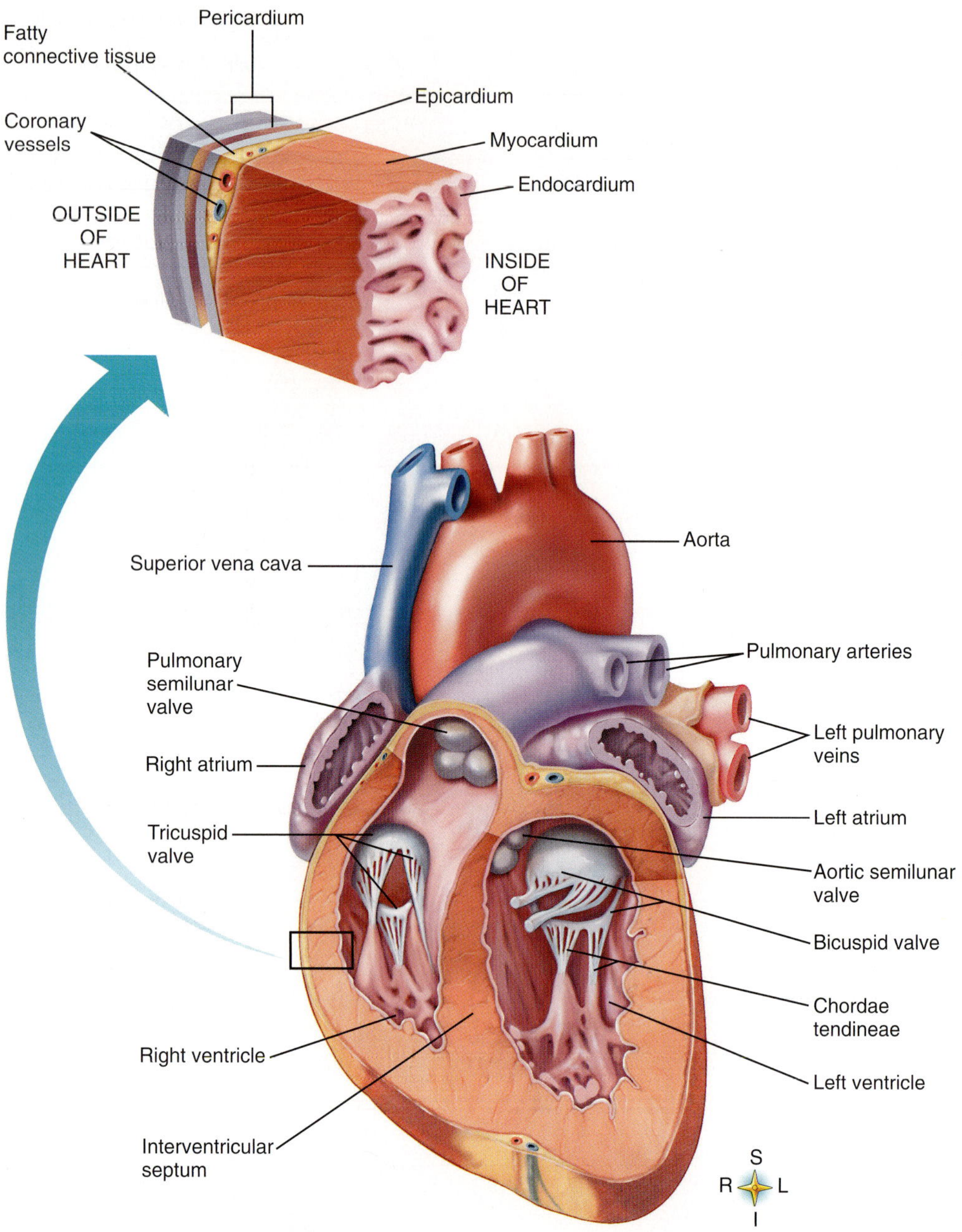

FIGURE 12-2 Layers of the heart and pericardium. (Modified from Thibodeau GA, Patton KT: *The human body in health and disease,* ed 4, St Louis, 2005, Mosby.)

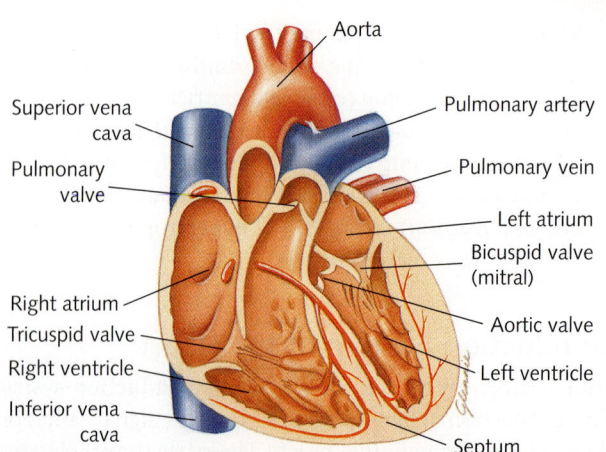

FIGURE 12-3 Chambers of the heart and the large vessels. (From Gerdin J: *Health careers today,* ed 4, St Louis, 2007, Mosby.)

Heartbeat

A **heartbeat** consists of the heart contracting (**systole**) S_1 and the heart relaxing (**diastole**) S_2. Together, the systole and diastole that produce the heartbeat are called the **cardiac cycle.** The measurement of the two parts of the cardiac cycle gives a blood pressure reading (e.g., 120/80 mm Hg). In this cycle, both atria contract together, filling the ventricles. As the atria relax, both ventricles contract and then relax. The heart therefore acts as a two-sided pump.

The sound "lubb-dupp" heard through a **stethoscope** can provide clues to health professionals about the functioning of a person's heart valves. The "lubb" sound is the ventricles contracting (systole) and the cuspid valves closing. The "dupp" sound appears to be the closing of the semilunar valves. If these sounds are not heard or do not sound the way described, this may indicate a valve malfunction. An abnormal heart

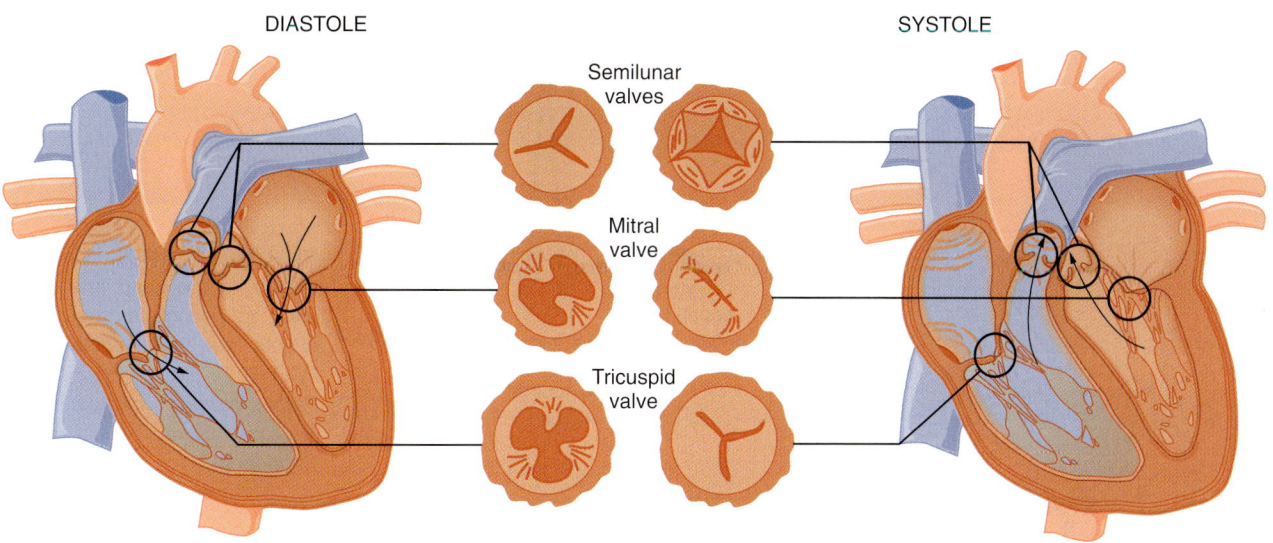

FIGURE 12-4 Valves of the heart. (From Black JM, Hawks JH: *Medical-surgical nursing: Clinical management for positive outcomes*, ed 8, St Louis, 2009, Saunders.)

sound caused by backflow of blood through the heart valve is called a **murmur.**

Cardiac Cycle

Four structures make up the conduction system and carry out the cardiac cycle: the sinoatrial node, atrioventricular node, atrioventricular bundle (bundle of His), and Purkinje fibers (Figure 12-5).

- The **sinoatrial (SA) node** is the natural "pacemaker" of the heart, and all electrical cardiac impulses are generated from this point. The modified cardiac muscle fibers are located in the right atrial wall near the opening or sinus of the superior vena cava. The SA node initiates an electrical impulse to the AV node with each heartbeat, which causes the walls of the atria to contract and forces the blood into the ventricle.
- The **atrioventricular (AV) node** is located in the lower left portion of the right atrium, near the point of contact between the right atrial and right ventricular septa. The AV node sends the electrical impulse to the bundle of His.
- The **atrioventricular bundle,** also known as the **bundle of His,** receives the impulse and sends it to two branches located on each side of the septum between the ventricles.
- **Purkinje fibers** extend along the outer walls of the ventricles. As the impulse passes through these fibers, the ventricles contract.

If the SA node fails to initiate an impulse, the AV node can begin the heartbeat. However, the heartbeat will be uncoordinated, and the circulation of blood throughout the body will be inadequate. In addition, several factors can influence the force of contraction and the rate of contraction such as drugs, hormones, and nerve stimulation. The term **stroke volume** refers to the amount of blood pumped by the ventricles in one beat. **Cardiac output** is the amount of blood pumped by the heart in 1 minute.

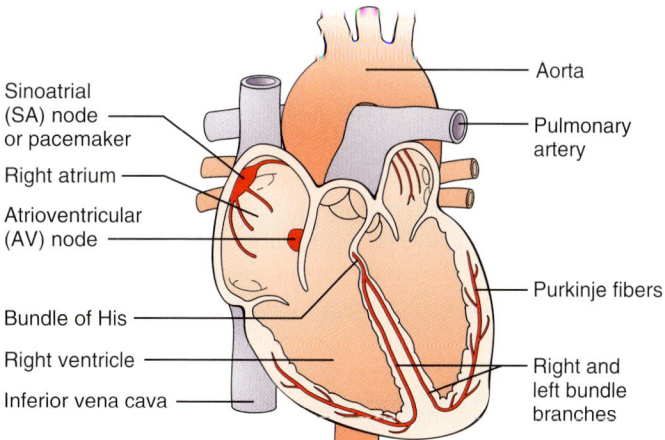

FIGURE 12-5 Conduction system of the heart. (Modified from Buck CJ: *Step-by-step medical coding, 2008 edition*, St Louis, 2008, Saunders.)

As you can see, medical assistants must be able to distinguish between normal and abnormal heart sounds. The complete cardiac cycle can be recorded on an **electrocardiogram (ECG)** (Figure 12-6), which is discussed in detail in Chapter 36.

Nerve Supply of the Heart

The **autonomic nervous system (ANS)** carries signals to the cardiac muscle, smooth muscle, and glandular epithelial tissue. The ANS is divided into two divisions, the **sympathetic** and **parasympathetic** divisions. Usually, the effects of the two systems are **antagonistic:** one inhibits while the other stimulates the area. Sympathetic nerve fibers within the heart act to

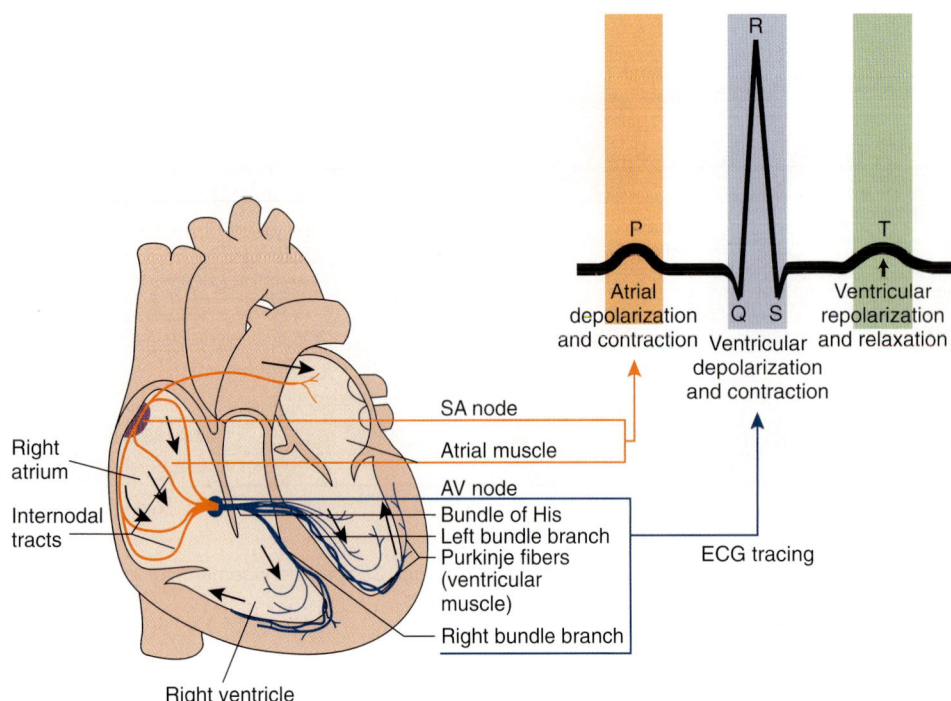

FIGURE 12-6 Conduction system in the heart and relationship to electrocardiogram. The events are indicated by letters: *P, Q, R, S,* and *T*. (From Gould B: *Pathophysiology for the health professions*, ed 4, St Louis, 2009, Saunders.)

accelerate or speed up the heart rate, whereas parasympathetic fibers, contained within branches of the vagus nerve, depress or slow down the heart rate.

Disorders of the conduction system include various **arrhythmias** (deviation from the normal heart rhythm), a **heart block** (occurs when an impulse is slowed or stopped at a certain point of the conduction process), and **flutter** (a rapid but regular heart contraction of the heart). For example:

> *Sinus bradycardia:* Heart rate less than 60 beats per minute.
> *Sinus tachycardia:* Heart rate between 100 and 160 beats per minute.
> *Atrial flutter:* Atrial arrhythmia that discharges impulses at 260 to 400 beats per minute.
> *First-degree atrioventricular block:* Block in which every impulse from the SA node is conducted to the ventricles.

Blood Supply

In order for the heart and the body to function, there must be a constant blood supply. Subsystems of the circulatory system are the pulmonary, coronary, and systemic circulations.

Pulmonary Circulation

Pulmonary circulation moves blood from the heart to the lungs and returns it to the heart again (Figure 12-7). The right side of the heart contains **deoxygenated blood** to be sent to the lungs for oxygenation (the pulmonary circuit). The left side of the heart contains oxygenated blood collected from the lungs to be supplied to the entire body (systemic circulation).

- *Right atrium:* Oxygen-deficient blood from the limbs, trunk, and brain enters the right atrium through two large veins, the superior and inferior venae cavae. The contraction of the right atrium forces the blood into the right ventricle through the tricuspid valve.
- *Right ventricle:* The right ventricle fills with blood, which is forced out by the contraction of the ventricle. The tricuspid valve closes and opens the pulmonary semilunar valve into the pulmonary artery. Blood is then pumped into both lungs.
- *Lungs:* The oxygen-deficient blood flows through the arteries and arterioles, finally reaching the lung capillaries. Here, the blood takes in needed oxygen that was inhaled and discards **carbon dioxide (CO_2)** to be exhaled. The oxygenated blood leaves the capillaries, moves through the venules, and flows back toward the left atrium of the heart in the pulmonary veins.

Systemic Circulation

Systemic circulation is the movement of oxygenated blood through the heart and back out to body tissues.
- *Left atrium:* Blood with high oxygen content enters the left atrium and is pumped to the left ventricle through the mitral valve, also called the bicuspid valve.
- *Left ventricle:* As the left ventricle fills, it contracts and pumps blood out through the largest artery in the body, the aorta. This closes the mitral valve and opens the aortic semilunar valve. The eventual backflow of blood against the valve closes the aortic valve.
- *Aorta:* The aorta distributes oxygen-rich blood to arteries and capillaries throughout the body. The aorta first moves up (ascending aorta), then arches back and continues down (descending aorta) the body in front of the spinal column.

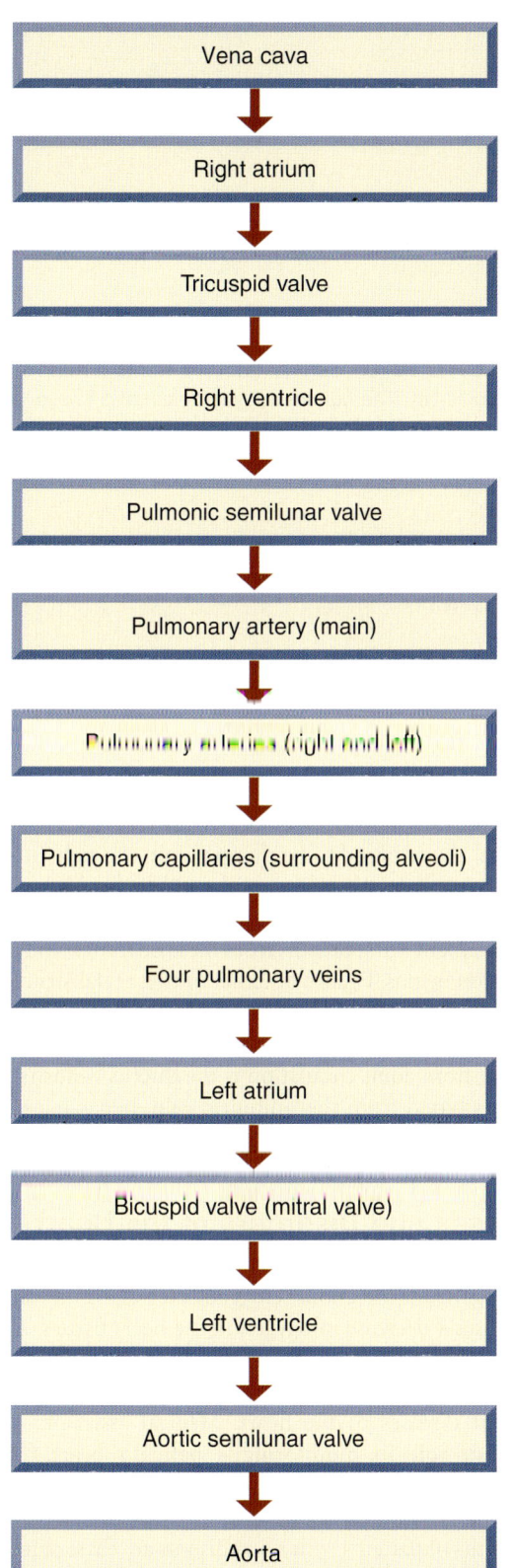

FIGURE 12-7 Blood flow through the heart and pulmonary circulation. (Modified from Herlihy B, Maebius NK: *The human body in health and illness,* ed 3, St Louis, 2007, Saunders.)

The aorta has several branches of arteries that carry blood to all body tissues (Figure 12-8).

Both ventricles contract at the same time, allowing the right atrium to fill with oxygen-poor blood and the left atrium to fill with oxygen-rich blood. When this cycle is complete, it begins again. In systemic circulation, blood flows into the arteries, through arterioles, and to the capillaries, which deliver oxygen and nutrients to the cells and collect CO_2 and cell waste. The deoxygenated blood moves through the venules, to the veins, and then back to the heart. In pulmonary circulation, deoxygenated blood flows through the arteries to the capillaries to give off CO_2 and picks up oxygen to be sent to the left atrium by the pulmonary veins.

Coronary Circulation

As briefly described in the section on heart valves, **coronary circulation** is the circulation of blood through the heart. Let us pick up where we left off, in the aorta, and see how the heart receives its blood supply.

- *Aorta:* Oxygen-rich blood leaves the left ventricle through the aorta. As the aorta leaves the heart, it first branches into the right and left **coronary arteries.**
- *Coronary arteries:* These arteries originate behind two of the three leaflets of the aortic semilunar valve and supply the heart muscle with blood rich in oxygen and other nutrients. Remember that although the blood is in the chambers of the heart, it only supplies a small amount of nourishment to the endocardium. The coronary arteries feed the myocardium and other heart layers. If a coronary artery or its branches become blocked, the heart muscle is deprived of oxygen (**ischemia**), causing death of tissue (**infarction**).

The left coronary artery further branches off to supply blood to the anterior portion of the right and left ventricles (left **anterior descending artery**) and to the left atrium and left ventricle (**circumflex artery**) (Figure 12-9).

The right coronary artery also branches off to form the **posterior descending artery,** which nourishes the left and right ventricles, and the **marginal artery,** which supplies the right atrium and the right ventricle.

Coronary artery blockages are causes of myocardial infarction (MI; heart attack) and are the sites of coronary bypass surgery, angioplasty, and stent placement to keep these arteries open.

BRAIN AND HEPATIC PORTAL CIRCULATION

Although the pulmonic and systemic circulations are the main areas of the circulatory system, there are others that contribute a needed blood supply to vital organs. The first is the blood supply to the brain through two pairs of arteries, carotid arteries and vertebral arteries. The right common carotid artery branches from the brachiocephalic artery and the left common carotid artery stems from the aortic arch. These arteries **bifurcate** (split into two branches) and become the internal and external carotid arteries. The **external carotid arteries** provide

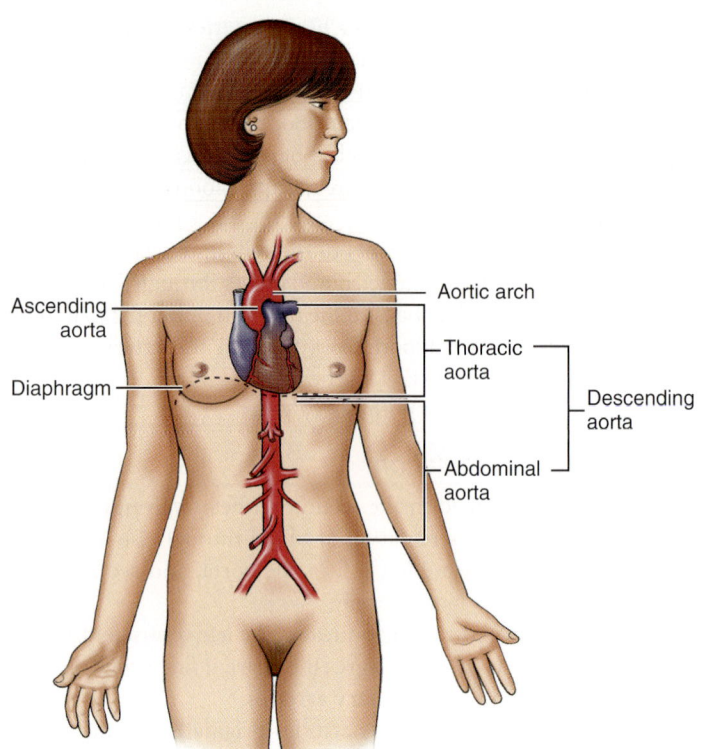

FIGURE 12-8 Segments of the aorta. (From Herlihy B, Maebius NK: *The human body in health and illness,* ed 3, St Louis, 2007, Saunders.)

a blood supply to the neck, face, and scalp, whereas the **internal carotid arteries** supply blood to the base of the brain and networks within various parts of the brain. The **vertebral arteries** arise from the subclavian arteries and move toward the brain. They join together within the brain to form the basilar artery that supplies blood to the brainstem and cerebellum. Branches of these arteries connect (**anastomose**) to form a circle of arteries referred to as the **circle of Willis**. This anastomosis provides a detour for arterial blood if an obstruction occurs, whereas the blood supply to the heart has no alternative route.

The hepatic portal circulation refers to the route of blood flow through the liver. It is comprised of the portal vein, hepatic veins, and the hepatic artery. This type of circulation carries blood rich in nutrients from the digestive organs to the liver where they are needed for metabolism.

The **portal vein** carries blood from the digestive organs (e.g., stomach, pancreas, intestines, and gallbladder) to the liver. The hepatic artery carries blood rich in oxygen to the liver, and the hepatic veins remove blood from the liver and transport it to the inferior vena cava. The hepatic portal system removes excess glucose and stores it as glycogen until needed and removes/detoxifies substances, such as alcohol and drugs, before they enter the rest of the system.

Fetal Circulation

Coronary circulation is different in the fetus. The fetal heart receives its oxygen from the placenta. Only a minute amount of blood enters the lungs of a fetus to nourish the lungs' cell tissue. When this occurs, an opening called the **ductus arteriosus** connects the pulmonary artery with the aorta. The **foramen ovale,** an opening located in the septum between the atria, allows blood to be pumped into the right atrium to the left atrium to the left ventricle and to the body without passing through the lungs that are not yet functioning. At birth, an infant's first breath closes these openings, and normal circulation begins. Failure of either of these fetal structures to close appear as a congenital heart defect and surgical intervention is necessary. The final feature of fetal circulation that is different from adult circulation is the **ductus venosus,** which conducts blood from the umbilical vein, bypassing the liver to the inferior vena cava.

Diseases and Disorders of the Heart

Heart disease can occur at birth (congenital) or can develop at any age from infections, clogged arteries, or any situation that causes a decrease in oxygen to the heart tissues. A **cardiologist,** a specialist who treats diseases of the heart, or an **internist,** a physician who specializes in internal medicine, can treat diseases of the heart. Medical assistants play an important role in monitoring a patient's heart function. Taking a health history and performing a physical assessment are key factors in diagnosing cardiovascular disease. Common complaints of patients with heart disease are chest pain, shortness of breath, increased pulse, heart palpitations, and intolerance to exercise.

Box 12-1 describes common signs and symptoms of heart disease, and Box 12-2 defines diagnostic tests and procedures for heart disease. Table 12-1 provides a cardiac drug classification, and Table 12-2 describes disorders of the heart.

Text continued on p. 211

BOX 12-1
Common Signs and Symptoms of Heart Disease

Angina pectoris	Condition characterized by short attacks of substernal pain that radiates to the left shoulder and arm; provoked by exertion and relieved by rest
Asystole	Cardiac standstill; absence of heartbeat
Bradycardia	Slow heart rate (less than 60 beats/min)
Claudication	Pain and weakness in the legs when walking because of inadequate blood supply; subsides with rest
Hypertension	Blood pressure greater than 140/90 mm Hg; considered a warning of more serious disease
Palpitation	Skipping or racing heartbeat felt by the patient
Prehypertension	Blood pressure between 120/80 and 140/90 mm Hg
Tachycardia	Rapid heart rate (more than 100 beats/min)

BOX 12-2
Diagnostic Tests and Procedures for the Heart

Arteriography, angiography	X-ray of the arteries after injection of radiopaque dye
Cardiac catheterization*	Procedure that visualizes heart activity and measures pressure within the heart chambers using catheterization of the heart
Echocardiography	Use of ultrasonic waves directed through the heart to obtain a visual picture of the heart structure while in motion (Figure 12-10)
Electrocardiography (ECG)	Tracing of the electrical activity of the heart
Holter monitor	Portable electrocardiograph that is worn for 24 hours to record a person's heart activity during normal daily activities
Stress testing	Test that measures heart activity under controlled physical activity (usually while walking on a treadmill)
Venography	X-ray of veins after injection of radiopaque dye

*A type of angiography.

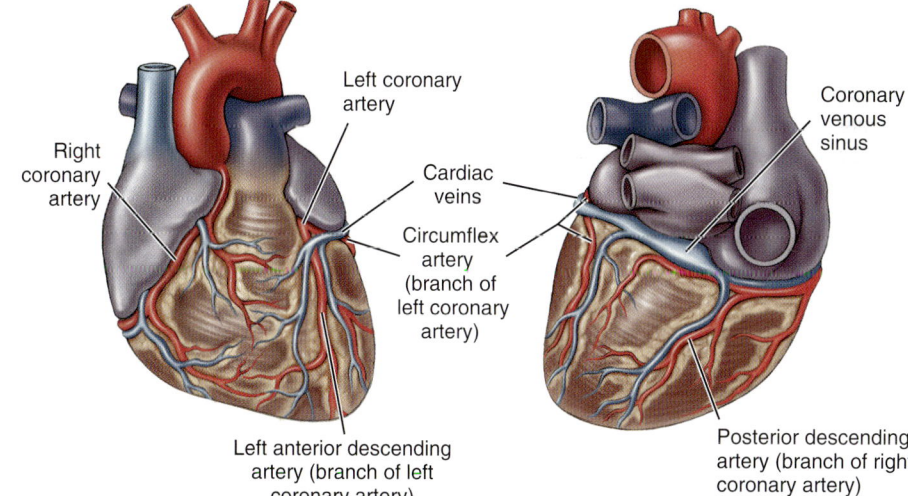

FIGURE 12-9 Blood supply to the myocardium through the coronary blood vessels. (From Herlihy B, Maebius NK: *The human body in health and illness*, ed 3, St Louis, 2007, Saunders.)

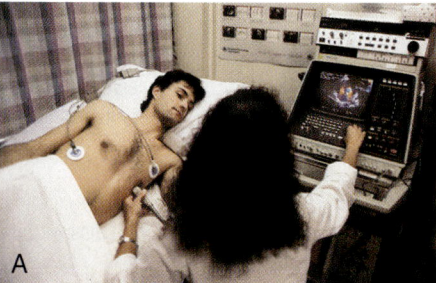 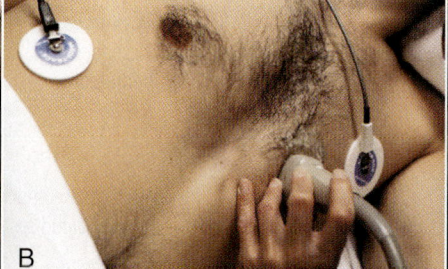 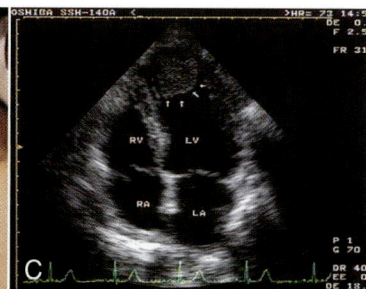

FIGURE 12-10 **A** and **B**, Echocardiography. **C**, Echocardiographic image showing a large apical thrombus. *RV*, Right ventricle; *LV*, left ventricle; *RA*, right atrium, *LA*, left atrium. (From Ballinger PW, Frank ED: *Merrill's atlas of radiographic positions and radiologic procedures*, ed 9, St Louis, 1999, Mosby.)

TABLE 12-1

Cardiac and Blood-Related Drug Classifications

Drug Classification	Common Generic (Brand) Names
Angiotensin-converting enzyme (ACE) inhibitors Relax blood vessels and improve cardiac output	captopril (Capoten) enalapril (Vasotec)
Antianginal drugs Relax blood vessels and reduce myocardial oxygen consumption	nitroglycerin (Nitrostat) isosorbide dinitrate (Isordil)
Antiarrhythmic drugs Strengthen heartbeat by improving heart muscle tone	procainamide (Pronestyl) disopyramide (Norpace)
Anticoagulants Prevent formation of blood clots	warfarin (Coumadin) heparin (Panheprin)
Beta blockers Lessen heart rate and increase the force of heart contractions	atenolol (Tenormin) metoprolol (Lopressor)
Calcium channel blockers Lessen myocardial oxygen demand by slowing the flow of calcium to smooth muscle cells	nifedipine (Procardia) diltiazem (Cardizem)

TABLE 12-2

Diseases and Disorders of the Heart

Disease and Description	Etiology	Signs and Symptoms	Diagnosis	Therapy	Interventions
DISORDERS OF HEART STRUCTURE					
Congenital Heart Disease Incomplete formations of heart structures during fetal development.					
Atrial septal defect (ASD) Abnormal opening that allows oxygenated blood from left atrium to flow into right atrium	Unknown: abnormal embryonic development; incomplete closure of foramen ovale	*Small defect:* fatigue, shortness of breath *Large defect:* **cyanosis,** dyspnea, **syncope**	Auscultation: murmur Chest x-ray ECG MRI	Surgical closure of opening	Emotional support for family
Patent ductus arteriosus Occurs after birth between the pulmonary artery and aorta	Failure of ductus arteriosus to close after birth	*Small defect:* asymptomatic *Large defect:* slow weight gain, dyspnea, decreased exercise tolerance	Auscultation: murmur Bounding pulse in lower extremities Chest x-ray	Surgical ligation of the ductus	Emotional support for family
Tetralogy of Fallot Includes four defects occurring at birth: 1. VSD 2. Pulmonary **stenosis** 3. Transposition of aorta to right 4. Hypertrophy of right ventricle	Unknown; abnormal embryonic development	Tachypnea, tachycardia, dyspnea, cyanosis, **hypoxia**	Auscultation: murmur Chest x-ray MRI ECG Polycythemia, increased hematocrit	Surgical interventions to repair the heart defects	Emotional support for family; provide family with necessary information to maintain child's health (e.g., nutrition, immunizations)
Coarctation of the aorta Narrowing of aorta causing a decrease in blood flow (Figure 12-11)	Unknown; possibly environmental or drug ingestion by mother	Pulmonary edema, pallor, cyanosis, dyspnea, tachycardia	Physical examination: x-rays, blood tests, cardiac catheterization	Surgical techniques to repair abnormality Prophylactic antibiotics	Encouragement to cope with disease process

TABLE 12-2

Diseases and Disorders of the Heart—cont'd

Disease and Description	Etiology	Signs and Symptoms	Diagnosis	Therapy	Interventions
INFLAMMATION OF THE HEART					
Bacterial endocarditis Acute (ABE) or subacute (SBE) disease of heart lining and valves (Figure 12-12)	Secondary infection	Fever, fatigue, heart murmurs, splenomegaly	Blood tests: CBC, ESR, cultures Echocardiogram	Antibiotic therapy, bedrest, nutritional support	Instructions on need for taking prescribed **prophylactic** (preventive) antibiotics before dental work or invasive procedures
Myocarditis Inflammation of myocardium (heart muscle)	Secondary infection or chronic drug or alcohol use	Palpitations, fatigue, dyspnea, fever, chest tenderness Blood work reveals increased WBC, ESR, and cardiac enzymes	Blood tests: CBC, ESR, cardiac enzymes Ventricular enlargement Chest x-ray Extreme cases require myocardial biopsy	Antibiotic therapy, bedrest, medications to stabilize arrhythmia	Encouragement to take medication; encourage proper nutrition to assist with tissue repair
Pericarditis Inflammation of the membranes covering the heart (pericardium)	Idiopathic or secondary infection	Fever, malaise, chest pain that increases with inspiration or heartbeat, dyspnea, tachycardia	Auscultation: grating sound Blood tests: CBC, ESR, cardiac enzymes, cultures Changes on ECG tracings	Antibiotic therapy Surgical drainage (pericardiocentesis) Medication to reduce fever, pain, and inflammation	Encouragement to follow through with medication regimen, rest, and proper nutrition
HEART MUSCLE DAMAGE					
Myocardial infarction Death of myocardial tissue caused by lack of oxygen (ischemia) to the tissue (Figure 12-13)	Coronary artery that supplies blood to the myocardium is blocked or occluded **(occlusion)**	Persistent and intense pain in left chest, shoulder, and jaw not related to exertion **Diaphoresis** (profuse sweating), pallor, hypotension, dyspnea, light-headedness	Patient history, ECG, and blood work: cardiac enzymes	Immediate hospitalization and treatment Stabilizing heart rhythm and minimizing damage to heart muscle	Call 911 for emergency help; keep patient calm, administer oxygen if ordered by a physician, and start CPR if necessary
VALVE DISORDERS					
Valvular Heart Disease May be congenital or caused by plaque. Figure 12-14 shows valves involved in heart disease.					
Mitral valve prolapse When valve flaps do not close properly (valvular insufficiency) (Figure 12-15)	Chordae tendineae may lengthen during contraction, causing valve not to close tightly	Patient may be asymptomatic (showing no symptoms); fatigue, fainting, and dyspnea have been reported	Auscultation: murmur Echocardiogram verifies nonclosure of valve ECG shows PVC	Depends on severity of symptoms; in severe cases, valve reconstruction or replacement is needed	Encourage patient to use antibiotics as prescribed by physician for dental or other invasive procedures
Stenosis Valve flaps harden, or scar tissue forms on flaps, keeping blood from flowing to the next chamber	Rheumatic fever or other group A beta-hemolytic streptococcus	Dyspnea and fatigue; cyanosis in extreme conditions	Cardiac murmur on auscultation and results of echocardiogram	Anticoagulants to prevent formation of thrombi Medications (e.g., diuretics) to reduce heart's workload	Patient teaching about foods low in sodium

Mitral stenosis is a common **sequela** of rheumatic fever
Tricuspid stenosis causes resistance from right atrium to right ventricle and leads to lung congestion

CBC, Complete blood count; *CPR*, cardiopulmonary resuscitation; *ECG*, electrocardiogram; *ESR*, erythrocyte sedimentation rate; *MRI*, magnetic resonance imaging; *PVC*, premature ventricular contraction; *VSD*, ventricular septal defect; *WBC*, white blood cell count.

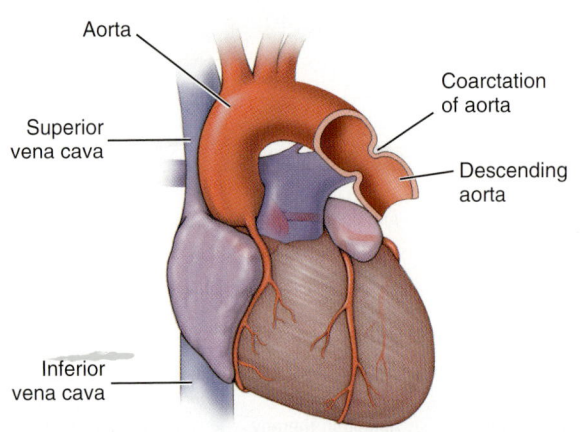

FIGURE 12-11 Coarctation of the aorta. (From Shiland BJ: *Mastering healthcare terminology,* ed 2, St Louis, 2006, Mosby.)

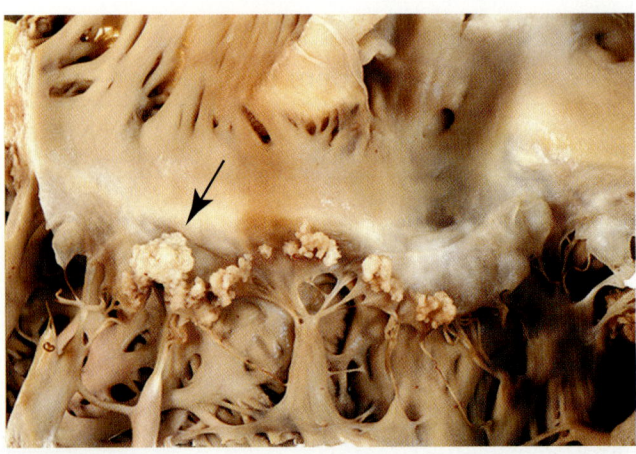

FIGURE 12-12 Acute bacterial endocarditis (ABE). Note how the heart valve is covered with large, irregular growths or vegetation *(arrow)*. (From Damjanov I, Linder J: *Anderson's pathology,* ed 10, St Louis, 1996, Mosby.)

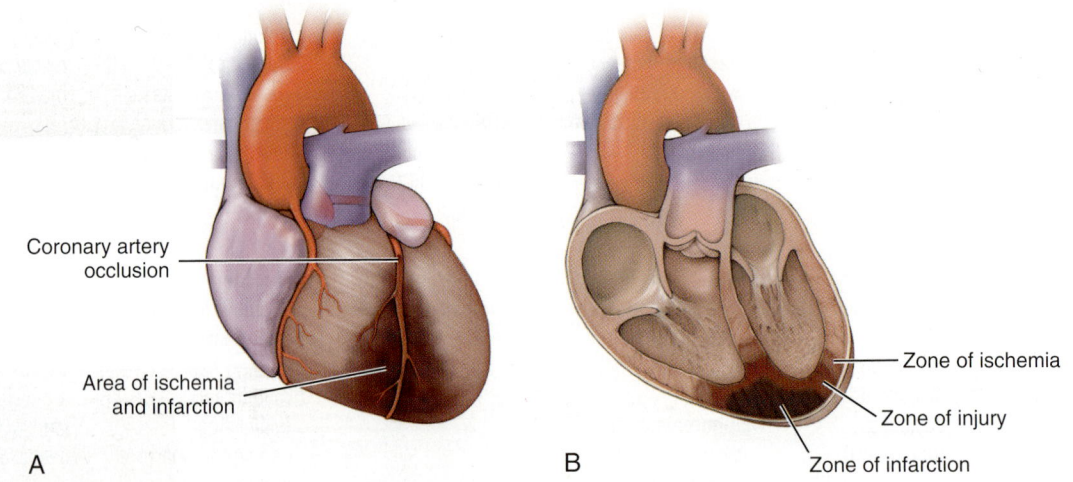

FIGURE 12-13 A, Ischemia and infarction produced by coronary artery occlusion. **B,** Myocardial infarction shown in a cross section of the heart (ventricles only).

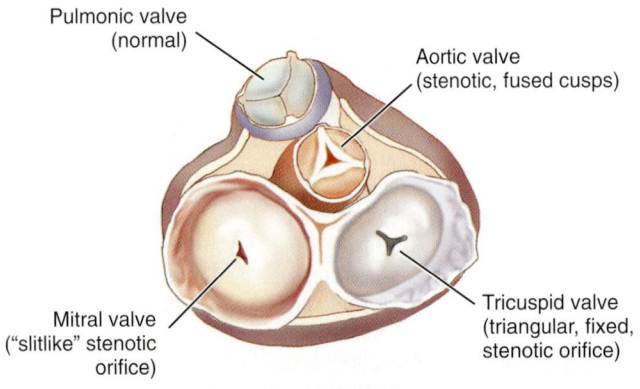

FIGURE 12-14 Valvular heart disease: disorders of aortic, mitral, and tricuspid valves. (From Shiland BJ: *Mastering healthcare terminology,* ed 2, St Louis, 2006, Mosby.)

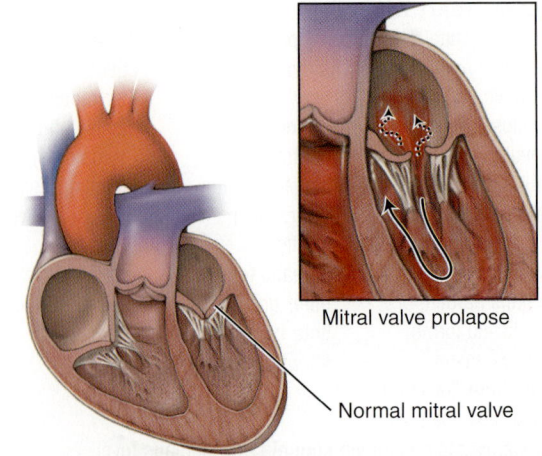

FIGURE 12-15 Mitral valve prolapse. (Modified from Shiland BJ: *Mastering healthcare terminology,* ed 2, St Louis, 2006, Mosby.)

PATIENT-CENTERED PROFESSIONALISM

- *How does understanding the structure and function of the heart's chambers and valves make it easier for the medical assistant to understand the heart's conduction system?*
- *How does understanding the structure and function of the heart help you to observe and report a patient's signs and symptoms? In what other ways does this knowledge help medical assistants provide better care to patients?*
- *How do pulmonary, coronary, and systemic circulations work together to provide a constant blood supply to all body parts?*

BLOOD VESSELS

You now know how blood and nutrients are circulated into, out of, and within the heart. Oxygenated blood from the lungs is circulated throughout the entire body, and deoxygenated blood is returned to the lungs (Figure 12-16). Blood and nutrients are also circulated throughout the entire body. **Blood vessels** are the elastic tubelike channels through which the blood circulates. The **diameter** of a blood vessel can increase in size (**vasodilate**) or decrease in size (**vasoconstrict**) in response to nerve stimulation and certain medications.

There are three types of blood vessels: arteries, veins, and capillaries (Figure 12-17). Knowing the normal structure and function of blood vessels can help you understand the disorders of these vessels.

Arteries

An **artery** is a *macroscopic* (large enough to be seen with the naked eye) blood vessel. Arteries take blood away from the heart, most of which is oxygenated. Exceptions to this are the pulmonary artery and the umbilical artery in the fetus, which carry deoxygenated blood. The artery must withstand the strong pressure caused by the contractions of the ventricles. Small arteries are called **arterioles**. Arterioles carry blood to the capillaries.

Table 12-3 lists the major arteries of the body and provides a comparison between pulse point and pressure point. Figure 12-18, *A*, shows the major arteries of the body.

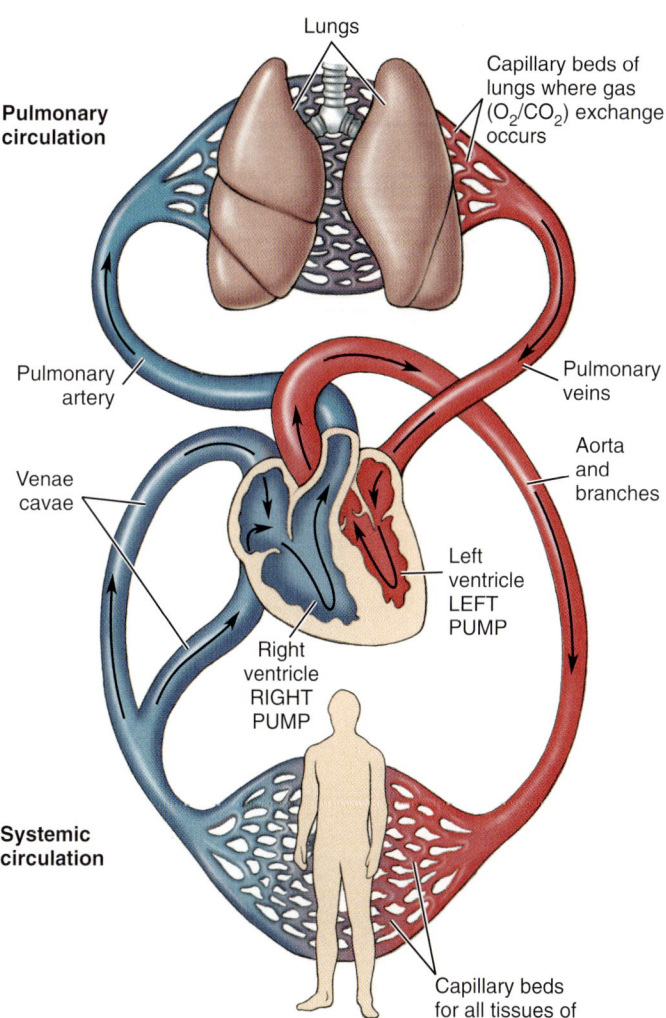

FIGURE 12-16 Pulmonary and systemic blood circulation. (From Herlihy B, Maebius NK: *The human body in health and illness,* ed 3, St Louis, 2007, Saunders.)

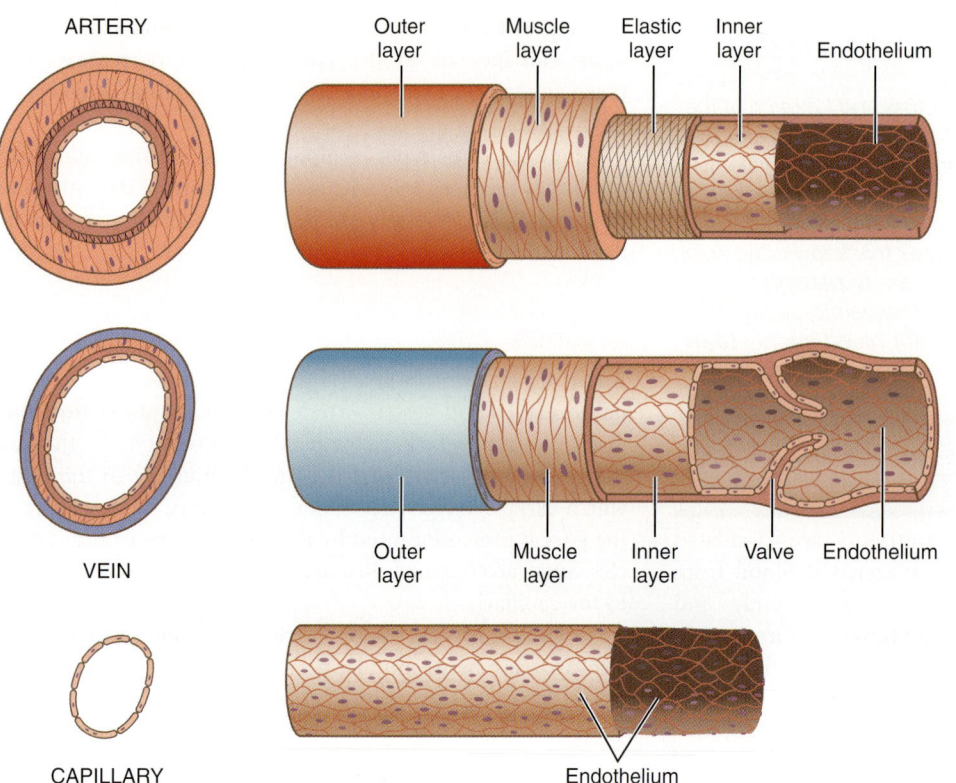

FIGURE 12-17 Blood vessels. Note the differences in the vessel walls among an artery, vein, and capillary. (Modified from Chabner DE: *The language of medicine,* ed 8, St Louis, 2007, Saunders.)

TABLE 12-3

Main Arteries of the Body

Artery	Location	Significance	Pulse Point	Pressure Point
Radial	Thumb side of wrist	Used to check pulse; supplies blood to lower arm	X	
Temporal	Front of ear	Used in an emergency to check for pulse; supplies blood to brain	X	X
Carotid	Each side of neck	Used to check adult pulse for CPR; supplies blood to head and neck	X	X
Aorta	After leaving the left ventricle, arches then bends over left lung, descends into thorax, and passes down trunk of the body	Main artery of the body		
Brachial	Inside of arm at bend of elbow	Used to check blood pressure and pulse in children for CPR; supplies blood to upper arm	X	X
Popliteal	Behind knee	Used to check for blood supply to lower leg; supplies blood to muscles of thigh, leg, and foot	X	
Dorsalis pedis	Upper surface of foot	Used to check for blood supply to lower extremities; supplies blood to muscles of foot and toes	X	
Subclavian	Behind collarbone	Supplies blood to vertebral column, spinal cord, ear, and brain		X
Femoral	Upper groin area	Pulse site; major artery of thigh	X	X

CPR, Cardiopulmonary resuscitation.

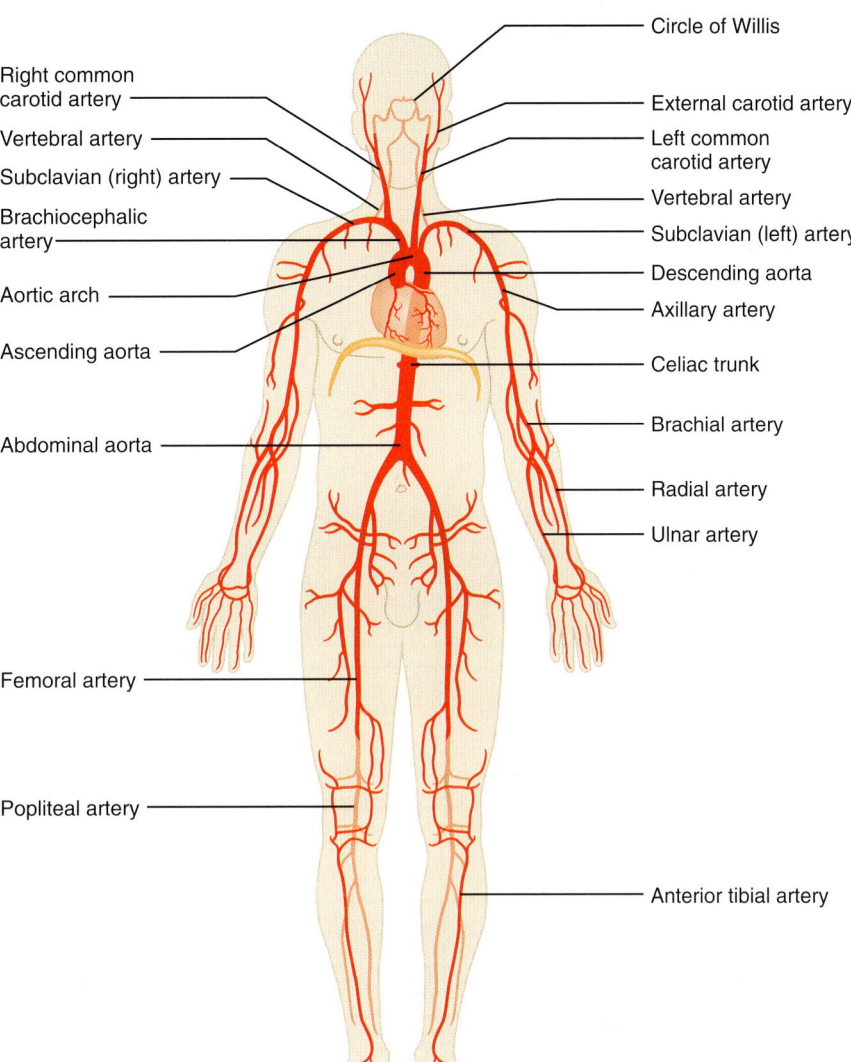

FIGURE 12-18 A, Arteries of the body.

FOR YOUR INFORMATION

As a person ages the heart muscle works harder to pump the same amount of blood throughout the body. Blood vessels become less elastic (arteriosclerosis) and hardened fatty deposits may have formed on the walls of the arteries (atherosclerosis), thus narrowing (stenosing) the passageway through the blood vessels. The loss of elasticity and the formation of fatty deposits make the arteries stiffer, therefore causing the heart to work harder to pump blood through them. The end result is high blood pressure (hypertension).

Veins

A **vein** is also a macroscopic blood vessel. However, a vein carries blood toward the heart, most of which is deoxygenated, and has less pressure than an artery. Exceptions to this are the pulmonary vein and the umbilical vein, which carry oxygenated blood. Small veins are **venules.** Venules take blood from the capillaries to the veins. Figure 12-18, *B,* shows the major veins of the body.

Veins are thinner and less elastic than arteries, so they give way under pressure. Blood moves through veins because of muscular action. Veins have one-way valves that force blood to flow forward. When a valve is damaged, the blood pools in that area, and the vein becomes twisted and swollen (**varix,** plural **varices**), resulting in a *varicose vein* (Figure 12-19).

PATIENT-CENTERED PROFESSIONALISM

- Why is it important for the medical assistant to know both the pulse sites and the pressure points of major arteries?
- What is the benefit to patients when medical assistants have a solid understanding of the structure and function of the blood vessels?

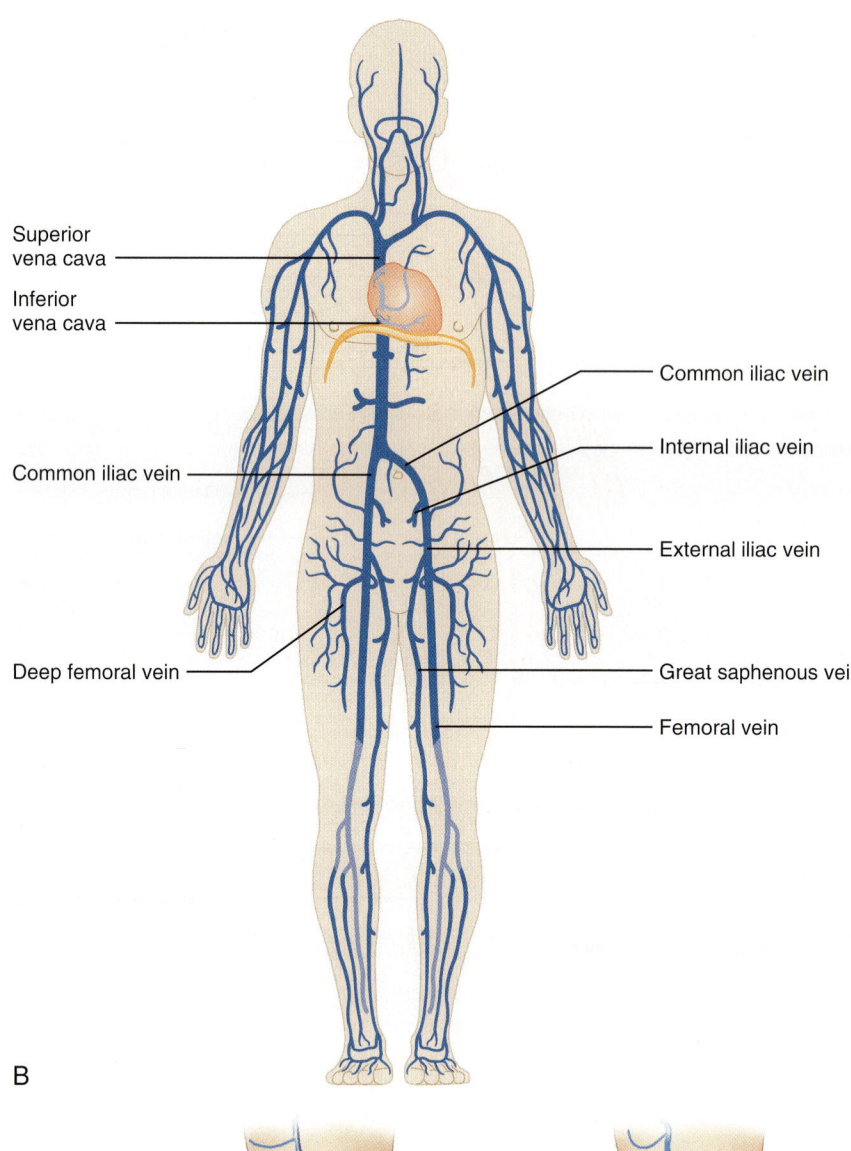

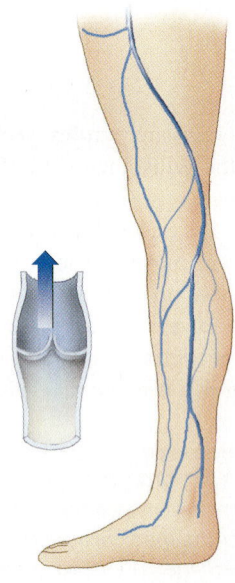
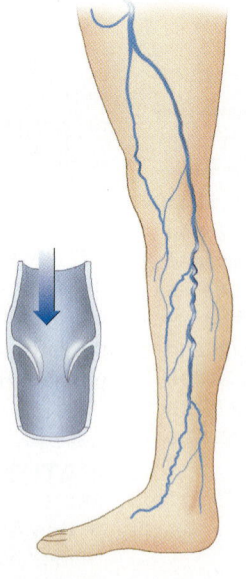
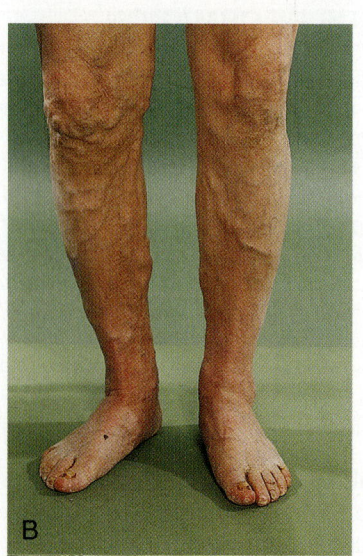

FIGURE 12-18, cont'd **B,** Veins of the body. (Modified from Buck CJ: *Step-by-step medical coding, 2008 edition*, St Louis, 2008, Saunders.)

A Normal Veins — Functional valves aid in flow of venous blood back to heart

Varicose Veins — Failure of valves and pooling of blood in superficial veins

B

FIGURE 12-19 **A,** Normal veins versus varicose veins. **B,** Varicose veins. (**A** modified from Leonard PC: *Building a medical vocabulary,* ed 6, Philadelphia, 2005, Saunders; **B** from *Mosby's dictionary of medicine, nursing and health professions*, ed 7, St Louis, 2006, Mosby.)

Capillaries

A **capillary** is a *microscopic* (too small to be seen with the naked eye) connecting blood vessel that carries blood from arterioles to venules. Capillaries are found in every body tissue. Body tissues are nourished with oxygen and nutrients as blood passes through the capillaries. Waste products, gases, and water leave cells and enter the capillaries and are returned in blood back toward the heart through the venules.

Disorders of Blood Vessels

Disorders of the blood vessels occur when the vessels do not function properly (Table 12-4).

CONCLUSION

The circulatory (cardiovascular) system is responsible for moving blood and lymph throughout the body. The heart follows a systematic pattern. If the conduction system is "firing" correctly, the heart contracts and blood is pumped to the body tissues. If a valve is not functioning correctly, however, all of the blood does not reach the body tissues. For good health, the heart must be structurally sound and be able to function at maximum capacity. If the lungs are diseased, the efficiency of the heart is affected, proving again that one system is dependent on another.

TABLE 12-4
Disorders of Blood Vessels

Disease and Description	Etiology	Signs and Symptoms	Diagnosis	Therapy	Interventions
ANEURYSM "Bulging out" **(dilation)** of a blood vessel caused by weakness of the wall (Figure 12-20)	Often congenital Episodes of inflammation or plaque buildup in a vessel can produce a weakness in the vessel wall	*Insidious* (without symptoms) or sudden onset Symptoms depend on location and size; as the wall increases in size, back or abdominal pain may be present Cerebral **aneurysm** may rupture, or headache may develop	Often found during routine physical exam, abdominal palpation, or x-ray studies for another disease	Surgical intervention to repair vessel	Potentially life-threatening emergency
CONGESTIVE HEART FAILURE Occurs when the heart muscle is unable to pump blood efficiently, causing the heart to enlarge and the lungs to fill with blood	Causes include coronary artery disease, chronic hypertension, valve disorders, heart attack, and congenital defects	Pulmonary edema, shortness of breath, dyspnea on exertion, dry cough, restlessness, tachycardia	Patient history, swelling of extremities, chest x-ray (enlarged heart), ECG, increased heart rate, distended neck veins	Medications (diuretics, cardiotonics), diet low in sodium, fluid restrictions	Encourage rest, decreased fluids, and frequent, small meals
ATHEROSCLEROSIS Progressive thickening of inner walls of arteries caused by breakdown of endothelium; replaced by soft fatty material in vessel, leading to occlusion Reduces blood supply to tissues	Buildup of fatty plaque caused by heredity, diet high in cholesterol-producing foods, and smoking	Vertigo (dizziness), hypertension, and dyspnea are common	Screening tests: cholesterol, triglyceride, and lipid levels Hypertension Decreased blood flow	Dietary restriction of saturated fats and foods high in cholesterol Smoking prohibited (causes blood vessels to **constrict**)	Instructions for a low-fat diet; encouragement of daily exercise; stopping tobacco smoking

TABLE 12-4
Disorders of Blood Vessels—cont'd

Disease and Description	Etiology	Signs and Symptoms	Diagnosis	Therapy	Interventions
ARTERIOSCLEROSIS Hardening of the arteries; arteries become brittle as a result of atrophy of muscular and elastic tissues	Accumulation of lipids caused by diet high in cholesterol; faulty carbohydrate metabolism; genetic factors	Intermittent **claudication,** skin temperature cool, bluish discoloration to extremities	Arteriogram, elevation in blood pressure	Exercise, vasodilators, treatment for skin infections	Encourage patient to follow diet low in fat and cholesterol, to exercise, and to rest
RAYNAUD DISEASE Brought on by temporary constriction of arterioles in the skin	Idiopathic; cold or stress	Pain and numbness in fingers, hands, or feet	History of numbness and paleness of area	Minimizing exposure to cold, vasodilators, application of warmth	Restricting tobacco smoking; avoiding stress
PHLEBITIS Inflammation of walls of a vein *Thrombophlebitis:* Clot forms in a vein secondary to **phlebitis** (Figure 12-21) *DVT:* Thrombosis of a deep, rather than a superficial, vein	Infections and trauma to an area; could be idiopathic but may occur after an injury	Pain and tenderness in affected area Swelling, redness, and warmth over area	History of events leading up to symptoms; venography	Analgesics, bedrest, and anticoagulants with use of support stockings	Instruct patient about no massaging of affected areas (may lead to release of a clot, or **thrombus**)
EMBOLUS Clot that travels	**Embolus** breaks off from a thrombus lodged in a blood vessel Emboli can also be composed of air, fat, or tissue	Severe pain in area of emboli; if a major artery is blocked to an extremity, the area becomes numb, pale, and cool to the touch	Pain in the area, especially calf of the leg Dyspnea, arrhythmias	Must be immediate to prevent the loss of life or tissue Anticoagulant therapy with possible surgical intervention	Bedrest
VARICOSE VEINS Abnormal occurrence of swollen and twisted veins of the legs and anus (hemorrhoids)	Valves in veins are defective; caused by prolonged standing or sitting	Legs: fatigue, pain, cramps; swelling of ankles Anus: rectal bleeding, possible protrusion from anus	Clinical inspection, history of prolonged sitting or standing	Wearing of elastic support hosiery Elevation of legs when edema occurs Removal of twisted veins (vein stripping) Use of astringents and warm soaks for hemorrhoids	Legs: patient teaching if job requires standing or sitting for long periods; moving around to improve circulation Anus: eating diet high in fiber; increasing fluid intake; using stool softeners

DVT, Deep vein thrombosis; *ECG,* electrocardiogram.

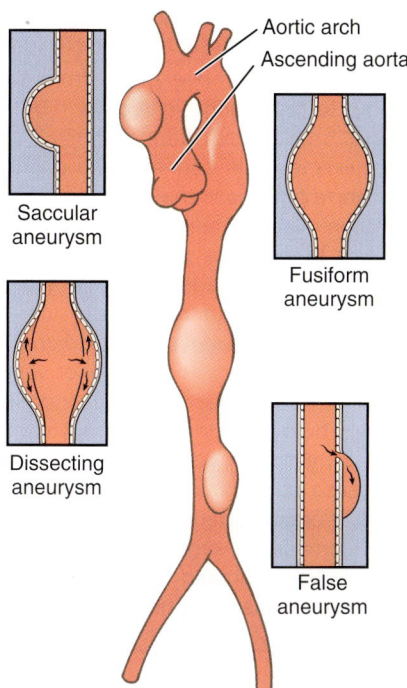

FIGURE 12-20 Types of aortic aneurysm. (Modified from Frazier MS, Drzymkowski JW: *Essentials of human diseases and conditions,* ed 4, St Louis, 2009, Saunders.)

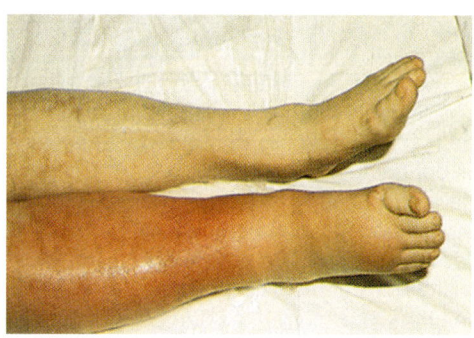

FIGURE 12-21 Thrombophlebitis. (From Lewis SM: *Medical-surgical nursing: assessment and management of clinical problems,* ed 5, St Louis, 2000, Mosby.)

Chapter Summary

Reinforce your understanding of the material in this chapter by reviewing the curriculum objectives and key content points below.

1. **Define, appropriately use, and spell all the Key Terms for this chapter.**
   - Review the Key Terms if necessary.
2. **Name the components of the cardiovascular system.**
   - The heart pumps the blood through blood vessels throughout the body to deliver oxygen to all body parts and to remove wastes.
   - The blood also carries hormones to target organs and removes excess fluids from the body.
3. **Identify the four cardiac chambers and describe the function of each.**
   - Two atria and two ventricles make up the heart.
   - The atria hold blood while the ventricles pump blood out of the heart to the lungs and body tissue.
4. **Locate the four cardiac valves of the heart and describe the function of each.**
   - The tricuspid valve is located between the right atrium and the right ventricle.
   - The pulmonary semilunar valve is located in the right ventricle allowing blood to move to the lungs.
   - The mitral (bicuspid) valve is located between the left atrium and left ventricle.
   - The aortic semilunar valve is located in the left ventricle allowing blood to move to the body.
   - Cardiac valves prevent regurgitation of blood to the atria when the ventricles contract or back into the ventricles after exiting to the lungs or body.
   - The valves open and close to regulate direction of blood flow.
5. **List the sequence of actions that takes place in the conduction system.**
   - The cardiac cycle begins with an electrical impulse in the sinoatrial (SA) node, travels to the atrioventricular (AV) node, to the bundle of His, and ends at the Purkinje fibers.
   - The conduction system generates the heartbeat sound.
   - Electrocardiograms (ECGs) record the electrical impulses of the complete cardiac cycle.
6. **Explain the importance of being able to recognize normal heart sounds.**
   - Valve malfunctions, for example, can often be identified by hearing an abnormal heartbeat.
7. **Identify the two divisions of the autonomic nervous system (ANS) that are responsible for modulating nerve conduction within the heart.**
   - The sympathetic nerve fibers within the heart act to speed up the heart rate.
   - The parasympathetic nerve fibers slow down the heart rate.
   - The effects of the two systems are antagonistic to one another.

8. **Trace the circulation of the blood from the heart to the lungs.**
   - The right atrium contracts and forces blood into the right ventricle through the tricuspid valve.
   - The right ventricle fills with blood that is forced out by the contraction of the ventricle.
   - The tricuspid valve closes, and the pulmonary semilunar valve opens into the pulmonary artery.
   - Blood is pumped into both lungs.
9. **Trace the circulation of blood to the heart (coronary circulation).**
   - Blood leaves the heart through the aorta and branches off into the right and left coronary arteries.
   - The left coronary artery supplies blood to the anterior portion of the heart, and the right coronary artery supplies blood to the posterior portion of the heart.
   - Coronary arteries supply the heart muscle with oxygen and nutrients.
10. **Trace the movement of oxygenated blood through the heart and back out to the body tissues.**
    - Blood with high oxygen content enters the left atrium from the lungs.
    - Blood is pumped to the left ventricle when the left atrium contracts.
    - Blood is pumped from the left ventricle to the aorta and out to the body tissues.
11. **Trace the oxygenated blood supply to the brain.**
    - Blood circulates to the brain through the carotid and vertebral arteries.
    - The right common carotid artery branches from the brachiocephalic artery and the left carotid artery stems from the aortic arch.
    - These arteries split into branches and become the internal and external carotid arteries.
    - The external carotid arteries supply the neck, face, and scalp.
    - The internal carotid arteries supply blood to the base of the brain and various parts of the brain.
    - The vertebral arteries arise from the subclavian arteries and move toward the brain to form the basilar artery.
    - The basilar artery supplies blood to the brainstem and cerebellum and connects to form the circle of Willis.
12. **Discuss the function of the hepatic portal system.**
    - The function of the hepatic portal system is to carry blood rich in nutrients from the digestive organs to the liver and remove the excess glucose from the blood and store it in the liver as glycogen until needed.
    - The portal vein carries blood from the digestive organs to the liver.
    - The hepatic artery carries blood rich in oxygen to the liver.
    - The hepatic veins remove blood from the liver and transport it to the inferior vena cava.
13. **Explain fetal heart circulation.**
    - The ductus arteriosus connects the pulmonary artery with the aorta to bypass the lungs.
    - The foramen ovale, located in the septum between the atria, allows blood to be pumped into the right atrium to the left atrium to the left ventricle and to the body without passing through the lungs.
    - The ductus venosus conducts blood from the umbilical vein, bypassing the liver to the inferior vena cava.
14. **List seven forms of heart disease and describe the risk factors, etiology, signs and symptoms, diagnosis, therapy, and interventions for each.**
    - Heart disease can occur at birth or at any age from infections, clogged arteries, and other situations that cause a decrease in oxygen to the heart tissues.
    - Medical assistants should be familiar with the symptoms of heart disease and heart attack.
    - Refer to Table 12-2.

Blood Vessels

15. **List three types of blood vessels and describe the function of each.**
    - Arteries carry oxygenated blood away from the heart.
    - Veins carry deoxygenated blood toward the heart.
    - Capillaries connect blood from the arterioles to the venules, allowing nourishment, removal of wastes, and gas exchange at the cell level.
16. **List eight disorders of the blood vessels and describe the etiology, signs and symptoms, diagnosis, therapy, and interventions for each.**
    - Refer to Table 12-4.
17. **Analyze a realistic medical office situation and apply your understanding of the cardiovascular system to determine the best course of action.**
    - Understanding the normal physiology of the cardiovascular system will help you understand how a disease process affects this system.
18. **Describe the impact on patient care when medical assistants have a solid understanding of the structure and function of the heart and blood vessels.**
    - Medical assistants who understand the structure and function of the heart and blood vessels will be better prepared to assist with medical procedures, communicate clearly to patients, and perform effective patient teaching.

PRACTICAL APPLICATIONS

If you have accomplished the objectives in this chapter, you will be able to make better choices as a medical assistant. Take another look at this situation and decide what you would do.

Dr. Kim Kea will examine Mr. Stan Baleaut later today as a routine follow-up for high blood pressure and possible coronary artery disease. Mr. Baleaut tells Erin, the medical assistant, that he has some left arm pain and also has been having some heart palpitations and wants Dr. Kea to check this. As Erin takes Mr. Baleaut's blood pressure, she obtains a reading of 150/88 mm Hg and a pulse rate of 92 beats/min. Dr. Kea examines Mr. Baleaut and orders a stat ECG as a way of ruling out a diagnosis of MI. As Erin is completing the ECG, Mr. Baleaut has several questions about vital signs and ECGs. Erin needs to educate him in several areas.

Mr. Baleaut wants to know the following:
1. What causes systolic blood pressure and diastolic pressure, and what is happening when each pressure is measured?
2. What is the pulse rate measuring?
3. What is the route of the conduction system through the heart?
4. Why was the Holter monitor Mr. Baleaut has worn in the past necessary when he had an ECG?
5. What is a myocardial infarction, and what symptoms does Mr. Baleaut need to know?
6. What is congestive heart failure, and what symptoms does Mr. Baleaut need to know?

WEB SEARCH

1. **Research the various forms of heart disease, including current diagnostic tests and treatments for each.** Heart disease is classified by abnormal heart structures during fetal development, inflammation of the heart muscles and blood vessels, damage caused by faulty valves, and diseased heart muscle tissue. To better understand the diagnosis and treatment of heart disease, a medical assistant needs to be aware of current diagnostic tests and current treatments.
   - **Keywords:** Use the following keywords in your search: American Heart Association, heart disease, heart attack, cardiology.

WORD PARTS: Circulatory System

HEART
Combining Forms

mediastin/o	mediastinum
ox/o	oxygen
thorac/o	chest
cardi/o	heart
endocardi/o	endocardium
myocardi/o	myocardium
pericardi/o	pericardium
atri/o	atrium
sept/o	septum; partition; divider
ventricul/o	ventricle; cavity
pulmon/o	lung
valv/o, valvul/o	valve
aort/o	aorta

Prefixes

epi-	above, on
peri-	around
tri-	three

Suffix

-ium	membrane

BLOOD VESSELS
Combining Forms

angi/o	vessel (usually blood)
arter, arteri/o	artery
arteriol/o	arteriole
phleb/o	vein
vas/o, vascul/o	vessel
varic/o	varicose vein

Prefix

de-	down; reversing

Suffixes

-ole	small
-ule	small

CIRCULATION, BLOOD SUPPLY, AND CONDUCTION SYSTEM
Combining Forms

coron/o	crown
scop/o	to examine; to view
steth/o	chest

Suffixes

-capnia	carbon dioxide
-scope	instrument used for viewing or listening

ABBREVIATIONS: Cardiovascular System

AED	automatic external defibrillator
ASD	atrial septal defect
AV	atrioventricular
CAD	coronary artery disease
CHF	congestive heart failure
DVT	deep vein thrombosis
ECG/EKG	electrocardiography
ECHO	echocardiography
HTN	hypertension
MI	myocardial infarction
MR	mitral regurgitation
MVP	mitral valve prolapse
NSR	normal sinus rhythm
PAC	premature atrial contraction
PVC	premature ventricular contraction
SA	sinoatrial

Blood, Lymphatic, and Immune Systems

13

evolve http://evolve.elsevier.com/klieger/medicalassisting

In Chapter 12, you were able to trace the movement of blood through the heart, to the lungs, and out to the other body systems through a network of blood vessels that work together to sustain life. By understanding the function and composition of blood, you will begin to recognize what a complex transport medium blood is and how it performs vital pickup and delivery services for the body. In addition, this chapter introduces two other systems: the lymphatic system and the immune system. These two systems are not typically considered "body systems" because their functions are carried out by specific cells, tissues, and organs within the circulatory system. Their most important functions are to maintain fluid balance and immunity. Therefore they play an important role in sustaining human life.

LEARNING OBJECTIVES

You will be able to do the following after completing this chapter:

Key Terms

1. Define, appropriately use, and spell all the Key Terms for this chapter.

Blood

2. List the eight components of blood plasma.
3. List three types of blood cells and describe the function of each.
4. List the four blood types and explain the importance of compatibility.
5. Explain the importance of Rh factor as it relates to pregnancy and transfusions.
6. List nine diseases of the blood and describe the etiology, signs and symptoms, diagnosis, therapy, and interventions for each.

Lymphatic System

7. List the four divisions of the lymphatic system and describe the function of each.
8. List four diseases of the lymphatic system and describe the etiology, signs and symptoms, diagnosis, therapy, and interventions for each.

Immune System

9. List the immune system's three lines of defense and describe each.

10. Distinguish between *natural* (inborn) immunity and *acquired* immunity and give an example of each.
11. List three diseases of the immune system and describe the etiology, signs and symptoms, diagnosis, therapy, and interventions for each.
12. Describe the considerations associated with the testing of AIDS patients.

Patient-Centered Professionalism

13. Analyze a realistic medical office situation and apply your understanding of the blood and lymphatic system to determine the best course of action.
14. Describe the impact on patient care when medical assistants have a solid understanding of the structure and function of the blood, lymphatic, and immune systems.

KEY TERMS

The Key Terms for this chapter have been organized into sections so that you can easily see the terminology associated with each aspect of the blood, lymphatic, and immune systems.

Blood

antibodies
erythrocytes
formed elements
hematopoiesis
hemolysis

leukocytes
plasma
stem cell
thrombocytes

Continued

Erythrocytes
biconcave
erythropoiesis
erythropoietin
hemoglobin
macrophages
metabolism
red blood cells (RBCs)
reticulocyte

Leukocytes
agranulocytes
basophils
differential count
eosinophils
granulocytes
leukocytosis
leukopenia
lymphocytes
microorganism
monocytes
neutrophils
phagocytes
phagocytosis
white blood cells (WBCs)

Thrombocytes
coagulation
coagulation factors
fibrin
fibrinogen
hemostasis
platelets
prothrombin
thrombin

Blood Types and Rh Factor
ABO blood groups
agglutinate
agglutination
antigen
donor
recipient
Rh factor
transfusions
type and crossmatch
universal donor
universal recipient

Blood Diseases
ecchymosis
petechiae
protozoa
serum

Lymphatic System
edema
interstitial fluid
lingual tonsils
lymph
lymph nodes
lymphatic vessels
lymphatics
lymphoid organs
mastectomy
palatine tonsils
pharyngeal tonsils
pharynx
spleen
T lymphocytes
thymosin
thymus gland
tonsils

Immune System
acquired immunity
active immunity
allergens
anaphylactic shock
artificially acquired immunity
attenuated
B lymphocytes
genetic immunity
histamines
immunity
interferons
natural acquired immunity
nonspecific immunity
passive immunity
pathogens
resistance
specific immunity
urticaria
vaccination

PRACTICAL APPLICATIONS

Read the following scenario and keep it in mind as you learn about the blood, lymphatic, and immune systems in this chapter.

Pierce Fisher has come to the health clinic today to see Dr. Giffin for a routine physical examination. Pierce tells Lisa, the medical assistant, he has been having episodes of dizziness and has some pain in his RLQ. Lisa notices that while Pierce's blood pressure is WNL, his temperature and pulse are elevated. Dr. Giffin examines Pierce and orders a stat CBC with a differential count to rule out a diagnosis of appendicitis. As Lisa is completing the blood draw, Pierce has several questions about his blood work and what it can tell the physician about his condition.

When Pierce's blood results come back, would you be able to tell what the results indicate?

FUNCTIONS OF THE BLOOD

Another component of the circulatory system is the blood itself. The function of blood is to transport oxygen and nutrients throughout the body and carry off wastes. Blood is important to our bodies in the following ways:

1. Blood takes oxygen from the lungs and nutrients from the digestive system to the body tissue.
2. Blood carries waste products away from the cells and to the kidneys and lungs for excretion.
3. Blood aids in regulating body temperature.
4. Blood distributes various hormones and chemicals throughout the body.

An average adult has 4 to 6 L of blood. The *pH* (degree of acidity or alkalinity of a substance) of blood is 7.4, or slightly alkaline. Whole blood is divided into two parts: the plasma (liquid matrix) and the formed elements (blood cells) (Figure 13-1). Blood is made up of approximately 55% plasma and 45% formed elements, depending on each individual. Understanding the normal structure and function of blood, as well as the different types of blood diseases, requires knowledge of these two components.

COMPOSITION OF THE BLOOD

Plasma

A pale-yellow fluid, **plasma** is about 90% water. The remaining 10% is composed of nutrients, electrolytes, gases, clotting factors, **antibodies** (substances that produce immunity), waste products, and hormones (Table 13-1).

Blood Cells

Blood is considered a tissue because it contains many types of cells. The blood cells are the **formed elements** of the blood and are composed of **erythrocytes** (red blood cells), leuko-

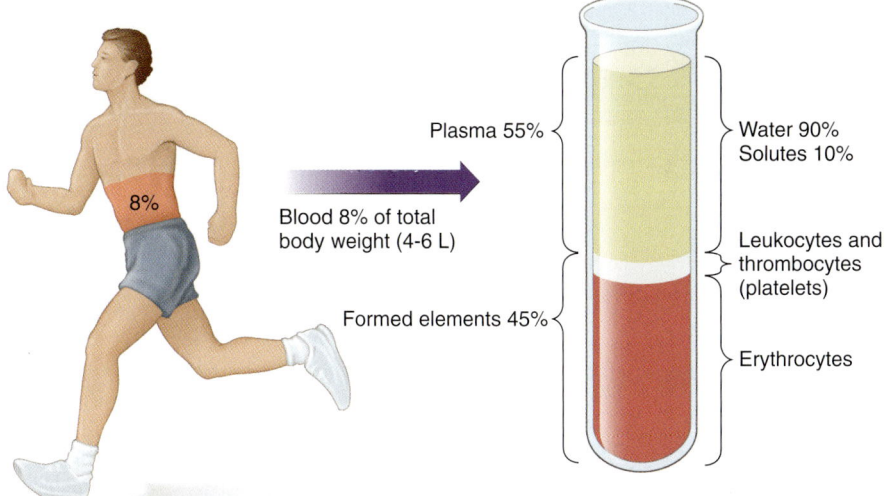

FIGURE 13-1 Approximate components of blood. (Modified from Applegate EJ: *The anatomy and physiology learning system*, ed 3, St Louis, 2006, Saunders.)

TABLE 13-1

Substances Carried in the Blood

Category	Substances
Nutrients	Carbohydrates
	Proteins
	Fats
Electrolytes	Chloride (Cl^-)
	Potassium (K^+)
	Calcium (Ca^{++})
	Sodium (Na^+)
	Bicarbonate (HCO_3^-)
	Phosphate (PO_4)
Gases	Carbon dioxide (CO_2)
	Oxygen (O_2)
Proteins	Globulins
	Albumin
Clotting factors	Fibrinogen
	Prothrombin
Waste	Urea
	Uric acid
	Amino acids
Other	Antibodies
	Hormones
	Enzymes

BOX 13-1

Stem Cell

A stem cell has the ability to produce specialized cells for various tissues of the body (e.g., heart, brain, liver, etc.). There are two types:

Embryonic stem cell: Stem cells obtained from aborted fetuses or leftover fertilized eggs from in vitro fertilization. Stem cells derived from embryos can replicate any cell in the body.

Adult stem cell: Stem cells specific to blood, intestines, skin, and muscle; cannot replicate all types of cells; they are present in children as well as adults.

Stem cell research is controversial. You can learn more about the various sides of this issue by researching on the Internet.

Erythrocytes

Red blood cells (RBCs) are the most numerous of the blood cells. The human body has about 5 million RBCs per cubic millimeter of blood. RBCs have a **biconcave** disk shape that makes it easier for them to "piggyback" oxygen. As blood flows through the body tissues, it releases the oxygen to be used in cellular **metabolism** (energy production).

RBCs contain **hemoglobin,** which is an iron-containing protein that carries both oxygen and carbon dioxide and provides the erythrocyte with its red color (Figure 13-4). A healthy diet contains enough iron to ensure that adequate hemoglobin formation takes place. Vitamin B_{12} and folic acid are also necessary for normal RBC production.

Erythropoiesis is the process of RBC formation. This process begins in the bone marrow (Figure 13-5). **Erythropoietin** (a hormone) is released from the kidney when the oxygen concentration is low in the blood. This stimulates the bone

cytes (white blood cells), and **thrombocytes** (platelets) (Figure 13-2). Blood cells, which are produced (**hematopoiesis**) in the bone marrow, are found mostly in the flat and irregular bones and in lymphoid tissue (lymph nodes, spleen, and thymus gland). All blood cells produced in the bone marrow originate from the same type of cell, the **stem cell** (Box 13-1). The stem cell differentiates into the erythrocyte, leukocyte, and platelet (Figure 13-3). See Appendix C for normal blood values.

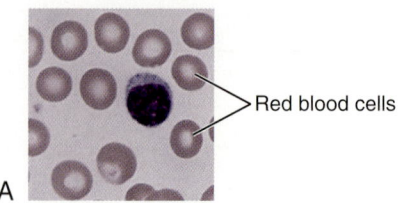

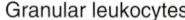

Granular leukocytes

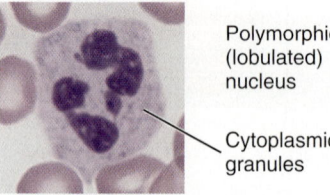

Agranular leukocytes

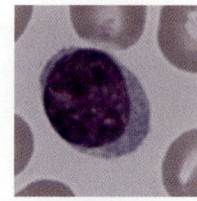

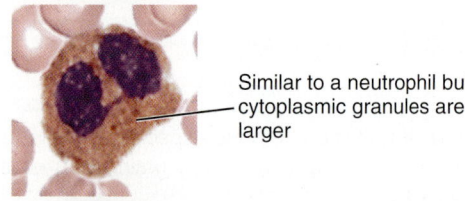

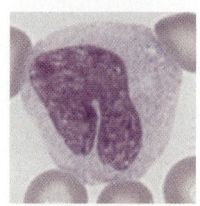

FIGURE 13-2 Formed elements in blood. **A,** Erythrocytes. **B,** Leukocytes. **C,** Platelets. (Modified from Carr JH, Rodak BF: *Clinical hematology atlas*, ed 3, St Louis, 2009, Saunders.)

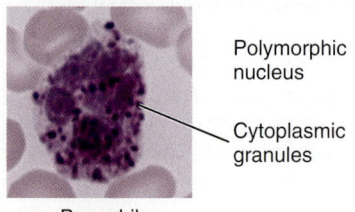

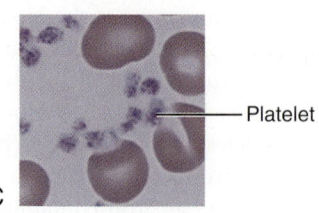

marrow to produce more erythrocytes. As the oxygen in the blood increases, this process subsides. An immature erythrocyte is referred to as a **reticulocyte.** As it matures, the RBC loses its nucleus, thus giving it more surface area to carry oxygen. The RBC erythrocyte count is normally between 4.5 and 5.5 million, depending on gender, and the RBC measures 7 to 8 μm in diameter. The life span of an RBC is 120 days. As the erythrocytes age and become fragile, their hemoglobin is recycled and the **macrophages** destroy them in the liver and spleen, which is a process referred to as **hemolysis.**

Leukocytes

White blood cells (WBCs) have a nucleus and are less numerous than erythrocytes. Leukocytes range from 4500 to 11,000

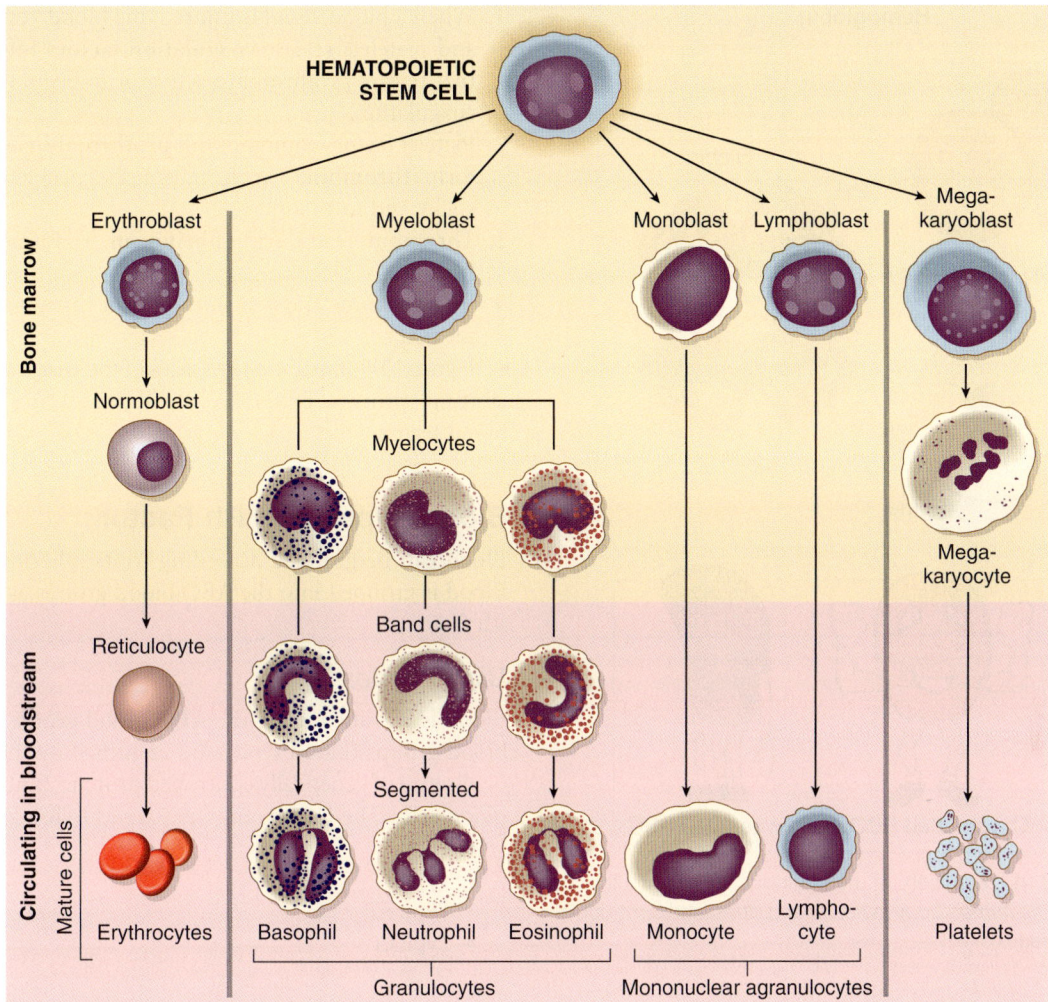

FIGURE 13-3 Development of the formed elements in blood. (From Chabner DE: *The language of medicine,* ed 8, St Louis, 2007, Saunders.)

per cubic millimeter of blood. WBCs act as scavengers, and their numbers increase during an infection or allergic reaction. This process of engulfing and digesting foreign material is called **phagocytosis.**

There are five types of WBCs, which can be differentiated by their staining properties observed through the use of a microscope. Some WBCs (**neutrophils, basophils,** and **eosinophils**) have **granulocytes** in their cytoplasm. Other WBCs are **lymphocytes** and **monocytes,** which are **agranulocytes.** Table 13-2 compares the properties of the five leukocytes.

When a physician orders a **differential count** (diff), the physician wants to know what percentage of each type of WBC is present in the blood. It also reveals any abnormal or immature cells. An increase or decrease in differential cells is helpful to the physician in the diagnosis of disease. For example, when leukocytes increase in number (usually above 11,000 per cubic millimeter of blood) the condition is referred to as **leukocytosis. Leukopenia** is a condition in which the number of WBCs is under 5,000 per cubic millimeter of blood.

FOR YOUR INFORMATION

Neutrophils are first responders to the site of an acute infection. A rapid production of additional neutrophils to fight the infection may not allow enough time for the neutrophils to mature. A reported "shift to the left" indicates the increased presence of immature neutrophils (bands) relative to the mature ones (segs), thus indicating an infection.

Thrombocytes

Platelets are fragments of cells that vary in shape and size and do not have a nucleus. Their function is to stop bleeding by forming a clot to help maintain **hemostasis** (prevention of blood loss) (Figure 13-6). Thrombocytes range from 250,000 to 400,000 per cubic millimeter of blood and are 2 to 5 μm in diameter.

An injury to a blood vessel causes a chain reaction that results in clot formation, as follows:

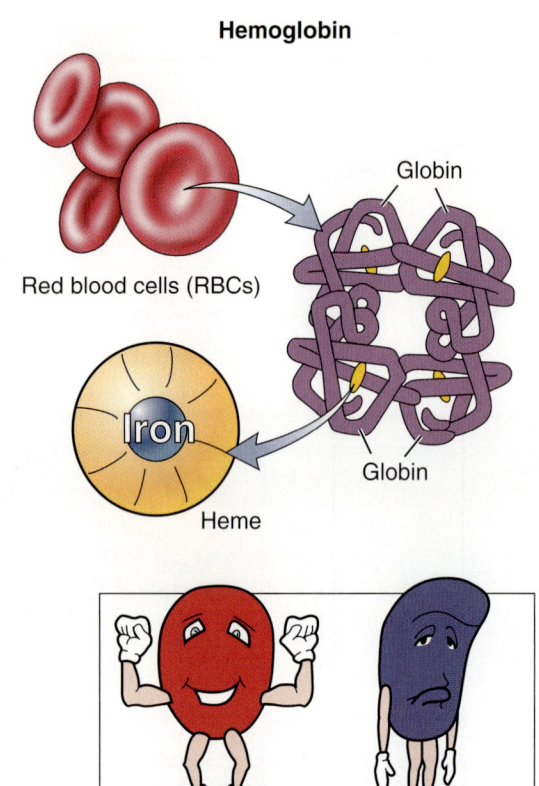

FIGURE 13-4 Function of hemoglobin. (From Herlihy B, Maebius NK: *The human body in health and illness,* ed 3, St Louis, 2007, Saunders.)

1. When a blood vessel is injured, the blood vessel constricts, and platelets release **coagulation factors** into the plasma that release prothrombin activator to begin the process of coagulation.
2. Platelet factors combine with **prothrombin** and calcium to form **thrombin,** which causes the platelets to become sticky and form a plug.
3. Thrombin reacts with **fibrinogen** to form a gel called **fibrin.**
4. RBCs become trapped in the fibrin threads, and a clot is formed.

Figure 13-7 illustrates the stages of the **coagulation** (blood-clotting) process. Box 13-2 lists abbreviations for common blood terms.

Blood Types and Rh Factor

Blood can be grouped according to its inherited properties. Blood is grouped into the ABO blood groups as well as by its Rh factor.

Blood Types

Blood is classified using the **ABO blood group** system. ABO blood groups (blood types) are identified by the presence of or absence of genetically controlled proteins (**antigens**) on red blood cells. The four blood types are as follows:
- Type A
- Type B
- Type AB
- Type O

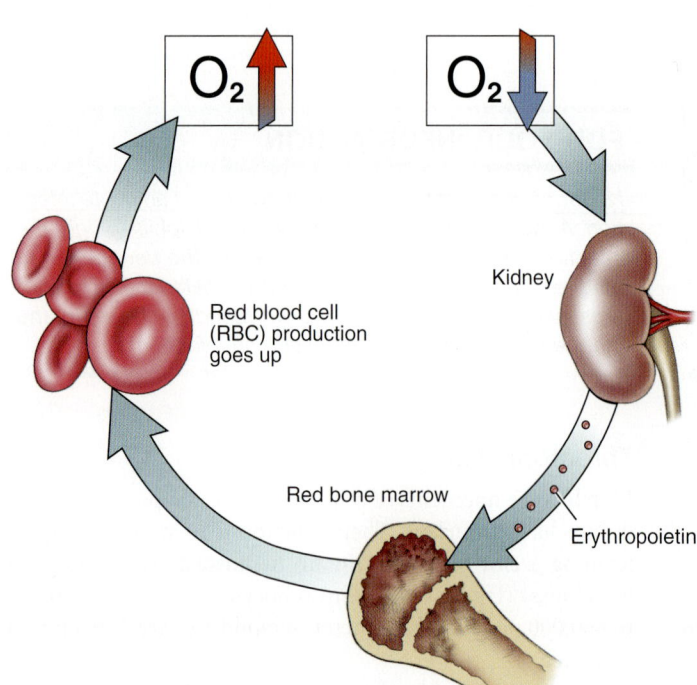

FIGURE 13-5 Regulation of red blood cell production by erythropoietin and oxygen (O_2). (From Herlihy B, Maebius NK: *The human body in health and illness,* ed 3, St Louis, 2007, Saunders.)

TABLE 13-2

Leukocytes

Cell Type and Description	Percent Present	Function	Size and Shape of Nucleus	Granule Staining Properties
GRANULOCYTE **Neutrophils (also called segs)** Considered **phagocytes**: first responders to an acute infection or damaged site; engulf microbes by phagocytosis. Their numbers increase significantly during an acute infection. Diameter of 10-15 μm. NOTE: A band is an immature neutrophil whose nucleus has not segmented. Range 0%-5%	55%-70%	Phagocytosis	3-5 lobes or segments	Pink
EOSINOPHILS Protect the body by reacting to the release of histamine during an allergic reaction. They also provide a defense against parasitic worms. Diameter of 12-17 μm.	1%-3%	Allergic reactions	2 lobes or segments	Orange-red
BASOPHILS Increase in response to allergic reactions. When basophils enter the tissue, they release histamine and heparin. Histamine dilates blood vessels to increase blood flow, and heparin inhibits the formation of blood clots. Diameter of 10-14 μm.	<1%	Allergic reaction Inflammatory response	2 lobes or U-shaped	Dark blue
AGRANULOCYTE **Lymphocytes** Work to activate the immune system. As the body is invaded by a **microorganism** (bacteria/virus), the lymphocytes multiply and form a plasma cell that makes a specific antibody. The antibody trips the immune system into action. Diameter of 6-12 μm.	25%-30%	Immunity	Large, almost fills cells	Nucleus dark blue
MONOCYTES First line of defense in the inflammatory process. Enter damaged tissues and become macrophages that continue the process of digesting cellular debris that was begun by the neutrophils. Diameter 12-20 μm.	3%-8%	Phagocytosis	U-shaped, surrounded by cytoplasm	Nucleus medium blue

BOX 13-2

Abbreviations for Common Blood Terms

Ab	antibody
Ag	antigen
CBC	complete blood count*
DIFF, diff	differential count
Hct, crit	hematocrit†
Hgb	hemoglobin; grams in 100 mL of blood
plat	platelet
PT	prothrombin time
PTT	partial thromboplastin time
RBC	red blood cell; RBC count
WBC	white blood cell; WBC count

*Number of RBCs, WBCs, and platelets per cubic millimeter of blood; includes Hct, Hgb, and cell volume measurements.
†Percentage of packed RBCs in a given volume of blood expressed as a percentage.

Table 13-3 shows a person with type B blood born with type B antigens and anti-A antibodies on the RBCs. Not all blood types are compatible. Care must be taken to give blood **transfusions** of the same blood type as the person receiving the transfusion. Death for the **recipient** can result when antibodies in the recipient's blood plasma join to the antigens in the person's blood causing the RBCs of the **donor** to **agglutinate** (clump together). As Table 13-3 shows, a person with type B blood can receive blood from a person with B or O. People with type O blood have neither A nor B antigens that can cause **agglutination** with A or B antigens; therefore they are considered **universal donors**. A person with type AB blood can receive A, B, AB, and O; people in this group are considered **universal recipients** because these people have no antigens to combine with the antibodies. Compatible blood types are determined by performing a **type and crossmatch** on both the donor's and the recipient's blood.

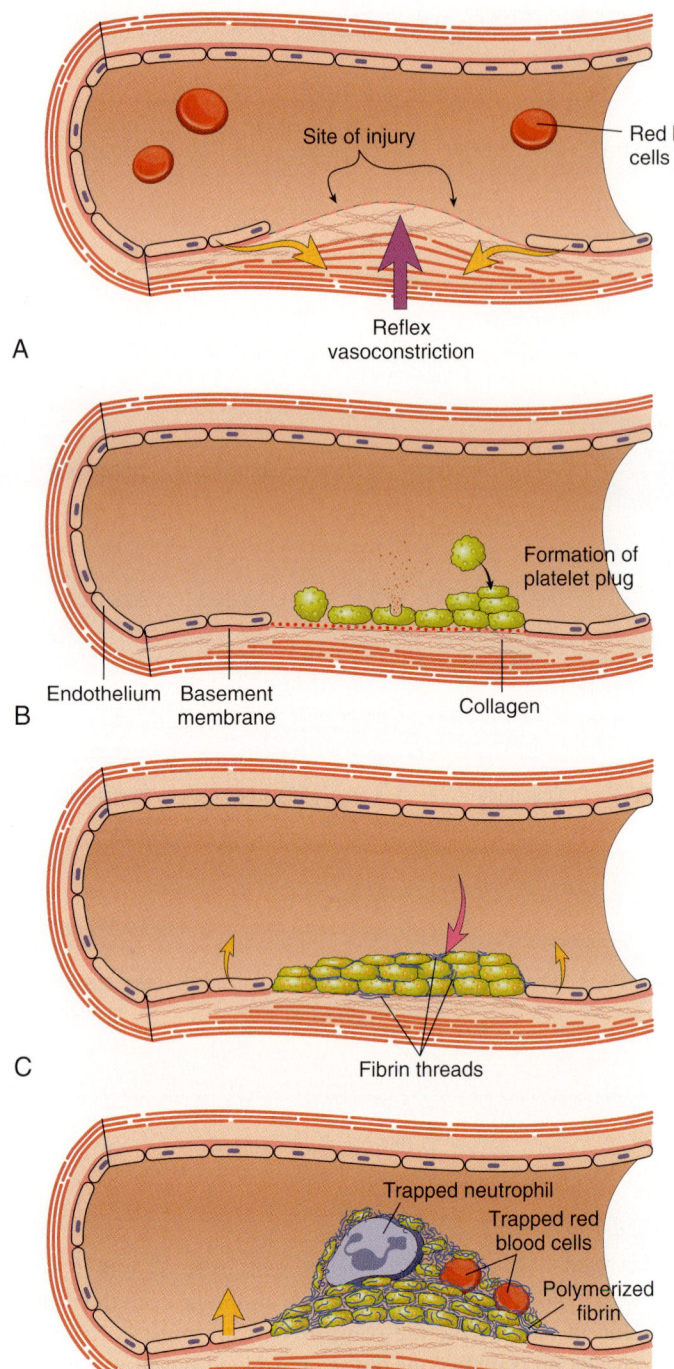

FIGURE 13-6 Process of hemostasis. (Modified from Kumar V et al: *Robbins and Cotran: pathologic basis of disease*, ed 7, Philadelphia, 2005, Saunders.)

Rh Factor

The **Rh factor** (rhesus factor) is another type of antigen that may be found on RBCs. If the Rh factor is found on the blood cells, this is recorded as Rh positive (+). Failure to have the Rh antigen registers as Rh negative (−).

Figure 13-8 shows the dangers of a baby born to an Rh-negative mother and Rh-positive father. If the baby is Rh positive, the mother's RBCs will stimulate the mother's blood to form anti-Rh antibodies. The next pregnancy with an Rh-positive baby could cause **hemolysis** of the baby's RBCs (hemolytic disease of the newborn [HDN]). It may also lead to death of the unborn fetus (*erythroblastosis fetalis*).

Diseases of the Blood

As in the heart and blood vessels, diseases also affect the blood (Table 13-4). Some blood diseases are associated with one of the three types of blood cells; others relate to incompatibility between blood types or Rh factors.

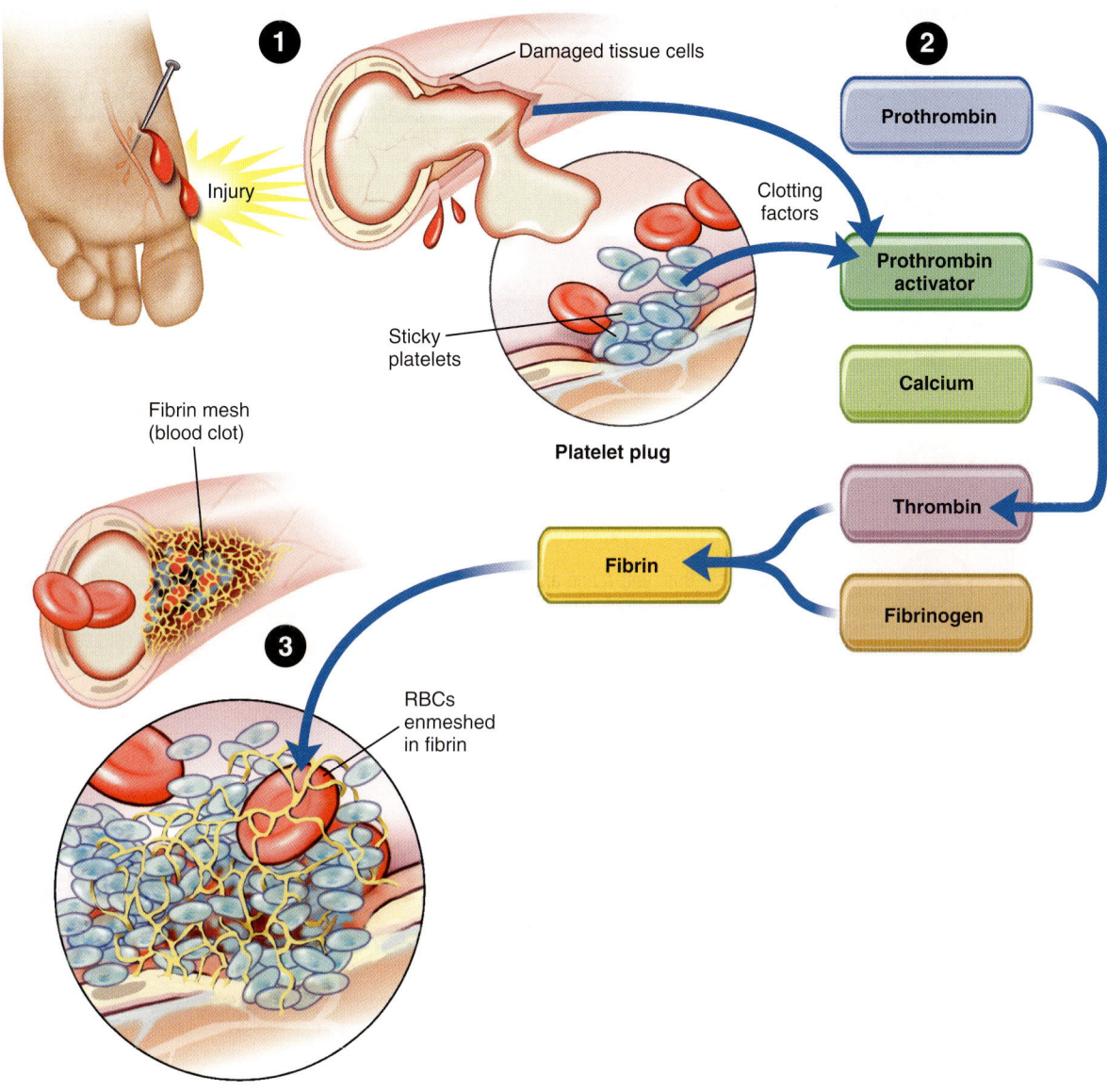

FIGURE 13-7 Process of blood clotting: (1) release of clotting factors from both injured tissue cells and sticky platelets at the injury site (which form a temporary platelet plug; (2) series of chemical reactions that eventually result in the formation of thrombin; and (3) formation of fibrin and trapping of red blood cells to form a clot. (Modified from Thibodeau GA, Patton KT: *The human body in health and disease,* ed 4, St Louis, 2005, Mosby.)

PATIENT-CENTERED PROFESSIONALISM

- Why is it necessary to understand the structure and function of each formed element of the blood? Explain the significance of each type of blood cell in a complete blood count (CBC).
- Explain the importance of knowing each parent's Rh factor before an infant's birth.
- How does blood typing affect a donor's and a recipient's ability to donate or receive blood?
- How is patient care affected by the medical assistant's understanding of blood cells, Rh factor, and blood typing?

LYMPHATIC SYSTEM

The final component of the circulatory system is the lymphatic system. The lymphatic system is an interconnected system of spaces and vessels between body tissues and organs. It filters out organisms that cause disease, produces certain WBCs, and generates antibodies, all without the help of a pump (unlike the blood, which has the heart). The lymphatic system is also important for the distribution of fluids and nutrients in the body because it drains excess fluids and protein so that tissues do not swell. Understanding the structure and function of the lymphatic system will help you understand the diseases that affect this system.

TABLE 13-3
Blood Types

Blood Type	Antigen (RBC Membrane)	Antibody (Plasma)	Can Receive Blood From	Can Donate Blood To
A (40%)	A antigen	Anti-B antibodies	A, O	A, AB
B (10%)	B antigen	Anti-A antibodies	B, O	B, AB
AB* (4*)	A antigen, B antigen	No antibodies	A, B, AB, O	AB
O† (46%)	No antigen	Both anti-A and anti-B antibodies	O	O, A, B, AB

*Type AB: universal recipient.
†Type O: universal donor.

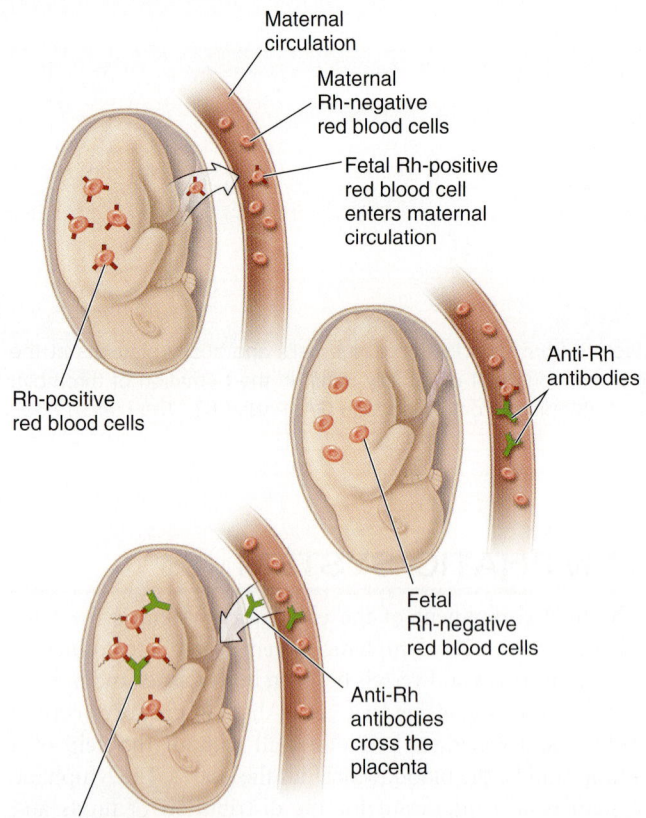

FIGURE 13-8 Erythroblastosis fetalis. (Modified from Thibodeau GA, Patton KT: *Anatomy and physiology*, ed 6, St Louis, 2007, Mosby.)

TABLE 13-4

Diseases and Conditions of the Blood

Disease and Description	Etiology	Signs and Symptoms	Diagnosis	Therapy	Interventions
DISEASES RELATED TO RBCs					
Anemia: Disease diagnosed by certain elements missing in the blood					
Iron deficiency anemia Low levels of iron in the blood	Chronic anemia with RBCs lacking sufficient iron for chronic blood loss Decreased iron intake Malabsorption	Pallor, fatigue, weakness	Laboratory tests show decrease in RBCs, Hgb, Hct Decreased serum iron and serum ferritin (**serum** is plasma minus clotting factors)	Diet with adequate iron-containing foods and correction of underlying cause (e.g., bleeding)	Reinforce the treatment plan and answer patient's questions
Pernicious anemia Megaloblastic anemia resulting in decrease of hydrochloric acid and deficiency of the intrinsic factor needed for vitamin B_{12} absorption	Genetic predisposition	Complaints of weakness; beefy, red tongue; tingling or numbness in limbs	Laboratory tests to rule out other anemias; gastric analysis	Vitamin B_{12} replacement and iron supplement	Encourage a well-balanced diet, including foods high in vitamin B_{12}
Malaria Caused by **protozoa** of the genus *Plasmodium*	Transmitted by an infected mosquito or blood products Mosquito injects spores into the wound, which settle in the liver	Chills, fever, headache, fatigue, sweating Signs of ruptured RBCs	Patient history of travel to the tropics, use of intravenous drugs, or recent blood transfusion Blood smear identifying parasite	Medication therapy for acute attacks	Eliminate breeding source for mosquitos Person should seek prophylactic treatment if traveling to known infested area
Septicemia Blood poisoning: systemic infection caused by a pathogenic organism	Complication of another infection	Patient's current complaints, including prior infections	Laboratory tests: positive blood cultures, CBC, BUN, PT, PTT	Antibiotic therapy for causative agent	Provide emotional support to family and patient; answer questions and explain course of treatment
Vitamin K deficiency Bleeding disorder caused by insufficient vitamin K (needed for blood to clot)	Inability to absorb vitamin K from foods	Poor blood coagulation	Laboratory tests, including PT	Vitamin K given parenterally	Diet high in vitamin K if malabsorption problem can be corrected
Polycythemia Overproduction of RBCs by the bone marrow	Unknown; high incidence in Jewish men	Weakness and fatigue with complaints of headache, dizziness, and double vision	Blood tests show increased RBCs	Possible splenectomy or phlebotomy to reduce RBCs	Removal of a pint of blood

Continued

TABLE 13-4
Diseases and Conditions of the Blood—cont'd

Disease and Description	Etiology	Signs and Symptoms	Diagnosis	Therapy	Interventions
DISEASES RELATED TO WBCs					
Leukemia					
Uncontrolled WBC (leukocyte) production interfering with normal blood cell production (leukocytosis) Forms include acute lymphocytic, chronic lymphocytic, acute myelogenous, and chronic myelogenous leukemia	Unknown	Fatigue, dyspnea on exertion, weight loss, and swollen cervical lymph nodes	Elevated WBCs Decreased RBCs, Hgb, Hct Tumor markers assist in determining type of leukemia	Medication therapy to induce remission (chemotherapy)	Assist patient with coping; encourage good nutrition and rest
DISEASES RELATED TO PLATELETS					
Thrombocytopenia					
Decreased clotting capabilities of the blood	Idiopathic or secondary to another disease	**Petechiae** and **ecchymosis** on the skin; easy bruising; bleeding from nose and gums	Rule out other platelet disorders through blood tests	Medication to induce platelet production	Instruct patient in ways to reduce injury and bleeding
DISEASES RELATED TO INCOMPATIBILITY					
Erythroblastosis fetalis					
Hemolytic disease of the newborn	Results from Rh incompatibility between mother and fetus	Cyanosis	Tests to confirm Rh compatibility (e.g., Coombs test, ABO typing)	Possible intrauterine transfusion Immune globulin (RhoGAM) to mother to provide passive immunity in future pregnancies	Prenatal care; tests before delivery to determine compatibility of Rh between mother and father

BUN, Blood urea nitrogen; *CBC*, complete blood count; *Hct*, hematocrit; *Hgb*, hemoglobin; *PT*, prothrombin time; *PTT*, partial thromboplastin time; *RBCs*, red blood cells; *WBCs*, white blood cells.

Structure

The lymphatic system has four components: (1) the lymphatic vessels, (2) the lymphatic fluid, (3) the lymph nodes, and (4) the lymphoid organs.

Function

Lymph is formed when blood plasma filters out of the spaces between the cells of the tissue. Most of this tissue fluid (**interstitial fluid**) reenters the blood through the capillary walls. The remaining tissue fluid enters the lymph capillaries and becomes lymph. The sole purpose of lymph is to return proteins, fats, hormones, and other needed substances back to the blood.

FOR YOUR INFORMATION

The lymphatic system becomes less effective as we age. T cells become less responsive to antigens and antibody levels do not rise as quickly after antigen exposure; therefore an increased susceptibility to viral and bacterial infections occurs. Vaccinations for acute viral diseases (e.g., influenza) are strongly recommended.

Lymphatic Vessels

The lymphatic system accomplishes the return of elements to the blood by way of four lymphatic vessels: (1) lymph capillaries, (2) lymphatics, (3) the thoracic duct, and (4) the right lymphatic duct.

Lymphatic vessels are found in all tissues and organs of the body that contain blood vessels.
- The lymph capillaries, like blood capillaries, unite to form larger vessels called **lymphatics**, which have valves to prevent backflow of lymph.
- The function of the lymphatics is to carry all materials not needed in the tissue spaces from the tissues through the vessels back to the subclavian veins.
- The lymphatics continue to spread out and form larger vessels (much like venules to veins) until they meet and form two main channels, the thoracic duct and the right lymphatic duct (Figure 13-9).
- The *thoracic duct* receives lymph from the left side of the body and all of the structures below the diaphragm, and the *right lymphatic duct* collects lymph from the remaining quadrant on the right side.

Lymph circulation, unlike blood circulation, flows only once through the lymphatic vessels and enters the blood (Figure 13-10). Even though the drainage of lymph is continuous, it is possible for fluid to accumulate in tissue spaces. When this happens, **edema** (swelling) results.

Lymph Nodes

Lymph nodes are small, oval-shaped bodies of lymphoid tissue. Lymph nodes vary in size from a pinhead to an almond and run along the course of the lymphatics. Nodes are usually found in groups or chains at the sides of the larger blood vessels, although they can stand alone. Lymph nodes contain lymphocytes and macrophages that serve as filters to kill foreign materials such as microorganisms or abnormal cells.

The function of the lymph nodes is twofold: (1) produce lymphocytes and monocytes and (2) serve as filters guarding against the spread of infection.

Lymphoid Organs

The **lymphoid organs** consist of the spleen, tonsils, and the thymus gland (Figure 13-11).

Spleen

The **spleen**, located in the upper left quadrant, has the following three functions:

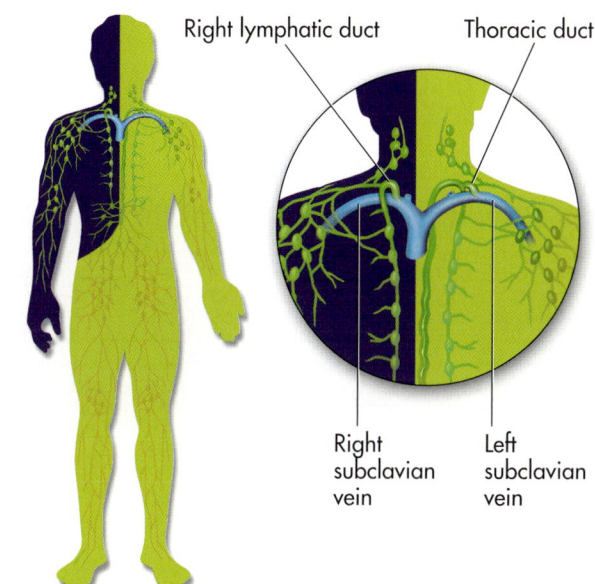

FIGURE 13-9 Areas of the body that are drained by the main lymphatic ducts. The right lymphatic duct drains lymph from the upper right quadrant of the body into the right subclavian vein. The thoracic duct drains lymph from the rest of the body into the left subclavian vein. (Modified from Thibodeau GA, Patton KT: *The human body in health and disease,* ed 4, St Louis, 2005, Mosby.)

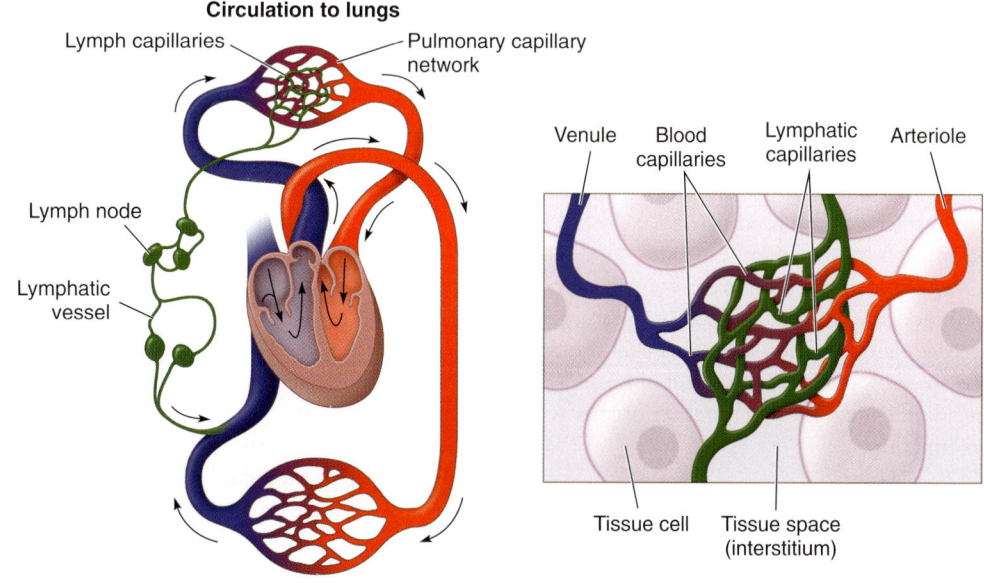

FIGURE 13-10 Relationship of the lymphatic vessels to the circulatory system. (Modified from Shiland BJ: *Mastering healthcare terminology,* ed 2 St Louis, 2006, Mosby.)

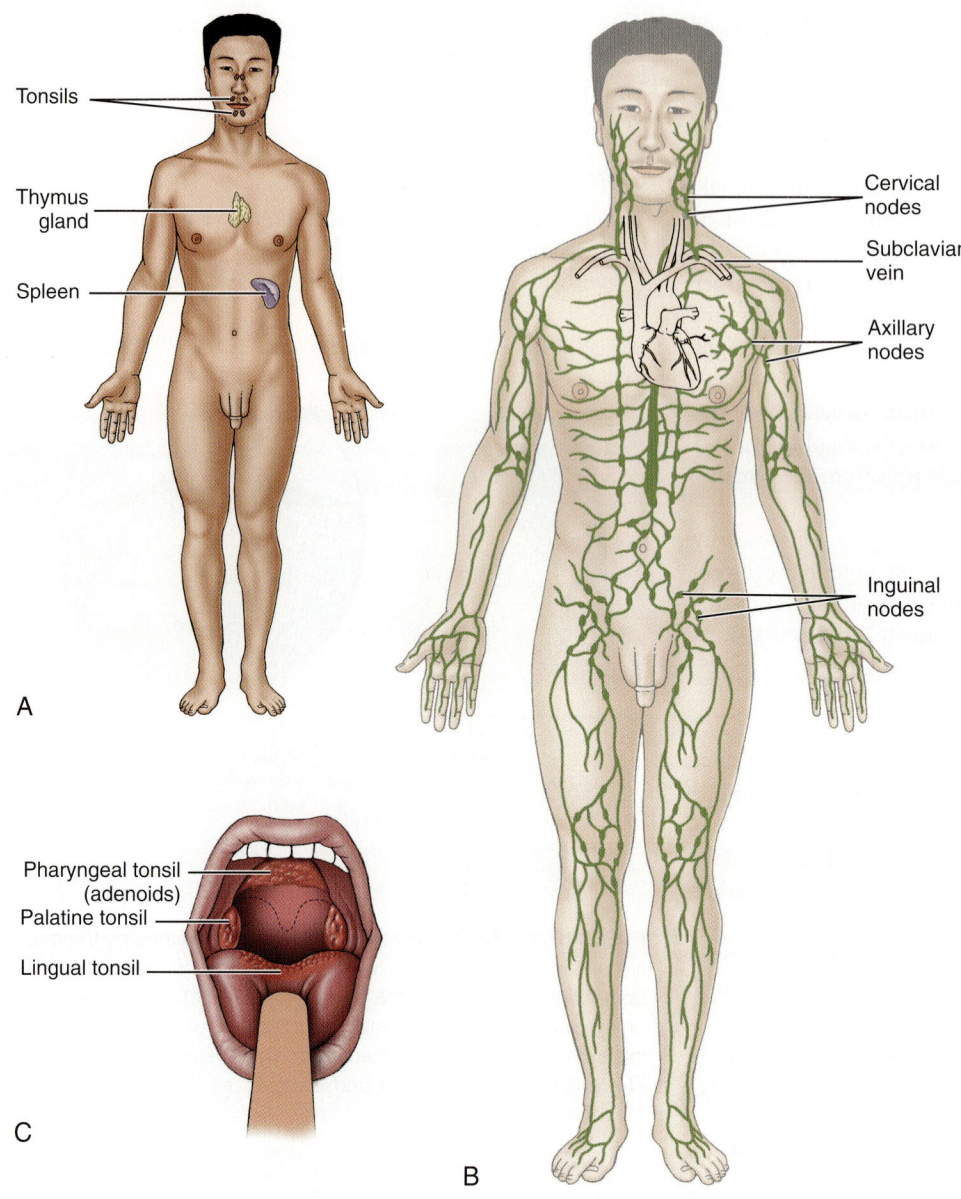

FIGURE 13-11 Lymphoid tissue locations. **A,** Lymphoid organs. **B,** Distribution of lymph nodes. **C,** Tonsils. (Modified from Herlihy B, Maebius NK: *The human body in health and illness,* ed 3, St Louis, 2007, Saunders.)

1. Storage of red blood cells until needed
2. Destruction and removal of worn out erythrocytes and platelets
3. Production of lymphocytes and monocytes by the spleen's lymphoid tissue

The spleen is a blood reservoir and can store about a pint of blood and release it quickly back into circulation when needed, such as after strenuous exercise or a hemorrhage. If the spleen is removed as a result of trauma (e.g., motor vehicle accident, injury), other internal organs will compensate for its function.

Tonsils

Tonsils are lymph nodes located in the **pharynx** (throat), nasal cavity, and at the back of the tongue (Figure 13-11, *C*). They are responsible for preventing bacteria from entering the body through the throat and for filtering tissue fluids in the mouth and nasal cavities. These often increase in size with throat and ear infections. The **pharyngeal tonsils** (adenoids) are located in the posterior wall of the nasopharynx. The **palatine tonsils** are in the lateral walls of the oropharynx, and the **lingual tonsils** are located on the surface and on the back of the tongue.

Thymus Gland

The **thymus gland** is located behind the sternum, on top of the heart, and just below the thyroid gland. The thymus gland is most active in the first few months after birth to establish the infant's immune system. The thymus secretes a hormone called **thymosin** that helps with the development of **T lymphocytes** (responsible for attacking viruses). The thymus is extremely sensitive to sex hormones, and after puberty the thymus gland gradually atrophies (decreases in size) and is

TABLE 13-5
Diseases of the Lymphatic System

Disease and Description	Etiology	Signs and Symptoms	Diagnosis	Therapy	Interventions
DISEASES RELATED TO LYMPH DRAINAGE					
Elephantiasis (lymphedema) Caused by inadequacy or inability of lymph to drain from limbs (Figure 13-12) Complication after **mastectomy** if lymphatics are removed	Obstruction or removal of lymph nodes	Affected limb swollen	Patient history; examination and lymphangiography to confirm site of blockage; history of surgical removal of lymphatics	Elevation of affected part	Encourage patient to wear prescribed elastic support garments
LYMPHOMAS					
Hodgkin's disease Chronic, progressive cancer of lymphoid tissue	Unknown	Swelling in cervical lymph nodes; fever, night sweats, weight loss	Lymph node biopsy	Radiation therapy in conjunction with chemotherapy	During treatment, encourage nutrition and provide support
Non-Hodgkin's lymphoma Neoplasm disease of lymphoid tissue	Unknown	Painless lymphadenopathy Complaints of fatigue, malaise, fever, and night sweats	Lymph node biopsy	Radiation to primary site combined with chemotherapy drugs	During treatment, follow through with procedures and maintain nutrition
Infectious mononucleosis Acute viral infection involving lymphatic tissue, usually in cervical region	EBV; transmitted through saliva	Fatigue, fever, sore throat, lymphadenopathy	Clinical presentation, mono laboratory tests CBC with differential: lymphocytes and monocytes <50%; elevated titer for EBV (monospot)	Based on symptoms Increased fluids during fever; antipyretic medications and antibiotics and steroids for secondary infections	Encourage good nutrition and rest

CBC, Complete blood count; *EBV,* Epstein-Barr virus.

replaced with fat and connective tissue. This event makes the body defense system more vulnerable to infection as a person ages. For example, people in their 70s have a harder time fighting off disease because the thymus is so small it can no longer produce a good supply of T cells. Stress hormones also negatively affect thymus function.

Diseases of the Lymphatic System

Diseases of the lymphatic system relate to the drainage of lymph as well as the drainage of lymph nodes and the tissue itself (Table 13-5).

PATIENT-CENTERED PROFESSIONALISM

- Why do medical assistants need to understand the function of the lymphatics?
- How is the lymphatic system important to the healthy functioning of the human body?

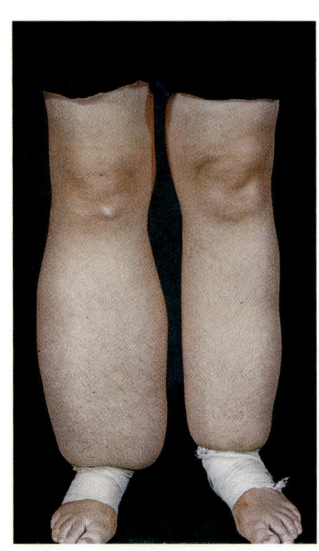

FIGURE 13-12 Lymphedema. This patient had bound her feet so that she could wear shoes. (From Black JM et al: *Medical-surgical nursing: clinical management for positive outcomes,* ed 8, St Louis, 2009, Saunders.)

IMMUNE SYSTEM

The lymphatic system plays an important role in protecting our bodies from diseases. The immune system aids in fighting the diseases that occur in the body. Daily, our bodies are exposed to harmful disease-producing bacteria (**pathogens**). The immune system provides **immunity,** the ability to counteract the toxic effects of many microorganisms.

Lines of Defense

The immune system has three lines of defense to resist the effects of microorganisms on the body: (1) physical and chemical barriers, (2) nonspecific immunity, and (3) specific immunity.

Physical and Chemical Barriers

Barriers prevent microorganisms from entering the body and include the following types:
- *Physical:* Skin and the membranes lining body passages
- *Chemical:* Sweat, tears, saliva, mucus

Nonspecific Immunity

Nonspecific immunity is a response from cells that surround and digest microorganisms, as well as from chemicals (e.g., histamine, certain antibodies) that help destroy bacteria. Furthermore, **interferons** are produced by cells infected with a virus, and T cells block the virus' ability to reproduce. Nonspecific immunity depends on intact skin and mucous membranes, chemical barriers produced by the body, and reflex actions (Figure 13-13).

The process of acquiring nonspecific immunity consists of the following:
1. Swelling, redness, warmth, and fever stimulate phagocytosis
2. Pain occurs in the area of an infection
3. An increased blood flow attracts white blood cells to the infected area
4. Phagocytes destroy invading bacteria (infection)
5. Nonspecific immunity is produced

For example, phagocytosis of bacteria by WBCs is a type of nonspecific immunity.

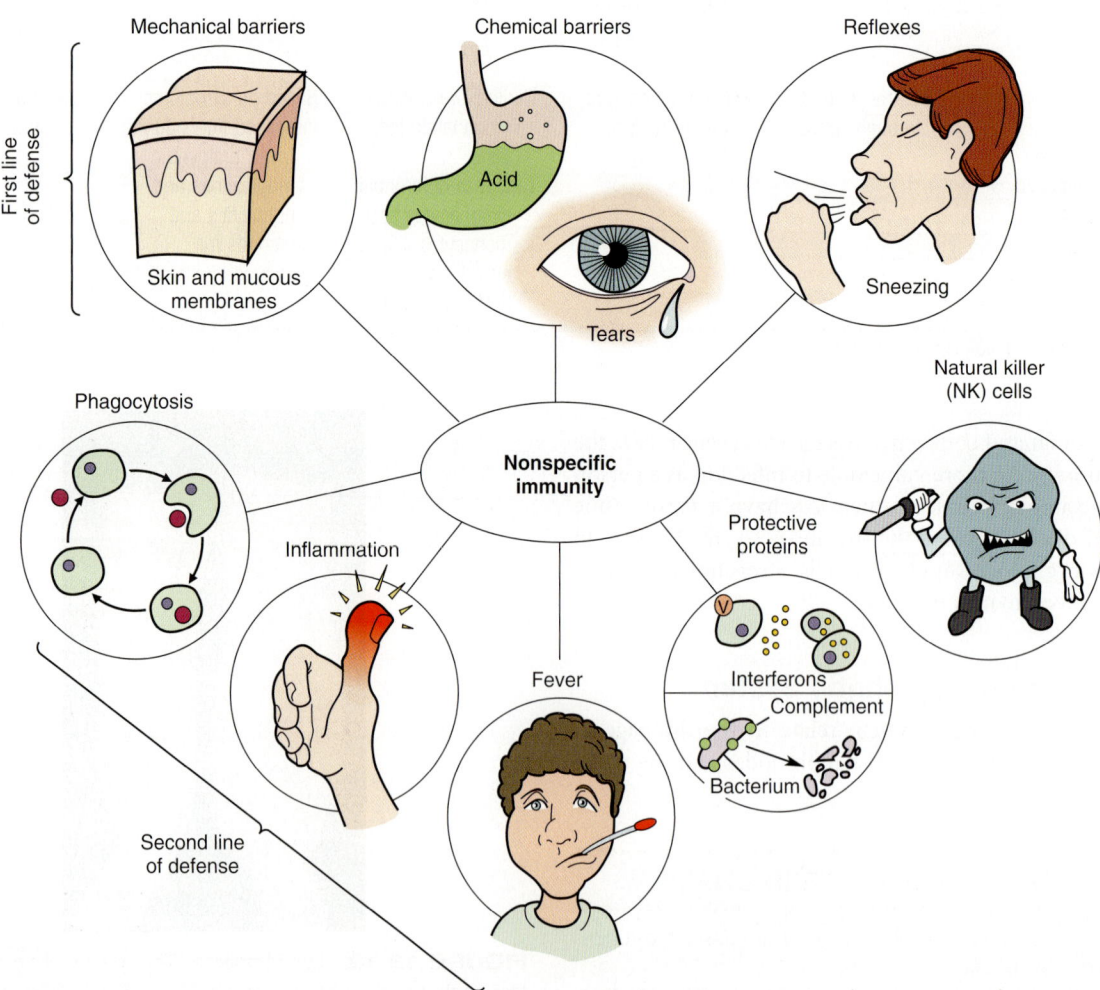

FIGURE 13-13 Process of nonspecific immunity. (From Herlihy B, Maebius NK: *The human body in health and illness,* ed 3, St Louis, 2007, Saunders.)

Specific Immunity

Specific immunity is selective for a particular type of disease or microorganism. It comes from two types of lymphocytes. The T lymphocytes (T cells) attack the foreign body directly. The **B lymphocytes** (B cells) multiply rapidly when an antigen is introduced, resulting in the production of antibodies. These antibodies remain in the blood and provide long-term immunity.

The process of acquiring specific immunity is as follows:
1. The immune system recognizes, attacks, destroys, and "remembers" each type of microorganism that enters the body.
2. Antibodies and specialized cells are produced that bind to and inactivate microorganisms when the body is attacked again.

Types of Immunity

There are two main types of immunity: genetic (inborn) immunity and acquired immunity (Figure 13-14).

Genetic Immunity

Genetic immunity, or natural (inborn) immunity, occurs when a person is born with a **resistance** to a specific disease (e.g., foot-and-mouth disease). This is species specific.

Acquired Immunity

Acquired immunity occurs either through a natural process of having a disease or an artificial process such as vaccination (Figure 13-15).

Natural acquired immunity occurs when the body produces its own antibodies after having the disease (**active immunity**) (e.g., chickenpox) or after the antibodies pass through the placenta or mother's milk and provides immunity (**passive immunity**).

Artificially acquired immunity is considered active when a person is immunized or given a **vaccination,** which is a sample of the disease in a weakened **attenuated** state (e.g., measles, mumps). In response the body produces antibodies that fight off the disease when exposed. Passive artificial immunity occurs when antibodies developed in one organism are injected into another organism (e.g., rabies, tetanus) as with giving gamma globulin.

Diseases of the Immune System

Even though the immune system defends the body against disease, it is also susceptible to disease. For example, an allergy is a hypersensitivity of the immune system to antigens. Antigens that create an allergic response are called **allergens.** Repeated exposure to an allergen causes the antigen-antibody response that causes the release of **histamines** and other inflammatory substances. This response usually causes symptoms such as a runny nose, irritated conjunctiva, and **urticaria** (hives). Occasionally the response to allergens may cause constriction of the airways, decrease in blood pressure, and irregular heart rhythms. These reactions can progress to a life-threatening condition called **anaphylactic shock.** The person would need immediate treatment, usually with an injection of epinephrine and inhalation therapy. Table 13-6 provides additional immune system diseases. A person's immune system sometimes will produce antibodies (immunity) against its own *(auto)* normal tissue. Two autoimmune diseases are *rheumatoid arthritis* and *lupus erythematosus.* Varied symptoms can occur such as joint pain, skin rash, and fever.

Special Considerations for AIDS Patients

Acquired immunodeficiency syndrome (AIDS) is a disease that has affected millions of people worldwide. AIDS patients are prone to opportunistic infections that arise because of the weakened immune system. Box 13-3 lists some common illnesses of the AIDS patient.

A patient must give consent before having the *human immunodeficiency virus* (HIV) antibody test. Most states require HIV counseling both before and after the test is given. Most also require that the test results be given in person (e.g., never leave a message), whether the results are negative or positive. The responsibility of this counseling lies with the physician or a trained HIV counselor.

A patient's medical record cannot be marked or coded in any manner on the outside to identify that an HIV test

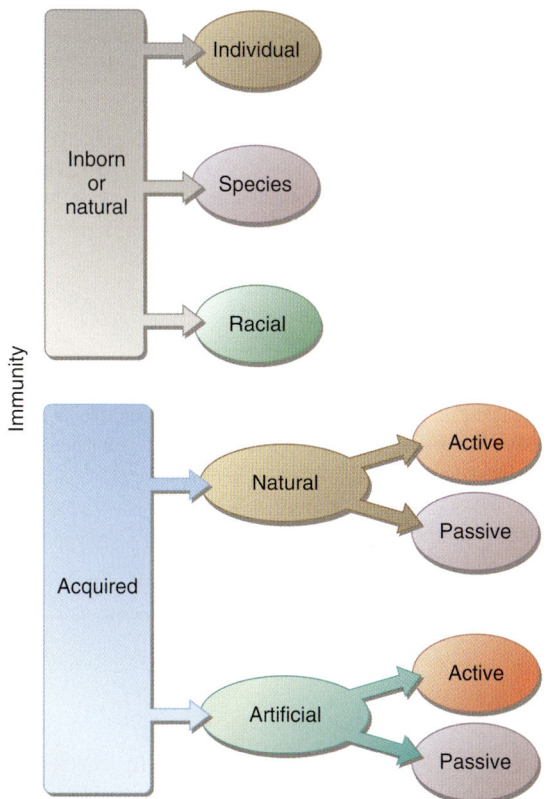

FIGURE 13-14 Different types of immunity. (Modified from Chester GA: *Modern medical assisting,* Philadelphia, 1998, Saunders.)

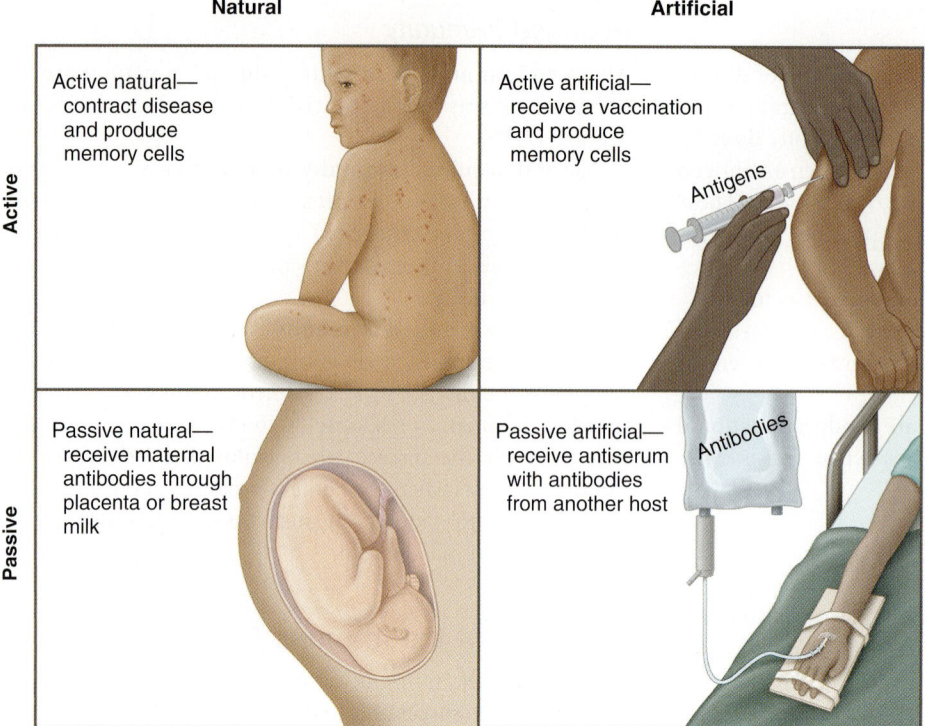

FIGURE 13-15 Types of acquired immunity. (Modified from Applegate EJ: *The anatomy and physiology learning system,* ed 3, St Louis, 2006, Saunders.)

TABLE 13-6

Diseases of the Immune System

Disease and Description	Etiology	Signs and Symptoms	Diagnosis	Therapy	Interventions
LUPUS ERYTHEMATOSUS					
Chronic inflammatory disorder that affects the connective tissues in various parts of the body	Autoimmune reaction (body produces antibodies) against own cells, which suppresses the body's natural immunity and damages tissues	Anorexia, weight loss, malaise, abdominal pain, rash, polyarthralgia (arthralgia of multiple joints)	Patient history and rash; CBC with differential; erythrocyte sedimentation rate, serum electrophoresis; C-reactive protein	Reduce stress; avoid sunlight. Nonsteroidal drug therapy, with short-term use of corticosteroids during acute episodes	Encourage use of sunscreen and stress reduction.
ACQUIRED IMMUNODEFICIENCY SYNDROME (AIDS)					
Caused by virus that attacks entire immune system; transmitted through body fluids	HIV attacks helper T cells, which interferes with immune system's ability to protect body from infection (Figure 13-16)	Persistent cough; weight loss, oral lesions; appearance of lesions on face and upper torso (Kaposi's sarcoma)	Patient history, positive HIV blood test; *Pneumocystis carinii* infection, candidiasis, or biopsy of lesion	Medications for opportunistic infections; antiviral therapy	Nutritional and emotional support

CBC, Complete blood count; *HIV,* human immunodeficiency virus.

was performed. All results are privileged and may not be disclosed except as provided by law. Currently, all 50 states require reporting of AIDS cases, without the patient's consent, to the Centers for Disease Control and Prevention (CDC) or to the state's health department. Since each state has its own reporting requirements, it is best to check in your particular state for information. Patients with HIV infection or AIDS have the same rights as people with other life-threatening illnesses and should be treated with dignity and respect.

BOX 13-3

Diseases and Infectious Agents Common to AIDS Patients

BACTERIAL
Pneumocystis carinii pneumonia
Mycobacterium tuberculosis

PARASITIC
Toxoplasma gondii (brain lesions)
Cryptosporidium
Microsporidia

VIRAL
Cytomegalovirus (retinitis)
Herpes zoster (shingles)
Herpes simplex

FUNGAL
Thrush *(Candida albicans)*
Cryptococcal meningitis
Histoplasmosis
Coccidioidomycosis

MISCELLANEOUS
Kaposi's sarcoma
Lymphomas

PATIENT-CENTERED PROFESSIONALISM

- How does genetic or natural immunity differ from acquired immunity, and why do medical assistants need to understand this?
- When a person is HIV positive, they may not develop AIDS. Why is it important to understand the disease and how it can be transmitted?
- How can medical assistants improve the care they provide to AIDS patients?

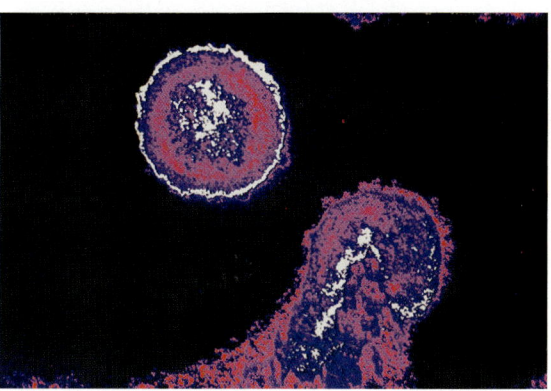

FIGURE 13-16 The human immunodeficiency virus (HIV). (From Shiland BJ: *Mastering healthcare terminology,* St Louis, 2003, Mosby.)

CONCLUSION

The cardiovascular system is responsible for moving blood and lymph throughout the body. The condition of the blood and lymph is crucial to the body to maintain homeostasis. Blood tissue contains both plasma and formed elements—the blood cells and platelets. RBCs transport oxygen, nutrients, and carbon dioxide. WBCs help the body resist infections and clean up injured tissues. Platelets provide a means for the body to prevent a loss of essential body fluids.

The lymphatic system acts to balance fluids by collecting lymph from the bloodstream, removing contaminants, returning the cleaned lymph back into the bloodstream, and thus preventing the spread of disease. The immune system is made up of many cells and tissues contained within the body's network of systems. It plays an important role in defending the body against disease.

Medical assistants need to understand the structure and function of the entire cardiovascular system so they can understand the related disease processes. Providing the best patient care means knowing first the normal and then the abnormal condition of the body's systems.

Chapter Summary

Reinforce your understanding of the material in this chapter by reviewing the curriculum objectives and key content points below.

1. **Define, appropriately use, and spell all the Key Terms for this chapter.**
   - Review the Key Terms if necessary.
2. **List the eight components of blood plasma.**
   - Blood plasma is the liquid portion of the blood.
   - Water, nutrients, electrolytes, gases, clotting factors, antibodies, waste products, and hormones are all components of blood plasma.
   - Blood is approximately 55% plasma and 45% formed elements (RBCs, WBCs, and platelets).
3. **List three types of blood cells and describe the function of each.**
   - Erythrocytes are red blood cells (RBCs); they are the most numerous and contain hemoglobin, which carries oxygen.
   - Leukocytes are white blood cells (WBCs); they help fight disease.
   - Thrombocytes are platelets; they help stop bleeding by forming clots.
4. **List the four blood types and explain the importance of compatibility.**

- Blood types are A, B, AB, or O; a person cannot receive blood that has a different antigen than the recipient's blood has.
- A type and crossmatch must be performed to ensure compatibility of the donor's and the recipient's blood.
- A transfusion of incompatible blood causes agglutination, and death can result for the recipient.

5. **Explain the importance of Rh factor as it relates to pregnancy and transfusions.**
   - Care must be taken in a pregnancy if the mother is Rh negative and the father is Rh positive.
   - A blood incompatibility results if people are exposed to a different Rh factor or blood group than their own. A mother will form antibodies against a fetus if the baby's blood is Rh positive and the mother is Rh negative.

6. **List nine diseases of the blood and describe the etiology, signs and symptoms, diagnosis, therapy, and interventions for each.**
   - Diseases of the blood affect all three types of blood cells. Blood incompatibility will cause life-threatening medical situations.
   - Refer to Table 13-4.

7. **List the four divisions of the lymphatic system and describe the function of each.**
   - Lymph is formed when blood plasma filters out of the spaces between the tissue cells.
   - The lymphatic vessels carry substances from the tissues not needed by the body.
   - The lymph nodes produce lymphocytes and monocytes and filter out harmful and unwanted substances.
   - The lymphoid organs function to filter, produce blood cells, and store RBCs until needed.

8. **List four diseases of the lymphatic system and describe the etiology, signs and symptoms, diagnosis, therapy, and interventions for each.**
   - Cancer can affect the lymphatic system and provide a means for cancer to metastasize.
   - Refer to Table 13-5.

9. **List the immune system's three lines of defense and describe each.**
   - Physical barriers include the skin and membranes, and chemical barriers include body fluids (sweat, tears, saliva, and mucus).
   - Nonspecific immunity is the body reacting to eliminate the effects of microorganisms and other toxic substances.
   - Specific immunity is the body producing antibodies for long-term immunity against a particular microorganism or disease.

10. **Distinguish between natural (inborn) immunity and acquired immunity and give an example of each.**
    - Genetic immunity occurs when a person is born with a resistance to a specific disease (e.g., foot-and-mouth disease).
    - Acquired immunity occurs either naturally (e.g., having measles) or artificially (e.g., vaccination) to protect the body against a specific disease.

11. **List three diseases of the immune system and describe the etiology, signs and symptoms, diagnosis, therapy, and interventions for each.**
    - A compromised immune system allows opportunistic infections to occur.
    - Refer to Table 13-6.

12. **Describe the considerations associated with the testing of patients with acquired immunodeficiency syndrome (AIDS).**
    - Counseling before and after testing for the human immunodeficiency virus (HIV) is required.
    - Results of the test must be given in person.
    - There must be no special marking on the outside of the patient chart, and the confidentiality of the patient must be respected.

13. **Analyze a realistic medical office situation and apply your understanding of the blood and lymphatic systems to determine the best course of action.**
    - Understanding the normal physiology of the blood and lymphatic systems will help you understand how a disease process affects this system.

14. **Describe the impact on patient care when medical assistants have a solid understanding of the structure and function of the blood, lymphatic, and immune systems.**
    - Medical assistants who understand the physiology of the blood, lymphatic, and immune systems will be better prepared to assist with medical procedures, communicate clearly to patients, and perform effective patient teaching.

PRACTICAL APPLICATIONS

If you have accomplished the objectives in this chapter, you will be able to make better choices as a medical assistant. Take another look at this situation and decide what you would do.

Pierce Fisher has come to the health clinic today to see Dr. Giffin for a routine physical examination. Pierce tells Lisa, the medical assistant he has been having episodes of dizziness and has some pain in his RLQ. Lisa notices that while Pierce's blood pressure is WNL, his temperature and pulse are elevated. Dr. Giffin examines Pierce and orders a stat CBC with a differential count to rule out a diagnosis of appendicitis. As Lisa is completing the blood draw, Pierce has several questions about his blood work and what it can tell the physician about his condition.

When Pierce's blood results come back, would you be able to tell what the results indicate?

1. What does the CBC measure, and why did the physician order a differential count?
   The blood tests return with the following results: "Hgb 14.6; Hct 46.1; WBCs 20,000; RBCs 5.3; Segs 75, Bands 1%, Eos 0%, Basos 0%, Mono 2%, Lymphs 22%, and Platelets 350,000."
2. Which of these results are abnormal, and which indicate a possible acute infection?

WEB SEARCH

1. **Research blood doping.** Some athletes, seeking a competitive edge, may resort to blood doping. What information do you need to have in order to discourage athletes from following this practice?
   - **Keywords:** Use the following keywords in your search: Blood doping, Illegal sports practices.
2. **Research current facts about blood and blood banking.** In society there are many myths about blood donation and receiving blood. It is important for the medical assistant to be knowledgeable about key facts concerning transfusions and donation.
   - **Keywords:** Use the following keywords in your search: American Association of Blood Banks, transfusion, blood donation.
3. **Research the incidence of anemia in the United States.** People who suffer from certain diseases are more likely to develop anemia. In addition, specific groups of people who are not suffering from disease may also be at risk. Medical assistants need to understand the incidence of anemia to provide better care to patients.
   - **Keywords:** Use the following keywords in your search: anemia, National Center for Health Statistics, incidence of anemia.

WORD PARTS: Blood, Lymphatic, and Immune Systems

BLOOD
Combining Forms

bas/o	base
coagul/o	clotting
cyt/o	cell
eosin/o	rosy, red
erythr/o	red
granul/o	granules
hem/o	blood
hemat/o	blood
hemoglobin/o	hemoglobin
leuk/o	white
phag/o	eat
thromb/o	clot

Suffixes

-cytosis	abnormal condition
-emia	blood condition
-globin	protein
-lytic	pertaining to destruction
-osis	abnormal condition
-penia	deficiency
-phage	eat
-poiesis	formation

LYMPHATIC AND IMMUNE SYSTEM
Combining Forms

immun/o	protection
lymph/o	lymph
splen/o	spleen
thym/o	thymus gland

Prefixes

ana-	again
inter-	between

ABBREVIATIONS: Lymphatic and Immune System

AIDS	acquired immunodeficiency syndrome
ELISA	enzyme-linked immunosorbent assay; test to detect anti-HIV antibodies
HD	Hodgkin's disease
HISTO	Histoplasmosis; fungal infection seen in AIDS patients
HIV	Human immunodeficiency virus; causes AIDS
HSV	Herpes simplex virus
KS	Kaposi's sarcoma

Respiratory System

14

evolve http://evolve.elsevier.com/klieger/medicalassisting

All humans need oxygen to survive. Our bodies use oxygen to extract energy from our food to support our cells, tissues, organs, and systems. We bring oxygen into our bodies by breathing. The process of breathing oxygen (O_2) in and carbon dioxide (CO_2) out is called *respiration* and is carried out by the respiratory system. This process also depends on the proper functioning of the circulatory system because this exchange of gases (O_2 for CO_2) occurs when the blood is transported to the lungs for absorption of oxygen and oxygen is distributed to the body cells through the blood vessels.

As with the cardiovascular system and all other body systems, it is very important that medical assistants understand the normal structure and function of the respiratory system so that they can better understand disease processes in this system.

LEARNING OBJECTIVES

You will be able to do the following after completing this chapter:

Key Terms
1. Define, appropriately use, and spell all the Key Terms for this chapter.

Structure and Function of the Respiratory System
2. List the two divisions of the respiratory system and identify the function of each.
3. Explain the purpose (function) of the respiratory system.
4. List the four main structures in the upper respiratory tract and describe the function of each.
5. List the four main structures in the lower respiratory tract and describe the function of each.

Breathing
6. Explain the difference between internal and external respiration.
7. List the two areas of the brain that control respiration, and identify which area regulates respiration subconsciously and which regulates respiration consciously.
8. Explain the importance of pulmonary function tests such as spirometry in the diagnosis of respiratory problems.

Respiratory Diseases and Disorders
9. List 10 common signs and symptoms of respiratory diseases and disorders.
10. List six common diagnostic tests for respiratory disease and describe the use of each.
11. List eight upper respiratory diseases and briefly describe the etiology, signs and symptoms, diagnosis, therapy, and interventions for each.
12. List 12 lower respiratory diseases and briefly describe the etiology, signs and symptoms, diagnosis, therapy, and interventions for each.

Patient-Centered Professionalism
13. Analyze a realistic medical office situation and apply your understanding of the respiratory system to determine the best course of action.
14. Describe the impact on patient care when medical assistants have a solid understanding of the structure and function of the respiratory system.

KEY TERMS

The Key Terms for this chapter have been organized into sections so that you can easily see the terminology associated with each aspect of the respiratory system.

Structure and Function of the Respiratory System
expiration
inspiration
lower respiratory tract
respiration
upper respiratory tract

Continued

Upper Respiratory Tract
Nose
cilia	nostrils
nasal septum	paranasal sinuses

Pharynx and Larynx
adenoids	nasopharynx
esophagus	oropharynx
laryngopharynx	palatine tonsils
larynx	pharynx (throat)

Lower Respiratory Tract
Trachea
epiglottis	trachea
thoracic	

Bronchi
bronchi	bronchioles

Alveoli
alveoli	surfactant
alveolus	

Lungs
diaphragm	inhalation
exhalation	lungs
hilum	pleura

Breathing
Ventilation Process
atmospheric pressure	internal (cellular) respiration
external (lung) respiration	phrenic nerve
intercostal muscles	ventilation

Regulation of Respiration
brainstem	medulla oblongata
cerebral cortex	pons

Respiratory Measurement
cardiopulmonary resuscitation (CPR)	spirometer
dead spaces	tidal volume
pulmonary function tests (PFTs)	

Respiratory Diseases and Disorders
Signs and Symptoms
aphonia	hypoxia
apnea	pneumothorax
asphyxia	pulmonary edema
clubbing	rales
dysphonia	rhonchi
dyspnea	sputum
hemoptysis	stridor
hemothorax	wheezes

Diagnostic Tests and Procedures
arterial blood gases (ABGs)	lung scan
bronchoscopy	magnetic resonance imaging (MRI)
chest x-ray	pulse oximetry
computed tomography (CT) scan	ultrasonography

Upper Respiratory Disorders
croup	pharyngitis
epistaxis	rhinitis
influenza	sinusitis
laryngitis	upper respiratory infection (URI)
pertussis	

Lower Respiratory Disorders
asthma	lung cancer
atelectasis	pleurisy
avian influenza (H5N1)	pneumonia
bronchitis	pulmonary embolism
bronchodilators	severe acute respiratory syndrome (SARS)
chronic obstructive pulmonary disease (COPD)	sudden infant death syndrome (SIDS)
emphysema	tuberculosis (pulmonary)

PRACTICAL APPLICATIONS

Read the following scenario and keep it in mind as you learn about the respiratory system in this chapter.

Mr. Chazara, who has a long history of smoking both cigarettes and cigars, has been diagnosed with COPD with constriction of the bronchi. He is dyspneic with stridor and wheezing. When he is seen by the physician, an order is written for spirometry testing. The testing is positive for a mild loss of vital capacity and for a moderate decrease in forced expiratory volume. Because of the decreased lung capacity, an order is also written for measurement of ABGs. In addition, Mr. Chazara has sinus congestion and a productive cough, but he has no fever; he needs medications for the congestion and the loss of lung function.

Do you understand the cause of Mr. Chazara's symptoms? Would you be able to explain the need for these tests to him?

STRUCTURE AND FUNCTION OF THE RESPIRATORY SYSTEM

It is important to understand the basic structure of the respiratory system as well as its purpose, or function.

Structure

The respiratory system is divided into the following two sections (Figure 14-1):

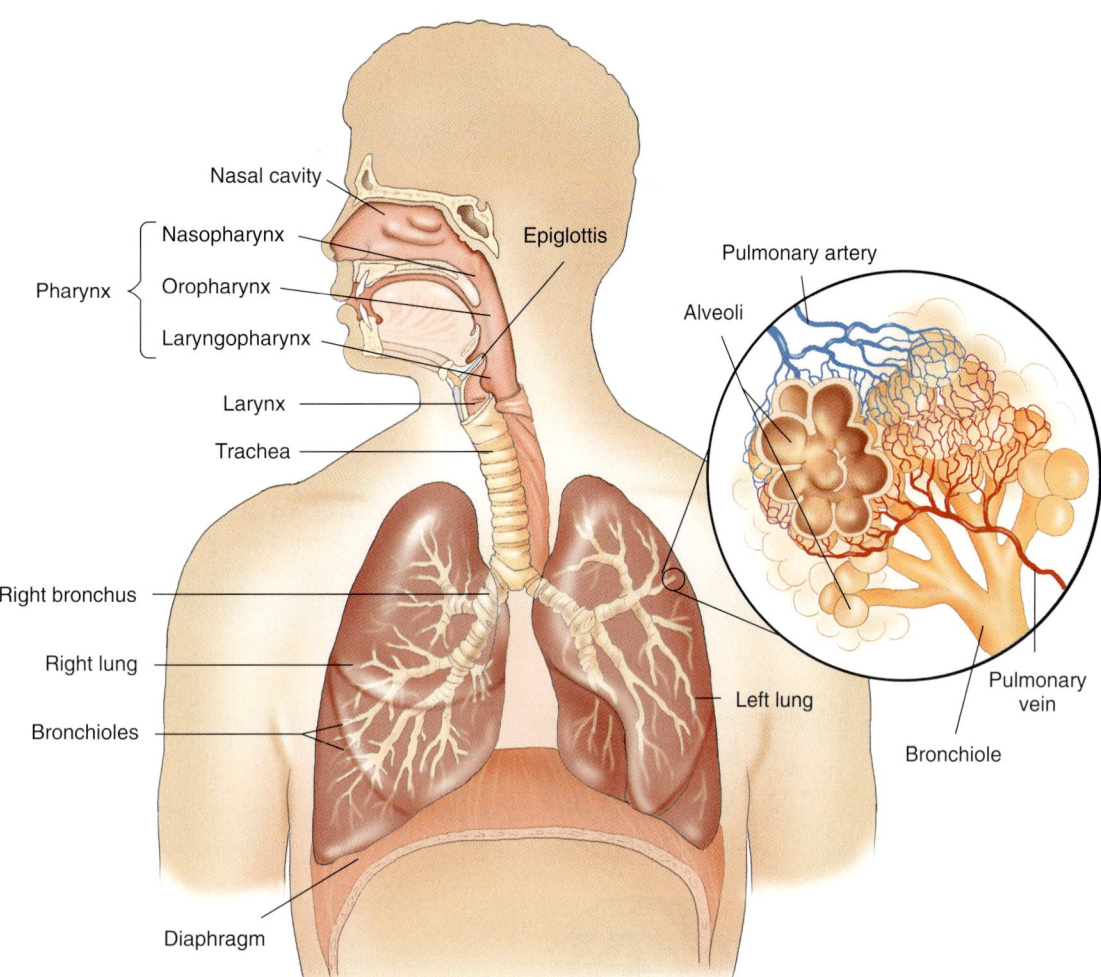

FIGURE 14-1 Structures of the respiratory system: upper and lower respiratory tracts. (From Leonard PC: *Building a medical vocabulary*, ed 6, St Louis, 2005, Saunders.)

- **Upper respiratory tract:** the nose, sinuses, pharynx (throat), and larynx ("voice box")
- **Lower respiratory tract:** the trachea ("windpipe"), bronchi, alveoli, and lungs

Function

The respiratory system provides oxygen (O_2) to the blood that is used for the manufacture of energy in the cells. It also removes and eliminates carbon dioxide (CO_2), a waste product, from the blood. This exchange process is ongoing and depends on the proper functioning of the organs that make up the upper and lower respiratory tracts. The lungs function to maintain the acid-base balance within the body through the exchange of oxygen and carbon dioxide. When the two tracts of the respiratory system work together, air is taken in and travels to the lungs, where O_2 is transferred to the blood and CO_2 is removed and expelled to the outside. This body process of inhaling O_2 (**inspiration**) to the lungs and exhaling CO_2 (**expiration**) is **respiration.**

PATIENT-CENTERED PROFESSIONALISM

- The respiratory system has two main functions. Why is it important for the medical assistant to understand the structure and function of the respiratory system?
- Knowing that the circulatory and respiratory systems work together to supply cells with the necessary oxygen and to remove metabolic wastes, how would the patient's respiratory system be affected if the heart was not able to pump blood efficiently?

UPPER RESPIRATORY TRACT

The upper respiratory tract warms, moisturizes, and cleans the air that is taken in during inspiration. This is accomplished through the four structures in the upper respiratory tract: the nose, sinuses, pharynx, and larynx (Figure 14-2).

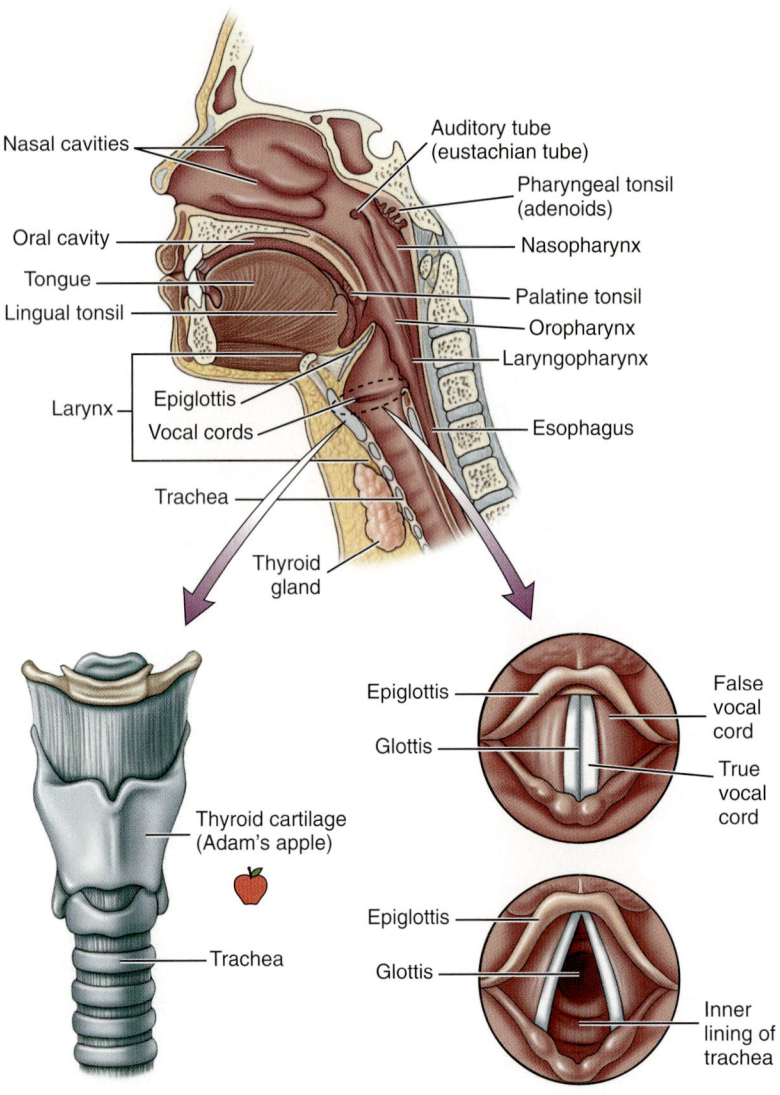

FIGURE 14-2 Organs of the upper respiratory tract. (From Herlihy B, Maebius NK: *The human body in health and illness,* ed 3, St Louis, 2007, Saunders.)

Nose

The nose performs two functions: (1) registers the sense of smell and (2) acts as a passageway for air. The nose is composed of bone and cartilage covered by skin and lined by a mucous membrane. The **nostrils** (nares) form the entrance to the nasal passages. Hairs are located at the entrance to filter out particles. The nasal cavities are separated by a partition, the **nasal septum.** Besides cartilage, the nose is comprised of several facial bones: the *ethmoid bone, vomer, palatine bone,* and the *hard palate.* The nasal passages and respiratory tract are lined with a mucous membrane that contains many microscopic hairlike projections (**cilia**) responsible for trapping dust and bacteria as air is inhaled to prevent their passage to the lungs.

Sinuses

The **paranasal sinuses** are basically air-filled cavities in the bones of the skull. They are lined with ciliated mucous membrane. As air passes through these cavities, it is warmed, cleaned, and moisturized.

There are four pairs of paranasal sinuses that drain into the nose (Figure 14-3), as follows:
1. Frontal sinuses
2. Maxillary sinuses
3. Ethmoidal sinuses
4. Sphenoidal sinuses

Pharynx

When air is inhaled through the nose, it passes through the paranasal sinuses where it is moistened and through the **pharynx** (throat) to the trachea. Air also passes through the mouth and into the pharynx when food is consumed. If a person breathes through the mouth when the nasal passages are clogged (e.g., during a common cold), the air is not filtered or moistened.

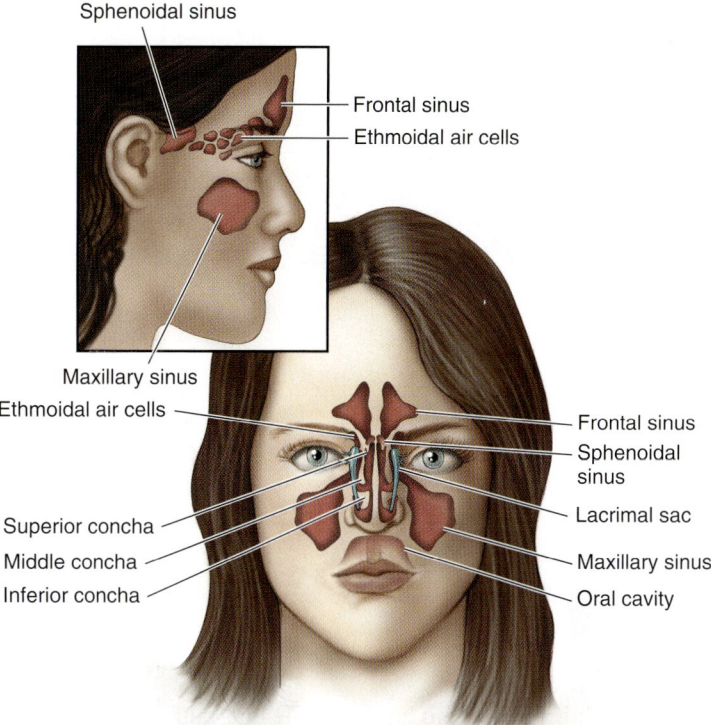

FIGURE 14-3 Paranasal sinuses. (Modified from Thibodeau GA, Patton KT: *The human body in health and disease,* ed 4, St Louis, 2005, Mosby.)

Essentially, the pharynx is a passageway for air and food. It is divided into three sections: the nasopharynx, oropharynx, and laryngopharynx.

The **nasopharynx,** the upper portion behind the nasal cavity, extends from the posterior nares to the soft palate. The **adenoids** are located in the nasopharynx.

The **oropharynx,** the middle portion behind the mouth, extends from the soft palate to the upper portion of the epiglottis. The oropharynx contains the palatine tonsils. The **palatine tonsils** are located on either side of the soft palate in the oropharynx. The tonsils are lymphatic tissues that filter out bacteria and viruses, preventing their entry into the respiratory tract. The tonsils are important for filtering organisms in children, but as people age, these tissues atrophy.

The **laryngopharynx** is the lower portion behind the larynx. This area ends above the larynx and branches into the larynx and the **esophagus** at the epiglottis.

FOR YOUR INFORMATION

"Pharynx" and "larynx" are frequently mispronounced. Note they both end in "-ynx."
Pharynx is pronounced "**fair** inks" (not "fair nicks").
Larynx is pronounced "**lair** inks" (not "lair nicks").

PATIENT-CENTERED PROFESSIONALISM

- Why is it important that the air we breathe is filtered, warmed, and humidified before its passage into the pharynx?
- What happens when cold air passes over the vocal cords?

Larynx

Located at the top of the trachea is the **larynx** ("voice box"), which holds the vocal cords and is surrounded by several pieces of cartilage for support. The thyroid cartilage is the largest and is referred to as the *Adam's apple* (see Figure 14-2). In addition to guarding the entrance to the trachea, the function of the larynx is to produce sound. Sound is produced when air passes over the vocal folds (cords). Tightened cords produce a high-pitched sound, and relaxed cords produce a low-pitched sound. If air is pushed out of the lungs more forcefully, the voice will be louder. If there is less pressure, the voice will be softer. The nose, sinuses, and mouth also influence the sound of the voice.

LOWER RESPIRATORY TRACT

The lower respiratory tract takes the air that was warmed, moisturized, and cleaned in the upper respiratory tract and moves it to the lungs, where O_2 can be exchanged for CO_2. This is accomplished through the four structures in the lower respiratory tract: the trachea, bronchi, alveoli, and lungs.

Trachea

The **trachea** ("windpipe") is a tube located in the front of the esophagus. It is composed of C-shaped rings of cartilage that prevent it from collapsing (Figure 14-4). The trachea extends from the larynx to the level of the **thoracic** vertebrae and divides into two tubes (bronchi), one for each lung. The **epiglottis** is attached to the base of the tongue. When a person swallows, the epiglottis moves over the trachea so that food or

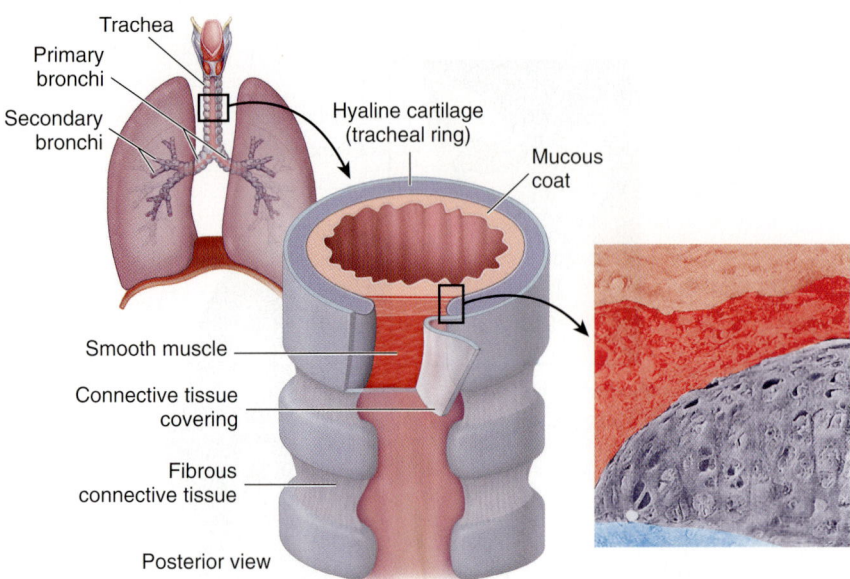

FIGURE 14-4 Cross-section of the trachea. Scanning electron micrograph shows the tip of one of the C-shaped cartilage rings. (Modified from Thibodeau GA, Patton KT: *The human body in health and disease,* ed 4, St Louis, 2005, Mosby.)

drink does not mix with air and enter the lungs through the trachea.

Bronchi

Air leaves the trachea and enters the **bronchi** (Figure 14-5). The main function of the bronchi is to provide a passageway through which air can reach the lungs.

The bronchi are composed of smooth muscle and have C-shaped rings of cartilage similar to the trachea. The right bronchus is shorter and at less of an angle than the left bronchus. Because of its size and position, foreign bodies entering the trachea often lodge in the right lung.

The bronchi branch into smaller tubes or branches (**bronchioles**) as they enter the lungs.

Alveoli

At the end of the bronchioles are tiny air sacs called **alveoli**. The walls of each **alveolus** (singular form of alveoli) are surrounded by capillaries that carry on the exchange of O_2 and CO_2 in the blood. These microscopic structures are numerous and lined with a membrane covered by **surfactant**. Surfactant is a fatty substance that lines the air sacs. It reduces the surface tension in the alveoli, thus reducing the chance for collapse when air moves in and out during respiration (Figure 14-6). Lack of adequate amounts of surfactant at birth, especially in a premature infant, results in *respiratory distress syndrome (RDS)*.

Lungs

The cone-shaped **lungs** are spongy and expandable. They are covered by a thin double-layered sac, the **pleura**, and are protected by the rib cage. The parietal pleural membrane lines the chest cavity, allowing the lungs to move easily within the chest cavity. The lungs are located in the thoracic cavity and each lung is divided into lobes. The *right lung* has three lobes (superior, middle, and inferior) and is slightly larger than the left lung. The *left lung* has only two lobes (upper and lower) because it shares thoracic cavity space with the heart (see Figure 14-5). The apex (top) of each lung extends just above the first rib and the base is the lower portion of the lung. The **hilum** is located in the midline area between the lungs where nerves, lymphatic tissue, blood vessels, and the bronchial tubes enter and exit.

The main muscle of breathing, the **diaphragm**, is located below the lungs. During inspiration, the diaphragm moves down and expands the volume of the thoracic cavity; during expiration, the cavity volume is reduced by the diaphragm moving upward.

The main function of the lungs is the exchange of O_2 and CO_2 with each respiration.

PATIENT-CENTERED PROFESSIONALISM

- What type of specialist would a patient with chronic breathing problems visit?
- What happens when the diaphragm becomes irritated?

BREATHING

Ventilation is the cyclical process of moving air into and out of the lungs, also referred to as *breathing* (respiration). If patients are unable to breathe on their own, mechanical assistance (ventilator) can be provided. Understanding the ventilation process and how the body regulates respiration, as well as ways to measure respiration, is important.

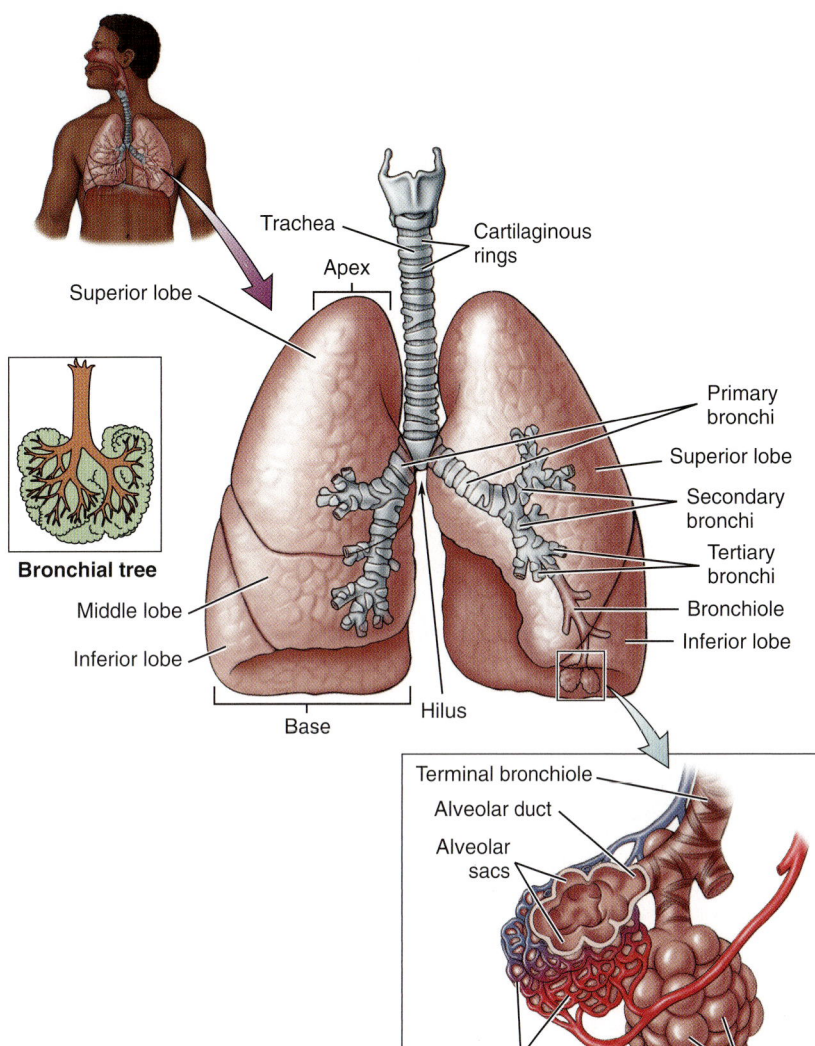

FIGURE 14-5 Trachea and bronchial tree (bronchi, bronchioles, and alveoli). (From Herlihy B, Maebius NK: *The human body in health and illness,* ed 2, St Louis, 2007, Saunders.)

Ventilation Process

When **atmospheric pressure** (pressure of the outside air) is greater than the pressure within the lung, inspiration occurs (Figure 14-7, *B*). When pressure within the lungs is greater than that of the air outside, air leaves the lungs and moves outward (expiration) (Figure 14-7, *C*). Atmospheric pressure remains constant, but pressure changes occur in the thoracic cavity (chest) and the lungs with each **inhalation** and **exhalation**. Figure 14-8 illustrates the mechanism of inhalation and exhalation.

Air is breathed in (inspiration) when the diaphragm is stimulated by the **phrenic nerve,** causing it and the **intercostal muscles** in the chest wall to contract. A vacuum is therefore created within the chest cavity. When these muscles relax, expiration occurs as the lungs expand to fill the cavity, forcing air out.

Remember, respiration is the exchange of O_2 and CO_2 gases among air, blood, and cells. Two types of respiration take place during ventilation, as follows:

- **External (lung) respiration** is the exchange of O_2 for CO_2 within the alveoli, or "lung breathing."
- **Internal (cellular) respiration** is the exchange of O_2 for CO_2 within the cells.

Without external respiration, cellular respiration cannot be accomplished.

FOR YOUR INFORMATION

The incidence of emphysema and chronic bronchitis increase as we age, mainly due to environmental changes. As a person ages the immune system is not as effective and diminishes a person's ability to fight off respiratory infections (e.g., pneumonia). As with the circulatory system (blood vessels), structural changes occur with the loss of elasticity in the alveoli.

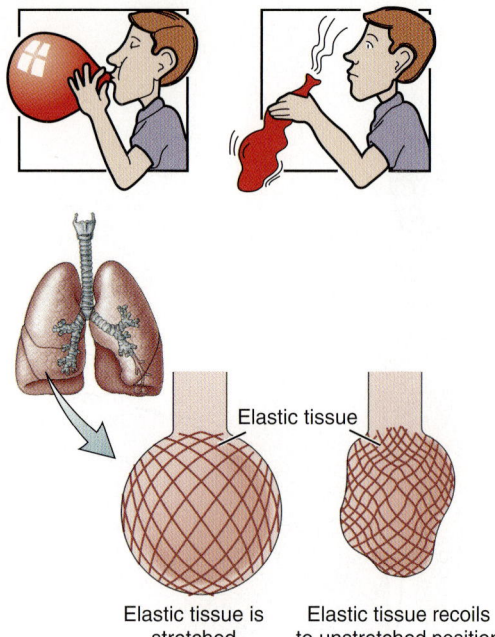

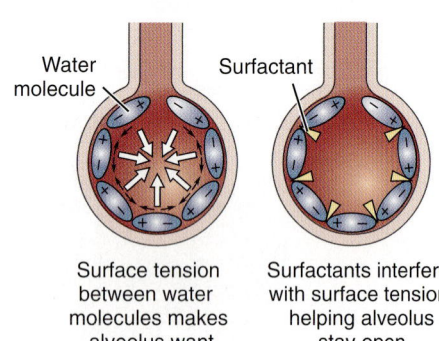

FIGURE 14-6 A balloon is made of elastic fibers that remain expanded as long as air pressure maintains tension, similar to the alveolus. Surface tension would collapse the alveolus, but pulmonary surfactants decrease surface tension, preventing the alveolus from collapsing. (From Herlihy B, Maebius NK: *The human body in health and illness,* ed 3, St Louis, 2007, Saunders.)

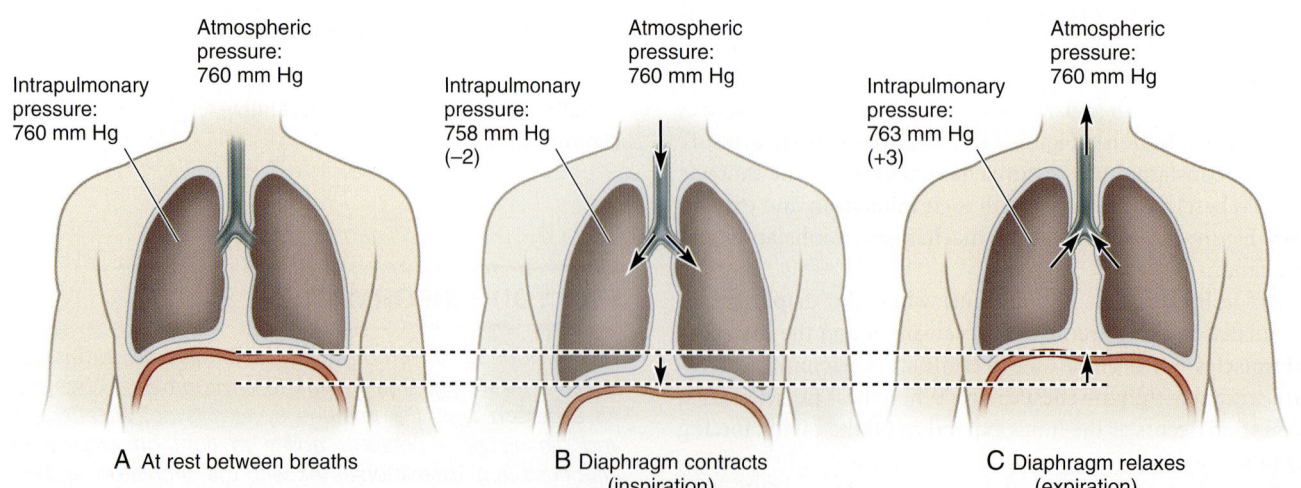

FIGURE 14-7 Pressures in pulmonary ventilation (breathing). (Modified from Applegate EJ: *The anatomy and physiology learning system,* ed 3, St Louis, 2006, Saunders.)

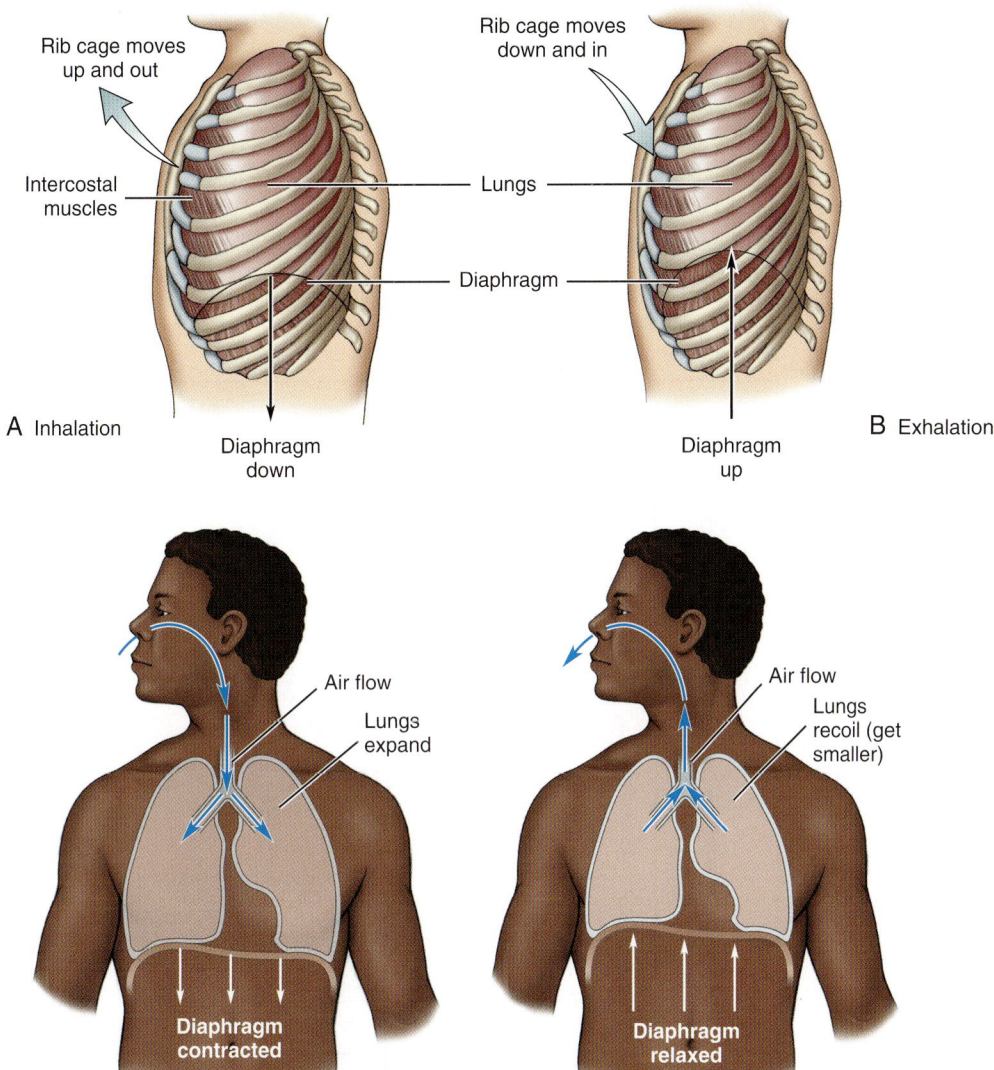

FIGURE 14-8 Inhalation and exhalation. (Modified from Herlihy B, Maebius NK: *The human body in health and illness,* ed 3, St Louis, 2007, Saunders.)

Regulation of Respiration

As you have learned, the process of respiration is necessary to maintain the proper levels of oxygen and carbon dioxide in the body tissues.

At the top of the spinal cord is the **brainstem.** Two components of the brainstem cause respiration to function *unconsciously* (automatically or involuntarily): the **pons** and **medulla oblongata.** The pons modifies and helps control breathing patterns, and the medulla is the main control center of breathing. Also, involuntary control of respiration is caused by the concentration of CO_2 in the blood. Respiration can also be controlled *consciously* or *voluntarily* (e.g., holding your breath or taking a long, slow, deep breath). Conscious control of respiration occurs in the **cerebral cortex.**

Respiratory Measurement

Health professionals measure ventilation for many reasons. For example, ventilatory function might be measured to check for an obstruction of airflow such as asthma, a tumor, or a swallowed object. Ventilation is also assessed to assist in the diagnosis of other respiratory diseases. Because the amount of air exchanged during respiration is related to the atmosphere and the resistance to airflow, measuring airflow and lung capacity can provide information about a patient's respiratory process.

Pulmonary function tests (PFTs) measure lung capacity (Table 14-1). Remember, PFTs do not diagnose a specific respiratory disease but identify the presence of pulmonary impairment. Several different diseases may cause a test result to be abnormal. One PFT used in many medical offices is *spirometry* (Figure 14-9). A **spirometer** is used to determine the **tidal volume,** or the amount of air inhaled and exhaled (e.g., air moved in and out of the lungs) during normal respiration.

When exhalation occurs after a normal breath, the air remaining in the lungs is considered *reserve volume.* Keep in mind that some air also remains in the upper respiratory tract,

TABLE 14-1

Pulmonary Function Tests (PFTs)*

Volume or Capacity	Definition	Amount
Tidal volume (TV)	Amount of air taken into and out of the lungs during respiration	500 mL
Residual volume (RV)	Amount of air that remains in the lungs after a maximal expiration	1200 mL
Inspiratory reserve volume (IRV)	Amount of air that can be forcibly inhaled after a normal inhalation	3000 mL
Expiratory reserve volume (ERV) ERV = FRC − RV	Amount of air that can be forcibly exhaled after a normal exhalation	1100 mL
Vital capacity (VC)	Amount of air that can be exhaled after maximum inhalation	4600 mL
Total lung capacity (TLC)	Total amount of air in the lung after maximum inhalation	—
Functional residual capacity (FRC)	Amount of air remaining in the lungs after normal expiration	5800 mL

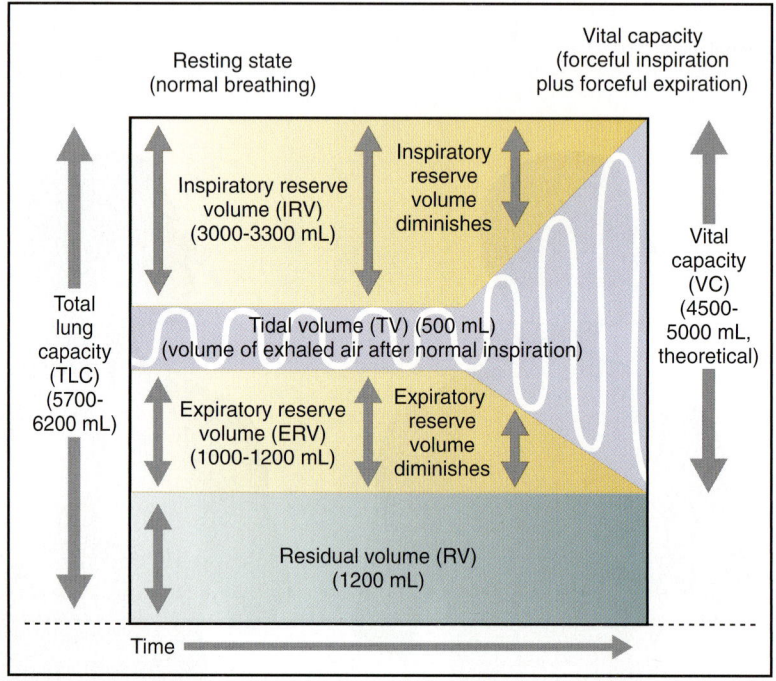

Figure from Gerdin J: *Health careers today,* ed 4, St Louis, 2007, Mosby.
*PFT measurements can be used to diagnose respiratory problems and to monitor patients' lung function.

bronchi, and bronchioles in **dead spaces.** This air never reaches the alveoli. It contains oxygen that is invaluable during **cardiopulmonary resuscitation (CPR).**

PATIENT-CENTERED PROFESSIONALISM

- *The lungs maintain the acid-base balance of the body by altering the rate and depth of respiration in response to changes in blood pH. What happens if the acid-base balance in the body is disrupted?*
- *Why is it important for the medical assistant to understand how respiration is regulated?*

RESPIRATORY DISEASES AND DISORDERS

Pulmonologists, otolaryngologists, and allergists specialize in treating diseases or conditions affecting the respiratory tract. Respiratory diseases and disorders can be classified according to the area affected: upper respiratory or lower respiratory tract. Many upper respiratory diseases are infectious and are responsible for lower respiratory diseases. Persons with a cold or the flu may also experience inflammation and swelling of the mucous membranes; these common symptoms are referred to as an **upper respiratory infection (URI).**

Respiratory disease usually causes the person's respiratory rate to increase in an attempt to get more air to the lungs. This causes the heart to work harder to supply the body's tissues with oxygen. Drugs may be prescribed to treat respiratory problems (Table 14-2).

Medical assistants need to be able to recognize the common signs and symptoms of and the diagnostic tests for the different types of respiratory disease.

- Study Box 14-1 to familiarize yourself with the signs and symptoms.
- Study Box 14-2 to learn about common diagnostic tests.

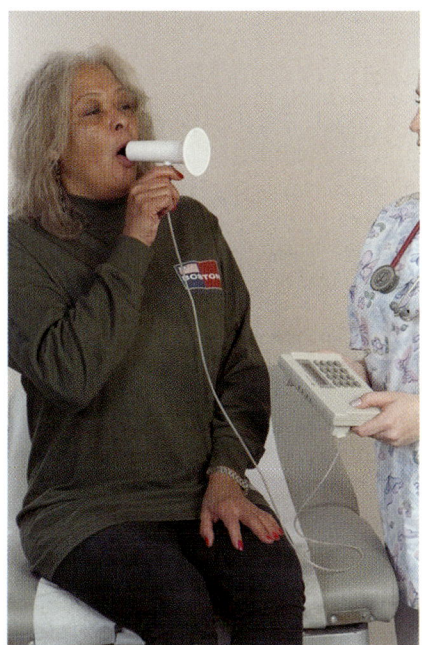

FIGURE 14-9 Spirometry uses a computer to measure the amounts of air taken in and exhaled.

TABLE 14-2
Respiratory Drug Classifications

Drug Classification	Common Generic (Brand) Names
Antihistamines	
Block histamine release; histamine constricts bronchial muscle.	fexofenadine (Allegra)
	loratadine (Claritin)
Antitussives	
Suppress the cough reflex.	dextromethorphan (Vicks Formula 44)
	codeine (Robitussin A-C)
Bronchodilators	
Relax bronchi.	albuterol (Proventil)
	theophylline (Theo-Dur)
Decongestants	
Reduce congestion or swelling of mucous membrane.	phenylephrine (Neo-Synephrine)
	oxymetazoline (Afrin)
Expectorants	
Promote expulsion of mucus from respiratory tract.	guaifenesin (Robitussin)
	iodinated glycerol (Organidin)

BOX 14-1
Common Signs and Symptoms of Respiratory Disease

Aphonia	Loss of ability to produce sounds
Apnea	Periodic cessation of breathing
Asphyxia	Insufficient intake of O_2
Atelectasis	Incomplete lung expansion; lung collapse
Clubbing	Abnormal enlargement of ends of fingers caused by low blood oxygen (Figure 14-10)
Dysphonia	Hoarseness; difficulty speaking
Dyspnea	Difficulty breathing
Hemoptysis	Spitting of blood from respiratory tract
Hemothorax	Blood in pleural cavity (Figure 14-11, *A*)
Hypoxia	Inadequate oxygen in tissues
Pneumothorax	Accumulation of air or gas in pleural space (Figure 14-11, *B*)
Pulmonary edema	Fluid in the lungs; common complication of cardiac disorders
Rales	Crackling sounds heard during inspiration
Rhonchi	Loud, low-pitched bubbling sounds heard during inspiration or expiration
Sputum	Mucus coughed up from the lungs
Stridor	High-pitched breathing heard during inspiration and associated with obstructed airway
Wheezes	High-pitched musical sounds caused by narrowing of respiratory passages; heard mainly during expiration

- Study Table 14-3 to understand the diseases of the upper and lower respiratory tracts.

New respiratory diseases continue to surface as more people share the same space. Severe acute respiratory syndrome (**SARS**) is a viral disease that apparently originated in China in 2003 (Box 14-3). Most of the cases that occurred in the United States were among travelers who had been to parts of the world where SARS was a problem.

PATIENT-CENTERED PROFESSIONALISM

- When the respiratory system is assessed for signs of disease, what methods are used?
- Why is it important for the medical assistant to understand the various diagnostic tests used to evaluate lung function?
- How can the medical assistant's understanding of the diseases of the respiratory system improve the care the patient receives at the medical office?

Text continued on p. 258

BOX 14-2

Diagnostic Tests and Procedures for the Respiratory System

Arterial blood gases (ABGs)	Measurement provides levels of oxygen and carbon dioxide in arterial blood to evaluate acid-base balance
Bronchoscopy	Endoscopic procedure used to visually examine the bronchial tubes (Figure 14-12)
Chest x-ray	Radiographic method used to visualize the lungs (Figure 14-13)
Computed tomography (CT) scan	Series of x-ray pictures taken at different angles, forming a composite, cross-sectional view of the organ or area of interest
Lung scan	Nuclear scanning test used to detect a blood clot
Magnetic resonance imaging (MRI)	Technique of visualizing soft tissues of the body by applying an external magnetic field that causes the hydrogen atoms in different body environments to release energy that is transformed into an image
Pulse oximetry	Test to measure the amount of oxygen in arterial blood
Ultrasonography	Technique that uses high-frequency sound waves to produce an image of the interior structure of a hollow organ

TABLE 14-3

Diseases and Disorders of the Respiratory System

Disease and Description	Etiology	Signs and Symptoms	Diagnosis	Therapy	Interventions
UPPER RESPIRATORY TRACT					
Croup — Acute respiratory disorder in children	Caused by a virus and usually follows an upper respiratory infection	Hoarseness, fever, barklike cough	Physical examination, presenting symptoms	Bedrest, antibiotic therapy, fluid intake, antipyretics, humidification	Encourage patients to seek treatment for respiratory infections
Epistaxis — Nosebleed	Cause could be trauma to nose, secondary condition resulting from sinusitis, rhinitis, nasal irritation, and hypertension	Blood loss from nostrils	Observation of episode	Find site of bleeding; initial action is to press nostrils together and apply cold compresses to area above nose and to back of neck	Keep air humidified in dry climates
Influenza — Flu; viral infection of upper respiratory tract	Caused by viruses transmitted by coughing, sneezing, and personal contact	Onset is sudden, with chills, fever, cough, muscle aches, and upper respiratory involvement	Based on patient's symptoms and knowledge of outbreaks in area	Rest, fluid intake, analgesics, antipyretics	Avoid giving aspirin because of its link with Reye syndrome in children
Laryngitis — Inflammation of larynx and vocal cords	Bacterial or viral infection; also caused by chemical irritants or complication of upper respiratory condition	Presentation of symptoms, including lack of voice; complaints of malaise	Examination of pharynx	Rest voice; use of antibiotics if bacterial infection is the cause	Avoid irritating substances (e.g., smoke, extreme air temperature, alcohol)
Pertussis — Whooping cough	Bacterial infection (*Bordetella pertussis*)	Gradual onset of fever and dry cough progressing to severe cough in rapid successions; cough with whooping inspiration	History of contact with infected person; increased white blood cells, with culture of identifying bacteria in secretions	Antibiotics, adequate fluid intake, nutrition	Receive immunizations beginning at age 2 months through age 2 for pertussis

TABLE 14-3
Diseases and Disorders of the Respiratory System—cont'd

Disease and Description	Etiology	Signs and Symptoms	Diagnosis	Therapy	Interventions
Pharyngitis Inflammation of throat	Bacterial or viral infection	Complaints of sore throat and difficulty swallowing	Physical examination, appearance of reddened throat	Analgesics and antipyretics, warm saline gargles; antibiotics for bacterial infection	Encourage patient to follow treatment plan to avoid secondary infection
Rhinitis Common cold	Viral infection (usually rhinovirus)	Mild chills and fatigue within a day, mild sore or scratchy throat, congestion, clear rhinorrhea (runny nose), cough, headache; sinus pain and pressure are common early symptoms	Physical examination and presentation of characteristic symptoms	Rest, fluid intake; antibiotics have no role in treatment of viral rhinitis; decongestants and pain relievers relieve symptoms but do not shorten duration of illness	Encourage rest and symptomatic treatment, if necessary
Sinusitis Inflammation of paranasal sinuses	Bacterial or viral infection	Swollen and tender area over affected cavity; low-grade fever with rhinorrhea and possible drainage	Culture of drainage, x-rays of sinus	Antibiotic for bacterial infection and drainage of affected sinus as needed	Encourage patient to follow treatment plan to avoid complications (e.g., permanent damage to mucosal lining)
LOWER RESPIRATORY TRACT					
Asthma Occurs when the bronchi and bronchioles contract	Cause could be in response to allergen, drug, exercise, or stress	Wheezing, dyspnea, complaints of chest tightness	Clinical evaluation to confirm patient's complaints; pulmonary function studies (PFTs)	**Bronchodilators**	Encourage patient to avoid triggering agents; early treatment for upper respiratory infection (URI)
Bronchitis Inflammation of bronchial mucous membranes	Caused by irritants, bacteria, or viral infection	Dry, hacking cough with mucus	Type of cough and sputum; chest x-rays to rule out other disorders	Antibiotic therapy with increased fluid intake; bedrest	Obtain treatment for URI
Chronic obstructive pulmonary disease (COPD) Combination of respiratory diseases, including chronic bronchitis, asthma, and emphysema	Various causes (e.g., viral, long-term smoking, exposure to pollutants)	Patient unable to ventilate the lungs adequately	Prior patient history of other obstructive pulmonary diseases	Medications, including bronchodilators and antibiotics; avoidance of respiratory irritants	Provide supportive care
Emphysema Results in abnormal distention and destruction of alveoli	Risk factors include irritants that cause chronic inflammation to alveolar sacs (e.g., smoke, pollution)	Chronic cough, dyspnea, shortness of breath, complaints of fatigue	History of smoking; barrel chest, clubbed fingers; PFTs	Bronchodilators and exercise to promote ventilation and cardiac function; oxygen therapy on low setting to correct hypoxia	Encourage patient to have flu and pneumonia vaccines; provide supportive care and answer questions about fluids and nutritional needs

TABLE 14-3

Diseases and Disorders of the Respiratory System—cont'd

Disease and Description	Etiology	Signs and Symptoms	Diagnosis	Therapy	Interventions
Lung cancer Malignant neoplasm of lung tissue	Risk factors include tobacco smoking, exposure to carcinogenic particles, pollutants, and genetic disposition	Coughing caused by tumor stimulation of nerve ending, hemoptysis, dyspnea, hoarseness, shortness of breath on exertion, edema of upper torso	Chest x-rays; needle biopsy of lung tissue, sputum analysis, bronchoscopy	Radiation therapy and chemotherapy to reduce size of tumor; possible surgery to remove section of lung (lobectomy) or entire lung (pneumonectomy)	Provide supportive care; encourage increased fluid and nutritional intake; provide palliative care for pain
Pleurisy Inflamed pleural surfaces of lungs	Injury to pleura (e.g., trauma, pneumonia)	Sudden onset of pain in the chest area aggravated by breathing and coughing	Auscultation detects rales; x-rays reveal an effusion	Pain medication; antipyretics for fever; bedrest, increased fluid intake, nutritional balance	Show patient how to splint the chest area when coughing to decrease discomfort
Pneumonia Inflammation of lung tissues	Caused by bacteria, chemical irritant, or virus	Often begins as URI, and progresses with chills, dyspnea, and purulent sputum	Culture of sputum; blood work shows excess of white blood cells; x-rays, PFTs	Broad-spectrum antibiotics; analgesics for pain; rest, increased fluid intake, nutritional balance	Encourage patients, especially elderly persons, to have influenza and pneumonia vaccines
Pulmonary embolism A clot dislodges and obstructs the pulmonary vascular branch either partially or completely	*Thrombus* from a deep vein injury or long-term immobility (e.g., wheelchair bound, long air flights) moves to the lungs; can also be postoperative complication	Shortness of breath, tachycardia, possible low-grade fever, warm and tender area in lower extremities	Patient history, predisposing condition (e.g., chronic lung disorder, long bone fracture, history of vascular insufficiency); lung scan, chest x-ray	Maintain adequate cardiovascular and pulmonary function; oxygen therapy as needed; anticoagulants to prevent formulation of clots	Encourage rest until stabilized; encourage deep-breathing exercises; remind patient to report abnormal bleeding (e.g., epistaxis, petechiae, occult blood in stool and urine, large bruises); stress importance of taking medications
Sudden infant death syndrome (SIDS) Sudden, unexplained death of an infant	Unknown; theory suggests relation to brainstem defect at birth	Infant found dead in crib	Autopsy	None	Provide psychological and emotional support for family; for infants at risk, use home monitoring device; position infants on back, without pillows or soft bedding, for sleeping
Tuberculosis (pulmonary) Bacterial infection of lungs, although bacteria can affect other areas of body; mandatory reporting to county public health office	*Mycobacterium tuberculosis* is primary agent; spread by aerosol droplets	Insidious onset; complaints of malaise, afternoon fever, weight loss, cough, hemoptysis; night sweats	Chest x-ray; positive tuberculin test or positive sputum culture	Antibiotic therapy, bedrest, adequate fluid intake with improved nutrition	Isolate infected persons; preventive measures; drug treatment plan

BOX 14-3
Respiratory Disease Update

The epidemic strain of *severe acute respiratory syndrome* (SARS) that caused the deaths of at least 774 people in 2003 has not been a problem since April 2004. The Centers for Disease Control and Prevention (CDC) and the World Health Organization (WHO) continue to monitor the situation globally.

In mid 2003 outbreaks of the **avian influenza** *(H5N1)* began in southeast Asia, and by July 2005 the virus had spread along the migratory routes of wild water fowl.

These diseases both cause lung failure.

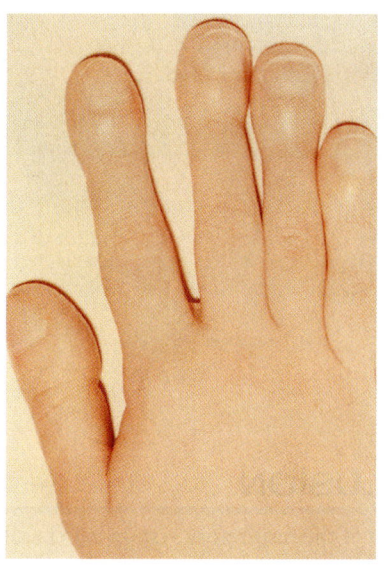

FIGURE 14-10 Clubbing. (From Zitelli BJ, Davis HW: *Atlas of pediatric physical diagnosis,* ed 4, St Louis, 2002, Mosby.)

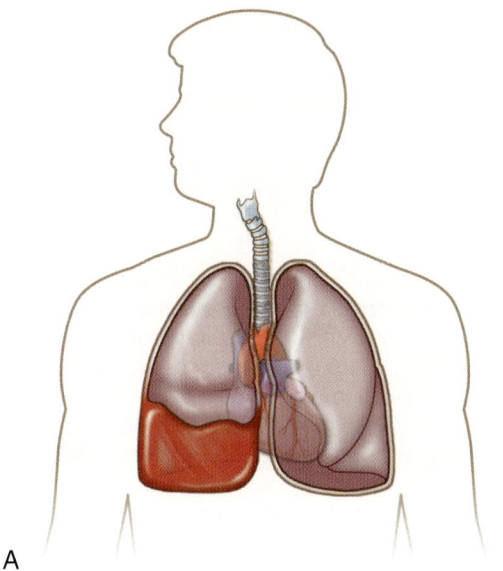

A

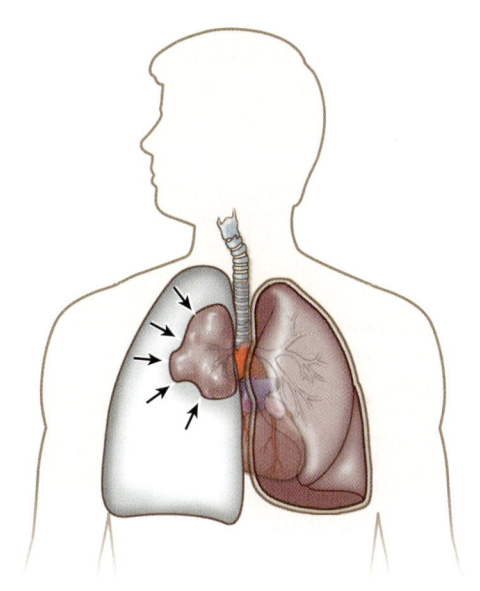

B

FIGURE 14-11 A, Hemothorax. Blood below left lung causes lung to collapse. **B,** Pneumothorax. Lung collapses as air gathers in pleural space. (Modified from Shiland BJ: *Mastering healthcare terminology,* ed 2, St Louis, 2006, Mosby.)

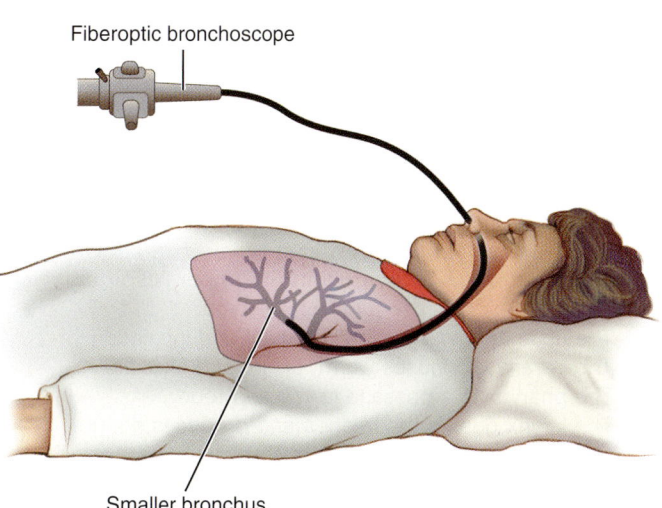

FIGURE 14-12 Bronchoscopy. (Modified from Shiland BJ: *Mastering healthcare terminology,* ed 2, St Louis, 2006, Mosby.)

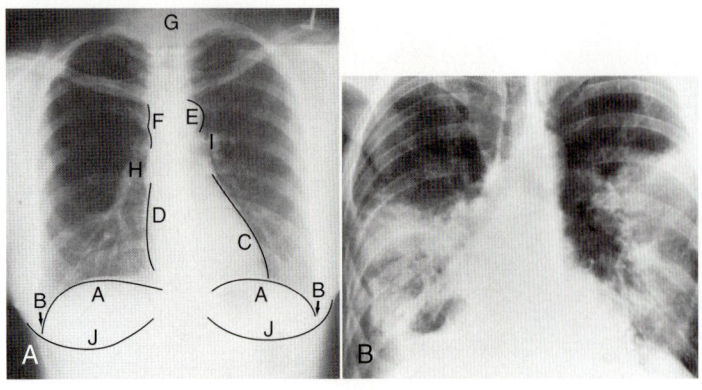

FIGURE 14-13 **A,** Normal posteroanterior (PA) chest x-ray. (Backward "L" in upper right corner is placed on film to indicate left side of patient's chest.) *A,* Diaphragm; *B,* costophrenic angle; *C,* left ventricle; *D,* right atrium; *E,* aortic arch; *F,* superior vena cava; *G,* trachea; *H,* right bronchus; *I,* left bronchus; *J,* breast shadows. **B,** X-ray showing lung of patient with pneumonia. (**A** From Black JM et al: *Medical-surgical nursing: clinical management for positive outcomes,* ed 8, St Louis, 2009, Saunders; **B** From Black JM et al: *Medical-surgical nursing: clinical management for positive outcomes,* ed 6, Philadelphia, 2001, WB Saunders.)

CONCLUSION

The function of the respiratory system is to breathe in air and exchange gases so that O_2 can be supplied to and CO_2 removed from body tissues. In addition, the respiratory system warms, filters, and humidifies the air we breathe. The nerve impulses from the brain interact with the diaphragm, larynx, and the lungs to coordinate external and internal respiration. Cardiac disorders greatly affect how well the respiratory system works, and the functioning of the respiratory system depends on the proper functioning of the circulatory system. This is another example of how one system impacts the functioning of other systems and allows the body to maintain homeostasis. With a good understanding of the structure and function of the respiratory system, you will be better able to work with patients experiencing respiratory problems.

Chapter Summary

Reinforce your understanding of the material in this chapter by reviewing the curriculum objectives and key content points below.

1. **Define, appropriately use, and spell all the Key Terms for this chapter.**
   - Review the Key Terms if necessary.
2. **List the two divisions of the respiratory system and identify the function of each.**
   - The upper and lower respiratory tracts contain the structures that work together to enable respiration.
   - The upper respiratory tract takes in air, warms it, humidifies it, and cleans it, then begins to move air through the respiratory system.
   - The lower respiratory tract is where the exchange of gases (O_2 and CO_2) takes place.
3. **Explain the purpose (the function) of the respiratory system.**
   - The respiratory system, by exchanging O_2 and CO_2 through internal and external respiration, provides the body with the nutrients it needs to function and eliminate wastes from the body.
4. **List the four main structures in the upper respiratory tract and describe the function of each.**
   - The nose aids in the sense of smell and inhalation.
   - The paranasal sinuses warm, clean, and filter air.
   - The pharynx is a passage for air and food.
   - The larynx guards the trachea and produces sound.
5. **List the four main structures in the lower respiratory tract and describe the function of each.**
   - The trachea allows the passage of air to the bronchi.
   - The bronchi allow passage of air to the lungs.
   - The lungs are responsible for the process of respiration.
   - The alveoli exchange O_2 and CO_2.
6. **Explain the difference between internal and external respiration.**
   - Respiration is the process of exchanging gases (O_2 and CO_2).
   - Internal respiration takes place at the cellular level, whereas external respiration takes place in the lungs.
7. **List the two areas of the brain that control respiration, and identify which area regulates respiration subconsciously and which regulates respiration consciously.**
   - Breathing is involuntary, or controlled subconsciously without thought or effort by the pons and medulla in the brainstem.
   - Breathing can also be consciously controlled (e.g., taking a purposeful deep breath) by the cerebral cortex.
8. **Explain the importance of pulmonary function tests (PFTs), such as spirometry, in the diagnosis of respiratory problems.**
   - PFTs are designed to measure respiration and are invaluable in the diagnosis of many problems such as obstruction of airflow by tumor, asthma, or a foreign object.
   - Spirometry measures the air taken in during normal inhalation and released on exhalation.

9. **List 10 common signs and symptoms of respiratory diseases and disorders.**
   - Recognizable signs and symptoms help pulmonologists, otolaryngologists, and allergists diagnose problems of the respiratory system.
   - Refer to Box 14-1.
10. **List six common diagnostic tests for respiratory disease and describe the use of each.**
    - Scientific advances have created technology that is capable of measuring and producing images that aid in the diagnosis of respiratory problems.
    - Refer to Box 14-2 and Table 14-1.
11. **List eight upper respiratory diseases and briefly describe the etiology, signs and symptoms, diagnosis, therapy, and interventions for each.**
    - The diseases and disorders of the respiratory system can be classified according to the division affected: upper respiratory or lower respiratory.
    - Refer to Table 14-3.
12. **List 12 lower respiratory diseases and briefly describe the etiology, signs and symptoms, diagnosis, therapy, and interventions for each.**
    - Upper respiratory diseases are infectious and can be responsible for lower respiratory diseases.
    - Refer to Table 14-3.
13. **Analyze a realistic medical office situation and apply your understanding of the respiratory system to determine the best course of action.**
    - Understanding the normal physiology of the respiratory system will help you understand how the disease process affects it.
14. **Describe the impact on patient care when medical assistants have a solid understanding of the structure and function of the respiratory system.**
    - Medical assistants who understand the physiology of the respiratory system will be better prepared to assist with medical procedures, communicate clearly to patients, and perform effective patient teaching.

PRACTICAL APPLICATIONS

If you have accomplished the objectives in this chapter, you will be able to make better choices as a medical assistant. Take another look at this situation and decide what you would do.

Mr. Chazara, who has a long history of smoking both cigarettes and cigars, has been diagnosed with COPD with constriction of the bronchi. He is dyspneic with stridor and wheezing. When he is seen by the physician, an order is written for spirometry testing. The testing is positive for a mild loss of vital capacity and for a moderate decrease in forced expiratory volume. Because of the decreased lung capacity, an order is also written for measurement of ABGs. In addition, Mr. Chazara has sinus congestion and a productive cough, but he has no fever; he needs medications for the congestion and the loss of lung function.

Do you understand the cause of Mr. Chazara's symptoms? Would you be able to explain the need for these tests to him?

1. What is the cause and effect of long-term cigarette and cigar smoking on the lungs?
2. What does the diagnosis of COPD mean?
3. What effect does the upper respiratory infection of sinus congestion and the productive cough have on COPD?
4. Why would you expect Mr. Chazara to be dyspneic with stridor and wheezing? Explain what each of these medical terms means.
5. What is spirometry testing?
6. What do increased residual volume and decreased vital capacity indicate?
7. Why would a bronchodilator be prescribed?
8. Why would an expectorant rather than an antitussive be prescribed?
9. Why would ABG measurements be ordered?

WEB SEARCH

1. **Research current status of diseases of the respiratory system.** A medical assistant is expected to be familiar with respiratory disorders and to be able to chart the patient's signs and symptoms.
   - **Keywords:** Use the following keywords in your search: avian influenza, Legionnaires' disease, SARS, American Lung Association.

WORD PARTS: Respiratory System

STRUCTURE AND FUNCTION
Combining Forms
alveol/o	alveoli
bronch/o, bronchi/o	bronchi
laryng/o	larynx, "voice box"
nas/o	nose
pharyng/o	pharynx, throat
pneum/o	lung
pulmon/o	lung
rhin/o	nose
trache/o	trachea, "windpipe"

Prefixes
ex-	out, away from
in-	in, inside

Suffixes
-ation	process
-pnea	breathing

UPPER RESPIRATORY TRACT
Combining Forms
adenoid/o	adenoids
tonsil/o	tonsils

Suffixes
-phonia	voice

LOWER RESPIRATORY TRACT
Combining Forms
bronch/o, bronch/i	bronchus
bronchiol/o	bronchiole
phren/o	diaphragm
pleur/o	pleura

Suffixes
-oxia	level of oxygen

BREATHING
Combining Forms
spir/o	breathing

ABBREVIATIONS: Respiratory System

ABGs	arterial blood gases
ARDS	adult respiratory distress syndrome
CA	cancer
COPD	chronic obstructive pulmonary disease
CPR	cardiopulmonary resuscitation
CXR	chest x-ray
LLL	left lower lobe
LUL	left upper lobe
PFT	pulmonary function test
RLL	right lower lobe
RML	right middle lobe
RUL	right upper lobe
SIDS	sudden infant death syndrome
SOB	shortness of breath
TB	tuberculosis
URI	upper respiratory (tract) infection

Digestive System

15

evolve   http://evolve.elsevier.com/klieger/medicalassisting

All people need nutrients, water, and electrolytes to live. The digestive system, also known as the *gastrointestinal system,* is responsible for providing these life-sustaining elements to our bodies. Although we can make eating choices, such as whether to eat an apple or a candy bar for a snack, the process of digesting that snack once eaten is handled unconsciously by the components of our digestive system.

The body systems depend on each other to function properly. For example, the digestive system takes food through the pharynx and strives to keep it out of our trachea so that our airway is not blocked and we do not choke. As a medical assistant, you need to comprehend the proper functioning of the digestive system so you can better understand the diseases and disorders that affect it. This understanding will make you a more knowledgeable and effective medical assistant.

LEARNING OBJECTIVES

You will be able to do the following after completing this chapter:

Key Terms
1. Define, appropriately use, and spell all the Key Terms for this chapter.

Structure and Function of the Digestive System
2. Explain the purpose of the digestive system.
3. List the four stages of the digestive process.
4. List the eight distinct areas of the digestive tract through which food passes during digestion.

Digestive Organs
5. Explain the role of the mouth in digestion.
6. Locate three structures in the mouth important to the digestive process.
7. Identify the pharynx and explain its role in digestion.
8. Locate the esophagus and explain its role in digestion.
9. Explain the role of the stomach in digestion.
10. Locate the peritoneum, sphincters, and fundus within the stomach.
11. Explain the role of the small intestine in digestion.
12. Locate the three main parts of the small intestine.
13. Explain the role of the large intestine in the digestive system.
14. Name and locate the four subdivisions of the large intestine.
15. Locate the rectum and explain its role in the digestive system.
16. Locate the anal sphincter and explain its role in the digestive system.

Accessory Organs
17. Name and locate the three accessory organs to the digestive system and describe the role of each in digesting nutrients.

Metabolism
18. Distinguish between anabolism and catabolism.

Diseases and Disorders of the Digestive System
19. List six diseases of the mouth and briefly describe the etiology, signs and symptoms, diagnosis, therapy, and interventions for each.
20. List two disorders of the esophagus and briefly describe the etiology, signs and symptoms, diagnosis, therapy, and interventions for each.
21. List five disorders of the stomach and briefly describe the etiology, signs and symptoms, diagnosis, therapy, and interventions for each.
22. List three disorders of the small intestine and briefly describe the etiology, signs and symptoms, diagnosis, therapy, and interventions for each.
23. List four disorders of the large intestine and briefly describe the etiology, signs and symptoms, diagnosis, therapy, and interventions for each.
24. List a disorder of the rectum and anal canal and briefly describe its etiology, signs and symptoms, diagnosis, therapy, and interventions.
25. List three diseases of the liver and briefly describe the etiology, signs and symptoms, diagnosis, therapy, and interventions for each.

26. List three disorders of the accessory organs to the digestive system and briefly describe the etiology, signs and symptoms, diagnosis, therapy, and interventions for each.

Patient-Centered Professionalism

27. Analyze a realistic medical office situation and apply your understanding of the digestive system to determine the best course of action.
28. Describe the impact on patient care when medical assistants have a solid understanding of the structure and function of the digestive system.

KEY TERMS

The Key Terms for this chapter have been organized into sections so that you can easily see the terminology associated with each aspect of the digestive system.

Structure and Function of the Digestive System

absorption
alimentary canal
digestion
elimination
gastrointestinal (GI) tract
ingestion

Digestive Organs
Mouth

bolus
buccal
mandible
maxilla
mouth
uvula

Tongue

deglutition
frenulum
mastication
taste buds
tongue

Ducts of Salivary Glands

enzyme
parotid gland
saliva
sublingual gland
submandibular gland

Teeth

bicuspids
canines
deciduous teeth
incisors
molars
permanent teeth

Pharynx and Esophagus

epiglottis
esophagus
peristalsis

Stomach

body
cardiac region
chyme
emulsification
fundus
gastrin
lipase
lower esophageal sphincter (LES)
mesentery
omentum
pepsin
peritoneum
pyloric sphincter
pylorus
rugae
sphincters
stomach
vagus nerve

Small Intestine

bile
duodenum
hepatic portal system
ileum
jejunum
lacteals
small intestine
villi

Large Intestine

ascending colon
cecum
colon
descending colon
large intestine
McBurney's point
sigmoid colon
transverse colon
vermiform appendix

Rectum

defecation
fecal
feces
rectum

Anal Canal

anal canal
anal sphincter
anus

Accessory Organs and Their Components

cholecystokinin
common bile duct
cystic duct
gallbladder
hepatic duct
insulin
liver
pancreas
pancreatin
secretin

Metabolism

anabolism
catabolism
metabolism

Digestive Diseases and Disorders
Signs and Symptoms

ascites
constipation
diarrhea
dyspepsia
dysphagia
emesis
flatulence
hematemesis
idiopathic
jaundice
malaise
melena
nausea
plaque
polyps
regurgitation

Diseases and Disorders

appendicitis
caries
celiac sprue
cholecystitis
cholelithiasis
Crohn disease
diverticulitis
esophagitis
gastric ulcer
gastritis
gastroenteritis
gastroesophageal reflux disease (GERD)
gingivitis
glossitis
hemorrhoids
hepatitis
hiatal hernia
Hirschsprung disease
intussusception
lactose intolerance
mumps
pancreatitis
pyloric stenosis
stomatitis
thrush
ulcerative colitis
Vincent infection
volvulus

PRACTICAL APPLICATIONS

Read the following scenario and keep it in mind as you learn about the digestive system in this chapter.

Saril Paratel, age 69, was brought to the physician's office with fever and pain in the RLQ of her abdomen. The pain has lasted for 3 days and has become progressively worse over the last 36 hours. The pain originally started in the umbilical area, but over time it moved to McBurney's point. Last night, Saril had nausea and vomiting. She has not had a bowel movement for 4 days. She had dyspepsia for several days before this episode of pain. She has also noticed that fatty foods tend to cause flatulence with some pain in her RUQ, radiating into her back at the right shoulder. No history of hematemesis is given, but malaise has been present for several weeks. When asked about diarrhea, Saril answers that her stools 5 days ago were soft, formed, and frequent; so yes, she had diarrhea. The WBC count ordered by the physician is reported as 15,600 WBCs with a differential of 67% neutrophils, 6% bands, 25% lymphs, 0% basos, 1% monos, and 1% eos. The physician refers Saril to a surgeon because he wants her to be evaluated for possible appendicitis and to rule out the cause of the RUQ pain.

Would you understand all of the terminology here? Would you be able to explain these findings to Saril if she had questions?

Function

The process of digestion consists of both the physical breakdown and the chemical breakdown of complex food into simpler substances. This is done so that the food nutrients can be absorbed into the bloodstream and then used by the body tissues, or those not needed can be eliminated from the body. The digestive organs, accessory organs, and their secretions allow the gastrointestinal (GI) system to move nutrients through four stages: (1) **ingestion,** (2) **digestion,** (3) **absorption,** and (4) **elimination.**

Structure

The **alimentary canal** (digestive tract) is a muscular hollow tube that extends from the mouth to the anus and measures approximately 30 feet. The digestive tract, or **gastrointestinal (GI) tract,** can be divided into several distinct areas and digestive organs through which nutrients pass during digestion. In addition, accessory organs secrete substances that aid in this process (Figure 15-1).

STRUCTURE AND FUNCTION OF THE DIGESTIVE SYSTEM

When learning about the body, it is often best to examine the "big picture," or the whole system, before the parts. The function and structure of the whole organ system can shed light on why each part works the way it does.

FOR YOUR INFORMATION

The digestive system is affected more by changes in other systems than by direct changes in the digestive system. For example, the reduction in bone mass and calcium content within the skeletal system eventually leads to dental problems (e.g., erosion of tooth sockets and receding gums that can lead to tooth loss, dental caries). Taste sensations diminish because of a decrease in taste receptors, and olfactory sensitivity can lead to dietary changes that affect the entire body. A slowdown of intestinal motility from a decrease in the surface area in the intestines also may lead to a problem. The decrease of the flow of secretins from the stomach, pancreas, liver, and small intestine leads to a decline in the system's ability to digest and absorb nutrients properly. Smooth muscle tone decreases, slowing the peristaltic process and causing a loss in sphincter control.

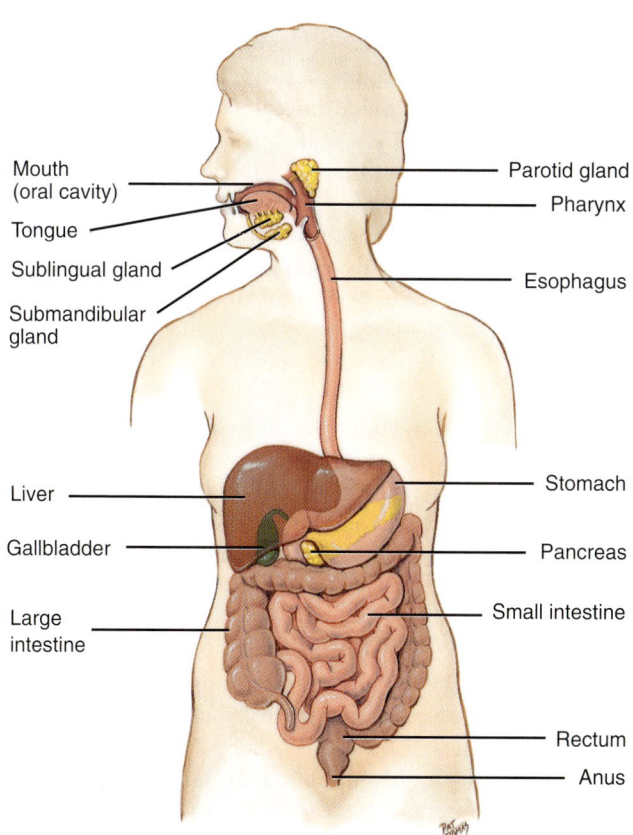

FIGURE 15-1 Organs of the digestive system. (Modified from Applegate EJ: *The anatomy and physiology learning system,* ed 3, St Louis, 2006, Saunders.)

> **PATIENT-CENTERED PROFESSIONALISM**
>
> - The organs of the digestive system are divided into two categories: those of the GI tract and those of accessory organs of digestion. Why is it important for the medical assistant to understand their general function in digestion and absorption of nutrients?

DIGESTIVE ORGANS

Now that you know the function and structure of the digestive system as a whole, it is time to explore the parts. Nutrients pass through eight distinct areas and digestive organs during digestion: the mouth, pharynx, esophagus, stomach, small intestine, large intestine, rectum, and anal canal.

Mouth

The **mouth** (oral cavity) is where food and nutrients first enter the digestive system. In the mouth, food is tasted and physically broken up by the teeth and mixed with saliva, which breaks the food down further with chemicals. When food is chewed and mixed with saliva, it becomes a semiliquid form known as a **bolus** (chewed food). Finally, the food is swallowed.

The oral cavity contains the tongue, duct openings of the salivary glands, and the teeth (Figure 15-2, *A*). It is an oval-shaped cavity that communicates with the pharynx. A cheek forms the cavity on each side (**buccal** refers to the cheek). The lips protect the front of the mouth. The soft and hard palate form the roof of the mouth, and the tongue forms most of the floor of the mouth. Hanging from the middle of the lower portion of the soft palate is the **uvula**, a fingerlike projection that directs food toward the esophagus to aid in swallowing. The **maxilla** forms the upper jaw, and the **mandible** forms the lower jaw to hold the teeth.

Tongue

The **tongue** is the organ for the sense of taste and assists in **mastication** (chewing), **deglutition** (swallowing), digestion, and talking. The **taste buds,** located on the tongue, allow us to taste sweet, sour, salt, and bitter. The tongue is anchored to the floor of the mouth by the **frenulum** and the hyoid bone.

Ducts of the Salivary Glands

The ducts of the salivary glands empty into the mouth (Figure 15-2, *C*). These glands secrete approximately 1500 milliliters (mL), or 1½ liters (L), of **saliva** daily. The **parotid gland, submandibular gland,** and **sublingual gland** emit secretions that mix with secretions of the small glands on the floor of the mouth. The parotid gland is the largest of the salivary glands. **Mumps** is a viral infection of the parotid gland that can have complications involving the ovaries and testes. Postadolescent males who contract the disease may become sterile. Saliva lubricates the mouth to enhance the swallowing of food and contains an **enzyme** called *amylase*. Carbohydrate digestion actually begins in the mouth and is assisted by a substance called *ptyalin*.

Teeth

Two sets of teeth develop during life. The first set is the **deciduous teeth** ("baby teeth"). There are 20 baby teeth, 10 in each jaw: four **incisors**, two **canines**, and four **molars**. These teeth eventually fall out. The second set of teeth is called the **permanent teeth**. Permanent teeth replace the baby teeth. There are 32 permanent teeth, 16 in each jaw: 4 incisors, 2 canines, 4 **bicuspids**, and 6 molars. Figure 15-2, *B*, illustrates the longitudinal section of a tooth.

Pharynx

When the bolus is swallowed, it enters the pharynx. As the bolus is being moved through the pharynx, an involuntary reaction occurs that causes the **epiglottis** (flap) to close over the trachea, causing the bolus to enter the esophagus and not the trachea (Figure 15-3). As food enters the esophagus from the pharynx, a process called **peristalsis** causes wavelike smooth muscle contractions that push food down to the stomach.

Esophagus

The **esophagus,** a muscular tube 9 to 10 inches long, connects to the pharynx at its upper end and with the stomach at its lower end. The esophagus carries food mixed with saliva from the mouth to the stomach by way of peristalsis but is collapsed when food is not being transported. The esophagus does not produce digestive enzymes or absorb food. Its sole purpose is to move food along the digestive tract.

Stomach

The esophagus passes through the diaphragm to connect to the **stomach**. The **peritoneum,** a serous membrane, provides protection for the digestive organs. There are two folds of the peritoneum: the omentum and mesentery. The **omentum** hangs in front of the stomach and intestines, and the **mesentery** attaches itself to the small and large intestines, joining them to the posterior abdominal wall for stabilization of the organs.

The esophagus ends in the upper portion of the stomach (Figure 15-4). The stomach is saclike and serves as a receptacle for food. It is located in the regions of the *epigastric, umbilical,* and *left hypochondriac* areas of the abdomen (refer to the body areas covered in Chapter 11).

The stomach has the following two **sphincters** guarding the entrance and exit of the stomach:
- The **lower esophageal sphincter (LES),** or cardiac sphincter, allows food to pass into the stomach. The LES prevents food from reentering the esophagus as food is converted into **chyme** (a liquid substance) by gastric juices.

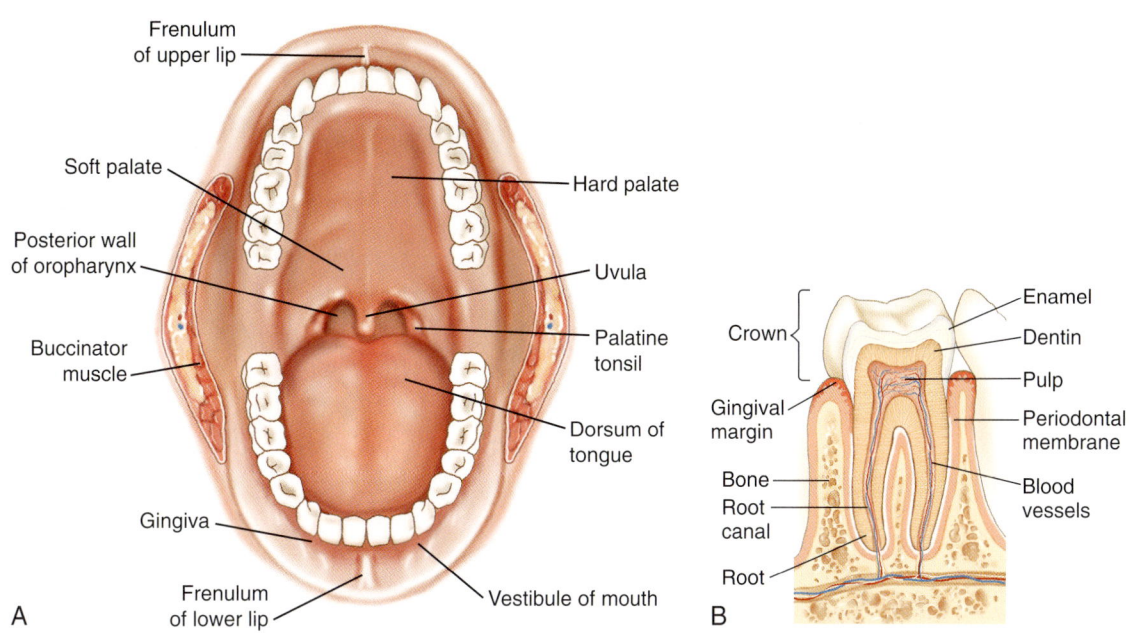
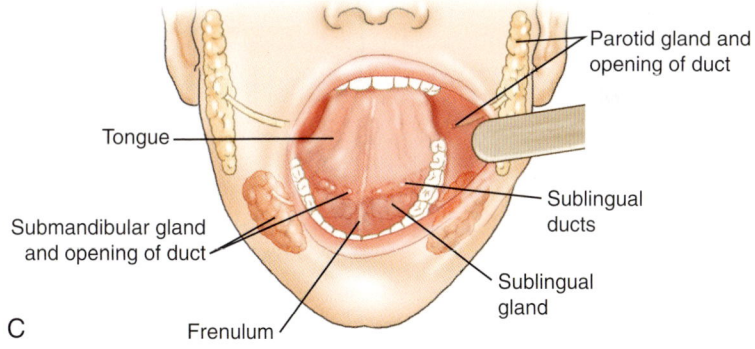

FIGURE 15-2 **A,** Structures in the mouth. **B,** Cross-section of a tooth. **C,** Location of the salivary glands. (From Leonard PC: *Building a medical vocabulary*, ed 6, St Louis, 2005, Saunders.)

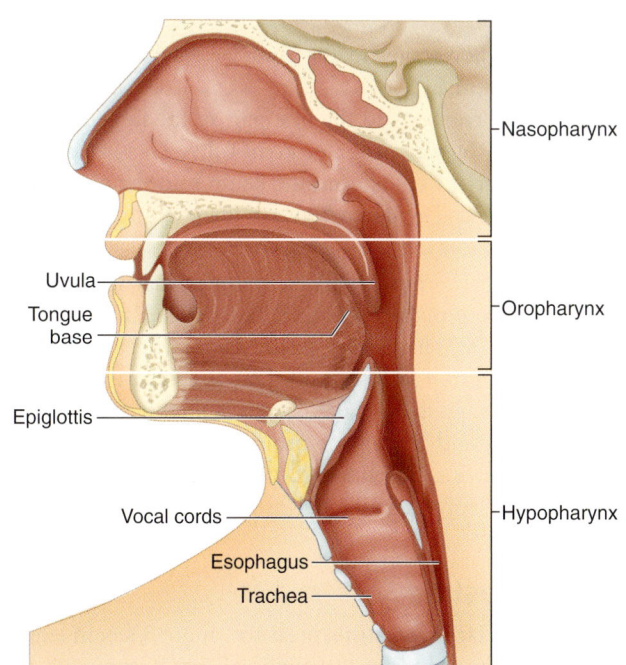

FIGURE 15-3 Food travels from the mouth to the pharynx to the esophagus. (From Goldman L, Ausiello D: *Cecil medicine*, ed 23, Philadelphia, 2008, Saunders.)

- The **pyloric sphincter** allows chyme to exit into the small intestine. The pyloric sphincter keeps food in the stomach until it has been processed and is ready to enter the small intestine as chyme.

The stomach has four different sections, as follows:

1. **Cardiac region:** Area surrounding the LES through which food enters the stomach from the esophagus.
2. **Fundus:** Upper expanded portion of the stomach beside the cardiac region.
3. **Body:** Middle portion of the stomach.
4. **Pylorus:** Bottom portion of the stomach.

The internal lining of the stomach is made up of a mucous membrane that contains folds, referred to as **rugae**. As the stomach fills with food and expands, the folds disappear. The stomach changes food from a semisolid (bolus) to a semifluid substance (chyme). Food remains in the stomach for 1 to 4 hours where it is churned to break it down into useable molecules. **Gastrin,** a digestive hormone, is released when food (mostly protein) enters the stomach. This action stimulates the secretion of gastric juices. The release of gastric juices containing hydrochloric acid and enzymes is controlled by the **vagus nerve** and enzymes. Hydrochloric acids assist to activate the enzyme **pepsin** for protein breakdown, absorption of iron, and elimination of bacteria. Gastric juices contain the

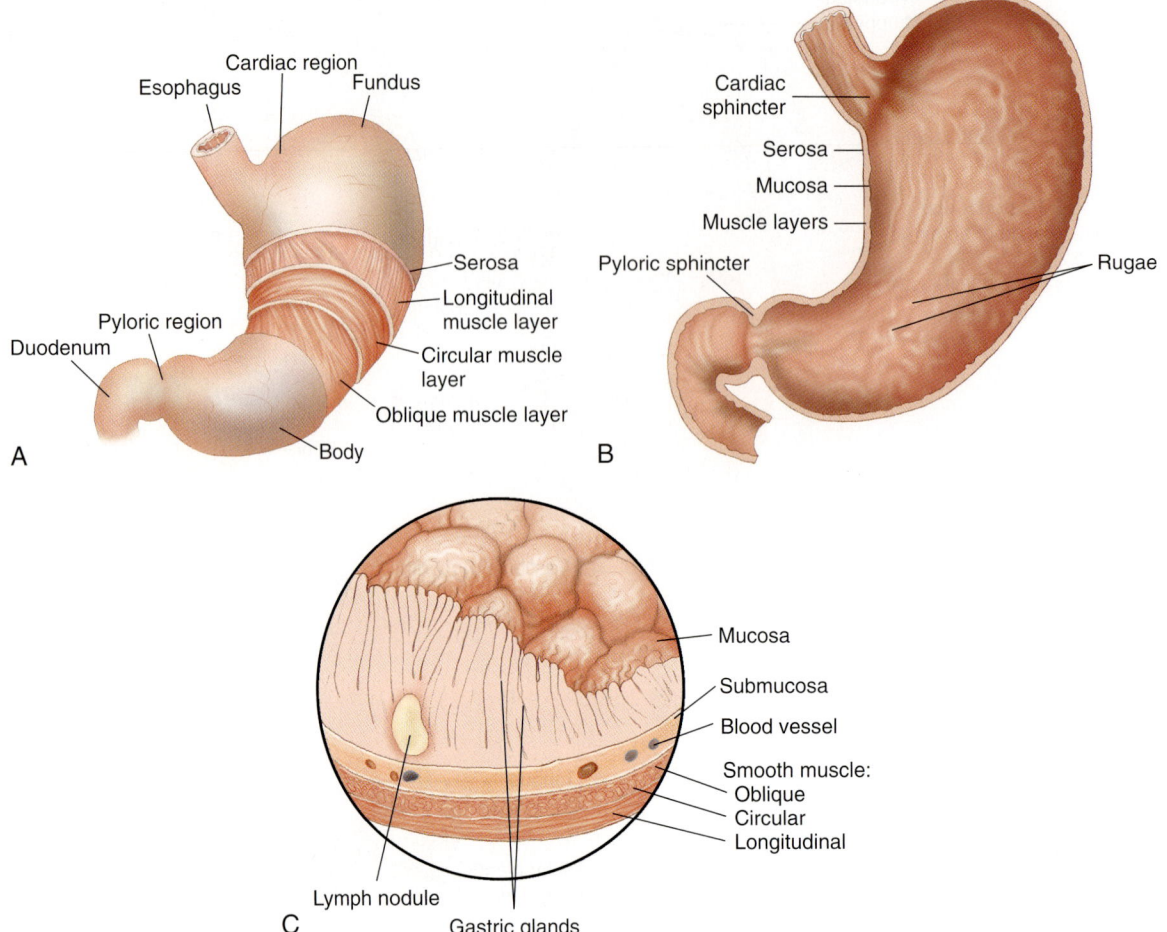

FIGURE 15-4 The features of the stomach. (From Leonard PC: *Building a medical vocabulary,* ed 6, St Louis, 2005, Saunders.)

enzyme **lipase** to aid in the breakdown of fats (**emulsification**). **Gastroenteritis** occurs when extensive inflammation and irritation occur in the lining of the stomach and intestine and is a symptom of many digestive disorders.

Small Intestine

As the chyme exits the stomach through the pyloric sphincter, it enters the **small intestine.** The small intestine is a hollow tube approximately 23 feet long and is located in the abdominal cavity. It is divided into three parts, as follows:

1. The **duodenum** begins at the pyloric sphincter of the stomach; it is only about 10 inches long. **Bile,** which breaks down fats, leaves the gallbladder, and pancreatic juices for sugar breakdown are excreted through ducts into the duodenum. As the duodenum begins to turn downward, it becomes the jejunum.
2. The **jejunum** extends between the duodenum and the ileum; it is about 8 feet in length. Within the jejunum are **villi,** finger-like projections that contain capillaries allowing nutrients to be absorbed by the blood, and **lacteals** that return nutrients to the lymphatic system (Figure 15-5). This process is called *absorption.* After nutrients are absorbed they travel to the liver by way of the **hepatic portal system.**
3. The **ileum** connects to the first part of the large intestine, the **cecum,** by way of the *ileocecal valve.* This valve allows waste material to pass from the ileum into the cecum, but not vice versa. The ileum between the jejunum and cecum is about 12 feet long.

The small intestine produces enzymes that break down sugars, including maltase, sucrase, and lactase. **Lactose intolerance** occurs when there is a deficiency of lactase. Lactase enables digestion of lactose, so if there is a lactase deficiency, lactose is not digested. The enzymes *peptidase* for proteins, *lipase* for fats, and *trypsin* for proteins are also produced in the small intestine. In addition, the small intestine absorbs nutrients, electrolytes, and vitamins.

Large Intestine

The **colon,** or **large intestine,** measures about 5 feet in length. The colon's functions are to (1) absorb water, minerals, and remaining nutrients; (2) synthesize and absorb B-complex vitamins; (3) allow for the formation of vitamin K; and (4) transport solid waste products out of the body.

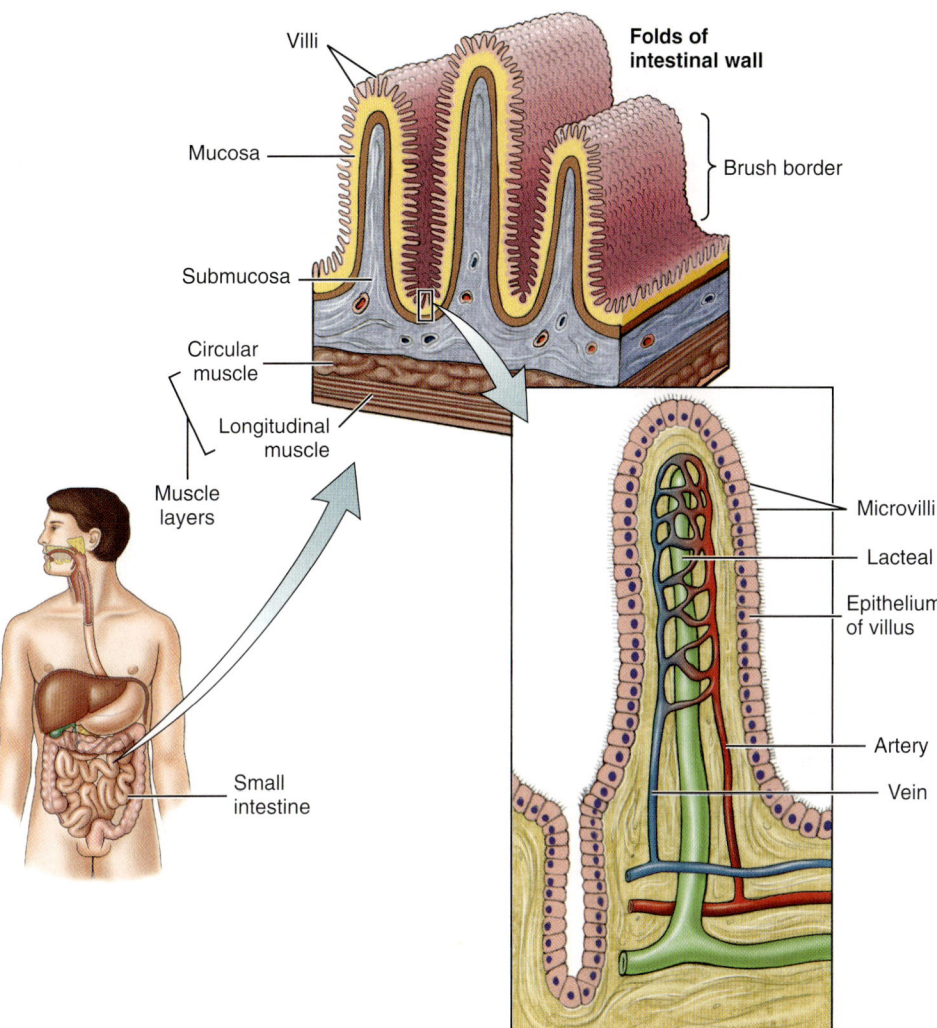

FIGURE 15-5 The small intestine. Folds of the intestinal wall showing the villi. *Inset,* A single villus. (From Herlihy B, Maebius NK: *The human body in health and illness,* ed 3, St Louis, 2007, Saunders.)

The **vermiform appendix** is attached to the cecum at the junction of the small intestine. The function of the appendix has been debated, but some believe that it breeds intestinal flora (bacteria) that break down food substances into waste products. Others, however, think it no longer serves a purpose. The colon is subdivided into four parts, as follows (Figure 15-6):

1. The **ascending colon** travels up (vertical) the right side of the body toward the lower part of the liver.
2. The **transverse colon** moves across the abdomen, below the liver and stomach, and above the small intestine.
3. The **descending colon** travels down the left side of the body and connects to the sigmoid colon.
4. The **sigmoid colon** is the S-shaped structure that joins to the rectum.

Rectum

The **rectum** is continuous with the sigmoid colon and measures about 5 inches in length. It stores all nondigestible wastes until they leave the system as **feces** (adjective form is **fecal**); this process is known as **defecation**.

Anal Canal

The rectum terminates at the **anal canal,** which is about 1½ inches in length. The **anal sphincter** is a ring of muscle at the opening of the **anus.** The sphincter keeps the anus closed until a stool (feces) needs to pass. Stool collects in the rectum and pushes on the walls of the rectum. This pressure causes the anal sphincter to relax, allowing stool to pass out of the body through the anus.

Figure 15-7 shows the entire digestive process of a carbohydrate, protein, and fat.

PATIENT-CENTERED PROFESSIONALISM

- *Food is prepared for use by cells in five basic activities: (1) ingestion, (2) movement, (3) mechanical and chemical digestion, (4) absorption, and (5) defecation. How does each of these basic activities aid in digestion?*
- *How does it impact patients when medical assistants understand how food is digested?*

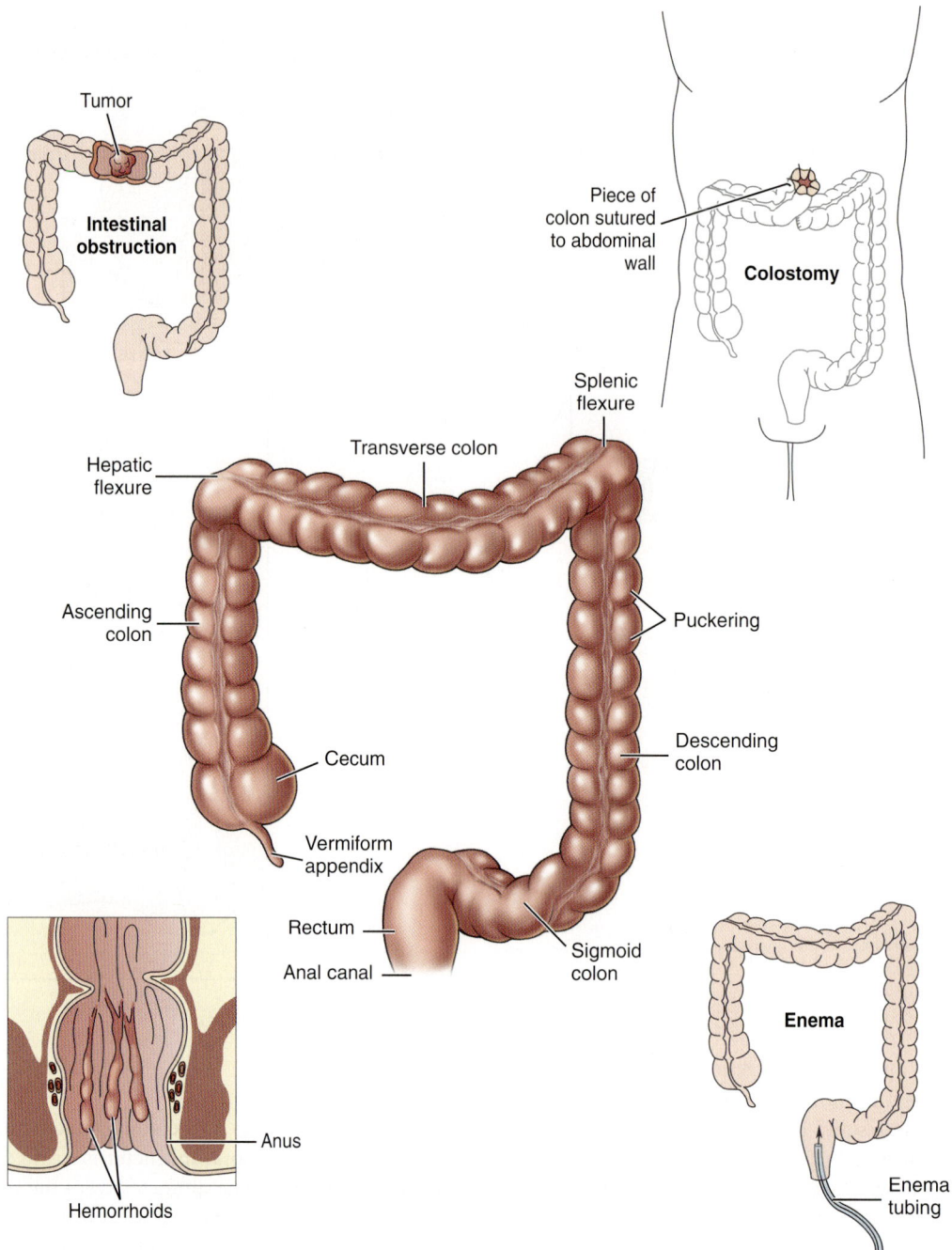

FIGURE 15-6 The large intestine, as well as some clinical conditions and procedures affecting the large intestine. (From Herlihy B, Maebius NK: *The human body in health and illness,* ed 3, St Louis, 2007, Saunders.)

ACCESSORY ORGANS

The salivary glands (covered in the mouth section), liver, gallbladder, and pancreas are not part of the digestive tract, but they have a role in digestive activities. They all secrete substances that help break down nutrients into a form that is usable by the body. They are considered accessory organs.

The liver, gallbladder, and pancreas all empty their secretions into the duodenum (Figure 15-8). It is in the duodenum that the final breakdown of nutrients takes place. The final step depends on the deposit of secretions from the accessory organs. Table 15-1 lists digestive secretions with their role in digestion. Digestive enzymes play a large role in chemical digestion, but selective hormones also contribute to the process. For example, when chyme, containing fatty contents and proteins, enters the duodenum, the hormone **cholecystokinin** stimulates the gallbladder to secrete bile and stimulates the pancreas to secrete a pancreatic juice rich in digestive enzymes. **Secretin** is another hormone that stimulates the pancreas to secrete bicarbonate ions to neutralize acid chyme in the duodenum. Both hormones are produced in the mucosal lining of the small intestine.

Digestive System CHAPTER 15 269

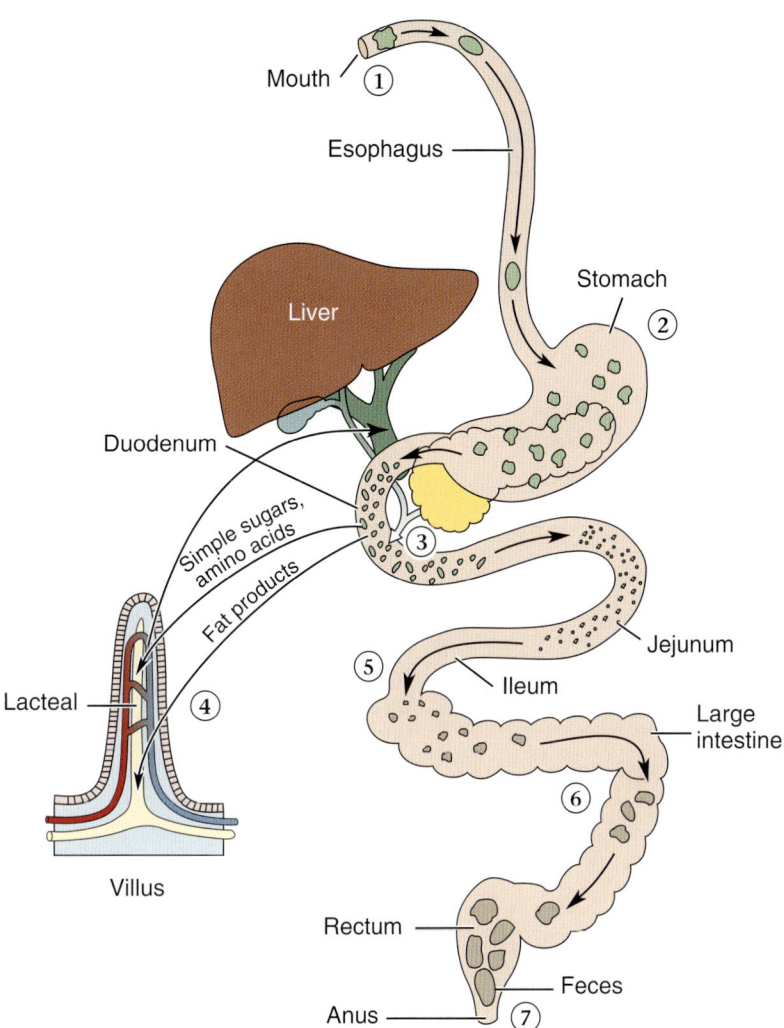
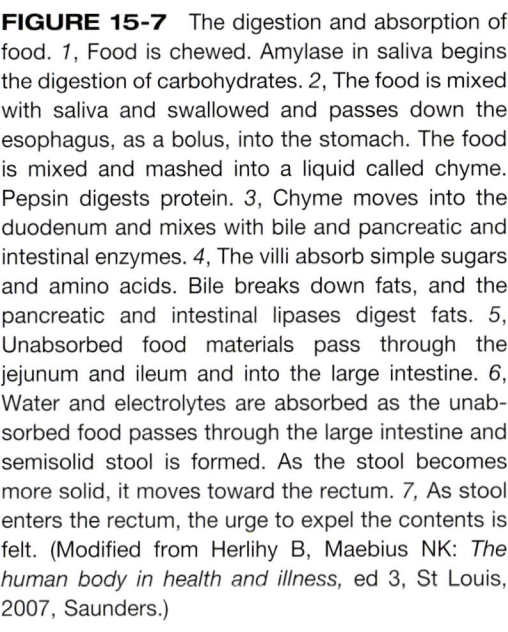

FIGURE 15-7 The digestion and absorption of food. *1,* Food is chewed. Amylase in saliva begins the digestion of carbohydrates. *2,* The food is mixed with saliva and swallowed and passes down the esophagus, as a bolus, into the stomach. The food is mixed and mashed into a liquid called chyme. Pepsin digests protein. *3,* Chyme moves into the duodenum and mixes with bile and pancreatic and intestinal enzymes. *4,* The villi absorb simple sugars and amino acids. Bile breaks down fats, and the pancreatic and intestinal lipases digest fats. *5,* Unabsorbed food materials pass through the jejunum and ileum and into the large intestine. *6,* Water and electrolytes are absorbed as the unabsorbed food passes through the large intestine and semisolid stool is formed. As the stool becomes more solid, it moves toward the rectum. *7,* As stool enters the rectum, the urge to expel the contents is felt. (Modified from Herlihy B, Maebius NK: *The human body in health and illness,* ed 3, St Louis, 2007, Saunders.)

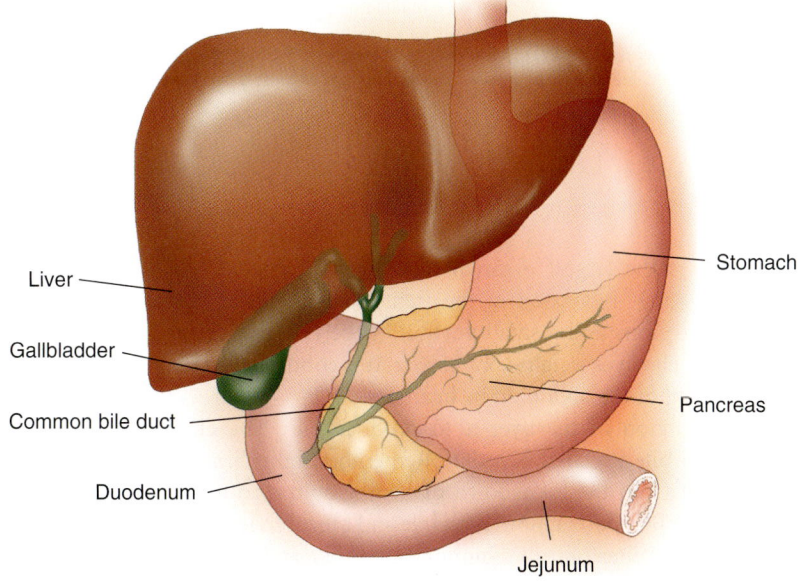

FIGURE 15-8 The liver, gallbladder, and pancreas. (From Leonard PC: *Building a medical vocabulary,* ed 6, St Louis, 2005, Saunders.)

TABLE 15-1

Digestive Secretions

Digestive Juice	Source	Substance	Functional Role*
Saliva	Salivary glands	Mucus	*Lubricates bolus of food; facilitates mixing of food*
		Amylase	**Enzyme; begins digestion of starches to disaccharide**
		Sodium bicarbonate	**Increases pH (for optimum amylase function)**
		Water	*Dilutes food and other substances; facilitates mixing*
Gastric juice	Gastric glands	Pepsin	**Enzyme; digest proteins to partially digested proteins**
		Hydrochloric acid	**Denatures proteins; decreases pH (for optimum pepsin function)**
		Intrinsic factor	**Protects and allows later absorption of vitamin B_{12}**
		Mucus	*Lubricates chyme; protects stomach lining*
		Water	*Dilutes food and other substances; facilitates mixing*
Pancreatic juice	Pancreas (exocrine portion)	Proteases (trypsin, chymotrypsin, collagenase, elastase, other carboxypeptidases, aminopeptidases, etc.)	**Enzymes; digest proteins and polypeptides to peptides and amino acids**
		Lipases (lipase, phospholipase, etc.)	**Enzymes; digest lipids to fatty acids, monoglycerides, and glycerol**
		Colipase	**Coenzyme; helps lipase digest fats**
		Nucleases	**Enzymes; digest nucleic acids (RNA and DNA)**
		Amylase	**Enzyme; digests starches**
		Water	*Dilutes food and other substances; facilitates mixing*
		Mucus	*Lubricates*
		Sodium bicarbonate	**Increases pH (for optimum enzyme function)**
Bile	Liver (stored and concentrated in gallbladder)	Lecithin and bile salts	*Emulsify lipids*
		Sodium bicarbonate	**Increases pH (for optimum enzyme function)**
		Cholesterol	Excess cholesterol from body cells, to be excreted with feces
		Products of detoxification	From detoxification of harmful substances by hepatic cells, to be excreted with feces
		Bile pigments (mainly bilirubin)	Products of breakdown of heme groups during hemolysis, to be excreted with feces
		Mucus	*Lubricates*
		Water	*Dilutes food and other substances; facilitates mixing*
Intestinal juice (succus entericus)	Mucosa of small and large intestine	Mucus	*Lubricates*
		Sodium bicarbonate	**Increases pH (for optimum enzyme function)**
		Water	*Small amount to carry mucus and sodium bicarbonate*
		Sucrase	**Enzyme; digests sucrose (cane sugar) to glucose and fructose**
		Lactase	**Enzyme; digests lactose (milk sugar) to glucose and galactose**
		Maltase	**Enzyme: maltose to glucose**

Modified from Thibodeau GA, Patton KT: *Anatomy and physiology,* ed 6, St Louis, 2007, Mosby.
***Boldface type** indicates a chemical digestive process; *italic type* indicates a mechanical digestive process.

Liver

The **liver** is the largest organ in the digestive system (see Figure 15-8). It is located in the right hypochondriac and epigastric regions and a small portion of the left hypochondriac area. The liver weighs about 55 oz. It is connected to the anterior wall of the abdomen by ligaments.

One function of the liver is to produce bile. The chief pigment in bile is called *bilirubin.* Remember, bilirubin is a by-product from the breakdown of hemoglobin during red blood cell (RBC) destruction. Both bile and bilirubin leave the body in feces. When bilirubin cannot leave the body, it remains in the bloodstream and causes a yellowish discoloration to the skin and sclera. The main function of bile is the digestion and absorption of fat. Other functions of the liver include the following:

- Metabolizes carbohydrates, fats, and proteins
- Manufactures blood proteins
- Removes toxins, bacteria, and worn-out red blood cells
- Removes waste products from the blood *(detoxification)*
- Manufactures cholesterol
- Stores vitamins A, B_{12}, D, E, and K
- Forms antibodies
- Stores simple sugars

It should be noted that drug metabolism occurs most often in the liver. Therefore it is necessary to regularly monitor that the patient has adequate liver function. Failure of the liver to metabolize medications adequately will result in drug toxicity.

Gallbladder

The bile produced by the liver travels to the gallbladder through the **hepatic duct** for storage. Bile leaves the gallbladder as needed through the **cystic duct.** The hepatic duct and the cystic duct join together and form the **common bile duct.** This duct enters the duodenum just below the pylorus.

The **gallbladder** is a pear-shaped sac about 4 inches long and is lodged under the liver. Its main function is to store bile until needed for digestion. When a meal including fat begins digesting in the stomach, a message is sent to the gallbladder via the nervous system, causing it to contract (squeeze). When this happens, bile enters the duodenum to complete the digestion of fat.

Pancreas

The **pancreas** is divided into three sections: head, body, and tail. It lies behind the stomach and in front of the first and second lumbar vertebrae. The pancreas produces **pancreatin,** which is used in protein breakdown in the duodenum, and **insulin,** which is used in maintaining blood glucose levels.

PATIENT-CENTERED PROFESSIONALISM

- Nutrients are the substances in food that are used as an energy source to fuel the needs of the body. What importance do accessory organs play in the digestive process?
- How might the medical assistant's ability to explain the importance of accessory organs to patients benefit their care and treatment?

METABOLISM

Metabolism is the change, both physical and chemical, that food nutrients undergo after absorption in the small intestine. The process of metabolism consists of two phases: anabolism and catabolism.

- **Anabolism** (buildup) is considered the "constructive" phase of metabolism because smaller molecules or simple substances are converted to larger molecules or more complex substances (e.g., amino acids converted to proteins).
- **Catabolism** (breakdown) is the opposite of anabolism. Catabolism is the "destructive" phase of metabolism in which larger molecules are converted into smaller molecules (e.g., glycogen converted to pyruvic acid). This process releases energy and is measured in calories. The energy released is used for cell growth and heat production.

Carbohydrates, fats, proteins, and other materials are metabolized to produce the energy needed to keep the body functioning.

PATIENT-CENTERED PROFESSIONALISM

- Metabolism is how the body uses the nutrients absorbed from the food we eat. Why is it important for the medical assistant to understand this process?
- How do anabolism and catabolism differ? What is a situation in which you might need to explain this difference to a patient?

DISEASES AND DISORDERS OF THE DIGESTIVE SYSTEM

Diseases of the digestive tract can be either *acute* (sudden and severe) or *chronic* (of longer duration or recurring). An internist or a gastroenterologist can treat diseases of the digestive tract.

Drugs may be prescribed to treat digestive problems (Table 15-2).

Medical assistants need to be able to recognize the common signs and symptoms of and the diagnostic tests for the different types of digestive system disorders and diseases.

- Study Box 15-1 to familiarize yourself with the common signs and symptoms.
- Study Box 15-2 to learn about common diagnostic tests.
- Study Table 15-3 to understand the diseases and disorders that affect the digestive system.

Text continued on p. 276

TABLE 15-2

Digestive Drug Classifications

Drug Classification	Common Generic (Brand) Names
Antacids Buffer or absorb hydrochloric acid (HCl) in the stomach	calcium carbonate (Tums) aluminum and magnesium (Maalox)
Antidiarrheals Provide relief from intestinal cramping and diarrhea	diphenoxylate (Lomotil) loperamide (Imodium)
Antiemetics Prevent or alleviate nausea and vomiting	meclizine (Antivert) prochlorperazine (Compazine)
Cathartics (stimulating laxatives) Cause evacuation of the bowel by stimulating nerves in the intestines resulting in increased peristalsis	senna (Senokot) bisacodyl (Dulcolax)
Laxatives Cause evacuation of the bowel by increasing the bulk of the feces, softening the stool, or lubricating the intestinal wall	methylcellulose (Citrucel) psyllium (Metamucil)
Anti-ulcer agents Prevent or alleviate symptoms of ulcers	esomeprazole (Nexium) lansoprazole (Prevacid)
Antispasmodics Prevent spasms or colic-type actions in the stomach or intestines	dicyclomine (Bentyl) belladonna alkaloids (Donnatal)

BOX 15-1

Common Signs and Symptoms of Digestive Disease

Anorexia	Loss of appetite
Ascites	Accumulation of fluid in the peritoneal cavity caused by an obstruction of the portal (liver) circulation
Colic	Acute abdominal pain
Constipation	Difficulty in defecation caused by hard, compacted stool
Diarrhea	Frequent bowel movements of loose, watery stools
Dyspepsia	Difficult digestion; uncomfortable feeling after eating (e.g., heartburn, bloating, nausea)
Dysphagia	Difficulty swallowing
Emesis	Expulsion of stomach contents; vomiting
Flatulence	Digestive gas
Guarding	Moving away from or flinching when a tender area of the abdomen is touched
Hematemesis	Vomiting of blood
Jaundice	Yellowish discoloration of skin caused by excessive bilirubin in the blood
Melena	Black, tarry feces caused by free blood in the intestines
Nausea	Inclination to vomit
Polyps	Usually benign growths attached to the mucosal lining of the colon
Regurgitation	Reflux of stomach acids and food into the esophagus
Rigidity	Stiff or "boardlike" abdomen
Vomiting	Forceful expulsion of stomach contents; emesis; "throwing up"

PATIENT-CENTERED PROFESSIONALISM

- The digestive system provides nutrients for the body through many processes. Diseases and disorders of this system can interfere with this process. Why is it important for the medical assistant to understand what signs and symptoms may be present in a patient with a digestive disorder or disease?

BOX 15-2

Diagnostic Tests and Procedures for the Digestive Tract

Abdominal x-ray	Detects and evaluates tumors and other abdominal disorders (flat plate of the abdomen).
Barium enema	Barium sulfate is introduced through the rectum for imaging the lower bowel (lower GI series).
Barium swallow	Oral ingestion of barium sulfate suspension for imaging the esophagus (upper GI series).
Cholecystography	Contrast study done by oral ingestion of an iodine preparation; imaging of the gallbladder occurs at various intervals.
Endoscopy	Visualization of the GI tract using an endoscope (Figure 15-9).
Colonoscopy	Visualization of the large intestine.
Laparoscopy	Endoscopic examination of the interior of the peritoneal cavity.
Sigmoidoscopy	Endoscopic examination of the sigmoid colon.

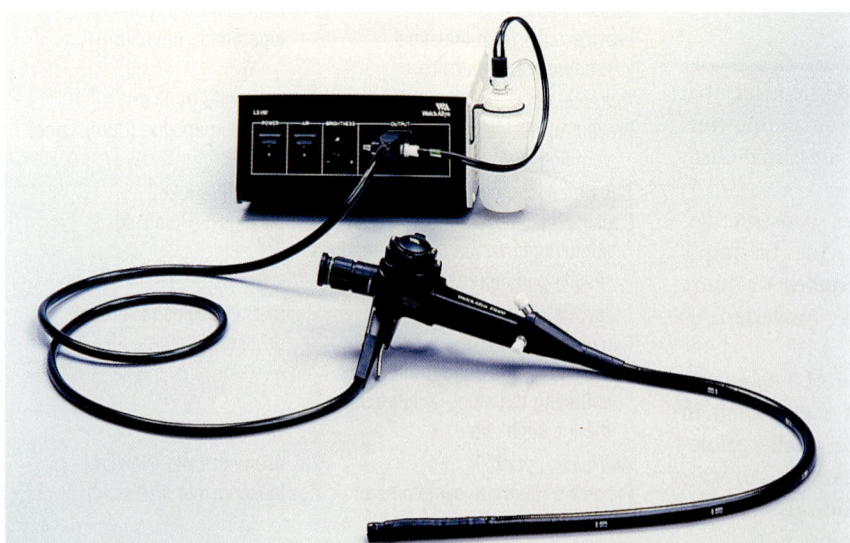

FIGURE 15-9 Endoscopy allows the physician to see inside the body. (Courtesy Welch Allyn, Skaneateles Falls, NY.)

TABLE 15-3

Diseases and Disorders of the Digestive System

Disease and Description	Etiology	Signs and Symptoms	Diagnosis	Therapy	Interventions
MOUTH					
Gingivitis — Infection of gums	Caused by **plaque** around base of teeth	Gums red and inflamed; gums bleed easily	Dentist confirms by oral examination	Removal of plaque and antibiotic therapy	Educate about proper brushing and flossing techniques
Stomatitis — Infection of mucous lining of mouth	Viral infection (herpes simplex)	Sudden onset; mouth pain, fever, tenderness of mucosa of mouth	Oral inspection: gums swollen, ulcerations of mouth and throat; viral smear	Symptom relief, including topical anesthetic medications for viral infections	Encourage oral hygiene, including saline or hydrogen
Vincent infection ("trench mouth") — Painful ulcerations of mucous lining of mouth	Secondary infection to gingivitis	Painful ulcerations of gums, excessive salivation, bad breath	Oral exam: bleeding gums, ulcerations	Antibiotic and surgery to repair gums	Emphasize good oral hygiene
Thrush — Fungal infection of mouth	Caused by the yeast *Candida albicans*	Pale-yellow patches in mouth	Oral exam and laboratory culture	Antifungal medication	Stress good oral hygiene
Caries — Tooth decay caused by bacteria and plaque	Bacteria break down sugars in foods; process produces acid, which causes enamel to erode	Toothache	Oral exam with x-ray	Removal of decay	Emphasize good oral hygiene and regular teeth cleaning
Glossitis — Inflammation of tongue	Streptococcal infection, vitamin B deficiency, anemia, chronic irritation (e.g., loose dentures, smoking)	Swollen tongue, painful chewing, painful tongue without swelling	Clinical presentation, culture of tongue	Antibiotics, topical anesthetic or analgesics for pain	Stress good oral hygiene and treatment of underlying causes
ESOPHAGUS					
Gastroesophageal reflux disease (GERD) — Backup of gastric juices into esophagus	Poor cardiac sphincter function resulting in heartburn	Belching, burning sensation in chest and mouth	Patient history and upper GI series to detect erosion and esophageal abnormalities	Head of bed elevated 4 to 6 inches; medication to inhibit gastric juice production	Limit alcohol consumption; lose weight and minimize tobacco use
Esophagitis — Inflammation of esophagus	Reflux of gastric acid causing chemical ingestion	Burning in chest area; pain following eating or drinking	Patient history and upper GI series to detect abnormalities	Bland diet to reduce acid production; medication to promote healing	Diet instruction: consume small meals; avoid spicy foods, caffeine, and alcohol
STOMACH					
Gastritis — Inflammation of stomach	Causative agent could be *Helicobacter pylori*, bacteria from spoiled food, drugs causing irritation (e.g., aspirin), or stress	Abdominal pain, heartburn	Visualization through gastroscopy Presenting signs and symptoms	Medications (e.g., antacid and those that reduce acid secretions) and antibiotics if causative agent is *H. pylori*	After finding source, if emotional stress, reduce stressful activities
Gastric ulcer — Lesion of mucosal lining of stomach or intestine	Breakdown of mucosal lining, by stomach acids or *H. pylori*	Epigastric pain	Past history and physical exam; upper GI series; endoscopy; gastric analysis	Rest, medications (antibiotics, antacids), surgery	Initiate lifestyle changes to reduce stress, thus reducing acid

Continued

TABLE 15-3

Diseases and Disorders of the Digestive System—cont'd

Disease and Description	Etiology	Signs and Symptoms	Diagnosis	Therapy	Interventions
Pyloric stenosis Narrowing of pyloric sphincter	Developmental error of sphincter muscle	Projectile vomiting	Clinical evaluation	Surgical intervention	None
Hiatal hernia Protrusion of stomach through diaphragm into chest cavity	Congenital defect in diaphragm	Heartburn when reclining; chest pain and discomfort in chest cavity if overweight	X-ray, upper GI series	Symptoms relieved through medication and lifestyle changes	Lose weight if overweight; smaller meals, sit up straight after eating
SMALL INTESTINE					
Celiac sprue Malabsorption disease with mucosal damage to small intestine caused by gluten (wheat) intolerance	Immunological reaction to protein	Anorexia, abdominal distention, intestinal bleeding	Biopsy of small intestine to verify villi destruction; symptoms abate on gluten-free diet	Gluten-free diet; corticosteroid treatment in some cases	Encourage adherence to diet
Intussusception Telescoping of one part of intestine into another; usually in ileocecal area (Figure 15-10)	*Adults:* cause may be tumors or polyps *Infants:* cause unknown	*Adults:* obstructive symptoms *Infants:* Cry and draw up legs; fever, vomiting	Medical history and x-ray studies of abdomen; laboratory studies show occult blood in stool; barium enema	Surgical intervention, restoration of electrolyte levels	Provide dietary education
Crohn disease Chronic inflammation of ileum	Unknown; theory of autoimmune disease	Chronic diarrhea; cramping abdominal pain	Patient history, barium enema and x-ray studies of abdomen; colonoscopy	Medical management: supplemental support, medications to relieve diarrhea, corticosteroids to reduce inflammation	Stress need for rest; encourage support group
LARGE INTESTINE					
Hirschsprung disease (megacolon) Chronic dilation of colon	Unknown	Severe abdominal distention; failure to thrive; explosive, watery diarrhea	Family history; rectal biopsy shows absence of ganglion in wall of colon and rectum	Low-residue diet; surgery to remove impaired section of colon	Provide family with support group information
Appendicitis Inflammation of vermiform appendix	Blockage of appendix allowing bacteria to multiply	Abdominal pain in RLQ, nausea, vomiting, fever, constipation	Symptoms of patient drawing up of knees in response to palpation of RLQ **(McBurney's point)**	Surgical removal	Ensure medical treatment for symptoms No laxatives
Ulcerative colitis Inflammation of mucosa of colon and rectum	Unknown	Bloody diarrhea, abdominal cramping, mucus-containing stools	Clinical symptoms (weight loss, fever, malaise)	Minimize food selections; medications: antidiarrheal and steroidal	Early treatment and diet free of food that is irritating to patient
Diverticulitis Inflammation of small out-pouches (diverticula) in colon	Blockage of diverticulum causing bowel bacteria to multiply	Fever; pain in left lower abdomen that abates after defecation	Sigmoidoscopy, colonoscopy; guaiac testing and elevated ESR	High residue diet, being careful to avoid seeded fruit and vegetables; rest, medication	Stress need for adherence to diet restrictions

TABLE 15-3

Diseases and Disorders of the Digestive System—cont'd

Disease and Description	Etiology	Signs and Symptoms	Diagnosis	Therapy	Interventions
Volvulus Colon twisting on itself (Figure 15-11)	Abnormal embryonic development	Abdominal pain, nausea, vomiting	Clinical symptoms and GI series (upper and lower)	Surgical intervention	Provide postsurgical diet
RECTUM AND ANAL CANAL					
Hemorrhoids Dilated veins in rectum and anus (internal or external position)	Swollen veins caused by blockage or pressure	Rectal pain, itching, protrusion, or bleeding	Inspection and proctoscopy to visualize internal lesions	Prevention of straining and constipation; diet high in fiber, increased water intake; medications as ordered by physician	Encourage adherence to fluid intake and diet high in fiber Stool softener as needed
LIVER					
Hepatitis A Inflammation of liver caused by viral infection	Oral contact with feces from infected person (e.g., through prepared food), drinking contaminated water, eating contaminated shellfish	Jaundice, fatigue, abdominal pain, loss of weight, diarrhea	Antibody testing "A" positive; clinical symptoms	Management of symptoms; avoidance of alcohol	Vaccine for prophylaxis, immunoglobulin after prophylaxis; provide prevention education
Hepatitis B Inflammation of liver caused by viral infection	Blood-borne pathogen transmitted through contact with infected person's blood or body fluids*	Jaundice, fatigue, abdominal pain, weight loss, diarrhea	Antibody testing "B" positive; clinical symptoms	Management of symptoms; avoidance of alcohol	Vaccine; use standard precautions in occupation; provide prevention education
Hepatitis C Inflammation of liver caused by a viral infection	Blood-borne pathogen transmitted through contact with infected person's blood†	Jaundice, fatigue, abdominal pain, weight loss, diarrhea	Antibody test for "C"; clinical symptoms	Medication for chronic symptoms; avoidance of alcohol	No vaccine; follow standard precautions (avoid sharing drug and tattooing equipment, toothbrushes, razors); provide prevention education
PANCREAS					
Pancreatitis Inflammation of pancreas	Excessive alcohol consumption; bile duct obstructed with gallstones; **idiopathic**	Sudden onset of severe abdominal pain, especially in epigastric area; abdominal distention with vomiting, fever, and tachycardia	Medical history; blood enzymes: amylose level increased	Symptomatic (surgical if obstructed bile duct)	Patient must avoid consuming large amounts of alcohol Diet low in fat

TABLE 15-3
Diseases and Disorders of the Digestive System—cont'd

Disease and Description	Etiology	Signs and Symptoms	Diagnosis	Therapy	Interventions
GALLBLADDER					
Cholecystitis Inflammation of gallbladder	Irritation of gallbladder caused by gallstone becoming lodged in cystic duct	Sudden onset of pain in mid-epigastric area or RUQ that radiates to back in right shoulder area	Ultrasonography and x-rays; elevated series levels of phosphatase	Antibiotic therapy or surgical intervention if antibiotics not adequate	Educate about low-cholesterol diet and weight management to prevent formation of gallstones
Cholelithiasis Gallstones of calcium or cholesterol in gallbladder or lodged in common bile duct	Gallstones leave the gallbladder and cause obstruction in bile duct or fill gallbladder causing irritation	Jaundice in severe cases; sudden onset of pain in mid-epigastric area or RUQ that radiates to back of right shoulder area	Ultrasonography and x-rays	Surgical intervention; lithotripsy; can be treated medically with medications to dissolve stones	Provide diet management to reduce the risk of forming gallstones

GI, Gastrointestinal; *RLQ*, right lower quadrant; *ESR*, erythrocyte sedimentation rate; *RUQ*, right upper quadrant.
*For example, sharing drug equipment, unprotected sex, and occupational exposure (e.g., needle sticks).
†For example, sharing drug equipment, blood transfusions before 1992, and occupational exposure; formerly known as *non-A, non-B hepatitis*.

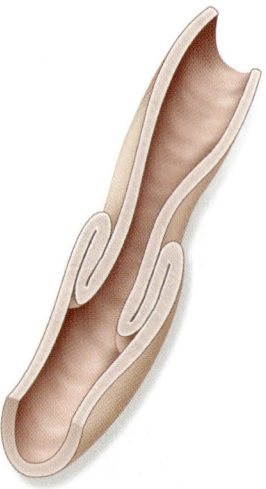

FIGURE 15-10 Intussusception. (Modified from Frazier MS, Drzymkowski JW: *Essentials of human diseases and conditions,* ed 3, Philadelphia, 2004, Saunders.)

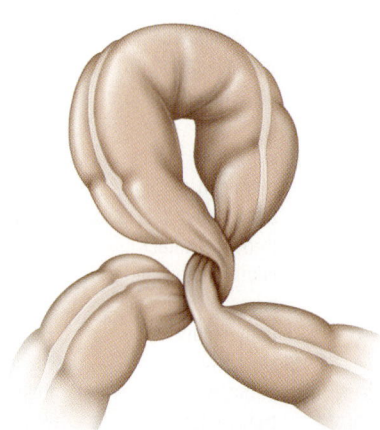

FIGURE 15-11 Volvulus. (Modified from Frazier MS, Drzymkowski JW: *Essentials of human diseases and conditions,* ed 3, Philadelphia, 2004, Saunders.)

CONCLUSION

The organs of the digestive system all work together to break food down to a form that can be used by the body cells. The digestive process is responsible for transport of food and wastes, physical and chemical breakdown, absorption of nutrients and water, and elimination of wastes. The digestive system keeps the body in balance by maintaining adequate hydration to include electrolytes and nutrition.

When the digestive system functions properly, it not only performs its tasks but also helps support the other systems of the human body. Medical assistants who are familiar with the structure, function, and pathophysiology of the digestive system are better prepared to deliver high-quality care to the patients they interact with in the medical office.

Chapter Summary

Reinforce your understanding of the material in this chapter by reviewing the curriculum objectives and key content points below.

1. **Define, appropriately use, and spell all the Key Terms for this chapter.**
   - Review the Key Terms if necessary.
2. **Explain the purpose of the digestive system.**
   - The digestive system changes the food and drink we ingest so that our bodies can use the energy from this intake.
   - After absorbing all the nutrients possible, the digestive system eliminates body waste.
3. **List the four stages of the digestive process.**
   - The digestive and accessory organs allow the gastrointestinal (GI) system to ingest, digest, absorb nutrients, and eliminate waste.
4. **List the eight distinct areas of the digestive tract through which food passes during digestion.**
   - The GI tract can be divided into eight distinct areas: the mouth, pharynx, esophagus, stomach, small intestine, large intestine, rectum, and anal canal.
5. **Explain the role of the mouth in digestion.**
   - The mouth is where food enters the digestive system. Food is masticated by the teeth, mixed with saliva and enzymes to help with the digestive process, and transported down the esophagus on its way to the stomach.
   - Food that has been chewed and mixed with saliva is called a bolus.
6. **Locate three structures in the mouth important to the digestive process.**
   - The mouth contains the tongue, duct openings of the salivary glands, and the teeth.
   - Saliva for digestion is secreted by the salivary glands, which lie outside the mouth but empty into the mouth.
   - The teeth are used for mechanical tearing of food.
7. **Identify the pharynx and explain its role in digestion.**
   - The pharynx (throat) is a long tubelike structure that transports food and liquid to the esophagus for digestion.
   - The bolus enters the pharynx as it is swallowed.
   - The epiglottis closes over the trachea during swallowing, which causes the bolus to enter the esophagus, and not the trachea.
8. **Locate the esophagus and explain its role in digestion.**
   - The esophagus lies behind the trachea and transports food into the stomach. It is flat except when food is being swallowed.
   - The esophagus carries the bolus to the stomach by the process of peristalsis.
9. **Explain the role of the stomach in digestion.**
   - The stomach serves as a short-term storage area for food being digested.
   - The stomach is where many chemicals and enzymes are mixed with food. Digestion starts in the stomach, especially the digestion of proteins.
   - The stomach slowly releases a thick near-liquid mass called chyme into the small intestine for more digestion and absorption.
10. **Locate the peritoneum, sphincters, and fundus within the stomach.**
    - The fundus is the top portion of the stomach.
    - Two sphincters guard the entrance and exit of the stomach: the cardiac sphincter at the esophagus, and the pyloric sphincter at the small intestine.
    - The peritoneum is a serous membrane that provides protection for the digestive organs.
11. **Explain the role of the small intestine in digestion.**
    - The small intestine aids in the breakdown of sugars, proteins, and fats.
12. **Locate the three main parts of the small intestine.**
    - The duodenum begins where the stomach ends.
    - The jejunum contains villi that allow nutrients to be absorbed by the blood.
    - The ileum connects to the cecum (first part of the large intestine).
13. **Explain the role of the large intestine in the digestive system.**
    - The colon absorbs water, minerals, and remaining nutrients in addition to synthesizing and absorbing B-complex vitamins.
    - The colon allows vitamin K to form.
14. **Name and locate the four subdivisions of the large intestine.**
    - The colon can be subdivided into the ascending, transverse, descending, and sigmoid colons.
    - The ascending colon travels up the right side of the body toward the lower part of the liver.
    - The transverse colon moves across the abdomen, below the liver and stomach, and above the small intestine.
    - The descending colon travels down the left side of the body and connects to the sigmoid colon.
    - The sigmoid colon joins to the rectum.
15. **Locate the rectum and explain its role in the digestive system.**
    - The rectum is almost at the end of the digestive system to store waste until it can leave the system as feces.
16. **Locate the anal sphincter and explain its role in the digestive system.**
    - The anal sphincter regulates defecation by allowing fecal material (waste) to be expelled.
17. **Name and locate the three accessory organs to the digestive system and describe the role of each in digesting nutrients.**
    - The liver, gallbladder, and pancreas all secrete important substances that aid in digestion.
    - The liver is located in the right hypochondriac and epigastric regions and produces bile that helps digest fats.
    - The gallbladder lies underneath the liver and stores bile until needed to further the digestive process.
    - The pancreas lies behind the stomach and in front of the first and second lumbar vertebrae. It is both an

endocrine and exocrine organ and produces pancreatin and insulin.

18. **Distinguish between anabolism and catabolism.**
    - Metabolism is the physical and chemical change nutrients undergo after absorption that involves both anabolism and catabolism.
    - Anabolism is the buildup of smaller molecules to nutrients the body needs.
    - Catabolism is the breakdown of larger molecules so the by-products can be used for cell energy.

19. **List six diseases of the mouth and briefly describe the etiology, signs and symptoms, diagnosis, therapy, and interventions for each.**
    - Diseases of the mouth may affect teeth, tongue, gums, or the mucous lining of the mouth.
    - Review Table 15-3.

20. **List two disorders of the esophagus and briefly describe the etiology, signs and symptoms, diagnosis, therapy, and interventions for each.**
    - Disorders of the esophagus often involve the backup, or reflux, of gastric juices (acids).
    - Review Table 15-3.

21. **List five disorders of the stomach and briefly describe the etiology, signs and symptoms, diagnosis, therapy, and interventions for each.**
    - Disorders of the stomach, as with other disorders of the digestive system, may be acute or chronic.
    - Review Table 15-3.

22. **List three disorders of the small intestine and briefly describe the etiology, signs and symptoms, diagnosis, therapy, and interventions for each.**
    - Review Table 15-3.

23. **List four disorders of the large intestine and briefly describe the etiology, signs and symptoms, diagnosis, therapy, and interventions for each.**
    - Review Table 15-3.

24. **List a disorder of the rectum and anal canal and briefly describe its etiology, signs and symptoms, diagnosis, therapy, and interventions.**
    - Review Table 15-3.

25. **List three diseases of the liver and briefly describe the etiology, signs and symptoms, diagnosis, therapy, and interventions for each.**
    - Hepatitis is recognized in several forms; hepatitis A, B, and C are the most frequently diagnosed types.
    - Review Table 15-3.

26. **List three disorders of the accessory organs to the digestive system and briefly describe the etiology, signs and symptoms, diagnosis, therapy, and interventions for each.**
    - Disorders of the accessory organs may involve inflammation and problems with gallstones.
    - Review Table 15-3.

27. **Analyze a realistic medical office situation and apply your understanding of the digestive system to determine the best course of action.**
    - Understanding the normal physiology of the digestive system will help in understanding how the disease process affects this system.

28. **Describe the impact on patient care when medical assistants have a solid understanding of the structure and function of the digestive system.**
    - Medical assistants who understand the physiology of the digestive system will be better prepared to assist with medical procedures, communicate clearly to patients, and perform effective patient teaching.

PRACTICAL APPLICATIONS

If you have accomplished the objectives in this chapter, you will be able to make better choices as a medical assistant. Take another look at this situation and decide what you would do.

Saril Paratel, age 69, was brought to the physician's office with fever and pain in the RLQ of her abdomen. The pain has lasted for 3 days and has become progressively worse over the last 36 hours. The pain originally started in the umbilical area, but over time it moved to McBurney's point. Last night, Saril had nausea and vomiting. She has not had a bowel movement for 4 days. She had dyspepsia for several days before this episode of pain. She has also noticed that fatty foods tend to cause flatulence with some pain in her RUQ, radiating into her back at the right shoulder. No history of hematemesis is given, but malaise has been present for several weeks. When asked about diarrhea, Saril answers that her stools 5 days ago were soft, formed, and frequent; so yes, she had diarrhea. The WBC count ordered by the physician is reported as 15,600 WBCs with a differential of 67% neutrophils, 6% bands, 25% lymphs, 0% basos, 1% monos, and 1% eos. The physician refers Saril to a surgeon because he wants her to be evaluated for possible appendicitis and to rule out the cause of the RUQ pain.

Would you understand all of the terminology here? Would you be able to explain these findings to Saril if she had questions?

1. What gastrointestinal organs are found in the RLQ?
2. Where is McBurney's point?
3. What is appendicitis?
4. What is hematemesis, and why would this be important in this case study?
5. What is the difference between emesis and regurgitation?
6. Did Saril really have diarrhea? Explain your answer.
7. What did the WBC count indicate?
8. How did the WBC differential confirm that Saril might have appendicitis?
9. What organs of digestion are found in the RUQ?
10. What disease processes might be seen with RUQ pain that radiates into the right back at the shoulder with associated flatulence?

WEB SEARCH

1. **Research the stomach and its disorders.** Consider that stress or nervousness can cause an upset stomach. Investigate the physiology of digestion and how gastric secretions are regulated.
   - **Keywords:** Use the following keywords in your search: digestion, gastric secretions, stomach.
2. **Research the liver and its disorders.** The liver has several major functions and can malfunction for many reasons. Investigate the different forms of hepatitis and causes of cirrhosis and treatments.
   - **Keywords:** Use the following keywords in your search: liver, hepatitis, cirrhosis, liver transplant.

WORD PARTS: Digestive (GI) System

MOUTH
Combining Forms

cheil/o	lip
dent/i, dent/o	teeth
dips/o	thirst
gingiv/o	gums
gloss/o, lingu/o	tongue
mandibul/o	mandible
maxill/o	maxilla
odont/o	teeth
or/o	mouth
sial/o	saliva
sialaden/o	salivary gland
staphyl/o	uvula; clusters
stomat/o	mouth

Suffix

-ase	enzyme

PHARYNX

pharyng/o	throat, pharynx

ESOPHAGUS AND STOMACH
Combining Forms

esophag/o	esophagus
gastr/o	stomach
prote/o	protein
vag/o	vagus nerve

Suffixes

-clysis	washing out
-emesis	vomiting
-pepsia	digestion
-phage	eat or swallow
-phagia	eating or swallowing
-stalsis	contraction

INTESTINES, RECTUM, AND ANAL CANAL
Combining Forms

an/o	anus
append/o, appendic/o	appendix
bil/i	bile
cec/o	cecum
col/o, colon/o	large intestine; colon
diverticul/o	diverticular
duoden/o	duodenum
enter/o	small intestine
fung/i	fungus
glyc/o	sugar
ile/o	ileum
jejun/o	jejunum
lact/o	milk
lip/o	fats
myc/o	fungus
proct/o	anus, rectum
prote/o	protein
py/o	pus
pylor/o	pylorus
rect/o	rectum
sigmoid/o	sigmoid colon
top/o	place or position

Suffixes

-cele	swelling of; hernia
-ose	sugar
-pexy	surgical fixation

ACCESSORY ORGANS
Combining Forms

hepat/o	liver
cholecyst/o	gallbladder
chol/e	bile
choledoch/o	common bile duct
cyst/o	bladder or sac
pancreat/o	pancreas

ABBREVIATIONS: Digestive (GI) System

ac	before meals (Latin *ante cibum*)
ALT	alanine transaminase; liver enzyme test
AST	aspartate transaminase; liver enzyme test
BaE, BE	barium enema
GA	gastric analysis
GI	gastrointestinal
IC	irritable colon
IVC	intravenous cholangiogram
NPO, npo	nothing by mouth (Latin *nulle per os*)
SGOT	serum glutamic-oxaloacetic transaminase (AST)
SGPT	serum glutamic-pyruvic transaminase (ALT)
pc	after meals (Latin *post cibum*)

Nervous System

16

evolve   http://evolve.elsevier.com/klieger/medicalassisting

The nervous system is the body's communication and control system. This complex system organizes and controls voluntary and involuntary activities of the body and enables all our body systems to work together. The brain is the control center of the nervous system. It sends and receives messages through a system of nerves that functions similar to a highway system. The spinal cord can be thought of as the interstate highway. It branches off into smaller and smaller bunches of nerves (highways, main streets, and side streets). In this way, our brains can send messages to and receive messages from any part of the body.

The brain sends and receives messages based on what we hear, see, taste, smell, and touch, and it allows us to react to what we sense. For example, if we see a ball coming at us, our brain helps us react by catching it or moving out of the way. This communication allows homeostasis to be maintained in the body.

To best understand the functioning of the nervous system, you need to know about its structure, the diseases and disorders that affect it, and how the sensory system communicates with it.

LEARNING OBJECTIVES

You will be able to do the following after completing this chapter:

Key Terms
1. Define, appropriately use, and spell all the Key Terms for this chapter.

Structure and Function of the Nervous System
2. Describe the organization of the nervous system and identify its two main divisions.
3. Explain the role of neurons and neuroglia in a nerve impulse.
4. Describe a synapse and explain its function.

Central Nervous System
5. List the main divisions of the central nervous system (CNS).
6. Identify the parts of the brain and briefly describe the function of each.
7. Explain the purpose of cerebrospinal fluid (CSF).
8. List the cranial nerves and describe their function.
9. List the spinal nerves and describe their function.

Peripheral Nervous System
10. List the main divisions of the peripheral nervous system.
11. Describe the functions of the sympathetic and parasympathetic nervous systems.
12. List and briefly describe six types of reflex actions.

Diseases and Disorders of the Nervous System
13. List and describe nine types of signs and symptoms of neurological disease.
14. List six types of diagnostic tests and procedures for neurological disease and describe the use of each.
15. List 11 diseases and disorders of the nervous system and briefly describe the etiology, signs and symptoms, diagnosis, therapy, and interventions for each.

Mental Health
16. Describe the twofold testing process used to determine mental health disorders.
17. List and describe seven common signs and symptoms of mental disorders.
18. List four types of tests and procedures used to diagnose mental disorders and briefly describe each.
19. List and briefly describe 20 mental health disorders.

Patient-Centered Professionalism

20. Analyze a realistic medical office situation and apply your understanding of the nervous system to determine the best course of action.
21. Describe the impact on patient care when medical assistants have a solid understanding of the structure and function of the nervous system.

KEY TERMS

The Key Terms for this chapter have been organized into sections so that you can easily see the terminology associated with each aspect of the nervous system.

Structure and Function of the Nervous System
Nerve Cells and Nerve Impulses

glial cells	neuroglia
nerve	neuron

Neurons

axon	myelinated
cell body	nerve fibers
dendrites	neurilemma
ganglion	nodes of Ranvier
integrative neurons (interneurons)	sensory (afferent) neurons
motor (efferent) neurons	sheath
myelin sheath	

Neuroglia

astrocytes	microglia cells
ependymal cells	oligodendroglia cells

Nerve Impulses

dermatome	receptors
nerve impulse	stimulus
neurotransmitters	synapse
plexus	

Divisions of the Nervous System

brain	central nervous system (CNS)
peripheral nervous system (PNS)	

Central Nervous System

arachnoid	dura mater
pia mater	

Brain

antidiuretic hormone (ADH)	gyri
brainstem	hypothalamus
cerebellum	linear
cerebrospinal fluid (CSF)	medulla oblongata
cerebrum	meninges
cortex	midbrain
cranial nerves	occipital lobe
diencephalon	oxytocin
epidural space	parietal lobe
equilibrium	pituitary gland
fissures	pons
frontal lobe	spatial
subarachnoid space	thalamus
subdural space	ventricles
sulcus	viscera
temporal lobe	

Spinal Cord

spinal column	spinal nerves
spinal cord	

Peripheral Nervous System

autonomic nervous system (ANS)	somatic nervous system

Autonomic Nervous System

"fight-or-flight" response	parasympathetic nervous system
homeostasis	sympathetic nervous system

Somatic Nervous System

abdominal reflex	patellar reflex
Achilles reflex	plantar reflex
Babinski reflex	reflex
corneal reflex	

Diseases and Disorders of the Nervous System

Alzheimer disease	meningitis
amyotrophic lateral sclerosis (ALS, Lou Gehrig disease)	multiple sclerosis (MS)
	neurologist
cerebrovascular accident (CVA, stroke)	Parkinson disease
	shingles (herpes zoster)
chronic fatigue syndrome	tic douloureux (trigeminal neuralgia)
encephalitis	
epilepsy	transient ischemic attack (TIA)

Signs and Symptoms

amoebae	insidious
aphasia	Kernig sign
ataxia	numbness
diplopia	pain
gait	paralysis
headache	predisposing factors
hemiparesis	seizures
hemiplegia	vertigo

Mental Health

akathisia	general anxiety disorder
amnesia	hallucination
antisocial	histrionic
attention deficit hyperactivity disorder (ADHD)	Munchausen syndrome
	narcissistic
autism	obsessive-compulsive disorder (OCD)
bipolar disorder	
catatonia	paranoid
conversion	post-traumatic stress disorder (PTSD)
delirium	
delusion	psychiatry
delusional disorder	psychosis
dementia	schizoid
depression	schizophrenia

Diagnostic Procedures for the Nervous System

angiography
computed tomography (CT) scan
electroencephalography (EEG)
electromyography (EMG)
electroneuromyography
lumbar puncture (spinal tap)
magnetic resonance imaging (MRI)
myelography
nerve conduction studies
positron emission tomography (PET) scan

PRACTICAL APPLICATIONS

Read the following scenario and keep it in mind as you learn about the nervous system in this chapter.

Sally Jones, age 72, complained of dizziness with a loss of sensation on the left side that lasted only for a few minutes over the past few weeks. She also had a headache that lasted only during the paresthesia. She has a long history of moderately controlled hypertension for which she has taken antihypertensives, "When I thought about them." Dr. Smith was concerned that she might be having TIAs. He prescribed a vasodilator and a mild analgesic for the headache when he saw her last week. Today she was brought to the emergency room with sudden left-sided hemiplegia and a headache but no aphasia. Except for the hypertension, Ms. Jones has been in relatively good health for her age. On admission, her blood pressure was 210/120 and she was semialert. Dr. Smith ordered a CT scan, which showed an infarct to the right frontotemporal lobes. Ms. Jones was admitted to the hospital for observation and possible treatment.

Do you understand what an infarct is, and how Ms. Jones's earlier symptoms relate to it?

NERVOUS SYSTEM STRUCTURE AND FUNCTION

The nervous system is the main communication and control system of the body, allowing the other body systems to function. The nervous system organizes and controls both the voluntary and the involuntary activities of the body by means of electrical impulses. Medical assistants need to understand the structure and function of the nervous system, including its cells and nerve impulses and two major divisions, the **central nervous system (CNS)** and the **peripheral nervous system (PNS).** This understanding will help you recognize how the nervous system is able to control the body's activities and maintain homeostasis.

Nerve Cells and Nerve Impulses

The nervous system is made up of nerves. A **nerve** is a bundle containing the fibers of many neurons and microscopic blood vessels. Nerves are protected by connective tissue and run to and from various organs and tissues in the body. As with every other body system, the smallest structural piece of the nervous system is the cell. These cells enable the whole system to function through electrical impulses that allow them to respond to stimuli.

Nerve Cells

There are two distinctive types of cells in the nervous system: neurons and neuroglia.

Neurons. The functional unit of the nervous system is the **neuron.** A neuron is a specialized unit that receives and transmits messages in the form of nerve impulses. Neurons carry these impulses throughout the CNS.

Neurons are classified into three areas according to their function.

TYPE OF NEURON	FUNCTION
Sensory (afferent) neurons	Transmit nerve impulses to the CNS from both within and outside the CNS.
Motor (efferent) neurons	Transmit impulses from the CNS to the muscles and glands of the body.
Integrative neurons (interneurons)	Conduct impulses between the afferent to the efferent neurons. Located within the brain and spinal cord.

Neurons respond to stimuli by conducting impulses. Each neuron has the following parts:

- A **cell body** (main part of the cell) contains a nucleus and projections called axons and dendrites (Figure 16-1). A group of cell bodies along the path of a nerve is a **ganglion.**
- The **axon** is attached to the cell body and carries impulses to other neurons and body tissues. A neuron has one axon with several branches. The larger the diameter of an axon, the faster the nerve impulses travel. An axon can be enclosed in a covering, or **myelin sheath,** which is not continuous. The separate parts are called the **nodes of Ranvier,** and the spaces consist of a layer of fats and proteins. Bundles of axons are **nerve fibers** and appear as white matter if **myelinated.** Not all axons are myelinated; unmyelinated axons appear as gray matter. **Neurilemma** is a continuous **sheath** around the myelin sheath.
- **Dendrites** function to receive nerve impulses. Dendrites pick up stimuli and carry the stimuli to the cell body. Each neuron has one or more dendrites that resemble tree branches. The tips of the dendrites are referred to as "receptors" because they receive stimuli.

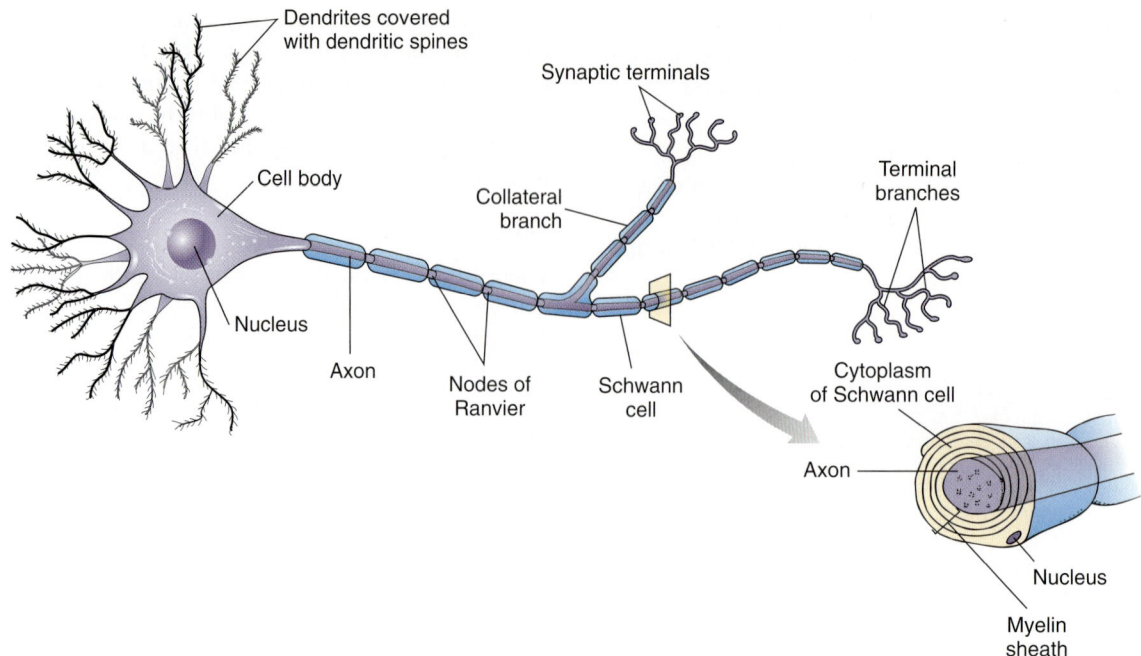

FIGURE 16-1 Structure of a neuron: dendrites, cell body, axon, and axon terminals. Structure surrounding the axon is the myelin sheath. Nodes of Ranvier are the spaces between the myelin. (From Solomon EP: *Introduction to human anatomy and physiology*, ed 3, St Louis, 2009, Saunders.)

Neuroglia. The **neuroglia,** or **glial cells,** are the most numerous of the nerve cells and are mainly located within the CNS. The neuroglias are responsible for the support, protection, insulation, and nourishment of the neurons. They do not carry nerve impulses. The different types of neuroglia are classified by their function.

TYPE OF GLIAL CELL	FUNCTION
Astrocytes	The most abundant type of the nerve cells; "star shaped." Astrocytes filter harmful substances from the blood circulating through the brain, forming the protective blood-brain barrier. They also transport water and salts between capillaries and neurons.
Ependymal cells	Line the cavities of the brain and assist in the formation of cerebrospinal fluid.
Microglia cells	Responsible for engulfing and destroying microorganisms and cellular waste in nervous tissue.
Oligodendroglia cells	Responsible for producing the myelin sheath for neurons in the CNS.

Figure 16-2 illustrates the various types of neuroglial cells.

Nerve Impulses

A **nerve impulse** starts when a **stimulus** (change in environment) acts on **receptors** (located on distal ends of dendrites). The stimulus must be strong enough to be sensed and appropriate for a particular neuron. For example, heat stimulates temperature receptors on the skin and sound waves stimulate the auditory nerve; neither receptor would respond to the other stimulus.

The nerve impulse occurs as follows (Figure 16-3):
1. The nerve is at rest.
2. An adequate stimulus occurs, and the impulse (a tiny electrical pulse) is generated.
3. The impulse travels along a myelinated axon and jumps from node to node.
4. The impulse reaches the end of the axon and moves to the muscle or gland.

When the impulse arrives at the end of the axon, there is a gap between it and the next neuron (or muscle or gland cell, depending on where the impulse is going). This gap is called a *synapse.*

Synapse. A **synapse** is a microscopic space (1/100,000 of an inch wide) between the end of one neuron and the start of the next neuron. When a nerve impulse reaches the end of a neuron, the synapse helps information transmit from one neuron to another. The electrical impulse in the neuron triggers the release of chemicals (**neurotransmitters**) that carry the impulse across the junction to the next neuron (Figure 16-4). After the impulse is transmitted across the synapse, another chemical is released so the neuron can reset itself allowing it to fire an impulse again if necessary.

Divisions of the Nervous System

As mentioned, the two main divisions of the nervous system are the CNS, which includes the brain and spinal cord, and

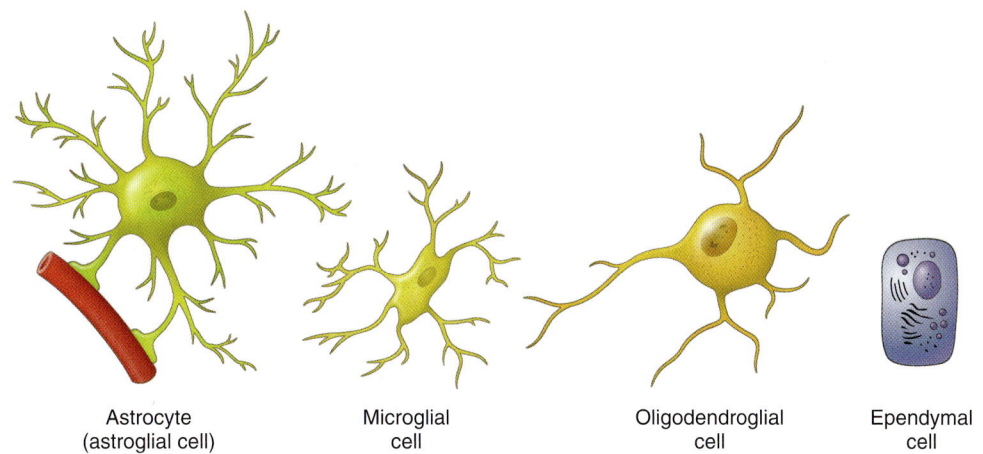

FIGURE 16-2 Neuroglial cells and an ependymal cell. (Modified from Chabner DE: *The language of medicine,* ed 8, St Louis, 2007, Saunders.)

the PNS, which consists of a series of nerves that connect the CNS with the various tissues of the body (Figure 16-5).

Central Nervous System

The **brain** and the **spinal cord** are protected by a membrane (**meninges**) with the following three layers (Figure 16-6):
1. The **dura mater** is a thick covering located closest to the skull and vertebral column and contains veins that drain blood from the brain
2. The **arachnoid** ("spiderweb") membrane, the middle layer, provides weblike space for the fluid between the second and third layers.
3. The **pia mater,** the thin membrane closest to the brain and **spinal column,** contains blood vessels to supply blood to the brain.

Box 16-1 lists protective layers and coverings for CNS structures.

Brain. The brain is a complex organ that fits inside the skull. It contains billions of neurons and has millions of synaptic connections. The brain is protected by the skull, which is made of several cranial bones, including the following:
1. Frontal
2. Parietal
3. Temporal
4. Sphenoid
5. Ethmoid
6. Occipital

As noted earlier, three-layered membranous coverings called *meninges* protect the brain. These tissues are continuous and also cover the spinal cord. The spaces between each layer are as follows:
- The **epidural space** is located outside the dura mater between the dura mater and vertebrae and skull and contains fat that acts as a cushion to absorb trauma.

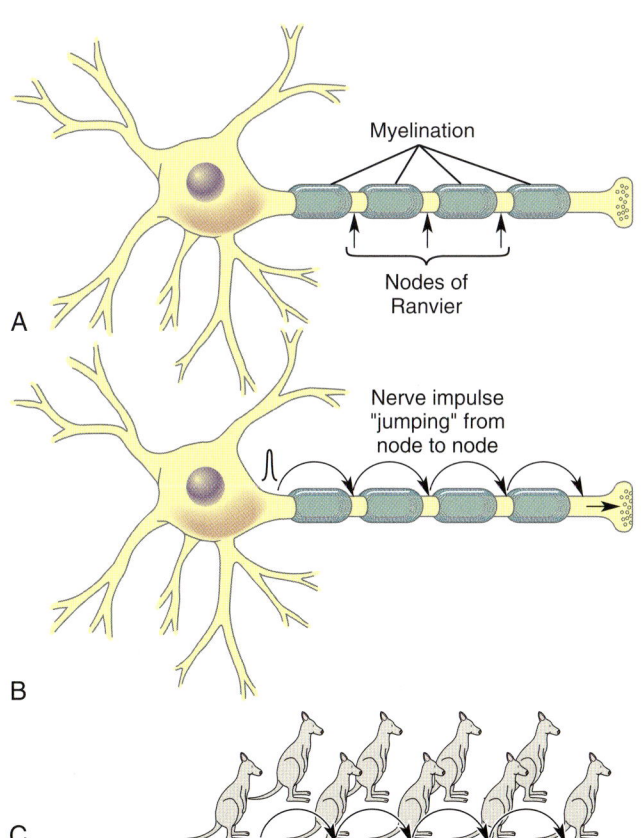

FIGURE 16-3 How nerve impulses work. **A,** Myelinated axon, showing exposed axonal membrane at the nodes of Ranvier. **B,** Nerve impulse jumps from node to node toward the axon terminal. Jumping allows the nerve impulse to travel the length of the axon very fast. **C,** Jumping of nerve impulse resembles the jumping or hopping of a kangaroo. Think of how much faster a kangaroo can move by jumping rather than walking. (From Herlihy B, Maebius NK: *The human body in health and illness,* ed 3, St Louis, 2007, Saunders.)

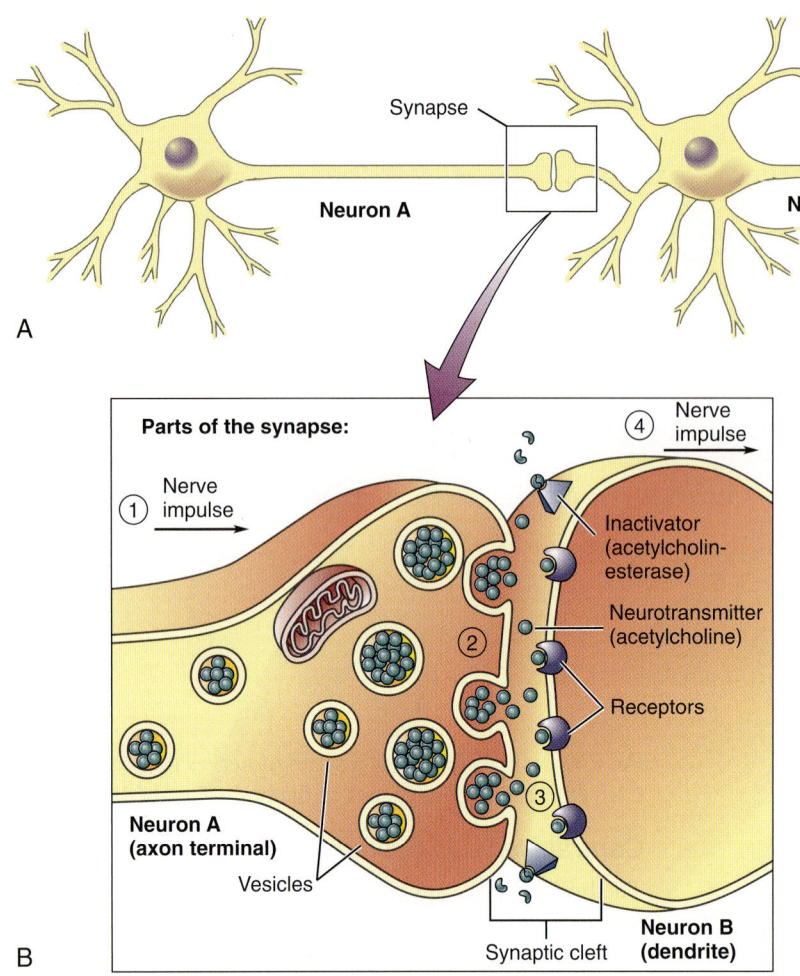

FIGURE 16-4 **A,** Synapse is located in the space between neuron *A* and neuron *B*. **B,** Parts of the synapse include the neurotransmitters, inactivators, and receptors. *1,* The nerve impulse travels along neuron A to its axon terminal where it causes the vesicles to merge, or fuse, with the membrane of the axon terminal *(2).* The vesicles open and release neurotransmitter into the synaptic cleft. *3,* The neurotransmitter diffuses across the synaptic cleft and binds to the receptor sites of neuron B, causing a new nerve impulse in the dendrite of neuron B, which travels toward the cell body and axon of neuron B *(4).* (From Herlihy B, Maebius NK: *The human body in health and illness,* ed 3, St Louis, 2007, Saunders.)

BOX 16-1

Protection of Central Nervous System Structures

Brain	Covered by cranial bones in skull; further protection by meninges and cerebrospinal fluid
Cranial bones, vertebrae	Lined with meninges
Nerve tissue	Protected by fluid, meninges, and bones
Spinal cord	Surrounded by vertebrae and cerebrospinal fluid

- The **subdural space** is located between the dura mater and arachnoid membrane and contains a serous fluid for lubrication.
- The **subarachnoid space** is located between the pia mater and arachnoid membrane and contains **cerebrospinal fluid (CSF),** which serves as a cushion to protect the brain and spinal cord.

CSF is a sterile, watery fluid that is a combination of lymphocytes, protein, sugar, chlorides, and interstitial fluid. CSF is formed by separation of fluid from blood in the choroid plexuses (capillaries) into the ventricles of the brain. It circulates through the ventricles and into the subarachnoid spaces of the brain and spinal cord and then is absorbed back into the blood. The amount of circulating CSF in the average adult is about 140 mL.

The 12 pairs of cranial nerves originate on the undersurface of the brain, mostly from the brainstem. The brain is divided into four main sections: cerebrum, diencephalon, brainstem, and cerebellum (Figure 16-7).

Cranial Nerves. There are 12 pairs of **cranial nerves** attached to the brain (Figure 16-8). The cranial nerves are numbered by Roman numerals in sequence of their origin (Table 16-1). The three types of nerve fibers represented are (1) motor (efferent—from CNS to body), (2) sensory (afferent—from body to CNS), and (3) mixed (sensory and motor). Use a mnemonic device to memorize the correct order of the cranial nerves. Let the first letter of each word be associated with a cranial nerve. For example:

On	I	Finn	VII
Old	II	And	VIII
Olympus	III	German	IX
Towering	IV	Viewed	X
Tops	V	Some	XI
A	VI	Hops	XII

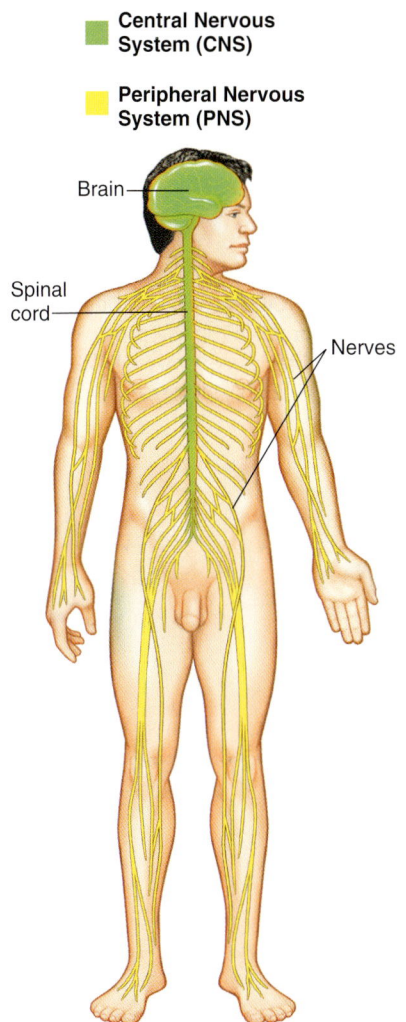

FIGURE 16-5 Major anatomical features of the human nervous system include the brain, the spinal cord, and each of the individual nerves. The brain and spinal cord make up the central nervous system (CNS), and all the nerves and their branches make up the peripheral nervous system (PNS). (From Thibodeau GA, Patton KT: *Anatomy and physiology*, ed 6, St Louis, 2006, Mosby.)

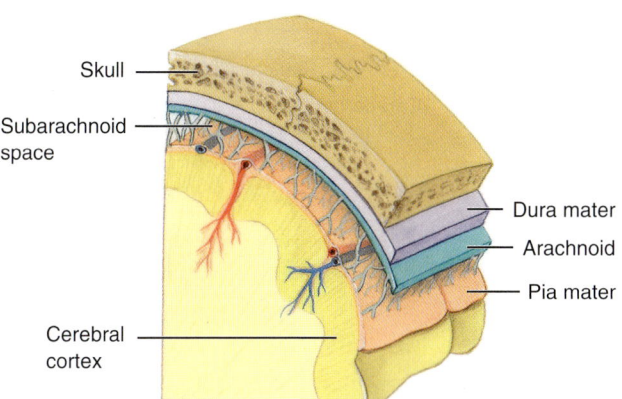

FIGURE 16-6 Protective layers of central nervous system (CNS). The three layers of meninges are the dura mater, arachnoid membrane, and pia mater. Cerebrospinal fluid (CSF) circulates within the subarachnoid space. Note the arachnoid villi projecting into dural sinus for drainage of CSF. (From Applegate EJ: *The anatomy and physiology learning system*, ed 3, St Louis, 2006, Saunders.)

Cerebrum. The **cerebrum** is the largest portion of the brain. It controls functions associated with thinking and voluntary activity. The outer portion of the cerebrum is the **cortex** (processes information), white soft matter covered in gray matter and arranged in folds or convolutions called **gyri**. The deeper folds, or grooves, are **fissures,** or sulci. The cortex contains the areas that allow humans to learn. The higher brain functions of learning, such as reasoning, memory, and abstract thought, also occur in the cortex.

The cerebrum is divided into right and left hemispheres that are separated by a longitudinal fissure, or **sulcus.** The right hemisphere controls the left side of the body. It is responsible for auditory and tactile perception, creative functions, and **spatial** orientation feelings. The left hemisphere controls the right side of the body. It controls language, hand movements, and **linear** thought. A band of nerve fibers (*corpus callosum*) connects the cerebral hemispheres. Each hemisphere has four lobes (Figure 16-9), as follows:

1. The **frontal lobe** controls voluntary muscles, speech, and judgment.
2. The **parietal lobe** controls sensory function such as pain, touch, and temperature interpretation.
3. The **temporal lobe** controls hearing, smell, and taste.
4. The **occipital lobe** controls vision.

There are four **ventricles** in the brain. The ventricles, which contain the choroid plexus, are small cavities responsible for the continual production of CSF, which cushions the nerve tissue of the brain and spinal cord. The ventricles align with the subarachnoid spaces and central lining of the spinal cord (Figure 16-10).

The emotional part of the brain is referred to as the *limbic system*. It is a group of structures interconnected throughout the cerebrum and the diencephalon. The limbic system is involved with various states of emotions, feelings, and with memory.

Diencephalon. The **diencephalon** is located under the cerebrum. It encases the third ventricle of the brain and includes the thalamus and hypothalamus.

The **thalamus** is composed of gray matter (unmyelinated nerve tissue) and is located between the cerebrum and midbrain. Its function is to relay messages from the eyes, ears, and skin by monitoring sensory stimuli, including touch and pressure sensations, to the brain. The messages are sent to the appropriate area in the cortex of the cerebrum. The thalamus has also been associated with the emotional states of pleasant and unpleasant sensations, and it is the brain's center for the perception of pain.

The **hypothalamus** is below the thalamus and connects to the CNS by controlling the activities of the "master gland," or **pituitary gland,** thus forming a link between the nervous and endocrine systems. The hypothalamus produces hormones that signal the anterior pituitary gland to release its hormones

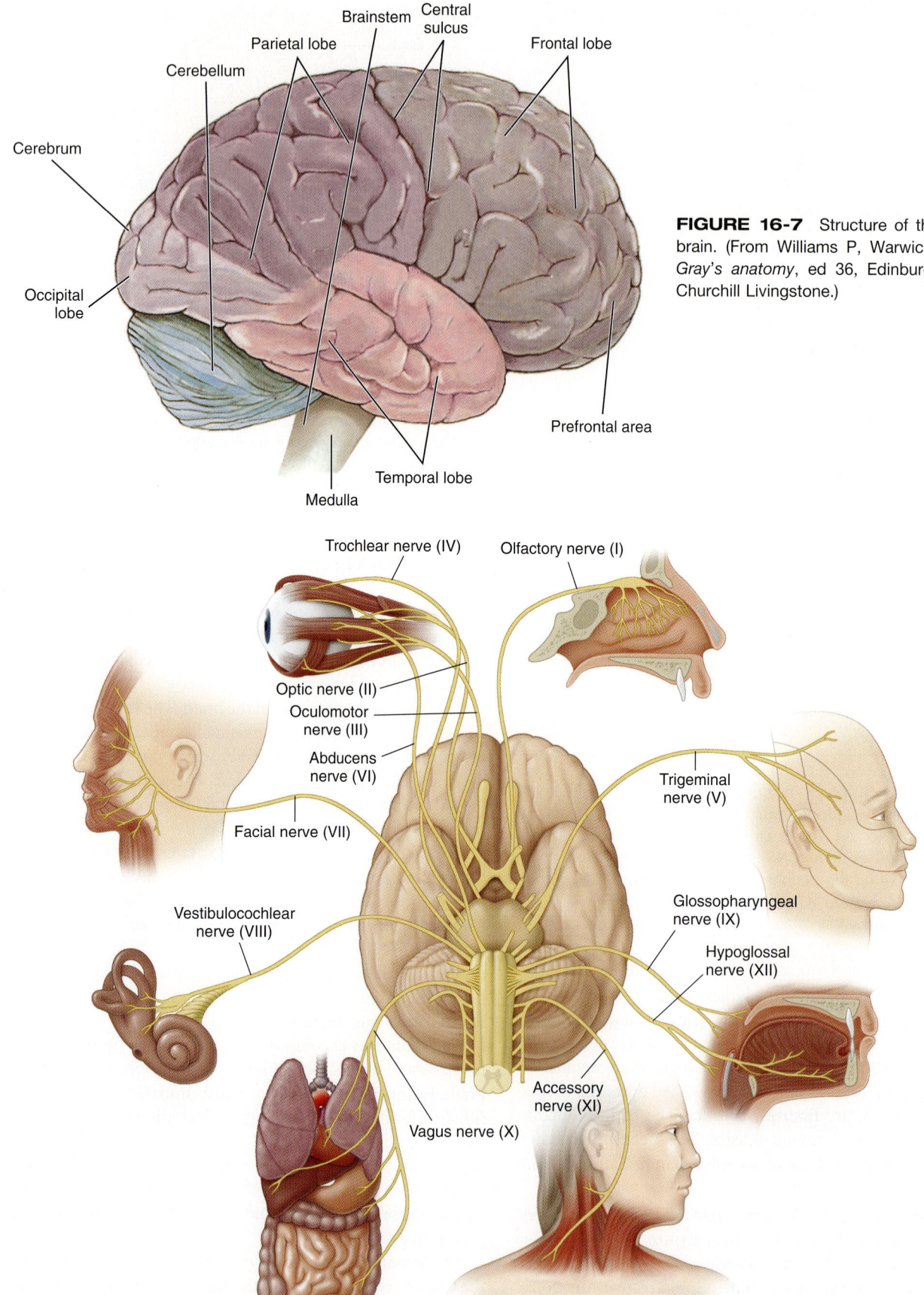

FIGURE 16-7 Structure of the human brain. (From Williams P, Warwick R, eds: *Gray's anatomy*, ed 36, Edinburgh, 1980, Churchill Livingstone.)

FIGURE 16-8 Undersurface of the brain showing attachments of the cranial nerves. (Modified from Thibodeau GA, Patton KT: *The human body in health and disease*, ed 4, St Louis, 2005, Mosby.)

TABLE 16-1

Cranial Nerves

Number	Name	Type	Conduct Impulses	Function
I	Olfactory	Sensory	From nose to brain	Olfaction (sense of smell)
II	Optic	Sensory	From eye to brain	Vision
III	Oculomotor	Motor	From brain to eye muscle	Controls upper eyelid muscles, eye movements, regulation of pupil size, and accommodation for close vision
IV	Trochlear	Motor	From brain to external eye muscle	Controls movement of external eye muscles
V	Trigeminal	Mixed	From brain to skin and mucous membrane of head From teeth to brain From brain to chewing muscle	Controls chewing movements Sensation around the eye Sensation from eye to upper jaw and throat Sensation in mandibular region
VI	Abducens	Motor	From brain to external eye muscles	Controls eye movement
VII	Facial	Mixed	From taste buds of tongue to brain From brain to face muscle	Controls taste, facial muscles; controls secretion of tears and saliva
VIII	Vestibulocochlear (Auditory)	Sensory	From ear to brain	Senses of equilibrium (balance) Hearing
IX	Glossopharyngeal	Mixed	From throat and taste buds to brain From brain to throat muscles and salivary glands	Controls taste (posterior third of tongue); salivation; controls swallowing muscles; blood pressure sensation
X	Vagus	Mixed	From throat, larynx, and organs in thoracic and abdominal cavities to brain From brain to muscles of throat and to organs in thoracic and abdominal cavities	Controls swallowing muscles
XI	Spinal (Accessory)	Motor	From brain to shoulder and neck muscles	Controls some shoulder movements Controls some head movements
XII	Hypoglossal	Motor	From brain to muscles of tongue	Controls tongue muscles (swallowing and speech)

into the blood for circulation. The hypothalamus also produces the hormone **oxytocin** for uterine contractions during and after childbirth and **antidiuretic hormone (ADH)** for fluid balance in the body. These two hormones are stored in the posterior pituitary gland, and their release is controlled by nerve stimulation when needed.

The hypothalamus further regulates the autonomic nervous system. This system is responsible for the involuntary activities of the internal organs (**viscera**) such as those associated with digestion and blood circulation. Body temperature, sleep cycles, appetite, thirst, and some emotions (e.g., fear, anger, pain, or pleasure) are also controlled by the hypothalamus.

Brainstem. The **brainstem** has three parts: the midbrain, pons, and medulla oblongata (Figure 16-11).

The **midbrain** is made up of nerve tissue that connects the lower portion of the cerebrum to the pons. CSF passes from the third ventricle to the fourth ventricle in the back portion of the brainstem. Cranial nerves III and IV originate in the midbrain, which serves as a center for visual and auditory reflexes. Visual reflexes include dilation and constriction of the pupil in response to light. The auditory reflex involves movement of the head in response to sound.

The **pons,** the middle section of the brainstem, acts as a bridge between the brain and spinal cord. Cranial nerves VI, VII, VIII, and X originate in the pons, which controls areas of the face, hearing, balance, blood pressure, and heart rate. Besides relaying information (sensory and motor) the pons plays a role in regulating patterned breathing (e.g., rate and rhythm).

The **medulla oblongata** is the lowest portion of the brainstem. It continues into the spinal cord. The white matter forms tracts that cross from one side of the body to the other. The gray matter contains cranial nerves IX to XII and some reflex areas. The medulla is responsible for involuntary movements such as heart and respiratory rate, vasoconstriction, swallowing, coughing, sneezing, hiccupping, and vomiting.

Cerebellum. The **cerebellum** is situated below the cerebrum and is often referred to as the "little brain." The cerebellum is composed of both gray and white matter and has two hemispheres, like the cerebrum. Connected to the brainstem by white fibers, the cerebellum controls the skeletal muscles for fine motor skills and coordination of voluntary muscle groups. The cerebellum is also responsible for maintenance of **equilibrium** (balance) and posture.

Spinal Cord. The **spinal cord** is a long bundle of nerves that conducts impulses to and from the brain. It also serves as a reflex center to receive and transmit messages through nerve fibers. It extends from the medulla to the end of the lumbar vertebrae. The center area is composed of gray matter and the exterior portion is white matter (myelinated nerve fibers covered with fatty membrane) (Figure 16-12). The white matter contains the ascending (sensory—afferent) and descending (motor—efferent) tracts (fiber bundles) that carry impulses to and from the brain.

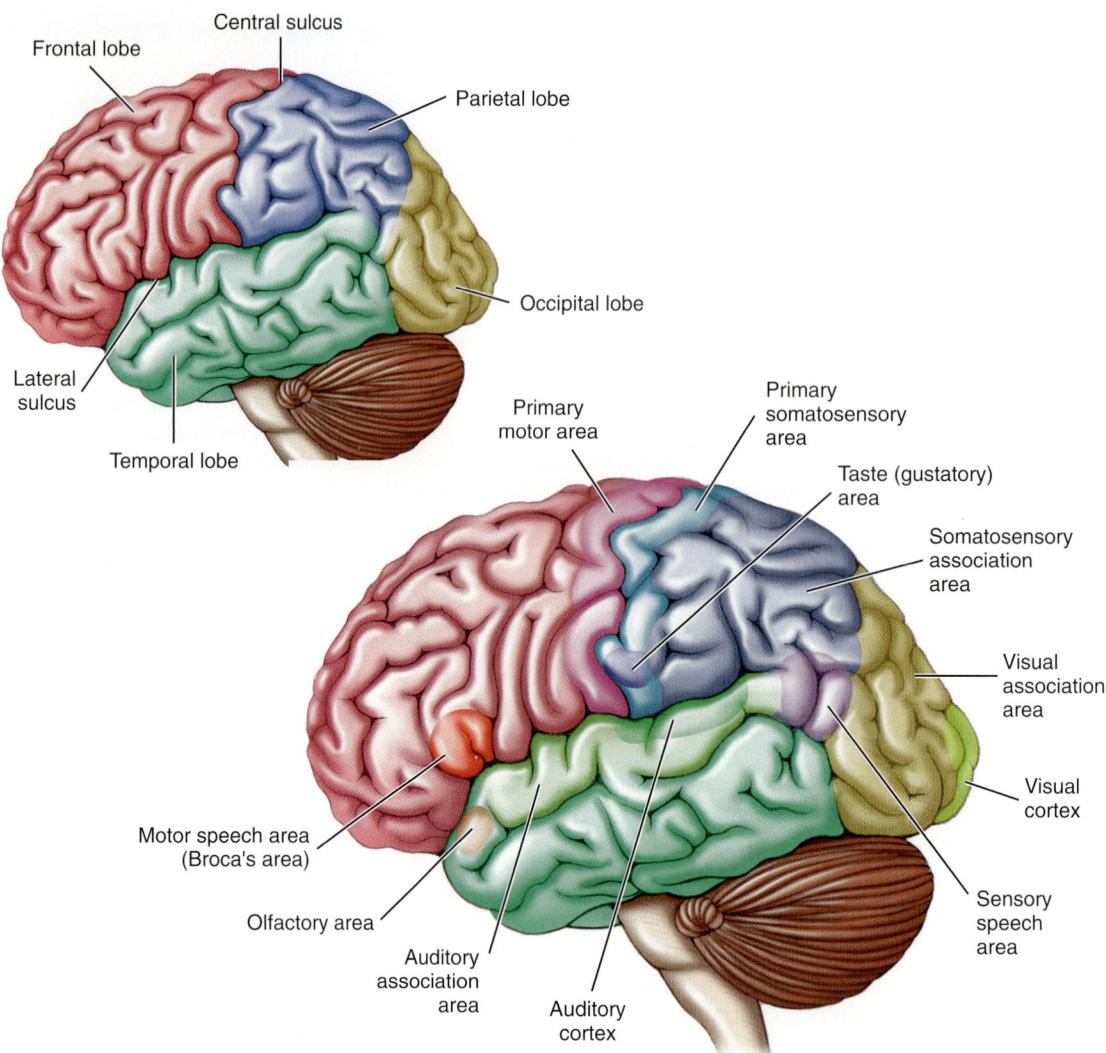

FIGURE 16-9 *Upper left,* Lobes of the cerebrum: frontal, parietal, temporal, and occipital. *Lower right,* Functional areas of the cerebrum. (From Herlihy B, Maebius NK: *The human body in health and illness,* ed 3, St Louis, 2007, Saunders.)

Spinal Nerves. There are 31 pairs of **spinal nerves** grouped according to spinal areas: eight cervical (C1 to C8), 12 thoracic (T1 to T12), five lumbar (L1 to L5), five sacral (S1 to S5), and one coccygeal (one pair). As the spinal nerves leave the spinal cord, they branch out and reorganize to form a network or **plexus** (Figure 16-13). Spinal nerves function to conduct impulses between the spinal cord and body parts not supplied by the cranial nerves. Areas of the skin supplied by a single spinal nerve are referred to as a **dermatome.** Each pair joins the spinal cord by the anterior (ventral) root, which carries motor impulses away from the spinal cord toward muscles or glands. The posterior (dorsal) root carries sensory impulses into the spinal cord (Figure 16-14).

Peripheral Nervous System

The PNS provides information to the CNS by way of both sensory and motor activity outside the CNS. If you stub your toe, the message that your toe hurts travels from the toe up the leg to the spinal cord and informs the brain. The cranial nerves and the spinal nerves are the PNS and are classified according to their origin. The autonomic nervous system controls the involuntary actions of smooth muscles, cardiac muscles, and glands (Figure 16-15). Another part of the PNS is the **somatic nervous system,** which transmits impulses to the skeletal muscles and is responsible for voluntary response to external stimuli by reflex action.

FOR YOUR INFORMATION

BRAIN FREEZE

Have you ever wondered why you get a headache when you consume a cold drink (e.g., iced coffee, slurpees) or eat ice cream too fast? It occurs because the blood vessels in the stomach constrict when they come in contact with a cold fluid. The pain that you feel in your head is not really occurring in your head at all. The sensation of pain is really diverted from your stomach to a nerve in your head which is responsible for receiving this type of sensation.

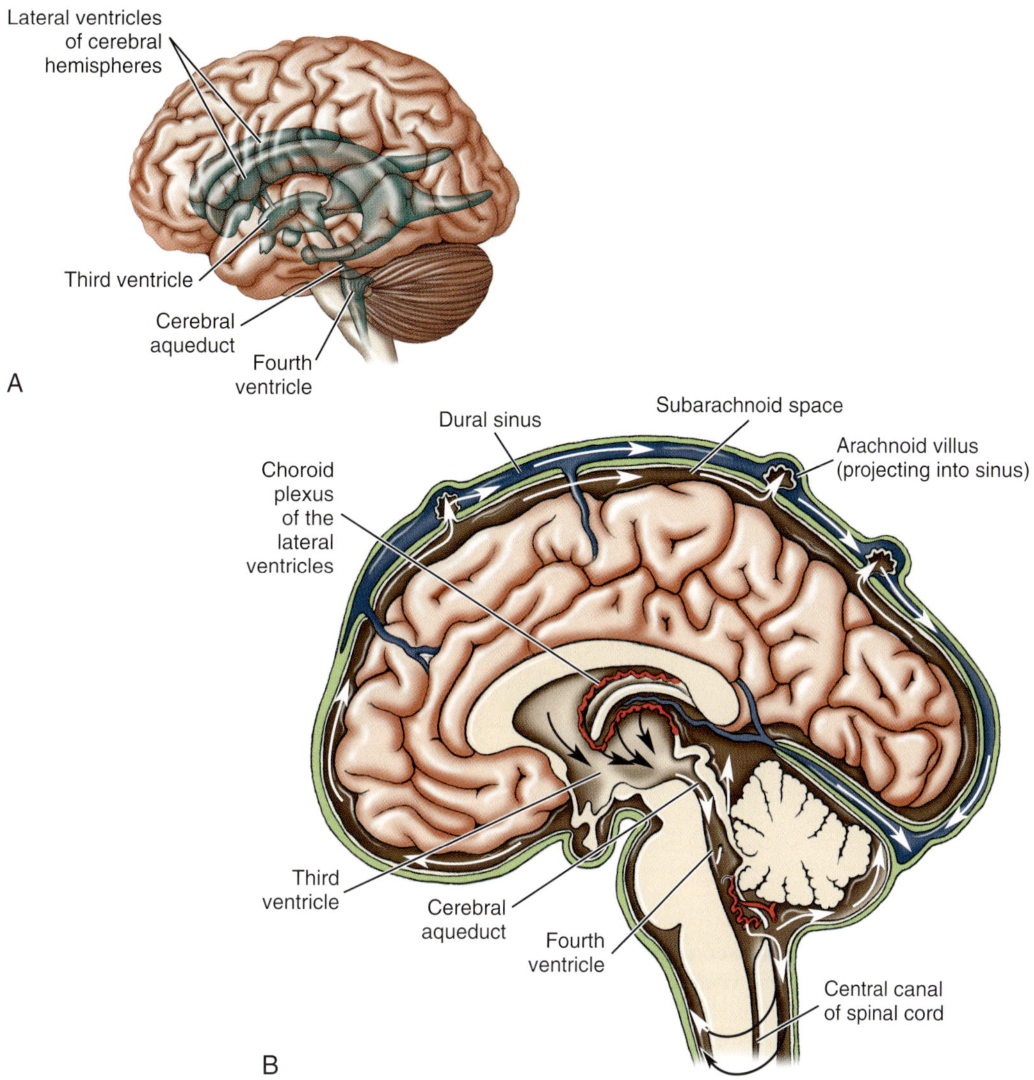

FIGURE 16-10 Cerebrospinal fluid (CSF): formation, circulation, and drainage. **A,** CSF forms within lateral, third, and fourth ventricles of the brain. **B,** CSF flows down through the central canal of the spinal cord to the base. CSF also flows from fourth ventricle into subarachnoid space surrounding the brain. CSF flows into arachnoid villus, which protrudes into the dural sinuses. CSF diffuses across membrane of the villus into dural sinuses, where it mixes with venous blood. Blood in the sinuses drains CSF away from brain and into the veins. (From Herlihy B, Maebius NK: *The human body in health and illness,* ed 3, St Louis, 2007, Saunders.)

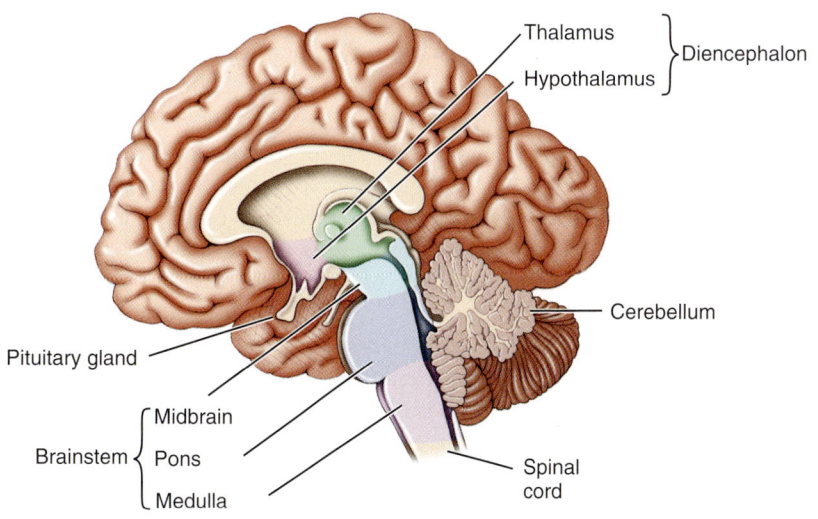

FIGURE 16-11 Diencephalon and brainstem. Diencephalon consists of the thalamus and hypothalamus. Note relationship between hypothalamus and pituitary gland. Brainstem is composed of the midbrain, pons, and medulla. (From Herlihy B, Maebius NK: *The human body in health and illness,* ed 3, St Louis, 2007, Saunders.)

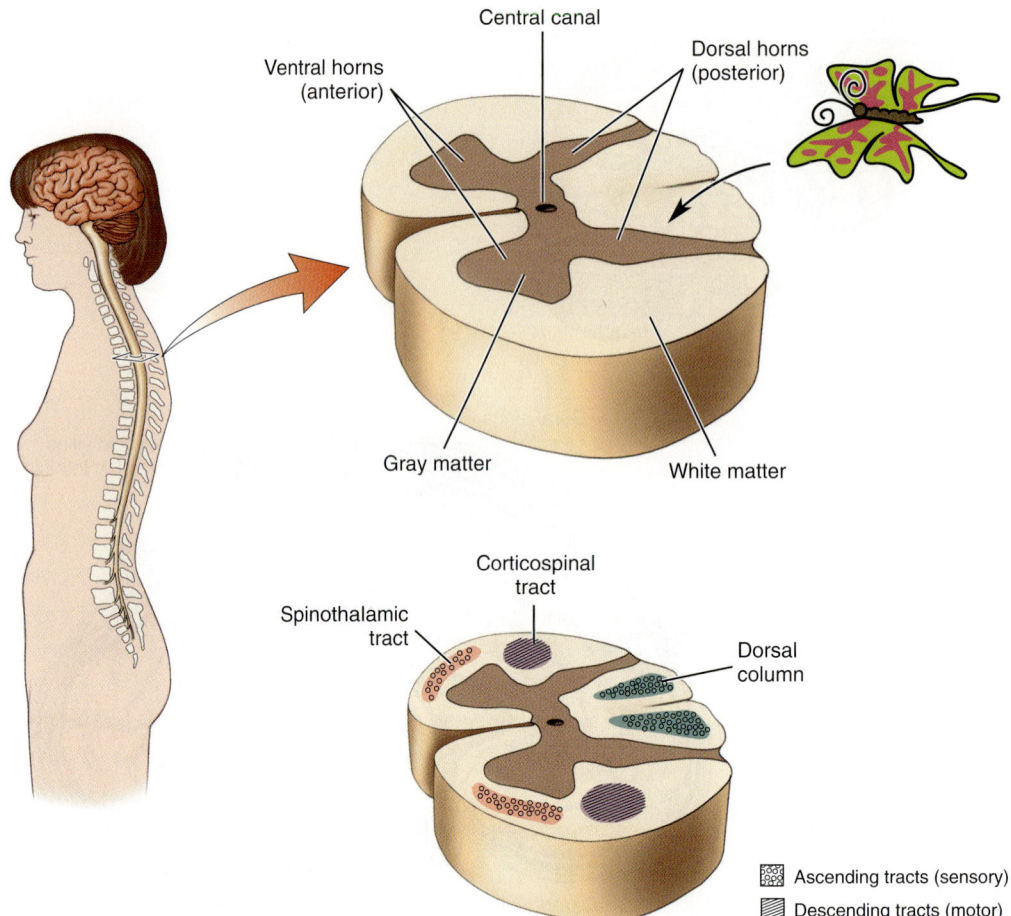

FIGURE 16-12 Cross-sections of spinal cord showing inner gray matter ("butterfly") and outer white matter. The butterfly wings (gray matter) are called the *dorsal horns* and *ventral horns.* The central canal is a hole in the middle of the spinal cord. The white matter shows the location of several tracts. (From Herlihy B, Maebius NK: *The human body in health and illness,* ed 3, St Louis, 2007, Saunders.)

Autonomic Nervous System. The **autonomic nervous system** (**ANS**) is controlled by the CNS, mainly the cerebral cortex, hypothalamus, and medulla. The CNS also oversees the involuntary activity of the heart, glandular secretions, and involuntary muscle actions. There are two divisions to the ANS: the sympathetic nervous system and the parasympathetic nervous system (Table 16-2).
- The **sympathetic nervous system** is responsible for the body's response to stress or any perceived emergency situations. The "**fight-or-flight**" **response** requires the body to respond quickly, thus allowing the use of maximum exertion.
- The **parasympathetic nervous system** returns the body to a state of balance, or **homeostasis,** and is responsible for maintaining normal activities of the body (e.g., digestion).

Somatic Nervous System. The somatic nervous system is the voluntary movement of skeletal muscles caused by the stimuli of sensory neurons. When a stimulus is transmitted through a sensory neuron to the CNS, it crosses a synapse to a motor neuron, and an appropriate message is sent to the skeletal muscle to respond or act. This process may be a **reflex.**

TABLE 16-2
Comparison of Sympathetic and Parasympathetic Actions

Organ	Sympathetic	Parasympathetic
Blood vessels	Dilate to increase blood flow to brain, heart, lungs, and skeletal muscles	No effect
Bronchial tubes	Dilate to increase breathing	Constrict to decrease breathing
Heart	Strength and rate increase	Rate decreases
Intestines	Activity decreases	Activity increases
Iris of eye	Pupil dilates	Pupil constricts
Liver	Activates conversion of glycogen to glucose	No effect
Sweat glands	Increased sweating	Normal secretions

A reflex is an involuntary response of an individual to a given type of stimulation to a given area. Several somatic reflexes cause the skeletal muscles to contract or a glandular secretion to react. Physicians test reflexes during a physical examination.

Nervous System **CHAPTER 16** 293

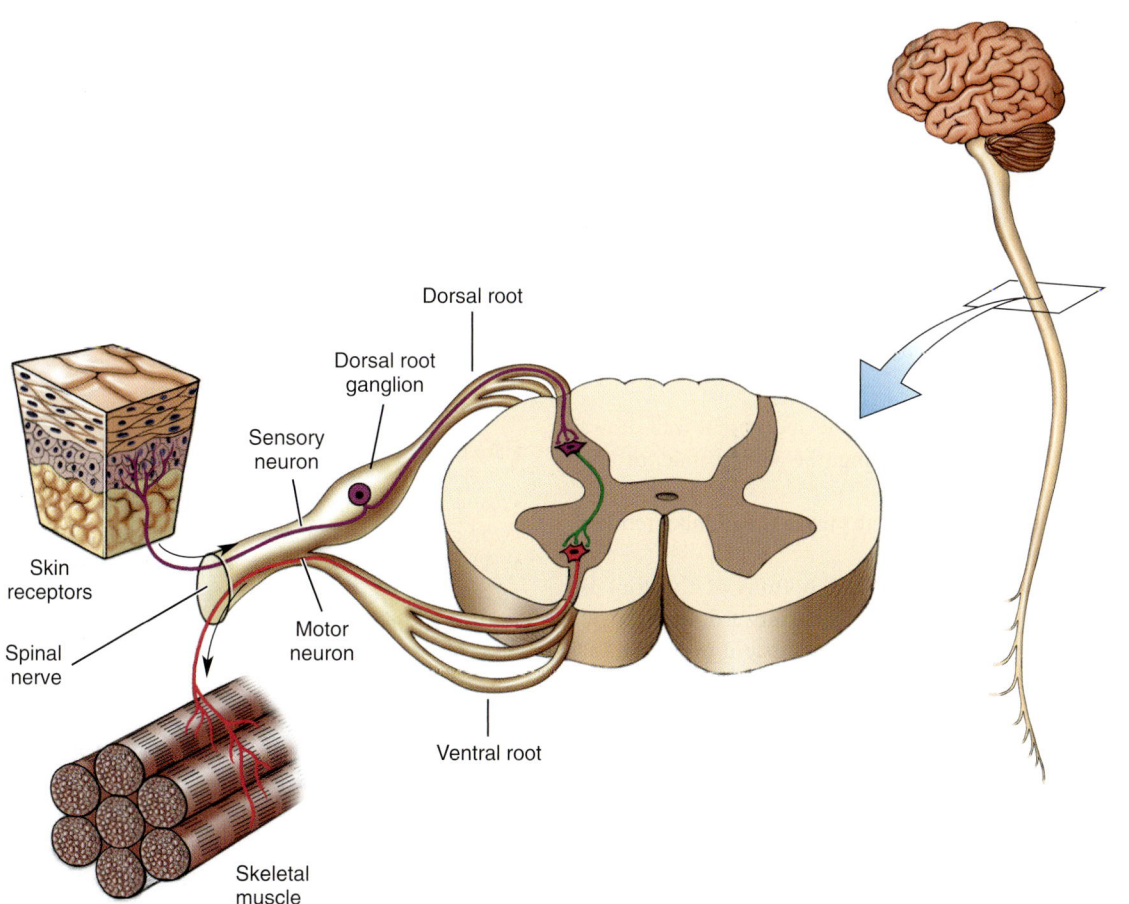

FIGURE 16-13 Spinal nerves (31 pairs): eight cervical, 12 thoracic, five lumbar, five sacral, and one coccygeal. Spinal cord ends at first lumbar vertebra *(L1);* cauda equina (extension of lumbar and sacral nerves) extends the length of the spinal cavity. Three major nerve plexuses (networks): cervical plexus, brachial plexus, and lumbosacral plexus. (From Applegate EJ: *The anatomy and physiology learning system*, ed 3, St Louis, 2006, Saunders.)

FIGURE 16-14 Attachment of spinal nerves to spinal cord. Spinal nerves contain both sensory and motor fibers. Sensory neurons attach to spinal cord at the dorsal root; motor neurons attach to spinal cord at the ventral root. (From Herlihy B, Maebius NK: *The human body in health and illness,* ed 3, St Louis, 2007, Saunders.)

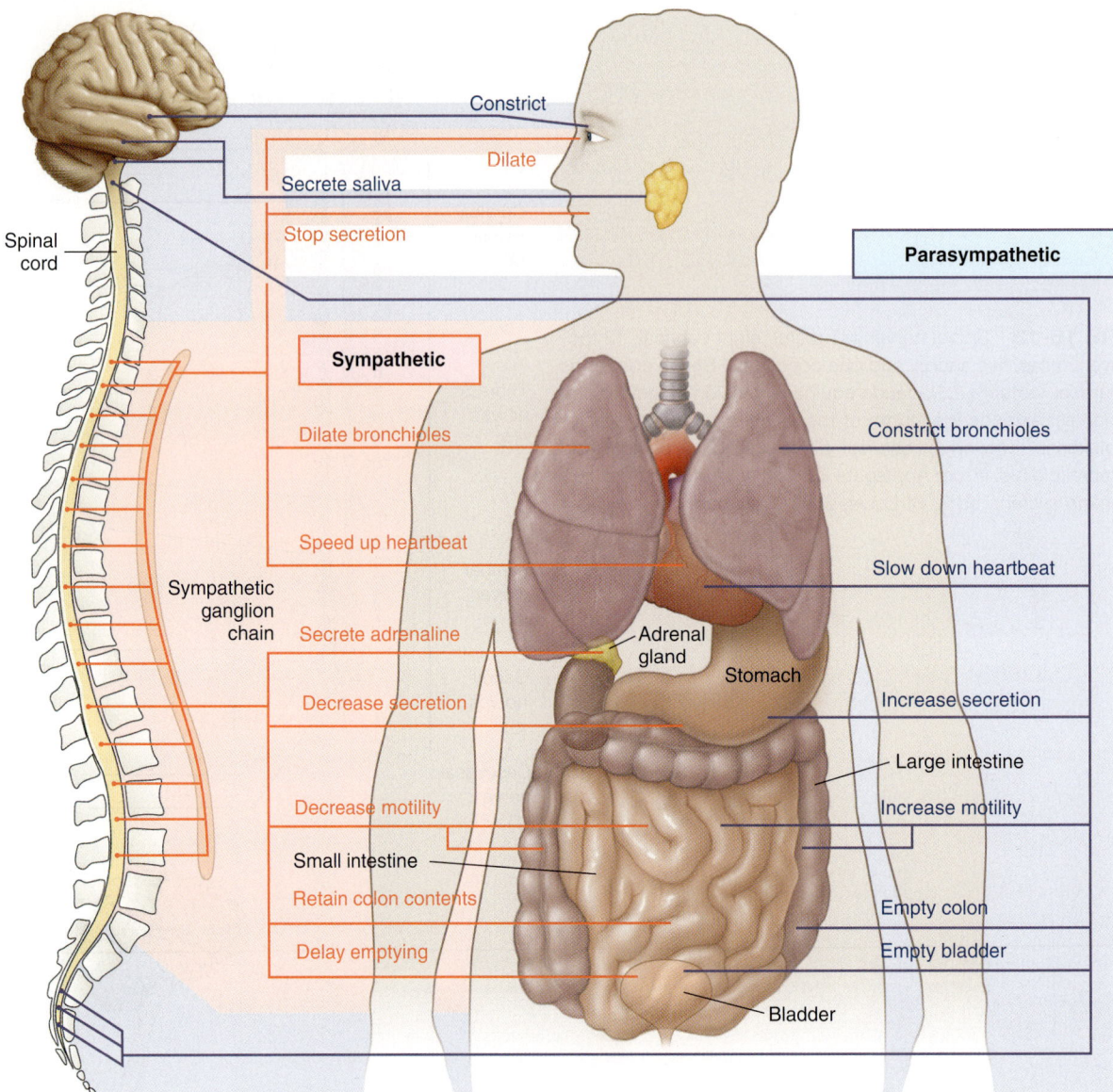

FIGURE 16-15 Innervation of major target organs by the autonomic nervous system (ANS). (Modified from Thibodeau GA, Patton KT: *The human body in health and disease,* ed 4, St Louis, 2005, Mosby.)

- **Abdominal reflex** occurs when the abdominal wall draws inward in response to stroking the lateral side of the abdomen.
- **Achilles reflex** (ankle jerk) occurs when the Achilles tendon is tapped and the foot extends.
- **Babinski reflex** occurs when the bottom of the foot is stroked upward. The great toe extends outward, and the rest of the toes curl. This is normal in infants but disappears at age 1½ years and is considered abnormal after this age.
- **Corneal reflex** occurs when the cornea is touched; the eye blinks or shuts in response.
- **Patellar reflex** (knee-jerk response) occurs when the patellar tendon is tapped and the lower leg extends outward (Figure 16-16).
- **Plantar reflex** occurs when the bottom of the foot is stroked and toes flex.

PATIENT-CENTERED PROFESSIONALISM

- *Why is it important for the medical assistant to understand the structure and function of the nervous system?*
- *Why is it important to know the difference between the CNS and the PNS and how each division depends on the other to function properly?*

DISEASES AND DISORDERS OF THE NERVOUS SYSTEM

As in other disease processes, listening to the patient's chief complaint, evaluating their present and past medical history, and performing a physical examination will help diagnose a neurological disease. A **neurologist** medically treats diseases

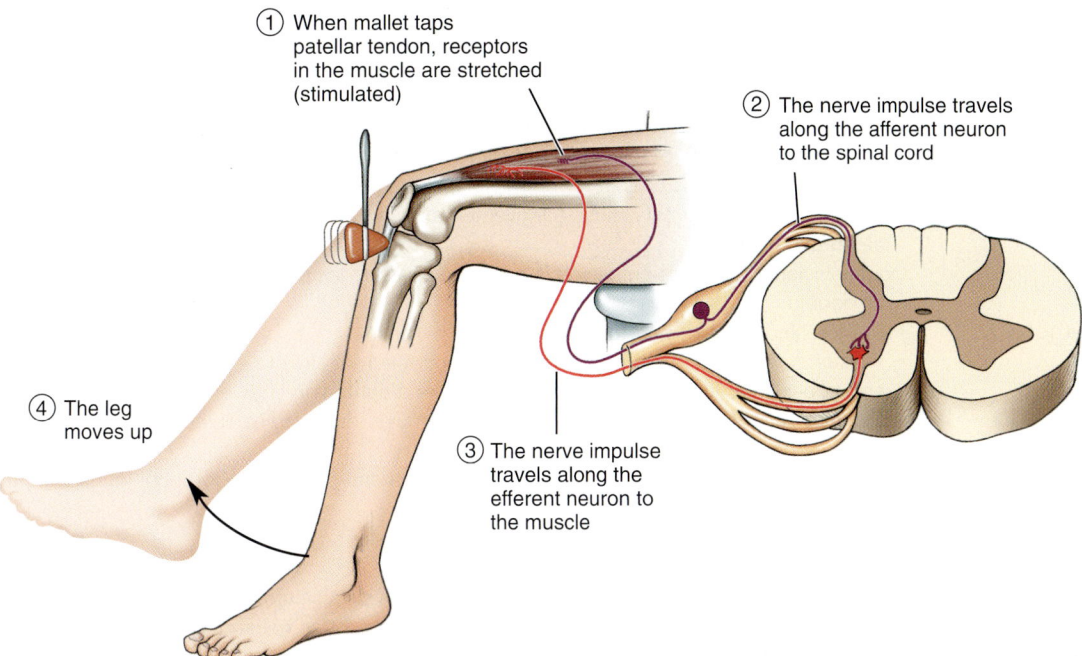

FIGURE 16-16 Knee-jerk reflex, illustrating four components of the reflex arc: *1,* stimulation of receptor; *2,* transmission of signal (sensory) toward spinal cord along afferent neuron; *3,* transmission of signal away from cord (motor) along efferent neuron; *4,* motor response of effector organ (e.g., contraction of skeletal muscle, which jerks leg upward). (From Herlihy B, Maebius NK: *The human body in health and illness,* ed 3, St Louis, 2007, Saunders.)

of the nervous system. Drugs may be prescribed to treat neurological diseases (Table 16-3).

Medical assistants need to be able to recognize the common signs and symptoms of and diagnostic tests for the different types of neurological diseases.
- Study Box 16-2 to familiarize yourself with the common signs and symptoms.
- Study Box 16-3 to learn about common diagnostic tests.
- Study Table 16-4 to understand the diseases that affect the nervous system.

Maintaining Nervous System Health

Maintaining the health of the nervous system is important. Many ways are available to enhance the health of this system, as follows:
- Adequate diet with special attention to vitamins A, C, and B-complex, as well as protein and carbohydrates for energy.
- Avoidance of substances that have an adverse affect on the nervous system (e.g., alcohol, drugs, carbon monoxide, and nicotine).
- Immediate treatment of infections and injuries to minimize loss of nerve function.
- Genetic counseling for parents of children with inherited disorders of the nervous system.
- Screening of newborns for phenylketonuria (PKU).

Text continued on p. 302

TABLE 16-3
Nervous System Drug Classifications

Drug Classification	Common Generic (Brand) Names
Analgesics Relieve pain by blocking pain impulses	meperidine (Demerol) propoxyphene (Darvon)
Anticonvulsants Prevent or reduce the severity of seizures	clonazepam (Klonopin) carbamazepine (Tegretol)
Antimigraine agents Relieve symptoms of migraine headaches	sumatriptan (Imitrex) zolmitriptan (Zomig)
Antiinfectives Reduce central nervous system infections	ceftazidime (Fortaz) ceftriaxone (Rocephin)
Antiparkinsonian agents Relieve or reduce tremors	benztropine (Cogentin) amantadine (Symmetrel)
Anti-Alzheimer agents Slow progression of disease	donepezil (Aricept) tacrine (Cognex)
Hypnotics Produce sleep	zolpidem (Ambien) secobarbital (Seconal)
Sedatives Decrease activity or excitability without causing sleep	phenobarbital (Solfoton) butabarbital (Butisol)
Anesthetics Cause loss of responsiveness to sensory stimulation	midazolam (Versed) sufentanil (Sufenta)
Vasodilators Produce relaxation of blood vessels	isosorbide dinitrate (Isordil) nitroglycerin (Nitrostat)

BOX 16-2

Signs and Symptoms of Neurological Disease

Aphasia	Inability to communicate through oral or written speech because of damage to the speech center (left hemisphere, left side of brain); an aphasic patient may be able to understand oral and written communication but is unable to formulate words to respond
Ataxia	Inability to control voluntary muscle movements because of damage to cerebellum or motor area of cerebral cortex
Diplopia	Double vision, blurred vision; vision is hampered by images not being in focus or images appearing as double
Headache	Pain or aching of or around the head (Figure 16-17) • *Tension headaches* result from long-term contraction of skeletal muscles around face, neck, scalp, and upper back; occur bilaterally; and feel "like a tightening shower cap" • *Cluster headaches* occur unilaterally; involve an eye, temple, cheek, and forehead; start during sleep; and can last for several weeks • *Migraine headaches* are a sudden throbbing, unilateral pain with photophobia, nausea, and vomiting
Numbness, tingling	Loss of sensation, or feeling of needles piercing the skin
Pain	Localized discomfort
Paralysis	Temporary or permanent loss of function, sensation, and voluntary movement • **Hemiplegia** is paralysis of only one side of the body, often caused by stroke • *Paraplegia* is paralysis of lower trunk and extremities resulting from spinal cord injury • *Quadriplegia* is paralysis involving both upper and lower extremities
Seizures (convulsions)	Disturbances of electrical activity of the brain • Box 16-4 lists the various types of seizures
Vertigo	Dizziness

BOX 16-3

Diagnostic Tests for Central Nervous System (CNS)

Lumbar puncture (spinal tap) (Figure 16-18)	Removal of cerebrospinal fluid (CSF) through needle inserted between third and fourth lumbar vertebrae; measures pressure in CNS, examines contaminants (e.g., blood, bacterial) in CSF
Electroencephalography (EEG) (Figure 16-19)	Electrical impulses from brain recorded as tracings through electrodes attached to patient's scalp; measures the brain's electrical activity
Computed tomography (CT) scan (Figure 16-20)	Better visualization of ventricles, subarachnoid space, and brain abnormalities (e.g., blood clot, tumors, or cysts) than with standard radiography
Magnetic resonance imaging (MRI)	Used to view the soft tissue; therefore tumors in the gray or white matter of the CNS are easier to capture
Angiography	Requires injection of radiopaque contrast medium (dye) into a blood vessel; series of x-rays shows abnormalities of the blood vessels of the brain
Myelography	Used to view structures around spinal cord; dye injected into subarachnoid space at third and fourth lumbar vertebrae; x-rays taken of patient in multiple positions
Electroneuromyography	Used to test and record neuromuscular activity by electrical stimulation
Electromyography (EMG)	Record of muscle activity; aids in diagnosing neuromuscular problems
Nerve conduction studies	Electrical impulses stimulate peripheral nerves; measure velocity of the impulse generated

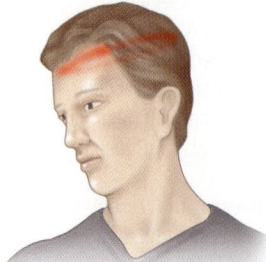
Muscle contraction headache

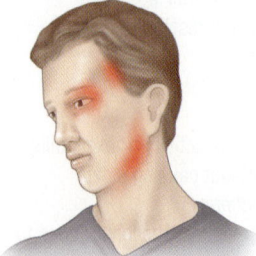
Cluster headache

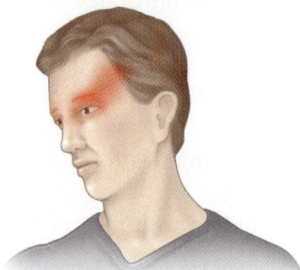
Migraine headache

FIGURE 16-17 Types of headache. *Shaded areas,* Regions of most intense pain. (Modified from Leonard PC: *Building a medical vocabulary,* ed 6, St Louis, 2005, Saunders.)

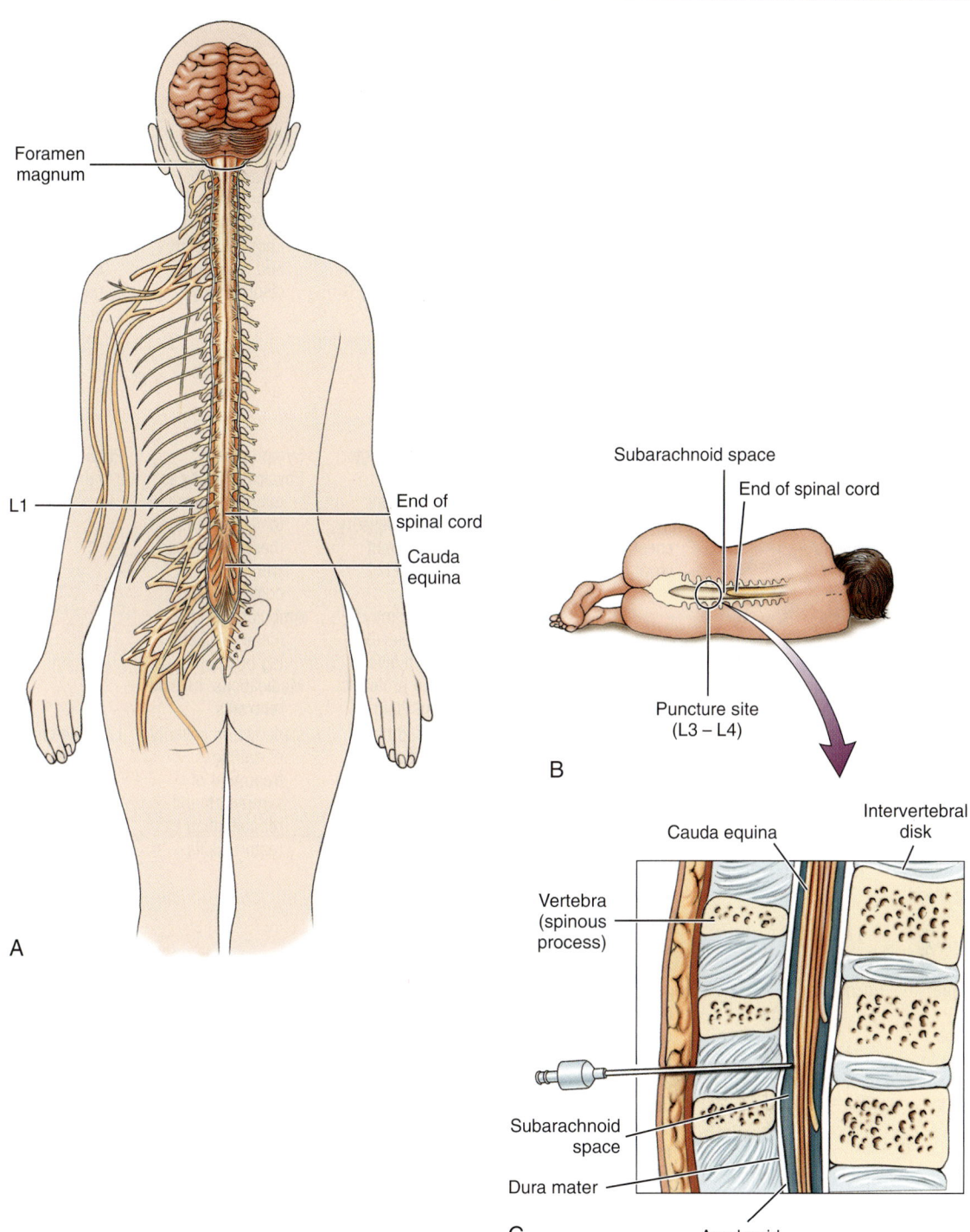

FIGURE 16-18 **A,** Location of spinal cord, which extends from foramen magnum of occipital bone to first lumbar vertebra *(L1)*. The cauda equina descends from base of the spinal cord *(L1)* to bottom of the spinal cavity. **B,** Note that spinal cord is shorter than spinal cavity. **C,** Telescoped area shows lumbar puncture (spinal tap). Needle is inserted into subarachnoid space between L3 and L4 vertebrae. Note that patient is lying so that the vertebral column is flexed; this position separates vertebrae and eases needle insertion. (From Herlihy B, Maebius NK: *The human body in health and illness,* ed 3, St Louis, 2007, Saunders.)

TABLE 16-4

Diseases and Disorders of the Nervous System

Disease and Description	Etiology	Signs and Symptoms	Diagnosis	Therapy	Interventions
Alzheimer disease Presenile dementia of chronic brain degeneration focusing on intellectual areas of brain; atrophy of both frontal and occipital lobes	Unknown; theories relate to gene disorders, aluminum poisoning, autoimmune disease, and viral infection Increased production or decrease in clearance of brain protein amyloid beta (A beta)	Confusion, disorientation, short-term memory failure, inability to carry out purposeful activities	Evaluation to rule out other dementia disorders; mental status exam, CT scan, MRI, EEG	Treat symptoms; administer medications to improve memory and behavioral disorders	Encourage family to provide a structured and supportive environment that ensures safety; family needs support and counseling
Amyotrophic lateral sclerosis (ALS), Lou Gehrig disease Motor neuron disease in which muscles of extremities atrophy and weaken	Unknown; theories include genetics, metabolic problems, and environmental agents	Weakness in hands and forearms that spreads to rest of body Eventual paralysis of chest muscles and vocal cords	Evidence of motor neuron involvement without sensory involvement Abnormal EMG results Blood test may show elevated protein levels Elevated protein in spinal fluid	Symptomatic Physical therapy to maintain muscle tone; speech therapy to assist with communication Ambulatory aids (cane, walkers, leg braces) Medications: muscle relaxants	Provide supportive help for family
Cerebrovascular accident (CVA, stroke) Blood vessel ruptures, or clot occludes blood vessel, decreasing blood flow to brain (Figure 16-21)	Deposits of cholesterol in arteries causing occlusion, or weakness in a blood vessel wall that ruptures and causes hemorrhage	Numbness or muscle weakness of face or limb, inability to move a limb or side of body **(hemiparesis)**; inability to speak, sudden severe headache, blurred or double vision, confusion, memory loss	Diagnosed by symptoms and neurological examination, CT scan, and EEG	Depends on severity of damage; treatment of symptoms and rehabilitation to restore skills	Lifestyle changes: diet, exercise, weight management, and decrease in smoking and alcohol consumption to guard against future strokes; awareness of at-risk factors: race, age, gender, and family history
Chronic fatigue syndrome Chronic disease that appears to be viral in nature and affects the entire body	Unknown	Impairment of short-term memory or concentration; sore throat; tender cervical and axillary nodes; pain without stiffness or redness; fatigue unrelated to exertion	History; patient complains of four or more symptoms for 6 months or longer	Gradual exercise program to increase over time; rest when fatigue is at its worst	Emotional support
Encephalitis Infection of tissues of brain and spinal cord	Viral invasion from bite of mosquito, ticks, or **amoebae** infestation from water Some forms spread by nasal secretions or open lesions	Fever, headache, low energy, drowsiness, irritability, restlessness	History of exposure, positive **Kernig sign,*** muscle weakness CSF pressure elevated with WBCs and proteins present	Antibiotic drugs for secondary infection; sedatives for restlessness; corticosteroids to reduce swelling Maintenance of fluids, nutritional needs, and rest	Onset within 24 hours of exposure, so immediate medical attention is critical, and prophylactic treatment for family is necessary
Epilepsy Disorder caused by abnormal electrical activity in brain resulting in seizures (see Box 16-4)	Idiopathic in some cases; in other cases, caused by trauma at birth, lesions and tumors, some metabolic disorders, and toxic substance exposure	Seizure activity	Clinical history, physical exam; CT, MRI, PET, cranial x-rays, and EEG to observe brain activity	Anticonvulsant drug therapy; surgery when underlying problem is organic	During a seizure, move potentially harmful objects away from patient; do not attempt to restrain patient; educate about disease, myths, misconceptions, and importance of following prescribed drug therapy

TABLE 16-4

Diseases and Disorders of the Nervous System—cont'd

Disease and Description	Etiology	Signs and Symptoms	Diagnosis	Therapy	Interventions
Meningitis Inflammation of brain and spinal cord coverings	Usually of bacterial origin Spread through droplet contact	Fever, severe headache, stiff neck, vomiting	Results of CSF examination and cultures of respiratory tract and blood	Antibiotic agents for causative agent; analgesics for headaches and muscle aches; maintain fluid, electrolyte, and nutritional balance	Identify source; institute appropriate precautions for infective materials Vaccine for college-age students
Multiple sclerosis (MS) Chronic progressive disease caused by degeneration of myelin sheath, which is replaced with scar tissue	Unknown, but autoimmune response suspected	Onset **insidious** (gradual) with paresthesias of extremities or muscle weakness, ataxia, dizziness (vertigo), double or blurred vision (diplopia)	Elevated CSF pressure Studies indicate slowed nerve conduction; lesions may be apparent on CT and MRI	Medication therapy for muscle spasms; corticosteroids to minimize acute attacks Rest and therapy to adjust to progressive loss of function in ADLs	Provide psychological support for family and patient
Parkinson disease Slowly progressive degenerative disorder characterized by resting tremor, pill rolling of fingers, and shuffling gait; pathogenic changes in basal ganglia and depletion of dopamine	Idiopathic	Fine, slowly spreading resting tremor; shuffling of feet when walking; muscle rigidity and weakness	Clinical manifestations include impaired postural reflexes, resting tremors, and **gait** (way of walking) involvement	Symptomatic approach: medications to reduce tremors and muscle rigidity; physical therapy to maintain muscle tone; and occupational therapy to maintain ADL skills	Encourage supportive environment
Shingles (herpes zoster) Acute inflammation of dorsal root ganglia	Dormant virus from chickenpox attacks dorsal root; activated by stress, trauma, and immune disorders	Pain and rash along a dermatome, especially in intercostal area (Figure 16-22)	Clinical evidence includes fever, malaise, and vesicles above affected dermatome, with pain, burning, and itching	Medications for pain and itching; antiviral agents for immuno-compromised patients	Rest and nutritional status need to be maintained
Tic douloureux (trigeminal neuralgia) Neuralgia of fifth cranial nerve	Unknown	Severe facial pain, especially when chewing and when exposed to cold temperatures	Tests to rule out sinus or tooth infections; symptoms include burning facial pain that occurs quickly and lasts 1 to 15 minutes	Medications to relieve discomfort; microsurgery to decompress nerve; radiosurgery to deaden nerve root	Nutritional needs must be maintained; encourage food high in calories and nutrients that require less chewing; small, frequent meals are preferred
Transient ischemic attack (TIA)† Temporary stoppage of blood to brain; "mini-stroke"	Stems from plaque emboli that block arteries in neck or vascular spasm in neck region	Temporary confusion, slurred speech, muscle weakness on one side of the body, blurred vision or diplopia that gradually subsides	Clinical history with confirming results from ultrasound of carotid or vertebral arteries	Medications to prevent plaque buildup and clot formation; surgery in patients with 70% blockage	TIAs could be warning sign of stroke

ADLs, Activities of daily living; *CSF*, cerebrospinal fluid; *CT*, computed tomography; *EEG*, electroencephalography; *EMG*, electromyography; *MRI*, magnetic resonance imaging; *PET*, positron emission tomography; *WBCs*, white blood cells.

*Kernig sign occurs when a patient is in a supine position, with leg flexed at the knee and hip, and is unable to straighten the leg fully.

†**Predisposing factors** include heart disease, diabetes mellitus, and hypertension.

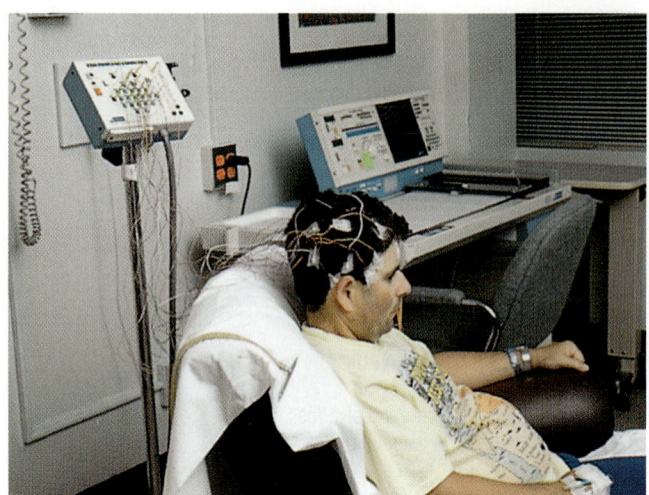

FIGURE 16-19 Electroencephalography (EEG). Electrodes are attached to patient's head; patient usually remains quiet with closed eyes during EEG procedure. In certain tests, prescribed activities may be requested. (From Chipps EM, Clanin NJ, Campbell VG: *Neurologic disorders,* St Louis, 1992, Mosby.)

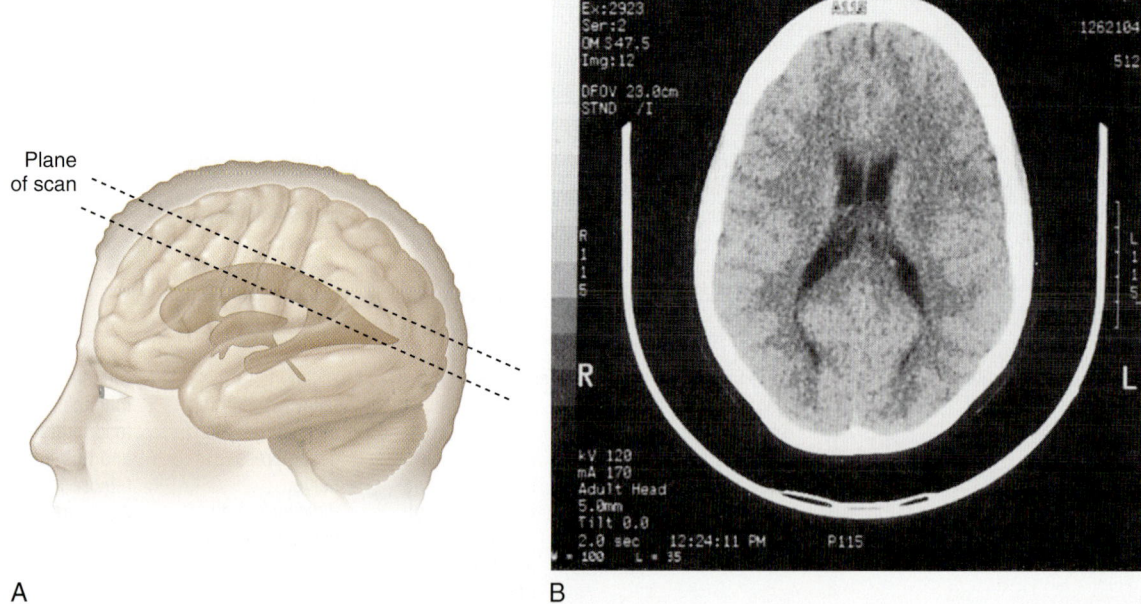

FIGURE 16-20 Computed tomography (CT) of brain. **A,** CT scans are taken at various cross sections of brain. **B,** Tomogram of plane in *A* shows a normal brain. (From Polaski AL, Tatro SE: *Luckmann's core principles and practice of medical-surgical nursing,* Philadelphia, 1996, Saunders.)

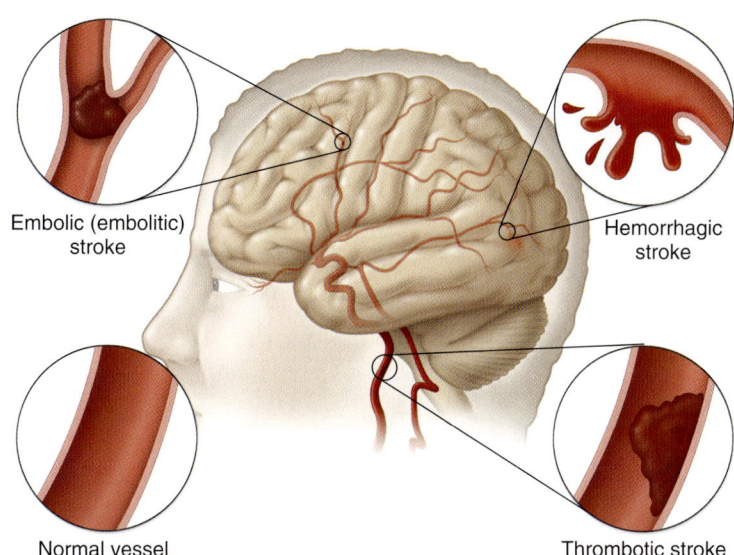

FIGURE 16-21 Types of stroke. Cerebrovascular accident (CVA), commonly referred to as a stroke, is a disruption in the normal blood supply to the brain. *Embolic* strokes are caused by emboli that break off from one area of the body and travel to the cerebral arteries. *Thrombotic* strokes are caused by plaque deposits that have built up on the interior of a cerebral artery, gradually blocking it. *Hemorrhagic* strokes are caused by a cerebral arterial wall rupture. (Modified from Leonard PC: *Building a medical vocabulary,* ed 6, St Louis, 2005, Saunders.)

BOX 16-4

Types of Seizures

PARTIAL SEIZURES
- Occur in defined areas of the brain and cause specific symptoms.
- Involve involuntary muscle contractions of one body part (e.g., face, hand, arm).

Simple Partial Motor Seizure
- Localized motor seizure (e.g., starts at thumb, spreads to hand, then to arms).
- Activities spread to adjacent areas of the brain.
- Patient does not lose consciousness.

Simple Partial Sensory Seizure
- Patient experiences distorted sense of being, including hallucinations, tingling, flashing lights, and dizziness.

Complex Partial Seizure
- Partial motor seizure that progresses to purposeless behavior (e.g., smacking lips, patting body parts).
- An *aura* (a sense of something about to happen) may precede onset of the seizure.
- Mental confusion may follow the seizure.

GENERALIZED SEIZURES
- Affect the electrical activity of the brain in a general manner.

Petit Mal Seizure (Absence Seizure)
- Change in patient's level of consciousness.
- Characterized by rolling or flickering of the eyes or lids, blank stare, and slight facial movements.
- Usually occurs in children and lasts 1 to 10 seconds.
- Person is unaware of the seizure activity.

Myoclonic Seizure
- Marked (identified) by brief, involuntary muscle jerks that can occur in rhythmic patterns.
- Loss of consciousness is brief.

Grand Mal Seizure (Tonic-Clonic Seizure)
- Begins with an outcry as air leaves the lungs and passes over vocal cords.
- Patient falls to ground and loses consciousness.
- Movements are first *tonic* (stiffening of muscles), then *clonic* (relaxing of muscles).
- Incontinence, labored breathing, and angina may follow.
- After seizure, which lasts 2 to 5 minutes, patient may experience confusion and muscle soreness and may fall into a deep sleep.

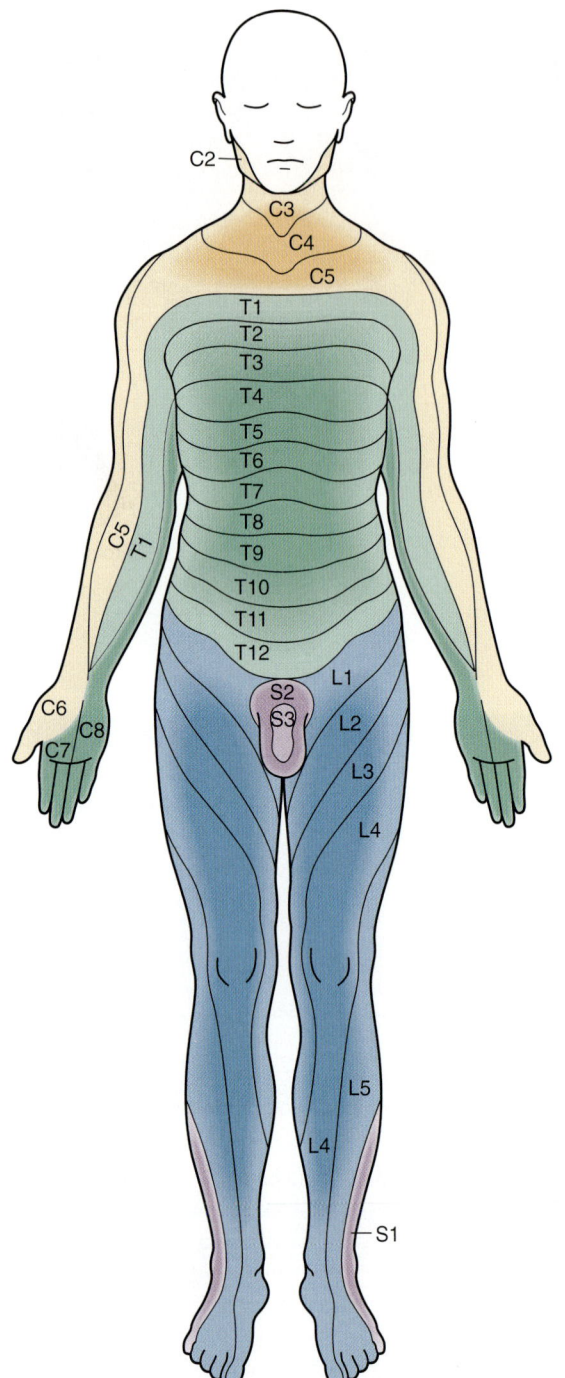

FIGURE 16-22 Major nerves of the body: dermatomes. Each dermatome (segment) is named for the spinal nerve that serves it. Shingles pain follows the nerve pathways. (From Marx J et al: *Rosen's emergency medicine: concepts and clinical practice,* ed 6, Philadelphia, 2006, Mosby.)

Dysfunctions of the nervous system adversely affect the patient's ability to think, reason, and carry out activities of daily living (ADLs). The nervous system allows individuals to act on input from their senses; without proper functioning of the system, ADLs can become difficult or even impossible.

FOR YOUR INFORMATION

Changes in the nervous system related to aging are numerous. The neurons in the brain decrease and memory becomes less efficient, thus requiring more time to remember a task. A general slowing of nerve conduction occurs; therefore reflexes tend to be slower, which affects coordination. A decrease in ankle-jerk reflex may affect balance.

PATIENT-CENTERED PROFESSIONALISM

- Why is it important for the medical assistant to be aware of the different nervous system disorders, including signs and symptoms, diagnostic tests, treatments, and general health maintenance of the nervous system?
- How can your ability to understand and explain this information benefit patients?

MENTAL HEALTH

The brain is the main control center of the body; thus when something is wrong with its structure or functioning, the patient's mental health can be affected by neurological symptoms. Some mental illnesses are directly linked to structural or chemical problems in the brain. Others are inherited, and for some mental disorders the cause is unknown.

Mental illnesses are psychological and behavioral and involve a wide range of problems in thought and function. Mental health evaluation begins with observation. Before diagnosing a mental health disorder, the patient is evaluated for signs of organic illness. When a physiological reason is not evident, possible psychological impairment becomes the focus.

Detecting Mental Health Disorders

Disorders of mental health are sometimes difficult to understand and diagnose. In fact, mental disorders are often misdiagnosed and go untreated. Symptoms may vary from mild behavioral changes to severe personality disturbances. Most often, symptoms are subtle and may not be noticed in the early developmental stages. **Psychiatry** is the medical science that deals with the origin, diagnosis, prevention, and treatment of developmental and emotional components of physical disorders. Drugs may be prescribed to treat mental disorders (Table 16-5).

Types of Mental Health Disorders

As with the other nervous system problems, medical assistants need to be able to recognize the common signs and symptoms

TABLE 16-5
Mental Health Drug Classifications

Drug Classification	Common Generic (Brand) Drugs
Alcohol deterrents Discourage use of alcohol	disulfiram (Antabuse)
Antidepressants Relieve symptoms of depressed mood	fluoxetine (Prozac) paroxetine (Paxil)
Antimanics Control mental disorders characterized by euphoria	lithium (Lithobid) chlorpromazine (Thorazine)
Antipsychotics Control psychotic symptoms	fluphenazine (Prolixin) risperidone (Risperdal)
Anxiolytics Relieve symptoms of anxiety	alprazolam (Xanax) lorazepam (Ativan)

BOX 16-5
Common Signs and Symptoms of Mental Health Disorders

Akathisia	Inability to remain calm
Amnesia	Inability to remember
Catatonia	Immobility from emotional rather than physical cause
Delirium	Confused, unfocused, and agitated behavior
Delusion	Persistent belief in an untruth
Hallucination	Unreal sensory perception
Psychosis	Impaired perception of reality

BOX 16-6
Diagnostic Tests and Procedures for Mental Health Status

Mental status examination	Assessment of patient's appearance, affect, thought processes, cognitive function, insight, and judgment
Laboratory tests	Complete blood count (CBC) with differential, blood chemistry profile, thyroid function panel, sexually transmitted disease (STD) screening
Imaging	CT scan, MRI, **positron emission tomography (PET) scan**

Psychological testing
- *Bender-Gestalt test* measures visuomotor and spatial abilities
- *Rorschach (inkblot) test* measures ability to integrate intellectual and emotional factors
- *Minnesota Multiphasic Personality Inventory (MMPI)* measures personality characteristics through forced-choice questions
- *Wechsler Adult Intelligence Scale (WAIS)* measures verbal and performance intelligence quotient (IQ)

of and diagnostic tests for the different types of mental health disorders.
- Study Box 16-5 to familiarize yourself with the common signs and symptoms of mental health disorders.
- Study Box 16-6 to learn about common diagnostic tests and procedures. Note that tests to determine the disorders are twofold: (1) physiological testing to identify if the origin is organic, including laboratory tests, electrocardiogram (ECG), brain scan, and magnetic resonance imaging (MRI), and (2) psychological testing, including personality testing and other tests as appropriate for the presenting symptoms.

PATIENT-CENTERED PROFESSIONALISM

- Why is it important for medical assistants to be aware of their biases concerning mental health and mental disorders affecting their patients?
- How do these biases affect the care that patients receive?

CONCLUSION

The nervous system impacts every other system of the body. The brain and spinal cord play a vital role in generating and transmitting information and impulses throughout the rest of the body.

Understanding the nervous system is crucial to providing effective care for and communicating clearly with patients of all ages. The growth and development of individuals affect the nervous system. The effects of aging on the nervous system vary; after age 50, people lose an estimated 1% of their neurons. When interacting with elderly patients, keep in mind that normal changes in the nervous system with aging are not the same as Alzheimer disease or dementia. Many individuals reach old age with no signs or symptoms of mental impairment.

Assessment of a patient's mental function is important because it may show changes that are consistent with organic brain disease. Assessment also allows the medical assistant to decide if the patient has the capacity to understand treatment guidelines. Your knowledge of the nervous system will likely be used every day. Whether you are asking patients questions, assisting with medical procedures, or performing other clinical or administrative functions, your understanding of this important and complex body system will impact the care that your patients receive.

BOX 16-7

Information Concerning Mental Health Disorders

DEVELOPMENTAL DISORDERS
Autism: Disorder characterized by preoccupation with inner thoughts; marked (noticeable) unresponsiveness to social contact.
Attention deficit hyperactivity disorder (ADHD): Characterized by inability to focus attention for short periods or to engage in quiet activities, or both.

SUBSTANCE-RELATED DISORDERS
Alcoholism: Physical and mental dependence on regular intake of alcohol.
Drug abuse: Use of legal or illegal drugs that cause physical, mental, or emotional harm and dependence.

ORGANIC MENTAL DISORDERS
Dementia: Irreversible impairment of intellectual activities.
Alzheimer disease: Progressive degeneration of frontal lobe of brain.

PSYCHOSES
Schizophrenia: Characterized by disturbances in thought content, perception, sense of self, and both personal and interpersonal relationships.
Delusional disorder: Characterized by false beliefs that include grandiose and persecutory delusions.

MOOD DISORDERS
Depression: Feeling of persistent sadness accompanied by insomnia, loss of appetite, and inability to experience pleasure.
Bipolar disorder: Disorder marked by severe mood swings from hyperactivity *(mania)* to sadness *(depression)*.

ANXIETY DISORDERS
General anxiety disorder: General feeling of apprehension brought on by episodes of internal self-doubt.
Obsessive-compulsive disorder (OCD): Disorder that interferes with daily functioning and is characterized by obsessive thoughts and compulsive actions (e.g., fear of germs leading to repeated cleaning).
Posttraumatic stress disorder (PTSD): Impairment that affects activities of daily living and is expressed as severe anxiety following a trauma.

SOMATOFORM DISORDERS
Conversion: Resolution of psychological conflict through loss of body function (e.g., paralysis, blindness).
Munchausen syndrome: Disorder characterized by intentional presentation of false symptoms that may include self-mutilation to obtain medical care.

PERSONALITY DISORDERS
Paranoid: Feeling a sense of being exploited or harmed without a credible basis.
Schizoid: Showing indifference to social relationships.
Antisocial: Exhibiting behavior that shows a disregard for the rights of others.
Narcissistic: Exhibiting behavior that lacks empathy and sensitivity to the needs of others.
Histrionic: Showing excessive attention-seeking tendencies.

Chapter Summary

Reinforce your understanding of the material in this chapter by reviewing the curriculum objectives and key content points below.

1. **Define, appropriately use, and spell all the Key Terms for this chapter.**
   - Review the Key Terms if necessary.
2. **Describe the organization of the nervous system and identify its two main divisions.**
   - The nervous system organizes and controls both the voluntary and the involuntary activities of the body by means of electrical impulses.
   - The central nervous system (CNS) and peripheral nervous system (PNS) work together to send information throughout the body.
3. **Explain the role of neurons and neuroglia in a nerve impulse.**
   - Neurons carry impulses throughout the CNS.
   - The neuroglial cells are responsible for the support, protection, insulation, and nourishment of the neurons but do not carry nerve impulses.
4. **Describe a synapse and explain its function.**
   - A synapse is a microscopic space between the end of one neuron and start of the next neuron.
   - Synapses help transmit information from one neuron to another.
   - Neurotransmitters are released to send the impulse across the synapse. They prevent continuous stimulation of nerve transmission, allowing nerves to rest.

5. **List the main divisions of the CNS.**
   - The CNS is made up of the brain and spinal cord.
6. **Identify the parts of the brain and briefly describe the function of each.**
   - Membranous coverings called meninges protect the brain.
   - The cerebrum controls functions associated with thinking and voluntary activities.
   - The diencephalon includes the thalamus, which relays messages from several parts of the body and monitors sensory stimuli, and the hypothalamus, which controls the activities of the pituitary gland and produces hormones to control the release or limit the production of the hormones.
7. **Explain the purpose of cerebrospinal fluid (CSF).**
   - CSF cushions and protects the nervous tissue of the brain and spinal cord.
8. **List the cranial nerves and describe their function.**
   - There are 12 pairs of cranial nerves attached to the brain. Refer to Table 16-1.
   - Cranial nerves consist of motor (efferent), sensory (afferent), and mixed (sensory and motor) fibers.
9. **List the spinal nerves and describe their function.**
   - There are 31 pairs of spinal nerves.
   - Spinal nerves are grouped by location: cervical, thoracic, lumbar, sacral, and coccygeal.
   - Each pair of nerves transmits impulses to or from the spinal cord. Each forms a dermatome.
10. **List the main divisions of the PNS.**
    - The autonomic nervous system (ANS) and the somatic nervous systems are parts of the PNS.
11. **Describe the functions of the sympathetic and parasympathetic nervous systems.**
    - The sympathetic and parasympathetic nervous systems are parts of the ANS.
    - The sympathetic nervous system is responsible for the body's response to stress ("fight or flight").
    - The parasympathetic nervous system returns the body to a state of balance.
12. **List and briefly describe six types of reflex actions.**
    - A reflex is an involuntary response to a given type of stimulation to a specific area.
    - Types of reflexes include abdominal (abdominal wall draws inward), Achilles (ankle jerk), Babinski (toe curl), corneal (eye blink), patellar (knee jerk), and plantar (toe flex).
13. **List and describe nine types of signs and symptoms of neurological disease.**
    - Refer to the Key Terms.
    - Diet, avoidance of dangerous substances, immediate treatment of infections and injuries, genetic counseling, and screening of newborns for phenylketonuria (PKU) are all ways to prevent neurological disease.
14. **List six types of diagnostic tests and procedures for neurological disease and describe the use of each.**
    - Refer to Box 16-3.
15. **List 11 diseases and disorders of the nervous system and briefly describe the etiology, signs and symptoms, diagnosis, therapy, and interventions for each.**
    - Refer to Table 16-4.
16. **Describe the twofold testing process used to determine mental health disorders.**
    - Tests for mental health disorders include physiological tests for body impairment and psychological tests for mental dysfunction.
17. **List and describe seven common signs and symptoms of mental disorders.**
    - Refer to Box 16-5.
18. **List four types of tests and procedures used to diagnose mental disorders and briefly describe each.**
    - Refer to Box 16-6.
19. **List and briefly describe 20 mental health disorders.**
    - Refer to Box 16-7.
20. **Analyze a realistic medical office situation and apply your understanding of the nervous system to determine the best course of action.**
    - By understanding the nervous system, you are more prepared to understand patients' perceptions and tailor education to their ability to comprehend.
21. **Describe the impact on patient care when medical assistants have a solid understanding of the structure and function of the nervous system.**
    - With effective communication and a good understanding of nervous system physiology, the medical assistant can successfully encourage patients to follow their prescribed treatment plan.

PRACTICAL APPLICATIONS

If you have accomplished the objectives in this chapter, you will be able to make better choices as a medical assistant. Take another look at this situation and decide what you would do.

Sally Jones, age 72, complained of dizziness with a loss of sensation on the left side that lasted only for a few minutes over the past few weeks. She also had a headache that lasted only during the paresthesia. She has a long history of moderately controlled hypertension for which she has taken antihypertensives, "When I thought about them." Dr. Smith was concerned that she might be having TIAs. He prescribed a vasodilator and a mild analgesic for the headache when he saw her last week. Today she was brought to the emergency room with sudden left-sided hemiplegia and a headache, but no aphasia. Except for the hypertension, Ms. Jones has been in relatively good health for her age. On admission, her blood pressure was 210/120 and she was semialert. Dr. Smith ordered a CT scan, which showed an infarct to the right frontotemporal lobes. Ms. Jones was admitted to the hospital for observation and possible treatment.

Do you understand what an infarct is, and how Ms. Jones's earlier symptoms relate to it?

1. What is a TIA? Why was that a precursor to the condition for which Ms. Jones was admitted to the hospital?
2. Why were the dizziness, loss of sensation, and the headache over the past few weeks important in making a diagnosis of TIA?
3. Why did Dr. Smith give Ms. Jones vasodilators?
4. What is paresthesia? Aphasia? Hemiplegia?
5. Why was the control of blood pressure important in the prevention of illness?
6. Why is there paralysis on the left side of the body when the right side of the brain is involved? Why does Ms. Jones not have aphasia?
7. Why did Dr. Smith order a CT scan rather than MRI?
8. What is a common name for the disease process for which Dr. Smith is treating Ms. Jones?
9. Knowing the infarct is in the frontal and temporal lobes, you would expect Ms. Jones to have what type of problem?

WEB SEARCH

1. **Research stroke.** Stroke is the third leading cause of death in the United States. To understand stroke better, a medical assistant needs to be aware of the various factors that contribute to stroke and to understand the treatment.

- **Keywords:** Use the following keywords in your search: stroke, CVA, aphasia, brain attack, American Stroke Association.

WORD PARTS: Nervous System

STRUCTURE AND FUNCTION
Suffixes

-esthesia	sensation, feeling
-kinesia	movement
-lepsy	seizure
-lexia	reading
-paresis	partial paralysis
-phasia	speech
-plegia	paralysis

Combining Forms

dendr/o	tree
gangli/i, ganglion/o	ganglion
gli/o	neuroglia
neur/o, neur/i	nerve

CENTRAL NERVOUS SYSTEM
Combining Forms

alges/o	sensitivity to pain
arachn/o	spider; arachnoid membrane
caud/o	tail
cerebell/o	cerebellum
cerebr/o	cerebrum
cortic/o	cortex
dur/o	dura mater
encephal/o	brain
medull/o	medulla oblongata
mening/o, meninge/o	meninges
myel/o	spinal cord; bone marrow
narc/o	stupor; sleep
pia	tender
pyr/o	fire; temperature increase; fever
radicul/o	root of a spinal nerve
rhiz/o	root
somn/o, somn/i	sleep
thalam/o	thalamus
ventricul/o	cavity

Prefixes

hemi-	half
quadri-	four
semi-	half

MENTAL HEALTH
Combining Forms

ment/o	mind
phren/o	mind; diaphragm
psych/o	mind
schiz/o	split

Suffixes

-phobia	irrational fear
-mania	excited state; excessive preoccupation

ABBREVIATIONS: Nervous System

ALS	amyotrophic lateral sclerosis
ANS	autonomic nervous system
CNS	central nervous system
CSF	cerebrospinal fluid
CVA	cerebrovascular accident
EEG	electroencephalogram
LP	lumbar puncture
MS	multiple sclerosis
PNS	peripheral nervous system
REM	rapid eye movement
TIA	transient ischemic attack

17 Sensory System

evolve   http://evolve.elsevier.com/klieger/medicalassisting

The body has millions of sensory receptors that interface between the nervous system and the internal and external environments. These receptors fall into two main categories: general sense organs and special sense organs. The most numerous are the general sense organs that produce the somatic (body) senses (e.g., touch, temperature, pressure, vibration, and body position) and initiate reflexes necessary for maintaining homeostasis. Special sense organs produce vision, balance (equilibrium), taste (gustation), hearing, and smell (olfaction) and initiate reflexes needed for homeostasis.

LEARNING OBJECTIVES

You will be able to do the following after completing this chapter:

Key Terms
1. Define, appropriately use, and spell all the Key Terms for this chapter.

Sensory System
2. Explain the purpose of the sensory system.
3. List and describe the five main senses.
4. List the five general sensations.
5. Name the organs and structures of the sensory system and describe the function of each.
6. List and describe seven common signs and symptoms of eye disease and four signs of ear disorders.
7. List six diagnostic tests and procedures for eye disease and four tests for ear disorders and explain the use of each.
8. List 12 eye diseases and 7 ear disorders and describe the etiology, signs and symptoms, diagnosis, therapy, and interventions for each.

Patient-Centered Professionalism
9. Analyze a realistic medical office situation and apply your understanding of the sensory system to determine the best course of action.
10. Describe the impact on patient care when medical assistants have a solid understanding of the structure and function of the sensory system.

KEY TERMS

The Key Terms for this chapter have been organized into sections so that you can easily see the terminology associated with each aspect of the nervous system.

Sensory System
equilibrium	proprioception
olfaction	tactile

Taste
gustatory receptors	papillae

Vision
accommodation	refraction
optic nerve	

Eyeball
anterior cavity	macula lutea
aqueous humor	opaque
canals of Schlemm	ophthalmoscope
choroid	optic disc (blind spot)
ciliary body	posterior cavity
cones	pupil
cornea	retina
fovea centralis	rods
iris	sclera
lens	vitreous humor

Continued

Eye Muscles	
extrinsic muscles	rectus
intrinsic muscles	suspensory ligament
oblique	

Accessory Organs	
canthus	conjunctiva

Eye Diseases	
amblyopia	glaucoma
astigmatism	hordeolum (stye)
cataract	hyperopia (farsightedness)
chalazion	myopia (nearsightedness)
conjunctivitis (pinkeye)	nystagmus
diplopia	presbyopia (old eyes)
dacryoadenitis	ptosis
esotropia	strabismus (cross-eye)
exophthalmia	xerophthalmia
exotropia	

Related Eye Terms	
Amsler grid	gonioscopy
exophthalmometer	ophthalmologist
fluorescein angiography	slit-lamp examination
fluorescein staining	tonometry

Hearing

auditory	middle ear
inner ear	outer ear

Outer Ear	
cerumen	pinna (auricle)
external auditory canal	tympanic membrane (eardrum)

Middle Ear	
eustachian tube	oval window
incus (anvil)	round window
malleus (hammer)	stapes (stirrup)
ossicles	

Inner Ear	
cochlea	organ of Corti
labyrinth	

Sound	
audiometry	pitch
decibels (dB)	

Ear Disorders	
deafness	otitis media
mastoiditis	otosclerosis
Ménière disease	presbycusis
otitis externa (swimmer's ear)	tinnitus

Related Ear Terms	
otolaryngologist	Rinne test
otoscopy	Weber test

Equilibrium

motion sickness	vestibular apparatus
semicircular canals	vestibule

PRACTICAL APPLICATIONS

Read the following scenario and keep it in mind as you learn about the sensory portion of the nervous system in this chapter.

Bob DeMarce, age 42, complained of vertigo, tinnitus, and a sensation of fullness of the right ear for the last month. He states that each episode did not follow a certain event. He denies any ear pain, fever, headache, or nausea.

Past medical history includes a recent ear infection that was treated with amoxicillin for 10 days. On examination, Dr. Bailey finds that the tympanic membrane is dull and inflamed. It is decided that Mr. DeMarce has had otitis media that failed to resolve.

Do you understand what otitis media is, and how Mr. DeMarce's earlier symptoms relate to it?

SENSORY SYSTEM

The senses allow the body to respond to both internal and external stimuli. Senses are needed to maintain homeostasis, protect the body from harm, and conduct pleasure or pain. Each sense (e.g., taste, vision, or smell) has a sensory system with receptors that allow it to transmit impulses to the central nervous system (CNS) for interpretation. The main senses include taste, smell (**olfaction**), vision, hearing, and balance. General sensations include pain, touch (**tactile**), pressure, temperature, and **proprioception** (Box 17-1 and Figure 17-1).

Taste

The tongue is a movable muscular organ that consists of two halves united in the center. **Papillae** cover the tongue and contain capillaries and nerves. The taste buds are distributed on the surface of the tongue and throughout the mouth, especially the soft palate. Each taste bud is made up of **gustatory receptors** that relay impulses to the brain. They are stimulated only if the substance to be tasted is in a solution. The four different kinds of taste buds and their separate locations on the tongue (Figure 17-2) are as follows:

1. *Sweet* taste: located near the tip of the tongue.
2. *Sour* taste: located on both sides of the tongue.
3. *Salty* taste: located near the tip of the tongue.
4. *Bitter* taste: located at the back of the tongue.

Smell

The sense of smell is accomplished by the olfactory nerve. Branches containing receptors are located throughout the upper part of the nasal cavity and the upper third of the septum (Figure 17-3). Nasal sensations of cold, heat, pain, and pressure are produced by the trigeminal nerve.

The sense of smell is closely related to the sense of taste. When the sense of smell is decreased (e.g., person has a cold), the sense of taste also diminishes. Olfactory nerves become

BOX 17-1

General Sensations*

- *Pain* is a reaction to tissue damage and therefore acts as a protective function of the body. Pain receptors are distributed throughout the body and react to release of chemicals when the tissue is damaged, when oxygen fails to reach tissue, or when tissues are stretched or deformed.
- *Touch* and *pressure* (tactile) receptors are located in the skin, subcutaneous tissue, and deep tissue and respond to pressure and vibration. Tactile receptors are most concentrated in the lips and fingers.
- *Temperature* receptors detect hot and cold. Cold receptors are stimulated at 10° to 25° C and heat receptors at 25° to 45° C. Both types of receptors adapt to the heat or cold, and therefore the sensation fades after 20 to 30 minutes *(accommodation)*.
- *Proprioception* receptors are found in muscles, tendons, joints, and inner ear and function to maintain balance and to create awareness of one's sense of position in space.

*See also Figure 17-1.

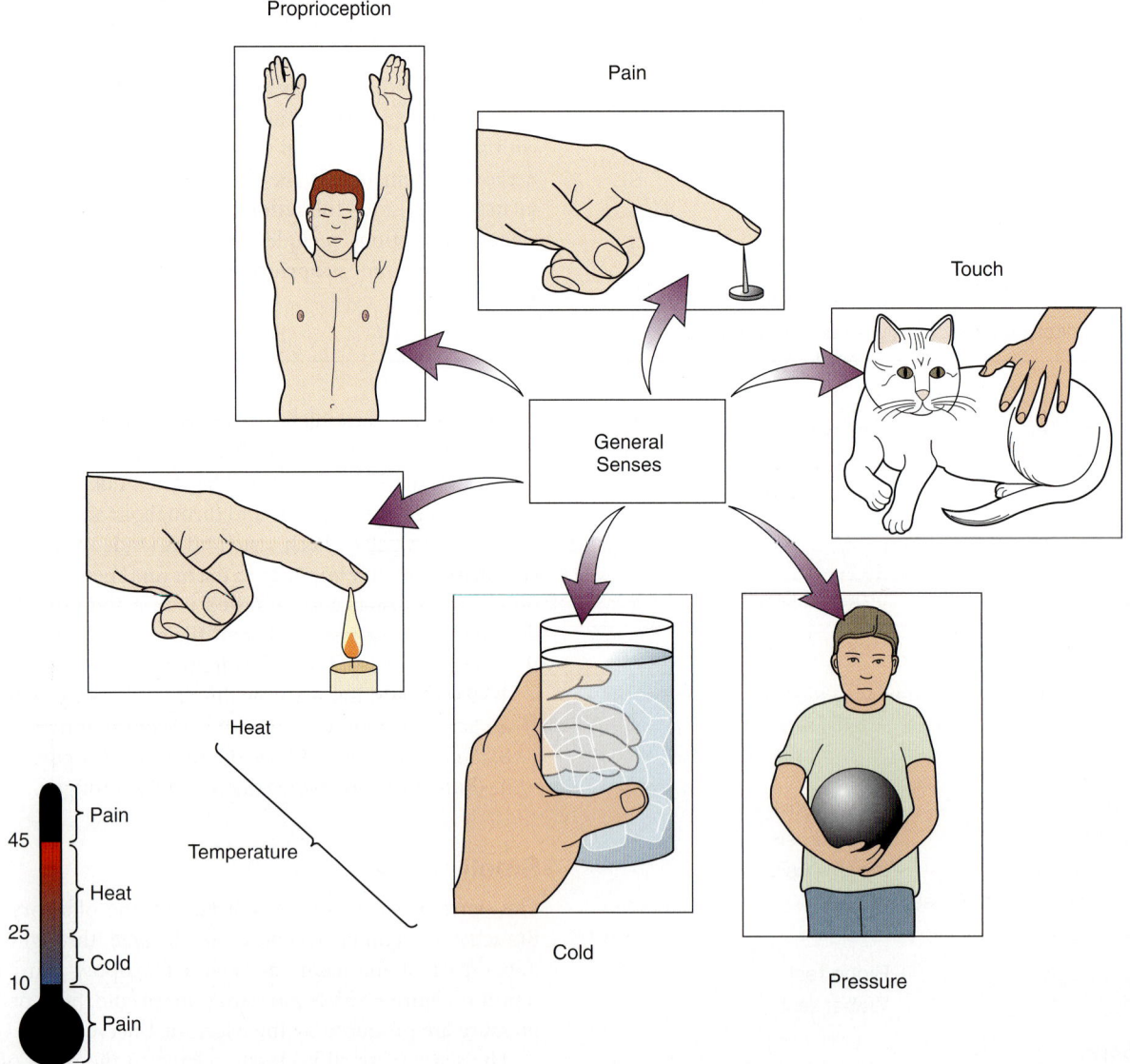

FIGURE 17-1 General senses: pain, touch, pressure, temperature, and proprioception. (From Herlihy B, Maebius NK: *The human body in health and illness,* ed 3, St Louis, 2007, Saunders.)

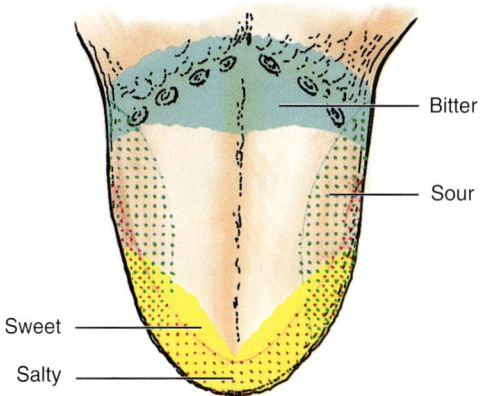

FIGURE 17-2 Sense of taste in the tongue (gustatory sense). Taste buds located on specific areas of tongue identify four taste sensations: bitter, sour, salty, and sweet. (From Applegate EJ: *The anatomy and physiology learning system*, ed 3, St Louis, 2006, Saunders.)

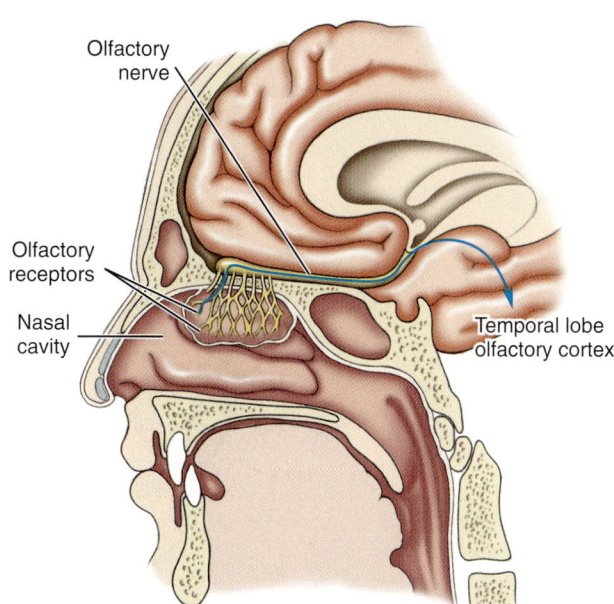

FIGURE 17-3 Sense of smell: the nose. The olfactory (smell) receptors are chemoreceptors and are located in the upper nose. Sensory information is transmitted through the olfactory nerve to the temporal lobe of the cerebrum. (From Herlihy B, Maebius NK: *The human body in health and illness,* ed 3, St Louis, 2007, Saunders.)

less sensitive after detecting the same odor over time, which is why it is harder to smell your laundry soap, bath soap, or shampoo if you use the same type over a long period.

Vision

The eye and other organs work together to provide vision.

Eye Structure and Function

The eye is the receptor organ of vision, providing us with three-dimensional sight. The eye receives light rays and sends the impulses to the **optic nerve.** The optic nerve carries impulses to the brain, where they are interpreted for sight. Each eye is located in a bony orbital cavity within the skull for protection.

Eyeball. The eyeball is a round, hollow structure about an inch in diameter. It is composed of three layers: the sclera, choroid, and retina. There are two cavities within the eye: the **anterior cavity** and the **posterior cavity** (Figure 17-4, *A*).

1. The **sclera,** or white of the eye, is the outermost layer. It is a fibrous protective tissue that maintains the shape of the eye, is the attachment site for the extrinsic eye muscles, and protects the other layers. The **cornea** is avascular and does not contain blood vessels, so light rays are allowed to penetrate.
2. The **choroid** is the middle layer and is **opaque.** It contains many blood vessels and is attached to the retina. The other parts of the middle layer are the iris and the ciliary body.
   - The **iris** lies beneath the cornea and is in front of the **lens.** The opening in the center of the iris is the **pupil.** The iris contains the eye color, and the pupil is a radial muscle that dilates or constricts to regulate the amount of light that enters the eye.
   - The **ciliary body** contains the ciliary muscle, which controls the shape or curvature of the lens and allows for near and far vision, a process called **accommodation.**
   The ciliary body also forms the aqueous humor that flows in front of the eye.
3. The **retina,** the third and innermost layer, lines the interior of the eyeball. The retina contains the **rods** and **cones** that are photoreceptors sensitive to light. Proper sight requires that light rays bend (**refraction**) as they pass through the eye structures to the retina. The optic nerve branches out within the retina to collect the impulses given off by the rods and cones and transmits them to the brain.
   - The rods are responsible for sight in dim light and peripheral vision, and are sensitive to black and white.
   - The cones are responsible for sight in bright light and are sensitive to color.

Between the cornea and the iris and between the iris and the lens is the anterior cavity and posterior cavity (Figure 17-4, *B* and *C*) filled with fluid (humor). The **aqueous humor** helps to maintain a constant pressure within the eye in the anterior cavity and provides nourishment to the cornea. Aqueous humor leaves the cavity by way of the **canals of Schlemm** (Figure 17-4, *C*) and into the bloodstream.

Directly behind the lens is the posterior chamber filled with **vitreous humor,** a clear, jellylike substance that maintains the shape of the eye and gives the retina support. Together the lens, vitreous humor, and the aqueous humor allow light rays to bend (refract) (Figure 17-4, *B*).

When the physician views the retina through the **ophthalmoscope,** a yellow disc (**macula lutea**) is seen.

The macula is responsible for the central and detailed vision needed to read, drive, recognize faces, watch television,

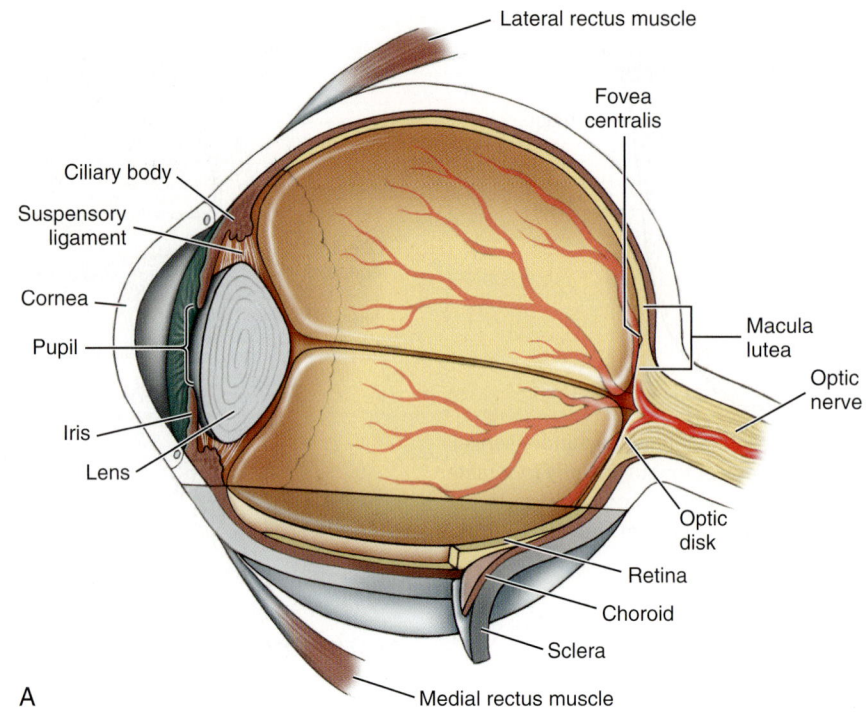

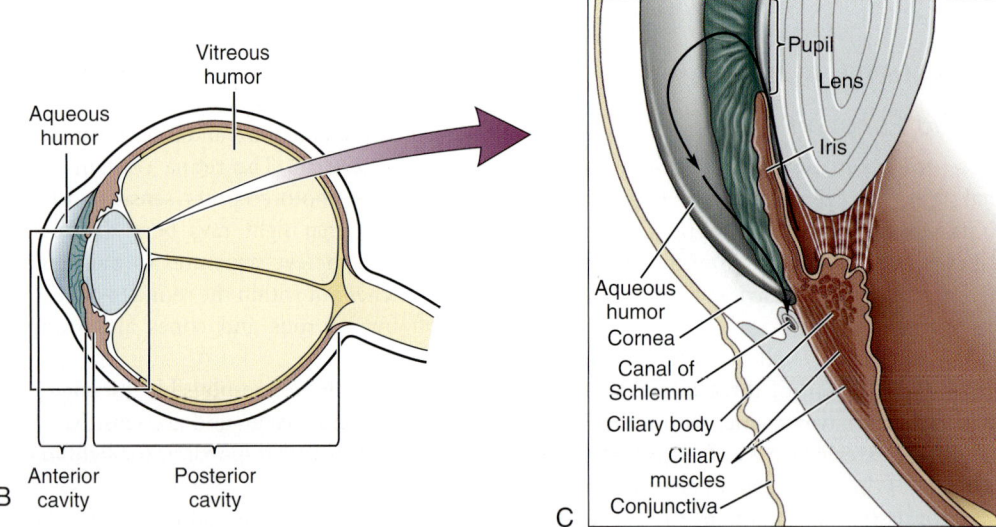

FIGURE 17-4 **A,** Structure of the eyeball. **B,** Cavities and fluids. Posterior cavity lies between retina and lens; it is filled with vitreous humor. Anterior cavity lies between lens and cornea. **C,** Note flow of aqueous humor from ciliary body to canal of Schlemm *(arrow).* (From Herlihy B, Maebius NK: *The human body in health and illness,* ed 3, St Louis, 2007, Saunders.)

sew, and do other tasks. Within the disc is the **fovea centralis** that contains only the cones for color vision. To the side of the fovea is a pale disc called the **optic disc,** or **blind spot.** There are no rods or cones in this area and thus no visual reception.

Eye Muscles. Six different **extrinsic** skeletal muscles allow the eye to move and anchor the eye in place. There are four **rectus** (straight) muscles—superior, inferior, medial, and lateral—and two **oblique** (angled) muscles—superior and inferior (Figure 17-5 and Table 17-1). The **intrinsic muscles** within the iris are smooth involuntary muscle, and this controls the amount of light entering the pupil and allows for close vision.

Accessory Organs. Besides the eye, additional organs help us to see. The visual accessory organs include the eyebrows, eyelids, eyelashes, lacrimal apparatus, and extrinsic eye muscles (Figure 17-6).

- The *eyebrows* are small patches of coarse hair above the eyes. The brows shade the eyes from sunlight and keep perspiration (sweat) from falling into the eyes.

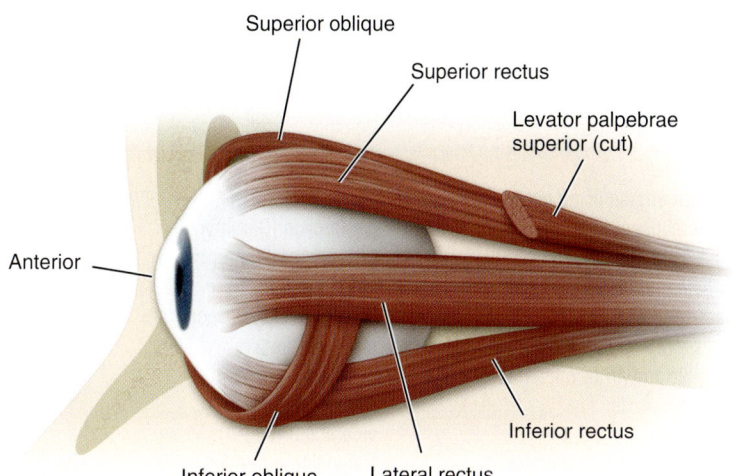

FIGURE 17-5 Muscles of the eye. (Modified from Chester GA: *Modern medical assisting,* Philadelphia, 1998, Saunders.)

TABLE 17-1
Eye Muscles

Muscle	Function	CN
EXTRINSIC		
Superior rectus	Elevates or rolls the eyeball upward	III
Inferior rectus	Depresses or rolls the eyeball downward	III
Medial rectus	Moves or rolls the eyeball toward the middle	III
Lateral rectus*	Moves or rolls the eyeball to the side or laterally	VI
Superior oblique*	Depresses or rolls the eyeball to the side or laterally	IV
Inferior oblique	Elevates or rolls the eyeball upward	III
INTRINSIC		
Ciliary	Allows the **suspensory ligament** to relax and the lens to become more convex for close vision	III
Iris, circular	Constricts the pupil to allow less light to enter the eye	III
Iris, radial	Dilates the pupil to allow more light to enter the eye	III

CN, Cranial nerve.
*Lateral rectus and superior oblique are controlled by CNs other than CN III.

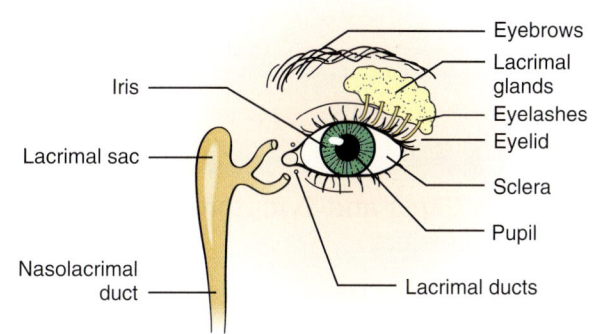

FIGURE 17-6 Visual accessory organs: eyebrows, eyelids, eyelashes, and lacrimal apparatus. Tears are secreted by the lacrimal gland, wash over the surface of the eye, and drain into the lacrimal sac and finally into the nasolacrimal duct. Crying floods the system, causing tears to flow. (Modified from Buck CJ: *Step-by-step medical coding, 2008 edition*, St Louis, 2008, Saunders.)

- The *eyelids* are protective folds covering the eyes. The lids protect the eye from excessive light and foreign matter by blinking. The area where the upper and lower lids meet is called the **canthus**. The **conjunctiva** is a mucous membrane that lines the underside of the eyelid and protects the exposed area of the eyeball.
- The *eyelashes* line the edge of the eyelid and serve to trap foreign objects (e.g., dust). The lashes protrude from oil-producing sebaceous glands on the edge of the lid.
- The *lacrimal apparatus* is composed of the lacrimal gland and tear ducts. The lacrimal gland secretes tears that drain into nasolacrimal ducts. Tears function to lubricate, cleanse the eye surface, and keep the eye from becoming dry. The enzyme *lysozyme* is present in tears and acts as an antiseptic agent by destroying foreign organisms.
- The *extrinsic eye muscles* are discussed in Table 17-1.

FOR YOUR INFORMATION

The effects of aging on the eyes are a decrease in the production of tears, thinning retinas, and yellowing lenses. The reduction of nerve activity to the eyes along with the fact that the iris stiffens making the pupil less responsive to light changes affects accommodation.

Eye Diseases

Diseases of the eye may be present at birth or may appear as the body ages. An **ophthalmologist** treats disorders of the eye. Drugs may be prescribed to treat diseases of the eye (Table 17-2).

Medical assistants need to be able to recognize the common signs and symptoms of and diagnostic tests for the different types of eye disorders.

TABLE 17-2

Eye Drug Classifications

Drug Classification	Common Generic (Brand) Drugs
Antifungals Reduce effects of fungal infection	natamycin (Natacyn)
Antiinfectives Destroy bacteria	gentamicin (Garamycin) tetracycline (Achromycin)
Antiinflammatories Reduce inflammation	ketorolac (Acular) dexamethasone (Decadron)
Antiseptics Prohibit growth of bacteria (prophylaxis)	silver nitrate 1% boric acid (Blinx)
Antivirals Treat infections of the eye	vidarabine (Vira-A) trifluridine (Viroptic)
Antiglaucoma agents Reduce intraocular pressure by increasing drainage of aqueous humor or decreasing its production	pilocarpine (Pilocar) apraclonidine (Iopidine)
Topical anesthetics Prevent eye pain	tetracaine (Pontocaine) proparacaine (Kainair)

BOX 17-2

Common Signs and Symptoms of Eye Disorders

Amblyopia	Dull or dim vision caused by disease
Diplopia	Seeing double
Dacryoadenitis	Inflammation of lacrimal gland
Esotropia	Turning inward of one or both eyes
Exophthalmia	Protrusion of the eyeballs
Exotropia	Turning outward of one or both eyes
Xerophthalmia	Dry eye

BOX 17-3

Diagnostic Tests and Procedures for the Eye

Amsler grid	Assesses central vision (macular degeneration)
Fluorescein angiography	Traces pathway through vessels of retina after injection of dye
Fluorescein staining	Assesses for abnormalities of cornea after drops of dye instilled into eye
Gonioscopy	Visualizes angle of anterior chamber (glaucoma)
Slit-lamp examination	Examines various layers of the eye
Tonometry	Measures intraocular pressure (glaucoma)

- Study Box 17-2 to familiarize yourself with the common signs and symptoms.
- Study Box 17-3 to learn about common diagnostic tests.
- Study Table 17-3 to understand the diseases that affect the eye.

Hearing

The ear is the major organ of hearing. It picks up sound waves and sends the impulses to the **auditory** center of the brain in the temporal region. Transmission of sound waves in the **outer ear** occurs through air; in the **middle ear**, it occurs through bone; and in the **inner ear**, it occurs through fluid. The inner ear also functions to maintain balance, **equilibrium,** and awareness of position.

Ear Structure and Function

The ear consists of three parts: the outer ear, middle ear, and inner ear (Figure 17-9).

Outer (External) Ear. The outer ear is the visible part of the ear and a canal that connects to the middle ear.

- The **pinna,** or **auricle,** is the projecting part of the ear. It is the flap of skin and cartilage on the outside of the head.
- The **external auditory canal** extends from the auricle to about 4 cm into the skull and ends at the tympanic membrane. Air vibrations are guided through the canal to the tympanic membrane.
- The **tympanic membrane,** or **eardrum,** is a thin membrane that completely separates the outer ear from the middle ear, with skin on the outside and a mucous membrane on the inside. The eardrum vibrates when struck by sound waves.

Middle Ear. The middle ear is a cavity in the temporal bone that is full of air. It is connected to the nasopharynx (throat) by the eustachian tube. The middle ear contains three small bones, or **ossicles,** that conduct sound waves. Because of their shapes, these bones form a movable chain between the eardrum and the **oval window.**

The **malleus (hammer), incus (anvil),** and **stapes (stirrup)** amplify sound waves across the middle ear to the inner ear when the eardrum vibrates. The oval window permits the passage of the sound waves from the ossicles to the inner ear. The **round window** is located below the oval window and separates the middle and inner ear. The round window bends as the stapes pushes the oval window, preventing pressure buildup in the inner ear.

The **eustachian tube** that links the ear and the nasopharynx regulates pressure in the middle ear to equalize the pressure on both sides of the eardrum. When sudden pressure changes occur (e.g., flying), swallowing helps to equalize the pressure. Children are more prone to ear infection because the eustachian tube connects to the throat horizontally. As a child grows, the angle increases, leaving less access for bacteria to enter the ear from the throat.

Inner Ear. The inner ear contains receptors for sound waves to permit hearing and maintain equilibrium. The inner ear, called the **labyrinth,** is composed of a bony outer shell and a membranous lining. Three major structures contain receptors for sound waves for hearing and for maintaining equilibrium.

TABLE 17-3

Diseases and Disorders of the Eye

Disease and Description	Etiology	Signs and Symptoms	Diagnosis	Therapy	Interventions
Cataract Opacity of lens of eye	*Senile cataracts:* in elderly; chemical changes in lens *Congenital cataracts:* in newborns; errors of metabolism *Traumatic cataracts:* trauma allows humor to invade lens capsule	Complaints of gradual vision loss; glare or poor vision in bright sunlight or night driving	Visual acuity test supports complaint of vision loss; **slit-lamp examination** identifies lens opacity and apparent cloudy lens on examination	Surgical lens extraction and lens implant to correct vision	Avoid activities after eye surgery that would increase eye pressure (e.g., bending over, straining with coughing, bowel movements, or lifting)
Chalazion Small mass on eyelid caused by inflammation and blockage of gland	Obstruction of gland duct in eyelid	Nontender, small cyst on eyelid	Visual examination	Warm compresses to open gland and antibiotic eye drops to prevent infection	Provide proper instructions for using warm compresses to prevent cross-contamination
Conjunctivitis (pinkeye) Conjunctiva becomes inflamed (Figure 17-7, C)	Irritation caused by allergies or viral or bacterial infection	Complaints of eye pain, photophobia, burning, itching, and crusting	Inspection of eye shows discharge, tearing, and hyperemia; culture and sensitivity tests of discharge identify organism	Topical antibiotic	Illustrate proper handwashing techniques to minimize spread of infection to family members; emphasize not to share towels, washcloths, or pillows
Glaucoma Aqueous humor does not drain properly, and intraocular pressure increases and compresses choroid layer, diminishing blood supply to retina	Can be found in families because of narrow channel between iris and cornea	May be insidious and progress slowly, therefore asymptomatic; dull morning headache, aching in eyes, loss of peripheral vision, seeing halos around lights, decrease in visual acuity; may also be acute with severe eye pain	**Tonometry** is used to measure intraocular pressure; slit-lamp exam for anterior eye structures	Medications to reduce aqueous humor production and promote outflow of humor; in extreme cases, laser surgery to enhance aqueous humor outflow	Encourage following treatment regimen to decrease risk of total blindness
Hordeolum (stye) Localized infection in eyelid (Figure 17-7, B)	Hair follicle in eyelid becomes infected with staphylococcal organism	Painful swelling of eyelid	Culture and sensitivity of exudate	Warm compresses 4 times daily; ophthalmic antibiotic drops or ointment	Instruct patient to use clean compress for each application; dispose of or launder it separately; caution not to squeeze stye or rub eye (could spread infection)
Ptosis Upper eyelid unable to remain open (Figure 17-7, A)	*Congenital:* levator muscles fail to develop *Acquired:* age, swelling, neurogenic factors, thiamine deficiency (alcoholism)	One eyelid covers iris partially or completely	Clinical inspection to determine cause may include glucose tolerance test to verify presence of diabetes, ophthalmic examination to rule out trauma or foreign body	If severe ptosis exists, surgical intervention is needed to resect levator muscles	Ensure patient is aware of increased risk for injury and perceptual and sensory alterations

TABLE 17-3
Diseases and Disorders of the Eye—cont'd

Disease and Description	Etiology	Signs and Symptoms	Diagnosis	Therapy	Interventions
Strabismus (cross-eye) Movements of eyeball not coordinated (Figure 17-7, D)	May occur from trauma or eye muscle imbalance	Eyes deviate inward, upward, or outward	Neurological examination to determine if cause is muscular or neurological	Patching normal eye to force affected eye to focus straight, strengthening muscle; surgical intervention to shorten muscle	Stress need for follow-up care; patient teaching for instilling eye medications if used after surgery
Macular degeneration *Dry:* Light-sensitive cells in the macula degenerate and die *Wet:* Abnormal blood vessels forming and leaking under the retina	Deterioration of cells in the macula (a small area in the center of the retina)	Images become distorted or blurry, black spots, images blotted out in the center with only the periphery able to be seen	Vision test and ophthalmoscopy detects spots of cellular waste material that form at the back of the eye *Amsler grid* detects changes in central vision	*Dry:* Cannot restore lost acuity, studies show certain vitamins and minerals may reduce, slow down, or stop further vision loss *Wet:* Laser treatments to stop bleeding and photodynamic therapy (PDT)	Counseling to help patient learn how to live with condition, and support network Vision aids (e.g., magnifying machines to read newsprint)

ADDITIONAL EYE CONDITIONS
Astigmatism: Refraction error caused by abnormal curvature of cornea and lens (Figure 17-8, C)
Hyperopia (farsightedness): Occurs when light rays form behind retina (Figure 17-8, B)
Myopia (nearsightedness): Occurs when light rays focus in front of retina (Figure 17-8, A)
Nystagmus: Rapid, involuntary, rhythmic movement of the eyeball
Presbyopia (old eyes): Occurs when the lens loses its ability to change shape during accommodation for close objects

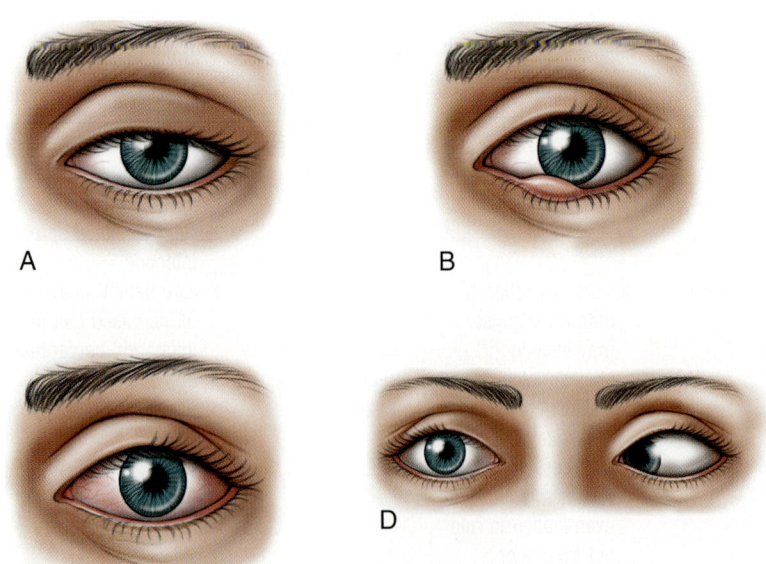

FIGURE 17-7 **A,** Ptosis of eyelid; droopy eyelid. **B,** Hordeolum, or stye. **C,** Conjunctivitis, or pinkeye. **D,** Strabismus. Note that eyeball deviates from the midline. (Modified from Herlihy B, Maebius NK: *The human body in health and illness,* ed 3, St Louis, 2007, Saunders.)

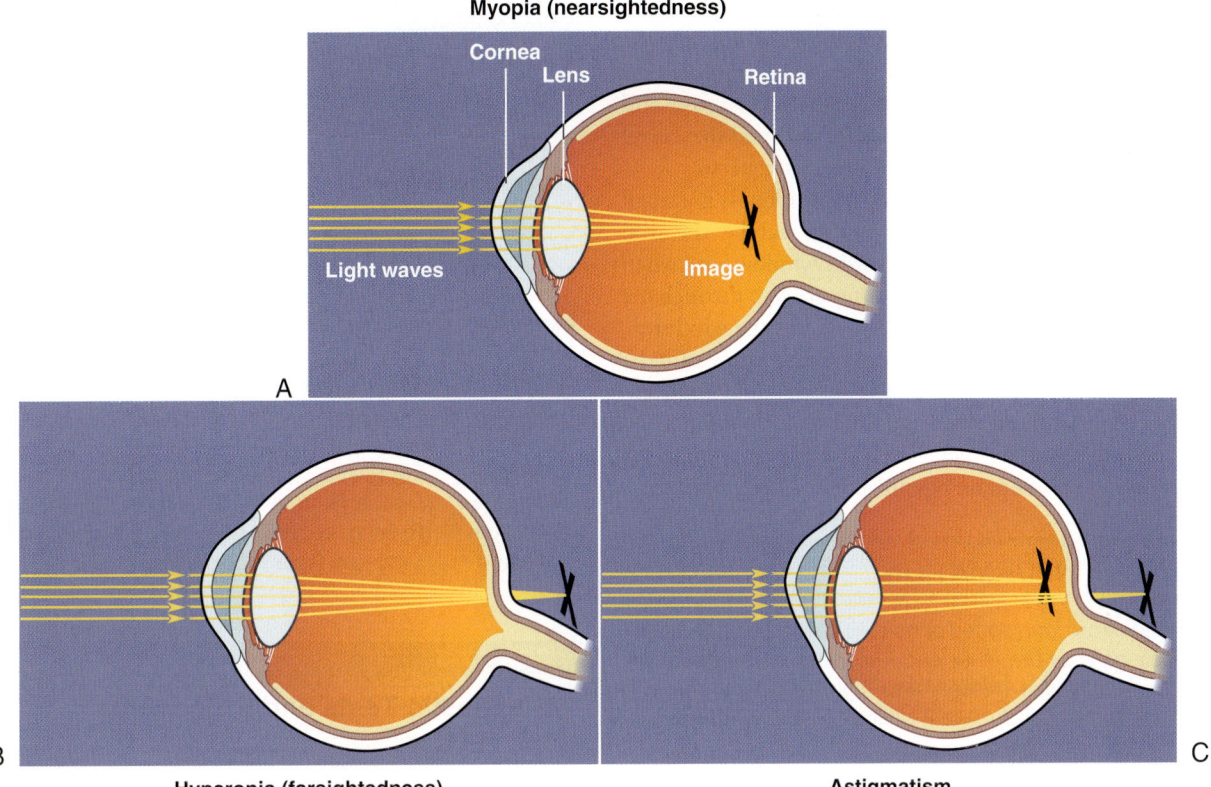

FIGURE 17-8 **A,** Myopia, or nearsightedness. **B,** Hyperopia or farsightedness. **C,** Astigmatism. (From Herlihy B, Maebius NK: *The human body in health and illness,* ed 3, St Louis, 2007, Saunders.)

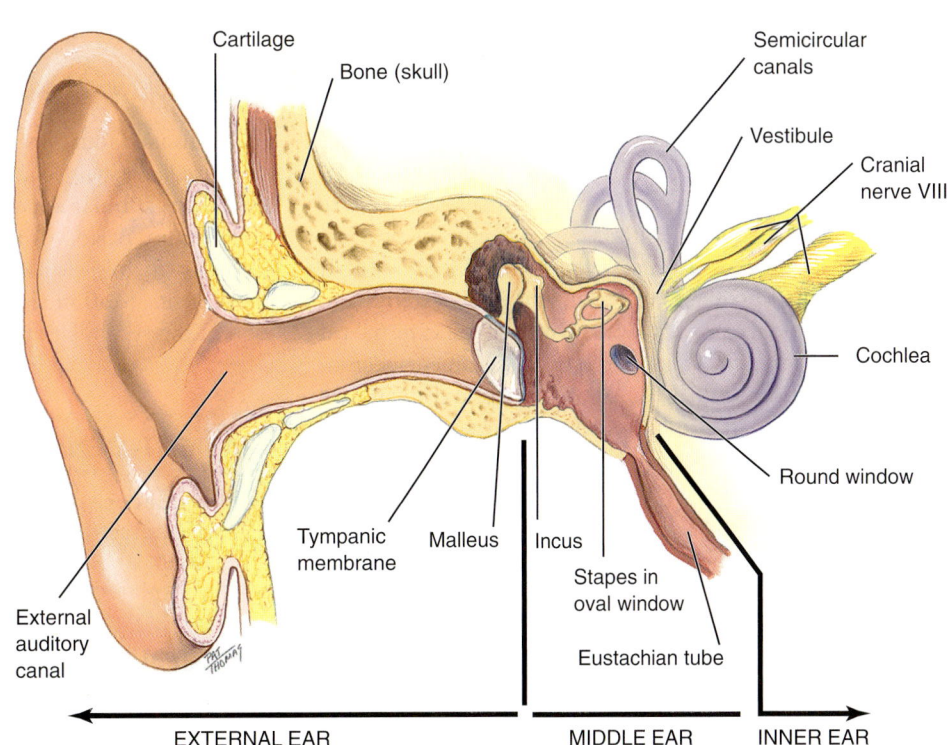

FIGURE 17-9 Three divisions of the ear (external, middle, and inner) and their structures. (From Jarvis C: *Physical examination and health assessment,* ed 5, St Louis, 2008, Saunders.)

1. The **cochlea** lies below the vestibule and is shaped like a snail shell. On the floor is the receptor for hearing, the **organ of Corti**. This receptor is made of tiny hairs. As fluid moves through the cochlea, the hairs move and initiate sensory nerve impulses (sound waves) that travel through the cochlear nerve to the acoustic nerve.
2. The **vestibule** controls the sense of position. It is a small chamber separated from the middle ear by the oval window. The stapes rests against the window, and when the sound waves are picked up, they are sent through the fluid in the inner ear by vibrating against the window.
3. The **semicircular canals,** located above the vestibule, control equilibrium. The canals contain liquid and hairlike cells that bend when the fluid is set in motion by body and head movements. The impulses are sent to the brain to help maintain equilibrium, or body balance.

FOR YOUR INFORMATION

Hearing loss from loud sound or noise is the result of damage to the hair cells of the inner ear. The walls of the auditory canals thin, eardrums thicken, and high frequency sounds are difficult to hear and make it difficult to follow conversations in a crowded room.

Sound

When sound waves vibrate, they create a **pitch.** The number of times a sound wave vibrates is referred to as *frequency,* and from this, pitch is determined. The greater and higher the frequency of sound waves, the higher is the pitch. The loudness of a sound is determined by the height of the sound waves and intensity of the vibration. Sound is measured in **decibels (dB).** The human ear hears up to 140 dB. If sound is higher than this, pain is experienced. **Audiometry** measures sounds heard by the human ear.

Ear Disorders

Disorders of the ear may occur at birth or may be associated with heredity, noise pollution, or age. A common problem seen in the medical office, especially in children and elderly patients, is a buildup of earwax **(cerumen)** in the external ear. Cerumen is produced by the sweat glands of the external ear to aid in protecting the canal. If too much cerumen accumulates, hearing can be impaired. An **otolaryngologist** can treat disorders of the ears, and an *audiometrist* evaluates hearing loss. Drugs may be prescribed to treat conditions of the ear (Table 17-4).

Medical assistants need to be able to recognize the common signs and symptoms of and diagnostic tests for the different types of ear disorders.
- Study Box 17-4 to familiarize yourself with the common signs and symptoms of auditory disorders.
- Study Box 17-5 to learn about common diagnostic tests and procedures.
- Study Table 17-5 to understand the diseases that affect the ear.

TABLE 17-4

Ear Drug Classifications

Drug Classification	Common Generic (Brand) Drugs
Antiinfectives Treat bacterial infections	neomycin, polymyxin B (Cortisporin), chloramphenicol (Pentamycetin)
Ceruminolytics Soften and break down earwax	carbamide peroxide (Murine ear drops; Cerumenex)

BOX 17-4

Common Signs and Symptoms of Ear Disorders

Otalgia	Ear pain
Otorrhea	Discharge from the auditory canal
Tinnitus	Ringing, buzzing, or a roaring sound in the ears
Vertigo	Dizziness (spinning sensation)

BOX 17-5

Diagnostic Tests and Procedures for the Ear

Audiometry	Measures how well a person hears various frequencies of sound
Otoscopy	Views the tympanic membrane and various parts of the outer ear
Rinne test	Compares bone conduction and air conduction of sound using a tuning fork
Weber test	Determines if a hearing loss is caused by conductive loss or sensorineural loss

Equilibrium

As mentioned, our sense of equilibrium is controlled by the semicircular canals located above the vestibule in the inner ear. The **vestibular apparatus** is involved in body balance, or equilibrium. Balance is related to maintaining the position of the body (mainly the head) with respect to gravity and sudden movements. **Motion sickness** is caused by excessive stimulation of the vestibular apparatus.

PATIENT-CENTERED PROFESSIONALISM

- *How does being knowledgeable about the sensory system and diseases affecting this system make the medical assistant a valuable asset in the medical office?*

CONCLUSION

The structure and function of the sensory system enable us to detect changes taking place through our sensory receptors. The five main senses are located throughout the head to

TABLE 17-5

Diseases and Disorders of the Ear

Disease and Description	Etiology	Signs and Symptoms	Diagnosis	Therapy	Interventions
Ménière disease Buildup of excess fluid in semicircular canals, with excess pressure on canals, vestibule, and cochlea	Unknown	Hearing loss, vertigo, **tinnitus**	Series of hearing tests; diuretic between tests reduces pressure in ear; if patient improves, diagnosis is confirmed; electrocochleography and MRI to rule out brain lesions	Medications, including diuretic and antivertigo drugs; in severe cases, shunt used to drain excess fluid to CSF	Encourage a diet low in sodium; Instruct patient to avoid sudden position changes
Mastoiditis Inflammation of lining of mastoid cells	Bacterial infection; often a complication of otitis media	Dull earache, low-grade fever, swelling of ear canal, discharge, hearing loss	X-rays confirm the diagnosis, and audiometric testing confirms hearing loss	Antibiotic therapy	Answer patient's questions and concerns about hearing loss; encourage compliance with prescribed treatment
Deafness *Conduction:* Interference with passage of sound waves from outside to inner ear	Impacted cerumen; foreign bodies; inflammation; damage to tympanic membranes (chronic otitis media)	Inability to respond to external stimuli from outer ear; tinnitus may be first symptom noticed by patient	Patient history, audiometry testing	Remove source	Answer patient's questions and concerns about hearing loss; provide information on support groups available
Sensorineural: Loss of function of cochlea or acoustic nerve	Brain tumor; **otosclerosis** (loss of vibrations) due to damaged ossicles; nerve damage; loud noise	Inability to respond to external stimuli from outer ear; tinnitus may be first symptom noticed by patient	Patient history, audiometry testing	Reduce further damage by removing source if known; use of ear protectors in areas with high noise levels	Answer patient's questions and concerns about hearing loss; provide information on support groups available
Otitis externa (swimmer's ear) Inflammation of outer ear	Common causes: allergy, bacteria, fungi, viruses, trauma	Pain or itching and swelling in ear canal	Direct examination of ear canal; culture of drainage	Analgesics for discomfort; antibiotics for causative agent	Encourage proper cleaning and drying of external ear and avoidance of allergic substance
Otitis media Inflammation of middle ear	Bacterial or viral infection	Complaint of severe earache; fever, vomiting, fullness in ears	Clinical evaluation: erythematous eardrum on examination	Possible surgery to insert tubes to drain fluid from eardrum if bulging; antibiotics to control infective agent; antihistamines to reduce fluids; antipyretics for fever and pain	Encourage general cleaning of ears to prevent buildup of moisture that can harbor microorganisms

Presbycusis: Progressive hearing loss occurring in old age

CSF, Cerebrospinal fluid; *MRI,* magnetic resonance imaging.

include vision, hearing, taste, smell, and equilibrium. The general senses are located throughout the body and respond to touch, pressure, temperature, pain, and position. Disorders of the sensory system are most often associated with the aging process, environmental factors, injury, and birth defects. Our life experiences are driven by our sensory system. How our body responds to changes in the environment depends on both our internal and external receptors.

Chapter Summary

Reinforce your understanding of the material in this chapter by reviewing the curriculum objectives and key content points below.

1. **Define, appropriately use, and spell all the Key Terms for this chapter.**
   - Review the Key Terms if necessary.
2. **Explain the purpose of the sensory system.**
   - The senses allow the body to respond to both internal and external stimuli.
   - The senses protect the body from harm, maintain the body in homeostasis, and transmit pleasure and pain.
3. **List and describe the five main senses.**
   - The five main senses are taste, smell, vision, hearing, and balance (equilibrium).
4. **List the five general sensations.**
   - General sensations include pain, touch (tactile), pressure, temperature, and proprioception.
5. **Name the organs and structures of the sensory system and describe the function of each.**
   - Papillae in the mouth allow us to taste sweet, sour, salty, and bitter.
   - The nose filters the air we breathe and transmits perceived fragrance and odor. The sense of smell is closely related to the sense of taste.
   - The eye refracts light for visual perception.
   - The ear is responsible for both sound and equilibrium.
6. **List and describe seven common signs and symptoms of eye disease and four signs of ear disorders.**
   - Refer to Box 17-2 for the eye and Box 17-4 for the ear.
7. **List six diagnostic tests and procedures for eye disease and four tests for ear disorders and explain the use of each.**
   - Refer to Box 17-3 for the eye and Box 17-4 for the ear.
8. **List 12 eye diseases and 7 ear disorders and describe the etiology, signs and symptoms, diagnosis, therapy, and interventions for each.**
   - Refer to Table 17-3 for eye diseases and Table 17-5 for ear diseases.
9. **Analyze a realistic medical office situation and apply your understanding of the sensory system to determine the best course of action.**
   - By understanding the sensory system, you are more prepared to understand patients' perceptions and tailor education to their ability to comprehend.
10. **Describe the impact on patient care when medical assistants have a solid understanding of the structure and function of the nervous system.**
    - With effective communication and a good understanding of sensory system physiology, the medical assistant can successfully encourage patients to follow their prescribed treatment plan.

PRACTICAL APPLICATIONS

If you have accomplished the objectives in this chapter, you will be able to make better choices as a medical assistant. Take another look at this situation and decide what you would do.

Bob DeMarce, age 42, complained of vertigo, tinnitus, and a sensation of fullness of the right ear for the last month. He states that each episode did not follow a certain event. He denies any ear pain, fever, headache, or nausea.

Past medical history includes a recent ear infection that was treated with amoxicillin for 10 days. On examination, Dr. Bailey finds that the tympanic membrane is dull and inflamed. It is decided that Mr. DeMarce has had otitis media that failed to resolve.

Do you understand what otitis media is, and how Mr. DeMarce's earlier treatment relates to it? The symptoms of Ménière disease, a disorder of the inner ear, mimic some of those present with otitis media.

1. How are otitis media and Ménière disease similar? How are they different?
2. Why were the vertigo, tinnitus, and a sensation of fullness over the past month important in making a diagnosis of otitis media?
3. What is Ménière disease, and what other symptoms does it present?
4. What type of diagnostic tests would be done to confirm a diagnosis of Ménière disease?
5. What would be the recommended lifestyle changes for Mr. DeMarce?

WEB SEARCH

1. **Research dry eye syndrome (DES).** DES is the most common eye disorder, affecting approximately 20% of the population. To understand DES better, a medical assistant needs to be aware of the various factors that contribute to DES and to understand the treatments that are available.
   - **Keywords:** Use the following keywords in your search: dry eye syndrome, DES.

2. **Research the many types of eye diseases that can be treated with laser surgery.** There are two different ways that ophthalmic lasers (thermal and photodisruptive lasers) are used to treat eye diseases.
   - **Keywords:** Use the following keywords in your search: Argon and krypton laser, YAG, ophthalmic laser.

WORD PARTS: Sensory System

SENSORY SYSTEM
Suffixes

-algesia	pain
-esthesia	sensation
-geusia	sense of taste
-osmia	sense of smell

VISION
Combining Forms

blephar/o	eyelid
chori/o, choroid/o	choroid
corne/o	cornea
cycl/o	ciliary body, ciliary muscle
dacry/o	tear; lacrimal apparatus
ir/o, irid/o	iris
kerat/o	cornea; horny tissue
lacrim/o	tear; lacrimal apparatus
lent/i	lens
ocul/o, ophthalm/o	eye
opt/o, optic	vision
phak/o, phac/o	lens
pupill/o	pupil
retin/o	retina
scler/o	sclera

Suffix

-opia	vision

HEARING
Combining Forms

audi/o	hearing
acous, acus	sound, hearing
cochle/o	cochlea
labyrinth/o	labyrinth
myring/o	tympanic membrane
ot/o	ear
staped/o, stapedi/o	stapes
tympan/o	tympanic membrane
vestibul/o	vestibule

Suffixes

-acusis	hearing
-otia	ear condition

ABBREVIATIONS: Nervous System

EYE AND VISION

OD*	*oculus dexter;* right eye
OS*	*oculus sinister;* left eye
OU*	*oculus uterque;* both eyes

EAR AND HEARING

AD*	*auris dextra;* right ear
AS*	*auris sinister;* left ear
AU*	*auris uterque;* both ears
ENT	ear, nose, throat
EENT	eyes, ears, nose, throat

*Not recommended for current charting but will appear when reviewing medical records prior to 2004.

18 Skeletal System

evolve http://evolve.elsevier.com/klieger/medicalassisting

The skeletal system is more than a group of bones. Our skeleton interconnects with other body systems to make us "whole." As a medical assistant, you need to understand the structure and function of the skeletal system to distinguish between proper and improper functioning. In addition, knowing skeletal system function enriches your understanding of the way all body systems work together to keep us in homeostasis; for example, the skeletal system functions closely with the muscular system to provide support for the body. To understand this system fully, you need to know about the formation of bone and cartilage, the axial and appendicular divisions of the skeleton, the structure and function of joints, and the diseases and disorders that affect the skeletal system.

LEARNING OBJECTIVES

You will be able to do the following after completing this chapter:

Key Terms
1. Define, appropriately use, and spell all the Key Terms for this chapter.

Skeletal System Function
2. List the five major functions of the skeletal system.
3. Describe how bone tissue is formed.
4. Explain how bones grow.
5. Describe the basic structure of bones.
6. List the four types of bone shapes and give an example of each.
7. Explain how bones repair themselves.

Axial and Appendicular Skeleton
8. Differentiate between the axial and the appendicular divisions of the skeleton.
9. Name and locate the bones of the skull.
10. Name the divisions of the spinal column and indicate the number of bones in each division.
11. Locate the sternum and describe how the ribs join to it.
12. List the three types of upper extremity bones.
13. List the bones of the lower extremities.

Articulations
14. Describe three types of joints.
15. List the three parts of a movable joint and describe the function of each part.
16. Name and describe the six types of movable joints.
17. Describe the structure and function of a ligament and a tendon.
18. Describe the four main types of movement.

Diseases and Disorders of the Skeletal System
19. List and describe the four types of signs and symptoms of skeletal disease.
20. List nine types of diagnostic tests and procedures for the skeletal system and describe the use of each.
21. List four types of injury to the bones and joints and briefly describe the etiology, signs and symptoms, diagnosis, therapy, and interventions for each.
22. List two types of bone infection and briefly describe the etiology, signs and symptoms, diagnosis, therapy, and interventions for each.
23. List two bone deficiency diseases and briefly describe the etiology, signs and symptoms, diagnosis, therapy, and interventions for each.
24. List five other bone diseases and briefly describe the etiology, signs and symptoms, diagnosis, therapy, and interventions for each.
25. List two bone neoplasms and briefly describe the etiology, signs and symptoms, diagnosis, therapy, and interventions for each.
26. List three joint diseases and briefly describe the etiology, signs and symptoms, diagnosis, therapy, and interventions for each.
27. List two congenital disorders of the skeletal system and briefly describe the etiology, signs and symptoms, diagnosis, therapy, and interventions for each.

Patient-Centered Professionalism

28. Analyze a realistic medical office situation and apply your understanding of the skeletal system to determine the best course of action.
29. Describe the impact on patient care when medical assistants have a solid understanding of the structure and function of the skeletal system.

KEY TERMS

The Key Terms for this chapter have been organized into sections so that you can easily see the terminology associated with each aspect of the skeletal system.

Function of the Skeletal System

cartilage	parathyroid hormone (PTH)
hematopoiesis	skeletal system
joint	stem cells

Bone and Cartilage

Bone Cells

Achilles tendon	osteoblasts
collagen	osteoclasts
medullary cavity	osteocytes

Bone Development

epiphyseal plate (growth plate)	ossification

Bone Structure

bone marrow	foramen
bone matrix	haversian system
compact bone	hyaline cartilage
elastic cartilage	lamellae
fibrous cartilage	sinus

Bone Types

Long Bones

cancellous bone	long bones
diaphysis	metaphysis
epiphysis	periosteum

Short, Flat, and Irregular Bones

flat bones	short bones
irregular bones	

Axial Skeleton

axial skeleton	hyoid bone
cranium	trunk

Skull

articulate	occipital bone
auditory meatus	paranasal sinuses
ethmoid bone	parietal bones
fontanels	pituitary gland
foramen magnum	sella turcica
foramina	sphenoid bone
frontal bone	sutures
frontal sinuses	temporal bones
maxillary sinus	

Facial Bones

hard palate	nasal conchae
lacrimal bones	palatine bones
mandible	vomer bone
maxillae	zygomatic bones
nasal bones	

Spinal Column

atlas	spinous process
axis	thoracic vertebrae
cervical vertebrae	thorax
coccyx	vertebra
lumbar vertebrae	vertebral column
sacrum	

Ribs

body	ribs
costal cartilage	sternum
false ribs	true ribs
floating ribs	xiphoid process
manubrium	

Appendicular Skeleton

appendicular skeleton

Upper Extremities

Shoulder

acromion process	process
clavicles	scapulae
pectoral girdle	

Upper Arm

humerus	olecranon process

Lower Arm

radius	ulna

Wrist

carpals	wrist

Hand

metacarpal	phalanges

Lower Extremities

Pelvic Girdle

acetabulum	ischium
erect	pelvic girdle
ilium	pubis

Femur and Patella

condyles	patella
femur	trochanters
head	

Lower Leg

fibula	tibia

Ankle

calcaneus	navicular
cuboid	talus
cuneiform	tarsal

Continued

Lower Extremities—cont'd
Foot

longitudinal arch	transverse arch
metatarsals	

Articulations
articulations

Joint Structure and Function

amphiarthroses	ligaments
articular cartilage	pivot joints
ball-and-socket joints	saddle joints
bursa	synarthroses
condyloid joints	synovial cavity
diarthroses	synovial fluid
gliding joints	tendons
hinge joints	

Movement

abduction	flexion
adduction	inversion
circumduction	pronation
eversion	rotation
extension	supination

Diseases and Disorders of the Skeletal System
orthopedic

Signs and Symptoms

ostealgia	osteonecrosis
osteitis	

Diagnostic Tests and Procedures

arthrography	myelogram
arthroscopy	radiography
bone density testing (BDT)	rheumatoid factor (RF) test
bone scan	serum calcium (Ca)
computed tomography (CT)	

Bone and Joint Injuries

closed reduction	open reduction
comminuted fracture	reduction
compound fracture	simple fracture
dislocation	spiral fracture
fractures	sprain
greenstick fracture	strain
impacted fracture	subluxation

Bone Infections

debrided	tuberculosis
osteomyelitis	

Bone Deficiencies

osteomalacia	rickets

Miscellaneous Bone Diseases

kyphosis	Paget disease
lordosis	scoliosis
osteoporosis	

Bone Neoplasms

carcinomas	osteomas
metastasized	sarcomas

Joint Diseases

ankylosis	gouty arthritis (gout)
arthritis	osteoarthritis
bursitis	rheumatoid arthritis (RA)
carpal tunnel syndrome	tophi
crepitation	

Related Skeletal Terms

ergonomic	palliative

Congenital Disorders

spina bifida	talipes

PRACTICAL APPLICATIONS

Read the following scenario and keep it in mind as you learn about the skeletal system in this chapter.

When she was 33 years old, Celia was injured in a skiing accident. She had a simple fracture of the distal end of the tibia and into the tarsals in her left leg. The fracture was located at the epiphyseal line. She also subluxated her knee in the same accident. The fracture was repaired with a closed reduction. After wearing a long leg cast for 8 weeks, an arthroscopy was performed on the knee to be sure the tendons and ligaments had not been torn or stretched because Celia was having difficulty bearing weight at that time. Before the arthroscopy, an arthrogram was performed on the knee and was negative; the arthroscopy was also negative. Over time, Celia seemed to recover from the fracture and had no problems until recently.

Celia is now 50 years old and has pain in her left ankle attributed to arthritis. She has also been diagnosed with early osteoporosis based on results of a bone density scan. The physician ordered analgesics for arthralgia and vitamin D and calcium supplements for osteoporosis. While talking with Steve, the medical assistant, Celia expresses concern that the osteoporosis and arthritis will only progress as she ages. She also has questions about some of the medical terms the physician used in speaking with her.

If you were in Steve's place, would you be prepared to discuss Celia's concerns and answer her questions?

FUNCTION OF THE SKELETAL SYSTEM

The **skeletal system** is the bony framework of the body and is made up of 206 bones with cartilage and other connective tissue to support bones. Bone is a combination of both living tissues, such as bone cells and blood cells and nonliving substances, including water and minerals. **Cartilage** is a nonvascular connective tissue that bends but does not break. Cartilage is located between most bones and also gives shape to some parts of the body (e.g., nose, ears).

The bones within the skeletal system perform five major functions. Each one is important for maintaining homeostasis and for optimal body function.

1. *Support.* The skeleton supports body structures and provides shape to the body.
2. *Protection.* The internal organs of the body are soft, and the skeleton provides protection against external trauma. The skull protects the brain, and the sternum and rib cage protect the heart and lungs.
3. *Movement.* The skeleton allows the muscles to move. Muscles are attached to the skeleton, and when they contract, movement occurs. Without this attachment, the muscles would be motionless. Bones serve as levers, which allow the weight of the muscle to move and function. When bones meet, they form a **joint.** A joint may be movable, slightly movable, or immovable.
4. *Mineral storage.* Bones serve as a place for the storage and release of minerals (e.g., calcium, phosphorus). As blood is filtered in the kidneys, phosphates are excreted in the urine and the calcium is retained. Homeostasis of blood calcium levels depends on the ability of calcium to move between blood and the bones. When calcium levels in the blood increase above normal, calcium is deposited in the bones. When the concentration decreases, calcium is withdrawn from bones and enters the blood. Proper levels of calcium in the bloodstream are maintained in the blood by the **parathyroid hormone (PTH)** and calcitonin produced by the thyroid gland. Low levels of calcium in the blood lead to irregular blood clotting, muscle spasms, and lack of essential nutrient absorption and can affect the digestive process.
5. *Blood formation.* Red marrow is found in the ends of most long bones and is responsible for the manufacture of blood cells. Do you remember from Chapter 13 how blood is formed? The red bone marrow produces **stem cells,** from which all blood cells are formed. The red blood cells carry oxygen, the white blood cells protect against infection, and the platelets are used in clotting. This process of blood cell formation is called **hematopoiesis,** which is a process within the skeletal system.

Together, bones, joints, and connective tissue form the basic framework of the body. Before learning the names of bones, it is important to understand their formation, development, and structure.

PATIENT-CENTERED PROFESSIONALISM

- *Why is it important for the medical assistant to understand the basic function of the skeletal system?*

BONE AND CARTILAGE

Bone and cartilage begin to form in early fetal development. Bone cells develop and form the different types of bones in the skeletal system. These cells continue to be active, and bone development and repair occur throughout the life span.

Bone Cells

In early fetal development, either cartilage or membranous tissue forms where the bones will eventually be. The long bones develop from cartilage and the flat and other bones from membranous tissue. Three main types of cells are involved in the formation of bone tissue: osteoblasts, osteoclasts, and osteocytes.

Osteoblasts are bone-building cells that develop in the bone's center with a network of blood vessels. Calcium and other minerals mix with the osteoblasts and fibers to create a strong protein substance called **collagen.** As a person grows, osteoblasts, found in the periosteum in layers of calcium, form on the outside of the bone. The osteoblasts stop synthesizing matrix and become embedded in the bone, at which point these cells become osteocytes.

Osteoclasts are bone-reabsorbing cells or bone-destroying cells that appear in the middle of bone. As these cells erode and hollow out the central cavity of a bone, a **medullary cavity** is formed. This cavity is where bone marrow is deposited in long bones (Figure 18-1, *A*).

Osteocytes are mature bone cells that are made up of organic and inorganic material and are found in the bone matrix. The organic material is jelly-like and allows the bones to be flexible; the inorganic material is mostly mineral salts of calcium and gives bone its hardness.

Bone Development

Bone formation, or **ossification** (calcification), begins about the eighth week of embryonic development, when cartilage is replaced with both osteoblasts and osteoclasts. For us to move effectively, our bones must be light. As the osteoblasts build new bone tissue, our bones grow and become heavier. The osteoclasts break down bone to make the hollow cavity larger as we grow so that the bones will still be strong but not too heavy. This activity permits bones to grow in length and diameter. Bone tissue formation and destruction continues throughout the life span. As a child develops, ossification occurs at a faster rate than bone reabsorption (resorption), but at about age 40 years, this process reverses and bone loss exceeds bone growth, leading to softening of bones and a greater chance for fractures.

Bone Structure

Bone tissue is a specialized form of dense connective tissue and is made up of osteocytes and collagen. The **bone matrix** is a mixture of collagen fibers and chemicals and is considered the cement that holds the bone together.

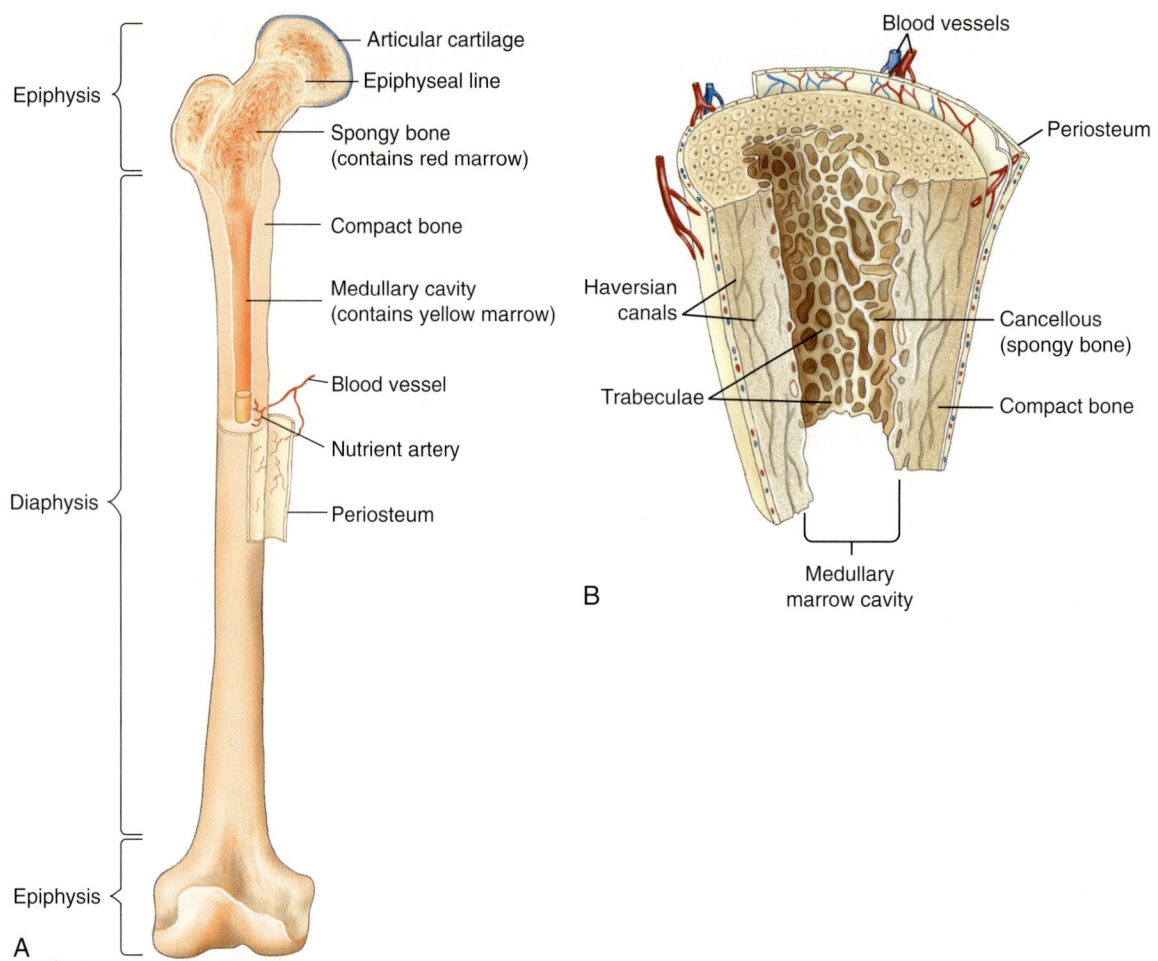

FIGURE 18-1 A typical long bone, partially sectioned. **A,** Major features of a long bone. Diaphysis is the long, main portion of a bone. Epiphyses are the knoblike ends of the bone. The outer part is compact, dense bone. The inner part is spongy and contains large spaces filled with bone marrow. **B,** Cross-section showing the haversian canals. (From Leonard PC: *Building a medical vocabulary*, ed 6, St Louis, 2005, Saunders.)

When various mineral salts (e.g., calcium, phosphorus) bind with the bone matrix, it becomes hardened (calcified). As bone begins to harden, it forms layers called **lamellae.** These structures are arranged in different patterns depending on bone type.

The bone receives its nutrition and has its waste removed through the **haversian system** (Figure 18-1, *B*). This structural unit has canals of veins, arteries, and lymph vessels that penetrate the bone matrix. The veins remove waste from the osteocytes, and the arteries transport nutrients to the bone.

Bone Marrow

There are two forms of **bone marrow** contained within the structure of bone: yellow and red. Both yellow and red marrow are made up of connective tissue and blood vessels.
- *Red marrow* is responsible for the manufacture of red and white blood cells.
- *Yellow marrow* is composed mostly of fat cells and produces some white blood cells.

Cartilage

Cartilage is connective tissue attached to bone and does not contain mineral salts. Therefore cartilage is more flexible. Its role in the skeletal system is to provide a smooth surface and cushioning between bones. Unlike bone, cartilage does not have blood vessels. The three forms of cartilage are hyaline, elastic, and fibrous.
- **Hyaline cartilage** covers the ends of bones and makes up structures such as the larynx, nose, and trachea.
- **Elastic cartilage** is very flexible and is constructed of elastic fibers. The outer ear is a good example of elastic cartilage.
- **Fibrous cartilage** connects bones to other bones at joints and serves as a protective cushion, as with the discs between the vertebrae in the spine.

Bone Surface Markings

Bones have markings (depressions or openings) that serve to provide a connection point for structures to make contact or

TABLE 18-1
Bone Surface Markings

Markings	Description	Example
Fossa	A depression or hollow space in a bone for attachments	Olecranon fossa (see Figure 18-10)
Foramen	Hole or opening in a bone through which blood vessels and nerves can pass	Foramen magnum (see Figure 18-6)
Sinus	Air-filled cavity in a bone	Frontal sinus of skull
Fissure	Narrow opening between parts of a bone that allows blood vessels or nerves to pass	Superior orbital fissure (see Figure 18-4, *A*)
Condyle	Large, rounded, knuckle-like prominence that forms a joint with another bone	Mandibular condyle (see Figure 18-4, *B*)
Tuberosity	Large, rounded, roughened process that attaches muscles and ligaments to the bone	Tibial tuberosity (see Figure 18-12)
Fontanel	Space between skull bones at birth filled with dense fibrous connective tissue	Anterior fontanel between frontal and parietal bones (see Figure 18-5)

a space through which blood vessels, ligaments, and nerves can pass (Table 18-1).

Bone Types

Bones are of different shapes and sizes depending on their location in the body and how they are used. Movement is determined by a bone's shape and joint structure. Bones are classified into four types according to their shape: long, short, flat, and irregular (Figure 18-2).

1. **Long bones** are found in the upper and lower extremities (arms and legs) and include the femur, fibula, tibia, humerus, radius, and ulna. Long bones of the lower extremities determine a person's height.
2. **Short bones** appear in the wrist (carpals) and ankle (tarsals).
3. **Flat bones** are found in the skull (e.g., frontal, parietal), ribs, and scapula.
4. **Irregular bones** make up the spinal column (vertebrae), the sphenoid and ethmoid bones of the skull, the sacrum, the coccyx, the patella (kneecap), and the mandible.

Long Bones

Long bones have compact bone tissue along the length of the bone for added strength and spongy bone at the ends for

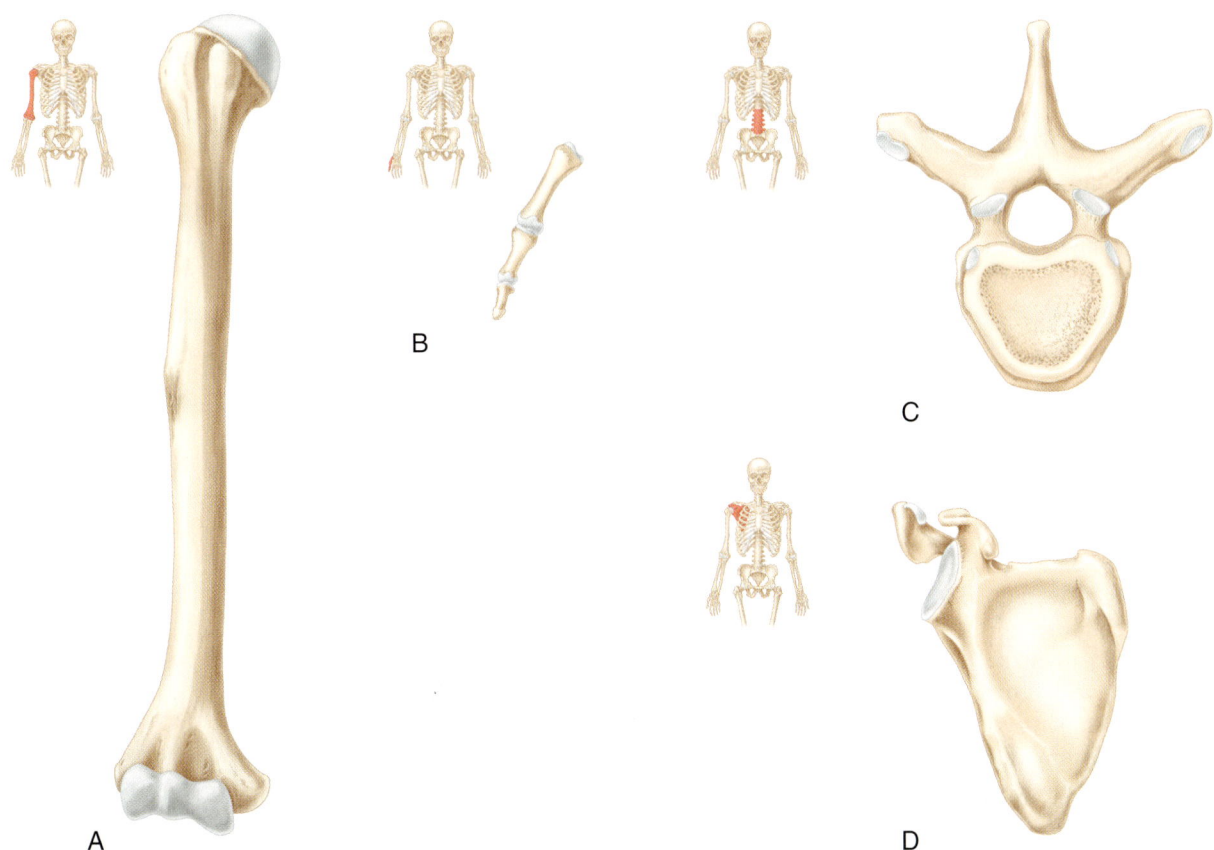

FIGURE 18-2 Examples of bone types include **(A)** long bones (humerus), **(B)** short bones (phalanx), **(C)** irregular bones (vertebra), and **(D)** flat bones (scapula). (From Thibodeau GA, Patton KT: *Anatomy and physiology*, ed 6, St Louis, 2007, Mosby.)

growth and flexibility (see Figure 18-1, *A*). The long bones are more complex in their structure than the other three bone types.

Long Bone Regions. A typical long bone has the following three distinct regions:

- **Diaphysis:** Main shaft (1) of the long bones.
- **Epiphysis:** Expanded ends (2) of long bones are filled with red bone marrow, which produces erythrocytes. The **epiphyseal plate** (layer of cartilage), or **growth plate,** is located where the epiphysis meets the metaphysis.
- **Metaphysis:** Flared ends (2) of long bones between the epiphyses and the diaphysis. During childhood, it grows, and around 18 to 25 years of age, it stops growing, and ossifies into solid bone.

Long Bone Structure. At one or both ends of a long bone, articular cartilage acts as a cushion to minimize wear and tear on the bone's end. **Cancellous** (spongy) **bone** tissue is attached to this cartilage and is the site for bone growth at the epiphysis (epiphyseal plate). These growth centers disappear as a child matures and appear as thin lines on x-rays. The bone matrix forms compact bone, which provides strength along the shaft of the bone. The shaft is filled with yellow marrow, which produces white blood cells and stores fat, and the cancellous bone contains red marrow for red and white blood cell production. The **periosteum** (covering on bone's outer surface) follows the bone pattern to each end. Muscles and tendons intertwine with fibers of the periosteum and anchor muscles, tendons, and ligaments to the bone. The periosteum provides the bone with the necessary nutrition to continue functioning as living tissue.

Short, Flat, and Irregular Bones

The short, flat, and irregular bones have spongy (cancellous) bone in the center and dense bone, or **compact bone,** on the outside. As in long bones, the spongy bone of the skull, ribs, and sternum are filled with red marrow.

Bone Repair

Bones are extremely strong, but with enough force, they can be broken (fractured). Inactive osteoblasts located under the periosteum are activated to repair bone after an injury.

As we age, osteoclasts are more active than osteoblasts. This causes the bones to be brittle because the central bone core is enlarging, but the outer surface of bone is not forming. Proper nutrition is especially important in maintaining bone density and health, as follows:

- Proper calcium intake (e.g., green leafy vegetables, dairy foods) is a requirement for proper ossification to take place in both bone growth and bone repair.
- Vitamin D allows calcium to be absorbed in the bloodstream and then deposited in the bones. It also acts as a stimulant to the osteoblasts to form new bone. Fresh vegetables and fish oils are a good source of vitamin D, but the best source is sunshine. As the sun's rays come in contact with the skin, the body forms vitamin D.

> **PATIENT-CENTERED PROFESSIONALISM**
>
> - Why is it important for the medical assistant to understand bone formation?
> - How does aging affect the body's ability to repair bones?

AXIAL AND APPENDICULAR SKELETON

The skeletal system is divided into two groups: the axial skeleton, comprising the bones of the head and **trunk,** and the appendicular skeleton, or bones of the upper and lower extremities and the girdles that attach these bones (Figure 18-3 and Box 18-1).

Axial Skeleton

The **axial skeleton** comprises the bones of the skull (cranium, facial bones, and bones of the ear), the spinal column, the ribs, the sternum, and the **hyoid bone.** The tongue is attached to the hyoid bone, which is located in the neck.

Skull

Twenty-two irregularly shaped bones form the skull. The **cranium** is actually a fusion of eight cranial bones with the vital function of protecting the brain and the remaining 14 are facial bones. Within the skull's framework are large spaces or cavities called **paranasal sinuses.** These air-filled spaces are lined with a mucous membrane (see Chapter 14). Sinuses serve to lighten the skull and they warm and moisten air entering the body.

Cranium. The cranial bones protect the brain from injury (Figure 18-4). The floor of the cranium provides a place for the brain to rest. In the adult cranium, these flat bones are

---

BOX 18-1

Bones of the Axial and Appendicular Skeleton

AXIAL SKELETON

Skull	
—Cranium	8
—Facial	14
—Ear	6
Hyoid	1
Spinal column	26
Sternum and ribs	25
SUBTOTAL	80

APPENDICULAR SKELETON

Upper extremities (shoulders, arms, hands)	64
Lower extremities (pelvis, legs, feet)	62
SUBTOTAL	126
TOTAL BONES	206

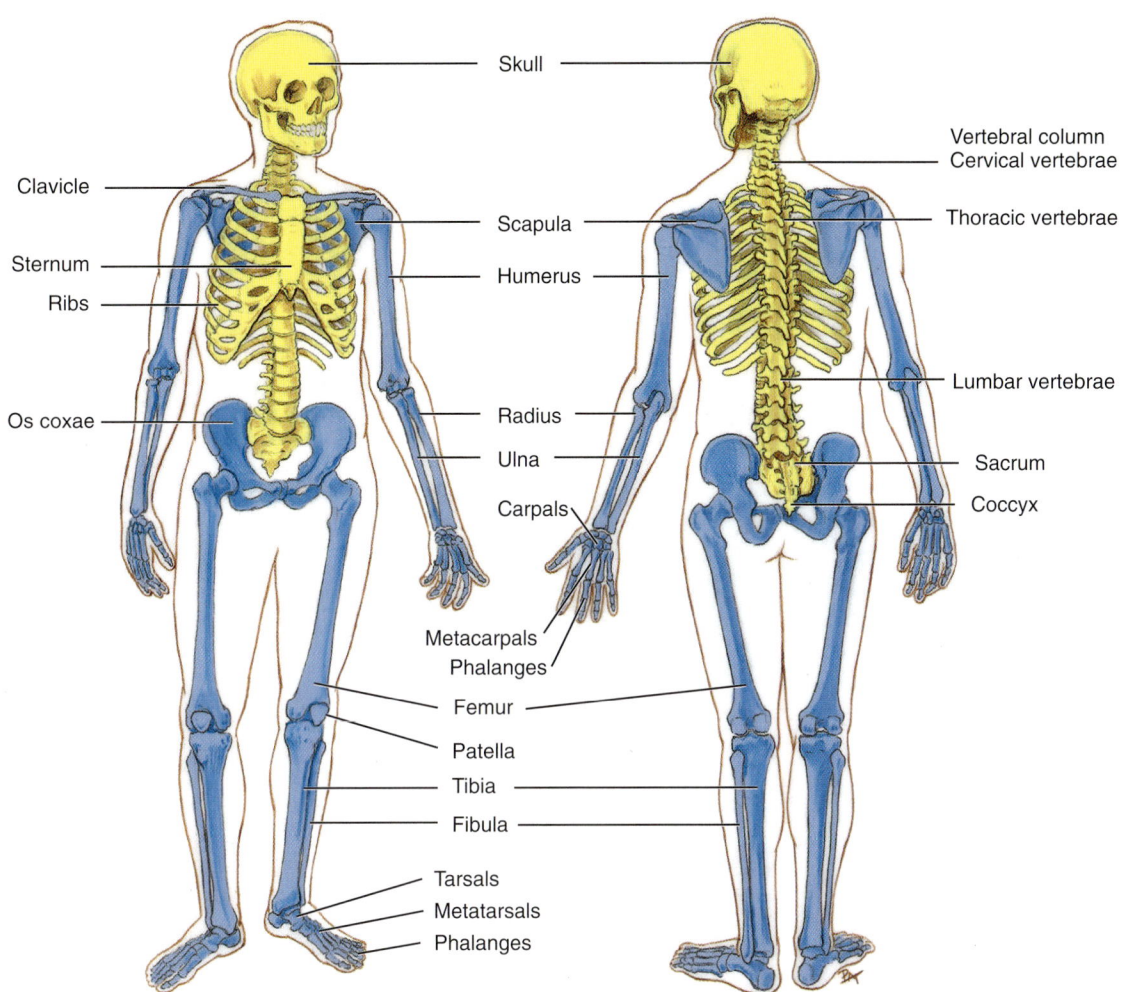

FIGURE 18-3 Divisions of the skeleton with major bones identified. Yellow = axial skeleton. Blue = appendicular skeleton. (From Applegate EJ: *The anatomy and physiology learning system*, ed 3, St Louis, 2006, Saunders.)

joined together (**articulate**) to form immovable joints called **sutures.** The cranial bones of an infant are not ossified or joined together completely at birth, allowing for the skull to be compressed during the birth process. **Fontanels,** or *soft spots,* are located between the cranial bones and close by ossification at about 18 months of age (Figure 18-5).

The frontal bone forms the front of the cranium, and the left and right parietal bones form the upper sides and top of the skull. The occipital bones form the back of the skull, and the temporal bones (left and right) form the lower sides of the skull. The ethmoid and sphenoid bones add to the floor of the cranium and support the nasal cavity and eye orbit areas.

- The **frontal bone** forms the forehead and extends from the top of the eye orbits (sockets) to the top of the head, where it joins the parietal bones. Located in the space above the eye sockets are the **frontal sinuses.** These air-filled spaces are lined with a mucous membrane.
- The two **parietal bones** give shape to the top of the cranium and extend to the sides. They articulate with other cranial bones (occipital, temporal, frontal, and some of sphenoid). These bones form the top and sides of the cranium.
- The **occipital bone** forms the back part of the cranial floor and is the covering for the back portion of the brain. This bone has a large opening (**foramen magnum**) in its base where the spinal column joins the skull. All throughout the cranial bones are smaller openings (**foramina**) through which the cranial nerves and blood vessels can pass.
- The **temporal bones** come together on each side of the cranium at the parietal area. This area contains the middle and inner ear structures. The **auditory meatus** (opening of the ear) is in the temporal bone.
- The **sphenoid bone** and **ethmoid bone** are located behind the nose and eye sockets. The sphenoid bone is the middle portion of the cranial floor. When looking down on the cranial floor, the sphenoid bone resembles a bat with outstretched wings; it serves to hold the cranial bones in place. Within the upper portion of the sphenoid bone is a bony projection called the **sella turcica** that houses the **pituitary gland** (Figure 18-6). The ethmoid

330 SECTION III Anatomy and Physiology

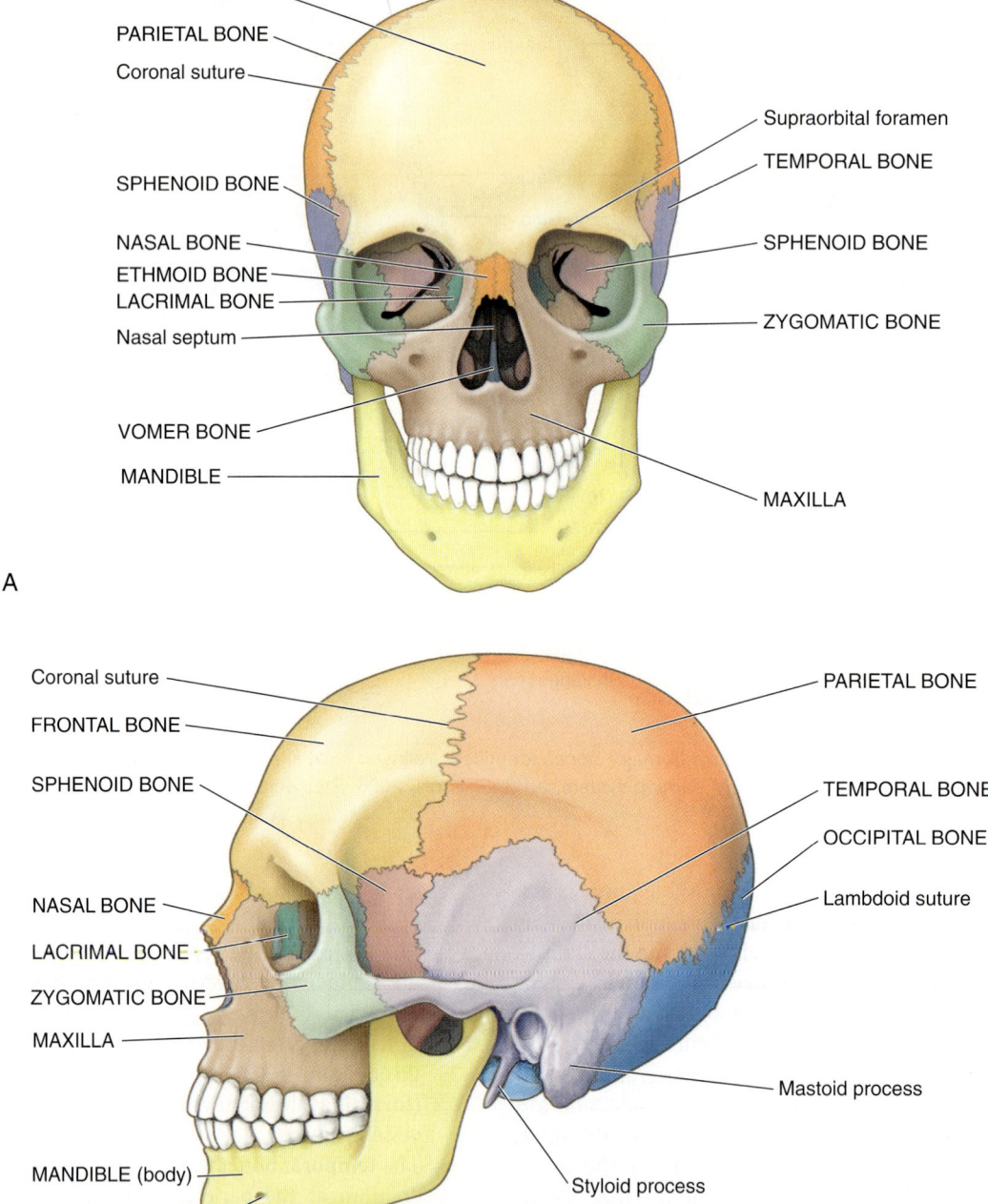

FIGURE 18-4 **A,** Anterior view of skull. **B,** Lateral view of skull. (Modified from Applegate EJ: *The anatomy and physiology learning system,* ed 3, St Louis, 2006, Saunders.)

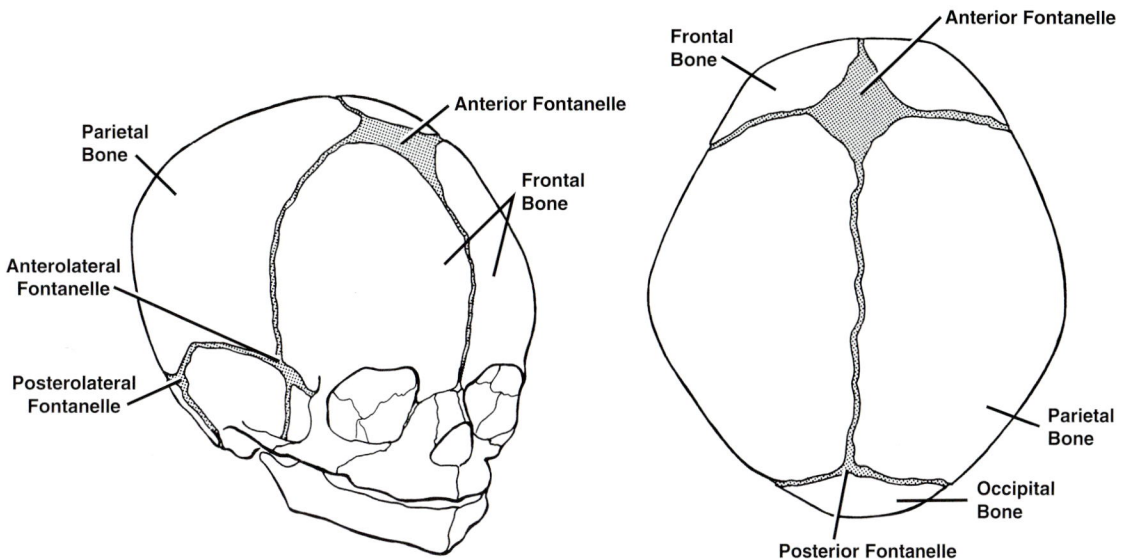

FIGURE 18-5 Fontanels (or fontanelles) in infant skull. Two largest fontanels are the anterior fontanel and posterior fontanel. (From Cummings C et al: *Cummings otolaryngology: head and neck surgery,* ed 4, Philadelphia, 2005, Mosby.)

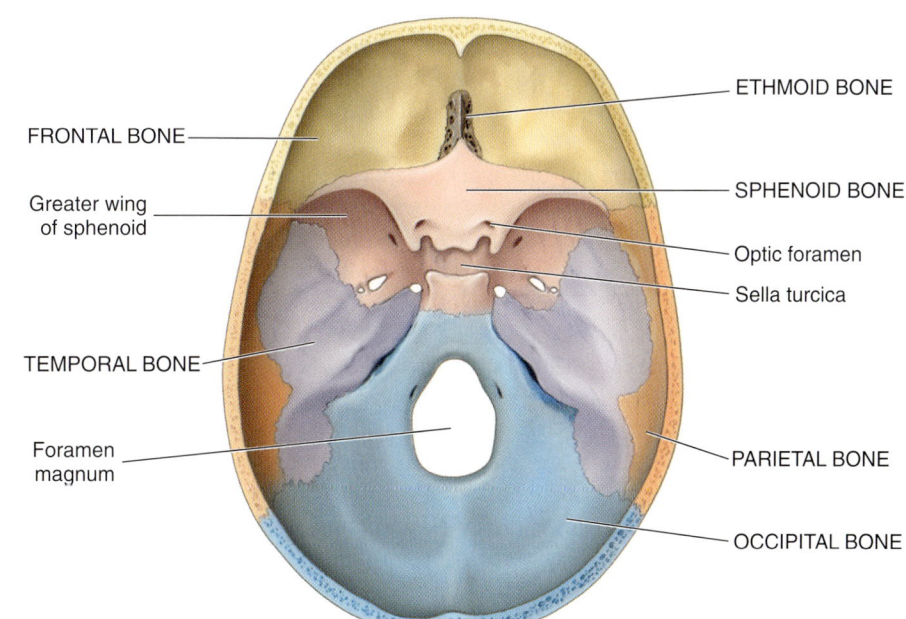

FIGURE 18-6 Cranial floor of skull as viewed from above. (Modified from Applegate EJ: *The anatomy and physiology learning system,* ed 3, St Louis, 2006, Saunders.)

bones form most of the bony area between the nasal cavity and the eye orbits.

Facial Bones and Surrounding Area. The facial bones are located in the anterior portion of the cranium (see Figure 18-4). These irregularly shaped bones protect the sense organs (e.g., eyes, nose) and give form to the face.

- The largest bone in the face is the **mandible** (lower jawbone). The mandible is movable and is used in chewing.
- The six smallest bones in the temporal area are found in the ear. The hammer (malleus), anvil (incus), and stirrup (stapes) are responsible for hearing (see Chapter 17).
- The mandible and the two **maxillae** (upper jawbones) join together to form the mouth. The maxillae are fused together to form the upper jaw and the **hard palate** (roof of the mouth). If this fusion does not take place normally during fetal development, a cleft palate results.
- Contained within each maxilla is a sinus cavity, the **maxillary sinus,** that comes together with the nasal cavity.
- The two **nasal bones** are located side by side and are attached to the maxillae to form the bridge of the nose.
- The **vomer bone** forms the lower wall between the nostrils, or nasal septum.

- The **zygomatic bones** (cheekbones) attach to the maxillae and form the lower portion of the eye orbits and the high portion of the cheekbones.
- The **lacrimal bones** are within the eye orbits and alongside the nose. These bones help form the walls of the nasal cavity and contain the tear ducts.
- The **palatine bones** are behind the hard palate and help form the walls of the nasal cavity and the floor of the eye orbits.
- The **nasal conchae** are above the roof of the mouth and the walls of the nasal cavities.

Because of their proximity to the face, the ethmoid bones with the 14 facial bones help to shape the face. Ligaments from the temporal bone and the mandible suspend the hyoid bone that is a movable base for the tongue and the attachment point for the neck muscles used during swallowing.

Spinal Column

The spinal column, or **vertebral column,** is a flexible, curved, segmented structure composed of vertebrae that are stacked on one another. The spinal column is a series of small bones that supports the head and provides attachments for the ribs. It also encases and protects the spinal cord.

The bones of the spinal column are named according to their location and are numbered from the top, proceeding downward. The five major divisions of the spinal column are as follows:

1. The **cervical vertebrae** are the upper seven vertebrae located in the neck. The first vertebra is the **atlas,** which supports the head. The occipital bone fits into the atlas and allows the head to nod. The second cervical vertebra is the **axis,** which serves as a pivot when the head turns from side to side (Figure 18-7).
2. The next 12 vertebrae are the **thoracic vertebrae,** located in the **thorax** (chest). The posterior portion of each of the 12 rib pairs is attached to these vertebrae.
3. The next five vertebrae are the **lumbar vertebrae,** located in the lower portion of the back. These vertebrae support the weight of the entire body and thus are heavier and larger than other vertebrae.
4. The **sacrum** begins as five separate vertebrae and eventually fuses together to form a wedge-shaped bone located between the two hipbones.
5. The **coccyx,** or tailbone, is the lowest part of the spine. The four coccygeal bones fuse together as one bone in the adult.

Vertebrae. Each **vertebra** has an opening (foramen) in the center that allows the spinal cord to pass through, and protects it at the same time. Adults have 26 vertebrae, and children have 33 vertebrae. In children, the five bones of the sacrum and the four bones of the coccyx fuse together to form one bone each in the adult (Figure 18-8). Ligaments that allow movement forward, backward, and sideways join each vertebra to one another. Discs of cartilage called *intervertebral discs* separate the vertebrae from one another. These discs act as shock absorbers to cushion and protect the vertebrae. Toward the front of each vertebra, except the first two, is a weight-bearing, drum-shaped structure called the **spinous process** (see Figure 18-7). The projections (processes) toward the body serve as attachment sites for the ribs.

Sternum and Ribs

The thoracic vertebrae, sternum, and ribs support the chest (thorax) area. The bones of the thorax serve to protect the heart, lungs, and other vital organs (Figure 18-9).

Sternum. The **sternum** (breastbone) is divided into the following three parts:
- Manubrium (upper portion)
- Body (middle portion)
- Xiphoid process (lower tip)

The **manubrium** joins with the clavicle (collarbone) and the first rib. The next nine ribs are attached to the **body** of the sternum by cartilage. The **xiphoid process** forms an attachment for the diaphragm and abdominal muscles.

Ribs. There are 12 pairs of **ribs.** All ribs are attached to the spinal column posteriorly but not all attach to the sternum. The first seven pairs attach to the sternum directly by **costal cartilage;** these ribs are known as **true ribs.** The next three pairs are referred to as **false ribs** because they are connected indirectly to the sternum (costal cartilage is attached to the seventh rib and not directly to the sternum). The remaining two pairs are called **floating ribs** because they are attached only to the vertebrae and not to the sternum.

Appendicular Skeleton

The **appendicular skeleton** includes bones of the upper extremities (shoulders, arms, wrists, and hands) and bones of the lower extremities (hips, legs, knees, ankles, and feet).

Upper Extremity

The upper extremity bones include the **pectoral girdle** (shoulder), upper and lower arm, wrist, and hand.

Shoulder. The shoulder girdle consists of two **clavicles** (collarbones) and two **scapulae** (shoulder blades). The bones of the shoulder girdle attach the arms to the axial skeleton. The clavicles are long bones situated in the front of the body and are above the first pair of ribs. The pectoral girdle does not attach to the vertebrae. One end of the clavicle is joined to the top of the sternum, and the other end attaches to the scapula. The clavicle and the sternum join together at the sternoclavicular joint (Figure 18-10).

The scapula is a flat, triangular-shaped bone. Where the clavicle and the scapula come together is not considered a joint but a **process** (projection on a bone). The **acromion process** is where the lateral ridge of the scapula and the clavicle join and is a site for muscle attachment.

Upper Arm. The upper arm bone is called the **humerus** and is the largest long bone in the upper extremity. The humerus fits into the shoulder and forms a joint with the scapula and with the bones of the forearm. The humerus joins the bones of the elbow at the **olecranon process** (commonly called the "funny bone"). When this area is hit, a pronounced unpleasant ("funny") sensation is felt because the ulnar nerve is stimulated.

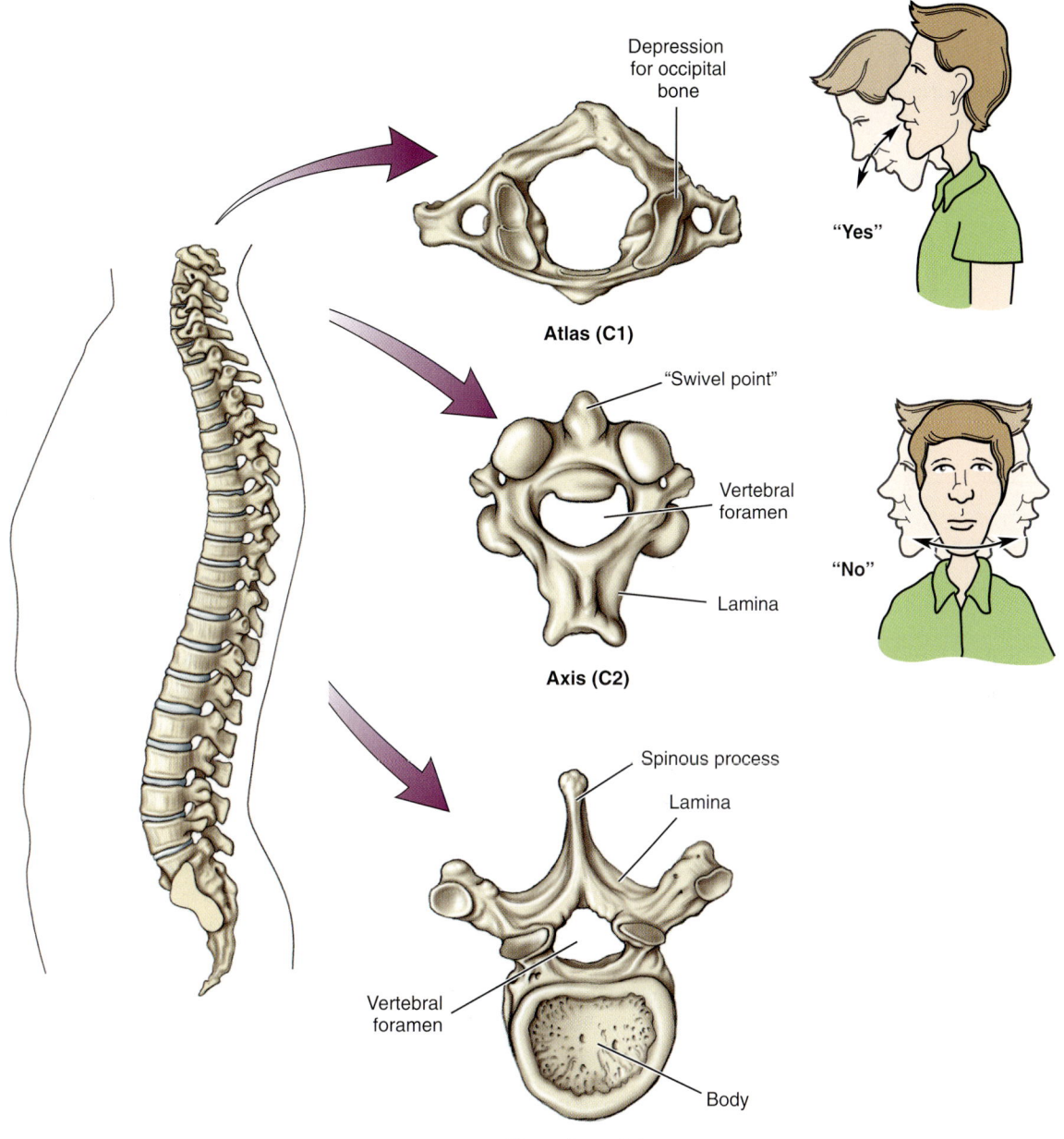

FIGURE 18-7 Structure of a vertebra: atlas (C1), axis (C2), and thoracic vertebrae. (From Herlihy B, Maebius NK: *The human body in health and illness,* ed 3, St Louis, 2007, Saunders.)

Lower Arm. The forearm consists of the **radius** and the **ulna**. The radius lies on the thumb side (medial) and the ulna on the side by the little finger (lateral).

Wrist. The **wrist** has eight small bones called **carpals** (including scaphoid, lunate, triquetrum, pisiform, trapezium, trapezoid, capitate, and hamate). These bones are arranged in two rows of four each and are bound together by ligaments to allow movement.

Hand. The **metacarpal** bones form the hand. The distal ends of these bones form the "knuckles" (metacarpophalangeal [MP] joint). These bones articulate with the **phalanges** or bones of the finger. The thumb only has a distal and a proximal phalanx, whereas the other fingers have three phalanges, including a middle phalanx.

Lower Extremity

The lower extremity includes the bones of the pelvic girdle (hipbone), femur (thigh), patella (kneecap), tibia and fibula (lower leg), tarsal (ankle), and foot (metatarsals and phalanges).

Pelvic Girdle. The **pelvic girdle** brings together the two hipbones and the sacrum and coccyx. The lower extremity is attached to the axial skeleton by the pelvic bones. The pelvic bones include the **ilium** (upper portion), **ischium** (lowest portion), and **pubis** (joins the hipbones together) in adulthood. The bones of the pelvic girdle support the legs when the body is **erect** (upright) and protect the lower abdominal organs and the female reproductive organs. The hipbones

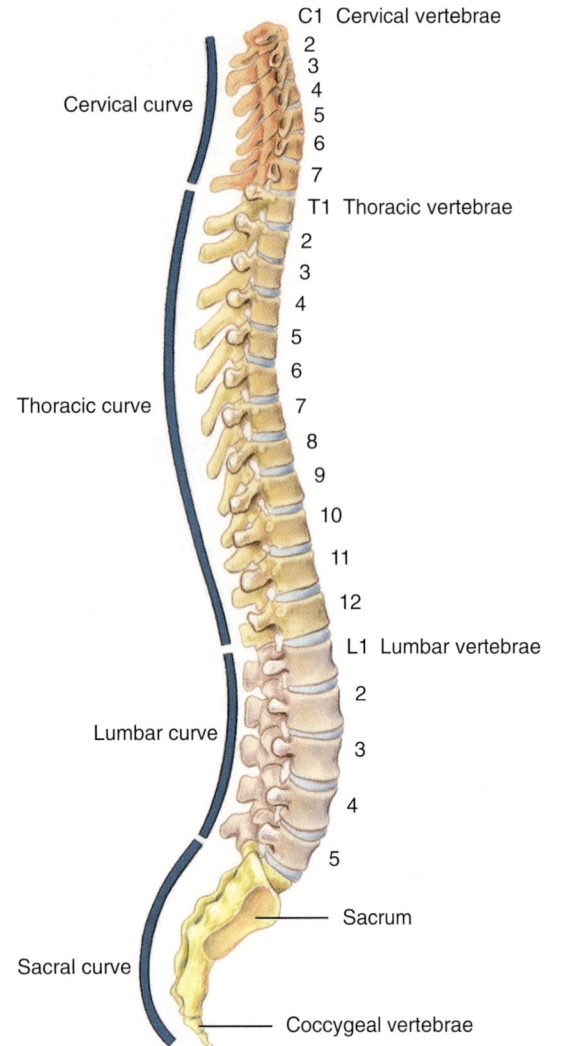

FIGURE 18-8 Vertebral column. (From Applegate EJ: *The anatomy and physiology learning system*, ed 3, St Louis, 2006, Saunders.)

form the **acetabulum,** a socket where the femur joins the pelvic girdle (Figure 18-11).

Femur. The **femur** (thighbone) is the longest and strongest bone in the body. The **head** (rounded projection) of the femur joins the pelvic bones at the acetabulum and forms a ball-and-socket joint similar to that in the shoulder. There are two bulges below the head of the femur called the greater and lesser **trochanters** that serve as attachments for muscles. At the distal end of the femur are two small bulges called the lateral and medial **condyles,** projections that fit into a bone and form a joint. The condyles of the femur join with the condyles on the tibia to form the knee joint.

Patella. The **patella** (kneecap) is an irregularly shaped bone positioned in front of the knee joint to protect this joint (Figure 18-12).

Lower Leg. The lower leg bones are the tibia and the fibula. The **tibia** is larger and stronger than the fibula and is located in the center of the lower leg. Proximally the tibia joins the femur behind the patella, and distally it joins the fibula and anklebone. Because it is situated at the front of the lower leg, the tibia is referred to as the "shinbone." The **fibula** is smaller and positioned more laterally. The distal portion of the fibula helps to form the ankle joint (see Figure 18-12). The fibula gives stability to the long bones of the leg to keep the body upright and stable.

Ankle. The seven **tarsal** bones (anklebones) include the **talus, calcaneus** (heel bone), **navicular, cuboid,** and three **cuneiform** bones.

Foot. The **metatarsals** are the long bones of the foot and are numbered from one to five, starting with number one on the medial side. The phalanges (toes) are similar to the fingers. There are three phalanges in each toe, except the "big" or great toe, which has only two phalanges, like the thumb.

The feet must endure the entire weight of the body and therefore must have good support. There are two arches on

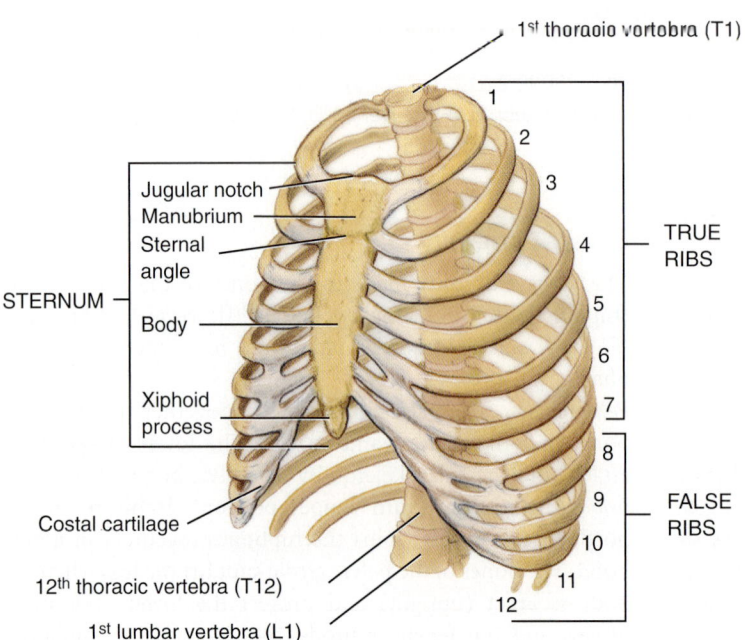

FIGURE 18-9 Thoracic cage. (From Applegate EJ: *The anatomy and physiology learning system*, ed 3, St Louis, 2006, Saunders.)

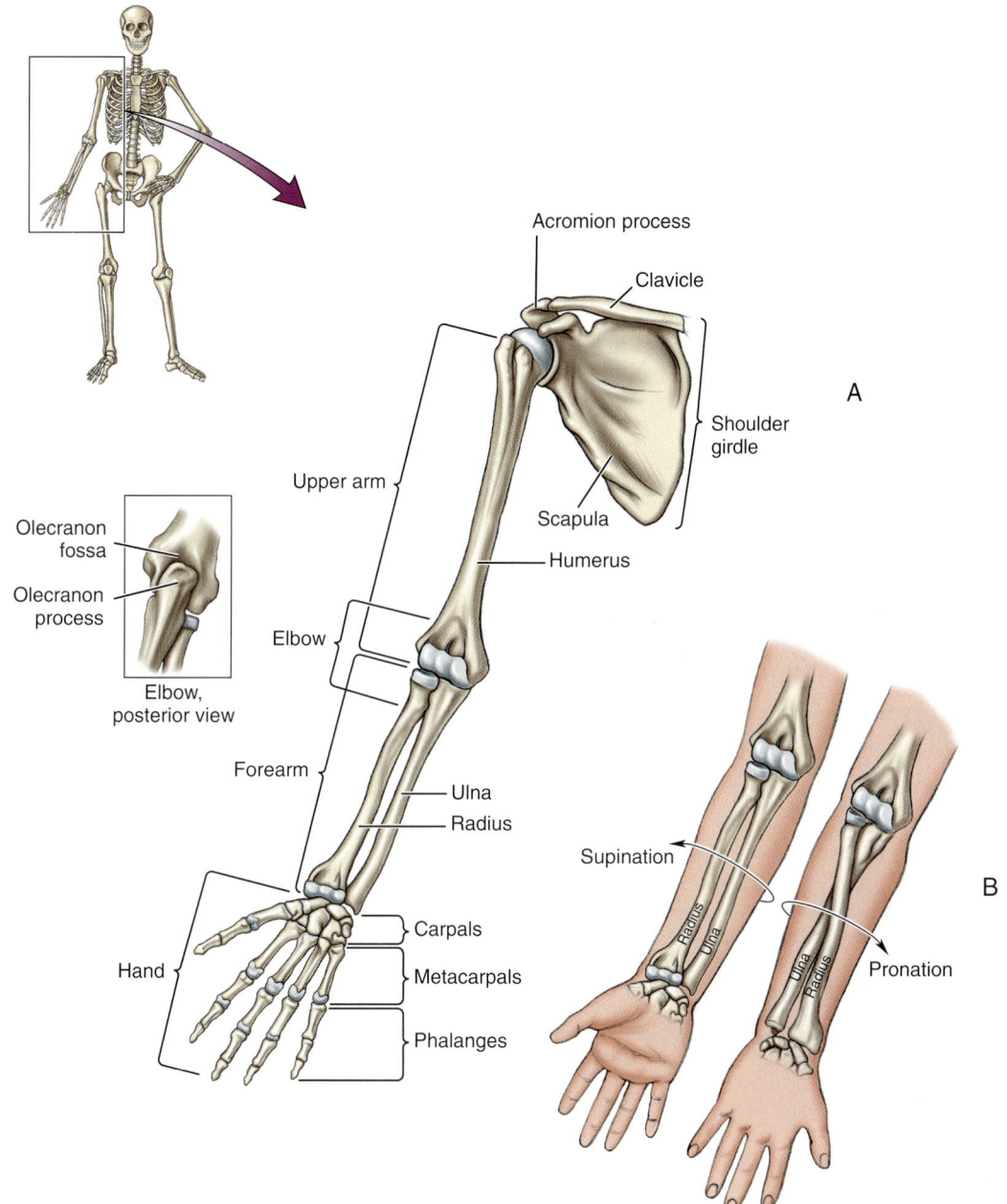

FIGURE 18-10 Bones of the upper limb. **A,** Shoulder girdle, upper arm, lower arm (forearm), and hand. **B,** Position of radius and ulna during supination and pronation. (From Herlihy B, Maebius NK: *The human body in health and illness,* ed 3, St Louis, 2007, Saunders.)

each foot that assist in adding the needed strength to support a person's body weight. The first is the **longitudinal arch,** which stretches from the calcaneus bone to the phalanges. The second arch goes from side to side or across the foot and is the **transverse arch** (Figure 18-13).

PATIENT-CENTERED PROFESSIONALISM

- *How would the medical assistant explain the difference between the two major divisions of the skeletal system to a patient?*

ARTICULATIONS

Articulations are joints where two or more bones come together. Articulations allow for body movement. You need to understand the structure and function of joints and how movement occurs.

Joint Structure and Function

To understand the different types of joints, it is best to classify them by how much movement the joint allows. There are three types of joints: the synarthrosis (no movement),

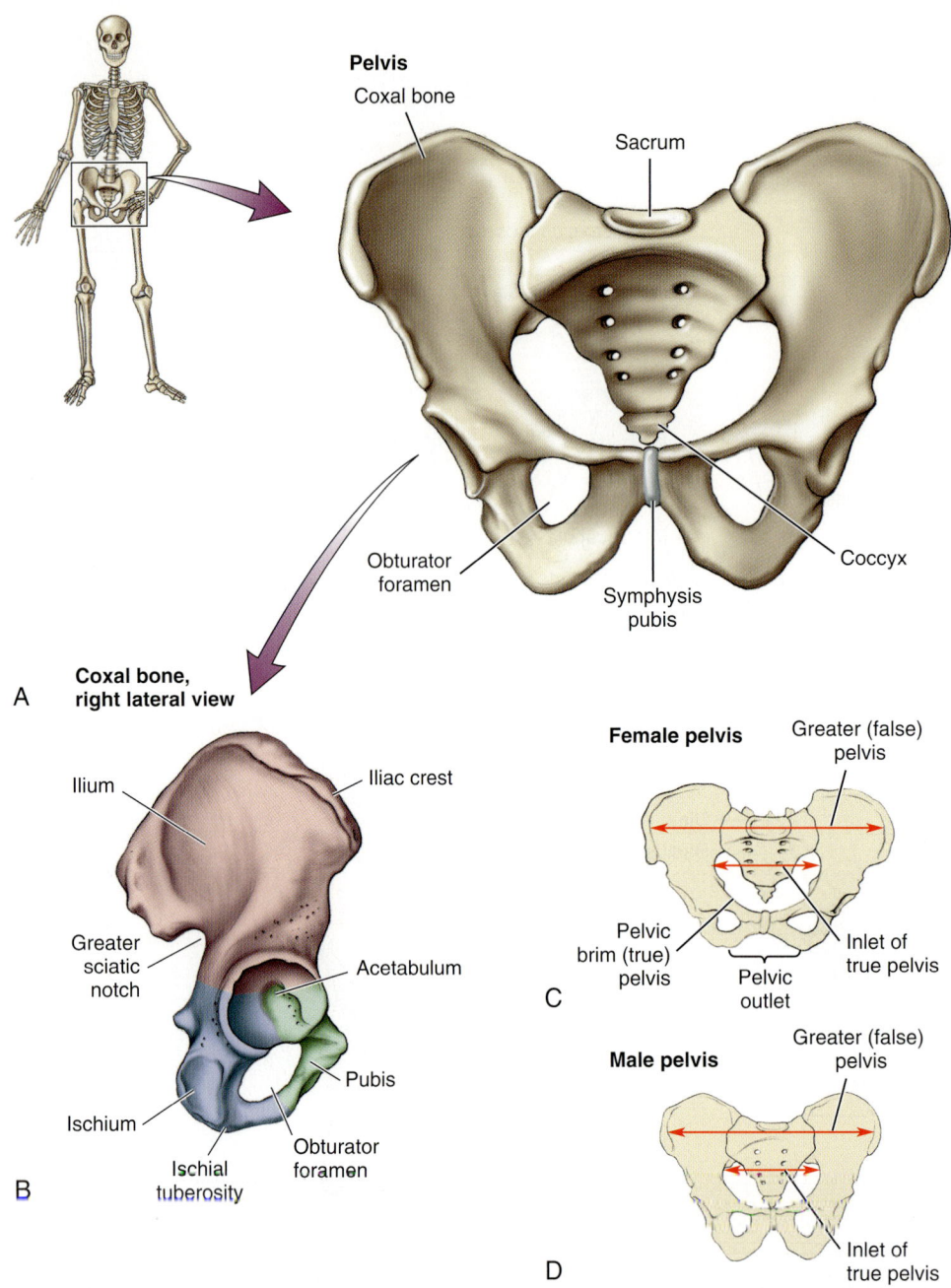

FIGURE 18-11 **A**, Bones making up the pelvic cavity. **B**, Coxal bone (ilium, ischium, and pubis). **C**, Female pelvis. **D**, Male pelvis. (From Herlihy B, Maebius NK: *The human body in health and illness,* ed 3, St Louis, 2007, Saunders.)

amphiarthrosis (slight movement), and diarthrosis (free movement).
- **Synarthroses** have a thin layer of dense fibrous connective tissue that unites the skull bones. The joints between the cranial bones, the sutures, are an example of a joint with no movement.
- **Amphiarthroses** are connected by cartilage, a strong tissue that only allows for slight movement. The symphysis pubis and the intervertebral discs between the vertebrae are good examples of a slightly movable joint.
- Most articulations in the body are **diarthroses,** meaning freely movable, such as the hip or shoulder joint.

Movable Joints

To understand movable joints, you must know their components, the types of movable joints, and how connective tissues aid in joint movement.

Components

A movable joint has three important parts: articular cartilage, bursa (fluid-filled sac), and joint cavity (synovial).
- **Articular cartilage** is a slippery type of cartilage that covers the surfaces of two bones that come together. This covering prevents the ends of the bones from touching and also absorbs jolts.

Skeletal System **CHAPTER 18** 337

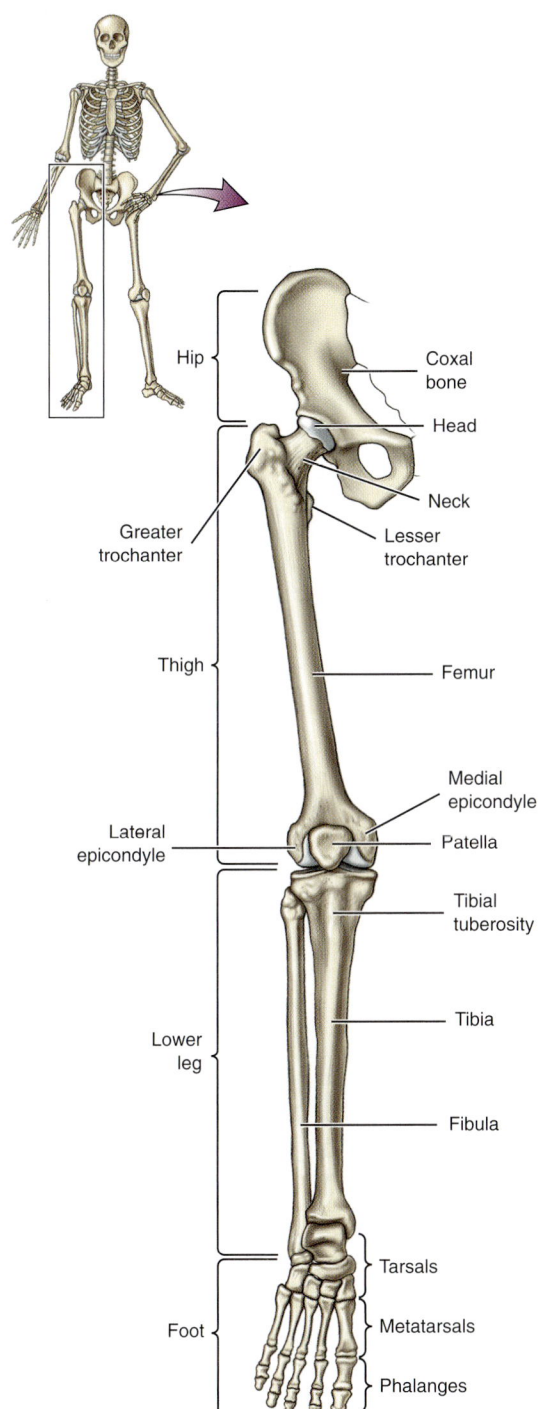

FIGURE 18-12 Bones of the lower limb. (Modified from Herlihy B, Maebius NK: *The human body in health and illness,* ed 3, St Louis, 2007, Saunders.)

- A **bursa** is a capsule made up of a tough, fibrous connective tissue and filled with synovial fluid. The bursa acts as a cushion between the moving parts of the joint.
- A **synovial cavity** is filled with **synovial fluid,** which reduces the friction caused by joint movement. As a person ages, the synovial fluid is not secreted as quickly, and the articular cartilage hardens.

Types

There are six types of diarthrosis articulations (Figure 18-14), as follows:
1. **Ball-and-socket joints** allow the widest range of movement. One bone with a ball-shaped head fits into the socket of the second bone. Examples include the hip and shoulder joints.
2. **Hinge joints** move only in one direction, similar to a hinged door. Examples include the knees and elbow joints (Figure 18-15).
3. **Pivot joints** allow for rotation. Examples include the wrist, ankle, bones of the forearm, and the movement between the atlas and the axis in the cervical vertebrae.
4. **Saddle joints** have saddle-shaped bones that fit into a concave-convex socket. An example is the movement of the thumb.
5. **Gliding joints** allow flat surfaces to move across each other. Examples are the vertebrae of the spinal column and carpal bones.
6. **Condyloid joints** are oval-shaped bones that fit into an elliptical cavity. An example is the wrist joint, where the radius and the carpal bones join.

Connective Tissues

Ligaments are bands of connective tissue that attach bones to bones. In some cases ligaments continue completely through a joint to provide added strength, as in the knee joint. **Tendons** are connective tissues that connect muscles to bones. Tendons provide the power needed to move the joints. Tendons are longer, often wider, and stronger than ligaments.

Movement

The chief function of movable joints is to allow the body to change position, providing motion to the body. There are four main types of movement, as well as several combinations of movements. Flexion, extension, abduction, and adduction describe the change in position of the body parts. Figure 18-16 illustrates various forms of joint movement.
- **Flexion** is a bending motion that brings two neighboring bones closer together. Examples include bending the forearm toward the shoulder and bending the fingers to close the hand.
- **Extension** is the opposite of flexion and results from an increase in the angle of the bones. Examples include straightening the forearm and straightening the fingers when opening the hand.
- **Abduction** occurs when an extremity is moved away from the body. An example is moving the arms away from the sides of the body (abduction = away).
- **Adduction** occurs when movement goes toward the midline of the body. An example is moving the arms back to the sides of the body (adduction = toward).

Other types of movement that involve combinations of these four movements include rotation and circumduction.

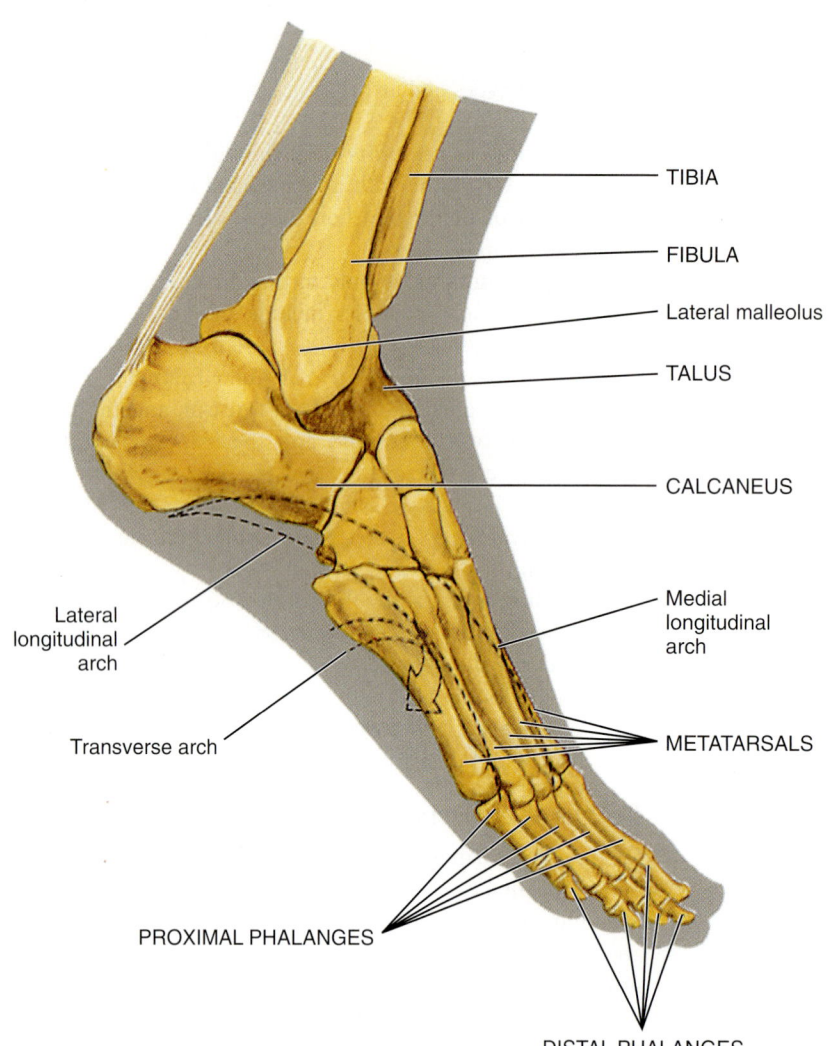

FIGURE 18-13 The bones of the right foot (lateral view). As indicated in the figure, the tarsal and metatarsal bones form several arches that help the foot support the weight of the body. (From Solomon EP: *Introduction to human anatomy and physiology*, ed 3, St Louis, 2009, Saunders.)

- **Rotation** occurs when one bone moves or turns on its own axis, as when turning the head from side to side. The forearm can turn the palm upward (**supination**) or turn the palm downward (**pronation**). The ankle can turn the sole inward (**inversion**) or turn the sole outward (**eversion**), away from the body. The foot is bent away from the body in *plantar flexion* and toward the body in *dorsiflexion*.
- **Circumduction** is a combination of flexion, abduction, extension, and adduction, in that order. To perform this movement, (1) put your head on your right shoulder, (2) move your head forward with your chin on your chest, (3) put your head on your left shoulder, and (4) drop your head backward. Another way to illustrate circumduction is to stand erect with arms outstretched at your sides, then draw an imaginary circle with your arms.

PATIENT-CENTERED PROFESSIONALISM

- Why is it important for the medical assistant to understand both the structural and the functional classifications of joints?

DISEASES AND DISORDERS OF THE SKELETAL SYSTEM

Disorders of the skeletal system can be due to an injury, inflammation, a congenital abnormality, or malformation of cells. Structures that are affected are bones, joints, and connective tissue. The treatment of **orthopedic** disorders (disorders involving bones or joints) can be short or long term. Table 18-2 lists skeletal drug classifications used in orthopedic therapy.

You need to be able to recognize the common signs and symptoms of and the diagnostic tests for the different types of skeletal disorders.

- Study Box 18-2 to learn about the common signs and symptoms.
- Study Box 18-3 for common diagnostic tests and procedures.
- Study Table 18-3 to learn about the diseases and disorders that affect the skeletal system.

In addition to being affected by various diseases and disorders, the bones and joints may undergo various injuries such as dislocation, subluxation, sprains, and fractures.

Text continued on p. 345

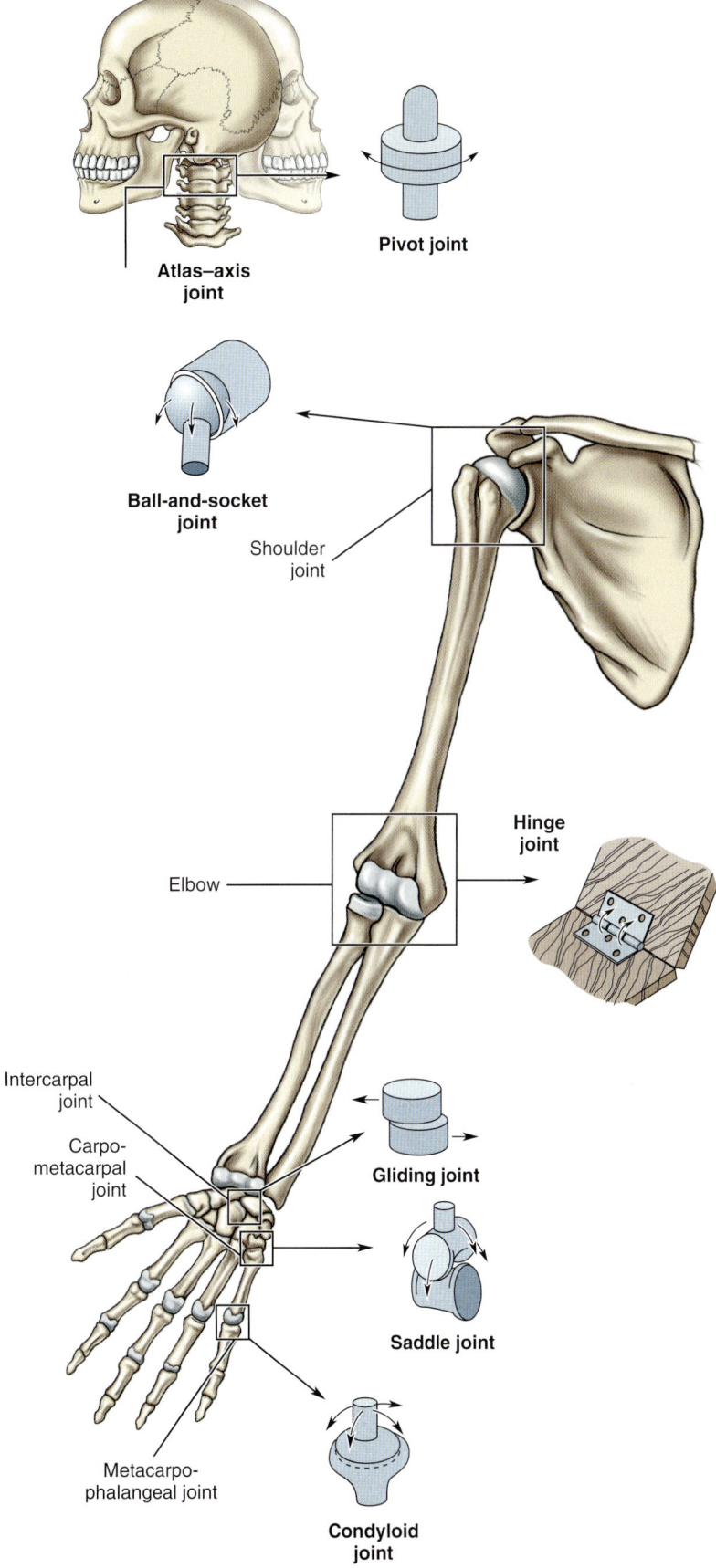

FIGURE 18-14 Freely movable joints (diarthroses): ball-and-socket, hinge, gliding, saddle, condyloid, and pivot joints. (From Herlihy B, Maebius NK: *The human body in health and illness,* ed 3, St Louis, 2007, Saunders.)

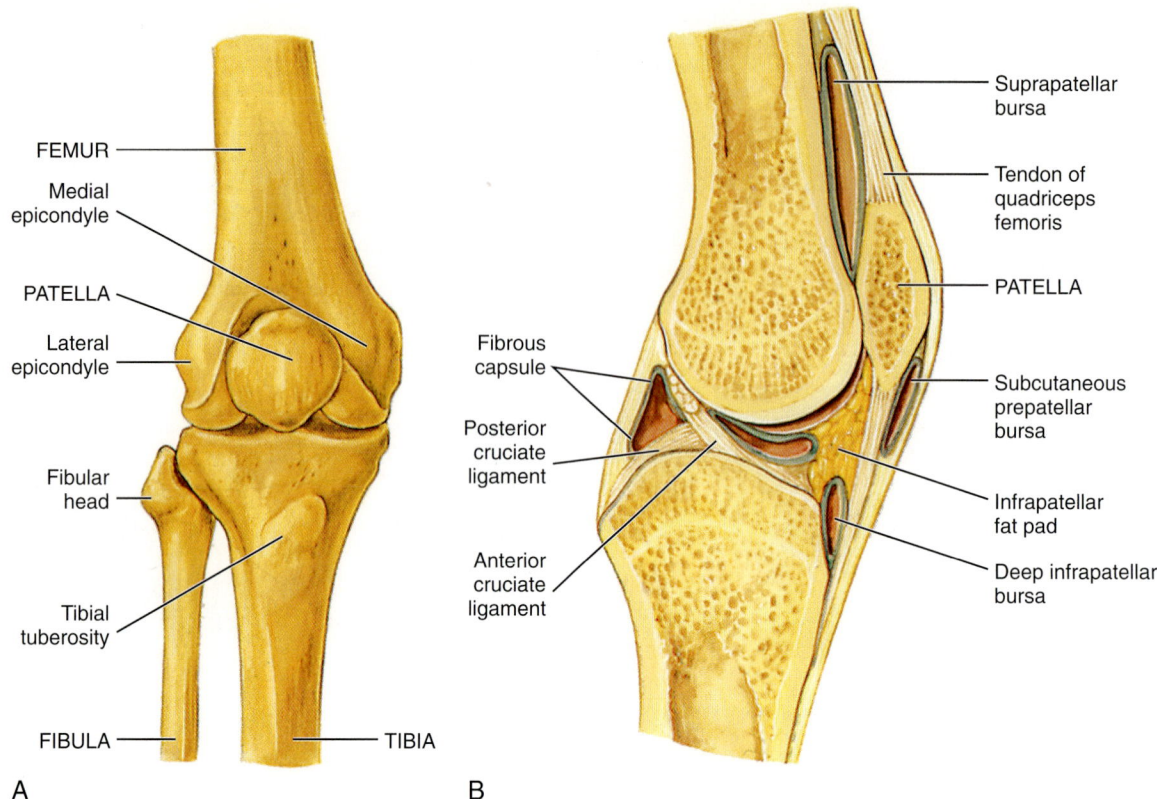

FIGURE 18-15 Structure and contents of a synovial joint (knee). **A,** Anterior view of the knee joint. **B,** Sagittal view of the knee joint. (From Solomon EP: *Introduction to human anatomy and physiology*, ed 3, St Louis, 2009, Saunders.)

TABLE 18-2
Skeletal Drug Classifications

Drug Classification	Common Generic (Brand) Drugs
Analgesics	ketorolac tromethamine (Toradol)
Relieve pain	acetaminophen (Tylenol)
Antiarthritics	celecoxib (Celebrex)
Relieve symptoms of arthritis	valdecoxib (Bextra)
Antigout agents	probenecid (Benemid)
Treat gout	allopurinol (Zyloprim)
Antiinflammatories	naproxen (Naprosyn)
Relieve and control inflammation	nabumetone (Relafen)
Osteoporotics	alendronate (Fosamax)
Prevent osteoporosis	estradiol (Estrace)

BOX 18-2
Common Signs and Symptoms of Skeletal Disease

Ostealgia	Pain within the bone
Osteitis	Inflammation of the bone
Osteonecrosis	Death of bone tissue
General complaints	Joint stiffness, swelling, decrease in bone mass, and immobility

BOX 18-3
Diagnostic Tests and Procedures for the Skeletal System

Arthrography	X-ray of a joint
Arthroscopy	Visual examination of a joint with an arthroscope
Bone density testing	BDT; radiologic test that determines bone density
Bone scan	Use of nuclear medicine to detect pathologies of bone
Computed tomography (CT)	CT scan; imaging technique that records transverse planes of body
Myelogram	X-ray of spinal canal done after injection of contrast medium
Radiography	Imaging technique using x-rays or gamma rays to make film records (x-rays, radiographs) of internal structures of body

LABORATORY TESTS

Rheumatoid factor (RF) test	Identifies presence of rheumatoid factor in the blood (as an indication of rheumatoid arthritis)
Serum calcium (Ca)	Measures the amount of calcium in the blood

TABLE 18-3

Diseases and Disorders of the Skeletal System

Disease and Description	Etiology	Signs and Symptoms	Diagnosis	Therapy	Interventions
BONE DISEASES					
Infections of the Bone Infections can enter the bone through an open fracture, blood transmission, or an adjacent infection.					
Osteomyelitis Infection of bone marrow and bone	Usually *Staphylococcus aureus;* bacteria can already exist in bloodstream or can enter at open fracture site	Sudden onset of pain and fever over affected bone; malaise	Blood cultures or wound culture of infection site	Antibiotic therapy; affected bone must be immobilized and dead bone tissue **debrided**	Encourage immediate attention to fractures and good skin care; discourage using coat hanger or knitting needles to scratch area under cast
Tuberculosis Infectious pulmonary disease that can affect other areas (e.g., musculoskeletal system)	*Mycobacterium tuberculosis* infection from lungs spreads to bone	Joint pain, swelling, tenderness, and limited motion; weight loss, fatigue, and fever with chills; night sweats and nonproductive cough	Positive Mantoux test indicates past infection; sputum culture smear is positive for acid-fast bacillus	Antibiotic therapy; rest	Reinforce long-term medical follow-up to prevent recurrence
Deficiencies of the Bone Deficiencies of calcium and phosphorus in the blood do not allow normal bone formation. Bones become soft and deformed because of the inability of bones to bear weight.					
Rickets Bone disease caused by a lack of vitamin D in children	Inability of body to absorb vitamin D; nutritional deficiency	Bones are soft due to lack of calcification	Physical exam	Adequate calcium, vitamin D, and exposure to sunlight; if cause is lack of absorption of needed minerals and vitamins, underlying disease must be treated	Encourage diet therapy with high-calcium foods or foods fortified with vitamin D; encourage "plenty of sunshine"
Osteomalacia Bone disease of adults; deficiency of calcium and vitamin D	Insufficient storage or utilization of vitamin D	Weight-bearing bones cannot hold their shape, so height is reduced; bones ache	Blood and urine analysis to estimate levels of calcium and phosphorus; skeletal films show areas of decalcification	Calcium supplements; vitamin D–fortified foods	Provide dietary instruction on foods high in calcium and vitamin D
Miscellaneous Bone Diseases Some bone diseases can result from hormonal imbalances and loss of bone activity (e.g., patient confined to bed).					
Osteoporosis More bone cells destroyed than made; decrease in bone density leaves bones porous	Decrease of bone cell production; often considered idiopathic	Spontaneous bone breaks; lower back pain	Bone density scans indicate decrease in bone density, especially in spine and pelvis; blood tests for phosphorus and calcium levels	Supplements of vitamin D and calcium; Analgesics to relieve pain; possible hormone therapy	Encourage daily walking or some form of physical activity, to include weight-bearing exercise

TABLE 18-3

Diseases and Disorders of the Skeletal System—cont'd

Disease and Description	Etiology	Signs and Symptoms	Diagnosis	Therapy	Interventions
Paget disease Slow, progressive inflammatory disease of bone tissue	Unknown	Bone swelling in long bones, dull pain in affected bone, or patient may be asymptomatic; hearing loss is possible	Skeletal films and bone marrow biopsies; blood studies to detect increased levels of alkaline phosphatase in blood and hydroxyproline in urine, caused by high rate of bone turnover	Dietary increase of protein, calcium, and supplements of vitamin D	Encourage patient to follow diet therapy
Scoliosis Lateral curvature of spine (Figure 18-17, *B*)	Idiopathic; or possible congenital defect, poor posture, or bone overgrowth	Onset insidious; fatigue and backache are frequent complaints	Physical examination and spinal x-rays	Physical therapy, exercise, back braces; possible surgery	Encourage good posture
Lordosis (swayback) Severe inward curvature in lumbar area (Figure 18-17, *C*)	Idiopathic	Onset insidious	Physical examination and spinal x-rays	Physical therapy, exercise, back braces	Encourage good posture
Kyphosis (hunchback) Forward curvature in thoracic area of spine (Figure 18-17, *A*)	Idiopathic	Onset insidious; fatigue and backache are frequent complaints	Physical examination and spinal x-rays	Physical therapy, exercise, back braces	Encourage good posture

Bone Neoplasms

Tumors of the bone usually cause pain and can cause fractures. A primary malignant tumor or sarcoma affects the ends of the bone. Secondary tumors are **carcinomas** that have **metastasized**.

Disease and Description	Etiology	Signs and Symptoms	Diagnosis	Therapy	Interventions
Osteomas Benign bone tumors; giant cell tumors occur at ends of long bones	Unknown	Bone pain, described as dull and localized	Bone biopsy; skeletal x-rays	Surgery to remove tumor	Provide follow-up rehabilitation if necessary
Sarcomas Malignant bone tumors of bone marrow and cartilage cells	Unknown	Bone pain, described as dull and localized	Skeletal film shows tumor that begins at epiphysis of long bones	Radiation and surgery; sometimes, amputation of extremity is necessary	Encourage follow-up rehabilitation

JOINT DISEASES

Arthritis

The inflammation of one or more joints usually accompanied by pain and stiffness. **Arthritis** is often a symptom of other diseases.

Disease and Description	Etiology	Signs and Symptoms	Diagnosis	Therapy	Interventions
Rheumatoid arthritis (RA) Chronic inflammatory joint disease that affects connective tissue and joints (Figure 18-18)	Idiopathic; women are most often affected	Acute inflammation of connective tissues; synovial membrane thickens and **ankylosis** results (bones fuse together); cartilage between joints gradually degenerates and is replaced by calcium	Joints appear swollen and painful; blood test to confirm positive rheumatoid factor	Antiinflammatories and analgesics to reduce discomfort and maintain joint motion	Treatment is life-long; encouragement of support group involvement can be positive for patient

TABLE 18-3

Diseases and Disorders of the Skeletal System—cont'd

Disease and Description	Etiology	Signs and Symptoms	Diagnosis	Therapy	Interventions
Osteoarthritis Cartilage on end of bones softens, and bones rub against each other	Unknown	Gradual onset, with aching joints the major symptom; **crepitation** (bone cracking or creaking) heard on movement	Skeletal x-rays show changes in bone and joint formation	Long-term **palliative** approach is usually taken. Analgesics for pain; antiinflammatories to reduce swelling; sometimes paraffin treatments on hands	Encourage activity to reduce stiffness
Gouty arthritis (gout) Result of uric acid not being metabolized	Failure of body to remove uric acid crystals that have been overproduced (metabolic), or kidneys fail to filter out normal production properly	Sudden onset of joint pain, especially great toe; other joint areas (wrists, ankles, knees) can also be affected; due to inactivity, **tophi** (calcified deposits) may occur at joint	Blood test shows increased urate crystals; erythrocyte sedimentation rate (ESR), white blood count, and urinalysis indicate hyperuricemia	Bedrest and immobilization of affected area should be ordered; applications of heat or cold, drug therapy, and diet restrictions also should be tried	To lessen recurrence of attacks, patient needs to be encouraged to follow a specific diet and increase fluid intake
Other Joint Diseases					
Bursitis Acute inflammation of bursa	Overuse of joint; arthritic changes	Swelling in joint area accompanied by pain; local inflammation and increased pressure during motion around a joint	Physical examination and x-ray to determine if swelling is caused by calcium deposits at site	Hot and cold applications, drug therapy, possible steroid injections at site	Encourage patient to follow treatment, avoid excessive stress on area, report signs of infection; physical therapy
Carpal tunnel syndrome Compression of median nerve in wrist	Occupational hazard for people who perform repetitive motions	Pain, numbness, burning in one or both hands (on thumb side especially)	Medical history; tingling sensation when median nerve tapped	Rest affected wrist(s); **ergonomic** devices to relieve stress to wrist; in extreme cases, surgery indicated	Short breaks between activities to rest wrists, or use wrist rests devised for computer keyboards and mouse pads
CONGENITAL DISORDERS Congenital disorders of the skeletal system are caused by a malformation of bone during embryonic development.					
Talipes (clubfoot) Deformity of one or both feet (Figure 18-19)	Unknown	Talus deformed, **Achilles tendon** shortened, and calcaneus flattened, causing foot to be bent	Obvious at birth	Corrective surgery	Encourage follow-up care by caregivers to include daily foot exercises, splint application, and special shoes
Spina bifida Spinal column in lumbar and sacral areas does not close completely	During first trimester, neural tube does not close properly; often caused by decreased folic acid levels in mother	*Spina bifida occulta:* signs may be subtle (e.g., hair tuft at end of spinal area, slight skin dimpling); *meningocele:* saclike structure protrudes from spinal area	If problem suspected, amniocentesis to detect high levels of acetylcholinesterase; ultrasound can detect spinal structure abnormalities during first trimester	*Meningocele:* surgery to correct defect; supportive measures; opening cannot be repaired	Ensure genetic counseling and good prenatal care

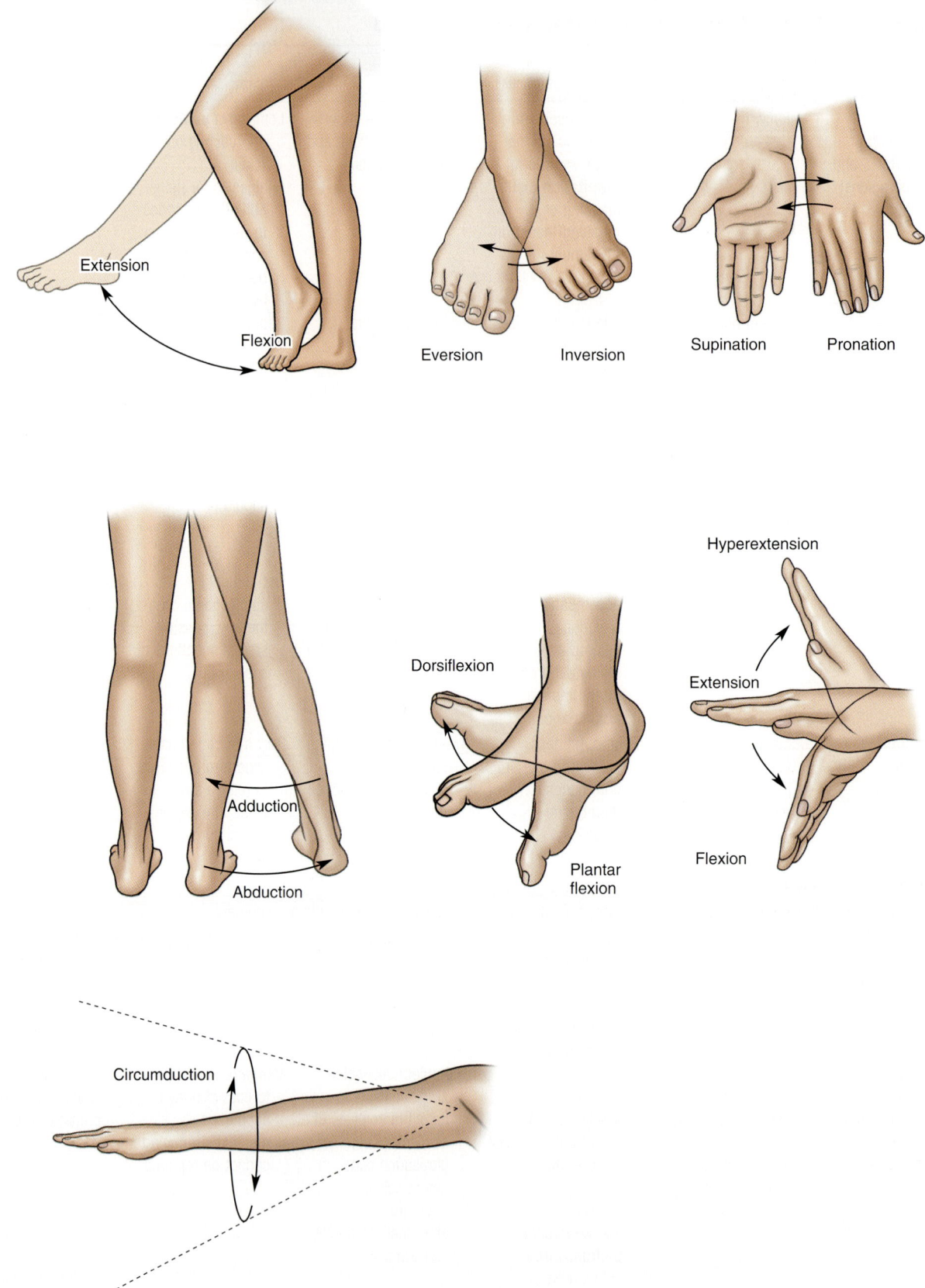

FIGURE 18-16 Types of joint movements. (From Herlihy B, Maebius NK: *The human body in health and illness,* ed 3, St Louis, 2007, Saunders.)

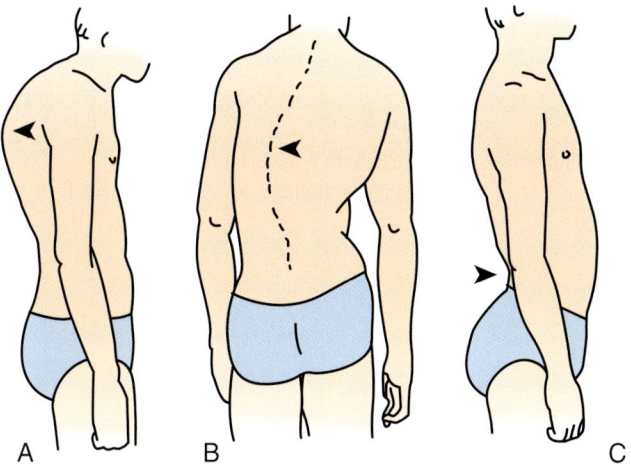

FIGURE 18-17 Abnormal curvatures of vertebral column. **A,** Kyphosis. **B,** Scoliosis. **C,** Lordosis. (From Black JM et al: *Medical-surgical nursing: clinical management for positive outcomes,* ed 8, St Louis, 2009, Saunders.)

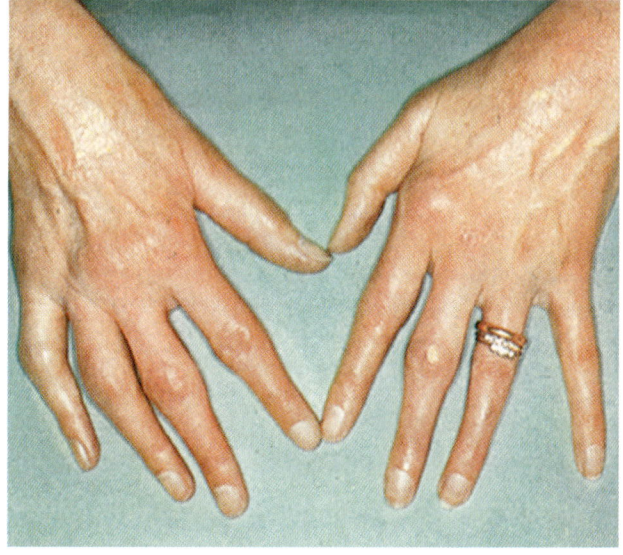

FIGURE 18-18 Rheumatoid arthritis. (From Wilson SF, Giddens JF: *Health assessment for nursing practice,* ed 2, St Louis, 2001, Mosby.)

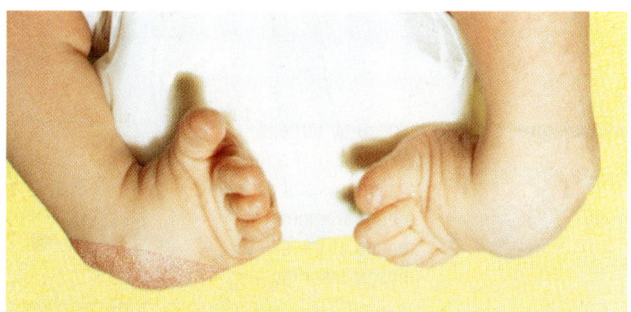

FIGURE 18-19 Talipes. (From Zitelli BJ, Davis HW: *Atlas of pediatric physical diagnosis,* ed 4, St Louis, 2002, Mosby.)

Dislocation is the displacement of a joint from its proper position. A dislocation of a bone could cause the surrounding ligaments to tear or stretch. Returning the bones to their original position is referred to as a **reduction.**

Subluxation is a partial dislocation of a joint (e.g., neck injury) that may be caused by sudden movement or trauma.

Sprains occur when the ligaments around a joint are stretched, torn, or ruptured. **Strains** occur when muscles and tendons are stretched beyond their capacity.

Fractures, or bone breaks, are the most common skeletal injury. Besides the break in the bone, the surrounding tissues are injured and blood vessels may be broken. Repairing a break when the skin has not been punctured by the fracture or does not require surgical opening is called a **closed reduction.** This type of repair requires realigning the bone, a cast, and rest. When a bone breaks and protrudes through the skin, however, the repair requires surgery to clean the wound and remove possible bone fragments before casting; this is called an **open reduction.** Broken bones that do not protrude through the skin may still require an open reduction (surgery) if the bone is so fragmented that it requires surgical screws or pins (internal fixation) to hold it together for healing. This can only be done through an incision. The most common types of fractures are **simple, compound, greenstick, spiral, comminuted,** and **impacted** (Table 18-4).

PATIENT-CENTERED PROFESSIONALISM

- Why must a medical assistant have a basic knowledge of disorders that affect the skeletal system?

FOR YOUR INFORMATION

Bones of the skeleton become thinner, relatively weaker, and slightly osteopenic as a person ages as a result of inadequate ossification. Most affected are the epiphyses, vertebrae, and the jaw resulting in fragile limbs, reduction in height, loss of teeth, and or chewing ability.

CONCLUSION

The skeletal system is a collection of bones and connective tissue working together to form the framework of the body. Bones come together to allow the body to be mobile and flexible. Some bones have cartilage on their ends. Bursae filled with synovial fluid are found in joints to absorb shock.

You may have been surprised to discover that in the earliest stages of bone development, the fetal skeleton is entirely cartilage. How many other systems did you find that interact with the skeletal system? The obvious answer is the muscular system

TABLE 18-4

Types of Fractures

Fracture	Definition	Illustration	Fracture	Definition	Illustration
Closed, or **simple**	Broken bone is contained within intact skin and can be easily reduced		**Pathological**	Results from weakening of bone by disease	
Open, or **compound**	Skin is broken near fracture and thus open to external environment, resulting in potential for infection		**Nondisplaced**	Bone ends remain in alignment	
Longitudinal	Fracture extends along length of the bone		**Displaced**	Bone ends are out of alignment and must be reduced to alignment	
Transverse	Fracture extends across the bone; produced by direct force applied perpendicularly to a bone		**Spiral**	Have long, sharp, pointed bone ends; produced by twisting or rotary forces	
Oblique	Produced by a twisting force with an upward thrust; fracture ends are short and run at an oblique angle across the bone		**Compression**	Bones compress on each other to cause fractures; produced by transmitted forces that drive bones together	
Greenstick	Produced by compression or angulation forces in long bones of children younger than age 10 years; bone is cracked on one side and intact but stretched on the other due to softness		**Avulsion**	Produced by forceful contraction of a muscle against resistance, with a bone fragment tearing at the site of muscle insertion	

TABLE 18-4
Types of Fractures—cont'd

Fracture	Definition	Illustration	Fracture	Definition	Illustration
Comminuted	Bone has multiple fragments and fracture is produced by severe, direct violence		**Depression**	Bone fragments (usually in the skull) are driven inward	
Impacted	Bones are pushed inside each other; produced by strong forces that drive bone fragments firmly together				

From Chester GA: *Modern medical assisting*, Philadelphia, 1998, Saunders.

---

but remember, you need nerve impulses to make the muscles work to move the bones. In addition, the endocrine system's parathyroid hormone (PTH) is needed to raise blood calcium, and the integumentary system is needed for vitamin D synthesis. As you can see, the skeletal system is no different from the other body systems, in that it interacts with and depends on other systems. Understanding the structure and function of the skeletal system is an important step in becoming a successful medical assistant.

FOR YOUR INFORMATION

An orthopedist (MD) specializes in bone, joint, and muscle disorders.
A *physiatrist* (MD) specializes in physical and sports medicine, as well as rehabilitation from skeletal injuries.
A *chiropractor* treats disorders originating from misalignment of the spine.
A *Doctor of Osteopathy* (DO) treats by changing the position of the bones and using traditional medicine.
A *podiatrist* specializes in diagnosing and treating disorders of the foot.
A *rheumatologist* diagnoses and treats diseases of connective tissue.

Chapter Summary

Reinforce your understanding of the material in this chapter by reviewing the curriculum objectives and key content points below.

1. **Define, appropriately use, and spell all the Key Terms for this chapter.**
   - Review the Key Terms if necessary.
2. **List the five major functions of the skeletal system.**
   - The skeletal system supports the body, protects internal organs, enables movement, stores minerals, and forms blood.
3. **Describe how bone tissue is formed.**
   - Fetal bone begins as cartilage. During the process of ossification (bone formation), osteoblasts produce bone cells (osteocytes) that replace the cartilage.
   - Osteoclasts work to enlarge bones from the inside cavity and remove bone debris.
4. **Explain how bones grow.**
   - Ossification begins in the embryonic stage, when osteoblasts and osteoclasts combine to replace cartilage.

- Bones grow outward from the epiphyseal plates at both ends of the bone. Bones lengthen and harden as a child grows.
- Good nutrition (calcium and vitamin D) is important for strong bones.
- Ossification slows as people age, and bones often become soft (osteomalacia) or brittle and porous (osteoporosis).

5. **Describe the basic structure of bones.**
   - Bone tissue is nonliving tissue made up of fluids and collagen (the bone matrix) that holds the bone together. As bone hardens, it forms lamellae.
   - Bone marrow is within the bones. There are two types of bone marrow: yellow and red. Bone marrow is responsible for the manufacture of blood cells.
   - Cartilage is attached to bone and is flexible.
   - Bone surface markings provide a connection point or a space for nerves, blood vessels, and ligaments to connect to other surfaces.

6. **List the four types of bone shapes and give an example of each.**
   - Long bones are the most complex type of bone and define height (e.g., the femur).
   - Short bones are numerous as in the ankle and wrist.
   - Flat bones protect major organs and act as attachment points for muscles from the front and back of the body (e.g., the sternum).
   - Irregular bones make up the spinal column, bones of the skull, and the jaw.

7. **Explain how bones repair themselves.**
   - Osteoblasts and osteoclasts are activated to repair bone during an injury.
   - Calcium and vitamin D are necessary for proper ossification to take place in bone growth and repair.

8. **Differentiate between the axial and the appendicular divisions of the skeleton.**
   - The axial skeleton includes the bones of the head and trunk.
   - The appendicular skeleton includes the bones of upper and lower extremities.

9. **Name and locate the bones of the skull.**
   - There are 22 irregularly shaped bones and flat bones that form the skull.
   - Refer to Figure 18-4.

10. **Name the divisions of the spinal column and indicate the number of bones in each division.**
    - There are five major divisions of the spinal column.
    - Cervical vertebrae (C1-C7) are located in the neck.
    - Thoracic vertebrae (T1-T12) are in the thorax (trunk) area.
    - Lumbar vertebrae (L1-L5) are in the lower back.
    - The sacrum (S1-S5) begins with five bones, which fuse and become one.
    - The coccyx, the last part of the spinal column, has four bones that fuse to become one (tailbone).

11. **Locate the sternum and describe how the ribs join to it.**
    - The sternum is the breastbone and is located in the midline of the chest cavity.
    - The sternum is divided into three parts: manubrium, body, and xiphoid process.
    - Some ribs attach to the sternum directly with cartilage, others attach indirectly, and others are not attached to the sternum at all.

12. **List the three types of upper extremity bones.**
    - The upper extremity includes the bones of the pectoral girdle, the upper and lower arm, and the wrist and hand.

13. **List the bones of the lower extremities.**
    - The lower extremities include the bones of the pelvic girdle, the femur, patella, tibia and fibula, tarsal, and foot.

14. **Describe three types of joints.**
    - Joints allow for body movement.
    - Diarthroses allow for free movement.
    - Synarthroses are joined by dense fibrous tissue and do not allow any movement.
    - Amphiarthroses are connected by cartilage and allow only slight movement.

15. **List the three parts of a movable joint and describe the function of each part.**
    - Movable joints have articular cartilage, bursa, and synovial cavity.
    - Articular cartilage fits over the end surface of bones and prevents the bones from touching and wearing away.
    - Bursa is a fibrous sac filled with synovial fluid located in some joints.
    - Synovial fluid in the synovial cavity or capsule acts as a lubricant to reduce friction between joints.

16. **Name and describe the six types of movable joints.**
    - Each of the six types of joints provides for a different type of motion.
    - Ball-and-socket: One bone with a ball fits into the socket of a second bone allowing for circumduction.
    - Hinge: Moves in only one direction.
    - Pivot: Allows for rotation.
    - Saddle: Saddle-shaped bones fit into a concave-convex socket.
    - Gliding: Flat surfaces move across each other.
    - Condyloid: Oval-shaped bones fit into an elliptical cavity.

17. **Describe the structure and function of a ligament and a tendon.**
    - Ligaments are bands of connective tissue that attach bones to bones.
    - Tendons are bands of connective tissue that connect muscle to bone.

18. **Describe the four main types of movement.**
    - Flexion, extension, abduction, and adduction allow the body to change position and move.
    - Flexion is the bending motion that brings two bones together.
    - Abduction is movement of a bone away from the midline of the body.
    - Extension occurs when the angle of two bones is increased.
    - Adduction is movement of a bone toward the midline of the body.
    - Circumduction is a combination of flexion, abduction, extension, and adduction.

19. **List and describe the four types of signs and symptoms of skeletal disease.**

- Ostealgia, osteitis, osteonecrosis, and other general complaints are common signs and symptoms of skeletal disease.
- Refer to Box 18-2.

20. **List nine types of diagnostic tests and procedures for the skeletal system and describe the use of each.**
    - Refer to Box 18-3.

21. **List four types of injury to the bones and joints and briefly describe the etiology, signs and symptoms, diagnosis, therapy, and interventions for each.**
    - Dislocation is the displacement of a joint from its position.
    - Subluxation is a partial dislocation caused by sudden movement or trauma.
    - Sprains occur when the ligaments around a joint are stretched, torn, or ruptured.
    - Fractures are bone breaks.
    - Refer to Table 18-4.

22. **List two types of bone infection and briefly describe the etiology, signs and symptoms, diagnosis, therapy, and interventions for each.**
    - Refer to Table 18-3.

23. **List two bone deficiency diseases and briefly describe the etiology, signs and symptoms, diagnosis, therapy, and interventions for each.**
    - Refer to Table 18-3.

24. **List five other bone diseases and briefly describe the etiology, signs and symptoms, diagnosis, therapy, and interventions for each.**
    - Refer to Table 18-3.

25. **List two bone neoplasms and briefly describe the etiology, signs and symptoms, diagnosis, therapy, and interventions for each.**
    - Refer to Table 18-3.

26. **List three joint diseases and briefly describe the etiology, signs and symptoms, diagnosis, therapy, and interventions for each.**
    - The cause of arthritis is unknown, but joints become immovable and symptoms are often seen with other diseases.
    - Use of ergonomic devices and proper posture when working or typing can help prevent carpal tunnel syndrome.
    - Bursitis often results from repetitive motion in sports (e.g., tennis, baseball, golf).
    - Refer to Table 18-3.

27. **List two congenital disorders of the skeletal system and briefly describe the etiology, signs and symptoms, diagnosis, therapy, and interventions for each.**
    - Refer to Table 18-3.

28. **Analyze a realistic medical office situation and apply your understanding of the skeletal system to determine the best course of action.**
    - Medical assistants need to be able to answer patients' questions about bones and injuries to the skeletal system.
    - Understanding the skeletal system enables medical assistants to communicate with patients confidently and clearly.

29. **Describe the impact on patient care when medical assistants have a solid understanding of the structure and function of the skeletal system.**
    - Understanding the structure and function of the skeletal system allows medical assistants to perform their duties more efficiently and effectively.

PRACTICAL APPLICATIONS

If you have accomplished the objectives in this chapter, you will be able to make better choices as a medical assistant. Take another look at this situation and decide what you would do.

When she was 33 years old, Celia was injured in a skiing accident. She had a simple fracture of the distal end of the tibia and into the tarsals in her left leg. The fracture was located at the epiphyseal line. She also subluxated her knee in the same accident. The fracture was repaired with a closed reduction. After wearing a long leg cast for 8 weeks, an arthroscopy was performed on the knee to be sure the tendons and ligaments had not been torn or stretched because Celia was having difficulty bearing weight at that time. Before the arthroscopy, an arthrogram was performed on the knee and was negative; the arthroscopy was also negative. Over time, Celia seemed to recover from the fracture and had no problems until recently.

Celia is now 50 years old and has pain in her left ankle attributed to arthritis. She has also been diagnosed with early osteoporosis based on results of a bone density scan. The physician ordered analgesics for arthralgia and vitamin D and calcium supplements for osteoporosis. While talking with Steve, the medical assistant, Celia expresses concern that the osteoporosis and arthritis will only progress as she ages. She also has questions about some of the medical terms the physician used in speaking with her.

If you were in Steve's place, would you be prepared to discuss Celia's concerns and answer her questions?

1. What is a simple fracture?
2. What is a closed reduction?
3. What is subluxation of a joint?
4. Where is the tibia? Where are the tarsals?
5. What type bone is the tibia? What type of bones are the tarsals?
6. Why would a fracture at the epiphysis be important in a child or young adult?
7. What is an arthrogram? Arthroscopy?
8. Why would a bone scan be used in diagnosing osteoporosis?
9. Why would analgesics be ordered for arthritis?
10. What is arthralgia?
11. Why would vitamin D and calcium supplements be ordered for osteoporosis?
12. What are the dangers for Celia if the osteoporosis progresses?

WEB SEARCH

1. **Research how weight-bearing activities, such as walking or moderate weightlifting, help build and retain bone mass.** Bone has the ability to alter its strength in response to mechanical stress by increasing the disposition of mineral salts and production of collagen fibers. Removing mechanical stress weakens bone through loss of bone minerals and collagen reduction.
   - **Keywords:** Use the following keywords in your search: weight-bearing exercise, bone formation.
2. **Research homeostatic imbalances of the skeletal system.**
   - **Keywords:** Use the following keywords in your search: hormone replacement therapy; osteoporosis, Paget disease, herniated disc.

WORD PARTS: Skeletal System

STRUCTURE
Combining Forms

calci/o	calcium
chondr/o	cartilage
my/o, muscul/o	muscle
oste/o	bone

Suffixes

-blast	immature embryonic form
-clast	to break
-cyt/o	cell

AXIAL SKELETON
Combining Forms

crani/o	cranium
mandibul/o	lower jaw
maxill/o	upper jaw
cervic/o	neck
spin/o, rachi/o	spine
spondyl/o, vertebr/o	vertebrae
clavicul/o	clavicle (collarbone)
lumb/o	lower back
cost/o	ribs
stern/o	sternum

Prefix

syn-	joined; together

APPENDICULAR SKELETON
Combining Forms

ankyl/o	Stiff or crooked
burs/o	bursa
calcane/o	heel bone
carp/o	wrist
coccyg/eo	coccyx (tailbone)
femor/o	femur (thighbone)
fibul/o	fibula
humer/o	humerus (upper arm)
ili/o	ilium
ischi/o	ischium

ARTICULATIONS
Combining Forms

arthr/o	joint
articul/o	joint articulation

Prefixes

ab-	away from
ad-	toward

SKELETAL DISEASE
Suffixes

-malacia	softening
-sarcoma	malignant tumor from connective tissue

ABBREVIATIONS: Skeletal System

BK	below knee
C1, C2, etc.	first cervical vertebra, second cervical vertebra, etc.
CTS	carpal tunnel syndrome
DJD	degenerative joint disease
Fx	fracture
Jt	joint
L1, L2, etc.	first lumbar vertebra, second lumbar vertebra, etc.
OA	osteoarthritis
RA	rheumatoid arthritis
ROM	range of motion
T1, T2, etc.	first thoracic vertebra, second thoracic vertebra, etc.
Tx	treatment

19 Muscular System

evolve http://evolve.elsevier.com/klieger/medicalassisting

Muscle weight is almost 50% of a person's total body weight, which means if you weigh 150 pounds (lbs), you have 75 lbs of pure muscle. There are more than 600 skeletal muscles in the human body. Muscles are the parts of our body that allow us to move; without muscles, body movement would be similar to the movement of a puppet. Like the bones, muscles also protect the vital organs of the body. Muscles are classified by their structure and location. All muscle activity is influenced by the nervous system. Muscles perform their function by alternating their contracting and relaxing activities. Muscles work in teams to pull, but muscles cannot push. As one muscle of the team pulls to work, the other muscle of the team is relaxing to prepare for work.

Understanding these facts about the muscles in the human body and how they function helps medical assistants provide better care for patients.

LEARNING OBJECTIVES

You will be able to do the following after completing this chapter:

Key Terms
1. Define, appropriately use, and spell all the Key Terms for this chapter.

Function and Structure of Muscles
2. State the three functions of muscle and explain the importance of each.
3. Explain the basic structure of muscle.
4. Describe the structure and function of tendons.

Muscle Contraction and Muscle Tissue
5. Explain how a muscle contracts.
6. Identify and define the two types of muscle.
7. Briefly describe the three types of muscle tissue.
8. List four characteristics of muscle tissue.

Principal Skeletal Muscles
9. List seven ways muscles can be named.
10. Locate and identify the main skeletal muscles of the body.

Diseases and Disorders of the Muscular System
11. List seven common signs and symptoms of muscular system disorders.
12. List two common diagnostic tests for muscular disease and describe the use of each.
13. State the two most common muscular disorders seen in the physician's office.
14. List two muscular diseases and briefly describe the etiology, signs and symptoms, diagnosis, therapy, and interventions for each.

Patient-Centered Professionalism
15. Analyze a realistic medical office situation and apply your understanding of the muscular system to determine the best course of action.
16. Describe the impact on patient care when medical assistants have a solid understanding of the structure and function of the muscular system.

KEY TERMS

The Key Terms for this chapter have been organized into sections so that you can easily see the terminology associated with each aspect of the muscular system.

Muscle Function

adenosine triphosphate (ATP)	lactic acid
antagonistic	muscle tone
atonic	synergistic
flaccid	tonus

Continued

Structure of Muscles and Tendons

Achilles tendon	ligament
aponeurosis	myoglobin
fascia	tendon
hamstrings	

Muscle Contraction

acetylcholine	neuromuscular junction
cholinesterase	synapse
isometric contraction	tetany
isotonic contraction	

Muscle Types

cardiac	irritability
contractility	skeletal
elasticity	smooth
extensibility	striated
involuntary	voluntary

Principal Skeletal Muscles

abductors	levators
adductors	mandible
deltoid	mastication
depressors	origin
extensors	prime mover
fixators	rotators
flexors	sphincters
insertion	

Diseases and Disorders of the Muscular System

atrophy	myalgia
contusion	myasthenia gravis
cramps	myositis
fibromyalgia	spasms
fibromyositis	sprain
hernia	strain
muscular dystrophy	torticollis (wryneck)

Related Diagnostic Terms

electromyography (EMG)	magnetic resonance imaging (MRI)

PRACTICAL APPLICATIONS

Read the following scenario and keep it in mind as you learn about the muscular system in this chapter.

Tommy, age 18, has been playing sports since childhood. He has used weights to increase and strengthen the muscles of his body. Tommy has often wondered just how the muscles of his body work to make him move and what happens when one muscle contracts. He knows that some muscles are involuntary and some are voluntary.

Two days ago, Tommy was skiing when he fell and twisted his left ankle. The emergency room physician told him that he had strained and sprained his ankle. In explanation, the physician also said that the extensors in the ankle had the greatest injury and that the contusion was going to become worse if Tommy did not keep ice on the ankle overnight. Because of the severity of the injury, Tommy was to see an orthopedist the next morning. The orthopedist has ordered antiinflammatories and muscle relaxants.

Tommy now has some new questions for the medical assistant about muscles, what the antiinflammatories will do, and what this might have done to his muscles had he been older.

Would you be able to answer Tommy's questions?

FUNCTION AND STRUCTURE OF MUSCLES

Knowing the function and structure of muscles in the body allows you to better understand the problems that can affect the muscular system.

Muscle Function

The three main functions of muscles are to (1) cause movement, (2) provide support, and (3) produce heat and energy.

Movement

Our bodies move in many ways. Types of body movements include moving from place to place (conscious or voluntary), reaction of the pupil to light (unconscious or involuntary), and even internal movement such as digestion, respiration, and heartbeat (unconscious or involuntary).

Muscles are specialized and contract when stimulated. When a muscle contracts, its fibers shorten; this produces movement. Muscles can only pull bones; they cannot push them. Most of the muscles of the body are arranged in **antagonistic** pairs, meaning that when one muscle moves in one direction (prime mover), its antagonist causes movement in the opposite direction (e.g., biceps versus triceps). Muscles can also be arranged in **synergistic** pairs. The muscles in either of these muscle pairs work together to bring about movement.

Support

Even when people are not moving, their muscles are in a state of partial contraction known as **muscle tone.** Muscle tone is an unconscious action resulting from nerve stimulation that keeps muscles in a state of readiness. A person's muscle tone dictates his or her posture. Muscle tone allows the abdominal muscles to hold the internal organs in place so that posture can be maintained for long periods with little or no evidence of fatigue. **Tonus** is the slight tension in the muscle that is always present, even when at rest. A person is said to be **flaccid** or **atonic** when muscle tone is lacking. Flaccid muscles do not provide the necessary support and ability of movement that is needed for the body to respond to stimuli.

Heat Production

Our bodies maintain an average body temperature of 98.6° F or 37° C. Temperatures above or below this range may indicate illness. The contraction of muscles that produces a person's body heat occurs in the following two ways:
- Chemical energy is used to make muscles contract. Some of this energy is lost as heat.
- The *aerobic* (occurring or living only in the presence of oxygen) and *anaerobic* (living in the absence of oxygen) reactions in muscles also produce heat.

Before a muscle contracts, it receives a nerve impulse. Skeletal muscles require energy to move, and **adenosine triphosphate (ATP)** is used for this process. When ATP generated in cellular respiration breaks down, the muscle fibers shorten. When a muscle runs out of ATP, the buildup of **lactic acid** (waste product) causes the tired and sometimes burning feeling of muscle fatigue.

Structure of Muscles and Tendons

You first learned about cells and tissues in Chapter 11. This section discusses the specific tissue types that make up muscles and tendons.

Muscle Structure

Skeletal muscles are bundles of long muscle fibers (muscle cells). They are specialized to *contract* (shorten) when given a stimulus and to *relax* (return to their original position) when the stimulus subsides. The larger the muscle, the greater is the number of fibers involved. Each group of fibers is held together and protected by connective tissue, which is covered by a fibrous sheath called **fascia** that covers, supports, and separates muscles. The fascia contains the muscle's blood, lymph, and nerve supply. Muscles are red because they contain **myoglobin,** a red pigment, and have a rich blood supply.

Tendon Structure

A **tendon** is a white cordlike structure made up of collagenous fibers that connects muscles to bone. Tendons are strong and very flexible. There are many tendons in the body; several important ones are listed here. Severe damage to major tendons can necessitate surgical repair.
- The **Achilles tendon,** the strongest tendon in the body, attaches the calf muscle to the calcaneus.
- The **hamstrings** are tendons located behind the knee. They are responsible for extending (straightening) the hips and flexing (bending) the knees.
- The **aponeurosis** is a wide, flat connective tissue that connects muscle to bone.

MUSCLE CONTRACTION

Muscle contraction enables movement, posture, and heat production. Some muscles contract and relax on our command (voluntary muscles); others do this independent of the person's control (involuntary muscles).

When one or more muscles in a group contract, or pull, the other muscles of the group relax. This contraction produces movement. When the bone is ready to be pulled back to the original position, the muscles switch roles: the contracting muscles relax and the previously relaxed muscles contract.

Before a skeletal muscle can contract, the muscle must be stimulated by nerve impulses. Where the muscle fiber and the nerve ending meet is called a **neuromuscular junction** (area where **synapse** occurs). **Acetylcholine** is released at this junction. This chemical is used by the nerve endings to send an impulse across the synapse to the muscle, which causes the next muscle to contract. The enzyme **cholinesterase** breaks down excess acetylcholine and thus stops the overstimulation of the muscle.

Contraction is controlled by the central nervous system (CNS), which includes the brain and the spinal cord. Voluntary muscle contractions are initiated in the brain while the spinal cord initiates involuntary movement. Skeletal muscles are able to produce varying levels of contractile force, thus preventing the muscle fibers from tearing. Smooth muscles contract in response to calcium levels.

> **PATIENT-CENTERED PROFESSIONALISM**
>
> - Why is it important for the medical assistant to understand the structure and function of the muscular system?
> - Why is it important to understand the function of tendons?

Types of Contractions

To be effective, muscles must contract in a smooth and sustained movement. When an individual lifts a heavy object, the muscles shorten and thicken as they contract. This is known as **isotonic contraction** (Figure 19-1, *A*). If that same individual pushed against the wall or tried to move an immovable object, no movement would occur. In this situation, muscle length would not change, but muscle tension would increase. This type of muscle contraction is known as **isometric contraction** and is often used to strengthen muscles (Figure 19-1, *B*).

Abnormal contractions are not smooth or sustained and are not useful.
- A *twitch* is a jerky response to a stimulus. If our muscles only twitched instead of moving smoothly, we would not be able to perform many fine motor tasks such as writing, buttoning, or zipping.
- A **tetany** is another form of abnormal contraction. This type of contraction is caused when the muscle is stimulated in a series of "rapid fire" impulses. In this situation each muscle fiber is not working with other fibers to respond to the stimulus but instead is working

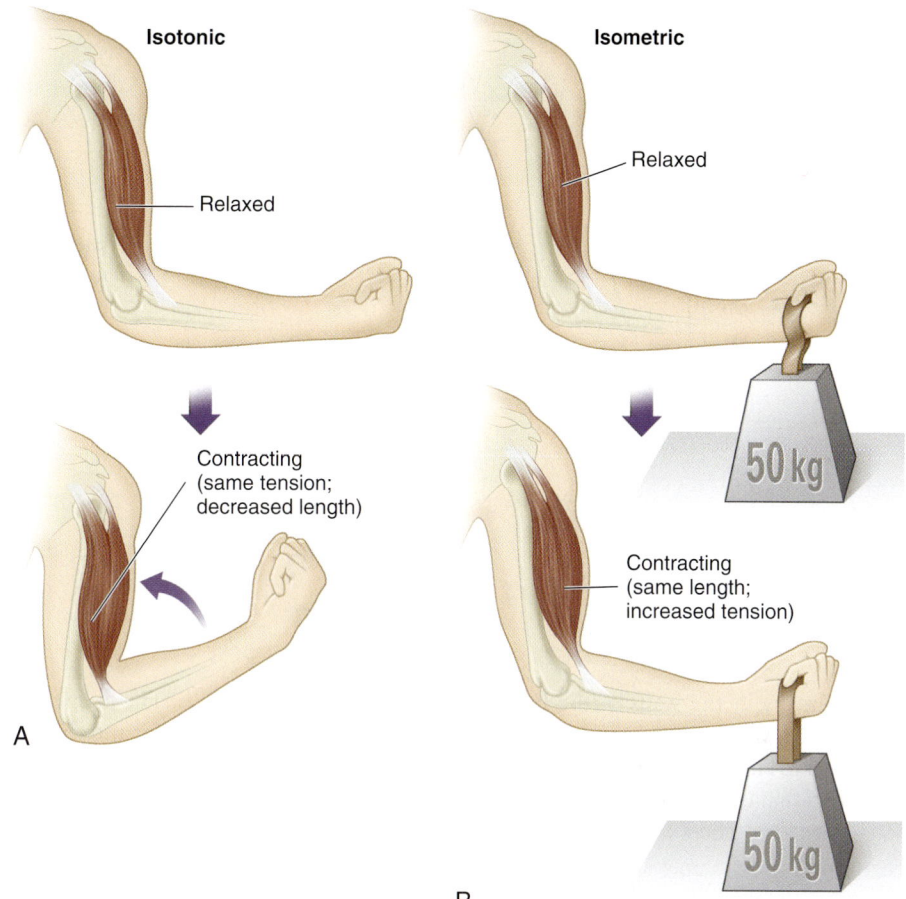

FIGURE 19-1 Muscle contraction types. **A,** Isotonic contractions produce movement. **B,** Isometric contractions do not produce movement. (Modified from Thibodeau GA, Patton KT: *The human body in health and disease,* ed 4, St Louis, 2005, Mosby.)

individually to cause the muscle to remain contracted at all times.

TYPES OF MUSCLE AND MUSCLE TISSUE

There are two main categories of muscles:
1. Voluntary
2. Involuntary

Voluntary and involuntary muscles are made up of one of the three types of muscle tissue (Figure 19-2):
1. Skeletal, also called "striated" or "voluntary"
2. Smooth, also called "involuntary" or "visceral"
3. Cardiac, striated in appearance but involuntary or smooth muscle in function

Voluntary Muscles

Voluntary muscles are so named because people can move these muscles when they want or can choose to hold them still. People have conscious (voluntary) control over these muscles. For example, you can voluntarily flex the biceps and triceps of your upper arm.

Skeletal muscles are voluntary muscles that attach to the bones of the skeleton and allow body movement. Under the microscope these muscle tissues appear **striated,** or "zebra striped," because they have light and dark bands of muscle fibers. These bands act to reinforce the tissue so that the fibers do not rupture during heavy lifting.

Involuntary Muscles

Involuntary muscles are muscles that people cannot control. These muscles work on their own without conscious stimulus. The diaphragm, a respiratory muscle of breathing, and the myocardium, the main muscle of the heart, are examples of involuntary muscles. They contract *involuntarily* in a rhythmic pattern to maintain breathing and heartbeat.

There are two types of involuntary muscle tissue: cardiac and smooth.
- **Smooth** muscle tissue (visceral muscle tissue) is nonstriated and is involuntary. This type of muscle makes up most of the organs of the body. For example, your stomach muscle is composed of smooth muscle tissue. They work without you thinking about them.
- **Cardiac** muscle has the same action as smooth muscle, so it is also involuntary. However, its microscopic appearance is striated. Cardiac muscle differs from the other muscles because microscopically it appears to be growing branches. The only place cardiac muscle is

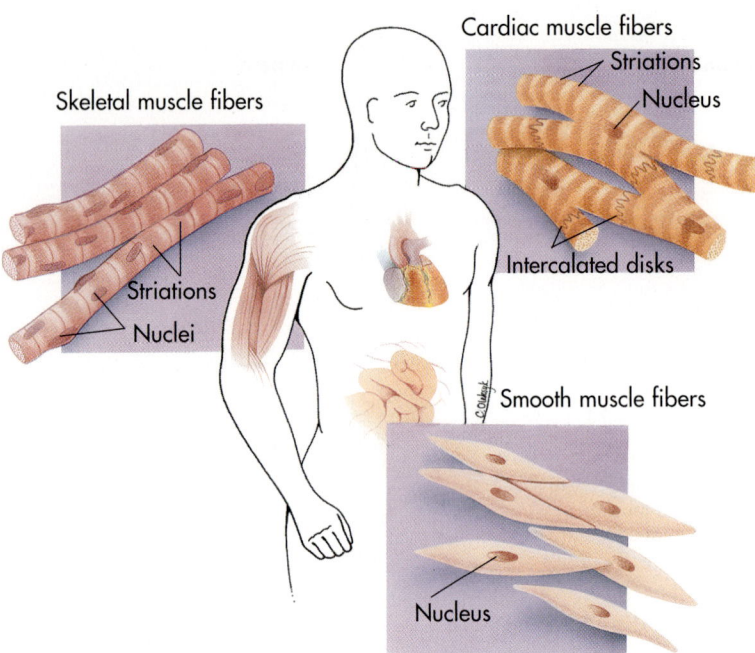

FIGURE 19-2 The three muscle types: skeletal (voluntary), smooth (involuntary), and cardiac (involuntary). (From Thibodeau GA, Patton KT: *The human body in health and disease*, ed 4, St Louis, 2005, Mosby.)

found is in the walls of the heart. The cardiac muscle must function as a complete unit instead of individual fibers. This is accomplished because of the *intercalated discs* that connect its fibers. When one fiber contracts, *all* connected fibers contract.

Characteristics of Muscle Tissue

Muscle tissue is unique in its structure and function and has the following four major characteristics:
1. **Contractility,** the ability of a muscle to shorten and thicken when given proper stimulation.
2. **Extensibility,** the ability of a muscle to stretch.
3. **Elasticity,** the ability of a muscle to return to its original length after stretching.
4. **Irritability,** the ability of a muscle to respond to stimulation.

PATIENT-CENTERED PROFESSIONALISM

Why must the medical assistant understand the principles of how muscles contract and the characteristics of muscle?

PRINCIPAL SKELETAL MUSCLES

You need to become familiar with the major skeletal muscles and groups. To better understand these muscles, it helps to understand why muscles are named the way they are.

Naming of Muscles

Every muscle in your body has a name. Four general categories are used to name the types of muscle, as follows:

1. The **prime mover,** or agonist, is the muscle responsible for movement when a group of muscles is contracting at the same time.
2. *Antagonists* are muscles that oppose or reverse the movement of the prime mover.
3. *Synergists* are muscles that help prime movers by stabilizing the movement.
4. **Fixators** are specialized synergists that stabilize the origin (nonmoving bone or muscle) of a prime mover so more tension is used to move the insertion bone.

In addition to names for "types" or "categories" of muscles, individual muscles all have names based on one or more characteristics of their function or structure.

Origin and Insertion

Muscles can be named for their origin and insertion. Where a muscle begins or is attached to a bone is its **origin.** Where it ends is its **insertion** point. Muscle origin is a fixed attachment, meaning it does not move, and muscle insertion is more movable. For example, the sternocleidomastoid muscle helps to rotate the head. It starts at the sternum and clavicle (origin) and ends at the mastoid process of the temporal bone (insertion) (Figure 19-3).

Location and Associated Bone

Muscles can also be named for their location, or the bone with which they are associated. Muscles are named by their location according to where the muscle is located in the body or near what organ. For example, the frontalis muscles overlie the frontal bones of the skull.

Size

Muscles named for their size indicate if they are large or small, narrow or wide. One example is the gluteus maximus, or

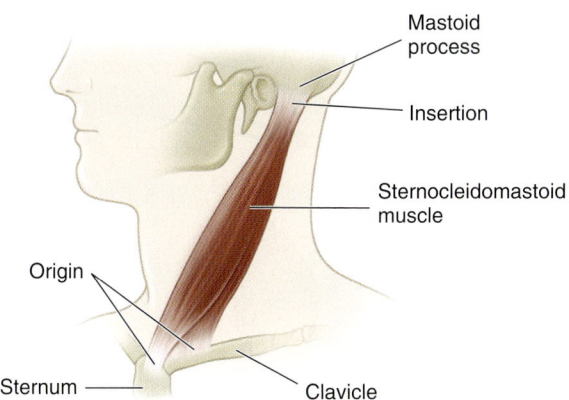

FIGURE 19-3 Sternocleidomastoid muscle. (Modified from Shiland BJ: *Mastering healthcare terminology,* ed 2, St. Louis, 2006, Mosby.)

buttock muscle. The gluteus maximus is the largest muscle in the body; the word *maximus* is Latin for "large."

Shape

Some muscle shapes are represented in their name. For instance, the **deltoid** muscle of the shoulder looks like an upside-down Greek letter D, called delta (δ).

Fiber Direction

Muscles may also be named for the direction of their fibers. Fiber direction can be vertical, horizontal, slanted, or crosswise (oblique), and the muscle group's name reflects the direction. The external oblique, a slanted muscle across and to the side of the abdomen and torso, is an example.

Number of Attachment Points

Muscles can be named for their number of attachment points, or origins (Figure 19-4). Naming of this type identifies how well the muscle is anchored to the bone. A prefix may be used to indicate the number of attachments. Examples include the biceps brachii (*bi* = two attachments), triceps brachii (*tri* = three attachments), and quadriceps femoris (*quad* = four attachments).

Use and Action

Finally, muscles can be named for the action of the muscle. For example, the flexors are responsible for flexing or bringing a body part toward the body. Muscles can also be named for their common use (Figure 19-5).

Actions of a muscle are typically indicated by the suffix *-or*. Examples are as follows:

- **Abductors** move a bone away from the midline. *Deltoid* moves the arm out to the side.
- **Adductors** move a bone toward the midline. *Pectoralis major* of the chest and *latissimus dorsi* of the back are used in swimming.
- **Levators** lift a bone. *Levator labii superioris* elevates the upper lip.

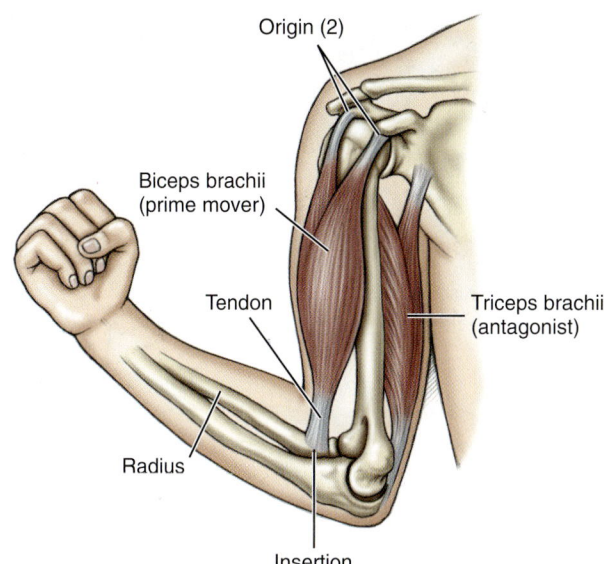

FIGURE 19-4 Origin and insertion points of a muscle. (From Herlihy B, Maebius NK: *The human body in health and illness,* ed 3, St Louis, 2007, Saunders.)

- **Depressors** lower a bone. *Subclavius* of the chest depresses the clavicle when lowering the forearm.
- **Flexors** bend a joint. *Biceps brachii* of the upper arm flexes the arm.
- **Extensors** straighten a joint. *Triceps brachii* of the upper arm extends the arm.
- **Rotators** move a joint on its axis. *Serratus anterior* under the arm rotates the scapula when throwing a ball.
- **Sphincters** are ringlike muscles that close an opening. *External anal* keeps the anal canal closed.

Muscles can have more than one action. For example, the *pectoralis major* muscle can flex, adduct, and rotate the arm.

Location of Major Muscles

Figure 19-6 illustrates the main muscles of the body from both the anterior view *(A)* and the posterior view *(B).*

Muscles of the Head

The main muscles of the head are those of facial expression and chewing (Table 19-1).
- *Muscles of expression* control a person's reaction to fear, joy, pain, and grief.
- *Muscles of chewing* or **mastication** control the lower jaw **(mandible).**

Muscles of the Neck

The neck muscles are slanted or diagonal and extend upward and downward. These muscles allow for rotation, flexion, and extension of the head and scapula (see Table 19-1).

Muscles of the Chest

The chest muscles control breathing. Table 19-1 highlights the thoracic wall muscles.

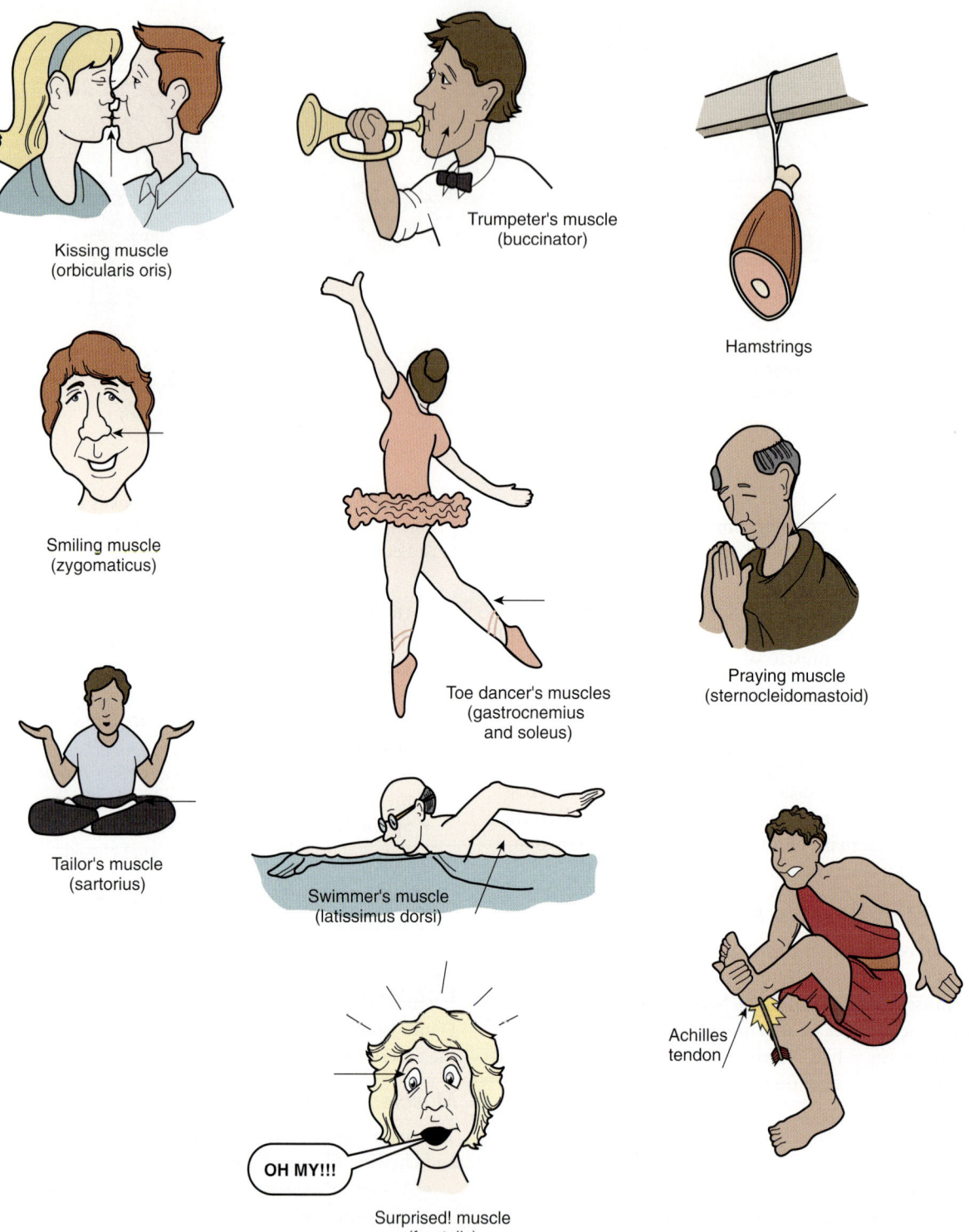

FIGURE 19-5 A variety of special muscles named for their common use. (Modified from Herlihy B, Maebius NK: *The human body in health and illness,* ed 3, St Louis, 2007, Saunders.)

TABLE 19-1

Skeletal Muscles

Muscle	Description	Origin to Insertion	Action

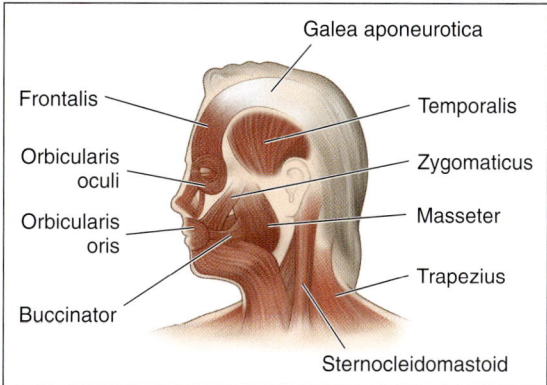

MUSCLES OF FACIAL EXPRESSION

Muscle	Description	Origin to Insertion	Action
Frontalis	Flat muscle that covers forehead	Cranial aponeurosis to eyebrows	Raises eyebrows
Orbicularis oculi	Circular muscle around eye	Maxilla and frontal bones to eyelid	Blinks and closes eye
Orbicularis oris	Circular muscle of mouth	Maxilla and mandible to lips	Closes and protrudes lips
Buccinator	Horizontal cheek muscle	Mandible and maxilla to skin around mouth	Flattens cheek
Zygomaticus	Diagonally from corner of mouth to cheekbone	Zygomatic bone to corner of mouth	Raises corner of mouth

MUSCLES OF MASTICATION

Muscle	Description	Origin to Insertion	Action
Temporalis	Fan-shaped muscle over temporal bone	Temporal bone to mandible	Closes jaw
Masseter	Covers lateral aspect of jaw	Zygomatic arch to mandible	Closes jaw

NECK MUSCLES

Muscle	Description	Origin to Insertion	Action
Sternocleidomastoid	Straplike muscle of neck	Sternum and clavicle to temporal bone	Flexes neck; rotates head
Trapezius	Large triangular muscle on posterior neck and shoulder	Occipital bone and spines of thoracic vertebrae to scapula	Extends neck; moves scapula

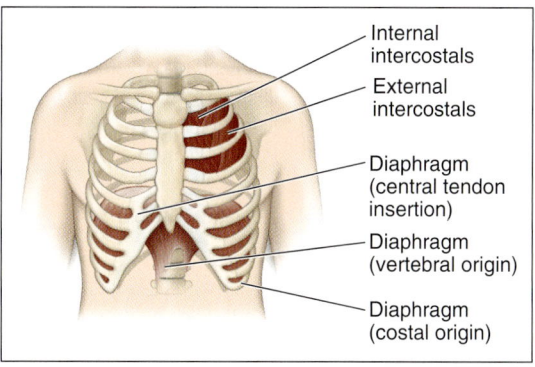

THORACIC WALL MUSCLES

Muscle	Description	Origin to Insertion	Action
External intercostals	Short muscles between ribs in the intercostal spaces	Ribs to rib below origin	Inspiration
Internal intercostals	Short muscles between ribs in the intercostal spaces	Ribs to rib above origin	Forced expiration
Diaphragm	Dome-shaped muscle between thorax and abdomen	Interior body wall to diaphragm	Inspiration

TABLE 19-1

Skeletal Muscles—cont'd

Muscle	Description	Origin to Insertion	Action

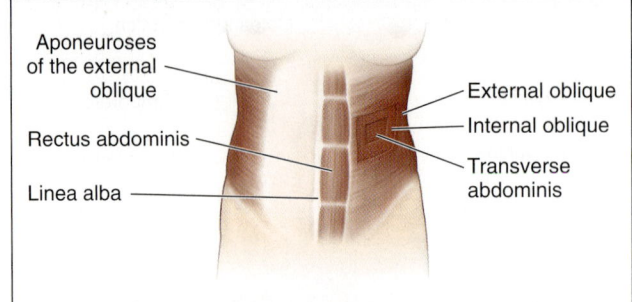

ABDOMINAL WALL MUSCLES

Muscle	Description	Origin to Insertion	Action
External oblique	Largest superficial abdominal wall muscle	Last eight ribs to iliac crest	Compresses abdomen
Internal oblique	Under external oblique	Iliac crest to lower ribs	Compresses abdomen
Rectus abdominis	Long straight muscle	Pubic bone to sternum and fifth to seventh ribs	Flexes vertebral column

SHOULDER AND ARM MUSCLES

Muscle	Description	Origin to Insertion	Action
Trapezius	Muscle on posterior neck and shoulder	Occipital bone to scapula	Adducts, elevates, and rotates scapula
Pectoralis major	Fan-shaped muscle that covers anterior chest (over heart area)	Sternum and clavicle to humerus	Adducts and flexes arm
Latissimus dorsi	Large, flat muscle of lower back region	Vertebrae to humerus	Adducts and rotates arm
Deltoid	Thick muscle that forms contour of shoulder	Clavicle and scapula to humerus	Abducts arm
Rotator cuff	Four muscles that form cuff over proximal humerus	Scapula to humerus	Rotates arm
Triceps brachii	Posterior compartment of arm that has three heads of origin	Humerus and scapula to ulna	Extends forearm
Biceps brachii	Anterior compartment of arm	Scapula to radius	Flexes and supinates forearm

LOWER EXTREMITY MUSCLES

Muscle	Description	Origin to Insertion	Action
Iliopsoas	Located in groin	Ilium and lower vertebrae to femur	Flexes hip
Gluteus maximus	Largest and most superficial muscle of buttocks	Ilium, sacrum, and coccyx to femur	Extends thigh
Gluteus minimus	Smallest and deepest of buttock muscles	Ilium to femur	Abducts and rotates thigh
Adductor muscles	Form muscle mass at medial side of each thigh	Pubis to femur	Adduct thigh

KNEE JOINT MUSCLES

Muscle	Description	Origin to Insertion	Action
Sartorius	Long, straplike muscle that lies obliquely across thigh; longest muscle in body	Ilium to medial tibia	Flexes thigh; rotates leg
Quadriceps femoris	Group of four muscles that forms fleshy mass of anterior thigh	Femur; except for rectus femoris, which originates on ilium to tibial tuberosity through patellar tendon	Extends knee; rectus femoris also flexes thigh
Hamstrings: Biceps femoris Semimembranosus Semitendinosus	Large fleshy muscle mass in posterior thigh; can be felt at back of knee	Ischial tuberosity to proximal tibia	Flexes leg; extends thigh

ANKLE AND FOOT MUSCLES

Muscle	Description	Origin to Insertion	Action
Tibialis anterior	Superficial muscle of anterior leg	Tibia to first metatarsal	Dorsiflexes foot
Soleus	Forms curved calf of leg	Tibia and fibula to Achilles tendon by way of calcaneus	Plantar-flexes foot

From Chester GA: *Modern medical assisting*, Philadelphia, 1998, Saunders.

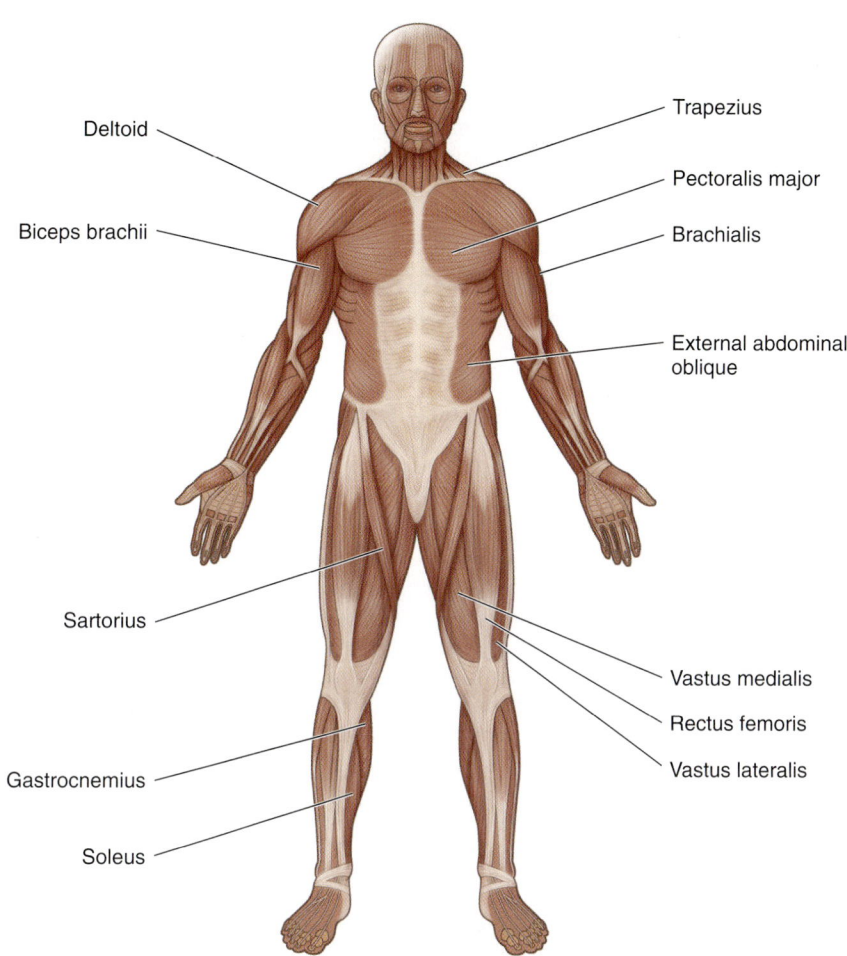
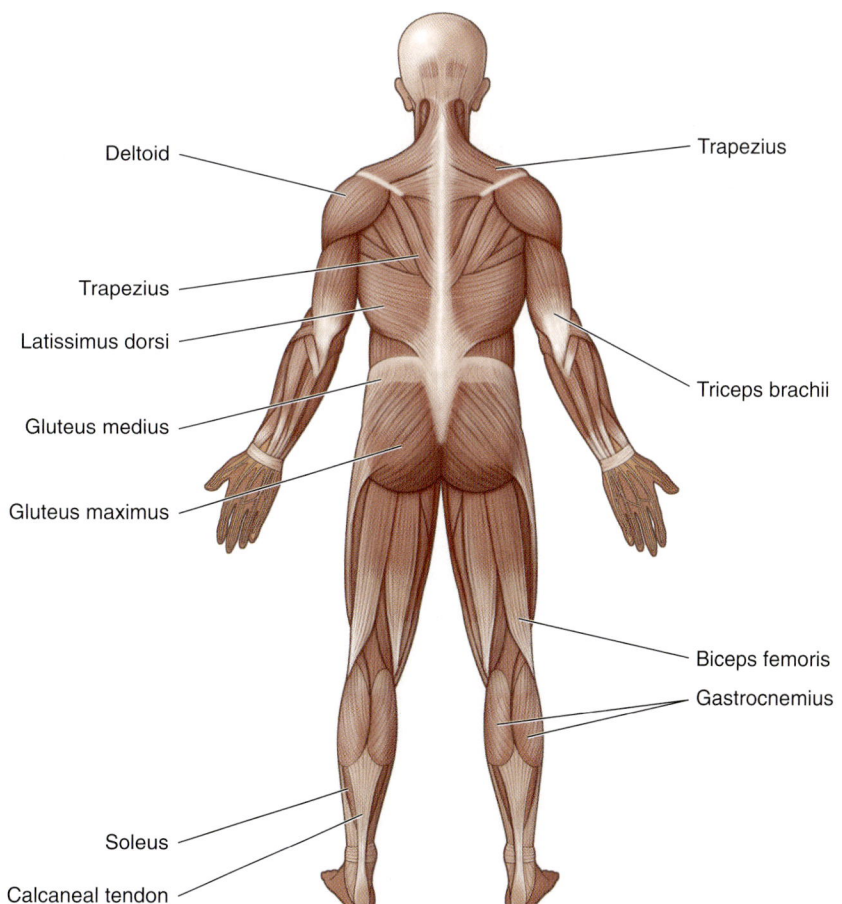

FIGURE 19-6 Muscles of the body. **A,** Anterior view. **B,** Posterior view.

Muscles of the Abdomen

Muscles of the abdomen control the movement of the abdominal wall and the pelvis. The abdominal muscles also assist in peristalsis, digestion, and elimination. Table 19-1 lists the three major muscles of the abdomen.

Muscles of the Upper Extremities

The muscles of the upper extremities move the shoulder, arm, forearm, wrist, hand, and fingers (see Table 19-1).

Muscles of the Lower Extremities

The lower extremity muscles assist in moving the thigh, knee, leg, ankle, foot, and toes (see Table 19-1).

PATIENT-CENTERED PROFESSIONALISM

Muscle names are not chosen at random. There are many factors associated with naming muscles, including their shape, location, closeness to bones, action, and size.
- *Why is it important for the medical assistant to learn about the relationship between the muscle and these factors?*

DISEASES AND DISORDERS OF THE MUSCULAR SYSTEM

Muscle disorders disrupt normal movement of the body. Several types of physicians treat muscle disorders. An *orthopedist* specializes in bone, joint, and muscle disorders. A *rheumatologist* diagnoses and treats diseases of the connective tissue and muscles. A *physiatrist* specializes in rehabilitative medicine, often needed after sports injuries. Muscle injuries (sprains and strains) and inflammatory conditions are some of the most common disorders seen in the medical office. Aging also causes a progressive loss of skeletal muscle and a decrease in strength, therefore making elderly persons more susceptible to falls. Box 19-1 provides information about this age-related muscle loss.

FOR YOUR INFORMATION

Aging affects the muscular system dramatically. There is a significant reduction in the size and strength of skeletal muscle because muscle fibers decrease in number and are smaller in diameter as we age. Muscle fibers contain less ATP, glycogen reserves, and myoglobin. Blood flow to active muscles decreases because the cardiovascular performance decreases.

BOX 19-1

Sarcopenia, Osteoporosis' Counterpart

In 1988, Dr. Irwin Rosenburg put a name to the skeletal muscle loss experienced by the aging population. "Sarcopenia," a deficiency of skeletal muscle, is as serious a health threat as osteoporosis (bone loss that leaves bones weak and easy to break). Sarcopenia robs aging people of muscle, leaving them weak and frail. Often, people do not even notice the loss until they are unable to do simple tasks such as walking or lifting themselves from a chair.

Sarcopenia involves not only losing strength and endurance but also gaining fat tissue. As muscle tissue disappears, fat takes its place. Remaining muscle fibers are weaker and do not contract as well, fatigue easier, and do not generate heat or burn calories.

Lack of exercise seems to worsen the effects of sarcopenia. Resistance training, such as weightlifting, places a burden on the muscles that they are not used to handling. The muscles respond by increasing in size. As muscles adapt, the weight is increased and the built-up muscle increases. Even though sarcopenia is a normal part of aging, failure to address the body's need for exercise will result in exaggerated muscle loss.

Muscle Injuries and Infection

Injuries to the skeletal muscles can result from overuse or trauma. Two common injuries are sprains and strains. People often use the terms interchangeably, but they are actually two different types of injuries. Muscle **strains** involve overstretching or tearing of muscle fibers. A **sprain** is an injury involving the stretching or tearing of a **ligament** or joint. Inflammation can be associated with these types of injuries. Inflammation may respond to treatment quickly, but a tear in the muscle may require several weeks of healing before the muscle repairs itself, often with fibrous tissue and thus forming scars.

- Stress-induced muscle tension can result in **myalgia** and stiffness in the neck.
- A **hernia** develops when a visceral organ (e.g., stomach or intestines) bulges (protrudes) through a weakness in the muscular wall (abdominal or inguinal). Surgical repair is required, or blood circulation to the intestines may be impaired, resulting in tissue necrosis (death).
- **Torticollis** (**wryneck**) is a condition in which a shortened sternocleidomastoid muscle can cause the head to tilt to the affected side (Figure 19-7). Torticollis may result from a congenital defect, birth canal trauma, a CNS disorder, or an accident.

Tetanus and trichinosis are two muscle diseases caused by organisms that enter the body through open wounds or improperly cooked meat.

- *Tetanus* ("lockjaw") is caused by the bacterium *Clostridium tetani,* which enters the body through a

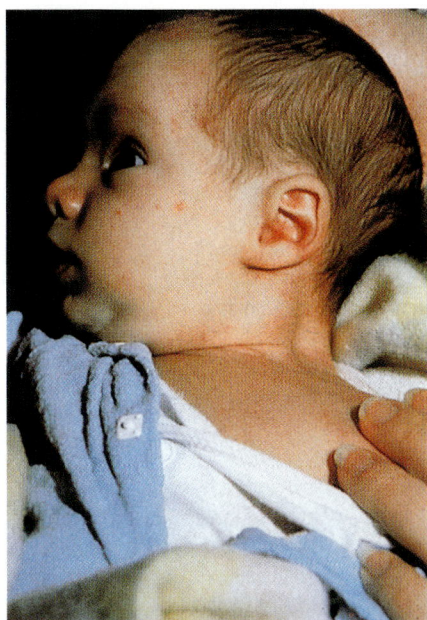

FIGURE 19-7 Torticollis. (From Zitelli BJ, Davis HW: *Atlas of pediatric physical diagnosis,* ed 4, St Louis, 2002, Mosby.)

TABLE 19-2
Muscle Drug Classifications

Drug Classification	Common Generic (Brand) Drugs
Analgesics/antiinflammatories Treat pain and inflammation	oxycodone ASA (Percodan) hydrocodone APAP (Vicodin) diclofenac sodium (Voltaren) etodolac (Lodine)
Skeletal muscle relaxants Treat localized spasms from muscle injury	cyclobenzaprine (Flexeril) carisoprodol (Soma)
Anticholinesterase Inhibits release of cholinesterase, allowing acetylcholine to accumulate; this increases muscle strength and function	ambenonium (Mytelase) neostigmine (Prostigmin)

BOX 19-2
Common Signs and Symptoms of Muscle Disease

Fibromyositis	Muscle and tendon inflammation
Contusion	Bruise resulting from internal bleeding and inflammation
Cramps	Painful muscle **spasms** (involuntary muscle twitches) or contractions
Myalgia	Muscle pain
Myositis	Muscle inflammation
Strain	Overstretching or tearing of a muscle
General complaints	Pain or tenderness, fatigue, malaise, muscle weakness, and fever

BOX 19-3
Diagnostic Tests and Procedures for the Muscles

Electromyography (EMG)	EMG records strength of muscle contraction resulting from electrical stimulation to muscle
Magnetic resonance imaging (MRI)	Magnetic properties of MRI used to record detailed information about internal structures
Muscle biopsy	Removal of muscle tissue for microscopic examination

deep, open wound. The organisms release a toxin that causes stiffness and rigidity of the muscles, especially in the jaw.
- *Trichinosis* is caused by a parasite found in uncooked meat, especially pork. The parasite enters the digestive tract and deposits larvae into the muscle tissue.

Drugs may be prescribed to treat muscle problems (Table 19-2). Medical assistants need to be able to recognize the common signs and symptoms of and the diagnostic tests for the different types of muscle system disease.
- Study Box 19-2 to familiarize yourself with the common signs and symptoms.
- Study Box 19-3 to learn about common diagnostic tests.
- Study Table 19-3 to understand the two major diseases that affect the muscular system.

PATIENT-CENTERED PROFESSIONALISM

- *Why is it important for the medical assistant to understand the pathophysiology, signs and symptoms, diagnostic tests, and treatments for disorders of the muscular system?*

CONCLUSION

The muscular system is crucial to maintaining our movement, posture, and body heat. However, it does not function alone. Muscles provide movement, but they work together to achieve coordinated movement only when the bones, joints, and nerves interact with the muscles. Muscles react to a stimulus by pulling toward it, away from it, rotating, and so on. Muscles are best studied by grouping them according to their specific function or location, by understanding how they are named, and by considering their type. As with the other body systems, a good understanding of the muscular system can help medical assistants perform more competently and communicate more clearly, resulting in more effective care for patients.

TABLE 19-3
Diseases and Disorders of the Muscular System

Disease and Description	Etiology	Signs and Symptoms	Diagnosis	Therapy	Interventions
Myasthenia gravis Progressive weakening and **atrophy** of muscles	Autoimmune disease affecting normal transmission of nerve impulses	Muscle weakness, usually starting with facial muscles and eye	Clinical symptoms, especially ptosis of eyelids; blood tests, chest x-rays, EMG; injection of anticholinesterase (improves muscle strength temporarily)	Symptomatic and supportive; thymectomy if tumor is involved; drug therapy: corticosteroids, pyridostigmine (Mestinon)	Encourage patient to rest and follow drug therapy as prescribed by physician
Fibromyalgia Syndrome that causes chronic pain in muscles and soft tissue surrounding joints	Unknown	Patient complains of dull, aching muscle pain throughout the body, especially in neck and shoulder area; other complaints include stiffness, fatigue, depression, and disturbed sleep	Patient history; on examination, physician will apply moderate amount of pressure in specific areas (tender points)	Patient education; low-impact exercise (e.g., walking, swimming), NSAIDs, sometimes antidepressants	Provide emotional support
Muscular dystrophy Group of X-linked genetic disorders characterized by progressive atrophy of symmetrical muscle groups	Unknown	Loss of muscle strength without neuronal involvement leading to progressive deformity	Elevations of muscle enzymes in the blood (CPK or CPK MM), but definitively by muscle biopsy	Supportive measures such as physical therapy and orthopedic procedures to minimize the deformity	Genetic counseling

CPK, Creatine phosphokinase; *EMG,* electromyography; *NSAIDs,* nonsteroidal antiinflammatories.

Chapter Summary

Reinforce your understanding of the material in this chapter by reviewing the curriculum objectives and key content points below.

1. **Define, appropriately use, and spell all the Key Terms for this chapter.**
   - Review the Key Terms if necessary.
2. **State the three functions of muscle and explain the importance of each.**
   - Muscles enable movement, both voluntary and involuntary, and they provide support for bones and organs.
   - Muscles create body heat to maintain internal temperature.
   - Muscles help other body systems function (e.g., digestive muscles, respiratory muscles).
3. **Explain the basic structure of muscle.**
   - Muscle tissue consists of bundles of long muscle fibers.
   - Connective tissue holds the fibers in the bundles.
   - A fibrous sheath covers, supports, and separates muscles.
4. **Describe the structure and function of tendons.**
   - Tendons are strong, white cordlike structures made up of collagenous fibers.
   - Tendons connect muscle to bone.
5. **Explain how a muscle contracts.**
   - Nerve impulses stimulate muscles to make them contract.
   - Muscles can only pull; they cannot push.
   - Effective muscle movements are smooth and can be sustained.
6. **Identify and define the two types of muscle.**
   - Muscles can be voluntary or involuntary.
   - Voluntary muscles are consciously moved.
   - Involuntary muscles move on their own to support their various body systems (e.g., heart, breathing).

7. **Briefly describe the three types of muscle tissue.**
   - Involuntary muscles are either smooth (nonstriated) or cardiac and make up organs or cardiac muscle, which appears striated and works as one unit in the heart.
   - Voluntary muscles are made up of skeletal muscle tissue and allow for lifting, moving, and bending. Voluntary muscles move the skeleton and the face.
8. **List four characteristics of muscle tissue.**
   - Muscle tissue is contractible, extensible, elastic, and "irritable" to varying degrees.
9. **List seven ways muscles can be named.**
   - Muscles can be named for their origin and insertion, location, size, shape, fiber direction, attachment points, and type of action.
10. **Locate and identify the main skeletal muscles of the body.**
    - Review Figure 19-6 and Table 19-1.
11. **List seven common signs and symptoms of muscular system disorders.**
    - Review Box 19-2.
12. **List two common diagnostic tests for muscular disease and describe the use of each.**
    - Electromyography (EMG) is a procedure that records the electrical activity of the muscles.
    - Magnetic resonance imaging (MRI) uses magnetic properties to record detailed information about internal structures and soft tissue.
    - Review Box 19-3.
13. **State the two most common muscular disorders seen in the physician's office.**
    - Myalgia and some form of muscle strain or sprain brought on by stress, trauma, or overexertion are most often seen.
14. **List two muscular diseases and briefly describe the etiology, signs and symptoms, diagnosis, therapy, and interventions for each.**
    - Review Table 19-3.
15. **Analyze a realistic medical office situation and apply your understanding of the muscular system to determine the best course of action.**
    - A medical assistant's understanding of the muscular system can be helpful when the assistant is working with patients who have injured muscles.
16. **Describe the impact on patient care when medical assistants have a solid understanding of the structure and function of the muscular system.**
    - Knowing how the muscles interact with each other and work in pairs helps medical assistants understand how they help to move the body and how injuries can occur.
    - A good understanding of the muscular system also reinforces for medical assistants the importance of following the prescribed treatment plan.

PRACTICAL APPLICATIONS

If you have accomplished the objectives in this chapter, you will be able to make better choices as a medical assistant. Take another look at this situation and decide what you would do.

Tommy, age 18, has been playing sports since childhood. He has used weights to increase and strengthen the muscles of his body. Tommy has often wondered just how the muscles of his body work to make him move and what happens when one muscle contracts. He knows that some muscles are involuntary and some are voluntary.

Two days ago Tommy was skiing when he fell and twisted his left ankle. The emergency room physician told him that he had strained and sprained his ankle. In explanation, the physician also said that the extensors in the ankle had the greatest injury and that the contusion was going to become worse if Tommy did not keep ice on the ankle overnight. Because of the severity of the injury, Tommy was to see an orthopedist the next morning. The orthopedist has ordered antiinflammatories and muscle relaxants.

Tommy now has some new questions for the medical assistant about muscles, what the antiinflammatories will do, and what this might have done to his muscles had he been older.

Would you be able to answer Tommy's questions?
1. How do muscles work to make the body move?
2. How do you define "synergistic muscles"?
3. How do you define "antagonistic muscles"?
4. What do voluntary muscles do in the body?
5. Define involuntary muscles.
6. What is the difference between a sprain and a strain?
7. What are the signs of a sprain?
8. Why would antiinflammatories and muscle relaxants be ordered?
9. If Tommy were older, what would the physician expect the aging process to have done to Tommy's skeletal muscles?
10. What are isotonic and isometric movements?

WEB SEARCH

1. **Research treatments available for the neuromuscular disease amyotrophic lateral sclerosis (ALS).** Progressive muscular atrophy occurs when nerve impulses are not generated.

- **Keywords:** Use the following keywords in your search: Charcot syndrome, Lou Gehrig disease, ALS.

WORD PARTS: Muscular System

Combining Forms

fasci/o	fascia
kines, kinesi/o	movement
muscul/o	muscle
my/o	muscle
ten/o, tendin/o	tendon
ton/o	tone

Suffixes

-asthenia	weakness
-trophy	nutrition

ABBREVIATIONS: Muscular System

ALS	amyotrophic lateral sclerosis
DTR	deep tendon reflex
EMG	electromyography
lig	ligament
NSAID	nonsteroidal antiinflammatory drug
OT	occupational therapy
PT	physical therapy

Urinary System

20

evolve http://evolve.elsevier.com/klieger/medicalassisting

The urinary system eliminates waste in our bodies and also maintains water and chemical balance, keeping our bodies in homeostasis. The urinary system depends on the other body systems to carry out its functions. For example, when you need to urinate, your bladder sends a message to the brain, letting it know of this need; thus the brain controls urination. Also, the digestive system creates fluid waste products that need to be eliminated by the urinary system, and muscles contract and relax to move waste products through the body and allow urine to exit the body.

Actually, as with the other body systems, the urinary system interacts in some way with all the body's other systems. Knowing the structure and function of all body systems, including the urinary system, will help medical assistants to understand the disease process. Their patients will receive the benefits of this understanding.

LEARNING OBJECTIVES

You will be able to do the following after completing this chapter:

Key Terms
1. Define, appropriately use, and spell all the Key Terms for this chapter.

Major Functions of the Urinary System
2. State the five major functions of the urinary system.

Urinary System Structure
3. Identify and locate the four major structures in the urinary system.
4. Describe the structure and main functions of the kidneys.
5. Explain the purpose of urine and describe urine formation.
6. Explain the structure of a nephron and its function in the kidney.
7. Describe the structure and function of the ureters.
8. Describe the structure and function of the urinary bladder.
9. Describe the structure and function of the urethra.

Diseases and Disorders of the Urinary System
10. List 13 common signs and symptoms of urinary system disorders.
11. List seven common diagnostic tests for urinary disease and describe the use of each.
12. List six urinary diseases and disorders and briefly describe the etiology, signs and symptoms, diagnosis, therapy, and interventions for each.
13. Explain the purpose of dialysis and list two types.

Patient-Centered Professionalism
14. Analyze a realistic medical office situation and apply your understanding of the urinary system to determine the best course of action.
15. Describe the impact on patient care when medical assistants have a solid understanding of the structure and function of the urinary system.

KEY TERMS

The Key Terms for this chapter have been organized into sections so that you can easily see the terminology associated with each aspect of the urinary system.

Major Functions of the Urinary System
azotemia
erythropoietin
excretory system
renin
uremia
urinary system

Continued

Structure of the Urinary System
Kidneys

aldosterone	loop of Henle
antidiuretic hormone (ADH)	medulla
Bowman's capsule	nephrons
calyces	pyramids
capsule	renal artery
cortex	renal pelvis
filtration	retroperitoneal
glomerulus	solutes
hilum	urea
kidneys	urine

Ureters

renal calculi	urinary reflux
ureters	

Urinary Bladder

micturition	urinary bladder
micturition reflex	urination
rugae	voiding
trigone	

Urethra

meatus	urethra
semen	

Diseases and Disorders of the Urinary System
Signs and Symptoms

albuminuria	ketonuria
anuresis	nocturia
bacteriuria	oliguria
diuresis	polydipsia
dysuria	polyuria
enuresis	proteinuria
frequency	pyuria
glycosuria	retention
hematuria	urgency
incontinence	

Diagnostic Tests and Procedures

blood urea nitrogen (BUN)	nephrologist
creatinine clearance test	renal computed tomography
cystoscopy	urinalysis
intravenous pyelography (IVP)	urologist
kidneys, ureters, and bladder (KUB)	

Diseases and Disorders

acute renal failure (ARF)	interstitial cystitis
chronic renal failure (CRF)	polycystic kidney
cystitis	pyelonephritis
glomerulonephritis	renal failure

Related Urinary Terms

dialysis	kidney transplant
diuretics	peritoneal dialysis
hemodialysis	

PRACTICAL APPLICATIONS

Read the following scenario and keep it in mind as you learn about the urinary system in this chapter.

Juanita is a regular patient in the medical office and has been in good health most of her life. At her office visit, she complains of pain in the flanks of her legs, in her lower abdomen, and in her back under her ribs. She also says that she has had burning and frequency of urination that has become progressively worse over 2 weeks. Furthermore, she says when she has to go to the bathroom, she has to hurry or she will not make it. The burning is not on the perineum but occurs as she starts the flow of urine. These symptoms have only made her incontinence worse, and she now has nocturia.

When asked if she can pinpoint anything new in her hygiene routine, Juanita states that she has been using a new perfumed soap on a regular basis to take her bath. On obtaining a urinalysis, hematuria is present. In addition, white blood cells are found on the microscopic examination. The physician has prescribed medications for treating what he has diagnosed as "urinary cystitis." Juanita would like to talk to the medical assistant to ask some questions.

Would you be able to answer Juanita's questions?

MAJOR FUNCTIONS OF THE URINARY SYSTEM

The **urinary system,** an **excretory system** ("excrete" means to separate and eliminate waste from the blood, tissues, and organs), performs five major functions. An easy way to remember these functions is with the acronym "FREPS," as follows:

1. **Filtration** filters toxic wastes out of the bloodstream for removal from the body (products of cell metabolism, excess salts, and urea).
2. **R**eabsorption (resorption) retains essential elements (water, sugar, and salts) that the body needs to maintain pH and homeostasis.
3. **E**xcretion excretes the waste products outside the body by way of the urethra.
4. **P**roduction of **erythropoietin** (a hormone that stimulates red blood cell production in the red bone marrow) is activated when the kidneys do not receive enough oxygen.
5. **S**ecretion of **renin** (enzyme needed for blood pressure regulation). If a person's blood pressure is insufficient to allow filtration in the glomerulus, renin is released into the blood and activates the blood protein *angiotensin,* which raises the blood pressure by causing the blood vessels to constrict.

Maintaining the proper water and electrolyte balance within the body is essential to good body homeostasis. Water, salts, and other substances are lost through urination, perspiration, digestion, and the respiratory process. If the body is to function properly, a normal balance of water and electrolytes must be maintained.

The pH scale ranges from 0 (very acidic) to 14 (very alkaline). The normal pH of urine is 6.5, or slightly acidic. When this system does not work as it should, toxins and nitrogen-containing waste materials build up in the bloodstream, and **uremia** or **azotemia** may occur.

PATIENT-CENTERED PROFESSIONALISM

- Why is it important for the medical assistant to understand all the functions of the urinary system?

STRUCTURE OF THE URINARY SYSTEM

The urinary organs consist of a pair of kidneys that secrete urine and two ureters that transport the urine from each kidney to the urinary bladder, in which urine is stored until the urethra carries it outside the body (Figure 20-1).

Kidneys

The **kidneys** are main organs of the urinary system and are crucial to the proper functioning of our bodies.

Location

The kidneys are located in the dorsal aspect of the body (**retroperitoneal**), about 1½ to 2 inches above the waist in the

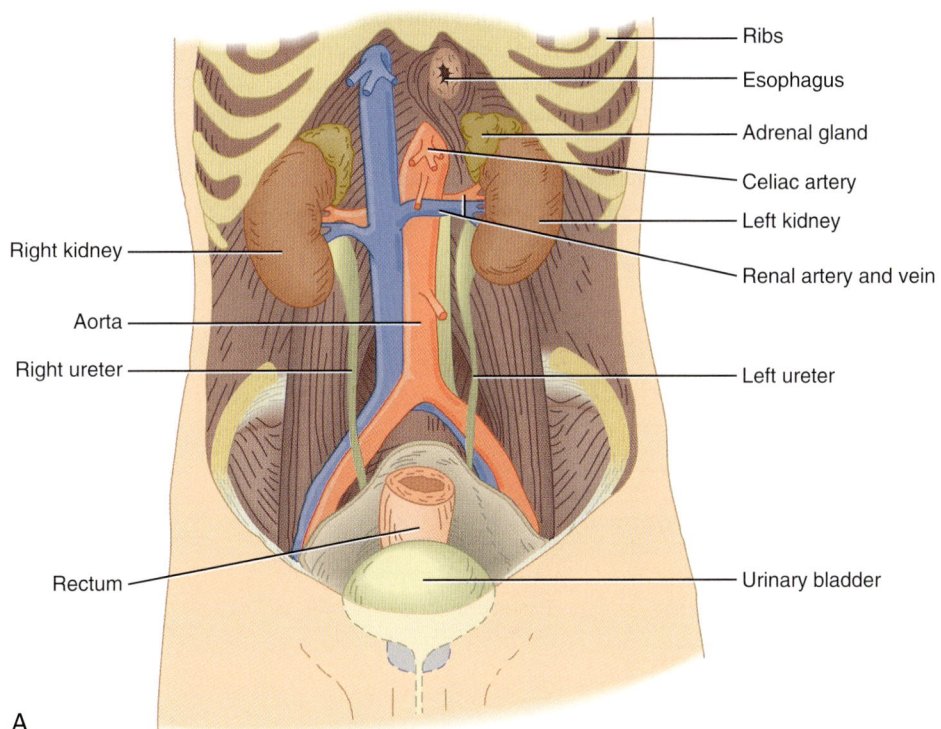

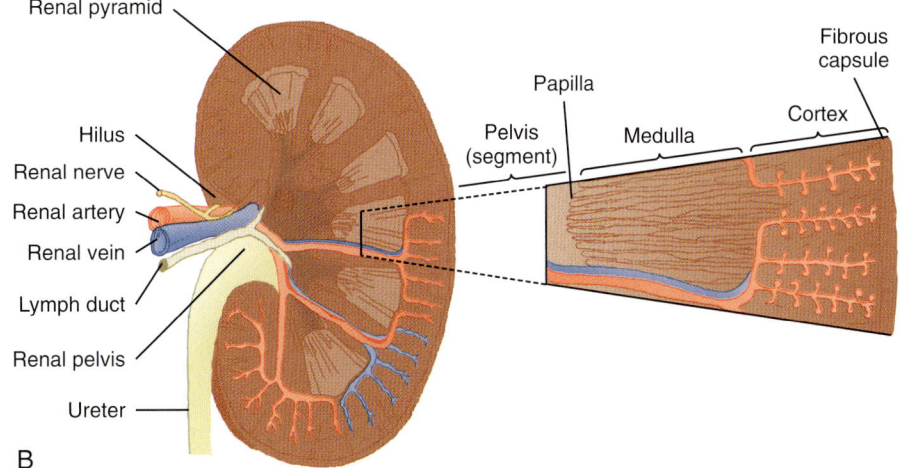

FIGURE 20-1 The urinary system. **A,** Anatomical relationship of the kidneys and related structures. **B,** Anatomy of the kidney. (Modified from Black JM et al: *Medical-surgical nursing: clinical management for positive outcomes,* ed 8, St Louis, 2009, Saunders.)

lumbar area on either side of the spinal column and are protected by the ribs. To find your kidneys, try the following:
- Stand up and put your hands on your hips (with your thumbs pointing toward your back).
- Move your hands up until you can feel your ribs.
- Your thumbs should be located at your kidneys.

Located on top of each kidney is an adrenal gland, as discussed further in Chapter 22. The adrenal glands release **aldosterone,** a hormone that maintains the balance of sodium and chloride ions in the blood. The right kidney is positioned slightly lower than the left kidney because the liver pushes the right kidney downward. The kidneys are held in place by bands of connective tissue and cushioned by fat deposits. A condition known as *renal ptosis* (sagging or prolapse of the kidney) occurs in very thin people as a result of inadequate fatty cushions.

Function

Metabolic wastes are excreted mainly by the kidneys, but as mentioned in previous chapters, the lungs, skin, and digestive tract also dispose of metabolic wastes (Figure 20-2). The kidneys also regulate the water-salt balance of the body fluids and maintain the body's pH.

The main function of the kidneys is to filter **urea** and other waste products from the blood. This process allows for the production of **urine.** Urine is composed of 95% water and 5% solid wastes. These wastes include nitrogenous wastes and some electrolytes (e.g., sodium, potassium). Daily production of urine is 1.5 to 2.5 L. Kidney failure, or **renal failure,** occurs if the kidneys produce less than 30 mL of urine per hour.

Urine Composition. Urine concentration and volume are controlled by actions of the following factors:
- *Renin.* When the filtration process of the kidneys declines, specialized cells within the kidneys release renin. Renin is an enzyme that reacts with a blood protein to form a substance that stimulates the adrenal gland to secrete aldosterone.
- *Aldosterone.* The release of aldosterone causes increased sodium reabsorption and concentrated urine.
- **Antidiuretic hormone (ADH).** A drop in blood pressure causes the posterior pituitary gland to secrete ADH, which causes increased water reabsorption. This process results in urine that is concentrated because of decreased urination and increased blood pressure (because more fluid is found in blood vessels).

Urine Formation. Urine formation occurs in the nephron when blood enters the kidney. Blood enters through the **renal artery,** which subdivides into smaller branches (arterioles) that take blood to Bowman's capsule and circulate it through the **glomerulus,** a cluster of capillaries that allows for filtration

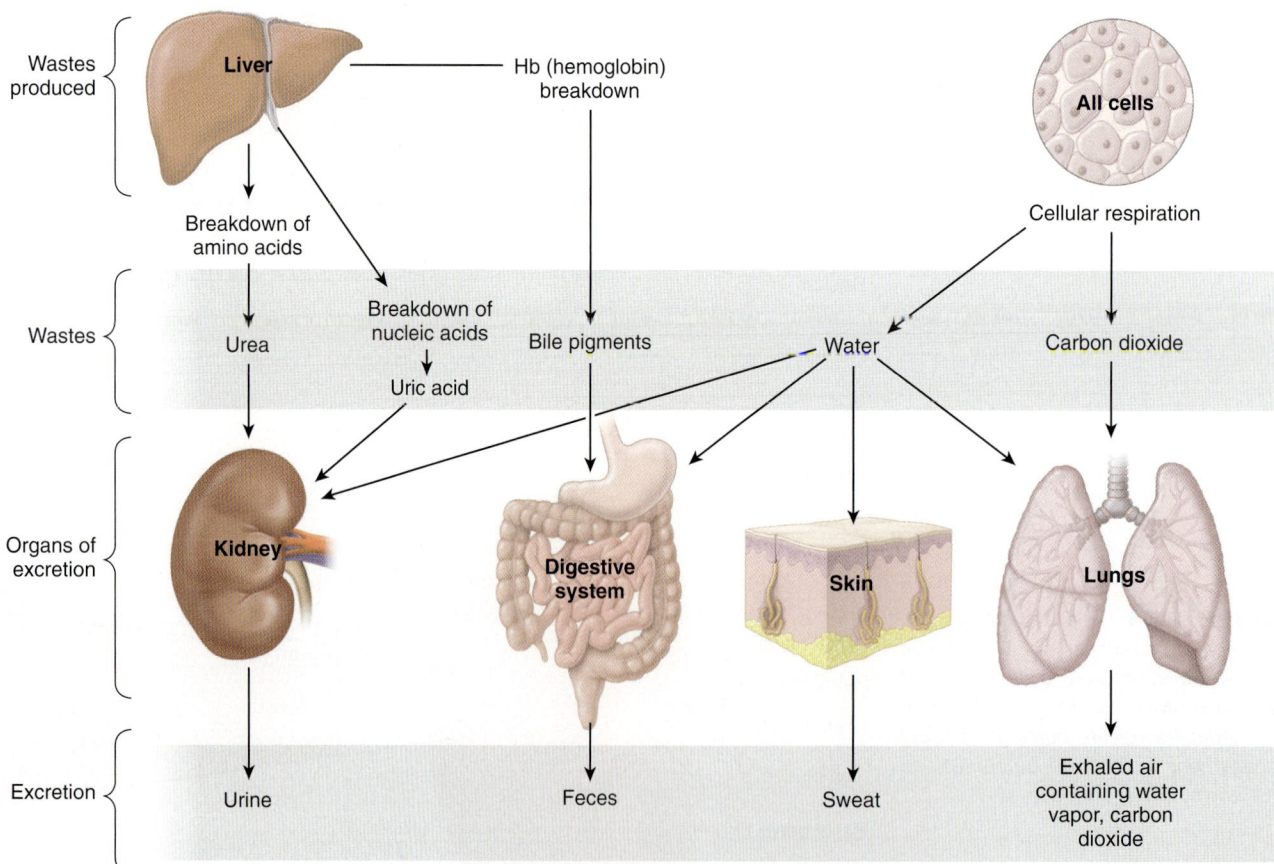

FIGURE 20-2 Wastes containing nitrogen are produced by the liver and transported to the kidneys. The kidneys excrete these wastes in the urine. (Modified from Solomon EP: *Introduction to human anatomy and physiology,* ed 3, St Louis, 2009, Saunders.)

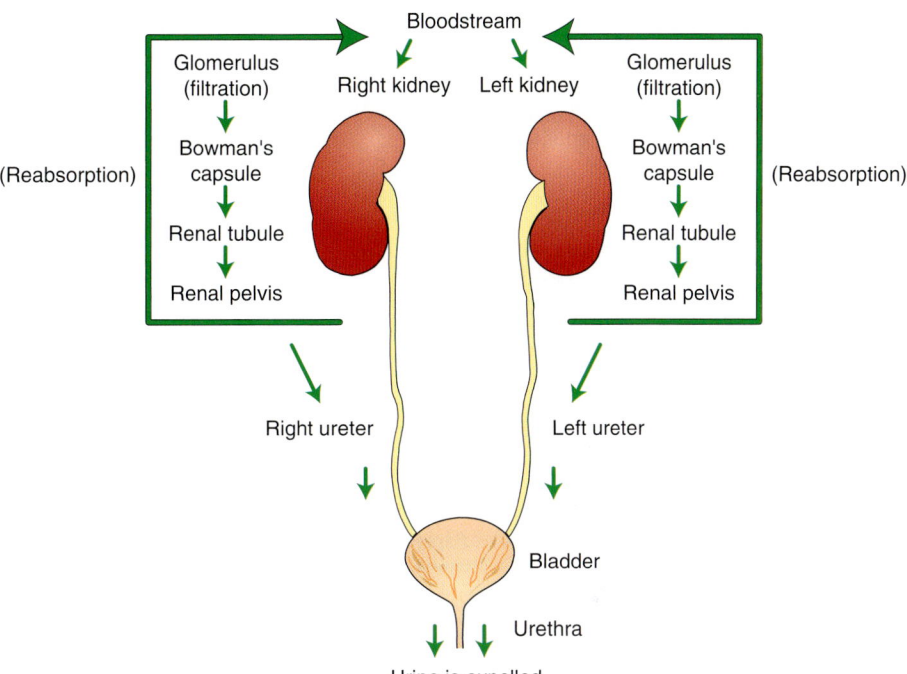

FIGURE 20-3 Diagram of the process of forming and expelling urine. (From Leonard PC: *Building a medical vocabulary*, ed 6, St Louis, 2005, Saunders.)

of fluids. Blood pressure forces small molecules (e.g., water, electrolytes, nutrients, and waste materials) out of the blood, through the glomerulus, and into the renal tubule. This process is called **filtration**. Within the renal tubules, water, electrolytes, and nutrients needed by the body are reabsorbed by the cells and returned to the blood. Toxins are then carried out with the remaining fluid, and urine is formed (Table 20-1 and Figure 20-3).

Structure

It is important to understand the external, internal, and microscopic structure of the kidney.

External Structure. If you have ever seen a kidney bean or a bean-shaped swimming pool, you have a good idea of the shape of a kidney. It is about 5 cm (2 inches) wide and 10 cm (4 inches) long, with a thickness of 2.5 cm (1 inch)—about the size of a fist. Each kidney is held in a fibrous **capsule**. The median side of each kidney has a depression called the **hilum**, or *hilus*, where the blood vessels, ureter, and nerves enter and exit the kidney.

Internal Structure. The kidney has three main areas: the cortex, medulla, and renal pelvis.

- The **cortex** is the outer layer. It is located next to the fibrous capsule (forms the outside of the kidney) and appears granular because it contains filters.
- The **medulla** is the inner layer. It is divided into sections shaped like triangles, called **pyramids**. The pyramids have collecting tubules that empty into the renal pelvis, the main collecting area for urine. The cuplike edges of the renal pelvis closest to the pyramids (called the **calyces**) collect urine formed in the kidneys.
- The **renal pelvis** narrows to form the ureter, which empties into the bladder.

TABLE 20-1

Urine Formation Process

Pressure	Process	Types of Molecules
Filtration	Blood pressure forces small molecules from glomerulus into Bowman's capsule	Water, glucose, proteins, salts, urea, creatinine, uric acid
Reabsorption (resorption)	Selective molecules are returned to blood	Water, glucose, proteins, salts
Secretion of toxins	Molecules continue through nephrons to collecting ducts	Uric acid, creatinine, ammonia, salts
Reabsorption of water	Water and salts return to nephrons to be excreted	Water, salts
Excretion	Wastes are excreted into collecting ducts in the form of urine	Water, salts, urea, uric acid, ammonia, salts, creatinine

Microscopic Structure. The main functioning units of the kidney are the **nephrons** (Figure 20-4). Each kidney consists of about 1 million nephrons. A nephron is a microscopic unit responsible for filtering waste products from the blood. The nephrons are funnel shaped, with a single coiled tube that twists into various shapes. At the beginning of the tube is a cup-shaped (or C-shaped) capsule called **Bowman's capsule**. This structure surrounds the glomerulus, a group of capillaries responsible for filtering the blood. The filtered blood enters a series of tubules and ends with the collecting tubule, which empties into the renal pelvis that empties urine into the bladder. It is through this tubular system that nutrients and

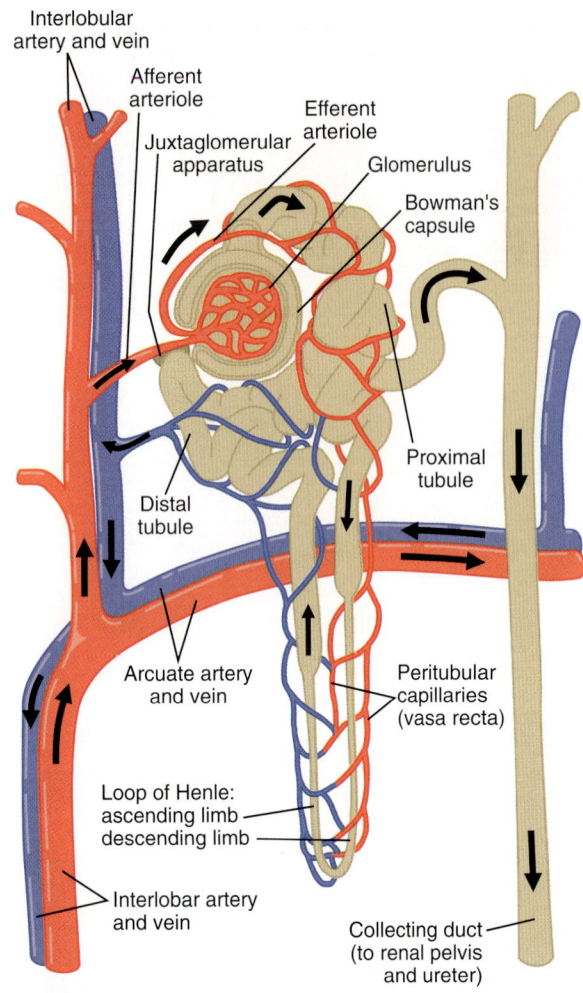

FIGURE 20-4 The nephron unit. (From Black JM et al: *Medical-surgical nursing: clinical management for positive outcomes,* ed 8, St Louis, 2009, Saunders.)

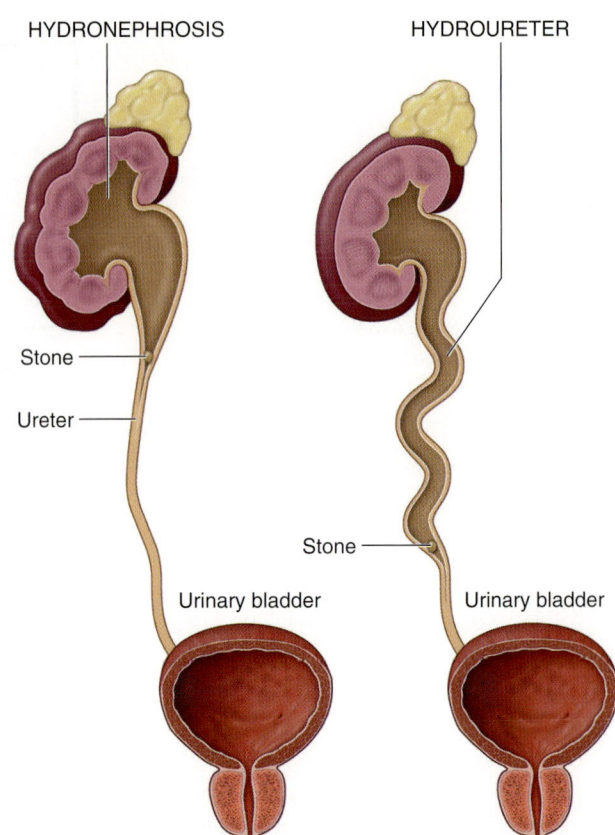

FIGURE 20-5 Hydronephrosis is the dilation of the renal pelvis and calyces that result from anatomical or functional processes interrupting the flow of urine (e.g., a stone in the upper part of the ureter). Hydroureter is caused by a stone in the lower part of the ureter and if untreated can lead to hypertension, loss of renal function, and sepsis. (Modified from Chabner DE: *The language of medicine,* ed 8, St Louis, 2007, Saunders.)

electrolytes are reabsorbed into the blood. The **loop of Henle** is an important part of this tubular collection system, reabsorbing **solutes** (especially sodium), and diluting the urine by osmosis (see Figure 20-3). The peritubular capillaries around the tubule are important in the resorption of fluids around the nephrons.

Ureters

There are two **ureters.** Each is about 25 cm (10 inches) long and carries urine from the renal pelvis to the urinary bladder by peristalsis. The ureters are muscular tubes, so even if a person is lying down, urine can travel through the ureters to the bladder. The bladder compresses against the ureter opening, which prevents urine from backing up into the ureters.

When the urine flows from the bladder back into the ureter during urination, **urinary reflux** occurs. This abnormal condition may result from a congenital defect, obstruction within the bladder, or a urinary infection. Because of the solutes in urine, some people tend to form kidney stones, or **renal calculi.** The calculi are washed into the ureter by urine. When a calculus or urolith is too large, it cannot pass through the ureter, causing obstruction (Figure 20-5). This causes severe pain in the flank and into the groin.

Urinary Bladder

The **urinary bladder** is a hollow muscular sac shaped like a balloon. The bladder wall is arranged in folds called **rugae** that allow the bladder to stretch as it fills. This ability to stretch allows the bladder to hold approximately 1000 mL of urine. The bladder is located in the ventral area of the pelvic cavity, just behind the pelvic bone. Its main function is to store urine until a reflex contraction causes urine to exit the body through the urethra. This usually occurs when the bladder has at least 250 mL of urine.

The process of excreting urine is called **urination, micturition,** or **voiding.** This process occurs when the two sphincters (ring-shaped muscles) open and allow urine to leave the bladder. The upper sphincter muscle is located below the bladder and works by involuntary control. The lower sphincter is under conscious control. The **micturition reflex** occurs when the stretch receptors located in the wall of the bladder transmit a nerve impulse and initiate the urge to expel urine. The **trigone** is the triangular area within the bladder that is formed by the entrance site of the ureters and the exit site of the urethra.

Urethra

The **urethra** extends from the bladder to the outside of the body. The urethral opening to the outside of the body is the **meatus.** The male urethra is longer (about 8 inches) than the female urethra and expels both urine and **semen** from the body. The female urethra only excretes urine. The female's urethra is shorter (about 1½ inches long) and closer to the vagina and anus, which explains why women have more lower urinary tract infections (UTIs) than males.

FOR YOUR INFORMATION

URETER VERSUS URETHRA
- There are two ureters; an easy way to remember this is to note that there are two "e"s in the word "ureter."
- There is one urethra; an easy way to remember this is to note that there is only one "e" in "urethra."

PATIENT-CENTERED PROFESSIONALISM

- Why would it be important for the medical assistant to ask a patient with renal disease about daily input and output of fluids?

DISEASES AND DISORDERS OF THE URINARY SYSTEM

Diseases and disorders of the urinary system may be caused by infections, malignant and benign tumors, or congenital abnormalities. Cardiac (e.g., hypertension) and endocrine (e.g., diabetes) problems, stones in the urinary tract, and trauma to the urinary system can also lead to urinary disorders. **Urologists** treat diseases and disorders of the urinary system. A **nephrologist** treats diseases of the kidneys.

Drugs may be prescribed to treat urinary problems (Table 20-2). As a medical assistant, you need to be able to recognize the common signs and symptoms of and diagnostic tests for the different types of urinary system disorders and diseases.
- Study Box 20-1 to familiarize yourself with the common signs and symptoms.
- Study Box 20-2 to learn about common diagnostic tests.
- Study Table 20-3 to understand the diseases and disorders that affect the urinary system.
- Study Box 20-3 to learn about dialysis and kidney transplantation.

Text continued on p. 378

TABLE 20-2
Urinary Drug Classifications

Drug Classification	Common Generic (Brand) Drugs
Antihypertensives Reduce blood pressure	lisinopril (Zestril) clonidine (Catapres)
Antibacterials Combat microorganisms; first-line drugs in treatment of UTIs	sulfisoxazole (Gantrisin) trimethoprim-sulfamethoxazole (TMP-SMZ) (Septra DS)
Antiseptics Prophylaxis; second-line of defense	cinoxacin (Cinobac) nitrofurantoin (Macrobid) for treatment of UTIs
Diuretics Increase urination	furosemide (Lasix) chlorothiazide (Diuril)
Antispasmodics Genitourinary muscle relaxant	flavoxate (Urispas) oxybutynin (Ditropan)
Analgesics Provide anesthetic effect on lining of urinary tract	phenazopyridine (Pyridium) pentosan (Elmiron)

UTIs, Urinary tract infections.

BOX 20-1
Common Signs and Symptoms of Urinary Disease

Albuminuria	Presence of large amounts of protein; usually a sign of renal disease or heart failure; also called **proteinuria**
Anuresis	Stopping of urine production or output of less than 100 mL per day
Bacteriuria	Bacteria in urine
Diuresis	Increased urine production
Dysuria	Painful or difficult urination
Enuresis	Involuntary discharge of urine after the age when bladder control is expected, especially at night; bedwetting
Frequency	Need to urinate often, without increased daily output
Glycosuria	Presence of glucose in the urine
Hematuria	Presence of blood in the urine
Incontinence	Inability to retain urine because of the loss of sphincter control
Ketonuria	Presence of ketones in the urine
Nocturia	Excessive urination at night
Oliguria	Diminished amount of urine output
Polydipsia	Excessive thirst (often seen in diabetic patients)
Polyuria	Excretion of abnormally large amounts of urine
Pyuria	Presence of pus in the urine
Retention	Inability to empty the bladder fully
Uremia	Large amount of urea and other nitrogenous wastes in the blood
Urgency	Feeling of need to urinate immediately

BOX 20-2

Diagnostic Tests and Procedures for the Urinary System

Blood urea nitrogen (BUN)	BUN measures amount of nitrogenous waste in the circulatory system
Creatinine clearance test	Measures rate at which nitrogenous waste is removed from the blood by comparing its concentration in the blood and urine over a 24-hour period
Urinalysis	Physical, chemical, and/or microscopic examination of the urine

NORMAL VALUES
Glucose: Negative
Bilirubin: Negative
Ketones: Negative
Specific gravity: 1.1 to 1.25 ± 0.05
Blood: Negative
pH: 4.5 to 8
Protein: Negative
Urobilinogen: 2 mg/dL
Nitrites: Negative
Leukocytes: Negative

Renal computed tomography	Imaging that shows a transverse view of the kidney
Intravenous pyelography (IVP)	Imaging of the KUB with a contrast medium
Kidneys, ureters, and bladder (KUB)	Imaging of the KUB without a contrast medium
Cystoscopy	Visual examination of the urinary bladder using a cystoscope (Figure 20-6)

TABLE 20-3

Diseases and Disorders of the Urinary System

Disease and Description	Etiology	Signs and Symptoms	Diagnosis	Therapy	Interventions
Glomerulonephritis Inflammation of glomeruli	Can be idiopathic or following group A beta hemolytic streptococcus infection	Decreased urine output, protein in urine (proteinuria), hematuria, back pain, edema, increased blood pressure	Clinical examination, urinalysis, and blood tests showing elevated BUN; x-rays to include KUB	Antibiotic therapy, rest, sodium restrictions, and **diuretics** to control edema (swelling)	Interventions depend on the cause of the condition
Renal failure Progressive loss of nephrons resulting in loss of renal function **Acute renal failure (ARF)** occurs suddenly from trauma (any condition that damages the kidneys) **Chronic renal failure (CRF)** occurs with long-term inability to excrete waste products	Decreased blood flow to kidney caused by obstruction of urine flow, toxins, or prior kidney disease	Urine reduction, lethargy, weakness, increased blood pressure	Blood studies to include increased BUN, creatinine, and potassium levels; hemoglobin and hematocrit decreased; radiographic studies to include IVP and sonograms of kidney	Monitoring fluids, sodium, and potassium intake to prevent system overload; nutritional therapy to provide for protein replacement; dialysis and possible kidney transplant (see Box 20-3)	Encourage support by family to maintain diet and fluid restrictions
Pyelonephritis Inflammation of renal pelvis and nephrons including connective tissue of kidneys	Bacterial infection from bladder travels through one or both ureters to kidney	Rapid onset of fever, chills, nausea, and vomiting; lower back pain	Urine specimen has a strong odor, blood, and pus; x-rays show enlarged kidneys	Antibiotic therapy with increased fluid intake and bedrest	Encourage follow-up evaluations after initial episode treated to evaluate renal function

TABLE 20-3
Diseases and Disorders of the Urinary System—cont'd

Disease and Description	Etiology	Signs and Symptoms	Diagnosis	Therapy	Interventions
Renal calculi Kidney stones made of mineral salts found in urinary tract. Stones may move into ureters	Unknown cause, although excessive amounts of calcium and uric acid in blood have been attributed to stone formation	Onset of sudden and severe pain in lower back accompanied by urinary frequency; patient may complain of nausea, vomiting, hematuria, fever, and chills	Family history, urinalysis, KUB, IVP, urogram	Remove calculi through lithotripsy (Figure 20-7) or surgery if it does not pass; provide medications for discomfort and infection; diet modifications and increased fluid intake; straining urine to catch the stone and analyze its composition	Encourage patient to avoid causative factors in diet
Polycystic kidney Kidney tissue is replaced with marblelike cysts (Figure 20-8)	Hereditary disease that presents itself in late adolescence or adulthood	Patient has impaired renal function with complaints of lower back pain, hematuria, and high blood pressure	Clinical presentation with positive results for blood, protein, and pus; x-rays show enlarged kidneys	Dialysis and/or kidney transplant; management of urinary tract infections and hypertension	Maintain follow-up care
Cystitis Inflammation of urinary bladder (UTI)	*Females:* Entry of bacteria via urinary meatus to urethra, caused by fecal contamination, and effects of sexual intercourse *Males:* Obstructive causes (e.g., strictures, enlarged prostate) Less common as a reaction to certain drugs, irritants (e.g., feminine hygiene spray, long-term catheter use)	Dysuria, frequency, urgency, nocturia; also, suprapubic pain, hematuria, low grade fever	Urine culture to detect presence of bacteria and sensitivity testing to determine correct antimicrobial drug	Antibiotic therapy, antispasmodics, and increased fluid consumption	Encourage patient to finish antibiotic therapy and drink fluids to promote renal blood flow and flush out bacteria in the urinary tract; also, encourage patient to urinate frequently (every 2-3 hours) and empty bladder completely on urination
Interstitial cystitis (painful bladder syndrome)	Unknown	*Females:* Chronic urinary urgency with or without pelvic pain	Rule out other heath conditions; urinalysis, C&S, bladder wall biopsy, cystoscopy to view bladder wall for ulcerations, potassium sensitivity test (PST)	Oral medication (Elmiron); antidepressants of the tricyclic group to help reduce hyperactivity of nerves within the bladder wall; antihistamines to reduce allergy symptoms and analgesics for pain relief.	Provide emotional support and encouragement for bladder training. Diet modifications: acid foods, alcohol, spices, chocolate, and caffeinated beverages. Exercise and discontinue smoking

BUN, Blood urea nitrogen; *C&S*, culture and sensitivity; *IVP*, intravenous pyelogram; *KUB*, kidneys, ureters, and bladder; *UTI*, urinary tract infection.

BOX 20-3

Dialysis and Kidney Transplantation

DIALYSIS

Dialysis is used to cleanse the blood of toxins brought on by acute renal disease or end-stage renal disease (ESRD). The process is continued until the problem is corrected or a kidney transplant can be performed. Dialysis can be used indefinitely, but it is not a cure. Dialysis allows the body to maintain the proper fluid, electrolyte, and acid-base balance. There are two methods used to clean the blood: **hemodialysis** and **peritoneal dialysis.**

Hemodialysis

A machine called an *artificial kidney* filters the patient's blood of impurities and returns the blood to the patient's body. A catheter is surgically implanted in the patient's artery, usually in the nondominant arm. The patient's blood passes through a semipermeable membrane in the machine. This procedure takes about 4 hours and must be done on an average of three times a week. The benefit of hemodialysis is that the patient is dialyzed by a professional, and the risk of infection is lower than with self-performed dialysis.

Peritoneal Dialysis

Peritoneal dialysis can be done with minimal equipment and in the patient's home. A catheter is surgically implanted in the patient's peritoneal cavity. A dialyzing solution is passed through the peritoneum and later drained. The procedure takes about 30 minutes and is done four times a day, 7 days a week. It can also be done every night during sleep for patients meeting certain criteria. The benefit of peritoneal dialysis is that the patient does not need to travel to a dialysis center on a regular basis. However, this type of dialysis must be done daily.

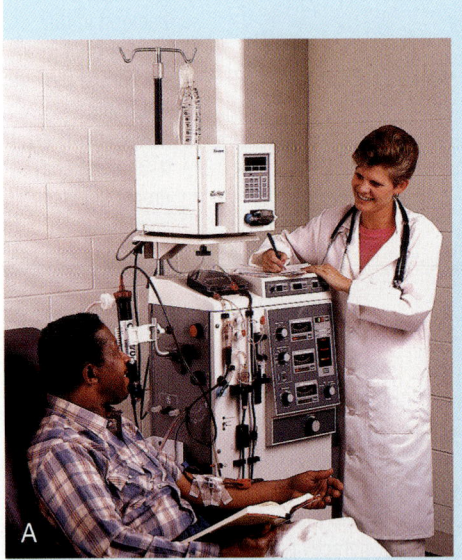
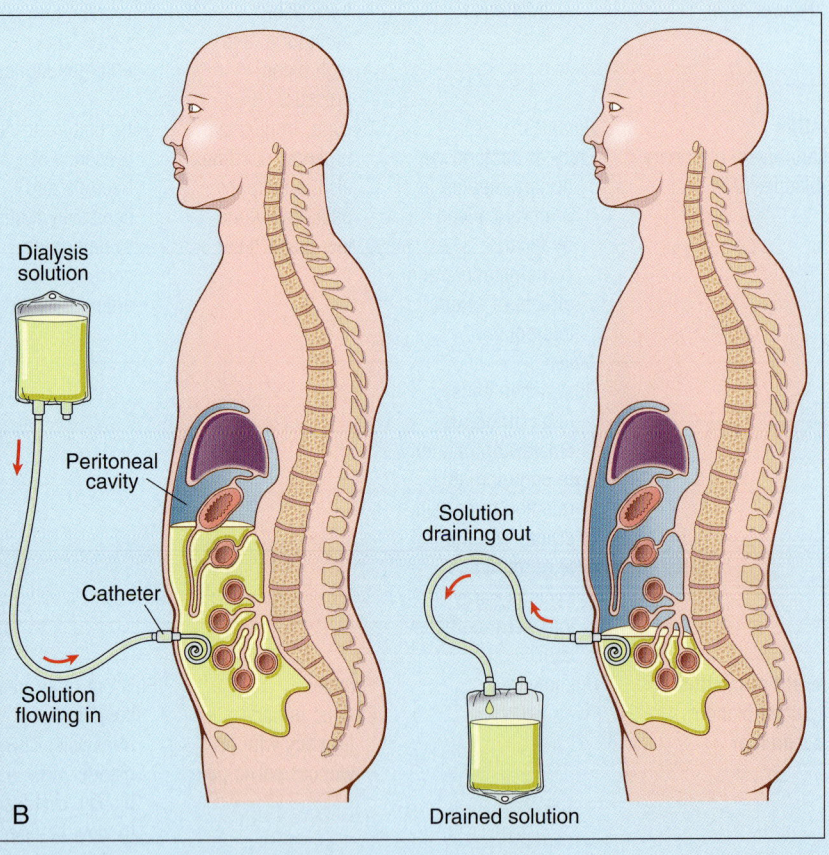

A, Hemodialysis. **B,** Peritoneal dialysis.
(From Chabner DE: *The language of medicine,* ed 8, St Louis, 2007, Saunders.)

Urinary System **CHAPTER 20** 377

BOX 20-3
Dialysis and Kidney Transplantation—cont'd

KIDNEY TRANSPLANTATION
A person with ESRD can have a **kidney transplant** if a suitable donor is found. Blood and tissue typing must be done carefully to avoid rejection of the donated organ. A transplant is having a donor's kidney surgically implanted in the patient (recipient). The recipient requires lifelong *immunosuppressive* medication to prevent organ rejection and antibiotics to prevent infection.

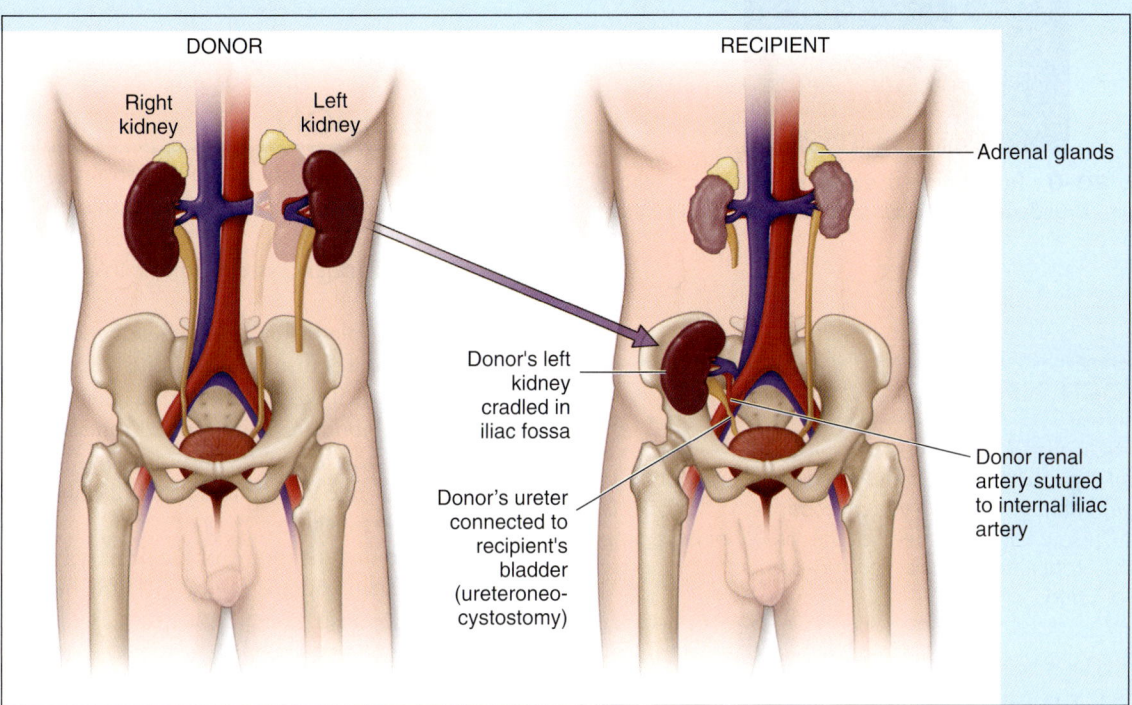

(Modified from Chabner DE: *The language of medicine*, ed 8, St Louis, 2007, Saunders.)

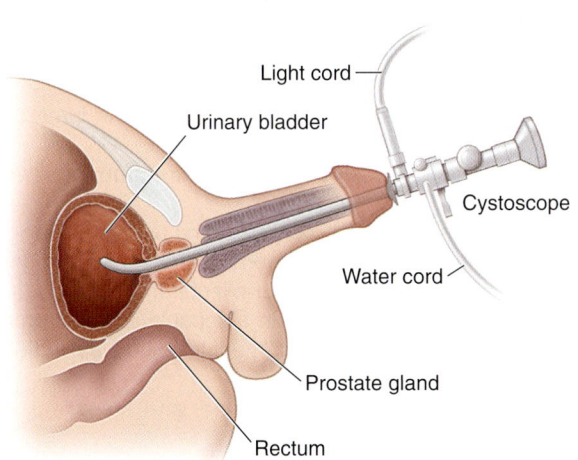

FIGURE 20-6 Cystoscopy. (Modified from LaFleur-Brooks M: *Exploring medical terminology: a student-directed approach*, ed 7, St Louis, 2009, Mosby.)

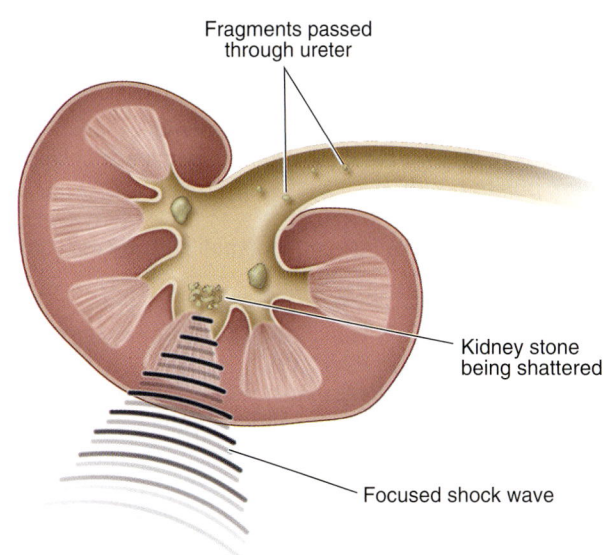

FIGURE 20-7 Lithotripsy. (Modified from LaFleur-Brooks M: *Exploring medical terminology: a student-directed approach*, ed 5, St Louis, 2000, Mosby.)

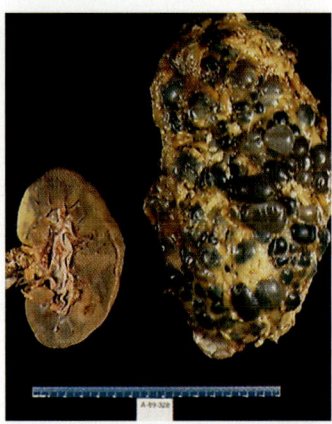

FIGURE 20-8 Polycystic kidney *(right)* and normal kidney *(left).* (From Brundage DJ: *Renal disorders*, St Louis, 1992, Mosby.)

FOR YOUR INFORMATION

Age-related changes in the urinary system include a significant decrease in functional nephrons, a reduction in glomerular filtering, and a lowered response to the effects of ADH. These changes, as well as the loss of muscle tone within the sphincter muscle, can cause an involuntary leakage of urine.

PATIENT-CENTERED PROFESSIONALISM

- What are the benefits to patients when medical assistants understand the diseases and disorders that affect the urinary system?
- How does understanding the signs and symptoms and diagnostic tests associated with urinary disease allow the medical assistant to provide better care to patients?

CONCLUSION

The urinary system maintains the homeostatic balance of the body's fluids by removing unwanted wastes from the blood, maintaining fluid balance, and regulating pH. The other structures of the urinary system either transport or store urine once it is formed.

The nephrons play a key role in the function of the urinary system. Blood passes through the kidneys approximately 300 times each day. As it passes through, the nephrons "clean" all of the blood in about 45 minutes and send about 6 cups of urine to the bladder every day. It is amazing to consider that less than half of one kidney is capable of doing all the work usually done by two kidneys.

With a solid understanding of the urinary system, medical assistants can help patients follow their treatment plans and maintain homeostasis.

Chapter Summary

Reinforce your understanding of the material in this chapter by reviewing the curriculum objectives and key content points below.

1. **Define, appropriately use, and spell all the Key Terms for this chapter.**
   - Review the Key Terms if necessary.
2. **State the five major functions of the urinary system.**
   - Filters toxins from the blood.
   - Reabsorbs essential substances the body needs.
   - Excretes waste products from the body.
   - Produces erythropoietin.
   - Secretes renin.
3. **Identify and locate the four major structures in the urinary system.**
   - The structure of the urinary system includes two kidneys, two ureters, a urinary bladder, and a urethra.
   - The two kidneys are retroperitoneal in the lumbar area protected by the ribs. A ureter exits each kidney and enters the bladder. The urethra exits the bladder and carries urine outside the body.
4. **Describe the structure and main functions of the kidneys.**
   - The kidney is a main organ of the urinary system.
   - The kidneys clean the blood by filtering out nitrogenous wastes and reabsorbing nutrients and water.
   - The kidney is enclosed in a capsule and has an outer layer (cortex), inner layer (medulla), and a collection site (renal pelvis).
5. **Explain the purpose of urine and describe urine formation.**
   - Urine is produced in the kidneys and carries waste products out of the body.
   - Blood enters the kidney through the renal artery, enters Bowman's capsule, and flows through the glomerulus, where the blood is filtered.
   - The filtered blood enters the renal tubules, where needed nutrients and water are reabsorbed by the cells.

- From the renal tubules, urine enters the renal pelvis for collection and further transport to the ureters for eventual exit from the body.

6. **Explain the structure of a nephron and its function in the kidney.**
   - The nephron is the basic filtering unit of the kidney.
   - Review Figure 20-3 and 20-4 for the pathway of the filtering process.

7. **Describe the structure and function of the ureters.**
   - The ureters are tubes leading from each kidney to the bladder.
   - Ureters force urine into the bladder with peristaltic movements of their muscular walls.

8. **Describe the structure and function of the urinary bladder.**
   - The urinary bladder is an expandable reservoir and holds urine until it can be released.
   - Sphincter muscles of the bladder work under conscious and unconscious control.

9. **Describe the structure and function of the urethra.**
   - The urethra is a single tube leading from the bladder to the outside of the body.
   - The male urethra is longer than the female urethra and is used for urine excretion and reproductive purposes.
   - The female urethra is shorter than the male urethra and only secretes urine.

10. **List 13 common signs and symptoms of urinary system disorders.**
    - Refer to Box 20-1.

11. **List seven common diagnostic tests for urinary disease and describe the use of each.**
    - Refer to Box 20-2.

12. **List six urinary diseases and disorders and briefly describe the etiology, signs and symptoms, diagnosis, therapy, and interventions for each.**
    - Refer to Table 20-3.

13. **Explain the purpose of dialysis and list two types.**
    - Dialysis cleanses the blood of toxins brought on by acute or end-stage renal disease.
    - Hemodialysis uses an artificial kidney machine to filter the patient's blood.
    - Peritoneal dialysis passes a special solution through the patient's peritoneum to cleanse the blood.

14. **Analyze a realistic medical office situation and apply your understanding of the urinary system to determine the best course of action.**
    - Knowledge of the urinary system and its terminology and processes can help medical assistants address patient concerns and support the physician's instructions.

15. **Describe the impact on patient care when medical assistants have a solid understanding of the structure and function of the urinary system.**
    - Medical assistants who understand the urinary system are better able to communicate with patients concerning problems and treatment of the urinary system and why it is so important to follow the physician's prescribed treatment plan.

PRACTICAL APPLICATIONS

If you have accomplished the objectives in this chapter, you will be able to make better choices as a medical assistant. Take another look at this situation and decide what you would do.

Juanita is a regular patient in the medical office and has been in good health most of her life. At her office visit, she complains of pain in the flanks of her legs, her lower abdomen, and her back under her ribs. She also says that she has had burning and frequency of urination that has become progressively worse over 2 weeks. Furthermore, she says when she has to go to the bathroom, she has to hurry or she will not make it. The burning is not on the perineum but occurs as she starts the flow of urine. These symptoms have only made her incontinence worse, and she now has nocturia.

When asked if she can pinpoint anything new in her hygiene routine, Juanita states that she has been using a new perfumed soap on a regular basis to take her bath. On obtaining a urinalysis, hematuria is present. In addition, white blood cells are found on the microscopic examination. The physician has prescribed medications for treating what he has diagnosed as "urinary cystitis." Juanita would like to talk to the medical assistant to ask some questions.

Would you be able to answer Juanita's questions?

1. Why do women have inflammation of the urinary tract more often than males?
2. What is hematuria? What is pyuria?
3. Would you expect Juanita to have pyuria since she has hematuria?
4. What is incontinence?
5. What is the difference between incontinence and enuresis?
6. What is the name of the symptom that is used to describe the feeling of the need to urinate immediately?
7. Why are urinary antiseptics used in treating urinary cystitis after antiinfectives have been prescribed?
8. What is urinary frequency?
9. What is nocturia?

WEB SEARCH

Diseases that affect the kidney are numerous. To be effective with patient teaching, the medical assistant needs to be aware of causes, treatments, and medications available.
1. **Research kidney disease** to better understand the disease process, underlying causes, medications, complications, and treatments.

- **Keywords:** Use the following keywords in your search: kidney disease, chronic kidney disease, kidney failure, dialysis, Medline.

WORD PARTS: Urinary System

URINARY TRACT
Combining Forms

cyst/o	bladder
noct/i	night
olig/o	scanty
ureter/o	ureter
urethr/o	urethra
vesic/o	bladder

KIDNEY
Combining Forms

azot/o	urea; nitrogen
cali/o, calic/o	calyx
cortic/o	cortex
glomerul/o	glomerulus
lith/o	stone
medull/o	medulla; middle
nephr/o	kidney
pyel/o	renal pelvis
ren/o	kidney
ur/o	urine; urinary tract

ABBREVIATIONS: Urinary System

ADH	antidiuretic hormone
ARF	acute renal failure
BUN	blood urea nitrogen
C&S	culture and sensitivity
CRF	chronic renal failure
HD	hemodialysis
IVP	intravenous pyelogram
KUB	kidneys, ureters, and bladder
UA	urinalysis
UTI	urinary tract infection

Reproductive System

21

evolve   http://evolve.elsevier.com/klieger/medicalassisting

The main purpose of the reproductive system is to enable the creation of new life through offspring, in other words, to allow humans to have children and "keep the species going." The human reproductive system contains the organs, tissues, and body structures that enable procreation. The reproductive system also produces important hormones needed by our bodies. Reproductive organs and structures can be affected by diseases and disorders that can cause illness and even infertility (inability to produce offspring).

Many other body systems influence the function of the male and female reproductive systems. The body must be in homeostasis for all these systems to function properly and to sustain and create life. Medical assistants need to understand the structure and function of the male and female reproductive systems, as well as the diseases and disorders that can affect these systems. It is also important to understand how human development occurs.

LEARNING OBJECTIVES

You will be able to do the following after completing this chapter:

Key Terms
1. Define, appropriately use, and spell all the Key Terms for this chapter.

Reproductive System
2. List the two main functions of the human reproductive system.
3. Name the reproductive cells produced by the male and female gonads.

Male Reproductive System
4. Trace the pathway that sperm follow through the five major structures of the male reproductive system, beginning with the testes and ending with the urethra.
5. Describe the two main functions of testosterone.
6. Differentiate between the primary and secondary male sex characteristics.
7. Explain the purpose of semen.
8. List seven common diagnostic tests for diseases and disorders of the male reproductive system and describe the use of each.
9. List five disorders of the male reproductive system and briefly describe the etiology, signs and symptoms, diagnosis, therapy, and interventions for each.

Female Reproductive System
10. List, identify, and describe the seven parts of the female reproductive system.
11. Describe the function of the hormones estrogen and progesterone.
12. Describe the function of the hormones prolactin and oxytocin.
13. Describe the function of follicle-stimulating hormone and luteinizing hormone.
14. Explain what happens in the five key stages of the menstrual cycle.
15. Explain what occurs during menopause.
16. List five common diagnostic tests for diseases and disorders of the female reproductive system and describe the use of each.
17. List nine disorders of the female reproductive system and briefly describe the etiology, signs and symptoms, diagnosis, therapy, and interventions for each.

Human Development
18. Explain how sperm fertilize eggs.
19. Distinguish among a zygote, an embryo, and a fetus.
20. Describe the major changes that occur in each of the three trimesters of pregnancy.
21. Describe the four stages of the birth process.
22. List five disorders of pregnancy and briefly describe the etiology, signs and symptoms, diagnosis, therapy, and interventions for each.

Sexually Transmitted Diseases

23. List three practices for preventing the spread of sexually transmitted diseases (STDs).
24. List seven STDs and briefly describe the etiology, signs and symptoms, diagnosis, therapy, and interventions for each.

Patient-Centered Professionalism

25. Analyze a realistic medical office situation and apply your understanding of the human reproductive system to determine the best course of action.
26. Describe the impact on patient care when medical assistants have a solid understanding of the structure and function of the male and female reproductive systems.

KEY TERMS

The Key Terms for this chapter have been organized into sections so that you can easily see the terminology associated with each aspect of the reproductive system.

Function and Structure of the Reproductive System

gametes
gonads

Male Reproductive System

androgen
bulbourethral gland
circumcision
Cowper's gland
cryptorchidism
ejaculation
ejaculatory duct
epididymis
erection
foreskin
genitourinary tract
glans penis
hydrocele
impotence
insemination
orchitis
penis
prepuce
prostate gland
scrotum
semen
seminal vesicles
seminiferous tubules
spermatozoa
sterility
testes
testosterone
urethra
vas deferens

Diseases and Disorders of the Male Reproductive System

benign prostatic hyperplasia (BPH)
epididymitis
prostatic cancer
prostatitis
testicular cancer

Female Reproductive System

areola
Bartholin's glands
body
breast
cervix
endometrium
estrogen
fallopian tubes
fundus
graafian follicle
labia majora
lactiferous ducts
mammary glands
myometrium
nipple
ovaries
ovum
perimetrium
perineum
uterus
vagina
vulva

Reproductive Cycle and Hormones of Reproduction

atrophy
corpus luteum
follicle-stimulating hormone (FSH)
hot flashes
human chorionic gonadotropin (hCG)
luteinizing hormone (LH)
mammograms
menarche
menopause
menses
ovulation
oxytocin
progesterone
prolactin

Abnormalities of Menstrual Cycle

amenorrhea
dysmenorrhea
menorrhagia
metrorrhagia

Diagnostic Tests and Procedures

cervicography
colposcopy
conization
dilation and curettage (D&C)
hysterosalpingography
mammography
Pap smear
pelvimetry
ultrasonography

Diseases and Disorders of the Female Reproductive System

candidiasis
endometriosis
fibrocystic disease of breasts
infertility
ovarian cysts
pelvic inflammatory disease (PID)
premenstrual syndrome (PMS)
prolapse of uterus
toxic shock syndrome (TSS)
uterine fibroids

Human Development

amniotic sac
chorion
embryo
episiotomy
fertilization
fetus
gestation
labor
last menstrual period (LMP)
parturition
placenta
postpartum
pregnancy
prenatal
umbilical cord
zygote

Disorders of Pregnancy

abruptio placentae
ectopic pregnancy
gestational diabetes
placenta previa
pregnancy-induced hypertension (PIH)
toxemia

PRACTICAL APPLICATIONS

Read the following scenario and keep it in mind as you learn about the reproductive system in this chapter.

Valerie has called her gynecologist for her annual Pap smear. The receptionist wants to be sure that Valerie did not make her appointment during the time of her menses. Her menarche was at age 14. She has taken oral contraceptives in the past. She is now approaching age 50 and has excessive bleeding with each menstrual period. Her LMP was a week ago, and she is to have the Pap smear with her physical examination today. The medical assistant asks Valerie if she does monthly BSEs. Dr. Jones started ordering a mammogram for Valerie on a yearly basis at age 35 because of a family history of fibrocystic disease of the breasts. Valerie asks Dr. Jones about taking HRT since she seems to be approaching menopause and has PMS with each menstrual period. Dr. Jones replies that she will discuss this with Valerie after the Pap smear report has returned.

Do you understand why the various aspects of Valerie's appointment were handled the way they were?

FUNCTION AND STRUCTURE OF THE REPRODUCTIVE SYSTEM

Before studying the male and female reproductive systems individually, you need to know a few general principles about the function and structure of the reproductive system.

Basic Function

The two main functions of the male and female reproductive systems are producing offspring and producing hormones. Offspring are necessary to ensure the survival of a species. Hormones function to develop the male and female secondary sex characteristics (e.g., body hair, voice) and assist in regulating the normal activity of the female reproductive system (e.g., pregnancy, lactation).

Basic Structure

Both men and women have sex glands, or **gonads,** that produce reproductive cells, or **gametes** (e.g., egg and sperm cells). The female's gonads, or ovaries, produce eggs, and the male's gonads, or testes, produce sperm. When a male and a female each contribute one of these specialized sex cells containing a portion of their own genetic information, the two sex cells fuse and then divide to form a new and unique individual.

PATIENT-CENTERED PROFESSIONALISM

- How would you use the facts about the function and structure of each reproductive system to explain the role that hormones play in reproduction?

MALE REPRODUCTIVE SYSTEM

In males, the reproductive system and the urinary system both use the urethra to pass body fluids, that is, semen and urine (Figure 21-1). In the male, this system is often referred to as the **genitourinary tract.**

The four main organs of the male reproductive system are the testes, excretory ducts, accessory glands, and external genitalia.

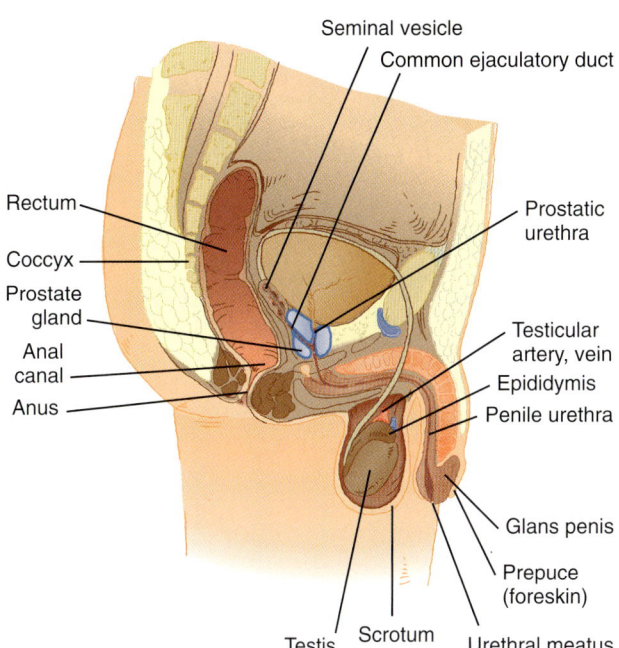

FIGURE 21-1 Male reproductive organs. (Modified from Black JM et al: *Medical-surgical nursing: clinical management for positive outcomes,* ed 8, St Louis, 2009, Saunders.)

Testes

Sperm cells (**spermatozoa**) are produced at a rate of 300 million per day in the bilateral **testes.** The testes are located in the **scrotum,** which is located outside the body (Figure 21-2). The testes develop within the abdominal cavity and usually descend into the scrotum 2 months before birth. Sometimes, one or both testes do not descend and remain in the abdomen. This condition is called **cryptorchidism,** or undescended (hidden) testes (Figure 21-3). To remain viable, sperm cannot withstand normal body temperature, which is why the testes are located outside the body in the scrotum. Cryptorchidism results in **sterility** (the inability to produce children) if corrective surgery is not performed. Beginning in puberty, sperm are formed constantly in the coiled **seminiferous tubules** within the testes. Another condition of the testes is **orchitis,** which presents as an inflammation of one or both testes accompanied by pain and swelling.

Scrotal swelling caused by an accumulation of fluid is a **hydrocele.** Two common reasons that this occurs are a structural defect present at birth (congenital) and the nonabsorption of fluid produced by the serous membrane lining the scrotum.

Testosterone

The testes (and adrenal gland) secrete the male hormone **testosterone.** Testosterone is the most familiar **androgen.** Testosterone is not secreted continuously in males. It is mainly secreted prenatally and then not again until puberty. During the prenatal period, testosterone determines the gender of the fetus and forms the male reproductive organs properly; it also

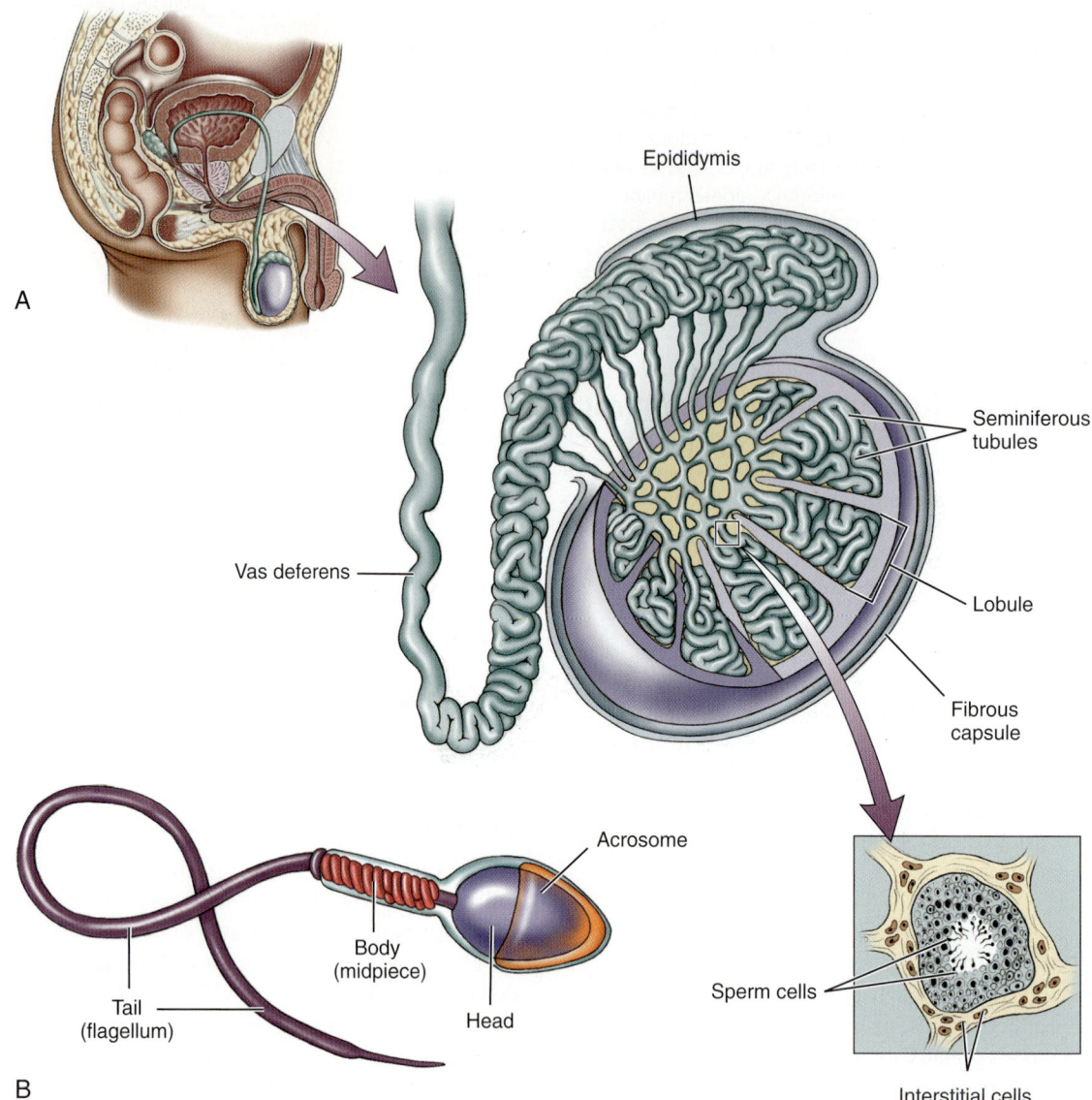

FIGURE 21-2 **A,** Male gonad. Note the connection with epididymis and vas deferens. **B,** Structure of a sperm. (From Herlihy D, Maebius NK: *The human body in health and illness,* ed 3, St Louis, 2007, Saunders.)

enables reproduction. Testosterone is then secreted continuously from puberty throughout the rest of the male's life.

Male Sex Characteristics

Testosterone is responsible for the development of both primary and secondary sex characteristics in the male. Primary sex characteristics in males include the following:
- Growth of the penis and scrotum
- Growth and activity of internal reproductive structures

Secondary sex characteristics in males include the following:
- Deepening of the voice
- Muscular development
- Growth of pubic, facial, and underarm hair

A male adolescent's growth spurt and acne problems are brought on by the increase of testosterone.

Excretory Ducts

Sperm cells leave the testes and travel through several ducts to reach a large coiled duct, the **epididymis.** Mature sperm are stored in the epididymis. Sperm leave the epididymis by way of a bilateral tube called the **vas deferens.** (This duct is cut during a vasectomy to halt the travel of the sperm past the epididymis.) The vas deferens joins with the seminal vesicles to form the **ejaculatory duct.** Just before the ejaculatory duct reaches the **prostate gland** that surrounds the urethra, each duct enlarges to form an *ampulla.* The ampulla stores sperm until ejaculation. Sperm can remain fertile in the ampulla for up to 42 days. After entering the prostate gland, the ejaculatory duct joins the **urethra,** which courses through the penis to the outside of the body.

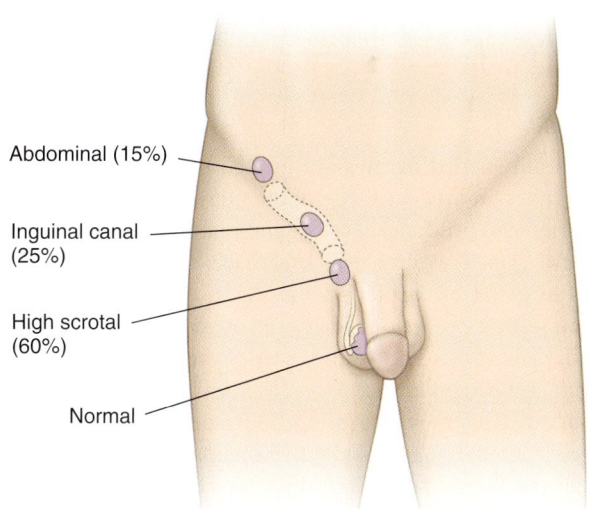

FIGURE 21-3 In cryptorchidism, the testis is not in the scrotum but may be found in the inguinal canal or abdominal cavity. Percentages indicate incidence of cryptorchidism in specific areas of the body. (Modified from Damjanov I: *Pathology for the health-related professions,* ed 3, Philadelphia, 2006, Saunders.)

PATHWAY OF SPERM: Testes → Epididymis → Vas deferens → Ejaculatory duct → Urethra

TABLE 21-1
Male Reproductive Drug Classifications

Drug Classification	Common Generic (Brand) Drugs
Anti–benign prostatic hyperplasia drugs Inhibit production of androgen hormones; used to treat obstruction of urinary flow	terazosin (Hytrin) doxazosin (Cardura)
Testosterone	fluoxymesterone (Halotestin)
Hormone replacement drug	methyltestosterone (Testred)
Benign prostatic hypertrophy	finasteride (Proscar)

Accessory Glands

The sperm cells mix with the fluids of the following three central glands:
- Seminal vesicles
- Prostate gland
- Bulbourethral (Cowper's) glands

This mixture is referred to as **semen.** The purpose of semen is to carry the sperm into the female reproductive tract during intercourse and to provide nourishment for the sperm.

The **seminal vesicles** produce a mucuslike fluid that provides nutrition and energy for the mobile sperm. This fluid accounts for 60% of the semen volume. The prostate gland wraps around the urethra and creates a milky, alkaline fluid that neutralizes the acidity of the urethra and vaginal secretions so that more sperm survive. The **bulbourethral gland,** or **Cowper's gland,** secretes a thick, mucous fluid into the urethra that acts as a lubricant.

External Genitalia

The **penis** has a long shaft that is suspended from the front and sides of the pubic arch and contains the urethra. It is composed of three layers of spongy vascular tissue and is covered with skin. At the end of the penis, a slight thickening of tissue forms the **glans penis.** The skin is folded doubly at the end of the penis to protect the glans penis and is called the **foreskin,** or **prepuce. Circumcision** is a procedure performed to remove this foreskin.

Erection and Ejaculation

The penis delivers semen, which contains the sperm, into the female reproductive tract (**insemination**) during sexual intercourse. When a male is sexually aroused, nerve impulses stimulate the arteries of the penis to dilate. Blood fills the layers of spongy tissue that compress against the wall of the veins, not allowing the blood to leave. This causes the penis to become erect and firm (**erection**). When the level of sexual excitement reaches its peak, secretions stored in the seminal vesicles, prostate gland, and ejaculatory ducts, along with sperm, are forcibly expelled through the urethra (**ejaculation**). The engorgement in the penis then lessens, and it returns to normal size. **Impotence** is the inability to have or sustain an erection during sexual intercourse (erectile dysfunction). This should not be confused with sterility, which is the inability to produce sperm.

Diseases and Disorders of the Male Reproductive System

Diseases and disorders of the male reproductive system can cause pain and inflammation, problems with urination, and even sterility. A *urologist* treats both urinary and reproductive disorders in men. As with the other body systems, drugs may be prescribed to treat problems of the male reproductive system (Table 21-1).

Medical assistants need to be able to recognize the common signs and symptoms of and the diagnostic tests for the disorders and disease conditions that affect the male reproductive system.
- Study Box 21-1 to learn about common diagnostic tests and procedures.
- Study Table 21-2 to understand the diseases and disorders that affect the male reproductive system.

BOX 21-1

Diagnostic Tests and Procedures for the Male Reproductive System

Digital rectal examination (DRE)	Insertion of gloved finger into rectum to palpate prostate
LABORATORY TESTS	
FTA-ABS	Fluorescent treponemal antibody absorption test; test to diagnose syphilis
PSA	Prostate-specific antigen; blood test for prostatic cancer
Gram stain	Used to diagnose gonorrhea
Sperm analysis	Count and analysis for number and health of spermatozoa
Ultrasonography	High-frequency sound waves to examine testes for abnormalities
VDRL	Venereal Disease Research Laboratories; test to screen for syphilis

Summary Points

- The male reproductive system functions to produce, maintain, and transport sperm.
- The testes are responsible for the production of spermatozoa and the secretion of testosterone.
- Testosterone is responsible for the secondary sex characteristic changes in the male at the onset of puberty.

PATIENT-CENTERED PROFESSIONALISM

- *Can you distinguish between the essential organs and the accessory organs of the male reproductive system?*
- *How would you describe the role of testosterone in development of both the primary and the secondary sex characteristics in the man?*

FEMALE REPRODUCTIVE SYSTEM

The male reproductive system enables the fertilization of the egg, and the female reproductive system produces the egg and carries offspring through pregnancy and childbirth. The female reproductive organs are located in the lower abdomen, and the whole reproductive system is almost entirely hidden within the pelvis. Medical assistants need to have a good understanding of the female reproductive organs and cycle, as well as the diseases and disorders that affect this system.

Reproductive Organs

The female reproductive system has two ovaries (which produce the eggs, or ova), two fallopian (uterine) tubes, one uterus, one vagina, and the external genitalia. Two breasts are accessory organs used to provide milk to offspring after childbirth.

Ovaries

The almond-shaped **ovaries** are located near the end of the uterine tubes and on each side of the uterus. The function of the ovaries is to produce, develop, and mature the egg (Figure 21-4). All eggs a woman will ever have are present in her ovaries at birth. At ovulation the egg is expelled from the **graafian follicle** on the outside of the ovary and is swept into the fallopian tube. The ovaries also secrete the hormones estrogen and progesterone.

Estrogen. **Estrogen** is one of the hormones that stimulate changes in the female reproductive organs and the development of the female secondary sex characteristics. Similar to testosterone in men, the amount of estrogen secreted increases during puberty in women at 9 to 12 years of age. Secretion of both estrogen and progesterone declines at ages 45 to 55.

Progesterone. Progesterone is produced by the corpus luteum after ovulation to prepare the uterus for pregnancy. Should pregnancy occur, the placenta takes over to produce enough progesterone to maintain the pregnancy.

Female Sex Characteristics. Estrogen is responsible for the development of both primary and secondary sex characteristics in women. Female primary sex characteristics include the following:

- Growth of sex organs and breasts
- Growth and activity of internal reproductive organs

Female secondary sex characteristics include the following:

- Widening of the pelvis
- Deposit of body fat in hips and thighs
- Growth of pubic and underarm hair

Fallopian Tubes

The bilateral **fallopian tubes** are each about 4 inches long. At ovulation, the egg travels from an ovary to the uterus through the fallopian tube. The fingerlike projections at the end of the tubes sweep the egg dropped from the ovary into the fallopian tube. When fertilization of an egg does happen, it occurs here. After fertilization, the egg usually continues to travel to the uterus and attach itself to the uterine wall for the pregnancy. An **ectopic pregnancy** will result if the fertilized egg attaches to the fallopian tube (or other site outside the uterus) instead and continues to develop there, resulting in tube rupture and miscarriage. This is an obstetrical emergency. When a sperm does not fertilize an egg, the egg degenerates and becomes part of the secretions of the vaginal tract.

Uterus

The **uterus,** or womb, is a hollow, pear-shaped organ located between the bladder and the rectum. It has the following three parts:

- The **fundus,** which is the top of the uterus above the fallopian tubes.

TABLE 21-2

Diseases and Disorders of the Male Reproductive System

Disease and Description	Etiology	Signs and Symptoms	Diagnosis	Therapy	Interventions
Benign prostatic hyperplasia (BPH) Enlargement of prostate gland; common in men after age 50	Hormonal and metabolic changes brought on by aging	Difficulty in starting urination, weak stream of urine, urinary frequency, or inability to empty bladder completely	Patient history, rectal examination, IVP	Symptomatic, to include medications and surgery (TURP)	Encourage patient to have regular prostate examinations
Prostatitis Infection of prostate	Bacterial infections	Pain and burning on urination, lower back pain, fever, muscular pain or tenderness, urinary frequency	Urinalysis, C&S, rectal examination	Antiinfectives, increased fluids, analgesics	Encourage patient to seek medical attention for UTI
Epididymitis Inflammation of epididymis	Bacterial infection, trauma, mumps, prolonged use of indwelling catheter	Fever, malaise, pain, groin and scrotal tenderness	Physical examination, urinalysis, C&S, increased WBCs in blood and urine	Antiinfectives, analgesics, rest, scrotal support	Encourage early treatment of UTIs
Prostatic cancer Cancer of prostate	Unknown	Urinary frequency, difficulty urinating, urinary retention	Rectal examination, blood test for PSA, biopsy, CT scan, ultrasonography	Hormonal therapy, surgical removal of prostate gland; advanced stages may require orchiectomy (surgical removal of testis) and chemotherapy	Encourage men over 50 to have an annual physical examination to include PSA test
Testicular cancer Cancer in one or both testicles	Unknown	Painless lump in testicle	Patient history of mumps, inguinal hernia during childhood; palpation of testes by physician; biopsy	Surgical treatment (orchiectomy) with possible radiation and chemotherapy	Encourage patient to perform monthly testicular self-examination
Hydrocele Fluid-containing sac within the scrotum	Congenital, usually a result of patent processus vaginalis, but inflammation and blockage of venous or lymphatic flow may produce the condition	Painless cystic mass in the scrotum	Physical examination and transillumination	Some are self-limiting, others may require aspiration as a temporary measure, treatment of the underlying condition, or surgical removal	Reassure the patient

C&S, Culture and sensitivity; *CT,* computed tomography; *IVP,* intravenous pyelography; *PSA,* prostate-specific antigen; *TURP,* transurethral resection of prostate; *UTI,* urinary tract infection; *WBCs,* white blood cells.

- The **body,** which is in the middle of the uterus below the fundus.
- The **cervix,** or neck, which is the lower portion of the uterus and extends into the vagina.

The uterus has three layers: the **perimetrium,** a serous layer; the **myometrium,** a thick muscular layer; and the **endometrium,** the vascular layer. The uterus is held in place by ligaments and is suspended from the abdomen to allow for growth in pregnancy. The uterus receives the **ovum,** or egg, from the fallopian tube. If this egg is fertilized, it will normally attach to the uterus for development.

Vagina

The **vagina** is a tube that descends from the uterus to the vulva (external genitalia). The vagina is in front of the rectum and

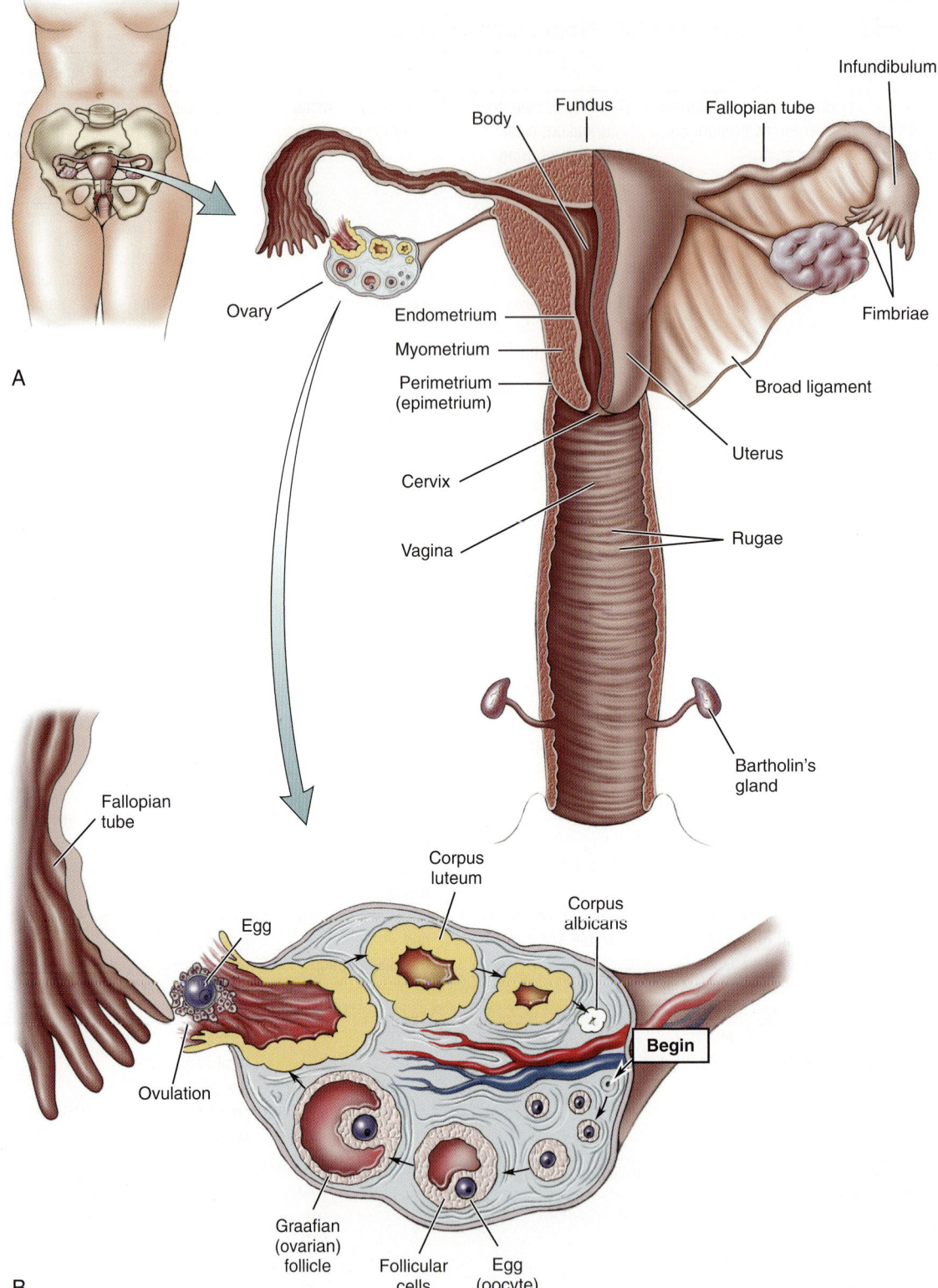

FIGURE 21-4 **A,** Female reproductive organs. **B,** Maturation of ovarian follicle. (From Herlihy B, Maebius NK: *The human body in health and illness,* ed 3, St Louis, 2007, Saunders.)

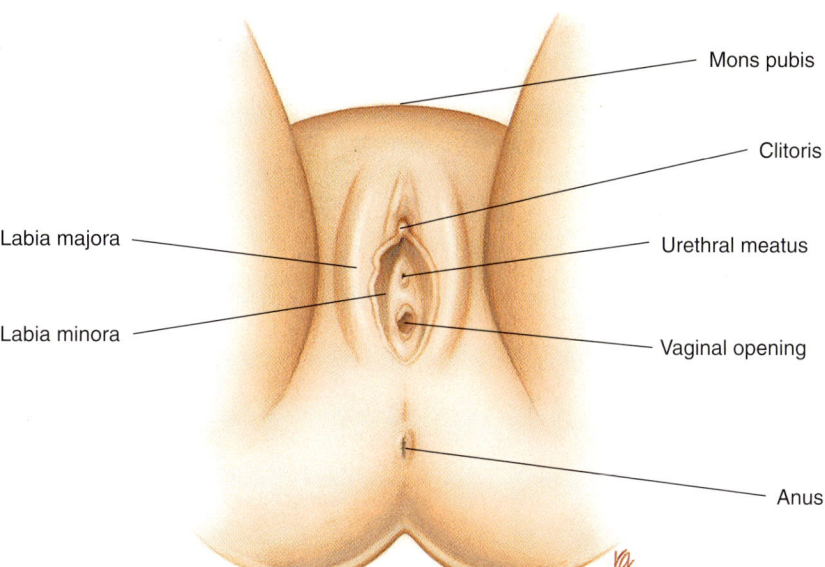

FIGURE 21-5 Female external genitalia, or vulva. (From Gerdin J: *Health careers today,* ed 4, St Louis, 2007, Mosby.)

behind the bladder. It is the organ where sperm enters and the baby emerges.

Vulva

The **vulva** is the external genitalia. It includes the *mons pubis,* **labia majora,** *labia minora,* the *clitoris,* and the *vestibule* and glands (Figure 21-5). The vestibule contains the openings of the urethra and the vagina. On either side of the vaginal opening is a pair of **Bartholin's glands** responsible for lubrication of the vaginal opening.

Perineum

The **perineum** is the external surface of the pelvis floor between the vaginal opening and the anus. This is the area that may be surgically incised (**episiotomy**) to allow for easier passage of the infant during childbirth.

Mammary Glands

The **mammary glands** are located within the **breast** and consist of lobes of glandular units that produce milk. In the center of each breast is a **nipple.** The **lactiferous ducts** transport the milk to the nipple. Surrounding the nipple is a dark-colored skin called the **areola.** Hormones regulate the function of the mammary glands.

Reproductive Cycle and Hormones of Reproduction

At puberty, when the reproductive organs are mature enough to respond to the estrogen secretions, the ovaries and uterus begin monthly menstruation cycles. A woman's reproductive cycles continue from puberty to menopause.

Menstrual Cycle

As puberty approaches, the anterior pituitary gland is stimulated by gonadotropin-releasing hormone (GnRH) to secrete **follicle-stimulating hormone (FSH)** and **luteinizing hormone (LH).** The five key phases in the menstrual cycle are as follows:

1. FSH causes the egg to ripen in the graafian follicle.
2. During this time the follicle secretes estrogen, which prepares the endometrium for the implantation of the fertilized egg.
3. LH starts **ovulation** (release of the egg from the ovary) and turns the follicle into the **corpus luteum.**
4. The corpus luteum releases progesterone and estrogen to thicken the uterine wall for pregnancy.
5. If fertilization does not occur, the hormonal levels decrease, the endometrium sheds, and the **menses,** or menstrual flow, begins.

A typical menstrual cycle lasts 28 days. The first day of menstruation is day 1 of the cycle, which will typically last about 5 days. Ovulation occurs 14 days before the next cycle (Figure 21-6). **Menarche** is the first menstrual cycle a woman experiences. Abnormalities of the menstrual cycle are listed in Box 21-2.

Menopause

The menstrual cycle happens every month from puberty until **menopause,** or the "change of life," which signals the end of a woman's reproductive life. As a woman approaches age 50, the ovaries' secretion of hormones (estrogen and progesterone) decreases, and the menstrual cycle becomes irregular and eventually stops. The resulting decrease in estrogen levels can bring about **hot flashes** (sensations of warmth), loss of bone density, depression, night sweats, and unexplained headaches. The lining in the vagina thins, and the breasts and vulva **atrophy** (lose muscle strength and decrease in size). These changes occur gradually over 5 to 7 years.

Hormones

In addition to estrogen, FSH, and LH, other hormones are important to the reproductive cycle.

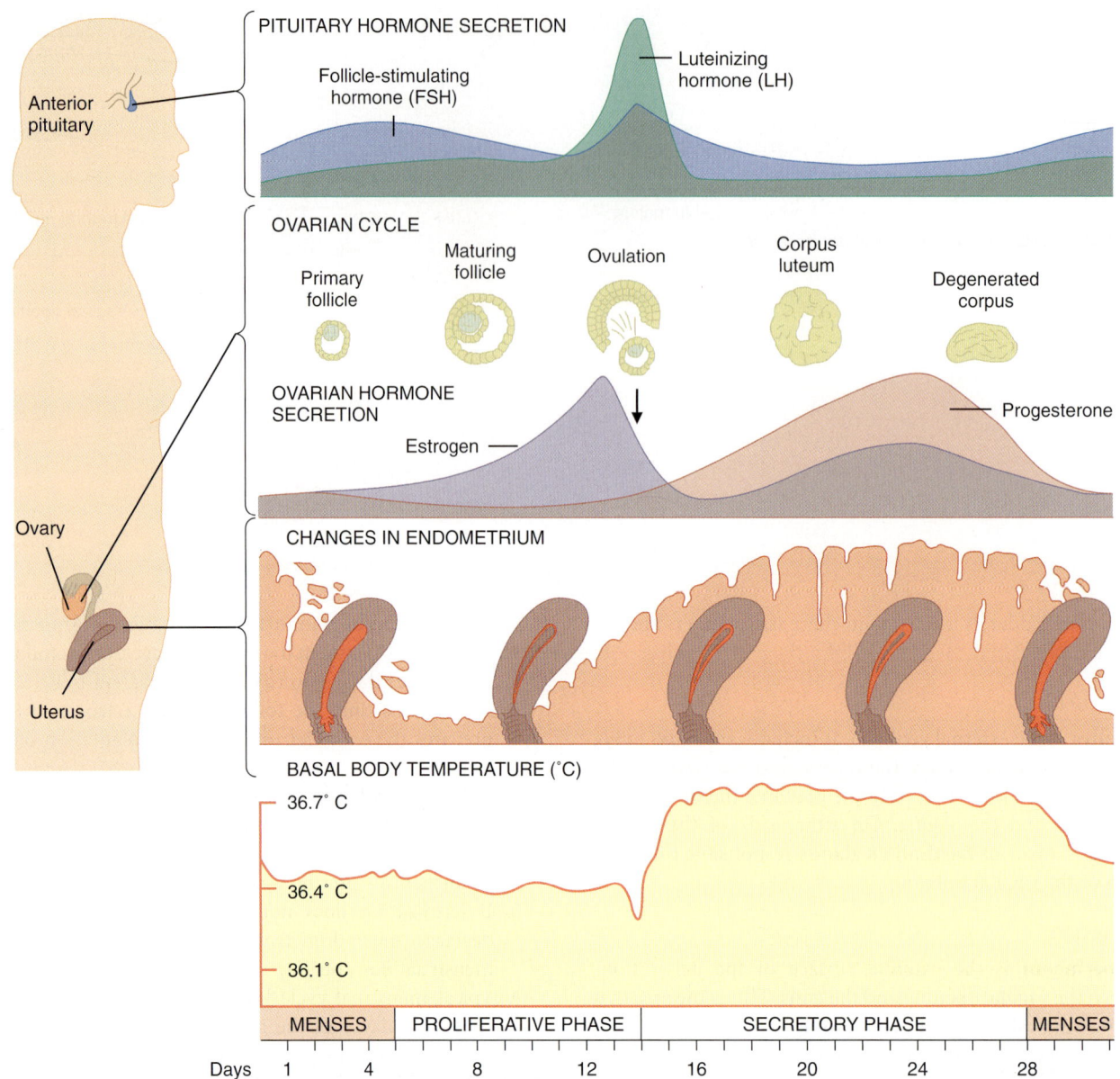

FIGURE 21-6 Menstrual (uterine) cycle. Note hormonal control of the menstrual cycle and the effects on the ovaries *(center)* and endometrium *(bottom)*. (From Black JM et al: *Medical-surgical nursing: clinical management for positive outcomes,* ed 8, St Louis, 2009, Saunders.)

BOX 21-2	
Abnormalities of Menstrual Cycle	
Amenorrhea	Absence of menstrual cycle
Dysmenorrhea	Painful menstrual cycle
Metrorrhagia	Bleeding between menses
Menorrhagia	Abnormally long or excessive bleeding during menses

Estrogen and **progesterone** aid in the development of glandular tissue, **prolactin** stimulates milk production, and **oxytocin** allows for the stimulation of uterine contractions for labor and postpartum and the expulsion of milk. **Human chorionic gonadotropin (hCG),** sometimes referred to as the "pregnancy hormone," is produced in large amounts by the ovaries (and later by the placenta) starting in early pregnancy. A pregnancy is detected by the presence of hCG, which is only produced during pregnancy and therefore is the basis of most pregnancy tests.

Diseases and Disorders of the Female Reproductive System

As with the male reproductive system, diseases and disorders in the female reproductive system can cause pain and inflammation, or even **infertility** (inability to become pregnant). A *gynecologist* treats diseases and disorders of the female repro-

TABLE 21-3
Female Reproductive Drug Classifications

Drug Classification	Common Generic (Brand) Drugs
Estrogen	estradiol (Estrace)
Hormonal replacement	conjugated estrogens (Premarin)
Oral contraceptives (OCs)	mestranol/norethindrone (Ortho-Novum)
Prevent pregnancy	norethindrone/estradiol (Tri-Norinyl)
Estrogen and progestin combinations, or either used separately	
Ovulation stimulants	clomiphene (Clomid)
Induce ovulation	danazol (Danocrine)
Progestins	megestrol (Megace)
Menopause	medroxyprogesterone (Provera)

BOX 21-3
Diagnostic Tests and Procedures for the Female Reproductive System

Cervicography	Photographic procedure using special camera to image entire cervix
Colposcopy	Visual inspection of vagina and cervix using a colposcope
Conization	Removal of cone-shaped section of cervix for biopsy
Dilation and curettage (D&C)	Dilation (or dilatation) of cervical opening and scraping of uterus to remove endometrial tissue
Hysterosalpingography	Imaging procedure using a contrast medium to visualize uterus and fallopian tubes
Mammography	X-ray of breasts for early detection of breast cancer
Pap smear	Papanicolaou test; cells are removed from cervix and vagina for microscopic analysis
Pelvimetry	Measurement of birth canal
Ultrasonography	High-frequency sound waves used to image the pelvic area

ductive system. A gynecologist who is a *fertility specialist* may be needed to ascertain the cause of the infertility and provide treatment that will result in a successful pregnancy. Drugs may be prescribed to treat problems in the female reproductive system (Table 21-3). Breast self-examination (BSE), along with regular health checkups and **mammograms,** can play a vital role in the early detection of breast cancer. Therefore patients are encouraged to perform a BSE at least monthly and at least 1 week after the menstrual cycle. You will learn more about BSE, mammograms, pelvic examinations, and Pap smears in Chapter 39.

Medical assistants need to be able to recognize the common signs and symptoms of and the diagnostic tests for the disorders and disease conditions that affect the female reproductive system.

- Study Box 21-3 to learn about common diagnostic tests and procedures.
- Study Table 21-4 to understand the diseases and disorders that affect this system in females.

Summary Points

- The female reproductive system produces ova on a regular monthly basis after puberty for the purpose of fertilization.
- Hormones regulate the cyclic menstrual process.
- The process of ovulation continues from puberty to menopause.

PATIENT-CENTERED PROFESSIONALISM

- *Can you distinguish between the essential organs and the accessory organs of the female reproductive system?*
- *How would you describe the role of estrogen in development of both the primary and the secondary sex characteristics in the woman?*
- *As puberty approaches, the anterior pituitary gland secretes hormones to begin the menstrual cycle. What role does each hormone play?*

FOR YOUR INFORMATION

The reproductive systems of both sexes are affected by the decrease in hormone levels as aging occurs. Women are affected when the decrease in hormone levels results in the cessation of ovulation and menstruation between the ages of 45 to 55. Circulating testosterone levels decline in men between the ages of 50 to 60, resulting in a gradual reduction in sexual activity.

HUMAN DEVELOPMENT

The female menstrual cycle occurs to produce eggs. You know what happens when these eggs are not fertilized: menses. Conception occurs when an egg is fertilized by the male's sperm, and pregnancy results. It is important to understand the prenatal development stages, as well as what happens during the birth process.

Prenatal Development Stages

Pregnancy, or **gestation,** is the time it takes for **prenatal** development. A human's gestational period is usually 266 days from the time fertilization takes place. When calculating the due date, 280 days is used because this represents the

TABLE 21-4

Diseases and Disorders of the Female Reproductive System

Disease and Description	Etiology	Signs and Symptoms	Diagnosis	Therapy	Interventions
Candidiasis Fungal infection (Candida) of vagina	Candida albicans; glycosuria; antibiotic, birth control, and steroid therapy	Severe itching, "cottage cheese" discharge; no odor present	Pelvic examination, culture testing	Fungal creams or suppositories	Encourage patient to seek treatment
Pelvic inflammatory disease (PID) Infection that involves fallopian tubes and surrounding tissue, resulting in scarred tissue; leads to sterility	Bacterial infection that travels from vagina through cervix, uterus, and fallopian tubes and into pelvic cavity	Fever, chills, malaise, foul-smelling discharge, back pain, pain in lower pelvic and abdominal areas	Pelvic examination, Gram stain, ultrasonography to check for abscess	Antibiotics, analgesics, bedrest	As directed by physician, provide patient education and encourage patient to seek treatment
Endometriosis Growth of endometrial tissue outside uterus and in pelvic cavity	Unknown; misplaced endometrial tissue implants on pelvic organs and irritates surrounding tissue	Dysmenorrhea before and after menstruation; constant pain in lower abdomen, vagina, and back; heavy menses	Pelvic examination, laparoscopy	Hormone replacement for women of childbearing age; tissue shrinks during menopause, pregnancy, and when nursing; hysterectomy in severe cases	Provide literature on pain management alternatives if supported by physician
Fibrocystic disease of breasts Chronic, noncancerous condition characterized by round lumps or cysts in breast tissue that cause pain and tenderness	Unknown; seems to be familial	Lumps or cysts occur in one or both breasts; breasts are tender on palpation and pain may be present	Palpation and mammography to rule out malignant neoplasm; biopsy as needed	Decrease caffeine consumption; possible fluid aspiration from cysts	Encourage patient to perform monthly BSE and have yearly mammography
Prolapse of uterus Displacement of uterus into vagina	Pelvic floor muscles weaken from childbirth or old age	Discomfort, backache, stress incontinence, or inability to urinate	Pelvic examination; visible on inspection	Weight loss; surgery to strengthen muscles of pelvic floor	Encourage patient to seek medical attention
Toxic shock syndrome (TSS) Septic infection caused by staphylococcal bacteria (Staphylococcus aureus)	Unknown	High fever, rash, and decrease in blood pressure; untreated, TSS can result in death	Patient history of tampon use, patient symptoms, and increased liver enzyme levels	Intravenous replacement of fluids; antibiotics to treat infection	Encourage patient to seek immediate treatment
Uterine fibroids Smooth muscle tumors within uterus; usually benign	Unknown	Pelvic pain, feeling of pressure, urinary frequency, abnormal bleeding, heavy or prolonged bleeding	Patient history, pelvic examination, ultrasonography	D&C	Provide emotional support
Ovarian cysts Fluid-filled sacs that form in the ovaries	Physiological cysts caused by normal function of ovary or neoplastic cysts	Painless swelling in the lower abdomen, urinary retention, and vaginal bleeding	Patient history, ultrasonography	Large cysts are drained or removed by laparoscopy	Provide emotional support

TABLE 21-4
Diseases and Disorders of the Female Reproductive System—cont'd

Disease and Description	Etiology	Signs and Symptoms	Diagnosis	Therapy	Interventions
Premenstrual syndrome (PMS) Combination of physical and emotional symptoms that appear before start of menstrual flow and stop with its onset	High estrogen levels that cause symptoms related to retention of fluid	Complaints of tension and irritability, headache, fatigue, restlessness, depression, breast tenderness, and joint pain	Patient history, pelvic examination	Relief of symptoms; decrease intake of sodium, moderate exercise, analgesics, decrease caffeine intake	Provide emotional support
Cervical cancer	Neoplasm associated with HPV; growth of malignant cells in the lining of the cervix	Often nonexistent; bloody vaginal discharge, metrorrhagia (pelvic and/or abdominal pain)	Positive Pap smear, pelvic examination, colposcopy (biopsy)	*Stage 0-1:* removal of abnormal cells; surgical interventions: • Cryotherapy: cells frozen • LEEP: electricity is passed through a loop of wire to slice off abnormal tissue • Cone biopsy: wedge of tissue removed • Laser surgery: laser light source used to remove diseased tissues *Late stage:* full or partial hysterectomy; radiation and or chemotherapy	

BSE, Breast self-examination; *D&C*, dilation and curettage; *HPV*, human papillomavirus; *LEEP*, loop electrosurgical excision procedure.

---

beginning of the **last menstrual period (LMP).** The gestation period for humans is 38 to 42 weeks, with the average being 40 weeks (Figure 21-7). This is considered to be a *full-term* pregnancy. The gestation period is broken into three *(tri-)* stages, or *trimesters.*

First Trimester

The first trimester includes the first day of the last menses and extends until 12 weeks of gestation. When **fertilization** (conception) occurs, the fusion of the sperm and egg forms a **zygote.** The zygote moves through the fallopian tubes, dividing several times as it progresses toward the uterus. The zygote has all the DNA, or genetic material from the male and female, needed to create a person. The zygote eventually divides to form an **embryo.** When the embryo reaches the uterus, about the seventh day, it implants high in the uterine wall.

As the embryo implants into the endometrium of the uterus, several membranes develop to support, protect, and provide nourishment to the developing embryo. The **amniotic sac** develops and fills with fluid to protect and cushion the embryo. All major body systems are developed during the first 8 weeks of the embryo's growth.

The embryo receives nutrition and oxygen through the **placenta.** The placenta is an organ that is formed from the outermost layer surrounding the embryo, the **chorion.** The placenta functions by taking oxygen and nutrients from the mother's blood to the embryo. Waste products from the embryo move from the embryo through the placenta into the mother's blood. The embryo and the placenta are connected by the **umbilical cord.** Within this cord are two arteries and a vein. The hormone hCG is responsible for the corpus luteum release of large amounts of estrogen and progesterone that maintain the endometrium. A positive pregnancy test confirms the presence of hCG in urine or blood.

After the eighth week of pregnancy, the embryo is called a **fetus** and is about 1 inch long. The fetus continues to grow and develop.

Second Trimester

The second trimester begins at the end of the first 12 weeks. The fetus starts to grow faster and is now about 4 inches long. Movement is felt about the fifth month (20 weeks). Accelerated growth and tissue specialization occur during this trimester. For example, the brain (cerebrum) develops further, and

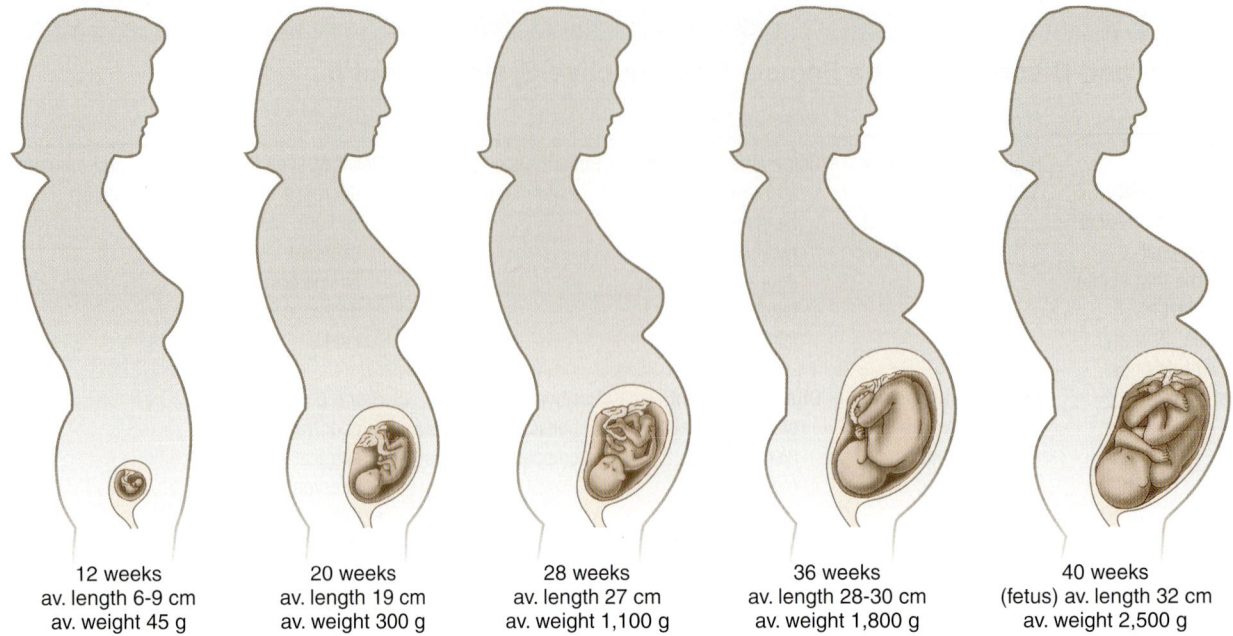

FIGURE 21-7 Fetal growth during pregnancy (*av.,* average; *cm,* centimeters; *g,* grams). (From Hunt SA: *Saunders fundamentals of medical assisting*—revised reprint, St Louis, 2007, Saunders.)

the vital centers in the brain for breathing and body temperature regulation are working. At 24 weeks the fetus is 10 to 12 inches in length.

Third Trimester

The third trimester begins at the end of week 28. During this period the fetus is very active and gains weight and grows quickly. A baby is considered "full-term" after the thirty-eighth week.

Birth Process

Parturition, or **labor,** is the physical process of the uterus expelling the fetus and the placenta. Labor is the process that forces the fetus and placenta from the uterus. Figure 21-8 shows the birth process. Labor occurs when the hormone oxytocin is secreted from the posterior pituitary gland, causing uterine contractions. Labor is divided into four stages, as follows:
- *Stage 1:* Cervical dilation and effacement occur with the onset of regular and forceful uterine contractions. The amniotic sac ruptures. Ends when the cervix is fully dilated and effaced.
- *Stage 2:* Crowning occurs, and the fetus is expelled, usually headfirst. The umbilical cord is clamped and cut when the baby's body has completed the passage through the birth canal. Ends with the birth of the baby.
- *Stage 3:* Detachment of the placenta and fetal membranes occurs and they are expelled, usually within 15 minutes after birth. Ends with the birth of the placenta.
- *Stage 4:* The mother begins the first stages of body changes 6 hours **postpartum.**

Within 1 minute after birth and again at 5 minutes after birth, the newborn is evaluated using a system called an *Apgar score* (Box 21-4). Heart rate, respiration, muscle tone, response to stimuli, and color are rated 0, 1, or 2 on a scale. The five ratings are added together to obtain one score. The maximum score is 10. A score less than 7 indicates that the newborn needs medical attention. The Apgar score has proved to be an accurate gauge of potential problems in the neonatal period but is not a predictor of the infant's growth and development or the quality of the infant's health after the neonatal period.

Disorders of Pregnancy

Occasionally, complications occur during pregnancy that could be life threatening to the mother, the fetus, or both. Complications can occur at any time during the gestational period. A *miscarriage* (spontaneous abortion) is the loss of the fetus before the twentieth week, and a *stillbirth* occurs after 20 weeks. Either of these conditions can result in great physical and emotional trauma for the mother, and one or both parents may be referred for counseling or support from community sources or other health care providers (e.g., social workers, fertility specialists). Table 21-5 lists disorders that can occur during pregnancy.

Summary Points

- Prenatal development is a two-phase process: (1) the embryonic period is the first 8 weeks of gestation, and (2) the fetal stage lasts from the end of the embryonic period until birth. This process occurs during the three trimesters of pregnancy.

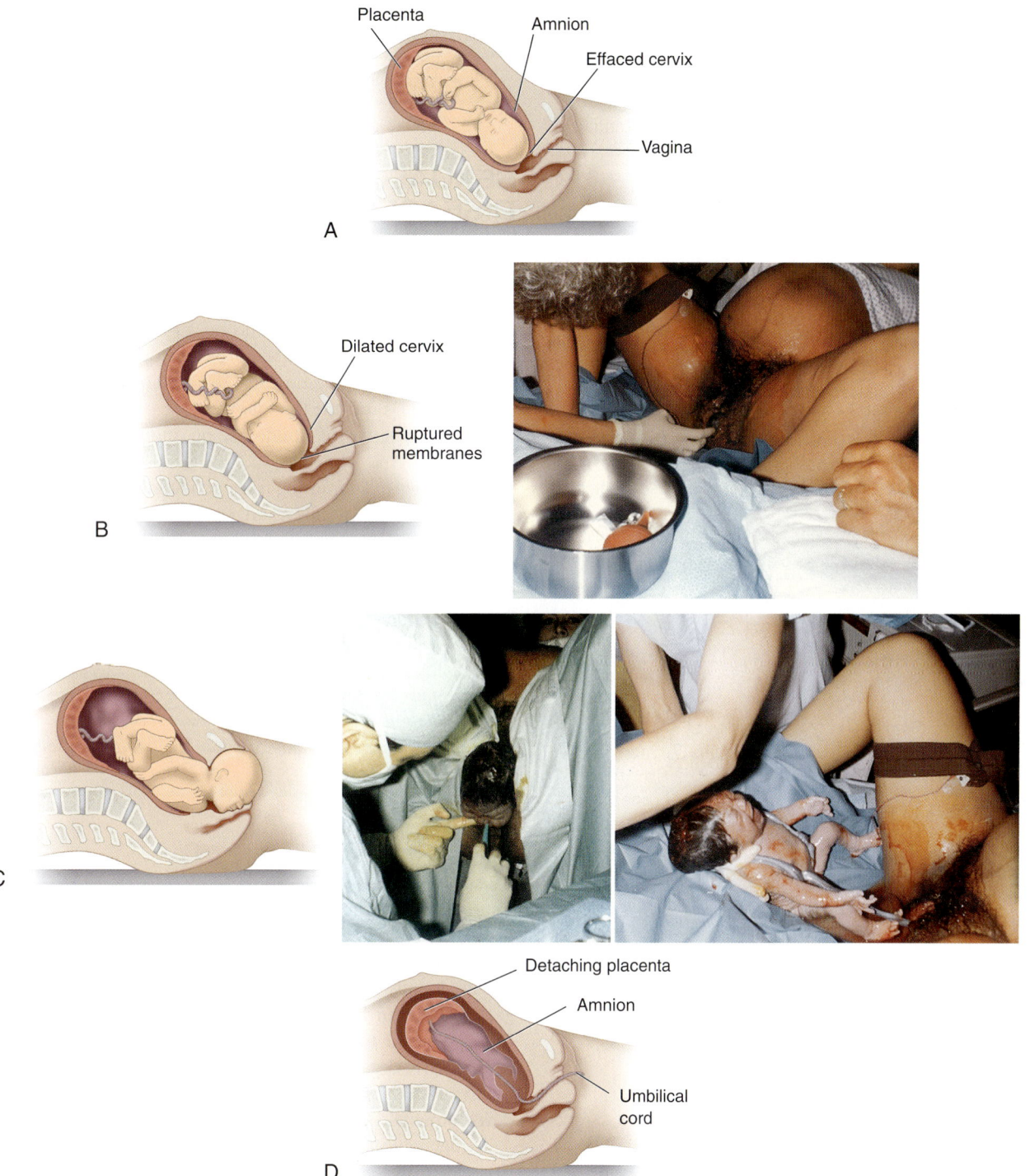

FIGURE 21-8 Process of childbirth. **A,** Before labor begins. **B,** Dilation stage. **C,** Expulsion stage. **D,** Placental stage. (From Applegate EJ: *The anatomy and physiology learning system,* Philadelphia, 1995, Saunders.)

BOX 21-4

Apgar Score

Within 1 minute after birth and again at 5 minutes, the general condition of all infants is assessed according to a standard scale developed by physician Virginia Apgar in 1958. The Apgar score is an assessment of the infant at birth and is used as a guide for subsequent care. Five specific areas are assessed separately and then summed together for a total score:

1. Heart rate
2. Respiratory rate
3. Muscle tone
4. Reflex irritability
5. Color

- A total score of 10 is perfect and indicates the infant is in the best possible condition.
- A total score of 7 to 9 is considered good, and the newborn usually requires no treatment.
- A total score of 4 to 6 indicates the infant needs close observation.
- A total score lower than 4 indicates the newborn requires immediate attention and possible placement in a neonatal intensive care unit.

Sign	Score (Points)		
	0	1	2
Heart rate	Absent	Below 100	Over 100
Respiratory rate	Absent	Slow, irregular	Good, crying
Muscle tone	Limp	Slow reflex of extremities	Active motion
Reflex, irritability (response to catheter in nose or slap to sole of foot)	No response	Grimace	Cough or sneeze; cry and withdraw foot
Color	Blue, pale	Body pink; extremities blue	Overall pink

- Labor occurs in four stages: (1) the cervix dilates; (2) the fetus is pushed through the birth canal to the outside; (3) the placenta and fetal membranes are expelled; and (4) the mother's body begins changing back to its prepregnancy state.

PATIENT-CENTERED PROFESSIONALISM

- *How would you summarize the gestation period?*

SEXUALLY TRANSMITTED DISEASES

Sexually transmitted diseases (STDs) range from easily treated infections to life-threatening diseases (Table 21-6).

Prevention of STDs is of great concern in the United States today. Persons with more than one sexual partner are more likely to contract an STD, and a person can have *concurrent* (more than one at one time) STDs. Methods to prevent the spread of STDs include the following:

- Safe sex (use of condoms, no indiscriminate sexual activity)
- Abstinence (refraining from sexual intercourse)
- Not reusing needles and syringes (use of disposable syringes and not sharing syringes)

The public should be educated on safe sex practices. In addition, all sexual partners must be treated when a diagnosis has been made.

PATIENT-CENTERED PROFESSIONALISM

- *Can you assess the value or importance of preventing the spread of STDs?*

CONCLUSION

Reproduction is the process of producing offspring to ensure a species' survival. Hereditary traits are passed from one generation to the next through reproduction. The male and the female gonads (testes in males, ovaries in females) produce gametes (sperm in males, eggs in females) and the sex hormones needed to develop and sustain the function of the reproductive organs and related structures. The female reproductive system is designed to carry the offspring through its developmental stages until childbirth.

Understanding the structure and function of the reproductive system, as well as the diseases and disorders that affect the male and female reproductive systems and pregnancy, will better prepare medical assistants to provide high-quality care to patients in the medical office.

TABLE 21-5

Disorders of Pregnancy

Disease and Description	Etiology	Signs and Symptoms	Diagnosis	Therapy	Interventions
Toxemia, or **pregnancy-induced hypertension (PIH)** Toxic condition that produces high blood pressure and proteinuria *Preeclampsia:* Hypertension with proteinuria or edema after 20 weeks' gestation *Eclampsia:* Hypertension and proteinuria with seizures	Unknown	Sudden weight gain with edema of face and extremities; patient complains of headaches, dizziness, nausea, and vomiting; in severe cases, patient may have seizures	Patient symptoms, increase in electrolyte levels, blood albumin, increased blood pressure, proteinuria	If fetus is mature enough for delivery, labor is induced; if not, hospitalization, bedrest, and medications to reduce blood pressure	Encourage patient to follow salt restrictions and continue with prenatal care
Ectopic pregnancy Fertilized egg implants outside uterus; usually in fallopian tubes	Unknown; fertilized egg does not follow normal progression to uterus because of tube stricture	Sudden onset of severe lower abdominal pain	Pelvic examination, ultrasonography, enlarged uterus	Surgery to terminate pregnancy	Encourage patient to seek immediate medical attention
Abruptio placentae Premature separation of placenta from uterine wall, either partially or completely	Unknown; trauma; use of illegal stimulants (e.g., cocaine)	Sudden abdominal pain, vaginal bleeding, and fetal activity decreases; mother must have immediate medical attention	Pelvic ultrasonography, if time allows; otherwise, clinical symptoms	Treatment for shock; surgical intervention	Encourage early and continual prenatal care
Placenta previa Attachment of placenta implants in lower portion of uterus	Unknown	Painless vaginal bleeding	Vital signs: shock Fetal heart rate decreases: decreased blood supply	Control of hemorrhaging; surgical intervention	Encourage early and continued prenatal care
Gestational diabetes Pregnant woman unable to metabolize carbohydrates; develops during latter part of pregnancy (24-28 weeks)	Risk factors are obesity, age over 30 years, and family history of diabetes	Classic symptoms of diabetes (e.g., excessive thirst, frequency of urination)	Routine screening for glucose on prenatal visits, with elevated levels above normal; glucose tolerance test week 20-24 of pregnancy	Controlled diet of carbohydrates; constant monitoring of blood glucose levels	Encourage patient to seek early and continued prenatal care; provide patient education

TABLE 21-6
Sexually Transmitted Diseases

Disease	Causative Organism	Transmission	Signs and Symptoms	Treatment	Complications
AIDS	HIV	Sexual contact; exposure to blood or blood products; mother to fetus; exposure to body fluids	*Active stage:* rash, cough, night sweats, malaise, swollen lymph nodes *Asymptomatic stage:* no symptoms, but test for HIV antigens is positive *Full active stage:* swollen lymph nodes, diarrhea, oral candidiasis, weight loss, fatigue, skin rash, fever; infections include pneumonia *(Pneumocystis carinii)* or Kaposi's sarcoma	No cure, but drug treatment improves survival	Neurological impairment
Chlamydial infection	*Chlamydia trachomatis*	Sexual contact; mother to fetus during vaginal delivery	Purulent vaginal discharge, genital pain, dysuria	10-day course of antibiotics (tetracycline, erythromycin)	Sterility, PID
Genital herpes	HSV-2	Sexual contact; mother to fetus during vaginal delivery	Genital soreness, ulcerations, pruritus, erythema; vesicles around genitals or anus that erupt for about 10 days	No known cure; treatment with antiviral (acyclovir) makes outbreaks less severe	
Genital warts	HPV	Sexual contact	Raised growths in or near penis, vagina, or rectum; painless but may itch	External treatments include removal by acid application, freezing, or burning	If left untreated, HPV could cause cervical or penile cancer
Gonorrhea	*Neisseria gonorrhoeae*	Sexual contact; mother to fetus during vaginal delivery	Yellow purulent discharge from genitourinary tract, painful and frequent urination, and painful genital area; or may be asymptomatic	Antibiotics (penicillin, amoxicillin, tetracycline)	Sterility, cystitis, endocarditis, arthritis, PID, ectopic pregnancy
Syphilis	*Treponema pallidum* (spirochete)	Sexual contact; mother to fetus via placenta; blood transfusion if donor in early stage and undiagnosed	*Primary stage:* genital lesions, enlarged lymph nodes *Secondary stage:* lesions of skin and mucous membranes, with generalized symptoms of headache and fever *Latent stage:* asymptomatic	Antibiotics, usually penicillin	Central nervous system disturbances, cardiovascular damage, psychosis
Trichomoniasis	*Trichomonas vaginalis*	Sexual contact	Itching with severe protozoal infection; frothy, gray-green, foul-smelling discharge from vaginal area	Antibiotics	Sterility, PID

AIDS, Acquired immunodeficiency syndrome; *HIV*, human immunodeficiency virus; *HPV*, human papillomavirus; *HSV-2*, herpes simplex type 2; *PID*, pelvic inflammatory disease.

Chapter Summary

Reinforce your understanding of the material in this chapter by reviewing the curriculum objectives and key content points below.

1. **Define, appropriately use, and spell all the Key Terms for this chapter.**
   - Review the Key Terms if necessary.
2. **List the two main functions of the human reproductive system.**
   - The human reproductive system serves to produce offspring.
   - Hormones are produced by the male and female reproductive systems for various body functions and traits.
3. **Name the reproductive cells produced by the male and female gonads.**
   - The male gonads are the testes, and they produce sperm.
   - The female gonads are the ovaries, and they produce eggs.
   - Gametes are the sex cells (ova and sperm) produced by the gonads.
4. **Trace the pathway that sperm follow through the five major structures of the male reproductive system, beginning with the testes and ending with the urethra.**
   - Semen passes through the genitourinary tract in the male.
   - Sperm travels from the testes to the epididymis to the vas deferens to the ejaculatory duct and finally to the urethra.
5. **Describe the two main functions of testosterone.**
   - The testes secrete testosterone.
   - Testosterone determines gender in the embryo and forms the male reproductive organs; it also enables reproductive function.
6. **Differentiate between the primary and the secondary male sex characteristics.**
   - Sex characteristics distinguish one sex from the other.
   - Primary sex characteristics are directly related to reproduction (e.g., development of the male reproductive organs).
   - Secondary sex characteristics are masculine but not directly related to reproduction (e.g., hair growth, deepening of voice, and enlarged muscles).
7. **Explain the purpose of semen.**
   - Semen is the (fluid) vehicle that transports the sperm from the male to the female reproductive system.
8. **List seven common diagnostic tests for diseases and disorders of the male reproductive system and describe the use of each.**
   - Review Box 21-1.
9. **List five disorders of the male reproductive system and briefly describe the etiology, signs and symptoms, diagnosis, therapy, and interventions for each.**
   - Review Table 21-2.
10. **List, identify, and describe the seven parts of the female reproductive system.**
    - The ovaries are almond-shaped organs that produce ova and hormones.
    - The bilateral fallopian tubes transport the fertilized or unfertilized egg to the uterus.
    - The uterus is a hollow muscular organ that holds fertilized eggs for development during pregnancy.
    - The vagina connects the uterus to the vulva and is the passageway for giving birth.
    - The vulva is the external female genitalia.
    - The perineum is the external surface of the pelvic floor; an episiotomy, if necessary, is performed in this area during delivery.
    - The mammary glands produce milk in each breast and are regulated by estrogen and progesterone.
11. **Describe the function of the hormones estrogen and progesterone.**
    - Estrogen aids in development of the reproductive organs and secondary sex characteristics and is responsible for ovulation.
    - Progesterone prepares the endometrium for pregnancy and also stimulates it to shed, causing menses, when pregnancy does not occur.
    - Estrogen and progesterone work together to regulate the menstrual cycle.
12. **Describe the function of the hormones prolactin and oxytocin.**
    - Prolactin stimulates milk production.
    - Oxytocin allows for the expulsion of milk and induction of labor.
13. **Describe the function of follicle-stimulating hormone (FSH) and luteinizing hormone (LH).**
    - FSH causes the ovum to ripen in the graafian follicle.
    - LH starts ovulation and turns the follicle into the corpus luteum.
14. **Explain what happens in the five key stages of the menstrual cycle.**
    - The menstrual cycle typically lasts 28 days and is repeated from puberty until menopause.
    - The first menstrual cycle is menarche.
    - The key stages of the menstrual cycle follow:
      a. FSH causes the egg to ripen in the graafian follicle.
      b. The follicle secretes estrogen to prepare the endometrium for implantation of the fertilized egg.
      c. LH starts ovulation and turns the follicle into the corpus luteum.
      d. The corpus luteum releases the hormones progesterone and estrogen to thicken the uterine wall for pregnancy.
      e. If fertilization has not occurred, the hormone levels decrease, the endometrium sheds, and menses begins.
15. **Explain what occurs during menopause.**
    - Menopause signals the end of a woman's reproductive life.

- The amount of hormones secreted by the ovaries decreases between ages 45 and 55, and menses eventually cease.

16. **List five common diagnostic tests for diseases and disorders of the female reproductive system and describe the use of each.**
    - Refer to Box 21-3.

17. **List nine disorders of the female reproductive system and briefly describe the etiology, signs and symptoms, diagnosis, therapy, and interventions for each.**
    - Review Table 21-4.

18. **Explain how sperm fertilize eggs.**
    - Fertilization occurs when a sperm penetrates an egg.

19. **Distinguish among a zygote, an embryo, and a fetus.**
    - A fertilized egg is a zygote.
    - Cell division develops the zygote into an embryo for the first 8 weeks of gestation.
    - After 8 weeks and until birth, the embryo is termed a *fetus*.

20. **Describe the major changes that occur in each of the three trimesters of pregnancy.**
    - The first trimester is the first 12 weeks of gestation. The zygote has divided enough to form an embryo and is implanted high in the uterine wall. The amniotic sac and placenta have developed to nourish and protect the embryo. All major body systems in the embryo are developed during the first trimester. After 8 weeks the embryo becomes a fetus.
    - The second trimester begins at the end of 12 weeks. The fetus starts to grow faster, and movement begins about the twentieth week. Accelerated growth and tissue specialization occur in this trimester.
    - The third trimester begins at the end of 28 weeks. The fetus is very active, gains weight, and grows quickly.

21. **Describe the four stages of the birth process.**
    - The hormone oxytocin causes the uterine contractions of labor.
    - The four stages are (1) cervical dilation and effacement; (2) crowning and expelling of the fetus; (3) expelling of the placenta and fetal membranes; and (4) changing of the mother's body back to its prepregnancy state.

22. **List five disorders of pregnancy and briefly describe the etiology, signs and symptoms, diagnosis, therapy, and interventions for each.**
    - Review Table 21-5.

23. **List three practices for preventing the spread of sexually transmitted diseases (STDs).**
    - Disease prevention is the most effective way to slow the spread of STDs.
    - To prevent the spread of STDs, encourage safe sex, abstinence, and not reusing needles and syringes.

24. **List seven STDs and briefly describe the etiology, signs and symptoms, diagnosis, therapy, and interventions for each.**
    - Review Table 21-6.

25. **Analyze a realistic medical office situation and apply your understanding of the human reproductive system to determine the best course of action.**
    - Understanding the male and female reproductive systems and the diseases and disorders that affect them will help when providing patient education and treatment.

26. **Describe the impact on patient care when medical assistants have a solid understanding of the structure and function of the male and female reproductive systems.**
    - Miscommunication and errors are less likely to occur when medical assistants understand the structure and function of the body system related to the patient's visit.

PRACTICAL APPLICATIONS

If you have accomplished the objectives in this chapter, you will be able to make better choices as a medical assistant. Take another look at this situation and decide what you would do.

Valerie has called her gynecologist for her annual Pap smear. The receptionist wants to be sure that Valerie did not make her appointment during the time of her menses. Her menarche was at age 14. She has taken oral contraceptives in the past. She is now approaching age 50 and has excessive bleeding with each menstrual period. Her LMP was a week ago, and she is to have the Pap smear with her physical examination today. The medical assistant asks Valerie if she does monthly BSEs. Dr. Jones started ordering a mammogram for Valerie on a yearly basis at age 35 because of a family history of fibrocystic disease of the breasts. Valerie asks Dr. Jones about taking HRT since she seems to be approaching menopause and has PMS with each menstrual period. Dr. Jones replies that she will discuss this with Valerie after the Pap smear report has returned.

Do you understand why the various aspects of Valerie's appointment were handled the way they were?

1. Why is it important that Valerie not make her appointment for her Pap smear during the time of menses?
2. What are the five stages of the menstrual cycle?
3. What is menarche? Are menstrual periods regular immediately following menarche?
4. What is HRT? What classifications of medications are given for HRT? For oral contraception?
5. What is BSE, and when should this typically be done?
6. What is fibrocystic disease of the breast? Why are mammograms and BSE important with this condition?
7. What is PMS?
8. What are the signs of menopause?

WEB SEARCH

1. **Research advances in antenatal medicine.** Before birth, medicine permits extensive diagnosis and treatment of disease in the fetus.

- **Keyword:** Use the following keyword in your search: antenatal medicine.

WORD PARTS: Reproductive System

MALE REPRODUCTIVE SYSTEM
Combining Forms

andr/o	male
epididym/o	epididymis
orchi/o, orchid/o	testis
prostat/o	prostate gland
semin/i	semen; seminal vessel
scrot/o	scrotum
spermat/o	spermatozoa; sperm cells
test/o	testis
vas/o	vessel; vas deferens
vesicul/o	seminal vesicle

FEMALE REPRODUCTIVE SYSTEM
Combining Forms

cervic/o	neck, cervix
colp/o, vagin/o	vagina
episi/o, vulv/o	vulva
gynec/o	female, women
hyster/o, metr/o, uter/o	uterus
mamm/o, mast/o	breast
men/o	menses
oophor/o, ovari/o	ovary
ov/o, ovul/o	egg
salping/o	fallopian

HUMAN DEVELOPMENT
Combining Forms

amni/o	amniotic
embry/o	embryo
fet/o	fetus
gravida	pregnant woman
nat/i	birth
para	given birth
toc/o	labor

ABBREVIATIONS: Reproductive System

MALE REPRODUCTIVE SYSTEM

BPH	benign prostatic hypertrophy
GU	genitourinary
TUR, TURP	transurethral resection of the prostate

FEMALE REPRODUCTIVE SYSTEM

BCP	birth control pill
BSE	breast self-examination
D&C	dilation (widening) and curettage (scraping)
FBD	fibrocystic breast disease
FSH	follicle-stimulating hormone
G	gravida (pregnant)
GYN	gynecology
hCG	human chorionic gonadotropin
HRT	hormone replacement therapy
IUD	intrauterine device (for contraception)
LH	luteinizing hormone
LMP	last menstrual period
OB	obstetrics, obstetrical
OCs	oral contraceptives ("birth control pills")
PMS	premenstrual syndrome

SEXUALLY TRANSMITTED DISEASES

GC	gonococcal bacteria
PID	pelvic inflammatory disease
STD	sexually transmitted disease
VDRL	Venereal Disease Research Laboratories; blood test for syphilis and other STDs

22 Endocrine System

evolve http://evolve.elsevier.com/klieger/medicalassisting

The endocrine system works with the nervous system to maintain homeostasis (balance) in the body. The glands and organs in the endocrine system help maintain homeostasis by regulating and controlling various body functions through the synthesis and secretion of hormones. Functions controlled and regulated by the endocrine system include growth and development, absorption of nutrients, metabolism, fluid balance, reproduction, and reactions to injury. *Endocrinology* is the study of the endocrine system. Diseases and disorders of the endocrine system are often caused by too much or too little hormone secretion or by the body's inability to use a hormone in the way it was meant to be used.

Medical assistants need to be familiar with the function of the endocrine system, its major glands, the organs containing endocrine tissue, the process of regulating hormones, and the diseases and disorders that affect this system.

LEARNING OBJECTIVES

You will be able to do the following after completing this chapter:

Key Terms
1. Define, appropriately use, and spell all the Key Terms for this chapter.

Endocrine System Function
2. Explain the two main functions of the endocrine system.
3. Compare and contrast *endocrine* and *exocrine* glands.

Major Endocrine Glands
4. Identify and locate the seven major endocrine glands.
5. List the hormones and primary function of each of the seven major endocrine glands.

Endocrine Activity in Cells and Organs
6. Describe prostaglandins, and explain how they differ from proteins and steroid hormones.
7. Name two hormone-secreting organs, and identify the hormones they secrete.

Regulation of Hormones
8. Define feedback, and explain how it keeps the body in homeostasis.

Diseases and Disorders of the Endocrine System
9. List 17 common signs and symptoms of endocrine system disease.
10. List 14 common diagnostic tests and procedures for endocrine system disease and describe the use of each.
11. List 10 endocrine diseases and disorders and briefly describe the etiology, signs and symptoms, diagnosis, therapy, and interventions for each.

Patient-Centered Professionalism
12. Analyze a realistic medical office situation and apply your understanding of the endocrine system to determine the best course of action.
13. Describe the impact on patient care when medical assistants have a solid understanding of the structure and function of the endocrine system.

KEY TERMS

The Key Terms for this chapter have been organized into sections so that you can easily see the terminology associated with each aspect of the endocrine system.

Endocrine System Function
endocrine glands
exocrine glands
homeostasis
hormone
target organ

Major Endocrine Glands
Pituitary Gland

antidiuretic hormone (ADH)	oxytocin
hypophysis	sella turcica
pituitary gland	

Thyroid and Parathyroid Glands

calcium tetany	parathyroid hormone (PTH)
parathyroid glands	thyroid gland

Adrenal Gland

adrenal glands

Adrenal Cortex

adrenal cortex	cortisol
aldosterone	glucocorticoids
androgens	mineralocorticoids
corticoids	steroid

Adrenal Medulla

adrenal medulla	norepinephrine
epinephrine	

Pancreas

glucagon	islets of Langerhans
insulin	pancreas

Endocrine Activity in Cells and Organs

melatonin	thymosin
pineal gland	thymus
prostaglandins	

Regulation of Hormones

feedback	positive feedback
negative feedback	

Diseases and Disorders of the Endocrine System

endocrinologist	hyposecretion
hypersecretion	

Signs and Symptoms

anorexia	hypoglycemia
exophthalmia	hypokalemia
goiter	hyponatremia
hirsutism	paresthesia
hypercalcemia	polydipsia
hyperglycemia	polyphagia
hyperkalemia	polyuria
hypernatremia	tetany
hypocalcemia	

Diagnostic Tests and Procedures

A_{1c}	radiography
computed tomography (CT)	radioimmunoassay (RIA)
fasting blood sugar (FBS)	thyroid function tests (TFTs)
glucose tolerance test (GTT)	total calcium
hormone level test	ultrasonography
magnetic resonance imaging (MRI)	urine glucose
radioactive iodine (RAI) uptake scan	urine ketones

Diseases and Disorders
Pituitary Gland

acromegaly	dwarfism
diabetes insipidus	gigantism

Thyroid Gland

cretinism	Graves disease
exophthalmos	myxedema
goiter	

Adrenal Glands

Addison disease	Cushing syndrome
Conn's syndrome	

Pancreas

diabetes mellitus

PRACTICAL APPLICATIONS

Read the following scenario and keep it in mind as you learn about the endocrine system in this chapter.

Juliette, age 4 years, cannot drink enough water and has to void frequently. Her mother says that Juliette eats all the time but is losing weight. She is also lethargic. At times her mother thinks that Juliette's breath has a fruity odor, although she does not chew fruit-flavored gum or eat fruit-flavored candy. After checking Juliette, Dr. Jay tells the mother that Juliette may have diabetes mellitus. Dr. Jay wants to do further testing as quickly as possible and orders a fasting blood sugar, which comes back elevated. Dr. Jay follows this with a glucose tolerance test (GTT). When the GTT is abnormally high, Dr. Jay prescribes insulin for Juliette.

Do you understand why Dr. Jay diagnosed Juliette with diabetes mellitus, and why she ordered the tests she did?

ENDOCRINE SYSTEM FUNCTION

The endocrine system is a group of glands that secrete **hormones** that regulate various body functions (Figure 22-1 and Table 22-1). These hormones are secreted directly into the bloodstream by glands that are referred to as "ductless glands" (endocrine).

The ductless endocrine glands should not be confused with the exocrine glands. **Exocrine glands** have ducts and include the sweat, sebaceous, and mammary glands, as well as glands that secrete digestive enzymes. **Endocrine glands** do not have ducts to carry the secreted hormones; instead, they secrete their hormones directly into the bloodstream. To help you distinguish between the two types, keep in mind that *endo* means "within," whereas *exo* means "outside"; *crine* means to "separate" or "secrete."

When hormones are secreted, receptors within the **target organ** cause the organ to react to the hormone. The hormone

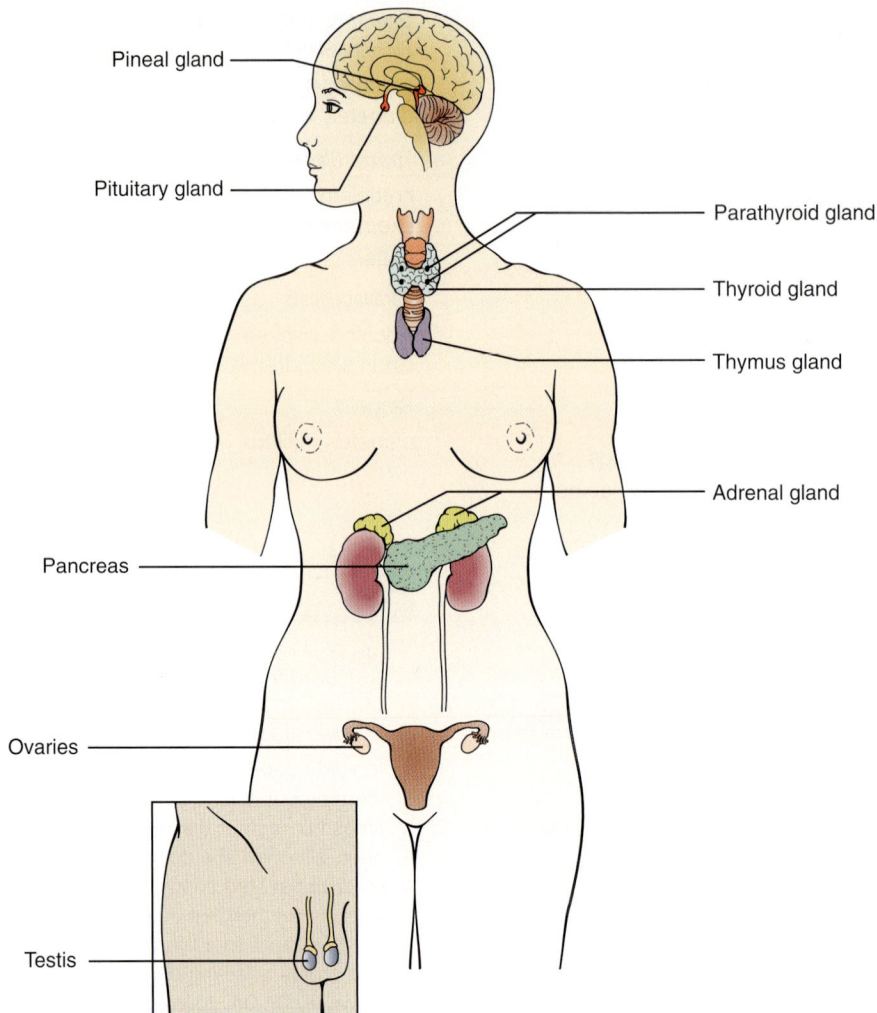

FIGURE 22-1 Major endocrine glands of the body. (From Buck CJ: *Step-by-step medical coding, 2008 edition*, St Louis, 2008, Saunders.)

fits into the cells of the target organ like a key in a lock. The hormonal action can promote growth, influence behavior, assist in reproductive activity, and even control metabolism. The production of a hormone can be controlled by the action of other hormones, feedback, or by nerve stimulation. Thus the two main functions of the endocrine system are (1) to regulate body functions by means of hormones and (2) to help maintain **homeostasis.**

FOR YOUR INFORMATION

CHARACTERISTICS OF HORMONES
- One hormone can influence production and concentration of other hormones.
- Growth, development, and personality are all affected by hormones.
- Most hormones are steroids, or proteins, with defined functions.

PATIENT-CENTERED PROFESSIONALISM

- *Compare and contrast how the nervous system and the endocrine system work to control homeostasis.*
- *Beside signals from the nervous system, what else causes hormones to be secreted?*

MAJOR ENDOCRINE GLANDS

Pituitary Gland

The **pituitary gland,** or **hypophysis,** is a small gland about the size of a pea held in the **sella turcica,** which is a depression in the sphenoid bone in the cranial cavity. The pituitary gland connects to the hypothalamus and is under its control. The hypothalamic hormones that are released from the hypothalamus act on various target cells within the pituitary gland. For example:

TABLE 22-1
Hormones and Primary Function of Major Endocrine Glands

Hormone	Target Tissue	Primary Function
PITUITARY GLAND		
Anterior Lobe		
Growth hormone (GH)	Bone and soft tissue	Promotes muscle tissue and long bone growth
Thyroid-stimulating hormone (TSH)	Thyroid gland	Stimulates thyroid gland to produce hormones for growth as well as other body functions
		Stimulates thyroxine production
Adrenocorticotropic hormone (ACTH)	Adrenal cortex	Stimulates secretion of steroids from adrenal cortex (adrenocortical hormones)
		Helps in stressful situations
Gonadotropins		
Follicle-stimulating hormone (FSH)	Gonads	Stimulates growth and hormone activity of testes and ovaries
Luteinizing hormone (LH)	Follicle cells of ovaries	Promotes ovulation
	Interstitial cells of testes	Stimulates testosterone secretion
Prolactin (PRL)	Mammary glands	Promotes growth of breast tissue and milk production
Melanocyte-stimulating hormone (MSH)	Melanocytes	Increases skin pigmentation
Posterior Lobe		
Antidiuretic hormone (ADH; vasopressin)	Kidney's collecting ducts	Responsible for water reabsorption in the kidney and its return to circulation
		Stimulates blood vessel constriction
Oxytocin (OT)	Uterus	Causes contractions of uterus during childbirth and milk secretion
	Mammary glands	
THYROID GLAND		
Thyroxine and triiodothyronine	Most cells	Increase body cell metabolism and leads to normal development of body systems
Calcitonin	Bone	Regulates calcium levels in the blood
PARATHYROID GLAND		
Parathyroid hormone (PTH; parathormone)	Bone	Regulates calcium levels in bones and blood
	Kidneys	Increases calcium levels in the blood
	Digestive system	
ADRENAL GLAND		
Adrenal Cortex		
Cortisol (glucocorticoids)	Most cells	Helps in carbohydrate metabolism
		Active during stress
		Depresses inflammatory and immune response
Aldosterone (mineralocorticoids)	Kidney tubules	Regulates sodium and water balance, and thus blood volume and pressure
Androgens, estrogens, and progestins (gonadocorticoids)	Ovaries or testes	Influence secondary sex characteristics
Adrenal Medulla		
Epinephrine and norepinephrine (catecholamines)	Skeletal muscle	Increased heart rate, glycogen breakdown, blood glucose, and blood pressure
	Cardiac muscle	Active during stress
	Blood vessels	
	Liver	
	Adipose tissue	
PANCREAS (Islets of Langerhans)		
Insulin	General	Decreases blood sugar levels
		Takes glucose into cells and stores as glycogen
Glucagon	Liver	Increases blood sugar by stimulating liver to release stored glycogen to become glucose
	Adipose tissue	
OVARIES		
Estrogen	Most cells	Helps in development of secondary sex characteristics in women
	Reproductive structures	
Progesterone	Uterus	Prepares and maintains the uterus in pregnancy
	Breast	
TESTES		
Testosterone	General	Helps in development of secondary sex characteristics in men
	Reproductive structures	
THYMUS		
Thymosin	General	Stimulates maturation of T-lymphocytes

When growth hormone–releasing hormone (GHRH) is released from the hypothalamus, it stimulates the release of growth hormone into the bloodstream from the anterior pituitary gland.

The pituitary gland is divided into anterior and posterior lobes (Figure 22-2). The pituitary gland is considered the "master gland" because it secretes several hormones that control other endocrine glands and because it affects both growth and development.

Anterior Lobe

The anterior lobe of the pituitary gland produces growth hormone, thyroid-stimulating hormone (TSH), adrenocorticotropic hormone (ACTH), and follicle-stimulating hormone necessary for the formation of ova and sperm (see Table 22-1).

Posterior Lobe

The posterior lobe of the pituitary gland is responsible for the secretion of **oxytocin** and **antidiuretic hormone (ADH).** Oxytocin is responsible for the contractions of the uterus during labor and after childbirth and the stimulation of milk production. ADH regulates the fluid balance in the body by controlling resorption of water and thus urine production.

Thyroid Gland

The **thyroid gland** is located in the neck on both sides of the trachea and larynx (just like a bow tie). The thyroid gland needs iodine to produce the thyroid hormones. The thyroid secretes three hormones: calcitonin, thyroxine (thyroxin, T_4), and triiodothyronine (T_3). These hormones stimulate the metabolic rate and promote growth. How much thyroid hormone is secreted depends on the anterior pituitary gland receiving a message (feedback) that the levels of the hormone are low in the blood, or a message that adequate amounts of hormone have been secreted and no more is needed. TSH is secreted from the anterior pituitary to promote production and secretion of the thyroid hormones.

Parathyroid Gland

There are four **parathyroid glands** located within connective tissue surrounding the thyroid gland. They secrete **parathyroid hormone (PTH),** or parathormone, which regulates the amount of circulating calcium and phosphorus in the blood and tissue fluid. PTH increases levels of calcium by stimulating release of calcium from the bones and the decrease of phosphorus, reabsorption of calcium from the kidney tubules, and absorption of vitamin D from the intestine. If calcium levels become too high, calcitonin is released from the thyroid gland to stop calcium removal from the bones (Figure 22-3).

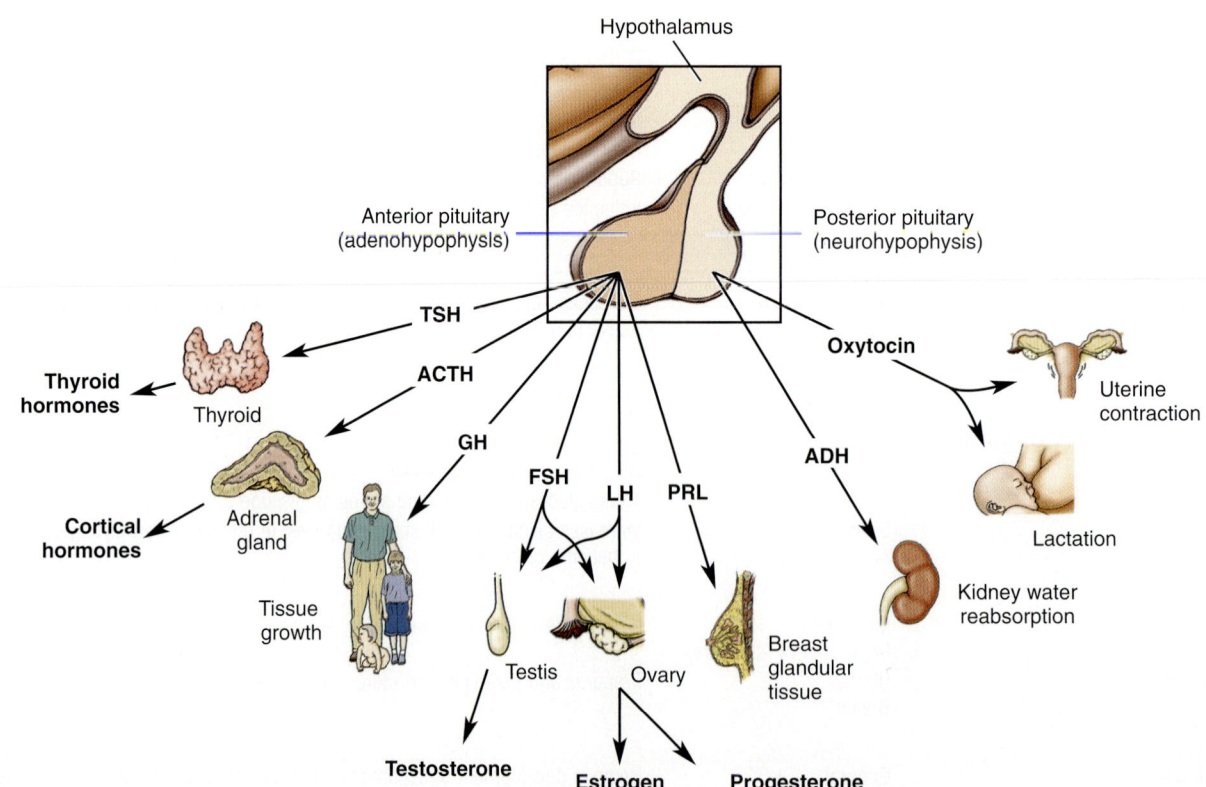

FIGURE 22-2 Pituitary gland. Hormones secreted by anterior and posterior lobes of pituitary gland along with their target organs. (Modified from Herlihy B, Maebius NK: *The human body in health and illness,* ed 3, St Louis, 2007, Saunders.)

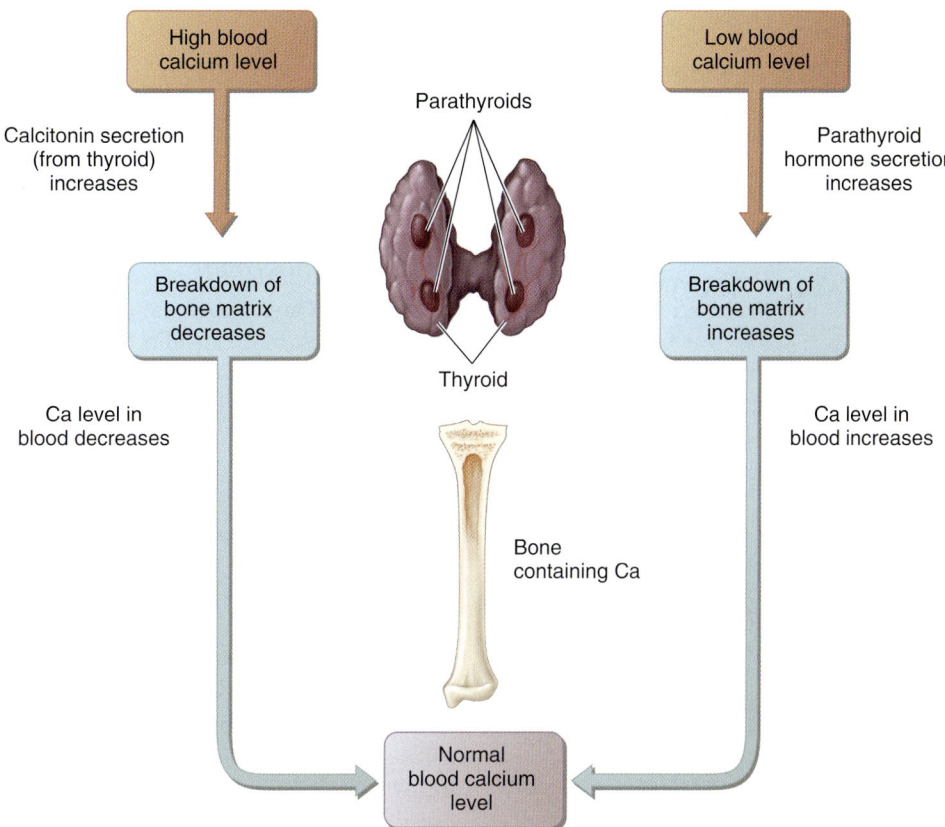

FIGURE 22-3 Regulation of blood calcium levels. (Modified from Thibodeau GA, Patton KT: *Anatomy and physiology*, ed 6, St Louis, 2007, Mosby.)

If the phosphorus levels are too high, calcium is released as feedback. A person having a thyroidectomy with parathyroid involvement needs to be monitored for muscle spasms (**calcium tetany**) that result from abnormal calcium levels in the blood.

Adrenal Gland

There are two **adrenal glands** located above the kidneys. Their structure, like that of the kidney, has an outer portion, the cortex, and an inner portion, the medulla. Both areas secrete hormones designed to assist the body in times of stress and also control metabolic rate.

Adrenal Cortex

The **adrenal cortex** secretes multiple hormones that are classified as corticosteroids or **steroids.** Steroid hormones pass through the cell membrane, enter the nucleus of a cell, and form a protein that produces specific effects in the target cell. For example, estrogen is a steroid hormone, and its production in a female adolescent will cause breast development. Box 22-1 identifies the short- and long-term effects of steroids when taken at high levels to build muscle mass and strength.

FOR YOUR INFORMATION

THE DANGERS OF STEROIDS

Steroids are synthetic forms of testosterone. Testosterone has two main effects: anabolic, which promotes muscle building, and androgenic, which is responsible for male traits (e.g., facial hair). Steroids used by athletes are modified to minimize the androgenic effects, but some effects remain.

HOW THEY WORK
- Blood carries steroid to muscle cells.
- Steroid attaches to cell and is drawn in by a receptor.
- Receptor and steroid bind to genes.
- Builds amino acids into new protein (for muscles).

Corticosteroids, or **corticoids,** are steroid hormones synthesized from cholesterol by the adrenal cortex. Types of corticoids include glucocorticoids, mineralocorticoids, and corticotropins.

Glucocorticoids promote the release of glucose from glycogen and provide extra energy in a stressful situation. These hormones also aid in reducing inflammation. However, if too

BOX 22-1

Short-Term and Long-Term Side Effects of Steroid Use

SHORT-TERM SIDE EFFECTS

Men	Women
Impotence	Facial hair growth
Reduced sperm count	Menstrual cycle changes
Shrinking of testes	Breast reduction
Breast development	Increased appetite
Baldness	Deepened voice
Higher voice	

LONG-TERM SIDE EFFECTS

Side effects can show up years after steroid use.
- Aggression and depression
- Increased risk of stroke
- Acne
- Voice change
- Elevated blood pressure
- Heart attack
- Increased LDL levels
- Liver damage (tumors)
- Weight gain, bloating
- Weakened tendons
- Blood clots
- Decreased growth development in teenagers

LDL, Low-density lipoprotein.

---

much hormone is produced for long periods, such as during prolonged stressful periods, glucocorticoids act as an immunosuppressant to the body. This lessens the body's ability to fight infections. **Cortisol** is the main glucocorticoid. A deficiency of cortisol, known as **Addison disease,** causes an increased melanin production, thus giving an individual a tanned appearance.

The **mineralocorticoids** control sodium, potassium, and water balance mainly through action on the kidneys. **Aldosterone** is the main mineralocorticoid. The kidneys are stimulated to excrete potassium and retain sodium.

Some sex steroids, particularly **androgens** and estrogens, are also produced by the adrenal cortex (as well as by the gonads). As discussed in Chapter 21, these hormones regulate secondary sex characteristics.

Adrenal Medulla

The **adrenal medulla** secretes two hormones (also called *catecholamines*): **epinephrine** and **norepinephrine.** These hormones increase during stressful situations, which enables the body to react as necessary. Normally, the adrenal gland secretes these hormones in small amounts to maintain balance within the system. When a person becomes anxious, nerve stimulation causes the medulla to secrete additional amounts of hormones to handle stress.

Pancreas

As discussed in Chapter 15, the **pancreas** has a major function in the digestive process as an exocrine gland and also serves as an endocrine gland. The islets of Langerhans in the pancreas play a key role in the production of hormones used to regulate blood sugar.

Islets of Langerhans

The **islets of Langerhans** scattered throughout the pancreas produce the hormone **insulin** and cause the secretion of the hormone **glucagon** (Figure 22-4). These hormones work to keep the blood sugar levels of the blood in balance. Insulin stimulates the breakdown of glucose so it can be stored as glycogen in the liver. When glucose is needed by the body, glucagon stimulates the liver cells to convert glycogen to glucose. Insulin acts as the key for cells to use glucose for energy.

Ovaries and Testes

Hormone production and the functions of the ovaries and testes (gonads) were discussed in Chapter 21. The hormone *estrogen* is secreted by the female gonad, the ovary; therefore the ovary is an endocrine gland as well. It assists with maturation of the egg, stimulates growth of blood vessels in the uterus in preparation of egg implantation, and is responsible for the development of the secondary sex characteristics in the female adolescent (Box 22-2). *Progesterone,* another hormone, promotes the storage of glycogen, further enhances the uterine wall for implantation, and is also responsible for the secretory cells of the mammary glands.

In males the main hormone secreted by the male gonad (the testes) is *testosterone.* Testosterone is responsible for the maturation of sperm and development of secondary sex characteristics at puberty (see Box 22-2).

PATIENT-CENTERED PROFESSIONALISM

- *Why is it necessary for the medical assistant to know the major endocrine glands and their structure and function and to understand the overall effects of hormones on the body?*
- *How can this knowledge affect the care that patients receive?*

ENDOCRINE ACTIVITY IN CELLS AND ORGANS

In addition to the endocrine glands, other organs and body cells can stimulate hormone activity. Prostaglandins are produced by many of the body's cells, and the pineal gland and thymus are two organs that produce important hormones.

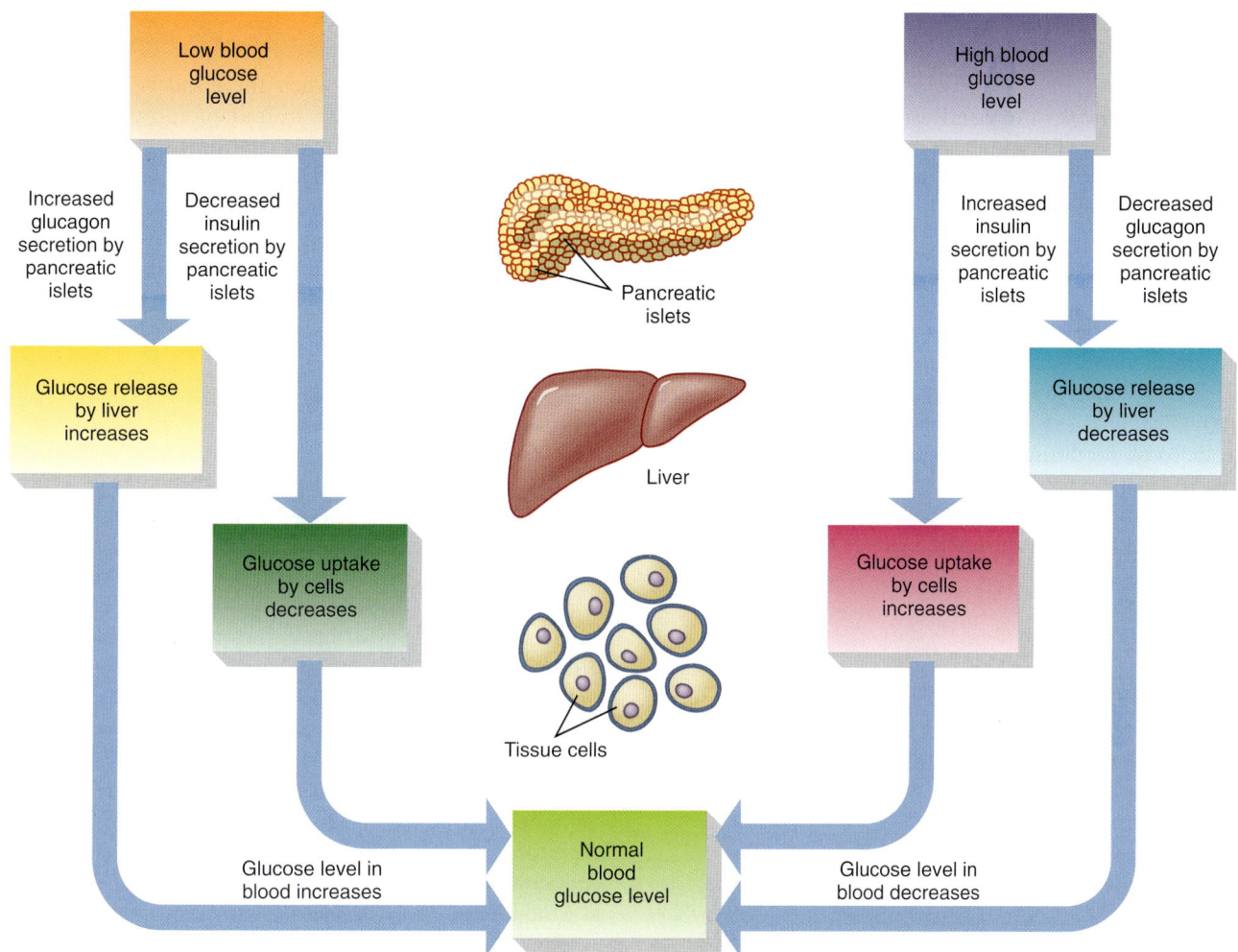

FIGURE 22-4 Regulation of blood glucose levels by the pancreas: Many other hormones, such as growth hormone, cortisol, and others, also influence blood glucose levels. (Modified from Thibodeau GA, Patton KT: *Anatomy and physiology*, ed 6, St Louis, 2007, Mosby.)

BOX 22-2

Secondary Sex Characteristics

MALE
Growth of all reproductive organs
Growth of facial and body hair
Growth of larynx, causing deepening of voice
Growth of skeletal muscles and closure of growth plate in long bones

FEMALE
Growth of duct system of mammary glands
Growth of uterus
Fatty deposits on hips and thighs
Closure of growth plate (epiphyseal disc) in long bones, stopping growth

Body Cells

Many body cells produce **prostaglandins**. Prostaglandins are short-lived hormone-like substances responsible for the regulation of blood pressure, a person's pain threshold, inflammation, and blood clotting.

Prostaglandins are not proteins or steroid hormones. Instead, they are lipids that mimic hormones. Prostaglandins are sometimes referred to as "local hormones." Proteins and steroid hormones from the endocrine glands circulate in the blood to "target" tissues, whereas prostaglandins act on adjacent (local) cells. Prostaglandins are similar to hormones but are not classified as hormones; hormones are produced by specialized cells grouped together in endocrine glands, but prostaglandins are produced by cells all over the body. They are formed and then released from cell membranes in response to a particular stimulus. Prostaglandins cause inflammation and fever and can intensify pain, so prostaglandin-inhibiting medications and therapy are used to reduce pain, fever, and inflammation.

The pineal and thymus glands stimulate the release of prostaglandins that are found in all cell membranes.

The kidneys, stomach, and small intestine also produce hormones and are discussed in their respective chapters.

Pineal Gland

The **pineal gland** is a small, cone-shaped organ in the brain that secretes **melatonin.** Onset of puberty in response to natural light has been attributed to melatonin, and melatonin is responsible for diurnal (day/night) cycles. Supplemental use of melatonin seems to induce sleep and relaxation. An overproduction of melatonin may be responsible for a type of depression that occurs during the winter months when daylight is limited.

Thymus

The **thymus** gland is both an endocrine gland and a lymphatic organ. The thymus gland secretes **thymosin,** which is important for the immune system to function properly. As a person ages, this secretion decreases and the gland changes to fat and connective tissue.

PATIENT-CENTERED PROFESSIONALISM

- How do prostaglandins (local hormones) differ from other hormones released in the body?

REGULATION OF HORMONES

The regulation of hormone secretion by the endocrine glands is accomplished by either negative or positive feedback. **Feedback** allows the body to stay in homeostasis by responding to either increased or decreased levels of a particular hormone in the blood. Feedback effects can be negative or positive.

Negative Feedback

As an example of negative feedback, consider how PTH regulates the concentration of calcium in the blood. A slight decrease in blood calcium triggers the parathyroid gland to increase its secretion of PTH, which causes calcium to leave the bones and enter the bloodstream. When the calcium level rises above what is needed, a feedback mechanism slows or inhibits the secretion of PTH (see Figure 22-3). Therefore the feedback effects respond negatively to the stimulus; that is, a **negative feedback** occurs. Negative feedback is the decrease of a stimulation when that stimulus is no longer needed (e.g., the condition has been met).

Positive Feedback

Positive feedback occurs when the gland is stimulated to increase hormone secretion instead of turning it off. For example, the onset of labor occurs because hormones are released that promote contractions of the uterus until the newborn is delivered. Once delivery occurs, the hormone level decreases, and the contractions stop. Positive feedback increases a stimulus to produce a needed action.

PATIENT-CENTERED PROFESSIONALISM

- How does feedback work?

DISEASES AND DISORDERS OF THE ENDOCRINE SYSTEM

Diseases of the endocrine system are often the result of an underproduction (**hyposecretion**) or an overproduction (**hypersecretion**) of a particular hormone. The effects of the disease can be seen in early childhood or may not be a problem until adulthood. An **endocrinologist** is a specialist who treats disorders of the endocrine system. Medications may be prescribed to treat endocrine disorders (Table 22-2).

As with the other nervous system problems, medical assistants need to be able to recognize the common signs and symptoms of and diagnostic tests for the different types of endocrine system diseases.

- Study Box 22-3 to familiarize yourself with the common signs and symptoms.
- Study Box 22-4 to learn about common diagnostic tests and procedures.
- Table 22-3 lists information concerning different types of endocrine system disease.
- Table 22-4 summarizes endocrine organs and disorders.

TABLE 22-2

Endocrine Drug Classifications

Drug Classification	Common Generic (Brand) Drugs
Corticosteroids	prednisone (Deltasone)
Treat those with inadequate ACTH, allergic disorders, respiratory disease, and osteoarthritis	hydrocortisone (Solu-Cortef)
Insulin replacement therapy (antidiabetic drugs)	glimepiride (Amaryl)
	pioglitazone (Actos)
Supplement or replace insulin when pancreatic function is impaired	insulin (Humulin, Novolin)
Thyroid hormone replacement	levothyroxine (Synthroid)
Treat hypothyroidism	liotrix (Thyrolar)
Antithyroid drugs	methimazole (Tapazole)
Treat hyperthyroidism	propylthiouracil (PTU)
Posterior pituitary replacement hormones	oxytocin (Pitocin)
Treat deficiencies of oxytocin and ADH	vasopressin (Pitressin Synthetic)

ACTH, Adrenocorticotropic hormone; *ADH,* antidiuretic hormone.

BOX 22-3

Common Signs and Symptoms of Endocrine Disease

Anorexia	Lack of appetite
Exophthalmia	Protrusion of eyeballs from their orbits
Goiter	Enlargement of thyroid gland not caused by a tumor
Hirsutism	Abnormal hairiness, especially in women
Hypercalcemia	Increase of calcium in the blood
Hyperglycemia	Increase of glucose in the blood
Hyperkalemia	Increase of potassium in the blood
Hypernatremia	Increase of sodium in the blood
Hypocalcemia	Deficiency of calcium in the blood
Hypoglycemia	Deficiency of glucose in the blood
Hypokalemia	Deficiency of potassium in the blood
Hyponatremia	Deficiency of sodium in the blood
Paresthesia	Abnormal touch sensation (e.g., prickling)
Polydipsia	Excessive thirst
Polyphagia	Excessive appetite
Polyuria	Excessive urination
Tetany	Continuous muscle spasms caused by an abnormal level of calcium in the blood

FOR YOUR INFORMATION

The endocrine system shows few functional changes with advancing age except for the rise in reproductive hormone levels at puberty and the decline in concentration of reproductive hormones at menopause in women. The effects of aging are more related to the changes in target organs and tissues that affect the body's ability to respond to hormonal stimulation rather than any decrease in the amount of circulating hormones.

PATIENT-CENTERED PROFESSIONALISM

- Why is it important for the medical assistant to be knowledgeable about the signs and symptoms of and diagnostic tests for diseases of the endocrine system?

CONCLUSION

The homeostatic state of the body is closely regulated by the nervous system and the endocrine system. The endocrine glands secrete hormones when stimulated. These hormones, when released, act on the intended target tissue by attaching themselves to the specialized receptors in the tissue. Think of each hormone as being a key: when it gets to the right lock

Text continued on p. 417

BOX 22-4

Diagnostic Tests and Procedures for the Endocrine System

Computed tomography (CT)	Scan used to test for bone density, hypoparathyroidism, and the size of the adrenal gland
Magnetic resonance imaging (MRI)	Imaging used to check for change in size of soft tissue (e.g., pituitary, pancreas, hypothalamus)
Radiography	X-ray imaging; done to detect changes in bone thickness and density
Ultrasonography	Ultrasonic recording that allows for visualization of deep structures (e.g., pancreas)
Radioactive iodine (RAI) uptake scan	Used to detect thyroid's ability to concentrate and retain iodine

LABORATORY TESTS

Hemoglobin A_{1c} (A1c)	Blood test that measures average blood glucose level over 3-month period (Box 22-5)
Fasting blood sugar (FBS)	Fasting glucose test; blood test that indicates amount of glucose present after a period of fasting
Glucose tolerance test (GTT)	Blood test that measures the body's ability to break down a concentrated glucose solution over a period of time
Hormone level test	Blood test that measures the amount of ADH, cortisol, growth hormone, and PTH in the blood
Radioimmunoassay (RIA)	Nuclear medicine test that detects hormone levels in the blood through use of radionuclides
Thyroid function tests (TFTs)	Blood test to assess the amount of T_3, T_4, and calcitonin circulating in the blood
Total calcium	Blood test that measures the amount of calcium
Urine glucose	Urine specimen tested for presence of glucose
Urine ketones	Urine specimen tested for ketones, which could indicate diabetes mellitus or hyperthyroidism

ADH, Antidiuretic hormone; *PTH,* parathyroid hormone.

BOX 22-5

Glycosylated Hemoglobin A_{1c} (A1c) Test

WHAT IS IT?
The A1c is a blood test that determines a person's average blood sugar over the past 3 months.

HOW IS THIS POSSIBLE?
Red blood cells have an average life span of 120 days. This test measures the "glucose coating" of a sample of hemoglobin. As the hemoglobin travels through the bloodstream, it picks up glucose that is in the blood; the more glucose in the blood, the more glucose that attaches to the hemoglobin.

WHY IS THIS IMPORTANT?
The A1c test provides information for long-term diabetic control. This information, plus a patient's day-to-day blood glucose levels, helps the physician design and revise a diabetic treatment plan that will work for the patient. Keeping a patient's blood sugar as close to normal as possible decreases the risk for development or worsening of diabetic complications. It is recommended that a diabetic patient have an A1c test two to four times a year.

WHAT IS A GOOD RANGE?

4% to 6%	Nondiabetic range
6% to 7%	Diabetic management plan is working well; it is unlikely that changes will be made to the patient's medication, exercise, or diet regimen
7% to 8%	Diabetic management plan is serving the patient well; regimen will remain the same unless the patient has too many low or too many high blood sugar readings
8% to 10%	Diabetic management plan needs to be reviewed and changes made to medication, diet, or exercise program
>10%	Diabetic management plan requires continued monitoring and adjustments; the higher the A1c results, the greater the chance that the patient will develop complications

TABLE 22-3

Major Diseases of the Endocrine System

Disease and Description	Etiology	Signs and Symptoms	Diagnosis	Therapy	Interventions
PITUITARY GLAND					
Dwarfism Undergrowth of bone and body tissues in children	Deficiency or lack of GH in childhood caused by tumor or unknown factors	Growth retardation, sexual immaturity, thyroid gland dysfunction	Clinical observation and low blood hormone levels; x-rays to determine presence of tumor	Replacement of GH and other hormones found to be deficient	Provide emotional support for child and family
Gigantism Overgrowth of body tissue before puberty, including long bones	Oversecretion of GH, may be caused by tumor in anterior pituitary gland	Accelerated growth of long bones; delayed mental and sexual development	Clinical observations; elevated GH blood levels; x-rays show pituitary tumor	Radiation of pituitary gland or surgical reduction	Support child or family
Acromegaly In adult with excessive GH secretion; overgrowth of bones and soft tissue of hands, feet, and face (Figure 22-5)	Excessive production of GH	Excessive overgrowth of soft tissue and the bones of the hands, feet, and face after puberty	Clinical presentation includes thickening of face, hands, and feet; blood GH level elevated; x-rays show tumor and bone thickening	Stop GH secretion by using radiation or surgical intervention to reduce size of pituitary	Provide emotional support

TABLE 22-3
Major Diseases of the Endocrine System—cont'd

Disease and Description	Etiology	Signs and Symptoms	Diagnosis	Therapy	Interventions
THYROID GLAND					
Childhood					
Cretinism Underproduction of thyroid hormone in childhood causing low metabolic rate, slow growth, and mental retardation	Underdevelopment of thyroid in utero; congenital factors	Swollen face, enlargement of lips, swollen and protruding tongue; stunted growth	Blood test shows low T_4 with elevated thyrotropin levels	Replacement of appropriate thyroid hormone	Educate about lifetime hormone replacement therapy
Adulthood					
Goiter (simple) Enlargement of thyroid caused by inadequate thyroid synthesis or lack of iodine in diet (Figure 22-6)	Often associated with iodine deficiency; inherited defects	Patient may complain of respiratory distress, dysphagia, and syncope	Clinical observation of irregular enlargement and stridor caused by tracheal compression; normal blood levels of thyroid hormone	Reduce hyperplasia through iodine administration, radioiodine therapy, or partial thyroidectomy	Encourage patient to report symptoms of hypothyroidism
Graves disease Overproduction of thyroid hormone; chief symptom is **exophthalmos**, or protrusion of eyeballs (see Figure 22-6)	Unknown; possible autoimmune response	Extreme nervousness, profuse sweating, flushed skin, hand tremors, increased appetite with weight loss, enlarged thyroid gland	Clinical presentation, past history, and elevated T_3 and T_4 levels	Drug therapy to suppress thyroid hormone production	Encourage follow-up supervision and regular thyroid hormone testing
Myxedema Underactive thyroid secretion; face appears swollen with dry and waxy appearance	Acquired impaired ability of thyroid gland to produce T_4	Decreased body temperature and pulse; weight gain; skin thickening; hair thins and falls out; tongue, hands, and feet increase in size	Retardation of physical and mental capabilities; low levels of T_4, thyrotropin, or both	Replacement of T_4 with medications	Encourage follow-up; educate about lifetime treatment
ADRENAL GLANDS					
Addison disease Deficiency of adrenocortical hormones	Autoimmune response causing destruction of adrenal glands	Muscular weakness, loss of appetite, fatigue, darkening of pigmentation, hypotension, low blood sugar, low sodium and high potassium blood levels, low metabolic rate	Low blood and urine levels of cortisol; elevated potassium, BUN, lymphocyte, and eosinophil levels	Hormone replacement therapy; control of salt intake; diet therapy includes increased proteins and carbohydrates	Encourage patient to follow diet, reduce stress, and avoid infection
Conn's syndrome Primary hyperaldosteronism	Tumor of the portion of the adrenal cortex responsible for secreting mineralocorticoids	Headaches, fatigue, nocturia, and excessive thirst	Hypernatremia, hypokalemia and hypertension	Fluid restriction and correction of electrolytes Potassium sparing diuretics such as spironolactone may be helpful	Low sodium diet and restricted fluids Blood pressure should be closely monitored

TABLE 22-3
Major Diseases of the Endocrine System—cont'd

Disease and Description	Etiology	Signs and Symptoms	Diagnosis	Therapy	Interventions
Cushing syndrome (disease) Adrenal cortex oversecretes ACTH, resulting in obesity, weakness, excessive hair growth, hypertension, and hyperglycemia (Figure 22-7)	Tumor of adrenal cortex or excessive secretion from pituitary gland; long-term use of corticosteroids	Fatigue, muscular weakness, fat deposits in back and abdomen, edema of feet and face	Clinical presentation of "moon face," buffalo hump, and obesity of trunk; serum cortisol levels elevated	Depends on cause; suppression of ACTH by drug therapy or reduction of tumor	Encourage lifetime following of prescribed therapy
PANCREAS					
Hypoglycemia Low plasma glucose level	*Reactive* type occurs 2-4 hours after a meal high in carbohydrates *Fasting* type occurs when person has not had adequate food or carbohydrates *Induced* type occurs when person with diabetes uses too much insulin without proper food intake; insulin use by nondiabetic; overuse of drugs or alcohol	Sweating, anxiety, tremors, tachycardia, palpitations, sudden fatigue, dizziness, behavioral changes or visual disturbances	Diagnostic tests for plasma levels of glucose and insulin (elevated insulin level and low plasma glucose level)	Dependent on cause; nutritional consultation	Encourage patient to follow diet (e.g., small, frequent meals with simple carbohydrates and minimize ingestion of complex carbohydrates)
Diabetes mellitus (DM) Main disease of insulin-producing pancreas (Figure 22-8 and Box 22-6)	Unknown, but linked to heredity	Hyperglycemia with glycosuria, polyuria, polyphagia, polydipsia, fatigue, and weight loss	Diagnostic tests of blood and urine and symptoms	Diet therapy and exercise; daily monitoring of blood and urine; medications to control glucose levels	Encourage patient to follow prescribed diet, exercise routine, and drug therapy

Insulin-Dependent Diabetes Mellitus
When an insulin deficiency occurs because of lack of insulin production, it is referred to as insulin-dependent diabetes (IDDM), juvenile-onset diabetes, or type 1 DM. Type 1 usually develops before age 20 years. Number of insulin-producing beta cells is decreased, causing insulin deficiency.

Non–Insulin-Dependent Diabetes Mellitus
When the pancreas cannot make sufficient quantities of insulin or the target cells in the body cannot use the insulin secreted, the disease is referred to as non–insulin-dependent diabetes (NIDDM), adult-onset diabetes, or type 2 DM. The pancreas produces insufficient amounts of insulin for all cells, but the target cells simply cannot use it. Type 2 usually occurs in overweight individuals after age 40 years.

ACTH, Adrenocorticotropic hormone; *BUN*, blood urea nitrogen; *GH*, growth hormone.

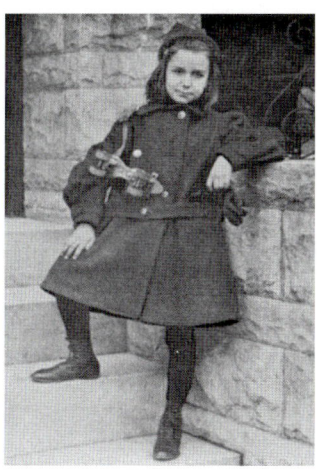 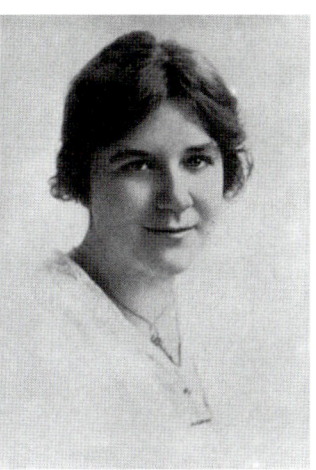 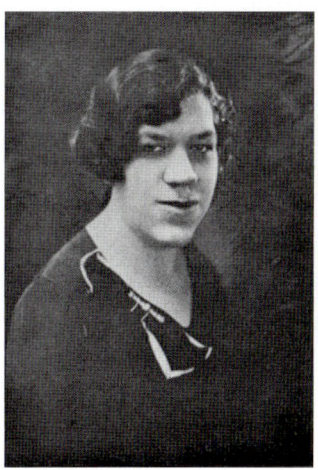 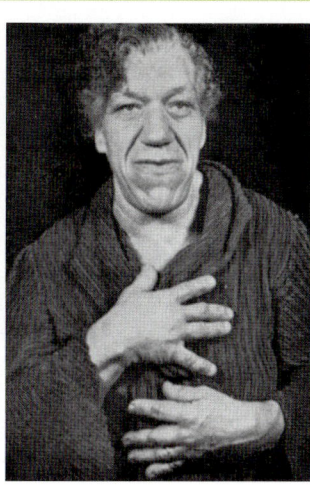

FIGURE 22-5 Progression of acromegaly. (From Ignatavicius DD, Workman ML: *Medical-surgical nursing: critical thinking for collaborative care*, ed 4, Philadelphia, 2002, Saunders.)

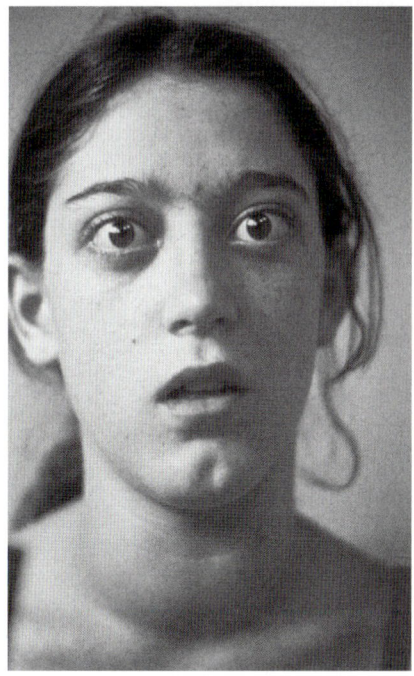

FIGURE 22-6 Classic Graves disease. Clinical features include a goiter and exophthalmos. (From Kliegman R et al: *Nelson textbook of pediatrics*, ed 18, Philadelphia, 2007, Saunders.)

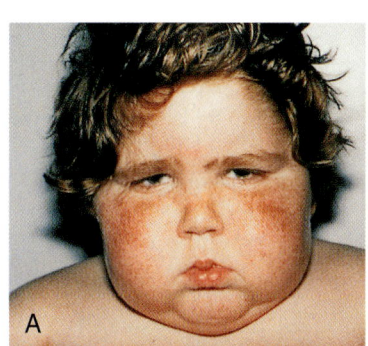 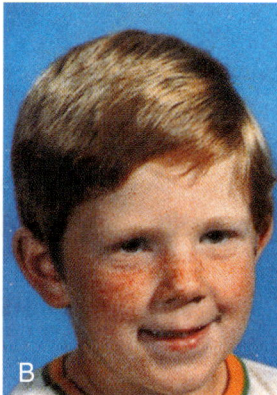

FIGURE 22-7 Cushing syndrome (disease). **A,** When first diagnosed. **B,** Four months after treatment. (From Thibodeau GA, Patton KT: *Anatomy and physiology*, ed 6, St Louis, 2007, Mosby.)

TABLE 22-4

Overview of Endocrine Hormones and Disorders

Gland	Hormone	Overproduction	Underproduction
Anterior pituitary	Growth hormone (GH)	Gigantism (child) / Acromegaly (adult)	Dwarfism (child)
Posterior pituitary	Antidiuretic hormone (ADH)	Syndrome of inappropriate secretion of ADH (SIADH)	Diabetes insipidus
Adrenal cortex	Aldosterone, cortisone, Cortisol	Cushing syndrome	Addison disease
Adrenal medulla	Epinephrine, norepinephrine	Pheochromocytoma	—
Thyroid	Thyroid hormones T_3 and T_4	Graves disease	Cretinism (child)
Pancreas	Insulin	Hypoglycemia	Diabetes mellitus
Parathyroid	Parathyroid hormone (PTH)	Bone degeneration	Tetany

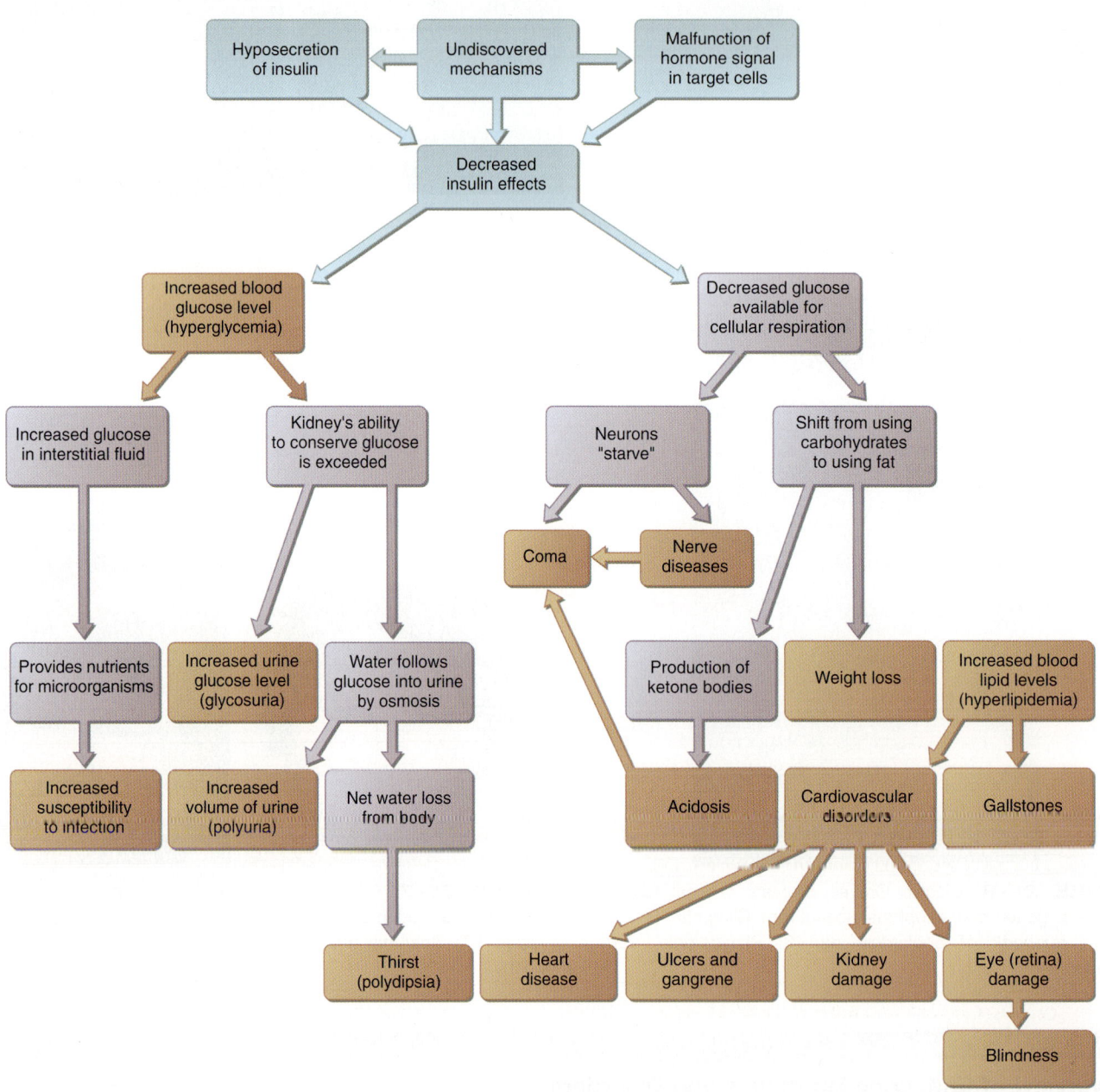

FIGURE 22-8 Signs and symptoms of diabetes mellitus (highlighted) result from decreased insulin effects. (Modified from Thibodeau GA, Patton KT: *Anatomy and physiology,* ed 6, St Louis, 2007, Mosby.)

> **BOX 22-6**
>
> **Warning Signs of Diabetes Mellitus***
>
> | TYPE 1 | TYPE 2 |
> |---|---|
> | Frequent urination | Frequent urination |
> | Excessive thirst | Excessive thirst |
> | Excessive hunger | Excessive hunger |
> | Weight loss | Overweight |
> | Unexplained irritability | Drowsiness |
> | Unexplained weakness and fatigue | Blurred vision |
> | | Numbness and tingling in hands and feet |
> | | Slow healing, yeast infections, and itching |
>
> *The onset of diabetes in adults occurs gradually, and therefore mild symptoms go undetected for years.
> Type 1 = IDDM; type 2 = NIDDM (see Table 22-3).

(target tissue), action occurs. Actions include response to stress, utilization of stored starch to produce energy, growth and repair of tissue, maintenance of proper pH for body fluids, and reproduction.

An inadequate amount of a hormone (e.g., insulin) or a lack of response by the target tissue (e.g., pancreas) creates symptoms, which the physician interprets to form a diagnosis (e.g., diabetes; see Box 22-6 for the warning signs of types 1 and 2 diabetes mellitus).

Chapter Summary

Reinforce your understanding of the material in this chapter by reviewing the curriculum objectives and key content points below.

1. **Define, appropriately use, and spell all the Key Terms for this chapter.**
   - Review the Key Terms if necessary.
2. **Explain the two main functions of the endocrine system.**
   - The endocrine system serves to regulate body functions through hormones and keeps the body in homeostasis.
3. **Compare and contrast endocrine and exocrine glands.**
   - Endocrine glands have no ducts and secrete directly into the bloodstream.
   - Exocrine glands have ducts and their secretions are transported outside the body.
   - Exocrine glands include sweat, sebaceous, and mammary glands.
4. **Identify and locate the seven major endocrine glands.**
   - Endocrine glands of the body include the pituitary, thyroid, parathyroid, and adrenal glands; the pancreas; and the male and female gonads.
5. **List the hormones and primary function of each of the seven major endocrine glands.**
   - Refer to Table 22-1.
6. **Describe prostaglandins, and explain how they differ from proteins and steroid hormones.**
   - Prostaglandins are chemical mediators and are considered to be "local" hormones.
   - Prostaglandins are produced by cells throughout the body.
7. **Name two hormone-secreting organs, and identify the hormones they secrete.**
   - The ovaries secrete estrogen for development of secondary sex characteristics in the female, and progesterone, which prepares the uterus for pregnancy.
   - The pancreas secretes insulin, which regulates blood glucose.
8. **Define feedback, and explain how it keeps the body in homeostasis.**
   - Positive or negative feedback serves to increase or decrease hormone activity as needed to keep the body in balance (homeostasis).
9. **List 17 common signs and symptoms of endocrine system disease.**
   - Refer to Box 22-3.
10. **List 14 common diagnostic tests and procedures for endocrine system disease and describe the use of each.**
    - Refer to Box 22-4.
11. **List 10 endocrine diseases and disorders and briefly describe the etiology, signs and symptoms, diagnosis, therapy, and interventions for each.**
    - Refer to Table 22-3.
12. **Analyze a realistic medical office situation and apply your understanding of the endocrine system to determine the best course of action.**
    - Understanding the diseases and disorders that affect the endocrine system enables the medical assistant to work with patients more effectively.
13. **Describe the impact on patient care when medical assistants have a solid understanding of the structure and function of the endocrine system.**
    - Patient care is optimized when the medical assistant understands the endocrine system. You will be better able to provide teaching instructions to patients when you know the importance of hormones functioning properly and how this assists in homeostasis.

PRACTICAL APPLICATIONS

If you have accomplished the objectives in this chapter, you will be able to make better choices as a medical assistant. Take another look at this situation and decide what you would do.

Juliette, age 4 years, cannot drink enough water and has to void frequently. Her mother says that Juliette eats all the time but is losing weight. She is also lethargic. At times her mother thinks that Juliette's breath has a fruity odor, although she does not chew fruit-flavored gum or eat fruit-flavored candy. After checking Juliette, Dr. Jay tells the mother that Juliette may have diabetes mellitus. Dr. Jay wants to do further testing as quickly as possible and orders a fasting blood sugar, which comes back elevated. Dr. Jay follows this with a glucose tolerance test (GTT). When the GTT is abnormally high, Dr. Jay prescribes insulin for Juliette.

Do you understand why Dr. Jay diagnosed Juliette with diabetes mellitus, and why she ordered the tests she did?

1. What type of diabetes mellitus would you expect Juliette to have at age 4?
2. What is the difference between *IDDM* and *NIDDM*?
3. Are the symptoms listed for Juliette typical of those found with diabetes?
4. What are the medical terms for being hungry all the time, having excessive thirst, and having to void often?
5. What other specific treatment will be needed to keep Juliette's blood sugar level lowered?
6. What is the term for an elevated blood sugar level? What is the term for sugar in urine?
7. What is a fasting blood sugar (fasting glucose test)? What is a GTT?
8. What glands and hormones are associated with diabetes insipidus?
9. What is positive feedback? Negative feedback? Why are these important in the endocrine system?

WEB SEARCH

1. **Research the role hormones have in the aging process.** Dehydroepiandrosterone (DHEA) is produced by the adrenal cortex. In young adults, the level is very high, but a decline is noticed in people as they age.

- **Keywords:** Use the following keywords in your search: DHEA, aging, hormones.

WORD PARTS: Endocrine System

Combining Forms

adren/o	adrenal gland
adrenocortic/o	adrenal cortex
calc/o	calcium
crin/o	secrete
endo	within
glyc/o	sugar
hypophys/o	pituitary gland
iod/o	iodine
kal/i	potassium
lact/o	milk
natr/o	sodium
parathyroid/o	parathyroid gland
pituitar/o	pituitary gland
thyr/o, thyroid/o	thyroid gland
trop/o	to stimulate

Suffixes

-crine	secrete
-dipsia	thirst
-physis	growth
-tropic	stimulating
-tropin	that which stimulates

ABBREVIATIONS: Endocrine System

ACTH	adrenocorticotropic hormone
ADH	antidiuretic hormone
Ca	calcium
DI	diabetes insipidus
DM	diabetes mellitus
FBS	fasting blood sugar
GH	growth hormone
GTT	glucose tolerance test
IDDM	insulin-dependent diabetes mellitus
K	potassium
LH	luteinizing hormone
Na	sodium
NIDDM	non–insulin-dependent diabetes mellitus
OT	oxytocin
PRL	prolactin
T_3	triiodothyronine
T_4	thyroxine
TFT	thyroid function test
TSH	thyroid-stimulating hormone

Integumentary System

23

evolve http://evolve.elsevier.com/klieger/medicalassisting

The skin, along with the hair, nails, and sweat glands, makes up the **integumentary system.** The skin is the largest of the body systems and provides protection against the environment. The skin is also involved with body temperature regulation, sensory perception, and elimination of toxins. The condition of people's skin reflects their general health, and skin changes throughout a person's life (Table 23-1). The physician evaluates the patient's skin **turgor** (normal tension in the skin) as part of the patient's physical assessment. The integumentary system is very important in working with the other body systems to maintain homeostasis. **Dermatology** is the study of the skin.

LEARNING OBJECTIVES

You will be able to do the following after completing this chapter:

Key Terms
1. Define, appropriately use, and spell all the Key Terms for this chapter.

Function and Structure of the Integumentary System
2. List the three main functions of the skin.
3. Explain how the body is able to maintain a constant temperature.
4. Identify the three layers of the skin and describe the structure and function of each.
5. Identify the three types of substructures of the skin and explain the function of each.

Damage to the Skin
6. List and briefly describe nine common skin lesions.
7. Define actinic keratosis, basal cell carcinoma, malignant melanoma, and squamous cell carcinoma and determine how to identify each.
8. List four treatment options for malignant skin lesions.
9. Explain the difference between *open* and *closed* wounds.
10. List and describe the three phases of wound healing.
11. Distinguish between a partial-thickness and a full-thickness burn as a means to assessing the depth of a burn.
12. Explain the purpose and use of the "rule of nines."

Diseases and Disorders of the Integumentary System
13. List and describe seven signs and symptoms of skin disease.
14. List five types of diagnostic tests and procedures for the skin and describe the use of each.
15. List 10 diseases and disorders of the integumentary system and briefly describe the etiology, signs and symptoms, diagnosis, therapy, and interventions for each.

Patient-Centered Professionalism
16. Analyze a realistic medical office situation and apply your understanding of the integumentary system to determine the best course of action.
17. Describe the impact on patient care when medical assistants have a solid understanding of the structure and function of the integumentary system.

KEY TERMS

The Key Terms for this chapter have been organized into sections so that you can easily see the terminology associated with each aspect of the integumentary system.

dermatologist	integumentary system
dermatology	turgor

Structure of the Skin

albinism	melanin
dermis	subcutaneous layer
epidermis	whorls
keratin	

Substructures of the Skin

Hair

follicle	shaft
root	

Continued

Substructures of the Skin—cont'd
Glands
acne	sebaceous glands
comedo	sebum
pore	sudoriferous glands

Nails
cuticle	nail body
free edge	nail root
lunula	nails

Damage to the Skin
Lesions
cyst	polyp
fissure	pustule
lesions	ulcer
macule	vesicle
papule	wheal

Skin Lesions
actinic keratoses	malignant melanomas
basal cell carcinomas	nevus
benign	squamous cell carcinomas
malignant	

Wounds
abrasion	laceration
closed wound	maturation phase
contusion	open wound
granulation phase	puncture
incision	wound
inflammatory phase	

Burns
first-degree burns	"rule of nines"
full-thickness	second-degree burns
partial-thickness	third-degree burns

Diseases and Disorders of the Integumentary System
Signs and Symptoms
abscess	excoriation
alopecia	furuncle
carbuncles	ichthyosis
cicatrix	keloid
crust	petechiae
decubitus ulcer	pruritus
diaphoresis	purpura
ecchymosis	ulcer
eczema	urticaria
erosion	vitiligo

Diagnostic Tests
blood antibody titer	tissue scrapings
skin biopsy	Tzanck test
skin test	Wood's light examination

Diseases and Disorders
cellulitis	erythema
dermatitis	herpes simplex
impetigo	scabies
Lyme disease	scleroderma
onychomycosis	tinea
pediculosis	warts (verrucae)
psoriasis	

PRACTICAL APPLICATIONS

Read the following scenario and keep it in mind as you learn about the integumentary system in this chapter.

Marilyn was taking a shower 2 weeks ago and found a large black mole on her shoulder. At first she ignored it, but after talking with her friend, she decided that she should see her family practice physician. This physician sent her to Dr. Nelson, a dermatologist, who diagnosed her lesion as a possible malignant melanoma. Dr. Nelson asked Marilyn if she had any pruritus, a fissure, or any crusting of the lesion. As Dr. Nelson examined Marilyn's shoulder, he noticed petechiae, ecchymosis, and purpura. When asked about these findings, Marilyn told the physician that the mole had itched and she had scratched the area in her sleep. On her leg was a furuncle that was inflamed, hot, and appeared to have a pus formation. On completing the physical examination, Dr. Nelson noticed that Marilyn had the tendency to keloid formation based on the appearance of her appendectomy scar.

Marilyn had quite a few questions for the medical assistant about the meaning of some of the terms used by Dr. Nelson. Marilyn left the dermatologist's office with surgery scheduled for removal of the melanoma in 2 days. Would you be able to answer Marilyn's questions?

FUNCTION AND STRUCTURE OF THE INTEGUMENTARY SYSTEM

Functions of the Skin

The skin serves three main functions to maintain homeostasis in the body: protection, temperature regulation, and sensation.

Protection

The skin protects the body and is the first line of defense against bacterial invasion. The skin is constantly exposed to heat, cold, and toxic substances. It can be scraped, bruised, or cut, but when the body is in a healthy state, skin can heal itself. The skin prevents excessive loss of electrolytes and fluids so the body and skin do not totally dry out. Melanin provides protection from the harmful effects of ultraviolet (UV) rays by providing pigment to the skin. When exposed to the sun's UV rays, the skin manufactures vitamin D, which is needed for the absorption of calcium.

TABLE 23-1
Life Cycle of the Skin

Texture	Flexibility	Glands	Healing
CHILDREN			
Smooth Unwrinkled	Very elastic and flexible	Few sweat glands (rely on increased blood flow to cool the body)	Rapid
ADULTS			
Skin reacts to the environment; can toughen if too much sun exposure	Flexibility and elasticity continue unless exposed to harmful external environment	Well-developed sebaceous and sweat glands Increased sweat production, thus body odor Increased sebum production leads to acne formation	Heals readily unless an underlying disease process is present
OLDER ADULTS			
Toughened Less elastic	Wrinkled	Decreased sebaceous and sweat gland activity Body loses ability to cool itself effectively	Slow

Temperature Regulation

The ability of the body to maintain a constant body temperature is important to the functioning of other processes in the body. For example, many chemical reactions take place in the body. These reactions depend on the action of certain enzymes. Without a constant body temperature, enzymes do not function properly. To maintain a constant body temperature, the body must balance the amount of heat it produces with the amount it loses. To prevent heat loss, the blood vessels within the skin constrict, causing "goose bumps." This "goose flesh" (*cutis anserina*) prevents heat loss by not allowing body heat to escape through blood vessels near the skin. When the body temperature rises above the normal range, the skin's capillaries dilate, and the sweat glands increase their secretions. This allows the body to maintain a constant body temperature because the sweat that is generated will cool hot skin (Figure 23-1).

Sensation

Within the skin are sensory receptors that detect pain, heat, cold, and pressure. When stimulated, these receptors make it possible for the body to respond to changes in both the external and the internal environment.

PATIENT-CENTERED PROFESSIONALISM

- Why is it important for the medical assistant to understand the function of the skin?

Structure of the Skin

The skin is composed of the epidermis, dermis, and subcutaneous layer (Figure 23-2).

Epidermis

The **epidermis** is the thin upper layer of the skin. The outer cells of the epidermis are filled with **keratin**, a waterproof protein that toughens the skin. As new cells are produced, they move to the top. The top layer of the epidermis is composed of flat (scalelike) dead cells. The top layer is shed and replaced constantly.

The epidermis is full of ridges that fit snugly over the papillae on top of the dermis. These ridges form the **whorls** (coils or spirals) or patterns that are known as fingerprints.

Some cells within the epidermis produce **melanin**, which provides color to the skin and protects against the sun's UV rays. The more melanin a person has, the darker his or her skin. A person unable to form melanin will have very white skin with no pigmentation, which is a condition called **albinism**. Figure 23-3 illustrates the many factors that contribute to a person's skin color.

Dermis

The **dermis** is thicker than the epidermis and lies beneath it. The dermis is composed of connective tissue and contains blood vessels, nerve endings, hair follicles, lymph vessels, and sweat glands. The connective tissue is mostly collagen fibers; these fibers provide for the elasticity and strength of the skin. The dermis adds support and nourishment to the skin.

Subcutaneous Layer

The **subcutaneous layer** lies below the dermis and consists mainly of adipose tissue and loose connective tissue. It attaches the skin to muscles and other tissue. This layer acts as a shock absorber for organs and conserves the body's heat.

Substructures of the Skin

Several important substructures are located within the skin. The hair, specific glands, and nails are all part of the integumentary system.

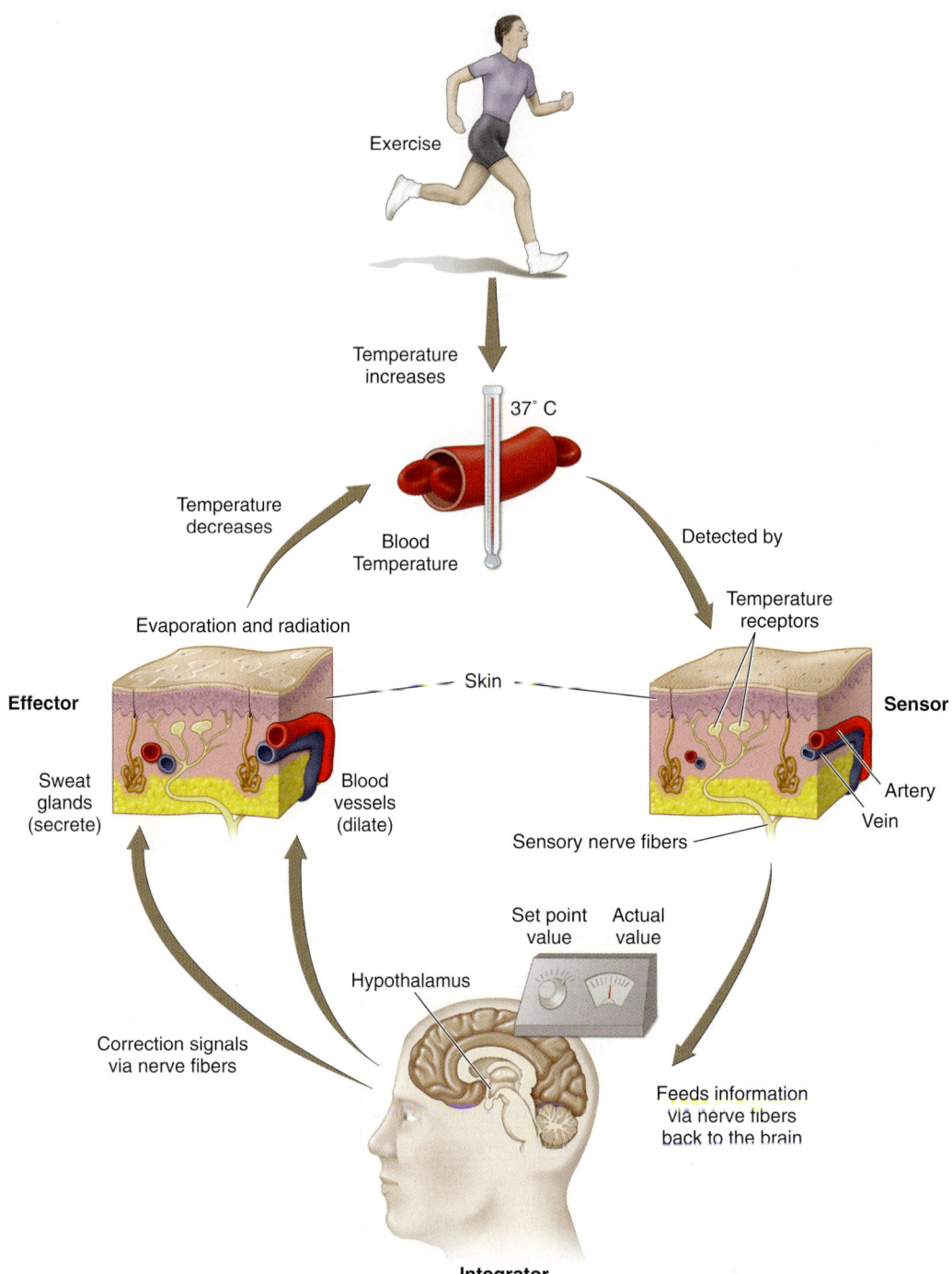

FIGURE 23-1 Role of the skin in homeostasis of body temperature. (Modified from Thibodeau GA, Patton KT: *Anatomy and physiology,* ed 6, St Louis, 2007, Mosby.)

Hair. Hair is distributed over the body except on the palms of the hands and soles of the feet. Hair develops within a **follicle** and grows from within the deep layers of the skin. Hair protects the skin. It is composed of nonliving material, mostly keratin. The **shaft** of the hair is the part you can see extending from the skin and it does not contain nerves. The **root** lies below the surface.

Glands. There are several types of glands in the skin, including sweat glands and oil glands (Figure 23-4).

The **sudoriferous glands,** or sweat glands, are small, coiled glands. Sweat glands maintain body temperature by releasing sweat, a watery fluid with dissolved body salts. Sweat evaporates to cool the body. Sweat glands are numerous in the hands, feet, and underarms (axilla). Sweat is released through pores. A **pore** is the duct opening that provides a pathway for fluid to leave the body.

The **sebaceous glands,** or oil glands, are located around hair follicles. Oil glands release **sebum** (oil) that lubricates the

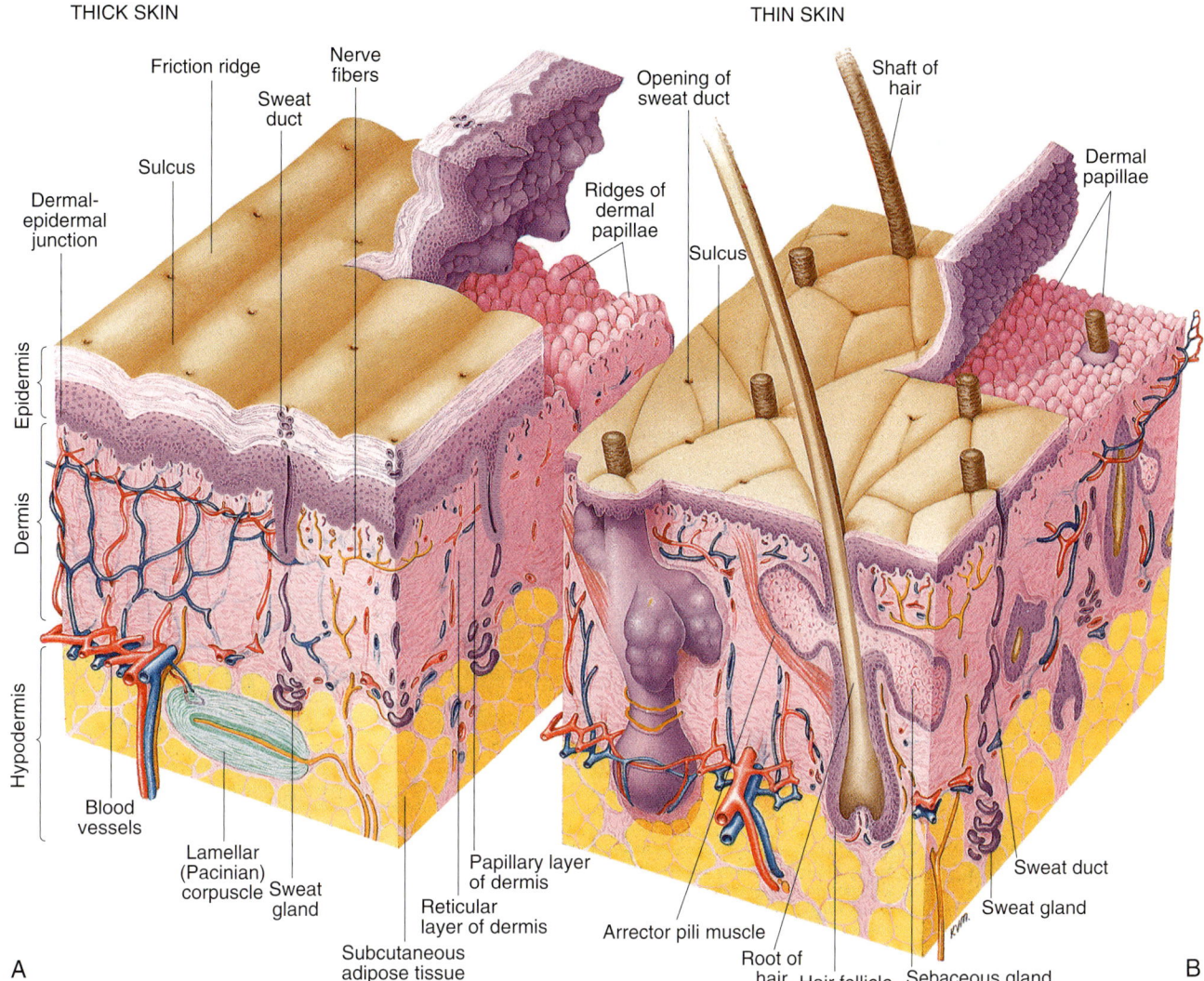

FIGURE 23-2 Structure of the skin. **A,** Thick skin is found on the palms and on the soles of the feet. **B,** Thin skin is found on most other body surfaces. (From Black JM et al: *Medical-surgical nursing: clinical management for positive outcomes,* ed 8, St Louis, 2009, Saunders.)

skin and hair. This prevents drying by minimizing water loss. Sebum also functions to inhibit the growth of certain bacteria. The activity of these glands increases at puberty because of increased hormone production in the body. This overstimulation can lead to **acne,** which occurs when the ducts of the glands become blocked. Once blocked, the sebum combines with dead cells and a *blackhead,* or **comedo,** forms or the comedo may be pustular *(whitehead).* The blackened area is actually a collection of melanin not dirt. When the duct ruptures, a *pimple* forms.

Nails. **Nails** protect the ends of the fingers and toes. They develop from epidermal cells and consist mainly of hard keratin. The nails appear pink because of the rich blood supply to the area. The **lunula,** or half-moon shape, is at the base of the nail and is white. The **cuticle** is a narrow band of epidermis at the base and sides of the nail. Under the cuticle lies the nail root. The **nail body** is the fingernail that covers the nail bed, and the part that extends out is referred to as the **free edge** (Figure 23-5).

PATIENT-CENTERED PROFESSIONALISM

- *Why is it important for the medical assistant to understand basic skin structure and substructure?*

DAMAGE TO THE SKIN

The skin provides protection for our bodies, but it can be damaged in the process. Lesions, wounds, and burns are ways in which the skin can be damaged.

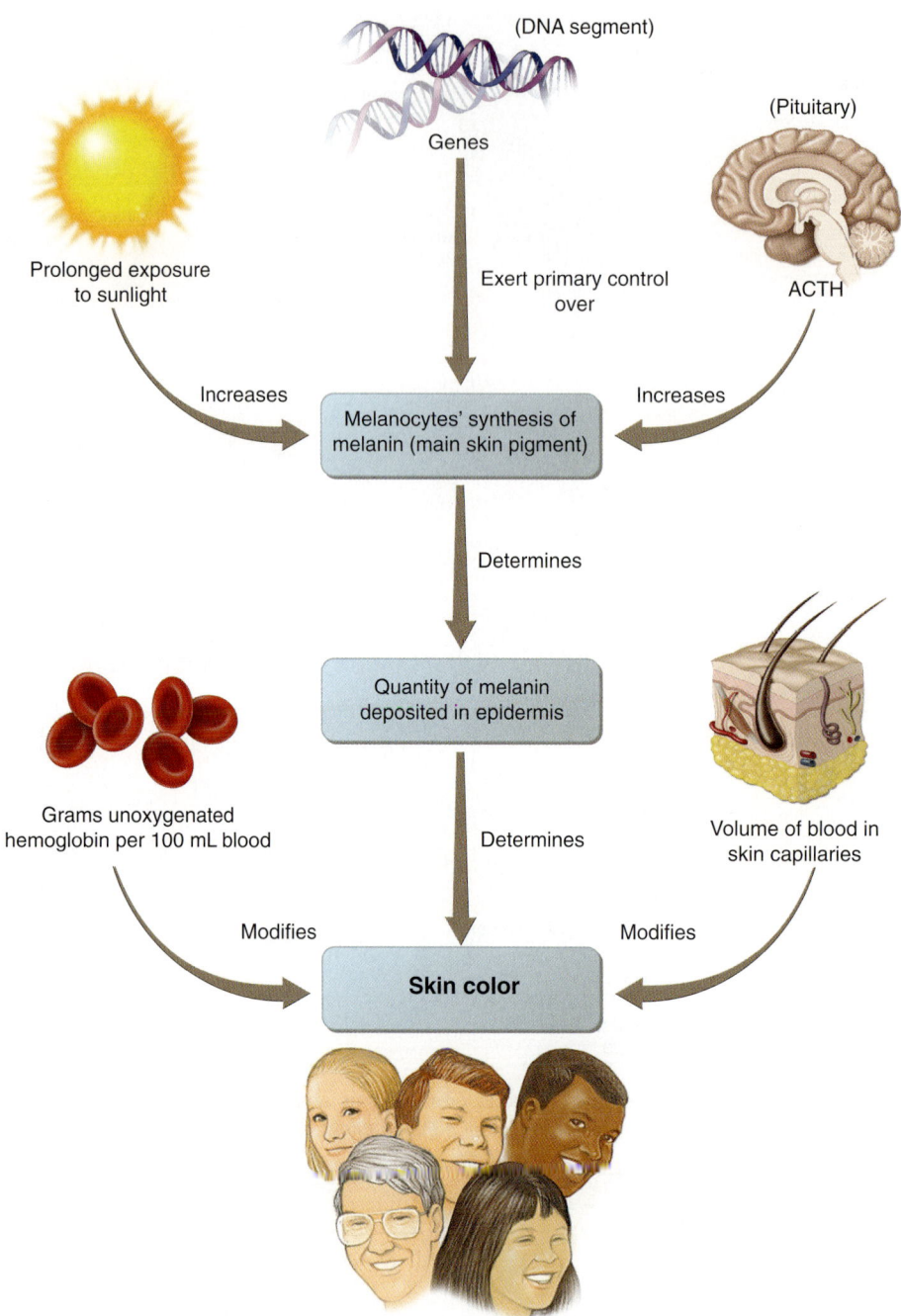

FIGURE 23-3 How genes affect skin color. (Modified from Thibodeau GA, Patton KT: *Anatomy and physiology,* ed 6, St Louis, 2007, Mosby.)

Lesions

Lesions are changes in the skin caused by an underlying disease or trauma that alters the basic structure of the skin. A skin lesion is any visible abnormality of the tissues. Common lesions include the following (Figure 23-6):
- **Cyst:** Thick-walled sac that contains fluid or semisolid material (e.g., sebaceous cyst).
- **Fissure:** Split or crack in the skin (e.g., anal fissure is a split in the anus).
- **Macule:** Flat, discolored area (e.g., freckle, age spot).
- **Papule:** Small, solid, raised area of the skin, less than 1 cm (e.g., pimple).
- **Polyp:** Stalklike growth from a mucous membrane (e.g., nasal polyps, intestinal polyps) that is often precancerous.
- **Pustule:** Small, raised area of the skin containing pus (e.g., acne).
- **Ulcer:** Erosion of the skin (bedsore).

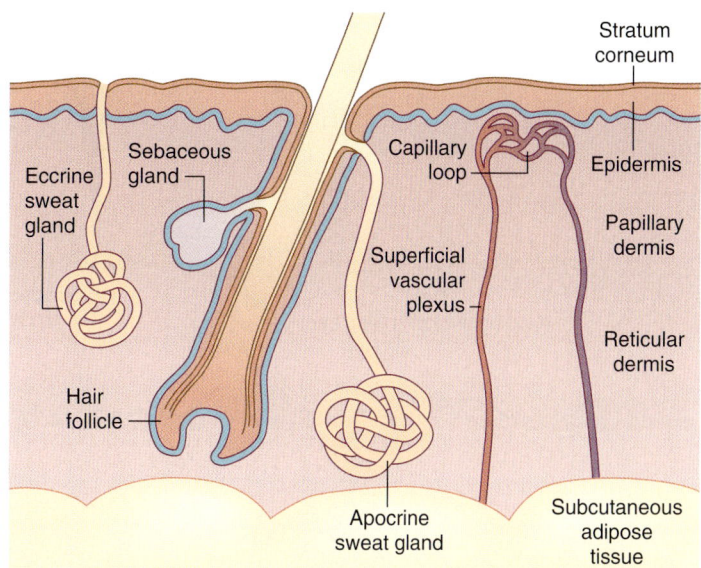

FIGURE 23-4 Glands of the skin. (From Goldman L, Ausiello D: *Cecil medicine*, ed 23, Philadelphia, 2008, Saunders.)

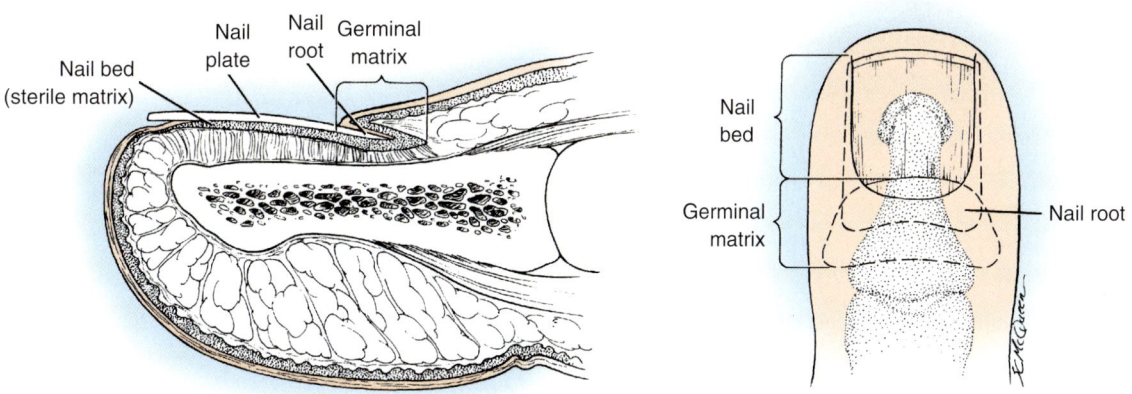

FIGURE 23-5 The nail. (From Canale ST, Beaty J: *Campbell's operative orthopaedics*, ed 11, Philadelphia, 2008, Mosby.)

- **Vesicle:** Blister; a collection of clear fluid under the skin (e.g., herpes or burn).
- **Wheal:** Slightly elevated central area surrounded by a pale red area (e.g., insect bite).

Precancerous Skin Lesions

Actinic keratoses are precancerous skin growths. This type of lesion is caused by prior sun exposure. Actinic keratoses are slightly scaly papules that appear pinkish to reddish. If left untreated, these lesions spread into the dermis to become squamous cell carcinomas (Figure 23-7).

Malignant Skin Lesions

Some types of skin lesions are **malignant,** or cancerous. Examples include basal cell carcinoma, malignant melanoma, and squamous cell carcinoma.

Basal Cell Carcinoma

Basal cell carcinomas are malignant skin lesions that appear as raised, flesh-colored papules with blood vessels around the edges. These lesions are slow growing, with local destruction and usually without metastasis (spreading). These lesions can appear anywhere in sun-exposed areas but usually appear on the face, nose, and neck (Figure 23-8).

Malignant Melanoma

Malignant melanomas are the most dangerous of all skin cancers. They can appear anywhere on the body. This type of cancer often develops from a **nevus,** or mole or birthmark. The danger of this form of cancer is that it can *metastasize* (spread) to any organ.

Figure 23-9 shows a typical malignant melanoma. Figure 23-10 shows a typical **benign** mole. Table 23-2 compares the appearance of a benign nevus to a malignant melanoma. The

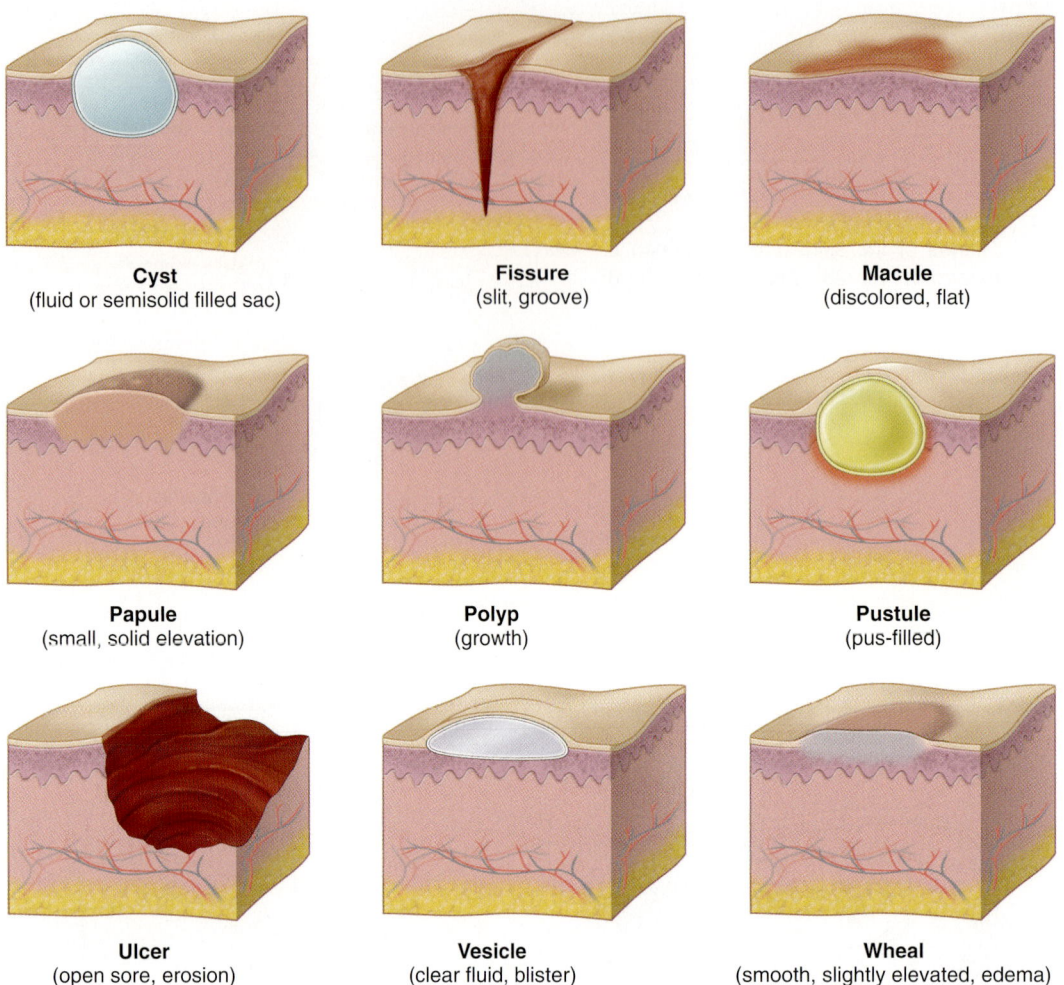

FIGURE 23-6 Common skin lesions. (Modified from Chabner DE: *The language of medicine,* ed 8, St Louis, 2007, Saunders.)

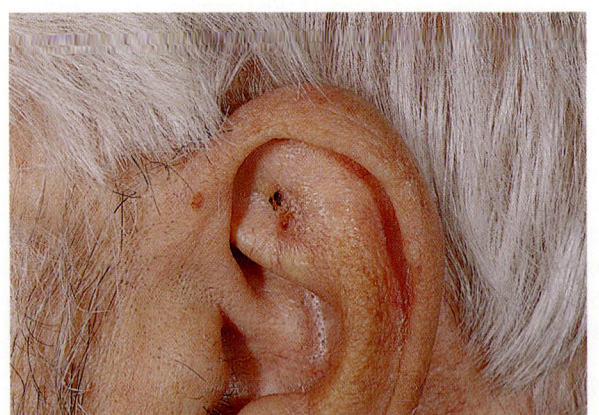

FIGURE 23-7 Actinic keratosis. (From Callen JP et al: *Color atlas of dermatology,* ed 2, Philadelphia, 2000, Saunders.)

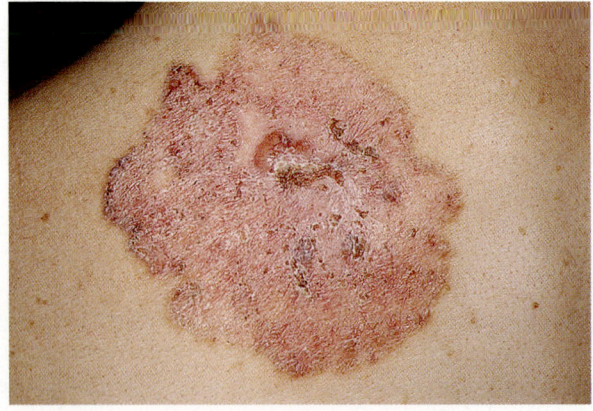

FIGURE 23-8 Superficial basal cell epithelioma. (From Callen JP et al: *Color atlas of dermatology,* ed 2, Philadelphia, 2000, Saunders.)

TABLE 23-2

Benign Mole versus Malignant Melanoma ("ABCDE Rule")

Characteristic	Benign Mole	Malignant Melanoma
Asymmetry	Symmetrical; each half is mirror image of other half	Asymmetrical Lopsided in appearance
Border	Outlined by a defined border	Outline irregular
Color	Shades of brown color are even	Black Uneven mixture of brown and black In extreme cases, white
Diameter	<6 mm (¼ inch)	>6 mm
Elevation	Flat or raised mole that does not change	Flat mole becomes raised above the skin or rough in surface; change in thickness, cracks in surface, bleeding

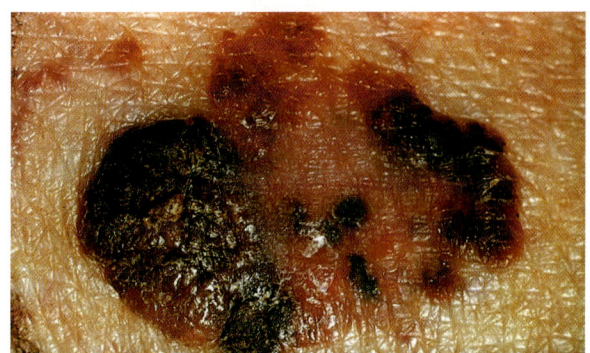

FIGURE 23-9 Malignant melanoma. (From Kumar V et al: *Robbins and Cotran: pathologic basis of disease,* ed 7, Philadelphia, 2004, Saunders.)

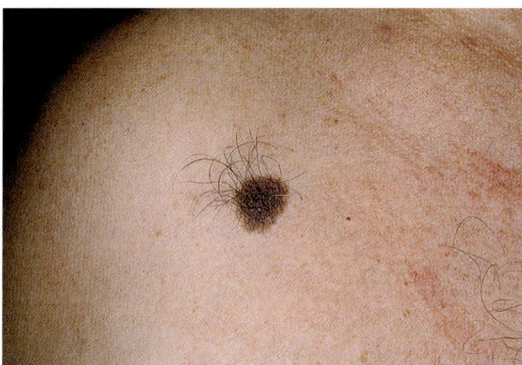

FIGURE 23-10 Congenital melanocytic nevus (benign mole). (From Callen JP et al: *Color atlas of dermatology,* ed 2, Philadelphia, 2000, Saunders.)

characteristics of a melanoma are easy to remember with the following "ABCDE rule" of self-examination:
- *A*symmetrical (uneven) in appearance. If an imaginary line is drawn through the middle of a melanoma, it will not produce matching halves.
- *B*orders are uneven. The edges of a melanoma appear irregular or scalloped.
- *C*olor changes appear. The area changes from two or more shades of black, brown, red, white, or blue.
- *D*iameter of a melanoma tends to grow faster than normal moles.
- *E*levation or thickness increases in a melanoma.

Pathophysiologists recognize that genetic predisposition is a factor in forming melanomas. They also cite exposure to UV radiation as a contributing factor for common skin cancers. UV rays damage the deoxyribonucleic acid (DNA) in skin cells, causing a change during mitosis that produces cancer cells.

Squamous Cell Carcinoma

Squamous cell carcinomas are skin cancers that appear as firm papules with ulcerations (Figure 23-11). They can also look like a thick, rough, wartlike growth; a scaly red patch with irregular borders; or an open sore that crusts or bleeds.

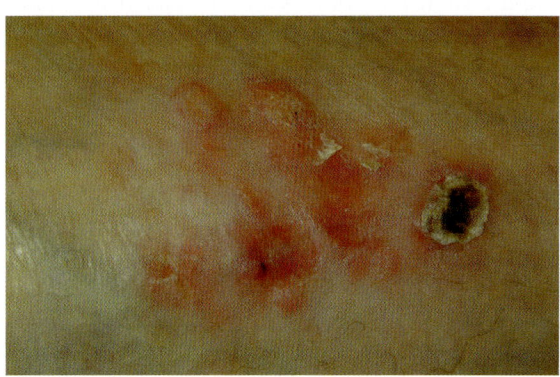

FIGURE 23-11 Squamous cell carcinoma. (From Townsend C et al: *Sabiston's textbook of surgery,* ed 18, Philadelphia, 2008, Saunders.)

This type of cancer can appear anywhere on the body but most notably on the lower lip, scalp, forehead, face, top of the ears, and back of the hands.

Therapy

Treatment options for malignant skin lesions vary but include the following:

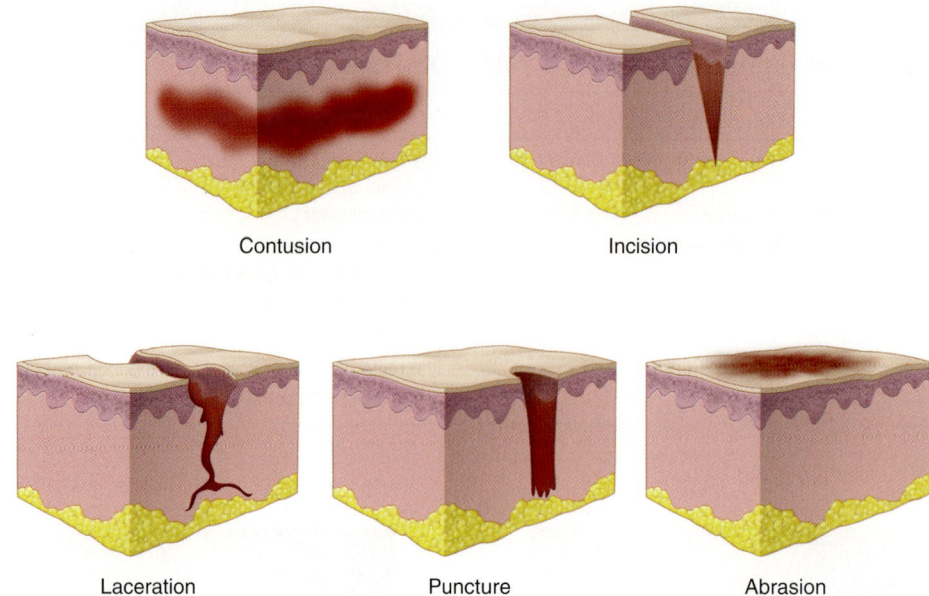

FIGURE 23-12 Types of wounds.

- *Cryosurgery:* Use of liquid nitrogen to burn off tissue by freezing.
- *Topical chemotherapy:* Use of chemicals to destroy tissue.
- *Excision:* Surgical removal of tissue.
- *Radiation:* Use of radiation to destroy tissue.

Wounds

A **wound** is some form of break in the skin. Wounds may be intentional (e.g., surgical incision) or accidental (e.g., stepping on a nail protruding from a board). Wounds are considered to be either open or closed, based on whether the skin has been broken.

Closed Wound

A **closed wound** occurs when damage is done to the tissues beneath the skin without a visible break in the skin. An example of a closed wound is a **contusion,** which occurs when blood vessels rupture and blood seeps into the tissue, giving the area under the skin a mottled, dark appearance, as with a bruise. Injuries to the musculoskeletal system often produce a contusion (e.g., sprains, strains, or fractures).

Open Wound

Open wounds occur when the skin is damaged and the tissue below is exposed. The four basic types of open wounds are as follows (Figure 23-12):
- An **incision** is a smooth cut into the skin (e.g., surgical incision).
- A **laceration** is a wound where the tissue edges are irregular (e.g., knife wound).
- A **puncture** is a wound made by a sharp object that pierces the skin (e.g., stepping on a nail).
- An **abrasion** is a wound in which the epidermis is scraped off (e.g., scraping a knee on the sidewalk when rollerblading).

Healing Process

Wound healing is the body's natural process of regenerating dermal and epidermal tissue. When a wound is sustained, a set of predictable events occurs to repair the tissue damage. These events or phases do overlap but can be separated into three phases:
- *Phase 1* is the **inflammatory phase,** and this phase begins when the skin is damaged. A blood clot forms and stops blood from flowing. The blood supply to the damaged area increases, allowing white blood cells and nutrients to aid in the healing process.
- *Phase 2* is the **granulation phase** or *proliferation phase.* This phase allows flesh to begin forming collagen, a protein that adds strength to the repairing tissue. A capillary supply forms to create a blood supply to the newly formed tissue.
- *Phase 3* is the **maturation phase.** Tissue continues to form and eventually hardens to form scar tissue. Scar tissue does not have nerve tissue or a blood supply and may have a raised or "puckered" appearance when healed.

Burns

A burn is damage to the skin caused by heat or severe cold, chemicals, electricity, or radiation. Burns are classified according to their depth and their surface area. Depth classifications include the following (Figure 23-13, *A*):
- **Partial-thickness** burns can be divided into first- and second-degree burns.

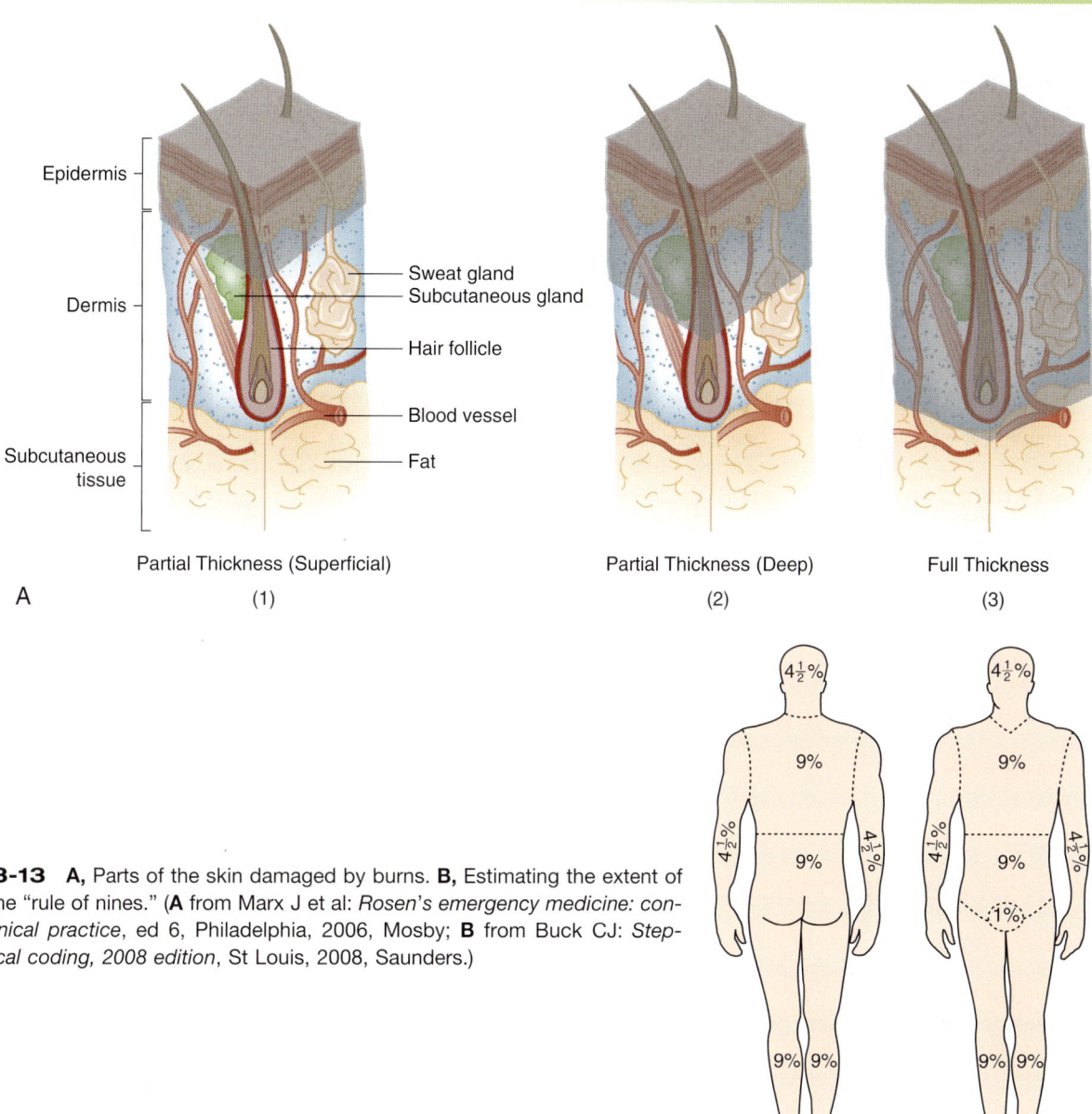

FIGURE 23-13 **A,** Parts of the skin damaged by burns. **B,** Estimating the extent of burns using the "rule of nines." (**A** from Marx J et al: *Rosen's emergency medicine: concepts and clinical practice*, ed 6, Philadelphia, 2006, Mosby; **B** from Buck CJ: *Step-by-step medical coding, 2008 edition*, St Louis, 2008, Saunders.)

First-degree burns involve only the epidermis, which appears reddened, with slight pain. A mild sunburn and brief contact with a hot object (e.g., iron, stove) are examples of first-degree burns.

Second-degree burns involve both the epidermis and the dermis. Damage to tissue is greater, and the area is blistered and severely swollen. Examples include severe sunburn and burns caused by hot liquids (e.g., coffee) or chemicals.

- **Full-thickness** burns are referred to as third-degree burns.

  Third-degree burns destroy the epidermis and dermis. There is deep tissue destruction and less pain because of nerve destruction. The skin appears charred or white. Examples include burns from electric shocks, flames, or chemicals.

A burn patient's total body surface (TBS) or body surface area (BSA) is evaluated according to the "**rule of nines**" (Figure 23-13, *B*). By dividing the body into regions and assigning a number related to 9, a burn area can be assessed. Thus, when an accident victim is described as "burned over 90% of his body," this is the percentage of the TBS involved in the burn. When determining treatment, the physician assesses the depth of the burn, the BSA of the burn, and the particular body parts involved. Burns on the face, neck, and genital areas are especially painful to treat. First-degree burns over 50% of the body's extremities may not be as difficult to treat as third-degree burns over 25% of the body that include the facial and neck area.

TABLE 23-3

Integumentary (Skin) Drug Classifications

Drug Classification	Common Generic (Brand) Drugs
Anesthetics (local) Block pain at site where administered	lidocaine (Xylocaine) procaine (Novocain)
Anti-acne drugs Treat acne vulgaris	tetracycline (Achromycin) tretinoin (Avita)
Antifungals Inhibit the growth of fungi	ciclopirox (Loprox) clotrimazole (Lotrimin)
Antiinfectives Inhibit growth of microorganisms on skin	mupirocin (Bactroban) neomycin (Neosporin)
Antipsoriatics Treat the effects of psoriasis	anthralin (Anthra-Derm) methotrexate (Methotrexate)
Antivirals Inhibit the effects of herpes simplex	acyclovir (Zovirax) penciclovir (Denavir)
Burn preparations Treat burned tissue	nitrofurazone (Furacin) mafenide (Sulfamylon)
Corticosteroids Act against inflammation	amcinonide (Cyclocort) hydrocortisone (Cort-Dome)
Keratolytics Remove warts, corns, and calluses	salicylic acid (Compound W) cantharidin (Verr-Canth)
Scabicides, pediculicides Kill parasites and destroy eggs	lindane 1% (Scabene) 5% permethrin (Elimite)
Antipruritics Temporarily relieve itching	diphenhydramine (Benadryl) hydroxyzine pamoate (Vistaril)

PATIENT-CENTERED PROFESSIONALISM

- *Tissue damage can occur in several ways. Why must the medical assistant be aware of methods to prevent skin damage?*
- *How does this awareness translate to better patient care?*

DISEASES AND DISORDERS OF THE INTEGUMENTARY SYSTEM

Diseases and disorders of the integumentary system are often exhibited as alterations of surface skin tissue. Conditions of the skin may be caused by bacteria, parasites, fungi, or viruses, or may have no apparent known cause. A **dermatologist** can treat diseases and conditions of the integumentary system, and drugs may be prescribed to treat these disorders (Table 23-3).

As a medical assistant you need to be able to recognize the common signs and symptoms of and the diagnostic tests for the different types of skin disorders and diseases.
- Study Box 23-1 to familiarize yourself with the common signs and symptoms.
- Study Box 23-2 to learn about common diagnostic tests and procedures.
- Study Table 23-4 to understand the diseases and disorders that affect the integumentary system.

BOX 23-1

Common Signs and Symptoms of Skin Disease

Abscess	Localized collection of pus that occurs on the skin or any body tissue
Alopecia	Loss of hair; baldness
Carbuncles	Large abscesses that involve connecting furuncles
Cicatrix	Scar formation
Crust	Dried serum, blood, and pus; scab
Decubitus ulcer	Pressure sore; caused by decreased circulation to tissue, which leads to death of tissue and bacterial infection
Diaphoresis	Excessive sweating
Ecchymosis	Collection of blood under the skin; skin has blue-black appearance
Eczema	Most common inflammation of the skin; accompanied by papules, vesicles, and crusts; usually an underlying condition of another disorder
Erosion	Destruction of the surface layer of skin
Excoriation	Removal of surface epidermis by scratching, burn, or abrasion
Fissure	Split or crack in the skin
Furuncle	Abscess that occurs around a hair follicle
Ichthyosis	Dry, scaly skin condition; skin has appearance of fish scales
Keloid	Overgrowth of fibrous tissue at site of scar tissue
Petechiae	Flat, pinpoint red spots
Pruritus	Severe itching
Purpura	Small hemorrhages into the skin and tissues
Ulcer	Erosion of the epidermis and dermis
Urticaria	Hives; raised areas that are smooth and cause itching
Vitiligo	Loss of pigment in the skin in patches; milk-white patches

FOR YOUR INFORMATION

Age-related changes affecting the skin are numerous. Both the epidermis and dermis thin and become less elastic, therefore leaving the skin more prone to injury and infection. The skin repairs itself slowly, and recurring infections are a possibility. Vitamin D production declines, causing muscle weakness and a reduction in bone strength. The blood supply to the dermis declines, and a decrease in both sebum and sweat gland production all leave the skin drier, therefore more wrinkles. Age spots and skin tags occur more often, and nails grow slower. Because of the decline in sweat gland activity the body cannot lose heat as quickly, thus making the elderly more prone to heat stroke. A decrease in melanocyte activity leaves the hair follicles grey or white.

BOX 23-2

Diagnostic Tests and Procedures for the Skin

Tissue scraping	Identifies bacterial or fungal disease
Skin biopsy	Removes section of lesion for pathological examination (Figure 23-14)
Wood's light examination	Detects skin infections (usually fungal) by using UV light filtered through a special type of glass (Figure 23-15)
Blood antibody titer	Blood test that indicates whether a person has or has had an infection
Tzanck test	Microscopic examination of skin lesions to screen for herpes virus
Skin test	Determines the reaction of the body to an allergen

- *Intradermal:* Subcutaneously injecting the patient with an allergy extract.
- *Patch:* Small patch of paper impregnated with suspected allergen is placed on the skin.
- *Scratch:* Minute amount of solution containing the suspected allergen is placed on a scratched area of the skin.

UV, Ultraviolet.

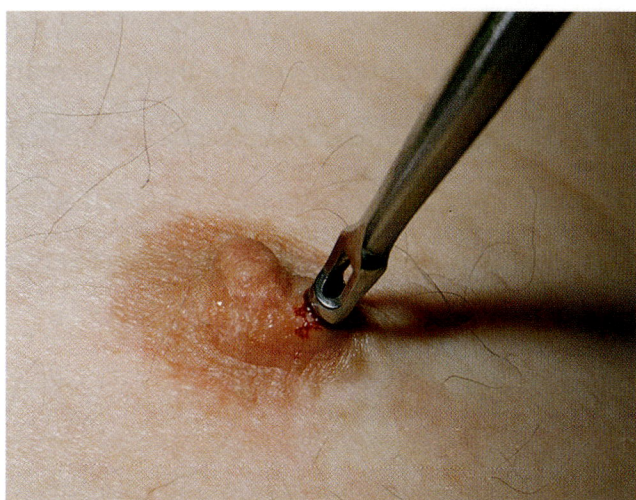

FIGURE 23-14 Punch biopsy. (From Habif TP: *Clinical dermatology,* ed 4, St Louis, 2004, Mosby.)

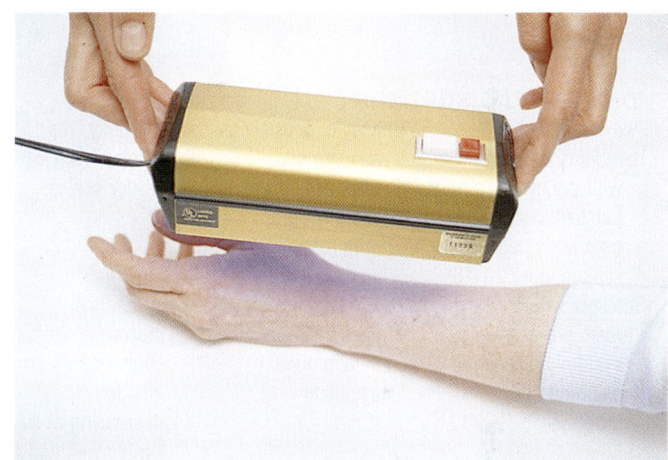

FIGURE 23-15 Wood's lamp. (From Wilson SF, Giddens JF: *Health assessment for nursing practice,* ed 4, St Louis, 2009, Mosby.)

PATIENT-CENTERED PROFESSIONALISM

- *Why should the medical assistant be aware of the causes of skin disorders?*

CONCLUSION

The skin is the body's protective covering, and along with the hair, nails, and glands, the skin makes up the integumentary system. The skin provides support and protection and plays an important role in maintaining homeostasis. The appearance of the skin (color, texture, and temperature) is an indicator of a person's physical condition. Diseases and disorders of the skin can be diagnosed and treated using several different methods.

Understanding the structure and function of the integumentary system is important in understanding how it works with the other body systems to maintain homeostasis. This understanding will help you provide better care to the patients who come to the physician's office with skin diseases or disorders.

TABLE 23-4

Diseases and Disorders of the Integumentary System

Disease and Description	Etiology	Signs and Symptoms	Diagnosis	Therapy	Interventions
BACTERIAL INFECTIONS					
Cellulitis Infection of skin and subcutaneous tissue caused by microorganisms (Figure 23-16)	Usually *Streptococcus* or *Staphylococcus* bacteria that enter skin through a cut or lesion	Redness of skin **(erythema)** with edema; area is hot and tender to the touch	Clinical symptoms of affected limb; blood culture	Antibiotic therapy; affected area is elevated and kept immobile; warm compresses applied to affected area to increase blood circulation; analgesic usually prescribed for discomfort	Encourage patient to pay attention to skin care after scratches and other seemingly minor injuries
Impetigo Infection causes pustules that rupture and form crusts (Figure 23-17)	Causative bacteria are either *Streptococcus* or *Staphylococcus aureus*	Small pustular lesions that appear on face, legs, and arms; spreads easily, especially after scratching an infected area	Clinical appearance and Gram stain of exudates	Use of antibiotics on affected areas	Encourage good hygiene, especially handwashing
IDIOPATHIC DISORDERS					
Psoriasis Hereditary **dermatitis** with dry, scaly, silvery patches, usually on both arms, legs, and scalp (Figure 23-18)	Unknown; possibly an autoimmune response, stress, allergies, and pregnancy	Thick, flaky, red patches with white, silvery scales	Clinical presentation reveals obvious symptoms	UV light therapy, steroid creams, and antihistamines	Provide emotional support for patient
Scleroderma Chronic progressive systemic disease of skin and body systems	Unknown; possibly from an autoimmune condition	Skin hardens (becomes leathery); some organs are affected by decreasing in size; joints swell and are painful	Physical examination, patient history, skin biopsy, and x-ray studies	Palliative Physical therapy to maintain strength of muscle tone	Provide emotional support for patient
PARASITIC DISEASES					
Lyme disease Skin disease that also affects joints and connective tissues	Caused by a spirochete that is transmitted by a bite from a deer tick	Red, itchy rash with bull's-eye appearance; joint pain and malaise	Physical examination, patient history, lesions; blood sample drawn for titer level	Removal of tick; antibiotics and medications for joint pain and fever	Provide emotional support for patient
Scabies Skin disorder caused by itch mite *(Sarcoptes scabiei)*	Mite spreads from person to person by close physical contact	Pruritus and rash in affected area	Visual examination of affected area	Removal of mites by shampoos, application of creams, and topical steroid preparations for itching	Provide support to family and encouragement to treat patient's environment (e.g., bedding, comb, brush)
Pediculosis Skin disorder caused by lice *(Pediculus humanus)**	Caused by lice and spread by human contact or sharing of personal items	Rash; presence of nits (eggs) on hair shaft, skin, or clothing	Visual examination	Prescription shampoo with repeat application in 7 to 10 days	Provide emotional support

TABLE 23-4
Diseases and Disorders of the Integumentary System—cont'd

Disease and Description	Etiology	Signs and Symptoms	Diagnosis	Therapy	Interventions
FUNGAL INFECTIONS					
Tinea Skin infection caused by fungus; classified according to body region affected	Direct contact with fungus or spores	Clinical presentation of patient; usually, scaly lesions and itching	Appearance and location of lesions; culture of lesions	Topical and oral antifungal medications as indicated	Encourage good hygiene
Tinea corporis: affects body; also called "ringworm" (Figure 23-19) *Tinea pedis:* affects feet; also called "athlete's foot" (Figure 23-20) *Tinea unguium:* affects nails; also called **onychomycosis** *Tinea cruris:* affects genital region; also called "jock itch" (Figure 23-21) *Tinea faciei:* affects face (Figure 23-22) *Tinea capitis:* affects scalp (Figure 23-23)					
VIRAL INFECTIONS					
Herpes simplex Skin infection caused by virus; "cold sores," "fever blisters" (Figure 23-24)	Caused by HSV-1	Blisters appear on lips, inside of mouth, and occasionally in nose; lesions usually at the junction of mucous membranes and skin	Physical examination	Antiviral medications; topical antivirals to heal and relieve pain	Encourage good handwashing because virus can be spread by contact
Warts (verrucae) Contagious epithelial growths (Figure 23-25)	Caused by HPV; spread by contact with skin shed from a wart	Elevated growths of epidermis	Visual examination	Surgical excision; cryosurgery	Emotional support

HPV, Human papillomavirus; *HSV-1*, herpes simplex virus type 1; *UV*, ultraviolet.
*P. humanus capitis: head lice; *P. humanus corporis:* body lice; *Phthirus pubis:* pubic lice.

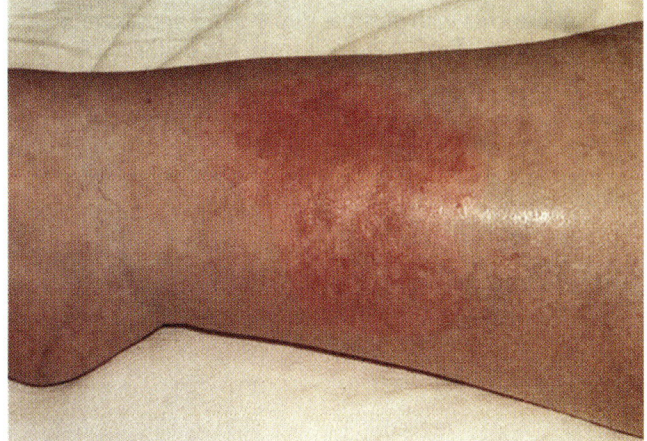

FIGURE 23-16 Cellulitis of the lower leg. (From Wilson SF, Giddens JF: *Health assessment for nursing practice,* ed 4, St Louis, 2009, Mosby.)

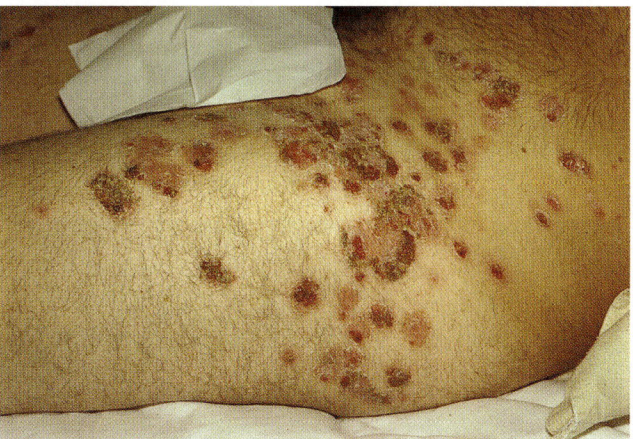

FIGURE 23-17 Impetigo. (From Cohen J, Powderly W: *Infectious diseases,* ed 2, St Louis, 2004, Mosby.)

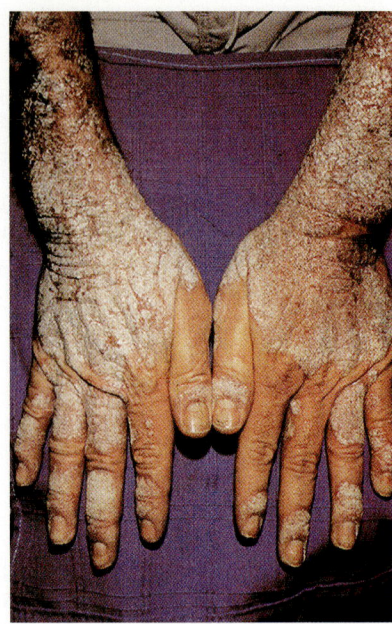

FIGURE 23-18 Psoriasis. (From Hill MJ: *Skin disorders,* St Louis, 1994, Mosby.)

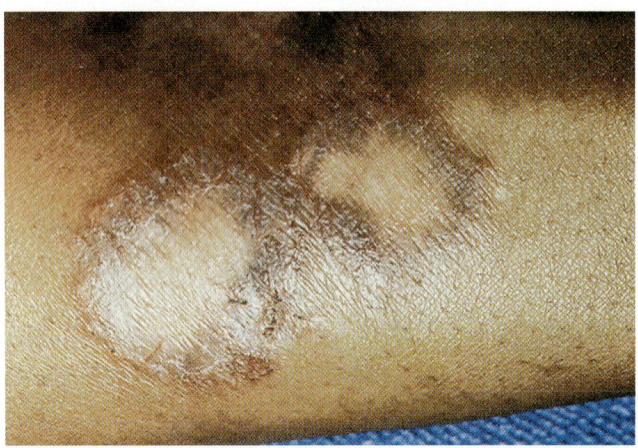

FIGURE 23-19 Tinea corporis. (From Hill MJ: *Skin disorders,* St Louis, 1994, Mosby.)

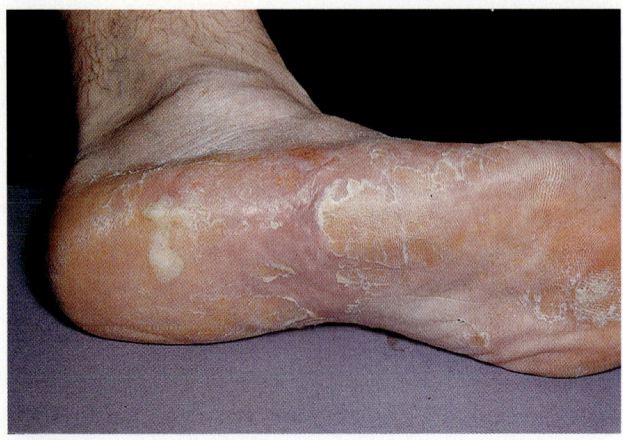

FIGURE 23-20 Tinea pedis resulting from *Trichophyton rubrum* infection. (From Cohen J, Powderly W: *Infectious diseases,* ed 2, St Louis, 2004, Mosby.)

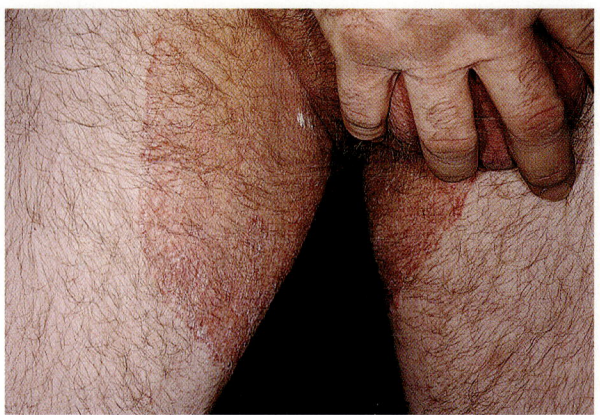

FIGURE 23-21 Tinea cruris. (From Callen JP et al: *Color atlas of dermatology,* ed 2, Philadelphia, 2000, Saunders.)

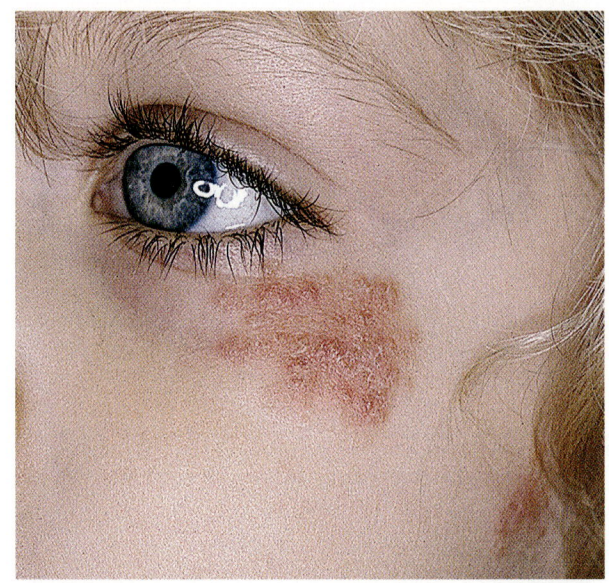

FIGURE 23-22 Tinea faciei. (From Callen JP et al: *Color atlas of dermatology,* ed 2, Philadelphia, 2000, Saunders.)

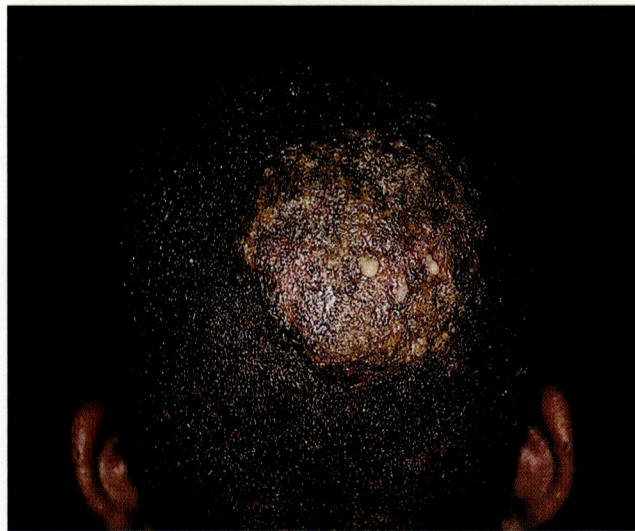

FIGURE 23-23 Kerion (nodular swelling with pustules) form of tinea capitis. (From Callen JP et al: *Color atlas of dermatology,* ed 2, Philadelphia, 2000, Saunders.)

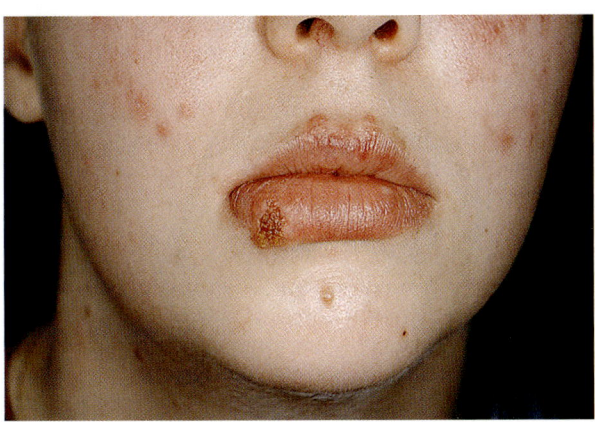

FIGURE 23-24 Herpes simplex infection. (From Callen JP et al: *Color atlas of dermatology,* ed 2, Philadelphia, 2000, Saunders.)

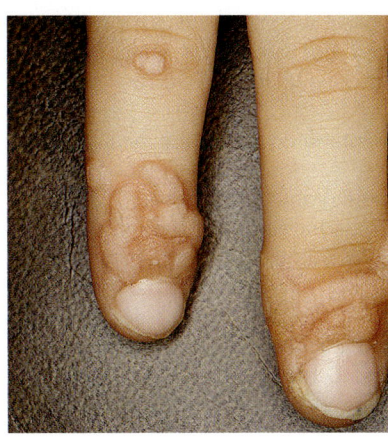

FIGURE 23-25 Verrucae (warts). (From Callen JP et al: *Color atlas of dermatology,* ed 2, Philadelphia, 2000, Saunders.)

Chapter Summary

Reinforce your understanding of the material in this chapter by reviewing the curriculum objectives and key content points below.

1. **Define, appropriately use, and spell all the Key Terms for this chapter.**
   - Review the Key Terms if necessary.
2. **List the three main functions of the skin.**
   - The skin serves to protect the body, regulate temperature, and detect sensations.
3. **Explain how the body is able to maintain a constant temperature.**
   - Enzymes do not function properly without a constant body temperature.
   - When the body becomes too cold, heat loss can be prevented by "goose bumps."
   - When the body becomes too hot, sweating cools the body.
4. **Identify the three layers of the skin and describe the structure and function of each.**
   - The epidermis and the dermis are the two upper layers of the skin.
   - The epidermis is the thin upper layer of flat, dead cells. This layer protects the skin against the sun's ultraviolet (UV) rays.
   - The dermis is thicker than the epidermis and contains the blood vessels, nerve endings, hair follicles, lymph vessels, and sweat glands.
   - The subcutaneous layer is mainly fatty adipose tissue and loose connective tissue and is located beneath the dermis. It provides shock absorption for organs and conserves heat.
5. **Identify the three types of substructures of the skin and explain the function of each.**
   - Hair protects the skin.
   - Sweat glands help maintain body temperature; oil glands prevent drying by reducing water loss.
   - Nails protect the ends of fingers and toes.
6. **List and briefly describe nine common skin lesions.**
   - Cysts are sacs filled with fluid or semisolid material.
   - Fissures are splits or cracks in the skin.
   - Macules are flat, discolored areas.
   - Papules are small, solid, raised areas of the skin.
   - Polyps are stalklike growths from a mucous membrane.
   - Pustules are small, raised areas of the skin that contain pus.
   - Ulcers are erosions of the skin.
   - Vesicles are blisters, collections of clear fluid under the skin.
   - Wheals are slightly elevated white areas of skin surrounded by a pale red area.
7. **Define actinic keratosis, basal cell carcinoma, malignant melanoma, and squamous cell carcinoma and determine how to identify each.**
   - Actinic keratoses are precancerous growths that are scaly papules.
   - Basal cell carcinomas are slow-growing malignant skin lesions that can appear anywhere on sun-exposed skin.
   - Malignant melanomas are a type of skin cancer with black coloring that can appear anywhere on the body and will metastasize.
   - Squamous cell carcinomas appear as firm papules with ulcerations.
   - Use the "ABCDE rule" to check for skin cancer.
8. **List four treatment options for malignant skin lesions.**
   - Cryosurgery, topical chemotherapy, excision, and radiation are some of the treatments for malignant skin lesions.
9. **Explain the difference between open and closed wounds.**
   - In an open wound the skin is damaged, and the tissue below is exposed.

- In a closed wound the tissues beneath the skin are damaged, but there is no visible break in the skin.

10. **List and describe the three phases of wound healing.**
    - Blood clotting occurs in the inflammatory phase.
    - Collagen is added, and a capillary supply is formed during the granulation phase.
    - Scar tissue forms during the maturation phase.

11. **Distinguish between a partial-thickness burn and a full-thickness burn as a means of assessing the depth of a burn.**
    - First- and second-degree burns are considered partial-thickness burns.
    - Third-degree burns are considered full-thickness burns.
    - Emergency medical assistance is needed for second- and third-degree burns.

12. **Explain the purpose and use of the "rule of nines."**
    - The "rule of nines" is a method of assessing the surface area involved in burns.
    - Treatment is based on the severity of the burn and total body surface (TBS) involved.

13. **List and describe seven signs and symptoms of skin disease.**
    - Refer to Box 23-1.

14. **List five types of diagnostic tests and procedures for the skin and describe the use of each.**
    - Refer to Box 23-2.

15. **List 10 diseases and disorders of the integumentary system and briefly describe the etiology, signs and symptoms, diagnosis, therapy, and interventions for each.**
    - Refer to Table 23-4.

16. **Analyze a realistic medical office situation and apply your understanding of the integumentary system to determine the best course of action.**
    - Medical assistants must understand the terminology and processes associated with the integumentary system so that they can provide better care to patients.

17. **Describe the impact on patient care when medical assistants have a solid understanding of the structure and function of the integumentary system.**
    - Medical assistants who understand the physiology of the integumentary system are better able to work with patients who come to the office for diseases and disorders of the skin.

PRACTICAL APPLICATIONS

If you have accomplished the objectives in this chapter, you will be able to make better choices as a medical assistant. Take another look at this situation and decide what you would do.

Marilyn was taking a shower 2 weeks ago and found a large black mole on her shoulder. At first she ignored it, but after talking with her friend, she decided that she should see her family practice physician. This physician sent her to Dr. Nelson, a dermatologist, who diagnosed her lesion as a possible malignant melanoma. Dr. Nelson asked Marilyn if she had any pruritus, a fissure, or any crusting of the lesion. As Dr. Nelson examined Marilyn's shoulder, he noticed petechiae, ecchymosis, and purpura. When asked about these findings, Marilyn told the physician that the mole had itched and she had scratched the area in her sleep. On her leg was a furuncle that was inflamed, hot, and appeared to have a pus formation. On completing the physical examination, Dr. Nelson noticed that Marilyn had the tendency to keloid formation based on the appearance of her appendectomy scar.

Marilyn had quite a few questions for the medical assistant about the meaning of some of the terms used by Dr. Nelson. Marilyn left the dermatologist's office with surgery scheduled for removal of the melanoma in 2 days.

Would you be able to answer Marilyn's questions?

1. What is the etiology of a malignant melanoma?
2. How do the signs of a malignant melanoma differ from those of a benign lesion?
3. What is pruritus? Fissure? Crusting?
4. What are petechiae? What is ecchymosis? Purpura?
5. What is the difference between a furuncle and a carbuncle?
6. Why would the physician be concerned that Marilyn had a history of keloids?
7. What are the stages of the healing process that you could expect Marilyn to have after surgery?
8. What is a closed wound? Give two examples.
9. What is an open wound? Give two examples.

> **WEB SEARCH**
>
> 1. **Research skin cancers to learn more about origins and the predisposition of the skin to cancer.** Discover how skin type, sun exposure, family history, age, and immunologic factors play a role in the development of skin cancers.
>
> - **Keywords:** Use the following keywords in your search: skin cancer, basal cell carcinoma, squamous cell carcinoma, malignant melanoma, and melanoma.

WORD PARTS: Integumentary System

Combining Forms

albin/o	white
cutane/o	skin
derm/o, dermat/o	skin
diaphor/o	sweat
hidr/o	sweat
histi/o	tissue
ichthy/o	fish; scalelike
kerat/o	horny, hard; keratin
melan/o	black; dark
myc/o	fungus
onych/o	nail (finger or toe)
seb/o	oil; sebum
trich/o	hair
xanth/o	yellow
xer/o	dry

ABBREVIATIONS: Integumentary System

BSA	body surface area
Bx	biopsy (removal of tissue for examination)
Decub	decubitus ulcer (bedsore)
Derm	dermatology
I&D	incision and drainage
TBS	total body surface
Ung	ointment
UV	ultraviolet (light)

24 The Medical Office

evolve http://evolve.elsevier.com/klieger/medicalassisting

The success of a medical practice depends on the organization and efficient functioning of the medical office. All staff members have a responsibility for quality patient care, whether it is provided directly or indirectly. The medical assistant is directly involved in how smoothly medical office tasks are accomplished. Understanding effective facilities management; office equipment use, purchase, and maintenance; supply inventory control; office management; policy and procedures manuals; and community resources available will help medical assistants keep the medical office running smoothly and provide the best environment for patient care.

LEARNING OBJECTIVES

You will be able to do the following after completing this chapter:

Key Terms
1. Define, appropriately use, and spell all the Key Terms for this chapter.

Facilities Management
2. Define facilities management and explain its importance to the medical office.
3. Explain the impact of HIPAA legislation on the management of office facilities.
4. Explain the impact of the Americans with Disabilities Act (ADA) on the physical structure of the medical office.
5. List two functions of the reception area.
6. Design a plan for a medical office reception area that reflects HIPAA and ADA regulations and incorporates the seven considerations for a reception area.
7. Describe the daily and weekly maintenance of the reception area.

Office Equipment
8. List six types of office equipment and explain how each is used in the medical office.
9. Demonstrate the procedure for preparing, sending, and receiving a fax.
10. Explain why inventory records are kept.
11. Assess the advantages and disadvantages of leasing versus buying office equipment.
12. Demonstrate the correct procedure for maintaining office equipment.

Supplies
13. Differentiate between capital and noncapital goods.
14. List three factors to be considered when establishing an inventory control system.
15. Demonstrate the correct procedure for creating and maintaining an inventory and ordering system.

Office Management
16. Explain the importance of teamwork in the medical office.
17. Describe the five steps in planning for a meeting.
18. Differentiate between an *agenda* and an *itinerary*.

Policy and Procedures Manuals
19. Explain the purpose of policy manuals and procedures manuals.

Community Resources
20. Explain why it is important for medical assistants to be aware of the community resources available in their area.
21. Demonstrate the correct procedure for gathering community resources.

Patient-Centered Professionalism
22. Analyze a realistic medical office situation and apply your understanding of the medical office to determine the best course of action.
23. Describe the impact on patient care when medical assistants have a solid understanding of all aspects of a well-planned and well-maintained medical office.

KEY TERMS

- advocate
- agenda
- Americans with Disabilities Act (ADA)
- back-ordered
- breach of confidentiality
- capital goods
- disclaimer
- disposable goods
- facilities management
- facsimile
- fax machine
- Health Insurance Portability and Accountability Act (HIPAA)
- inventory records
- invoice
- itinerary
- lead time
- noncapital goods
- notebook computers
- order quantity
- outsourced
- packing slip
- personal digital assistants (PDAs)
- policy manual
- postage meter
- preventive maintenance
- procedures manual
- purchase order
- reorder point
- safety stock
- vendor
- warranty card

PRACTICAL APPLICATIONS

Read the following scenario and keep it in mind as you learn about the planning and maintenance of a medical office in this chapter.

Janine is a new member of the office staff. She has not had any training in the medical assisting field, but she has been working as a receptionist in a loan office. On her first day at work, Janine is assigned to work at the front desk with the receptionist. As the patients for the day come in, she asks many personal questions about each patient and then proceeds to tell the receptionist what she knows about each patient. When told to be sure the names of the patients have been obliterated from the sign-in sheet, she uses a yellow highlighter. As she answers the phone, everyone in the office can hear her conversations. Janine immediately rearranges the large plants in the reception area, and now a plant is partially blocking the doorway.

A fax from a surgeon arrives for Dr. Lopez, and Janine places it on the front counter next to the sign-in sheet until she has a chance to give it to Dr. Lopez. When asked to move the fax, Janine replies that it would "definitely be easier" if the fax was just placed next to the front window rather than in the back room so she would not have to walk so far. Also, Janine does not understand why the office needs a dedicated line for the fax machine. Why not just have the fax line connected to the multiline telephone at the front desk?

Janine was asked to leave a week later after she refused to maintain the equipment. As the office personnel looked for the manuals for the new equipment that had been purchased, no manuals could be found; when she was contacted, Janine admitted to discarding them.

What would you tell Janine about why she was asked to leave her job at the medical office?

FACILITIES MANAGEMENT

The concept of maintaining the atmosphere and physical environment of an office is called **facilities management**. Facilities management in the medical office is the responsibility of all staff members. The atmosphere and environment of the medical facility send a nonverbal message to the patients and even staff; this should be a positive message, not a negative one. Attention to decor of the reception room and its cleanliness and a pleasant patient greeting can lift the spirits of patients and make their waiting time more agreeable.

When planning for, improving, or maintaining a medical office, several legal considerations must be taken into account (e.g., HIPAA, ADA), and available guidelines can help create a good reception area environment for patients.

Health Insurance Portability and Accountability Act

The **Health Insurance Portability and Accountability Act (HIPAA)** was enacted by the U.S. Congress in 1996. Title I of HIPAA protects health insurance coverage for employees and their families when they change or lose their jobs. In essence, Title I prohibits any group health plan from creating eligibility rules or assessing premiums for individuals in the plan based on health status, medical history, or disability. Also, Title I limits restrictions that a group health plan can place on benefits for preexisting conditions. A limit of 12 months is allowed for preexisting conditions unless the individual had coverage before enrolling in the new plan. Title II requires the establishment of national standards for electronic health care transactions and national identifiers for providers, health insurance plans, and employers. Also addressed in Title II is the security and privacy of health information. It provides guidelines for health care providers and insurance carriers for administrative procedures concerning the following issues:

- Electronic transfer of claims
- Disclosure of patient information
- Privacy and security issues to protect the privacy of a patient's health care information

Protected information includes all demographic or health information that identifies or can potentially identify an individual.

HIPAA puts a new focus on how day-to-day operations are handled. For example, business associates (staff) should sign a confidentiality agreement that states they agree to comply with the medical office's privacy regulations (Box 24-1). The office environment must be arranged in a manner that protects the privacy of the patient and his or her information. For example, computer monitors need to be positioned so that no unauthorized individuals can see the screen containing private patient information. As you explore the administrative aspects of the medical office, you will learn how these guidelines affect the medical assistant's role in maintaining the patient's right to confidentiality.

BOX 24-1

Example of Confidentiality Agreement*

It is the purpose of Sunshine Medical Practice to protect the confidentiality of the medical records and privacy of all its patients, as mandated by the HIPAA legislation.

The patient has a legal right to privacy concerning his or her medical information and medical records. It is the obligation of Sunshine Medical Practice to uphold that right. For this reason, no member of this office to whom patient medical information or medical records is available may in any way violate this confidentiality except with the written consent of the patient and in accordance with the policy of Sunshine Medical Practice and the rules and regulations of the State of Florida.

I have read the above statement and agree to abide by its contents.

SIGNATURES:
Employee: _____ Date _____
Witness: _____ Date _____

*Medical staff must sign a confidentiality agreement that requires them to protect the confidentiality of their patients' medical information.

BOX 24-2

Facilities Management Requirements to Meet ADA Requirements

ENTRANCE
Access
1. Width of area leading to the door of the building must be 36 inches wide, slip resistant, and made of a stable material.
2. Ramps longer than 6 feet must have two railings, 34 to 36 inches high. The width of the ramp must not be less than 36 inches.
3. Elevators and ramps must be available to all public areas.

Doors
1. Door must be 32 inches wide and the door handles no higher than 48 inches.
2. Door handles and interior doors must open easily.

INTERNAL
Restrooms
1. Identification of the restroom must include a tactile (braille) sign.
2. Door width must be 32 inches wide.
3. Access for wheelchairs into the stalls requires a width of at least 5 feet by 5 feet.
4. Sinks, soap dispensers, and hand dryers must be easily accessible and able to be operated with a closed fist.

FOR YOUR INFORMATION

BREACH OF CONFIDENTIALITY

Breach of confidentiality *occurs, for example, when a sign-in sheet that requests the patient to identify the reason for the visit to the medical office is used for unauthorized reasons, breaking the patient's right to privacy.*

Americans with Disabilities Act

The **Americans with Disabilities Act (ADA)** also affects the physical structure of the medical office. The architectural standards and alterations portion of the ADA requires that physically accessible routes and fixtures be available to all who enter the facility. People in wheelchairs and those with other types of disabilities must be able to enter, exit, and safely move about the building. This includes having ramps and making sure the size of door openings accommodates wheelchairs. Corridors must be wide enough to allow wheelchairs, walkers, and gurneys to turn, and lavatory sinks and toilets must be accessible to all. Box 24-2 provides examples of requirements that must be met for a medical office to be ADA compliant.

Reception Area

The medical office, including the reception area, must be designed to protect patient privacy, as well as allow access to all individuals. It is important to keep in mind the main functions of the reception area when considering its design and maintaining it.

Function

The reception area serves two main functions: providing a place to greet patients on arrival and providing an area for patients to wait until they can see their health care provider.

Design

A patient's first impression of a medical facility and its staff is often influenced by the condition of the reception area. Cluttered, unkempt reception areas are unprofessional. Because of this, the reception area should be well maintained for the *aesthetic* (pleasant to look at or experience) comfort, as well as the physical comfort, of the patient. Small reception areas may become a concern later; thus prior coordination with a builder is essential.

Every attempt should be made to create a comfortable, welcoming environment (Figure 24-1). Considerations for making the reception area more pleasant for patients include the following:

- The colors in the area should be calming (e.g., soft colors).
- Chair cushions and carpet in the waiting area should not be of the same color, since older patients might have difficulty distinguishing where one ends and the other begins. The use of contrasting colors makes the distinction clear.
- The lighting should be adequate to allow patients to read. Soft lighting from either table and floor lamps

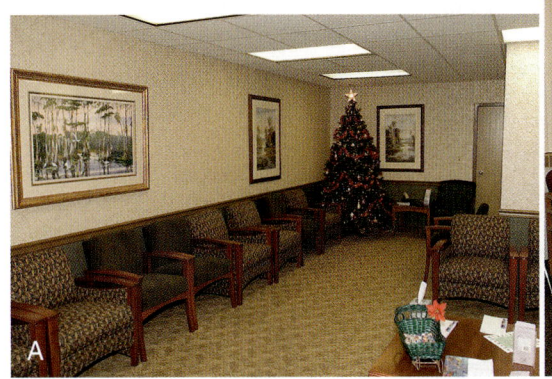
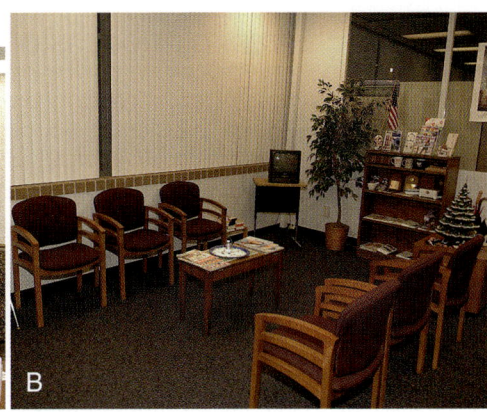

FIGURE 24-1 Waiting areas in medical offices.

or wall sconces creates a pleasant atmosphere for patients. However, once again overhead lighting of significance helps the patients to see more clearly than dim lighting.
- Furniture needs to be comfortable, and there should be enough seating to accommodate peak times in office scheduling. Single-seating arrangements are used most often because choosing an empty seat on a sofa next to a stranger may not be comfortable for patients. Medical practices that treat patients with incontinence problems (e.g., urology, pediatrics) should select materials that can repel stains and odor.
- The placement of plants can soften the institutional look of a medical office. They also act as a noise barrier. Keep in mind that any plants or flowers in the medical setting should be artificial because some patients have allergies.
- Updated window treatments and artwork create a professional image for the waiting area.
- The temperature should not be above 73° F, and good air exchange is important.
- Reading materials or other appropriate materials should be provided to occupy patients while they wait and continually exchanged for current literature.

The selection of reading material available to patients and guests should include current magazines and reading material for children. Pamphlets concerning health maintenance and various organizations (e.g., American Diabetes Association, insurance companies) are also appropriate and must be kept current.

Some offices add a fish tank or have piped-in music to provide a sense of calm to the waiting area. A TV with special programming channels on health maintenance can occupy the patient's time while waiting. Specialty offices may require additional touches to accommodate their patients. For example, the furniture in a pediatrician's office must be durable and safe to accommodate active children and easy to disinfect. There should be a place for controlled activity, including quiet toys (e.g., puzzles), and children's reading materials should be available (Figure 24-2). A TV and VCR or DVD player with age-appropriate movies also works well in the pediatric setting.

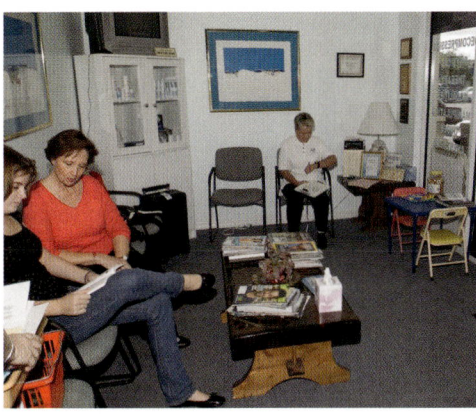

FIGURE 24-2 Children's play area in medical office waiting area.

Maintenance

The medical assistant is responsible for keeping the reception area neat and orderly throughout the day. The reception area should be checked for neatness often during the day, but especially before the office opens and when returning from lunch. The room needs to be straightened again at the end of the day. This lessens the time spent refreshing the area in the morning before opening. A professional cleaning staff is often hired to clean the office completely at least weekly (e.g., floors, dusting, and windows).

NOTE: OSHA requires that all exit routes are clearly marked and easily accessible when needed to make an emergency exit. Also, electrical equipment should be safely plugged in and extension cords properly used.

FOR YOUR INFORMATION

OFFICE MAINTENANCE AND HIPAA

The HIPAA Privacy Rule does not consider a cleaning service a "business associate" because the work they perform does not involve the use or disclosure of protected health information. However, if the service was hired to shred documents that contain protected health information, a business associate relationship may exist, and the service would be bound by the HIPAA guidelines.

PATIENT-CENTERED PROFESSIONALISM

- What is the purpose of a confidentiality agreement?
- How can the medical assistant make certain that the medical office is accommodating for all patients?

OFFICE EQUIPMENT

Medical assistants handle office equipment daily by using, evaluating, and maintaining it and training others in its use. Because of this, assistants must keep up with technological advances. Office equipment continues to become smaller in size, larger in capacity, and faster in processing speed. These advances and good organizational skills assist the office staff in completing time-consuming tasks more quickly. Equipment manuals provide instructions for use, as well as troubleshooting guidelines for equipment malfunctions.

Typical office equipment includes the fax machine, photocopy machine, telephone system, mailing equipment, and computers. Medical assistants also need to know (1) what information should be kept in the equipment inventory records about each piece of office equipment, (2) the difference between leasing and buying equipment, and (3) how each piece of equipment is maintained to prolong its efficiency.

Types of Equipment

Fax Machine

Using **facsimile** communication *(fax transmission)* is a fast, reliable, and inexpensive (the cost of a phone call) way to send information. A *dedicated phone line* may be used to operate the fax machine, which does not interfere with incoming patient phone lines. This line permits faxes to be sent and received 24 hours a day. Medical records, medication refill approvals, correspondence (e.g., referrals, reports), insurance information, and laboratory and x-ray results can be faxed. A medical assistant should fax information only when necessary and only at the physician's direction. Always verify the patient has a signed and dated "release of information authorization" form in their medical chart.

To protect patient privacy and confidentiality, documents should be faxed only to *secured* areas, where privacy is assured and there is no general patient or visitor traffic. In addition, confirmation should be requested that the documents have been received by the party for whom they were intended. Legal concerns with regard to the HIPAA Privacy Rule for fax use are listed in Box 24-3.

The **fax machine** scans each page, translates the information to electronic impulses, and electronically transmits an exact copy (facsimile) of the original document from one location to another using a telephone line or from a modem to a fax machine. An all-in-one machine can photocopy, scan, and fax a single document (Figure 24-3). Each of the many brands of fax machines works somewhat differently, but the basic process is similar from machine to machine.

BOX 24-3
Legal Concerns When Faxing Patient Information

Legal Issues	Resolution
1. Confidentiality	Need "authorization to release records" form signed by patient or legal guardian and dated.
2. Information	Fax only the minimum medical information needed to accomplish the task, and never fax financial information about the patient.
3. Location	Only fax information to secure areas in a physician's office, nursing station, or pharmacy.

Does the HIPAA Privacy Rule allow patient medical information to be faxed to another physician's office?

Yes; the new rule allows physicians to disclose protected health information to another physician's office for treatment purposes as long as reasonable and appropriate administrative, technical, and physical safeguards are in place. For example, the sender must confirm that the fax number to be used is in fact the correct one for the physician's office and that the fax machine is in a secure location to prevent unauthorized access to the information. Good business practices to follow include making certain the person to whom the fax is addressed is waiting for it and not allowing faxes to sit in the machine, where unauthorized people can view them.

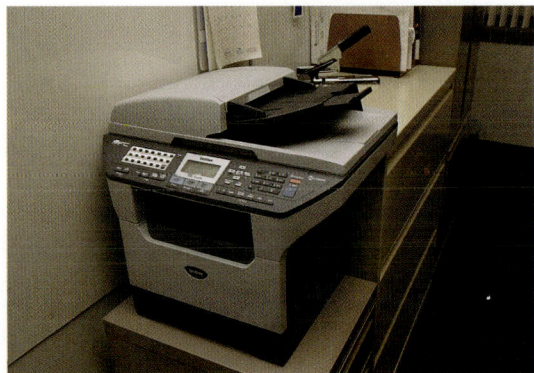

FIGURE 24-3 Typical all-in-one fax machine, scanner, and photocopier.

A cover sheet should be used because it provides protection (by covering potentially sensitive information) and precedes the document to be faxed (Figure 24-4). It should include the name and fax number of the sender and the receiver, number of pages being sent, and the telephone number to call if a problem occurs during the transmission. Also, cover sheets must include a **disclaimer** to protect the privacy of the patient (e.g., HIPAA mandates). For example, the disclaimer might read "This Fax is only for Dr. Right. No one else is entitled to read the enclosed. If received in error, notify the sender (555-9876), then destroy the document or delete the transmission).

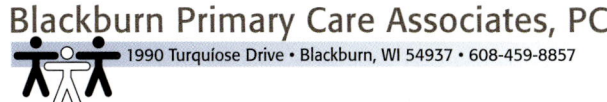

FIGURE 24-4 Example of cover sheet for fax transmittal.

Facsimile transmittal

Blackburn Primary Care Associates, PC
1990 Turquoise Drive • Blackburn, WI 54937 • 608-459-8857

To: P.J. Morales, M.D.   **Fax:** 007-555-6655

From: Blackburn   **Date:** 10/21/20XX

Re: Referral Information   **Pages (including coversheet):** 2

CC:

☐ Urgent   ☒ For Review   ☐ Please Comment   ☐ Please Reply   ☐ Please Recycle

The information contained within this fax transmission contains confidential information. If this transmission has been received in error, notify the sender by calling 555-9876. Then, destroy by shredding or delete this transmission.

The cover page and document are inserted into the machine, the telephone number of the receiving machine is dialed, and the "send" button is pressed.

Procedure 24-1 provides general instructions for using a fax machine. Older fax machines operate with "thermal" paper instead of bond paper. When a fax is received on thermal paper, it must be photocopied because the printing on thermal paper will fade over time.

Photocopy Machine

After the telephone, the photocopier is the most frequently used piece of equipment in the medical office. Its purpose is to duplicate a document by taking a picture and transferring it to a piece of paper using a heat process. Copies of medical records, medical reports, insurance claims, correspondence, and other medical documents can be made quickly and easily. The medical assistant must remove all medical documents from the photocopier after copies have been made.

Features available for photocopiers include enlarging, reducing, collating, and stapling capabilities; color and black and white options; and two-sided copying. Paper and toner supplies are needed to keep the copier functional. As with fax machines, many brands of copy machines are available, with each operated according to the individual manufacturer's instructions. To make a photocopy, the original document is prepared by removing paper clips, staples, and flags (self-adhesive). The document is then correctly placed, usually face down, on the glass (or fed into the document feeder—face up or face down, depending on the manufacturer's instructions). The desired paper size (usually defaults to $8\frac{1}{2} \times 11$) and the number of copies to be processed is selected, and the "start" button is pressed. A budgetary consideration is to minimize the practice of making extra copies "just in case" that are thrown away later.

Telephone Equipment

As a medical assistant you should be familiar with the various types of telephone equipment that may be used in the office.

Multiple telephone lines are standard in most offices today (Figure 24-5). A typical multiline telephone has six buttons. Four are for incoming and outgoing calls, one is an intercom button, and the other is to place a caller on hold. When the telephone rings, you need to identify which line is ringing (the incoming call is typically indicated by a flashing light). To answer the call, the button that corresponds to the flashing light is pressed. In larger offices, calls may be handled through a switchboard.

You may be asked to provide input when the office is considering updating the telephone system. Important factors to consider include the following:

- *Ease of expansion.* As a practice grows, the system should be equipped to have telephone lines added easily. A multi-practitioner medical practice typically has four lines available initially.
- *Ease of use for the staff.* A complicated system could result in lost calls.
- *Dedicated telephone lines.* Having separate telephone lines for the fax machine and on-line Internet services leaves the telephone lines open for patient calls.
- *Special features:*
  1. *Call forwarding* can be used to forward calls to other departments (e.g., billing, prescription refill, or laboratory).
  2. *Conference calling* can be used to have a three-way conversation with consulting physicians and patients' families. *Teleconferencing* is an extension of a conference call with the inclusion of cameras, speaker phones, and television monitors with the phone provider networking all phones together.
  3. The *privacy button* is for the physician to use when speaking without being interrupted.
  4. The *repeat call* (or *redial*) feature redials the last number called up to 30 minutes previously.
  5. *Caller ID* allows the person answering the phone to see the telephone number of the person who is calling.

PROCEDURE 24-1 Prepare, Send, and Receive a Fax

TASK: Correctly send and receive information by fax, maintaining confidentiality according to HIPAA guidelines.

EQUIPMENT AND SUPPLIES
- Cover sheet
- Document(s) to be faxed
- Pen
- Fax machine

SKILLS/RATIONALE

1. **Procedural Step.** Gather equipment and supplies.
   Rationale. This provides for efficient use of time.
2. **Procedural Step.** Prepare the fax to send.
   a. Obtain the document to be faxed. Check the file for a signed and dated "release of information" authorization form.
   When patient information is to be faxed, such as to another physician or to an attorney, a signed and dated "release of information" authorization form must be on file in the patient's medical record. A patient may give permission to release all of his or her information or may limit what information is to be released to a specific visit, time frame, or condition.
   b. Obtain the information of the intended recipient.
   Verify that you have the correct fax number. If the faxed document is to be read only by the intended recipient, a telephone call should be made to the recipient in advance of the document being faxed to ensure that the recipient is available to receive the fax and is waiting at the fax machine for its arrival.
   Rationale. Medical records are highly confidential. Every effort should be made to ensure that the information being faxed is sent to the correct party.
   c. Create a medical facility cover sheet.
   The medical facility may already have a "template" for a fax cover sheet; if not, a template or cover sheet will need to be created. A fax cover sheet must contain areas for the following information (see Figure 24-4):
   (1) Sender information: company name, company telephone number, name of person sending the fax. Company address and fax number may also be included.
   (2) Receiver information: company name, company fax number, name of person receiving the fax (Attention:). Company address and telephone number may also be included.
   (3) Number of pages to be faxed, description of fax contents (Re:), notice of confidentiality. A short message to the receiver may be included.
   d. Prepare the cover sheet.
   Using either your computer or a black or dark-blue ink pen (never pencil), fill in the required information on the form as illustrated in Figure 24-4. *Never* send a fax without a cover sheet.
   e. Prepare the document.
   Documents being faxed should not be on colored paper. If a document is on colored paper, a copy should be made and lightened before faxing. Documents must be free of staples and paper clips.
   Rationale. A fax machine will interpret colored paper as having a black background, and when the fax is received, it will be too dark to be read. Staples and paper clips "jam" the machine.
3. **Procedural Step.** Send the fax.
   a. Place the cover sheet and document into the fax machine according to the manufacturer's instructions.
   Read the manufacturer's instructions for the operation of your facility's fax machine.
   NOTE: Usually an imprint of a document appears in the sending tray illustrating whether the document is to be face up or face down.
   Rationale. The correct process for fax machines may vary slightly from manufacturer to manufacturer. For example, some fax machines may require that the documents are inserted face up, whereas others are face down.
   b. Dial the telephone fax number of the recipient. When documents are placed face down, write the receiver's fax number on the back of the last document.
   Before pressing the start button to send the fax, check the display window to ensure the correct number has been entered. If the number is incorrect, press the "clear" or "reset" button, then reenter the correct number. Remember to include the area code as needed.

Continued

PROCEDURE 24-1 Prepare, Send, and Receive a Fax—cont'd

Rationale. Writing the receiver's number on the last page of the documents to be sent helps the sender to enter the correct fax number.

c. Press "start."

d. When the document has completely processed through the machine, press the button to receive a receipt.

If the number rings busy, some fax machines will redial the number at timed intervals. If the fax is not transmitted, the receipt will indicate this. Verify that the number is correct before resending the document. Some machines will automatically print out a receipt.

NOTE: A good business practice is to set the fax machine to automatically generate a receipt (verification form).

e. Remove the document from the machine, and attach the receipt to the document.

The document and the receipt should be returned to the file where originally obtained. If this is a newly created document, a file should be created.

4. **Procedural Step.** Receive the fax.

a. On receipt of a fax, immediately remove the document from the machine.

Your facility will be the recipient of confidentially faxed documents. All documents should be delivered to the intended recipients, with the cover sheet in place, and should not be read by unauthorized personnel. Authorized personnel, such as medical assistants, may read the document and determine what actions should be taken.

b. Determine the intended recipient of the document.

A faxed document is considered as equally valid as an original document and should be treated as the original document would be.

c. Deliver the document to its intended recipient or review for action.

Occasionally a fax will be intended for only the physician to view. The fax should be delivered personally to the physician and should not be read by any other party.

d. Perform the action or file the document.

If the fax is a laboratory report, for example, the action taken would be to "pull" the patient's medical record, attach the faxed lab results to the front, and deliver to the physician for review. Once the fax has been reviewed and the physician has indicated reading the report, the fax is inserted in the patient's medical record and the patient's medical record is filed.

NOTE: Although it is rare, some fax machines may still use "thermal" paper. Documents received on this type of paper must be photocopied because the images fade in approximately 1 year.

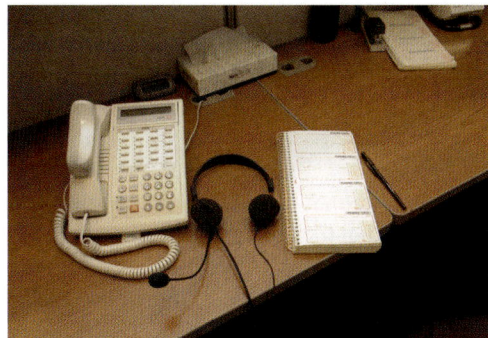

FIGURE 24-5 Multiline telephone systems are a common feature in medical offices. A headset can be attached to the telephone.

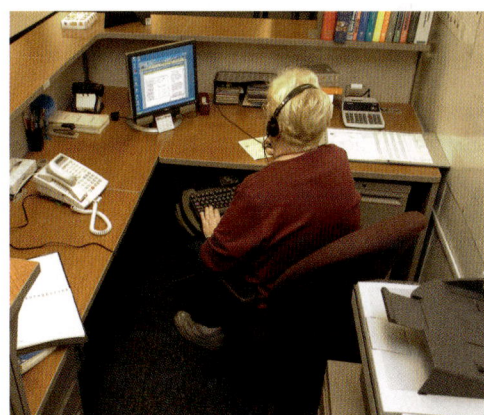

FIGURE 24-6 Telephone headset leaves the hands free and facilitates good body posture.

6. *Speaker phone* is a feature that allows the phone to be used without the phone being held next to the face and ear. It enables a small group of people near the phone to hear the conversation and to be heard when they speak. Care must be taken not to use the speaker phone function when patient information may be overheard by unauthorized people.

7. A *headset* allows you to use both hands while speaking on the phone (Figure 24-6).

A telephone system can be programmed to have an automated menu (e.g., "If you want to make an appointment, press 1; for a prescription refill, press 2"). The menu should always have an option to press for immediate personal assistance in the event the call is an emergency. Physicians and office managers routinely carry cellular phones and pagers to maintain a link to the medical office.

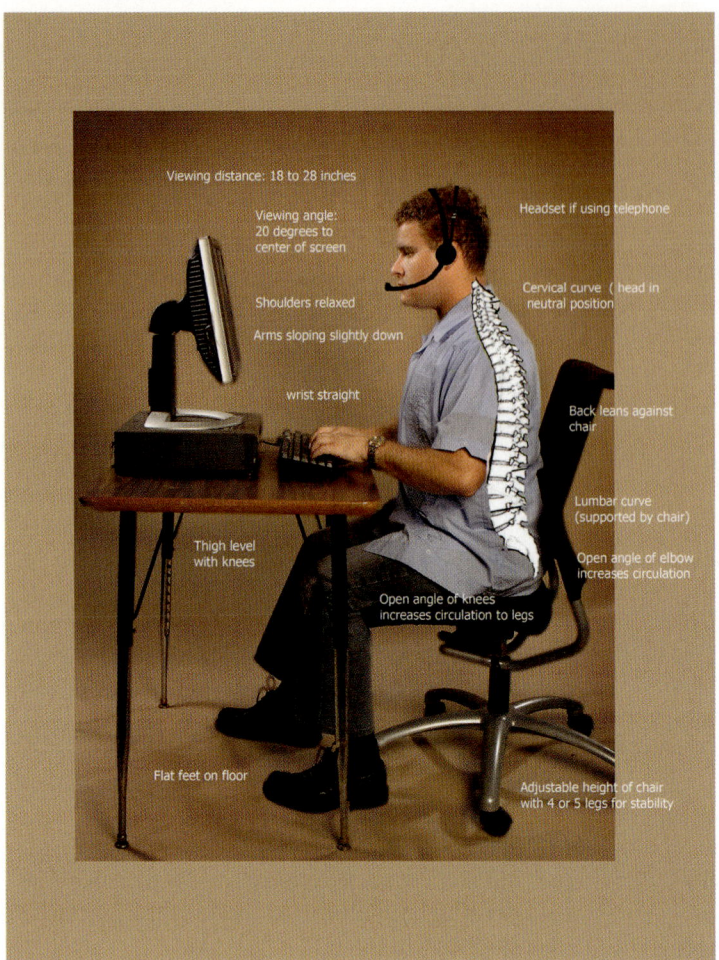

FIGURE 24-7 Example of a computer workstation that illustrates the concept of ergonomics.

Answering Systems

A medical office usually closes for lunch, at the end of the business day, and sometimes for staff meetings. A system must be in place to handle patient calls during these periods. Two methods are routinely used: an answering service and an answering machine or a voice mail system.

Answering Service. An answering service is a business entity that handles patient calls during hours the medical practice is closed. If the physician needs to respond to the caller, the answering service will page the physician. In some cases the call will be forwarded to the physician's location. At other times a message will be taken and given to the medical assistant when the office reopens.

Answering Machine. Answering machines are often found in a small medical office setting. When the staff is leaving the office, the machine should be turned "on." The message should identify the name of the office, what to do in case of an emergency, and what information is needed for a nonemergency call. When the office reopens, messages should be retrieved immediately and calls returned as soon as possible.

Voice Mail. Voice mail is a computerized answering service that automatically answers a call, plays a prerecorded greeting, and then records a message from the caller. Voice mail is typically part of the telephone system and not a separate piece of equipment. Messages can be retrieved, replied to, saved, deleted, and even forwarded to someone else.

Computers

Computers can organize, store, and process information and are an essential part of the modern medical office. As a medical assistant you need to understand many of the computer's functions and must be able to use it efficiently. Computers are discussed in more detail in Chapter 25.

Placement in the Office. Considerations in the placement of a computer in the office include (1) privacy requirements, to ensure screens containing financial and medical information cannot be viewed by others; (2) amount of desk space, allowing adequate space for the monitor, keyboard, and peripheral equipment; and (3) proximity of electrical outlets. Also, the computer must be ergonomically positioned to avoid injury to the user (Figure 24-7). *Ergonomics* is the science of adjusting the work environment (e.g., workstations, equipment) to prevent injuries. For example, proper positioning of the computer monitor, keyboard, and chair can reduce the risk of wrist, arm, back, and eye strain. Box 24-4 discusses computers and health-related issues.

BOX 24-4

Computers and Health Related Issues

Musculoskeletal disorders (MSDs), also referred to as repetitive strain injuries (RSI), are injuries of the muscles, nerves, tendons, ligaments, and joints caused by prolonged keyboarding, mouse usage, or continued shifting between the mouse and keyboard. Included in this classification of injuries are the following:
- *Tendonitis of the wrist.* Inflammation of the tendon as a result of repetitive motion or stress on the tendon. Symptoms include extreme pain that extends from the forearm to the hand and tingling in the fingers.
- *Carpal tunnel syndrome (CTS).* Inflammation of the nerve that connects the forearm to the palm of the wrist. Symptoms include burning pain when the nerve is compressed and numbness and tingling in the thumb.

Another health-related condition caused by computer usage is *computer vision syndrome (CVS).* Symptoms include sore, tired, burning, itching, or dry eyes; blurred or double vision; headache or sore neck; difficulty shifting focus from display device (monitor) and documents; color fringes or after-images when looking away from the monitor; and increasing sensitivity to light.

Techniques to reduce computer-related health issues include the following:
- Take frequent breaks (every 30 to 60 minutes) during computer work to exercise hands and arms (e.g., stand up, walk around, or stretch).
- Every 10 to 15 minutes, close your eyes and rest them for at least 1 minute.
- Adjust the lighting.
- When wearing corrective lenses, have an adjustment made to accommodate computer viewing.
- Viewing distance should be 18 to 28 inches (arm's length).

FOR YOUR INFORMATION

COMPUTERS AND HIPAA

If a patient can view medical information simply by glancing at a computer screen, the HIPAA regulation has been violated. To avoid this, the computer screen needs to be angled away from a patient's view. Computer screens should never face a reception area or a corridor. Patients should go directly from the reception area to the examination area. This avoids having a patient wandering around a restricted area.

Mobile Computers. Physicians are routinely using **notebook computers** to store patient information and the smaller **personal digital assistants** (**PDAs**) to keep appointments, phone numbers, addresses, to-do lists, notes, and other important information they need to have "on hand." This type of computer should not be left in the exam rooms, or in places where patient information may be viewed by an unauthorized person.

Mailing Equipment

In a large medical practice the fastest way to process mail is by using a **postage meter.** A postage meter is a postage providing system that is leased to the user by an authorized provider. An advantage to this type of postage system is that it prints variable postage according to the mail characteristics and mail service needed, except periodicals. Postage can be printed on adhesive strips for use on large envelopes or packages; for regular-size envelopes, the postage can be placed directly onto the envelope. Before printing postage, the material to be mailed should be weighed. The two types of postage scales are the *mechanical* scale, which uses springs to balance the scale, and the *digital* scale, which has a computer chip. Mechanical scales are the least expensive, but the spring often stretches after long-term usage. Digital scales, however, can be recalibrated easily if needed.

To use a postage meter, the medical assistant should make certain the correct date is set, weigh the envelope, and select the correct rate according to postal regulations. Next, the envelope is fed through the letter-sealer base of the machine, where postage is automatically applied and the letter is sealed. After this, the letter is ready for mailing. Remember, envelopes and packages without enough postage will be returned by the United States Postal Service (USPS). Sending mail with too much postage is a wasteful practice and should not be done.

If a mass mailing is to leave the office (e.g., statements), the postage rate would be the same on all envelopes, so time is saved in processing. The advantage of using a metered mail system is that it does not need to be postmarked by the post office and therefore moves on to its destination faster. It is important to remember that the letter-sealer portion of the equipment can be purchased, but the meter must be leased. Only authorized manufacturers can lease postage meters and they are held responsible by the USPS for meter control, operation, replacement, and maintenance. When the meter runs low on postage, the meter box can be taken to the local post office for additional postage. Some postage meter companies have toll-free numbers to call; postage can then be charged to an office credit card and updated automatically.

Equipment Inventory Records

The purpose of maintaining **inventory records** is to document the physical assets of the medical office. Information kept about an item should include the following:
- Product name and model
- Description of the item
- Location in office
- Date of purchase (original receipt if possible)
- Purchase price
- Place of purchase
- Serial number or inventory number
- Service agreement

This information can be used for *depreciation* purposes or an insurance claim in the case of fire or theft and is useful when determining possible updates and repair needs. This information should be placed in a safe location, away from possible damage or loss.

Lease versus Buy

As a medical assistant, you need to understand how purchasing decisions are made in a medical office. An important decision facing the medical office is whether major office equipment should be purchased or leased. Leasing has definite advantages and disadvantages that should be considered. The type of practice and the needs of the practice are major factors in decision making.

Buying a product gives ownership to the practice and allows the owners the freedom to use the equipment as they see fit.

Leasing requires an agreement that outlines conditions for the use of the equipment and requires an initial up-front fee followed by monthly payments. There are different types of lease agreements, and each must be considered carefully.

For example, mailing equipment (letter-sealer) can be bought, but because postage rates are under government control, a postage meter must be leased.

Advantages of Leasing

- Leasing equipment that requires excessive use, needs to be replaced frequently, or requires costly repairs saves the medical practice money in the long run because replacement and repairs are often included in the terms of the lease.
- Leasing technical equipment that needs to be frequently updated will be less expensive for the practice because some lease agreements provide frequent equipment updates at no additional cost to the office.
- The initial cost to buy an item may be a sizable cash drain on the facility, and since leasing requires less cash up front, it may be a favorable alternative.

Disadvantages of Leasing

- The practice does not own the leased equipment.
- Lower interest rates on purchase agreements may make purchasing the equipment a better choice for the facility.
- Leased equipment cannot be sold because it is not owned by the practice.
- Leasing can be more expensive than buying over a period of time because of overuse fees or higher payments.

Maintaining Equipment

Both administrative and clinical office equipment, whether leased or owned, must be maintained to keep it in working condition. Lawsuits as a result of alleged faulty equipment can be averted if a formal maintenance program is in place. It is also essential to keep records on preventive and corrective measures taken. These records can be kept on a computer or in card files and should include dates of inspection and repair. Procedure 24-2 provides guidelines for establishing a maintenance program for all office equipment. It is best if one person is assigned the responsibility of this task. Preventive maintenance needs to be performed by the medical staff, and warranties may protect against faulty or damaged equipment.

Preventive Maintenance

Preventive maintenance is the action taken by the medical office to identify potential failures and to avoid a breakdown of equipment (similar to having regular vehicle inspections). For example, if a door gasket on an autoclave is replaced at regular intervals before it becomes brittle, the machine will operate at optimum capacity. The equipment inventory records provide a baseline to begin the process.

Many equipment companies offer preventive maintenance agreements or service agreements on purchased equipment. *Maintenance agreements* are contracts that provide for regular maintenance service at defined intervals or on an as-needed basis. The purpose of a maintenance agreement is to prevent or minimize breakdowns. *Service agreements* provide for labor costs and usually a discounted price on parts for a set time. These agreements are usually based on 1 year of service, with renewal as an option. As with all contracts, these should be secured in a locked, fireproof cabinet. It is important that the telephone number for service be kept in an easily accessible area, in case there is a need for repair. Some offices elect to attach the contact number to the equipment.

Warranties

A **warranty card** accompanies most major equipment purchases. The purpose is to provide protection for the buyer against defective items. To activate the warranty, the card must be filled out (registered) and returned to the manufacturer. Warranties guarantee that the equipment will be free from defect for a certain period after purchase (e.g., 90 days). When an item is misused, vandalized, or mistreated, the warranty is voided. An extended warranty is often offered on major pieces of equipment. This protects the buyer from paying for replacement parts and labor. When the warranty period is over, the warranty card can be discarded. Management must take care in contracting this type of coverage, as it could be prohibitive.

PATIENT-CENTERED PROFESSIONALISM

- Why must the medical assistant be aware of how to operate all office equipment and have good organizational skills?
- How would you describe the lease versus buy option?
- Once equipment is acquired, what administrative functions should be done in the office?
- How does more efficiency in the medical office translate to better service and care to patients?

PROCEDURE 24-2 Maintain Office Equipment

TASK: Create an office document that identifies office equipment and allows for product information and maintenance data to be recorded.

EQUIPMENT AND SUPPLIES

- List of office equipment to include all administrative and medical equipment, such as:

Computer(s)	Electrocardiograph machine
Telephone system	Glucometer
Transcription machine	Cholesterol machine
Fax machine	Electronic thermometer(s)
Photocopy machine	Sigmoidoscope
Postage meter	Ultrasound equipment
Postage scale	X-ray equipment
Printer	

- Maintenance, service, and warranty agreements
- List of office repair and supply companies
- File folder(s)
- Computer with spreadsheet and word-processing software
- Pen or pencil

SKILLS/*RATIONALE*

1. **Procedural Step. Create a document to list office equipment used in the facility.**
   Separate the list into administrative and clinical equipment. Identify the required data of each piece of equipment and vendor.
   Rationale. This establishes a "template" that can be used electronically or that can be photocopied and kept on file to be referred to as maintenance is required.

2. **Procedural Step. Create a file folder for administrative equipment and one for clinical equipment.**
   Files can also be created by vendor, by type of equipment, or for each individual piece of equipment.
   Rationale. This provides the facility with a complete list of all office equipment in one place. Depending on the amount and type of equipment, folder selection is one that best suits the needs of the office.

3. **Procedural Step. Attach any maintenance, service, or warranty agreements to each piece of product information about the equipment.**
   Using correct filing procedures, alphabetically file by vendor name, or alphabetically file by type of equipment.
   Rationale. This allows for quick access to each piece of equipment's information for accurate and efficient documentation of maintenance or repairs.

4. **Procedural Step. Create a maintenance log for each piece of equipment. Attach each maintenance log on the left inside cover of the main file folder.**
   Print the name of the piece of equipment in the top right-hand corner. List the manufacturer, identification number, date of purchase, and purchase price directly below the name.
   Rationale. This establishes a beginning record of all equipment used by the facility.

5. **Procedural Step. Physically inspect each piece of equipment.**
   Ensure that each piece of equipment is in proper working order and is calibrated as mandated by the manufacturer. Look for frayed cords, broken parts, and improper functioning. Note on the maintenance log the date and the status of the equipment (e.g., "works correctly and calibrated to manufacturer's standards," "performs function but LED readout does not register," or "not working and needs repair").
   Rationale. This provides the facility with a beginning status report of all equipment. As new equipment is purchased, a file can be established and a maintenance log started.

6. **Procedural Step. Determine the manufacturer's recommended time frame for maintenance.**
   Since some pieces of equipment require routine maintenance, a schedule should be established to have a technician "service" the equipment on a regular basis. (You may want to create a "tickler" file to remind you that maintenance is required.) Other office equipment will only require maintenance if the equipment is not working properly. In this case, the service agent can be called and an appointment set for repair.
   Rationale. Following this procedure will ensure that all office equipment is in good repair and working whenever it is needed.

Continued

> **PROCEDURE 24-2** Maintain Office Equipment—cont'd
>
> 7. **Procedural Step.** Document all maintenance and repairs on the maintenance log, and keep all receipts of repairs or maintenance in the folder along with the agreements.
>
>   *Rationale.* Keeping all documentation together in one place for each piece of equipment provides a complete overview of the equipment's history.

SUPPLIES

All medical offices use supplies, the items used in patient care and administrative procedures. Supplies can be identified as being disposable, capital, or noncapital.

- **Disposable** (expendable, nondurable, or consumable) **goods** are used then discarded. For example, tongue blades and other medical supplies, housekeeping items, and office supplies are all disposable goods.
- **Capital** (durable) **goods** are usually expensive and expected to be permanent or to last several years (e.g., autoclaves, examination tables, office furniture, and surgical instruments).
- **Noncapital goods** are reusable but are less costly than capital goods (e.g., blood pressure equipment, scales).

An inventory must be kept of all supplies, and care must be taken when ordering, receiving, paying for, and storing them.

Supply Inventory

To avoid running out of needed supplies, one person in the medical office should be designated to handle supplies management. Often, a medical assistant is responsible for the inventory and maintenance of supplies and for initiating requests for supplies, or one medical assistant may be responsible for clinical supplies and another for office supplies. A system to handle this responsibility must be chosen to fit the needs of the office.

If the supply cabinet is well organized and a habit is developed to check supplies at least weekly, a shortage of items can be avoided. Dividing items into categories (administrative and clinical) and urgency of need (vital to office operation or incidental use only) makes the process easier. It is also important to know which suppliers require advance notice for orders (e.g., supplier for letterhead that must be custom printed with information about the practice) and the expected time for delivery. All order information should be documented so ordering can be accomplished if the designated person is not available.

Ordering

A set method for ordering supplies should be established. The following factors should be considered when establishing an inventory control system (Figure 24-8).

- **Reorder point:** Minimum quantity of a supply to be on hand. When this quantity is reached a supply should be reordered. Establishing a reorder point is based on how much an item is used, the time it takes from ordering an item to receiving the item, how much **safety stock** or extra items are on hand, and the time before the next inventory.
- **Order quantity:** Optimal quantity of a supply to be ordered at one time.
- **Lead time:** Amount of time it takes to receive an order once placed.

To be effective, an ordering system must be designed for the needs of the office. One system used requires supplies be preprinted on inventory control cards or forms.

ITEM	MINIMUM QUANTITY ON HAND	AMOUNT ON SHELF	DATE INVENTORY TAKEN
2X2 NS GAUZE SQ	6 BAGS		
2X2 ST GAUZE SQ	6 BOXES		
EXAM TABLE PAPER	12 ROLLS		

FIGURE 24-8 Example of inventory control system.

If several supplies are needed from a **vendor,** a **purchase order** is usually initiated. A purchase order gives the name, address, and telephone number of both the vendor and the medical office. A preassigned number is stamped on the purchase order. To order items, the medical assistant needs to list the name, product number, quantity, unit of order, unit price, and the extended price of each line item. In some situations, either the office manager or the physician will need to authorize the purchase of items. Procedure 24-3 provides general instructions for ordering supplies and maintaining inventory control.

Receiving

When an order is received, a **packing slip** is included. The packing slip lists all items ordered, the items sent, and the number of items **back-ordered** (out-of-stock items). When the order is received, the packing slip should be signed and dated. The packing slip(s) must be compared to the original purchase order(s). This prevents items being added to an order and the office being charged later for items not received. Each item should be checked against the packing slip for size, style, amount, and condition. When completed, the packing slip is attached to the purchase order, and the inventory card is updated to reflect the addition of these items in stock. Any errors found must be reported to the vendor immediately.

Payment

The vendor sends an invoice either with the order or separately to let the office know the total charges for the order. The statement shows the summary of the order or account activity.

Invoice. An **invoice** is a form prepared by the vendor describing the products sold by item number, the quantity, and the price. The invoice is considered a source document and is used for paying the vendor. When received, the invoice should be dated, compared against the packing slip to verify that items were received, and signed, indicating the order is correct and payment should be made. If the order is incorrect and does not agree with the packing slip, it should be noted on the invoice.

Statement. The vendor produces a statement giving the purchase order number, date items sent, and total cost of all items sent to the buyer. The statement should be compared to the invoice to make sure only items received have been billed. The office management should pay only after the invoice has been checked for accuracy and the statement shows the same amount. If the office has only one order from the source, the invoice sent with the order will be used for payment. Statements for a set time may include information from several orders made.

Storage Control

Guidelines for storing supplies include the following:
1. Supplies should be kept in an area that is clean, dry, and well lit. It is best to establish an area for administrative supplies and one for clinical supplies (Figure 24-9).
2. It is helpful if cabinets are labeled to indicate specific items stored inside.
3. When placing the items on the shelf, newer items should be placed in the back to help with rotation of supplies.
4. Always follow the manufacturer's instructions for storage (e.g., refrigeration, protection from light).
5. Items that have an expiration date can be marked with a highlighter to indicate they need special attention.
6. Shelves should be labeled to identify items on each shelf, which is especially helpful for new employees. An empty space indicates an item is out of stock.
7. Always be sure items have been properly handled in shipment, especially items requiring refrigeration.

PATIENT-CENTERED PROFESSIONALISM

- *What steps can be taken to make certain that medical supplies are available in the office?*

OFFICE MANAGEMENT

The medical office must be managed effectively to ensure that the staff have the equipment and supplies they need and that they are able to perform their duties. In addition, office records and documents must be stored in such a way that they can be easily retrieved when needed. Meetings and travel should be planned with careful attention to detail. Effective management will eliminate time spent correcting mistakes and save the time of the other office staff involved.

Personnel

Staffing in a medical office requires the office manager to evaluate the needs of each department. Each area is responsible for a variety of duties, and it is important for all personnel to have a good understanding of their responsibilities and those of the other team members. The office manager and the physician should foster the approach that makes employees understand that they play an important part in the quality of patient care. Understanding how your work contributes to the overall success of the practice is important.

A valued employee will develop effective working relationships with other employees so that together they can achieve the goals of the medical practice. The office team is made up of individuals with varied backgrounds and experiences, which influences perception and values. The success of the medical office is built on cooperation and team effort. The health care team must have a common purpose to work together effectively. The goals of the employee and the employer cannot be in conflict; quality patient care must be the common goal.

Office conflicts can be kept to a minimum by applying the following concepts learned about human relations:

PROCEDURE 24-3 Inventory Control: Ordering and Restocking Supplies

TASK: Create an inventory system for nondurable supplies used in the physician's office or clinic.

EQUIPMENT AND SUPPLIES
- Supply list
- File box
- Supply inventory order cards: 3 × 5 or 5 × 7 index cards or work papers
- Blank divider cards for file box
- Pen or pencil
- List of vendors

SKILLS/*RATIONALE*

1. **Procedural Step. Create a list of all disposable supplies used in the facility.**
   Separate the list into "administrative" or "clinical" supplies.
   Rationale. This establishes a "template" that can be used electronically or that can be photocopied and kept on file to be referred to at each inventory period.

2. **Procedural Step. Place a divider card (A-Z).**
   On a file card, neatly print the name of the vendor with the address, telephone number, fax number, and e-mail address. If you have a specific contact person or sales representative, list that name.
   Rationale. This provides the facility with a complete list of all vendor information.

3. **Procedural Step. File the completed vendor cards behind the appropriated A-Z divider cards.**
   Using correct filing procedures, alphabetically file by vendor name or alphabetically file by type of supplies purchased from the vendor.
   Rationale. This allows for quick access to each vendor's information for accurate and efficient ordering of supplies.

4. **Procedural Step. Create an inventory card for each disposable supply item on the supply list.**
   Print the name of one disposable item on each inventory card in the upper left-hand corner of the card. Print the name of the vendor in the lower left-hand corner of the card. Directly below the item's name, print the product identification number.
   Rationale. This establishes a record of all items used by the facility.

5. **Procedural Step. Enter the unit price.**
   The "unit price" is the smallest quantity the vendor accepts as a minimum order and the current price of the item. In pencil, print these numbers directly beneath the vendor name (e.g., $2.50 each, 100 per box, 1 box $76.29, 1 carton $158.00). Also enter the possible price breaks on given items that will save money when bought in certain quantities.
   Rationale. This indicates how the item is to be ordered. By writing this information in pencil, the medical assistant will be able to update the inventory cards as price changes occur.

6. **Procedural Step. Establish the reorder point.**
   The "reorder point" is the minimum number of items the facility should keep on hand. Typically, this is half the quantity that is ordered at a time (e.g., 12 units are ordered at a time; when the inventory reaches 6, a new order is placed). Write this number directly beneath the product identification number listed in Step 4 or on the inventory list.
   Rationale. When supplies on hand fall to or below this number, more of the item must be ordered from the vendor, according to office established reorder amounts.

7. **Procedural Step. Inventory all items on the inventory list, noting the date the inventory was taken. Check expiration dates on all supplies if available and remove from the shelf if expired.**
   Count each item the facility currently has available (see Figure 24-8).
   Rationale. Some items require an exact number (e.g., print cartridges for the computer printer), whereas other items will be counted by box (e.g., 7 boxes of small, powder-free latex gloves). Each facility will establish its own guidelines for how often supplies should be inventoried (e.g., once a week, monthly, every 2 months). Expired items cannot be used for patient care. The office should have a written protocol for the disposition of outdated items.

8. **Procedural Step. Write the current number on hand (in stock) next to the item on the supply list.**
   Example: Small, powder-free latex gloves—5 boxes.
   Rationale. This establishes a baseline for determining what needs to be ordered.

9. **Procedural Step. Compare the quantity on hand to the reorder point on the inventory control card or supply list.**
   Example: The facility has 5 boxes in the cabinet; the reorder point is 7 boxes. Small gloves need to be ordered.

Continued

PROCEDURE 24-3 Inventory Control: Ordering and Restocking Supplies—cont'd

Items that are below the minimum standards should be highlighted on the supply list.
Rationale. This provides a quick visual reference and establishes which items will need to be ordered.

10. **Procedural Step.** Locate the inventory control card for each item that is highlighted.
Rationale. This provides you with each vendor's information, as well as all item inventory cards from the same vendor in one stack.

11. **Procedural Step.** Order supplies.
Telephone, fax, or e-mail the order to each vendor. When an order has been placed, indicate the date ordered on the inventory card, amount ordered, and unit price.
Rationale. This provides the facility with an ongoing record of how much is being ordered and how often.

12. **Procedural Step.** When the order is received, indicate the date and quantity received.
When unpacking the supplies, check each item received against the packing slip. Note any back-ordered items, missing items, or price changes.
Rationale. This keeps your inventory control cards current with up-to-date prices and allows for follow-up of the back-ordered items.

13. **Procedural Step.** Refile the cards in alphabetical order by item, when the complete order has been received, and the information recorded.
Inventory control cards with back-ordered items should be flagged using a metal tab or "sticky note."
Rationale. This ensures that the card will be available for use at the next ordering period. Flagging the cards that contain back-ordered items allows for follow-up.

14. **Procedural Step.** Restock the items.
Place new items on the shelf behind the currently stocked supplies.
Rationale. Most medical supplies have an expiration date. Placing the new supplies on the shelf behind the supplies already stocked ensures that the oldest supplies will be used first, and that supplies are not being thrown away because they were pushed back on the shelf and expired before they could be used.

NOTE: It is not acceptable to be out of any item that the physician may require to treat a patient.

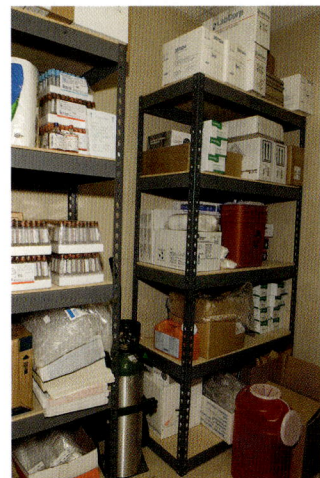

FIGURE 24-9 Example of a storage area for clinical supplies.

- A team member must be willing to accept others who have a different point of view.
- Good listening can help avoid conflicts that result from a lack of understanding.
- Cooperation with other employees is necessary to attain the goals of the practice.
- Accepting the appropriate share of job responsibility is important in maintaining a pleasant work environment for all personnel.

FOR YOUR INFORMATION

PROFESSIONALISM

Professionalism includes not only doing what is expected but also taking the time to see what needs to be done.

Insurance Records

All insurance policies related to the medical practice should be listed, logged, and filed in a fireproof cabinet. Insurance policies may include life insurance, health and accident coverage, vehicle insurance, property insurance, disability insurance, and malpractice insurance. The log should include the policy number, effective date, expiration date, and insurance company name, phone number, and contact person. Policies should be kept in a locked, fireproof cabinet or a bank safety deposit box.

Having the policies protected and accessible makes it easy to file claims if needed. Policies that protect the physician or office against liability should never be discarded, even when they expire. A lawsuit could be filed against the practice, and the policy in effect at the time of the incident is the one that would cover the costs.

Logistical Planning

At some time in any type of medical practice, a medical assistant will be asked to arrange a meeting or travel for employees.

Meetings

Whether the meeting is *external* (outside the office such as a medical association meeting) or *internal* (within the medical office such as a meeting of office employees), attention to detail is necessary. External meetings require that the vital information needed for planning the meeting (e.g., day, time, length, and location) be obtained in advance.

Planning for external and internal meetings includes the following steps:

Step 1: Once the day and time have been selected, a meeting room at the desired location should be secured. If the meeting room is not familiar, a diagram of the room is helpful. This provides room size, room arrangement, proximity to eating places, and available audiovisual aids needed for the meeting.

Step 2: An **agenda** should be prepared that sets the tone for an effective meeting. Agendas include information such as the length of the meeting, topics to be covered, their order, and the individual responsible for each topic.

Step 3: Once the agenda is set and distributed to the attendees, materials required for the meeting need to be assembled (duplicate copies, charts, paper, pencils, or audiovisual equipment).

Step 4: At least 5 days before the meeting, all participants should receive a reminder notice or telephone call. At this time questions can be answered as to availability of parking and location of other necessary facilities.

Step 5: The final responsibility is to check the meeting room, including seating arrangements, temperature control, lighting, and a person to handle last-minute problems.

Internal meetings (e.g., office staff only) are less formal and more relaxed but still need to be conducted in a professional manner. The tone of the meeting should encourage participation by all staff members. Interoffice meetings should be held regularly to improve and maintain office communication and to identify and resolve potential problems.

Minutes. The "minutes" from a meeting serve as a reminder of what occurred and allow for task follow-up. A medical assistant may be asked to record the events of a meeting. It is important that the minutes always reflect the agenda. The date, place, time, and names of those attending and absent are noted. The items discussed are written in the same order as the agenda, even if discussed out of order. The minutes should be typed and signed by the person transcribing them as soon as possible. The minutes should be kept in a notebook composition book and placed in a secure place.

Travel

Making travel arrangements for the physician or other staff members can be simplified if it is approached as assembling pieces of a puzzle. Close attention to detail and careful planning cannot eliminate problems but will minimize them. If arrangements are to be made regularly, an experienced travel agent can be helpful. The Internet has made it easy for individuals to make arrangements on their own. No matter what method is chosen, basic preliminary information must be gathered, as follows:

- The dates of travel
- Means of transportation (i.e., airplane, train)
- Hotel reservations
- Number of people traveling
- Car rental, if required

After all the arrangements have been made, an **itinerary** can be prepared. An itinerary describes the overall trip and indicates what is scheduled to happen each day. The departure point with the exact day and time, the flight and seat number, and hotel accommodations with confirmation and telephone numbers are items also included on an itinerary.

> **PATIENT-CENTERED PROFESSIONALISM**
>
> - Why must office management make the health care team understand that they play an important role in quality patient care?
> - How should insurance policies be stored?
> - What is the difference between an *agenda* and an *itinerary*?

POLICY AND PROCEDURES MANUALS

An office **policy manual** explains the day-to-day operations of the medical office and provides general information that affects all employees. Examples of the need for office policies include employee responsibilities, job descriptions, dress code, office hours, jury duty, vacation time, benefits, and "calling in sick." The policy manual provides a reference for new employees and serves as a guide to clarify expectations of experienced staff members. The expectations of all employees with regard to HIPAA regulations and the Privacy Rule must be explained in the policy manual or a separate manual. Particular attention must be paid to any contracted services (outsourcing) (e.g., insurance billing, transcription). The work performed by these agencies must be audited by office personnel as they would audit their own work, and a policy must be written describing who will be responsible for auditing **outsourced** work and the criteria to be used. Self-audits are useful since they help minimize recurrent errors in billing and/or procedures. Scheduling in-house audits can limit abuse, errors, or fraud.

A **procedures manual** contains specific instructions on how procedures are to be performed, including calibration and operation of equipment.

Manuals provide a basis for setting priorities. Box 24-5 provides information on how a policy regarding patient information could be combined with procedural information. Tasks should be identified to clarify what has immediate priority and what may be routine (to determine whether something can be postponed or must be done immediately).

Once manuals are created, time should be spent annually updating and using them as a reference. All employees are required to read both the policy manual and the procedures manual and sign and date that they have done so. If they have

> **BOX 24-5**
>
> ## Example of Policy and Procedure for HIPAA Regulation
>
> This example shows how a medical office could write a policy for disclosure of protected patient health information* and could include the procedure for carrying out this function.
>
> **POLICY**
>
> It is the policy of Sunshine Medical Practice to protect the privacy of patient health information, as mandated by HIPAA legislation. Therefore the amount of information accessible in response to a request for information is limited to the minimum amount needed to perform a specific type of work or to complete a function.
>
> **PROCEDURE**
>
> 1. Define why an individual would need patient health information.
>   a. Providing patient care
>   b. Purposes of billing for patient care
>   c. Legal issues (addressed in a separate policy and procedure)
> 2. Requests for patient information are solely limited to individuals who need the information to carry out patient care duties.
>   a. Physicians, nurse practitioners, physician's assistants, medical assistants
>   b. Ancillary personnel (e.g., pharmacy, laboratory, or radiology)
> 3. Determine the reason for which the information would be needed.
>   a. Request of patient
>   b. Purposes of treatment or billing
>   c. Laboratory or pharmacy services needing additional information to provide care
>   d. Determining health care compliance and utilization
>
> *Each medical facility will determine its own policies and procedures for release of protected patient health care information.

questions about any policy or procedure, they need to clarify them with office management at that time. As procedures change or new equipment is purchased, procedures manuals should be revised. Self-audits can also correct procedures that have become redundant or burdensome.

Development

Development of a procedures manual begins with a list of all procedures done in the medical practice. Each step listed for a procedure should be in the order that it is performed, similar to the procedures in this textbook. All instruments and supplies needed for the procedure should be listed. It is helpful for a tray setup to have a photo included with the procedure. Once a procedure is learned, it is not necessary to refer to the procedure manual unless changes occur, but new or temporary employees may find the manual useful. All employees should date and initial that they have read the manual and understand what is expected of them.

Maintenance

Maintaining and updating the manuals is important for continuity. All staff members should be involved in keeping procedures current. Updates could come from new regulations passed by the federal government, journals, and even textbooks. If a policy or procedure is revised, the date of the revision should be noted, and all employees should initial that they have reviewed the revision.

Enforcement

A written description of job expectations is important so that all employees understand their responsibilities. By having written guidelines, an employee can be held accountable for job duties.

Normally, employees are first notified verbally that they have violated set policy or procedure. This verbal notification needs to be documented in the employee's personnel file. If the *infraction* occurs again, the second warning is in written form, noting the date, time, and circumstances of the second infraction. At this time the employee should be counseled that continuation of the infraction could lead to dismissal. Documentation of the counseling session must be signed by the office manager and the employee, and then placed in the employee's personnel file.

If these documentation steps are taken, when an employee is dismissed for failure to follow policy or procedure, the employee cannot deny knowledge of a set policy or procedure being in place or claim that he or she had no previous warnings that the policy or procedure had been violated.

Marketing

Marketing tools may also be developed using elements of the office's policy and procedures manuals. Marketing tools may include brochures, web pages, press releases, or even seminars and classes for other medical professionals or the community. Any marketing tools should promote the medical office's expertise and skill and can also highlight important policies of the office. Market strategies are numerous and are used to increase the medical practice's visibility in the community.

> **PATIENT-CENTERED PROFESSIONALISM**
>
> - *If you were a new employee, how would you use the policy manual and the procedures manual?*
> - *What questions could you ask in an interview about the medical office's manuals?*

COMMUNITY RESOURCES

A medical practice frequently needs to refer a patient to an agency for assistance. For example, a patient may need counseling, support, or access to social services. Some agencies will provide assistance on a sliding scale based on income and the

ability to pay, whereas others may be free of charge. Typical referral agencies are as follows:
- Family and marriage counseling
- Behavioral counseling
- Substance abuse counseling
- Genetic counseling
- Financial and legal counseling
- Easter Seals
- March of Dimes
- Society for the Blind
- American Heart Association
- Homeless shelters
- Child abuse and domestic violence agencies
- Food banks
- Support groups by condition
- Hospice
- Assisted living facilities
- Meals on Wheels
- Medical transport

The names and telephone numbers of these agencies should be kept readily available for a patient's use. Professional organizations can provide additional information to patients about their illness; for example, a patient with hypertension might be interested in information from the American Heart Association, and a patient with nutrition or weight concerns may benefit from contact with the American Dietetic Association.

Each community typically has a network of support groups for various diseases. These groups will provide the patient with encouragement and the emotional support necessary to follow the treatment regimen and will sometimes assist with transportation. Often the local newspaper lists the various support groups available, with meeting days and times. Procedure 24-4 provides criteria for locating a community resource for a patient's specific need.

The patient trusts that you will ensure that they are treated fairly when looking for assistance. Whether you like it or not the patient sees you as their **advocate,** a trusted voice that looks out for their welfare. What issues are important to you? Is the expansion of the Family and Medical Leave Act to include paid leave an issue that is important to you? Could you become an advocate to expand affordable child care for working parents? How do you plan on promoting or supporting the issues of your patients?

PATIENT-CENTERED PROFESSIONALISM

- *Why is it important for the medical assistant to be aware of community resources available for patients?*

CONCLUSION

The organization of a medical office is the responsibility of all staff members. The reception area is important for the smooth functioning of the medical office and should be designed and maintained with the patient in mind. The office should adhere to HIPAA and ADA guidelines to protect patient confidentiality, regulate how patient information can be disclosed, and provide physical access to all patients. To create an environment that benefits patients and staff and meets the requirements, all staff must pay close attention to how they perform their duties.

The needs of the patients and the size of the practice will dictate the type and functionality of equipment needed and the amount of supplies to keep on hand. Keeping accurate inventory records for supplies and equipment assists those responsible for updating equipment and ordering supplies to maintain an efficient workflow within the office.

Office management requires that all medical office personnel understand the importance of structure in meetings, accurate travel arrangements, secure insurance records, and being actively aware of policy and procedures in the medical facility. Being part of a medical office team requires that each individual maintain a professional work ethic and attitude.

Patients may require additional assistance from community agencies. It is beneficial if the medical office has the names and phone numbers of organizations in the area to help patients make contact.

Medical offices can be efficient and can provide quality patient care only when everyone works together.

PROCEDURE 24-4 Develop and Maintain a Current List of Community Resources

TASK: Gather information from your local telephone book, library, and newspaper or search the Internet, and create a reference document (fact sheet) to identify community resources for patient use.

EQUIPMENT AND SUPPLIES
- Local phone book
- Local or regional newspaper
- Internet access
- Computer with spreadsheet and word-processing software
- Pen or pencil

SKILLS/RATIONALE

1. **Procedural Step.** Research the following resources available in your area using the local phone book, local or regional newspaper, local library, or Internet:
   - Council on Aging
   - Hospice services
   - Civic organizations
   - Social services
   - American Heart Association
   - American Red Cross
   - American Cancer Society
   - Public Health Department
   - Various support groups (e.g., cancer, diabetes, Alzheimer's disease, Alcoholics Anonymous)
   - Local agricultural service extension for dietary help

   Rationale. Becoming familiar with the available resources in your area will help you provide community resource referral information to your patients.

2. **Procedural Step.** Create a list of each resource available. Include a telephone number, address, contact person, hours of operation, and what types of services each agency provides.

   Rationale. This provides the facility with a comprehensive list of all available resources and provides a patient with choices of organizations.

3. **Procedural Step.** Key the information gathered into a document using either a word-processing or spreadsheet software program. Double-check your information for accuracy. Print a hard copy and save an electronic file on the computer or some type of external device (e.g., flash drive, jump drive).

   Rationale. By printing a hard copy, you will have a quick reference guide that can be photocopied and given to a patient. A copy can also be kept near the phone to refer to as needed when providing recommendations to patients who call the office for a referral. Saving the document allows for updating.

4. **Procedural Step.** Update the information routinely. This can be done quarterly, semi-annually, or annually. Information should also be updated whenever new information or resources are discovered.

   Rationale. This keeps your resource list current. By keeping this information on the computer, you can retrieve the document easily, correct information quickly, and provide your patients with up-to-date information.

Chapter Summary

Reinforce your understanding of the material in this chapter by reviewing the curriculum objectives and key content points below.

1. **Define, appropriately use, and spell all the Key Terms for this chapter.**
   - Review the Key Terms if necessary.
2. **Define facilities management and explain its importance to the medical office.**
   - Facilities management is the concept of maintaining the physical environment of an office.
   - Maintaining the atmosphere and physical condition of the medical office is the responsibility of the staff.
3. **Explain the impact of HIPAA legislation on the management of office facilities.**
   - The Health Insurance Portability and Accountability Act (HIPAA) provides mandates for health care providers and insurance carriers about the release of private patient information.

- Medical offices have confidentiality agreements that all staff must sign.

4. **Explain the impact of the Americans with Disabilities Act (ADA) on the physical structure of the medical office.**
   - Medical offices must be designed to provide access to all individuals, including those with disabilities.

5. **List two functions of the reception area.**
   - The reception area is where patients are greeted on arrival and checked in for services.
   - Patients wait in the reception area until their health care provider can see them.

6. **Design a plan for a medical office reception area that reflects HIPAA and ADA regulations and incorporates the seven considerations for a reception area.**
   - Light, color, furniture, plants, window treatments, and temperature should be considered when planning an effective reception area.
   - Patient confidentiality must be maintained at all times.
   - Refer to Box 24-2.
   - Age-appropriate activities and materials should be provided in the reception area to give patients something to do while they wait.
   - The reception area should be welcoming, clean, and professional.

7. **Describe the daily and weekly maintenance of the reception area.**
   - The reception area should be straightened several times each day and refreshed before opening each morning.
   - A professional cleaning staff usually does a thorough cleaning at least weekly.

8. **List six types of office equipment and explain how each is used in the medical office.**
   Medical assistants need to know how to use the following:
   - Fax machines for transmitting and receiving patient information.
   - Photocopy machines for copying patient records and insurance cards.
   - Telephone systems for patient communication.
   - Answering systems for taking messages when the office is not available to patients.
   - Office computers for patient accounts.
   - Postage meters for mailing correspondence, claims, and statements.

9. **Demonstrate the procedure for preparing, sending, and receiving a fax.**
   - Refer to Procedure 24-1.

10. **Explain why inventory records are kept.**
    - Inventory records are used in maintaining an adequate supply for use in the office, for depreciation purposes, and in case of fire or theft.
    - Inventory records are also useful when purchasing updated equipment.

11. **Assess the advantages and disadvantages of leasing versus buying office equipment.**
    - Leasing is essentially "renting" equipment for the office; it is not owned.
    - Leasing may be more convenient for maintaining and updating equipment.
    - Buying equipment conveys ownership.
    - Buying equipment may be more costly to cash flow.
    - The best method for each medical office depends on the type and needs of the practice.

12. **Demonstrate the correct procedure for maintaining office equipment.**
    - Review Procedure 24-2.
    - Equipment that is properly maintained can be used for its lifetime with fewer problems.
    - Service or maintenance agreements can be purchased to help maintain equipment.
    - Warranties protect the buyer against defective items for a period of time after purchase.

13. **Differentiate between capital and noncapital goods.**
    - Capital (durable) goods are expected to be permanent or to last a long time.
    - Noncapital goods are reusable but not as expensive as capital goods, with a shorter life span than capital goods.

14. **List three factors to be considered when establishing an inventory control system.**
    - Reorder point, order quantity, and lead time must be considered when establishing an inventory control system.

15. **Demonstrate the correct procedure for creating and maintaining an inventory and ordering system.**
    - Refer to Procedure 24-3.

16. **Explain the importance of teamwork in the medical office.**
    - The entire office staff must share the common goal of providing quality care to patients.

17. **Describe the five steps in planning for a meeting.**
    - Secure a meeting room for the correct time and date.
    - Prepare and distribute an agenda to meeting participants.
    - Assemble materials needed for the meeting.
    - Reminder phone call or e-mail notice should be sent 5 days before the meeting.
    - Check the meeting room; assign a detail person for last-minute problems.
    - Meetings may be *internal* (inside the office) or *external* (out of the office).
    - Meeting minutes need to be typed as soon as the meeting is over and filed in a secure location.

18. **Differentiate between an agenda and an itinerary.**
    - An agenda includes information about the length of the meeting, topics to be covered, their order, and the individual(s) responsible for each topic.
    - An itinerary describes an overall trip and what will happen each day. It includes the departure point, flight and hotel information, and ground transportation.

19. **Explain the purpose of policy manuals and procedures manuals.**
    - A policy manual explains the day-to-day operations of the medical office and provides general information that affects all employees.
    - A procedures manual contains specific instruction on how procedures are to be performed.

20. **Explain why it is important for medical assistants to be aware of the community resources available in their area.**

- Patients may need assistance from community agencies for health maintenance.
- Information from organizations about their illness may benefit patients.

21. **Demonstrate the correct procedure for gathering community resources.**
    - Review Procedure 24-4.
22. **Analyze a realistic medical office situation and apply your understanding of the medical office to determine the best course of action.**
    - The medical assistant must protect patient confidentiality at all times.
    - A thorough understanding of the reasons behind the guidelines for effective front office functioning is necessary.
23. **Describe the impact on patient care when medical assistants have a solid understanding of all aspects of a well-planned and well-maintained medical office.**
    - A good impression of the practice is formed when the medical office is planned, maintained, and running smoothly.

PRACTICAL APPLICATIONS

If you have accomplished the objectives in this chapter, you will be able to make better choices as a medical assistant. Take another look at this situation and decide what you would do.

Janine is a new member of the office staff. She has not had any training in the medical assisting field, but she has been working as a receptionist in a loan office. On her first day at work, Janine is assigned to work at the front desk with the receptionist. As the patients for the day come in, she asks many personal questions about each patient and then proceeds to tell the receptionist what she knows about each patient. When told to be sure the names of the patients have been obliterated from the sign-in sheet, she uses a yellow highlighter. As she answers the phone, everyone in the office can hear her conversations. Janine immediately rearranges the large plants in the reception area, and now a plant is partially blocking the doorway.

A fax from a surgeon arrives for Dr. Lopez, and Janine places it on the front counter next to the sign-in sheet until she has a chance to give it to Dr. Lopez. When asked to move the fax, Janine replies that it would "definitely be easier" if the fax was just placed next to the front window rather than in the back room so she would not have to walk so far. Also, Janine does not understand why the office needs a dedicated line for the fax machine. Why not just have the fax line connected to the multiline telephone at the front desk?

Janine was asked to leave a week later after she refused to maintain the equipment. As the office personnel looked for the manuals for the new equipment that had been purchased, no manuals could be found; when she was contacted, Janine admitted to discarding them.

What would you tell Janine about why she was asked to leave her job at the medical office?

1. In many ways, Janine has broken confidentiality in the medical office as required by HIPAA. Name three ways in which she has done this.
2. What is HIPAA, and how does it affect patient care?
3. Why is a multiline phone system important in a medical office?
4. What special features should be considered when deciding on a phone system for the medical office?
5. How is the ADA important in the medical office? What are three of the design features that are important for patient safety?
6. How did Janine make Dr. Lopez's office dangerous for a person with a physical disability?
7. Why is it important to keep manuals that are sent with new equipment?
8. Would you want Janine to be a fellow employee in a medical office with you? Defend your answer.

WEB SEARCH

1. **Research the topic of risk management to better understand the medical assistant's responsibility in preventing accidents in the work environment.** Risk management should be approached from a proactive standpoint. To prevent accidents, careful planning, identification, analysis, management, and tracking are necessary. Every employee must take ownership in minimizing the patients' exposure to risk.
    - **Keywords:** Use the following keywords in your search: risk management, risk concepts, accident prevention.

25 Computers in the Medical Office

evolve http://evolve.elsevier.com/klieger/medicalassisting

Mention technology and most people think of computers. Every facet of our lives has some computerized component (e.g., appliances, televisions, and cars), and the medical office is no different. A computer in a medical office allows the medical assistant to prepare documents (e.g., letters, memos), schedule patient appointments, process patient's insurance claims, post charges and payments to the patient's accounts, send e-mails, and browse the internet.

As a medical assistant, you may become the primary operator of a computer system in your medical office. In many medical offices, computers are now being used for practice management and management of patient accounts. Computers are designed to help you do your job more efficiently. Understanding the computer equipment and different types of software used is an important part of your duties. Computers are becoming more prevalent in medical offices today, and this trend will continue.

Computer skills will give you an edge when looking for employment, and these skills will make you a valuable resource in the medical office. The first step in obtaining these skills is to understand the functions, components, and use of computers, as well as the tasks that can be done more efficiently by using practice management software in the medical office.

LEARNING OBJECTIVES

You will be able to do the following after completing this chapter:

Key Terms
1. Define, appropriately use, and spell all the Key Terms for this chapter.

Functions of the Computer
2. List four main functions of a computer system.
3. List four uses of a computer system in the medical practice.

Components of the Computer
4. List the eight main components of a computer system.

Basics of Computer Use
5. Define "network" and list three types of networks.
6. Explain the importance of maintaining network security and list three safeguards for medical office computer use.
7. Demonstrate how to access a website on the Internet.
8. Differentiate between a "directory" and a "search engine" and explain the advantages and disadvantages of each.
9. List five ways a word-processing document can be changed.
10. List three ways a spreadsheet can be used in the medical practice.
11. Explain the purpose of a database.

Computer Systems in Medical Practice Management
12. List three things to check before installing practice management software onto the office computer system.
13. List four important office tasks that can be completed with practice management software.
14. Explain the importance of backing up medical office data regularly.

Patient-Centered Professionalism
15. Analyze a realistic medical office situation and apply your understanding of computers in the medical office to determine the best course of action.
16. Describe the impact on patient care when medical assistants understand the essentials of computers and their use in the medical practice.

Computers in the Medical Office **CHAPTER 25** 461

KEY TERMS

- backed up
- bit
- booted up
- browser
- byte
- CD-ROM
- central processing unit (CPU)
- cold boot
- cursor
- database management
- default
- encounter form
- flash drive
- floppy disk
- font
- guarantor
- hard drive
- hardware
- host
- initialized
- ink-jet printer
- interface
- Internet service provider (ISP)
- keyboard
- laser printer
- menus
- microprocessor
- modem
- monitor
- motherboard
- mouse
- network
- optical character recognition (OCR)
- password
- patient
- PDA
- peripherals
- point
- practice management
- printer
- prompt
- random-access memory (RAM)
- read-only memory (ROM)
- scanner
- search engine
- software
- sound card
- spreadsheet
- tape backup
- toggle key
- touch screen
- trackball
- tutorial
- URL
- user ID
- warm boot
- wizards
- word processing
- zip drive

PRACTICAL APPLICATIONS

Read the following scenario and keep it in mind as you learn about the use of computers in the medical office.

Dr. Santos has just hired Terrell, a medical assistant, to transfer demographic and insurance data from the current paper records to the computerized patient accounting system. Terrell's assignment is to ensure that all the information on current patients is up-to-date in the computer and that the latest updates and additions to the computer program are installed. As each new patient arrives at the office, Terrell has the duty of obtaining information for the data entry. He then must be sure that the appointment has been scheduled into the computer so that medical notes and insurance information will be available as needed. Kate, an established patient, comes to the office and sees the new computer system in operation. Terrell explains that the office is becoming more technologically advanced and that the computer will be used to schedule appointments, store transcription, and manage patient accounts in the future.

Would you be prepared to use the computer to perform data entry, scheduling, and other medical office tasks?

FUNCTIONS OF THE COMPUTER

A computer is an electronic device that converts data into information. Since a computer does not communicate through spoken or written words, it uses a series of *0s* and *1s* to describe data to represent information. A **bit** is the smallest unit of data and is an abbreviation for binary digit. A **byte** is a string of bits used to represent a character, digit, or symbol. It is usually 8 bits. Computers function to take in (input), process, generate (output), and store information, as follows:

1. *Input.* Any information that is entered into the computer is done by using an input device (add-on component; e.g., mouse, keyboard, microphone, scanner).
2. *Processing.* The computer takes the data entered and performs a variety of tasks according to the software program being used.
3. *Output.* When data leave the computer through the monitor, speakers, printer, modem, and so on, information is provided to the user.
4. *Storage.* Computers have the capacity to store data on the hard drive, compact disks (CDs), disks (i.e., floppy disks, zip drives), and other devices and media for future use.

In the medical practice, computers handle both administrative and clinical tasks, as follows:

- In an administrative function, computers aid in patient billing, appointment scheduling, maintaining patient accounts, processing insurance claims, and database management (Figure 25-1).
- In the hospital clinical setting, a patient's entire medical record can be stored and accessed by computer. Some physician offices generate and store a patient's medical transcription in the computer, as well as laboratory reports and reports for ancillary services. Typically, **practice management** software can generate in-house reports of a patient's entire clinical history, including dates of services, diagnoses, procedures, and the name of the attending physician for each visit.

The technical advances of the computer affect everyone who works in health care. The type of computer chosen

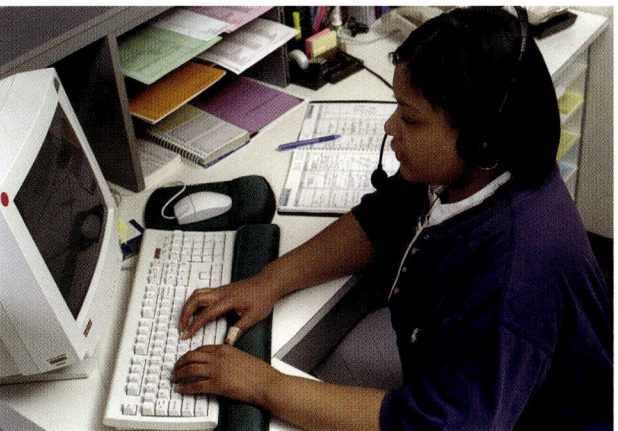

FIGURE 25-1 A medical assistant uses the computer to enter patient information.

depends on the needs of the facility or the practice. Many computers are used in hospitals because a hospital requires that large amounts of data be processed very rapidly and that all departments be wired (connected) so they can access the data they need. In a small medical practice, only one computer may be sufficient to handle the needs of the practice. Laptops are gaining popularity over bulky desktop models.

> ### PATIENT-CENTERED PROFESSIONALISM
>
> - How would the medical assistant make effective use of the computer in a medical office setting?

COMPONENTS OF THE COMPUTER

A *component* is a part. The computer has several types of parts, or components. **Hardware** is the mechanical devices and physical components of a computer system such as the CPU, hard drive, other internal disk drives, and memory (internal hardware). Hardware can also be outside of the computer; this type of hardware is called a "peripheral." **Peripherals** are electronic devices that can be attached to the computer, other than the standard input-output devices such as the monitor, keyboard, and mouse. These external components include speakers, microphones, printers, digital cameras, and modems. These devices often require special software packages called *drivers*. These are usually included at the time of purchase with the software package and other devices (external storage media, scanners, speakers, and microphones). Figure 25-2 shows some of the various components of a computer system.

Hardware is the basic computer equipment, and **software** (computer program) is the "intelligence" of a computer. The software program installed tells the computer what to do or how to interact with the user and how to process the user's data. A computer without software is like a CD player without a CD. Without software, the user can only turn the computer on and off.

The following sections describe eight basic hardware parts in a computer system.

Central Processing Unit

The **central processing unit (CPU)** is responsible for interpreting and executing software instructions. Within the framework of the CPU is the **microprocessor** (CPU chip found on the main board) that controls and coordinates many functions of the computer (e.g., speed of processing). The CPU is the "brain" of the computer and is responsible for basic processing operations. The CPU retrieves instructions and data from RAM (electronic circuit that holds data and programs), processes those instructions, and then places the results back into RAM so they can be displayed or stored. The CPU contains memory to process mathematical

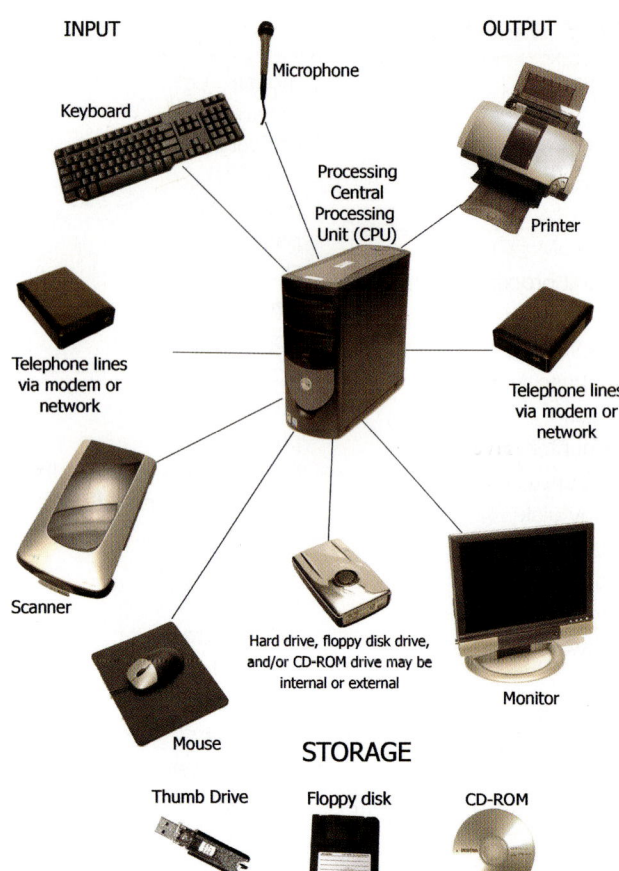

FIGURE 25-2 Components of a computer system.

calculations and compare data and runs the software programs by processing the data. Software programs are loaded into RAM when the processor needs to run them. When trying to remember the multiple functions of the CPU use the acronym CALM.
- **C** for control
- **A** for arithmetic
- **L** for logic
- **M** for memory

Several specific types of memory in a computer are connected directly to the CPU.

Random-Access Memory

Random-access memory (RAM) is the read and write memory that the CPU can use for temporary storage when the computer is working. The more RAM a computer has, the more programs it can handle.

Read-Only Memory

Read-only memory (ROM) is a permanent type of memory that contains instructions to the CPU on how to set itself up when the system is initially turned on, or **booted up.** The ROM contains information about the general configuration of the machine that does not change. A **cold boot** occurs when the power is first supplied to the computer. A **warm boot** occurs when the system has been active, then "freezes up," and the operator must restart the computer. This can be done by pressing the "reset" button on the computer or with a combination of keystrokes (e.g., Ctrl, Alt, and Delete).

Storage Devices

A storage device, such as the hard drive and floppy disk or CD-ROM, allows for additional data storage and provides a means for the CPU to process more data. Storage capacity is measured in *megabytes* (MB) or *gigabytes* (GB) with 1000 MB equaling 1 GB.

Hard Drive

The **hard drive** is the main device a computer uses to store programs information and data for the long term. The hard drive is a fixed rigid disk housed inside the CPU that contains the operating system. It holds more data than a floppy and is more expensive. **Backing up** the hard drive means copying data from the hard drive to another form of storage device.

Floppy Disks Versus Flash Drives

Floppy disks are secondary storage devices that store information for or from your computer (see Figure 25-2). The original floppy disk was 5¼ inches square and was very flimsy and "floppy." Currently a floppy disk, or *diskette,* is about 3½ inches square and is enclosed in a hard plastic shell. When diskettes are used for auxiliary storage, they must be formatted (**initialized**) to hold data. Many new computers do not have floppy drives; the drives must be purchased separately.

Flash drives (memory sticks, jump drives, travel drives, USB drives, or thumb drives) are replacing floppy disks as an easy method for transferring data between systems. They plug into the *USB* (Universal Serial Bus) *port* on a computer. These storage devices come in a variety of memory sizes (e.g., 64 MB to 16 GB) and are small enough to fit on a key chain.

CD-ROMs

A **CD-ROM** holds more data than a floppy disk or flash drive but not as much as a hard drive (see Figure 25-2). CD-ROMs, DVDs, and recordable CDs have become the primary distribution medium for software. Most disks are "read only," which means the computer can retrieve information from the disk but cannot place information on it. Developments in technology improved disks to allow writing and rewriting data. CD-Rs can be recorded on, and CD-RWs (rewritable) can be recorded on, erased, and reused many times.

External Storage Devices

External storage devices, such as **zip drives** or **tape backups,** have high storage capacity (e.g., 600 GB). Hospitals and large practices generate and store huge volumes of data, some of which would be impossible to replace should a computer catastrophe occur. For this reason, practice managers are diligent about safeguarding their data by having backups done on a daily basis. Many practice management systems offer the possibility of backing up data "offsite," with storage there as well.

Motherboard

The **motherboard** is the main circuit board that contains memory chips (programmed by people), power supply, and vital components for processing. Components, such as a CD-ROM drive, hard drive, video, and **sound cards** (internal components for multimedia functions such as sound and animation), are connected to the motherboard. If this important part of the system breaks, the system is said to have "crashed." The motherboard allows processing and storage to interact with each other.

Mouse

The **mouse** is a pointing device that can either be connected to the computer or be independent (wireless). Some computers use a **trackball,** or *touch pad,* that performs the same function as a mouse. The mouse functions to move a **cursor** (pointer) around the screen and allows the user to click on document parts, website links, and so on. The arrow keys also help to move the cursor around.

Keyboard

A **keyboard** is used to input data (by typing) and has various command keys on the keyboard that direct the computer to perform a variety of different functions, such as Home; Delete; Page Up; and up, down, and side arrows (Box 25-1.) The standard keyboard has the same alphabetical arrangement as a typewriter, with the addition of 12 function keys (F1 through F12) that can accomplish preset keystroking shortcuts. Box 25-2 lists common special function keys. Several of these special keys are considered to be **toggle keys.** These keys allow the user to switch from one mode of operation to another. For example, pressing the insert key allows the user to switch between the insert function and the typeover mode; the same is true with the Caps Lock key, which allows the user to move from lower case to upper case letters.

BOX 25-1

Special Function Keys

- **Function keys (F1-F12):** Initiate commands or complete tasks in application programs
- **Alt, Ctrl, and Shift:** Used with function keys; extend number of possible functions; provide keyboard shortcuts to some commands
- **Esc:** Backs out of a program or menu
- **Print screen:** Used alone or with Alt key to place the screen onto the clipboard
- **Arrow keys:** Moves the cursor around on the screen in the direction of that key's arrow.
- **Page Up/Down, Home, and End:** Moves from one place to another quickly in a document or screen.

BOX 25-2

Common Special Keys

- **Alphanumeric keys:** Used for data entry; resemble a typewriter keyboard layout.
- **Caps Lock:** Used to switch between uppercase and lower case letters.
- **Backspace:** Used to delete characters to the left of the cursor.
- **Delete (Del):** Used to delete characters to the right of the cursor or removes the character that the cursor is on.
- **Enter:** Used at the end of a paragraph or to enter commands.
- **Insert:** Used to move between typeover and insert mode.
- **Shift:** Used to produce uppercase letters or symbols.
- **Tab:** Used to move the cursor for defined intervals, usually five spaces.

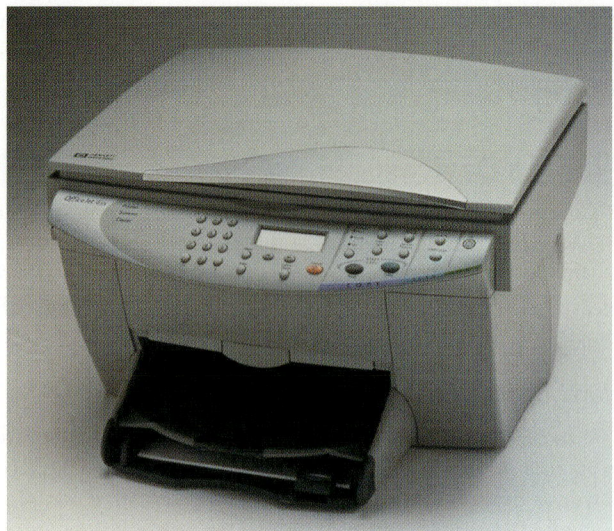

FIGURE 25-3 Laser printer.

Monitor

A **monitor** is similar to a television screen and provides instant visual feedback. It displays what has been entered into the computer; therefore it is an output device. When a patient asks about his or her account balance, the patient's name is entered and the CPU retrieves the data and displays the information on the screen. Monitors are rated by size and number of dots, or *pixels*. The smaller and more numerous the dots, the finer and more detailed are the images on the screen. When data is seen on the screen, it is referred to as a soft copy.

Printers

Printers are output devices that reproduce information onto paper. A printed copy is referred to as a *hard copy*. The type of printer required depends on the user's need for speed, print quality, and type of paper used. The most popular types of printers for medical offices tend to be ink-jet and laser printers. "Dot matrix" printers were used frequently in the past and may still be used in some offices to process insurance claim forms.

- **Ink-jet printers** are quieter than dot matrix printers. Ink-jet printers form characters on the paper by imprinting ink in the shape of letters. This type of printer can print text, color, and graphics.
- **Laser printers** produce high-quality copies at high speeds (Figure 25-3). Some laser printers can print color, and almost all laser printers can print graphics and text.

Modems

Modems allow computers to communicate with each other and with the Internet over phone lines, digital subscriber lines (DSL), or cable networks. These devices can be located within the computer or they can be a separate item. Modems have the capacity to transmit faxes and e-mail. All offices should have a dedicated line for the modem.

Other Auxiliary Input Devices

Optical Character Recognition

The **optical character recognition** (**OCR**) computer system scans and reads typewritten characters. The checkout at the grocery store uses this type of system. Third-party payers often use OCR to "read" CMS-1500 claim forms during processing.

Touch Screen

With a **touch screen,** a light pen or human touch is used to point to words, diagrams, or symbols. Many clinical settings are converting to the touch screen form of charting that is already being used in hospitals.

Scanner

A **scanner** uses a light source similar to a photocopier to copy a picture or document placed on its bed (glass plate) and sends it through the modem or cable to a computer. The item scanned into data format is a reproduction of the original and can be viewed on the monitor, saved, printed, or used in other ways.

PDA

The **PDA** (personal digital assistant) is increasing in popularity. Initially designed as a personal organizer, it has evolved over the years to be much more. PDAs are small portable computers, or microcomputers, that are less powerful than PCs. There are two basic types of handheld devices that fit into the palm of the hand. One type has a miniature keyboard and touch screen and the other uses a *stylus* (point device shaped like a pen) to touch the screen and write in data by hand. PDAs are designed to complement PCs. A physician can use a PDA to access a patient's chart, pharmacy and medical information, financial data, and medical references.

> **PATIENT-CENTERED PROFESSIONALISM**
>
> - Why is it important for the medical assistant to understand the basic components of a computer system?

BASICS OF COMPUTER USE

To use a computer effectively a person must tell the computer what tasks to perform, but the information provided by the computer must be interpreted correctly. Sometimes the information comes from the user. A **prompt** message may ask the user to enter some type of data (e.g., "Enter patient name"). A sequence of prompts is used to develop an **interface** (connection) between the user and the computer. Many software packages use **wizards,** a sequence of screens that directs users through multiple steps to help them to add hardware or software.

Menus were developed to allow the novice to be able to use various options without having to remember specific commands. For example, when a menu tab is clicked (e.g., File), the menu appears on the screen, or "drops down," and gives a list of options. When using a program, the Help button on the menu bar is available to instruct the user in various functions. A **tutorial,** on the other hand, is a step-by-step guide that self-teaches generic skills needed to use software.

When first learning to use a computer, many people find that "trial and error" is a good way to learn. Practice helps improve your skill with the mouse, as well as helping you understand how to use the various functions available. This section provides an overview of some essentials of computer use, including networks and security, Internet use, word processing, spreadsheet use, and database management.

Networks and Security

When computers are interconnected to exchange information, this is referred to as a **network.** There are three basic types of networks, as follows:

- *Local area network (LAN):* A group of computers and other devices that are connected within the same building.
- *Wide area network (WAN):* A group of computers connected between buildings, cities, and even countries.
- *Intranet:* An organization's internal network, using either LAN or WAN. An intranet is not accessible to the public or those outside the organization. Typical information accessible within the intranet is the policy and procedures manuals, office forms, hospital information, and internet links to various medical sites.

To gain access, networks require a **user ID** (combination of letters and numbers that serves to identify the user) and a **password** (a special set of characters known only to the user and the person who assigned the password) to protect and secure data. This limits those who have access to specific data.

In a medical setting, Health Insurance Portability and Accountability Act (HIPAA) regulations require strict adherence to maintaining the confidentiality of the patient's medical record. In its regulation, HIPAA provides a minimum standard by using a format that is global for anyone sending or receiving electronic information over computer lines via a modem. Each medical software program manufactured follows this HIPAA format. The HIPAA regulations regarding privacy of medical information were enacted to make certain that the privacy of patient information is secure (Box 25-3).

In addition to HIPAA regulations, three other safeguards for protecting patient privacy with regard to computers are as follows:

1. Point the computer screen away from the public.
2. Use *screen savers* to cover information if the computer is not used in a set period.
3. Place printers and fax machines in a secure area away from the general public.

Internet Use

The largest WAN that exists is the Internet, a global network that connects computers together. The Internet is the largest electronic library. Physicians often retrieve articles from medical databases to keep current with medical advancements in their field of practice (Figure 25-4). Each computer connected to the Internet is a **host** and is independent of the others. An **internet service provider** (**ISP**) is a company that provides a host access to the Internet (e.g., Earthlink, America Online). Each user is given an address specific to his or her computer.

Messages are transmitted over the Internet when a **URL** (address) is entered into the **browser.** Common browser programs include Netscape Navigator and Microsoft Internet Explorer. For example, when the URL http://www.cdc.gov is entered, the home page for the Centers for Disease Control and Prevention (CDC) appears. An explanation of each part of the address follows:

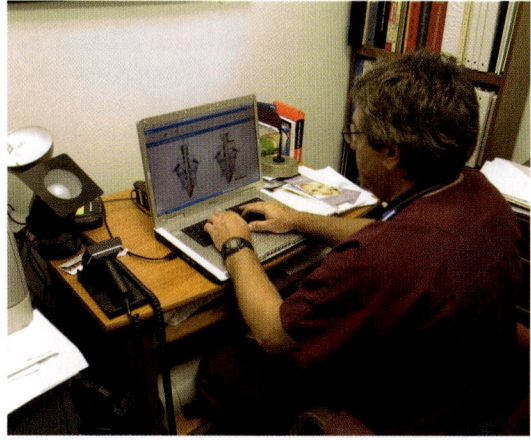

FIGURE 25-4 A physician can use the internet to research up-to-date information.

BOX 25-3

Computer and Network Security

As more patient information is stored on computers, shared on computer networks that can often be accessed from a physician's home, and sent electronically to third-party payers, security and privacy have become national priorities. Several legal and regulatory measures can impact health care organizations and the way they maintain security of electronically recorded and stored patient information.

These measures include federal regulations, as well as guidelines from professional organizations and accrediting agencies such as the Joint Commission (JCAHO). The most comprehensive regulation is provided by the Health Insurance Portability and Accountability Act (HIPAA) of 1996, which protects patient privacy by requiring the creation of uniform standards for electronic transmission of health information. The process of developing and adopting standards has progressed more slowly than expected. Standards have been developed in several areas. Once they are formally adopted, organizations have 24 months to demonstrate compliance. Five standards have been adopted, as follows:

1. Electronic transmission of financial (claims-processing) information
2. Use of standard code sets
3. Use of national provider identifiers (NPIs)
4. Use of employer identification numbers (EINs)
5. Confidentiality and security protection measures to establish and enforce security within an organization, measures to maintain security of the physical parts of a computer system where data is stored, measures to control access to data, and measures to protect information and restrict access to electronically transmitted data

Health care providers must become aware of these standards and must ensure that their facilities conform to them.

In addition, within a medical office, each individual who uses the computer should have a unique *password,* which should be changed on a regular basis. The password is a set of alphanumerical characters that allows the user to *log on* (enter) the system or specific parts of the computer system. Individuals should not share their passwords with others.

Each individual should have access to only the types of information and applications that fall within his or her scope of work and responsibility. System security should be designed in such a way that each security level permits access to only the applications and databases each individual needs to perform his or her tasks. Each specific application should know which individuals are authorized to use it.

If a practice uses a service bureau to prepare documents, all documents, in paper or electronic form, should be returned to the practice at the end of the contractual period.

Modified from Hunt SA: *Saunders fundamentals of medical assisting*—revised reprint, St Louis, 2007, Saunders.

BOX 25-4

Common Internet Domains

.com	Commercial site; operated by VeriSign Global Registry Services.
.net	Network site; operated by VeriSign Global Registry Services.
.gov	Government site; reserved exclusively for the U.S. government; operated by the U.S. General Services Administration.
.edu	Educational site; reserved for postsecondary institutions accredited by an agency on the U.S. Department of Education's list of Nationally Recognized Accrediting Agencies; registered only through EDUCAUSE.
.org	Noncommercial site; .org is *intended* to serve the noncommercial community, but all are eligible to register; operated by Public Interest Registry.
.mil	Military site; reserved exclusively for the U.S. military; operated by the U.S. Department of Defense Network Information Center.

- *cdc.gov*—The *domain name* that indicates the name of the system or location of the computer: "cdc" is the name, and ".gov" is the domain in which the name is registered. Common domains are listed in Box 25-4.

Browsers and websites contain **search engines** that allow a user to enter a topic, word, or group of words into a text box. When this is done, the search engine will search the Internet for matches. A list of matches will appear, and the user can click on each listing to reference the information provided. Common search engines are Google.com, Dogpile.com, and Webcrawler.com. There are even search engines specifically for medical and health-related searches (e.g., Mayo Clinic, MedAlert).

Box 25-5 provides more information about effectively conducting a search on the Internet.

FOR YOUR INFORMATION

PRIMARY METHOD OF INTERNET ACCESS IN 2006
- **Dial-up:** 8.7%
- **Cable:** 50%
- **DSL:** 39.7%
- **Satellite Internet:** 1.6%

Word Processing

Medical offices use computers to produce written correspondence, reports, forms, and other documents. **Word processing** is a system of entering and editing text that requires interaction between a person and a computer. Word processing improves business communications by using automated equipment to produce letters, memos, and reports.

- *http (hypertext transfer protocol)*—the protocol is the way computers exchange information on the Internet.
- *www (World Wide Web)*—A graphical interface for the Internet made up of Internet servers that provide access to documents, which in turn lead to other documents.

BOX 25-5

Effective Research on the Internet

The Internet is a valuable tool for locating information if you understand how to use it effectively. Two key methods of researching the Internet involve using directories and search engines.

USING DIRECTORIES (BROWSING)
A *directory* is a group of categories (subjects). Using a directory, you can select a topic of interest by clicking on it. Selecting a broad category will take you to a listing of subcategories. Selecting a subcategory will take you to a list of topics in that subcategory. You can keep narrowing down until you have pinpointed the topic you want to research. As you narrow down, the topics become more and more specific to your interest.

Advantages
- Directories are created and maintained by a person, business, or organization in an attempt to provide quality sites that will be most useful and to "weed out" the unhelpful sites.
- If you do not fully understand the organization of your topic, general directories are a good place to start.

Disadvantages
- Directories contain fewer sites than search engine searches because they have been organized manually and attempt to provide only quality sites. However, some quality sites may have been missed and may not be included.
- The directory is only as good as the person, business, or organization that established and maintains it.

USING SEARCH ENGINES (KEYWORD SEARCHING)
A search engine allows the user to "key in" a word or phrase of interest. The search engine looks for matches to these words in all the websites in its database. The search results are prioritized (usually by which words are closest to what the user entered in order and form) and displayed as a list of "hits." Many people do not realize, however, that search engines do not cover all websites on the Internet. Therefore it is a good idea to always use several different search engines. Different search engines produce different results, and something not found on one search engine may be found on another. Some search engines have "advanced" options that allow you to enter more specific criteria for the search. Also, if you are unable to find what you are looking for in the first 20 to 30 hits, vary your keywords and search again.

Advantages
- Search engines are very helpful when looking for specific terminology, topics, or information.
- Search engines are also helpful when looking for specific websites or information on organizations or institutions.
- Other online sources (e.g., newspapers, journals, other web-based publications) can often be found easily using search engines.

Disadvantages
- Search engines allow you to enter keywords, not provide context. For example, entering "cold" would produce more results than necessary. Entering "cold medicine" or "common cold," however, would narrow the search by providing context.
- Search engines often produce many results. The user should not assume that the first result is the best; several searches may have to be performed using different keywords and different search engines.

EVALUATING THE INFORMATION
Directories and search engines are great places to start your research. However, your research is not complete until you have verified the credibility of the sources of information. Anyone can publish information on the Internet, and some people or groups may be motivated to publish information that is not true or that is distorted.

Ask yourself the following questions about the websites you use for research:
1. Who created the website? Is it part of a library, university, or government website? Was it created by an individual who wants to express his or her opinions or sell something? Why is this information being provided?
2. Could the information be biased?
3. Are sources of data and information given? (Does the website specify where it received its information?) If so, are these sources unbiased and credible?
4. Can the information presented on the site be found on other websites about this topic? Is the information comparable? Always check to be certain you are using credible sources.

Word processing software programs allow the user to merge individual paragraphs into one paragraph; insert an address, date, and salutation; and many other document preparation functions. When a person begins keying in the text of a document, typing errors are a minor concern. After completion the software allows the user the flexibility to improve the quality of the document by using the spell-check program, change the **font** and **point** (character style and size), and change the format (e.g., double or single spacing). Remember, however, that these useful features do not eliminate the need for careful review of the document. Another advantage of word processing is the capability of reusing documents. An example of reusing a document is the resume. It can be retrieved, updated periodically, printed, and stored until needed again.

Spreadsheets

Spreadsheet software aids in manipulating numerical data for financial management, as in setting up a budget. A grid of rows and columns is displayed on the screen. Numbers can be entered and a mathematical formula assigned. The computer automatically calculates the result. The advantage is medical practices can set up their own formulas or use the built-in formula functions. Spreadsheets can be used for many purposes in the medical office, especially financial applications and reports (e.g., accounts payable, profit and loss, payroll, budget management).

Database Management

Software for **database management** helps the user work with facts and figures comparable to those kept on file cards or in a Rolodex. The program stores, organizes, and locates the files when needed to review or update. If a patient moves, the software searches for his or her record from the database file and changes it according to the input entered. Patient records can be located easily and stored with little effort using a database. A medical office computer database also stores information about providers, insurance carriers, procedural and diagnostic codes, charges, and payment information. This information provides a link between related pieces of information and helps to process paperwork (e.g., insurance forms).

PATIENT-CENTERED PROFESSIONALISM

- Why must the medical assistant follow established security measures concerning the use of computers?

COMPUTER SYSTEMS IN MEDICAL PRACTICE MANAGEMENT

Many software packages are available for the medical practice. Medical software is not limited to administrative functions. For example, some software programs insert laboratory reports directly to the patient's electronic medical record (EMR). Software has been developed to allow the physician to write prescriptions, thus minimizing medical errors by alerting the physician if the drug prescribed interacts with other medications and eliminating errors from poor handwriting. Mastering the tasks in any program takes practice and patience. The key to understanding the workings of a program is to begin by reviewing the operating manual, which discusses special features, prompts, menu selection, and keys that assist the user in navigating through the software. New users will have to be familiar with the latest version of *Windows* (or the current operating system being used on the computer system) and have a basic understanding of keyboarding and medical practice management. Experienced users can focus on the operating functions of the program. Understanding these features will help the user be more productive. Some software companies will provide inhouse, onsite training for all staff members.

Choosing a Software Program

With so many types of practice management software on the market today, choosing a new computer system for the medical practice can be a daunting task. If this becomes your responsibility, first organize the facts, then proceed as follows:

1. Obtain input from the physicians and staff as to which functions and capabilities are needed by the system to handle office functions.
2. Determine the office budget; what is the practice willing to spend for the system?
3. Inquire among other practices what type of system they are using. Are they satisfied with it? Does it still fit their needs? Would they purchase it again? Why or why not?
4. If possible, visit other offices to see their systems in use. Ask the staff how complicated the system is to use. Ask what features they like and which ones they dislike.
5. Ask for competitive bids from any company whose product interests you.
6. Determine what type of training they offer: inhouse, at their site, or one-on-one?
7. Ask what other features are included in the contract: periodic updates (e.g., CPT and ICD-9-CM codes every year), service maintenance, and training.
8. Ask if the medical practice can lease or must buy the program. Can the practice lease with an option to buy?

After assembling the facts, discuss the options with the physicians and make a decision. Remember to save all the paperwork used in making the choice.

Program Installation and Setup

Before practice management software can be installed, certain *software requirements* must be met. The software usually is on a CD and accompanied by installation instructions. The installer must be certain the following features are available:

- Windows-compatible computer (if this is the operating system the software requires; most of these programs are Windows compatible)
- Minimum amount of RAM needed for the software
- Enough hard-drive space
- Updated operating system (e.g., Microsoft Windows, Mac OS, OS/2)

After the program is installed, the basic sequence of setup might proceed as follows:

1. Enter practice information (e.g., address, tax ID number, and practice type).
2. Enter provider information. This information, besides demographic information, must include the physician's license information, Social Security and DEA numbers,

and the option box to indicate that the provider's signature is on file. This is used on the CMS-1500 insurance form, Box 31.
3. Enter insurance company data to include demographics and type (e.g., Blue Cross).
4. Enter patient data to include demographics, birth date, gender, Social Security number, and insurance information, including a guarantor. A **patient** is the person who receives medical treatment; a **guarantor** is the person who guarantees to pay for the treatment.
5. Enter the procedural codes (CPT) and diagnostic codes (ICD) most frequently used by the practice, and renew and update yearly. Optional information to add is code description and standard fee.
6. Enter billing information. This portion is the medical practice's greatest asset. This function manages transactions, general billing forms, and statements.
7. Enter other features if available such as electronic claim processing, collection letters, and managed care referral generation.

This list provides basic information, but vendors often have a tutorial for their programs or they may provide on-the-job training.

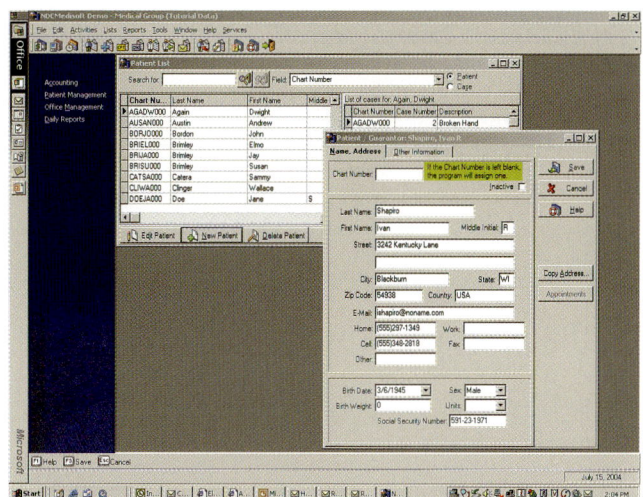

FIGURE 25-5 It is essential to enter information on new and established patients accurately into the computer system because this will impact claims filed with the patient's insurance company.

Tasks

Many tasks can be performed with medical office management software. The tasks vary, depending on the brand purchased. However, some common tasks of medical practice software are entering new patients, scheduling, insurance processing, and generating reports.

New Patient Entry

Entering new patients is done either when opening a new practice or when adding a patient to an existing practice. A common way to enter a new patient is as follows:
1. Select *new patient* from the file menu.
2. Enter all patient information in the appropriate fields.
3. Select *save* from the file menu.

At this point, the computer will assign an account number to this newly registered patient (Figure 25-5).

Typical information required in the patient window are the patient's name, address, telephone number, insurance information, employment information, birth date, gender, and Social Security number.

Scheduling

An appointment scheduler is usually included in a practice management program (Figure 25-6). Patient scheduling reports can be generated to include daily, weekly, and monthly reports. These reports typically include patient name, account number, date of service, attending physician, diagnosis code, procedure code, and charge, possibly with additional information. The program usually allows for listing by the type of appointment that is scheduled. An appointment date or a range of dates can be used to generate a report for a particular provider (Figure 25-7), a particular CPT code, or a diagnosis.

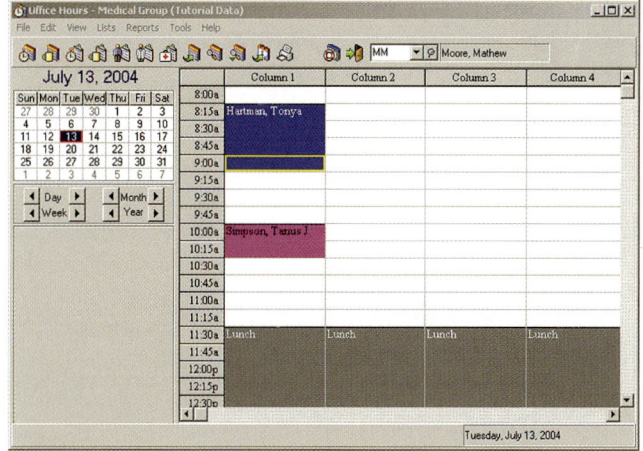

FIGURE 25-6 Booking more than one 15-minute time slot for Dr. Moore's patients allows for appointments of varying lengths. Longer appointments would probably require an hour on the schedule.

This information can be used to manage appointment or surgery scheduling. Chapter 26 provides additional information about scheduling patient appointments using the medical office computer system.

Insurance Processing

Most programs allow for easy accessibility to patient billing and insurance information. This allows the medical practice to post charges and payments at any time. Using the information on the **encounter form,** the diagnosis and procedures performed are entered into the patient's account; this posts the charges for the claim (Figure 25-8). After this new information has been entered, pressing *enter* should **default** the claim to the primary insurance listed for the patient's account.

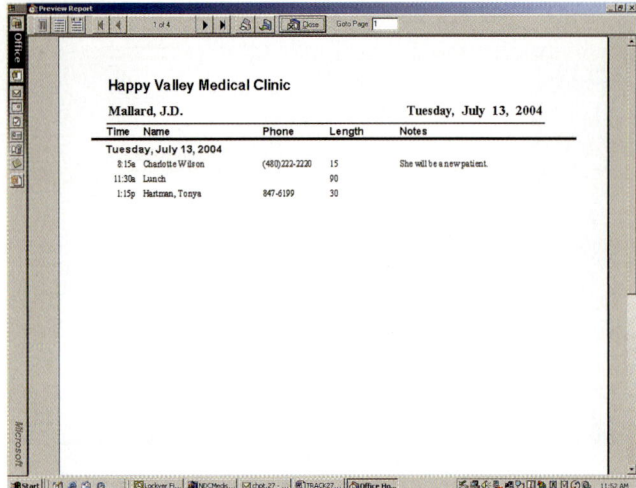

FIGURE 25-7 Computers can generate a "clinic list" of all appointments scheduled for a particular day, for a range of dates, or by provider or office site.

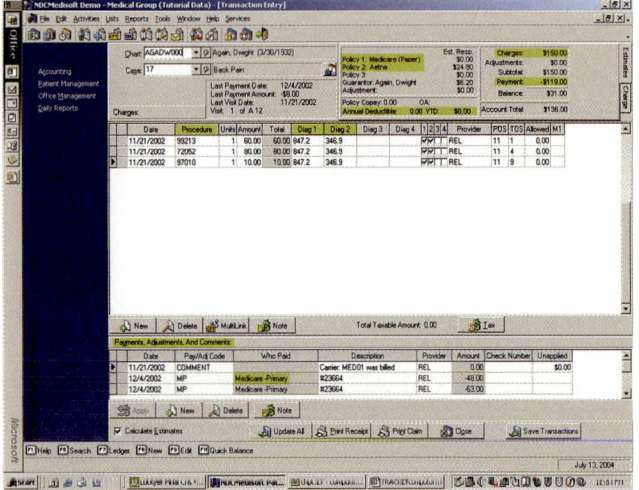

FIGURE 25-8 Codes and charges from the encounter form are posted to the patient's account on the transaction entry screen. This screen also provides relevant information about the current status of the patient's account.

This claim will then drop into the insurance queue, and the next time an insurance billing cycle is run, it will automatically be included (Figure 25-9).

Report Generation

The "reports" feature of any practice management program allows the medical practice to manage their cash flow, budget, and staff. "Aging" reports, transaction reports, end-of-quarter and end-of-year reports, and "productivity by physician" reports all help track the finances of the practice and are useful for planning staff increases, budgets, equipment purchases, and hiring of new physicians (Figure 25-10).

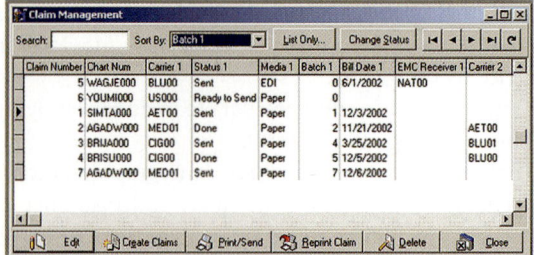

FIGURE 25-9 The claim management screen provides an electronic history of each claim. It functions as an "insurance tracking log."

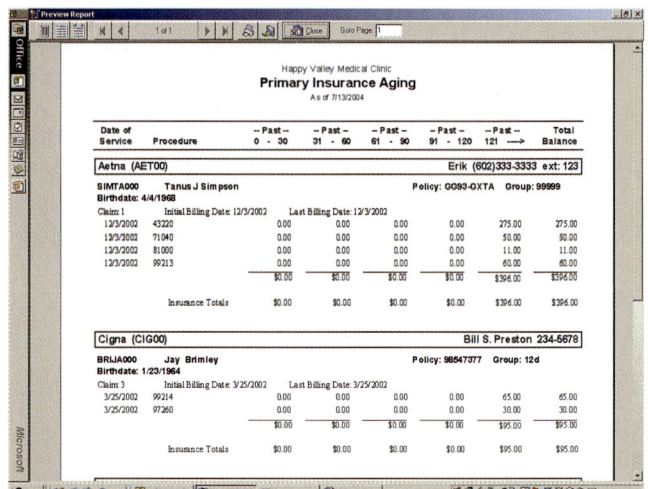

FIGURE 25-10 "Primary Insurance Aging" reports help determine which accounts need personal attention and collection efforts.

Backup and Exit

Protecting the data on the hard drive is a major priority because it contains so much data necessary to maintaining patient and practice records. A tape backup was once used by practices to prevent the overwhelming task of trying to reconstruct lost data. If the system crashed, the data from the backup tape could be copied to the hard drive. Currently, a CD is often used to read and write the data and save it for use if the system crashes. Some systems permit offsite data backup and storage.

To safeguard the data files of the practice, the files should be updated at the end of each workday. The backup files should be removed from the office at close of business or placed in a fireproof site in case of fire. If the hard drive were destroyed, without backup, all data would have to be reentered. Once the activities of the day have been **backed up,** the user can exit the program (Figure 25-11).

PATIENT-CENTERED PROFESSIONALISM

- *Why is it important for the medical assistant to understand how practice management software functions?*

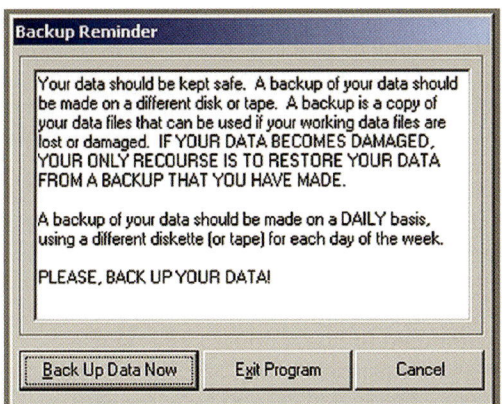

FIGURE 25-11 Daily backups prevent permanent loss of data should a system failure occur.

CONCLUSION

Computers continue to become smaller in size, larger in capacity, faster in processing, and lower in cost. Still, the newest computer software and hardware cannot solve all office problems. The computer is only as good as the person managing the system. A responsible individual who knows how to use the technology to perform office tasks will make the equipment perform in an efficient and effective manner. Remember that although computers may improve the speed and accuracy with which office tasks can be performed, these systems do not reduce the need for good communication, organization, and time management skills. A computer system makes the medical office run more smoothly, but only when it is operated by a capable, competent medical assistant whose focus is providing the best possible service and care to patients.

Chapter Summary

Reinforce your understanding of the material in this chapter by reviewing the curriculum objectives and key content points below.

1. **Define, appropriately use, and spell all the Key Terms for this chapter.**
   - Review the Key Terms if necessary.
2. **List four main functions of a computer system.**
   - Computer systems input, process, generate, and store information.
3. **List four uses of a computer system in the medical practice.**
   - Computer systems in medical practices aid in patient billing, appointment scheduling, database management, and report generation for fiscal practice management.
4. **List the eight main components of a computer system.**
   - Eight components of a computer system are the CPU, motherboard, mouse, keyboard, monitor, printers, modems, and other auxiliary input and output devices.
5. **Define "network" and list three types of networks.**
   - A network is a group of computers interconnected to exchange information.
   - Local area network (LAN) is a group of computers within the same building.
   - Wide area network (WAN) is a group of computers that connect computers between buildings, cities, and countries.
   - Intranets are internal networks within organizations using either LAN or WAN.
6. **Explain the importance of maintaining network security and list three safeguards for medical office computer use.**
   - HIPAA guidelines require certain standards to protect the security and privacy of patient information transmitted or accessed over networks.
   - Safeguards to protect electronic patient information include passwords so that patient information is available only on a "need to know" basis, an audit trail so that access to the information can be traced through passwords, and screen savers so that patient information does not remain open on an inactive screen.
7. **Demonstrate how to access a website on the Internet.**
   - Entering an Internet address into a browser window is one way to access a desired website page.
8. **Differentiate between a "directory" and a "search engine" and explain the advantages and disadvantages of each.**
   - A directory is a listing of categories that can be used for browsing; a search engine is used to locate websites based on keywords.
   - Directories can be advantageous because they contain prescreened sites (so their listings tend to be more useful), and they are a good starting point to organize a search. Directories can be disadvantageous because some useful sites may be missing since the sites are prescreened. Also, a directory is only as good as the organization that maintains it.
   - Search engines can be advantageous because they are helpful when searching with specific terminology since searches are keyword generated, and they provide links to other useful online sources (e.g., journals). Search engines can be disadvantageous because they require a refined use of terms, and they often produce too many results.
   - Always perform your Internet searches using more than one directory or search engine to ensure you are obtaining more varied results.
   - Always check the credibility of the websites that you use for research.
9. **List five ways a word processing document can be changed.**

- Word processing allows users to move text and delete or add sections of text, perform spelling and grammar checks, merge individual paragraphs into one paragraph, change the font and point of the type, and change the format and spacing of the document.
10. **List three ways a spreadsheet can be used in the medical practice.**
    - Spreadsheets can be used to generate payroll, estimate budgets, and generate other financial reports (e.g., profit and loss statements, accounts receivable).
11. **Explain the purpose of a database.**
    - The purpose of a database is to store large amounts of related information. For example, each patient's pertinent information in the database can be added, stored, retrieved, updated, or deleted as needed.
    - Databases allow users to manipulate data for various purposes.
12. **List three things to check before installing practice management software onto the office computer system.**
    - Before installing software, it is important to be sure the office computer has the appropriate operating system, amount of RAM, and amount of hard drive space.
13. **List four important office tasks that can be completed with practice management software.**
    - New patient entry and patient record updating, scheduling, insurance processing, and report generations are tasks that can be performed with practice management software.
14. **Explain the importance of backing up medical office data regularly.**
    - It is critical to back up medical office data in case the data on the computer are lost because of fire or damage to the hard drive.
15. **Analyze a realistic medical office situation and apply your understanding of computers in the medical office to determine the best course of action.**
    - Medical assistants must be able to understand and operate medical office computer systems.
    - Medical assistants must stay up-to-date with the changes in technology.
16. **Describe the impact on patient care when medical assistants understand the essentials of computers and their use in the medical practice.**
    - Patient care is enhanced because of increased productivity within the office. All information about the patient is located in one place and, with authorization, can be shared with other health care providers.

PRACTICAL APPLICATIONS

If you have accomplished the objectives in this chapter, you will be able to make better choices as a medical assistant. Take another look at this situation and decide what you would do.

Dr. Santos has just hired Terrell, a medical assistant, to transfer demographic and insurance data from the current paper records to the computerized patient accounting system. Terrell's assignment is to ensure that all the information on current patients is up-to-date in the computer and that the latest updates and additions to the computer program are installed. As each new patient arrives at the office, Terrell has the duty of obtaining information for the data entry. He then must be sure that the appointment has been scheduled into the computer so that medical notes and insurance information will be available as needed. Kate, an established patient, comes to the office and sees the new computer system in operation. Terrell explains that the office is becoming more technologically advanced and that the computer will be used to schedule appointments, store transcription, and manage patient accounts in the future.

Would you be prepared to use the computer to perform data entry, scheduling, and other medical office tasks?

1. What functions would you expect to be accomplished by the computer?
2. What administrative tasks can be done on a computer?
3. What clinical tasks can be done on the computer?
4. How can a computer assist the health care professional who wants more information on uncommon diseases?
5. How is word processing used in a physician's office?
6. What is meant by "backing up" a computer? Why is backing up at the end of the day so important?
7. What are the three types of networks? Which would you expect to find in a small private practice? Which would you probably find in a medical practice that has multiple sites over a large area?
8. What is the importance of HIPAA in regard to computer use?

WEB SEARCH

1. **Research medical software products using the Internet.** As a worldwide computer network, the Internet provides access to a variety of resources. Finding additional information concerning the different types of software available for use in a medical office is a valuable tool for the student.

- **Keywords:** Use the following keywords in your search: medical practice management software, Lytec, Medi-Soft, Medical Manager.

26 Medical Office Communication

evolve http://evolve.elsevier.com/klieger/medicalassisting

The daily functioning of a medical practice relies on good communication skills. As you have learned in previous chapters, effective communication involves excellent skills not only in speaking and listening but also in conveying nonverbal and written messages. Medical assistants and other health professionals must use effective communication skills in such daily activities as:

- Greeting patients
- Speaking with patients and other professionals on the telephone
- Scheduling appointments
- Corresponding with patients and other health professionals in writing

When applying effective communication skills in these areas, health professionals must meet patient expectations for professionalism, as well as HIPAA regulations on how patient information can be communicated or disclosed (Box 26-1).

LEARNING OBJECTIVES

You will be able to do the following after completing this chapter:

Key Terms
1. Define, appropriately use, and spell all the Key Terms for this chapter.

Greeting Patients
2. Describe how a warm, professional greeting affects patients.
3. Demonstrate the correct procedure for giving patients verbal instructions on how to locate the medical office.
4. Explain the purpose of the medical practice information booklet.
5. Demonstrate the correct procedure for constructing a patient information brochure.

Managing the Telephone
6. Describe how a medical assistant's tone of voice affects telephone conversations.
7. List 12 guidelines for telephone etiquette and explain the importance of each.
8. Demonstrate the correct procedure for answering a multiline telephone system.
9. Explain the considerations for screening incoming calls.
10. Explain the importance of a triage (protocol guidelines) manual.
11. Describe the process of placing a caller on hold when needed.
12. List the seven types of information documented when taking a phone message.
13. List three types of outgoing calls that administrative medical assistants may make.

Scheduling Appointments
14. Explain the importance for patients, medical assistants, and physicians of managing office appointments efficiently and consistently.
15. Demonstrate the correct procedure for preparing and maintaining the office appointment book.
16. List one method of blocking off, or reserving, time *not* to be used for patient scheduling.
17. Explain the considerations for canceling a patient appointment.
18. List 10 abbreviations commonly used in scheduling appointments.
19. Demonstrate the correct procedure for scheduling a new patient for an office visit.
20. List six appointment-scheduling techniques and explain the advantages and disadvantages of each.
21. List two special problems that can occur in scheduling appointments and explain what can be done to prevent each.
22. Explain the purpose of an appointment reminder.

23. Demonstrate the correct procedure for scheduling a patient for outpatient diagnostic testing.

Handling Mail

24. Explain why it is important to sort incoming mail.
25. List four classifications of U.S. mail.
26. List eight special services offered by the post office that can help medical offices track, insure, and receive delivery confirmation for the mail they send.
27. Demonstrate the correct preparation of an envelope.

Managing Written Correspondence

28. Explain the proper use of a letter and a memo in medical office communication.
29. List nine guidelines for preparing effective written communication in the medical office.
30. Identify proofreader's marks used to edit written correspondence.
31. Demonstrate the correct procedure for composing, keying, and proofreading a business letter and preparing the envelope.
32. Demonstrate the correct procedure for composing a memo.
33. Describe the format used to prepare a manuscript based on clinical research performed in the office.
34. List seven types of medical office reports and describe the purpose of each.

Patient-Centered Professionalism

35. Analyze a realistic medical office situation and apply your understanding of medical office communication to determine the best course of action.
36. Describe the impact on patient care when medical assistants have a solid understanding of communication in the medical office.

KEY TERMS

abstract	memo
autopsy report	modified-block format
certified mail	modified-wave scheduling
cluster scheduling	necropsy
consultation reports	new patients
discharge summary	open-hour scheduling
double booking	operative report
emergency	patient information brochure
established patients	progress notes
full-block format	proofreading
history and physical (H&P) report	radiology report
	registered mail
manuscript	streaming scheduling
matrix	time-specified scheduling
medical practice information booklet	transcriptionist
	wave scheduling

PRACTICAL APPLICATIONS

Read the following scenario and keep it in mind as you learn about the importance of communicating effectively in the medical office in this chapter.

Tara is a new medical assistant at a physician's office. Dr. Vickers has hired her to answer the phone and to greet patients as they arrive, as well as to assist with making appointments as needed. On a particularly busy day, the phone is ringing with two lines already on hold and a new patient arrives at the reception desk. Steve, the physician's assistant, asks Tara to make an appointment for another patient to see Dr. Vickers as soon as possible. Since the office makes appointments in a modified wave, Steve tells the patient to wait to be seen because Tara has found an opening in about a half hour. In all the confusion, Tara does not return to the patients who are on hold for several minutes, and one of the calls is an emergency. Furthermore, Tara is short-tempered with the new patient who has arrived at the office. Tara's frustration about the busy schedule she is expected to keep shows, and the new patient states that she is not sure that she has chosen the best physician's office for her medical care.

What effect will Tara's frustration have on this medical office? How would you have handled this situation differently?

GREETING PATIENTS

As a medical assistant, you may serve as a receptionist. The receptionist is the first person a patient sees in the medical office. Make sure the patient's first impression of you and the medical practice is positive. If a patient is calling for the first time to schedule an appointment, make sure the patient knows how to find the office. Procedure 26-1 shows how to use verbal instructions to give patients directions for locating the medical office.

As you recall from Chapter 24, the reception desk should be accessible to patients when they enter the office. In addition, the counter height needs to be high enough to maintain the confidentiality of patient information. You must keep several considerations in mind when greeting **new patients** and **established patients,** as well as other visitors to the medical office.

New Patients

Patients new to the medical office (first visit or first visit to the office in 3 years) need to feel welcome. Some practices will mail a "new patient packet" before the patient's first office visit. If forms have not been sent previously, give the new patient a pen and the forms that must be completed; these forms are discussed in Chapter 34. Explain the policies of the medical office, or give the patient a **medical practice information booklet,** or **patient information brochure,** that provides

BOX 26-1

HIPAA: the Privacy Rule and Security Rule

The Health Insurance Portability and Accountability Act (HIPAA) of 1996 mandates that the privacy and security of patient information be maintained in a confidential manner. This process begins when the individual arrives for their first appointment. Patients must be given detailed *written* information concerning their privacy rights. This includes the steps the practice will take to protect their privacy and how the medical practice will use patients' *protected health information* (PHI).

To document that the medical practice made an effort to comply with this regulation, the practice must obtain a written acknowledgment from the patient that he or she has reviewed these rights. Acknowledgment may be in the form of a signature or the patient's initials on the notice signifying that he or she has received the required information. If the patient declines to acknowledge receiving a *Notice of Privacy Practices*, this must be documented in the patient's chart. This documentation shows a good faith effort was made by the practice to inform the patient and details the reason for failure to accomplish this act and comply with the regulation.

Medical practices must also post a *Notice of Privacy Practices* in the office, usually in the reception area. Additional copies of the notice should be made available if a patient requests a copy. The regulation also requires medical practices to have a written policy and procedure in place for determining who has access to patient medical information. For example, the policy may state that the receptionist may view the names of the patients coming into the office but may *not* view patients' records.

To accommodate computerized information, two types of access codes (passwords) should be used. The first set would allow the receptionist to view the physician's schedule but would not allow the receptionist to view patient records. The second set would allow the physician, nurse, and medical assistant to view the patient records for the purpose of patient care. A tracking system that keeps detailed information of all staff members viewing a patient's medical record should be in place.

The HIPAA regulation also addresses the issues of sign-in sheets and calling the names of patients who are sitting in the waiting area.

Can a medical practice use patient sign-in sheets and call out the names of patients in the waiting room?

Yes; the practice can do both, as long as the information disclosed is appropriately limited. The Privacy Rule allows for *incidental disclosure* as long as appropriate safeguards are in place. For example, the sign-in sheet cannot contain confidential patient information (e.g., reason for the visit, medical problem). It is best to change used sheets with clean ones periodically during the day. Calling patients by name is still the most acceptable, courteous, and respectful way to "invite" patients into the examination area.

---

this information (Box 26-2). An information booklet or brochure should provide answers to nonmedical questions. Procedure 26-2 explains information necessary to construct a brochure. Figure 26-1 provides samples of various types of brochures used to provide information to a patient about a medical practice.

Let patients know that when they finish reviewing the brochure, you will be glad to answer any questions about the medical practice. In addition, inform patients that you are available to help them complete the forms, if necessary. Sometimes patients have trouble reading or seeing, and just handing them a form to be completed may be seen as uncaring. People unable to read are embarrassed to say so, and therefore they may not fill out the forms correctly. Some may not understand the questions being asked because of medical terminology used in the forms. Patients may not want to admit they need help or may be confused.

Helping patients with forms also saves time. Some offices have a private area set aside to answer questions and to fill out forms. This allows for minimal distractions and patient privacy.

Established Patients

Personalize the greeting when returning patients come into the office (e.g., "The doctor will be with you shortly, Ms. Jones; please make yourself comfortable in the reception

BOX 26-2

Patient Information Booklet

The patient information booklet (or brochure) communicates policies of the practice (e.g., payment must be made at the time of service). It clarifies appointment policies, office hours, prescription refill policies, and so on. It should avoid technical terminology and should be written as if the staff is speaking to the patient (e.g., "We want to make your medical care our number-one priority").

A patient brochure, or medical practice information booklet, should answer frequently asked questions, thus saving staff time by limiting the need to repeat information. This reduces telephone calls about office policies (e.g., office hours). The booklet invites the patient to be an active participant in his or her care.

---

area"). Remember, do not address a patient by their first name unless the patient has given you permission to do so. If other patients approach the desk while you are speaking with a patient, stop long enough to acknowledge their presence and tell them you will be available shortly. This lets them know that they are important as well and will receive your full attention. Every patient should be made to feel that he or she has the full attention of the office staff and that his or her needs have priority, no matter how busy the office is that day.

PROCEDURE 26-1: Give Verbal Instructions on How to Locate the Medical Office

TASK: Provide verbal instructions to a caller on how to locate the medical office.

EQUIPMENT AND SUPPLIES
- Telephone
- City map
- Pen or pencil

SKILLS/RATIONALE

1. **Procedural Step. Address the patient or caller in a polite and professional manner.**
   Rationale. The tone and pitch of your voice can promote a positive first impression of the office.

2. **Procedural Step. Ask the person, "Where will you be coming from?"**
   Rationale. This provides the medical assistant with a location on which to base directions. Find the location on a city map if needed. An Internet mapping service (e.g., MapQuest) may also be helpful in providing door-to-door directions.

3. **Procedural Step. Determine the most direct route to the medical office, with alternate routes if possible. Provide the person with major cross streets and landmarks.**
   Rationale. Providing the most direct route will save the patient or caller time and will lessen the likelihood of not finding the office. Having alternate routes, cross streets, and landmarks available will be helpful for people unfamiliar with the area. For example, "turn left on McCleary, take the next right onto Dearborne. Our parking lot is across the street from the bank." Keep in mind that the person may be driving, walking, or taking public transportation.

4. **Procedural Step. Allow the patient or caller sufficient time to write down the directions.**
   a. Repeat the directions back to the person, as needed, with a cheerful and pleasant tone.
   b. Ask the person to repeat the directions back to you if the location is somewhat difficult to find.
   Rationale. This provides excellent customer service and a favorable impression of the medical office.

5. **Procedural Step. Provide the caller with the office's phone number in case the person needs to call for further clarification of directions en route. If time permits, the medical assistant may mail written directions and a map to the patient before the appointment.**
   Rationale. Again, this provides excellent customer service and a favorable impression of the medical office. Written directions and a map may be included in the office's informational brochure, which is often mailed to new patients.

6. **Procedural Step. Ask the caller if they have any questions.**
   Rationale. Clarifies information provided and helps avoid any misunderstanding.

7. **Procedural Step. Politely end the call after answering any questions.**
   Rationale. This action displays a professional approach and provides a favorable impression of the office.

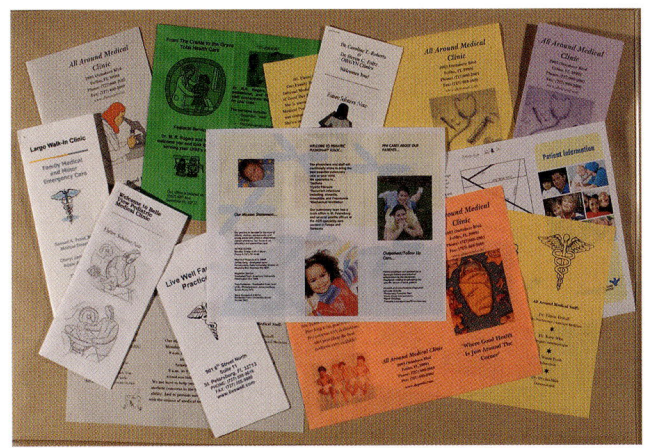

FIGURE 26-1 Brochures provide information to the patient about the various services that the medical practice offers and often answers frequently asked questions that the patient needs to understand.

PROCEDURE 26-2 Create a Medical Practice Information Brochure

TASK: Create a "mock" patient information brochure for a medical practice.

EQUIPMENT AND SUPPLIES
- Computer
- Software program that allows for brochure layouts
- Examples of local medical practice brochures and local medical office policies
- Pen or pencil

SKILLS/RATIONALE

1. **Procedural Step.** Determine the content information to include in the informational brochure to be provided to patients.
   Rationale. Provides an effective means to communicate with patients about office policies.
   Items for consideration may include:
   - Practice's philosophy statement
   - Goals of the practice
   - Description of the practice
   - Physical location of the office (address), including a map
   - Telephone numbers, e-mail address, web page
   - Office hours, day, and time
   - Names and credentials of staff members*
   - Types of services
   - Policy regarding appointment scheduling, no-shows, and cancellations
   - Payment options
   - Prescription refill policy
   - Types of insurance accepted
   - Referral policy
   - Release of records policy
   - Emergency protocols
   - Who to contact if the physician is unavailable
   - Frequently asked questions
   - Any special needs considerations
   - Personal information about the physician (e.g., area roots, special interests, and include special training and board certification)

2. **Procedural Step.** Write and key a short paragraph describing each of the topics to be included in the brochure. Proofread the keyed information.
   Rationale. The medical assistant can read the content and make corrections as needed. A brochure should never be sent out with incorrect information or "typos." Remember, this may be the first interaction a patient has with your office and an impression will be formed.

3. **Procedural Step.** Determine the layout of the brochure.
   a. The layout should be visually pleasing.
   b. Consider the placement of the office logo.
   c. Ensure that the name of the practice, address, and phone number are prominent.
   d. Some software programs have a brochure template that may work for creating this booklet. If a separate program is not available, any word processing program can be used.

4. **Procedural Step.** Have the office manager or physician approve the final draft.
   a. Make corrections as requested.
   b. The physician has final approval.

5. **Procedural Step.** Print the brochure.
   This may be done at the office if the office photocopier can provide quality copies. Otherwise, submit the brochure electronically to a printing company for professional-looking brochures.

*Some offices choose not to include this information.

Other Visitors

Occasionally, people other than patients, such as family members, sales representatives, and other physicians, may request to see the physician. If possible, answer questions concerning when the physician can see them, or assist them with making an appointment. The office should have a procedure to let the receptionist know which visitors the physician will see without an appointment. All visitors should be treated courteously.

> **PATIENT-CENTERED PROFESSIONALISM**
>
> - Why must the medical assistant greet patients and all visitors to the medical office in a professional manner?
> - Why is it important that the medical practice information brochure be structured to anticipate patients' most common nonmedical questions?

MANAGING THE TELEPHONE

Every caller who phones the medical office forms an impression of the physician and all health care workers in the office. In fact, people often form a mental picture of the person they are speaking with according to the way his or her voice sounds on the telephone. When people talk face to face, an impression is formed based on many factors. When talking on the telephone, a speaker's personality is projected by the voice alone. The receptionist's voice should be businesslike, courteous, pleasant, and friendly.

Telephone Voice

The quality of your voice is important because it is a major way to express your ideas to others. A person's voice tends to project that person's personality to listeners. The voice is a valuable tool to promote a professional image. You have probably heard this before, but it is true: if you smile while talking on the phone, callers can tell.

Tone

Your *tone*, or the sound of your voice, should be expressive and pleasant not monotone. The *pitch* (highs and lows) should be low because this projects and carries the voice better and tends to be calming. When emphasizing a word or important point, the pitch should be raised. Raising the inflection of the voice at the end of a sentence is useful because people tend to remember what they heard last.

Volume

The volume used when delivering a message must be appropriate for what is being said and for the physical condition of the patient. Speaking loudly is irritating to most patients. They may feel they are being spoken to rudely (e.g., "yelled at") or disrespectfully.

Clarity

You need to speak distinctly so that it will be easy for patients to understand your message. Patients also need to understand the terms used. Speak in lay terms (nontechnical terms); the message is lost if the patient does not understand the terminology. Pronounce words correctly, and ask patients to pronounce or spell their last name if you are unsure how to say it correctly.

Rate of Speed

If you speak too rapidly, you will not be well understood and waste time repeating yourself. Speaking too slowly causes your words to sound disconnected, which can also irritate the listener. Speaking too quickly or too slowly can make it difficult for the listener to follow the conversation, and the person may lose interest. Speaking clearly requires that you adjust your rate of speed according to the listener's needs.

Telephone Etiquette

The word *etiquette* essentially means "manners." Using good etiquette on the medical office telephone helps make a good impression on those who call. Good telephone manners reflect the qualities of pleasantness, promptness, politeness, and helpfulness. Guidelines for proper telephone etiquette follow. When making phone calls, always know the purpose of why the call is being made. You want to present a favorable impression on the patient that you are organized and capable of handling their needs. If you have told a patient you would return their call at a certain time, do it.

Before the Call

1. Prepare yourself by checking your body posture.
2. Make sure you have the supplies to take messages (pens, paper, message pad, appointment book, and watch to record time).

When Speaking with the Caller

1. Always identify yourself and the office so that callers know they have reached the correct number (e.g., "Good morning, Westside Medical Office, this is Lisa. How can I help you?"). Use a greeting that is going to give the caller the impression that the medical office staff is professional.
2. Be as courteous over the telephone as you would be with someone face to face.
3. Avoid slang terms and technical terms.
4. Listen attentively. Do not interrupt callers until they finish saying everything they want to say. If you speak too quickly, an important fact may be missed. Do provide feedback to let people know you are listening. Sound alert and helpful.
5. Think about how the caller feels. Be empathetic and show concern for what a patient is saying. The patient's needs are critical to the medical practice. Concentrate on what

> **BOX 26-3**
>
> **Handling Rude or Impatient Callers**
>
> - Stay calm and speak slowly. Getting angry will only make matters worse.
> - Be diplomatic and polite.
> - Show willingness to resolve the problem.
> - Think like the caller. Remember their problems or concerns are important.
> - Offer to have the office manager talk to the caller.

is being said, keeping in mind the patient needs to feel important.

6. Ask questions if you do not understand something.
7. Listen for overtones; much can be learned from a person's tone of voice and rate of speech (Box 26-3).
8. Take notes to help you remember the important points and to gain clarification, especially date and time.
9. Give clear explanations.
10. Try to avoid placing callers on hold. When it is necessary, ask the caller first, and thank the caller for holding when returning to the line. Be sure their time on hold is minimal.

When the Call Is Over

Leave the caller with a pleasant feeling when the conversation is finished (e.g., "Thank you for calling, Ms. Jones"). Remember that the first impression of the medical office staff will stay with the caller long after the call is over.

Incoming Calls

When the medical assistant uses proper telephone techniques, screening incoming calls becomes easier. Before picking up the receiver, discontinue any other conversations or activity (e.g., eating, chewing gum) that can be heard by the calling party. Procedure 26-3 explains the proper techniques for answering a multiline telephone in a medical office. When a caller requests to speak to "the doctor," the medical assistant can use these techniques to process the requests in a professional manner. Calls from other physicians should be put through to the physician promptly, if he or she is available.

Tact must be used when a caller requests to speak to the physician. The callers must never feel that the physician is trying to avoid them. It is best to acknowledge that the physician is not available or is with a patient before asking for the caller's identity. If the caller wants to hold for the physician, keep the caller informed about what is happening (e.g., "The doctor is still unavailable. Would you like to continue to hold?"). Always offer to take a message or ask "would you like me to transfer you to Ms. John's voicemail?"

Office policy should list the types of situations for which the medical assistant can interrupt the physician. Table 26-1 provides the protocol to be used as a guide when certain situations arise. Medical assistants are not permitted to exercise independent decisions and must limit their actions to preset protocols established by the physician. When this information is firmly and competently relayed, callers gain confidence in the office's ability to assist them. Often a new patient will call and request directions to the facility; it is important that this information be provided accurately and with clarity (see Procedure 26-1).

Placing the Caller on Hold

The telephone in a medical practice is in constant use. Most offices have more than one telephone line, and more than one call can come into the office at the same time. See Procedure 26-3 for a more detailed explanation of the process for putting a caller on hold.

Telephone Messages

When you take a message, certain information should be obtained (see Procedure 26-3 for details). Remember, always record what the patient tells you. Write the message in a duplicate telephone logbook. Give the original to the appropriate person for follow-up. Utilize copy messages that leave a copy within the message book, but always remember to tear out the original.

Outgoing Calls

You must also be prepared to place outgoing calls. Have all needed information available before making the call. Before dialing the number, always listen for a dial tone. Many times a call may be coming in to the office at the same time you are trying to dial out. In this case, a loud noise on the phone line will be heard. Outgoing calls that medical assistants may need to make include the following:

- Changing or confirming a patient's appointment.
- Making outpatient appointments or patient referrals.
- Ordering supplies or laboratory forms.
- Calling in prescriptions and/or refills.

Long-Distance Calls

When you need to call a person or company in a different state, it is important to know in which *time zone* the person or company is located. Figure 26-2 shows the time zones of the United States and Canada. For example, if you were in an office in Massachusetts and needed to make a call to Nevada, you would need to remember that Nevada is 3 hours *behind* Massachusetts in time. Therefore 9 AM in Massachusetts is 6 AM in Nevada. Some medical offices require that all long-distance phone calls be recorded in a long-distance telephone log (caller, time, and reason for calling). Check your office policy manual for any special considerations for long-distance calling.

Telephone Directory

At times you may need to look up a telephone number and use a telephone directory. The telephone directory's "white pages" list residential phone numbers and addresses in alphabetical order by residents' last names. The "yellow pages" list area businesses' contact information in alphabetical order by

PROCEDURE 26-3   Answer a Multiline Telephone System

TASK: Answer a multiline telephone system in a physician's office or clinic in a professional manner. Respond to a request for action, place a call on hold, transfer a call to another party, and accurately record a message.

EQUIPMENT AND SUPPLIES
- Telephone
- Appointment book
- Message pad
- Telephone emergency triage reference guide
- Physician referral sheet
- Pen or pencil
- Headset (optional)

SKILLS/RATIONALE

1. **Procedural Step. Answer the phone.**
   a. Smile before answering the phone.
      Rationale. The caller may not be able to see the smile but will hear it in your voice. Often, a telephone call to make an appointment is the first interaction the patient has with the office or clinic. Make the first impression a pleasant one.
   b. Answer the telephone by the third ring; speak directly into the transmitter, with the mouthpiece positioned 1 inch from the mouth.
      Rationale. Answering promptly conveys interest in the caller. The voice carries better when the mouthpiece is properly positioned.
   c. Speaking distinctly with a pleasant tone and expression, at a moderate rate, and with sufficient volume, identify the office and yourself. The greeting should start with the time of day (such as "Good morning" or "Good afternoon"), and a request to help should be included.
      Rationale. By speaking distinctly with a pleasant tone, at a moderate rate, and with sufficient volume, the caller will be able to understand what is being said. By identifying the facility and yourself, the caller will know that the correct number has been reached and to whom they are speaking.
      Example: "Good morning, Dr. Smith's office, this is Stacey speaking. How may I help you?"
   d. Verify the identity of the caller and request the caller's phone number.
      Rationale. This confirms the origin of the call and provides a phone number to return the call should it be disconnected or if the intended receiver of the call is unavailable.
   e. Provide the caller with the requested information or service, whenever possible.
      Medical assistants handle four types of calls on a routine basis:

      (1) **Appointments.** Because these are typically the most common phone calls made to the medical office, it is important to have the appointment book or electronic scheduling program easily accessible and near the telephone.

      (2) **Payment or account balance information.** If the medical facility does not have a separate department that handles these calls, it is best to have patient records close to the phone so that the medical assistant answering the phone has access.

      (3) **Physician referrals.** Most medical facilities have a physician referral list typed and located near the phone. The list should contain physicians, laboratories, hospitals, and other medical services frequently used by the physician in patient referrals.

      (4) **Emergencies.** Emergency calls may or may not be made to the medical facility. If this is a common occurrence for the practice, an emergency screening reference guide should be located near the phone. Along with the triage reference guide, emergency phone numbers for fire, police, poison control, and ambulance services should be readily accessible if 911 does not connect with these services in your area.
      Rationale. The medical assistant can handle many calls and conserve the time and energy of the physician or other staff members.
   f. If you are unable to assist the caller, transfer the caller to the person who can assist. First, ask if you may put the caller on hold. Wait for a response, and place the call on hold. Then transfer the call to the appropriate staff member. (**NOTE:** Some telephone systems allow you to immediately transfer the caller without placing him or her on hold.)

Continued

PROCEDURE 26-3 Answer a Multiline Telephone System—cont'd

Example: "I would like to transfer you to the accounting department. May I put you on hold? Thank you. Please hold."

NOTE: *Never* leave a caller on hold for more than 90 seconds. If the line is not answered within this time, return to the caller and ask to take a message. If the caller does not want to be put back on hold, ask the caller for a phone number at which the call can be returned.

2. **Procedural Step.** If more than one line is ringing at once, put a caller on hold:
   a. Answer the first line, and ask if you can put the caller on hold (remember to wait for a response).
   b. Answer the second line, and ask the caller to please hold (again, waiting for a response first).
   c. Return to the first call, and either help the caller or direct the call to the correct person, using the appropriate hold request, or ask for a phone number at which the call can be returned as soon as possible.
   d. Return to the second call, and repeat the process for subsequent incoming calls.
      Rationale. This ensures that all callers are treated with courtesy and respect.

3. **Procedural Step.** Take a message.
   a. Collect complete and accurate information that you can pass on to the party with whom the caller wishes to speak.
      Rationale. Complete, accurate information helps the person quickly and efficiently return the call and addresses the needs or concerns of the caller.
   b. Record the following information:
      (1) Recipient of the message.
         Rationale. When taking a telephone message, it is important to know to whom the message needs to be directed so that the message is received promptly.
      (2) Name of the caller. If you are unsure of the spelling of the caller's name or did not understand the caller, ask the caller to spell it for you.
         Rationale. When taking a telephone message, it is important to determine the relationship of the caller to the patient if the caller is someone other than the patient, to ensure that the caller has a legal right to ask questions or be given information about the patient.
      (3) Date and time the message is taken.
      (4) Urgency of the message.
         Rationale. It is important for the physician or other health professional to know if this situation must be handled immediately, as in an emergency.
      (5) Allergies. If no allergies exist, write "none" or "0" in the box. Allergy information is available in the patient's medical record but any changes need to be noted. (This information may be unnecessary if no drug therapy is needed for the patient.)
         Rationale. The condition reported may require a prescription.
      (6) Message content. Record exactly what the patient tells you.
         Rationale. The "heart" of the message includes the reason why the call was made and the caller's question for the physician or other allied health professional (or action the caller wants the physician to take).
      (7) Return phone number.
         Rationale. The person for whom the call was placed must have the phone number of the caller to return the call.
      (8) Pharmacy name and phone number. This information may be found in the patient's medical record.
         Rationale. Including the name and number of the patient's pharmacy in the message provides the physician

---

MESSAGE FROM

For Dr.	Name of Caller	Ref. to pt.	Patient	Pt. Age	Pt. Temp.	Message Date	Message Time	Urgent
Hughes			Roland Aiken	40+		10/13/xx	3:00 PM	No

Message: needs more Aldactazide (25mg tabs) — takes 1 daily   Allergies: 0

Respond to Phone #	Best Time to Call	Pharmacy Name / # Westside	Patient's Chart Attached	Patient's chart #	Initials
814-555-2010		814-555-9817	Yes		KJ

DOCTOR - STAFF RESPONSE

Doctor's / Staff Orders / Follow-up Action

OK - call to pharmacy JH
  # 30
  12 refills
  Sig: i po qam

Call Back	Chart. Mes.	Follow-up Date	Follow-up Completed-Date/Time	Response By:
Yes No	Yes No	/ /	/ /	

Product # 78-9156-Pkg, #78-9157-Pads, Bibbero Systems, Inc., Petaluma, CA.

Continued

PROCEDURE 26-3 Answer a Multiline Telephone System—cont'd

with a ready means of contacting the pharmacy should the need arise and ensures the correct pharmacy is called.

(9) Initials of message taker.
Rationale. For purposes of accountability and in case a question arises, the identification of the person taking the message needs to be indicated and should be recorded during the course of the phone call.

(10) Physician and staff response. This section of the form is completed by the individual to whom the message was directed. It is used whenever a telephone encounter with a patient results in, for example, the reporting of symptoms or a change in treatment. The provider writes in the action taken or to be taken (e.g., physician writes prescription that medical assistant will call in to pharmacy), call back (yes or no), chart message (yes or no), and follow-up date.
NOTE: If the medical assistant is assigned to make the follow-up call, the provider usually writes his or her initials immediately following the narrative. Sometimes both the provider and the medical assistant place their initials in the response box.
Rationale. Completing this portion of the form and placing it in the medical record is necessary after such calls, as this action must be documented in the medical record as part of the continuous record of care given.

4. **Procedural Step. Terminate the call in a pleasant manner, and replace the receiver gently.**
   a. Be sure to thank the caller and ask if there is anything further you can do to assist the caller before hanging up.
   b. It is best if the caller ends the call first. The proper language to end a call is to say, "Good-bye, Ms. Jones, and thank you for calling." It is never appropriate to say "bye-bye" or to use any other form of familiarization when ending a call.
   Rationale. Proper telephone technique is often the first impression a new patient has of the medical practice.

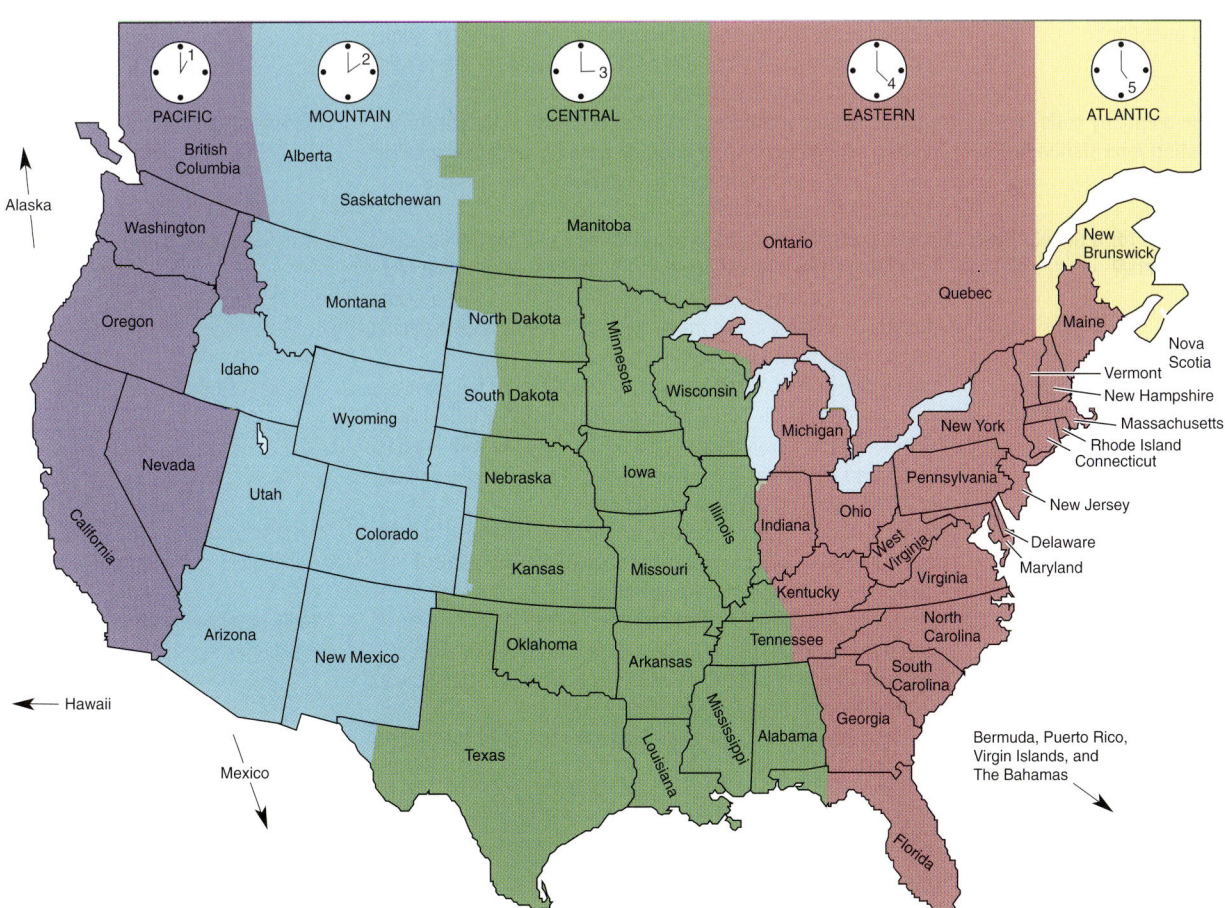

FIGURE 26-2 Time zones in the United States and Canada. (From Hunt SA: *Fundamentals of medical assisting—revised reprint,* St Louis, 2007, Saunders.)

TABLE 26-1
Protocol for Screening Telephone Calls

Type of Call	Action Taken by Medical Administrative Assistant	Call Handled by Whom
Patient requests appointment	If not a potential emergency, schedule appointment.	Medical administrative assistant
Patient requests prescription refill	Take a message with medication name and patient's pharmacy name and number. Send message with patient's medical record to physician.	Physician will call pharmacy if approved; clinical medical professional will phone patient to inform patient as to action taken by the physician (refilled or not refilled)
Patient asks to talk with physician or clinical medical professional because patient is ill or needs some medical information	Take a message, send message with patient's medical record to physician or clinical medical professional. (Depending on the severity of the patient's illness, the call may need to be transferred immediately to the physician or clinical medical professional.)	Physician or clinical medical professional
Patient is returning a call to the physician or clinical medical professional	Transfer call directly to physician or clinical medical professional as requested.	Physician or clinical medical professional
Another physician calls for the physician	Transfer call directly to physician as requested; no need to ask the reason for the call.	Physician
Outside laboratory calls with test results	Transfer call directly to individual requested by the laboratory.	Identified staff member
Patient is uncomfortable identifying the reason for calling	Ask the patient if the call is an emergency. If not, ask the patient if you can have the clinical medical professional return a call to the patient.	Clinical medical professional
Patient calls for test results	Take a message; send message with patient's medical record to physician or clinical medical professional.	Physician or clinical medical professional
Patient calls with insurance or billing question	After confirming the identity of the patient and if the patient is entitled to the information, answer the patient's question. Some information may not be able to be released over the phone and may need to be mailed directly to the patient's home.	Medical administrative assistant
Insurance company calls requesting information on a patient	Identify requested information and identity of caller. Usually, only limited information may be given over the phone, and the caller should send a written request for information that has been authorized by the patient.	Medical administrative assistant
Personal calls for a member of the office staff	Transfer directly to the staff member. If the call is for the physician and the physician is with a patient, notify the caller of that fact and ask if you should interrupt (i.e., "The doctor is with a patient right now; would you like me to interrupt?"). NOTE: Follow office protocol regarding physician interruptions.	Identified staff member
Administration calls for a member of the office staff	Transfer directly to the staff member. If the call is for the physician and the physician is with a patient, notify the caller of that fact and ask if you should interrupt (i.e., "The doctor is with a patient right now; would you like me to interrupt?"). NOTE: Follow office protocol regarding physician interruptions.	Identified staff member
Patient has a complaint	Attempt to handle the situation if at all possible; otherwise, take a message or transfer the call to the appropriate individual. If necessary, notify physician of complaint.	Medical administrative assistant or identified staff member
Patient has been poisoned	Immediately give caller telephone number of poison control center and obtain identification of patient. Poison control centers are properly equipped to handle poisonings in a rapid manner; assist with emergency help as appropriate.	Notify physician, and document call in patient's medical chart
Pharmaceutical sales representative wants appointment to give sales talk to physician and clinical medical professional	Make appointment under the guidelines established for the office.	Medical administrative assistant
Office supply sales representative	Take message and give to staff member chiefly responsible for buying office supplies.	Identified staff member

Modified from Potter BA: *Medical office administration; a worktext,* Philadelphia, 2003, Saunders.

the business (or business owner's) name and type of business. Yellow pages can also be found on the Internet. Some telephone directories contain a special section that lists local government or municipal contact information (city hall, public works, governmental offices, and schools). Many medical offices keep a list of frequently called telephone numbers (laboratories, local hospitals and pharmacies, and supply companies). This may be a printed list or a file stored on the office computer system.

PATIENT-CENTERED PROFESSIONALISM

- What telephone techniques would you use if you were responsible for answering the telephone at the medical office? What impact will this have on patients who call?
- Why must the medical assistant be aware of telephone etiquette? What are some general guidelines to follow?

SCHEDULING APPOINTMENTS

An administrative medical assistant is often the person who schedules appointments in the medical office. For consistency, it is best if only one person schedules the appointments, but this is not always possible, especially in a large practice. Although offices should have their own set of policies and procedures (which is important since these documents are used to train new personnel), some general principles apply when scheduling appointments effectively. Medical assistants need to understand the importance of effective scheduling, how to use the office appointment book, or the computerized scheduling feature of their practice management software and the techniques available for scheduling appointments. Remember, appointment scheduling needs to focus on the needs of the physician (e.g., time needs to be allotted for the physician to return phone calls, review patient laboratory results, meet with drug representatives, and to complete dictations of chart notes, letters, etc.). Also, the ability to schedule efficiently will require attention to the dynamics of the facility (e.g., number of examination rooms, availability of equipment, and time needed for procedures scheduled), and available resources (e.g., staff).

Effective Scheduling

Good scheduling management allows for efficient office functioning. The scheduling system chosen must be flexible enough to handle emergency situations, as well as the routine daily schedule. Patients do not find it acceptable to wait for long periods. Few patients are willing to wait longer than 20 minutes. Having an appointment schedule that accommodates the physician's preferences and commitments allows for a smoothly operating practice. Each office should have a standard for the time needed for each type of procedure so that the medical assistant can gauge the time needed for the appointment and assign appointments accordingly. Always advise patients of delays since this allows the patient the option of rescheduling an appointment, waiting, or returning later. It is not always necessary to provide the reason why the provider will be late.

Making the schedule flow smoothly can be a challenge for the medical office. It takes the cooperation of all staff members to make it happen. But effective scheduling is the backbone of an efficient medical practice.

Appointment Book

Many types of appointment books are used in medical offices today. Often, appointment books are spiral-bound, and each page is dated and contains a day of the week. The time allotted for appointments varies from every 10 minutes to every 60 minutes (Figure 26-3). The appointment book must be accurate because the daily workflow depends on its contents.

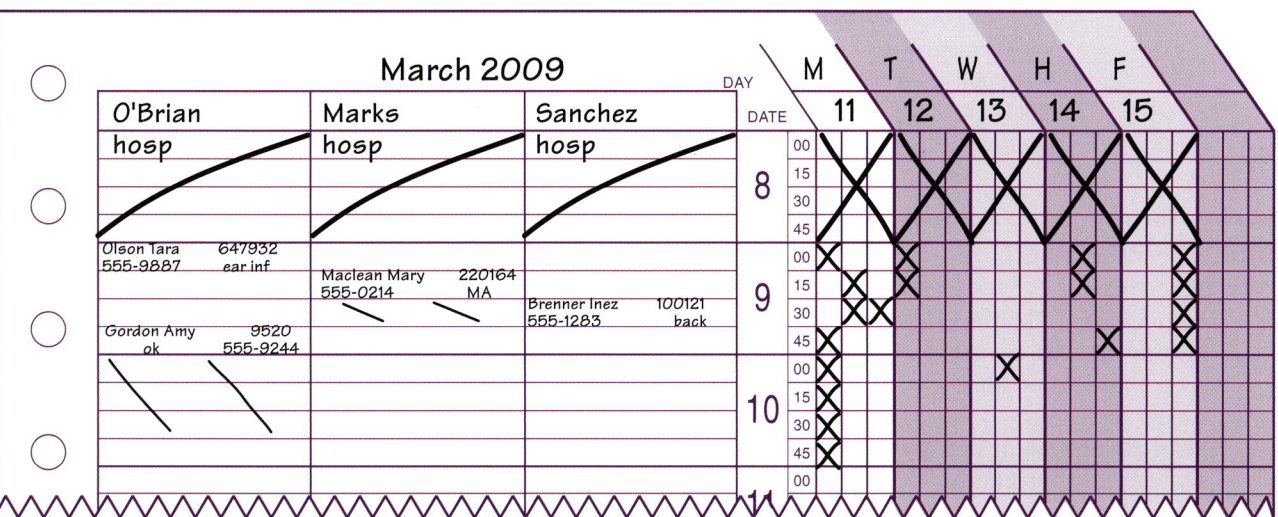

FIGURE 26-3 The appointment book allows appointments of differing lengths of time to be recorded (e.g., 15 minutes to 60 minutes), and time can be blocked off when a physician is not available to see patients. (Courtesy Bibbero Systems, Inc., Petaluma, CA; 800-242-2376; fax 800-242-9330; www.bibbero.com.)

Before appointments can be made, it must be determined when the physician is available. Most offices establish a **matrix** (reserved time) or develop some other format to block off time that is *not* to be used in patient scheduling. Using a slanted line or an "X" to mark off the nonpatient appointment periods informs staff about when the physician is not able to see patients. A brief statement explaining this notation is used (e.g., "hospital rounds"; see Figure 26-3). Open appointment times are indicated by the blank boxes in the grid. In an office of several providers, each may have their own appointment book. If providers are sharing examination rooms, the scheduling is critical.

Procedure 26-4 explains the process of establishing the matrix of an appointment book page and scheduling a patient appointment in detail. When appointments are entered, the patient's name and phone number are entered. If a patient is a "no-show" or cancels the day of the appointment, a notation next to the patient's name must be placed in ink. This documentation protects the medical practice in case of a lawsuit. The appointment book is a legal document; this is why most offices require that only black ink be used to write in it. Other important aspects of scheduling appointments include the use of computerized appointment systems and abbreviations in scheduling. Everyone in the office must be apprised of abbreviations made in the appointment books, so they may be aware of all notations in the book. It is important to remember that when a patient fails to appear for their appointment (no-show, or NS), the incident must appear in the patient's chart.

Computerized Appointments

Computerized systems for appointment scheduling offer medical assistants great flexibility. The system will search a particular physician's schedule and can also search other health providers in the medical practice to locate an available appointment time. The schedule can be printed daily (Figure 26-4). As with any computerized data, a backup system should be in place if the system fails. Electronic appointment books are very efficient in that they can mark all electronic health records (EHRs) for that day, or if the practice does not use EHRs, the computer can pull up all patients' names in alphabetical order for pulling the charts efficiently. The electronic appointment book prints out a grid that identifies the appointment times for each health care provider, allowing the schedule to be reviewed for the day.

Abbreviations

When an appointment is made, a reason should be recorded. Using an abbreviation allows the medical assistant to indicate the reason for the appointment without writing out the reason using complete words and sentences (e.g., "complete physical exam" is "CPE"). This is much quicker and also helps prevent spelling errors and hard-to-read explanations. Box 26-4 shows common abbreviations used for appointment setting.

PROCEDURE 26-4 Prepare and Maintain an Appointment Book

TASK: Establish the matrix of an appointment book page and schedule a new and established patient appointment.

EQUIPMENT AND SUPPLIES
- Appointment book
- Office policy for office hours and list of physician's availability
- Pencil
- Calendar

SKILLS/RATIONALE

1. **Procedural Step.**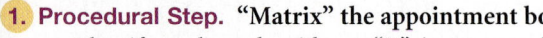
   a. Identify and mark with an "X" in an appointment book those times when the office is not open for patient care.
   b. Determine the hours that each physician will not be available for appointments.
   c. Block out time for emergency visits, and reserve time for unexpected needs.

   NOTE: This can be accomplished manually in an appointment book or electronically in a computer software program. (For the purposes of this procedure, this task is performed manually in an appointment book.)
   Rationale. Predetermined time(s) must be blocked out on the appointment book so that patients are not inadvertently scheduled to be seen during these times. "Matrixing" the appointment book

Continued

PROCEDURE 26-4 Prepare and Maintain an Appointment Book—cont'd

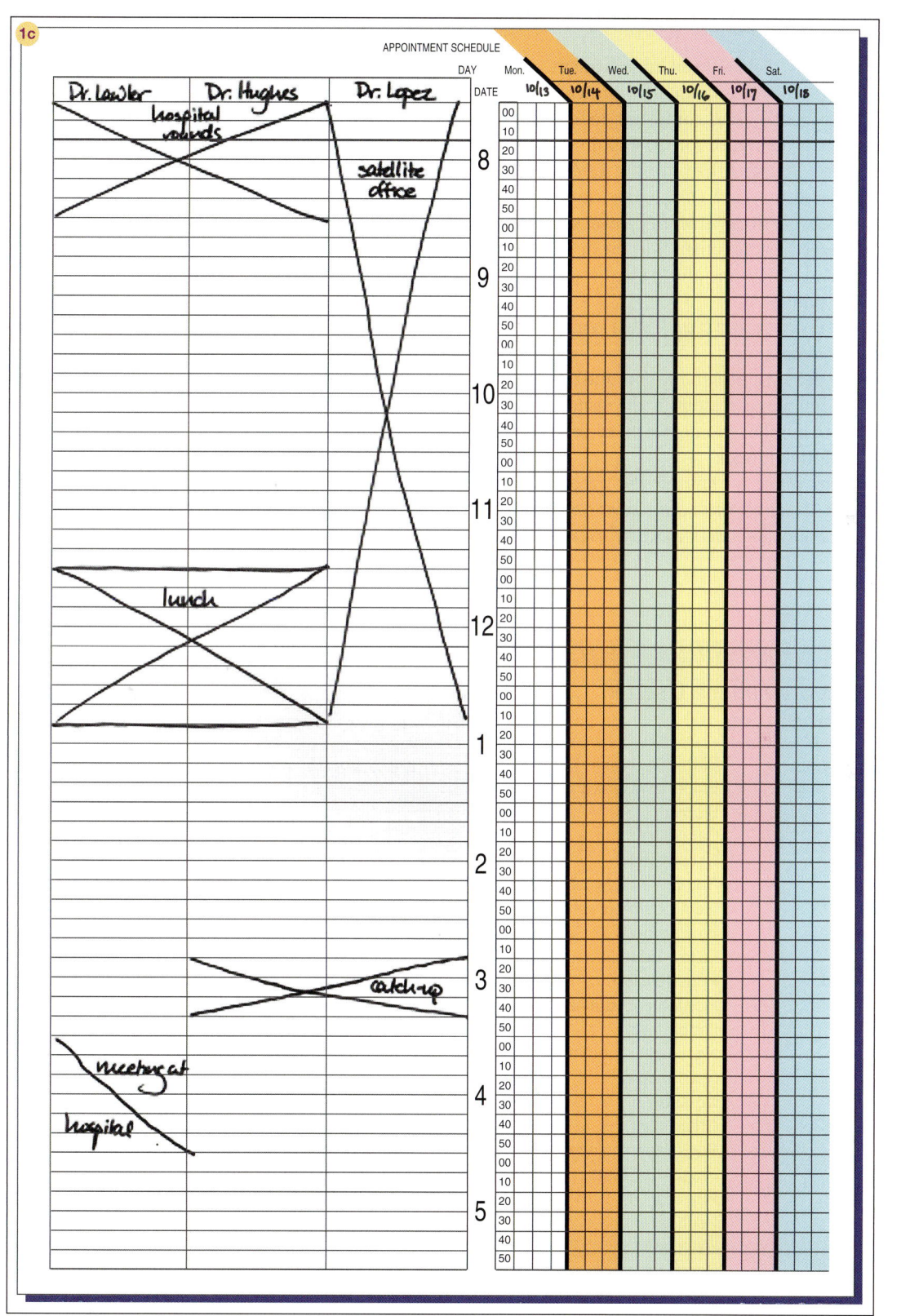

PROCEDURE 26-4 Prepare and Maintain an Appointment Book—cont'd

shows the available time slots that can be used for patient appointments.

2. **Procedural Step. Schedule an appointment.**
   a. When a patient requests an appointment time, identify the patient's chief complaint to determine the amount of time needed for the appointment.
      Rationale. The patient's chief complaint determines the amount of time required for the visit. Office policies should be established to provide standard procedure times for patient scheduling.
   b. Identify whether the patient is a new or an established patient and determine the patient's preference for date and time.
      Rationale. New patients often require a longer office visit than established patients.
   c. Once the patient agrees to the date and time, enter the patient's full name, reason for the visit, and patient's day phone number (home, work, or cell number) in the appointment book.
      Rationale. Writing in a reason for the visit allows the clinical assistant to prepare equipment and supplies needed for the visit. Writing in a telephone number allows for quick reference if the patient must be rescheduled for any reason. If the patient is new to the facility, write "NP" (new patient) after his or her name. Accommodating the patient's needs makes it more likely the patient will keep the appointment.

   NOTE: An appointment book is a legal document and can be subpoenaed as evidence in court. Because of this, appointments should be entered in ink. However, if a manual appointment book is kept, standard practice is to enter the appointments in pencil to allow for changes such as rescheduling. A record of no-show appointments should be kept and documented in patient records. A photocopy of the appointment page is accepted as a permanent record.

3. **Procedural Step. Complete an appointment card.**
   When the patient is required to come back for a follow-up appointment, make the patient an appointment card to include the date and time. If making an appointment by phone, repeat the date and time to the patient.
   Rationale. Appointment cards and repeating appointment information help the patient remember the appointment.

BOX 26-4
Common Abbreviations Used in Appointment Setting

BCP	Birth control pill
BP	Blood pressure check
Bx	Biopsy
Can	Cancelled
Cons	Consultation
CPE, CPX	Complete physical examination
ECG, EKG	Electrocardiography
FB	Foreign body
FU	Follow up (follow-up)
HTN	Hypertension
I&D	Incision and drainage
Lab	Laboratory
N&V	Nausea and vomiting
NP	New patient
NS	No-show
OV	Office visit
PAP	Pap (Papanicolaou) smear (test)
Pgt	Pregnancy test
PX	Physical
ReC, RECK	Recheck
Ref	Referral
RS	Reschedule
SOB	Shortness of breath
Surg	Surgery
S/R	Suture removal
URI	Upper respiratory infection
UTI	Urinary tract infection

Be careful when using abbreviations; all staff members must be knowledgeable about the abbreviations used and in agreement about their meaning and only use those that have been approved by the medical office.

New Patient Appointments

When a new patient calls the medical office for an appointment, you should obtain the following information:

1. *Name.* Obtain the patient's last name, first name, and middle initial. Ask the patient to spell the last name to avoid an error.
2. *Address.* Obtain the home address and the billing address, if different from the home address.
3. *Telephone number.* Obtain the telephone numbers for home, cellular phone, and work so that an appointment time can be confirmed, canceled, or changed.
4. *Purpose of the visit.* This information is necessary to schedule the correct length of time for the appointment.
5. *Referral.* If another physician is referring the patient, try to schedule the patient as soon as possible. The patient needs to bring any applicable documents to the appointment.
6. *Insurance coverage.* Insurance information can be verified to save time when the patient comes into the office.

Procedure 26-5 explains the process of scheduling new patients in detail, both manually and using the computer. Chapter 25 provides more information on using the medical office computer to perform scheduling and other tasks.

FIGURE 26-4 Computer-generated appointment schedule. (From Hunt SA: *Fundamentals of medical assisting—revised reprint,* St Louis, 2007, Saunders.)

Schedule for 10/13/XX for Dr. Howard Lawler

Time	Patient	Phone	Comments
8:00a	HOSPITAL ROUNDS		
8:20a	↓		
8:40a	↓		
9:00a	Wayne Harris	452-8117	New Patient; Complete Physical
9:20a	****************		
9:40a	Ella Jones	932-8174	recheck — cancel 8am 10/13
10:00a	Fred Linstatt	452-0667	recheck
10:20a	Mary Higgens	731-8241	recheck; URI 2 weeks ago
10:40a	Tina Leggett	932-0451	PE
11:00a			
11:20a	Tracey Jones	462-0157	2-yr PE; father Robert
11:40a	Keith Jones		3-yr PE
12:00p	LUNCH		
12:20p	↓		
12:40p	↓		
1:00p	↓		
1:20p			
1:40p			
2:00p	Winston Hill	648-0791	PE
2:20p			
2:40p			
3:00p			
3:20p			
3:40p			
4:00p	Meeting at hospital		
4:20p	↓		
4:40p	↓		
5:00p			
5:20p			
5:40p			

Established-Patient Appointments

An established patient is any patient who has been seen in the past 3 years by the physician or another physician in the practice, no matter what the locale (patients who have not been to the office in 3 years should be considered "new" patients). The following information is needed when established patients call:

1. *Telephone.* Obtain the telephone numbers for both home and work for the same reason as a new patient.
2. *Purpose of the visit.* This is obtained, as with the new patient, for scheduling purposes.
3. *Insurance information.* Ask if the patient's insurance information has changed.
4. *Demographic information.* Ask established patients if there has been any change in their home address.

Appointment Techniques

Medical assistants are often responsible for scheduling appointments. An office policy listing time periods for the various types of medical services allows the medical assistant to assign appointment times accordingly. Routine office visits require an average of 15 to 20 minutes when only basic equipment and staff are needed (Figure 26-5).

Each office must choose a method of scheduling appointments that fits the activities of the physician and needs of the office. Various techniques are used for scheduling patients.

Time-Specified

Time-specified scheduling gives each patient an appointment for a definite period (e.g., 10-10:15 AM). The medical assistant scheduling the appointment needs to know exactly why the patient is being scheduled. A 15-minute appointment is adequate for a follow-up visit, in most cases, but more time is needed for a well-patient visit.

Wave

Wave scheduling is not as structured as the time-specified system and allows for more flexibility. Wave scheduling is designed to self-adjust and avoid backups. This type of

490 SECTION IV Administrative Medical Assisting

PROCEDURE 26-5 Schedule a New Patient

TASK: Schedule a new patient for an office visit.

EQUIPMENT AND SUPPLIES
- Appointment book
- Telephone
- Pencil and paper

SKILLS/RATIONALE

1. **Procedural Step.** Obtain preliminary information.
   a. Name of the physician for whom to book the appointment.
   b. Purpose of the appointment.
   c. Scheduling preferences of the patient.

   Rationale. It is important to have this information so you can then locate and schedule an appropriate appointment time slot in the appointment book.

2. **Procedural Step.** Obtain the patient's demographic information and chief complaint.

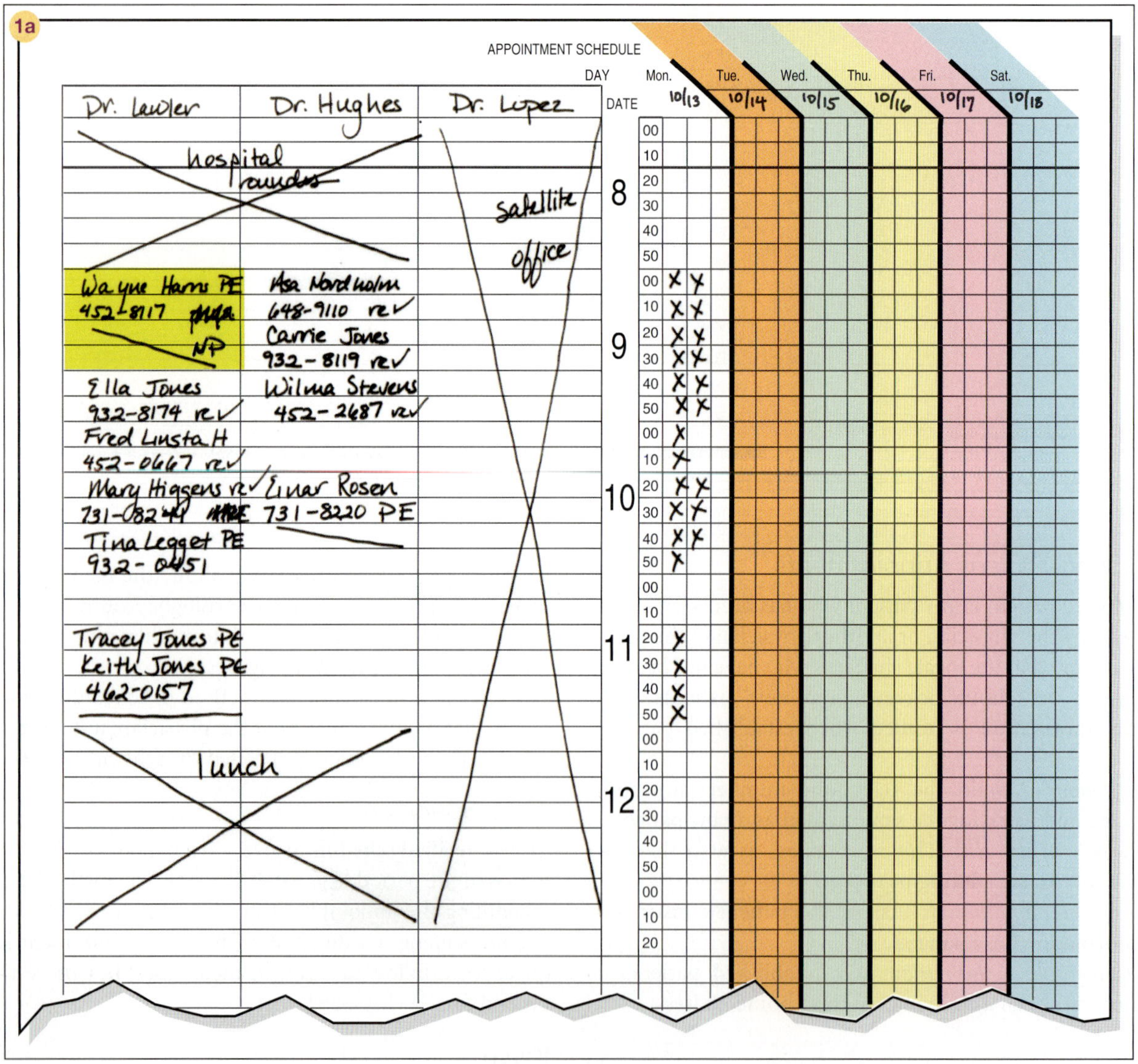

Continued

PROCEDURE 26-5 Schedule a New Patient—cont'd

  a. Patient's name (verify the spelling of the name).
  b. Patient's address.
  c. Patient's daytime phone number, including cell or work number.
  d. Patient's date of birth.
     Rationale. Not all the information, such as the address and date of birth, will be recorded in the appointment book. This information will be used to start the patient's medical record. However, it is important that this information is gathered at the time the first appointment is scheduled.
  e. Determine the new patient's chief complaint, and ask when the first symptoms occurred.
     Rationale. This information is needed to help determine the length of time needed for the appointment and the degree of urgency.

3. **Procedural Step. Determine whether the patient was referred by another physician.**
   Reference the patient history form for this information or ask the patient directly. You may need to request additional information from the referring physician, and your physician will want to send a consultation report and a thank-you letter.

4. **Procedural Step. Enter the appointment in the appointment book.**
   a. Search the appointment book for the first available appointment time and an alternate time. Offer the patient a choice of these dates and times. It is best to give the patient two appointment options: a morning appointment on one date and an afternoon appointment on another date.
      Rationale. Patients are better satisfied if they are given a choice.
   b. Enter the time agreed on in the appointment book, followed by the patient's daytime telephone number, reason for visit, and the abbreviation "NP."
      Rationale. Writing in a reason for the visit allows the clinical assistant to prepare equipment and supplies needed for the visit. Writing in a telephone number allows for quick reference if the patient must be rescheduled for any reason. "NP" establishes the new patient status.

5. **Procedural Step. Obtain additional information at the time the appointment is made.**
   a. Request insurance information and explain any financial policies at the time the appointment is made.
      Rationale. This ensures that the patient will be aware of the payment policy and that the office can verify insurance benefits before the appointment.
   b. Provide directions to the office, as well as any special parking instructions.
      Rationale. This provides for excellent customer service and relieves any patient anxiety about being able to find the medical facility (see Procedure 26-1).
   c. Repeat the day, date, and time of the appointment, and ask if the patient has any questions before ending the conversation.
      Rationale. This helps verify that the patient understands when the appointment is scheduled and allows the patient one more opportunity to ask questions or clarify the office payment policy.

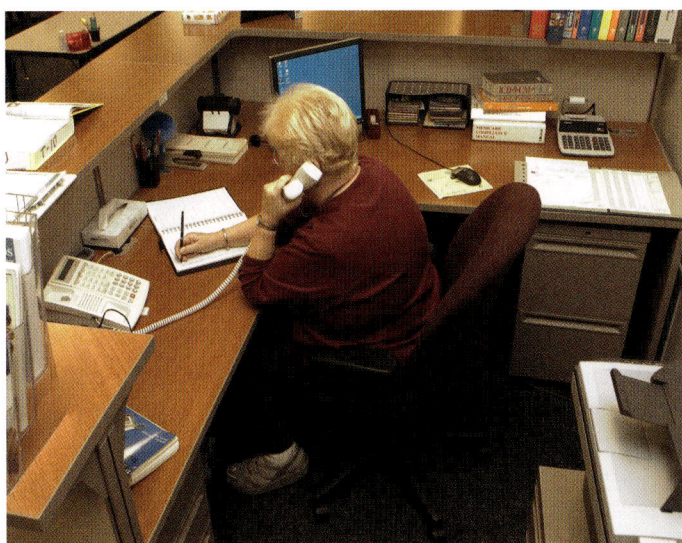

FIGURE 26-5 Medical assistant scheduling an appointment in an appointment book.

scheduling takes into account no-shows and late arrivals. Each hour block is divided into the average appointment time. For example, if the average amount of time used for each appointment is 15 minutes, four patients could be scheduled between 9 and 10 AM. In this case the four patients would be given an appointment time at the beginning of the hour (9 AM). Patients are seen in the order of their arrival. The idea behind the flexible appointment system is that each patient will not arrive at exactly the same time or require the entire time, and by the end of the hour, all patients will be seen and the schedule will be on track.

Modified Wave

As with the wave method, **modified-wave scheduling** is also based on the idea that each visit will not take the required time. However, instead of scheduling the entire group of patients at the beginning of the hour, the group is split in half. One half of the group is scheduled for the beginning of the hour and the remaining on the half hour. Thus, using the example given in the wave method, two patients would be given a 9 AM appointment and the other two would be given a 9:30 AM appointment. This allows time to catch up before the next hour begins.

Streaming

Streaming scheduling uses the concept of meeting the needs of the patient. Appointments are set according to why the patient is coming into the office, therefore allowing enough time for the procedure. In most cases, each time slot is broken into 15-minute intervals. A procedure needing an hour would use four time slots, but a procedure needing only 5 minutes (e.g., blood pressure check) would get one 15-minute slot and another patient needing only 5 minutes may be booked in the same slot. This type of booking accounts for the "in-and-out" patient and leaves enough slots open for emergencies.

Double Booking

Double booking is similar to wave scheduling, but instead of more than one patient scheduled at the beginning of the hour, two patients are scheduled to see the physician at the same time. This is similar to an airline selling more seats than available. The assumption is there will be cancellations and no-shows. This form of scheduling is helpful if a patient needs to be seen that day and has no appointment, but it often causes the office schedule to fall behind. This type of scheduling should not be done on a regular basis, and patients should be informed that they are being double-booked and that they will probably have to wait after arrival.

Cluster (Group) or Categorization

In **cluster scheduling,** several appointments for similar types of examinations are grouped. For instance, some medical offices will only do complete physical examinations the last Friday of the month or only on Fridays. Grouping specialty examinations allows the practice to meet patient demands and is a better use of resources. Often, specialty personnel (e.g., a nutritionist) must see these patients and the time they can be scheduled is limited.

Open Hour

Open-hour scheduling allows patients to be seen any time within a specified time frame on a first-come, first-served basis. This type of scheduling is typically used in walk-in clinics because of the steady flow of patients. An appointment book is often needed to establish a matrix and to mark which patient has arrived first. A disadvantage of this scheduling method is that patients may have to wait for a considerably long time, depending on the number of patients already there when they arrive.

Acute Needs

From time to time, patients call and request to see the physician the same day. The medical assistant will have to screen the patient to determine the urgency of the call and the need for an immediate office appointment. Office criteria should be developed to determine what constitutes an **emergency.** The physician or other supervisory medical staff must be available to help with the decision process. Some patients will be advised to go directly to the emergency room because of their condition. If a patient is scheduled to come in on an emergency basis, it usually means the patient is told to arrive at the end of the day, or to come in right away, but the patient may have to wait.

Some offices build a "buffer period" into their schedule to accommodate emergencies or walk-in patients. This buffer period is a designated flexible hour in the schedule that is used to meet the needs of patients while not disrupting the rest of the schedule. After all, patients cannot predict when they will become sick or injured. You will learn more about handling office emergencies in Chapter 46.

Special Circumstances

Problems that disrupt the scheduling process include "no-shows," cancellations, late arrival of patients, late arrival of the physician, and unexpected times when the physician is called away from the office. Inclement weather can make travel dangerous, resulting in cancelled appointments. An electrical power loss can cause a medical practice to close, resulting in the cancelling or rescheduling of appointments.

No-Shows and Cancellations. Patients sometimes fail to keep an appointment, or they cancel an appointment without rescheduling. "No-show" information needs to be noted in the appointment book and on the patient's medical record for legal purposes. Patients who do this chronically are "noncompliant with treatment."

Late Arrival of Patients. If a patient is repeatedly late for a scheduled appointment, scheduling the person at the end of the day helps alleviate the resulting delay.

Late Arrival or Unexpected Absence of Physician. Patients understand occasionally waiting for the physician, usually 20 minutes, but repeated lengthy waits result in agitation and stress. Patients should be notified if they will be required to wait more than 20 minutes. This shows respect for their time and allows them an opportunity to reschedule. Always notify patients if the physician will be delayed, and give an approximate time of the physician's arrival. Patients may take this opportunity to run an errand or make some phone calls. This reduces their stress and the resulting stress placed on the office staff.

Appointment Reminder

An appointment reminder card helps patients remember their next appointment. Many patients will carry the card in their wallet or purse for easy reference. It should be given to patients before they leave the office. If a new patient schedules an appointment, an appointment card can be sent with the patient information packet.

The appointment card takes many forms, but the information it contains is standard. The following information is imprinted on the card (Figure 26-6):
- Line to record patient's name
- Line(s) to record date and time of appointment
- Physician's name, address, and telephone number
- Sometimes, office policy concerning cancellations

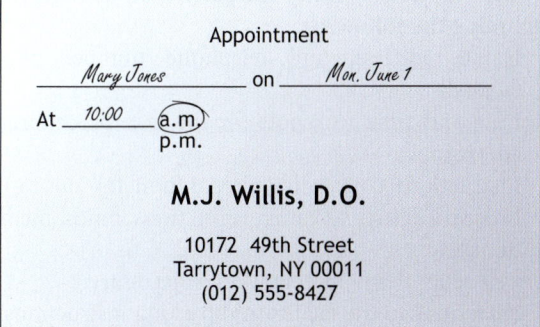

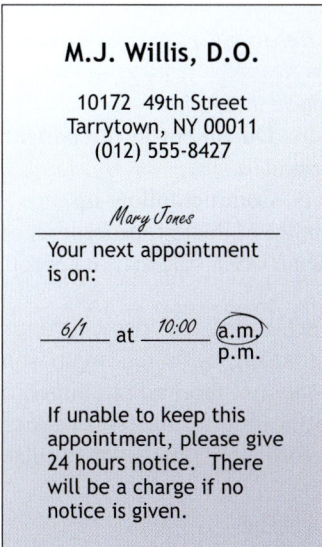

FIGURE 26-6 Appointment reminder card.

Another way to remind patients about upcoming appointments is with a phone call. The medical assistant may call each patient scheduled for an appointment the day before as a reminder. Be certain you have the permission of the patient to leave information such as appointment times on their answer machine. This could be a HIPAA violation if done without permission.

Scheduling Ancillary Appointments for Patients

Sometimes medical assistants schedule patients for surgery, consultations, referrals, physical therapy, x-rays, and outpatient diagnostic testing (Procedure 26-6). To make certain these things are done in a timely manner, the medical assistant will often call and schedule the appointment as a convenience for the patient. The medical assistant must be aware that each health care plan has its own requirements that must be met before providing an authorization number. Scheduling guidelines for ancillary appointments require that the medical assistant have all information readily available before calling for an appointment. For example, the patient should be consulted as to preference for day and time (e.g., "Friday mornings work best for me"). The patient's health record must be readily available before calling since pertinent information will be found within the chart (e.g., diagnosis, health insurance information). After scheduling the appointment the patient should be called to inform him or her of the day and time, as well as of any preparation need before the test (e.g., nothing to eat past midnight). All information about the appointment and the patient's notification must be documented in the patient's health record. Table 26-2 provides information the medical assistant must have available when making ancillary appointments or scheduling surgery for the patient.

PATIENT-CENTERED PROFESSIONALISM

- *Why is it important to follow established guidelines when scheduling patients? What are the established guidelines?*
- *How would you handle the situation of a physician being delayed for his afternoon appointments? How are patients affected by this situation?*
- *Why is it important to inform waiting patients of a provider's delay?*

HANDLING MAIL

Handling correspondence is an important administrative medical office duty. Incoming and outgoing medical office mail needs to be handled properly to make sure patients and office staff alike receive their correspondence. Setting protocol for the efficient handling of incoming and outgoing mail is key to an organized daily routine, which will include other

PROCEDURE 26-6: Schedule Outpatient and Inpatient Appointments

TASK: Schedule a patient for a physician-ordered diagnostic test or procedure, either in an outpatient or inpatient setting, or inpatient admission within the time frame requested by the physician, confirm the appointment with the patient, and issue all required instructions.

EQUIPMENT AND SUPPLIES
- Physician's order for either an outpatient or inpatient diagnostic test, procedure, or inpatient admission
- Name, address, and telephone number of diagnostic facility performing the test or the admitting facility
- Patient medical record
- Test preparation or preadmission instructions
- Telephone
- Pencil

SKILLS/RATIONALE

1. **Procedural Step. Schedule appointment using an order for an outpatient or inpatient diagnostic test, procedure, or admission and the expected time frame for results.**
   Rationale. A physician's order is required prior to scheduling diagnostic tests, procedures, or inpatient admissions. The urgency of receiving the test results, having procedures done, or patient care affects the timing of the appointment.

2. **Procedural Step. Secure approval for the procedure from the patient's insurance company.**
   Rationale. In some cases it is important to confirm that a patient's insurance benefits are valid and the needed procedure will be covered by the patient's insurance policy. This is accomplished by contacting the insurance company directly.

3. **Procedural Step. Determine patient availability.**
   a. Call the patient to determine the availability of dates and times before scheduling the appointment.
      Rationale. This ensures that the patient will be able to comply with all arrangements. The best practice is to obtain an alternate date and time as well.
   b. Pull the patient's record before calling to schedule the test or admission.
      Rationale. All of the patient's information, such as address, phone number, and insurance information, will be requested by the facility. Having the patient's record accessible before calling ensures the information is readily available.

4. **Procedural Step. Contact the facility and schedule the procedure, test, or admission.**
   a. Provide the facility with the information needed for arrangements.
      - Order the specific test or procedure needed, or inform the facility of the admitting order.
      - Provide the patient's diagnosis.
      - Give the patient's name, address, daytime telephone number, and date of birth.
      - Provide the patient's insurance information, including policy numbers and addresses.
      - Establish the date and time of the procedure or time of admission.
      - Determine any special instructions or requirements for the patient.
      - Notify the facility of any urgency for test or procedure results.

5. **Procedural Step. Notify the patient of arrangements, including the following:**
   a. Name, address, and telephone number of the facility.
   b. Date and time to report for the test, procedure, or admission.
   c. Instructions concerning preparation for the test or procedure (such as eating restrictions, fluids, medications, etc.).
   d. Tell what, if any, preparation is necessary.
   e. Directions to the facility and parking instructions.
   f. Ask the patient to repeat the instructions.
   g. Send written instructions to the patient, if applicable.
      Rationale. These details are provided to ensure that the patient understands the preparation necessary for the test and the importance of keeping the appointment.

6. **Procedural Step. Document in the patient's chart all information provided.**

7. **Procedural Step. Conduct follow-up.**
   a. Place a reminder of the test, procedure, or admission on the physician's desk calendar or appropriate tickler file.
   b. Record the scheduled test, procedure, or admission on an office tracking log for follow-up with the facility if the results are not received in a timely manner.
   c. Place the notification for the test or procedure in the patient's record and make it available to the physician.
      Rationale. This allows for timely follow-up of the results, which will impact patient care.

Table 26-2
Information Needed to Schedule Patients for Ancillary Services

Inpatient Elective Admission	Inpatient Direct Admission (Emergency from medical office)	Inpatient Procedure	Outpatient Admission	Outpatient Procedure
Patient demographics	Patient demographics	Patient demographics	Patient demographics	Patient demographics
Patient diagnosis	Patient diagnosis	Patient diagnosis	Patient diagnosis	Patient diagnosis
Physician admitting	Physician admitting	Physician admitting	Physician admitting	Physician admitting
Type of bed or floor	Type of bed or floor	Procedure room schedule	Type of bed or floor	Procedure room schedule
Insurance authorization	Insurance authorization	Insurance authorization	Insurance authorization	Insurance authorization
Patient preparation (fax admit orders to hospital on admission date)	Patient preparation (fax admit orders directly to designated floor)	Patient preparation (provide patient with instructions)	Patient preparation (fax admit orders to hospital on admission date)	Patient preparation (provide patient with instructions)
Preadmission testing		Preadmission testing	Preadmission testing	Preadmission testing
		Length of procedure		Length of procedure
		Anesthesia required		Anesthesia required
Notify patient of dates and other information	Notify physician	Notify patient of dates and other information	Notify patient of dates and other information	Notify patient of dates and other information

duties for the medical assistant. Medical assistants responsible for handling the mail should familiarize themselves with postal laws, regulations, and procedures. The United States Postal Service (USPS) website, www.usps.com, is a great resource for this information.

Interoffice mail, the mail coming from within the office or from other offices of the same practice, can be handled in a variety of ways, according to office protocol. This type of correspondence does not go through the USPS.

Incoming Mail

When mail arrives, it needs to be sorted into categories before being opened. Many different types of mail will be sent to the medical office: payments, insurance correspondence, journals, personal mail, magazines, brochures, and advertisements. The sorting of mail saves valuable time for the physician and office staff. Letters marked "Personal" are separated from other mail and delivered unopened to the person to whom they are addressed. If a "Personal" letter is accidentally opened, "Opened in error" should be noted on the envelope with the opener's initials.

The USPS classifies U.S. mail into several types, or classes (Box 26-5). Considerations for handling incoming mail include the following:
- First-class mail should be opened with a letter opener (to avoid damaging the contents), date-stamped, and inspected for signatures, enclosures, and complete addresses.
- Envelopes should be attached to the correspondence to which they belong, if the date of mailing might become an issue (e.g., legal notices, delinquent bill payments).
- Correspondence received from patients or other physicians regarding a patient's illness, laboratory reports, pathology reports, and operative reports should be attached to the patient's medical record and placed on the physician's desk.

BOX 26-5
U.S. Postal Service (USPS) Mail Classifications

- *First-class mail* includes all sealed or unsealed letters up to and including 13 oz (e.g., correspondence, statements). The maximum weight is 70 lbs, and the maximum size is 108 inches in length and girth combined. If the envelope is not standard size, then all four sides of the envelope should be marked First Class.
- *Bound and printed mail or standard mail* includes circulars and advertising materials that weigh less than 16 oz.
- *Media mail* includes library material, packages, and manuscripts weighing 1 to 70 lbs with a combined girth of 108 inches.

- When payments are received, the payment is entered in the daily journal and posted on the patient's ledger card or account by the appropriate person.
- Mail should be arranged according to importance and placed on the physician's desk (i.e., express mail, first-class mail on top).
- The physician will need to initial all papers that require proof that he or she has read them (e.g., laboratory reports, pathology reports). Initials signify that the physician has reviewed the material personally.

Outgoing Mail

Correspondence that leaves the medical office should be prepared properly. This helps ensure it will arrive at its destination quickly and will create a professional impression. General guidelines for properly preparing outgoing mail are as follows:
- Copies should be made of all correspondence, providing a record of what was sent, and filed in the patient's

record. The original letter and a typed envelope should be clipped together and placed on the physician's desk for signature.
- Use the appropriate handling method to send the mail (Box 26-6).
- Fold the letter or correspondence correctly before placing inside the envelope.
- Prepare the envelope properly.

These guidelines are discussed in detail in the following sections. The volume of mail leaving the office will increase when patient statements are sent out. As mentioned in Chapter 24, a postage meter reduces the time spent in stamping the envelopes and saves frequent trips to the post office to purchase stamps. The postage meter can be set for the proper class of mail and the correct amount and date.

Folding Letters

The folding and inserting of a letter will depend on the letterhead used and the envelopes provided. The letter should be face up and folded into thirds to fit into a #10 envelope (Figure 26-7). If a #6¾ envelope is used, the letter should be folded in half and then into thirds (Figure 26-8).

BOX 26-6

Special Handling Methods for Mail

Most medical office mail is sent first class, but certain items require special handling.
- **Registered mail** is used when items have a declared monetary value and are being sent via first-class mail. Registered mail can be insured for a maximum amount of $25,000. This option is available for First Class and Priority Mail.
- *Insured mail* is also used when items have a monetary value, but it is used for items valued at $400 or less and being mailed via First Class or Priority Mail.
- *Return receipt* is used when the medical office needs proof that an item mailed was received by the intended person. The recipient must sign the return receipt, which is returned to the sender, and this provides proof that the sender's mail was received.
- *Restricted delivery* is used when the item needs to be delivered only to a specific recipient. It can be used to help maintain patient privacy (e.g., delivery is restricted to only the patient, and no one else is authorized to receive the mail).
- **Certified mail** is used when it is necessary to prove that a letter was delivered and is available for Priority Mail. The recipient signs a return receipt to verify that the delivery was made. Certified mail is used for items that are considered urgent. It also provides proof that that an item was mailed. A letter sent to discharge a patient from the practice must be sent by certified mail. The receipt is kept with the patient's record.
- *Express mail* guarantees overnight delivery or second-day service within the United States. It is available 7 days a week for items up to 70 lbs and measuring 108 inches in combined length and girth.
- *Priority mail* is first-class mail weighing more than 13 oz and up to 70 lbs. It is the fastest method to have heavier mail delivered within 2 or 3 days. Priority mail rate over 13 oz is determined by zone and weight.
- *Mailgrams* are special services offered by both the U.S. Postal Service (USPS) and Western Union.

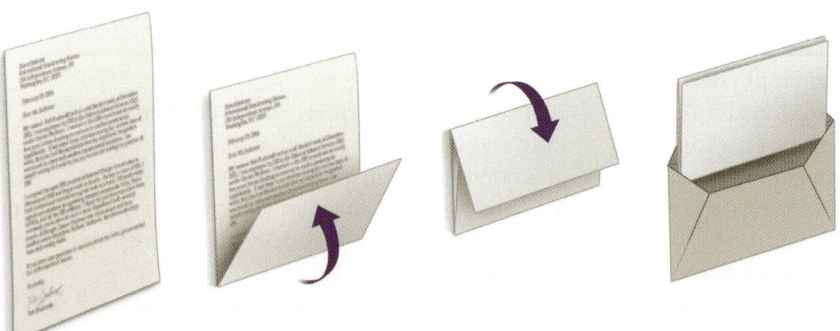

FIGURE 26-7 Method of folding a letter to place inside a #10 envelope. (From Young AP, Kennedy DB: *Kinn's the medical assistant,* ed 10, St Louis, 2007, Saunders.)

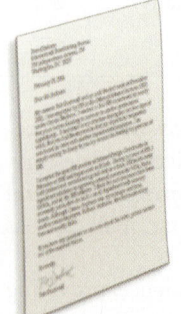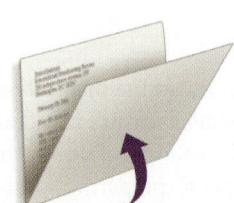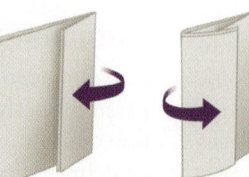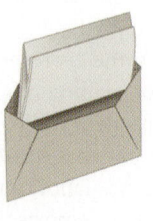

FIGURE 26-8 Method of folding a letter to place inside a #6¾ envelope. (From Young AP, Kennedy DB: *Kinn's the medical assistant,* ed 10, St Louis, 2007, Saunders.)

BOX 26-7

State Abbreviations for Mailing Addresses

AK	Alaska	MT	Montana
AL	Alabama	NC	North Carolina
AR	Arkansas	ND	North Dakota
AZ	Arizona	NE	Nebraska
CA	California	NH	New Hampshire
CO	Colorado	NJ	New Jersey
CT	Connecticut	NM	New Mexico
DC	District of Columbia*	NV	Nevada
DE	Delaware	NY	New York
FL	Florida	OH	Ohio
GA	Georgia	OK	Oklahoma
GU	Guam*	OR	Oregon
HI	Hawaii	PA	Pennsylvania
IA	Iowa	PR	Puerto Rico*
ID	Idaho	RI	Rhode Island
IL	Illinois	SC	South Carolina
IN	Indiana	SD	South Dakota
KS	Kansas	TN	Tennessee
KY	Kentucky	TX	Texas
LA	Louisiana	UT	Utah
MA	Massachusetts	VA	Virginia
MD	Maryland	VI	Virgin Islands*
ME	Maine	VT	Vermont
MI	Michigan	WA	Washington
MN	Minnesota	WI	Wisconsin
MO	Missouri	WV	West Virginia
MS	Mississippi	WY	Wyoming

*Not a state, but this abbreviation is used.

Envelope Preparation

When addressing an envelope, following simple guidelines helps the post office speed the mail to its destination.

1. A business letter envelope is $4\frac{1}{8} \times 9\frac{1}{2}$ inches (#10). The address should begin 14 lines from the top and 4 inches from the left edge of the envelope. This is the most common envelope used for correspondence.
2. A standard size envelope is $3\frac{5}{8} \times 6\frac{1}{2}$ inches (#$6\frac{3}{4}$). The address should begin 12 lines down from the top and 2 inches from the left edge.
3. Only use capital letters to start words throughout the address.
4. Do not use punctuation.
5. Use single spacing and block format.
6. Use two-letter abbreviation for state, district, or territory. State abbreviations of two letters without periods or spaces were developed to use with the *optical character reader* (OCR), which reads numbers, capitals, and small letters typed by machine or word processor. OCR has all post office locations and zip code numbers and can recognize the state abbreviation faster than the whole word. Box 26-7 provides a list of acceptable state abbreviations.
7. The last line in the address must have the city, state, and zip code. Using zip codes speeds mail to its destination. A zip code directory can be purchased at the post office or can be found on-line. It is important to recognize that only 27 characters are to be used in the last line, including spaces.
8. If mail is to be sent via special handling (e.g., registered mail), this needs to be identified in all-capital letters and placed below the stamp.

Figure 26-9 shows properly addressed envelopes.

NOTE: Envelopes can be processed by using the *envelope* and/or *label* function in a word processing program.

PATIENT-CENTERED PROFESSIONALISM

- Why is it important to sort the mail in a planned sequence?
- How important is it to follow USPS guidelines when addressing an envelope?
- How might patients be affected if mail is not handled efficiently?

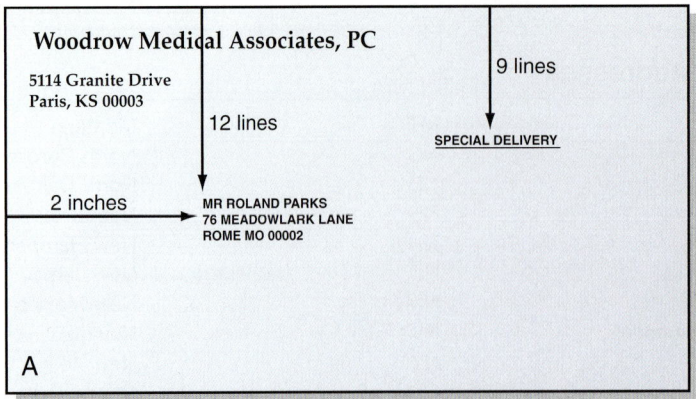

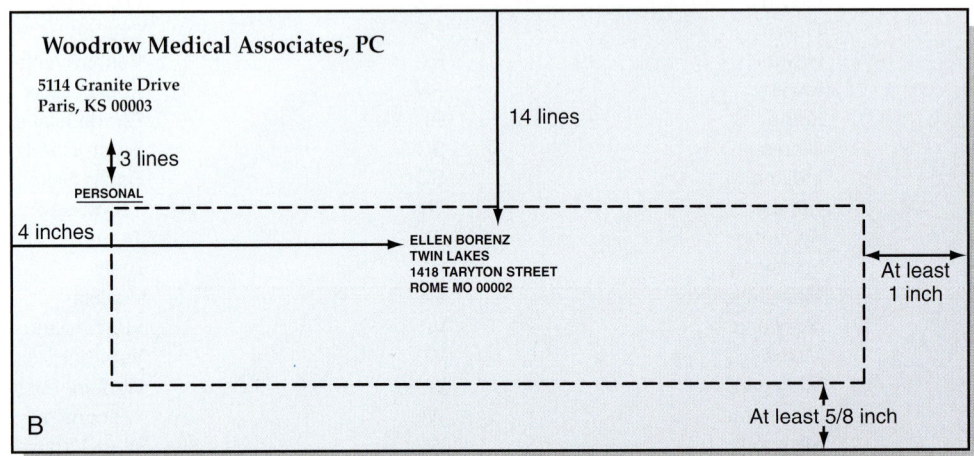

FIGURE 26-9 Correct format for addressing **A**, #6¾ envelope and **B**, #10 envelope.

MANAGING WRITTEN CORRESPONDENCE

All written correspondence from the medical office must create a good impression. It should be neat, in the correct format, professional and courteous in tone, and error-free. You need to understand the basic guidelines for effective written correspondence as well as the writing formats used for business letters, memos, and manuscripts.

Guidelines for Effective Written Correspondence

All written correspondence, whether sent within the office, out to patients, or to other organizations, needs to be written in a clear, concise, professional way. Basic guidelines for effective written correspondence are as follows:

1. Before writing, plan the message so that it meets the needs of the reader. The message should contain all the information the receiver needs to have, written in good grammatical style.
2. Present ideas positively (e.g., "Please feel free to call if I can be of assistance" instead of "If I can be of further help, please do not hesitate to let me know").
3. Include all essential information. Confusion or errors can result when a letter does not include all essential information. Often, time is wasted because a second letter needs to be written to add to or clarify the first communication.
4. Ensure clarity. Written communications need to be written clearly so that they cannot be misunderstood.
5. Write in an action-oriented style (e.g., "We will mail you the lab report" instead of "The lab report will be mailed to you"). Clear, direct writing is effective and efficient.
6. Use concrete or specific language (e.g., "a fever of 106.4° F" instead of "a high fever"). Confusion exists when general statements are used because the reader may have difficulty understanding the meaning.
7. Use proper sentence structure.
8. Use proper paragraph structure.
9. Edit and proofread messages carefully. Reviewing basic grammar, punctuation, capitalization, and word usage rules will assist in the editing process.

Proofreading

As you know, any communication a patient receives from the medical office creates an impression. Clear, well-organized, and accurate communication creates a good impression; communication that is not clear, organized, or accurate creates a negative impression. Before sending anything you write or type, you need to proofread it to be certain the document is free of errors. Some medical assistants proofread directly from the computer screen, scrolling line by line. Others prefer to print out the document and proofread the hard copy. Key points to remember when **proofreading** are as follows:

1. When reviewing a letter, pay close attention to the date, enclosure notation, and recipient's name.
2. Concentrate as you read, and check for keying errors. Even though most word processors have a spelling checker, it will not detect a miskeyed word if it is another word spelled correctly (e.g., mistakenly keying "spat" instead of "stat," or "two" instead of "too").
3. Use the correct word (e.g., affect/effect, advice/advise).
4. Check punctuation after proofreading for spelling and word usage.
5. Do not rely solely on "spell check"; always have a dictionary and Thesaurus handy.

Remember if you have misspelled words in your written communications, patients may also mistrust the quality of your skills.

Table 26-3 lists frequently used proofreading symbols and proofreader's marks. Always be sure to read over the printed copy of a document before sending it.

Letter and Memo Preparation

Medical office correspondence is often in the form of letters, memos, and electronic mail (e-mail, discussed in Chapter 7). Medical assistants need to use the correct form when using these types of correspondence.

Business Letters

A business letter includes the following elements:

1. *Date line.* The position of the date line on the page depends on the style of the letter used.
   - Typed three lines below the letterhead.
   - Written as month, day, and year (e.g., October 1, 2009, not 10/1/09).
   - Date the letter using the day it was dictated or written, not the day typed.
2. *Inside address.* When using letterhead, the inside address contains the name and address (with zip code and any suite numbers) to whom the letter is written. If not using letterhead, the name and address of the physician and medical office are also included and appear flush with the margin before the inside address.
   - Typed three to eight lines below the date line.
   - Place the person's name on the first line and the company's name on the second line.
   - Contains no more than five lines.
   - Single-space the address.
3. *Attention line.* May be used if a person's name is not known or is not stated on the first line of the inside address. The attention line is flush with the left margin of the letter.

4. *Salutation.* This is the opening greeting of the letter.
   - Typed two to four lines below the inside address.

> *Example:*
> QRS Insurance Company
> 41 Main Street
> Buxton, OR 11000
> (skip 2 lines)
> ATTENTION: Medical Director

   - If an "attention" line is used, type the salutation two spaces below the attention line.
   - Capitalize the first word, the title, and the surname. "Mrs." is used for married females; "Miss" or "Ms." may be a matter of personal preference.
   - Use a colon following the salutation (e.g., Dear Dr. Smith:).
   - Use "To Whom It May Concern" as a salutation in letters not addressed to any particular person.
5. Subject or regarding line.
   - Typed two lines below the salutation.
   - Should be short and to the point (e.g., Subject: Disability Evaluation).
6. *Body.* This is all the material between the salutation and the closing (the message).
   - Begins two lines below the salutation.
   - If the message is short, use double spacing; otherwise, single spacing is recommended.
   - Double space between paragraphs.
   - If entire body is double-spaced, use indentation with new paragraphs.
7. *Closing.* This is the "goodbye" of the letter.
   - Typed two lines below the last line of the message (e.g., "Sincerely yours,").
   - Box 26-8 shows examples of acceptable closings.
8. *Signature line.* This is the name and title of the person who signs the letter.
   - Typed four lines below the complimentary close.
9. *Reference notation.* This is used when a person does not type his or her own letter. If the writer's initials are included, they are in all-capital letters, followed by a slash mark or colon, and then followed by the typist's initials in lowercase letters (e.g., TLM/rgn or TLM:rgn).

BOX 26-8

Examples of Complimentary Closing in Business Letters

GREAT RESPECT
Respectfully yours
Yours respectfully
Very respectfully yours

FORMAL
Yours very truly
Very truly yours
Very cordially yours

LESS FORMAL
Sincerely yours
Yours truly
Yours sincerely

FRIENDLY
Cordially yours
Yours cordially

TABLE 26-3

Proofreading Marks

Symbol or Margin Notation	Meaning	Example
ℐ or ⌿ or ⁊	Delete	take it out
⌒	Close up	print as o̞ne word
⨌	Delete and close up	clo̸se up
∧ or > or ⋏	Insert	insert here (something)
#	Insert a space	put one here
eq #	Space evenly	space evenly where indicated
stet	Let stand	let marked text stand as set
tr	Transpose	change order the
[	Set farther to left	too far to the right
]	Set farther to right	too far to the left
¶	Begin a new paragraph	the same is true. ¶ In conclusion
sp	Spell out	set 5 lbs as five pounds
cap	Set in CAPITALS	set nato as NATO
lc	Set in lowercase	set South as south
ital	Set in *italic*	set oeuvre as *oeuvre*
bf	Set in **boldface**	set important as **important**
∨	Superscript or superior	∨ as in πr^2
∧	Subscript or inferior	∧ as in H_2O
⌃,	Comma	red, blue, and yellow
⌄'	Apostrophe	Calvin's lizard was green.
⊙	Period	The end is near ⊙
; or ;/	Semicolon	1, this; 2, that
: or ⊙⊙	Colon	is the following:
⌄' ⌄' or ⌄⌄	Quotation marks	He said, "I did it."
( )	Parentheses	Run (fast) now.

- Typed two lines below the signature line, flush with the left margin.
10. *Enclosure notation.* Informs reader of any enclosures, or additional items, included in the mailing (e.g., Enclosure: Resume). Make absolutely certain you have enclosed the information you noted.
- Indicate the number of enclosures (e.g., Enc: 5).
- Typed two lines below the last entry, flush with the left margin.
11. *Copy notation.* The courtesy "carbon" copy (CC) notation lists all the people receiving the letter in addition to the addressee.

- Typed two lines below the last entry, flush with the left margin.

Example:
CC: Audit cttee
Finance cttee

When letters are two or more pages long, the additional pages are printed on plain paper of the same quality and color as the letterhead used for the first page.

Procedure 26-7 explains the process of composing and proofreading business correspondence and preparing envelopes.

The letter in Figure 26-10, *A* illustrates the basic elements of a typical business letter in block-style format.

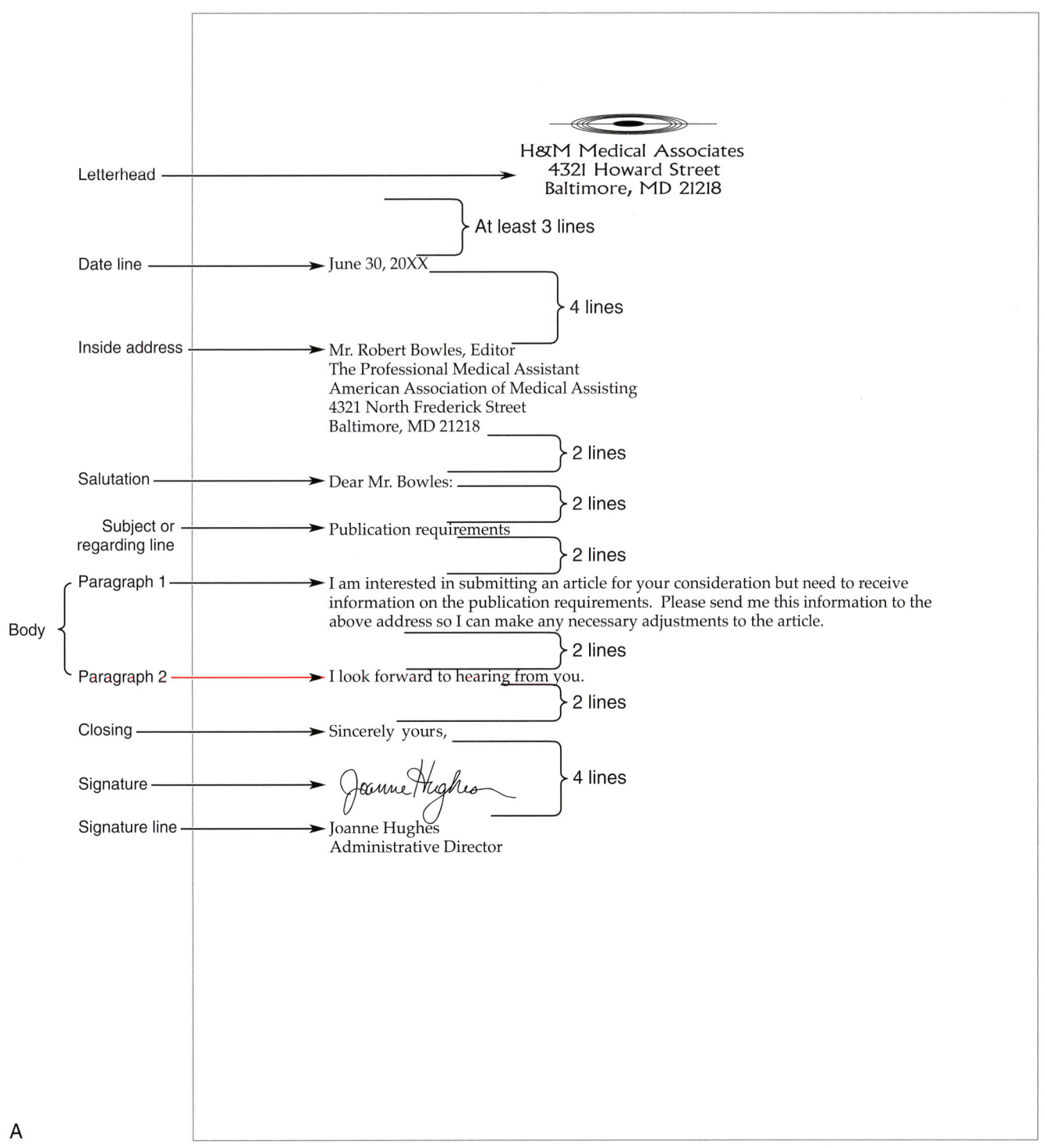

FIGURE 26-10 A, Elements of a business letter (block style in full-block format).

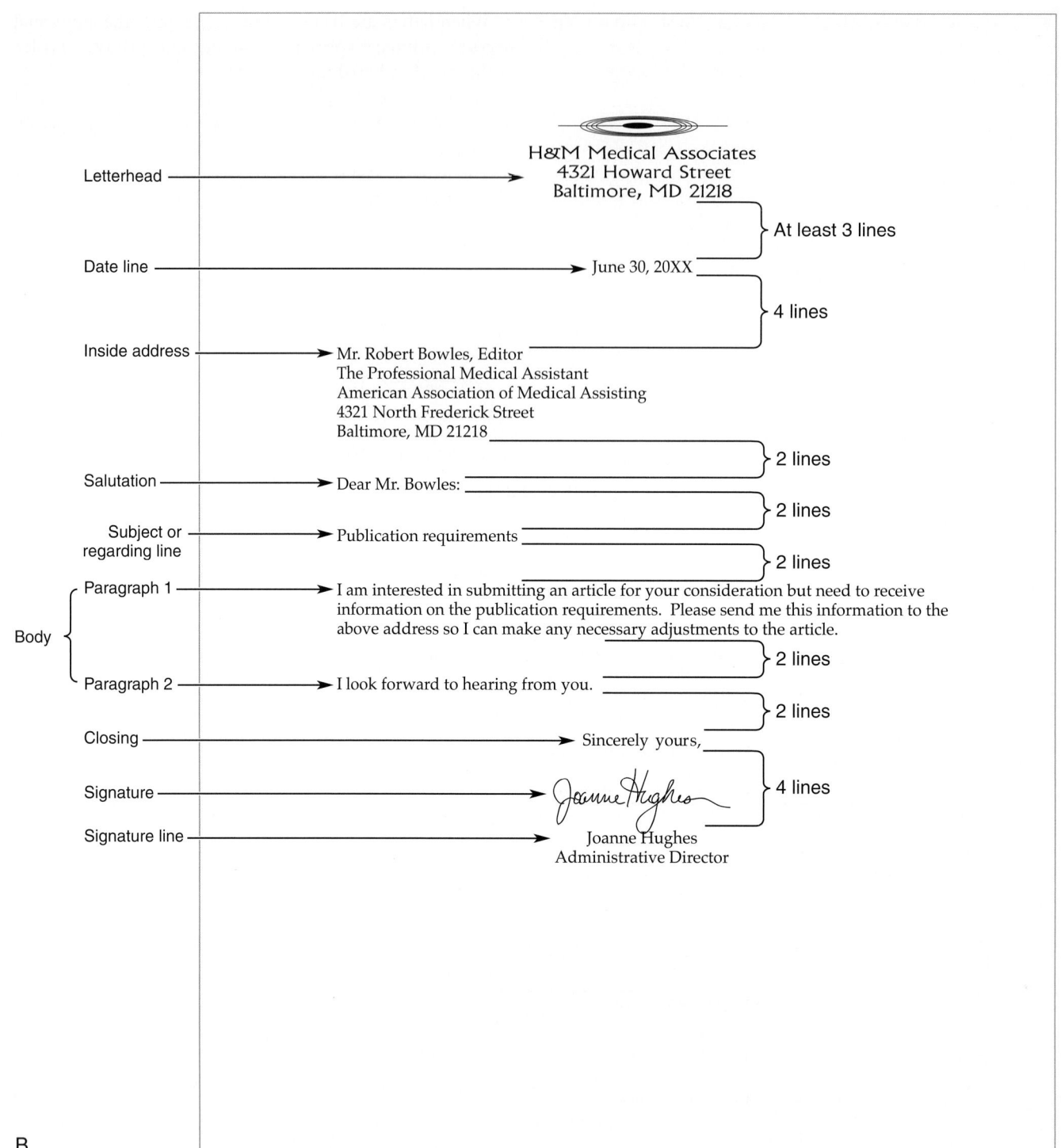

FIGURE 26-10, cont'd B, Elements of a business letter (modified-block format).

PROCEDURE 26-7

Compose Business Correspondence

TASK: Compose, key, and proofread a business letter using the guidelines of a common style.

EQUIPMENT AND SUPPLIES
- Word processor, computer with printer, or typewriter
- Paper
- Letterhead stationery
- Pen or pencil
- Envelope

SKILLS/RATIONALE

1. **Procedural Step. Assemble all needed equipment and supplies.**
   a. Determine the letter style.
   b. Obtain the name and address of the recipient.
   Rationale. This allows for efficient use of time and ensures the letter will be sent to the correct recipient.

2. **Procedural Step. Prepare a rough draft of the letter.**
   a. Use established business correspondence guidelines (see Figure 26-10).
   Rationale. This ensures that all topics are covered, that the appearance of the letter is professional, and that the correct format has been used. Working from a draft allows for quick corrections and ease of additions or rearrangement of information.
   b. Edit and proofread the draft carefully for grammatical, spelling, and punctuation errors. If the document was keyed, proofread for miskeyed information. (See Table 26-3 for correct use of proofreading marks.)
   Rationale. All business correspondence represents the image of the practice. No correspondence should be sent from the office with errors, as it will reflect poorly on the medical practice. Spelling errors and often grammatical and punctuation errors can be corrected through the "spell check" function of the word processor. Remember, however, that if a miskeyed term is an actual word, it will not be identified as an error. The spell check function of a word processor must never replace careful and thorough proofreading of a draft.
   c. Correct errors on the rough draft.
   If the rough draft was handwritten, the correspondence should now be keyed. If the rough draft was originally keyed, make corrections and save.

3. **Procedural Step. Prepare the final draft of the letter.**
   a. Set the correct line spacing and margins for attractive placement of the letter.
   b. Print a copy on plain paper and review for errors and overall appearance of the final draft.
   Rationale. This avoids wasting letterhead if you decide changes need to be made once you have reviewed the hard copy.
   c. Insert letterhead into the printer. Print a hard copy of the final draft.
   This is the copy of the correspondence that will be sent.
   d. Remove the completed document and sign it, or present it to the physician for his or her signature.
   If the document is written under the medical assistant's name, the medical assistant will sign it. Remember that the medical assistant can send out correspondence requesting information for the office. The physician should sign all other correspondence.

4. **Procedural Step. Print copy of the letter.**

5. **Procedural Step. Prepare the correspondence for mailing or electronic transmission.**
   a. Select the envelope size.
   b. Address the envelope according to postal OCR guidelines. (See Figure 26-9 for the correct method.)
   c. Tri-fold the letter with neat creases. (See Figures 26-7 and 26-8 for the correct method.)
   d. Insert the letter into the envelope. (See Figures 26-7 and 26-8 for the correct method.)
   e. Add postage.
   f. Mail the letter.
   Rationale. The appearance of the envelope is as important as the content. The envelope should be free of errors.
   NOTE: If the document is prepared for electronic transmission, the letter is sent as an e-mail attachment.

- **Full-block format** has all lines flush with the left margin, and punctuation at the end of the salutation and complimentary close is omitted. This type of formatting does not include indented paragraphs, which tend to slow a typist. This type of letter also appears more formal and businesslike.
- **Modified-block format** has all letter parts flush with the left margin. The date, closing, and signature lines are centered on the page. This type of format is more traditional and appears more balanced (Figure 26-10, *B*). The modified-block style letter with indented paragraphs of five spaces is a slight variation of this standard format.

There are other business letter styles, but currently, most correspondence is written in one of these two formats.

Memos

A **memo,** or memorandum, is written for employees within the medical office setting. Memos might provide details about an upcoming meeting or relay office policy decisions. The elements of a memo are simple and include the following:

1. *Heading.* The heading should include the name of the person receiving the memo, the sender's name, the subject, and the date. Figure 26-11 shows two different formats.
2. *Body.* The body of the memo should be typed, single-spaced, with double spacing between paragraphs.

Memo writing should be concise. Copies of all memos circulated to office staff should be filed alphabetically by subject or by date in a binder. Many offices require staff initials as proof that everyone concerned has read the memo. See Procedure 26-8 for more details about composing a memo.

Manuscript and Report Preparation

A **manuscript** is an article for a journal or other publication. You may be asked by the physician (provider) to type a manuscript describing clinical research performed in the office. In addition, you may be asked to type various kinds of procedure reports and records.

Manuscripts

A manuscript begins with an **abstract,** which provides a brief summary of each section of the manuscript. The margin settings depend on whether the document will be bound or unbound. An unbound manuscript will have a 1-inch margin all around. A bound edition will have a 1½-inch left margin to allow for binding. Each publisher or journal will have set guidelines for submission of papers to be published. Manuscripts often include but are not limited to the following sections: title, abstract, introduction, main discussion, materials and methods, results or findings and discussion, conclusion, acknowledgments, references, and appendices. Manuscripts accepted for publication must follow the strict style format set by the individual publisher.

Medical Reports

A detailed record of the patient's care is necessary every time a patient is seen in a hospital, outpatient clinic, or physician's office. This record is created when the health care provider dictates the results of tests, examinations, and procedures. Each facility will establish a format for the reports to satisfy auditing procedures and accrediting standards.

A medical office initiates the history and physical report, progress notes, and sometimes x-ray reports, whereas other report forms may be done by the hospital. Even so, it is important to be aware of the content of all types of reports because they are often copied to the medical office. Following are several types of basic medical reports used by facilities.

History and Physical Report. The **history and physical (H&P) report** is the primary document because it must be in the

Jones Medical Clinic

To: Office Staff
From: Sandy Wilton, Office Manager
Date: May 2, 20XX
Subject: Staff Meeting

On Monday, May 9, 20XX Justin Collman, a representative from the Alliance Corporation will be here to discuss the new pension and profit sharing plan.

The meeting will be held from 12 to 2 in the office library. The doctors will permit the office to be closed 2 hours, with the answering service on for patient calls. No office appointments or lab services are to be scheduled for this time.

The booklets describing the plan were mailed to each employee's home a week ago. Please read through the booklet and come prepared for any questions you might have concerning the plan.

If you are unable to attend this meeting for any reason, please notify me in advance. Thank you.

Jones Medical Clinic

To: Office Staff   Date: May 2, 20XX
From: Sandy Wilton, Office Manager   Subject: Staff Meeting

On Monday, May 9, 20XX Justin Collman, a representative from the Alliance Corporation will be here to discuss the new pension and profit sharing plan.

The meeting will be held from 12 to 2 in the office library. The doctors will permit the office to be closed 2 hours, with the answering service on for patient calls. No office appointments or lab services are to be scheduled for this time.

The booklets describing the plan were mailed to each employee's home a week ago. Please read through the booklet and come prepared for any questions you might have concerning the plan.

If you are unable to attend this meeting for any reason, please notify me in advance. Thank you.

FIGURE 26-11 Memo formats.

PROCEDURE 26-8 Compose a Memo

TASK: Compose, key, and proofread a memo.

EQUIPMENT AND SUPPLIES
- Word processor, computer with printer, or typewriter
- Paper
- Pen or pencil

SKILLS/RATIONALE

1. **Procedural Step.** Assemble all needed equipment and supplies.
   Rationale. This allows for efficient use of time and ensures the memo will be sent to the correct recipient(s).
2. **Procedural Step.** Create a memo form, or access a template file.
   Access a memo template from the word processing template file. If a template is not available for use, key a Memo Form using the guidelines below. Save the blank document for future use.
   NOTE: If using Microsoft Word, a memo template may be accessed and created by performing the following steps:
   - On the **File** menu, click **New**.
   - In the **New Document** task pane, under **New Form Template**, click **General Templates**.
   - Click the **Memos** tab.
   If you do not see the Wizard in the **Templates** dialog box, you might need to install it.
   - Follow the steps in the Wizard.
   NOTE: You can use the Memo Wizard to create a memo for printing, e-mail distribution, or faxing.
3. **Procedural Step.** Fill in the required data (see Figure 26-11).
   a. *Date:* When keying the date, use the same rules as if writing a business letter.
   b. *To:* List the names of all recipients. Names can be listed by hierarchy or alphabetically. If sending the memo to a group or department, the department or group name can be listed (e.g., All Employees, Department Managers) instead of listing individual names.
   c. *From:* List the name and title of the person sending the memo.
   d. *Subject:* Key a brief description of the purpose of the memo.
   e. *Body:* Key the memo message.
   NOTE: Salutations and closings are not used when sending memos.
4. **Procedural Step.** Ensure the format is correct.
   a. All lines of a memo are justified flush left.
   b. One-inch margins are used.
   c. The words *Date, To, From,* and *Subject* are double-spaced.
   d. The body is single-spaced, with double spacing between paragraphs.
5. **Procedural Step.** Distribute the memo.
   a. Proofread and edit the memo carefully using proofreader's marks (see Table 26-3).
   b. Make corrections as necessary.
   c. Print the memo from the computer and photocopy the required number of copies. Place a memo on each recipient's desk or in the person's "in-house" mailbox. Some facilities require the recipient to initial the memo and return it to the sender as an acknowledgment of receipt.
   NOTE: Memos can also be sent electronically in the form of e-mail or an e-mail attachment.

---

patient's medical record before treatment is initiated. In a hospital setting, the H&P must be transcribed within 24 hours of the patient's admission. Figure 26-12 provides an example of a history in full-block format. The H&P details the patient's past medical history, surgery, allergies, and social and family histories. A review of the patient's body systems is done as well. The history consists of subjective findings as related by the patient (e.g., chief complaint, symptoms), and the physical examination provides objective data as determined by the physician (e.g., vital signs, height, and weight).

Consultation Report. A physician specializing in a specific field of medicine provides **consultation reports.** The primary physician requests a consultation from another physician when his or her expertise in that disease process is needed. The consulting physician examines the patient and then dictates a report of the examination, opinions about a course of treatment, and prognosis. This report is sent to the referring physician.

Operative Report. Immediately after a surgical procedure, an **operative report** is dictated by the surgeon about the

```
                    ST. VINCENT'S HOSPITAL
                      153 West 11th Street
                     New York, NY 10011-0000

                       HISTORY AND PHYSICAL

        PATIENT: Gregory Williams              DATE: July 9, 20XX
        MEDICAL RECORD NO: 86-90-14
        PHYSICIAN: M. J. Willis, DO
```

CHIEF COMPLAINT: Gregory Williams, a 17-year-old white male, presented himself to the emergency room at 7:45 a.m. complaining that he had a pain in his abdomen, which started last evening and has persisted and worsened throughout the night.

DETAILS OF PRESENT ILLNESS: The pain was originally in the mid portion of his abdomen, but it gradually shifted and is mainly in his right lower quadrant. He had no nausea or vomiting. He ate a normal dinner, but he has had nothing by mouth since he awakened at 6:00 a.m. He did not sleep well during the night because of his discomfort. He has never had an attack like this before. His bowels have not moved. He has urinated twice without discomfort and with no effect on the abdominal pain.

PAST HISTORY: His only previous illnesses were tonsillitis, measles, and chickenpox with no complications or sequelae.

PHYSICAL EXAMINATION: Physical examination reveals a tall, thin, well-developed white male in obvious discomfort who is more uncomfortable when he moves. He is alert and answers all questions intelligently. His temperature was 99.4° F, pulse 100, blood pressure 110/78. Examination of his nose and throat were normal. Physical examination of his chest failed to show any abnormalities. Abnormal findings were primarily in the abdomen, without contact. His abdominal musculature seemed tense and he was holding himself tense. He was not breathing deeply. Excursions were flat. On abdominal palpation, his abdominal muscles were tense in the epigastrium and in the right lower quadrant. On palpation, he had severe tenderness and board-like rigidity in the lower right quadrant. Rebound tenderness was most pronounced in the right lower quadrant. Bowel sounds were not remarkable. On rectal examination, his rectum was clear and there was marked tenderness in his rectum, high on the right side. There were no hernias.

LABORATORY RESULTS: A blood count revealed a WBC of 16,000 with an increase in his differential. Urinalysis was normal.

IMPRESSION: On the basis of the blood count, history, and physical examination, a diagnosis of acute appendicitis was made and immediate operation was recommended. He agreed. Prior to operation, he had a physical examination by the surgical resident who found no contraindications to spinal anesthesia or an appendectomy.

PLAN: Gregory was admitted to the hospital and immediate appendectomy was performed.

M. J. Willis, D.O.

MJW: bp
D: 9/9/20XX
T: 9/10/20XX

FIGURE 26-12 Example of history and physical (H&P) report for patient with acute appendicitis admitted to hospital through emergency department. (Modified from Sloane S, Fordney MT: *Saunders manual of medical transcription,* Philadelphia, 1994, Saunders.)

procedure (Figure 26-13). Preoperative and postoperative diagnoses are included. The procedure done, any pathological specimens, the findings as a result of the procedure, and other personnel involved in the surgical procedure are included. All operative reports contain time anesthesia ensued, when the procedure ended, and when the patient was sent to recovery. This is primarily due to surgical suite costs.

Radiology Report. A **radiology report** describes the findings and the interpretation of all radiographs by a radiologist (Figure 26-14). Some x-ray images require a dye (contrast media), use of ultrasound, or sensitive x-ray film. Each radiology format will include the date, type of study done, ordering physician's name, age of the patient, and the findings. The report will be signed by the radiologist who interpreted the film and made a clinical judgment.

ST. VINCENT'S HOSPITAL
153 West 11th Street
New York, NY 10011-0000

OPERATIVE REPORT

PATIENT: Sharon Crawford   DATE: May 18, 20XX

MEDICAL RECORD NO: 74-34-65   ASSISTANT: Isaac Jones, M.D.

SURGEON: M. J. Willis, D.O.

ANESTHESIOLOGIST: Steven Holt, M.D.

PREOPERATIVE DIAGNOSIS: Carcinoma of the transverse colon.

POSTOPERATIVE DIAGNOSIS: Same

OPERATION: Colectomy. Colocolostomy.

PROCEDURE: Two weeks ago the patient was operated on at this hospital for an intestinal obstruction, which was due to a carcinoma of the transverse colon. A bar colostomy was performed. In the interim period, the colon was cleaned out proximally and distally. No other lesions were found.

The patient was placed on the operating table in a supine position. Anesthesia was begun with intravenous sodium Pentothal. An endotracheal tube was inserted and inhalation endotracheal anesthesia was continued throughout the operation. There was a functioning transverse colostomy in the right upper quadrant. The abdomen was doubly prepped and draped. Using sharp dissection the colostomy was freed from the skin of the abdomen. This merely freed the colostomy from the adhered abdominal skin. The abdomen was not entered. The colostomy wall was closed with interrupted silk sutures. Drapes were removed and a full new abdominal prep carried out.

The colon was freed with sharp dissection from the abdominal wall opening in the peritoneal cavity. This allowed the closed colostomy to drop into the peritoneal cavity.

The entire peritoneal cavity was examined. The liver was free of any tumor. The entire large and small bowel was examined. There was a 4 cm. irregular tumor in the mid-portion of the transverse colon encircling the colon. There was no evidence of any more tumor in the abdomen. The mesenteries were all clear of tumor. It was decided to resect en masse the tumor, the hepatic and splenic flexures, the transverse mesocolon and the omentum.

The omentum was freed, the midcolic artery was divided within 1 cm. of the superior mesenteric artery. The arcade of the hepatic flexure was divided where it came off the right colic artery. On the left side the arcade was divided at the left colic artery. Hemostasis was established. It was possible to bring the remaining right colon and left colon together in an end-to-end anastomosis. A very adequate anastomosis was made.

The rents in the mesentery were closed. Hemostasis was established. The wound was closed with interrupted silk sutures. The specimen was examined. There was adequate margin. No lymph nodes were noted.

The patient tolerated the procedure well and left the operating room in good condition. Patient discharged from the hospital with wound well healed and bowels moving satisfactorily.

M. J. Willis, D.O.

MJW: ssb
D: 5/18/20XX
T: 5/19/20XX

FIGURE 26-13 Example of operative report. (Modified from Sloane S, Fordney MT: *Saunders manual of medical transcription*, Philadelphia, 1994, Saunders.)

```
University Radiological Group, Inc.
1234 Main Street
Los Angeles, CA 90012-0000

NAME: Jane Doe  DOB: 03/17/50  RM/BD: 513301  EDP# 75033  ORD# 00034
REFERRING PHYSICIAN: John Smith, M.D.    PERFORMED BY CMK
DATE: 04/16/XXXX  TIME: 1735
MJ DATE: 04/17/XXXX  TIME: 1012
RADIOLOGIST: James Jones, M.D.
DATE AND TIME OF FINAL REPORT: 04/18/XX  1036
X-RAY# 000097959

EXAMINATION: CHEST PA & LATERAL

The heart size and contour are normal. There is streaky infiltration in the
left infraclavicular region extending back down toward the left hilar area.
There is somewhat similar interstitial infiltration in the projection of the 2nd
right anterior interspace. There are several smooth, rounded areas of
radiolucency within the infiltrate.

There are also interstitial infiltrations in the right, mid, and left paracardiac
regions.

The costophrenic angles are clear.

Impression: BILATERAL UPPER LOBE INFILTRATIONS WITH PROBABLE CAVITY
FORMATION WITH BRONCHOGENIC SPREAD TO THE RIGHT, MID, AND LEFT
LOWER LUNG FIELDS.

THE FINDINGS ARE MOST LIKELY ON THE BASIS OF TUBERCULOSIS, BUT THE
EXACT ETIOLOGY AND ACTIVITY MUST BE ESTABLISHED CLINICALLY.


_____
James Jones, M.D.


JJ/alb
D: 4/18/XX
T: 4/18/XX
```

FIGURE 26-14 Example of radiology report. (Modified from Sloane S, Fordney MT: *Saunders manual of medical transcription*, Philadelphia, 1994, Saunders.)

Discharge Summary. The **discharge summary** is a final progress note about a patient who is leaving the hospital. It is a comprehensive review of the patient's hospital stay. It also includes the patient's condition at discharge, postdischarge medications prescribed for the patient, discharge diagnosis, and instructions for follow-up care and office visits.

Autopsy Report. An **autopsy report** includes the preliminary diagnosis for a patient's cause of death, patient's medical history (if known), both internal and external examination impressions, and the results of microscopic examination of tissues. When a **necropsy** (autopsy) is done, the report should be part of the final medical record within 60 days.

Progress Notes. **Progress notes** are added to a patient's medical record each time the patient is treated. The physician records the patient's chief complaint, noting any significant aspect of the patient's condition, and the course of treatment, prescribed medications, and diagnosis. Progress notes are always recorded in chronological order, as are prescriptions, laboratory reports, and consultations (Figure 26-15).

> **ROLAND, SARA** MEDICAL RECORD NO: 678-99-08-02
>
> **SUBJECTIVE:**
> Mrs. Roland returns today for a followup of her incontinence. A review of the history with the patient today indicates that she has had stress-related incontinence for 1 or 2 years requiring the use of pads. Interestingly, the patient has had marked urinary frequency of one or two times every hour for the past 15 or possibly 20 to 25 years. She has also had nocturia two or three times a night for a long period of time. This may be somewhat worsened by the diuretics she is currently using, but I suspect that she may have had this even prior to diuretic therapy.
>
> **OBJECTIVE:**
> ABDOMEN: The physical examination today demonstrates a massively obese abdomen. There is a well-healed midline infraumbilical incision from prior hysterectomy.
>
> PELVIC: The pelvic examination demonstrates a mild cystocele and a moderate to severe rectocele. The speculum examination demonstrates no abnormalities, and the bimanual examination is not remarkable for tenderness or mass.
>
> A renal sonogram has been performed and demonstrates normal renal units bilaterally. The remainder of the abdominal sonogram is likewise unremarkable. Cystoscopy demonstrates slight descensus of the bladder neck. There is diffuse erythema throughout the bladder. Upon distention of the bladder, punctate glomerulations or hemorrhages developed. The remainder of the examination is unremarkable. No tumors or stones are appreciated. The trigone is normal. The cystometrogram demonstrates an increased residual urine of approximately 100 cc. The first sensation, however, is at 75 cc and by 200 to 250 cc, the patient has moderately severe urgency with a maximum volume threshold of only 250 cc, which is about half of the normal capacity. A Marshall test was then performed and does demonstrate definite stress-related urinary incontinence. The Bonnie, or O-Tip, test suggests urethral hypermobility with a resting angulation of 45°. With Valsalva, there is some worsening of this. The patient has definite correction of the stress-related incontinence with elevation of the bladder neck during examination.
>
> **ASSESSMENT:**
> Mrs. Roland does definitely have urethral hypermobility with stress-related urinary incontinence and a rectocele that is currently asymptomatic. Unfortunately, the patient also has severe detrusor instability, a decreased volume threshold, and changes in the bladder, which may indicate a mild form of interstitial cystitis. This would certainly explain her chronic history of frequency and her diminished bladder capacity.
>
> **PLAN:**
> I discussed the various treatment alternatives with the patient. Although a bladder neck suspension may correct the incontinence, she would still be left with urgency, frequency, and possibly an inability to void successfully and would, therefore, require intermittent catheterizations. For these reasons, I do not feel this patient is an ideal candidate for a bladder neck suspension. I will, therefore, try to treat her medically. First, I will concentrate on the urgency and the frequency. The patient was given a prescription of Ditropan, 5 mg p.o.t.i.d., p.r.n. for 1 month with refills. I will see her in 2 months. If she has had some response to this, I could consider adding Ornade to improve her bladder neck tone.
>
> D: 01-02-XX   T: 01-03-XX   Hal Griswold, M.D./mtf

FIGURE 26-15 Sample chart entry using SOAP (*s*ubjective, *o*bjective, *a*ssessment, *p*lan) format. (Modified from Sloane S, Fordney MT: *Saunders manual of medical transcription,* Philadelphia, 1994, Saunders.)

Medical Transcription

Occasionally, a medical assistant may be asked to perform the duties of a medical transcriptionist. A **transcriptionist** is a person who listens to recorded dictation and converts it to a written document. The process begins when the physician speaks into a machine (Dictaphone) and the information is recorded. The transcriptionist listens to the recorded information through a headset and keys it into a word processor (or types it using a typewriter). This action produces a printed document, which is proofread and edited.

PATIENT-CENTERED PROFESSIONALISM

- Why is it important for the medical assistant to develop good writing skills?
- Give an example of how a medical assistant's poor writing can negatively affect a patient.

CONCLUSION

A medical practice must make a good impression on patients and other people involved in its services. A good reputation is important for keeping current patients and attracting new patients. Effective communication in the medical office makes new patients feel welcome, helps established patients continue to feel important, and ultimately ensures good patient care by preventing misunderstandings and errors. In the same way, written correspondence should reflect the medical practice's high standards for patient care and effective communication. Communicating effectively with patients instills confidence and can even help ensure that patients will follow their treatment plans.

Good communication is not just something medical office professionals should "try" to do. It is something they *must* do to provide effective patient care.

Chapter Summary

Reinforce your understanding of the material in this chapter by reviewing the curriculum objectives and key content points below.

1. **Define, appropriately use, and spell all the Key Terms for this chapter.**
   - Review the Key Terms if necessary.
2. **Describe how a warm, professional greeting affects patients.**
   - A cheerful, sincere personal greeting will make patients feel welcome and put them at ease.
3. **Demonstrate the correct procedure for giving patients verbal instructions on how to locate the medical office.**
   - Review Procedure 26-1.
4. **Explain the purpose of the medical practice information booklet.**
   - All new patients should be given information about the practice's policies and services.
   - The booklet will answer questions that patients might not think to ask.
5. **Demonstrate the correct procedure for constructing a patient information brochure.**
   - Review Procedure 26-2.
6. **Describe how a medical assistant's tone of voice affects telephone conversations.**
   - A person's telephone voice projects the professional attitude of the medical office.
7. **List 12 guidelines for telephone etiquette and explain the importance of each.**
   - Using good telephone etiquette is important when promoting a positive image of the medical practice.
   - Review the lists under "Telephone Etiquette."
8. **Demonstrate the correct procedure for answering a multiline telephone system.**
   - Review Procedure 26-3.
9. **Explain the considerations for screening incoming calls.**
   - Incoming calls should be handled promptly and messages taken accurately to promote an efficient and effective medical office.
   - Emergency calls receive immediate priority.
10. **Explain the importance of a triage manual.**
    - Triage manuals (protocol guidelines) help the receptionist screen incoming calls and determine the level of urgency.
    - Refer to Table 26-1.
11. **Describe the process of placing a caller on hold when needed.**
    - Avoid placing callers on hold whenever possible.
    - Always ask permission before placing a caller on hold and wait for their answer.
    - Refer to Procedure 26-3.
12. **List the seven types of information documented when taking a phone message.**
    - It is very important to obtain the necessary information in a phone message so that the call can be returned.
    - Review Procedure 26-3.
13. **List three types of outgoing calls that administrative medical assistants may make.**
    - Confirming appointments, referrals to other physician offices, and ordering office supplies are examples of outgoing calls an administrative medical assistant may make.
    - Outgoing calls are necessary to confirm appointments and to assist in making outpatient appointments.
14. **Explain the importance for patients, medical assistants, and physicians of managing office appointments efficiently and consistently.**
    - Daily workflow depends on the accuracy of the appointment book.
    - Everyone's stress levels in the medical office are reduced when appointments are scheduled and managed effectively.
    - Patients appreciate an office that runs on time.
15. **Demonstrate the correct procedure for preparing and maintaining the office appointment book.**
    - Review Procedure 26-4.
    - Appointment books may be on paper or on the computer.
    - Appointment slots should be assigned according to the type of procedure to be done.
16. **List one method of blocking off, or reserving, time not to be used for patient scheduling.**

- Establishing a matrix is an effective way to block off time in the medical office schedule.
- Time may be blocked out for physician vacations, meetings, court appearances, and so on.

17. Explain the considerations for canceling a patient appointment.

The office may need to cancel patient appointments when:
- An emergency dictates the physician is needed elsewhere.
- Inclement weather makes traveling dangerous for patients and staff.
- Facility problems occur such as loss of electricity.

If a patient cancels an appointment:
- Make the rescheduling as convenient as possible for the patient.
- If this is a noncompliant patient pattern, it needs to be documented in the patient's record.

18. List 10 abbreviations commonly used in scheduling appointments.
- Using the correct abbreviation is vital.
- Abbreviations save time and space when keeping the schedule.
- Review Box 26-4.

19. Demonstrate the correct procedure for scheduling a new patient for an office visit.
- Review Procedure 26-5.
- Always follow the medical office's procedures for scheduling new and established patients.
- Complete name, address, telephone numbers, purpose of visit, name of referring physician, and type of insurance coverage are essential pieces of information.
- Inaccurate information gathered at the first new patient visit can generate multiple billing problems later.

20. List six appointment-scheduling techniques and explain the advantages and disadvantages of each.

There are many techniques used for scheduling, and the one chosen for the office setting should complement the available resources.
- *Time specified.* Every patient has an appointment for a definite time, so the office knows exactly how many patients to expect. The schedule runs smoothly as long as everyone shows up on time. Cancellations and no-shows leave time gaps in the schedule, resulting in underutilization of resources.
- *Wave.* Four patients are given appointments for 15-minute time slots (e.g., for 9 AM and all seen by 10 AM). Schedule is flexible and self-adjusts (eventually all four patients will be seen within the hour). If all four patients show up at exactly the same time, however, some will have to wait.
- *Modified wave.* Instead of the wave scenario, two patients are given appointments at the hour (e.g., 9 AM) and two patients at the half hour (e.g., 9:30 AM). All are seen within the hour (e.g., by 10 AM), but you are accommodating only two patients each half hour, so the patient load is better distributed than with wave. Again, late arrivals, cancellations, and no-shows will affect the schedule.
- *Stream.* Appointments are scheduled according to patient needs. When a patient needs less than 15 minutes for an appointment, another patient may also be booked into the same time slot for the same amount of time.
- *Double booking.* The time slot has two patients scheduled at the same appointment time, first come, first served. Double booking is the method least favored by patients because it often involves more waiting and patients feel rushed when they are with the physician. The advantage to the office is a "backup patient" in that time slot if the other patient scheduled cancels or is a no-show.
- *Cluster.* Several appointments for similar visits are grouped (e.g., all physicals on Fridays). This scheduling allows for better utilization of staff resources but is often inconvenient for the patient.
- *Open hour.* This method works best for walk-in clinics. No appointment is necessary; first come, first served. Advantages are patient convenience and often, evening and weekend hours. Disadvantage is not being able to predict the number of patients.

21. List two special problems that can occur in scheduling appointments and explain what can be done to prevent each.
- Cancellations and "no-shows" mean office resources are not being used optimally because the physician is waiting for the patients. No-shows should be documented in the patient medical record. Chronic late offenders should be scheduled at the end of the day, and confirming reminder calls should be made a day before the appointment.
- Emergency visits must fit into the schedule. Some offices will double book in this case or will have an allotted time in the schedule used only for emergencies.

22. Explain the purpose of an appointment reminder.
- Patients can be reminded of appointments with cards or phone calls.
- Appointment reminders minimize the number of missed appointments.

23. Demonstrate the correct procedure for scheduling a patient for outpatient diagnostic testing.
- Review Procedure 26-6.

24. Explain why it is important to sort incoming mail.
- Mail should be categorized when received according to order of importance to the recipient.
- Sorting mail in order of importance saves time for the physician.

25. List four classifications of U.S. mail.
- Understanding the classifications of mail will make it easier to process incoming mail and outgoing mail in the medical office.
- Review Box 26-5.

26. List eight special services offered by the post office that can help medical offices track, insure, and receive delivery confirmation for the mail they send.
- Special mailing services may be used depending on the type of item or correspondence being sent.
- Certified mail and return receipts must be filed in the patient chart for legal purposes.
- Review Box 26-6.

27. Demonstrate the correct preparation of an envelope.
- Envelope preparation should follow the post office guidelines to promote efficiency of delivery.
- Refer to Figures 26-7 to 26-9.

28. **Explain the proper use of a letter and a memo in medical office communication.**
    - Memos are used for interoffice communication.
    - Letters are used to communicate with those outside the medical office (patients, vendors, or other physicians).
29. **List nine guidelines for preparing effective written communication in the medical office.**
    - Plan the message.
    - Present the message positively.
    - Include all essential information.
    - Ensure clarity.
    - Use active, not passive voice ("action-oriented style").
    - Use specific language the reader will understand.
    - Use proper sentence structure.
    - Use proper paragraph structure.
    - Edit and proofread the message carefully before sending.
30. **Identify proofreader's marks used to edit written correspondence.**
    - Proofreader's marks help the proofreader see what needs to be corrected before the correspondence is sent.
    - All correspondence must be proofread before being sent out of the office.
    - Refer to Table 26-3.
31. **Demonstrate the correct procedure for composing, keying, and proofreading a business letter and preparing the envelope.**
    - Review Procedure 26-7.
    - Correct formatting of a business letter creates a good impression of the medical practice and its staff.
32. **Demonstrate the correct procedure for composing a memo.**
    - Review Procedure 26-8.
    - Memos should be clear and concise.
    - Memos are used for interoffice correspondence.
33. **Describe the format used to prepare a manuscript based on clinical research performed in the office.**
    - Manuscript preparation follows defined guidelines and styles set by individual publishers.
34. **List seven types of medical office reports and describe the purpose of each.**
    - History and physical (H&P) reports are initiated by the medical office before treatment begins.
    - Progress notes provide documentation of every patient encounter and are a record of the patient's current status, including chief complaint, course of treatment, and diagnosis.
    - Consultation reports contain information about the examination, opinions of treatment, and the patient's prognosis as rendered by a specialist or another physician asked for a second opinion.
    - Operative reports describe the surgical procedure and include pathological specimens, results, and personnel involved.
    - Radiology reports describe the findings and the interpretation of all radiographs.
    - Discharge summary is the final progress note of the patient's stay in the hospital.
    - Autopsy report includes both internal and external examination of tissues and probable cause of death.
35. **Analyze a realistic medical office situation and apply your understanding of medical office communication to determine the best course of action.**
    - How does the medical assistant's attitude and treatment of callers and patients affect the functioning of the practice?
36. **Describe the impact on patient care when medical assistants have a solid understanding of communication in the medical office.**
    - Patient perception of the medical practice is formed in part through the communication they receive.
    - Greeting patients, answering the telephone, scheduling appointments, and writing effectively will create a positive impression of the medical practice.

PRACTICAL APPLICATIONS

If you have accomplished the objectives in this chapter, you will be able to make better choices as a medical assistant. Take another look at this situation and decide what you would do.

Tara is a new medical assistant at a physician's office. Dr. Vickers has hired her to answer the phone and to greet patients as they arrive, as well as to assist with making appointments as needed. On a particularly busy day, the phone is ringing with two lines already on hold and a new patient arrives at the reception desk. Steve, the physician's assistant, asks Tara to make an appointment for another patient to see Dr. Vickers as soon as possible. Since the office makes appointments in a modified wave, Steve tells the patient to wait to be seen because Tara has found an opening in about a half hour. In all the confusion Tara does not return to the patients who are on hold for several minutes, and one of the calls is an emergency. Furthermore, Tara is short-tempered with the new patient who has arrived at the office. Tara's frustration about the busy schedule she is expected to keep shows, and the new patient states that she is not sure that she has chosen the best physician's office for her medical care.

What effect will Tara's frustration have on this medical office? How would you have handled this situation differently?

1. Why is the role of the receptionist so important in putting a patient at ease?
2. When answering the phone, what are the voice qualities that are important in making a good impression?
3. What are the guidelines necessary in answering multiline calls?
4. What information should be obtained from a patient when making appointments?
5. Why is a patient information booklet important for a new patient?
6. What is modified-wave appointment scheduling? What are the problems with this type of scheduling?
7. How should Tara have handled the callers placed on hold?

WEB SEARCH

Communication in the medical office is handled several ways. The telephone is an important tool when doing business. Creating good first impressions by using telephone techniques that make telephone conversations more effective is vital.

1. **Research additional theories on telephone techniques.** How a caller is treated provides the person with an impression about the capabilities of the medical practice.
   - **Keywords:** Use the following keywords in your search: telephone etiquette, phone etiquette.
2. **Research appointment scheduling.** For the medical office to operate smoothly, appointment scheduling must be done efficiently.
   - **Keywords:** Use the following keywords in your search: appointments, appointment quest, medical appointments.

27 Medical Records and Chart Documentation

evolve http://evlove.elsevier.com/klieger/medicalassisting

When health care professionals care for a patient, they must document what they observed and what medical services were provided. This information goes into a patient's chart, which contains the patient's medical record. The medical record includes not only examination and test results, procedures, diagnoses, and treatment plans but also information provided by the patient about his or her health and family history, current symptoms, and recent life changes. Medical records are confidential documents that must be filed carefully so the patient's information can be retrieved when needed. Handling medical records is an important part of a medical assistant's duties.

LEARNING OBJECTIVES

You will be able to do the following after completing this chapter:

Key Terms
1. Define, appropriately use, and spell all the Key Terms for this chapter.

Purpose and Contents of Medical Records
2. Explain the purpose of a medical record.
3. List the two types of medical records.
4. List three uses of the medical record.
5. Discuss the advantages and disadvantages of electronic medical records and a manual record system.
6. Explain how the medical record protects the legal interests of the patient, the health care provider, and the medical practice.
7. Demonstrate the correct procedure for pulling patient records.
8. Demonstrate the correct procedure for registering a patient.
9. List and describe seven basic forms used to start a new patient's medical record.
10. Demonstrate the correct procedure for creating a medical record for a new patient using alphabetical, color-coded tabs.
11. List five examples of forms that could be added to an established patient's medical record as care is provided.
12. Demonstrate the correct procedure for adding documents to an existing patient record.
13. Demonstrate the correct procedure for protecting the confidentiality of patients and their medical records.
14. Differentiate between *source-oriented* and *problem-oriented* records.
15. Describe where progress notes fit into the POMR format of organizing a patient's record and explain the acronym SOAP.

Charting in the Patient's Record
16. Explain the importance of documenting all services provided to the patient.
17. Identify specific actions as "Do"s or "Don't"s of charting in patients' medical records.
18. List the three steps for correcting an entry error in the patient's medical record.

Selecting a Filing System
19. State the three considerations for selecting a filing system.
20. State the three components of a filing system plan that should be recorded in detail in the office procedure manual.
21. Differentiate among vertical drawer, lateral open-shelf, lateral drawer, and movable lateral file cabinets.
22. List six supplies typically used with a manual filing system.

Filing Methods
23. List four methods of filing and briefly explain each.
24. Discuss the advantages and disadvantages of alphabetical filing.

25. List the areas addressed in the 10 rules for alphabetical filing.
26. Discuss the advantages and disadvantages of numerical filing.
27. Differentiate between *straight-number* filing and *terminal-digit* filing.

Basic Filing Procedures

28. List in order the five steps of preparing and filing medical records and briefly describe each.
29. Demonstrate the correct procedure for filing medical records using the alphabetical system.
30. Demonstrate the correct procedure for filing medical records using the numerical system.
31. Differentiate between *active* and *inactive* files.
32. Explain the need to purge files regularly in a medical practice.

Patient-Centered Professionalism

33. Analyze a realistic medical office situation and apply your understanding of charting and filing medical records to determine the best course of action.
34. Describe the impact on patient care when medical assistants understand the importance of accurate documentation and efficient filing of medical records.

KEY TERMS

acronym
active files
aging labels (year labels)
alphabetical filing
caption
charting
coding
conditioning
continuity of care
cross-reference
database
direct filing
electronic medical record (EMR)
entry
filing
guides
inactive files
indexing
indirect filing
key unit
labels
medical record
numerical filing
objective
out guides
plan
problem list
problem-oriented medical record (POMR)
progress notes
provider
purge
releasing
SOAP
sorting
source-oriented format
subjective
terminal-digit filing
tickler file
work-related injury

PRACTICAL APPLICATIONS

Read the following scenario and keep it in mind as you learn about medical records and chart documentation in this chapter.

Deanna is a new administrative medical-assisting extern at Dr. Juanea's office. Shirley, the office manager, asks Deanna to prepare a file for a new patient who will be seen tomorrow in the office. Shirley tells Deanna to be sure that she has color-coded the file folder and that the necessary forms have been included inside. In this office the medical records are problem-oriented and all records are SOAP format; both are new concepts to Deanna, who was taught to prepare source-oriented records. After Deanna has prepared the new patient's file, Shirley asks her to pull the necessary records for tomorrow's appointments from the lateral open-shelf file cabinet containing patient records filed in alphabetical order. As she pulls the records, Deanna is to annotate the patient list for tomorrow's schedule. With the assistance of Shirley, Deanna will also purge the inactive patient records.

Would you be able to perform these tasks?

PURPOSE AND CONTENTS OF MEDICAL RECORDS

Medical records are important to the functioning of a practice in many ways. It is important to understand their purpose, as well as what types of information, forms, and documentation are contained in a patient's medical record. A patient's medical record contains both administrative data (patient's name, age, sex, date of birth [DOB], insurance, consent for treatment, and a release form) and clinical data (diagnoses, therapeutic procedures, diagnostic testing results, and x-ray and operative reports).

Purpose

Medical records provide evidence of patient assessments, interventions, and communications. Since the medical record is a permanent and legal document, care must be taken to preserve its contents. File management begins when the patient is seen in the medical office and medical information is collected (e.g., family history, past history, and known allergies) and ends when the file is destroyed. The patient's record can be used for the following purposes:

- **Continuity of care** among health care providers
- Filing insurance claims
- Resolving legal matters such as lawsuits
- Future health issues of family and others

To serve its purpose, the patient's medical record must contain all the details about the patient's illness and care provided to the patient. In addition, remember that all information contained within the medical record is confidential. Only those involved in the care of the patient may discuss the patient's care. Financial information should never be placed in the patient's record because it is not information that is needed by health care **providers** for continuing care.

> **FOR YOUR INFORMATION**
>
> **DOCUMENTATION**
>
> *Keep this in mind:* **If it is not documented, it was not done.**
>
> The medical assistant must make certain all care provided, including any treatments and communications, is documented to protect the legal interests of the patient, medical practice, and the physician. Signature of the surgeon, physician, or provider is necessary to make this file legal.

Types of Medical Record Systems

Electronic Medical Record

In 2004, President Bush outlined a plan to encourage **electronic medical records (EMRs)** for Americans within 10 years. Even though several states formed *Regional Health Information Organizations (RHIO)* to create a unified network, the switch from paper charts to an EMR system has been slow. Two reasons for the delay have been the startup costs to convert to an electronic system and the time required for staff training. Progress may be forthcoming with the revision to the *Stark* anti-referral rule and anti-kickback statute by the U.S. Department of Health and Human Services (HHS) that allows hospitals to help physicians with the financial cost of EMR implementation. This change should move more physicians closer to a fully automated office.

Electronic medical records, also known as *Electronic Health Records (EHR), Personal Health Records (PHR), Electronic Patient Records (EPR),* are a complete electronic collection of an individual's health-related and personal data. These data combined with other EMR system functions related to clinical, financial, and front office management can be stored, analyzed, and distributed to health care providers to coordinate diagnosis and treatment, payers for reimbursement purposes, and so on.

Long identified as the biggest obstacle to coordination of quality patient care is the lack of access to patient information at critical times. The use of electronic medical records takes health care into the twenty-first century by decentralizing medical records and creates a system that connects physicians, hospitals, and pharmacies through a secured network. The EMR improves workflow efficiencies by allowing physicians to enter point-of-care clinical data (information) into a computer station or laptop in any facility where a patient is receiving treatment, provides timely access to patient information for other health care professionals, and reduces errors caused by illegible documentation. Typical information included within the EMR includes progress notes, radiology reports, and laboratory results.

The EMR is advantageous for the following reasons:
- All entries are legible.
- Reduces time spent on the data-collection process.
- The record can be accessed by multiple practitioners at the same time.
- Missing records do not become a problem.
- Once the information is entered into the computer, the record is instantaneously complete.
- Release of patient information to other providers and insurance companies is much easier.
- Reports are easy to generate.
- The maintenance and storage of paper records are eliminated.

Along with these benefits come responsibilities. Records must be protected by passwords to allow entry only on a "need to know" basis, and computer screens must be situated so that they are not in view of the general public. Many of the security systems and encryption protections used in the financial industry are being replicated for EMR use.

The disadvantages of EMRs, as mentioned earlier, are the startup costs and the extensive employee training. Other possible disadvantages are the numerous updates from fast-changing technology, computer viruses that can destroy data, system breakdowns that could cause loss of information, and security problems.

Manual Medical Records

Filing documents "by hand" is the most basic and oldest method of maintaining medical records. Small medical offices do well with this type of system since only a few people need access to the files; this system does not require extensive orientation. However, the records are prone to errors (e.g., misfiling), storage space becomes an issue as more records are acquired and others are purged, and the supplies are costly. As medical offices update their medical software for insurance billing and scheduling, the need to create a bridge to future EMRs will be evident.

Contents of Medical Health Records

Within each patient's medical record are several forms. The forms required for a specialty practice will vary according to the type of documentation required. The importance of these forms cannot be stressed enough because they provide the information needed to support the course of treatment (e.g., test results, consultation reports). Medical assistants need to be familiar with the type of information in a medical record, as well as the various forms a medical record may take.

Data Records

Before a patient comes to the office, the patient's file is "pulled" and an out guide is filed in its place (Procedure 27-1). If the patient is new, the patient is "registered" and a medical record is started with some basic forms (Procedure 27-2). The following are examples of information and forms included in standard file assembly:
- *Patient registration (or patient information) form* contains demographic and billing information (e.g., patient's complete name, date of birth, Social Security number, address, phone number, marital status, insurance carrier,

Medical Records and Chart Documentation CHAPTER 27

PROCEDURE 27-1 — Pull Patient Records for a Manual Record System

TASK: Before the start of the business day, pull patient records for the daily appointment schedule.

EQUIPMENT AND SUPPLIES
- Appointment book, appointment list
- Pen
- Tape
- Out guide
- Two-hole punch
- Patient records

SKILLS/RATIONALE

1. **Procedural Step.** Locate and review the day's appointment schedule in the appointment book.
2. **Procedural Step.** Generate the daily appointment list (type, photocopy, or print from the computer).
   Rationale. This provides all office personnel with a list of the appointments for the day, allowing each person to prepare for their part in providing for patients.
3. **Procedural Step.** Identify the full name of each scheduled patient and the reason for the visit.
   Rationale. The full name will be used in locating the patient's record from the office filing system.
4. **Procedural Step.** Pull the patients' records from the filing system; place a checkmark next to each patient's name on the appointment book as each record is pulled. Insert an out guide in its place, identifying user and date.
   Rationale. This determines that the correct records have been pulled and that none has been omitted.
5. **Procedural Step.** Review each record for completeness.
   Rationale. It is important that each record is thoroughly reviewed to ensure that all information has been entered correctly, that any previously ordered tests have been performed, and that the results have been returned and documented in the patient's record.
6. **Procedural Step.** Annotate the appointment list with any special considerations.
   Rationale. This alerts the physician or staff that special concerns must be addressed with the patient, such as needing to discuss scheduling a surgery or needing a copy of the patient's insurance card.
7. **Procedural Step.** Arrange all records sequentially by appointment time.
   NOTE: Some offices will arrange the schedule's patient records alphabetically. This is helpful when the patient cancels or arrives late or if another patient must be seen ahead of the scheduled time. Records are easier to access because you do not need to know the appointment time to find the record. How to organize records depends on the preference of the facility.
   Rationale. This provides an efficient and time-saving method of organizing the patient's record and ensures that everything is available for the physician before seeing the patient.
8. **Procedural Step.** Place the records in a specified location that is out of view from unauthorized persons.
   Rationale. Confidentiality of patient information must be ensured at all times, yet the records need to be in a convenient place.

and employer). This information is used for administrative office functions such as scheduling, insurance, filing, and billing statements (Figure 27-1).

- *Health history form* contains a collection of **subjective** information about the patient (e.g., description of current complaint in the patient's words, symptoms, or physical signs). This information can be obtained by the medical assistant during an interview or by having the patient fill out the form before the first appointment. It contains the chief complaint, details of the present illness, current illnesses, and social, occupational, and family history (Figure 27-2).
- *Consent to treat form* is a legal form that protects all health care personnel when caring for the patient by signifying that the patient has been informed of treatment risks and alternatives.
- *Consent to use and disclose health information form* is a form that must be signed before any patient information can be released (e.g., to the insurance company for payment).

PROCEDURE 27-2 Register a New Patient

TASK: Complete a registration form for a new patient, obtaining all required information for credit and insurance claims.

EQUIPMENT AND SUPPLIES
- Registration form (patient information form)
- Pen
- Clipboard
- Private conference area

SKILLS/RATIONALE

1. **Procedural Step.** Establish new patient status.
2. **Procedural Step.** Obtain and document the required information.
   a. Full name, birth date, name of spouse (if married)
   b. Home address, telephone number (include zip code and area code)
   c. Occupation, name of employer, business address, telephone number
   d. Social Security number and driver's license number, if any
   e. Name of referring physician, if any
   f. Name and address of person responsible for payment
   g. Method of payment
   h. Health insurance information
   i. Name of primary carrier (and secondary carrier, if applicable)
   j. Type of coverage
   k. Group policy number
   l. Subscriber number
   m. Assignment of benefits, if required

   Rationale. This information is necessary for credit and insurance claims.

3. **Procedural Step.** Review the entire form.
   Rationale. This helps to be certain that information is complete and legible.

4. **Procedural Step.** Request insurance card and make a photocopy of both sides.
   Rationale. This process verifies insurance information.

- *History and physical (H&P) form* is used by the physician to assess the patient's past problems and current state of health.
- *Progress notes* entered into the patient's record are used to update the status of the patient's health. Included with each **entry** (a written description of what care was provided for the patient) are the date and time, as well as the signature and credentials of the person charting. This is done each time the patient is seen by a health care provider. Progress notes include the patient's current symptoms (chief complaint) as documented by the medical assistant, vital signs, diagnosis if known, treatment plan, and evaluation of plan to date. These are all documented by the health care provider.
- *Medication log* is a list of the current medications taken by the patient. A notation should also be made to include over-the-counter (OTC) medications and herbal and natural preparations.

Forms added to an established patient's medical record as services are provided could include radiographic reports, laboratory reports, pathology reports, diagnostic procedures, consultation reports, and hospital reports, such as discharge summaries (Figure 27-3).

Procedure 27-3 outlines the creation of a patient file.

Procedure 27-4 shows how to add items to an established medical record. As each document is added to the patient's record, the latest information is always placed on top in chronological order because it indicates the patient's current status.

NOTE: If an established patient sees the physician for a **work-related injury,** a new file must be made because all health information before the injury is *not* to be made available to the employer.

NOTE: If any patient has a legal issue pending for or against your provider a new file must be made titled "Legal Chart" and only information related to the litigation is placed into the new chart.

Text continued on p. 524

REGISTRATION
(PLEASE PRINT)

GEORGE WHITE, M.D.
234 ANY STREET
SOMEWHERE, USA 50000
TELEPHONE: (123) 456-7890

Home Phone: _____

Today's Date: _____

PATIENT INFORMATION

Name _____ Soc. Sec.# _____
     Last Name   First Name   Initial

Address _____

City _____ State _____ Zip _____

Cell Phone _____ E-mail: _____ Fax #: _____

Single ____ Married ____ Widowed ____ Separated ____ Divorced ____ Sex M ____ F ____ Age ____ Birthdate _____

Patient Employed by _____ Occupation _____

Business Address _____ Business Phone _____

By whom were you referred? _____

In case of emergency who should be notified? _____ Phone _____
                                              Name   Relation to Patient

PRIMARY INSURANCE

Person Responsible for Account _____
                                Last Name   First Name   Initial

Relation to Patient _____ Birthdate _____ Soc. Sec.# _____

Address (if different from patient's) _____ Phone _____

City _____ State _____ Zip _____

Person Responsible Employed by _____ Occupation _____

Business Address _____ Business Phone _____

Insurance Company _____

Contract # _____ Group # _____ Subscriber # _____

Name of other dependents covered under this plan _____

ADDITIONAL INSURANCE

Is patient covered by additional insurance? ____ Yes ____ No

Subscriber Name _____ Relation to Patient _____ Birthdate _____

Address (if different from patient's) _____ Phone _____

City _____ State _____ Zip _____

Subscriber Employed by _____ Business Phone _____

Insurance Company _____ Soc. Sec.# _____

Contract # _____ Group # _____ Subscriber # _____

Name of other dependents covered under this plan _____

ASSIGNMENT AND RELEASE

I, the undersigned, certify that I (or my dependent) have insurance coverage with _____
                                                                                   Name of Insurance Company(ies)
and assign directly to Dr. _____ insurance benefits, if any, otherwise payable to me for services rendered. I understand that I am financially responsible for all charges whether or not paid by insurance. I hereby authorize the doctor to release all information necessary to secure the payment of benefits. I authorize the use of this signature on all insurance submissions.

_____   _____   _____
Responsible Party Signature   Relationship   Date

ORDER # 58-8425 • © 1996 BIBBERO SYSTEMS, INC. • PETALUMA, CALIFORNIA • TO REORDER CALL TOLL FREE: (800) 242-2376 OR FAX: (800) 242-9330   (REV. 12/06)

FIGURE 27-1 Example of information sheet for a new patient. (Form # 58-8425-P courtesy Bibbero Systems, Inc., Petaluma, CA; (800) 242-2376; fax (800) 242-9330; www.bibbero.com.)

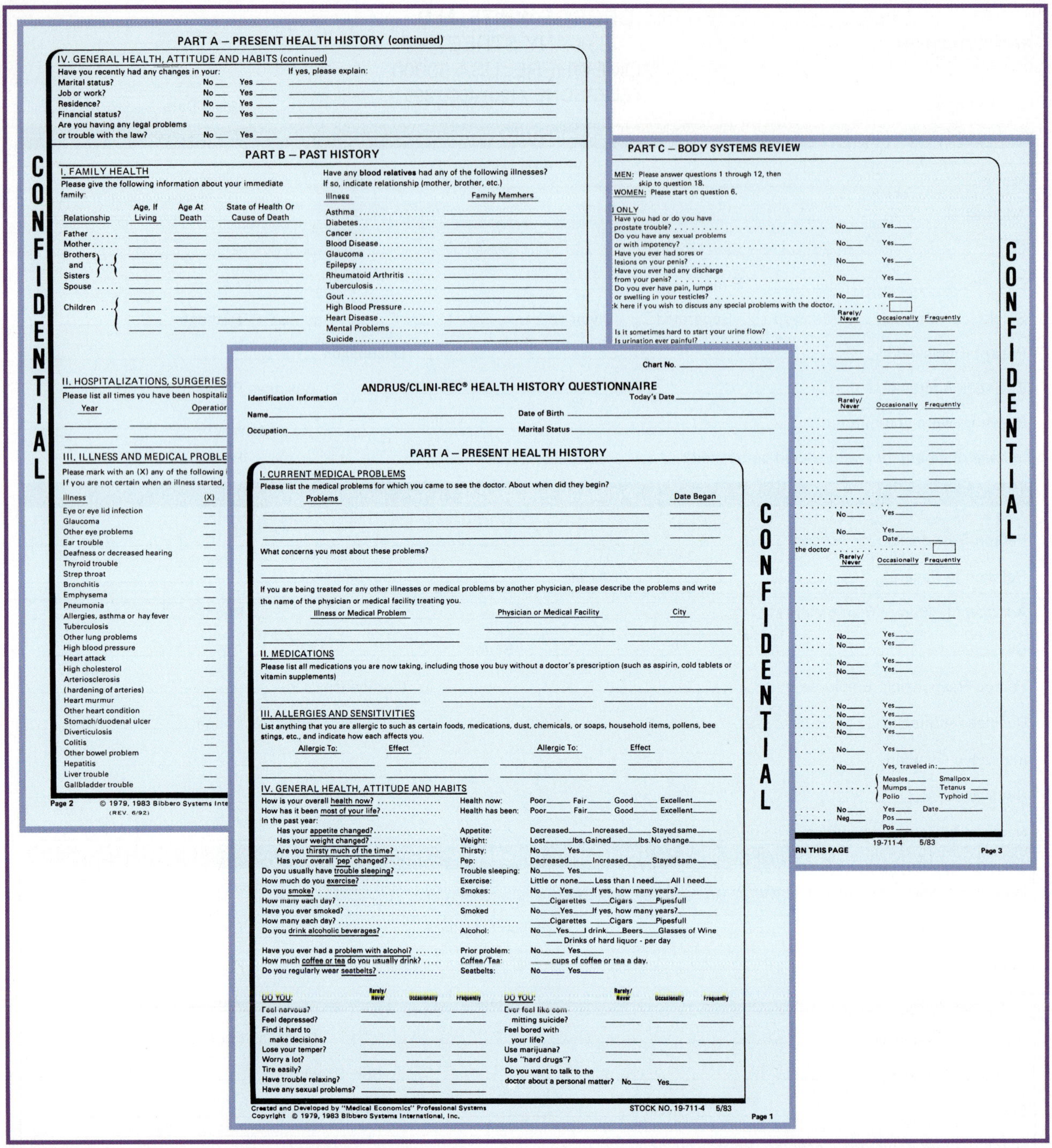

PART A – PRESENT HEALTH HISTORY (continued)

IV. GENERAL HEALTH, ATTITUDE AND HABITS (continued)

Have you recently had any changes in your: If yes, please explain:

Marital status? No ___ Yes ___

Job or work? No ___ Yes ___

Residence? No ___ Yes ___

Financial status? No ___ Yes ___

Are you having any legal problems or trouble with the law? No ___ Yes ___

PART B – PAST HISTORY

I. FAMILY HEALTH

Please give the following information about your immediate family:

Relationship	Age, If Living	Age At Death	State of Health Or Cause of Death
Father			
Mother			
Brothers and Sisters			
Spouse			
Children			

Have any **blood relatives** had any of the following illnesses? If so, indicate relationship (mother, brother, etc.)

Illness	Family Members
Asthma	
Diabetes	
Cancer	
Blood Disease	
Glaucoma	
Epilepsy	
Rheumatoid Arthritis	
Tuberculosis	
Gout	
High Blood Pressure	
Heart Disease	
Mental Problems	
Suicide	

II. HOSPITALIZATIONS, SURGERIES

Please list all times you have been hospitaliz

Year Operation

III. ILLNESS AND MEDICAL PROBLE

Please mark with an (X) any of the following

If you are not certain when an illness started,

Illness	(X)
Eye or eye lid infection	
Glaucoma	
Other eye problems	
Ear trouble	
Deafness or decreased hearing	
Thyroid trouble	
Strep throat	
Bronchitis	
Emphysema	
Pneumonia	
Allergies, asthma or hay fever	
Tuberculosis	
Other lung problems	
High blood pressure	
Heart attack	
High cholesterol	
Arteriosclerosis (hardening of arteries)	
Heart murmur	
Other heart condition	
Stomach/duodenal ulcer	
Diverticulosis	
Colitis	
Other bowel problem	
Hepatitis	
Liver trouble	
Gallbladder trouble	

Page 2 © 1979, 1983 Bibbero Systems Inte (REV. 6/92)

CONFIDENTIAL

PART C – BODY SYSTEMS REVIEW

MEN: Please answer questions 1 through 12, then skip to question 18.
WOMEN: Please start on question 6.

ONLY

Have you had or do you have prostate trouble? No___ Yes___

Do you have any sexual problems or with impotency? No___ Yes___

Have you ever had sores or lesions on your penis? No___ Yes___

Have you ever had any discharge from your penis? No___ Yes___

Do you ever have pain, lumps or swelling in your testicles? No___ Yes___

k here if you wish to discuss any special problems with the doctor. ☐

Rarely/Never Occasionally Frequently

Is it sometimes hard to start your urine flow?

Is urination ever painful?

Yes, traveled in: Measles Mumps Polio Smallpox Tetanus Typhoid

Yes___ Date___

RN THIS PAGE 19-711-4 5/83 Page 3

CONFIDENTIAL

Chart No. ___

ANDRUS/CLINI-REC® HEALTH HISTORY QUESTIONNAIRE

Identification Information Today's Date ___

Name ___ Date of Birth ___

Occupation ___ Marital Status ___

PART A – PRESENT HEALTH HISTORY

I. CURRENT MEDICAL PROBLEMS

Please list the medical problems for which you came to see the doctor. About when did they begin?

Problems Date Began

What concerns you most about these problems?

If you are being treated for any other illnesses or medical problems by another physician, please describe the problems and write the name of the physician or medical facility treating you.

Illness or Medical Problem | Physician or Medical Facility | City

II. MEDICATIONS

Please list all medications you are now taking, including those you buy without a doctor's prescription (such as aspirin, cold tablets or vitamin supplements)

III. ALLERGIES AND SENSITIVITIES

List anything that you are allergic to such as certain foods, medications, dust, chemicals, or soaps, household items, pollens, bee stings, etc., and indicate how each affects you.

Allergic To: Effect Allergic To: Effect

IV. GENERAL HEALTH, ATTITUDE AND HABITS

How is your overall health now? Health now: Poor___ Fair___ Good___ Excellent___

How has it been most of your life? Health has been: Poor___ Fair___ Good___ Excellent___

In the past year:

Has your appetite changed? Appetite: Decreased___ Increased___ Stayed same___

Has your weight changed? Weight: Lost___ lbs. Gained___ lbs. No change___

Are you thirsty much of the time? Thirsty: No___ Yes___

Has your overall 'pep' changed? Pep: Decreased___ Increased___ Stayed same___

Do you usually have trouble sleeping? Trouble sleeping: No___ Yes___

How much do you exercise? Exercise: Little or none___ Less than I need___ All I need___

Do you smoke? Smokes: No___ Yes___ If yes, how many years?___

How many each day? ___ Cigarettes ___ Cigars ___ Pipesfull

Have you ever smoked? Smoked: No___ Yes___ If yes, how many years?___

How many each day? ___ Cigarettes ___ Cigars ___ Pipesfull

Do you drink alcoholic beverages? Alcohol: No___ Yes___ I drink___ Beers___ Glasses of Wine ___ Drinks of hard liquor - per day

Have you ever had a problem with alcohol? Prior problem: No___ Yes___

How much coffee or tea do you usually drink? Coffee/Tea: ___ cups of coffee or tea a day.

Do you regularly wear seatbelts? Seatbelts: No___ Yes___

DO YOU:	Rarely/Never	Occasionally	Frequently
Feel nervous?			
Feel depressed?			
Find it hard to make decisions?			
Lose your temper?			
Worry a lot?			
Tire easily?			
Have trouble relaxing?			
Have any sexual problems?			

DO YOU:	Rarely/Never	Occasionally	Frequently
Ever feel like committing suicide?			
Feel bored with your life?			
Use marijuana?			
Use "hard drugs"?			

Do you want to talk to the doctor about a personal matter? No___ Yes___

CONFIDENTIAL

Created and Developed by "Medical Economics" Professional Systems
Copyright © 1979, 1983 Bibbero Systems International, Inc.
STOCK NO. 19-711-4 5/83 Page 1

FIGURE 27-2 General health history questionnaire. (Form # 19-711-4 courtesy Bibbero Systems, Inc., Petaluma, CA; (800) 242-2376; fax (800) 242-9330; www.bibbero.com.)

PROCEDURE 27-3

Initiate a Patient File for a New Patient Using Color-Coded Tabs

TASK: Set up and organize a file that contains the personal data necessary for a complete record and any other information required by the medical office for a new patient. This should be done using an alphabetical, color-coded filing system.

EQUIPMENT AND SUPPLIES
- File folder (end tab/top tab)
- A-Z color-coded tabs (self-adhesive)
- Blank file label (self-adhesive)
- Color-coded year label (annual age-dating label)
- Medical alert or other label types, as appropriate
- Forms:

Patient information
Assignment of benefits
Waiver
Treatment authorizations
Referral slips
Health history
Progress notes
Visit log
Ledger card/computer software program

Prescription flow sheet
Laboratory reports
Diagnostic reports
Consultation reports
Hospital discharge summaries
Surgery reports
Miscellaneous correspondence
Encounter form

SKILLS/RATIONALE

1. **Procedural Step.** Obtain and review a completed patient information form.
   Rationale. This document provides basic demographic and billing and insurance information. Reviewing the form verifies that personal data and insurance information are complete.

2. **Procedural Step.** Select the appropriate folder and place the completed and reviewed form on the left inside cover of the file, using the method preferred by the medical facility (see Figure 27-1).
   Rationale. Placing the patient information on the left inside cover of the medical file helps medical assistants and others using the file to find and verify information quickly and keeps demographic information separate from the medical record.

3. **Procedural Step.** Place a progress note form and prescription flow sheet on the inside right cover of the file with the progress note form on top. File additional forms in reverse chronological order, meaning the most recent on top, followed by the next most recent, and so forth. Label each form with the patient's name.
   Rationale. Documents typically included on the right inside cover of a file pertain directly to patient care. Filing these forms in reverse chronological order allows for the most current event or treatment to be on top and most easily accessible. Making certain the patient's name is on each form minimizes the chance of misfiling documents if a form/document falls out of the chart.

PROGRESS NOTES	Patient: Andrews, Sophia
	NKA
6/4/- -	S: Patient complains of bilateral temporal headaches for the past 2 days. Worse in evenings. OTC meds do not seem to help. Some visual blurring and nausea.
	O: T 98.6°F P 86. reg R 16 BP 168/98® /G.Chester, CMA (AAMA)
	A: Overall Exam WNL: Eyegrounds also WNL.: Heart and lungs clear to auscultation Diagnosis: Hypertensive cephalgia
3	P: 1) Lopressor 50 mg. Take 1 hs # 30 no refills/Rx to patient/G. Chester, CMA (AAMA) 2) Reduce salt intake Na diet to patient /G. Chester, CMA (AAMA) 3) Call if cephalgia not relieved within 4 days 4) Re-check in 7 months, appt given for 7-2-XX /G.Chester, CMA (AAMA) GC

4. **Procedural Step.** Create a file label.
   Indent three spaces from the left edge of the label on the second line from the top of the label, then type/key in the patient's last name and first name, followed by the middle initial and any title on the file label. This is referred to as *indexing order*. Some offices will include the date of birth (DOB).

Continued

PROCEDURE 27-3 Initiate a Patient File for a New Patient Using Color-Coded Tabs—cont'd

Rationale. By formatting the file folder labels the same way for each patient, using correct indexing order, filing is neater, more consistent, and more efficient and retrieving files is simpler.

5. **Procedural Step.** Attach the file label in the center of the file tab.
6. **Procedural Step.** Attach alphabetical, color-coded labels.
   Identify the first two letters of the patient's last name (e.g., "Jones" would be J and O) and apply on either the lower or upper portion of the end tab (depending on office policy), below the file label.
   NOTE: Some offices will also use the patient's DOB.
   Identify the first initial of the patient's first name and place this letter tab ¼ inch above the file label.
   NOTE: Some offices will not use the first initial.
   NOTE: Label placement can differ from office to office.
   Rationale. Using the first initial will assist in locating files, especially for patients with the same last name.

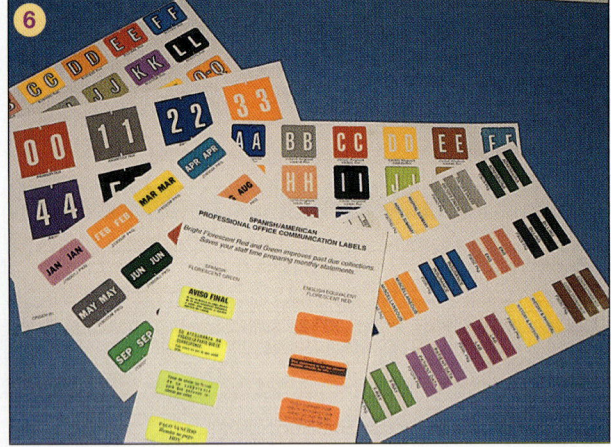

7. **Procedural Step.** Attach the current year "aging" label above the first-name initial tab.
   Rationale. The year label identifies the year in which the patient was last seen.
8. **Procedural Step.** Compile the file. Place the patient information, health history, and other forms in the patient's file.
9. **Procedural Step.** Attach a "Medical Alert" label on the front of the file.
   Rationale. If the patient has identified a medical condition (e.g., allergy, diabetes, pacemaker, etc.) on the patient information form, a medical alert label must be placed on the front of the file to alert all medical personnel.
10. **Procedural Step.** Prepare a ledger card or enter the patient information into a computerized management program.
    Rationale. A ledger card is basically a place to keep a record of all services and fees, insurance payments, patient payments, insurance adjustments, and to maintain the patient's current balance. A computer software program, such as Lytec or Medisoft, can automate this process.
11. **Procedural Step.** Attach an encounter form (superbill) to the outside of the patient's file.
    Rationale. This form is attached before the patient sees the physician and provides a place for the physician to indicate the charges for the visit.

Left Inside

Patient information sheet
Prescription sheet
Assignment of benefits
Visit log
Treatment authorizations and referral slips
HIPAA Consent form

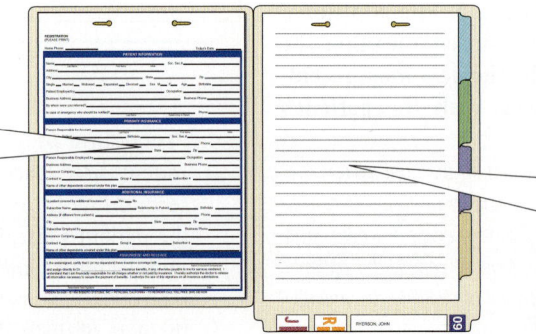

Right Inside

Progress notes
Most recent physical examination
Laboratory reports
Diagnostic tests
Consultations
Hospital discharge summaries
Surgery reports
Medical records from other facilities
Correspondence

FIGURE 27-3 Contents of a medical record. (Modified from Hunt SA: *Saunders fundamentals of medical assisting—revised reprint,* St Louis, 2007, Saunders.)

PROCEDURE 27-4

Add Supplementary Items to an Established Patient File

TASK: Add supplemental documents and progress notes to patient files, observing standard steps in filing while creating an orderly file that facilitates ready reference to any item of information.

EQUIPMENT AND SUPPLIES
- Patient file
- Assorted documents (e.g., H&P form and laboratory, diagnostic testing, and procedural reports)
- Stapler
- Clear tape
- Two-hole punch
- Alphanumerical sorter

SKILLS/*RATIONALE*

1. **Procedural Step. Retrieve the appropriate patient file from the file storage area.**
   Rationale. This ensures that supplemental forms are filed in the correct patient's file.

2. **Procedural Step. Condition the document.**
   Remove all extraneous materials such as paper clips or pins, mend any tears with tape, staple related pages together, and punch holes if needed.
   Rationale. Conditioning a document ensures that it is in good condition and is processed and ready to be filed. Leaving paper clips on documents causes the document to become attached to other nonrelated materials.

3. **Procedural Step. Release the document.**
   Be sure the document has been marked that it has been reviewed by the appropriate person and it is ready for filing. This mark may be a person's initials, a checkmark, or a "FILE" stamp.
   Rationale. Most medical offices have a policy that physicians need to review all reports and then initial them before they are filed. This helps ensure that the physician has seen the report and that it was not accidentally overlooked before filing.

4. **Procedural Step. Index and code the document.**
   Indexing refers to deciding where a document needs to be filed such as in a medical record or elsewhere (e.g., office accounting file). *Coding* refers to writing on or marking a document to indicate how it should be filed (e.g., by patient last name) once you have determined where it should be filed (indexing).
   Rationale. This ensures that the document is correctly filed for easy retrieval for future reference.

5. **Procedural Step. Sort documents for filing.**
   Arrange documents and papers in proper filing sequence before taking them to the filing storage area where they will be filed. Some offices will use a "desktop sorter" to facilitate this process. (A desktop sorter has a series of dividers between which papers are placed in filing sequence.) Sorters typically have different means of classification to allow you to sort in multiple ways (e.g., alphabetically, numerically, or days of the week).
   Rationale. The use of a sorter makes the filing process much more efficient because it saves the medical assistant time, and the sorting can be accomplished while sitting at a desk in between answering phones and greeting patients.

6. **Procedural Step. Open fasteners and file each document according to categories into the established patient's file, with the most recent document on top. Close fasteners to secure chart documents.**

7. **Procedural Step. Return the file to the storage cabinet.**
   Rationale. Adding documents to a file in reverse order ensures the most current information is readily accessible.

FOR YOUR INFORMATION

OWNERSHIP

The physician owns the medical record, but the patient owns the information. The Health Insurance Portability and Accountability Act (HIPAA) Privacy Rule gives the patient the right to examine and obtain a copy of their health information and request corrections. This rule requires health care providers to notify patients about their privacy rights, implement privacy policies and procedures, and secure patient records and information so they are not available to unauthorized personnel. See Box 27-1 for more information.

Procedure 27-5 explains the legal implications associated with confidentiality issues regarding patients and their medical records.

BOX 27-1

Documentation and HIPAA Regulations

1. If patient care is not documented, it is as though it did not happen.
2. Health Insurance Portability and Accountability Act (HIPAA) regulations protect the privacy of personal health records by limiting access to a patient's medical records.
3. HIPAA regulations require providers to issue a written statement to each patient informing them about how the patient's health information may be used.
4. Patients have a right to review their medical records, seek corrections, and/or receive a copy of their medical record.
5. The patient's "Protected Health Information" (PHI) cannot be revealed without the patient's consent, and only on a need-to-know basis. This includes written, verbal, and electronic communications of PHI.
6. Patient files must not be out in the open where a patient's name could be seen. Files must be held in a secure area away from view (e.g., in file holder facing backward).
7. When employees are away from their desk, patient information cannot be left on a computer screen or displayed by an open file left on the desk or a message book left open for viewing.
8. All patient appointment schedules must be in a secure location. Schedules cannot be taped to the wall in the examination room, hallway, or any place that another can view a patient's name.

Format Guidelines

There are still a large percentage of medical offices that continue to use a paper-based medical record. As technologies advance and the costs of computerized medical records become affordable, electronic records will become more prominent. Computerized methods are already becoming the norm in large facilities. Both types of medical records have the capabilities of either the source-oriented format or the problem-oriented format.

Stored medical paper-based charts can be shredded after they are scanned to computer disk/digital versatile disk (CD/DVD). Maintenance of methods to retrieve the charts is essential in the changing type of storage.

Source-Oriented Record. When a medical office uses the **source-oriented format** to organize a medical record, the record has dividers to separate the medical information. Each divider has a color tab with the heading of the section on it. When a document is added to a section, the most recently dated document is placed on top. Typical dividers include the following:

1. History and physical examination
   - Summary of family medical history, social history, patient's history of disease and injury
   - Objective observations regarding all activity of the patient
2. Progress notes
   - Current observations and patient's discussion of signs and symptoms
3. Medications
   - Current and OTC medications and herbal preparations
   - Description of body tissue sent to a laboratory
   - Results of patient's radiological study (e.g., x-ray, magnetic resonance imaging (MRI), computed tomography (CT) scan, or nuclear medicine)
   - Ancillary reports (e.g., laboratory, pathology, or radiology)
4. Operative reports
   - Detailed account of patient's surgical procedure, including types of incision and instruments and techniques used
5. Correspondence
   - Letters to the physician from the patient, consultations, referral reports, etc.

When a physician wants to review a specific report, the appropriate tab is located, and the report can easily be reviewed. The source-oriented format is used most frequently in medical offices and hospitals.

Problem-Oriented Record. The **problem-oriented medical record (POMR)** is arranged according to the patient's health complaint. Each complaint is seen as a problem or condition that needs further action (e.g., treatment, patient education). The following four stages are used to resolve a problem when using the POMR format of organizing a patient's health record:

1. A **database** (information source) is established. This is composed of subjective information (thoughts, feelings, ideas) and **objective** information (concrete facts) identified in the patient interview and obtained during the health history, chief complaint, present illness, physical examination, laboratory procedures, and diagnostic tests. This information will be stored in paper files or, in larger facilities where electronic charting is done, in a computer database.
2. Using the information provided by the database identifies a **problem list** (Figure 27-4). Each problem is given a specific number and is used when referring to all treatments performed and diagnostic testing conducted for the problem.

Medical Records and Chart Documentation CHAPTER 27 525

PROCEDURE 27-5: Maintain Confidentiality of Patients and Their Medical Records

TASK: Explain through role playing how confidentiality of patient issues and their medical records is maintained.

EQUIPMENT AND SUPPLIES
- Authorization form for "Release of Medical Records"

SKILLS/RATIONALE

1. **Procedural Step.** Select a partner to be a patient as you assume the role of the administrative medical assistant.
   Rationale. This provides you with the opportunity to interact one-on-one when explaining the procedures involved in maintaining patient confidentiality.

2. **Procedural Step.** Explain to the "patient" through role playing how the integrity of confidences shared in the office is maintained regarding the following medical office topics:
   a. Attorneys calling the office to gain information about a patient.
   b. Release of information about a minor.
   c. Advertising and media.
   d. Computerized medical records.
   Rationale. The partner should assume these roles and ask questions pertaining to each of the topics, providing you, the medical assistant, with the opportunity to explain each situation.

3. **Procedural Step.** Explain to the "patient" through role playing how confidences shared in the office are maintained regarding the following specialty topics:
   a. Child abuse.
   b. Sexually transmitted diseases (STDs).
   c. Sexual assault.
   d. Mental health.
   e. AIDS and HIV.
   f. Substance abuse.
   Rationale. The "patient" should assume roles and ask questions regarding these topics, providing you, the medical assistant, with the opportunity to explain each situation.

4. **Procedural Step.** Explain to the "patient" through role playing how the following situations regarding confidentiality issues are handled in the medical office:
   a. Subpoenaed medical records.
   b. HIPAA guidelines.
   c. Areas of mandated disclosure by state and federal regulations.
   Rationale. This provides you with the opportunity to practice explaining sensitive information with a patient and answering patient questions.

5. **Procedural Step.** Explain to the "patient" through role playing the "Patient's Bill of Rights."
   Rationale. This provides you with the opportunity to learn and comprehend patients' rights so that you are confident in presenting this information to a patient.

6. **Procedural Step.** Explain to the "patient" through role playing and complete an authorization form for release of medical records.
   Rationale. This provides you with the opportunity to understand how medical records are released so that you are confident in presenting this information to a patient.

7. **Procedural Step.** Place original release of medical records in the correspondence section of a patient's medical record.

8. **Procedural Step.** Document in the patient's chart that the release of information form was processed.

---

3. A **plan** of action is created for each problem. This may include laboratory and diagnostic tests, patient education, and treatment (e.g., starting medication regimen).

4. **Progress notes** follow each identified problem in a **SOAP** format (Figure 27-5). Progress notes start with each problem numbered and include the following four categories:
   - *Subjective data.* Information provided by the patient as to why he or she came to see the physician, referred to as the chief complaint (e.g., "I'm dizzy," "my stomach hurts").
   - *Objective data.* The objective information obtained through the physical examination and the review of symptoms, or any information that is observed (e.g., rash, fever).
   - *Assessment.* The assessment of the clinical diagnosis, or final diagnosis based on the information found from the chief complaint, the physical examination (e.g., physi-

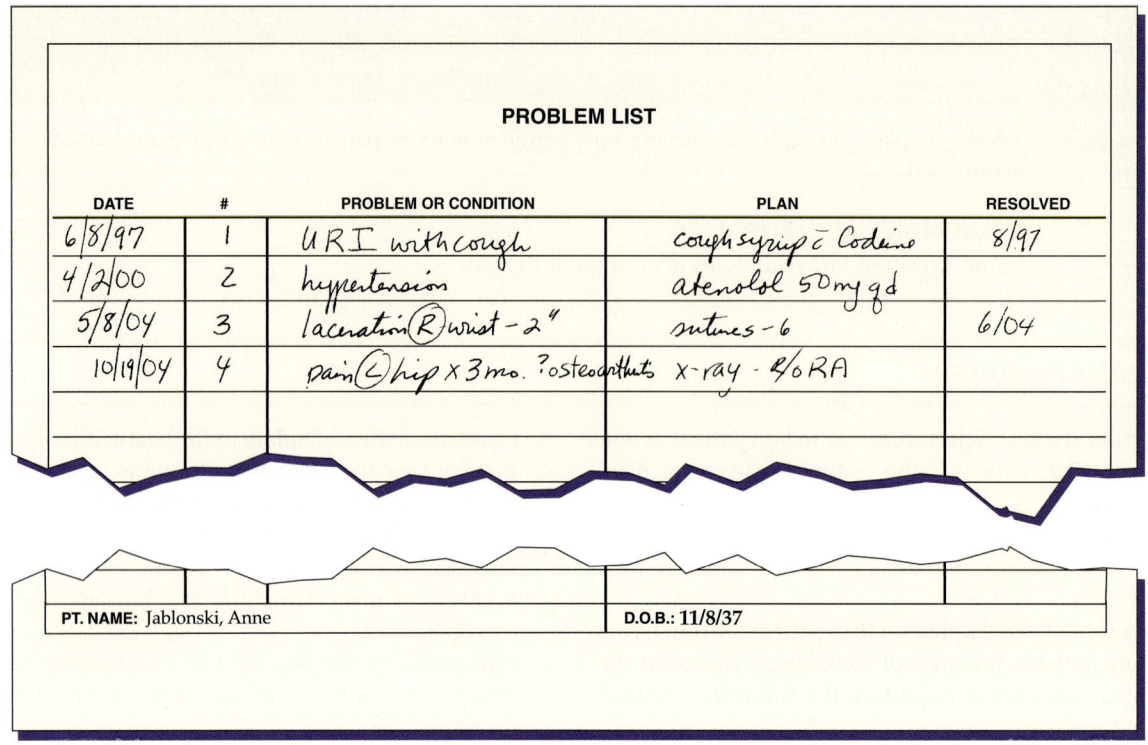

FIGURE 27-4 Example of a problem list. (Modified from Hunt SA: *Saunders fundamentals of medical assisting—revised reprint,* St Louis, 2007, Saunders.)

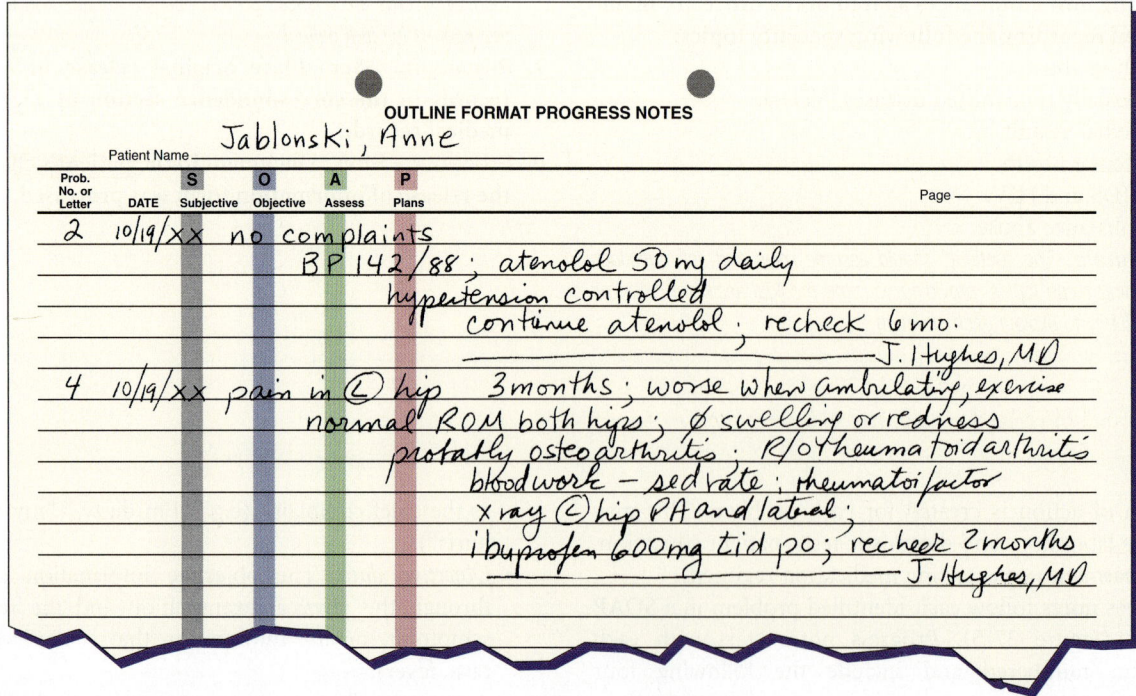

FIGURE 27-5 Example of SOAP charting related to a problem list. (Modified from Hunt SA: *Saunders fundamentals of medical assisting—revised reprint,* St Louis, 2007, Saunders.)

cian's conclusion of reported problem based on data presented), and the results of the laboratory and radiologic tests. Assessing all the information provided allows the physician to arrive at a diagnosis.
- *Plan.* The plan of action, or the treatment action to be taken (e.g., antibiotics for 7 days).

POMR formatting is extremely advantageous when more than one physician is (or will be) treating the patient because all information pertaining to a specific "problem" can be located in a concise format. Information that does not fit into the SOAP format can be written in paragraph form as a chart note within the progress note.

PATIENT-CENTERED PROFESSIONALISM

- What is the possible outcome if the legal, ethical, and moral standards of records management are not followed?
- What purpose do the various data forms serve?
- What formats are used for documentation in a patient's medical record?

CHARTING IN THE PATIENT'S RECORD

Charting is the process of documenting events in written form. It is an important part of the patient's care because it communicates the patient's condition and the care received. All office visits, telephone calls, and other interactions with the patient must be documented. Since the patient's record is a legal document, it is the medical practice's best defense against lawsuits and provides documentation for third-party payers. For these reasons, charting must be legible and accurate. Remember, if it was not documented it did not happen and if it was not signed it did not happen. Signatures are important to be able to identify the author, give credit, and maintain exacting information and who did it. Corrections to the record must be made according to established guidelines.

Guidelines

Charting must communicate that the patient has been provided quality care and medically necessary services. All services provided must be documented, even if the service is not billable; for example, phone calls made and diagnostic procedures scheduled are not billable, but they must be documented to show continuity of patient care.

The medical assistant frequently is responsible for recording results of procedures performed. When all members of the health care team document all relevant information in the medical record, patient care is improved and fully reimbursed and the provider is protected legally. See Box 27-2 for charting "do"s and "don't"s.

The ultimate goal is to provide accurate, legible, consistent, and concise entries. If an entry is illegible (paper-based), the

BOX 27-2
Charting "Do"s and "Don't"s

DO:
- Verify the name on the file before charting.
- Check to be certain the patient's name appears on each document page. The name should be in place prior to filing.
- Begin all entries with the date and time. Conclude with your signature and credentials.
- Use black ink because it is easier to photocopy.
- Use military time to avoid confusion (Box 27-3) if this is office policy.
- Chart all pertinent observations. Use patient quotes when possible.
- Write neatly and legibly, using proper grammar and approved abbreviations. (Wording must be accurate, clear, and concise.)
- Chart the plan of care and the physician's orders that were done, with the results and the patient's responses immediately after the procedure.
- Chart all patient teaching, precautions, and assessments of the patient's understanding.
- Chart patient's noncompliance or failure to follow treatment.
- Fill in all blank spaces and lines on a preprinted form, even if you only add "N/A" (not applicable) or draw a line through the space.
- Chart as soon as care is given; never wait and chart later.
- All entries must be signed.

DON'T:
- Rely on memory to chart important information.
- Criticize treatment in the notes.
- Draw conclusions or make assumptions.
- Add procedures done previously to the chart.
- Erase or alter chart notes in any way.
- Chart anything you did not see or do.
- Change the patient's wording.
- Use abbreviations that are not standard and approved by the office.
- Leave empty spaces at the end of a line.
- Skip lines between entries.
- Leave space before your signature.
- Guess at spelling.

fact that the service was provided cannot be established; it is as though it were never provided or documented at all and a misinterpretation of the procedure could result. Chart all entries in black ink because black ink photocopies the best. (Different offices may have different procedures; many facilities allow *only* black ink, whereas some institutions require blue ink because it also photocopies well and makes it easier to identify the "original" entry.)

All entries in a patient's record should begin with the date of the encounter. A line should be drawn at the end of the entry to the space for the signature to prevent information

BOX 27-3

Samples of Standard and Military Time

Standard	Military	Standard	Military
1:00 AM	0100	1:30 PM	1330
9:20 AM	0920	2:00 PM	1400
10:10 AM	1010	3:45 PM	1545
11:00 AM	1100	4:15 PM	1615
Noon	1200	Midnight	2400

A method used to convert military time into standard time is to subtract 2 from any given time after noon. Remove the first digit from the military time and subtract 2. For example:

1300 = 300 − 2 = 1 PM or After 12 noon, add 1200 to
1700 = 700 − 2 = 5 PM the hour and convert minutes 1:30 = 130 + 1200 or 1330

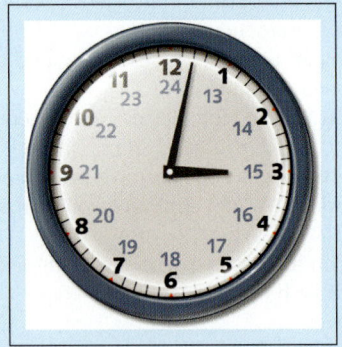

Illustration from Gerdin J: *Health careers today*, ed 3, St Louis, 2003, Mosby.

from being inserted at a later date. Each computer-based program has a method designed for their software.

Box 27-4 lists the charting information needed for complete documentation in a patient record.

Correction Procedures

When charting, the medical assistant may find it necessary to make corrections on the patient's paper-based medical record. *Never* use correction fluid (e.g., Wite-Out) or erase in the medical record. The proper way to correct an entry follows (Figure 27-6):

1. Draw a line through the error.
2. Insert the correction above the error.
3. In the margin, write "correction" or "corr" ("error" or "err" is also used), your initials (or first initial last name in full), and the date.

NOTE: The appropriate correction procedure may be subject to the medical practice's policy; some practices may require you to write your name in full when making a correction, not just your initials.

PATIENT-CENTERED PROFESSIONALISM

- Why is it important that the patient's medical record follow established guidelines?

SELECTING A FILING SYSTEM

When choosing a filing system for paper-based medical records, a medical office must determine what types and volume of documents will be filed. In most cases, more than one type of filing system will be used. For example, a *numerical* (numeric) system may be used for patient records, whereas an *alphabetical* (alphabetic) system may be used for business records; subject and geographical filing might be used for research or correspondence. Each method, with the exception of the numerical system, uses alphabetical concepts.

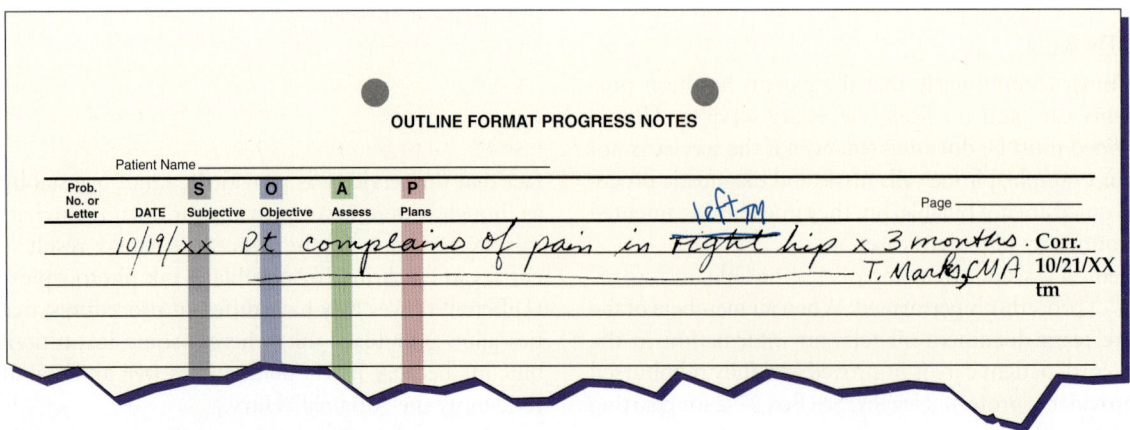

FIGURE 27-6 Example of appropriate way to correct a medical record. (Modified from Hunt SA: *Saunders fundamentals of medical assisting—revised reprint*, St Louis, 2007, Saunders.)

BOX 27-4

Charting Information Needed for Complete Documentation in the Patient Record

CHIEF COMPLAINT
Date
Time
Symptoms as told by the patient (in patient's own words, if possible)
Proper signature

PROCEDURE
Date
Time
Type (e.g., vital signs)
Results
Patient reaction
Proper signature

MEDICATIONS
Date
Time
Name of medication
Dosage given
Route
Site (if injection)
Patient reaction
Proper signature

SPECIMEN COLLECTION
Date
Time
Type/site (e.g., urine, blood)
Results
Proper signature

TO OUTSIDE
Test requested
Date sent
Place sent
Proper signature

DIAGNOSTIC AND LABORATORY TESTS
Date
Time
Type of test ordered
Schedule date (if known)
Place being performed
Proper signature

LABORATORY TEST RESULTS
Date
Time
Name of test
Results
From Outside (Telephone)
Record results on appropriate form
Laboratory report to physician for review, then filed with chart
Proper signature

PATIENT EDUCATION
Date
Time
Type of instructions
Signed form stating patient understood instructions and medical assistant to witness
Proper signature

MISSED APPOINTMENTS, TELEPHONE REQUESTS, PRESCRIPTION REFILLS
Date
Time
Situation (e.g., refill request, missed appointment)
Proper signature

When choosing a filing system, the practice needs to consider the following:
- Available space
- Available budget
- Potential volume of patient records
- Selection of supplies
- Types of storage equipment
- Type of filing system best suited to the medical practice's needs

Once selected, a plan must be made for the filing system, and details must be entered into the practice's policy and procedures manual. The plan should contain the following components:
- Maintenance of the system and records
- Retrieval of the records
- Security of all records held in the office

Equipment

Several styles of filing cabinets are used in the medical office. The selection of a filing cabinet depends on what types of records are to be stored. Table 27-1 compares four different types of filing cabinets. Files may also be stored with automated or computerized systems.

Automated Files

Automated files or rotary files can only be used in large facilities (e.g., hospitals) because of their cost and space requirements. The operator indicates the shelf needed, and the shelf is automatically moved into position by a motor, thereby eliminating the need for any pushing and pulling of cabinets and shelves.

TABLE 27-1

Types of Filing Cabinets

Type	Description	Advantages	Disadvantages	Example
Vertical (or drawer) file cabinet	Each drawer pulls out toward user Often used for business records and correspondence Typical cabinet holds about 700 files	Records are more protected in case of fire Records can be examined from above Usually locks	Requires more space when the drawer is pulled out Holds about 700 files, so use limited in a medical setting Danger of tipping if more than one drawer is open at once	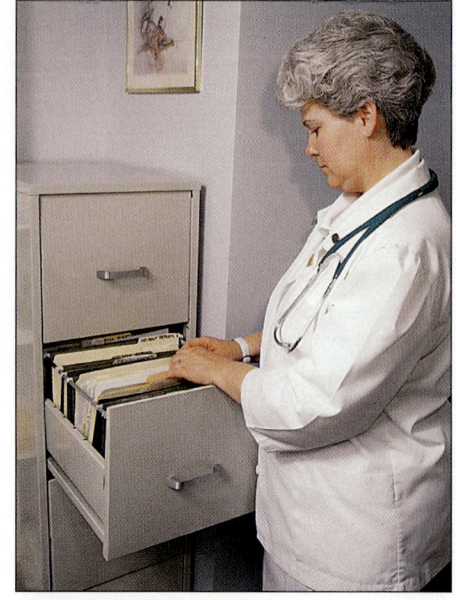
Lateral open-shelf file cabinet	Has stationary shelves and door cover that slides up and back into cabinet Files are removed by pulling them out laterally Usually holds about 1000 records	Patient records stored horizontally for quick retrieval Misfiling easily seen and corrected if color-coded system used; helps keep records in proper order Can be locked	Lateral open-shelf files require more room than vertical files	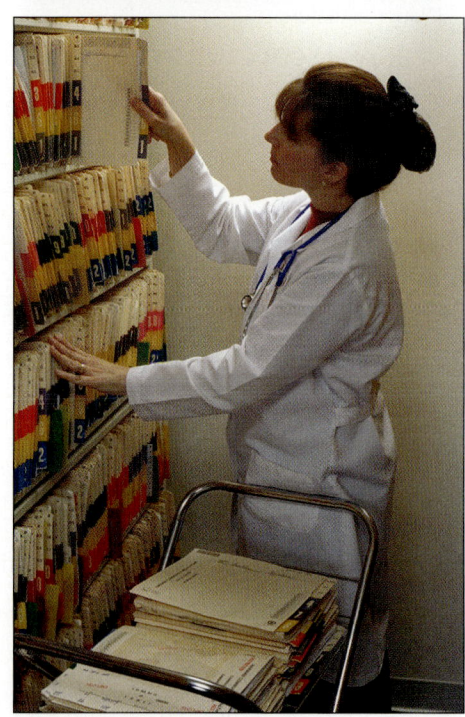

TABLE 27-1
Types of Filing Cabinets—cont'd

Type	Description	Advantages	Disadvantages	Example
Lateral drawer (or horizontal drawer) file cabinet	Has movable shelves that roll out sideways Patient records are filed from right to left Entire record label is visible Holds more records but requires more wall space than vertical file	Holds more records than vertical file cabinet Can be locked	More space is required for lateral or horizontal drawer file cabinets than for vertical cabinets	
Rotary (or movable lateral) file cabinet	Electronically or manually powered to rotate or move files in position to be accessed Maximizes use of space and holds large volume of records	Use of space is maximized Large volumes of records can be held	Provides less privacy and protection than file cabinets that can be closed completely and locked Normally kept in locked room	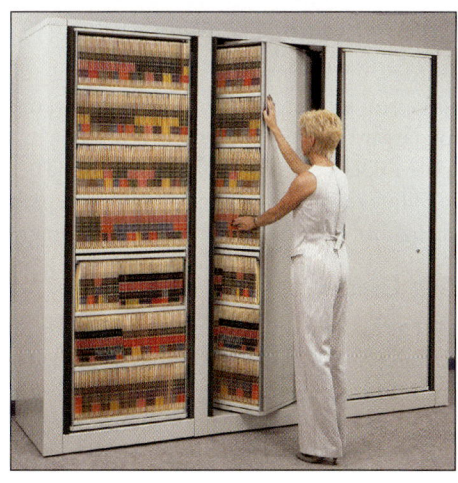

Vertical cabinet from Chester GA: *Modern medical assisting*, Philadelphia, 1998, Saunders. Lateral drawer cabinet courtesy Bibbero Systems, Inc., Petaluma, CA; (800) 242-2376; fax (800) 242-9330; www.bibbero.com. Rotary cabinet courtesy Mayline Group, Sheboygan, WI.

FOR YOUR INFORMATION

ISSUES OF CONFIDENTIALITY AND PRIVACY

The security of patient health care information, whether it is maintained on paper or through a computer network, presents confidentiality and privacy problems. As the health care industry continues its move toward linking institutions through communication networks, new confidentiality and privacy issues arise. A patient's health information will no longer be contained within the originating institution's health care facility but will travel among a multitude of facilities. Computerization increases the quantity and availability of data, thus raising a concern that demands for the data may be beyond the scope for which they were originally collected. State and Federal policies governing requirements for informed consent could be challenged because patients have limited access to their health record and may have little choice in consenting to its disclosure for certain purposes. The question then becomes: does Congress need to enact a detailed health information privacy law?

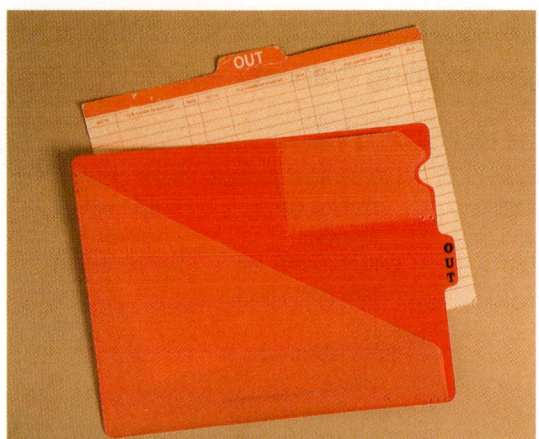

FIGURE 27-7 Out guides.

Filing Supplies

In addition to the physical filing cabinet or system itself, supplies are needed to hold, organize, and label documents, records, and forms.

Color-Coding/A-Z File Guides

Guides, or dividers, are used to separate file folders into sections and indicate a letter, number, or range of letters. Guides are larger than file folders and made of a material heavier than a file folder (e.g., fiberboard, pressboard). Their purpose is to facilitate record filing and retrieval by separating file space into recognizable and easily handled groupings.

Out Guides

Out guides are dividers of a different size and color than a file folder. Out guides should always be used when a file is removed from file storage. The out guide is placed in the space where the patient's record was filed. Its purpose is to allow the medical office to identify the precise location of a file and who has the file. Out guides should have a place to write the date, time, and name of the person removing the file. When used properly, out guides significantly reduce the time lost in locating missing files. Think of an out guide as a bookmark you place in a book that you are reading to save your place (Figure 27-7). If bar-coded labels are used, medical charts can be scanned to track the chart's location. This feature eliminates lost files that have not been signed out.

File Folders

File folders are used to contain patient documents. They can be purchased in several color and size selections. Tabs (full-cut, half-cut, third-cut, or fifth-cut) extend along the top edge or side edge and are used to indicate what is in the file with the addition of a label. The top-cut (tab) folder is stored in a vertical file cabinet, and the folder with the tab on the side is stored in a lateral cabinet.

File folders may be purchased with inside dividers and fasteners attached to the inside covers to hold documents. They can be purchased with half pockets located on the inside panel and be constructed for self-expansion with a reinforced spine.

File Labels

Labels are used to identify the contents of the file. Labels can indicate a patient's name or provide other information about the patient (e.g., allergy, advance directives) (Figure 27-8). The label has space for a **caption** (words that describe the contents, name of a person, or subject). Most labels are self-adhesive and should always be typed or computer-printed for clarity. An additional feature can include bar codes used for scanning and tracking medical charts.

Aging Labels

Aging labels (year labels) are adhesive, color-coded labels used to indicate the last year a patient was seen in the medical office. When pulling files for office appointments, always make sure the file has a current year label on it if appropriate. Current year labels are placed over the top of the outdated year label, so there is always only one year's date (label) visible on the file. The last two digits of the year are used. Aging labels help when purging files for inactive status.

Color-Coded Labels

A color-coding system consists of labels that indicate a number, a letter, or an *alphanumerical* (letters, numbers) character. An alphabetical or numerical color-coded system assigns each letter, number, or preprinted numbering sequence a different color. Subject files can also be color coded, with each subject area being assigned a different color. The advantage of using a color-coding system is that files can be retrieved faster and misfiled records are easy to see (Figure 27-9).

Medical Records and Chart Documentation CHAPTER 27 533

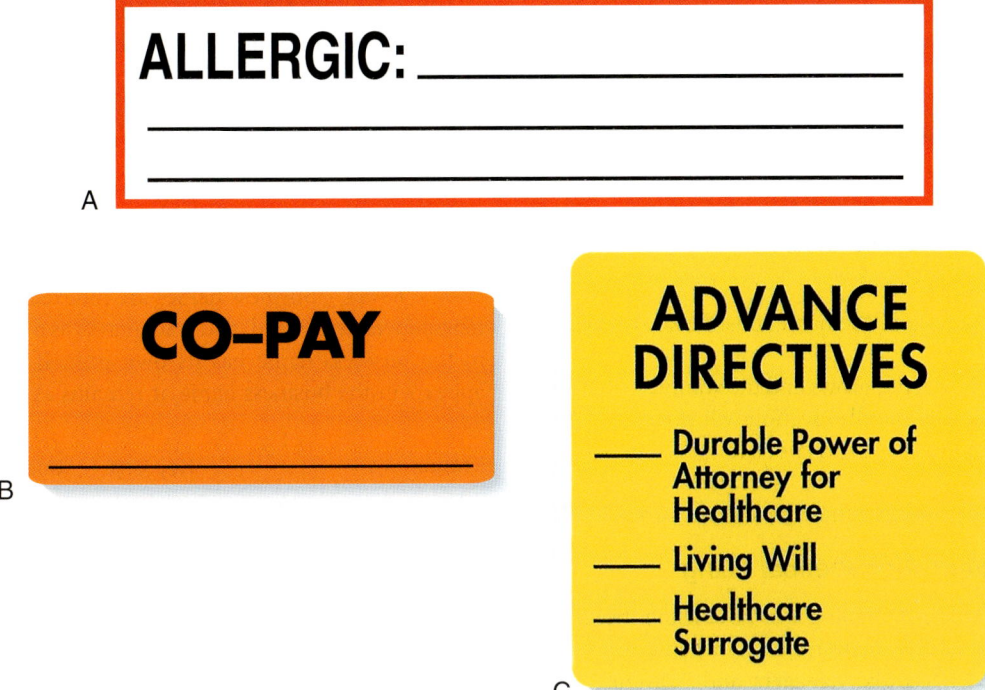

FIGURE 27-8 **A** to **C**, File labels allow the physician and medical staff to quickly see important information about the patient. (Labels **A** # 38-50701-1, **B** # 33-9052, and **C** # 38-50624 courtesy Bibbero Systems, Inc., Petaluma, CA; (800) 242-2376; fax (800) 242-9330; www.bibbero.com.)

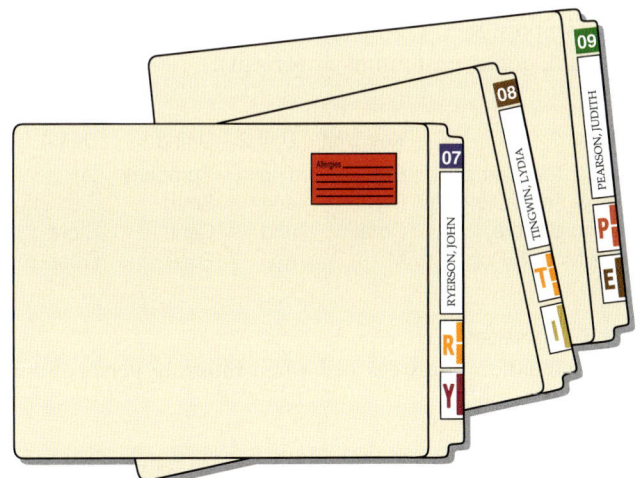

FIGURE 27-9 Color labels used for filing. In this case the alphabetical system is used: the first label indicates the first letter of the last name, and the second label indicates the second letter of the last name. Labels for the year of the patient's last visit are also color-coded. (Modified from Hunt SA: *Saunders fundamentals of medical assisting-revised reprint,* St Louis, 2007, Saunders.)

PATIENT-CENTERED PROFESSIONALISM

- What information is necessary when choosing a file storage system?
- What supplies are needed for a filing system?
- How can a well-organized filing system benefit the patients in the medical practice?

FILING METHODS

A medical office will select a filing method for patient and office records that meets the needs of the practice. Common filing systems are alphabetical, numerical, alphanumerical, and subject filing. Each has distinctive qualities that accommodate different record needs. Patient records are filed either by the patient's name or by a numerical method. Business records and correspondence can be filed alphabetically or by subject.

Alphabetical Filing

The **alphabetical filing** method uses letters of the alphabet to determine how files are arranged. Using the same sequence as the letters of the alphabet, files are organized by last names of people or names of businesses. This is the most common method of filing.

The **indexing** process is the determination of how a record will be filed. Each name is broken into units. All personnel responsible for filing activities must be consistent in their filing procedures. The office must determine how each piece of information is to be filed and not allow any deviation. This should be established in the medical practice's policy and procedures manual.

Advantages and Disadvantages

Alphabetical filing is the most common system used in small to medium-sized medical practices. It is considered a **direct filing** system because finding a patient file or business folder only requires knowing the correct name. As with any system, alphabetical filing has advantages and disadvantages.

Advantages
- Alphabetical filing is the easiest system to learn.
- Alphabetical filing allows for easy training of new staff members.
- Only one sorting is required.

Disadvantages
- The correct spelling of the name must be known to find a folder.
- As the medical practice grows and the volume of patients increases, each alphabetical section will expand, requiring periodic shifting of file sections in the file drawers or cabinets.
- Unauthorized personnel could have easier access to files.

Rules for Efficient Alphabetical Filing

The key objective to effective filing is to be able to retrieve the appropriate record or information quickly when it is needed. The Association of Records Managers and Administrators (ARMA) has established rules to assist in efficient alphabetical filing. Without specific rules, the filing process becomes inefficient. The purpose of indexing rules is to provide consistency among the office staff when filing information, whether it is business or patient related.

Read each rule and study the examples provided. Understanding how names are divided into the indexing units is the first step to alphabetical filing. If the **key unit,** or first unit (e.g., the first letter or character), is similar, move on to the second and succeeding units until a difference is apparent. For example, "Sanders" would be filed before "Santos" because "d" comes before "t" in the alphabet (*d* and *t* are the first letters in each name that are different). Before moving on to the next rule, fully understand the current rule.

Rule 1: Sequencing Order
Personal Names. Personal names are indexed accordingly:
- The last name is the key unit, or first unit.
- The first name or initial is the second unit.
- The middle name or initial is the third unit. In some medical offices the preference is to spell out the middle name.

NOTE: If an initial represents a unit, this initial will precede a unit consisting of a complete name beginning with the same letter (e.g., T. Jones would be filed before Tamara Jones). Keep in mind the rule that *nothing comes before something*—because no additional letter is immediately after the letter T. in T. Jones, this name would come before Tamara Jones, which has the letter *a* immediately after the T.

Name	Key Unit	Unit 2	Unit 3
Douglas A. Telle	Telle	Douglas	A
Amanda B. Telley	Telley	Amanda	B
John J. Telly	Telly	John	J

When a person's last name could be mistaken for the first name, a **cross-reference** folder should be made (e.g., Lee Wong).

Key Unit	Unit 2	
Wong	Lee	
Lee	Wong	See Wong, Lee

Business Names. Business names are indexed as written, using newspapers, letterhead, and trademarks as a guide. Each word in the business name has its own unit. If a person's name appears in the business name, it remains as written.

Name	Key Unit	Unit 2	Unit 3
Johnny Appleseed Farm	Johnny	Appleseed	Farm
Jumpin' Box Toys	Jumpin	Box	Toys

Rule 2: Miscellaneous Words and Symbols
Prepositions, articles, conjunctions, and symbols are considered separate indexing units.
- Prepositions: in, out, at, on, by, to, of, with.
- Articles: a, an, the (when appearing as the first word of a business name, articles are indexed last or discarded; articles have no significance in filing).
- Conjunctions: and, but, or, nor.
- Symbols: &, $, ¢, #, % (symbols are spelled in full—e.g., and, dollar, cent, number, percent).

Name	Key Unit	Unit 2	Unit 3	Unit 4
A Big Top Company	Big	Top	Company	(A)
Big & Small Clothing	Big	and	Small	Clothing
$ and ¢ Store	Dollar	and	Cent	Store
The Mom & Pop	Mom	and	Pop	(The)

Rule 3: Punctuation
All punctuation is disregarded when indexing personal and business names.

Name	Key Unit	Unit 2	Unit 3
Barney's Tea Room	Barneys	Tea	Room
Elaine C. Jones-Smith	JonesSmith	Elaine	C
Hide-Away Motel	HideAway	Motel	

Rule 4: Initials and Abbreviations
Personal. Initials, abbreviations of personal names, and nicknames are indexed as they are written.

Name	Key Unit	Unit 2	Unit 3
J. John Smith	Smith	J	John
Bill James Smith	Smith	Bill	James
Wm. James Smith	Smith	Wm	James

Business. Single letters representing a business or organization are indexed as written. If a single letter is separated by a space, each letter is indexed separately. An **acronym** (word formed from the first few letters of several words) is indexed as one unit. Television and radio station call letters are considered one unit.

Name	Key Unit	Unit 2	Unit 3	Unit 4
CNN	CNN			
S A C Furniture	S	A	C	Furniture
T & A Clinic	T	and	A	Clinic
IBM	IBM			

Rule 5: Titles

Personal and Professional Titles. Professional titles (Dr., Prof.), general titles (Mr., Ms., Mrs.), and professional, numerical, and seniority suffixes are always indexed last.

Name	Key Unit	Unit 2	Unit 3	Unit 4
James J. Jameston, MD	Jameston	James	J	MD
Ms. Joan Summers, CMA (AAMA)	Summers	Joan	CMA	Ms
Joseph K. Suthe, II	Suthe	Joseph	K	II
Senator Mary Toth	Toth	Mary	Senator	

Religious Titles. Religious titles not followed by a last name are indexed as written.

Name	Key Unit	Unit 2	Unit 3
Brother John	Brother	John	
Father John Jones	Jones	John	Father

Titles in Business Names. Titles used in the name of a business are indexed as written.

Name	Key Unit	Unit 2	Unit 3
Mr. Jay's Coffee	Mr	Jays	Coffee
Uncle Ben's China	Uncle	Bens	China

Rule 6: Prefixes

A foreign name that has a prefix or an article included is combined with the last name to become the key unit, without the use of spaces. However, using uppercase and lowercase letters is allowed for the articles.

Name	Key Unit	Unit 2
Robert de la Guard	delaGuard	Robert
Tom De Marce	DeMarce	Tom
Jerry Los Angel	LosAngel	Jerry
Saint John's Church	SaintJohns	Church
St. John's Rectory	SaintJohns	Rectory
Van der Mills' Clothing	VanderMills	Clothing

NOTE: "St." is indexed as if it were spelled out (as with "Saint" John's Rectory).

Rule 7: Numbers in Businesses

Numbers spelled out are indexed in the file alphabetically (e.g., "Five-Spot Shop" would come before "Two Brothers Restaurant"). Numbers expressed in digit form are indexed before alphabetical letters or words (as in "7 Eleven"). Arabic numerals (1, 2, 3) are filed *before* Roman numerals (I, II, III); thus in the file, the chart for "7 Eleven" would come before "II Club."

Name	Key Unit	Unit 2
7 Eleven	7	Eleven
II Club	II	Club
One Towing	One	Towing

Rule 8: Organizations and Institutions

Banks, colleges, hotels, schools, and so forth are indexed as written. The letterhead of the organization or institution provides the correct reference.

Name	Key Unit	Unit 2	Unit 3	Unit 4
1st Union Bank	1	Union	Bank	
First Atlantic Credit Union	First	Atlantic	Credit	Union
M.L.K. High School	MLK	High	School	
R.F.K. Institute of Art	RFK	Institute	of	Art

Rule 9: Identical Names

When names (whether personal or business) are identical, the filing order is determined by address. The following guidelines prevail:

- City name.
- State name (if cities are identical).
- Street name (if city and state names are identical).
- House or building numbers (if the above are identical).
- If street address and building names are included in the address, disregard the building name.
- Zip codes are never indexed.

Name	Key Unit	Unit 2	Unit 3	Unit 4	Unit 5	Unit 6	Unit 7
Mrs. Sally Fieds 67 Atkins Ave Albany, NY 32141	Fieds	Sally	Mrs	Albany	NY	Atkins	Ave
Mrs. Sally Fieds 63 Atkins Blvd Albany, NY 32147	Fieds	Sally	Mrs	Albany	NY	Atkins	Blvd

Because addresses may change frequently, most medical offices use the date of birth or Social Security number rather than addresses when names are identical, using year, month, and date. For example, the file of Mrs. Sally Fieds with a birth date of 7/12/74 would come before the file of Mrs. Sally Fieds with a birth date of 2/9/78. When using Social Security numbers, Mrs. Sally Fieds 190-xx-0106 would come before Mrs. Sally Fieds 206-xx-1789 in the file.

Name	Key Unit	Unit 2	Unit 3	Unit 4	Unit 5
James Smith Birth date: January 2, 1999	Smith	James	1999	January	2
James Smith Birth date: April 2, 2001	Smith	James	2001	April	2

Rule 10: Government Names

All government agencies are first indexed by United States Government, using "United" as the key unit, "States" as unit 2, and "Government" as unit 3, then the agency. The fourth and succeeding units are the main words in the name of the department.

Name	Key Unit	Unit 2	Unit 3	Unit 4	Unit 5
U.S. Government Department of the Treasury	United	States	Govern- ment	Treasury	Depart- ment

NOTE: The telephone book can be a good resource for help in finding the correct alphabetical filing.

Numerical Filing

In the **numerical filing** method, patient files are given numbers and arranged in numerical sequence. Medical assistants must consider the following two factors when using a numerical filing system:

1. How to assign the number.
2. How to file the records once the number is assigned.

Medical offices that have a large number of patient files may choose to keep medical records according to an assigned number. For example, the number may be assigned on the basis of the patient's Social Security number or the patient's order of registration as a new patient. The numerical system is an **indirect filing** method because a listing of patient names must be used to locate the correct number. This is an extremely difficult system because of issuing current numbers to old patients.

Advantages and Disadvantages

As with the alphabetical filing method, there are advantages and disadvantages to the numerical method.

Advantages
- Numerical filing is the most confidential system.
- Expansion is unlimited.
- Misfiled folders are easy to locate.
- It is easy to remove inactive files when numbers are assigned based on patient order of registration (because the age of the file will be apparent by its number).

Disadvantages
- To find a folder, the correct number must be known. This is accomplished by either using a password to access the patient's computerized file or having access to a master list of patients names that provides the patient's number. This makes locating every file a two-step process.
- A file list must be constantly updated and maintained.
- Numbers could be transposed without being detected.
- It is easy to misfile.

Methods

The two most common methods by which filing can be done numerically are straight-number filing and terminal-digit filing.

Straight-Number Filing. Straight-number filing is the most common form of numerical filing. File folders are filed in numerical sequence. Thus, files in straight-number filing would appear as #3456, #3457, #3458, and so on. When using straight-number filing, as the numbers increase, so do the files. The longer the number, the harder it may become to file because that area of numbers will be the highest concentration of newer patient files.

Terminal-Digit Filing. **Terminal-digit filing** organizes a number by the final digits of the number. The digits are usually separated into groups of two or three. For example, the file number 107654 can be separated into groups of twos. The last two digits (terminal digits) (54) identify the file drawer number; the second two digits (76) identify the number of the file guide; and the first two digits (10) provide the number of the file folder behind the file guide (Figure 27-10).

Subject Filing

Subject filing is most frequently used with correspondence or research. If the physician is starting a research project on hypertension, all correspondence on this subject will be labeled "hypertension." This allows all materials on a particular subject to be kept in one folder.

Color Coding

A color-coding system can be used with alphabetical or numerical filing and in combined alphanumerical files. Several companies offer color-coded tabs; the medical assistant must

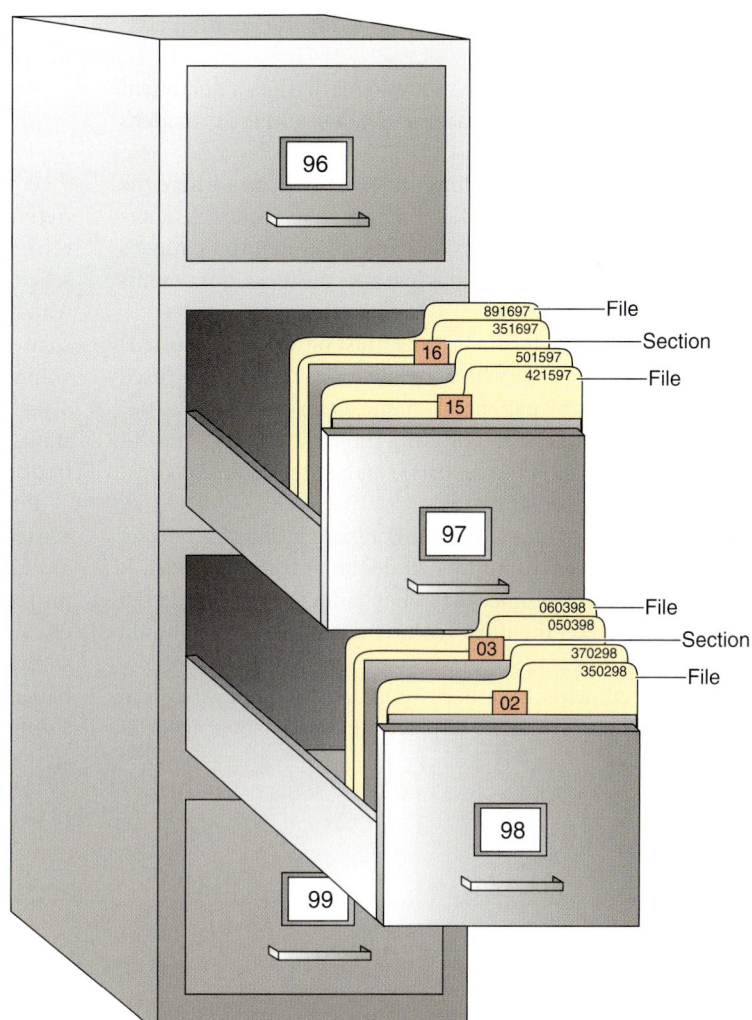

FIGURE 27-10 Vertical file cabinet, showing use of terminal-digit filing method.

follow the manufacturer's directions. Color coding makes filing easier and draws attention to misfiled folders.

TICKLER FILE

If the medical office does not use a computerized "reminder" system, an effective reminder aid is the **tickler file.** This type of file "tickles the memory" about upcoming events (e.g., license renewal, payments, and call-back appointments). A tickler file can be organized by putting the event to be remembered on a 3 × 5 card and placing it behind a numbered date guide. This system allows you to file reminders for any month of the year ahead on a year-round basis.

> **PATIENT-CENTERED PROFESSIONALISM**
>
> - Why is it important for everyone who handles patient files to understand the rules for each system?

REVIEW OF BASIC FILING PROCEDURES

Medical assistants need to be familiar with the basic steps for preparing and filing, as well as for purging and retaining files for maintenance.

Steps for Preparing and Filing

Preparing documents for filing involves the following steps:

Step 1: **Conditioning.** The files must be in good condition before they are filed. This requires removing all staples and paper clips, mending any torn edges on the document, and verifying that the patient's name appears on each page of a multiple-page document.

Step 2: **Releasing.** A file is "released" when a mark (e.g., checkmark, initials) is placed on the document indicating it should be filed. For example, releasing would occur after a physician has read a patient's laboratory report and checks it off for filing in the patient's record. The physician, or other authorized staff member, depending on the information classification, performs this step.

Some offices use a rubber stamp to mark when a document is ready for filing. It has a place for the date and the provider's initials.

Step 3: Indexing and **coding**. Indexing indicates where the document is to be filed, and coding provides a mark (underlining or highlighting) with the keyword (often the patient's last name). This action also separates business documents from patient information.

Step 4: **Sorting.** The documents must be arranged (sorted) for filing. An alpha sorter has tabs labeled A-Z and can be used to sort all papers by patient last name. Or, a document sorter with captions on the tabs indicating subject areas (e.g., laboratory reports, consultation reports) can be used to initially sort documents of a similar nature.

Step 5: **Filing.** Once this stage is reached, filing can occur. Filing is the process of putting all documents in the folder. It is important to remember that when a document is added to an established file, the most recently dated document should be placed on top.

After documents have been prepared for filing, they can either be filed immediately or placed in an alphabetical sorter for filing later.

Procedure 27-6 outlines the process for alphabetical filing.

Procedure 27-7 shows the process for numerical filing.

Purging and Retention

Active files are kept in a file cabinet where they are easy to retrieve. These medical files are for patients who are routinely scheduled for care. **Inactive files** are the files of patients who have not visited the practice within a certain time span (set by the practice). Some larger practices with a high volume of patients will **purge** (clean out) records every 1 or 2 years. Purging is the preparation of a file to go from active status to inactive status. Smaller practices may purge less frequently.

Purging depends on the amount of storage available and the turnover and volume of patients in the practice. These files are usually stored "off site," but they can also be placed on *microfiche* (a small sheet of film containing reduced images) or can be microfilmed to reduce storage space. New computer software programs are also available for scanning inactive patient records onto a computer (compact) disk (CD) for storage. This method is compact and cost efficient, and office staff can be easily trained to do this.

PROCEDURE 27-6 — File Medical Records Using the Alphabetical System

TASK: Correctly file a set of patient records using an established alphabetical filing system.

NOTE: Filing medical records by an alphabetical system is an activity related to the competency of organizing a patient's medical record.

EQUIPMENT AND SUPPLIES
- Patient files
- Alphanumerical sorter

SKILLS/*RATIONALE*

1. **Procedural Step.** Retrieve the appropriate patient files from the file storage area.
2. **Procedural Step.** Complete any documentation needed.
3. **Procedural Step.** Add any supplemental forms or records generated according to office procedure.
4. **Procedural Step.** Sort the files alphabetically, using a "desktop sorter" if possible.
   Rationale. The use of a sorter makes the filing process much more efficient because it saves the medical assistant significant time.
5. **Procedural Step.** Remove the files from the sorter and return the files to the storage cabinet, correctly filing them alphabetically into the appropriate sequence.
   Rationale. Specific indexing rules must be followed when filing, whether alphabetical or numerical. This ensures that the document is easy to retrieve for future reference.
6. **Procedural Step.** Verify that the filing location is correct by checking the record in front and in back of the record to be filed.

PROCEDURE 27-7 File Medical Records Using the Numerical System

TASK: Correctly file a set of patient records, using an established numerical filing system.

EQUIPMENT AND SUPPLIES
- Patient files
- Numerical sorter

TASK/RATIONALE

1. **Procedural Step.** Retrieve the appropriate patient files from the file storage area.
2. **Procedural Step.** Complete any documentation necessary.
3. **Procedural Step.** Add any supplemental forms or records generated according to office procedure.
4. **Procedural Step.** Sort the files numerically, using a "desktop sorter" if possible. The office filing system may be straight number or terminal digit.
   Rationale. The use of a sorter makes the filing process much more efficient because it saves the medical assistant significant time.
5. **Procedural Step.** Remove the files from the sorter, and return the files to the storage cabinet, correctly filing them into the appropriate numerical sequence.
6. **Procedural Step.** Remove out guide and either discard index card from pocket or cross-out the name of the person who had removed the file.

Depending on office file space, files are usually purged every year, or even monthly in large practices. Purging of medical records can also mean removing unnecessary old materials from the medical record such as paid insurance claims and unneeded notes (e.g., phoned-in laboratory results). Each office should have a policy indicating when files are to be removed from main file storage.

Most state statutes require that medical records be kept (retained) at least 7 years from the last information entry date. The American Medical Association (AMA) recommends keeping adult records for 10 years and keeping records for 3 years after a minor reaches the age of majority (which varies from state to state, usually age 18 or 21). If a file is to be discarded, the documents should be shredded or burned. This protects the confidentiality of its contents. Some medical offices contract with a business that provides this service. The outside service must follow the same guidelines for confidentiality of patient records as the medical office. Both the office and the outside service are bound by HIPAA guidelines. Files that chart patients' familial or inherited diseases should be kept indefinitely. Many organizations now realize keeping charts indefinitely may be the only way to determine disease-based information such as certain cancers (e.g., breast cancer, colon cancer, or prostate cancer). Human immunodeficiency virus/acquired immunodeficiency syndrome (HIV/AIDS) is a disease with limited history, and these charts must be retained for an unlimited time. Post-polio syndrome is a condition/sequela of a disease that is older than 60 years. The subsequent conditions of diseases that have been destroyed may have historical consequences in charting.

> **PATIENT-CENTERED PROFESSIONALISM**
> - What function does preparing documents serve?
> - What does purging documents accomplish?

CONCLUSION

Medical records are the confidential, legal documents used to record the health care services provided to an individual at a medical facility. Medical records are used in planning, coordinating, and evaluating a patient's care, as well as for protecting the interests of the patient, practice, and health care provider in case of lawsuit. Medical records contain historical information that is essential to the family, community, and country. Records that may indicate the progress of disease are pertinent to the continuum of care.

To handle the essential information and documentation in the medical record effectively and efficiently, medical assistants need to know how to generate, update, file, store, and maintain these records. Accuracy is necessary; if a service is not documented on the medical record, it is considered to have never happened. In order for patients to receive the best care possible, their medical records must be handled with as much diligence and competence as the services provided to them for care and treatment.

Chapter Summary

Reinforce your understanding of the material in this chapter by reviewing the curriculum objectives and key content points below.

1. **Define, appropriately use, and spell all the Key Terms for this chapter.**
   - Review the Key Terms if necessary.
2. **Explain the purpose of a medical record.**
   - A patient's medical record provides legal evidence of assessment, interventions, and communication between health care providers and the patient.
   - If a patient's care is not documented, it is considered not done.
3. **List three uses of the medical record.**
   - Laboratory reports, consultation letters, and other documentation provide information to support the course of treatment.
   - Medical records are used to track progress, file insurance claims, and to resolve legal matters such as lawsuits.
4. **List the two types of medical records.**
   - Electronic medical records (EMRs).
   - Manual medical records.
5. **Discuss the advantages and disadvantages of EMRs and a manual record system.**
   - Advantages: legible entries, reduces time, accessed by multiple practitioners, no missing records, easier release of information, makes report generation easier, and storage is not a problem.
   - Disadvantages: startup costs, extensive training technology updates, computer virus, and equipment breakdown.
6. **Explain how the medical record protects the legal interests of the patient, the health care provider, and the medical practice.**
   - The medical record is a legal document and is a record of the services provided, communications, and other interactions between the patient and the provider, the physician, or the medical facility.
   - The medical record can be used as evidence in a lawsuit.
7. **Demonstrate the correct procedure for pulling patient records.**
   - Review Procedure 27-1.
8. **Demonstrate the correct procedure for registering a patient.**
   - Review Procedure 27-2.
9. **List and describe seven basic forms used to start a new patient's medical record.**
   - The forms required for different types of practices may vary.
   - Typical forms included in the medical record are the patient information form, health history, consent to treat form, consent to use and disclose health information form, H&P form, progress notes, and medication log (list).
10. **Demonstrate the correct procedure for creating a medical file for a new patient using alphabetical, color-coded tabs.**
    - Review Procedure 27-3.
11. **List five examples of forms that could be added to an established patient's medical record as care is provided.**
    - Various radiographic reports, laboratory reports, diagnostic procedure reports, consultation reports from other physicians, and hospital reports (operative, pathology) could be added to an existing patient's medical record.
12. **Demonstrate the correct procedure for adding documents to an existing patient record.**
    - Review Procedure 27-4.
13. **Demonstrate the correct procedure for protecting the confidentiality of patients and their medical records.**
    - Review Procedure 27-5.
14. **Differentiate between source-oriented and problem-oriented records (POMRs).**
    - A source-oriented format organizes a patient's file into sections according to the source of the documents (e.g., x-ray reports, consultations).
    - A POMR is organized according to the patient's health problem.
15. **Describe where progress notes fit into the POMR format of organizing a patient's record and explain the acronym SOAP.**
    - The POMR is arranged according to the patient's health complaint. There are four components of the POMR: database, problem list, plan, and progress notes.
    - The progress notes are written in a SOAP format, which consists of subjective data, objective data, assessment, and plan.
16. **Explain the importance of documenting all services provided to the patient.**
    - All services provided to a patient must be clearly documented to receive reimbursement for care provided (prove medical necessity), establish a legal record of all treatment, and provide for continuity of care should the patient be transferred to other health care providers.
17. **Identify specific actions as "Do"s or "Don't"s of charting in patients' medical records.**
    Do:
    - Use direct quotations from the patient when possible.
    - Chart the plan of care, results, physician's orders, and patient's responses immediately after performing the procedure.
    - Chart all patient teaching, precautions, and assessment of patient understanding.
    - Make sure all charting entries are accurate and legible.
    - Use black ink.

Don't:
- Chart anything you have not personally witnessed or performed.
- Chart from memory.
- Chart your personal opinions about the patient or treatment rendered.
- Write carelessly or illegibly.
- Use correction fluid or erase any entries.

18. **List the three steps for correcting an entry error in the patient's medical record.**
    - Draw a line through the incorrect entry.
    - Insert the correction above the error, indicating a correction is being made.
    - Include the name or initials of the person making the correction with the date.

19. **State the three considerations for selecting a filing system.**
    - Volume of patient files.
    - Budget allocated for equipment purchase.
    - Space available for the equipment.

20. **State the three components of a filing system plan that should be recorded in detail in the office procedure manual.**
    - A plan must be made for the maintenance, retrieval, and security of all records held in the office. This plan should be indicated by office policy and procedure.

21. **Differentiate among vertical drawer, lateral open-shelf, lateral drawer, and movable lateral file cabinets.**
    - Vertical drawer: Each drawer pulls out toward you. Folders are filed front to back in the drawer and removed by lifting them up and out of the drawer.
    - Lateral open-shelf: Stationary shelves with a door cover that flips up and back. Folders are filed side to side and removed by pulling them out laterally.
    - Lateral drawer: Movable shelves that roll out sideways. Folders are filed from right to left and removed by pulling them out laterally.
    - Movable lateral file: Cabinets rotate manually or automatically for file selection.

22. **List six supplies typically used with a manual filing system.**
    - Cabinets
    - A-Z guides or numerical guides
    - Appropriate-size file folders
    - Out guides
    - Various types of alphanumerical labels
    - Special-alert labels (e.g., allergies, collection)

23. **List four methods of filing and briefly explain each.**
    - Alphabetical filing is by a patient's last name.
    - Straight-number filing is based on the entire number as the key unit.
    - Terminal-digit filing uses the last two digits of the patient's identifying number as the key unit for determining file placement.
    - Subject filing is used in research studies and is organized by subject matter.

24. **Discuss the advantages and disadvantages of alphabetical filing.**
    - Alphabetical filing is the easiest method to learn and only requires one sorting.
    - A disadvantage is that unauthorized personnel could have easier access to files.

25. **List the areas addressed in the 10 rules for alphabetical filing.**
    - Filing rules relate to sequencing order, miscellaneous words and symbols, punctuation, initials and abbreviations, titles, prefixes, numbers in businesses, organizations and institutions, identical names, and government names.
    - In general, if the key unit on more than one file is alike, move on to the second and succeeding units until a difference is apparent.

26. **Discuss the advantages and disadvantages of numerical filing.**
    - Numerical filing is the most confidential method, and expansion is unlimited.
    - A disadvantage is that the correct number must be known to find a folder, making locating a file a two-step process.

27. **Differentiate between straight-number filing and terminal-digit filing.**
    - Straight-number filing is the most common method, and files follow in whole-number sequence.
    - Terminal-digit filing organizes a number by its final digits.

28. **List in order the five steps of preparing and filing medical records and briefly describe each.**
    - Conditioning. Documents must be prepared by removing staples and paper clips.
    - Releasing. Documents must have a release mark, meaning they are ready to be filed.
    - Indexing and coding. Documents must be indexed according to their source (e.g., all laboratory reports) and coded according to how they will be filed (e.g., patient's last name).
    - Sorting. Documents must be sorted for filing.
    - Filing. Documents must be filed according to established procedure (e.g., alphabetical or numerical).

29. **Demonstrate the correct procedure for filing medical records using the alphabetical system.**
    - Review Procedure 27-6.

30. **Demonstrate the correct procedure for filing medical records using the numerical system.**
    - Review Procedure 27-7.

31. **Differentiate between active and inactive files.**
    - Active files are those currently in use.
    - Inactive files are those of patients not seen within a specified time span set by the medical practice.

32. **Explain the need to purge files regularly in a medical practice.**
    - Files are purged or moved from active status to inactive status to keep the main file storage area as up-to-date as possible and to allow for expansion of active files.

33. **Analyze a realistic medical office situation and apply your understanding of charting and filing medical records to determine the best course of action.**
    - Each medical office should have its own policies on how medical records should be charted, filed, stored, and purged.
    - Understanding how to create and maintain medical records helps the practice to run more efficiently and provides protection in legal matters. It also improves continuity of patient care by providing accurate documentation and accessibility to a patient's record.

34. **Describe the impact on patient care when medical assistants understand the importance of accurate documentation and efficient filing of medical records.**
    - Physicians use medical records to monitor patient treatment and progress; also, when patients are referred to other physicians, continuity of care transfers easily.
    - Medical records provide information needed to support the course of treatment and establish medical necessity; if they are inaccurate or incomplete, patient care is negatively affected.
    - Accurate medical records protect both the patient and the practice; they also help ensure that payment of insurance claims is timely.

PRACTICAL APPLICATIONS

If you have accomplished the objectives in this chapter, you will be able to make better choices as a medical assistant. Take another look at this situation and decide what you would do.

Deanna is a new administrative medical-assisting extern at Dr. Juanea's office. Shirley, the office manager, asks Deanna to prepare a file for a new patient who will be seen tomorrow in the office. Shirley tells Deanna to be sure that she has color-coded the file folder and that the necessary forms have been included inside. In this office the medical records are problem-oriented and all records are SOAP format; both are new concepts to Deanna, who was taught to prepare source-oriented records. After Deanna has prepared the new patient's file, Shirley asks her to pull the necessary records for tomorrow's appointments from the lateral open-shelf file cabinet containing patient records filed in alphabetical order. As she pulls the records, Deanna is to annotate the patient list for tomorrow's schedule. With the assistance of Shirley, Deanna will also purge the inactive patient records.

Would you be able to perform these tasks?

1. Why is the medical record necessary? What are its uses?
2. What is meant by "color-coding" a patient file?
3. What forms should Deanna be sure are in the new record?
4. What is meant by "problem-oriented" medical records?
5. What does SOAP mean?
6. What is a "source-oriented" patient record?
7. What are the advantages of open-shelf filing? What are the disadvantages?
8. Why is alphabetical filing advantageous? What are the disadvantages?
9. What will Deanna do to "annotate" a patient list?
10. What is "purging" a file or a record? Why should patient records be purged on a regular basis?

WEB SEARCH

1. **Research the topic of medical records to learn more about how private medical information has become.** The tradition of physician-patient privilege was the only protection of patient privacy for many years. HIPAA set a national standard for privacy for health information, but is it enough?
    - **Keywords:** Use the following keywords in your search: HIPAA, AHIMA, medical records, medical information, privacy rights.'

Financial Management

28

evolve http://evolve.elsevier.com/klieger/medicalassisting

The front-office duties and responsibilities of a medical assistant vary according to the type of medical practice. The person at the front desk typically is responsible for clerical and basic bookkeeping duties (computerized or manual). This requires accurate recording of the physician's charges and receipts for payment of services. The office manager usually prepares the payroll and handles accounts payable and accounts receivable. In most practices, the daily journals, disbursement records, and payroll records are forwarded to an accountant who completes the quarterly income and disbursement summaries for income tax purposes.

Even though others handle many financial aspects of the medical practice, it is important for you to understand basic bookkeeping and accounting principles and procedures. An understanding of the "big picture" will help you manage whatever "parts" of the system for which you may be responsible. Also, because fees, billing, and collection directly relate to patients, efficient handling of these aspects will improve patients' overall experience.

LEARNING OBJECTIVES

You will be able to do the following after completing this chapter:

Key Terms
1. Define, appropriately use, and spell all the Key Terms for this chapter.

Accounting Principles
2. State the accounting equation.
3. Explain the differences among assets, liabilities, and owner's equity.
4. Explain the difference between a debit and a credit.
5. List three types of assets in a medical office.
6. Demonstrate the correct procedure for establishing a petty cash fund, maintaining an accurate record of expenditures, and replenishing the fund as necessary.
7. Explain what an accounts receivable "aging" report shows.
8. Differentiate among the following financial statements: income statement, statement of owner's equity, and balance sheet.

Bookkeeping Procedures
9. List three types of forms used on a pegboard system to record the daily transactions.
10. List two advantages of using a pegboard (single entry) bookkeeping system.
11. Demonstrate the correct procedure for posting service charges and payments using the manual (pegboard) system.
12. List four advantages of using a computerized bookkeeping system.

Banking Procedures
13. List the five requirements of banks for checks being deposited and explain the importance of confirming these five items when accepting checks from patients.
14. Define "third-party" check, "postdated" check, and check "paid in full."
15. List seven security tips for check writing.
16. Differentiate between restrictive endorsement and blank endorsement.
17. Demonstrate the correct procedure for preparing a bank deposit.
18. List four methods of making deposits and briefly explain each.
19. Demonstrate the correct procedure for reconciling a bank statement.

Billing and Collections
20. List four ways in which a patient statement can be prepared.
21. Demonstrate the correct procedure for explaining professional fees before providing services.

22. Explain how an adjustment affects the balance of a patient's account and list four reasons why an adjustment might be made.
23. Describe the collection process, including the role of third-party payers.
24. Demonstrate the correct procedure for establishing payment arrangements on a patient's account.
25. List four guidelines for making telephone calls to collect debts.
26. Demonstrate the correct procedure for explaining a statement of account to a patient.
27. Demonstrate the correct procedure for collecting delinquent accounts.

Payroll Processing

28. List six laws that affect earnings and withholdings and briefly explain each.
29. Differentiate between gross wages and net pay.
30. List the three principal deductions from the employee's gross pay that are required by federal law.
31. List the four types of information in the employee earnings record.

Patient-Centered Professionalism

32. Analyze a realistic medical office situation and apply your understanding of medical office financial management to determine the best course of action.
33. Describe the impact on patient care when medical assistants have a solid understanding of the financial aspects of a medical office.

KEY TERMS

ABA number
accounting
accounting equation
accounts receivable (AR)
adjustment
aging report
asset
balance sheet
bank statement
blank endorsement
bookkeeping
co-insurance
co-payment
credit
daysheet
debit
debtor
dependents
deposit
deposit slip
employee earnings record
Employee's Withholding Allowance Certificate (Form W-4)
encounter form
endorse
exemption
Fair Debt Collection Act of 1977
Fair Labor Standards Act
Federal Employees' Compensation Act
Federal Insurance Contributions Act (FICA)
Federal Truth in Lending Act
Federal Unemployment Tax Act (FUTA)
fee schedule
financial statements
gross wages
income statement
ledger cards
liability
Medicare tax
net income
net loss
net pay
nonsufficient funds (NSF)
one-write system
owner's equity
payable
payee
payer
payroll
payroll register
pegboard
pegboard system
petty cash
postdated
professional discounts
qualified endorsement
receipt-charge slip
reconciled
restrictive endorsement
salary
special endorsement
statement
statement of owner's equity
statement-receipt
State Unemployment Tax Act (SUTA)
superbill/routing form
T-account
Tax Payment Act
transactions
voucher
wages
workers' compensation
write-off

PRACTICAL APPLICATIONS

Read the following scenario and keep it in mind as you learn about the financial aspects of a medical practice in this chapter.

Meredith is the office manager for a private physician. She is responsible for the financial management of the office. She is the person who tracks the assets and liabilities for the accountant and interprets "owner equity" so that the physician will know the net value of the practice. As part of her job description, Meredith also disburses petty cash. She makes sure that the vouchers with receipts attached and the cash on hand balance at the end of each workday. As each patient leaves the office, the payments for office visits are collected. The goal is to collect whatever is necessary from patients (co-payment, co-insurance) on the day of service. If patient receivables are current, outstanding insurance claims become the main focus for accounts receivable. Another one of Meredith's duties is to approve or disapprove of professional discounts and write-offs as fee adjustments. Finally, she generates collection letters and telephone calls for overdue and delinquent accounts.

Would you be able to perform these responsibilities in the medical office?

ACCOUNTING PRINCIPLES

Accounting is considered the "language" of business because it describes the activities of a business. Effective accounting records provide the medical practice with accurate and timely information regarding the financial activities and condition of the practice. The accounting process analyzes, classifies, records, summarizes, and interprets the **transactions** (financial activities) or activities of the business in financial terms. Accounting and bookkeeping are not the same activity.

Accounting involves the design and management of the financial operating system; it specifies how bookkeeping should be done. **Bookkeeping** is the basic process of recording the financial activities of the business.

Medical assistants need to understand the accounting equation, assets and liabilities, and the various types of financial statements used for medical office accounting.

Assets, Liabilities, and Equity

Assets, liabilities, and equity are three important accounting principles.

- *Assets.* A medical practice has many items of value. It acquires items, such as cash, equipment, and supplies, that will be used to conduct the daily activities of the practice. Anything of value that is owned by the medical practice is an **asset.** Assets have value because they can be used to acquire other items of value or be used to operate the medical practice. Even art or sculpture may be included in this asset.
- *Liabilities.* An amount owed by the medical practice is called a **liability.** Liabilities are debts and include what the business owes its creditors (e.g., business loans, charge accounts, or vendors).
- *Owner's equity.* The amount remaining after the liabilities are subtracted from the assets is called **owner's equity.** Owner's equity is the investment the physician or physicians have made in the medical practice. When a medical practice is being started, the owner puts an initial investment of cash into the practice. This infusion of cash increases the cash assets and owner's equity and funds the operation of the business.

Assets, liabilities, and equity are all a part of the accounting equation. A T-account is used to represent the accounting equation.

Accounting Equation

An equation that expresses the relationship among assets, liabilities, and owner's equity is called the **accounting equation.** The accounting equation is stated as follows:

$$\text{Assets} = \text{Liabilities} + \text{Owner's equity}$$

The total of the amounts on the left side of the equation (assets) will always be equal to the total of the amounts on the right side (liabilities + owner's equity).

For example, if the office pays $50 cash for medical supplies, the cash account decreases, but the medical inventory supply account increases by the same amount. This keeps the equation in balance because the total assets have remained the same and the liabilities and owner's equity remain unchanged.

$$\text{Cash} + \text{Medical supplies} = \text{Liabilities} + \text{Owner's equity}$$

Opening balance:

$$1000 + 500 = 600 + 900$$

After transaction:

$$(1000 - 50) + (500 + 50) = 600 + 900$$
$$950 + 550 = 600 + 900$$

Therefore each side of the equation is equal.

If the office had charged the $50 in medical supplies, how would the equation change and would it be in balance?

After transaction:

$$1000 + (500 + 50) = (600 + 50) + 900$$
$$1000 + 550 = 650 + 900$$

Instead of $50 being subtracted from cash, $50 was added to liabilities and the accounting equation is still in balance.

NOTE: Total assets and total liabilities have each increased by the same amount. Owner's equity cannot increase by increasing liabilities; it can increase only through the owner contributing more equity to the business or the business earning a profit.

T-Accounts

The accounting equation can be represented as a T, as shown in Figure 28-1. As seen with the previous example of the purchase of medical supplies, a transaction changes the balance of two different accounts in the accounting equation. When using the T-account, an amount recorded on the left side of the T is called a **debit** and an amount recorded on the right side is called a **credit.** The T-account is the basic tool used to analyze the effect of a transaction on accounts. A debit entry will *increase* the value of an asset account but will *decrease* a liability and owner's equity account.

Using the above example, T-accounts would appear as follows:

After transaction:

1000	+	500	=	600	+	900
		+50		+50		
1000	+	550	=	650	+	900
D C		D C		D C		D C
1000		500		600		900
		50		50		

Asset accounts (e.g., cash, equipment owned) have normal debit balances (D, left side), and liability and owner's equity accounts have normal credit balances (C, right side). Since

Assets	=	Liabilities + Owner's Equity
Left side		Right side

A

T-Account	
Left side	Right side
DEBIT SIDE	CREDIT SIDE

B

FIGURE 28-1 A, Accounting equation in T-account form. **B,** T-account showing the debit side *(left)* and credit side *(right)*.

asset accounts have normal debit balances, they increase on the debit side and decrease on the credit side. Liability and owner's equity accounts increase on the credit side and decrease on the debit side.

It is important to remember that each transaction will change the balance of at least two specific accounts, one on each side of the T-account. For example, disbursing cash will decrease cash (a credit). The other half of the transaction must be a debit that offsets the credit to the cash account. That debit can be an increase in an asset (e.g., increase in inventory) or a decrease in a liability (debit) that was paid through the original disbursement of cash (credit).

Types of Assets

Although the specific assets of a medical practice will vary, some types of assets are common to many medical practices: cash, accounts receivable, and miscellaneous assets such as property and equipment.

Cash

A medical practice receives cash for services rendered. This may be in the form of a payment from a patient (either full payment or a co-payment) or by the insurance company. Petty cash is another cash asset of the medical office.

Petty Cash. **Petty cash** is an amount of cash kept on hand used for making small payments for incidental supplies. Ideally, "cash control" (having a record of what money is spent and how) is best maintained when payments are made by check. Some expenses are small, however, and writing a check is not time- or cost-effective. In these situations, a separate cash fund for making small cash payments is maintained (the petty cash fund). Each office will decide on the actual dollar amount kept in the fund, but essentially, the fund should provide for small cash purchases for a month. The petty cash account is an asset and has a debit, or positive, balance. Remember only one person should be responsible for petty cash.

Each time a payment is made from the petty cash fund, a numbered form, or **voucher,** is prepared (Figure 28-2). The voucher shows the date and purpose of the withdrawal, to whom the money was paid, and the amount of the payment. Petty cash vouchers are kept in the petty cash box until the fund is replenished.

Every time petty cash is paid out, the transaction should also be recorded in the petty cash record (Figure 28-3). Employees requesting reimbursement from the petty cash fund should submit proof of their expenditures, such as a receipt, and it should be attached to the voucher. The amount in the petty cash box decreases with each payment. Eventually, the fund needs to be replenished. When reconciling a petty cash fund, the person responsible for the fund totals the vouchers, distributes the total into proper categories, and reimburses the fund for the amount of the vouchers to bring the cash balance back up to the original amount. Procedure 28-1 explains the process of accounting for petty cash.

Amount $ 42.00 No. 17

RECEIVED OF PETTY CASH

For 7/31/XXXX

Charge to Postage

Approved by Gail Landers

Received by Erica Taylor

FIGURE 28-2 Petty cash voucher. (Modified from Kinn ME, Woods MA: *The medical assistant,* ed 8, Philadelphia, 1999, Saunders.)

For example, if the amount initially put in the petty cash fund is $50.00, and at the end of the month the vouchers total $49.10 and $0.90 remains, there is no shortage or surplus of money in the petty cash fund. In this case a check is written for $49.10 and then cashed to bring the account back to $50.00.

However, if at the end of the month the voucher total is $48.00, but only $1.00 remains, this means there is a shortage of $1 in the fund. A shortage slip is made out to account for the missing money ($1.00), and a check is written for $49.00. The voucher total plus the shortage slip will account for the $49.00 check (see Procedure 28-3).

No.	Date	Description	Amount	Office Exp.	Auto.	Misc.	Balance
	04/01	FUND ESTABLISHED					50.00
1	04/02	POSTAGE DUE	.55	.55			49.45
2	04/08	PARKING FEE	6.00		6.00		43.45
3	04/10	DELIVERY CHARGE	2.32			2.32	41.13
4	04/25	STATIONERY SUPPLIES	3.38	3.38			37.75
		TOTAL	12.25				
		BALANCE	37.75	3.93	6.00	2.32	
	CK#	374	12.25				50.00

FIGURE 28-3 Petty cash record. (From Kinn ME, Woods MA: *The medical assistant,* ed 8, Philadelphia, 1999, Saunders.)

PROCEDURE 28-1 Manage an Account for Petty Cash

TASK: Establish a petty cash fund, maintain an accurate record of expenditures, and replenish the fund as necessary.

EQUIPMENT AND SUPPLIES
- Petty cash box or envelope
- Petty cash expense record
- Petty cash vouchers with receipts or list of petty cash expenditures
- Two blank checks
- Calculator
- Pen or pencil

SKILLS/RATIONALE

1. **Procedural Step.** Establish the amount needed in the petty cash fund.
2. **Procedural Step.** Write a check for the determined amount, and put the cash in the petty cash box or envelope.
   Rationale. This establishes a petty cash fund.
3. **Procedural Step.** Record the beginning balance to the petty cash record.
4. **Procedural Step.** Prepare a petty cash voucher for each amount withdrawn from the fund and attach a sales receipt or an explanation of the payment.
   Rationale. The vouchers, sales receipts, and explanations of payment will be used for audit purposes.
5. **Procedural Step.** Enter each expense in the petty cash expense record, allocating them to the correct disbursement categories. Calculate the new balance.
   Rationale. Bringing forward the new balance after each entry keeps the balance current and helps determine when it is time to restore the fund to its original balance.
6. **Procedural Step.** At the end of the month or when the fund balance has reached the established minimum, count the remaining currency in the petty cash box.
7. **Procedural Step.** Total all vouchers in the petty cash box.
8. **Procedural Step.** Add the voucher total to the amount in the petty cash fund. This should equal the original amount.
   Rationale. The total of the remaining cash and the total of the expense vouchers should equal the amount originally in the petty cash fund.
9. **Procedural Step.** Prepare a check for "cash" for the amount that was used for expenses (total of the vouchers). Enter the check number on the petty cash expense record.
   This check should be categorized in the disbursement journal by the categories on the petty cash receipt.
10. **Procedural Step.** After the replacement check is cashed, add the money back to the cash box.
11. **Procedural Step.** Record the amount added to the fund on the expense record.
12. **Procedural Step.** Bring the balance forward.
    NOTE: Petty cash is usually kept in a locked drawer or locked box; it is generally not kept at the front desk. Usually only one person on staff is responsible for petty cash. Change for patients should not be made from the petty cash fund; there should be separate funds for that purpose. Staff should never be permitted to borrow from petty cash.

Accounts Receivable

Accounts receivable (AR) are used to record patient transactions when an amount is still due (owed) to the office (e.g., when an insurance payment has not yet arrived). A charge to a patient's AR account will increase the account balance, and a payment or adjustment will decrease the balance. The information provided by the AR account assists in managing the cash flow of the practice. This account represents credit extended to the customer (e.g., how much money is owed to the practice by patients). Think of AR as an account that is for "collection of past services."

Aging of Accounts. An AR report that is beneficial to the financial success of the medical practice is the **aging report,** which shows the "age" of the debt, or how long the debt has gone unpaid. The following categories are used to identify accounts that are overdue:

- *Current:* These accounts include services that were provided within the month, and the accounts have not yet been sent an end-of-month statement.

- *0-30:* These accounts include services within the month and have been sent an end-of-month statement.
- *31-60:* These accounts reflect 2 months of billing services and need attention.
- *61-90:* These accounts have received 3 months of billing invoices, are long overdue, and may be sent to a collection agency.
- *Over 90:* These accounts are seriously overdue and should be in collection.

The longer an account "ages," the less likely the practice is to recover the amount due in full. Aging accounts should be done on a monthly basis to maintain control of the accounts receivable.

Miscellaneous Assets

Assets such as cash and accounts receivable in a medical office are easy to identify. However, a medical practice may own the property and the building where the medical office is located. The medical supplies, equipment, and furniture in the facility are all things of value owned by the business and are considered assets.

Types of Liabilities

Liabilities are debts owed by the medical practice. Liabilities are written as **payable** (e.g., notes payable, accounts payable, or wages payable). Think of a note payable as a "loan," accounts payable as "credit charges" (for inventory, supplies, and utilities), and wages payable as "money due to employees."

Financial Statements

Financial statements are reports that tell the owner (physician) the fiscal (financial) condition of the practice. The owner uses these statements to consider expansion of the practice, budget for additional staff and equipment, and make salary adjustments (Figure 28-4).

Income Statement

An **income statement** shows the results of income (revenues) and expenses over time, usually a month or year. The income statement shows money earned by the medical office and the expense of doing business. Another name for the income statement is a *profit and loss statement* or a *statement of income and expenses.* The income statement condenses the results of the activities into one figure, either **net income** or **net loss**. The income statement is prepared first so that the result (net income or loss) can be recorded in the statement of owner's equity, which is prepared next.

Statement of Owner's Equity

The **statement of owner's equity** reports the changes in the owner's financial interest during a reporting period and why the investment has changed. The net income or net loss amount is needed before the statement of owner's equity can be prepared. An investment or cash inflow to the medical practice will increase owner's equity, and withdrawals will decrease it. The ending balance (capital) on the statement of owner's equity is used on the balance sheet, so this statement must be prepared before the balance sheet.

Balance Sheet

The **balance sheet** reports the financial condition of a medical practice on a given date, usually the end of each month. It shows what the medical practice owns and owes, as well as the amount of owner's equity (capital). By reviewing the balance sheet with the income statement, the physician is able to assess the financial position of the practice.

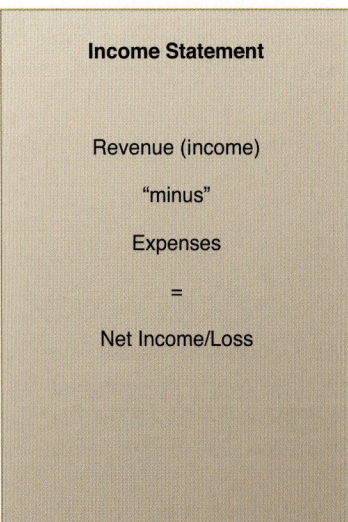
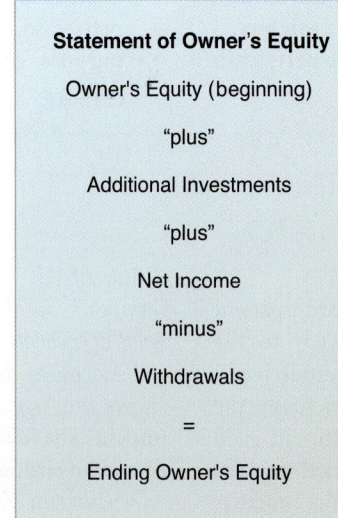
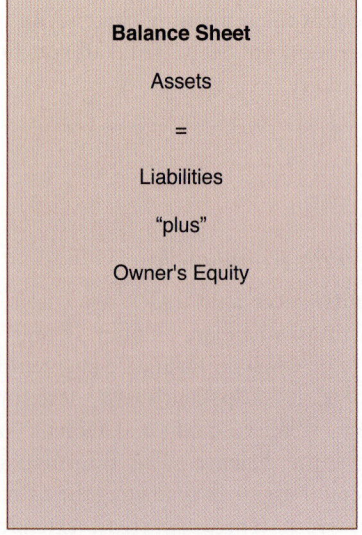

FIGURE 28-4 Financial statements: income statement, statement of owner's equity, and balance sheet.

PATIENT-CENTERED PROFESSIONALISM

- Why is it important for the medical assistant to understand basic accounting principles?
- If a medical assistant asked for a salary raise, which financial statements would provide information to the medical practice to make such a decision?

BOOKKEEPING PROCEDURES

Bookkeeping involves the systematic recording of financial business transactions. The person performing this function must understand the entire accounting system. A medical assistant performs bookkeeping tasks when recording all financial transactions on the daysheet or entering the information into a computerized management system. The recorded data are organized and reported on a timely basis so that appropriate financial statements can be prepared.

Many offices use a computerized patient accounting system for their daily bookkeeping tasks. Computerized bookkeeping is becoming increasingly common. Bookkeeping can also be done with the pegboard system.

Pegboard System

The **pegboard system,** or **one-write system,** is a type of recording system designed to increase the efficiency of recording daily transactions (Figure 28-5). It is used most often for three types of documents or forms: payroll, general ledgers, and accounts receivable. The **pegboard** is a special device used to write the same information on several forms at one time (Figure 28-6).

The name "pegboard" comes from the pegs along one side of the board. The forms used with this device have holes punched along one side. Each of the forms is placed on the pegs. Thus the lines on each form are aligned, one beneath the other, and information written will be correctly positioned on each form. When an entry is made on the form on the top page of the pegboard, the data is reproduced on all the other forms beneath it at the same time. This happens because the forms are printed on NCR, or no carbon required, paper, which is chemically treated to allow the transfer of entries from one sheet to another. Carbonized strips are on the form in specific places that must be recorded more than once. Remember that anything you write on the top sheet will show on the NCR sheets, so do not place miscellaneous papers or forms (e.g., phone messages) on top of the pegboard and write on them.

The pegboard has two major purposes: (1) it provides a solid writing base for writing on the forms by hand and (2) information is recorded on several forms at once, thus saving time and reducing the chance of error.

When a patient arrives for the scheduled office visit, the medical assistant attaches either the receipt-charge slip or the encounter form (superbill) to the pegboard to register the patient and then to the front of the patient's medical record. The physician completes the information on the form and returns the chart, with the form, to the front desk, where the medical assistant enters the dollar amount on the form from the **fee schedule** for all treatments. Daysheets, various charge forms, and ledger cards are used on the pegboard system, and the medical assistant needs to understand how to post service charges and payments using this system. (See Chapter 25 for illustrations of these procedures done on a computer.)

Daysheet

The **daysheet** acts as a journal for recording the day's activities. It provides a record of the patients seen, charges, and payments received on a daily basis (Figure 28-7). Each day, all

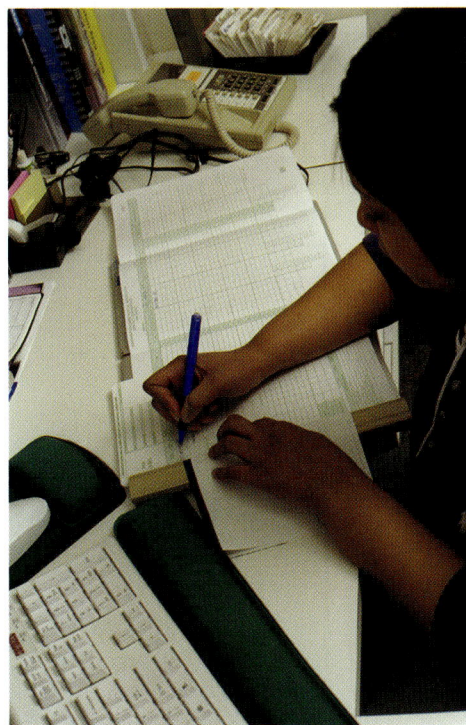

FIGURE 28-5 Medical assistant using pegboard system to record the day's activities.

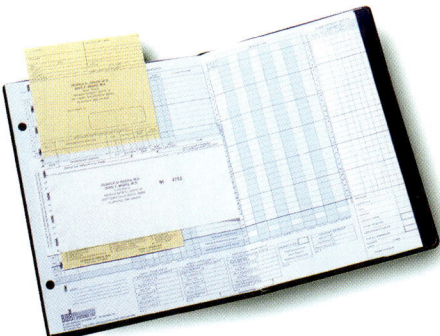

FIGURE 28-6 Use of a daysheet provides a record of patients seen, charges, and payments for a given day. (Courtesy Bibbero Systems, Inc., Petaluma, CA (800) 242-2376; fax (800) 242-9330; www.bibbero.com.)

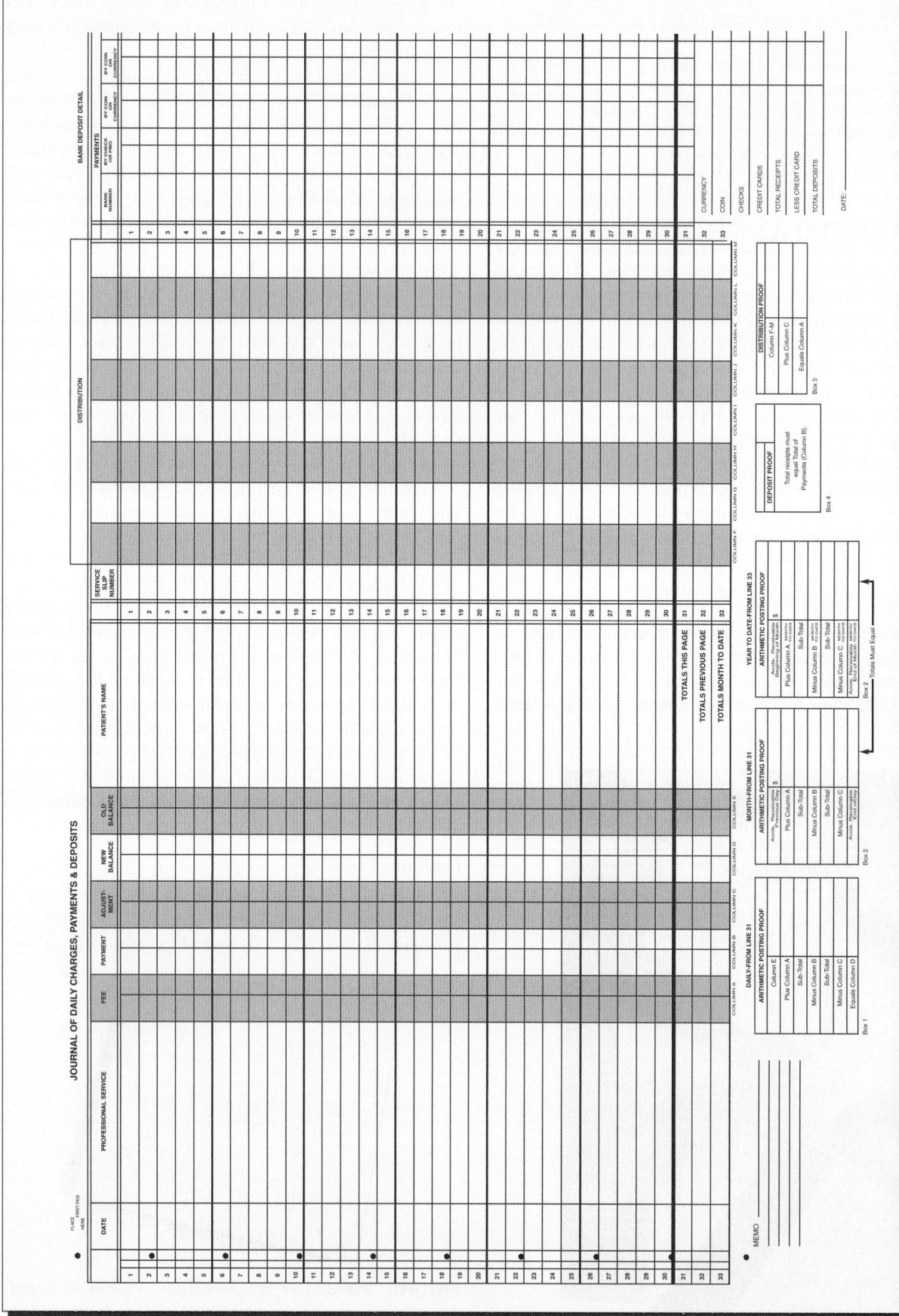

FIGURE 28-7 Sample daysheet used with a pegboard system. (Product No. 42-9029 courtesy Bibbero Systems, Inc., Petaluma, CA (800) 242-2376; fax (800) 242-9330; www.bibbero.com.)

columns of the daysheet are totaled and checked for accuracy. The daysheet lets the physician know the amount of money collected for the day and the amount still owed.

Charge Forms

Several types of charge forms are used in the medical office. Two common charge forms are the encounter form and the receipt-charge slip.

Encounter Form. The **encounter form,** or **superbill/routing form,** is a charge form that lists the ICD-9 and CPT codes most frequently used in the medical practice. (These codes are discussed in more detail in Chapter 29.) Figure 28-8 shows a completed encounter form. Note the blank spaces for adding codes and a space for the physician to indicate when the patient should return for follow-up. Also included is a financial box to list financial data such as outstanding balance. The encounter form should be updated frequently, so it is important not to order an inordinate amount each printing.

Receipt-Charge Slip. The **receipt-charge slip,** or **statement-receipt,** is a charge form with two parts. The right side is the *charge slip,* listing the previous balance, treatments, and the patient's name (statement). The left side lists financial data such as the charges for certain treatments, payments received (receipt), and the current balance (Figure 28-9). The left portion of this form is returned to the patient as a *receipt* for any payment given to the physician that day.

Ledger Cards

When arriving for a scheduled appointment, a new patient is asked to complete a patient information (registration) sheet. This completed data sheet provides the demographic and insurance information needed to prepare a patient ledger card (Figure 28-10).

Ledger cards contain demographics (name, address, and telephone number) about the patient, as well as important billing information. When the patient is provided treatment, the ledger card is inserted between the charge slip (the encounter form or statement-receipt) and the daysheet and the type of service and the charges are recorded (charges for each service should be listed on the physician's fee schedule). Payment is recorded, and the current balance is listed. The ledger card is a permanent record on each patient and contains the up-to-date status of the patient's account. Many offices photocopy the ledger cards and mail them to their patients as account statements.

Posting Payments

When a patient visits the medical office and makes a payment, it is recorded immediately. Payments may be in the form of check, cash, or credit card. Payments are also received electronically or in the mail from the insurance company, as well as from the patient at a later date.

Procedure 28-2 explains the process of posting service charges and payments to the patient's account.

Procedure 28-3 explains how to record charges and credits to the patient's account.

Immediate Payment by Credit Card. A patient may offer to pay for services with a credit card or debit card. The medical practice must have an agreement with the credit card company. The agreement indicates a service charge will be applied to each transaction made by the medical office. Often a flat fee or a small percentage of the total payment goes to the credit card company as per the agreement. When the payment is processed, the patient receives a hard copy of the transaction as a receipt. The transaction is posted on the ledger card, recording all information (credit card company, total amount, and date).

Payment by Mail. Payments from patients are sometimes received in the mail after the appointment. In this situation the ledger card is pulled and positioned on the appropriate line on the daysheet. The payments are posted on the ledger card and daysheet.

Payment from Third-Party Payers. Payments from insurance companies (third-party payers) usually do not cover the total amount, so the account must be adjusted after an insurance payment is received. Adjustments are made according to the agreement between the insurance company and the physician about how much can be charged for a service. For example, Medicare has specified "allowable" charges for services. When a physician agrees to accept Medicare patients, he or she must not charge more than the Medicare "allowable" amount. The difference between the physician's charge and the correct Medicare payment must be "adjusted" (deducted from) on the patient's account; the patient is not charged for this difference. (This process is explained further in the Billing and Collections section.)

Computerized Account Management

There are many computerized account management systems for medical offices. The procedures used are similar to those of the pegboard system. The current date is verified each morning because this is the date recorded when posting the business transaction of the medical office. An encounter form is attached to the patient's chart. When returned to the front desk, the patient's account is "pulled up" on the computer, the current charges are entered (posted), and payments and adjustments are made. A receipt can be printed for the patient. At the end of the workday, a daysheet (daily journal) can be printed and all entries verified. Computerized systems will automatically post the daily transactions to each patient's account and total all activities for the day.

Advantages of using various types of computerized systems include the following:

1. Claims to insurance companies can be submitted electronically (837 Professional claim), or a CMS-1500 form can be generated.
2. Reports of financial and billing information can be more detailed and printed easily. For example, a summary of all billing items for a patient can be provided to include current balance, an account ledger can provide transaction

Text continued on p. 557

552 SECTION IV Administrative Medical Assisting

Blackburn Primary Care Associates, PC
1990 Turquoise Drive
Blackburn, WI 54937
(608) 555-8857

Howard M. Lawler, MD 11
Joanne R. Hughes, MD 21
Ralph Garcia Lopez, MD 31
TAX ID NO. 00-00000000

GUARANTOR NAME AND ADDRESS	PATIENT NO.	PATIENT NAME	DOCTOR NO.	DATE
Darla Sissle 468 Maple Street Blackburn, WI 54937		Darla Sissle	21	6/5/XX
	DATE OF BIRTH	TELEPHONE NO.	INSURANCE	
			CODE / DESCRIPTION	CERTIFICATE NO.
	2/17/32	555-2075	CPC	21 - 58624

OFFICE - NEW
X	CPT	SERVICE	FEE
	99201	Prob Foc/Straight	
	99202	Exp Prob/Straight	
	99203	Detailed/Low	
	99204	Compre/Moderate	
	99205	Compre/High	

OFFICE - ESTABLISHED
X	CPT	SERVICE	FEE
	99211	Nurse/Minimal	
	99212	Prob Foc/Straight	
	99213	Exp Prob/Low	55
	99214	Detailed/Moderate	
	99215	Compre/High	

OFFICE - CONSULT
X	CPT	SERVICE	FEE
	99241	Prob/Foc/Straight	
	99242	Exp Prob/Straight	
	99243	Detailed/Low	
	99244	Compre/Moderate	
	99245	Compre/High	

PREVENTIVE CARE - ADULT
X	CPT	SERVICE	FEE
	99385	18-39 Initial	
	99386	40-64 Initial	
	99387	65+ Initial	
	99395	18-39 Periodic	
	99396	40-64 Periodic	
	99397	65+ Periodic	

GASTROENTEROLOGY
X	CPT	SERVICE	FEE
	45300	Sigmoidoscopy Rig	
	45305	Sigmoid Rig w/bx	
	45330	Sigmoidoscopy Flex	
	45331	Sigmoid Flex w/bx	
	45378	Colonoscopy Diag	
	45380	Colonoscopy w/bx	
	46600	Anoscopy	

CARDIOLOGY & HEARING
X	CPT	SERVICE	FEE
	93000	ECG (Global)	55
	93015	Stress Test (Global)	
	93224	Holter (Global)	
	93225	Holter Hook Up	
	93227	Holter Interpretation	
	94010	Pulm Function Test	
	92551	Audiometry Screen	

INJECTIONS & IMMUNIZATION
X	CPT	SERVICE	FEE
	86585	TB Skin Test	
	90716	Varicella Vaccine	
	90724	Flu Vaccine	
	90732	Pneumovax	
	90718	TD Immunization	
	90782	Injection IM*	
	90788	Injection IM Antibiot*	
		Injection joint*	
	SM MED MAJOR (circle one)		
FOR ALL INJECTIONS, SUPPLY DRUG INFORMATION			

REPAIR & DERMATOLOGY
X	CPT	SERVICE	FEE
	17110	Warts: #	
		Tags: #	
		Lesion Excis	
		Lesion Destruct	
SIZE CM: SITE:			
MALIG: PREMAL/BEN: (Check One Above)			
		Simple Closure	
		Intermed Closure	
SIZE CM: SITE:			
	10060	I&D Abscess	
	10080	I&D Cyst	

OTHER | **SUPPLIES/DRUGS***
DRUG NAME:
UNIT/MEASURE:
QUANTITY

DIAGNOSTIC CODES: ICD-9-CM

- ☐ 789.0 Abdominal Pain
- ☐ 795.0 Abnormal Pap Smear
- ☐ 706.1 Acne Vulgaris
- ☐ 477.0 Allergic Rhinitis
- ☐ 285.9 Anemia, NOS
- ☐ 281.0 Pernicious
- ☐ 411.1 Angina, Unstable
- ☐ 427.9 Arrhythmia, NOS
- ☐ 440.9 Arteriosclerosis
- ☐ 714.0 Arthritic, Rheumatoid
- ☐ 414.0 ASHD
- ☐ 493.90 Asthma, Bronchial W/O Status Ast.
- ☐ 493.91 Asthma, Bronchial W/ Status Ast.
- ☐ 466.1 Bronchiolitis, Acute
- ☐ 466.0 Bronchitis, Acute
- ☐ 727.3 Bursitis
- ☒ 786.50 Chest Pain ⟵
- ☐ 574.20 Cholelithiasis
- ☐ 372.30 Conjunctivitis, Unspecified
- ☐ 564.0 Constipation
- ☐ 496 COPD
- ☐ 692.9 Dermatitis, Allergic
- ☐ 250.01 Diabetes Mellitus, ID
- ☐ 250.00 Diabetes Mellitus, NID
- ☐ 558.9 Diarrhea
- ☐ 562.11 Diverticulitis
- ☐ 562.10 Diverticulosis

- ☐ 782.3 Edema
- ☐ 492.8 Emphysema
- ☐ V16.0 Family History of Diabetes
- ☐ 780.6 Fever of Undetermined Origin
- ☐ 578.9 G.I. Bleeding, Unspecified
- ☐ 727.41 Ganglion of Joint
- ☐ 535.0 Gastritis, Acute
- ☐ V72.3 Arrhythmia, NOS
- ☐ 748.1 Headache
- ☐ 550.90 Hornia, Inguinal, NOS
- ☐ 054.9 Herpes Simplex
- ☐ 053.9 Herpes Zoster
- ☐ 708.9 Hives/Urticaria
- ☐ 401.1 Hypertension, Benign
- ☐ 401.0 Hypertension, Malignant
- ☐ 402.90 Hypertension, W/O CHF
- ☐ 244.9 Hypothyroidism, Primary
- ☐ 380.4 Impacted Cerumen
- ☐ 487.1 Influenza
- ☐ 564.1 Irritable Bowel Syndrome
- ☐ 464.0 Laryngitis, Acute
- ☐ 454.9 Leg Varicose Veins
- ☐ 424.0 Mitral Valve Prolapse
- ☐ 412 Myocardial Infarction, Old
- ☐ 715.90 Osteoarthritis, Unspec. Site
- ☐ 620.2 Ovarian Cyst

- ☐ 614.9 Pelvic Inflammatory Disease
- ☐ 685.1 Pilonidal Cyst
- ☐ 462 Pharyngitis, Acute
- ☐ 627.1 Postmenopausal Bleeding
- ☐ 625.4 Premenstrual Tension
- ☐ 782.1 Rash
- ☐ 569.3 Rectal Bleeding
- ☐ 398.90 Rheumatic Heart Disease, NOS
- ☐ 431.9 Sinusitis, Acute, NOS
- ☐ 782.1 Skin Eruption, Rash
- ☐ 845.00 Sprain, Ankle
- ☐ 848.9 Sprain, Muscle, Unspec. Site
- ☐ 785.6 Swollen Glands
- ☐ 246.9 Thyroid Disease, Unspecified
- ☐ 463 Tonsillitis, Acute

- ☐ 474.0 Tonsillitis, Chronic
- ☐ 465.9 Upper Respiratory Infection, Acute
- ☐ 599.0 Urinary Tract Infection
- ☐ V03.9 Vaccination/Bacterial Dis.
- ☐ V06.8 Vaccination/Combination
- ☐ V04.8 Vaccination, Influenza
- ☐ 616.10 Vaginitis, Vulvitis, NOS
- ☐ 780.4 Vertigo
- ☐ 787.0 Vomiting, Nausea

RETURN APPOINTMENT
_7_ Days
___ Weeks
___ Months

Authorization Number:
▶ _____

BALANCE DUE
DATE OF SERVICE	CPT CODE	DIAGNOSIS CODE(S)	CHARGE

Place of Service:
☒ Office
( ) Emergency Room
( ) Inpatient Hospital
( ) Outpatient Hospital
( ) Nursing Home

TOTAL CHARGE $ 110
AMOUNT PAID $ 100
PREVIOUS BAL $ 100
BALANCE DUE $ 110

Check #: _____
(Circle Method of Payment)
CASH **CHECK** MC VISA

Physician's Signature
▶ *Joanne R. Hughes, MD*

FIGURE 28-8 Encounter form (superbill). (From Hunt SA: *Saunders fundamentals of medical assisting—revised reprint,* St Louis, 2007, Saunders.)

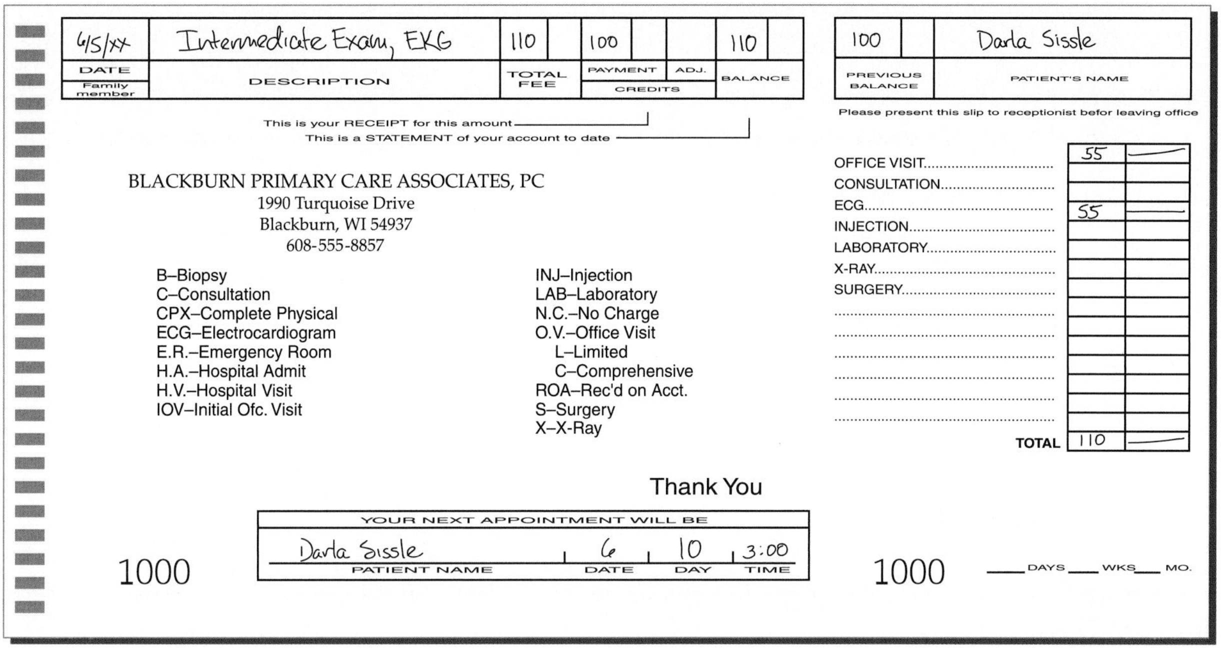

Financial Management **CHAPTER 28** 553

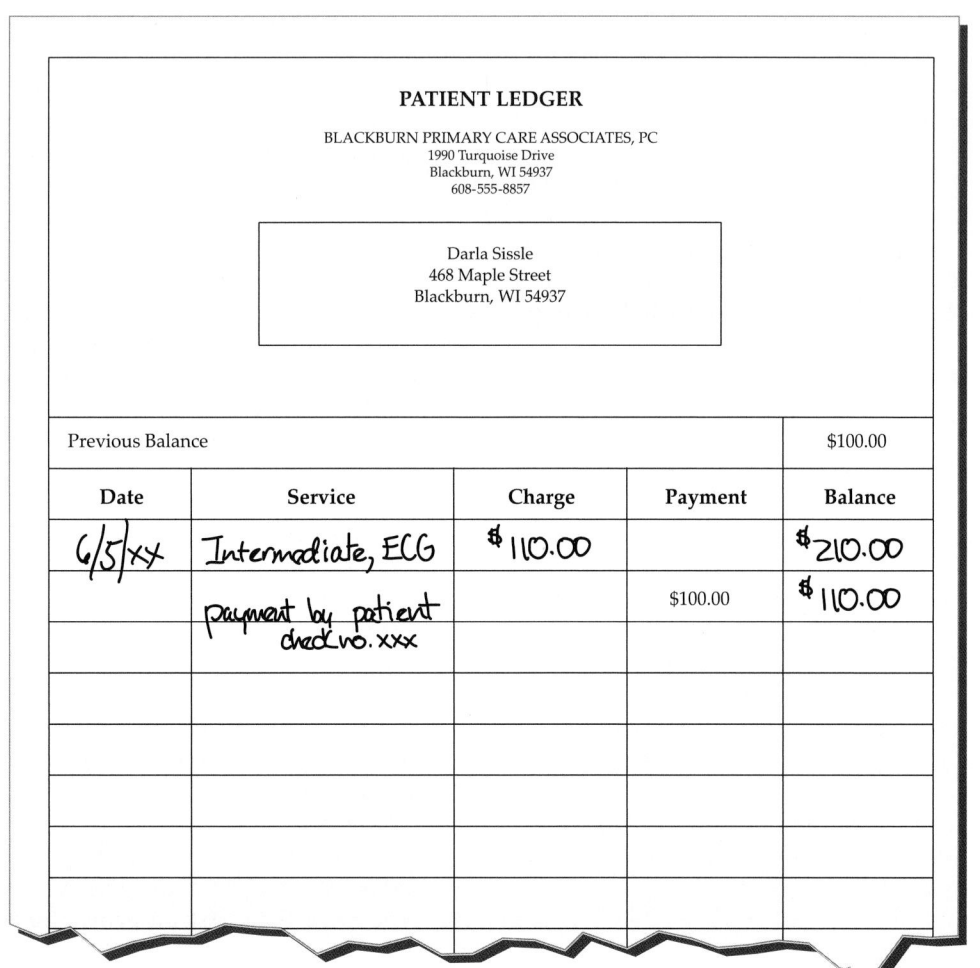

FIGURE 28-9 Receipt-charge slip for the pegboard system. (From Hunt SA: *Saunders fundamentals of medical assisting—revised reprint,* St Louis, 2007, Saunders.)

FIGURE 28-10 Patient account ledger. (From Hunt SA: *Saunders fundamentals of medical assisting—revised reprint,* St Louis, 2007, Saunders.)

PROCEDURE 28-2 Post Service Charges and Payments to the Patient's Account

TASK: Post service charges and payments to a daysheet and ledger card, and prepare a receipt.

EQUIPMENT AND SUPPLIES
- Pegboard/clipboard
- Calculator
- Pen, pencil
- Daysheet (daily journal)
- Receipts
- Ledger cards
- Encounter form
- Previous day's balance
- List of patients and services
- Fee schedule

SKILLS/*RATIONALE*

1. **Procedural Step. Prepare the pegboard:**
   a. Place a new daysheet on the board.
   b. Place a series of receipt-charge slips over the pegs aligning the top receipt with the first open writing line on the daysheet.
   OR
   a. Acquire a Journal of Daily Charges and Payment sheet.
   Rationale. This should be done every morning before scheduled appointments arrive so that the office is prepared to receive patients.

2. **Procedural Step. Using a pen, date the daysheet/daily journal sheet with the current date, then carry forward the balances from the previous day's financial activity.**
   To "carry forward" means to record the totals from the previous daysheet on the new sheet you have just prepared.
   Rationale. It is important that a ballpoint pen be used to ensure that the information is transferred through all layers of the pegboard system. Carrying forward balances ensures that all totals are current.

3. **Procedural Step. Pull ledger cards for patients scheduled for appointments that day.**

4. **Procedural Step. Align the ledger card.**
   When a patient arrives, insert the ledger card under the first receipt, aligning the first available writing line of the card with the carbonized strip on the receipt.
   Rationale. It is important to align the ledger card accurately with the receipt to ensure correct posting of information to the receipt, ledger card, and daysheet.
   OR
   Enter date on ledger card.

5. **Procedural Step. On the receipt-charge slip, enter the date and the patient's name.**
   Also enter on the daysheet/daily journal sheet any existing balance from the patient's ledger card in the Previous Balance column and the number of this receipt in the Receipt Number column. (If using a daily journal sheet, skip this latter action and move to Step 8.)

6. **Procedural Step. Detach the charge slip from the receipt and clip it to the patient's chart.**
   Rationale. The physician then can mark the slip to indicate the service(s) performed for the patient during the appointment.

7. **Procedural Step. Remove the ledger card from the pegboard.**
   Rationale. Removing the ledger card from the pegboard prepares you to be ready to make entries for other patients.

8. **Procedural Step. Complete the ledger card.**
   When the completed charge slip/encounter form is returned at the end of the visit, enter on it the appropriate fee(s) for the service(s) provided, using the office's fee schedule.

9. **Procedural Step. Locate on the pegboard the receipt with the number that matches the number on the patient's charge slip. (If using daily journal sheet, move to Step 12.)**
   Rationale. This is done to make certain it is the correct receipt.

10. **Procedural Step. Reinsert the patient's ledger card over the daysheet and under the correct receipt.**

11. **Procedural Step. Complete the receipt.**
    a. Enter the professional service code and services provided.
    b. Write the fee for the patient's visit on the receipt.
    Rationale. This will serve as the patient's receipt of services.

12. **Procedural Step. Ask the patient for payment; record the payment amount and the new balance for the patient's account.**

Continued

PROCEDURE 28-2 | **Post Service Charges and Payments to the Patient's Account—cont'd**

Rationale. This brings the patient's account up to date and provides current information for the patient.

13. **Procedural Step.** Remove the completed receipt from the pegboard and give the patient the receipt.
    OR
    Complete a receipt with appropriate information.
14. **Procedural Step.** Refile the ledger card according to office procedure.
15. **Procedural Step.** Repeat Steps 4 through 14 for each patient or receipt of payment for the day.
    If this sheet is filled during the day, prepare a new sheet and continue the day's activities. Then, at the end of the day, fill in the Total Sheet Numbers at the top of the form.
16. **Procedural Step.** At the end of the day, total all columns of the daysheet using a pencil until totals have been verified as accurate. This consists of two parts.

    a. Add up the amounts shown in columns A, B1, B2, C, and D, plus the total of the cash column, the total of the checks columns, and the total to deposit.
       Rationale. This determines the figures that need to be entered in the "Totals This Page" row.
    b. Add the figure in column A in the "Totals This Page" row and the figure in column A in the "Totals Previous Page" row. Do the same for columns B1, B2, C, and D.
       Rationale. This determines the figure that needs to be entered in the "Totals Month to Date" row.

17. **Procedural Step.** Write in ink the proof totals on the bottom of the daysheet and add the total number of pages in the Sheet Number space at the top of the daysheet page(s).

Figure courtesy Colwell, a division of Patterson Companies, Inc., St Paul, MN (800) 637-1140.

PROCEDURE 28-3 Record Adjustments and Credits to the Patient's Account

TASK: Record adjustments such as insurance payments, write-offs, professional discounts, and nonsufficient funds (NSF) using a pegboard/daily journal sheet.

EQUIPMENT AND SUPPLIES
- Pegboard/clipboard
- Calculator
- Pen, pencil
- Daysheet (daily journal)
- Ledger cards
- Previous day's balance
- List of patients and services
- Fee schedule

SKILLS/*RATIONALE*

Refer to the figure for Step 16 in Procedure 28-2 as you complete this procedure.

RECORDING ADJUSTMENTS

When an adjustment is necessary (e.g., insurance payment is less than charge based on contractual agreement; overpayment to account is made) the amount of the adjustment is entered in column B2.

To determine a new balance for the patient, add together the patient's previous balance and any current charges, then subtract from this sum any credits that appear in column B1, as well as the adjustment that shows in column B2. This produces the patient's new balance.

1. **Procedural Step. Pull the patient's ledger card and align it with the first available empty row on the daysheet.**
   Rationale. It is important to align the ledger card accurately to ensure correct posting of information to the ledger card and daysheet.
2. **Procedural Step. Fill out the ledger card, entering the date and the following information:**
   a. Notation of the payment.
   b. "Received on Account" (ROA) in the "Professional Services" area.
   c. Amount of the payment in the "Payment" column.
   d. Amount of the adjustment in the "Adjustment" column.
   e. New balance (calculated as stated above).
3. **Procedural Step. Refile the ledger card according to office procedure.**
4. **Procedural Step. Provide a refund if the patient's account has a credit balance (e.g., patient makes payment at time of service, then patient's insurance company is billed and makes subsequent payment).**
   a. To eliminate a credit balance, you must debit the account.
   b. Place the amount of the refund in the adjustment column in brackets, indicating it is a debit, not a credit adjustment.
   c. Write "Refund to Patient" in the description column.
   d. Write and mail a check to the patient in the amount of the refund.

RECORDING NONSUFFICIENT FUNDS

NSF situations are considered a "charge" and are accounted for on the daysheet in column A. Entering an NSF on the daysheet is similar to entering a charge for a professional service. If a notice of NSF is received in the mail, enter this information in column A by writing "NSF" in the "Professional Services" column. In column A, enter the sum of the returned check itself, plus any service charge your office makes for an NSF.

1. **Procedural Step. Pull the patient's ledger card and align it with the first available empty row on the daysheet.**
   Rationale. It is important to align the ledger card accurately to ensure correct posting of information to the ledger card and daysheet.
2. **Procedural Step. Fill out the ledger card, entering the date and the following:**
   a. Notation of "NSF" (including check number) in the "Professional Services" area.
   b. Amount of the NSF (check amount + service charge) in the "Fee" column.
   c. New balance.
3. **Procedural Step. Refile the ledger card according to office procedure.**
   NOTE: A receipt-charge slip is typically not used when entering an NSF on the daysheet.

Continued

PROCEDURE 28-3 Record Adjustments and Credits to the Patient's Account—cont'd

RECORDING COLLECTION AGENCY PAYMENT

When the medical practice is unable to collect on an account, it often turns it over to a collection agency. Some office policies write off the balance due, bringing the balance to zero. When the collection agency makes an agreement with the patient, an amount less than previously owed is usually settled on and the agency takes a percentage (40% to 60%) of those monies collected.

1. **Procedural Step.** Pull the patient's ledger card and align it with the first available empty row on the daysheet. A charge-receipt is not needed.

    Rationale. It is important to align the ledger card accurately to ensure correct positioning of the information to the ledger card and daysheet.

2. **Procedural Step.** Enter the patient's previous balance on the daysheet.

    Rationale. Once an account has been turned over to a collection agency the patient's account balance on account is written off to keep the accounts receivable balance accurate.

3. **Procedural Step.** Fill out the ledger card, entering the date and the following:
    a. Notation of "Reverse Collection" in the "Professional Services" area.
    b. Amount of the collection agency payment in adjustment column in brackets (debit).
    c. Amount of the payment in the payment column.
    d. Zero out any remaining balance by doing a credit adjustment.

    Rationale. Since this is not an original or new charge, the charge column is not used.

4. **Procedural Step.** Refile the ledger card according to office policy.

---

details with a procedure summary, and the program can capture payments and adjustments from both patient and insurance. Patient statements can be formatted to include prior balance, current activity, insurance pending amount, and aged patient balance.

3. Less room is needed for storage of paper records.
4. Entering data into one screen can automatically update other electronic forms.

> **PATIENT-CENTERED PROFESSIONALISM**
>
> - How is the pegboard system enhanced by the requirements used in bookkeeping?

BANKING PROCEDURES

The medical assistant responsible for administrative duties will receive payments for physician services in the form of cash, check, or credit card. When accepting a check for payment, the medical assistant must be aware of the basic check requirements necessary to make the payment valid. Sometimes the medical assistant may be asked to complete a check when purchasing office supplies or to complete a bank deposit at the end of the day. Understanding how to perform these duties correctly will make your job easier, whether these are your responsibilities or those of another medical assistant.

Checks

Although you may be familiar with writing checks, you should take a few precautionary steps when accepting and writing checks in the medical office. Understanding these precautions protects both the patient and the practice.

Accepting Checks

Checks received for medical services will be from a patient (personal check), an insurance company, or both. For example, a patient may make a co-payment with a check, and the portion of the service fee for which the insurance company is responsible can also be paid to the office in the form of a check. Medical assistants need to understand what information should be verified and follow office procedure on different types of checks. Checks with a "limited time" or "limited amount" must be deposited in a timely manner. "Not good after 90 days" and/or not written over the preprinted maximum dollar amount are examples of a "limited" check.

Check Requirements. When accepting a check for payment you must verify the following information:

1. *Correct provider name* (the **payee**). Check the spelling, as well as any credentials or titles (e.g., Rosa Parks Clinic; Pete Pierson, MD).
2. *Current date.* Check to verify that the date and year are correct and that the check is not **postdated** (a postdated check has a future date written on it).
3. *Correct amount.* Make sure the written amount on the check is the same as the number amount.
4. *Current address and phone number.* Verify that the demographic data (name, address) on the check match the patient's information on file.
5. *Affixed signature.* Verify that the person who signed the check (the **payer**) is listed on the check.

By confirming this information, you can prevent potential problems later with the bank or the patient.

Different Types of Checks. The medical office should have a written policy that states how the front desk is to handle "out-of-town" checks, third-party checks, and checks that are marked "paid in full."

- *Out-of-town checks* are written on an account in a bank that is not local. Some offices do not accept out-of-town checks.
- *Third-party checks* are "made out" to someone else but "signed over" to the medical practice. Third-party checks usually are not accepted because the medical office does not know the payer. An exception is an insurance check made out to the patient and endorsed by the patient to the medical practice.
- Checks marked *paid in full* should not be accepted unless the amount does cover the entire current balance. If the amount on a check that is marked "paid in full" does not cover the full amount, a notation above the endorsement should indicate that the payment is received toward an account balance.

Occasionally, the medical office receives other forms of payment such as the following:

- A *certified check* is stamped certified and the amount indicated on the check is held in the patient's account.
- A *cashier's check* is written by the bank to guarantee the check is good.
- *Traveler's checks* are purchased in defined amounts (e.g., $10, $20). When purchased, they are signed and signed again in front of the payee.
- *Money orders* are purchased at a bank or U.S. Postal Service for a specified amount. They are used to pay bills when the patient does not have a bank account.

Writing Checks

Payment by check provides the medical office with an excellent record of spending. By looking back at the checkregister (record of checks written, to whom, and for what amount), the physician or office manager can see where the money of the practice is going. Trends can be seen, and budgets prepared more easily. The cancelled check, when received from the bank with the bank statement, serves as a receipt and a permanent record. Most banks do not return cancelled checks each month but will return them on request. The bank does provide the check numbers on the bank statement, so they may be reconciled with the checkbook.

Different styles of checks include end-stub, wallet, and book styles. The type chosen for the medical practice depends on the needs and preferences of the person responsible for handling funds. Many physicians choose the end-stub style checks because they provide a place for recording important information about the payee or the reason the check was written.

The medical assistant may be required to fill out the necessary information on a check and then present it for an authorized signature (Figure 28-11). If you are asked to write checks, follow these security tips for check writing:

1. Only authorized office personnel may sign the check. Each authorized person must have a signature card on file at the bank.
2. The record portion of the end-stub style should be filled in before the check is completed.
3. All lines should be filled in closest to the left end of the line to prevent additions to the line. When the item written is completed, a long line should be added to fill out the line.

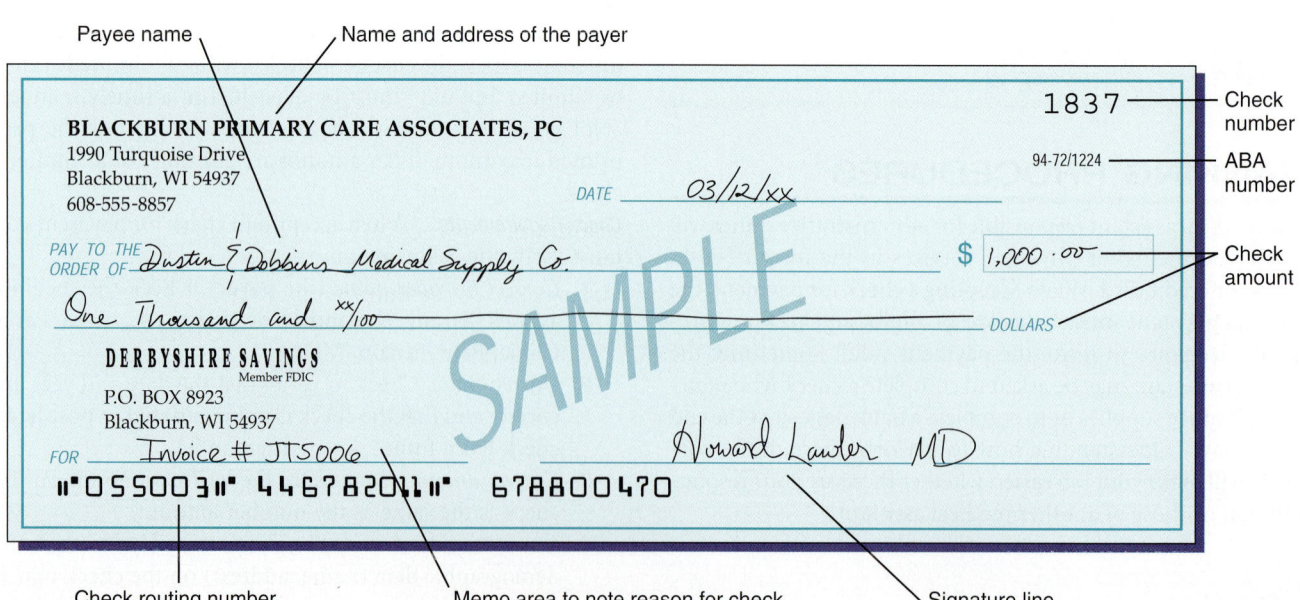

FIGURE 28-11 Completed check. (Modified from Hunt SA: *Saunders fundamentals of medical assisting—revised reprint,* St Louis, 2007, Saunders.)

Financial Management CHAPTER 28 559

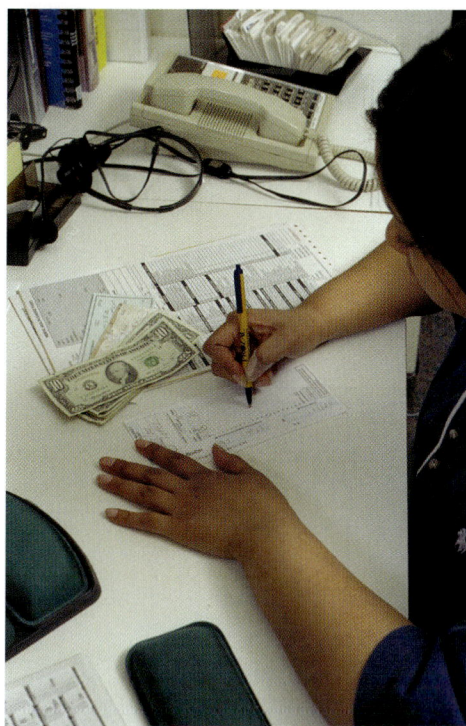

FIGURE 28-12 Accurate records reflect the competency of the staff. The medical assistant should use a calculator when adding numbers and should be careful not to transpose numbers when performing financial activities such as preparing deposit slips.

4. Check amounts are written with numbers and words. This eliminates misinterpreting the amount intended on the check.
5. Write the number amount in the box directly next to the dollar sign to reduce the chance of an additional number being added. Some medical offices use a check-writing machine that makes small perforations across the amount to prevent alterations.
6. Enter the cents as number of cents over the number one hundred (e.g., 10/100 for 10 cents).
7. Write the amount in words on the blank line that ends in "Dollars" *under* the line that starts with "Pay to the order of."

Deposits

A **deposit** is when money (cash or checks) is prepared and sent to a financial institution to be placed in an account. Deposits are usually made at the end of each business day (Figure 28-12). The medical assistant may be responsible for preparing or making deposits, so it is important to understand the concept of endorsement, how to use a deposit slip, and various deposit methods.

Endorsement

The physician or designated person must **endorse** the checks before they can be deposited. (Endorsing transfers all rights to another party, in this case the financial institution where

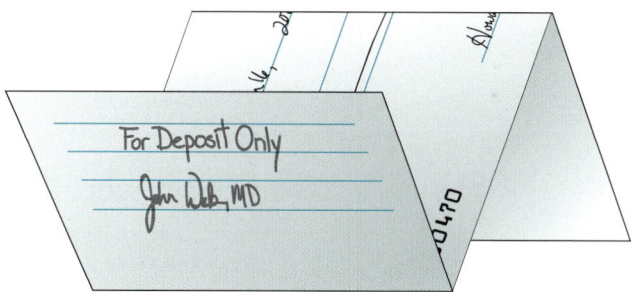

FIGURE 28-13 Physician's restrictive endorsement on the back of a check in the designated area.

the checks will be deposited.) This can be accomplished by having the physician sign each check in ink in the designated area on the back (Figure 28-13), or most often, the endorsement is obtained by stamping the back of each check with a specially designed stamp. Most medical offices prefer using a stamp because the check can be endorsed immediately on receiving the check for payment. The stamp can include the physician's signature with special instructions (e.g., "Alan Dean, M.D. For deposit to account of within named payee only").

- "For Deposit Only" is a form of **restrictive endorsement** because it limits what can be done with the check.
- A **blank endorsement** is when the payee (person to whom the check is written) signs only his or her name on the back of the check.
- A **special endorsement** includes words that specify to whom the endorser makes the check payable such as when a patient signs the back of an insurance check over to the medical practice for payment on their account (e.g., "Charlie Baker [patient] Pay to the order of Alan Dean, M.D.").
- Occasionally, a **qualified endorsement** is used to prevent future liability of the endorser. An attorney uses a qualified endorsement to accept a check on behalf of a client (e.g., "Paid in Full").

Deposit Slip

After the checks have been endorsed, a **deposit slip** is prepared. A deposit slip is completed each business day and is presented to the bank with the monies (cash, checks) so the deposit will be properly credited to the correct bank account. Most deposit slips are preprinted with the depositor's name, address, and the account number into which the money is being deposited. Most medical practices use deposit slips that are in duplicate form so a receipt can be kept for the deposit. Deposit slips are located at the end of the checkbook or may be separate documents in a book. They have a place for recording the date and columns in which to record the amount of cash (currency and coin) and individual checks (Figure 28-14).

When recording checks, the payer's name (name of the person who wrote the check) can be listed. Sometimes the **ABA number** (number assigned by the American Bankers Association to identify the payer's bank and location) is used. The ABA number is located on the upper right corner of each check as a whole number followed by a hyphen and ending

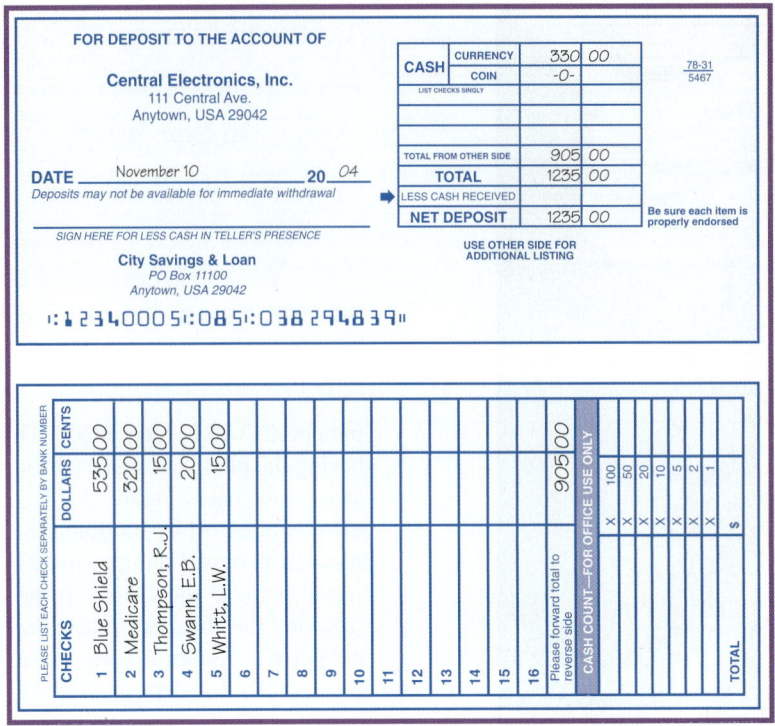

FIGURE 28-14 Front and back of a completed deposit slip. (From Young AP, Kennedy DB: *Kinn's the medical assistant,* ed 10, St Louis, 2007, Saunders.)

with a "fraction" (e.g., 94-72/1224). All credit card deposits are recorded on a separate deposit slip because they are deposited into a special account for this type of transaction.

Procedure 28-4 outlines the correct process for preparing a bank deposit.

Deposit Methods

Deposits can be made in several ways, including the following:
- *In person.* The deposit is handed to the teller, who in turn verifies the information contained on the deposit slip and provides a deposit receipt. Automated (or automatic) teller machines (ATMs) allow the deposit of monies into an account without a teller.
- *By mail.* This type of deposit is best used when the deposit consists only of checks. Special deposit forms are provided to the user by the bank, and a receipt can be made and later verified by the bank (Figure 28-15).
- *Electronic.* Electronic banking allows for all deposits to be made directly to a person's bank account. This is usually done by insurance companies that have made prior arrangements with the medical practice. The receipt of funds can be verified by viewing computerized banking records or through a statement sent to the medical office. Electronic banking also allows the medical office to have its liabilities (e.g., mortgage and lease payment, payments for vendors, or utilities) automatically deducted from its checking account.
- *Night deposit.* The bank provides the business with a key to the night depository and a special bank bag. The customer opens the locked drawer and places the bag into the drawer. The following morning, the bank verifies the deposit slip, credits the proper account, and forwards a deposit receipt to the customer.

No matter what deposit system is used, it is important to remember that the deposit receipt is a financial document and must be retained to verify a transaction. Good fiscal management requires daily deposits.

Statement Reconciliation

Each month the bank will mail a **bank statement** (statement of all banking activities for a set period) to the medical practice along with all canceled checks (Figure 28-16). Bank statements also list each deposit made, any service charges, interest received, and any other fees (e.g., ordering of checks, NSF checks). These statements must be **reconciled** monthly (put into agreement with the checkbook). Some banks provide this service by e-mail.

A bank statement is reconciled when the checks written on the medical practice's account are compared to those received by the bank. Any checks written or deposits deposited after the closing date of the bank statement are subtracted from or added to the balance. The bank reconciliation may be done on the back of the statement or on separate sheets of paper (Figure 28-17). Any errors found on the statement must be reported immediately to the bank. Procedure 28-5 shows how to reconcile a bank statement.

Text continued on p. 566

PROCEDURE 28-4: Prepare a Bank Deposit

TASK: Correctly prepare a bank deposit for the day's receipts and complete appropriate office records related to the deposit.

EQUIPMENT AND SUPPLIES
- Currency (cash and coin amounts)
- Checks for deposit (amounts for deposit)
- Deposit slip
- Endorsement stamp (optional)
- Deposit envelope

SKILLS/RATIONALE

Refer to Figure 28-14 throughout this procedure.

1. **Procedural Step. Organize currency, including coins.**
   Place bills in order with the largest denomination on top and arrange so that all bills are face up and in the same direction.
   Rationale. Organizing the currency facilitates processing of the deposit at the bank.

2. **Procedural Step. Accurately count and total the currency, then record the total on the bank deposit slip.**
   Record the individual pieces on the back of the deposit slip. (Write down the number of $20 bills, $10 bills, and so on.)

3. **Procedural Step. Prepare the checks that will be included in the deposit.**
   Endorse each check, using a restrictive endorsement.
   Rationale. To transfer the title and to protect the checks from loss or theft, a restrictive endorsement needs to be placed on the back side of each check.

4. **Procedural Step. Fill out the deposit slip.**
   a. List each check separately on the back of the deposit slip.
   b. Total the amount of the checks.
   c. Record the total on both the back and the front of the deposit slip.
   NOTE: Record the checks starting with the largest amount and ending with the smallest amount. Some practices prefer that checks be added to the deposit slip in the order they were received. Checks may be recorded using the payer's name, or if the bank prefers, the ABA number can be used instead (upper right corner of each check; see Figure 28-11).

5. **Procedural Step. Total the amount of currency and checks, and enter the total on the front of the deposit slip.**
   This figure will be entered as the net deposit if no cash is being withdrawn.

6. **Procedural Step. Record the total amount of the deposit in the office checkbook.**
   Rationale. This keeps the account accurate and allows for reconciliation of the balance.

7. **Procedural Step. Write the date of the deposit (that day's date) on the front of the deposit slip.**

8. **Procedural Step. Make a photocopy of the front and back of the deposit slip for the office record if a duplicate deposit slip was not made.**
   Rationale. This is important for purposes of verification of the deposit, should this become necessary.

9. **Procedural Step. Place the currency, checks, and completed deposit slip in an envelope or bank bag for transporting to the bank.**

Bank by Mail

Make your deposits in one easy step and get your receipt at the same time! Here's how:

1 Complete your personalized deposit slip as usual. Endorse the reverse side of all checks with the words "FOR DEPOSIT ONLY," sign your name and place your account number underneath. If you have an endorsement stamp, you may stamp the reverse side of each check.

2 In the detachable panel below, neatly print the name to which the deposit is to be credited, and write all applicable transaction information.

3 Peel back and remove the detachable panel. *This is your deposit receipt.* Please retain it as no other receipt will be mailed.

4 Be sure to place deposit slips, loan payment coupons, checks, etc. inside the envelope before mailing. DO NOT SEND CASH OR COIN in this envelope. Your deposit will appear on your monthly bank statement.

Please keep the detachable receipt for your records.

022000

☐ Please indicate if you wish to receive a supply of these envelopes for future deposits and we will mail them to you at the address on your receipt.

☐ Please indicate if this is a new address.

PLEASE DETACH AND RETAIN FOR YOUR RECORDS.

LIFT HERE

Bank of America

ACCOUNT NO.	AMOUNT	TRANSACTION ENCLOSED
________	$ ________	☐ Deposit for Checking Account
________	$ ________	☐ Deposit for Savings Account
________	$ ________	☐ Payment on Loan
________	$ ________	☐ Other________

TODAY'S DATE	TELEPHONE NO.	022000

NAME ________

ADDRESS ________ CITY/STATE/ZIP ________

THIS COPY IS FOR YOUR RECORDS. PLEASE REMOVE AND RETAIN.

FIGURE 28-15 Example of bank-by-mail deposit envelope. (Courtesy Valley Bank of Nevada, Las Vegas.)

0821-402054

#821

N 2

CALL (888) 555-2932
24 HOURS/DAY, 7 DAYS/WEEK
FOR ASSISTANCE WITH
YOUR ACCOUNT.

PAGE 1 OF 2   THIS STATEMENT COVERS: 6/22/XX THROUGH 7/22/XX

INTEREST CHECKING
0821-402054

SUMMARY

PREVIOUS BALANCE	252.10	MINIMUM BALANCE	142.55
DEPOSITS	68.74+	AVERAGE BALANCE	220.00
INTEREST EARNED	.18+	ANNUAL PERCENTAGE YIELD EARNED	.96%
WITHDRAWALS	109.55−		
CUSTOMER SERVICE CALLS	.00−		
INTERLINK/PURCHASE FEE	.00−	INTEREST EARNED 20xx	2.23
MONTHLY CHECKING FEE AND OTHER CHARGES	.00−		
▶ NEW BALANCE	211.47		

CHECKS AND WITHDRAWALS

CHECK	DATE PAID	AMOUNT	CHECK	DATE PAID	AMOUNT
202	7/05	15.05	203	7/15	94.50

DEPOSITS

	DATE POSTED	AMOUNT
CUSTOMER DEPOSIT	7/22	68.74
INTEREST PAYMENT THIS PERIOD	7/22	.18

BALANCE INFORMATION

DATE	BALANCE	DATE	BALANCE	DATE	BALANCE
6/22	252.10	7/05	237.05	7/15	142.55
				7/22	211.47

24 HOUR CUSTOMER SERVICE

EACH ACCOUNT COMES WITH 3 COMPLIMENTARY CALLS PER STATEMENT PERIOD.

CALLS TO 24 HOUR CUSTOMER SERVICE THIS STATEMENT PERIOD: 0

INTEREST INFORMATION

FROM	THROUGH	INTEREST RATE	ANNUAL PERCENTAGE YIELD (APY)
6/22	7/22	1.00%	1.01%

INTEREST RATE/APY AS OF 7/22/XX IF YOUR BALANCE IS

$ 0 - 4,999	.1.00%	1.01%
$ 5,000 - 9,999	.1.00%	1.01%
$ 10,000 AND OVER	.1.00%	1.01%

CALL 1-888-555-2932 IN CALIFORNIA ANYTIME FOR CURRENT RATES.

MEMBER FDIC

STATEMENT

FIGURE 28-16 Example of bank statement. (From Young AP, Kennedy DB: *Kinn's the medical assistant,* ed 10, St Louis, 2007, Saunders.)

THIS WORKSHEET IS PROVIDED TO HELP YOU BALANCE YOUR ACCOUNT

1. Go through your register and mark each check, withdrawal, Express ATM transaction, payment, deposit or other credit listed on this statement. Be sure that your register shows any interest paid into your account, and any service charges, automatic payments, or Express Transfers withdrawn from your account during this statement period.

2. Using the chart below, list any outstanding checks, Express ATM withdrawals, payments or any other withdrawals (including any from previous months) that are listed in your register but are not shown on this statement.

3. Balance your account by filling in the spaces below.

ITEMS OUTSTANDING	
NUMBER	AMOUNT
TOTAL	$

ENTER

The NEW BALANCE shown on this statement _____ $ _____

ADD

Any deposits listed in your register $ _____
or transfers into your account $ _____
which are not shown on this $ _____
statement. +$ _____

TOTAL _____ +$ _____

CALCULATE THE SUBTOTAL _____ $ _____

SUBTRACT

The total outstanding checks and
withdrawals from the chart at left _____ −$ _____

CALCULATE THE ENDING BALANCE

This amount should be the same
as the current balance shown in
your check register _____ $ _____

IF YOU SUSPECT ERRORS OR HAVE QUESTIONS ABOUT ELECTRONIC TRANSFERS

If you believe there is an error on your statement or Express ATM receipt, or if you need more information about a transaction listed on this statement or an Express ATM receipt, please contact us immediately. We are available 24 hours a day, seven days a week to assist you. Please call the telephone number printed on the front of this statement. Or, you may write to us at United Trust Company, P.O. Box 327, Anytown, USA.

1) Tell us your name and account number or Express card number.

2) As clearly as you can, describe the error or the transfer you are unsure about, and explain why you believe there is an error or why you need more information.

3) Tell us the dollar amount of the suspected error.

You must report the suspected error to us no later than 60 days after we sent you the first statement on which the problem appeared. We will investigate your question and will correct any error promptly. If our investigation takes longer than 10 business days (or 20 days in the case of electronic purchases), we will temporarily credit your account for the amount you believe is in error, so that you may have use of the money until the investigation is completed.

FIGURE 28-17 Reverse side of bank statement to be used for reconciling a checking account. (From Young AP, Kennedy DB: *Kinn's the medical assistant,* ed 10, St Louis, 2007, Saunders.)

PROCEDURE 28-5
Reconcile a Bank Statement

TASK: Correctly reconcile a bank statement with the checking account.

EQUIPMENT AND SUPPLIES
- Ending balance of previous statement
- Current bank statement
- Canceled checks for current month
- Checkbook stubs
- Calculator
- Pencil

SKILLS/RATIONALE

Refer to the figure below throughout this procedure.

1. **Procedural Step.** Compare the closing balance of the previous statement with the beginning balance of the current statement.
   a. Look on the previous statement where it states "New Balance."
   b. Look on the current statement where it states "Previous Balance."

   Rationale. These balances must be in agreement to continue with the reconciliation process.

2. **Procedural Step.** Compare the checks written with the items on the statement.

   Rationale. This verifies that the statement reflects the correct amounts.

   NOTE: Because most banks no longer send canceled checks back to their clients, the check register must be used for this comparison of check numbers to the statement.

Alan T. Slatkin, M.D.
BANK RECONCILIATION
JUNE 20XX

BALANCE PER BANK STATEMENT		$525.00
+ Deposit in Transit		
June 28	$291.47	
June 29	$94.21	$385.68
		$910.68
− Oustanding Checks		
#137 June 19	$200.00	
#145 June 27	$150.00	$350.00
		$560.68
BALANCE PER BANK STATEMENT		$575.68
Services Charge		$10.00
NSF Check		$5.00
ADJUSTED CHECKBOOK BALANCE		$560.68
PREPARED BY:		
DATE:		

Continued

PROCEDURE 28-5 Reconcile a Bank Statement—cont'd

3. **Procedural Step.** Place a checkmark (✓) in the reference area of the check register to reflect that these checks have cleared the bank.
   Rationale. This will help later when you need to identify the outstanding checks.
4. **Procedural Step.** List and total the outstanding checks from this statement, as well as any outstanding checks from previous bank reconciliations.
5. **Procedural Step.** Complete the bank statement reconciliation worksheet on the back of the bank statement, or apply the bank statement reconciliation formula.
   a. Enter the new balance from the current bank statement ("Bank statement balance").
   (This is the starting point for the formula.)
   b. Enter total amount of outstanding checks from the compiled list.
   NOTE: Do not include any certified checks as outstanding because their amount has already been deducted from the account.
6. **Procedural Step.** Reconcile deposits.
   Compare the check register and deposit slips to the bank statement to make sure that all deposits were made in the correct amount and to identify any deposits made that are shown in the check register, but not on the statement.
   Rationale. This verifies that the statement reflects the correct amounts.
7. **Procedural Step.** Add interest.
   If the office's checking account is an "interest-bearing" account:
   a. Add amount of the interest earned to the account deposit at this time.
   b. Add interest deposit to the check register.
8. **Procedural Step.** Update the bank statement reconciliation formula with any deposits that are in the check register but are not shown on the statement.
9. **Procedural Step.** Enter the corrected bank statement balance.
10. **Procedural Step.** Total any bank charges that appear on the bank statement and subtract them from the checkbook balance.
    Such charges may include service charges, automatic withdrawals, ATM, payments, and NSF checks.
    Rationale. This provides a corrected checkbook balance.
11. **Procedural Step.** If the checkbook balance and the statement balance do not agree, check the following items, then repeat the process as required:
    a. Check your arithmetic.
    b. Remember to include all the outstanding checks.
    c. Remember to record all deposits or interest earned; make sure you did not record anything twice.
    d. Make sure no figures are transposed. (If the amount of the error is divisible by 9, you may have done this.)
    e. Make sure you remembered to correct your checkbook balance at the time of the previous statement.

Figure modified from Chester GA: Modern medical assisting, Philadelphia, 1998, Saunders.

PATIENT-CENTERED PROFESSIONALISM

- If you were responsible for receiving payments from the patient made by check, what information would you verify?
- Why is it important for the medical assistant to be aware of how to do a bank deposit and reconcile a bank statement, even when this is not a typical duty?

BILLING AND COLLECTIONS

A patient is billed (sent a statement for the balance on the account) when all fees are not collected at the time of service or not paid by his or her insurance company after a claim has been filed. Patients with outstanding balances are billed monthly, even when an insurance claim is pending. Collection is the process of obtaining payment for services. "Aging" accounts that are "delinquent" with unpaid balances are sent to collection agencies for further attempts at payment for services already rendered.

Billing

A patient's **statement,** or bill of what is owed, can be prepared in the following ways:
- *Photocopy of ledger card.* This is the easiest method because the ledger card contains current account information. A window envelope is used to accommodate the folded statement. The statement is folded in such a way that the patient's name and address show through the window, so there is no need to address the envelope, which saves time.
- *Prepared statement.* A statement is prepared from the information included on the ledger card. This method is time-consuming because it requires not only typing the

information on a separate sheet of paper but also addressing the envelope.
- *Outside billing services.* This method requires that all patient-related financial records be given to an independent service to perform the billing process. Practices may find that this type of service, although expensive, allows for better cash flow. Many practices prefer this type of service to hiring full-time, in-house billing employees, who would require benefits.
- *Computerized billing.* Medical offices that are computerized have the advantage of being able to generate all statements from information in the patient accounts. Billing cycles can be run on demand, and more detailed financial reports can be generated for accounts receivable management.
- *E-statements.* Patients may wish to receive their statements via e-mail. The office can e-mail a statement of account to the patient with privacy issues addressed.

The statement should always contain a notice clearly stating the office's payment policy (e.g., payment due on receipt).

Fee Policy

A patient should always be informed of the fee policy of the office. Most offices have a sign in the reception area that states "payment is due at the time of service." If the patient is a "self-pay" (e.g., bill is paid by the patient not by insurance), an estimate of the total costs should be discussed before the appointment. If the patient has insurance, it is acceptable to ask for the patient's portion of the total cost, whether the deductible, the **co-insurance** (percentage of total charge not paid by insurance), or the **co-payment** (usually $10 to $20 per visit), at the time of service. Procedure 28-6 outlines the process of explaining professional fees before providing services.

The collection process begins with the patient's first visit and continues with each subsequent visit. New patients should be made aware of billing policies at the time the appointment is made to be ready to make payment and avoid embarrassment. Problems can arise later if the patient fails to make a payment on the day of service. Some practices will attach a finance charge if accounts are not kept up-to-date. The expla-

---

PROCEDURE 28-6: Explain Professional Fees Before Services Are Provided

TASK: Explain the physician's fees so that the patient understands his or her obligations before receiving services.

EQUIPMENT AND SUPPLIES
- Physician's fee schedule
- Surgical cost estimate
- Estimate of medical expenses form
- Private area for discussion

SKILLS/*RATIONALE*

1. **Procedural Step. Take the patient to a private area for discussion of fees.**
2. **Procedural Step. Display a professional attitude toward the patient during the discussion.**
   Demonstrate a willingness to provide answers and look for solutions to payment arrangements, ensuring the patient has a thorough understanding of what will be expected.
   Rationale. Discussing long-term medical fees is often stressful for the ill patient and requires the medical assistant to be professional, understanding, and caring while remaining firm.
3. **Procedural Step. Provide the patient with an estimate of anticipated fees before services are provided.**
   Emphasize that what is being discussed is an estimate and that the actual cost may be different based on what types of services are ultimately provided.
   Rationale. In cases involving surgery or long-term treatment (e.g., chemotherapy), patients are given an estimate of medical expenses. This informs the patient of what insurance benefits will or will not cover and if alternative payment arrangements need to be made.
4. **Procedural Step. Determine whether the patient has specific concerns that may hinder payment.**
   Rationale. This provides an opportunity for making special arrangements, if needed.
5. **Procedural Step. Make appropriate arrangements for a discussion between the physician and patient if further explanation is necessary.**

nation for this charge should be included in the brochure on office policy. Patients may have questions about their statements, and the medical assistant must be prepared to help explain billing.

Billing Cycles

Each medical office chooses a billing cycle that meets the needs of the medical practice. Two forms are generated by the billing department: the CMS-1500 claim form to the insurance company and the bill (statement) to the patient. Most funds come from insurance payments, so practices try to file claims within 1 or 2 days of the date of service. Now, especially with electronic claim filing, the turnaround time is much faster for claim settlement, which improves the practice's cash flow. Types of cycle billing include the following:
- *Daily.* This method is used if the practice is large and patient accounts are divided into small sections. Claims are generally sent out every day.
- *Weekly.* Claims to insurance companies may be sent in batches on a weekly basis (e.g., all the Blue Cross claims are run at the same time). Statements to patients can be spaced according to the alphabet and divided into four sections for the month. For example, statements A-F could be sent out the first week, G-M the next week, N-S the next, and T-Z the last week of the month. This type of billing spreads the return payments over the month for ease of posting and better cash flow.
- *Biweekly (or semimonthly).* Patient statements are sent every 2 weeks, or twice a month on the 15th and the 30th, with half sent on each date.
- *Monthly.* All the patient statements are sent together at the same time of the month, usually at the beginning of the month or last week of the month.

Fee Adjustments

The daysheet has a column for making adjustments. An **adjustment** is an amount that is added or subtracted from the physician's fee, changing the patient's account balance. To make an adjustment to a fee, only the ledger card and the daysheet are needed. Adjustments change the amount owed in patient accounts for various reasons, including discounts (credit), write-offs (credit), returned checks (debit), and overpayments (credit). Occasionally, an adjustment is needed for an incorrect charge because the service was not coded or documented correctly (usually the incorrect charge is voided [adjusted], and the correct charge or code is rebilled).

Professional Discounts

Professional discounts are sometimes given to other health care professionals and their families. If a professional discount is to be given, a note in the service column should indicate the reason for the discount (e.g., "courtesy" or "professional discount"). This includes accepting only what the insurance has paid, not asking the patient for the difference (co-insurance) if allowed, and not accepting co-payments. The amount is subtracted from the account balance. Many physicians no longer do this because insurance companies are not responsible for the entire fee if a discount has been applied. Their contention is that the discount is not applied for all their subscribers, only those who are health care professionals or family, and therefore is not equitable.

Write-offs

A **write-off** is done when a portion or the entire amount of the charges cannot be collected. If a patient has declared bankruptcy, the entire amount must be written off. Portions of fees may need to be written off if the physician's fee is above the "allowable" amount in an agreement with a third-party payer (insurance companies, Medicare, or Medicaid). Insurance payments are based on contracted amounts and usually cover only a portion of the service fee charged. Because of the contract, the balance remaining cannot be charged back to the patient. This may also be done for other reasons (e.g., bankruptcy) or when the person cannot pay the bill because of personal circumstances and the physician or representative subtracts an amount from the bill owed.

The amount written off is subtracted from the account balance. Money received from a collection agency (company that collects debts that are overdue and then keeps a "finder's fee," or percentage, of the amount collected) provides only for the office's percentage share; the agency's portion of the recovered balance is another example of a write-off.

Returned Checks

When a patient does not have enough funds in his or her bank account, a check may be returned for **nonsufficient funds (NSF).** If the check cannot be resubmitted to the bank, the amount of the returned check must be added back to the patient's account balance, along with any applicable fees charged by the practice's bank for the returned check.

Overpayments

Occasionally, a patient will overpay (pay more than the balance) on his or her account. This shows as a credit, or negative balance, on the ledger card because it is money owed to the patient. To avoid confusion the credit balance should be circled or placed in parentheses. If a refund is sent to the patient, the amount sent is debited to the account to bring the account balance to zero. Refunds should be made promptly.

If there is an overpayment by insurance companies or Medicare on an account, the check should be deposited and the company or Medicare informed; you will be advised by the entity where and how you should write a refund check. In this case, you will have a "paper trail" should there be any question. The original check is never returned.

Collection Process

Payment at the time of service allows the medical practice to control collection costs. Zero-balance accounts (patient accounts that are paid in full) do not have statements sent out monthly, which saves the practice the cost of preparing and mailing statements. Most often, however, full payment is not received at the time of service. A patient may make a co-payment, but the practice relies heavily on third-party payers. To be successful, a medical office should have written policies on payment, payment plans, and collection of overdue accounts.

The accounts receivable report details the age (length of time a patient's bill is left unpaid) of each account. When an account is not kept up-to-date, even after several statements have been mailed requesting payment, the medical practice must attempt to collect the overdue amounts in a professional manner. The office can make a call to the patient, mail a collection letter, or turn the account over to a professional collection agency. The longer the bill is unpaid, the harder it is to collect.

Payment Plans

One of the most sensitive areas in the medical office is following up with patients on an overdue account. Patients may face unexpected financial problems (e.g., loss of job, death of spouse, or divorce) and may need a plan to help them complete their financial obligation.

Payment plans allow the patient to pay the outstanding balance in two or three payments. If more time is needed, the office may include a finance charge. Finance charges may be applied if four or more payments are needed. As required by the **Federal Truth in Lending Act,** a "Truth in Lending" form should be completed in duplicate, with a copy in the patient's record and a copy to the patient (Figure 28-18). This document acts as a disclosure statement and includes the terms of the agreement, start and ending dates, financial charges, rate of interest, total payment due, and the patient's signature. This form is required for accounts requiring more than four payments, even if a finance charge is not added to the account, and must be kept on file for 3 years.

Procedure 28-7 explains how to establish a payment plan to assist a patient in paying for services on a large or overdue account.

Procedure 28-8 outlines how to explain the statement of account so that patients understand their obligations.

Telephone

When the medical assistant needs to contact the person responsible for an overdue account, good communication skills must be used. Even though the goal is to collect the money owed, goodwill must always be maintained. The **Fair Debt Collection Act of 1977** (see Chapter 4) specifies guidelines for collecting money owed. When contacting people to collect money owed to the medical office, you may not harass them with threats or abusive language. Also, contact must only be made during reasonable hours (e.g., 8 AM to 9 PM), and you may call only once a week. An office policy defining the correct approach is helpful (Box 28-1).

The following example of a medical office policy outlines what to do and say while on the phone with a patient who has a past-due account:

1. Listen to the patient's explanation as to why the account is overdue.

FIGURE 28-18 Disclosure statement: example of document for compliance with Federal Truth in Lending Act.

BOX 28-1

Sample Office Policy for the Collection of Debts

1. Calls can only be made between 8:00 am and 9:00 pm (considered normal waking hours).
2. When telephone contact has been made, no more than one call per week is allowed.
   a. Failure to reach the patient or other party does not allow for daily callbacks.
   b. Threats or other forms of harassment are always unacceptable.
3. If an employer requests that calls not be made to the patient's place of employment, calling the patient at work must be stopped.
4. Never threaten a patient.

- Identify if the patient was unhappy with the treatment provided. Notify the physician if this is the case.
- Identify financial problems (e.g., loss of job) that the patient may be having.

2. Agree on a payment plan.
3. Maintain the goodwill of the patient. A patient who is treated rudely will speak badly of the practice and may seek legal action.

PROCEDURE 28-7 Establish Payment Arrangements on a Patient Account

TASK: Establish a payment plan to assist a patient in paying for services on a large ("high-dollar") or overdue account.

EQUIPMENT AND SUPPLIES
- Patient's billing statement (ledger card and account information)
- Calendar
- "Truth in Lending" form
- Paper
- Private area for discussion

SKILLS/RATIONALE

1. **Procedural Step.** Determine that all information on the billing statement is correct.
2. **Procedural Step.** Discuss possible payment arrangements that are acceptable to the practice.
   Encourage the person responsible for the account to decide which option is most appropriate for his or her budget.
   Rationale. Better compliance can be expected when the person responsible for making the payment has contributed to the discussion and agreed to the best option.
3. **Procedural Step.** Determine when the first payment will be made.
4. **Procedural Step.** Prepare the "Truth in Lending" form, and have the person responsible for the account sign the form if the agreement requires more than four installments (see Figure 28-18).
   Rationale. A "Truth in Lending" form must be completed to be in compliance with federal regulations (Regulation Z).
5. **Procedural Step.** Explain any finance charges that will accrue on the account.
6. **Procedural Step.** Document the agreement by making notes attached to the ledger card.
   Rationale. Credit information is highly confidential and is not kept in the patient file. Attach information to the ledger card or keep separate files for patients' financial and credit information.

Documentation should be provided concerning the agreement made by the patient. These notes may be attached to the ledger card or filed in a "collections folder" but should never be included in the patient's medical record.

Collection Letter

If the person responsible for the account does not respond to notices on the statements or telephone messages to call the physician's office, a collection letter should be sent. The message in a collection letter needs to be clearly understood by the receiver (the patient). The wording needs to be firm but positive. Every effort to give the **debtor** (person owing money) an opportunity to pay should be offered. Provide the debtor with adequate time to respond. State the consequences of not following up on the request for payment. Box 28-2 provides suggestions on composing collection letters.

Collection Agency

The physician must make the decision to send an account to a collection agency after all other attempts have failed. If an account is sent to a collection agency, the medical practice can no longer send statements to the patient. The patient is to pay the collection agency directly once the physician has sent the account for collection. The collection agency will keep its share per an arranged percentage (usually 50% to 60%) and will forward the remaining amount to the physician's office on a contracted basis, usually either monthly or as payments are received from the patient.

The medical assistant may have to gather all data needed by the collection agency to proceed with a collection. If a debtor contacts the medical office about the process, the debtor must be instructed to contact the agency directly. If the debtor pays the medical office instead of the agency, the office needs to contact the agency. Care should be taken in choosing a collection agency, being sure the agency has the same ethical and business attitudes as the physician. Remember that the collection agency represents the physician's office to the patient.

Procedure 28-9 explains the process of collecting delinquent accounts.

PATIENT-CENTERED PROFESSIONALISM

- Why must the medical assistant be aware of the entire billing process to be effective in patient care?

PROCEDURE 28-8

Explain a Statement of Account to a Patient

TASK: Explain a statement of account to a patient who has questions so that the patient understands his or her obligations.

EQUIPMENT AND SUPPLIES
- Patient statement
- Patient information form
- Encounter form(s)
- Physician's fee schedule
- Private area for discussion

SKILLS/RATIONALE

1. **Procedural Step.** Determine that the patient has the correct statement and ask the patient what seems to be the problem.
   Rationale. It is possible that a patient has received the wrong statement. Therefore you need to make sure the statement belongs to the patient and that the insurance numbers, patient address, and patient telephone numbers that appear on the statement are all correct.

2. **Procedural Step.** Examine the statement for any possible errors.
   a. Compare the statement with the encounter form(s).
   b. Compare the statement to the fee schedule.
   Rationale. It is possible that an error has been made on the statement. For example, an incorrect charge may have been billed or a mathematical error may have occurred. Taking this step also demonstrates to the patient that his or her concerns are important to you as well and that you are willing to make adjustments should an error be found.

3. **Procedural Step.** Review with the patient each of the items that appears on the statement.

   a. The date of the service.
   b. The type of service rendered.
   c. The fee charged for the service.

4. **Procedural Step.** If an error is located, correct it immediately and apologize to the patient.
   Rationale. This assures the patient that you are a professional and promotes continued open communication.

5. **Procedural Step.** If there was no error and your discussions do not resolve the patient's concerns, make arrangements for a discussion between the physician and patient for further explanation to resolve the problem.
   Rationale. It is important to recognize when a conversation between the patient and physician is necessary to resolve the situation.

6. **Procedural Step.** If there was no error and the patient understands the statement, it is beneficial at this time to determine whether the patient has specific concerns that may hinder payment.
   Rationale. This provides an opportunity for making special arrangements, if needed.

PAYROLL PROCESSING

The **payroll** is the financial record of employees' salaries, wages, bonuses, net pay, and deductions. There are two main reasons for maintaining accurate payroll records. First, complete information is needed to compute the wages for each employee for a payroll period. Second, the data provide information for the government reports (e.g., Forms 8109 and 940) that all employers are required to complete. An employer is required by law to withhold certain amounts from an employee's check to pay for taxes. Payroll information is highly confidential and is handled only by authorized personnel.

Earnings and Withholding Laws

Federal laws and many state laws require the employer to deduct and collect specified amounts from employees' gross earnings (before deductions). Other laws address working conditions, hours, and earnings. Others relate to taxes that must be paid by the employer to provide specific employee benefits. The employer is responsible for sending required withholdings to the appropriate government agencies, along with reports verifying the figures, on a timely basis.

Fair Labor Standards Act

The **Fair Labor Standards Act,** or the Wage and Hour Law, specifies that employers engaged in interstate commerce (the exchange of goods or services between buyers and sellers in two or more states) must pay their hourly employees (employees paid by the hour) overtime at a rate of $1\frac{1}{2}$ times the regular rate (time-and-a-half) for hours worked in excess of 40 per workweek. The Fair Labor Standards Act provides that man-

BOX 28-2

Suggestions for Composing a Collection Letter

1. Your account has always been paid promptly in the past, so this must be an oversight. Please accept this note as a friendly reminder of your account due in the amount of $_____.
2. Since your care in this office in [March], we have had no word from you in regard to how you are feeling or regarding your account due. If it is impossible for you to pay the full amount of $_____ at this time, please call this office before [June 15] so that satisfactory arrangements can be worked out.
3. Medical bills are payable at the time of service unless special credit arrangements are made. Please send your check in full or call this office before [June 30].
4. If you have some question about your statement, we will be happy to answer it for you. If not, may we have a payment before the end of this month?
5. Unless some definite arrangement is made to reduce your balance of $_____, we can no longer carry your account on our books. Delinquent accounts are turned over to our collection agency on the 25th of the month.
6. Once established, a payment plan can be reinforced by recognizing the first remittance with a letter of acknowledgment:
   Thank you for the recent payment of $_____ on your account. We are glad to cooperate with you in this arrangement for clearing your account. We will look for your next check at about the same time next month and your final payment the following month.
7. When arranged by a telephone call, a payment schedule can be confirmed by a letter.
   As agreed on in our telephone conversation today, we will expect you to mail a payment of $50 on [February 10]; $50 on [March 10]; and the balance on [April 10]. If some emergency should prevent your making one of these payments on time, please notify us immediately by telephone.

"DO"S AND "DON'T"S

Do:
1. Individualize letters to suit the situation.
2. Design your early letters as mere reminders of debt.
3. Always imply that the patient has good intentions to pay, until lack of response over time proves otherwise.
4. Send letters with a firmer tone only after you have sent one or two friendly reminders.

Don't:
1. Use the same collection letter for a patient with good paying habits as for a patient known to neglect financial obligations.
2. Place any type of overdue notice on a postcard or on the outside of an envelope. This is an invasion of privacy.

Modified from Young AP, Kennedy DB: *Kinn's the medical assistant,* ed 9, Philadelphia, 2003, Saunders.

---

agement and supervisory employees are exempt from this regulation. These employees are referred to as "salaried" personnel. Provisions for the minimum wage (the minimum hourly amount an employee can be paid) and a normal workweek (e.g., "full time" equals 40 hours) are also included in this act. The minimum wage rate is adjusted periodically by Congress.

Social Security Tax

The federal Social Security law, or **Federal Insurance Contributions Act (FICA),** provides funds to support benefits for employees and their families. The FICA tax pays for retirement benefits for workers age 62 and older, dependents of the retired worker, and disability benefits. Both the employer and the employee pay the FICA tax. FICA tax requires withholding 6.2% of wages (first $106,800 of wages as of 2009, then Social Security tax not deducted for rest of year). FICA tax is a combination of the 6.2% Social Security tax and a 1.45% Medicare tax, both of which are also paid by the employer. These amounts may be periodically adjusted by the U.S. Congress.

Medicare Tax

The **Medicare tax** is collected to support Medicare, a federal health insurance program for people who have reached age 65. The tax rate is 1.45%, and this tax is withheld from the employee's pay earned all during the year. The employer matches the 1.45% of the tax collected from the employee.

Federal Income Tax

The **Tax Payment Act** requires employers not only to withhold income tax and then pay it to the Internal Revenue Service (IRS) but also to keep accurate records of the names, addresses, and Social Security numbers of persons employed. Records also need to be kept of the date of employment, gross earnings and withholdings, and the amounts and dates of payment for each employee.

Required Forms. Two forms used to report employee pay must be generated regularly, as follows:
1. The employer must submit quarterly reports (Form 941) to the IRS.

PROCEDURE 28-9 Prepare Billing Statements and Collect Past-Due Accounts

TASK: Process monthly statements and evaluate accounts for collection procedures.

EQUIPMENT AND SUPPLIES
- Patient ledger card
- Patient information form
- Collection form letters
- Computer
- Stationery and envelopes
- Collection agency commission requirements

SKILLS/*RATIONALE*

PREPARING BILLING STATEMENTS

1. **Procedural Step.** Determine the billing schedule for the medical practice.
   Rationale. Initially, consider the timing of when statements are prepared and sent out. Different offices send statements according to different schedules, including monthly billing and cycle billing.

2. **Procedural Step.** Assemble all the accounts that have outstanding balances (e.g., owe payment to the medical office).
   a. Review the new balance column on the patient's ledger card.
   b. Pull each one that shows an amount owed.

3. **Procedural Step.** Separate the accounts into two groups:
   a. Routine billing accounts.
   b. Past-due accounts.

PERFORMING ROUTINE BILLING

1. **Procedural Step.** Prepare ledger cards to serve as billing statements.
   Many medical practices use a photocopy of the patient's ledger card as the billing statement. Care is taken throughout the month in making entries on the ledger card so that when monthly statements are prepared, photocopying it for use as a statement is a quick process.

2. **Procedural Step.** Photocopy each ledger card and place in an envelope.
   The design of the patient ledger card for use as a statement allows for it to be used in a "window" envelope, thus saving the time needed to type the patient's mailing address.
   NOTE: The envelope used should be the "security" style to protect confidentiality of patient information.

3. **Procedural Step.** Print out computer-generated statements, if applicable.
   Medical practices that use computer software for management of patient accounts can easily print patient statements. The software provides a "report" function that allows for all accounts with outstanding balances to print out as individual statements. These statements are then folded and placed in a "window" envelope in the same manner as a photocopied ledger card.

COLLECTING PAST-DUE ACCOUNTS

1. **Procedural Step.** Gather all patient ledger cards with past-due balances.
   Patient ledger cards should be "flagged" when the patient's account reaches a past-due status of 30, 60, 90, or 120 days. Accounts can be placed in "tickler" files, or color-coded tabs can be placed directly on the ledger card to indicate the past-due statement.

2. **Procedural Step.** Separate accounts according to the action required:
   a. 30 days: friendly reminder.
   b. 60 days: stern letter.
   c. 90 days: letter stating the account will be turned over to a collection agency if not paid by a specified date.
   Rationale. Sorting the ledger cards into stacks of like accounts allows you to create form letters for each category. Once form letters are created and saved on the computer, patient names, dates, and amounts can be entered specific to each patient.

3. **Procedural Step.** Create the appropriate form letter for each account using company stationery, and mail to the patient.
   a. The "friendly reminder" letter can be included with a patient's statement on company letterhead and in a company envelope.
   b. The "stern letter" should be sent on company letterhead and sent in a plain envelope without the office's return address.
   c. The third and final letter should be sent on company letterhead in a company envelope and should be sent certified mail with return receipt requested.

4. **Procedural Step.** Turn the account over to the collection agency at the time specified.

Continued

PROCEDURE 28-9 Prepare Billing Statements and Collect Past-Due Accounts—cont'd

When the patient's account reaches 120 days (or the number of days determined by the practice) and the third and final letter has been sent and return receipt received, you must turn the account over to a collection agency, as stated in the final letter. This is required by law. All monies paid once the account has been sent to collection will be received by the collection agency and are subject to the commission agreement. You may not receive further payments by the patient. Any such payments made to the medical office must be immediately sent to the collection agency. If a patient calls the office wanting to discuss payment arrangements, you must refer these questions directly to the collection agency. The collection agency will send the office a statement of accounts paid and a check for monies collected, typically once a month or as contracted with the agency.

5. **Procedural Step.** Post payments received from the collection agency to the patient ledger card and daysheet.
Any balances that are left owing may be adjusted off the account (see Procedure 28-3). This is the physician's or office manager's decision, unless mandated by bankruptcy.

OTHER COLLECTION CIRCUMSTANCES
1. **On the death of a patient, collect any outstanding balances from the patient's estate.**
   a. A statement is sent to the patient's address by certified mail, return receipt requested.
   b. If you do not receive a response, you may contact the county probate clerk's office and file a claim against the estate.
2. **For a patient filing for bankruptcy, stop all collection efforts immediately (depending on the classification filed).**
   The medical office will be notified when a patient has filed for Chapter 11 bankruptcy. A representative from the office must attend the bankruptcy hearing or file a written proof of claim for payment. No further collection actions may be taken with Chapter 11. Medical bills are often the last claims to be paid. Most likely, no reimbursement will be paid, and any remaining balances must be adjusted off the patient's account.
   Chapter 13 bankruptcy requires that the patient pay a fixed amount that is divided between all creditors. No other collection actions may be taken.

Friendly reminder

On reviewing the office financial records, I have found that you have an outstanding balance of $_____. If there has been a billing error or if you have medical insurance that will cover the debt, please contact our office immediately so a correction can be made. Otherwise, please send a check so your account can be kept current.

Stern letter

You have not yet responded to my previous letter dated _____ regarding your outstanding bill at the office. If you are unable to pay the entire balance at this time, I would be glad to discuss various payment options with you. If you have already sent a remittance, I would appreciate you forwarding me a copy of the canceled check so I can make sure your account is corrected.

Turn over to collection agency

Your bill is now _____ months overdue and because you have neglected to contact the office we are now forced to refer your outstanding balance to a professional collection agency. We hope you contact the office or pay your bill by (date) so the referral is not necessary. This is the last notice you will receive from this office.

3

Figure modified from Chester GA: Modern medical assisting, Philadelphia, 1998, Saunders.

2. A yearly report must be sent to the employee (W-2 form). The W-2 form reflecting the previous year's activity must be sent to employees by the end of January of the following year or within 1 month of termination. Employees use W-2 forms to file their federal and state income taxes.

The amount of federal income tax withheld from an employee's wages depends on amount of total gross earnings and number of exemptions claimed. An **exemption** is the amount of an individual's earnings that is exempt from income taxes (nontaxable) based on the number of **dependents**. An employee is entitled to one personal exemption, plus an additional exemption for each dependent. Each employee has to fill out an **Employee's Withholding Allowance Certificate (Form W-4)**. If an employee fails to turn in the W-4 form, the employer will use the zero-deduction tables to calculate money to be withheld.

Tax Guide. Each year the employer receives an updated tax guide (*Circular E: Employer's Tax Guide*) that contains tables for federal income and FICA taxes, as well as the rules for depositing these taxes. This publication is also available at the IRS website. The wage tax-bracket tables cover all the variations of payroll periods (e.g., weekly, biweekly, semimonthly, and monthly). The tables are subdivided on the basis of married, single, and head-of-household persons. An easy way to determine the tax to be withheld from an employee's gross wages is to do the following:

1. Locate the correct table for pay period under married, single, or head of household.
2. Find the wage bracket in the first two columns of the table.
3. Find the column for the number of exemptions claimed.
4. Read down the exemption column until you see the appropriate wage-bracket line.

Federal Unemployment Tax Act

The **Federal Unemployment Tax Act (FUTA)** requires employers to pay 6.2% tax based on each employee's earnings. This tax benefits employees who become unemployed. The taxable wage base is the first $7,000. This means that for the purpose of computing tax, only the first $7,000 of a worker's wages for a calendar year are counted. The **State Unemployment Tax Act (SUTA)** is tied directly to FUTA; the amount of SUTA taxes paid may be offset (credited) against what the employer owes for the FUTA taxes. Not all states have state unemployment taxes, and the tax may be determined by the number of employees.

Workers' Compensation Insurance

Workers' compensation laws require employers to pay insurance that will reimburse employees for wage losses resulting from job-related injuries or reimburse families if work-related death occurs. Employers may be required to carry workers' compensation insurance, which they can purchase through a commercial insurance company. The **Federal Employees' Compensation Act** covers only federal government workers, but it sets the standard for workers' compensation laws in most states.

Earnings

Employees of the medical practice may be paid a salary or wage, depending on the type of work and the period covered. Money paid to a person for managerial or administrative services is referred to as **salary** (set amount of pay for a certain period such as 1 year). Money paid for either skilled or unskilled (no formal training) labor is called **wages** and is computed by multiplying the hourly pay rate by the number of hours worked. Deductions from total earnings (**gross wages** from either salaries or wages) are taken for the following reasons:

- Federal income tax withholding (required)
- State income tax withholding (required)
- FICA tax (required)
- Purchase of U.S. savings bonds (optional)
- Medical and life insurance premiums (optional)
- Contributions to a charitable organization (optional)
- Repayment of personal loans (optional)

The total earnings paid to an employee after payroll taxes and other deductions have been taken is called **net pay**. Net pay is calculated by subtracting total deductions from gross earnings.

Gross Pay

The first step to calculate the amount of an employee's paycheck is to determine the gross amount of wages earned by the employee. Using an hourly rate as a basis, it is necessary to know the rate of pay and the number of hours the employee has worked during the payroll period. The hours worked by an employee must be accurately maintained. If an hourly employee works overtime, the number of hours over 40 hours in a given week is calculated at time-and-a-half (if the practice falls under the Wage and Hour Law).

> For example, Lisa Fisher, a medical assistant, makes $10 an hour for a 40-hour workweek. Last week she worked 44 hours for Mediplace Clinic. Remembering that overtime for her is calculated at time-and-a-half, her gross pay can be calculated as follows:
>
> Regular time hours: 40 × 10 = $400
> Overtime earnings: 4 × 15 = $60
> Gross pay: $460
>   or
> Total time × Regular rate of pay: 44 × 10 = $440
> Overtime fee: 4 × 5 = 20
> (The 4 overtime hours are worth an additional $5 an hour at time-and-a-half = $15 an hour.)
> Gross pay: $460

Withholdings Required By Law

Federal law requires three principal deductions from the employee's gross pay, as follows:

1. The amount of *Social Security tax* deducted can be calculated either by multiplying the taxable wages by the Social Security rate (6.2%) or by referring to tax tables

found in the IRS publication, *Circular E: Employer's Tax Guide*.
2. The *Medicare tax* is applied to the same taxable wages at a rate of 1.45%.
3. A large portion of the federal government's revenue comes from the *federal income tax* that is withheld from the employee's gross pay. The rules and regulations change often. The best practice is to use a current edition of *Circular E*.

> For example, using the percentage method, the taxes for medical assistant Lisa Fisher can be computed as follows:
> $460 × 6.2% (Social Security) = Tax of $28.52
> $460 × 1.45% (Medicare) = Tax of $6.67
> When multiplying by a percentage, remember to convert it to a decimal first. To multiply $460 by 6.2%, you must first convert 6.2% to a decimal by multiplying by 100 (6.2 × 100 = 0.062):
> $460 × .062 = $28.52

Other Deductions

Many different types of deductions are made by agreement between the employee and the employer. Employee contributions to a retirement plan are based on total wages earned. Often, a deduction is made to share part of the cost of health insurance with the employer. In situations when an employee receives advances from the employer, the employee often repays the debt through payroll deductions.

Payroll Register

Employers are required to retain all payroll records showing payments and deductions. The **payroll register** shows information about the earnings and deductions of each employee for the pay period (Figure 28-19). It acts as a summary sheet showing all the data for each employee on a separate line. Regular, overtime, and total earnings are recorded in a payroll register from information on time cards. Amounts deducted

---

PAYROLL - PR9972
Langer Medical Office

QRTLY / ANNUAL PAYROLL REGISTER
04/01/XX - 06/30/XX

6:05 PM 07/06/XX
PAGE 1

	HOURS	GROSS	FICA WAGE	MEDI WAGE	FED TAX	FICA	MEDICARE	STATE TAX	DED AMT	NET AMT	CHECK NO.
0001 Anderson, Rhonda											
	80.00	692.00	692.00	692.00	41.52	42.90	10.34	21.34	14.36	561.54	4367
	80.00 @ 8.65000 = 692.00		REGULAR								
0002 Dunbar, Mario											
	80.00	2000.00	2000.00	2000.00	246.77	124.00	29.00	65.13	45.00	1490.10	4368
	80.00 @ 25.0000 = 2000.00		REGULAR								
0003 Ruiz, Selena											
	60.00	720.00	0.00	720.00	34.02	0.00	10.44	1.08	7.20	667.26	4369
	60.00 @ 12.0000 = 720.00		REGULAR								
0004 Nadich, Denise											
	80.00	1500.00	0.00	1500.00	222.69	0.00	21.75	28.23	15.00	1212.33	4370
	80.00 @ 18.7500 = 1500.00		REGULAR								

PAYROLL - PR9972
Langer Medical Office

QRTLY / ANNUAL PAYROLL REGISTER
04/01/XX - 06/30/XX

6:05 PM 07/06/XX
PAGE 2

	HOURS	GROSS	FICA WAGE	MEDI WAGE	FED TAX	FICA	MEDICARE	STATE TAX	DED AMT	NET AMT	CHECK NO.
CURRENT PAYROLL TOTALS											

TOTAL HOURS 300.00
GROSS WAGES 4912.00
FICA WAGES 2692.00   MEDICARE WAGES 4912.00
FEDERAL TAX 545.00
FICA 166.90   MEDICARE 71.53
STATE TAX 115.78
DEDUCTION AMT 81.56

NET AMOUNT 3931.23

FIGURE 28-19 Payroll register printed from a computerized payroll system.

for payroll taxes, health insurance, and other deductions are calculated and recorded in a payroll register, as are the total amount to be paid to each employee and the check number of each payroll check. Before checks are written for an employee's net pay, the calculations should be checked for accuracy.

Payroll Checks

The information used to prepare payroll checks is taken from the payroll register. A payroll check usually has a detachable stub to provide a summary of the earnings and deductions. Employees keep the pay stubs for their records of deductions and net pay received (Figure 28-20).

Employee Earnings Records

The details affecting payments made to an employee are recorded in the **employee earnings record.** This information is recorded each pay period. The record includes earnings, deductions, net pay, and accumulated earnings for the calendar year. Employee earnings records are used to complete the required tax forms at the end of the year.

Figure 28-21 summarizes the payroll process from calculation of earnings through generation of the employee earnings record.

PATIENT-CENTERED PROFESSIONALISM

- Why is it important for an employee to understand the regulations designed for the record keeping of payroll earnings?

CONCLUSION

Accurate and complete financial records help the medical practice stay in business and be successful. Medical assistants may be involved with some or all of the management of the practice's finances. Regardless of what financial responsibilities you may have in the medical practice, it is important that you understand the basic accounting and bookkeeping principles and procedures needed to manage the finances.

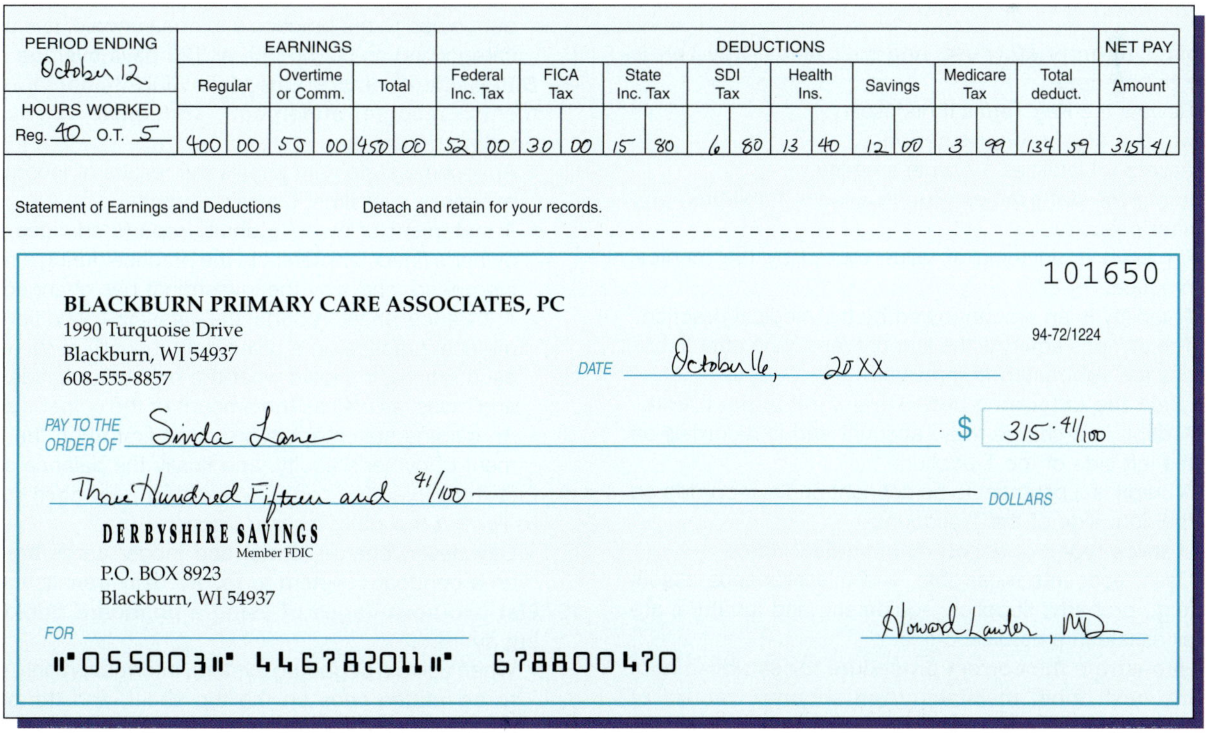

FIGURE 28-20 Paycheck with attached stub for employee to keep as a record. (From Hunt SA: *Saunders fundamentals of medical assisting—revised reprint,* St Louis, 2007, Saunders.)

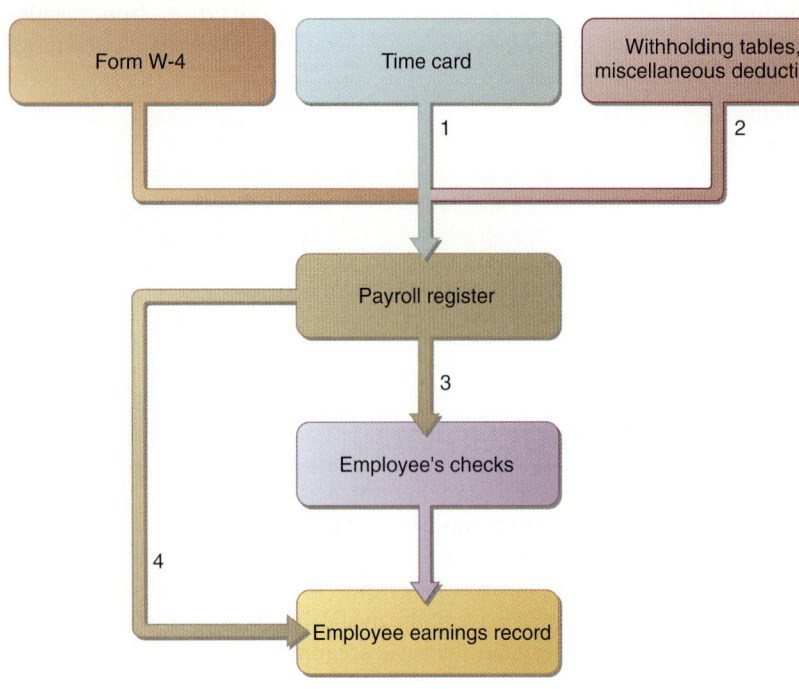

FIGURE 28-21 *1,* A time card is used to record all employee hours worked and to calculate regular, overtime, and total earnings. *2,* Payroll taxes are calculated using withholding tables and information on employee's W-4 form. Other deductions are taken as well. *3,* Payroll checks are written for the net pay for each employee. *4,* Information from the payroll register is recorded on each employee's earnings record.

Chapter Summary

Reinforce your understanding of the material in this chapter by reviewing the curriculum objectives and key content points below.

1. **Define, appropriately use, and spell all the Key Terms for this chapter.**
   - Review the Key Terms if necessary.
2. **State the accounting equation.**
   - Assets = Liabilities + Owner's equity.
3. **Explain the differences among assets, liabilities, and owner's equity.**
   - An asset is anything of value owned by the medical practice.
   - A liability is an amount owed by the medical practice.
   - The owner's equity is the amount remaining after liabilities are subtracted from assets.
4. **Explain the difference between a debit and a credit.**
   - A debit is a charge to an account and is recorded on the left side of the T-account.
   - A credit is a payment to an account and is recorded on the right side of the T-account.
5. **List three types of assets in a medical office.**
   - Cash, accounts receivable, and miscellaneous assets (e.g., property, supplies, equipment, and furniture) are all assets in a medical office.
6. **Demonstrate the correct procedure for establishing a petty cash fund, maintaining an accurate record of expenditures, and replenishing the fund as necessary.**
   - Review Procedure 28-1.
7. **Explain what an accounts receivable "aging" report shows.**
   - An accounts receivable aging report shows how long debt owed to the practice has gone unpaid. It is usually categorized as 30, 60, 90, or 120 days overdue.
8. **Differentiate among the following financial statements: income statement, statement of owner's equity, and balance sheet.**
   - An income statement shows the results of income and expenses over time, usually a month.
   - A statement of owner's equity reports changes in the owner's financial interest in the practice during a reporting period, and why the investment has changed.
   - A balance sheet reports the financial condition of a medical practice on a given date, usually at the end of each month. It shows what the medical practice owns and owes, as well as the amount of the owner's equity.
   - An income statement is prepared first, then the statement of owner's equity, and finally the balance sheet.
9. **List three types of forms used on a pegboard system to record the daily transactions.**
   - Daysheets, charge forms, and ledger cards are used on a pegboard system to record daily transactions.
10. **List two advantages of using a pegboard bookkeeping system.**
    - When using a pegboard system, information only needs to be written once on the top sheet, and the special paper allows the information to be transferred to the sheets below. The pegs keep all the forms in alignment.

- The pegboard provides a hard, flat surface on which to write forms by hand.
11. **Demonstrate the correct procedure for posting service charges and payments using the pegboard system.**
    - Review Procedure 28-2.
12. **List four advantages of using a computerized bookkeeping system.**
    - Computerized bookkeeping systems allow for single, electronic entry, as well as ease in storing data, printing reports, and submitting claims electronically.
13. **List the five requirements of banks for checks being deposited and explain the importance of confirming these five items when accepting checks from patients.**
    - Correct payee: the check must be made out to the health provider depositing the check.
    - Current date: postdated checks are not acceptable.
    - Correct amount: the word and number amount must agree on the face of the check.
    - Current address and phone number: the payer's information must agree with the office account information.
    - Affixed signature: the payer's signature should agree with the payer's name as it appears on the check.
    - The medical assistant should verify all information on the check before accepting it; otherwise, it may be refused by the bank for deposit.
14. **Define "third-party" check, "postdated" check, and check "paid in full."**
    - A third-party check is endorsed over to a third party (the doctor) who is not the original payee (such as the patient on an insurance check).
    - A postdated check is made out for a future date not the current date.
    - A check that is marked paid in full signifies that the payee will make no further attempt to collect any funds and that the account is considered closed ("paid in full").
    - Medical offices should have written policies to establish how these types of checks are handled.
15. **List seven security tips for check writing.**
    - Only authorized personnel should sign the check.
    - The record portion of the end-stub style should be filled in before the check is completed.
    - All lines should be filled in close to the left end of the line to prevent additions to the line. When the item written is completed, a long line should be added to fill out the line.
    - Check amounts are written with numbers and words, and the amounts should agree.
    - Write the number amount close to the dollar sign to reduce the chance of an additional number being added.
    - Enter the cents as "amount over 100" (e.g., 10 cents = 10/100).
    - Write the amount in words on the line under the "Pay to the Order of" space.
16. **Differentiate between restrictive endorsement and blank endorsement.**
    - A restrictive endorsement limits what can be done with the check (e.g., who can cash it, whether funds can be withdrawn, or whether the entire amount must be deposited).
    - A blank endorsement occurs when the payee (person to whom the check is written) signs only his or her name on the back of the check. When this is done, the check may be signed over to a third party.
17. **Demonstrate the correct procedure for preparing a bank deposit.**
    - Review Procedure 28-4.
18. **List four methods of making deposits and briefly explain each.**
    - Deposits can be made in person by presenting the deposit to a teller at the bank.
    - Deposits can be made by mail, with the bank returning the deposit receipt by mail.
    - Deposits can be made electronically, such as wire transfer of funds from one account to another, or one bank to another.
    - Deposits can be made by using the night deposit if the bank is closed for business when a deposit is made.
19. **Demonstrate the correct procedure for reconciling a bank statement.**
    - Review Procedure 28-5.
20. **List four ways in which a patient statement can be prepared.**
    - A patient statement can be prepared using a photocopy of the ledger card, a manually-prepared statement, an outside billing service, or done with computerized billing.
21. **Demonstrate the correct procedure for explaining professional fees before providing services.**
    - Review Procedure 28-6.
22. **Explain how an adjustment affects the balance of a patient's account, and list four reasons why an adjustment might be made.**
    - An adjustment can provide a debit or a credit to a patient account balance.
    - Professional discounts, write-offs for bankruptcy or insurance adjustments, returned checks, and overpayments are reasons for adjustments to patient accounts. Occasionally, accounts may also be adjusted because of an error in coding or documentation that results in an incorrect charge.
23. **Describe the collection process, including the role of third-party payers.**
    - When a patient receives services, a co-payment may be made, or the fee may be paid in full if the patient has no insurance.
    - If the patient is covered by insurance, the insurance company will pay its portion of the charges after a claim for the service is submitted. Depending on the insurance, the balance of the bill may then be collected from the patient, submitted to a secondary policy, or written off according to contractual agreements.
    - If an account remains unpaid over time, an attempt must be made to collect the fee.
24. **Demonstrate the correct procedure for establishing payment arrangements on a patient's account.**
    - Review Procedure 28-7.
25. **List four guidelines for making telephone calls to collect debts.**

- Calls can only be made during normal waking hours, usually 8 AM to 9 PM.
- Only one call may be made per week.
- If an employer requests that calls not be made to the employee's workplace, such calls must be stopped.
- Threatening or harassing patients is not permitted.

26. **Demonstrate the correct procedure for explaining a statement of account to a patient.**
    - Review Procedure 28-8.
27. **Demonstrate the correct procedure for collecting delinquent accounts.**
    - Review Procedure 28-9.
28. **List six laws that affect earnings and withholdings and briefly explain each.**
    - Fair Labor Standards Act: overtime for hourly employees set at time-and-a-half; minimum wage established; normal workweek of 40 hours.
    - Social Security tax: withheld to provide funds to retirement/support benefits for employees and their families.
    - Medicare tax: collected to support Medicare, the federal health insurance program for older people.
    - Tax Payment Act (federal income tax): employer withholds tax and pays it to the Internal Revenue Service.
    - Federal Unemployment Tax Act (FUTA): requires employers to pay tax based on each employee's earnings; to benefit employees who become unemployed.
    - Workers' compensation: requires employers to pay insurance that will reimburse employees for wage losses from job-related injuries or their families if death occurs on the job.
    - Employers must keep accurate records of deductions and withholdings from employee paychecks.
29. **Differentiate between gross wages and net pay.**
    - Gross wages are the earnings before any deductions have been taken.
    - Net pay is what an employee receives after deductions have been taken from gross earnings.
    - Net pay is calculated by subtracting total deductions from gross earnings.
30. **List the three principal deductions from the employee's gross pay that are required by federal law.**
    - Withholdings required by federal law include Social Security (FICA) tax, Medicare tax, and federal income tax.
31. **List the four types of information in the employee earnings record.**
    - Employee earnings records contain the gross earnings, deductions, net pay, and accumulated earnings for the calendar year for an employee.
32. **Analyze a realistic medical office situation and apply your understanding of medical office financial management to determine the best course of action.**
    - Medical assistants must understand how the finances in a medical practice are managed.
33. **Describe the impact on patient care when medical assistants have a solid understanding of the financial aspects of a medical office.**
    - Accurate and complete financial records help ensure that patients' questions and problems can be addressed swiftly, that their claims are paid by third parties in a timely manner, and that they are aware of the charges and the expectations for payment.

PRACTICAL APPLICATIONS

If you have accomplished the objectives in this chapter, you will be able to make better choices as a medical assistant. Take another look at this situation and decide what you would do.

Meredith is the office manager for a private physician. She is responsible for the financial management of the office. She is the person who tracks the assets and liabilities for the accountant and interprets "owner equity" so that the physician will know the net value of the practice. As part of her job description, Meredith also disburses petty cash. She makes sure that the vouchers with receipts attached and the cash on hand balance at the end of each workday. As each patient leaves the office, the payments for office visits are collected. The goal is to collect whatever is necessary from patients (co-payment, co-insurance) on the day of service. If patient receivables are current, outstanding insurance claims become the main focus for accounts receivable. Another one of Meredith's duties is to approve or disapprove of professional discounts and write-offs as fee adjustments. Finally, she generates collection letters and telephone calls for overdue and delinquent accounts.

Would you be able to perform these responsibilities in the medical office?

1. What are assets? What are liabilities?
2. Why is it important for a physician to be aware of the owner equity before spending money for new equipment?
3. What is petty cash, and how is it used by the medical office?
4. Why is it important for Meredith to complete a petty cash voucher each time that money is removed from the petty cash fund?
5. Why is it important to keep accounts receivable at a low level?
6. What are professional discounts?
7. What is a write-off?
8. How should a collection phone call be handled?

WEB SEARCH

1. To understand accounting principles better, **research the difference between cash-based accounting and the accrual method.** As you have learned, financial records provide a method for a business to monitor its financial status. Each method has advantages and different ways to record the same transaction.

- **Keywords:** Use the following keywords in your search: cash-based accounting, accrual accounting, cash vs. accrual accounting/method.

29 Medical Coding

evolve http://evolve.elsevier.com/klieger/medicalassisting

Coding involves transforming written or verbal descriptions into numbers. Coding, in itself, is not a new concept. Many routine activities of our lives involve some type of coding. When we go to a store, the merchandise we buy has a bar-code that is scanned at the checkout counter. When we mail a letter, we add a zip code to the address that allows the post office to sort and deliver our mail more quickly and efficiently. When you first begin to code, you may find the process challenging, but it is important to add to your coding knowledge whenever possible. The more familiar you become with medical terminology and the longer you work in a medical office, the easier it will become to perform diagnostic and procedural coding.

LEARNING OBJECTIVES

You will be able to do the following after completing this chapter:

Key Terms
1. Define, appropriately use, and spell all the Key Terms for this chapter.

Diagnostic Coding
2. Define diagnosis and diagnostic coding and describe the development of diagnostic coding.
3. State the original purpose for ICD codes and list the four current uses of the ICD system.
4. List six types of organizations and agencies that use ICD codes.
5. List six benefits to the medical assistant, facility, and patients when medical assistants understand how to code correctly.
6. Explain the format and structure of the *International Classification of Diseases* (ICD-9-CM) manual.
7. Explain the difference between Volume 1 and Volume 2 of the ICD-9-CM manual.
8. Explain what "main term" means and list the four items represented by main terms in ICD-9-CM coding.
9. Locate information in the volumes and appendices of the ICD-9-CM manual using main terms and subterms.
10. Differentiate between primary and principal diagnoses and between concurrent conditions and secondary conditions.
11. Locate the area of the CMS-1500 claim form where ICD-9 codes are entered.
12. Demonstrate the correct procedure for diagnostic coding to the highest degree of specificity.

Procedural Coding
13. Describe the development of procedural coding.
14. State the purpose of CPT coding.
15. List four types of organizations or agencies that use CPT codes.
16. Explain the format and structure of the *Current Procedural Terminology* (CPT-4) manual.
17. List the six sections of the CPT manual and the code number ranges for each section.
18. Locate information in the sections and appendices of the CPT manual.
19. Demonstrate the correct procedure for CPT coding to the highest degree of specificity.
20. Locate the area of the CMS-1500 claim form where CPT codes are entered.
21. Identify three factors used in Evaluation and Management (E/M) coding.
22. List the three key components on which the level of service in E/M coding is based.
23. List the four types of examination in E/M coding.
24. List the four types of medical decision making in E/M coding.
25. List three contributory factors that affect the choice of E/M codes.
26. List the seven steps for determining the correct E/M code.

Patient-Centered Professionalism
27. Analyze a realistic medical office situation and apply your understanding of diagnostic and procedural coding to determine the best course of action.

28. Describe the impact on patient care when medical assistants understand the importance of accurate, efficient diagnostic and procedural coding.

KEY TERMS

- acute
- appendices
- chief complaint (CC)
- chronic
- concurrent condition
- consultation
- contributory factors
- conventions
- coordination of care
- counseling
- diagnosis
- E codes
- eponym
- established patient
- examination
- greatest specificity
- guidelines
- history
- history of present illness (HPI)
- inpatient
- instructional terms
- key components
- main term
- medical decision making
- medical necessity
- modifiers
- morbidity rates
- mortality
- new patient
- outpatient
- pertinent past, family, and/or social history (PFSH)
- presenting problem
- primary diagnosis
- principal diagnosis
- referral
- review of systems (ROS)
- secondary condition (diagnosis)
- subjective findings
- V codes

PRACTICAL APPLICATIONS

Read the following scenario and keep it in mind as you learn about medical coding in this chapter.

Jenny, a medical assistant, is the insurance clerk in a large medical practice. She has been with the practice for 10 years and has gradually learned how to perform coding. She uses the ICD-9-CM codes and the CPT-4 codes daily. Phyllis, a long-term patient, was seen today with a chief complaint of a sore throat, influenza, and a chronic cough. Phyllis has diabetes mellitus and hypertension, as well as chronic obstructive pulmonary disease. The physician not only examined her respiratory tract and listened to her heart but also checked her other body systems. He also reviewed her symptoms and took a past history as it related to her presenting symptoms. In addition, the medical decision making was more complex for Phyllis because many medications used for cough contain sugar.

When Phyllis left the office, Jenny immediately began the process of coding her visit. Would you be able to code this visit?

DIAGNOSTIC CODING

Webster's New World Dictionary defines a **diagnosis** as "the act or process of deciding the nature of a diseased condition by examination of the symptoms." *Dorland's Illustrated Medical Dictionary* defines diagnosis as "the determination of the nature of a case of disease" based on signs, symptoms, and laboratory findings. Learning about the history and purpose of diagnostic coding, the ICD-9-CM manual, and the process of diagnostic coding will help you become a more successful medical assistant.

History and Purpose

To understand diagnostic coding, it is essential to know about the history of diagnostic coding, the groups who use it, and its importance.

History of Diagnostic Coding

In seventeenth century England, statistical information was gathered through a system known as the "London Bills of Mortality" (**mortality** is death from a particular disease). By 1937 this method of tracking information had evolved into another system called the "International List of Causes of Death."

The World Health Organization (WHO) put out a publication in 1948 that could be used to track both mortality and **morbidity rates** (the rate of disease, or proportion of diseased persons in a given population or locality). The WHO listing, called the International Classification of Diseases, paved the way for the current diagnostic coding manual used around the world today, the *International Classification of Diseases,* ninth revision (ICD-9), which was published in 1977.

The ICD-9 was already the accepted method of classifying diseases internationally when the U.S. National Center for Health Statistics (NCHS) decided to modify the statistical study with clinical information for better data. These modifications allowed morbidity data (from medical records, medical case reviews, and other medical care programs) to be classified for indexing, as well as for basic health statistics. The result of this modification was the *International Classification of Diseases,* ninth revision, *Clinical Modification* (ICD-9-CM). The ICD-9-CM (or "ICD-9") describes the precise clinical picture of each patient and provides specific information—more than what is needed for statistics and analyses of health care trends.

When the U.S. Congress passed the Medicare Catastrophic Coverage Act in 1988 (which was later repealed), ICD-9-CM coding became very important. This act mandated (as of April 1989) the use of ICD-9-CM codes on each Part B Medicare claim submitted by health care providers. Guidelines regarding the use of ICD-9-CM codes were published by the Health Care Financing Administration (HCFA), now the Centers for Medicare and Medicaid Services (CMS), and these guidelines went into effect in each state. The part of the act mandating the use of ICD-9-CM codes was not repealed, and the failure of a medical facility to use ICD-9-CM codes correctly could result in severe penalties (see introduction to ICD-9-CM for further historical information).

The ICD-9-CM manuals are printed by several publishers in varying formats. Some manuals are printed with only the first two volumes for use in outpatient facilities. Manuals printed with all three volumes are for hospital use only. The ICD-9-CM codes are updated yearly and published in three publications for coders to make updates in the coding books. NCHS and CMS are the federal agencies responsible for overseeing all changes and modifications to the ICD-9-CM. All medical offices should have the latest edition of the ICD-9-CM for accuracy in claims processing.

Purpose of ICD-9 System

The original purpose of the ICD system was to provide morbidity (sickness) statistics for WHO, but the system has expanded and currently is used in the following ways:

1. To provide mortality statistics for WHO and other information for agencies that compile health care statistics using ICD-9 diagnostic codes and track trends in incidence of disease and treatment.
2. To establish **medical necessity** and simplify the payment process for health care services.
3. To translate written medical terminology or descriptions into numbers to provide a universal, common language among third-party payers and health care providers.
4. To evaluate the patterns and appropriateness of how health care is used, as well as cost factors.

Users of ICD-9 Codes

Many different agencies and organizations use ICD-9 codes, including the following:

- Professional standards review organizations
- Physicians and other health care providers
- Government health care programs
- Medical insurance carriers
- Medical researchers
- Hospitals

Importance of Diagnostic Coding

Diagnostic coding is extremely important for the four current uses listed previously. In addition, accurate diagnostic coding is also crucial for the prompt payment of insurance claims. Every individual diagnosis (and procedure or service, as described in the procedural coding section) must be assigned a correct and complete code number.

Because of the complexity of diagnostic and procedural coding, a working knowledge of medical terminology and anatomy and physiology is essential. In today's computerized medical offices, frequently used codes can be preset in the program for ease of keying in the charges. However, you will still have to "translate" the written diagnosis on the encounter form into a code to enter into the computer. Thus all medical office personnel in charge of insurance claims should be familiar with the essentials of how to find a code in the coding manual. Medical assistants familiar with and competent in coding benefit themselves, the medical practice, and patients in the following ways:

- A medical assistant who is efficient in coding is more marketable. In fact, coders are currently in great demand.
- Coding skills provide the ability to review and update all codes used in the medical facility (at least annually), thus avoiding costly and time-consuming denial or delay of payment for claims.
- Accurate coding helps maximize the provider's third-party reimbursements.
- Accurate coding facilitates coding reviews and audits to prove compliance.
- Accurate and efficient coding helps ensure prompt payment of patient claims, saving patients and medical assistants the time and effort of follow-up on unpaid accounts and claims.

The ICD-9-CM Manual

In addition to understanding the history, purpose, and importance of the ICD-9-CM coding system, medical assistants need to be familiar with the ICD-9-CM manual. Keep in mind that several companies publish the ICD-9, and the format may differ somewhat from one publisher to another. However, the various publications are similar enough so that you can get a good idea of the format.

Originally, the ICD-9-CM was published as a three-volume set. Newer versions are available as a single book or a set of multiple volumes, depending on the publisher. Coders in a medical office or other outpatient setting use Volume 1 *(Tabular List of Diseases)* and Volume 2 *(Alphabetic Index of Diseases)* only, which are usually bound together in one manual. Volume 3 *(Procedures)* is mainly used in hospitals. ICD-9 is published annually and becomes effective October 1 of each year.

Introduction

The beginning pages of the ICD-9-CM manual, typically identified with Roman numerals, constitute an introduction and guide to using the ICD-9. This introductory information includes the following:

- A discussion of the history and background of the ICD-9-CM system
- Instructional steps for using the manual correctly
- A listing of official conventions, footnotes, symbols, and instructional notes
- A summary of code changes
- General guidelines for coding and reporting inpatient and outpatient diagnoses

Read and study these introductory topics carefully, paying particular attention to the guidelines, because these will assist you in coding to the **greatest specificity.** Never submit a claim with a three-digit code when a four-digit or five-digit code is available. Documentation must always support the code chosen. Coding to the greatest specificity is the goal because it reflects the most accurate, detailed diagnosis based on the documentation.

Conventions and Terminology. The introduction explains the **conventions** and terminology used in the ICD-9-CM manual. To interpret the language of the ICD-9, the medical assistant must become familiar with the abbreviations, punctuation, symbols, and instructional notes used throughout the manual. Box 29-1 lists ICD-9-CM coding conventions.

Main Terms. In ICD-9 coding, a **main term** represents one of the following:

- A disease (e.g., pneumonia, influenza, bronchitis)
- A condition (e.g., open wound, fatigue, fracture, injury)
- A noun (e.g., syndrome, disease, disturbance)
- An adjective (e.g., large, double)

The *Alphabetic Index* of the ICD-9-CM is organized by main terms. Identifying the main term allows the coder to locate the correct information and code number for a particular problem or condition.

BOX 29-1

International Classification of Diseases (ICD-9-CM): Coding Conventions, Symbols, and Terminology

ABBREVIATIONS

NEC **Not Elsewhere Classifiable** (in the codebook). All codes with this listing are to be used with *ill-defined terms*. Use only when a separate code describing the disease or injury is not listed in the code manual.
Example: Fibrosclerosis
710.8 Other specified diffuse diseases of connective tissue
Multifocal fibrosclerosis (idiopathic) **NEC**

NOS **Not Otherwise Specified** (by the physician). This abbreviation is the equivalent of "unspecified." It refers to a lack of sufficient detail in the physician's diagnostic statement to be able to assign a specific code.
Example: Malignant neoplasm of colon
153.9 Malignant neoplasm of colon, unspecified
Large intestine **NOS**

NOTE: The malignant portion of the colon needs to be stated in the medical record. Avoid using nonspecific codes, if possible. Ask the physician for more information so that a specific code may be used.

PUNCTUATION

[ ] **Brackets** are used in the *Tabular List* to enclose synonyms, alternative wordings, or explanatory phrases.
Example: 426.13 Other second-degree atrioventricular block
Mobitz (type) I **[Wenckebach's]**

( ) **Parentheses,** found in the *Tabular List* and *Alphabetic Index,* are used to enclose supplementary, descriptive words that do not affect the code assignment; referred
Example: 287.1 Qualitative platelet defects
Thrombasthenia **(hemorrhagic) (hereditary)**

Colons are used in the *Tabular List* after an incomplete term that needs one or more of the modifiers that follow to make it assignable to a given category.
Example: 112 Candidiasis
Includes: Infection by *Candida* species
Moniliasis

} **Braces** are used to enclose a series of terms, each of which is modified by the statement appearing at the right of the brace.
Example: 103.0 Pinta, primary lesions
Chancre (primary)
Papule (primary)   **of pinta** [carate]
Pintid

OFFICIAL GOVERNMENT SYMBOLS (MAY NOT BE USED IN ALL TEXTS)

◻ The **lozenge symbol,** printed in the left margin of the *Tabular List,* preceding a disease code in ICD-9-CM, indicates that the content of a four-digit code has been modified from the original ICD-9.
Example: 016.1 ◻ Tuberculosis of genitourinary system, Bladder

§ The **section mark symbol,** printed in the left margin preceding a code, denotes the placement of a footnote at the bottom of the page that is applicable to all subdivisions of that code.
Example: § 364.6 Cysts of iris, ciliary body, and anterior chamber

OTHER SYMBOLS—MAY CHANGE FROM PUBLISHER TO PUBLISHER AND ARE SHOWN TO ILLUSTRATE VARIOUS TYPES OF SYMBOLS THAT MAY BE ENCOUNTERED

[code] **Italicized (slanted) brackets** enclosing a code, used in Volume 2, the *Alphabetic Index,* indicate the need for another code.
Example: Microaneurysm, retina 362.14
Diabetic 250.5 **[362.01]**

● **Black circle** may signal a code is new to this revision.

[**Large bracket** may signal a new or revised code.

▲ **Black triangle** may signal a revised code.

④ ⑤ Either of these symbols signals that a *fourth* or *fifth*
☑ ☑ *digit is required* for coding to indicate the highest
4th 5th level of specificity.

NOTE: Other symbols may indicate male diagnosis only, female diagnosis only, newborn diagnosis only, pediatric diagnosis only, or adult diagnosis only.

From Fordney MT, French LL: *Medical insurance billing and coding: an essentials work text,* Philadelphia, 2003, Saunders.

Print Type. Bold and italic typefaces have special meaning in the ICD-9-CM manual.
- **Boldface type**

In Volume 1 *(Tabular List),* all titles and codes are printed in bold.

Example: **317**   Mild mental retardation

In Volume 2 *(Alphabetic Index),* only the main term is printed in bold.

Example: **Dermatitis**

- Italic typeface

In both volumes, italic type is used to highlight all exclusion notes and to identify codes that should not be used as the primary code for a condition or problem.

If you look up code 517.1 in Volume 1, you will see the diagnosis (rheumatic pneumonia) with italic instructions to *code first underlying disease (390).* This means that code 390 (rheumatic fever without mention of heart involvement) should be listed first on the claim form because it is the patient's primary problem or condition. The rheumatic pneumonia is a manifestation of the underlying problem—the rheumatic fever.

Instructional Terminology. Certain words and phrases have special meaning in the ICD-9-CM manual. Box 29-2 lists common **instructional terms** and their meaning.

Volume 2: Alphabetic Index

In most manuals, the introduction to the ICD-9-CM is followed by Volume 2 *(Alphabetic Index of Diseases),* then Volume 1 *(Tabular List of Diseases).* Essentially, Volume 2 is referenced before Volume 1 because it is an index to Volume 1. Volume 2 consists of an alphabetical listing of terms and codes with special tables, followed by two supplementary sections.

Section 1: Index to Diseases and Injuries. Section 1 of Volume 2 is the Index to Diseases and Injuries. This section allows users to look up main terms (from the diagnoses documented in the patient's chart) in the index. Box 29-3 shows the structure of this section.

Supplementary Sections. Two supplementary sections follow the *Alphabetic Index:*
- *Table of Drugs and Chemicals* (Section 2, Volume 2) is an alphabetical index to poisoning and external causes of adverse effects of drugs and other chemical substances.
- *Alphabetic Index to External Causes of Injury and Poisoning* (E Codes) is Section 3 of Volume 2. E codes classify environmental events, circumstances, and other conditions as the cause of injury and poisoning.

Special Tables. Two special tables are included alphabetically in Volume 2:

BOX 29-2

Instructional Terms Used in ICD-9-CM Manual

Includes. Further defines or clarifies the term listed and represents the most frequently used terms to serve as a guide.
See code category **461** in Volume 1 and Figure 29-1.

Excludes. Terms following "excludes" are not to be used with the listed code. Often the applicable code, or code range, is given.
See code category **461** in Volume 1 and Figure 29-1.

Use additional code. When you see this phrase, an additional code must be used to provide a more comprehensive picture of the diagnosis.
See code **330** in Volume 1.

Notes. Provide additional instructions or guidelines.
See code **305** in Volume 1.

See. Directs you to a more specific term under which the correct code can be found.
Look up "nonspherocytic hemolytic anemia" in Volume 2.

See also. Indicates additional information is available that may provide an additional diagnostic code.
Look up "Busquet's disease" in Volume 2.

See Category. Indicates you should review the entire category specified before assigning a code.
Look up "late effect of extradural abscess" in Volume 2.

Code first any underlying condition. Use additional code for any associated condition; provides guidance when more than one code must be used.
See Code **785.4**, gangrene.

BOX 29-3

ICD-9-CM: Structure of Volume 2, *Alphabetic Index*

Section 1: Index to Diseases and Injuries

Main terms	Appear in **boldface** type.
Subterms	Are indented two spaces to the right under the main terms.
Carry-over lines	Are indented more than two spaces from the level of the preceding line.
Modifiers	Appear in parentheses ( ).

- *Table of Hypertension* subdivides hypertensive diagnoses as "malignant," "benign," or "unspecified."
- *Table of Neoplasms* classifies neoplasms by body site, then as "malignant," "benign," "uncertain behavior," or "unspecified."

Volume 1: Tabular List

Volume 1 of ICD-9 is a numerical listing of the disease and injury codes and consists of 17 chapters (Table 29-1). After the *Tabular List* (at code 999.9) are the "V codes" and "E codes" tabular lists, then five official ICD-9 appendices.

Chapter Structure. The 17 chapters in Volume 1 list and describe all the numbers that can be assigned as codes. The

TABLE 29-1
ICD-9-CM: Chapters and Code Ranges

Chapter	Classification	Code Range
1	Infectious and Parasitic Diseases	001-139
2	Neoplasms	140-239
3	Endocrine, Nutritional & Metabolic Diseases, and Immunity Disorders	240-279
4	Diseases of the Blood and Blood-Forming Organs	280-289
5	Mental Disorders	290-319
6	Diseases of the Nervous System and Sense Organs	320-389
7	Diseases of the Circulatory System	390-459
8	Diseases of the Respiratory System	460-519
9	Diseases of the Digestive System	520-579
10	Diseases of the Genitourinary System	580-629
11	Complications of Pregnancy, Childbirth, and the Puerperium	630-677
12	Diseases of the Skin and Subcutaneous Tissue	680-709
13	Diseases of the Musculoskeletal System and Connective Tissue	710-739
14	Congenital Anomalies	740-759
15	Certain Conditions Originating in the Perinatal Period	760-779
16	Symptoms, Signs, and Ill-Defined Conditions	780-799
17	Injury and Poisoning	800-999

Alphabetic Index can help you pinpoint the most specific code from the *Tabular List* for a given diagnosis. The structure of these 17 chapters is as follows:

- *Sections* refer to the divisions of the *Tabular List*; sections are organized in groups of three-digit code numbers.
- *Categories* refer to the codes listed within a specific three-digit code section.
- *Subcategories* are groups of fourth-digit code numbers listed after three-digit categories. Any code with more than three digits requires a decimal point between the third and fourth digits (e.g., diabetes codes 250.xx).
- *Subclassifications* are fifth-digit code numbers listed after the fourth-digit code number of a three-digit category. (Five digits is the highest level of specificity for any code.)

Figure 29-1 is a copy of a page from Volume 1 (the *Tabular List*) of the 2004 ICD-9-CM manual. Note the format showing the section, category, subcategory, and subclassification.

Supplementary Classifications (V codes, E codes). The two supplementary classifications in Volume 1 of ICD-9-CM list V codes and E codes, which provide supplemental or additional information about the primary code(s). Generally, these codes do not stand alone, although the V code may, in some circumstances.

V Codes. The **V codes,** or Supplementary Classification of Factors Influencing Health Status and Contact with Health Services (V01 to V83), are located immediately after the last

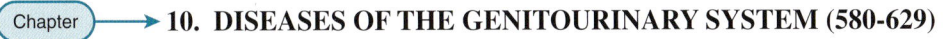

FIGURE 29-1 Example of the format from ICD-9-CM, Volume 1, *Tabular List of Diseases.* Note the format showing the section, category, subcategory, and subclassification. (From Buck CJ: *Step-by-step medical coding,* 2009 edition, St Louis, 2009, Saunders.)

tabular code, which is 999.9. When V codes are used to explain reasons for an office visit when a patient is not currently ill, the code may stand alone. Main terms may include the following:
- Examination
- Therapy
- Observation
- Tests
- Screening (for)
- Care (of)

V codes also show problems or situations that influence a patient's health status (but are not a current illness or injury), such as the following:
- Family history of asthma (F/H/O)
- Personal history of cancer (P/H/O)
- Transplant status (heart, lung, liver, kidney)
- Dialysis (abdominal or peritoneal)
- Chemotherapy

Reimbursement for V codes depends on the individual's insurance company's guidelines. Some insurers do not cover preventive or routine services (e.g., screening colonoscopy), and the service then becomes an out-of-pocket expense for the patient.

Examples of V codes:
V72.5   Routine chest x-ray film
V20.2   Well-baby examination
V72.31   Routine gynecological examination

E Codes. **E codes,** or Supplementary Classification of External Causes of Injury and Poisoning (E800 to E999), provide a classification of environmental events, circumstances, and conditions as the cause of injury, poisoning, and other adverse effects. Classifications include how an accident occurred, whether a drug overdose was accidental or intentional, and other circumstances that caused the injury or condition being coded. E codes are never used alone; they are used in addition to a code from the main chapters of ICD-9-CM that indicates the nature of the condition. Medical assistants should check insurance carriers' guidelines on how to handle E codes before submitting claims.

Examples of E codes:
E814.x   Motor vehicle traffic accident involving collision with pedestrian
E881.x   Fall on or from ladders or scaffolding
E906.0   Dog bite

Appendices. Volume 1 includes five **appendices** (A, B, C, D, and E) that appear in order at the end (Box 29-4).

The Diagnostic Coding Process

When a patient sees the physician for the initial visit, a medical **history** is normally taken. The health care provider (e.g., physician) or another member of the medical team conducts an in-depth interview with the patient and establishes the main reason for the visit, called the *chief complaint,* which is noted in the medical record as the *CC.* After performing a physical examination, the physician determines the *diagnosis,* which is generally noted in the record as the *Dx, Impression (Imp.),* or *assessment.*

As mentioned previously, diagnostic (ICD-9) coding involves converting verbal and written descriptions of medical diagnoses into a series of numbers of at least three digits. Sometimes one or two additional digits are added to define the patient's clinical condition more fully and bring the code to the highest level of specificity, based on the documentation.

BOX 29-4

ICD-9-CM: List of Appendices

Appendix A	Morphology of Neoplasms
Appendix B	Glossary of Mental Disorders
Appendix C	Classification of Drugs by American Hospital Formulary Service (AHFS) and their ICD-9-CM Equivalents
Appendix D	Classification of Industrial Accidents According to Agency
Appendix E	List of Three-Digit Categories

Examples of common diagnoses and associated ICD-9-CM codes:
Pneumonia, organism unspecified   486
Essential hypertension, benign   401.1
Tension headache   307.81

After the patient encounter, a claim form is completed to send to the third-party payer. The claim form lists the diagnoses (identified by the physician and documented in the medical record) in the form of ICD-9 codes. Medical offices often use the CMS-1500 (formerly HCFA-1500) claim form to file third-party claims (discussed further in Chapter 30).

A familiarity with Volumes 1 and 2 and conventions in the ICD-9-CM manual is most helpful as you learn how to perform diagnostic coding. To understand the process fully, however, you need to know the difference between primary and principal diagnoses, how to abstract from patient records, and how to pinpoint the right diagnostic code.

Primary vs. Principal Diagnosis and Other Terms

Medical assistants must understand the concepts of primary diagnosis versus principal diagnosis and secondary condition (or diagnosis) versus concurrent condition.
- A **primary diagnosis** is the condition considered as the patient's major health problem and is usually listed first in Block 21 on the CMS-1500 claim form (Figure 29-2). Up to three additional *concurrent* or *secondary* conditions can be listed on the claim form if they were treated during the

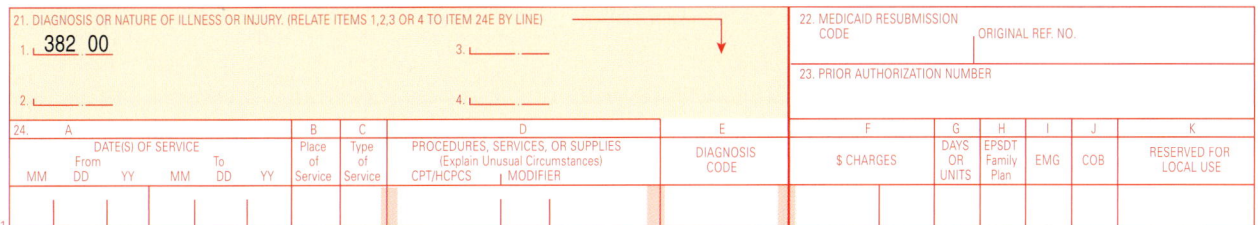

FIGURE 29-2 Diagnosis codes are entered into Block 21 of the CMS-1500 claim form. The primary diagnosis, "acute suppurative otitis media without spontaneous rupture of eardrum," has been entered onto line 1 (382.00). (From Fordney MT: *Insurance handbook for the medical office,* ed 10, St Louis, 2008, Saunders.)

same encounter. The physician's office or clinic will use primary diagnoses, even if the patient receives care from the office or clinic physician during a hospital stay.

- The **principal diagnosis** is the condition that is established to be chiefly responsible for triggering the admission of the patient to the hospital for treatment. Note that hospitals use a different claim form known as the UB-04. The UB-04 allows for the principal diagnosis and up to four concurrent conditions, ranked in the order of their severity. In some cases the primary and the principal diagnoses may be the same.
- A **concurrent condition** occurs at the same time as the primary diagnosis and affects the treatment or recovery from the condition. There may be one or more concurrent conditions during any encounter.
- A **secondary condition** (or diagnosis) is a disorder affecting the patient at the same time as the primary diagnosis but not necessarily affecting the prognosis of the primary condition. The order in which the secondary conditions appear on the claim form is not significant, but they must impact treatment and must be documented in order to be listed.

In addition to these special terms, you must also understand how to handle terms such as *probable, suspected,* and *rule out* in medical record statements.

> If a patient comes to the office complaining of chest pain and shortness of breath, a heart attack may be "probable" or "suspected." However, until it is established that the patient has actually had a heart attack, the medical assistant should only code the symptoms: chest pain and shortness of breath. If you submit a diagnosis code (e.g., the code for a heart attack) rather than one for the symptoms (chest pain, shortness of breath), the insurance carrier will include the heart attack diagnosis in the patient's history even though it has not been proved. This could cause problems for the patient in the future if he or she elects to change insurance companies because "heart attack" will show in the patient's history as a "preexisting" condition.
>
> The coding guidelines are different for inpatient coding. If you are doing inpatient coding, be certain to read the Inpatient Coding Guidelines in the front of the ICD-9-CM manual and follow established hospital coding guidelines. In most instances, conditions are automatically assumed to be **acute** if not specifically identified as **chronic**.

Abstracting Information from Patient Records

The medical assistant who handles claims submissions and coding must learn how to abstract information from the patient's medical record. This means reading the medical record carefully after a patient encounter to determine what diagnoses and symptoms have been identified and documented and then coding these diagnoses and symptoms to the highest degree of specificity. This ability, along with knowledge of reimbursement and coding guidelines, can be applied to the preparation of CMS-1500 claims, which result in the optimal payment that the medical record can support. Essentially, this means that the claim form reflects *all* services provided to the patient so that the physician or practice can be reimbursed for each appropriately.

Finding the Right Diagnostic Code

As previously mentioned, the *Alphabetic Index* (Volume 2) of the ICD-9-CM is organized by main terms printed in bold type for easy reference. Coders can use the *Alphabetic Index* to look up main terms and then use the *Tabular List* (Volume 1) to determine the exact code. Keep in mind that anatomical sites are not used for main terms in ICD-9 coding. A diagnosis of breast lump, for example, is found under "lump" rather than under the anatomical site "breast." Procedure 29-1 illustrates how to assign the proper ICD-9 code.

> **WARNING:** Never code directly from the *Alphabetic Index* alone because the diagnosis must be coded to the *greatest specificity* (which cannot be listed in the Index because of space restrictions). This can only be accomplished by examining the entire section for the diagnosis in the *Tabular List* (Volume 1).

ICD-9-CM Volume 3

Volume 3 is included in the ICD-9-CM manual only when it will be used specifically for hospital coding. Volume 3 contains the codes for procedures done for hospital inpatients only. These codes are not used for outpatient surgeries and procedures, office procedures, or recovery of the physician's fee for services (whether for inpatients or outpatients). Volume 3 codes represent the means for the hospital to receive reimbursement for their facility overhead involved in procedures

PROCEDURE 29-1: Diagnostic Coding

TASK: Assign the proper *International Classification of Diseases* (ICD-9-CM) code to the highest degree of specificity based on medical documentation for auditing and billing purposes.

EQUIPMENT AND SUPPLIES
- Current ICD-9-CM codebook
- Medical dictionary
- Patient's medical record

SKILLS/RATIONALE

1. **Procedural Step.** Identify the key term in the diagnostic statement.
   Rationale. The purpose is to determine the primary diagnosis, the main reason for the encounter. Keep in mind that the primary diagnosis should be coded first and then other official diagnoses. Check the document carefully; you should not code every diagnosis that is documented in the record but only the diagnosis or diagnoses that match the service or procedures provided. Never code conditions described as "rule out," "suspected," "probable," or "questionable." If no definitive diagnosis was made, code the symptoms as documented by the physician.

2. **Procedural Step.** Locate the diagnosis in the *Alphabetic Index* (Volume 2, Section 1) of the ICD-9-CM manual.

3. **Procedural Step.** Read and understand footnotes, symbols, or instructions.
   Rationale. Pay particular attention to the words "see" and "see also"; they are used to inform users of the ICD-9-CM manual that they should try another term in the Alphabetic Index to find what they are looking for. (See Box 29-1 for a thorough list of ICD-9-CM conventions.)

4. **Procedural Step.** Locate the diagnosis in the *Tabular List* (Volume 1).
   Rationale. The Tabular List is where you can locate any exclusions associated with the code and verify that the code you have identified is correct.

5. **Procedural Step.** Read and understand the inclusions and exclusions noted in the *Tabular List*.
   Rationale. Exclusions are terms or conditions that are not included with the code. They can help you to isolate a more specific ICD-9-CM code for the condition you are coding.

6. **Procedural Step.** Make certain you include fourth and fifth digits, when available.
   Rationale. Using fourth and fifth digits when available ensures that you code to the highest degree of specificity.

7. **Procedural Step.** Assign the code to the highest degree of specificity appropriate and document in the medical record.
   Rationale. If you have followed all the previous steps, you can facilitate accuracy in record keeping once you have assigned the diagnostic code.

8. **Procedural Step.** Ask yourself these final questions:
   a. Have you coded the diagnosis to the highest level of specificity?
   b. When you transferred the code to the patient form and to subsequent records and forms, did you record the code accurately?
   c. Are there any secondary diagnoses or conditions addressed during the encounter that need to be coded?

(housekeeping, utilities, ancillary staff). These codes are *not* used to recover the surgeon's fees for operating services; the surgeon uses CPT (procedural) codes for these fees.

Table 29-2 provides a basic overview of the coding resources that are used to perform diagnostic and procedural coding.

ICD-10-CM

Traditionally, WHO, which owns and publishes the disease classification, releases an updated version of ICD about every 10 years. ICD-10 is now available and is being used in some parts of the world. The intent of ICD-10 was to increase clinical detail and address information regarding previously classified diseases, as well as new diseases discovered since ICD-9. In ICD-10, conditions are grouped in the most appropriate way for general epidemiological purposes and evaluation of health care. Organizational changes, content improvements, and new features are added to ICD-10-CM, and the number of codes is significantly increased.

For more information on ICD-10-CM, visit the Centers for Disease Control and Prevention (CDC) and NCHS website: www.cdc.gov/nchs.

PATIENT-CENTERED PROFESSIONALISM

- *How does understanding the history and purpose of diagnostic coding better prepare the medical assistant for selecting the proper code?*

TABLE 29-2

Overview of Coding Resources

Resource	Description	Use
ICD-9-CM Volume 1 *Tabular List*	Contains code and description of diagnosis or condition	Inpatient use for diagnosis; outpatient use for diagnosis.
ICD-9-CM Volume 2 *Alphabetic Index*	Use main term to locate code, then check *Tabular List* for diagnosis	Inpatient use for diagnosis; outpatient use for diagnosis.
ICD-9-CM Volume 3	Procedure codes only	Used *only* for inpatient hospital surgeries and procedures; reimbursement for facility billing only, not for physician.
CPT-4	Procedure codes only	Used for physician/healthcare providers billing both inpatient and outpatient services.

PROCEDURAL CODING

Procedural coding is transferring medical services and procedures into code numbers. Procedures are coded using CPT codes. CPT stands for *Current Procedural Terminology*. The CPT code manual is sometimes referred to as CPT-4 because it is the fourth edition developed and published by the American Medical Association (AMA). CPT is used to code all procedures and services performed by physicians and other health care providers in an outpatient or clinical setting. The CPT code manual contains a systematic listing of all descriptive terms and corresponding identification codes used for reporting medical services. As with ICD-9-CM diagnosis codes, CPT codes are used on claim forms prepared and submitted to all third-party payers and government agencies involved in health care.

History and Purpose

As with diagnostic coding, medical assistants should know the history of CPT codes, the groups using it, and the importance of procedural coding.

History of Procedural Coding

The first CPT manual appeared in 1966 as a result of an effort by the AMA to create a method of accurately and universally identifying all medical and surgical procedures and services used throughout the United States. The AMA publishes a new volume of CPT codes every year to keep current with rapidly changing medical technology; new codes are added and some older codes are deleted or revised. Because of these annual changes, it is important that the medical assistant use the most recent CPT coding manual. The new CPT codes are published every October and go into effect January of the following year.

Purpose of CPT System

The CPT system provides an effective and reliable method of communication among health care providers and government programs (e.g., Medicare, Medicaid, TRICARE, and CHAMPUS), as well as patients and their private insurers.

Users of CPT Codes

As with the ICD-9 codes, many different agencies and organizations use CPT codes, including the following:
- Physicians and other health care providers
- Government health care programs (Medicare, Medicaid)
- Medical insurance carriers and managed care companies
- Medical education and research

CPT codes are part of the code standards selected by the Health Insurance Portability and Accountability Act (HIPAA) to describe services in electronic transactions.

Importance of Procedural Coding

CPT coding is used for claims processing and development of dependable guidelines in reviewing appropriate medical care. The uniform coding language of CPT is also applicable in medical education and research by providing a method of comparing how medical care is utilized, both locally and nationally. A five-digit number identifies the procedures and services in the CPT manual. By using these codes, the process of reporting procedures and services is simplified through the accurate identification of all medical care given by the health care provider.

CPT Manual

The CPT code manual lists and describes codes for services (e.g., office visits) and procedures (e.g., coronary bypass surgery). Symbols are used in the CPT manual to give the coder additional information about the codes. It is important for medical assistants to understand the organization and structure of the CPT manual so they will be able to locate information efficiently.

Symbols

Several important symbols are used in the CPT manual. Accurate coding of procedures cannot be accomplished without a thorough understanding of the symbols and conventions used in this coding system. Using correct codes when coding clinical procedures is critical. Besides selecting the five-digit code

> **BOX 29-5**
>
> ### Current Procedural Terminology: Symbols used in CPT Coding
>
> 1. Bullet (•) placed in front of the code number identifies *new codes* for procedures and services.
> 2. Triangle (▲) placed in front of a code indicates that the description for the code has been *changed or modified* since the previous edition. Changes may be additions, deletions, or revisions in code descriptions.
> 3. Plus (+) placed in front of a code indicates an *add-on code*. Add-on codes are never used alone; they are used in addition to another primary procedure or service code.
> 4. Circle with a line through it (Ø) identifies a *modifier -51 exempt code*. When coders see the Ø, it cautions them to check the primary procedure code to see what other procedures are included in that code before using the modifier -51 exempt code.
> 5. Horizontal triangles (►◄) placed at the beginning and the end of new or revised guidelines indicate changes in wording. *This symbol is not used for procedure description changes.*
> 6. Semicolon (;) is used to separate main and subordinate clauses in code descriptions to save space in the coding manual where a series of related codes are found.

> **BOX 29-6**
>
> ### Sections of the CPT Manual and Their Code Ranges
>
> 1. Evaluation and Management: 99201 to 99499
> 2. Anesthesiology: 00100 to 01999 and 99100 to 99140
> 3. Surgery: 10021 to 69990
> 4. Radiology (including Nuclear Medicine and Diagnostic Ultrasound): 70010 to 79999
> 5. Pathology and Laboratory: 80048 to 89356
> 6. Medicine (except Anesthesiology): 90281 to 99199 and 99500 to 99602

accurately, however, you must also be aware of the symbols and their meanings (Box 29-5).

Organization

The CPT manual is organized similar to the sequence of events a patient goes through from the onset of illness to recovery. It begins with an introduction and then contains sections for the various types of services and procedures performed. These sections begin with office visit codes and then progress to more specific procedures performed: anesthesia, surgery, radiology and laboratory procedures, medicines administered, and other nonsurgical services.

Introduction. The introduction of the CPT manual provides instructions for using CPT and also includes a listing of the sections and their numerical sequences (Box 29-6). In more recent CPT manuals, the AMA has included a section after the introduction that includes an illustrated anatomical and procedural review as a quick reference tool.

Evaluation and Management Section. The first section of the CPT manual is Evaluation and Management (E/M) services and is divided into broad categories such as office and hospital visits and consultations. All codes in this section begin with the numbers 99, not 00 as you might expect, because these codes are listed first. The E/M codes are placed in the front of the book because they are the most frequently used codes, as discussed later in this chapter.

Tabular List. The Anesthesia, Surgery, Radiology, Pathology/Laboratory, and Medicine sections follow the E/M section in the CPT manual. The Surgery section contains the largest number of codes. Anesthesia codes begin with 00, and the codes follow in order somewhat, ending with Medicine codes, which start with 90 and end with 99. In some places, numbers are missing between codes (e.g., Anesthesia code 00192, immediately followed by code 00210) to allow future code additions.

At the beginning of each section, **guidelines** to aid in the use of coding for that section are included. The medical assistant must read these guidelines for a better understanding of how to code the procedures and services within each section. The guidelines are different for each section of codes.

Appendices. The following five appendices are found after the *Tabular List* in the CPT manual:

Appendix A	List of all modifiers applicable to CPT coding
Appendix B	Summary of applicable additions, deletions, and revisions of codes
Appendix C	Clinical examples of correct usage of the codes
Appendix D	Summary of CPT add-on codes
Appendix E	Summary of CPT codes exempt from modifier "51"

Alphabetic Index. The last section in the CPT is the *Alphabetic Index*. Similar to the ICD-9-CM manual, the *Alphabetic Index* is organized by *main terms*. Each main term can stand alone, or it can be followed by modifying terms *(subterms)*. Main terms can be located using one of the following four categories:

1. Procedure or service (e.g., repair)
2. Organ or other anatomical site (e.g., breast)
3. Condition (e.g., pregnancy)
4. Synonyms, eponyms, or abbreviations (e.g., finger/digit/phalanx, Marshall-Marchetti-Krantz Procedure, ECG)

A main term may be followed by up to three indented terms that modify the main term. It is important to read the entire list when modifying terms are shown because these subterms affect the selection of the appropriate procedure.

Again, you should not code by the *Alphabetic Index* alone. After making the code selection in the *Alphabetic Index*, locate that code in the *Tabular List* and read the description(s). Then select the most appropriate code based on your documentation.

Procedural Coding Process

Procedures and services performed during a patient encounter are listed in the medical record, on the encounter form, and on the patient ledger card. Figure 29-3 shows a portion of a patient's medical record with the following procedures noted:

1. Puncture aspiration of left breast cyst
2. Pap smear

To code these procedures accurately, use the following basic steps:

Step 1. Identify the main term (as discussed previously). In the first procedure, the main term could be "breast" (the site)

Step 2. Locate the main term (breast) in the *Alphabetic Index*. Under the main term, note a series of subterms, also in alphabetical order, indicating possible procedures involving the breast. The correct subterm is "cyst," and the modifying term is "puncture aspiration." This tells you that possible codes are 19000 and 19001.

Step 3. Turn to the tabular (numerical) list, locate codes 19000 and 19001, and code to the greatest specificity. The patient had only one cyst, so 19000 is the correct code.

Step 4. Repeat this process for additional procedures. In the second procedure, Pap smear, "Pap" is an **eponym** and can be considered the main term. On locating Pap smear in the *Alphabetic Index*, you find three different code ranges (88141-88155, 88164-88167, and 88174-88175). In this case the correct code for a routine Pap smear would be 88150. Because multiple services are performed, the use of a modifier may be indicated on the secondary procedure.

The same answer can be reached by using the main term "aspiration" (the procedure). Read the index note to see "puncture aspiration" in that column, with subterm "cyst," then "breast." This takes you to the same code "range," 19000-19001. Remember that often there is more than one way to arrive at the same correct code.

CPT codes are entered into Block 24 of the CMS-1500 claim form (Figure 29-4).

Code Format in Tabular Section

The CPT manual uses indenting and semicolons to present information clearly.

Indenting. There are two types of code sets in the tabular section, as follows:

- *Stand-alone codes.* An example of a stand-alone code is 40810. Note the structure of the description after the code as it appears in the tabular list:

FIGURE 29-3 Example of a portion of a patient record noting procedures.

PHYSICAL EXAMINATION: Temp: 98.5, pulse: 66 and regular. B/P 126/82. Weight: 144 lb. Height: 62" Neck: Supple without thyroid enlargement or lymphadenopathy. Lungs: Clear without rales, rhonchi, friction rubs. Heart: Regular rate and rhythm. No murmurs heard. Abdomen: Soft and nontender without rebound, guarding, or tenderness. There is an approximate 2-cm mass in Lt breast, which, upon aspiration, revealed approximately 5 cc of brownish fluid. Pelvic examination revealed a normal cervix. Pap smear was done.

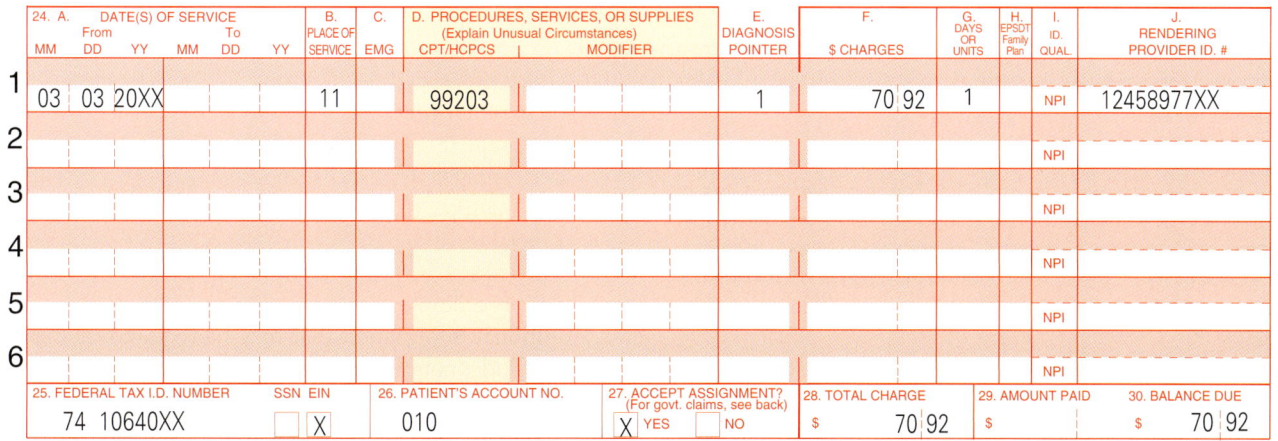

FIGURE 29-4 Procedure codes are entered into Block 24D of the CMS-1500 claim form. The service shown here is a new patient office visit. (From Fordney MT: *Insurance handbook for the medical office,* ed 10, St Louis, 2008, Saunders.)

40810	Excision of lesion of mucosa and submucosa, vestibule of mouth; without repair

- *Indented codes.* An example of an indented code is 40812. It simply reads "with simple repair," and these words are indented.

40810	Excision of lesion of mucosa and submucosa, vestibule of mouth; without repair
40812	with simple repair

The first code, 40810, has a complete description and can stand on its own. Code 40812 is only a partial description and cannot stand on its own. To make the code 40812 complete, you must use the first part of the description *before the semicolon* ("Excision of lesion of mucosa and submucosa, vestibule of mouth"), then use the partial description listed with code 40812. In other words, the complete description for code 40812 would read "Excision of lesion of mucosa and submucosa, vestibule of mouth; with simple repair." Simply stated, if the excision of the lesion is done without repair, the appropriate code is 40810. If the excision of the lesion is done with simple repair, the appropriate code is 40812.

Semicolons. The semicolon is critical when coding procedures. The words after the semicolon indicate alternative anatomical sites, alternative procedures, or a description of the extent of the procedure or service.

Coding to Greatest Specificity

To use the code that most completely and accurately describes the procedure or service performed, you must read the entire section and follow all guidelines and coding conventions in choosing the right code. Procedure 29-2 discusses how to locate a procedure code.

Modifiers

At times, the five-digit CPT code does not completely and adequately describe the procedure or service performed, and modifiers are used. **Modifiers** indicate that a procedure or service has been altered in some way or by some special circumstance but not in such a way that it has changed the procedure or service itself. Modifiers are composed of a hyphen and two digits.

An example of a modifier is "-50." This modifier indicates a bilateral procedure performed during the same session if the same procedure is performed on both paired body parts. If the patient had a therapeutic steroid injection in *both* arms for treatment of carpal tunnel syndrome, the code would be 20526-50.

If the CPT code description includes the word "bilateral," do not use modifier -50. The code itself includes the description and appending modifier -50 is redundant reporting.

More information and examples for use of modifiers can be found in the introduction section of the CPT manual. Appendix A in the back of the CPT manual lists all the modifiers, with descriptions and helpful notes.

Unlisted Procedures

Occasionally, you will encounter a service or procedure (e.g., experimental, seldom used, or newly approved) for which there is no code. When a procedure or service cannot be located in the CPT manual, an "unlisted procedure" code can be used. These codes end in -99 and are found at the end of each subsection.

Category III Codes

Category III codes are temporary codes used for new technology, services, and procedures. A listing of Category III codes follows the Medicine section in the CPT manual. If a Category III code is available, it should be used instead of an "unlisted procedure" code. Using Category III codes helps researchers and public health experts identify and track new treatments, technology, services, and procedures for clinical efficiency, utilization, and outcomes.

The format of Category III codes differs somewhat from that of regular CPT codes. Category III codes have four numerals followed by an alphabetical character. For example, "0009T" would be the Category III code for "endometrial cryoablation with ultrasonic guidance."

New Category III codes are released semiannually, and the full set of these codes is published in the next year's edition of the CPT manual. Codes in this section may or may not eventually become Category I codes incorporated into the main body of CPT. Category III codes are deleted after 5 years, when either they become Category I codes or the codes are no longer in use.

Special Reports

When a new, unusual, seldom-used, unlisted, or Category III procedure is used, a "special report" must normally accompany the claim. Such reports help insurance carriers determine the appropriateness of care and the medical necessity of the service or procedure provided. A special report should include the following:

- A complete description of the service or procedure performed
- The nature, extent, and need for the service or procedure
- The time, effort, and equipment necessary to perform the procedure or service

Additional information that may be required in a special report includes complexity of symptoms, final diagnosis, pertinent physical findings, diagnostic and therapeutic procedures, concurrent problems, and follow-up care. A special report is typically developed and dictated by the physician (or other health care professional).

PROCEDURE 29-2 Procedural Coding

TASK: Assign the proper *Current Procedural Terminology* (CPT) code to the highest degree of specificity based on medical documentation for auditing and billing purposes.

EQUIPMENT AND SUPPLIES
- Current CPT codebook
- Medical dictionary
- Patient's medical record

SKILLS/RATIONALE

1. **Procedural Step.** Read the introduction, guidelines, and notes before using the latest edition of the CPT codebook. New procedures added to the text are identified with the symbol "•" placed before the code number; the symbol "▲" signifies a revised procedure descriptor.
   Rationale. This familiarizes you with the codebook and any new changes.

2. **Procedural Step.** Review all services and procedures performed on the day of the encounter, including all medications administered and trays and equipment used.
   Rationale. Once you have identified all the services performed at the encounter, you can begin to code the services.

3. **Procedural Step.** Identify the main term in the procedure.

4. **Procedural Step.** Locate the main term in the *Alphabetic Index*. Review any subterms listed alphabetically under the main term.
   Rationale. This provides you with a set of codes to verify, narrowing the choice of the correct code even further. Review all descriptions within the section.

5. **Procedural Step.** Verify the code sets in the tabular (numerical) list. Select the code with the greatest specificity.
   Rationale. Selecting the code with the greatest specificity ensures that the procedures will be reimbursed to the highest degree.

6. **Procedural Step.** Determine if a modifier is required.
   Rationale. Modifiers must be assigned if a five-digit code does not completely and adequately describe the procedure or service performed. (See the introduction section of the CPT manual for a review of modifiers.)

7. **Procedural Step.** Assign the code.
   The following eight steps are focused on determining the level of Evaluation and Management (E/M) service.
   a. Identify if the patient is new or established.
   b. Determine where the patient is being seen.
   c. Determine whether the visit is a consultation or other special service.
   d. Determine whether the visit is a result of an illness or is a preventive medical service.
   e. Determine the level of history.
   f. Determine the level of examination.
   g. Determine the level of medical decision making.
   h. Assign the most accurate CPT code.
   Rationale. Following these eight steps allows you to code to the highest specificity.

8. **Procedural Step.** Ask yourself these final questions:
   a. Have you coded the diagnosis to the highest level of specificity?
   b. When you transferred the code to the patient form and to subsequent records and forms, did you record the code accurately?
   c. Are there any secondary diagnoses or conditions addressed during the encounter that need to be coded?

Evaluation and Management Coding

E/M is one of the more challenging aspects of CPT coding. The section in the CPT manual that deals with E/M codes is divided into broad categories, including "office or other outpatient services," "hospital inpatient services," and "consultations." Categories are further divided into two or more subcategories, with a few exceptions.

All subsections have information and guidelines, which should be studied thoroughly before attempting to select an E/M code. It is crucial for medical assistants to understand the vocabulary used in E/M coding, the three major factors in E/M coding, the levels of service, and contributory components before attempting to determine the correct E/M codes. In addition, thorough documentation of all services and procedures is necessary as proof if questions are asked by the insurance company.

Vocabulary

The medical assistant must become familiar with several common terms to use E/M coding accurately. First, there are two categories of patients: new and established.
- A **new patient** is a patient who has not received any professional services from the physician, or another physician of the same practice, within the past 3 years.

- An **established patient** is a patient who has received professional services from the physician, or another physician of the same practice, within the past 3 years. Patients who have been seen for the first time in the hospital or other setting and subsequently are seen in the office for follow-up care are considered established patients.

Other terms relate to admission.

- An **outpatient** is a patient who is being treated in the hospital or medical center for (typically) less than 24 hours. An outpatient can be admitted and discharged on the same day or subsequent days but within 24 hours.
- An **inpatient** is a patient who has been admitted to the hospital for a stay longer than 24 hours.

It is also important to know the terms related to the way time is spent during an office visit and how a patient was treated by a physician.

- **Counseling** requires that the health care provider conduct a discussion with the patient (or family members) regarding the patient's diagnosis, test results, recommended treatment, prognosis, and follow-up care.
- A **consultation** requires a health care provider to render a service at the request of another health care professional such as for a second opinion. Normally, a consultation consists of only one encounter to treat one illness by providing additional information, and the primary provider retains control over the patient's care. For example, a family practitioner seeing a patient for general health care may be unable to cure the patient's persistent bronchitis. The family practitioner suggests that the patient see a pulmonologist for an expert opinion. The pulmonologist may suggest further diagnostic studies or a change of medication. The primary care physician still retains control of the balance of the patient's overall health care.
- A **referral** is the transfer of a patient's care from one health care provider to another for a specific problem. For example, a family practitioner transfers the care of a patient to a cardiologist when the patient complains of symptoms that suggest heart abnormalities, but the family practitioner retains control of other medical care.

Finally, it is important to know what is meant by terms in the medical records. For example:

- The **chief complaint** (**CC**) is a statement (usually made by the patient in his or her own words) that describes the reason for the visit (e.g., "After I eat, I have a burning pain in the middle of my chest").

Three Factors

The following three factors must be determined before the process of E/M coding begins:

1. *Place of service.* You must determine where the service was provided. Was the service rendered in the provider's office? Inpatient hospital? Emergency department? Nursing home?
2. *Type of service.* Was the procedure or service an office visit, a consultation, hospital admission, or another type?
3. *Patient status.* Is the patient a new patient, established patient, outpatient, or inpatient?

Levels of E/M Service

Determination of the level of E/M service to be selected is based on three **key components:** history, examination, and the difficulty of medical decision making. In addition to these three key components, there may be contributing factors such as counseling, coordination of care, nature of the presenting problem, and time.

History. A history is **subjective findings** (information given by the patient). Four types of history are used to define specific E/M services, as follows:

1. *Problem Focused.* The problem-focused level of history taking usually consists of only a CC and a brief history of the illness or presenting problem, or **history of present illness** (**HPI**). *Example:* A 10-month-old child with a diaper rash.
2. *Expanded Problem Focused.* An expanded problem-focused history includes a chief complaint, a brief HPI, and a problem-pertinent **review of systems** (**ROS**). *Example:* A 21-year-old woman with recurrent urinary tract infection (UTI). No fever.
3. *Detailed.* A detailed history typically includes a chief complaint, an extended HPI, an extended ROS, and a **pertinent past, family, and/or social history** (**PFSH**). *Example:* The initial office visit of a 42-year-old male who presents with symptoms of headache, nasal congestion, fever, and a deep cough with purulent sputum for the past 4 days, worse at night. No nausea or vomiting. No shortness of breath. Patient does not smoke.
4. *Comprehensive.* A comprehensive history includes a chief complaint, an extended HPI, and a complete ROS and PFSH. *Example:* An 83-year-old woman who complains of shortness of breath (SOB), chest pain on exertion for the past week with loss of appetite, and intermittent blurred vision. Symptoms improve if she lies down for a while. No recent weight loss, cough, or muscle pain. All other systems are negative. The patient is a widow and lives alone. She does not smoke or drink alcohol.

Examination. There are also the following four types of **examination:**

1. *Problem Focused.* A problem-focused examination is limited to the affected body area or organ system. *Example:* The examination for the 10-month-old child with diaper rash would typically be limited to the perianal area only.
2. *Expanded Problem Focused.* An expanded problem-focused examination is limited to the affected body area or organ system and other symptomatic or related organ systems. *Example:* For the 21-year-old female with a recurrent UTI, the examination would probably focus on the genitourinary system.
3. *Detailed.* This extended examination involves the affected body areas and other organ systems that may be related or contributing to the problem. *Example:* For the 42-year-old male with headache, nasal congestion, fever, and cough with sputum, the examination would include all affected body systems (e.g., respiratory, cardiovascular).

4. *Comprehensive.* This extensive examination includes a complete single-organ system or general multisystem examination. *Example:* For the 83-year-old female with SOB, chest pain, and blurred vision, the examination would include most body systems because of the potential combination of serious problems.

Medical Decision Making. The E/M component of **medical decision making** examines the following three factors:

- The difficulty of establishing a diagnosis and selecting a treatment and management plan, as measured by the number of possible diagnoses and different management options considered.
- The amount and difficulty of reading and analyzing the necessary medical documents (e.g., diagnostic tests).
- The risk of significant complications, morbidity (disease) and mortality (death), significant co-morbidities, and possible management options.

The four types of medical decision making are as follows:

1. *Straightforward.* All three factors above are minimal.
2. *Low Complexity.* Low-complexity decision making consists of a limited number of diagnoses and management options, limited amount and complexity of data to be reviewed, and low risk of complications and morbidity and mortality if the condition were left untreated.
3. *Moderate Complexity.* At the moderate-complexity level, there are multiple diagnoses and management options, moderate amount and complexity of data to be reviewed, and moderate risk of complications and morbidity and mortality.
4. *High Complexity.* At the high-complexity level of medical decision making, there are extensive diagnoses and management options, extensive amount and complexity of data to be reviewed, and high risk of complications and morbidity and mortality.

Contributory Components. Three **contributory factors** affect the choice of E/M codes in most patient encounters: (1) *counseling* (explained earlier), (2) *coordination of care,* and (3) *nature of the presenting problem.* Another contributory component may be time. **Coordination of care** occurs when the health care provider consults with other providers or agencies in arranging and planning how to manage the patient's condition, with or without the patient being present. For example, a primary care physician who has a patient in a nursing home may call the nursing home to leave orders for new medications, may call another physician to request a consultation for the patient, or may call another facility for the patient's last radiology report.

A **presenting problem** is whatever symptom, illness, or injury caused the encounter. Box 29-7 describes the five types of presenting problems used in defining the E/M codes.

Time can be a contributory component but is not a factor in qualifying for a particular level of E/M service, *unless the provider spends more than 50% of the encounter in face-to-face counseling.* Time is never a factor in emergency room visits.

BOX 29-7

Five Types of Presenting Problems Used in Defining Evaluation and Management (E/M) Codes

MINIMAL
A problem that does not require the attention of a physician. The services are provided by an ancillary member of the staff (e.g., nurse, nurse practitioner, or physician's assistant), but the services require that a physician is on the premises.

SELF-LIMITED or MINOR
A problem that is transient in nature and is likely to run its course with management.

LOW SEVERITY
A problem in which the risk of morbidity and mortality is low without treatment and full recovery is expected.

MODERATE SEVERITY
A problem in which the risk of morbidity and mortality is moderate, with an increased probability of functional impairment without treatment.

HIGH SEVERITY
A problem in which the risk of morbidity and mortality is high to extreme, with a high probability of severe or prolonged functional impairment without treatment.

For inpatient visits, the term "unit/floor time" is used. *Unit/floor time* includes the time the physician spends examining the patient, communicating with the patient's family members and other professionals, and documenting and reviewing chart notes. The actual amount of time spent in counseling and coordination of care must be well documented in the patient's medical record. E/M codes for new and established patients have a suggested amount of time for physicians' face-to-face encounters, which can be used as a guide for choosing the correct code.

Determining the Correct E/M Code

Choosing the correct E/M code is a multistep process. Keep in mind that documentation in the medical record must fully support the level of service chosen.

All three key components (history, examination, and medical decision making) must meet or exceed the requirements listed in the CPT manual in order to report a particular level of service for new patients, initial hospital care, office or confirmatory consultations, and emergency department services. For reporting established patient services and follow-up care, only two of the three key components must be met or exceeded.

Appendix C in the CPT manual provides numerous clinical examples for many E/M services. The AMA provides these examples to assist the coder in choosing the correct E/M code level because of the combination of factors that can affect code selection in E/M coding.

Documentation Guidelines

The importance of complete and thorough documentation of information in the patient's medical record cannot be overemphasized. To be complete, the medical record must include proper documentation of all three key components required for E/M coding, plus the nature of the problem, the approximate amount of time spent with the patient, and the extent of counseling and coordination of care, if applicable. Medicare and other third-party payers have the right to audit providers' offices for carelessness in documentation and misuse of codes; a violation of the coding rules can result in substantial fines and penalties.

PATIENT-CENTERED PROFESSIONALISM

- List some similarities and differences between ICD-9-CM and CPT-4 coding, including those related to documentation requirements.

CONCLUSION

Coding is an important skill in any medical setting. For the medical practice to be reimbursed at the highest level that can be supported by the medical documentation, coding must be done accurately and efficiently. Inaccurate, inefficient coding not only will result in loss of money for the practice but also could result in legal problems and fines. Patients are affected when their claims are not reimbursed promptly by third-party payers and when they are continually billed for balances for which they are not responsible.

Effective diagnostic and procedural coding requires a good knowledge of medical terminology, a familiarity with the ICD-9-CM and CPT-4 manuals, the ability to extract information from medical records, and the discipline to read all explanations in the manuals completely to ensure the most specific code is chosen. Coding may not be easy at first, but the more practice you have, the more your coding skills will increase.

Chapter Summary

Reinforce your understanding of the material in this chapter by reviewing the curriculum objectives and key content points below.

1. **Define, appropriately use, and spell all the Key Terms for this chapter.**
   - Review the Key Terms if necessary.
2. **Define diagnosis and diagnostic coding, and describe the development of diagnostic coding.**
   - A diagnosis is the act or process of deciding the nature of a disease or condition by examination of the symptoms.
   - Diagnostic coding is the transformation of written or verbal descriptions of diseases and conditions into numbers.
   - The World Health Organization (WHO) published what was later to be called the *International Classification of Diseases* (ICD) in 1948 for the purpose of tracking morbidity and mortality worldwide.
   - ICD-9-CM is the clinical modification of this same system currently in use in the United States. The clinical modification makes the data more useful for health care utilization purposes.
   - ICD-10 is being used in some parts of the world, but ICD-10-CM has not yet been adopted for general use in the United States.
3. **State the original purpose for ICD codes and list the four current uses of the ICD system.**
   - The original purpose of the ICD coding system was to track morbidity and mortality statistics worldwide.
   - ICD-9 codes (a) provide health care statistics for tracking trends in morbidity and treatment, (b) establish medical necessity for reimbursement, (c) provide a common language for third-party payers and health care providers, and (d) evaluate the utilization of health care resources.
4. **List six types of organizations and agencies that use ICD codes.**
   - ICD codes are used by both public and private organizations and agencies, including professional standards review organizations, physicians and other health care providers, government health care programs, medical insurance carriers, medical researchers, and hospitals.
5. **List six benefits to the medical assistant, facility, and patients when medical assistants understand how to code correctly.**

   The medical assistant should become familiar with the format of the ICD-9 to facilitate accurate diagnostic coding.
   - Coding is a very marketable skill for a medical assistant.
   - Costly and time-consuming audits can be avoided by reviewing and updating codes annually.
   - Efficient coding helps avoid costly delays on claim turnaround.
   - Accurate coding can help maximize the facility's third-party reimbursements.
   - Accurate and efficient coding is important during coding reviews to prove compliance.
   - Prompt payment of claims can be ensured if there are no coding errors requiring resubmission of a claim or by filing a "clean claim."
6. **Explain the format and structure of the ICD-9-CM manual.**
   - The ICD-9-CM manual is divided into three volumes. Volume 1 is the *Tabular List*, and Volume 2 is the

Alphabetic Index. Volume 3 is only used by hospitals for coding inpatient procedures.
- Codes are listed in sections beginning with three-digit categories. Subcategories include a fourth digit, with subclassifications having a fifth digit for the code. Any code higher than a three-digit category has a decimal point before the fourth digit and the addition of the fifth digit, if indicated.

7. **Explain the difference between Volume 1 and Volume 2 of the ICD-9-CM manual.**
   - Volume 1 is the *Tabular List of Diseases* and contains all the codes in chronological order, starting with 001 and ending with 999.9.
   - Volume 2 is the *Alphabetic Index of Diseases* and usually comes first in the manual.
   - All coding should be done from Volume 1.

8. **Explain what "main term" means and list the four items represented by main terms in ICD-9-CM coding.**
   - The "main term" is the essence of the diagnosis. Main terms are broad, generic qualifications for codes. Use of subterms will aid in coding to "greatest specificity."
   - In ICD-9-CM coding, a main term represents a disease, a condition, a noun, or an adjective.

9. **Locate information in the volumes and appendices of the ICD-9-CM manual using main terms and subterms.**
   - Main terms appear in bold in the index.
   - Subterms are indented under the main term and provide further clarification or specification of the main term.

10. **Differentiate between primary and principal diagnoses and between concurrent conditions and secondary conditions.**
    - Medical assistants who do coding in a physician's office or clinic will use the primary diagnosis for outpatients.
    - Hospitals code the principal diagnosis for inpatients as the main diagnosis established after study.
    - Concurrent conditions may be present at the same time as the chief complaint and may affect the treatment or recovery from the chief complaint.
    - Secondary conditions occur at the same time as the chief complaint but do not necessarily affect the treatment and prognosis of the primary condition or chief complaint.

11. **Locate the area of the CMS-1500 claim form where ICD-9 codes are entered.**
    - ICD-9 codes are entered into Block 21 of the CMS-1500.

12. **Demonstrate the correct procedure for diagnostic coding to the highest degree of specificity.**
    - Review Procedure 29-1.

13. **Describe the development of procedural coding.**
    - The first *Current Procedural Terminology* (CPT) manual in 1966 was the result of efforts by the American Medical Association (AMA) to create a method of accurately and universally identifying all medical and surgical procedures and services used in the United States.

14. **State the purpose of CPT coding.**
    - CPT coding translates the services and procedures provided to a patient into numerical codes for common identification of services.
    - CPT provides an effective and reliable method of communication among health care providers and government programs (e.g., Medicare, Medicaid, TRICARE, and CHAMPUS), as well as patients and their private insurers.

15. **List four types of organizations or agencies that use CPT codes.**
    - CPT codes are used by public and private third-party payers, as well as physicians and researchers.

16. **Explain the format and structure of the CPT-4 manual.**
    - The CPT-4 manual is similar to the ICD-9-CM manual. In an alphabetical index (in the back of the manual), a code is identified under a main term and then subterms. A numerical tabular listing provides all the CPT codes with descriptions, divided by sections.

17. **List the six sections of the CPT manual and the code number ranges for each section.**
    - Evaluation and Management codes (99201-99499)
    - Anesthesia (00100-01999, 99100-99140)
    - Surgery (10021-69990)
    - Radiology (70010-79999)
    - Pathology and Laboratory (80048-89356)
    - Medicine (90281-99199, 99500-99602)

18. **Locate information in the sections and appendices of the CPT manual.**
    - Main terms are located in the index, which then refers to a range of codes in a specific section of the CPT manual.
    - Codes are chosen based on the documentation in the medical record.
    - Appendices A through E are located in the back of the manual, after Medicine.

19. **Demonstrate the correct procedure for CPT coding to the highest degree of specificity.**
    - Review Procedure 29-2.

20. **Locate the area of the CMS-1500 claim form where CPT codes are entered.**
    - CPT codes are entered into Block 24D of the CMS-1500.

21. **Identify three factors used in Evaluation and Management (E/M) coding.**
    - Factors used in E/M coding are place of service (hospital, nursing home, office), type of service (consultation, hospital discharge), and patient status (new or established patient).

22. **List the three key components on which the level of service in E/M coding is based.**
    - The three components are history, examination, and medical decision making.

23. **List the four types of examination in E/M coding.**
    - The four types of examination are problem focused, expanded problem focused, detailed, and comprehensive.

24. **List the four types of medical decision making in E/M coding.**
    - The four types of medical decision making are straightforward, low complexity, moderate complexity, and high complexity.

25. **List three contributory factors that affect the choice of E/M codes.**

- Three factors affecting E/M code choice are counseling, coordination of care, and nature of the presenting problem.
- Time can be a factor if the provider spends more than 50% of the encounter in face-to-face counseling.

26. **List the seven steps for determining the correct E/M code.**
    - To determine the correct E/M code, determine the patient's status, identify the type of service, identify the place of service, establish the level of history, establish the level of the examination, determine the level of medical decision making, and note the time element involved and other contributory factors. Then choose the correct E/M code.
    - Complete and accurate documentation of all three key components, plus the contributory factors (including time, if applicable), is critically important when selecting the correct code.

27. **Analyze a realistic medical office situation and apply your understanding of diagnostic and procedural coding to determine the best course of action.**
    - Coding must always be done to the highest degree of specificity.
    - Some situations may seem similar, but on closer examination, they might require very different codes, resulting in differing fees or reimbursement levels for the services provided.

28. **Describe the impact on patient care when medical assistants understand the importance of accurate, efficient diagnostic and procedural coding.**
    - ICD-9-CM and CPT-4 codes are used on claim forms for all third-party payers and government agencies involved in health care; claims are paid more quickly (and patients' account balances cleared) when claim forms are error free and contain the correct codes.

PRACTICAL APPLICATIONS

If you have accomplished the objectives in this chapter, you will be able to make better choices as a medical assistant. Take another look at this situation and decide what you would do.

Jenny, a medical assistant, is the insurance clerk in a large medical practice. She has been with the practice for 10 years and has gradually learned how to perform coding. She uses the ICD-9-CM codes and the CPT-4 codes daily. Phyllis, a long-term patient, was seen today with a chief complaint of a sore throat, influenza, and a chronic cough. Phyllis has diabetes mellitus and hypertension, as well as chronic obstructive pulmonary disease. The physician not only examined her respiratory tract and listened to her heart but also checked her other body systems. He also reviewed her symptoms and took a past history as it related to her presenting symptoms. In addition, the medical decision making was more complex for Phyllis because many medications used for cough contain sugar.

When Phyllis left the office, Jenny immediately began the process of coding her visit. Would you be able to code this visit?

1. Why is coding a medical visit so important and what is actually being accomplished by coding?
2. What part of the medical visit is coded using ICD-9-CM codes?
3. What part of the medical visit is coded using CPT codes?
4. What is a diagnosis?
5. What is the difference between Volume 1 and Volume 2 of the ICD-9-CM manual?
6. What is a chief complaint? Which of these symptoms is the chief complaint?
7. What is the primary diagnosis? Concurrent conditions? Secondary conditions?
8. Why are words such as "probable," "suspected," and "rule out" not used with outpatient diagnosis coding?
9. How would you code the CPT E/M code pertaining to the history above? How would you use CPT codes for the medical decision making?

WEB SEARCH

1. **Research ICD-10-CM to learn more about additions that address previously classified diseases.**
   - **Keywords:** Use the following keywords in your search: ICD-10-CM, NCHS.

Medical Insurance

30

evolve   http://evolve.elsevier.com/klieger/medicalassisting

One of every seven people in the United States is hospitalized each year, and many more see physicians for medical attention. This health care is expensive. In the past 15 years the overall cost of medical care has increased by more than 230%. Health insurance helps individuals and families pay their health care expenses. Without insurance, a large percentage of individual or family income would be eaten up, savings wiped out, and proper care neglected.

Even though health insurance is so important, about 45.5 million people, or 15% of U.S. residents, lack health coverage (Kaiser Family Foundation, 2007). Health insurance premiums rise every year, and many cannot afford to pay for health care coverage. This is a growing problem across the United States that deserves the attention of lawmakers, citizens, and health care professionals alike.

This chapter explains health insurance and reinforces why it is important for medical assistants to become familiar with the purpose of medical insurance, the roles of the involved parties, medical insurance policies and plans, third-party payers, and the importance and process of submitting accurate insurance claims.

LEARNING OBJECTIVES

You will be able to do the following after completing this chapter:

Key Terms
1. Define, appropriately use, and spell all the Key Terms for this chapter.

Overview of Health Insurance
2. Explain the need for medical insurance.
3. Describe how medical insurance originated in the United States.
4. List six factors responsible for the increases in health insurance premiums since the mid-1990s.
5. Describe two federal laws enacted to improve the availability of health insurance.
6. Explain how the "Patient Care Partnership" helps protect patient rights concerning their HMO plans.

Patient and Provider Roles in Medical Insurance
7. Explain why it is important for the health care team to treat patients as you would a "customer."

8. List five types of insurance choices available for eligible patients.
9. Explain "coordination of benefits" and how the "birthday rule" applies.
10. Describe the role of the physician and other members of the health care team in serving the patient.

Medical Insurance Policies and Plans
11. Differentiate between indemnity (fee-for-service) plans and managed care plans.
12. Explain the difference between PAR and non-PAR providers.
13. Compare and contrast PPO, HMO, and POS plans.
14. Describe the UCR, episode of care, capitation, RVS, and RBRVS methods of determining fees.
15. List five methods of cost containment used by third-party payers and the government.

Third-Party Medical Insurance
16. Define "private carrier" and give a well-known example.
17. Explain the difference between *group* and *individual* commercial policies.

18. Explain when third-party liability might apply.
19. Differentiate between Medicare and Medicaid.
20. Differentiate between TRICARE and CHAMPVA.
21. Differentiate between workers' compensation and disability income insurance.
22. Differentiate among Medi-Medi, Medigap, and MSP.
23. Demonstrate the correct procedure for applying managed care policies and procedures.
24. Describe how preauthorization works.

Medical Insurance Claim Cycle

25. Briefly describe the five phases of the medical insurance claim cycle.
26. Explain the purpose of a "release of information" (ROI) authorization.

Submitting Claims

27. Define "clean claim" and state its importance.
28. List two things medical assistants should check before preparing an insurance claim form.
29. Explain what should be done if a patient does not have insurance coverage or if a patient's insurance policy does not cover a procedure.
30. Demonstrate the correct procedure for accurately completing a CMS-1500 claim form.
31. List four advantages of submitting insurance claims electronically.
32. Describe the proper type, size, and color for entering information that can be recognized by OCR software.
33. Explain the purpose of a medical claims clearinghouse.
34. Describe the purpose and use of an insurance claims register.

Preventing Rejections and Delays

35. List five technical errors that could cause a claim to be rejected or delayed.
36. List four reasons a claim might be rejected and might not be eligible for resubmission.
37. List five actions that medical assistants can take to be proactive in claims completion and submission.

Claims Follow-Up

38. Define EOB and explain what should be done with it when received.

Patient-Centered Professionalism

39. Analyze a realistic medical office situation and apply your understanding of medical insurance to determine the best course of action.
40. Describe the impact on patient care when medical assistants understand the essentials of medical insurance and are capable of submitting clean claims to insurers.

KEY TERMS

- abuse
- allowable charges
- balance billing
- basic benefits
- beneficiary
- birthday rule
- capitation
- catastrophic disability
- CHAMPVA
- clean claim
- clearinghouse
- CMS-1500
- co-insurance
- comprehensive plans
- Consolidated Omnibus Reconciliation Act (COBRA)
- coordination of benefits (COB)
- co-payments
- cost containment
- curriculum vitae (CV)
- deductible
- dependent
- disability income insurance
- encounter form
- episode of care
- explanation of benefits (EOB)
- Federal Employee Compensation Act (FECA)
- fiscal intermediary
- fraud
- gatekeeper
- group policy
- group practice association
- guidelines
- Healthcare Common Procedure Coding System (HCPCS)
- Health Insurance Portability and Accountability Act (HIPAA)
- health maintenance organization (HMO)
- implied contract
- indemnity (fee-for-service) plan
- independent practice association (IPA)
- individual policy
- insurance claims register
- legislation
- major medical benefits
- managed care
- mandates
- Medicaid
- medical savings account (MSA)
- medically necessary
- Medicare
- Medicare Part D
- Medicare (as) Secondary Payer (MSP)
- Medigap
- Medi-Medi
- National Provider Identifier (NPI)
- network
- nonparticipating provider (non-PAR)
- optical character recognition (OCR)
- partial disability
- participating provider (PAR)
- Patient Care Partnership
- point-of-service (POS) plan
- preauthorization
- precertification
- preexisting condition
- preferred provider organization (PPO)
- premiums
- primary care physician (PCP)
- relative value scale (RVS)
- relative value units (RVUs)
- release of information (ROI)
- residual disability
- resource-based relative value scale (RBRVS)
- Social Security Disability Income Insurance (SSDI)
- sponsor
- subscriber
- Supplemental Security Income (SSI)
- third party
- total disability
- TRICARE
- usual, customary, and reasonable (UCR)
- veteran
- waiver
- workers' compensation

PRACTICAL APPLICATIONS

Read the following scenario and keep it in mind as you learn about medical insurance in this chapter.

Dr. Jay has hired Maria as his insurance clerk. Maria's previous experience was with household liability claims and coverage. She has not had experience with the CMS-1500 or with coding of medical conditions. She is not aware that the claim begins with the appointment and patient registration and ends with payment by the insurer. Jude Beck, a new patient of Dr. Jay, is seen in the office for what appears to be diabetes mellitus. An ECG, urinalysis, and blood test were done during the visit without checking with Mr. Beck's insurance first. In his notes, Dr. Jay states that he must "rule out diabetes mellitus," so Maria codes this as the "primary diagnosis" and sends the claim without a final diagnosis. When the results of the laboratory work are received, Dr. Jay documents in the medical record that the final diagnoses are dehydration and hypertension with tachycardia.

When the registration form was completed, Mr. Beck failed to check off which of his insurance companies is primary and which is secondary. In processing the claim, Maria sends it with a diagnosis of "diabetes mellitus" to one of the two insurance companies, which turns out to be the secondary insurer. The claim is denied because there is no EOB attached from the primary payer. Maria does not resubmit the claim to the company that is actually the primary carrier.

Could you explain to Maria what went wrong and how the claim should have been handled?

OVERVIEW OF HEALTH INSURANCE

Medical insurance impacts almost all aspects of the medical practice, from the information that must be collected from patients, to fees charged, to the processing and payment of insurance claims. Medical assistants, whether serving as medical insurance specialists or performing other duties, need a good understanding of the various aspects of medical insurance.

Definitions and Purpose

Webster's dictionary defines *insurance* as "coverage by contract whereby one party agrees to make compensation to another for certain incurred injuries, property loss, or damage by a specified unforeseen event or peril." *Health insurance* narrows down this "specified unforeseen event or peril" to expenses incurred from hospitalization and medical care for illness or injury. In either case, the purpose of medical insurance is to protect a **subscriber** or member (the person who is covered by the insurance policy agreement) by covering medical expenses as specified in the contract.

As discussed in Chapter 4, the physician-patient relationship is an **implied contract.** Insurance carriers are not a party to the implied contract between physician and patient but still play a part in the relationship, so they are considered a **third party** to the contract and are referred to as "third-party payers."

Historical Note

Although it dates back to the mid-1800s, health insurance did not become well known in the United States until later. In 1929, at Baylor University in Dallas, Texas, a group of school-teachers agreed to pay $6 a year in exchange for 21 days at the university hospital, if needed. This arrangement between the teachers and the hospital evolved later into the popular Blue Cross and Blue Shield programs.

Cost and Availability

The cost of medical insurance has skyrocketed in recent years. Some yearly premiums increase as much as 40% in 1 year. One recent *USA Today*/Kaiser Family Foundation survey found that in 2007 the average annual premium for employer-sponsored health insurance was $4,200 for single coverage and $12,700 for family coverage. During the 1970s and 1980s, health insurance costs remained fairly stable, but in the mid-1990s, premiums began to rise sharply, at about four times the rate of inflation. Reasons for these dramatic increases in health insurance premiums include the following:

- New medical technology
- Medical needs and demands of a longer-living population
- Overuse and misuse of medical services
- Consumer demands for easier and broader access to health care
- Public pressure to make health care a profitable business
- Federal and state mandates

More recently, experts blame **mandates** for increasing the cost of health insurance. Mandates can provide people with more options but will also drive up the price of health care. Federal mandates include a ban on "drive-through" deliveries, requiring a minimum time for new mothers to remain in the hospital after birth. Another mandate requires that any "cap" on mental health benefits be the same as the cap on physical health benefits. In 1965 there were only seven state-mandated insurance benefits. By 2000, there were almost 1,000 mandated benefits. Although people like these mandates, the result is that costs force premiums up and health insurance is no longer affordable for many Americans.

Although medical insurance is available to nearly everyone, 45.5 million Americans did not have health insurance coverage in 2007. The main reason is the high cost of coverage; these individuals and families simply cannot afford the premiums. Other reasons include ineligibility for employment-based insurance coverage and presence of a high-risk illness or physical condition. The groups most likely not to have health insurance coverage are young adults, certain minority groups, and older individuals under age 65.

The government has enacted **legislation** to improve the availability of health insurance. The **Consolidated Omnibus Reconciliation Act (COBRA)** enacted in 1985 requires employers with 20 or more employees to continue to offer coverage in their group health plan to certain former employees, retirees, spouses, and **dependent** children for up to 18 months in the event of voluntary or involuntary termination of employment. A covered spouse and dependents are eligible to continue coverage for up to 36 months. However, individuals are usually required to pay the premiums (at the group rate) plus a surcharge (up to 2%) to cover administrative costs.

The **Health Insurance Portability and Accountability Act (HIPAA)** was enacted in 1996 to improve health insurance availability for individuals who lose coverage as a result of job change or loss. This legislation is an attempt to ensure health insurance is "portable," reduce health care **fraud** and **abuse,** guarantee privacy and security of health information, and enforce standards for health information. HIPAA also does the following:

- Restricts an employer's or insurer's ability to use "preexisting condition" exclusions or limitations.
- Requires most employers and insurers to comply with certification training requirements.
- Restricts group health plans from discrimination on the basis of health status.

Health Care Reform

Most people believe that health care reform is a high priority. It is no secret that the massive and complex U.S. health care system is broken, but no one knows how to fix it. A tremendous amount of effort and money has been spent to find a solution, but little progress has been made. Some managed care programs resulting from this effort have had limited success. Readily available and affordable health insurance remains a controversial issue in the United States.

The "Patients' Bill of Rights," updated in 2003 by the American Hospital Association to the **Patient Care Partnership,** gave patients the right to sue their health maintenance organization (HMO) plans and was a direct result of problems with managed care organizations (e.g., HMOs). Some alarming stories have circulated about HMOs denying patients lifesaving treatments or forcing them to travel long distances to see HMO-approved physicians. Under this bill, new rules govern the following aspects of patient rights and managed care:

- Plan offerings
- Utilization review
- Internal and external appeals
- Grievance processes
- Formularies for prescription drugs
- Participation of plan enrollees in clinical trials
- Patient information
- How plans work with physicians (including incentive compensation arrangements)

PATIENT-CENTERED PROFESSIONALISM

- Why is it important for the medical assistant to understand costs associated with health care?
- Even though the federal government has enacted legislation to improve the availability of health insurance, why do you think so many Americans have no health insurance?

PATIENT AND PROVIDER ROLES IN MEDICAL INSURANCE

Patients, health care professionals, and insurance carriers must all interact to provide quality patient care and ensure payment. When each of these parties understands their role, the process is more efficient and effective.

The Patient Seen as Customer

In this age of rapid change in health care, marketing and consumer opinions now suggest that patients no longer be viewed as "patients" but as "customers." In the past, many people viewed the physician-patient relationship without question: "My doctor is the expert; I must do as he says if I am to get well." With the advent of the Internet, many people no longer take their doctor's word as final; they log on to the Internet and research symptoms, indications, procedures, and risks on their own. By putting the patient in the category of "customer," physicians must become "marketing" experts, in addition to being "healing" experts. Seeing patients as "customers" relates to the fact that practicing medicine is a business—a service. In business the goal is to attract and keep customers.

Patients also are beginning to realize that their insurance company controls much of their health care. Even if a physician thinks a patient should undergo a certain diagnostic test or surgical procedure, the insurance company may not agree. This can be frustrating to both the patient and the physician. Patients, physicians, and insurance companies must work together in order to deliver quality health care.

Health Insurance Choices

Patients are also the customers of health insurance organizations. The insurance marketplace offers many choices and opportunities for purchasing health insurance.

Employer-Sponsored Group Plans. Eligibility in an employer-sponsored group plan usually involves only a short waiting period, typically 30 days. Also, a group plan normally does not have restrictions on **preexisting conditions,** and **premiums** (or a portion of them) are often paid by the employer.

Government-Sponsored Programs. Examples of government-sponsored programs include Medicare, Medicaid, TRICARE, CHAMPVA, and workers' compensation. In these programs, individuals must meet federal and state guidelines for eligibility (see later discussion).

Medical Savings Account. A **medical savings account (MSA)** is only used to pay for medical care with pretax dollars. MSAs can be established for self-employed individuals and employer groups of 50 or fewer employees. If all the money in the MSA is not used, it may be permitted to grow tax free in the account for future medical expenses or retirement. If money is paid out for nonmedical expenses, the amount withdrawn will be taxed. Individuals with an MSA may be able to see any physician or visit any hospital they choose, or they may be restricted, depending on the policy. One drawback to MSAs is that the deductibles are typically high, as much as $5000 per year.

Private and Individual Policies. Eligibility for private or individual policies tends to be more rigidly controlled than most employer-sponsored group health plans. Younger people can usually qualify without a detailed physical examination. The applicant completes a questionnaire on medical and family history. Private policies often involve preexisting conditions and "riders" (additions to the policy), and premiums are normally much higher than with employer-sponsored plans.

Medigap and Supplemental Policies. Medigap and supplemental plans are designed for Medicare beneficiaries who want health care coverage in addition to Medicare. Eligibility requirements are not as strict with these policies because Medicare, as the primary insurer, tends to pay for many of the health care costs. Supplemental policies often pay all or part of Medicare deductibles and the balance of the allowable, **medically necessary** charges incurred.

Coordination of Benefits

When a patient is covered by more than one insurance policy, the **coordination of benefits (COB)** rules apply. This means that the individual's total reimbursement from both policies will be coordinated so as not to exceed the total cost of his or her medical care. Coverage by more than one insurance policy is less common now because of the excessive cost of health care. Such coverage is especially seen in the case of a minor child of divorced parents.

In COB cases the insurance specialist must be informed as to which plan is primary. Often, an employer-sponsored group plan is primary; however, if both plans fall under this category, the **birthday rule** applies for dependents. The birthday rule states the policy of the parent whose birthday comes first in a calendar year is primary for any dependent child or children, regardless of which parent is older. If the parents are separated or divorced with a court decree, the plan of the parent with custody of and financial responsibility for the child is primary, unless the divorce decree states otherwise. If the parents have joint custody, the plan of the parent with physical custody of the child at the time treatment begins is considered primary. It is important that the insurance specialist determines primary coverage before the beginning of treatment.

Health Care Team as Providers of Service

If patients are viewed as "customers," the health care team is considered the provider of quality "service" to them. The physician plays the leadership role in providing quality service to patients, and teamwork is essential.

Physician's Role

The physician's role in the health care team is vital. The physician should provide compassionate care and expert medical services that promote the personal health and total well-being of all patients. Patients often educate themselves about medical symptoms and problems now that Internet access is readily available. In addition, the media encourage the public to become better informed when choosing health care providers. As a result, physicians and other health care practitioners may provide prospective patients information about their training and qualifications, as follows:

- Proof of education, training, and experience, termed a **curriculum vitae (CV)**
- Quality of care, which can be measured in many ways. Some experts suggest using the following six points, or quality indicators, to compare health care providers:
  1. Credentials (credentialing, board certification, affiliations with hospitals or professionals, and clinical performance)
  2. Experience
  3. Range of services
  4. Participation in research and education
  5. Patient satisfaction
  6. Outcomes

Patients have a right to obtain information about the specialty, board certification, and hospital affiliations of physicians participating in their health care plans. With this information, patients can make better choices in selecting their health care professional. This also serves to strengthen the physician-patient relationship.

Teamwork

All health care providers must realize that patients are becoming better informed about health care and their choices. If physicians and their health care teams do not treat patients well, the patients will go elsewhere. Physicians and other health care professionals must use proven business tactics: get organized, see patients on time, explain problems and procedures thoroughly, ask and answer questions, and return phone calls promptly. The entire health care team must work together to provide the best care possible to patients.

PATIENT-CENTERED PROFESSIONALISM

- What is the advantage for the medical assistant of being aware of different health care programs?
- What is the advantage of an employer-sponsored group plan over a private or individual plan?

MEDICAL INSURANCE POLICIES AND PLANS

Medical assistants must understand the types of insurance policies, types of coverage, fee structures, and methods of cost containment. There are many different types of insurance policies and plans. The plans may vary but there are two general types, with terms and concepts that apply to all policies.

The two main types of insurance policies are indemnity (fee-for-service) plans and managed care plans. Each type of policy comes in several different forms.

Indemnity (Fee-for-Service) Plans

In the early 1980s the most common type of health insurance plan was the **indemnity (fee-for-service) plan.** Indemnity plans paid the individual or health care provider for covered services up to a set amount. Usually, the patient paid the health care provider and then submitted a claim form to the insurance company. If the provider was a participant in the insurance company's plan, the company paid the health care provider directly.

Indemnity plans are available from private insurance companies and nonprofit companies (e.g., Blue Cross/Blue Shield) and are still widely in use. Fee-for-service plans often have **basic benefits,** which usually pay hospital or medical bills. Types of insurance benefits coverage include basic hospital and medical, major medical, and comprehensive.

Basic hospital insurance covers the cost of hospital bills, and *basic medical insurance* pays for surgeon's fees, anesthesia services, the health professional's visits in the hospital, and office visits and procedures.

Major medical insurance coverage adds more insurance benefits for major illnesses (e.g., cancer) and injuries (e.g., multiple injuries as a result of an accident) beyond the basic benefits available. **Major medical benefits** usually have a **deductible** and/or **co-payments** (or **co-insurance**). The deductible is how much money a patient must pay "out of pocket" before the insurance company starts paying the bills. Usually, the deductible only has to be met once a year, whereas co-payments apply to all visits. After that, the insurance company pays all or a specified percentage of the medical bills, depending on the insurance policy.

Deductibles typically range from $100 to $5,000 per year, and premiums are inversely related to the deductible amount (e.g., the higher the deductible, the lower the premium). The patient then must pay the balance of the bills, which can be a co-payment (fixed fee, such as $15 or $20 per visit) or co-insurance (percentage of the cost, such as 10% or 20%). A common plan is the "80/20 policy"; after the deductible is paid, the insurer pays 80% of the **allowable charges,** and the insured (or patient) pays the remaining 20%.

Comprehensive plans have policies in which major medical and basic benefits apply. A typical indemnity insurance policy has a $100 to $1,000 deductible and an 80/20 co-insurance payment. This means that the patient pays the first $100 to $1,000 of health care expenses out of pocket. After that the insurance company pays 80% of *covered* expenses, and the patient pays the balance, or 20% of the charges. If the health care provider is a **participating provider (PAR),** which means the provider has a contractual agreement with the insurance company to accept the amount paid (after deductibles and co-payment are made), the provider must accept the amount paid by the insurance company as payment in full and cannot bill the patient more than the predetermined amount.

Box 30-1 explains the difference between a PAR and a **nonparticipating provider (non-PAR).** The following example shows the payment calculation for a patient covered by a private, commercial, fee-for-service insurance provider.

BOX 30-1

PAR versus Non-PAR

A practitioner becomes a *participating provider* (PAR) when he or she signs an agreement (contract) with the insurance carrier to comply with certain requirements. These requirements typically include but are not limited to the following:

- The provider will furnish *medically necessary* services.
- Provider services will be consistent with professionally recognized standards of health care.
- The provider will file claims for the patient.
- The provider will accept the carrier-determined *allowed amount* as payment in full and will not bill the patient for any difference between the allowed amount and the charged amount.

In return, the provider receives some amenities such as the following:

- The carrier will make payment directly to the provider.
- Assignment of benefits is automatic.
- Some carriers will furnish free CMS-1500 claim forms to PARs with preidentifying provider information.

A *nonparticipating provider* (non-PAR) has not signed an agreement with the insurance carrier. Although non-PARs must still furnish medically necessary services consistent with professionally recognized standards of health care, the following also apply:

- Non-PARs are not responsible for filing claims for patients (with the exception of Medicare).
- Non-PARs do not have to accept the carrier's payment as payment in full and may bill the patient for any difference between the actual charge and the carrier's allowed amount.

If the patient does not assign benefits, payment is sent to the policyholder and the non-PAR must collect the payment from the patient for services rendered.

> Alice Peterson is a new patient at the clinic today. Her insurance identification card indicates that she is covered under a Blue Cross/Blue Shield preferred provider organization (PPO) policy with a $500 deductible and a 90/10 co-insurance. The encounter form indicates charges for today's services total $210. The clinic is a PAR of this PPO. The medical assistant might ask Ms. Peterson if she has met her deductible, or the patient might volunteer this information. The least amount that should be collected from Ms. Peterson today would be 10% of the total charges, or $21. At this point the assistant might not know what Blue Cross/Blue Shield's allowable charge is for these services, but it will be indicated when the explanation of benefits is received.
>
> This breaks down mathematically as follows:
> a. If Ms. Peterson has not met any of her deductible, she would owe the entire $210 for today's service (because her deductible is $500 and this $210 would go toward meeting her yearly deductible).
> b. If Ms. Peterson has already met only $200 of her deductible, she still owes $300 on her deductible. Since today's charge is $210, it would still be applied to her deductible, and she would pay the entire amount to the provider. She has then met $410 of her deductible, with $90 still remaining to meet on the deductible.
> c. If Ms. Peterson has met her entire deductible, she would only owe 10% of the allowable charge. Assuming this physician charges the allowable amount, the amount Ms. Peterson owes today can be calculated as follows:
> 10% of $210 = 0.10 × $210 = $21

Note that the health care provider's charge often exceeds the amount allowed by the third-party payer, so when the contract reads that 80% of the *covered* charges will be paid, this does not mean that they will pay 80% of the caregiver's fee. The difference between the caregiver's fee and the third-party payer's allowed amount must be "adjusted," or written off the patient's account for a PAR provider. Figure 30-1 is an example of how deductibles and co-insurance affect a patient's payment.

Managed Care Plans

Managed care is a composite health care system in which hospitals and health care professionals organize a **network.** This network coordinates and arranges health care services and benefits for a group of individuals (usually referred to as "enrollees" or "members") for the purpose of managing cost, quality, and access to health care. A managed care organization is usually a corporation established under state and federal laws. This corporation hires employees (physicians, nurses, other health care providers) to provide health care to its enrollees. These employees are under contract with the managed care organization and, to some degree, take their orders from corporate management. The focus of these organizations is to "manage" the cost, quality, and access to health care—managed care. Enrollment in managed health care has become widespread. As of 2000, about 180 million Americans (almost 62% of the U.S. population) belonged to a managed care plan.

Three of the most common types of managed care are PPOs, HMOs, and POS plans.

Preferred Provider Organization

A **preferred provider organization (PPO)** is a health care delivery arrangement that offers insured individuals certain incentives if they choose health care providers from a list of those who are contracted with the PPO. Examples of the incentives offered to enrollees include lower deductibles and co-payments. PPO network providers, in turn, agree to charge their patients lower fees in exchange for this "preferred provider" status, which in turn should bring them a large patient base.

Health Maintenance Organization

A **health maintenance organization (HMO)** is an organization that provides a wide range of comprehensive health care services for plan participants at a fixed periodic payment, usually $10 to $25 (or more) a month. The patient pays this monthly fee and must use the HMO's physicians and facilities. HMO plans offer comprehensive health care coverage for lower premiums and co-payments than many indemnity plans, but participants have restrictions on their choice of health care providers.

HMOs are organized in two different ways: group practice and independent practice.

In a **group practice association,** HMO physicians and other health care services are housed in the HMO's own locations. The providers who practice at the HMO may be independent contractors or employees of the HMO. If the relationship is that of employer-employee, the type of group practice is called a *staff model HMO*. HMO members can receive services from any physician who is a member of the group. This physician is referred to as the patient's **primary care physician (PCP).** This PCP, or **gatekeeper,** is the person who must authorize patient referrals to specialists.

An **independent practice association (IPA)** establishes a contractual relationship with health care providers in private practice and hospitals to provide services to its members. Health care providers who participate in HMOs are typically paid a flat monthly amount for each patient enrolled in the HMO who has selected that provider as PCP. The physician receives the same amount each month for each patient whether the patient receives health care services during that month or does not. This method of payment is called **capitation;** this fee is based solely on the number of participants, not on services rendered to them.

Point-of-Service Plan

A **point-of-service (POS) plan** is an "open-ended" HMO option with more flexibility. This type of plan permits members to choose providers "out of network," but it is designed to encourage the use of in-network providers. Some POS plans are associated with increased cost, such as lower reimbursements and higher co-payments, when out-of-network is used.

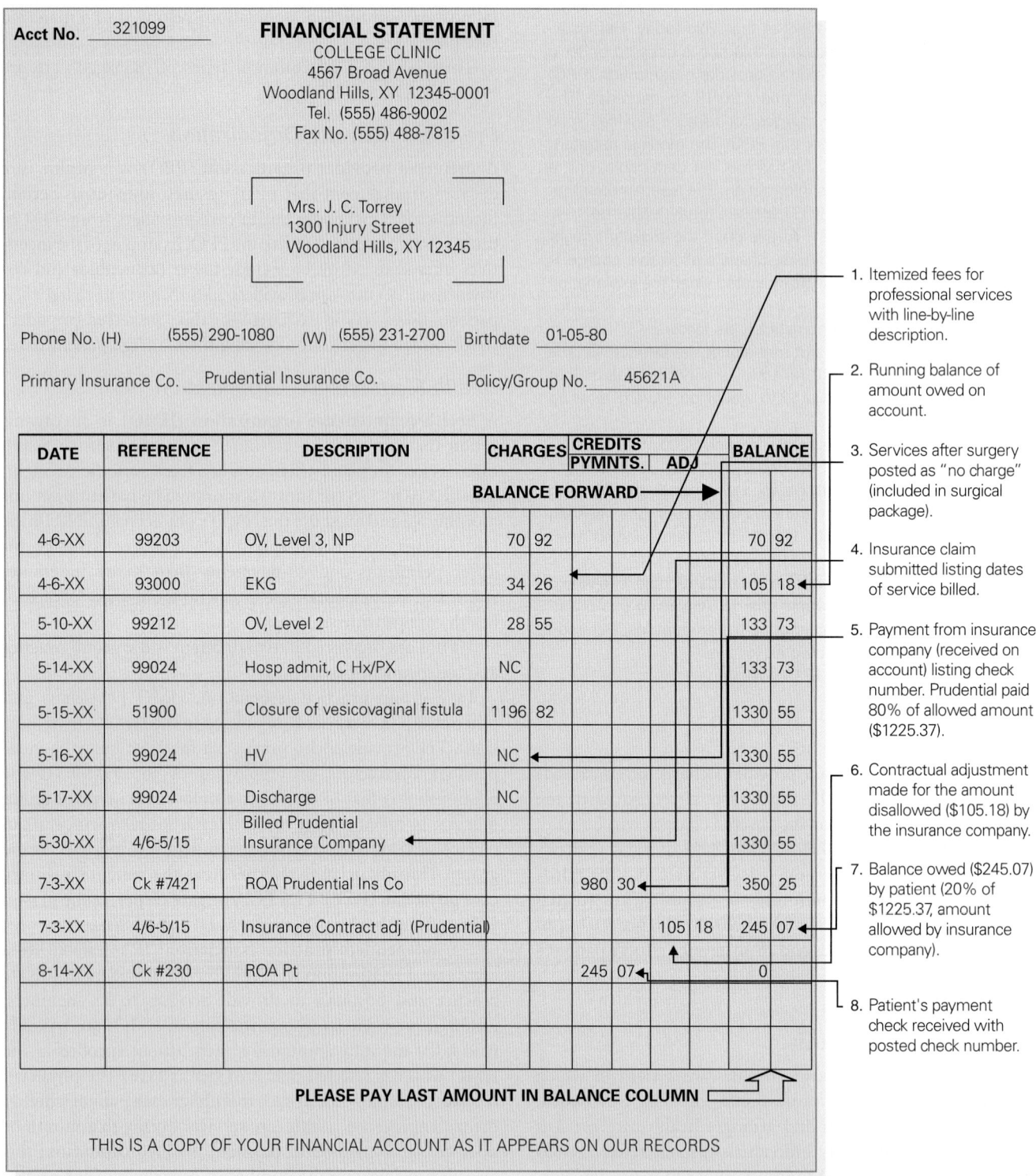

FIGURE 30-1 Ledger card illustrating posting of professional service descriptions, fees, payments, adjustments, and balance due. The participating provider's charges may be higher than the third-party payer's allowable amount, or covered charges. Note items 4, 5, 6, and 7 on this patient's ledger card. 51900 has a 90-day global–1 day preop included. Unless the admission day is the day the decision for surgery is made, that day is included in the fee for surgery. In this scenario, it would be fairly obvious the decision for surgery is not done on day of admission (Office visit 5/10/XX). (Modified from Fordney MT: *Insurance handbook for the medical office*, ed 10, St Louis, 2008, Saunders.)

Fee Structures

There are several methods by which physician's fees are determined with regard to medical insurance. Five methods of structuring fees are as follows:

1. Usual, customary, and reasonable
2. Episode of care
3. Capitation
4. Relative value scale
5. Resource-based relative value scale

Usual, Customary, and Reasonable

The phrase **usual, customary, and reasonable (UCR)** refers to the typically charged or prevailing fees for health services within a geographical area. A fee is generally considered to be *reasonable* if it falls within the parameters of the average, or commonly charged, fee for an identical or similar service within that specific geographical region.

Insurance companies establish UCR fees as follows:

- A "usual" fee is the fee that an individual health care provider most frequently charges for a specific procedure.
- A "customary" fee is the fee level determined by the administrator of a health care benefit plan from actual fees submitted for a specific procedure by other providers. This fee level establishes the maximum benefit payable for that procedure.
- A "reasonable" fee is the fee charged by a physician for a specific procedure that has been modified by complications or unusual circumstances. Therefore it may differ from the physician's usual fee or the benefit administrator's customary fee.

The concept of using UCR fees to determine how much to reimburse patients covered by insurance for specific treatment has been used by the insurance industry since the early 1960s. See Box 30-2 for more information about how UCR fees are determined.

Episode of Care

Episode of care is a term used to describe and measure the various health care services and encounters rendered in connection with a specific injury or period of illness. It is a tool for measuring the impact of health care services on cost and quality. An episode of care is defined as "a block of one or more medical services received by an individual during a period of relatively continuous contact with one or more providers of service in relation to a particular medical problem or situation." Episodes of care provide a comprehensive framework from which both the cost and the effectiveness of medical care can be examined. Many insurance companies are using episodes of care to profile provider costs, comparing one provider's costs to treat an episode to those of other providers in the same specialty treating episodes of the same condition.

The fee for an episode of care is a flat amount charged for a particular service or procedure. For example, a set amount is established for a complete hysterectomy, including preoperative and postoperative treatment, as well as the procedure itself. If complications occur, additional fees may be incurred.

Capitation

Introduced earlier, capitation is another managed care approach to keep health care costs down. Capitation creates a financial incentive to deliver health care using the most effective means: preventive health care. Healthy patients require less treatment for the same amount of money per month.

Capitated managed care systems offer an important opportunity to provide high-quality, cost-effective care. Capitated health care delivery systems, however, have strong incentives to avoid patient populations in need of care. This is especially true in the case of patients who are disabled, aged, or dying. This introduces an element of financial risk, which is familiar to insurance organizations, but of concern to hospitals and physicians, to whom these risks are transferred under capitation.

Relative Value Scale

The **relative value scale (RVS)** was pioneered by the California Medical Association in 1956 to help physicians establish rational, relative fees. Other states soon followed California's example. Hundreds of the most frequently performed procedures were compiled, given procedure numbers similar to those in the American Medical Association's *Current*

BOX 30-2

How Are UCR Fees Determined?

Usual, customary, and reasonable (UCR) fees are influenced by the fees that physicians charge in various geographical areas and by the size of the population. Heavily populated areas, where the cost of living is higher, usually have higher health care fees.

The Health Insurance Association of America (HIAA), an organization of 380 health insurance companies, surveys providers' fees periodically. This fee survey helps insurance companies set UCR fees. Insurance companies are not legally required to use HIAA's fee survey or any other information when setting UCR benefit levels. In fact, reimbursement calculations by private or commercial insurance companies are unregulated and uncontrolled.

Current UCR rates may be outdated despite HIAA's attempts to update fee data to keep up with changing information. It may take up to 2 years for providers to return HIAA's fee surveys, for HIAA to complete the data, and for member insurance companies and subscribers to receive it. Geographical differences may not be taken into account equitably when insurance companies set UCR rates. Although boundaries are usually set according to zip code, insurance companies are free to create boundaries as they choose. They may split a state in half or lump several small communities together to determine one boundary. If a large city and a small town are considered to be within the same boundary, large discrepancies in fees could exist.

Procedural Terminology (CPT) and assigned a unit value. The assigned unit value represented the value of that procedure in relation to other common procedures. Although no monetary value was placed on the units, many insurance companies used the RVS to determine benefits by applying a conversion factor that assigned a monetary value to the unit value.

In 1978 the Federal Trade Commission (FTC) interpreted the California RVS as a fee-setting instrument and prohibited its publication and distribution. This was an attempt by the FTC to make medical practice more competitive by ruling against the setting of fees and by encouraging physicians to advertise.

Resource-Based Relative Value Scale

The **resource-based relative value scale (RBRVS)**, a method of setting Medicare fees, is one of the outcomes of the Medicare Physician Payment Reform enacted in the Omnibus Budget Reconciliation Act of 1989 (OBRA '89). Since the beginning of Medicare, Part B of the program has paid physicians using a fee-for-service system based on customary, usual, and reasonable charges. The RBRVS, which was changed in 1992, consists of the following three components:

1. **Relative value units (RVUs).** Every service or procedure has three parts: physician work done, practice overhead (regional cost), and cost of malpractice insurance (regional cost). Each part is assigned an RVU.
2. *Geographic Practice Cost Indices* (GPCI). The GPCI is provided by the local Medicare carrier. Because practice overhead expense and malpractice insurance costs can vary significantly by region, "geographic adjusted factors" (GAFs) are applied to make the fees equitable nationwide.
3. *Conversion factor* (CF). The CF is a universal dollar amount applied to the RVUs (with the GPCI factored in) to establish the Medicare allowable charge. The CF changes every year and is published in the *Federal Register*.

The formula to calculate a Medicare fee follows:

$$RVU \times GAF \times CF = \text{Medicare allowable charge per service}$$

Professional liability and overhead components are computed by the Centers for Medicare and Medicaid Services (CMS).

The RBRVS fee schedule is designed to provide national uniform payments after being adjusted to reflect the differences in practice costs across geographical areas.

Cost Containment

Much effort has been made recently to contain the rising costs of health care. State and local governments as well as private third-party payers are developing methods to reduce benefit payments and costs associated with health care. **Cost containment** includes the following concepts:
- Preauthorization for inpatient hospitalization and certain other services
- Controlling the use of services
- Cost sharing
- Using nonphysician providers
- Verifying the "medical necessity" of services

Although the need to contain health care costs is urgent, there are pros and cons to cost containment. Cost containment activities affect health care systems in the following ways:

1. Cost containment can affect the quality of care received by patients.
2. Financial risk shifting changes the fundamental ethical basis of the health care system.
3. Cost containment can restrict access to types of services and service to minorities, underserved populations, and others who already have limited access to health care.

PATIENT-CENTERED PROFESSIONALISM

- Why must the medical assistant understand the different types of insurance policies?
- What is the advantage for the medical assistant who understands fee structure?
- What can the medical assistant do to help with cost containment in health care?
- What role do nonphysician providers play in health care today?

THIRD-PARTY MEDICAL INSURANCE

Types of third-party insurance programs include private commercial coverage, government programs, coverage for disabilities, and policies for additional, secondary coverage to primary policies.

Private Carriers

A private carrier is a provider of health insurance that a person can obtain through a group plan or as an individual. These policies are purchased through private (nongovernment) organizations whose sole business (commercial enterprise) is insurance.

Blue Cross and Blue Shield

Blue Cross/Blue Shield, commonly referred to now as "the Blues," is probably the best-known medical insurance program in the United States. Approximately one in four Americans is covered by these plans:

- Blue *Cross* covers hospital services. It originated in 1929 with the previously mentioned schoolteachers' agreement with Baylor University Hospital.
- Blue *Shield* covers physicians' services. It began in 1939, with members restricted to earning less than $3,000 per year and premiums costing $1.70 a month.

Previously a national program, Blue Cross/Blue Shield currently consists of many independent member companies, each serving specific geographical areas.

Other Commercial Carriers

Private commercial carriers offer different types of policies, including group and individual policies. Medical assistants need to understand these types of policies, as well as the effect of third-party liability.

Group Policies. A **group policy** is an insurance policy purchased by a company for its employees or purchased by a group representing similar professions such as farmers or professional engineers. Typically, these groups receive lower premiums than individual insurance policies because of a large pool of employees or members. There are often no "preexisting condition" limitations with this type of policy.

Group policies differ from one organization to another because policy benefits are often tailored according to the requirements of each particular group. With some employer-sponsored group plans, the employer pays a portion of the employee's monthly premium as a fringe benefit and the portion of the premium that is the employee's responsibility is deducted from the employee's paycheck.

Individual Policies. An **individual policy** is an insurance contract purchased by individuals who are not eligible for a group policy or who do not qualify for government-sponsored plans (e.g., Medicare, Medicaid). Premiums for individual policies typically are very costly, and the applicant must complete a comprehensive application form before acceptance. "Riders" (exclusion for specific illnesses or injuries treated previously) and noncoverage for preexisting conditions are common with individual policies.

In the past, a husband and wife or a parent and dependent who were both eligible for employer-sponsored group health insurance coverage could conceivably recoup benefits that exceeded the actual cost of medical treatment. Now, almost all insurance carriers include a COB clause in their policy. This clause coordinates benefits in such a way that total payment from both carriers can be no more than 100% of the cost for professional procedures or services. The insurance carrier that is considered "primary" is sent a claim first and pays according to the stipulations of the contract. After the primary carrier has paid, the **explanation of benefits (EOB)** from the primary carrier is forwarded to the secondary carrier for consideration of possible payment under their policy for the remaining charges.

Third-Party Liability

In certain situations, the patient's health insurance plan is not the primary coverage, as in an automobile accident. Block 10 on the CMS-1500 addresses third-party liability, and it is important that questions *a, b,* and *c* in this block are answered correctly (Figure 30-2). This helps the health insurance carrier establish whether another insurer is liable for payment. For example, if the patient had a work-related injury or illness, workers' compensation would be primary. If the patient tripped on a crumbling sidewalk in front of a store, the store's liability policy would probably be primary.

Government Payers

Several federal and state programs exist to pay for the medical costs of eligible people. These include Medicare, Medicaid, TRICARE and CHAMPVA, and workers' compensation.

Medicare

The **Medicare** program was developed in 1966, initially as a national health insurance program for elderly people. At present, people who qualify for Medicare benefits include those age 65 and older, those who are permanently disabled, and children and adults receiving dialysis for permanent or chronic kidney failure (or who have had a kidney transplant). Medicare is administered nationally by the Centers for Medicare and Medicaid Services (CMS), formerly the Health Care Financing Administration (HCFA). CMS is responsible for the operation of the Medicare program and for the selection of the regional insurance companies, called **fiscal intermediaries** (or *agents*), who process Medicare claims.

If the health care professional providing services to the Medicare beneficiary is a PAR, the Medicare payment is sent directly to the provider. However, a PAR must accept Medicare's reimbursement as payment in full (after the deductible and co-insurance have been met) and cannot bill the beneficiary for any balances (billing patients for the remaining balance after insurance has paid is called **balance billing**). Additionally, claims submitted by PARs are automatically *crossed over* (sent or transmitted) to supplemental insurers. Non-PARs can bill 115% of Medicare's *allowed* charge (called the "limiting charge"), and the payment is sent

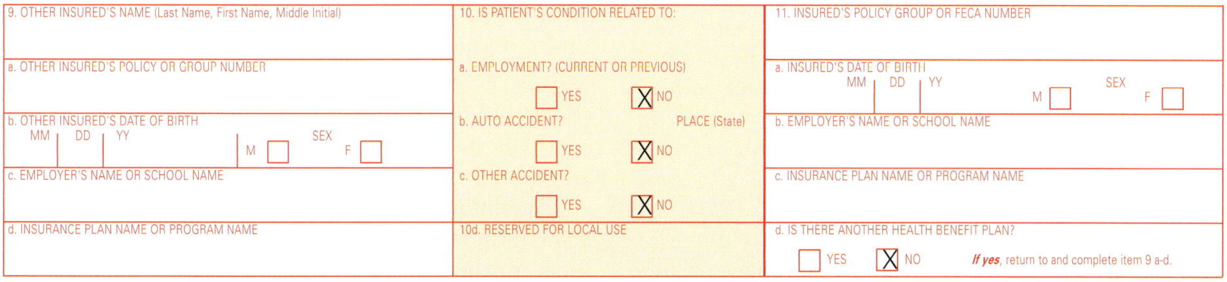

9. OTHER INSURED'S NAME (Last Name, First Name, Middle Initial)	10. IS PATIENT'S CONDITION RELATED TO:	11. INSURED'S POLICY GROUP OR FECA NUMBER
a. OTHER INSURED'S POLICY OR GROUP NUMBER	a. EMPLOYMENT? (CURRENT OR PREVIOUS) ☐ YES ☒ NO	a. INSURED'S DATE OF BIRTH MM DD YY SEX M ☐ F ☐
b. OTHER INSURED'S DATE OF BIRTH MM DD YY SEX M ☐ F ☐	b. AUTO ACCIDENT? PLACE (State) ☐ YES ☒ NO	b. EMPLOYER'S NAME OR SCHOOL NAME
c. EMPLOYER'S NAME OR SCHOOL NAME	c. OTHER ACCIDENT? ☐ YES ☒ NO	c. INSURANCE PLAN NAME OR PROGRAM NAME
d. INSURANCE PLAN NAME OR PROGRAM NAME	10d. RESERVED FOR LOCAL USE	d. IS THERE ANOTHER HEALTH BENEFIT PLAN? ☐ YES ☒ NO *If yes,* return to and complete item 9 a-d.

FIGURE 30-2 Block 10 of the CMS-1500 claim form is used to indicate whether third-party liability comes into play (e.g., workers' compensation, automobile insurance, or liability insurance). (From Fordney MT: *Insurance handbook for the medical office,* ed 10, St Louis, 2008, Saunders.)

to the beneficiary because patients seeing non-PARs normally pay for office visits at the time of service. Patients seeing non-PARs must file their own claim to any supplemental insurance carrier. Both PARs and non-PARs must submit all Medicare claims.

Medicare pays benefits only for procedures and services that are medically necessary. If there is a question about whether a particular service or procedure is covered, the medical assistant should consult the Medicare provider's manual, the CMS website, or the Local Medicare Review Policies (LMRPs). *Medicare Part B News* can be downloaded from the CMS website for up-to-date information on Medicare guidelines. Medicare also furnishes an annual fee schedule, which must be used when posting charges and filing claims for Medicare-eligible patients.

Medicare has three parts: Part A, Part B, and Part C. Parts A and B are the most widely known, and Part C was established in 1997 and became effective in 1999 to provide additional choices for beneficiaries. **Medicare Part D** is a federal program to subsidize the costs of prescription drugs for Medicare beneficiaries in the United States. It was enacted as part of the Medicare Prescription Drug, Improvement, and Modernization Act of 2003 and became effective in 2006.

Medicare Part A. Part A covers inpatient care in hospitals, critical care facilities, and skilled nursing facilities. It also covers hospice care and some home health care, if the patient (referred to as the **beneficiary**) meets certain conditions. When an individual qualifies for Social Security benefits at age 65, he or she is automatically enrolled in Part A, which is free if the individual worked and Medicare taxes were withheld from wages.

Medicare Part B. Part B helps pay for physicians' services (not routine physical examinations), outpatient hospital care, durable medical equipment (e.g., wheelchairs), clinical laboratory tests, and some other medical services. All persons eligible for Part A may enroll in Part B. However, a monthly premium is deducted from the individual's Social Security check to pay for Part B coverage. Each beneficiary must pay a deductible each year before Medicare begins paying benefits. After the deductible is met, Medicare will pay 80% of the allowable charge, and the beneficiary must pay 20%. The following example shows the payment calculation for a patient with Medicare Part B.

> Victor Edwards is a Medicare patient. The Medicare fee schedule lists $147.55 for the service performed today (the clinic is also PAR for Medicare). Mr. Edwards informs the medical assistant that he has met the Medicare deductible for the year. Therefore he would be responsible for 20% of today's bill.
> This can be calculated as follows:
> 20% of $147.55 = 0.20 × $147.55 = $29.51

Medicare Part C. Part C, called *Medicare Advantage,* allows individuals eligible for Parts A and B (except for those with end-stage renal disease) to choose to receive their Medicare benefits through a variety of plans, including the Medicare managed care plan and the Medicare private fee-for-service plans. Medicare Advantage plans provide care under contract to Medicare. They may provide benefits such as coordination of care or reduced out-of-pocket expenses. Some plans may offer additional benefits such as vision care, dental services, and prescription drugs. Medicare Advantage plans are now available in many parts of the United States.

Medicare Part D. Medicare Part D is available to anyone eligible for Medicare (Part A and/or Part B). Part D provides prescription drug coverage insurance through private companies approved by Medicare. Part D was designed to help people with Medicare lower their prescription drug costs, protect against future cost, and have greater access to medically necessary drugs.

Medicaid

In 1965, Congress passed Title 19 of the Social Security Act, setting up a combined federal-state program called **Medicaid.** Technically, Medicaid is not an insurance program. Rather, it is an assistance program that provides medical care for people with income below the national poverty level. Medicaid is funded by both federal and state governments and like Medicare is administered by a *fiscal intermediary,* which is a contracting organization that processes claims.

The federal government establishes certain guidelines at a national level for Medicaid eligibility, and individual states may authorize additional services or make additional groups eligible at the state level, based on their available funds. Therefore Medicaid programs vary from state to state.

The health care provider can choose to accept Medicaid patients or not, but providers cannot pick and choose which Medicaid patients they will treat. As with Medicare, physicians who accept Medicaid patients must agree to accept Medicaid reimbursement for *covered services* as payment in full (they cannot balance-bill). Eligibility requirements for Medicaid are set by each state within the federally mandated guidelines. Eligible groups are classified as categorically needy and medically needy (Box 30-3).

Under the Medicare program, once an individual qualifies at age 65, he or she has lifelong coverage. With Medicaid, however, eligibility must be reestablished on a month-to-month basis, except for patients who reside in long-term care (nursing home) facilities. After an individual applies for and is accepted into the Medicaid program, an identification (ID) card (or form) is issued showing the effective dates (Figure 30-3). Some states have replaced paper ID cards with plastic cards with magnetic strips, similar to a credit card. When a patient comes to the provider's office, the medical assistant swipes the card and receives immediate eligibility information. This automated *eligibility verification system* (EVS) has greatly improved the process of treating Medicaid patients.

In addition to verifying Medicaid eligibility, there is usually some form of preauthorization for certain types of care and for all inpatient services. Medical assistants should stay current with the rules and regulations and know what services require prior approval by the Medicaid program in their state. If a Medicaid recipient requests a noncovered service, the medical

BOX 30-3

Classification of Groups Eligible for Medicaid Benefits

CATEGORICALLY NEEDY

1. Families, pregnant women, and children
   a. Aid to Families with Dependent Children (AFDC)–related groups
   b. Non-AFDC pregnant women and children
2. Aged and disabled persons
   a. Supplemental Security Income (SSI)–related groups
   b. Qualified Medicare Beneficiaries (QMBs)
3. Persons receiving institutional or other long-term care in nursing facilities (NFs) and intermediate care facilities (ICFs)
   a. Medicaid beneficiaries
   b. Medi-Medi beneficiaries

MEDICALLY NEEDY

1. Medically indigent non-income and low-income individuals
2. Low-income persons losing employer health insurance coverage (Medicaid purchase of COBRA coverage)

---

assistant must ask that individual to sign a **waiver** stating that the patient understands that the service or procedure will not be paid by Medicaid and that the patient accepts financial responsibility. (For more information on Medicaid programs and state-to-state eligibility, visit the CMS website.)

TRICARE and CHAMPVA

TRICARE and CHAMPVA are the health care programs of the U.S. military.

TRICARE. TRICARE is the military's comprehensive health care program for active-duty personnel, eligible family members, retirees and family members under age 65, and survivors of deceased members of all U.S. uniformed services. Individuals who qualify for TRICARE are called beneficiaries, and the active-duty member is called a **sponsor.** The TRICARE program is managed by the military in partnership with civilian hospitals and clinics. It is designed to give eligible individuals access to high-quality health care at affordable prices. All military hospitals and clinics are part of the TRICARE program.

There are three options under the TRICARE program, as follows:

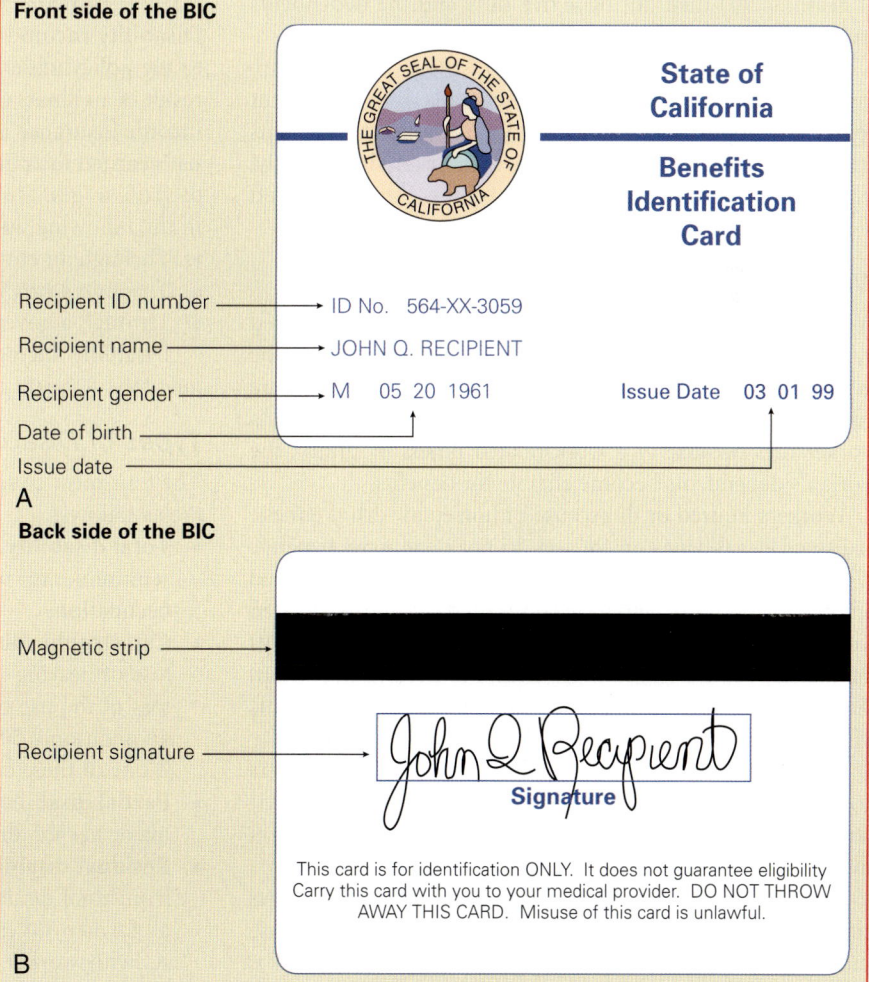

FIGURE 30-3 Example of **(A)** front and **(B)** back of identification card issued by Medicaid. Medicaid programs differ from state to state, thus cards (or forms) for identification may vary widely. (From Fordney MT: *Insurance handbook for the medical office,* ed 10, St Louis, 2008, Saunders.)

1. TRICARE Prime, similar to an HMO
2. TRICARE Standard, formerly known as the Civilian Health and Medical Program of the Uniformed Services (CHAMPUS), a traditional fee-for-service plan
3. TRICARE Extra, a PPO

To qualify for benefits under TRICARE, individuals must be eligible and must be listed in the Defense Enrollment Eligibility Reporting System (DEERS) computerized database of the Department of Defense. Those eligible for TRICARE include the following:

- Eligible family members of active-duty service members
- Military retirees and their eligible family members
- Surviving eligible family members of deceased active or retired service members
- Wards and preadoptive children
- Some former spouses of active or retired service members who meet certain length-of-marriage rules and other requirements

CHAMPVA. The Civilian Health and Medical Program of the Department of Veterans Affairs (**CHAMPVA**) is a health benefits program that provides coverage to the spouse or widow(er) and the children of a **veteran** who (1) is rated permanently and totally disabled because of a service-connected disability, (2) was rated permanently and totally disabled because of a service-connected condition at the time of death, *or* (3) died during active duty and the dependents are not otherwise eligible for TRICARE benefits.

Although the TRICARE and CHAMPVA programs are similar, CHAMPVA is completely separate, with a different beneficiary population than TRICARE. Although the benefits are comparable, the programs are administered separately, with significant differences in claim-filing procedures and preauthorization requirements.

Workers' Compensation

Workers' compensation is an insurance program authorized by federal and state law that requires employers to pay the medical expenses and loss of wages for workers who are injured on the job or who have job-related illnesses. Also, if a worker dies because of a work-related illness or injury, the worker's dependents become eligible for benefits.

Workers injured or ill because of horseplay, drunkenness, or use of illegal drugs on the job do not qualify for benefits. Workers with self-inflicted injuries or injuries that occurred off the job and those who have committed a crime or violated company policy also do not qualify. If a worker is injured off the job site while engaged in an errand or performing within the parameters of the worker's job responsibilities, benefits will probably be granted.

The **Federal Employee Compensation Act (FECA)** covers nonmilitary employees of the federal government. Its provisions are similar to those of other workers' compensation laws.

In *state workers' compensation* programs, individual states mandate the amount of coverage the employer must purchase and the benefits. The amount of the insurance premium is usually determined by the degree of risk associated with the job classification. For example, premiums for an accounting firm or bank would probably be substantially lower than for a construction company whose employees build skyscrapers. Some states do not make employers obtain workers' compensation insurance if they have fewer than three to five (depending on the state) full-time employees, or if they employ temporary workers, domestic help, child care personnel, or volunteers for charitable organizations. Each state sets up a state compensation board or commission to administer the laws and handle appeals.

Health care providers are required to accept the benefits paid by workers' compensation as payment in full. If the workers' compensation patient being treated by the provider is also a private patient of that medical facility, a separate medical record should be set up for the workers' compensation records, which typically do not adhere to the same confidentiality and privacy rules as those for private medical patients. Some states accept workers' compensation claims submitted on the CMS-1500; others have their own forms that must be used for submitting claims. The medical assistant should contact the workers' compensation carrier or the state workers' compensation office for guidelines in filing claims.

Disability Income Insurance

Disability income insurance is insurance that pays benefits to the policyholder if he or she becomes unable to work as a result of an illness or injury that is not work related. Disability income insurance is not designed to replace *all* of an individual's earned income, only a portion of it, usually 45% to 60% of gross wages. Disability income insurance can be provided in the following ways:

- Through an employer
- Through a private policy purchased by the individual
- Through a government-sponsored program (e.g., SSDI)

Disability income insurance coverage is basically either *long term* (2 years or more) or *short term* (less than 2 years).

Types of Disability

The four most common types of disability in insurance terms are as follows:

- **Total disability.** The individual is unable to perform the requirements of his or her occupation or of any occupation.
- **Catastrophic disability.** The individual has loss of speech, loss of hearing in both ears, loss of sight in both eyes, or loss of the use of two limbs. Some insurance policies pay an additional 50% of the monthly total disability amount if one of these catastrophic losses occurs.
- **Partial disability.** The individual can still perform part of his or her job duties.
- **Residual disability.** The individual has begun to recover from total disability but is not yet capable of performing all former duties or earning former wages.

As with workers' compensation, disability income insurance contracts typically exclude benefits in cases of self-inflicted injuries and injuries or illness caused by criminal conduct, acts of war, or military service.

Federal Disability Income Plans

There are two government disability income plans in the United States: SSDI and SSI.

Social Security Disability Income Insurance. **Social Security Disability Income Insurance (SSDI)** is a program for individuals who become disabled from injury or illness not associated with their employment. SSDI is administered by the Social Security Administration (SSA) and funded by FICA tax withheld from employee wages and matching employer contributions. An individual applying for SSDI benefits must have worked long enough to accumulate enough "credits" to qualify.

Supplemental Security Income. **Supplemental Security Income (SSI)** is similar to SSDI in that both programs are run by SSA, both offer disability benefits, and both use the same legal definition of "disability." However, the programs differ significantly in their financial qualifications and benefits.

Differences between SSDI and SSI.

1. *Benefit amounts.* SSDI benefits are calculated on the disabled worker's past earnings, whereas SSI benefits are fixed.
2. *Health care benefits.* Recipients of SSDI qualify for Medicare benefits 24 months after receipt of their first check. SSI recipients qualify for Medicaid benefits immediately.
3. *Effect of income and resources of others.* SSDI recipient benefits are not affected by unearned (nonwage) income, or income or support received from other sources, whereas benefits of SSI recipients may change (or stop) if the person receives such other income or support.

Secondary Policies

A secondary policy covers costs not paid by a primary policy (one that pays first). Secondary plans include Medi-Medi, Medigap, and Medicare Secondary Payer (MSP).

Medi-Medi

The Medicare-Medicaid Crossover Program, called **Medi-Medi** or *Care-Caid*, focuses on Medicare and Medicaid working together to serve low-income seniors. The Balanced Budget Act of 1997 provides states with block grants to help Medicare recipients pay Part B Medicare premiums. Beneficiaries with incomes between 120% and 135% of poverty level are entitled to full payment of Part B premiums, and those with incomes between 135% and 175% are eligible for a portion of the benefits. "Cost sharing" between these two programs allows enrollees to receive the care they need but otherwise might not be able to afford. Medicaid also pays for certain services not covered by Medicare such as prescription drugs, nursing home care, and other home care and community-based long-term care services.

Medigap

As mentioned earlier, most Medicare beneficiaries do not have to pay for their Medicare Part A coverage, but they do pay for Part B, which is deducted from their monthly Social Security checks. Also, Medicare does not pay for all medical expenses. As a result, many Medicare-eligible individuals purchase **Medigap** insurance, a secondary insurance policy. Medigap is a short name for *medical supplemental insurance*. Medigap is designed to fill some of the "gaps" in coverage left by Medicare. Private insurance companies, *not* the U.S. government, sell Medigap insurance.

To protect senior citizens, the federal government closely regulates Medigap insurance. There are 10 standardized Medigap plans, labeled "A" through "J." Plan A offers a very basic supplement to Medicare coverage; plan J offers much more comprehensive coverage but is also expensive. Every plan provides the same coverage through each insurance company; the only difference is the cost of that company's premium for that specific plan. This makes it easier for the elderly person to choose the right plan. He or she simply decides how much coverage is needed (plans A through J), then "shops around" to find the lowest premium.

A 65-year-old person enrolling in Medicare Part B for the first time has 6 months from the date Part B coverage takes effect to purchase a Medicare supplemental policy. During this time, the individual cannot be refused coverage because of age or any medical condition. Under law, everyone who wants to buy Medigap coverage must be enrolled, regardless of health. With Medigap insurance policies, applicants cannot be refused coverage because of "preexisting conditions." To qualify, the individual simply applies for a policy during the open enrollment period. Medigap plans can only be sold to individuals who are covered by the original Medicare fee-for-service plan.

Medicare Secondary Payer (MSP)

With **Medicare (as) secondary payer (MSP),** Medicare is not the primary payer because the Medicare beneficiary has another health insurance plan (typically an employer-sponsored plan) that must pay first. For example, if a Medicare beneficiary has a younger spouse who is still employed and carries insurance, the spouse's plan will be primary and Medicare becomes the secondary payer for the Medicare beneficiary.

CMS emphasizes that providers must investigate all options in each case to determine whether MSP applies. Medicare can be secondary to any of the following:
- Group health insurance
- Automobile or liability insurance
- Workers' compensation insurance
- Black lung benefits
- Veterans Affairs insurance
- Supplemental insurance
- HMO coverage
- United Mine Workers benefits

The medical assistant must investigate whether a Medicare beneficiary's second insurance is primary to Medicare, or vice versa (Table 30-1). Many medical offices have a questionnaire for the Medicare patient to complete to help determine this answer.

TABLE 30-1
Medical Insurance Coverage for Events/Patients with MSP

Event/Patient	Other Insurance Coverage	Primary Insurance	Secondary Insurance
Motor vehicle accident	Automobile liability; no-fault insurance	Liability policy	MSP
Accident on another person's property	Home owner's; business liability	Liability policy	MSP
Illness or injury in elderly employee or spouse (age 65 or older)	EGHP	EGHP	MSP
Illness related to black lung disease in current or former coal miner	Federal Black Lung Act (FECA); workers' compensation	FECA	Medicare does not apply
Illness or injury related to U.S. military service	Department of Veterans Affairs	Department of Veterans Affairs	MSP
Injury or illness in dependent of active-duty member of U.S. military	TRICARE	TRICARE	MSP
Illness or injury occurring on the job	Workers' compensation	Workers' compensation	Medicare does not apply
ESRD in current or former employee	Employer group coverage	Employer group coverage	MSP
Disability (except ESRD) in employee or dependent under age 65	Employer group coverage	Employer group coverage	MSP
Laid-off employee with continuation coverage (COBRA)	COBRA coverage	COBRA	MSP
Spouse of deceased employee with continuation coverage (COBRA)	COBRA coverage	COBRA	MSP

Modified from Fordney MT, French LL: *Medical insurance billing and coding: an essentials worktext*, Philadelphia, 2003, Saunders.
COBRA, Consolidated Omnibus Reconciliation Act; *EGHP*, Employee Group Health Plan; *ESRD*, end-stage renal disease; *FECA*, Federal Employee Compensation Act; *MSP*, Medicare (as) Secondary Payer.

Rules and Regulations

The medical assistant must be aware of many rules and regulations when working with patients who have various types of medical insurance. Most insurance carriers have their own guidelines for completing claims and submitting them for payment. It is important to follow these specific guidelines to receive maximum reimbursement. Also, deadlines for claims submission vary among third-party payers. Procedure 30-1 explains how to apply managed care policies and procedures.

It is helpful for medical assistants involved with submitting insurance claims to create a chart or a table listing the most common insurance carriers for the practice and noting the filing deadline for each. Claims with the shortest time limit might be completed first. Keep in mind, however, that all insurance claims must be submitted in a timely manner.

Preauthorization

Preauthorization (authorization in advance) is a procedure required by most managed health care and indemnity plans. Patients or medical assistants must often obtain preauthorization before a provider performs a specific procedure or treatment for a patient, typically inpatient hospitalization, multiple sessions of physical therapy, and certain diagnostic tests. Preauthorization pertains to medical necessity and appropriateness and does not necessarily guarantee payment. It is not a treatment recommendation or a guarantee that the patient will be insured or eligible for benefits when services are performed. Preauthorization works as follows:

1. The medical assistant contacts the health care plan, either by phone or in writing, and requests permission to perform the treatment or service proposed. The insurance company may ask the provider to stipulate the CPT and ICD-9-CM codes used for the patient's treatment.
2. The plan's representative then either authorizes the service or procedure or does not authorize it. Often, when a procedure or service is authorized, a specific identifying number or code is given, which must be noted on the claim form when billing for services.

Preauthorization is also used to identify members for case management or disease management programs. Approval or denial of requests for services is determined by review of all available related medical information and possibly a discussion with the requesting physician. Figure 30-4 shows an example of a treatment authorization request form.

Precertification

Precertification is the method used for determining in advance how much the patient's insurance policy will reimburse or pay for a particular service or procedure (e.g., hospitalization, surgery, diagnostic tests). The medical assistant will contact the benefits department of the patient's insurance company, giving the patient's insurance information (e.g., group number, subscriber ID number) and particulars of the procedure to be performed (e.g., date of admission, how many expected days in the hospital). The insurance company will ask for the CPT and ICD-9-CM codes for the services, as well

**Managed Care Plan
Treatment Authorization Request**

**TO BE COMPLETED BY PRIMARY CARE PHYSICIAN
OR OUTSIDE PROVIDER**

Health Net ☐   Met Life ☐
Pacificare ☐   Travelers ☒
Secure Horizons ☐   Pru Care ☐

Member No. 1357906

Patient Name: Louann Campbell   Date: 7-14-20XX

M ____ F _X_ Birthdate 4-7-1952   Home telephone number 555-450-1666

Address 2516 Encina Avenue, Woodland Hills, XY 12345-0439

Primary Care Physician Gerald Practon, MD   Provider ID# TC 14021

Referring Physician Gerald Practon, MD   Provider ID# TC 14021

Referred to Raymond Skeleton, MD   Address 4567 Broad Avenue

Woodland Hills, XY 12345-0001   Office telephone no. 555-486-9002

Diagnosis Code 724.2   Diagnosis Low back pain

Diagnosis Code 722.10   Diagnosis Sciatica due to herniated nucleus pulposus

Treatment Plan: Orthopedic evaluation of lumbar spine R/O herniated disc L4, 5

Authorization requested for procedures/tests/visits:

Procedure Code 99244   Description New patient consultation

Procedure Code _____   Description _____

Facility to be used: _____   Estimated length of stay _____

Office ☒   Outpatient ☐   Inpatient ☐   Other ☐

List of potential consultants (i.e., anesthetists, assistants, or medical/surgical):

Raymond Skeleton, MD - Orthopedic

Physician's signature _____

TO BE COMPLETED BY PRIMARY CARE PHYSICIAN

PCP Recommendations: See above   PCP Initials _____

Date eligibility checked 7-14-20XX   Effective date 1-15-20XX

TO BE COMPLETED BY UTILIZATION MANAGEMENT

Authorized _____   Not authorized _____

Deferred _____   Modified _____

Authorization Request# _____

Comments: _____

FIGURE 30-4 Example of managed care plan treatment authorization request form. The form has been completed by a primary care physician for preauthorization of a professional service by another provider. (Modified from Fordney MT, French LL: *Medical insurance billing and coding,* Philadelphia, 2003, Saunders.)

as the fee to be charged. They will then make a determination of benefits available under the patient's policy; for example, for a hysterectomy the company may pay 75% of the charges, with the patient responsible for the remaining 25%. Many physicians then ask the patient to pay in advance or to arrange a payment plan for the portion of the charge not covered by the patient's insurance benefits. See Procedure 30-1 for an example of how to obtain precertification from a health care provider.

Every surgeon's office checks carefully for both preauthorization and precertification.

PATIENT-CENTERED PROFESSIONALISM

- Why must the medical assistant be familiar with the basic guidelines of third-party payers?

PROCEDURE 30-1 Apply Managed Care Policies and Procedures

TASK: Obtain precertification from a patient's HMO for requested services or procedures. Obtain a referral from a patient's HMO for requested consultation or treatment.

EQUIPMENT AND SUPPLIES
- Photocopy of the patient's insurance identification card
- Patient's information form
- Patient's encounter form
- Patient's medical record
- Precertification form

SKILLS/RATIONALE

1. **Procedural Step. Gather the set of documents needed to provide the information necessary to obtain a managed care precertification.**
   These documents include the patient's medical record, insurance information, and a precertification form.

2. **Procedural Step. Review the gathered records.**
   Rationale. This step determines the service, test, or admission for which precertification is being sought from the patient's insurance provider, as well as locates any insurance-related information needed to complete the precertification form.

3. **Procedural Step. Complete the precertification/referral form.**
   a. Blanks 1 through 7 of the form indicate who is making the request for precertification/referral and for whom the request is being made.
   b. Blanks 8 through 14, the "Specialist Referral" section, can be used when a physician wants to refer a patient to another physician or specialist for consultation or treatment. It can also be used to request precertification for a specific procedure, test, or admission.
   c. Blanks 15 through 21 identify the specific procedure, test, or admission for which precertification is being requested.
   d. Blanks 22 through 25 of the form provide the fax number and items that will be completed by the insurance carrier.

4. **Procedural Step. Proofread the entire form to ensure it is accurate. Double-check identification numbers,** the spelling of names, and codes to be sure they are correct.
   Rationale. Good proofreading can save time and help keep precertification from being delayed or mistakenly denied.

5. **Procedural Step. Send (usually fax) the form to the insurance carrier for review and action.**
   In some cases, it is also possible to phone the insurance carrier to obtain precertification for a referral.
   After the form is completed and submitted, it is reviewed by the carrier. If precertification is granted, an authorization number is entered in the "Auth Number" item. If applicable, the "# of Visits" and the "Expiration Date" items will be filled in by the insurance carrier. In addition, the person from the insurance company responsible for approving the precertification enters his or her signature and phone number in the "Authorized SHHMO Signature" and "Phone #" items.

6. **Procedural Step. Wait for a response from the managed care organization.**
   If approved, the managed care organization will either return the completed form or provide you with an authorization number over the phone that you can write on the form yourself.

7. **Procedural Step. Process and place a copy of the completed form in the patient's medical record.**
   In the case of a referral, make a copy of the completed form for the patient's file. The patient will pick up the original completed form to take to the specialist.

Continued

PROCEDURE 30-1 Apply Managed Care Policies and Procedures—cont'd

③

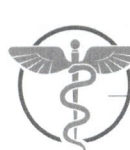

STANDARD HEALTHCARE HMO

PRE-CERTIFICATION REQUEST

Fill out form completely
Current clinical information, indicating medical necessity, must be faxed with authorization request form. Lack of this information will result in a delay in the authorization process.

Date: ____①____ Contact Person: ____②____

Office Phone Number: ____③____ Office Fax Number: ____④____

PATIENT DEMOGRAPHICS

Patient Name: ____⑤____ ID #: ____⑥____ PCP #: ____⑦____

SPECIALIST REFERRAL Referral Status: (Check One) In-Network ____ Out-of-Network ____ ⑧

Specialist Physician: ____⑨____ Referring Physician: ____⑩____

Diagnosis: ____⑪____ Reason for Referral: ____⑫____

Auth Number: ____⑬____ Expiration Date: ____⑭____

REQUEST FOR PROCEDURES, TESTING, AND ADMISSIONS
(In-Network and Out-of-Network)

Facility: ____⑮____ Physician: ____⑯____

Diagnosis: ____⑰____ Diagnosis Code(s): ____⑱____

Procedure Code(s): ____⑲____

Scheduled Date: ____⑳____ Mark One: __Inpatient __Outpatient __Ambulatory Surgery ㉑

Prior authorization is not required for referrals to chiropractors, podiatrists, and dermatologists, but they must be contracted providers for Standard Healthcare HMO plans. Diagnostic testing must be performed at a contracted facility.

Please forward completed form to: Standard Healthcare HMO Fax: 555-912-4415 ㉒

Auth Number: ____㉓____ # of Visits: ____㉔____ Expiration Date: ____㉕____

SHHMO APPROVAL COMPLETED BY: ____㉖____ Phone #: ____㉗____
(Authorized SHHMO Signature)

Use of this form does not guarantee eligibility of coverage and does not supersede any member benefit plan limitations or the provider's contractual limitations.

Confidentiality Note:
The information contained in this facsimile message may be legally privileged and confidential information intended only for the use of the individual or entity named above. If the reader of this message is not the intended recipient, you are hereby notified that any dissemination, distribution, or copying of this fax is strictly prohibited. If you have received this fax in error, please immediately notify the sender above and return the original message to us at the address below by the U.S. Postal Service. Thank you for your cooperation.

Customer Service:
Standard Healthcare HMO
1500 Summitt Avenue
Western, NY 99992
(555) 800-6000

MEDICAL INSURANCE CLAIM CYCLE

The medical insurance claim process, beginning with the patient's initial visit to the medical office and continuing through claims generation and payment, is referred to as a "cycle" (Box 30-4). The cycle goes through many steps before payment is received from the insurance carrier. Then, when the patient returns for the next visit, the process begins again.

Confidentiality

At every step in the cycle of an insurance claim, medical assistants must maintain patient confidentiality. In order for the provider's office to complete and submit a claim to the insurance carrier for reimbursement, confidential information must be given to this third party. Therefore, when a patient first comes to the medical facility, the patient typically signs a form that includes a statement giving the health care provider permission to disclose certain health information to the patient's insurance carrier. This form is referred to as a **release of information (ROI)** form. Some medical offices include a section for release of information on the patient information (registration) form; others use a separate form. An ROI form is usually valid for only 1 year, and the medical assistant must make sure that each patient has a current ROI in his or her medical record. In the case of Medicare, a patient can sign a "lifetime release of information," if it is worded correctly according to Medicare's guidelines (Figure 30-6).

As mentioned, Medicare and Medicaid claims must now be submitted electronically. Although electronic claims do have advantages over paper claims, many are asking if confidential medical information in electronic files can be safeguarded.

HIPAA has mandated specific guidelines for transmittal of electronic patient information, which all health care providers must adhere to and enforce.

PATIENT-CENTERED PROFESSIONALISM

- Why is it valuable for the medical assistant to understand the cycle of an insurance claim and understand the rules of confidentiality?

SUBMITTING CLAIMS

The goal of claims submission is to complete a claim correctly and as soon as possible after a service or procedure is performed. Claims must be submitted within the time limits dictated by the carrier ("timely filing"), and all submitted claims need to be "clean." A **clean claim** has no errors or omissions and is the best defense against delays or rejections. This assures the health care provider that everything possible has been done to receive maximum reimbursement (supported by the medical documentation) in a minimal time frame.

BOX 30-4

Insurance Claim Cycle

PHASE 1: PATIENT APPOINTMENT
The patient contacts the medical facility and schedules an appointment. This can be done by phone, in person, or by another provider's office.

PHASE 2: PATIENT REGISTRATION
The patient arrives at the office. Usually, there is some type of "signing in" process. The patient then completes a series of informational forms, presents his or her insurance identification card, and (if the patient is new to the practice) a medical record is created, or the medical record is obtained and updated as necessary.

PHASE 3: PATIENT EXAMINATION
The patient is escorted to the clinical area, where some type of examination and discussion takes place. This is sometimes called the "encounter phase." The patient meets the health care provider and members of the medical team who will list patient diagnoses and services on the encounter form (Figure 30-5). The health care provider may also note the charges and the approximate time of a follow-up appointment, if needed.

PHASE 4: PATIENT CHECKOUT
The patient is directed or escorted back to the reception area, where payment is made (depending on the policy of the medical practice) and a follow-up appointment is scheduled, if necessary.

PHASE 5: INSURANCE CLAIM PROCESSING
After the patient encounter is complete, the insurance claim process begins.
- Claims are generated either through data entry into patient-accounting software or by using a paper claim form. Caution must be taken so that the claim form is "clean"; that is, there are no errors or omissions and all coding is correct.
- Claims are submitted to the third-party payer either electronically or manually. For major third-party payers, such as Medicare and Medicaid, claims are forwarded to a fiscal intermediary, who has contracted to handle claims for these government payers. CMS has mandated that claims must be submitted electronically as of October 2003 (with some exceptions as specified by CMS).
- The third-party payer processes the claim and sends back an explanation of benefits (EOB) with payment.
- The medical assistant posts the payment to the patient's account and bills the patient for the balance, submits the balance to a second payer, or writes off the balance (e.g., PAR fee agreements for accepting assignment).

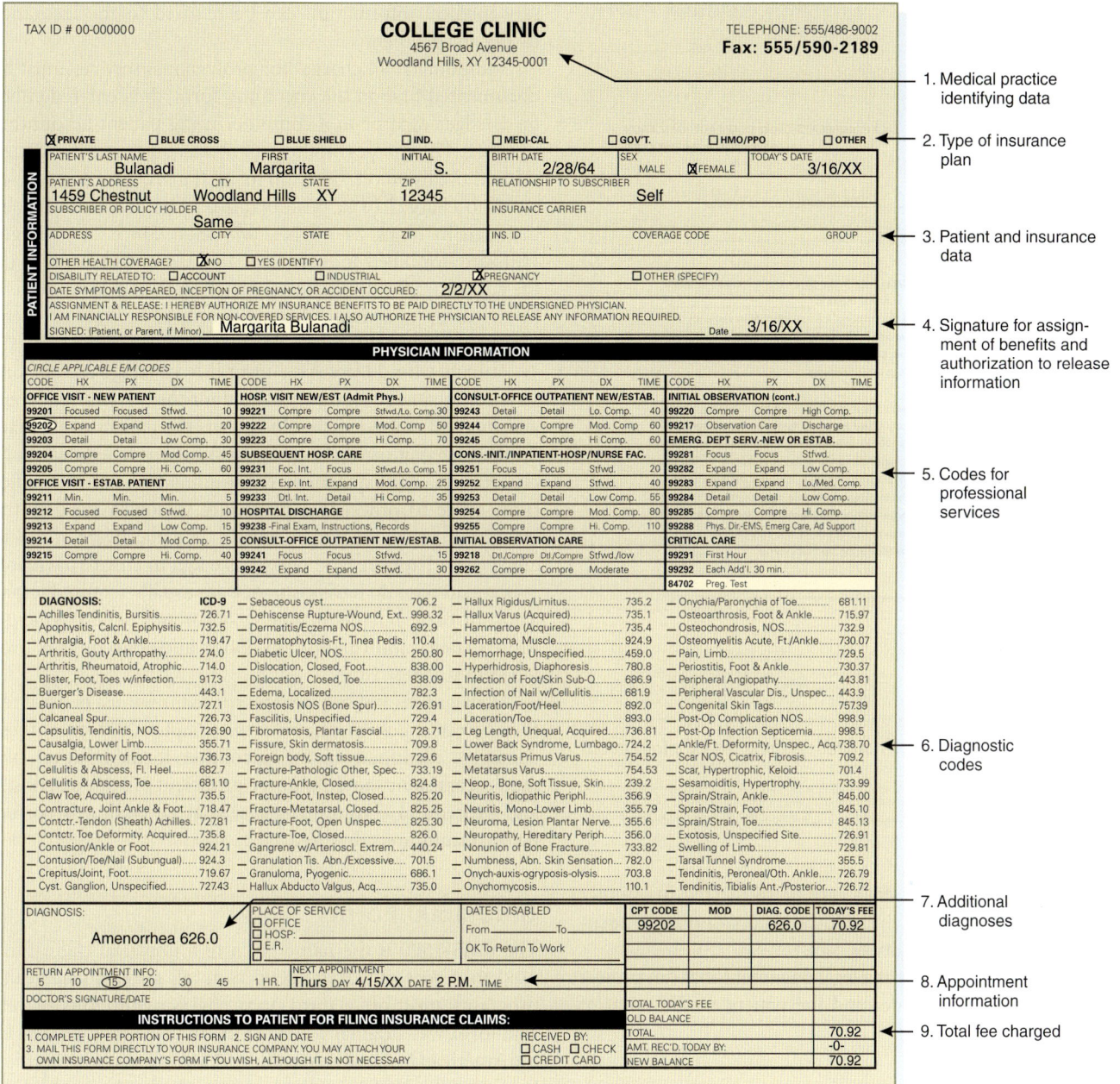

FIGURE 30-5 Encounter form; procedural codes for professional services are from *Current Procedural Terminology* (CPT) and diagnostic codes from *International Classification of Diseases,* ninth revision, *Clinical Modification* (ICD-9-CM). (In Fordney MT: *Insurance handbook for the medical office,* ed 8, Philadelphia, 2004, Saunders. Form courtesy Bibbero Systems, Inc., Petaluma, CA; (800) 242-2376; Fax (800) 242-9330; www.bibbero.com.)

The medical assistant therefore must understand the guidelines and requirements of each insurance carrier to attain this goal. Before submitting any claim the medical assistant should check the documentation for the claim and the guidelines of the patient's insurance carrier to be sure these agree.

Proper Documentation

All services, procedures, and diagnoses must be fully documented in the patient's medical record before being included on an insurance claim.

Documentation is the process of recording information, such as a patient's complaint, condition, treatment, and response to treatment, in the medical record, as discussed in Chapter 27. Documenting this information fully and accurately is one of the most important aspects of patient care. In addition to providing necessary information for third-party reimbursement by justifying the medical necessity of services and procedures, accurate documentation helps ensure the patient is receiving the best possible medical care, as follows:

1. Documentation provides information about the patient's complaint, condition, treatment, response to treatment,

Lifetime Release Form

Blackburn
Primary Care Associates, PC
1990 Turquoise Drive
Blackburn, XY 11111
(555) 608-8857

LIFETIME BENEFICIARY CLAIM AUTHORIZATION AND INFORMATION RELEASE

Patient Name: ____________________

Medicare ID Number: ____________________

I, __________(patient initials), request that payment of authorized Medicare benefits be made either to me or on my behalf to ______________ (physician/supplier). I authorize any holder of medical information about me to release to the Health Care Financing Administration/Centers for Medicare and Medicaid Services and its agents any information needed to determine these benefits or the benefits payable to related services.

I understand my signature requests that payment be made and authorizes release of medical information necessary to pay the claim. If other health insurance is indicated in Block 9 of the CMS-1500 claim form or elsewhere on other approved claim forms or electronically submitted claims, my signature authorizes the release of the information to the insurer or agency shown. In Medicare assigned cases, the physician or supplier agrees to accept the charge determination of the Medicare carrier as the full charge, and I am responsible only for the deductible, coinsurance, and noncovered services. Coinsurance and the deductible are based upon the charge determination of the Medicare carrier.

Patient's Signature: ____________________

Date: ____________

FIGURE 30-6 Example of lifetime "release of information" document for Medicare.

and progress. If a patient's care is transferred to another health care provider, the medical record serves as documentation for continuity of care.

2. Documentation serves as a legal document that can protect and defend the provider and the patient in the event of legal action.

Insurance Carrier Guidelines

Insurance **guidelines** represent organized instructions developed by specific third-party insurance carriers to assist health care providers in filling out the CMS-1500 (or other insurance claim forms). When these guidelines are followed, claims will be processed quickly and with maximum payment allowed by the insurance contract. It is important to remember that each major carrier has its own guidelines, and guidelines for the same carrier (e.g., Medicaid, workers' compensation, Blue Cross/Blue Shield) may differ from state to state.

Billing and Coding Requirements

Before preparing a claim, the medical assistant needs to make sure there is a valid ROI form on file for the patient whose claim is being prepared. A signature from the patient, or his or her parent or legal guardian, is required so that the necessary medical information can be released to the insurance carrier for payment.

Additionally, all charges for professional services must be documented first on the encounter form, then entered either on a ledger card or in a computer using patient-accounting software. The charges on the patient's account must be identical to those listed on the claim form. If a procedure or service was "no charge" (e.g., postoperative visit), it should not be included in Block 24 of the CMS-1500. Since "no charge" visits are not billed to insurance, they are coded "99024" on the encounter form for clinical history tracking. If the patient has made any payment, this also needs to be shown on the patient's account.

Patients who do not have insurance coverage are responsible for the entire amount charged for the services rendered, and medical assistants should inform the patient of this fact on the first visit or when the appointment is scheduled. Policies for collecting payment from uninsured patients differ from office to office. If a procedure is not covered by the insurance policy, the patient should be made aware of this in advance and appropriate measures taken to ensure payment.

Patients who do have insurance are usually required to pay a portion of the bill (deductible, co-insurance, or co-payment). More detailed information on billing and collections is provided in Chapter 28.

All diagnoses and services and procedures must be assigned the correct codes, as discussed in Chapter 29. Often, these codes are identified on the **encounter form;** however, the medical assistant should become proficient in both diagnostic and procedural coding to ensure that all coding is correct before claims are submitted.

CMS-1500 Form

The **CMS-1500** is the name given to a universal claim form used to report outpatient services to all government health programs; most other third-party payers require this as well. The form was originally created by HCFA and approved by the American Medical Association (AMA) Council on Medical Services. The HCFA-1500 was originally developed for submitting Medicare claims and was later adopted by many other private commercial insurance carriers to standardize the claims process. Since HCFA is now called CMS, the name of the form has been changed to "CMS-1500," but it is basically the same as the HCFA form.

The CMS-1500 has two sections: a top portion for patient or insured information (Blocks 1 through 13) and a bottom portion for physician or supplier information (Blocks 14 through 33). The form is printed in red ink to optimize the electronic scanning process that "reads" the entries. Figure 30-7 shows an example of the front of the CMS-1500 form; Figure 30-8 shows the back of the form.

Completing the CMS-1500 Form

Before you begin filling in the blocks of the CMS-1500, enter the name and address of the fiscal intermediary or the insurance carrier to whom the claim is being sent. This information

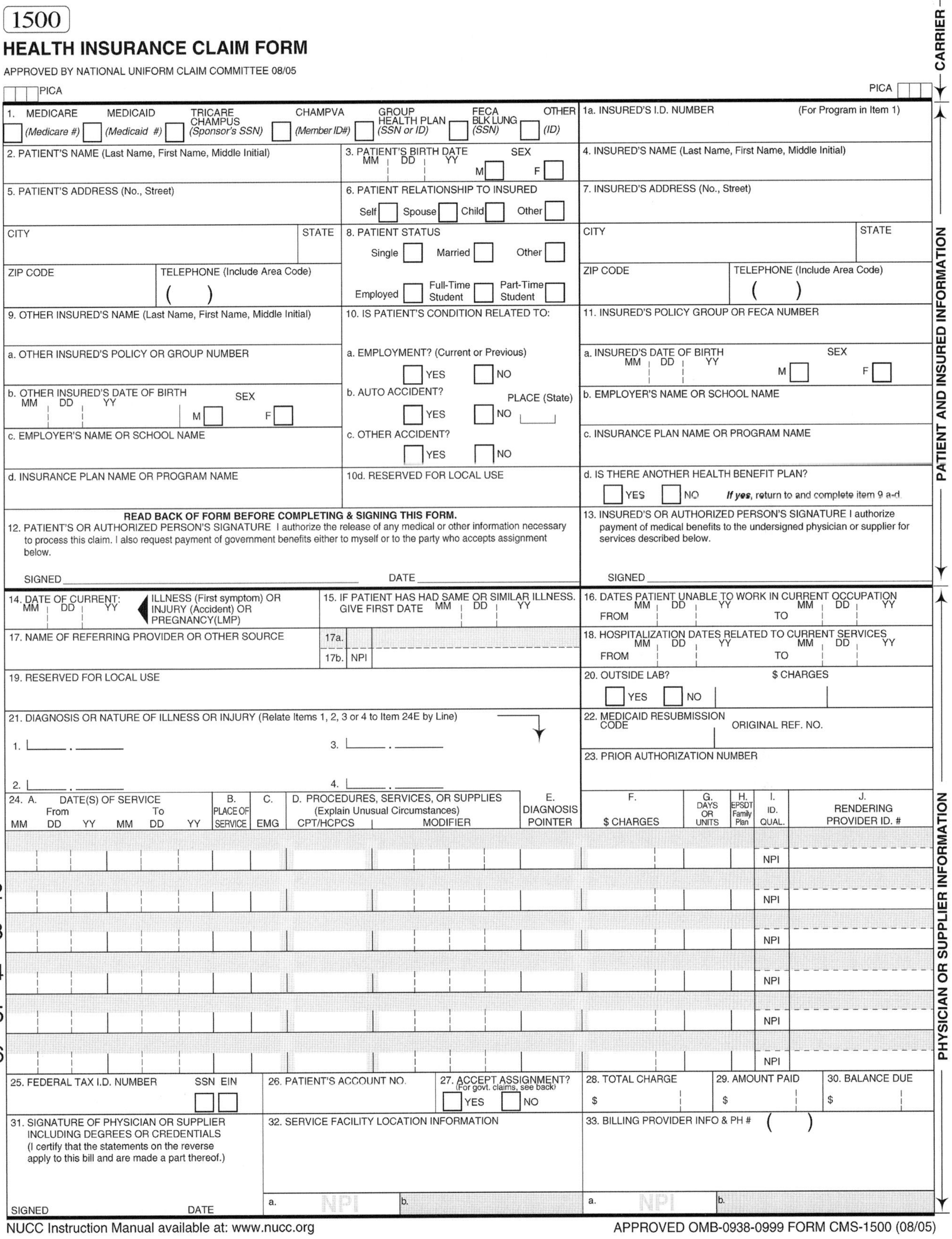

1500

HEALTH INSURANCE CLAIM FORM

APPROVED BY NATIONAL UNIFORM CLAIM COMMITTEE 08/05

PICA | PICA

CARRIER

1. MEDICARE (Medicare #) | MEDICAID (Medicaid #) | TRICARE CHAMPUS (Sponsor's SSN) | CHAMPVA (Member ID#) | GROUP HEALTH PLAN (SSN or ID) | FECA BLK LUNG (SSN) | OTHER (ID)

1a. INSURED'S I.D. NUMBER (For Program in Item 1)

2. PATIENT'S NAME (Last Name, First Name, Middle Initial)

3. PATIENT'S BIRTH DATE MM DD YY SEX M F

4. INSURED'S NAME (Last Name, First Name, Middle Initial)

5. PATIENT'S ADDRESS (No., Street)

6. PATIENT RELATIONSHIP TO INSURED Self Spouse Child Other

7. INSURED'S ADDRESS (No., Street)

CITY STATE

8. PATIENT STATUS Single Married Other

CITY STATE

ZIP CODE TELEPHONE (Include Area Code) ( )

Employed Full-Time Student Part-Time Student

ZIP CODE TELEPHONE (Include Area Code) ( )

9. OTHER INSURED'S NAME (Last Name, First Name, Middle Initial)

10. IS PATIENT'S CONDITION RELATED TO:

11. INSURED'S POLICY GROUP OR FECA NUMBER

a. OTHER INSURED'S POLICY OR GROUP NUMBER

a. EMPLOYMENT? (Current or Previous) YES NO

a. INSURED'S DATE OF BIRTH MM DD YY SEX M F

b. OTHER INSURED'S DATE OF BIRTH MM DD YY SEX M F

b. AUTO ACCIDENT? YES NO PLACE (State)

b. EMPLOYER'S NAME OR SCHOOL NAME

c. EMPLOYER'S NAME OR SCHOOL NAME

c. OTHER ACCIDENT? YES NO

c. INSURANCE PLAN NAME OR PROGRAM NAME

d. INSURANCE PLAN NAME OR PROGRAM NAME

10d. RESERVED FOR LOCAL USE

d. IS THERE ANOTHER HEALTH BENEFIT PLAN? YES NO *If yes*, return to and complete item 9 a-d.

READ BACK OF FORM BEFORE COMPLETING & SIGNING THIS FORM.

12. PATIENT'S OR AUTHORIZED PERSON'S SIGNATURE I authorize the release of any medical or other information necessary to process this claim. I also request payment of government benefits either to myself or to the party who accepts assignment below.

SIGNED DATE

13. INSURED'S OR AUTHORIZED PERSON'S SIGNATURE I authorize payment of medical benefits to the undersigned physician or supplier for services described below.

SIGNED

PATIENT AND INSURED INFORMATION

14. DATE OF CURRENT: MM DD YY ILLNESS (First symptom) OR INJURY (Accident) OR PREGNANCY(LMP)

15. IF PATIENT HAS HAD SAME OR SIMILAR ILLNESS. GIVE FIRST DATE MM DD YY

16. DATES PATIENT UNABLE TO WORK IN CURRENT OCCUPATION FROM MM DD YY TO MM DD YY

17. NAME OF REFERRING PROVIDER OR OTHER SOURCE

17a.

17b. NPI

18. HOSPITALIZATION DATES RELATED TO CURRENT SERVICES FROM MM DD YY TO MM DD YY

19. RESERVED FOR LOCAL USE

20. OUTSIDE LAB? YES NO $ CHARGES

21. DIAGNOSIS OR NATURE OF ILLNESS OR INJURY (Relate Items 1, 2, 3 or 4 to Item 24E by Line)

1. ___ . ___ 3. ___ . ___

2. ___ . ___ 4. ___ . ___

22. MEDICAID RESUBMISSION CODE ORIGINAL REF. NO.

23. PRIOR AUTHORIZATION NUMBER

24. A. DATE(S) OF SERVICE From MM DD YY To MM DD YY	B. PLACE OF SERVICE	C. EMG	D. PROCEDURES, SERVICES, OR SUPPLIES (Explain Unusual Circumstances) CPT/HCPCS MODIFIER	E. DIAGNOSIS POINTER	F. $ CHARGES	G. DAYS OR UNITS	H. EPSDT Family Plan	I. ID. QUAL.	J. RENDERING PROVIDER ID. #
1								NPI	
2								NPI	
3								NPI	
4								NPI	
5								NPI	
6								NPI	

25. FEDERAL TAX I.D. NUMBER SSN EIN

26. PATIENT'S ACCOUNT NO.

27. ACCEPT ASSIGNMENT? (For govt. claims, see back) YES NO

28. TOTAL CHARGE $

29. AMOUNT PAID $

30. BALANCE DUE $

31. SIGNATURE OF PHYSICIAN OR SUPPLIER INCLUDING DEGREES OR CREDENTIALS (I certify that the statements on the reverse apply to this bill and are made a part thereof.)

SIGNED DATE

32. SERVICE FACILITY LOCATION INFORMATION

a. NPI b.

33. BILLING PROVIDER INFO & PH # ( )

a. NPI b.

PHYSICIAN OR SUPPLIER INFORMATION

NUCC Instruction Manual available at: www.nucc.org

APPROVED OMB-0938-0999 FORM CMS-1500 (08/05)

FIGURE 30-7 Front side of CMS-1500 universal claim form.

BECAUSE THIS FORM IS USED BY VARIOUS GOVERNMENT AND PRIVATE HEALTH PROGRAMS, SEE SEPARATE INSTRUCTIONS ISSUED BY APPLICABLE PROGRAMS.

NOTICE: Any person who knowingly files a statement of claim containing any misrepresentation or any false, incomplete or misleading information may be guilty of a criminal act punishable under law and may be subject to civil penalties.

REFERS TO GOVERNMENT PROGRAMS ONLY

MEDICARE AND CHAMPUS PAYMENTS: A patient's signature requests that payment be made and authorizes release of any information necessary to process the claim and certifies that the information provided in Blocks 1 through 12 is true, accurate and complete. In the case of a Medicare claim, the patient's signature authorizes any entity to release to Medicare medical and nonmedical information, including employment status, and whether the person has employer group health insurance, liability, no-fault, worker's compensation or other insurance which is responsible to pay for the services for which the Medicare claim is made. See 42 CFR 411.24(a). If item 9 is completed, the patient's signature authorizes release of the information to the health plan or agency shown. In Medicare assigned or CHAMPUS participation cases, the physician agrees to accept the charge determination of the Medicare carrier or CHAMPUS fiscal intermediary as the full charge, and the patient is responsible only for the deductible, coinsurance and noncovered services. Coinsurance and the deductible are based upon the charge determination of the Medicare carrier or CHAMPUS fiscal intermediary if this is less than the charge submitted. CHAMPUS is not a health insurance program but makes payment for health benefits provided through certain affiliations with the Uniformed Services. Information on the patient's sponsor should be provided in those items captioned in "Insured"; i.e., items 1a, 4, 6, 7, 9 and 11.

BLACK LUNG AND FECA CLAIMS

The provider agrees to accept the amount paid by the Government as payment in full. See Black Lung and FECA instructions regarding required procedure and diagnosis coding systems.

SIGNATURE OF PHYSICIAN OR SUPPLIER (MEDICARE, CHAMPUS, FECA AND BLACK LUNG)

I certify that the services shown on this form were medically indicated and necessary for the health of the patient and were personally furnished by me or were furnished incident to my professional service by my employee under my immediate personal supervision, except as otherwise expressly permitted by Medicare or CHAMPUS regulations.

For services to be considered as "incident" to a physician's professional service, 1) they must be rendered under the physician's immediate personal supervision by his/her employee, 2) they must be an integral, although incidental part of a covered physician's service, 3) they must be of kinds commonly furnished in physician's offices, and 4) the services of nonphysicians must be included on the physician's bils.

For CHAMPUS claims, I further certify that I (or any employee) who rendered services am not an active duty member of the Uniformed Services or a civilian employee of the United States Government or a contract employee of the United States Government, either civilian or military (refer to 5 USC 5536). For Black-Lung claims, I further certify that the services performed were for a Black Lung-related disorder.

No Part B Medicare benefits may be paid unless this form is received as required by existing law and regulations (42 CFR 424.32).

NOTICE: Any one who misrepresents or falsifies essential information to receive payment from Federal funds requested by this form may upon conviction be subject to fine and imprisonment under applicable Federal laws.

NOTICE TO PATIENT ABOUT THE COLLECTION AND USE OF MEDICARE, CHAMPUS, FECA, AND BLACK LUNG INFORMATION
(PRIVACY ACT STATEMENT)

We are authorized by CMS, CHAMPUS and OWCP to ask you for information needed in the administration of the Medicare, CHAMPUS, FECA, and Black Lung programs. Authority to collect information is in section 205(a), 1862, 1872 and 1874 of the Social Security Act as amended, 42 CFR 411.24(a) and 424.5(a) (6), and 44 USC 3101:41 CFR 101 et seq and 10 USC 1079 and 1086; 5 USC 8101 et seq; and 30 USC 901 et seq; 38 USC 613; E.O. 9397.

The information we obtain to complete claims under these programs is used to identify you and to determine your eligibility. It is also used to decide if the services and supplies you received are covered by these programs and to insure that proper payment is made.

The information may also be given to other providers of services, carriers, intermediaries, medical review boards, health plans, and other organizations or Federal agencies, for the effective administration of Federal provisions that require other third parties payers to pay primary to Federal program, and as otherwise necessary to administer these programs. For example, it may be necessary to disclose information about the benefits you have used to a hospital or doctor. Additional disclosures are made through routine uses for information contained in systems of records.

FOR MEDICARE CLAIMS: See the notice modifying system No. 09-70-0501, titled, 'Carrier Medicare Claims Record,' published in the <u>Federal Register</u>, Vol. 55 No. 177, page 37549, Wed. Sept. 12, 1990, or as updated and republished.

FOR OWCP CLAIMS: Department of Labor, Privacy Act of 1974, "Republication of Notice of Systems of Records," <u>Federal Register</u>, Vol. 55 No. 40, Wed Feb. 28, 1990, See ESA-5, ESA-6, ESA-12, ESA-13, ESA-30, or as updated and republished.

FOR CHAMPUS CLAIMS: <u>PRINCIPLE PURPOSE(S):</u> To evaluate eligibility for medical care provided by civilian sources and to issue payment upon establishment of eligibility and determination that the services/supplies received are authorized by law.

<u>ROUTINE USE(S):</u> Information from claims and related documents may be given to the Dept. of Veterans Affairs, the Dept. of Health and Human Services and/or the Dept. of Transportation consistent with their statutory administrative responsibilities under CHAMPUS/CHAMPVA; to the Dept. of Justice for representation of the Secretary of Defense in civil actions; to the Internal Revenue Service, private collection agencies, and consumer reporting agencies in connection with recoupment claims; and to Congressional Offices in response to inquiries made at the request of the person to whom a record pertains. Appropriate disclosures may be made to other federal, state, local, foreign government agencies, private business entities, and individual providers of care, on matters relating to entitlement, claims adjudication, fraud, program abuse, utilization review, quality assurance, peer review, program integrity, third-party liability, coordination of benefits, and civil and criminal litigation related to the operation of CHAMPUS.

<u>DISCLOSURES:</u> Voluntary; however, failure to provide informaion will result in delay in payment or may result in denial of claim. With the one exception discussed below, there are no penalties under these programs for refusing to supply information. However, failure to furnish information regarding the medical services rendered or the amount charged would prevent payment of claims under these programs. Failure to furnish any other information, such as name or claim number, would delay payment of the claim. Failure to provide medical information under FECA could be deemed an obstruction.

It is mandatory that you tell us if you know that another party is responsible for paying for your treatment. Section 1128B of the Social Security Act and 31 USC 3801-3812 provide penalties for withholding this information.

You should be aware that P.L. 100-503, the "Computer Matching and Privacy Protection Act of 1988", permits the government to verify information by way of computer matches.

MEDICAID PAYMENTS (PROVIDER CERTIFICATION)

I hereby agree to keep such records as are necessary to disclose fully the extent of services provided to individuals under the State's Title XIX plan and to furnish information regarding any payments claimed for providing such services as the State Agency or Dept. of Health and Human Services may request.

I further agree to accept, as payment in full, the amount paid by the Medicaid program for those claims submitted for payment under that program, with the exception of authorized deductible, coinsurance, co-payment or similar cost-sharing charge.

SIGNATURE OF PHYSICIAN (OR SUPPLIER): I certify that the services listed above were medically indicated and necessary to the health of this patient and were personally furnished by me or my employee under my personal direction.

NOTICE: This is to certify that the foregoing information is true, accurate and complete. I understand that payment and satisfaction of this claim will be from Federal and State funds, and that any false claims, statements, or documents, or concealment of a material fact, may be prosecuted under applicable Federal or State laws.

According to the Paperwork Reduction Act of 1995, no persons are required to respond to a collection of information unless it displays a valid OMB control number. The valid OMB control number for this information collection is 0938-0999. The time required to complete this information collection is estimated to average 10 minutes per response, including the time to review instructions, search existing data resources, gather the data needed, and complete and review the information collection. If you have any comments concerning the accuracy of the time estimate(s) or suggestions for improving this form, please write to: CMS, Attn: PRA Reports Clearance Officer, 7500 Security Boulevard, Baltimore, Maryland 21244-1850. This address is for comments and/or suggestions only. DO NOT MAIL COMPLETED CLAIM FORMS TO THIS ADDRESS.

FIGURE 30-8 Back side of CMS-1500 universal claim form.

must appear in the upper right-hand margin of the claim form. If claims are being prepared manually using a typewriter, it is important that the form is lined up properly so that all information falls within the confines of the box or field dedicated to these data. It is also important that you follow OCR guidelines (discussed in the next section) when preparing paper claims.

Procedure 30-2 shows the process of completing each block in the CMS-1500 form. Keep in mind that the instructions serve only as a general guide and may differ from carrier to carrier and state to state. Medical assistants should keep specific instructions on file for each major payer to which they submit claims.

Electronic Claims

There are essentially two methods for claims submission: electronic and paper. Electronic claims may be submitted directly using the Internet or a dedicated phone line. Most government carriers and many commercial carriers require the provider to enroll with them and use their software before submitting claims electronically.

If the medical office uses computerized patient-accounting software, insurance claims are generated within the program. The medical assistant enters the necessary demographic and financial data into the computer and chooses a menu, and the claim is either printed out or sent to the carrier electronically. Electronic claims have the following advantages over paper claims:

1. Electronic claims are processed much faster, and reimbursement time is significantly shortened.
2. Electronic claims processing can reduce error rates and claims rejection because incorrect claims can be filtered out before submission.
3. Electronic claims submission reduces paperwork (e.g., copying, stuffing envelopes, and trips to the post office) and frees up staff for other work.
4. Electronic claims processing reduces postage and other material costs (e.g., forms).

Electronic claims filing has the following disadvantages:

1. Power outage or equipment malfunction is always a threat.
2. The initial outlay for computer equipment can be expensive.
3. Patient privacy is a concern, as discussed earlier.

Electronic claims submission involves the use of OCR software and in some cases, clearinghouses.

Optical Character Recognition

Optical character recognition (OCR) is a process whereby a specialized piece of electronic equipment scans printed documents using software that recognizes ASCII text (a universally recognized computer text file). A special bulb causes the preprinted red portion of the CMS-1500 to "disappear." The resulting image allows the software to "see" just the filled-in data, without the printed lines and text of the form obstructing the characters. For optimum OCR "reading," black text on a white background is recommended, with a standard type font (e.g., Times New Roman) in no less than 12 point. All data appearing on the CMS-1500 form should be in uppercase, and no punctuation should be used.

OCR scanning allows "paper" claims to be converted into electronic data.

Clearinghouses

A medical claims **clearinghouse** is an organization that receives claims from medical facilities, checks them for completeness and accuracy, and forwards them electronically to the proper carrier. If there is an error on a claim, the provider is notified, the error is corrected, and the claim is resubmitted. This helps ensure that most claims that reach the carrier are "clean."

Using the services of a clearinghouse has many advantages. All claims are sent to one location, thus eliminating the need for sending claims to multiple insurance carriers and using a variety of software packages. Clearinghouses are up to date with all current carrier guidelines. Claims with errors are rerouted back to the provider for correction before being sent to the insurance carrier, where payment would be delayed. The speed of electronic claims has greatly reduced the turnaround time for reimbursement and facilitates cash flow.

Clearinghouses do charge a nominal fee for each claim submitted, typically less than $1 per claim.

Processing Claims

When received at the insurance carrier's office, paper claims are scanned into a computer. The computer views the patient information, diagnosis and procedure codes, and the charges listed and matches this information to what is in the carrier's computer database. If errors are found, the claim is immediately rejected and returned to the provider's office. If clean, the claim continues on to be processed, and if the deductible has been met, a check is issued.

The information on electronic claims does not have to be scanned into the computer because it is transmitted as an electronic file. Other than that, the steps for processing electronic claims are about the same as for paper claims.

Tracking Claims

After the insurance claim is submitted to the third-party payer, the medical assistant should create some form of claims-tracking method for paper claims. Most computerized patient-accounting software programs have an insurance "aging" component built into the program, and it is a fairly simple task to generate aging reports or unpaid claim reports.

One efficient method of following up on paper claims is to create an **insurance claims register** or log. When a claim is submitted, the medical assistant notes the date filed, patient's name, name of the insurance carrier, and total amount of the charges listed on the claim. When payment

PROCEDURE 30-2 Complete the CMS-1500 Claim Form

TASK: Apply third-party guidelines and use a physician's fee schedule to complete an insurance claim form.

EQUIPMENT AND SUPPLIES
- Photocopy of the patient's insurance identification card
- Patient's information form
- Patient's encounter form
- Patient's medical record
- Physician's fee schedule
- CMS-1500 insurance claim form

SKILLS/RATIONALE

(Throughout this procedure, refer to Figure 30-7.)

1. **Procedural Step. Identify the patient's primary third-party payer, or the company or agency to which the claim will be submitted for payment.**
   You can identify the third-party payer by looking at the photocopy of the patient's insurance identification card (see Figure 30-3).

2. **Procedural Step. Enter the name and address of the third-party payer in the top right corner of the insurance form using all-capital letters and no punctuation.**

3. **Procedural Step. Complete the top half of the form.**
   Block 1: Check the type of health insurance coverage applicable to the claim.
   Block 1a: Enter the insured's ID number exactly as it appears on his or her insurance card. If the patient has Medicare coverage, enter the Medicare number. For CHAMPVA/TRICARE, the sponsor's Social Security number is used.
   Block 2: Enter the patient's name in the correct format: last name first, first name, then middle initial.
   Block 3: Enter the patient's date of birth using the "MM DD YYYY" format. Place an "X" in the appropriate gender box.
   Block 4: Enter the name of the insured (the policyholder) for commercial and Blue Cross/Blue Shield claims; enter "SAME" if the patient and the insured are the same person. If the insured's name is different from that of the patient, enter the last name, first name, and middle initial in this block. If there is insurance primary to Medicare, either through the patient's or spouse's employment or another source, list the name of the insured here. If Medicare is primary, this block should be left blank. For CHAMPVA/TRICARE, enter the sponsor's name.
   Block 5: Enter the patient's address and phone number. Enter the street address on the first line, the city and state on the second line, and the zip code and telephone number on the third line. Remember to use OCR guidelines (uppercase letters and no punctuation).
   Block 6: Indicate the patient's relationship to the insured. Check either "Self," "Spouse," "Child," or "Other." If Medicare is primary, then Block 6 is left blank.
   Block 7: Enter the insured's address if it is different from the patient's address. If the addresses are the same, then enter "SAME" in this block. Complete Block 7 only when Blocks 4 and 11 are completed. For Medicare and Medicaid claims, leave this block blank.
   Block 8: Enter the patient's marital status, as well as whether the patient is employed or a student.
   Block 9: If the patient has other medical insurance coverage, and he or she is not the insured, enter the insured's name and complete Blocks 9a to 9d. If there is no other insurance, leave Blocks 9a to 9d blank and proceed to Block 10. If there is secondary coverage, complete Blocks 9a to 9d. Block 9 is required to be completed if "yes" is marked in Block 11d.
   Block 10: Indicate to what the patient's condition is related. Its use is required. The appropriate boxes in Block 10 are checked to identify whether the patient's condition is related to his or her employment, an auto accident, or other accident. If any of the boxes in this block is checked "yes," it may indicate that the patient's health insurance is not primary and that other insurance, such as workers' compensation or an automobile insurance policy, may be primary.
   Block 11: Enter the insured's policy or group number. For commercial carriers, enter the group policy name/number from the patient's insurance ID card. This block is generally left blank for Medicaid claims. For insurance primary to Medicare, enter the insured's policy or group number. If Medicare is primary, the word "NONE" must appear in the block. Doing this indicates that Medicare is primary. For a claim to be considered for MSP, a copy of the primary payer's EOB must be included with the claim form.

Continued

PROCEDURE 30-2 Complete the CMS-1500 Claim Form—cont'd

Block 12: The patient or authorized person must sign and date this item. If a signature is on file, the words "SIGNATURE ON FILE" or "SOF" should be entered here. This block is left blank on Medicaid claims.

Block 13: The patient or authorized person should sign and date this item if he or she agrees that benefits are to be paid directly to the provider. If the patient's signature is already on file, "SIGNATURE ON FILE" or "SOF" may be entered here. For Medicare supplements and crossover claims, "SIGNATURE ON FILE" or "SOF" must also appear in this block. For Medicaid, leave blank.

4. **Procedural Step.** Complete the Physician/Supplier Section, the bottom half of the CMS-1500 form.

Block 14: Enter the date of the first symptoms of the current illness or date of injury. This information is required for accident or medical emergency claims. The date of the first symptom of the current illness, injury, or pregnancy is entered in this block only if documented in the medical record. If the claim is related to pregnancy, the date of the last menstrual cycle is entered. Caution should be used here, because an incorrect date may indicate a preexisting condition, and the claim will be rejected.

Block 15: Enter the date the patient was first treated for this condition. Completion of this block is optional, and it should be left blank on Medicare claims.

Block 16: If a patient is unable to work in his or her current occupation, and if this is a workers' compensation claim, enter the applicable dates into this block. Completion of this block is required for workers' compensation claims, but not for most other carriers.

Block 17: Enter the name of the referring (or ordering) physician, if applicable. If the physician orders a test or procedure that is performed by an ancillary health care provider, but the physician/source interprets the results, his or her **National Provider Identifier** (**NPI**) name must be entered here, and his or her NPI number must be entered into Block 17b.

Block 18: Enter the hospitalization dates related to the current services, if applicable, if the claim is for a related hospital admission and discharge. If the patient has not yet been discharged, leave the "To" box blank.

Block 19: This block is reserved for local use. In most cases, this block will be left blank. Some private payers require that the word "Attachments" be entered here when specific documentation accompanies the claim. There are circumstances on Medicare and Medicaid claims when information might be entered here. Must use NPI with any information submitted in this block. You will need to check with the local fiscal intermediary or the guidelines of the third-party payer for details.

Block 20: This block is used to indicate when outside laboratory services have been provided. If laboratory procedures are listed on the claim in Block 24 and these services were performed in the provider's facility, the "No" box in Block 20 is checked with an "X" or left blank. If laboratory work shown on the claim was done by an outside laboratory and billed by the provider, check the "Yes" box and enter the total amount of the charges. Some payers require that this block be left blank if no tests were done.

Block 21: This block is used to indicate the diagnosis or diagnoses. The patient's diagnosis (or diagnoses) is entered using ICD-9-CM codes. The primary diagnosis should be listed first, and all diagnosis codes should be coded to the highest level of specificity. Up to four codes (in priority order) can be entered in Block 21.

Block 22: Use this block for Medicaid resubmissions. Completion of this block is only required for replacement claims for Medicaid. In such cases, you would enter the appropriate 3-digit replacement code, followed by the 17-digit transaction control number of the most current incorrectly paid claim.

Block 23: This block can be completed in various ways. For private and commercial carriers and Medicaid, enter the 10-digit prior authorization number for those procedures requiring prior approval assigned by the peer review organization (PRO). To determine this, you would need to consult the specific guidelines for the payer to whom the claim is being submitted. If performing laboratory procedures covered by the Clinical Laboratory Improvement Act (CLIA), enter the 10-digit CLIA certification number in this block.

Block 24a through 24k: These blocks will be completed one row at a time for each service provided. In other words, complete the first row only of Block 24a, then for this same service, complete the first row only of Block 24b, and so on, until the entire first row of Blocks 24a to 24k has been filled out for the first service. Then go back and start entering the information for the second service provided in the second row of Blocks 24a to 24k. Fill out Block 24 in this manner so that you work with the information of only one service at a time.

Block 24a: The first date of service for the charge on this line should be placed in the "From" column. When a claim is for more than 1 day of the same service on a line item, the days must be in consecutive order. The last date of service is required in the "To" column. Enter the month, day, and year (in MM DD YYYY format) for each procedure, service, or supply. When "From" and "To" dates are shown for a series of identical services, enter the number of days or units in Block 24g.

Continued

PROCEDURE 30-2 Complete the CMS-1500 Claim Form—cont'd

Block 24b: The "Place of Service" code is entered here.

Block 24c: Labeled "EMG." For certain carriers, enter an "X" or "E" as appropriate if documentation indicates a medical emergency existed. Leave this block blank for Medicare claims.

Block 24d: Enter the procedure, service, or supply code using the appropriate five-digit CPT or **Healthcare Common Procedure Coding System (HCPCS)** code. A two-digit position modifier is entered when applicable. If an unlisted procedure code is used (codes ending in -99), a complete description of the procedure must be given. Use a separate attachment to do this.

Block 24e: Link the procedure/service code back to the diagnosis code in Block 21 by indicating the applicable number of diagnosis codes (1, 2, 3, or 4) to that line's procedure code.

Block 24f: Enter the charge for each listed procedure, supply, and service.

Block 24g: The number of days or units for the service(s), procedure(s), and supply(ies) is entered. This field is normally used for multiple visits, units of supplies, anesthesia minutes, or oxygen volume. If only one service is performed, enter the number "1."

Block 24h: This block is used for the Early and Periodic Screening Diagnosis and Treatment (EPSDT)/Family Plan. Leave this block blank for all claims with the exception of certain Medicaid claims. If this is applicable, enter the appropriate alphabetical referral code here.

Block 24i: Enter the ID qualifier 1C in the shaded portion.

Block 24j: Enter the rendering provider's NPI number in the lower unshaded portion. In the case of a service provided "incident to" the service of a physician or nonphysician practitioner, when the person who ordered the service is not the supervising provider, enter the NPI of the supervisor in the lower portion of this field.

Block 25: The provider's nine-digit federal tax identification number is entered, and the appropriate box checked. In the case of an unincorporated practice, the provider's Social Security number is entered and "SSN" is checked.

Block 26: Enter the patient's account number as assigned by the supplier's accounting system. If submitting the claim electronically, you are required to provide a patient account number.

Block 27: This block is used to indicate whether the provider accepts assignment of benefits. The appropriate box should be checked. If the supplier is a PAR, assignment must be accepted for all covered charges. For non-PARs, this can be left blank. For Medicaid, check "Yes."

Block 28: Total column 24f and enter the total charges in this field.

Block 29: Enter the total amount, if any, that has been paid by the patient. This block should be left blank if no payment has been made.

Block 30: This block is used for all private payers and when there is secondary insurance. The balance owing is entered as indicated on the encounter form or the EOB. Not required by Medicare.

Block 31: Enter the signature of the provider or representative, and the date the form was signed. The signature may be typed, stamped, or handwritten; however, the characters should not fall outside the block. When claims are transmitted electronically, a signed agreement must be on file in place of an actual signature on a paper claim form.

Block 32: Enter the name and address of the facility where the services were performed if other than the patient's home. Most third-party payers allow the word "SAME" to be entered into Block 32 if the place where services were provided is the same as the place entered in Block 33 (physician/supplier's billing name, address, zip code, and phone). If "yes" is checked in Block 20, enter the name and address of the laboratory that performed the outside laboratory service. Enter the NPI of the service facility in Block 32a.

Block 33: Enter the provider's billing name, address, zip code, and telephone number. Be aware that a missing phone number can cause the claim to be rejected. Enter the billing provider or group NPI number in 33a. Medicare does not require completion of 33b. Again, be sure to refer to third-party guidelines.

5. **Procedural Step.** **Review the claim.**
Before submitting the claim, it is important that you take the time to proofread the claim for accuracy and completeness. It is best to be proactive when working with claim forms. You must make every effort possible to produce a clean claim, rather than spending valuable time trying to fix a claim after problems have been discovered by the payer.

6. **Procedural Step.** **Submit the claim.**
Claims may be submitted manually, by mail, or electronically via a clearinghouse or directly to the payer.

Patient's Name Group/Policy No.	Name of Insurance Company	Claim Submitted		Follow-Up		Claim Paid		Difference
		Date	Amount	Date	Date	Date	Amt	
Davis, Bob	BC/BS	1-7-XX	319.37			2/28/00	294.82	24.55
Cash, David	BC	1-8-XX	268.08	2-10-00	3-10-00			
Smythe, Jan	Medicaid	1-9-XX	146.15	2-10-00				
Phillips, Emma	Medicare	1-10-XX	96.28	2-10-00				
Perez, Jose	Medi-Medi	1-10-XX	647.09	2-10-00				
Amato, Joe	TRICARE	2-1-XX	134.78	3-10-00				
Rubin, Billy	Aetna	2-4-XX	607.67	3-10-00				
Pfeifer, Renee	Travelers	2-10-XX	564.55	3-10-00				
Tam, Chang	Prudential	2-15-XX	1515.79					
Brown, Harry	Allstate	2-21-XX	121.21					
Park, James	BC	2-24-XX	124.99					

FIGURE 30-9 Insurance claims register used to track claims and follow-up on activity. (From Fordney MT, French LL: *Medical insurance billing and coding,* Philadelphia, 2003, Saunders.)

is received, the amount of reimbursement and the date received are recorded. Figure 30-9 shows an example of an insurance register.

The insurance register should be checked at least weekly. Any delinquent (past-due) claims should receive special attention such as a follow-up letter or a telephone call. After an appropriate time has elapsed (3 to 4 weeks), the medical assistant should notify the patient that no payment has been received from the insurance carrier, and a statement should be sent. It should not be the responsibility of the provider's office to continue to pursue payment from third-party carriers after an initial letter or phone call. Note that paper claims historically take two to three times longer to complete and process than electronic claims.

PATIENT-CENTERED PROFESSIONALISM

- *What can the medical assistant do to help the insurance specialist submit clean claim forms?*

PREVENTING REJECTIONS AND DELAYS

Submitting a Clean Claim

Submitting a clean claim is the best defense against rejection or delay of payment. Clean claims are usually paid on the first submission. Because of the many third-party payers with special requirements and guidelines, plus an increasing emphasis on documentation and accurate coding, submitting a clean claim needs special attention and care, even for the most experienced medical assistant.

Common Reasons for Rejections and Delays

Claims are often rejected or delayed because of technical errors, such as the following:

- Mechanical errors, such as transposed numbers and misspelled names
- Incorrect or missing patient or supplier information
- Incorrect or incomplete ICD-9-CM or CPT codes
- Claim not submitted in specified time limit
- Missing referrals or preauthorization numbers

In these situations, the medical assistant can usually correct the claim and resubmit it to the carrier. However, claim rejections can also result from issues over which the provider's office has no control and where resubmission is not normally an option such as the following:

1. The service or procedure is not a covered option of the insurance contract. Benefits are not available for this service, and it is an "out of pocket" expense for the patient. This can be predetermined by precertifying the procedure.
2. The service or procedure was performed because of a *preexisting* condition. Some patients are aware of "preexisting condition" clauses in their insurance contract and that services related to the specific diagnosis are not covered under the policy.
3. The service or procedure was not *medically necessary*. Any service not documented to the carrier's satisfaction as being medically necessary will be denied.

In the case of rejection because of one of these three reasons, the medical assistant should transfer the balance of the charge to the patient's responsibility and send the patient a bill.

Be Proactive

The medical assistant who is a successful medical insurance claims specialist should endeavor to become *proactive* in claims completion and submission, as follows:

- Obtain accurate and complete information from patients and keep this information current.
- Learn the requirements and guidelines of the major insurance carriers handled in the medical facility.
- Stay current on mandates for government-sponsored plans such as Medicare, Medicaid, and TRICARE/CHAMPVA.
- Attend conferences and seminars on compliance, coding, and medical record documentation.
- Create and maintain a current list of "hotline" phone numbers and contact names for all carriers for quick and accurate response to claims questions.

By putting forth extra effort to do your best in ensuring that all claims submitted are as accurate as possible, you will be rewarded by receiving minimal denials and maximum reimbursements. This can result in a considerable cost savings to the practice and improved cash flow.

- Dates of services rendered, claim received, and claim processed
- Type of service (may be coded)
- Charge for each service or procedure listed on the claim
- Amount the insurance carrier allowed on each charge
- Whether or not the patient or insured has met the deductible
- Patient's share of the charge (co-insurance/co-pay)
- Amount the carrier is (or is not) paying on the allowable charge
- How the amount reimbursement (or denial) was determined
- Reasons (codes) for denial or rejection of one or more services or procedures
- Any applicable notes that affect claims processing

If the EOB indicates an error on the claim that can be corrected, the medical assistant should correct and resubmit the claim as soon as possible. If the claim cannot be resubmitted (for the reasons listed previously), it is the patient's responsibility to follow up with the claim in most of these situations. Options open to the patient or insured include an appeal to the insurance carrier and a petition for review to the State Insurance Commissioner's office.

PATIENT-CENTERED PROFESSIONALISM

- What are the reasons for claims being rejected, and how can these situations be prevented?

PATIENT-CENTERED PROFESSIONALISM

- What happens if the medical office cannot interpret the EOB?

CLAIMS FOLLOW-UP

With every claim submitted, whether a payment is made or not, an EOB document is generated. Usually, both the provider and the patient receive a copy of the EOB (Figure 30-10).

Interpreting and evaluating the EOB help medical assistants determine the amount of the reimbursement or the reason for the denial. Medical assistants should become familiar with the process of interpreting EOBs so they can determine how much, if anything, the patient still owes, or if an error was made on the claim. No universal form is used for EOBs, so deciphering them can be challenging at first.

The EOB usually includes the following information in some form:

- Patient or insured's name and insurance identification number

CONCLUSION

The many private and government-sponsored insurance carriers may have different guidelines and policies to follow for claims submission. Medical assistants may work with insurance claims on a daily basis; thus it is important for them to understand the basic concepts of medical insurance and claims so they can ensure that the necessary information is accurate, up-to-date, well-documented, and handled properly.

Medical assistants who understand the concepts of medical insurance and the process of submitting a clean claim will be in demand in the job market. In addition, they can help the practice receive correct, timely payment for the services performed. Finally, because medical insurance can be complicated, knowledgeable medical assistants can better help patients with questions and problems concerning payment of services and claims.

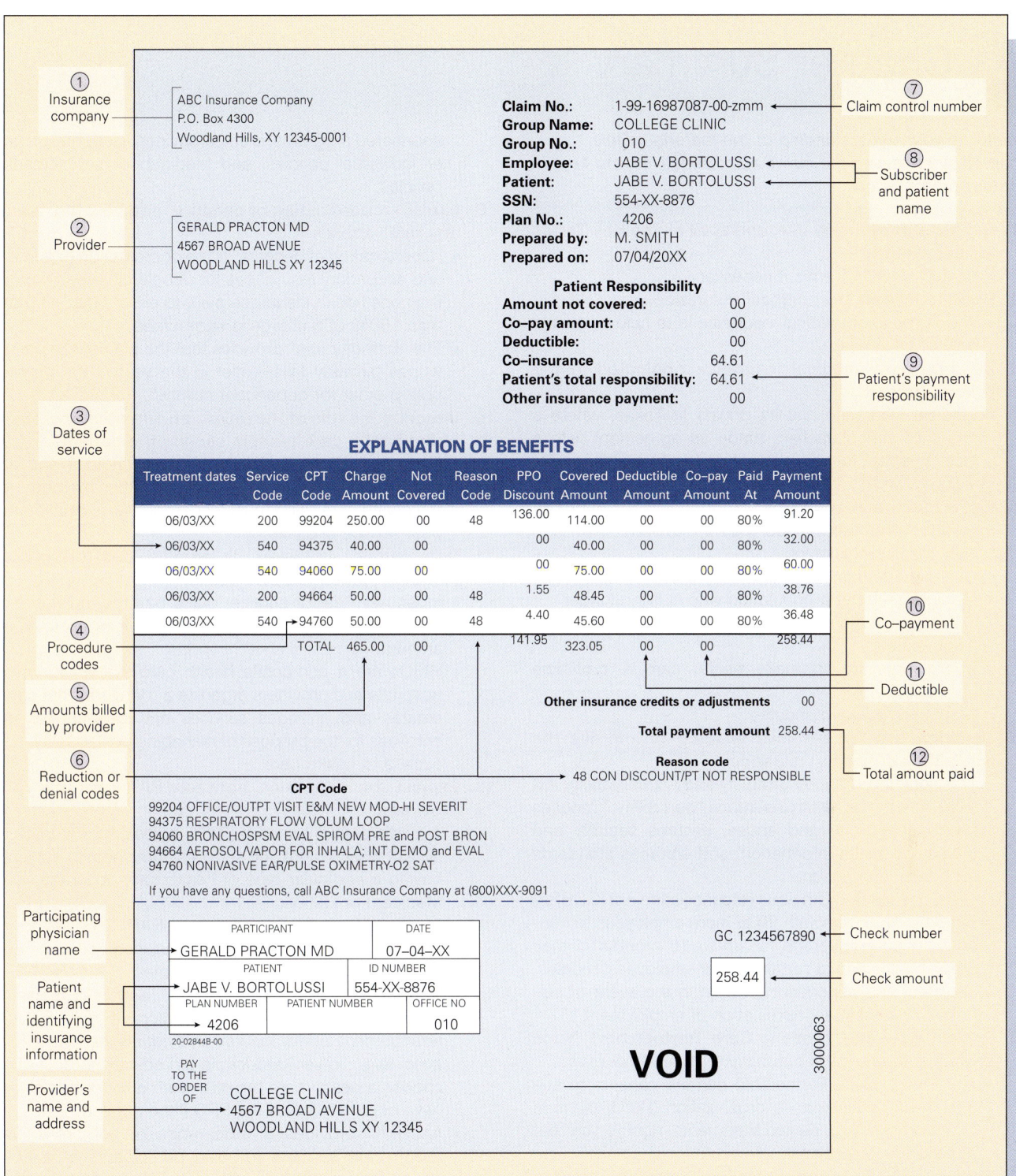

FIGURE 30-10 Example of "explanation of benefits" document. (From Fordney MT, French LL: *Medical insurance billing and coding,* Philadelphia, 2003, Saunders.)

Chapter Summary

Reinforce your understanding of the material in this chapter by reviewing the curriculum objectives and key content points below.

1. **Define, appropriately use, and spell all the Key Terms for this chapter.**
   - Review the Key Terms if necessary.
2. **Explain the need for medical insurance.**
   - The purpose of medical insurance is to help cover the cost of health care.
3. **Describe how medical insurance originated in the United States.**
   - Medical insurance has its origins in Texas, where a group of schoolteachers made an agreement with a local hospital to pay a monthly fee in exchange for visits.
4. **List six factors responsible for the increases in health insurance premiums since the mid-1990s.**
   - New medical technology
   - Overuse and misuse of medical services
   - Medical needs of a population who is living longer
   - Consumer demands for easier and broader access to health care
   - Public pressure to make health care a profitable business
   - State and federal mandates
5. **Describe two federal laws enacted to improve the availability of health insurance.**
   - The Health Insurance Portability and Accountability Act (HIPAA) ensures health insurance "portability," reduces health care fraud and abuse, ensures security and privacy of health information, and enforces standards for health information.
   - The Consolidated Omnibus Reconciliation Act (COBRA) requires employers with 20 or more employees to continue to offer coverage for up to 18 months in their group health plan to certain former employees, retirees, spouses, and dependent children in the event of voluntary or involuntary termination of employment.
6. **Explain how the "Patient Care Partnership" helps protect patient rights concerning their HMO plans.**
   - The Patient Care Partnership permits patients to sue their health maintenance organization (HMO) plans in certain cases (e.g., denied treatments, right to see "out of network" physicians).
7. **Explain why it is important for the health care team to treat patients as you would a "customer."**
   - Treating a patient as a "customer" places the emphasis on service, and health care providers need to compete for patients as does any business.
   - Patients are better informed and more aware of their rights and choices, and a patient can seek medical care from any number of qualified providers.
8. **List five types of insurance choices available for eligible patients.**
   - Insurance choices for eligible participants include employer-sponsored group plans, government-sponsored programs, medical savings accounts, private or individual policies, and Medigap or supplemental policies.
9. **Explain "coordination of benefits" and how the "birthday rule" applies.**
   - "Coordination of benefits" is the coordination of primary and secondary insurances for people covered by more than one health insurance plan, to ensure that no more than 100% of a charge is reimbursed.
   - The "birthday rule" provides that the plan of the parent whose birthday falls earlier in the year is the primary policyholder for dependent children.
10. **Describe the role of the physician and other members of the health care team in serving the patient.**
    - Because patients today have more choices and are better informed, the physician and other members of the health care team must work together to provide the best service possible.
11. **Differentiate between indemnity (fee-for-service) plans and managed care plans.**
    - Indemnity (fee-for-service) plans pay the individual or health care provider for covered services up to a set amount.
    - HMOs are a composite health care system in which hospitals and providers organize a "network" that coordinates and arranges services and benefits for the enrollees for the purpose of managing cost, quality, and access to health care.
12. **Explain the difference between PAR and non-PAR providers.**
    - A participating provider (PAR) agrees by contract to accept assignment for services furnished to patients having a particular type of health care coverage (e.g., Medicare or HMO).
    - A non-participating provider (non-PAR) chooses not to enter into a contract with the insurance company and therefore does not accept assignment.
13. **Compare and contrast PPO, HMO, and POS plans.**
    - A preferred provider organization (PPO) delivery arrangement offers insured individuals certain incentives (e.g., lower deductible or co-payment) if they choose a health care provider from a list of those who have contracted with the PPO ("the network").
    - An HMO provides a wide range of comprehensive health care services for plan participants at a fixed periodic payment to the physician, (e.g., $10 to $25 a month).
    - A point-of-service (POS) plan is an "open ended" HMO option with more flexibility. This type of plan permits members to choose "out of network" but does more to encourage in-network providers by paying a greater portion of the fee.
14. **Describe the UCR, episode of care, capitation, RVS, and RBRVS methods of determining fees.**
    - Usual, customary, and reasonable (UCR) refers to the commonly charged or prevailing fees for similar health services within a geographical area.

- Episode of care is used to describe and measure the various health care services rendered in connection with a specific injury or period (time frame) of illness.
- Capitation is a fee type used by some HMO models in which the provider is paid a specific fee per period (usually monthly) per enrollee, regardless of services provided.
- The relative value scale (RVS) is an established list of procedures and services with assigned unit values to aid in setting fees.
- The resource-based relative value scale (RBRVS) is used by Medicare to establish fees using RVS units, geographical indices, and a national conversion factor to arrive at a regionally specific fee for procedures.

15. **List five methods of cost containment used by third-party payers and the government.**
    - Requiring preauthorization for inpatient hospitalization, procedures, and certain other services.
    - Controlling the use of ancillary services (e.g., physical therapy, CT scans).
    - Cost sharing with the patient.
    - Using nonphysician providers (e.g., nurse practitioners, physician assistants).
    - Verifying the "medical necessity" of services.

16. **Define "private carrier" and give a well-known example.**
    - A private carrier is a provider of health insurance that a person can obtain through a group plan or as an individual. These policies are purchased through private (nongovernment) organizations whose sole business is insurance.
    - Blue Cross/Blue Shield is one of the first and most well known private carriers in the United States.

17. **Explain the difference between group and individual commercial policies.**
    - A group policy is an insurance policy that is purchased by a company for its employees or by an organization (e.g., union) for its members. Because of the large volume of subscribers, premiums are often lower, and the employer may pay a portion of the premium as a benefit.
    - Individual policies are policies purchased from the insurance company by individuals, without benefit of a group discount. Individual policies often have high premiums and high deductibles.

18. **Explain when third-party liability might apply.**
    - Third-party liability arises in situations such as automobile accidents or accidents in the workplace, when automobile insurance or workers' compensation insurance may be the primary insurer. Therefore the patient's health insurance may not be responsible for primary coverage.

19. **Differentiate between Medicare and Medicaid.**
    - Medicare is a federal assistance program that pays medical benefits to those age 65 and older, permanently disabled persons, and patients with end-stage renal disease. Once qualified for Medicare, the person has it for life.
    - Medicaid is a federal or state assistance program that provides medical care for persons whose income falls below the national poverty level. Medicaid is only available on a month-to-month basis, and the patient must requalify every 30 days.

20. **Differentiate between TRICARE and CHAMPVA.**
    - TRICARE is the U.S. military's comprehensive health care program for active-duty personnel, eligible family members, retirees and family members under age 65, and survivors of deceased members of all U.S. Uniformed Services.
    - CHAMPVA is a health benefits program that provides coverage to the spouse or widow(er) and children of a veteran who is permanently and totally disabled as a result of a service-related disability or who died during active duty.

21. **Differentiate between workers' compensation and disability income insurance.**
    - Workers' compensation is an insurance program that pays medical expenses and loss of wages for workers who are injured on the job or who have job-related illnesses.
    - Disability income insurance pays benefits to the policyholder if the person becomes unable to work as a result of an illness or injury that is not work related.

22. **Differentiate among Medi-Medi, Medigap, and MSP.**
    - Medi-Medi, Medigap, and MSP are secondary, supplementary insurance plans.
    - The Medicare-Medicaid Crossover Program (Medi-Medi) focuses on Medicare and Medicaid working together to provide health care services to low-income seniors.
    - Medigap insurance is secondary insurance sold by private companies and is designed to fill the "gaps" in Medicare benefits.
    - Medicare Secondary Payer (MSP) means Medicare is not the primary insurance. The patient is typically covered by an employer-sponsored plan first.

23. **Demonstrate the correct procedure for applying managed care policies and procedures.**
    - Review Procedure 30-1.

24. **Describe how preauthorization works.**
    - Preauthorization is the advance approval of a health plan that a requested treatment or procedure is medically necessary and appropriate and will be considered a "covered" service for policy benefits. Claims submitted without the proper preauthorization information will be denied.

25. **Briefly describe the five phases of the medical insurance claim cycle.**
    - Phase 1: Patient appointment is initial contact with medical office.
    - Phase 2: Patient registration; demographics must be correctly entered in patient's account.
    - Phase 3: Patient examination (encounter) is completed, and physician enters diagnosis and procedures or services on the encounter form.
    - Phase 4: Patient checkout; patient makes any follow-up appointment and payment as necessary.
    - Phase 5: Insurance claim processing is done by ledger card or computer.

26. **Explain the purpose of an ROI authorization.**
    - A release of information (ROI) is needed to permit the medical office to release personal information and health records to third parties (e.g., insurance companies, other physicians or facilities).

27. **Define "clean claim" and state its importance.**
    - A clean claim is one that has been submitted with no errors or omissions.
    - A clean claim is processed faster, and turnaround time for cash flow is better.
28. **List two things medical assistants should check before preparing an insurance claim form.**
    - Medical insurance claims are based on accurate and complete documentation of services in the medical record.
    - When completing the CMS-1500, the medical assistant should follow the guidelines of the specific insurance carrier to whom the claim is being sent.
29. **Explain what should be done if a patient does not have insurance coverage or if a patient's insurance policy does not cover a procedure.**
    - Patients with no insurance coverage should know in advance that they are expected to pay for services the day of the appointment.
    - If a patient's policy does not cover a specific procedure or service, many offices will expect all or a significant portion of the charge to be paid in advance or on the day of service.
    - Office policies for this may vary, but such an office policy should exist.
30. **Demonstrate the correct procedure for accurately completing a CMS-1500 claim form.**
    - Review Procedure 30-2.
    - The universal form used by most third-party payers for claims submission is the CMS-1500 (formerly the HCFA-1500).
31. **List four advantages of submitting insurance claims electronically.**
    - Electronic claims are processed faster.
    - Errors resulting in claims rejection are minimized.
    - Paperwork is reduced.
    - Postage and other material costs are eliminated.
32. **Describe the proper type, size, and color for entering information that can be recognized by OCR software.**
    - Type compatible with optical character recognition (OCR) is typically black type, 12 point, a "normal" font such as Times New Roman, and in all-capital letters using no punctuation.
33. **Explain the purpose of a medical claims clearinghouse.**
    - A medical claims clearinghouse serves as a "filter" for claims before they are submitted to third-party payers.
    - The clearinghouse scans each claim for errors or omissions and returns those with errors to the provider before submitting to the insurance carrier. Thus, claims passed by the clearinghouse on to the third-party payers are "clean" and will be processed sooner, with no resubmissions.
34. **Describe the purpose and use of an insurance claims register.**
    - An insurance claims register allows the medical assistant to track the status of all insurance claims submitted and enables easier follow-up of unpaid claims.
    - A computerized patient accounting system will automatically track claims once they are submitted to third-party payers.
35. **List five technical errors that could cause a claim to be rejected or delayed.**
    - Mechanical errors such as transposed numbers or letters.
    - Incorrect or missing patient information.
    - Incorrect or incomplete ICD-9-CM or CPT codes.
    - Claims submitted beyond the specified time limit.
    - Missing referrals or preauthorization numbers.
36. **List four reasons a claim might be rejected and might not be eligible for resubmission.**
    - Service or procedure is not a covered benefit of the policy.
    - Preexisting condition was excluded from the benefit pool.
    - Documentation does not prove medical necessity.
    - Preauthorization was not obtained.
37. **List five actions that medical assistants can take to be proactive in claims completion and submission.**
    - Obtain accurate information from the patient and keep it current.
    - Learn the requirements and guidelines of the specific carriers.
    - Keep up-to-date on government program mandates.
    - Attend conferences and seminars on coding, compliance, insurance, and medical record documentation.
    - Create a current list of "hotline" phone numbers and contacts for all your insurance carriers for quick and accurate response to claims questions.
38. **Define "EOB" and explain what should be done with it when received.**
    - The explanation of benefits (EOB) document, which is generated with every claim submitted, shows the method used to determine the amount of reimbursement or the reason for a denial of payment.
    - The medical assistant should become familiar with the various formats and how to interpret EOBs. After reviewing the EOB, the payment should be applied to the patient account balance. If no payment is made or a denial was received, the patient needs to be contacted and financial responsibility of the balance is transferred to the patient.
39. **Analyze a realistic medical office situation and apply your understanding of medical insurance to determine the best course of action.**
    - Although insurance companies and third-party payers have different policies and procedures for submitting claims, many similar general concepts apply when preparing and submitting all insurance claims.
40. **Describe the impact on patient care when medical assistants understand the essentials of medical insurance and are capable of submitting clean claims to insurers.**
    - Patients' insurance bills are paid more quickly when claims are submitted correctly and efficiently.
    - This benefits both the patient and the medical office.

PRACTICAL APPLICATIONS

If you have accomplished the objectives in this chapter, you will be able to make better choices as a medical assistant. Take another look at this situation and decide what you would do.

Dr. Jay has hired Maria as his insurance clerk. Maria's previous experience was with household liability claims and coverage. She has not had experience with the CMS-1500 or with coding of medical conditions. She is not aware that the claim begins with the appointment and patient registration and ends with payment by the insurer. Jude Beck, a new patient of Dr. Jay, is seen in the office for what appears to be diabetes mellitus. An ECG, urinalysis, and blood test were done during the visit without checking with Mr. Beck's insurance first. In his notes, Dr. Jay states that he must "rule out diabetes mellitus," so Maria codes this as the "primary diagnosis" and sends the claim without a final diagnosis. When the results of the laboratory work are received, Dr. Jay documents in the medical record that the final diagnoses are dehydration and hypertension with tachycardia.

When the registration form was completed, Mr. Beck failed to check off which of his insurance companies is primary and which is secondary. In processing the claim, Maria sends it with a diagnosis of "diabetes mellitus" to one of the two insurance companies, which turns out to be the secondary insurer. The claim is denied because there is no EOB attached from the primary payer. Maria does not resubmit the claim to the company that is actually the primary carrier.

Could you explain to Maria what went wrong and how the claim should have been handled?

1. Why is it important for the registration form to be completed accurately?
2. Why would the secondary insurance not pay for the claim before payment by the primary carrier?
3. What are the guidelines for coding a "rule out" diagnosis in the outpatient setting?
4. Why is preauthorization so important when dealing with insurance?
5. What is the implication for Mr. Beck of Maria not tracking the claims?
6. What is an "EOB"?
7. Why does the EOB of primary insurance need to be sent to the secondary insurance?
8. Why is a "clean claim" so important in obtaining insurance payment?

WEB SEARCH

1. **Research the different insurance carriers to learn more about the services and the different types of plans they offer.** Each insurance carrier appeals to an employer or an individual because of the services or plans offered, the cost, or both.

- **Keywords:** Use the following keywords in your search: Aetna, Blue Cross/Blue Shield, Cigna.

31 Infection Control and Asepsis

evolve http://evolve.elsevier.com/klieger/medicalassisting

Patients with infections and infectious disease regularly come to the medical facility for treatment. As the medical assistant goes from patient to patient performing clinical procedures, such as taking vital signs and assisting the physician, the potential for transmitting disease is high if the medical assistant does not follow protective measures such as handwashing, sanitization, and proper handling of medical waste. Thorough handwashing and/or use of alcohol rubs by all medical personnel before each patient contact is one of the most effective ways to combat **nosocomial infections.** Nosocomial infections are those that occur as a result of treatment in a health care facility (e.g., hospital, outpatient treatment center).

Infection control and medical and surgical asepsis are crucial in medical facilities to prevent the spread of disease and infection. Understanding and following the guidelines for breaking the "chain of infection" protects not only the patients and other health care workers in the facility but also the medical assistant.

LEARNING OBJECTIVES

You will be able to do the following after completing this chapter:

Key Terms
1. Define, appropriately use, and spell all the Key Terms for this chapter.

Infection Control
2. Explain why it is important for medical assistants to understand the basic principles of infection control.
3. Explain the difference between nonpathogenic and pathogenic microorganisms.
4. List the six requirements that must be present for microorganisms to grow.
5. List five classes of disease-causing microorganisms and give at least one example of a disease caused by each.
6. Describe the five parts of the "chain of infection," and give three examples of how this chain can be broken.
7. Define the roles of the CDC and OSHA regarding Standard Precautions.
8. Demonstrate the correct procedure for practicing Standard Precautions.
9. Demonstrate the correct procedure for properly disposing of biohazardous materials.
10. List the five responsibilities of employers to protect employees against exposure to potentially biohazardous materials, according to the OSHA Bloodborne Pathogens Standard.
11. List the six types of information found on an MSDS and explain how an MSDS supports the "right-to-know" law.

Medical Asepsis
12. Differentiate between *medical* asepsis and *surgical* asepsis.
13. Explain the difference between *normal* flora and *transient* flora.
14. List four methods of maintaining hand hygiene.
15. Demonstrate the correct procedure for handwashing for medical asepsis.
16. Demonstrate the correct procedure for hand sanitization using an alcohol-based hand rub.
17. Demonstrate the correct procedure for applying and removing nonsterile gloves.

Surgical Asepsis
18. Differentiate among sanitization, disinfection, and sterilization.
19. Demonstrate the correct procedure for sanitizing instruments.
20. Demonstrate the correct procedure for performing chemical sterilization of items.
21. Explain the basic purpose and function of an autoclave.

22. Demonstrate the correct procedure for wrapping items for the autoclave.
23. Demonstrate the correct procedure for performing steam sterilization of items in an autoclave.
24. Describe how the autoclave is maintained on a daily and monthly basis.
25. Explain the purpose of a chemical indicator, sterilization strip, and biological indicator.
26. List three factors that influence the shelf life of sterilized instruments.

Patient-Centered Professionalism

27. Analyze a realistic medical office situation and apply your understanding of infection control and asepsis to determine the best course of action.
28. Describe the impact on patient care when medical assistants understand how to prevent the spread of disease and exposure to potentially biohazardous materials in the medical office.

PRACTICAL APPLICATIONS

Read the following scenario and keep it in mind as you learn about infection control and medical and surgical asepsis in the medical office.

Janine is a new medical assistant in the office of Dr. McGee, a specialist in infectious diseases. Janine did her practical experience in a pediatric practice, often caring for children with viral and bacterial infections. As she begins her new employment, Janine asks to see the MSDSs and the current Exposure Control Plan. She also wants to know where the PPEs for her use are stored.

During patient care, medical workers often come in direct contact with many microorganisms, as Janine will in an office that specializes in infectious diseases. Janine's supervisor wants to be sure Janine is prepared to protect patients, other staff, and herself from infection. The supervisor reviews with Janine the importance of proper handwashing in infection control. Another important task for Janine will be performing both medical asepsis and surgical asepsis on a regular basis, so the supervisor assesses Janine's ability to perform these skills. The supervisor asks Janine what is done at the end of the day before leaving the office to break the cycle of infection. Janine responds that all medical workers should remove any garments that have been in direct contact with pathogens and nonpathogens and each person should carefully sanitize his or her hands.

Would you be prepared to take the necessary precautions to stop the spread of infection in the medical office?

KEY TERMS

aerobes
anaerobes
antiseptic hand rub
antiseptic handwash
autoclave
autoclave tape
bacilli
bacteria
biological indicator
carrier
Centers for Disease Control and Prevention (CDC)
chemical indicator
cocci
diplococci
direct contact
disinfection
engineering controls
exposure control plan
exposure incident
fungi
hand hygiene
handwashing
indirect contact
infection control
material safety data sheet (MSDS)
medical asepsis
method of transmission
microorganisms
nonpathogens
normal flora
nosocomial infection
Occupational Safety and Health Administration (OSHA)
parasites
pathogens
personal protective equipment (PPE)
protozoa
reservoir host
resident flora
rickettsiae
"right-to-know" law
route of entry
route of exit
sanitization
spirilla
spores
staphylococci
sterile
sterilization
sterilization strip
streptococci
surgical asepsis
surgical handwash
susceptible host
transient flora
viruses
work practice controls

INFECTION CONTROL

Because medical assistants or other health care providers may interact with patients who have infections or infectious disease, individuals must understand the basics of **infection control** so the spread of disease may be prevented and not passed to other patients and staff. Knowledge about microorganisms and how infection is spread from one person to another is necessary before the medical assistant performs any tasks in the medical office. The body has many natural defenses to prevent microbes from entering the body such as skin, tears, stomach acid, and cough reflex. Stopping the transmission of infectious diseases within the medical office can be accomplished by following simple guidelines. In addition, many regulations and guidelines are in place to help health care professionals prevent the transmission of infectious agents (microbes) and break the chain of disease transmission. The CDC and OSHA work to stop the spread of disease by establishing and enforcing these guidelines and regulations.

Microorganisms

Microorganisms are found in the air we breathe, on our skin, on everything we touch, and even in our food.

Microorganisms are so small that they can only be seen with a microscope. Fortunately, not all microorganisms are harmful.

Nonpathogens are not harmful and are not disease-producing microorganisms. They help keep a balance in the environment (e.g., decomposing materials) and in the body (e.g., breaking down food in the digestive tract). Nonpathogens also help to limit the growth of pathogens. Nonpathogens represent **normal flora** or **resident flora,** occurring naturally on the skin and in the body, and they fight off infection when they remain in their normal location. If a nonpathogenic organism is transported to an area outside its normal environment, it can become a disease-producing organism.

Pathogens are disease-producing microorganisms. When a pathogen invades a person who has a weakened immune system, an infection can occur, possibly leading to death. Even people who are healthy may become infected and may die, depending on the type of pathogen (e.g., a healthy person could contract HIV from having sex with someone infected with HIV). In most cases, however, people with weakened immune systems are more likely to acquire infection.

> **EXAMPLE OF A NONPATHOGEN BECOMING A PATHOGEN**
>
> *Escherichia coli* is a species of bacteria that live in the lower digestive tract. If they travel to the urinary tract, an infection occurs, as when females incorrectly wipe from back to front after toileting (instead of front to back). This can deposit rectal contaminants into the urethra, which may result in a urinary tract infection (UTI).

As with people, microorganisms must have certain conditions in order to grow (Box 31-1).

Disease-Causing Microorganisms

The medical assistant may be exposed to several classes of microorganisms on a daily basis (Table 31-1). By maintaining a healthy state, the body will often be able to resist an infection. Each class of microorganisms has its own unique characteristics. Pathogens can produce poisons (toxins) that react with the body tissues, whereas other types of microorganisms cause an allergic reaction or destroy cells.

Bacteria

Bacteria are single-celled microorganisms that multiply rapidly. Bacteria are classified according to shape and arrangement (Figure 31-1) and include the following:

- **Cocci** are round or spherical.
- **Diplococci** are cocci occurring in pairs (e.g., gonorrhea, meningitis).
- **Streptococci** are cocci occurring in chains (e.g., bacterial pneumonia, upper respiratory infection).
- **Staphylococci** are cocci arranged in clusters (e.g., acne, boils, or pus).
- **Bacilli** are rod shaped and occur singly, in pairs, and chains (e.g., typhoid, diphtheria, anthrax, and tuberculosis).

BOX 31-1

Growth Requirements for Microorganisms

1. *Nutrients.* All microorganisms need a food source, whether that source is alive or dead. Microorganisms use nitrogen and carbon to carry out their life functions. Although every type needs these two nutrients, the specific nutritional needs for different microorganisms vary.
2. *Darkness.* Most microorganisms prefer dark, moist conditions. Low light or no light is optimal for bacterial growth.
3. *pH.* The degree to which something is an acid or a base is referred to as its pH. A pH of 7 is neutral, greater than 7 is acidic, and less than 7 is basic. Microorganisms that prefer a neutral pH are called *neutrophiles*. Most pathogens are neutrophiles. Microorganisms that prefer an acidic environment are called *acidophiles* (e.g., yeasts, molds). Microorganisms that prefer a basic environment are called *alkalinophiles* (e.g., *Vibrio cholerae,* the cause of cholera).
4. *Temperature.* An ideal temperature for pathogens of the human body and most fungi is 98.6° F. Other pathogens prefer extremely warm temperatures (e.g., in hot springs) or colder temperatures (e.g., in ice cream and other dairy products).
5. *Oxygen and gases.* Depending on the type of microorganism, oxygen may be required. Microorganisms that need oxygen are called **aerobes.** Microorganisms that prefer anaerobic (oxygen-free) conditions are called **anaerobes.** Gangrene is the result of anaerobic microorganisms. Many microorganisms require carbon dioxide in their environment as well.
6. *Moisture.* Moisture is necessary for microorganisms to function and grow. Damp environments are ideal for most microorganisms.

Bacilli can form hard-walled capsules (**spores**) and are difficult to kill.

- **Spirilla** are spiral or corkscrew shaped (e.g., Lyme disease, syphilis).

To assist with identification, bacteria can also be grouped according to their staining properties. For example, gram-positive bacteria (*Staphylococcus aureus*) will stain purple and gram-negative bacteria (*Escherichia coli*) will stain red. Those bacteria not accepting a stain are spores, which means they have a protective covering that is resistant to disinfection and require sterilization to destroy them.

Rickettsiae

Rickettsiae are **parasites** that need a host to survive, so they cannot live outside the body. They are smaller than bacteria. They are carried by fleas, lice, ticks, and mites. When these insects bite, the rickettsiae can be transmitted into the human body (e.g., Rocky Mountain spotted fever).

Fungi

Fungi include yeast and molds and are either a single-cell or multicellular microorganisms (e.g., ringworm). They can live

TABLE 31-1
Common Disease-Causing Microorganisms

Type/Organism	Disease
BACTERIA	
Bacillus anthracis	Anthrax
Clostridium tetani	Tetanus (lockjaw)
Salmonella paratyphi*	Food poisoning
Neisseria gonorrhoeae	Gonorrhea
Streptococcus pyogenes	Streptococcal throat infection ("strep")
Staphylococcus aureus	Toxic shock syndrome (and others)
RICKETTSIAE AND SPIROCHETES	
Plasmodium vivax	Malaria
Rickettsia rickettsii	Rocky Mountain spotted fever
Borrelia burgdorferi	Lyme disease
FUNGI	
Trichophyton rubrum†	Tinea pedis (athlete's foot)
Trichophyton and *Microsporum*	Tinea capitis (ringworm of scalp)
Candida albicans	Thrush (candidiasis of mouth)
Histoplasma capsulatum	Histoplasmosis
PROTOZOA	
Entamoeba histolytica	Dysentery
Trichomonas vaginalis	Trichomoniasis
Toxoplasma gondii	Toxoplasmosis
Giardia lamblia	Giardiasis
VIRUSES	
Varicella-zoster virus	Chickenpox, herpes zoster (shingles)
Herpes simplex virus types 1 and 2	Herpes simplex
Human immunodeficiency virus (HIV)	Acquired immunodeficiency syndrome (AIDS)

**Salmonella enteritidis* serotype paratyphi A.
†Also *Trichophyton mentagrophytes* and *Epidermophyton floccosum*.

Protozoa

Protozoa (parasites) are single-celled animals found in contaminated water and decaying material (e.g., amoeba causes dysentery, malaria).

Viruses

Viruses can only reproduce if they are within a living cell. When viruses invade, they take over the cell and alter the genetic materials (e.g., DNA, RNA). They are the smallest of all microorganisms and are only visible when viewed under an electron microscope. Figure 31-2 shows the human immunodeficiency virus (HIV), which causes acquired immunodeficiency syndrome (AIDS). Since viruses (e.g., cold, flu) live within cells, they cannot be destroyed by disinfection methods.

Chain of Infection

Pathogens (disease-causing agents) follow a cycle, or "chain," to transmit disease from one person to another. The most common way for disease to enter the body is through a break in the skin or a compromised body system. Diseases can also enter the body from the nasal mucosa. If the person's immune system is functioning properly, the person may be able to fight off the disease process. Also, if any part of the chain is broken (e.g., microbes or germs are washed away from the hands), the disease cannot spread. If the body's defenses are weak, however, the microbes will invade. When a disease is spread from one person to another, the following chain of events occurs (Figure 31-3):

1. An infected person, known as the **carrier** or **reservoir host,** carries the disease-causing microbes (*causative agent— bacteria, viruses, protozoa, and so forth*).

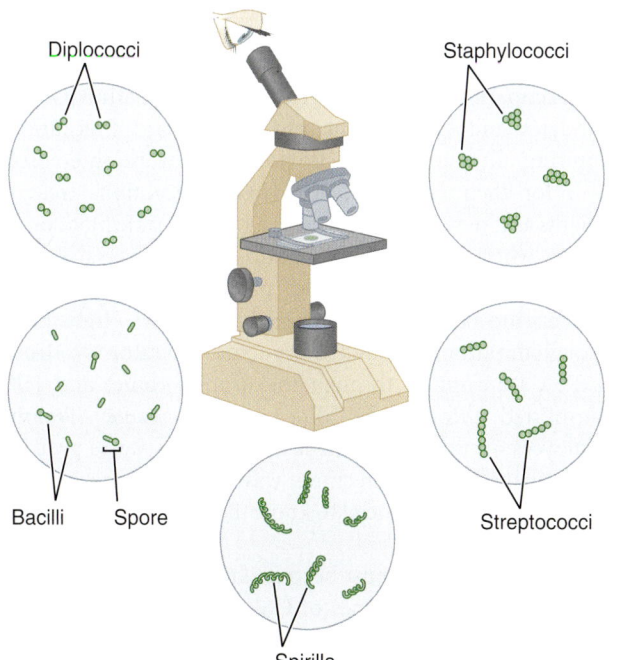

FIGURE 31-1 Bacteria are classified by their shape.

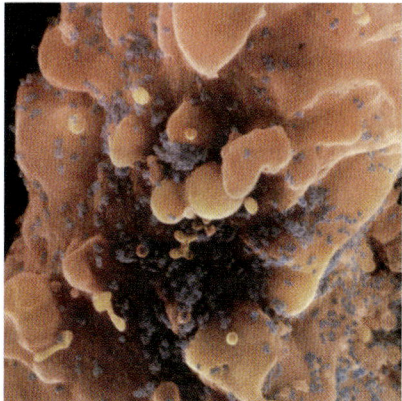

FIGURE 31-2 Human immunodeficiency viruses spread over neighboring cells when released from an infected white blood cell. The viruses are seen here in blue using an electron microscope. (From Thibodeau GA, Patton KT: *The human body in health and disease,* ed 4, St Louis, 2005, Mosby.)

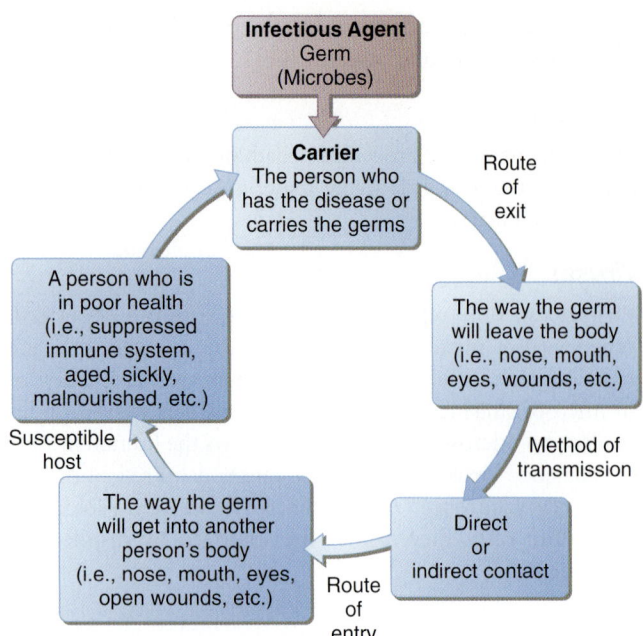

FIGURE 31-3 The cycle ("chain") of infection.

2. The microbes exit the body through urine, feces, saliva, blood, tears, mucous discharge, or other means. The method by which the germs leave the body is called the **route of exit**.
3. Another person is infected through **direct contact** (e.g., person-to-person contact or contact with body secretions) or **indirect contact** with contaminated substances (e.g., food, air, instruments). The mode by which the microbes travel to the susceptible host is called the **method of transmission**.
4. The microbes enter the other person's body through the nose, mouth (airborne—inhalation), eyes, or broken skin. The method by which the germs enter the person's body is called the **route of entry**.
5. The **susceptible host** (person, insect, or animal that can be infected by the microorganism) becomes a reservoir host if infected, and the chain of infection starts again. This is how disease can spread to many people.

Since pathogens grow and reproduce quickly, medical assistants must know how to keep disease-producing organisms from spreading. Hand sanitization is the most important method of preventing the spread of disease in the medical office. Good personal hygiene and the use of disposable gloves when handling potentially biohazardous materials are other methods that can break the chain of infection.

Centers for Disease Control and Prevention

The **Centers for Disease Control and Prevention (CDC)** is part of the U.S. Public Health Service and Department of Health and Human Services. In 1987 the CDC issued guidelines for protecting health care workers from blood-borne infections and HIV. These guidelines became known as "Universal Precautions." The CDC issued new guidelines in 1996 called "Standard Precautions" that apply to all clients and patients receiving treatment at health care facilities. The two most common carriers of microbes in a medical office setting are the staff and equipment used for patient treatments (e.g., stethoscope, examination table). Standard Precautions are designed to reduce the risk of transmission of microorganisms from both recognized and unrecognized sources of infection in a patient care setting (Figure 31-4 and Procedure 31-1).

Standard Precautions must be observed at **ALL TIMES** and for **ALL PATIENTS** regardless of age, gender, and diagnosis. Procedures for Standard Precautions cover the following areas:

- Body fluid classifications (e.g., blood, body fluids except sweat and tears, secretions, excretions, nonintact skin, and mucous membranes).
- Use of protective barriers to protect the health care worker from exposure to infectious materials, including protective eyewear, gowns, boots (shoe covers), masks, head covering, and gloves (Figure 31-5).
- Biohazard waste management, including use of proper containers for disposal of materials.

Infectious waste (any material that has the potential to carry disease) is mandated by law to be separated at the place of origin (e.g., medical office), labeled as to contents, and either decontaminated on site or removed by a commercially licensed biohazard waste management company. Procedure 31-2 gives detailed instructions for properly disposing of biohazardous waste.

Occupational Safety and Health Administration

The **Occupational Safety and Health Administration (OSHA)** mandates and enforces the use of Standard Precautions, requiring all employers to provide a safe working environment for their employees. Universal Precautions treat all patients as if they are infected with a transmissible bloodborne disease, whereas Standard Precautions are Universal Precautions plus transmission-based precautions. Examples of transmission-based diseases are tuberculosis, transmitted through the airborne route; severe acute respiratory syndrome (SARS), transmitted through the droplet route; and HIV, transmitted through the direct contact route. Training employees on the management of hazardous waste products and management of infectious waste is a requirement. All health care employees need to know that their working conditions are safe.

Medical assistants must become familiar with the biohazard symbols and guidelines of OSHA to protect themselves against exposure to bloodborne pathogens (note the symbols in Figure 31-4). Procedures using Standard Precautions are designed to minimize the risk of an infection being

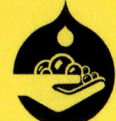
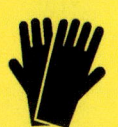
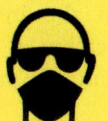
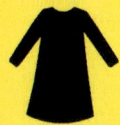

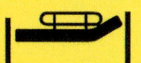
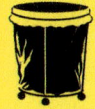
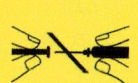

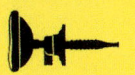
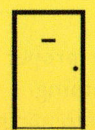

FIGURE 31-4 Standard Precautions for infection control. (Courtesy Brevis Corporation, Salt Lake City, UT.)

PROCEDURE 31-1: Practice Standard Precautions

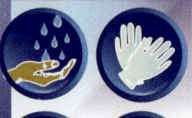
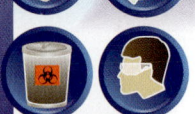

TASK: Identify and demonstrate the application of Standard Precautions in a real or simulated scenario, as assigned by the instructor. Develop an exposure and postexposure control plan or review the medical assisting department's plan and comment on its contents. Sign-off and date.

EQUIPMENT AND SUPPLIES
- Personal protective equipment (PPE): eyewear, gown, boots (shoe covers), mask, gloves
- Current Standard Precautions
- Biohazardous waste container
- Puncture-resistant sharps container

SKILLS/RATIONALE

1. **Procedural Step.** Assemble all necessary equipment.
   Rationale. It is important to have all supplies and equipment ready and available before starting any procedure to ensure efficiency.

2. **Procedural Step.** Select the appropriate PPE for the procedure assigned.
   Rationale. Understanding which barrier precautions must be used for every medical procedure is critical to ensure the highest level of protection is used to reduce the risk of transmission of microorganisms from both recognized and unrecognized sources of infection.

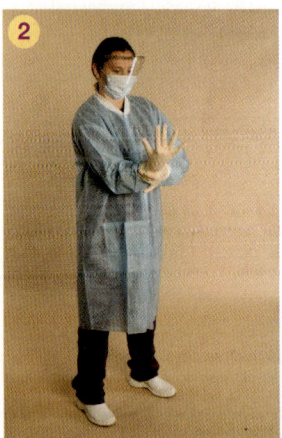

3. **Procedural Step.** Identify body substance isolation (BSI) procedures.
   Rationale. Depending on the type of microorganism suspected or the method of transmission, BSI procedures may be implemented.

4. **Procedural Step.** Apply transmission-based precautions as they apply to the assigned procedure.
   Rationale. Knowing whether the possible transmission of organisms is airborne, droplet, or direct or indirect contact helps to identify the BSI procedures required to prevent contamination.

5. **Procedural Step.** Describe Standard Precautions as they apply to all body fluids, secretions and excretions, blood, nonintact skin, and mucous membranes.

6. **Procedural Step.** Describe to the instructor the importance of continuing education as it relates to practices using Standard Precautions, including the following:
   a. Barrier protection
   b. Handwashing/hand sanitization
   c. PPE
   d. Needles, handling sharps
   e. Cleanup and disposal of contaminated items
   f. Identification and labeling of biohazardous material

7. **Procedural Step.** Develop an exposure and postexposure control plan or review department's and identify exposure control mechanisms in a simulated exposure event. Include the following areas:
   - Barrier protection
   - Environmental protection
   - Housekeeping controls
   - Safety training programs
   - Follow-up
   - Documentation
   - Material safety data sheet (MSDS)

   Rationale. Having a predetermined exposure control plan ensures that all medical personnel are routinely trained in preventing or handling incidents of contamination or have a resource to reference as needed.

8. **Procedural Step.** Demonstrate the proper use of the following exposure control devices:
   - Sharps containers
   - Eyewash stations
   - Fire extinguishers
   - Biohazardous waste containers

   Rationale. Practicing the proper use of each of these exposure control devices helps to ensure their correct use when working in a medical facility.

9. **Procedural Step.** Demonstrate proper documentation of Standard Precautions training.
   Cite the time requirement for the training or retraining record.

Continued

PROCEDURE 31-1 Practice Standard Precautions—cont'd

Rationale. OSHA regulations require proper documentation of all instances of Standard Precautions training for every employee each year as part of the facility's exposure control plan.

10. **Procedural Step.** **Demonstrate knowledge of the basic guidelines approved by OSHA and recommended by the CDC for a postexposure action plan, as follows:**
    a. Wash needle sticks, punctures, or lacerations with soap and water.
    b. Flush splashes to the nose, mouth, or skin with water.
    c. Irrigate eyes with clean water, saline, or sterile irrigants.
    d. Report the incident to the appropriate personnel.
    e. Follow all office exposure control policies regarding follow-up treatment, which may include vaccinations or chemoprophylaxis.

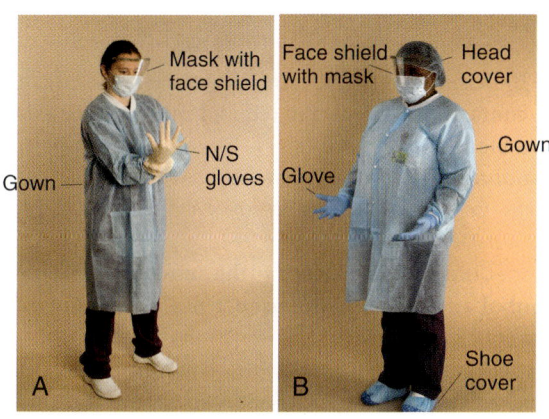

FIGURE 31-5 Personal Protective Equipment. **A,** Gloves, waterproof laboratory coat, and face shield. **B,** Addition of head covering and shoe covers to the PPE.

transmitted and thus protect the patient and the health care worker.

OSHA's *Occupational Exposure to Bloodborne Pathogens Standard* (1992) mandates that employers do the following (Box 31-2):

1. Develop an **exposure control plan** and provide annual training for all employees who perform tasks involving potential occupational exposure to bloodborne pathogens.
2. Implement **engineering controls** and **work practice controls**.
3. Provide employees with and train employees in the use of **personal protective equipment** (**PPE**). Depending on the type of practice, each employee may require specific PPE, which the employer must supply.
4. Follow established procedures for record keeping and reporting of all **exposure incidents,** including follow-up measures.
5. Communicate potential hazards to employees with the use of signs and labels.

PATIENT-CENTERED PROFESSIONALISM

- Why is it important for the medical assistant to understand infection control methods?
- How do infection control methods protect both employees and patients?
- Why must the medical assistant know the chain of infection?
- How would you describe the working relationship between the CDC and OSHA?

MEDICAL ASEPSIS

Medical asepsis is the process of making an area clean and free of infection-causing microorganisms. Procedures that involve body parts that are not normally "sterile" require medical asepsis (also called the "clean" technique) and not sterile asepsis. By following the guidelines established by the CDC, medical assistants can reduce the spread of infection. This protects both themselves and their patients. Medical aseptic techniques are designed to promote cleanliness and prevent contamination.

As mentioned, normal flora or resident flora refers to microorganisms on the epidermis and deeper layers of the skin that are usually nonpathogenic. **Transient flora** refers to microorganisms that grow on the surface of the skin and are picked up easily by the hands. These transient microorganisms can be pathogenic. The use of aseptic techniques in the medical office reduces the transfer of pathogens (Box 31-3). Hand hygiene and the use of gloves are important parts of medical asepsis.

Handwashing

One of the most effective ways to reduce pathogenic transmission is through frequent handwashing. Frequency, soap, friction, and warm running water are all necessary components of handwashing for effective infection control. Regular soap is sufficient, but the use of an antimicrobial soap is preferred for medical asepsis if contact with body fluids has occurred (Figure 31-8 and Procedure 31-3).

Text continued on p. 648

PROCEDURE 31-2 Properly Dispose of Biohazardous Materials

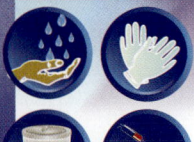

TASK: Identify waste classified as biohazardous and select appropriate containers for disposal. Assemble all equipment and demonstrate disposal of actual or simulated waste, following exposure control guidelines.

EQUIPMENT AND SUPPLIES
- Personal protective equipment (PPE)
- Current Standard Precautions
- Biohazardous waste container
- Sharps container

SKILLS/RATIONALE

1. **Procedural Step. Assemble all necessary equipment.**
   Rationale. It is important to have all supplies and equipment ready and available before starting any procedure to ensure efficiency.

2. **Procedural Step. Select the appropriate PPE for cleaning a blood spill.**
   Rationale. Understanding which barrier precautions should be used in every medical procedure is critical to ensure the highest level of protection.

3. **Procedural Step. Identify waste classified as "biohazardous."**
   a. Any item contaminated with blood or body fluids must be discarded in an appropriately labeled "biohazardous waste" container.

   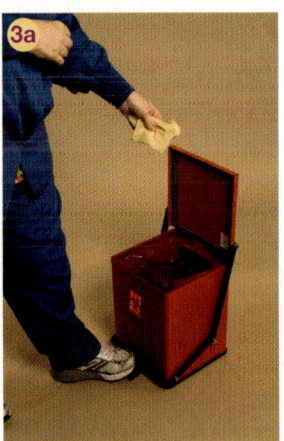

   b. All items used for a medical procedure but not saturated with blood or body fluids may be disposed of in regular waste containers (e.g., cotton ball with a small drop of blood).
   c. All sharp implements, such as needles, scalpel blades, and glass slides, must be discarded in a puncture-resistant sharps container.
   d. Biohazardous waste and puncture-resistant sharps containers are typically red and must be labeled with a biohazard symbol.
   Rationale. Selecting the appropriate container for disposal, for sharps, for general waste, and for laboratory specimens is critical to maintain infection control.

4. **Procedural Step. Identify the universal biohazard symbol and describe the proper use of the biohazardous spill cleanup kits.**
   Prepackaged kits are available to manage a variety of biohazardous waste spills. Be sure to check for expiration dates and rotate stock. Also, read the manufacturer's instructions for each kit and routinely provide all personnel with in-service training.
   Rationale. These kits should be purchased and kept on hand in case of biohazard emergencies.

5. **Procedural Step. Explain housekeeping safety controls.**
   a. All chemical containers or potentially hazardous materials containers must be properly labeled. When a label becomes unreadable, the contents of the container must be properly discarded and a new product purchased.
   b. Any spill of blood or body fluids and all counter or patient surfaces must be cleaned with a 1:10 bleach solution. Gloves must be worn during the cleaning and discarded in the appropriate biohazardous waste container on completion.
   c. Containers must never be filled more than two-thirds full. Never retrieve any item from a biohazardous waste container once it has been discarded.
   d. Biohazardous waste containers and puncture-resistant sharps containers must be removed from the medical facility by a commercially licensed biohazard waste management company.

Continued

Infection Control and Asepsis **CHAPTER 31** 645

PROCEDURE 31-2 **Properly Dispose of Biohazardous Materials—cont'd**

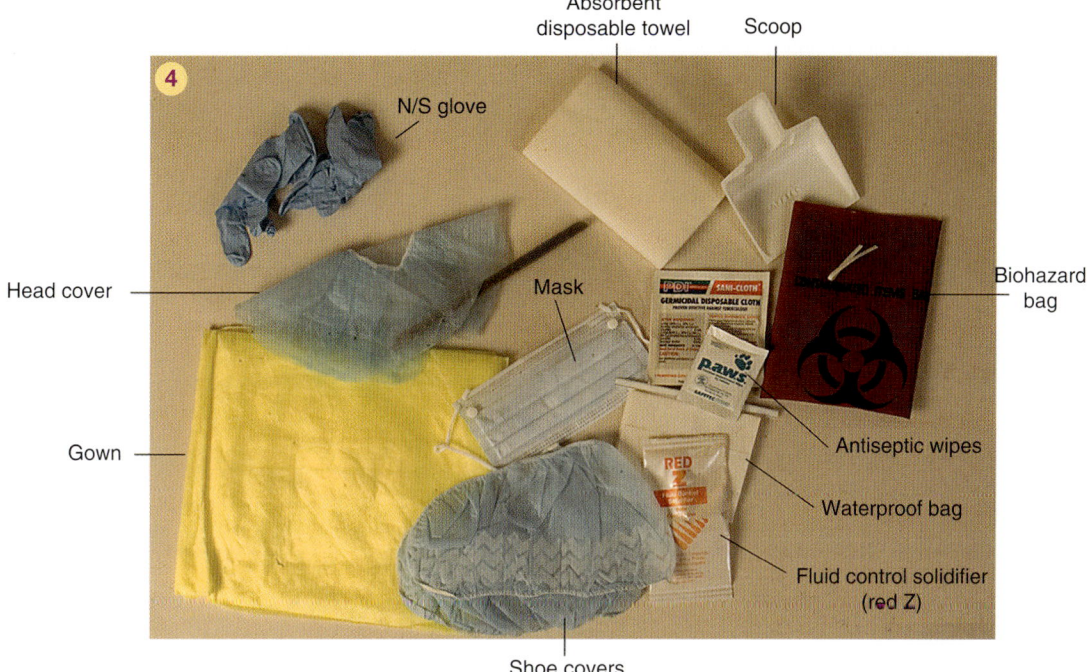

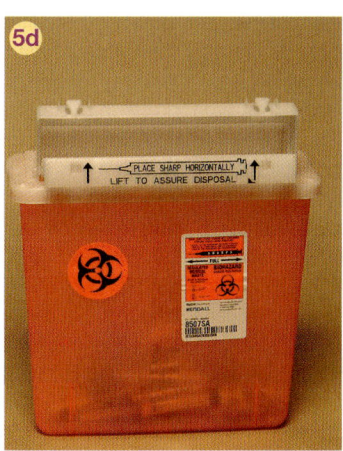

6. **Procedural Step.** Review material safety data sheets (MSDSs).
   a. MSDSs must be obtained and maintained for every chemical used in the medical facility. Many manufacturers supply MSDSs with every purchase of the product. For any chemical that does not come with an MSDS, an Internet search will typically locate one.
   b. Keep all MSDSs in one binder. Label the binder as such, and keep it in one location so that everyone in the office knows where to find it.

7. **Procedural Step.** Document the decontamination of equipment.
   A laboratory safety manual should be kept where all personnel can locate it. All decontamination of equipment must be recorded, including the type of decontamination, date, time, and person(s) who provided the decontamination. A written plan for preventing this type of decontamination in the future is worthwhile.

8. **Procedural Step.** Describe the importance of ongoing safety training.

BOX 31-2

Requirements of Employers: OSHA Bloodborne Pathogens Standard

EXPOSURE CONTROL PLAN
Each medical office must develop a written exposure control plan. The purpose of an exposure control plan is to identify tasks where there is the potential for exposure to blood and other potentially infectious materials. Creating an exposure control plan is considered an administrative control since it involves changing how or when employees do their job.
- A timetable must be published indicating when and how communication of potential hazards will occur.
- The employer must offer employees the hepatitis B vaccine within 10 working days of employment (at no cost to the employee). If employees sign a form to refuse the vaccine, they can change their mind at no cost to the employee.
- The employer must document the steps that should be taken in case of an exposure incident, including a post-exposure evaluation and follow-up, strict record keeping, implementation of engineering controls, provision for PPE, and general housekeeping standards. This plan must be posted in the medical office.
- There must also be written procedures for evaluating the circumstances of an exposure incident.
- Training records must be kept for 3 years.

ENGINEERING CONTROLS AND WORK PRACTICES
The employer must provide engineering controls or equipment and facilities that minimize the possibility of exposure. Engineering controls involve physically changing a work environment. Examples of engineering controls include the following:
- Providing puncture-resistant containers for used sharps.
- Providing needleless systems, eyewash stations, and biohazard labels.
- Providing handwashing facilities that are readily accessible.
- Equipment for sanitizing, decontaminating, and sterilizing.

The employer must also enforce work practice controls. Work practice controls also minimize the possibility of exposure by making sure employees are using the proper techniques while working. Examples include the following:
- Enforcing proper handwashing or sanitizing procedures.
- Enforcing proper technique for using and handling needles to prevent needle sticks.
- Enforcing proper techniques to minimize the splashing of blood.

PERSONAL PROTECTIVE EQUIPMENT
Employers must provide and employees must use PPE when the possibility exists of exposure to blood or contaminated body fluids. The use of PPE equipment is often essential but is generally the last line of defense after engineering controls, work practices, and administrative controls.

This equipment must not allow blood or potentially infectious material to pass through to the employee's clothes, skin, eyes, or mouth. Examples of PPE include the following:
- Gowns/laboratory coats (fluid resistant)
- Face shields
- Goggles
- Gloves
- Head cover and shoe covers

If an employee has an allergy to powder or latex, the employer must provide hypoallergenic or powderless gloves. The employee cannot be charged for PPEs.

EXPOSURE INCIDENT MANAGEMENT
An exposure incident is contact with blood or biohazard infectious material that occurs when doing one's job. When an exposure incident is reported, the employer must arrange for an immediate and confidential medical evaluation. The information and actions required are as follows:
- Documenting how the exposure occurred.
- Identifying and testing the "source" individual, if possible.
- Testing the employee's blood, if consent is granted.
- Providing counseling.
- Evaluating, treating, and following up on any reported illness.

Medical records must be kept for each employee with occupational exposure for the duration of employment plus 30 years.

COMMUNICATION OF POTENTIAL HAZARDS TO EMPLOYEES
A medical assistant will be exposed to hazardous chemicals on the job. OSHA classifies materials in the work environment according to the degree of hazard to health that they impose. In most cases, chemicals handled by medical assistants are not any more dangerous than those used in the home. However, exposure is likely to be greater, concentrations higher, and exposure time longer in certain procedures.

The **"right-to-know" law,** OSHA's hazard communication standard, states that each employee has a right to know what chemicals he or she is working with in the workplace. The right-to-know law is intended to make the workplace safer by making certain that all information regarding chemical hazards is known to the employee. OSHA publishes specific guidelines for method of storage, labeling, handling, cleaning spills, and disposing of the materials. This information is supplied in the **material safety data sheet (MSDS),** a fact sheet divided into nine sections, about a chemical that includes the following information (Figure 31-6):
- Identification of the chemical
- Listing of the physical and health hazards
- Precautions for handling
- Identification of the chemical as a carcinogen
- First-aid procedures
- Name, address, and telephone number of manufacturer

Many MSDS information sheets can be obtained in repositories on the Internet. An MSDS should be updated at least every 3 years. Employers must ensure that all products have an up-to-date MSDS when they enter the workplace.

Potential hazards are also communicated with labels and color. Any containers with biohazard waste must be orange (or reddish orange) and must display the biohazard symbol (Figure 31-7). These labels and colors alert employees to the risk of possible exposure.

PPE, Personal protective equipment.

BOX 31-3

Aseptic Techniques for the Medical Office

1. Sanitize hands before and after patient contact
2. Wear gloves when handling contaminated articles
3. Treat all substances as if they contained pathogens
4. Clean all equipment soon after patient use
5. Discard disposable equipment and supplies soon after patient use
6. Use protective covering (PPE) when there is a possibility of contaminating the uniform
7. Place all dressing material in a waterproof, red biohazard bag

PPE, Personal protective equipment.

MATERIAL SAFETY DATA SHEET (MSDS)

Date of Issue: 4/28/02
Date of Revision: 8/8/03

SECTION 1 IDENTIFICATION

CHEMICAL NAME: Glutaraldehyde	INFORMATION TELEPHONE NUMBER: 1 (800) 733-8690
TRADE NAME: Aldecide	EMERGENCY TELEPHONE NUMBER:
MANUFACTURER'S NAME: Brennan Corporation	1 (800) 331-0766
MFG. ADDRESS: P.O. Box 93	
CITY: Camden STATE: NJ ZIP: 08106	

SECTION 2 COMPOSITION OF INGREDIENTS

CAS NUMBER	CHEMICAL NAME OF INGREDIENTS	PERCENT	PEL	TLV
111-30-8	Glutaraldehyde	2.5	0.2 ppm	0.2 ppm
7732-18-5	Water	97.4	None	None
7632-00-0	Sodium Nitrite	<1	None	None

SECTION 3 PHYSICAL AND CHEMICAL PROPERTIES

BOILING POINT: 212° F	SPECIFIC GRAVITY (H_2O = 1): 1.004
VAPOR PRESSURE (mm Hg): 0.20 at 20° C	VAPOR DENSITY (AIR = 1): 1.1
ODOR: Sharp odor	pH: 7.5-8.5
SOLUBILITY IN WATER: Complete (100%)	MELTING POINT: n/a
APPEARANCE: Bluish-green liquid	FREEZING POINT: 32° F
EVAPORATION RATE: 0.98 (Water = 1)	ODOR THRESHOLD: 0.04 ppm

SECTION 4 FIRE AND EXPLOSION HAZARD DATA

FLASH POINT: Not flammable (aqueous solution)

FLAMMABILITY LIMITS: LEL: n/a   UEL: n/a

EXTINGUISHING MEDIA: n/a (aqueous solution)

SPECIAL FIRE FIGHTING PROCEDURES: n/a

UNUSUAL FIRE/EXPL HAZARDS: None

SECTION 5 REACTIVITY DATA

STABILITY: Stable

CONDITIONS TO AVOID: Avoid temperatures above 200° F.

INCOMPATIBILITY (MATERIAL TO AVOID): Acids and alkalines will neutralize active ingredient.

HAZARDOUS DECOMPOSITION BYPRODUCTS: None

HAZARDOUS POLYMERIZATION: Will not occur

FIGURE 31-6 Material safety data sheet (MSDS). **A,** Front.

MATERIAL SAFETY DATA SHEET

PAGE 2

SECTION 6   HEALTH HAZARD DATA

ROUTE OF ENTRY: **SKIN:** Yes   **EYES:** Yes   **INHALATION:** Yes   **INGESTION:** Yes

SIGNS AND SYMPTOMS OF OVEREXPOSURE:

SKIN: Moderate irritation. May aggravate existing dermatitis.

EYES: Serious eye irritant. May cause irreversible damage.

INHALATION: Vapors may be irritating and cause stinging sensations in the eyes, nose, and throat.

INGESTION: May cause irritation or chemical burns of the mouth, throat, esophagus, and stomach. May cause vomiting, diarrhea, dizziness, faintness, and general systemic illness.

CARCINOGENICITY DATA: **NTP:** No   **AIRC:** No   **OSHA:** No

SECTION 7   EMERGENCY FIRST AID PROCEDURES

SKIN: Wash skin with soap and water for 15 minutes. If irritation persists, seek medical attention.

EYES: Immediately flush with water for 15 minutes. Seek medical attention.

INHALATION: Remove to fresh air. If irritation persists, seek medical attention.

INGESTION: Do not induce vomiting. Give large amounts of water. Seek medical attention.

SECTION 8   PRECAUTIONS FOR SAFE HANDLING AND USE

SPILL PROCEDURES: Ventilate area and wear protective gloves and eye gear. Wipe with sponge, mop, or towel. Flush with large quantities of water. Collect liquid and discard it.

WASTE DISPOSAL METHOD: Container must be triple rinsed and disposed of in accordance with federal, state, and/or local regulations. Used solution should be flushed thoroughly with water into sewage disposal system in accordance with federal, state, and/or local regulations.

PRECAUTIONS IN HANDLING AND STORAGE: Store in a cool, dry place (59-86° F) away from direct sunlight or sources of intense heat. Keep container tightly closed when not in use.

SECTION 9   CONTROL MEASURES

VENTILATION: Adequate ventilation to maintain recommended exposed limit.

RESPIRATORY PROTECTION: None normally required for routine use.

SKIN PROTECTION: Wear protective gloves (butyl rubber, nitrile rubber, polyethylene, or double-gloved latex).

EYE PROTECTION: Wear safety goggles or safety glasses.

WORK/HYGIENE PRACTICES: Prompt rinsing of hands after contact. Handle in accordance with good personal hygiene and safety practices. These practices include avoiding unnecessary exposure.

FIGURE 31-6, cont'd   **B,** Back. (From Bonewit-West K: *Clinical procedures for medical assistants,* ed 7, St Louis, 2008, Saunders.)

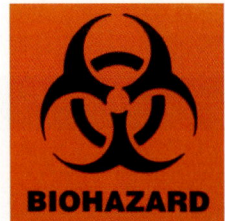

FIGURE 31-7   Biohazard warning label.

In 2002 the CDC published updated guidelines for "hand hygiene" in a health care setting. **Hand hygiene** is a general term that includes the following:
- **Antiseptic hand rub:** Applying an antiseptic (alcohol-containing) hand rub product to all surfaces of the hands. The effective amount varies with each product.
- **Handwashing:** Washing with plain soap and water.
- **Antiseptic handwash:** Washing hands with water and a soap containing an antiseptic agent (e.g., hexachlorophene).
- **Surgical handwash:** Washing with an antiseptic preparation for an extended time, following a certain protocol.

Infection Control and Asepsis **CHAPTER 31** 649

PROCEDURE 31-3 **Perform Proper Handwashing for Medical Asepsis**

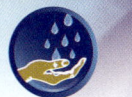

TASK: Prevent the spread of pathogens by aseptically washing hands, following Standard Precautions.

EQUIPMENT AND SUPPLIES
- Liquid antibacterial soap
- Nailbrush or orange stick
- Paper towels
- Warm running water
- Regular waste container

SKILLS/*RATIONALE*

1. **Procedural Step. Remove rings and watch (or push watch up on the forearm so the wrist is clear of any jewelry).**
   Rationale. The wearing of jewelry increases the number of microorganisms on the hands. Moving the watch up on the forearm provides complete access to fingers, hands, and wrists.

2. **Procedural Step. Stand close to the sink, without allowing clothing to touch the sink.**
   Rationale. The sink is considered contaminated. Reaching over the sink increases the risk of becoming contaminated by microorganisms.

3. **Procedural Step. Turn on the faucets, using a clean paper towel.**
   Rationale. The faucets are considered contaminated because they can contain bacteria.

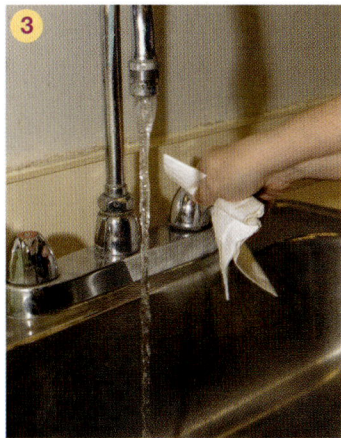

4. **Procedural Step. Adjust the water temperature to warm.**
   Rationale. Water that is too hot or too cold can cause chapping and cracking, therefore providing an entry point for pathogens. Warm water removes less of the protective oils on the hands, thus reducing the chance of chapping and cracking.

5. **Procedural Step. Discard the paper towel in the regular waste container.**
   Rationale. The paper towel is considered contaminated after touching the faucets and cannot be reused.

6. **Procedural Step. Wet hands and wrists under warm running water, and apply liquid antibacterial soap (using a paper towel to activate soap dispenser).** Keep the hands and forearms lower than the elbows at all times, being careful not to touch the inside of the sink, which is also considered to be contaminated.
   Rationale. By keeping the hands and forearms lower than the elbows, water flows from the least to the most contaminated area, rinsing bacteria and debris into the sink.

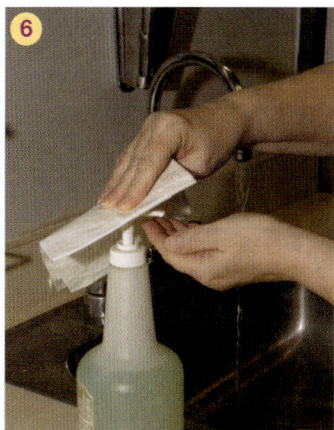

7. **Procedural Step. Work the soap into lather by rubbing the palms together using a circular motion.** Interlace fingers and rub the soap and water between the fingers a minimum of 10 times.
   Rationale. Rubbing the hands together in this manner causes friction, which dislodges microorganisms and other debris from the hands.

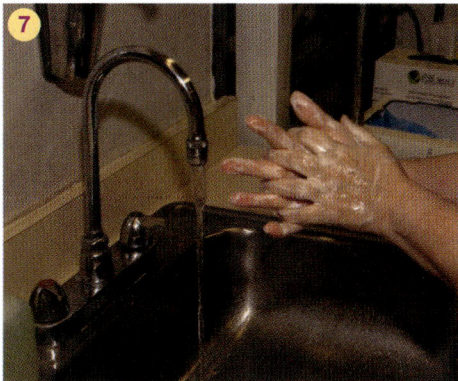

8. **Procedural Step. Clean the fingernails with a nailbrush or an orange stick.**

Continued

PROCEDURE 31-3 Perform Proper Handwashing for Medical Asepsis—cont'd

Rationale. Microorganisms collect underneath the fingernails; using a nailbrush or orange stick removes them without damaging the skin.

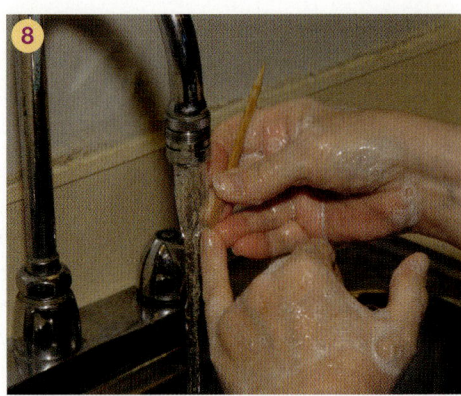

9. **Procedural Step.** Rinse hands thoroughly under warm running water, holding them in a downward position and allowing soap and water to run off the fingertips.
   Rationale. Rinsing hands in this manner allows microorganisms to run off the hands and into the sink rather than going back up the arms.

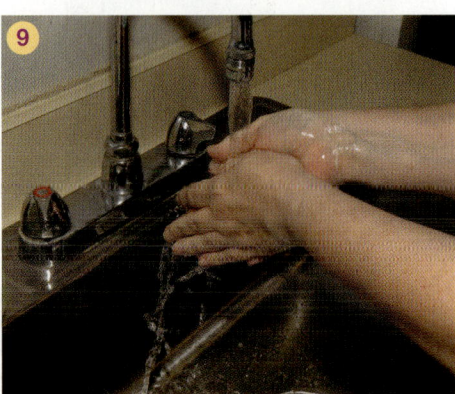

10. **Procedural Step.** Repeat the procedure if hands are grossly contaminated.
11. **Procedural Step.** Dry the hands thoroughly, from the fingers to wrists and forearm, and discard the paper towel.

Rationale. Drying the hands gently prevents them from becoming chapped. Make sure hands are dried completely; damp skin may also cause chapping.

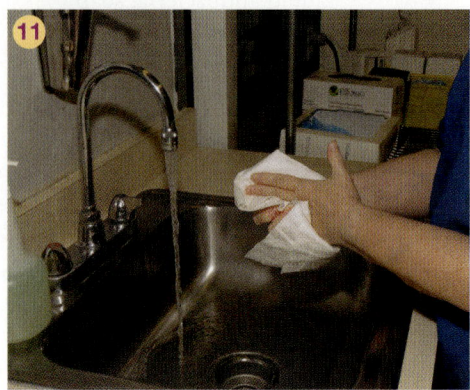

12. **Procedural Step.** Using a dry paper towel, turn the faucets off and discard the towel in the regular waste container.
    Rationale. Using a wet towel to turn off the faucets, which are considered contaminated, may allow for microorganisms to seep through the towel onto now clean hands.

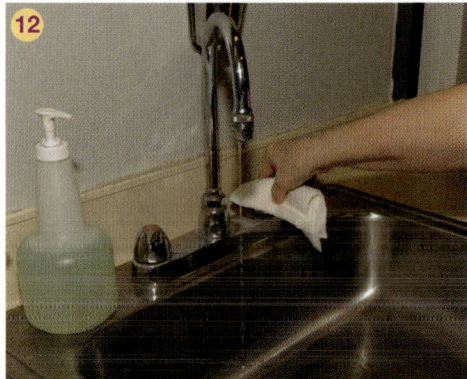

13. **Procedural Step. Clean the area around the sink.**
    Clean the sink area with a fresh paper towel to remove water and debris that may have splashed onto the work area during the handwashing procedure. Appropriately discard the paper towel.
    Rationale. Use several paper towels stacked together so that water and debris do not seep through and recontaminate clean hands.

Alcohol-Based Hand Rubs

The CDC recommends the use of alcohol-based hand rubs by all health care providers during patient care. These rubs significantly reduce the number of microorganisms on the skin, are fast acting (e.g., 15 to 20 seconds), and cause less skin irritation than regular handwashing techniques.

When hands are not visibly soiled, the CDC recommends the use of an alcohol-based hand rub for hand asepsis. Acceptable hand rubs are preparations containing 60% to 95% alcohol. The following are examples of clinical situations when an alcohol-based hand rub can be used:

1. Before and after patient contact.
2. Before applying gloves and after removing gloves.
3. After removal of gloves when minimal contact with body fluids or excretions, mucous membranes, wounds, and dressings has occurred.
4. When moving from a contaminated portion of the body (e.g., mouth) to a clean body site.
5. After contact with medical equipment used during patient care.

The hand rub lotion or gel is applied to the palm of the hand, using enough to wet both hands. Hands are rubbed together, covering the entire surface and including nails and the wrist area, until dry (Procedure 31-4).

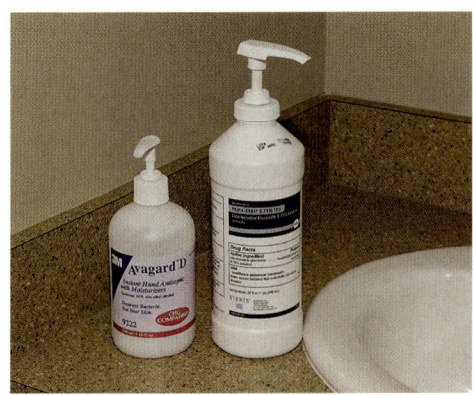

FIGURE 31-8 Antimicrobial soap and alcohol-based hand rubs.

The exact amount needed to reduce the bacteria on the hands varies from product to product. Therefore the manufacturer's instructions should be followed.

Gloves

Nonsterile disposable gloves are used when performing clean procedures (e.g., drawing blood) and when being exposed to contaminated substances (e.g., handling specimens). When applying the nonsterile gloves, you can touch both the inside and the outside of the glove. When removing the gloves after a procedure, you must be careful not to contaminate the hands and clothing (Procedure 31-5).

Gloves reduce hand contamination by an average of 75%. They also prevent cross-contamination and protect patients and health care providers from infection. Gloves must be applied before and changed after each patient encounter.

The medical assistant must remember that the use of gloves does not eliminate the need for hand hygiene, and the use of hand hygiene does not eliminate the need for gloves. Box 31-4 provides key components for hand hygiene compliance.

> **PATIENT-CENTERED PROFESSIONALISM**
>
> • Why must the medical assistant understand the need for proper hand sanitization and the use of gloves in a medical office setting?

PROCEDURE 31-4 **Perform Alcohol-Based Hand Sanitization**

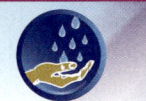

TASK: Prevent the spread of pathogens by applying an alcohol-based hand rub.

EQUIPMENT AND SUPPLIES
- Alcohol-based hand rub containing 60% to 95% ethanol or isopropanol (gel, foam, or lotion)

SKILLS/*RATIONALE*

1. **Procedural Step. Visibly inspect hands for obvious contaminants or debris.**
   Rationale. When hands are visibly dirty, contaminated with proteinaceous material, or visibly soiled with blood or other body fluids, they must be washed with either a nonantibacterial soap and water or an antibacterial soap and water.

2. **Procedural Step. Remove rings and watch or push watch up on the forearm so the wrist is clear of any jewelry.**
   Rationale. The wearing of jewelry increases the number of microorganisms on the hands. Moving the watch up on the forearm provides complete access to fingers, hands, and wrists.

3. **Procedural Step. When decontaminating hands with an alcohol-based hand rub, dispense an ample amount of the product into the palm of one hand.**
   Follow the manufacturer's recommendations regarding the amount of product to use.

4. **Procedural Step. Rub the hands together covering all surfaces of hands and fingers, up to ½ inch above the wrist.**

5. **Procedural Step. Rub hands together until hands are dry, approximately 15 to 30 seconds.**
   NOTE: Alcohol-based hand rubs will not replace the need for sinks or other hand hygiene supplies (e.g., soap, paper towels). Because health care workers may experience a "buildup" of emollients on the hands after repeated use of alcohol-based products, the CDC recommends washing hands with soap and water after 5 to 10 applications of gel.

PROCEDURE 31-5   Apply and Remove Clean, Disposable (Nonsterile) Gloves

TASK: Apply and remove disposable gloves properly.

EQUIPMENT AND SUPPLIES
- Alcohol-based hand rub
- Disposable gloves
- Biohazardous waste container

SKILLS/RATIONALE   STANDARD PRECAUTIONS ARE TO BE FOLLOWED.

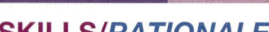

APPLYING GLOVES

1. **Procedural Step. Select the correct size and style of gloves.**
   Gloves should be selected by size so that they fit snugly but are not too tight. Select the style that best fits personal needs, such as latex or vinyl, with or without powder.

2. **Procedural Step. Sanitize hands as described in Procedure 31-3 or 31-4.**
   Rationale. "Gloving" is not a substitute for sanitizing the hands.

3. **Procedural Step. Apply gloves and adjust them to make sure they fit comfortably.**
   Rationale. A fit that is too tight can cause the glove to tear; a fit that is too tight or too loose can make it difficult to perform tasks effectively.

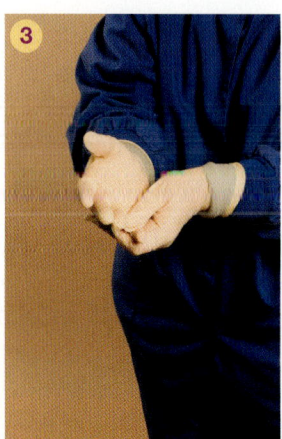

4. **Procedural Step. Inspect the gloves carefully for tears, holes, or punctures.**
   If you find a defect in a glove, you must remove, discard, and replace it. Because the defective glove has not yet come in contact with potentially biohazardous material, it can be disposed of in an ordinary waste receptacle.

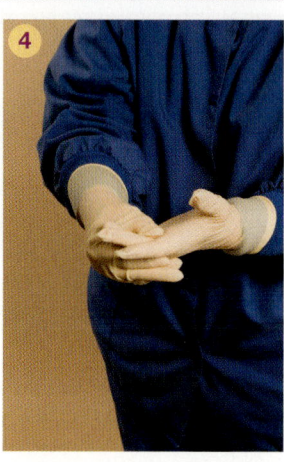

REMOVING GLOVES

You must remove gloves carefully to prevent contamination of your hands by the possible pathogens on the outside of the gloves.

1. **Procedural Step. Grasp the outside of one glove with the first three fingers of the other hand approximately 1 to 2 inches below the cuff.**
   Rationale. This helps to avoid touching a soiled glove to a clean hand. Touching the skin with the dirty glove could contaminate it.

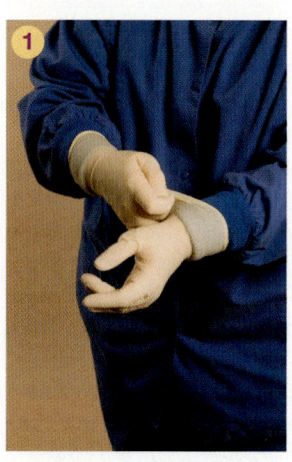

Continued

PROCEDURE 31-5 Apply and Remove Clean, Disposable (Nonsterile) Gloves—cont'd

2. **Procedural Step.** Stretch the soiled glove by pulling it away from the hand, and slowly pull the glove downward off the hand.

   As you pull the glove off, your arm should be extended away from your body, and your hands should be pointed downward. Remove the glove by turning it inside out.

   Rationale. Pulling the outside of the glove with your fingers curled under the cuff will cause it to turn inside out as it is removed. This will confine the contaminants that were on the outside surface to the inside of the removed glove. If the glove has not been torn or damaged during this step, it can touch your skin once it is inside out.

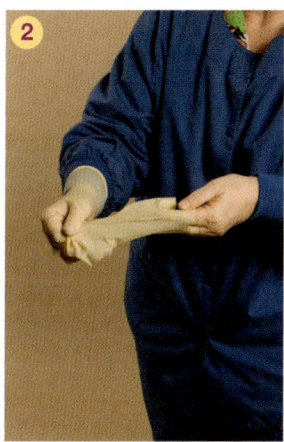

3. **Procedural Step.** As the glove is pulled free from the hand, ball it in the palm of the gloved hand.

   Rationale. Balling the glove into the still-gloved hand prevents loose fingers of the contaminated glove from accidentally touching a clean surface.

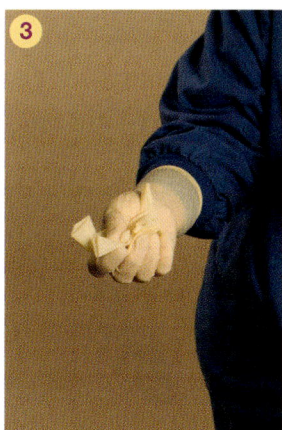

4. **Procedural Step.** Remove the other glove.

   While holding the soiled glove in the palm of the still-gloved hand, place the index and middle fingers of the ungloved hand inside the glove of the gloved hand, and turn the cuff downward, being careful not to touch the outside of the soiled glove.

   Rationale. This ensures that only clean skin touches clean skin.

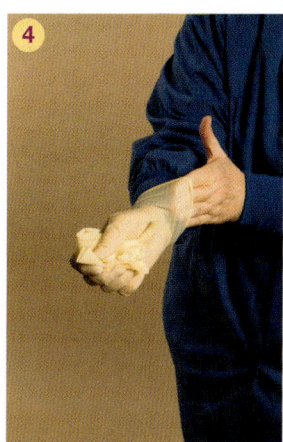

5. **Procedural Step.** Stretch the glove away from the hand, and pull the cuff downward over the hand and over the balled-up glove, turning it inside out with the balled glove inside.

   Rationale. By turning the glove inside out, all contaminated material is enclosed within the glove, reducing the chance of accidental contamination.

6. **Procedural Step.** Carefully dispose of the gloves in a marked biohazardous waste container.

   A red plastic biohazard bag is adequate for glove disposal, because gloves do not have any sharp edges that could puncture the bag.

   Rationale. Grossly contaminated gloves are considered hazardous even after the contamination has been contained to the inside.

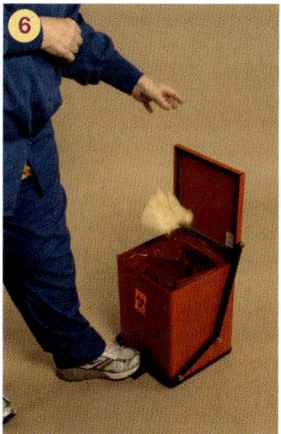

7. **Procedural Step.** Sanitize the hands.

   Always sanitize the hands after a procedure.

   Rationale. Remember that gloving is not a substitute for thorough hand sanitization.

> **BOX 31-4**
>
> ### Components for Hand Hygiene Compliance
>
> There are three important components for proper hand hygiene.
> 1. *Handwashing:* Wash hands with soap and water. Include contact with soap for at least 15 seconds, covering all surfaces (palm, back of hand, fingers, fingertips, and fingernails); rub to produce friction and turn off water without recontaminating the hands.
> 2. *Alcohol-based hand rub:* Use enough to cover all surfaces (palm, back of hand, fingers, fingertips, and fingernails). Rub until dry which ensures sufficient volume has been applied.
> 3. *Gloves:* Remove gloves using correct technique so the hands are not contaminated with a contaminated glove surface.

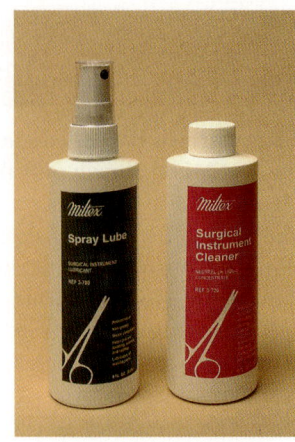

FIGURE 31-9 Commercially available surgical instrument care products.

SURGICAL ASEPSIS

Surgical asepsis is not the same as medical asepsis. **Surgical asepsis** is removing *all* microorganisms, both pathogenic and nonpathogenic, from an object. Surgical asepsis applies to all techniques used to maintain a sterile environment. To be considered **sterile,** an item must be free from all microorganisms, including spores.

Three main techniques are used to prevent the spread of infection in the medical office: sanitization, disinfection, and sterilization.

Sanitization

Sanitization reduces the number of microorganisms on an item and is the lowest level of infection control. Items that only touch the surface of the skin can be sanitized. Think of sanitization as a "good old-fashioned scrubbing." A brush, low-sudsing detergent, and hot water for rinsing are used. Sanitizing does not destroy all microorganisms or spores. Before an item can be disinfected or sterilized, however, it must be sanitized. Failure to remove organic material prevents the steam or chemical from penetrating the surface of the item.

Sanitization is the first step to clean and sterile instruments. The medical assistant should begin to sanitize instruments immediately after an instrument has been used or as soon as possible after use. When items containing contaminated materials (e.g., blood, mucus) are sanitized, the material is first rinsed with *cool* water. Cool water will not coagulate the protein in the contaminated material. A low-sudsing detergent with a neutral pH (Figure 31-9) should be used with a scrub brush to clean the instruments and to loosen any debris (Procedure 31-6). When possible, ultrasonic cleaning should be used for cleaning instruments, since it reduces the risk of injury by eliminating hand scrubbing, which can lead to accidental skin punctures. After scrubbing or ultrasonic cleaning, the instruments must be fully rinsed with clean or distilled water to remove any residue. Dry each instrument with a clean towel or paper towels.

Disinfection

Disinfection is the process of applying an antimicrobial agent to nonliving objects to destroy pathogens and is considered an intermediate level of infection control. Disinfection occurs when scrubbing or soaking an item with a chemical cleaning agent (e.g., 10% bleach solution, alcohol). Disinfection destroys or inhibits the activity of microorganisms, but it has no effect on spores.

Sterilization

Sterilization destroys all microorganisms, including spores. Sterilization occurs by using heat, steam under pressure, gas, ultraviolet (UV) light, or chemicals (Box 31-5). Any device

> **BOX 31-5**
>
> ### Methods of Sterilization
>
> **HEAT**
> **Steam under Pressure**
> - 250° F at 15 lbs of pressure for 20 to 30 minutes, depending on the type of item
>
> **Dry Heat**
> - 320° F for 1 to 2 hours, depending on the type of item
>
> **GAS**
> **Ethylene Oxide**
> - Used for heat-sensitive items
> - Exposure time of 1 to 3 hours
> - Items must be placed in an aerator to remove toxic residue from the packaging and item
>
> **SOLUTION (CHEMICAL AGENTS)**
> - Item(s) submerged in a chemical agent for 4 to 24 hours, depending on the item and agent used
>
> **RADIATION (ULTRAVIOLET)**
> - Used by manufacturers to sterilize items sensitive to steam and chemicals (e.g., plastics)

Infection Control and Asepsis **CHAPTER 31** 655

PROCEDURE 31-6 **Sanitize Instruments**

TASK: Properly sanitize contaminated instruments by cleansing with detergent and water to reduce the number of microorganisms, or by using an ultrasound cleaner.

EQUIPMENT AND SUPPLIES
- Disposable gloves
- Rubber (utility) gloves
- Fluid-resistant laboratory coat
- Laboratory safety glasses
- Stiff nylon brush
- Container to hold instruments
- Instrument cleaning solution, stain remover, and lubricant
- Ultrasonic cleaner
- Material safety data sheet (MSDS) for cleaning solution
- Towel

SKILLS/RATIONALE STANDARD PRECAUTIONS ARE TO BE FOLLOWED.

1. **Procedural Step. Review the MSDS for the chemical agent being used.**
   Rationale. Before beginning to work with any chemicals, first read the MSDS information to avoid injury or illness from improper handling of the chemical. It also provides first-aid information and recommendations if you should come in contact with chemicals.

2. **Procedural Step. Put on gloves, laboratory coat, and safety glasses.**
   Rationale. Personal protective equipment (PPE) must be used whenever there is a chance of contamination from body fluids, as when cleaning contaminated instruments.

3. **Procedural Step. Apply utility gloves over the disposable gloves.**
   Rationale. Utility gloves provide protection against accidental punctures or cuts from sharp instruments and should be worn when sharps are sanitized. Utility gloves also provide added protection to hands and wrists from harsh chemicals.

4. **Procedural Step. Mix cleaning solution for the instruments, following directions on the label. Alternately, prepare the ultrasound cleaning device, following the manufacturer's directions.**
   Rationale. Directions for mixing solutions may vary depending on the manufacturer. It is important to follow the specific directions on the bottle to ensure that the correct strength is used.

5. **Procedural Step. Remove contaminated instruments from the area, and place them in a covered container.**
   NOTE: If the instruments cannot be cleaned immediately after use, they should be soaked in a low-sudsing detergent.

6. **Procedural Step. Prepare instruments for sanitization by first separating out the sharp and delicate instruments.**
   Rationale. Separating sharp instruments from other instruments helps prevent the dulling of sharp edges and lessens the chance of accidental injury. Delicate instruments should also be separated to prevent them from being damaged. Delicate instruments are typically sanitized using the ultrasound cleansing method (see end of procedure).

7. **Procedural Step. Rinse all instruments under cool running water to remove organic material.**
   Instruments should be rinsed under cool to tepid water (approximately 100° to 110° F).
   Rationale. Hemostats and scissors and any hinged or ratcheted instruments must be open when rinsing and washing to allow for the removal of debris. Blood is more easily removed with cool water; hot water coagulates organic material, making it difficult to remove.

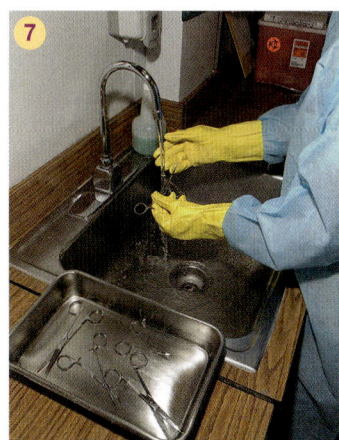

8. **Procedural Step. Using a scrub brush and cleaning solution, loosen any debris on the instruments.**
   a. Be sure to scrub all surfaces, including hinges and ratchets, and to scrub into the serrations.
   b. Remove any stains or rusting as needed with the appropriate chemicals or brush.
   c. Some sudsing of the cleaning solution should occur during this process; this helps to loosen debris and body fluids.
   d. Delicate instruments should be scrubbed carefully to prevent damage and personal injury.

Continued

PROCEDURE 31-6 Sanitize Instruments—cont'd

Rationale. Stains and rust prevent instruments from being free of microorganisms. If these cannot be removed, the instrument must be taken out of circulation and not used.

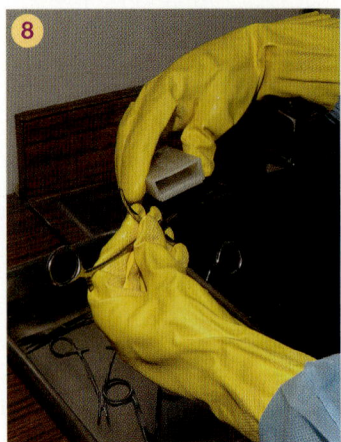

9. **Procedural Step. Rinse the instruments.**
   Using hot water, rinse the instruments to remove all soap and residue; this will allow for adequate sterilization. Allow the instruments to drain as much water as possible, and then place them on several layers of paper towels or a lint-free cloth towel.
   Rationale. Hot water must be used because it dries faster than cold water and helps prevent water spots on the instruments. Leaving soap or residue on the instruments will not allow the steam of autoclaving to penetrate properly to the surface of the instruments.

10. **Procedural Step. Dry each instrument with a paper towel.**
    Place the towel-dried instrument on a dry lint-free towel for additional air drying.
    Rationale. Instruments must be completely dry before wrapping for the autoclave. Dry instruments do not rust, do not form water spots, and do not dilute chemicals used for disinfection after sanitization.

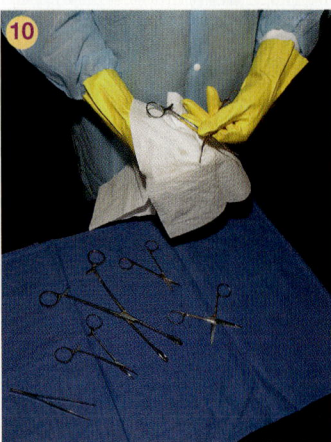

11. **Procedural Step. Dispose of the cleaning solution.**
    Once all instruments have been sanitized, the cleaning solution should be disposed and not reused.

12. **Procedural Step.** Once the instruments are completely dry, inspect them for defects and check for proper working condition.
    If a flaw is apparent, the instrument should be promptly and properly repaired, or discarded if repairs are not possible. A defective instrument should not be used until repairs have been completed. Care when handling instruments prevents problems with improper function on its next use.

13. **Procedural Step. Lubricate hinged instruments.**
    Once instruments have been dried and inspected, lubricate the hinges and ratchets.
    Rationale. Lubricating hinges and ratchets on instruments prolong their use and help them to function better.

14. **Procedural Step.** Discard any contaminated material, such as towels, in the appropriate biohazardous waste container.

15. **Procedural Step.** Remove and dispose of PPE as appropriate.
    NOTE: Instruments are now ready to be wrapped for autoclaving.

ULTRASONIC METHOD

1. **Procedural Step.** Prepare ultrasonic cleaning solution according to the manufacturer's instructions and pour into the machine.

2. **Procedural Step.** Separate the different types of metals (e.g., stainless steel, aluminum).

3. **Procedural Step.** Open hinged instruments and place them in the ultrasonic cleaner, completely covering them with solution.

4. **Procedural Step.** Turn on the ultrasonic machine and set the timer for the recommended period.

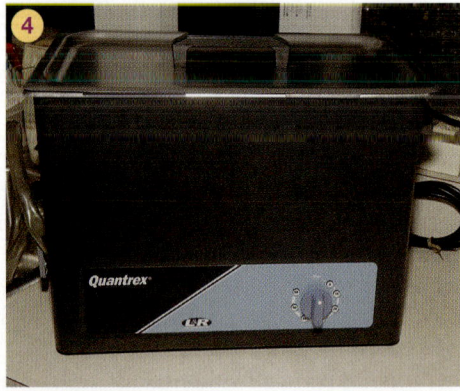

5. **Procedural Step.** Remove the instruments at the end of the cleaning cycle.

6. **Procedural Step.** Change the ultrasonic cleaner according to the manufacturer's instructions, keeping it covered between uses.

7. **Procedural Step.** Rinse instruments with warm water to remove soap residue.
   Rationale. Residue left on the instruments could cause staining of instruments.

8. **Procedural Step.** Dry instruments before sterilization to prevent water spots or rust from forming.

that enters a sterile body cavity (e.g., catheter, probe, or hemostat) and instruments that cut the skin (e.g., scalpel with blade, scissors) must be sterilized.

Gas autoclaves and chemical baths are used to sterilize equipment that would be damaged by heat and moisture. Procedure 31-7 explains the process of properly sterilizing an item using a chemical agent.

Steam Sterilization

An **autoclave** is used to produce steam under pressure. Steam sterilization is the primary method used to sterilize instruments in the medical office. Autoclaves can be automatic or manual (Figure 31-10).

Steam under pressure destroys microorganisms by causing them to explode. The primary conditions that must be met for steam sterilization to occur include the following:

- Pressure of 15 lbs
- Temperature of 250° to 270° F
- Time period per manufacturer's recommendations, depending on size of surgical pack or instruments

---

FOR YOUR INFORMATION

HOW DOES AN AUTOCLAVE WORK?

The outer chamber of the autoclave jacket creates a buildup of steam that is forced into the inner chamber. Items to be sterilized are placed in the inner chamber. When 15 lbs of pressure has been reached, the temperature will be maintained at 250° to 270° F. The autoclave has a pump that operates to remove all air from the chamber; only after all the air is removed can the correct pressure and temperature be reached. The items are then exposed to these conditions for a prescribed time.

The drying cycle is as important as the sterilizing cycle. When time has expired, the pressure is vented and the door opened ½ to ¾ inch to aid the drying process. Wetness can cause a break in sterility because moisture allows bacteria to grow. When dried, the items are carefully removed for storage.

The following ways are used to determine whether the items were exposed to conditions necessary for sterility:

- Disposable paper pouches usually have a thermal or **chemical indicator** embedded in the paper that changes colors when the package has been exposed to steam pressure and the correct temperature.
- A **sterilization strip,** or indicator strip, with an embedded chemical indicator is placed in the center of a dense pack. When the strip changes color, it signifies that the center of the pack was exposed to conditions necessary for sterility: pressure, temperature, and time (Figure 31-11, A).
- If a wrapper is used, **autoclave tape** is used to seal the package (Figure 31-11, C). Stripes on the tape have a chemical indicator that will change color when exposed to the correct steam pressure and temperature.
- The use of a **biological indicator** is the only true indicator that an item is sterile (Figure 31-12). A biological indicator is processed in the autoclave and then either sent to an outside laboratory to obtain results or processed in the office by using an incubation process. Successful test results identify that all bacterial spores have been killed.

Instruments used immediately can be placed in a perforated tray and sterilized unwrapped. A towel should be placed under the instruments to absorb moisture. Jars must be placed on their sides, and liquids are done separately.

Procedure 31-8 demonstrates how to wrap items correctly for the autoclave. Do not wrap items too tightly since inadequate sterilization may occur from improper wrapping.

Procedure 31-9 explains how to load an autoclave properly for the sterilization process. Providing adequate space between packs allows for proper steam circulation and drying. Overloading the sterilizer may cause sterilization failure.

Items that are packaged for sterilization can be used immediately or stored for later use. Items *flash sterilized (sterilized but not wrapped) must be used immediately.* How the item is wrapped and stored is also important. The medical assistant must be careful not to contaminate the article when opening the wrapping.

AUTOCLAVE MAINTENANCE

Daily cleaning of the autoclave requires the inner chamber and door gaskets to be wiped with a damp, lint-free cloth. Monthly, a mild detergent should be used to clean the autoclave, and it should be rinsed to remove any residue.

Wrapping Items for Sterilization

The items to be sterilized may be wrapped to maintain sterility. This is accomplished by using disposable paper wrappers, disposable paper pouches, or two 140-thread–count muslin wrappers. The wrapping material chosen must be permeable to steam (i.e., it must allow steam to pass through). The wrapping material must also be strong enough to hold together during the processing and handling stages.

FOR YOUR INFORMATION

HOW DOES A BIOLOGICAL INDICATOR WORK?

The biological indicator is a container with live spores that is placed in a load of items for sterilizing. It is placed in an area that steam may not penetrate if the autoclave is not working properly or if the items are improperly loaded. The front area by the door, the bottom shelves, and the back of the autoclave by the vent are all areas that may not receive the correct amount of steam. Once the biological indicator has been processed, it is usually sent to an independent laboratory with a control sample for testing. Lack of growth is a sign that the autoclave was functioning properly. The CDC recommends that an autoclave be tested using a biological indicator at least weekly.

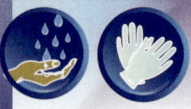

PROCEDURE 31-7 Perform Chemical Sterilization

TASK: Properly sterilize items using a chemical agent.

EQUIPMENT AND SUPPLIES
- Chemical agent, disinfectant
- Material safety data sheet (MSDS) for disinfectant solution
- Fluid-resistant laboratory coat
- Laboratory safety glasses
- Disposable gloves
- Utility gloves
- Stainless steel or glass container with cover
- Towels
- Articles to be disinfected
- Sterile transfer forceps

SKILLS/RATIONALE

STANDARD PRECAUTIONS ARE TO BE FOLLOWED.

1. **Procedural Step.** Review the MSDS for the chemical agent being used.
   Rationale. Before beginning to work with any chemicals, first read the MSDS information to avoid injury or illness from improper handling of the chemical. It also provides first-aid information and recommendations if you should come in contact with chemicals.

2. **Procedural Step.** Apply personal protective equipment (PPE).
   Rationale. PPE must be used whenever there is a chance of contamination from body fluids, as when cleaning contaminated instruments.

3. **Procedural Step.** Apply utility gloves over the disposable gloves.
   Rationale. Utility gloves provide protection against accidental punctures or cuts from sharp instruments and should be worn when sharps are sanitized. Utility gloves also provide added protection to hands and wrists from harsh chemicals.

4. **Procedural Step.** Mix disinfectant solution following directions on the label.
   Rationale. Directions for mixing solutions may vary depending on the manufacturer. It is important to follow the specific directions on the bottle to ensure that the correct strength is used.

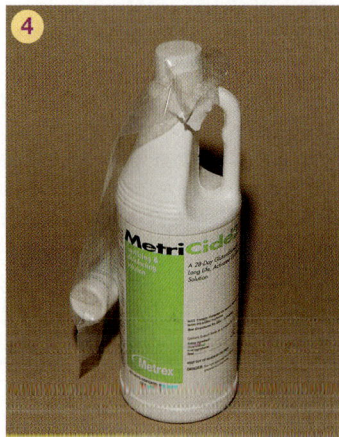

5. **Procedural Step.** Check the expiration date.
   Rationale. Loss of potency may result if solution is beyond expiration date.

6. **Procedural Step.** Pour sufficient quantity of disinfectant solution into a stainless steel or glass container with an airtight cover to allow for complete immersion of items to be disinfected.

Continued

Infection Control and Asepsis **CHAPTER 31** 659

PROCEDURE
31-7 **Perform Chemical Sterilization—cont'd**

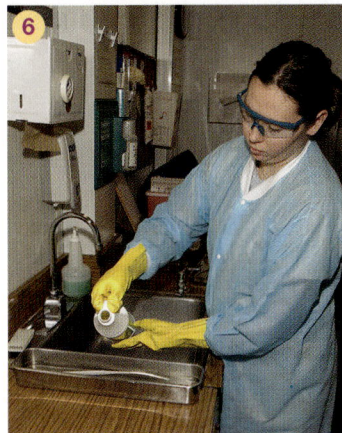

7. **Procedural Step.** Gather items to be disinfected. Prepare instruments by first separating out the sharp and delicate instruments.
   Rationale. Separating sharp instruments from other instruments helps prevent the dulling of sharp edges and lessens the chance of accidental injury. Delicate instruments should also be separated to prevent them from being damaged.
8. **Procedural Step.** Sanitize the items by following the steps in Procedure 31-6.
9. **Procedural Step.** Dry the items.
   Rationale. Placing items into the solution while still wet will dilute the solution and decrease its effectiveness.
10. **Procedural Step.** Place the items in the disinfectant chemical solution, making certain that the instruments are completely covered in the chemical agent.
    Rationale. Completely covering all items allows the chemical agent to reach all parts of the instrument.
11. **Procedural Step.** Place the airtight lid on the container.
    Rationale. Keeping the container covered prevents the escape of toxic fumes into the environment and prevents evaporation of the solution.

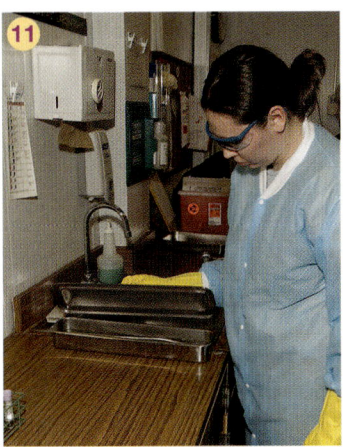

12. **Procedural Step.** Disinfect the items for the required time.

The length of time may vary with the type and strength of disinfectant being used. Exposure time may be from 20 minutes to 3 hours or longer. For example, items must be soaked for 1 to 4 hours in Cidex solution.
Rationale. The required time allows for the complete destruction of all microorganisms.
NOTE: Never add additional instruments to those already soaking since the length of disinfecting time will be affected.

13. **Procedural Step.** Before using them, remove the items from the chemical agent and rinse completely.
    This may be accomplished by lifting a stainless steel tray that fits inside the container out of the container and rinsing the items under running water or in a sterile, distilled-water bath.
    Rationale. This removes residue from the items, which could cause irritation to the tissues of the patient.

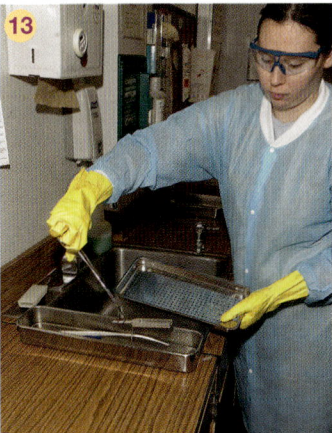

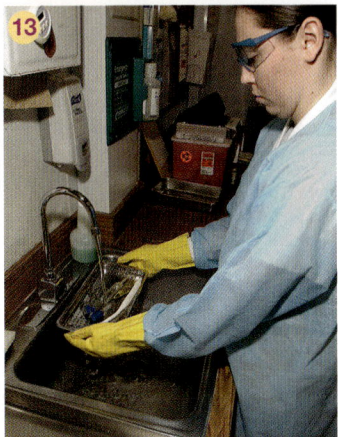

14. **Procedural Step.** Using sterile transfer forceps, remove the items from the tray for use.
15. **Procedural Step.** Dry items before use with a sterile towel.
16. **Procedural Step.** Remove gloves and sanitize the hands.
    NOTE: Change the solution in the container every 7 to 14 days or as recommended by the manufacturer.

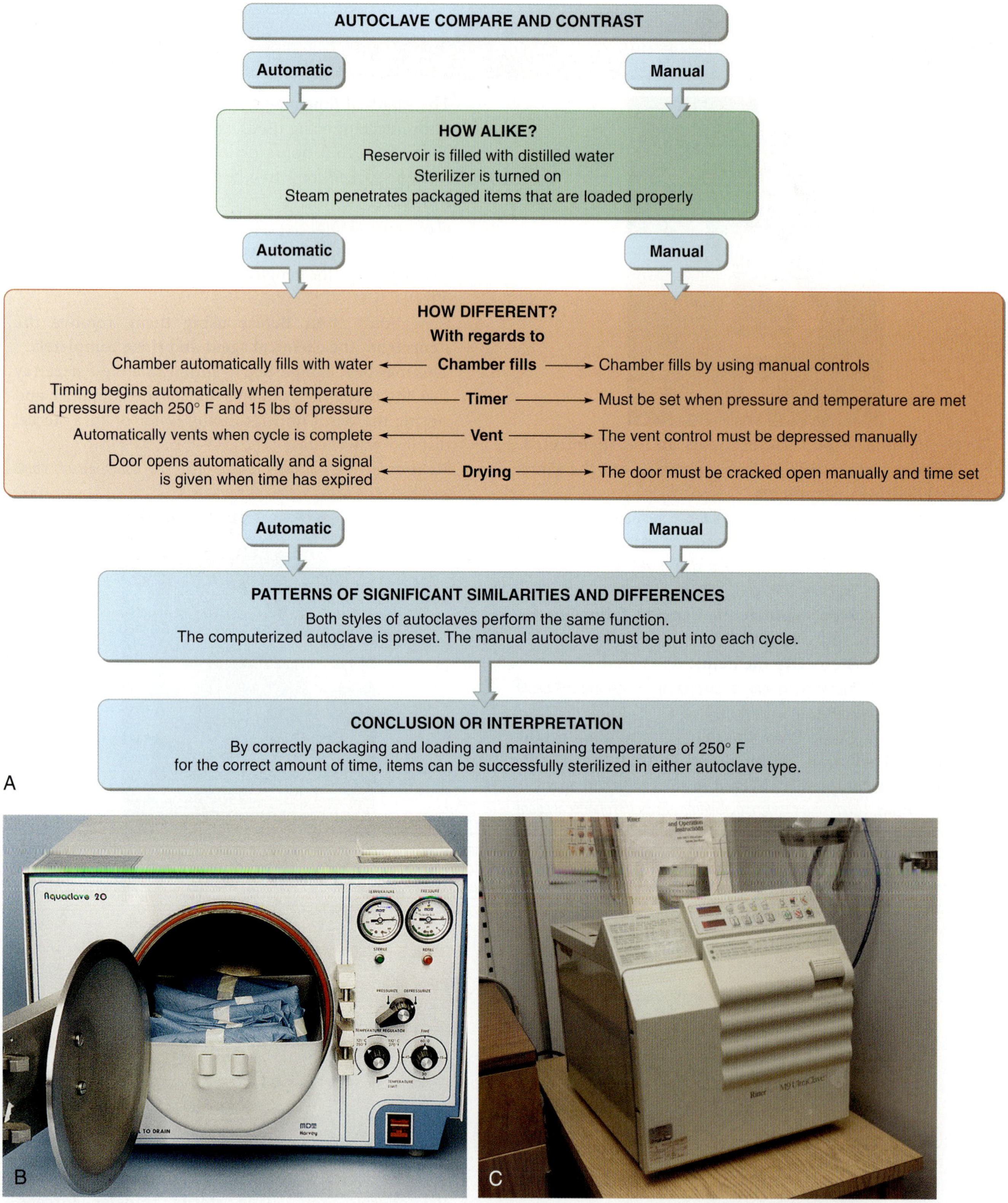

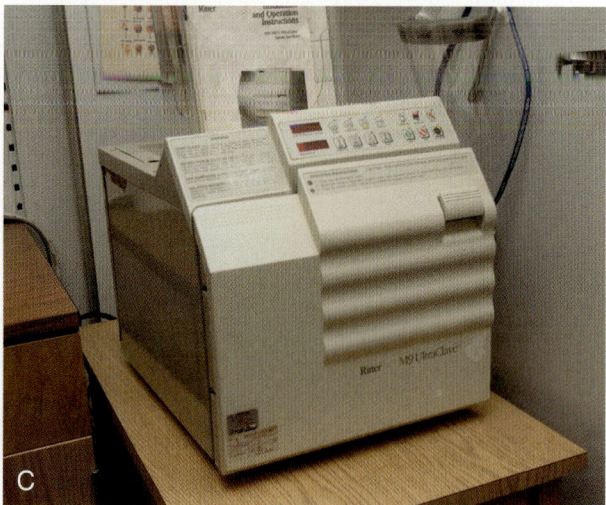

FIGURE 31-10 **A,** Comparison of automatic and manual autoclave operation. **B,** Manual autoclave: Aquaclave. **C,** Automatic autoclave.

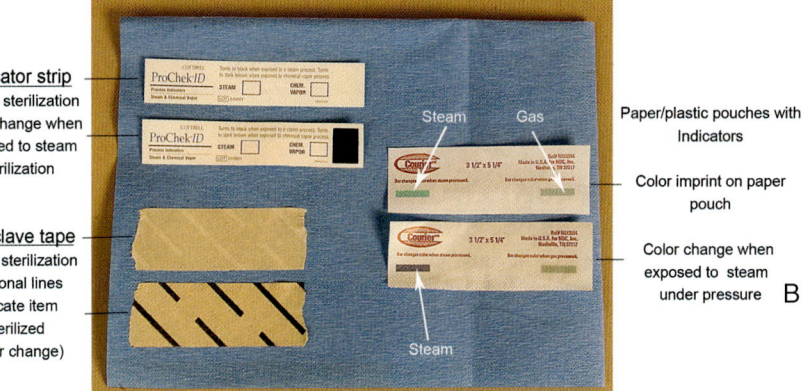

FIGURE 31-11 A, Sterilization strips, or chemical indicator strips, contain a heat-sensitive dye and change color when the sterilizer has maintained the proper parameters (e.g., correct temperature, pressure for the cycle, and for a certain period of time). **B,** Chemical indicator embedded in paper pouch. **C,** Autoclave tape. *Top,* Before the sterilization process. *Bottom,* Diagonal lines appear during autoclaving and indicate that the wrapper article has been sterilized.

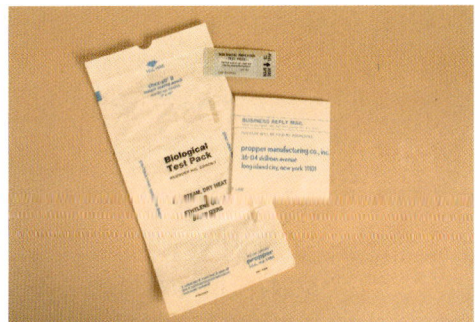

FIGURE 31-12 Biological indicator. A biological test pack includes two spore tests that are sterilized and one spore control that is not sterilized.

TABLE 31-2
Recommended Shelf Life of Sterilized Items Stored by Various Methods

Storage Method	Expiration
Linen wrapped, four-layer thickness	30 days
Paper	30 days
Nonwoven fabric	30 days
Linen wrapped, with tape-sealed dustcover	3 months
Plastic/paper combination, heat sealed	3 months
Plastic film, tape sealed	3 months
Linen wrapped, with heat-sealed dustcover	6 months
Plastic film, heat sealed	6 months to 1 year

Storage

Instruments can be prepared, sterilized, and stored for a certain period (30 days to several months) before use. The length of time an item can be stored (shelf-life) depends on the following (Table 31-2):
- Type of packaging material used.
- Number of thicknesses used.
- Number of times the item will be handled before being taken to the sterile field.
- Type of shelf where the item is stored (open or closed).
- Environment in the storage area (temperature, humidity, cleanliness).
- How the package is sealed (tape or heat seal).

When storing items, the sterilized package with the oldest date is placed in front. It is true that an item remains sterile until the integrity of the package is broken. For the purpose of providing guidelines, however, paper-wrapped or muslin-wrapped items remain sterile for 30 days, and paper and plastic pouches or tubing are considered sterile for 6 months to 1 year. Storage shelves should be dry, dust free, and covered. If a package is considered "nonsterile" (e.g., outdated, broken seal), the items must be totally reprocessed (resanitized or redisinfected) and rewrapped and resterilized.

PATIENT-CENTERED PROFESSIONALISM

- *Why is it important for the medical assistant to follow each part of the asepsis process when preparing an item for use in a procedure?*

CONCLUSION

The first chapter in the Clinical Medical Assisting section of this text covers infection control and asepsis because this knowledge is necessary before learning about the clinical procedures and duties of the medical assistant that may involve exposure to potentially hazardous materials and pathogens. Protecting patients and staff from the spread of disease is critical in a medical office. Medical assistants need to understand fully the guidelines of infection control and the medical and surgical aseptic techniques that can help them break the chain of infection.

By following the policies and procedures of the medical facility and adhering to the Standard Precautions issued by the CDC and mandated by OSHA, medical assistants help ensure that the medical office is a safe and healthy environment for all patients, workers, and visitors.

PROCEDURE 31-8 Wrap Instruments for the Autoclave

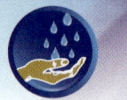

TASK: Wrap sanitized instruments for autoclaving.

EQUIPMENT AND SUPPLIES
- Autoclave wrapping material
- Autoclave tape
- Sterilization indicator strip
- Sterilization pouch
- Waterproof pen

INSTRUMENT PACK
- Ten 4 × 4–inch gauze squares
- 1 forceps
- 1 Kelly hemostat
- 1 S/S (sharp/sharp) operating scissors
- Or items designated by instructor

INDIVIDUAL PACK
- 1 small rake retractor
- Or items designated by instructor

SKILLS/RATIONALE

STANDARD PRECAUTIONS ARE TO BE FOLLOWED.

1. **Procedural Step.** Sanitize the hands.
2. **Procedural Step.** Assemble equipment and supplies.
   NOTE: For this procedure you will be wrapping a pair of forceps, a pair of operating S/S scissors, a pair of Kelly hemostats, and ten 4 × 4 gauze squares in autoclave wrap (instrument pack), as well as a small rake retractor (individual pack) in a sterilization pouch, or items designated by your instructor.

INSTRUMENT PACK
3. **Procedural Step.** Place the appropriate-size wrappers for the instruments pack item on a clean, flat surface in a diamond-shaped position.

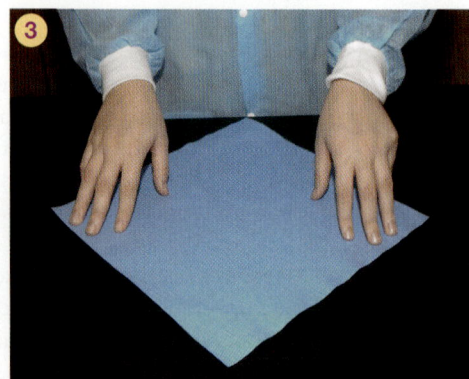

4. **Procedural Step.** Place the items for the instrument pack in the center of the wrapping material.
   If an instrument is being wrapped and it has a moveable joint, it should be opened. Place a 4 × 4 gauze square folded over the cutting edges of the scissors.
   Rationale. If instruments are closed, the steam may not seep into the hinges for complete sterilization. Instruments with sharp edges should have the edges covered with gauze squares to prevent the puncture of the package or injury to someone handling the pack. Placing a 4 × 4 gauze square over the cutting edge of the scissors also protects the instrument from becoming dull or damaged.

5. **Procedural Step.** Place a sterilization strip in the center of the pack (the most difficult place for steam to reach).
   NOTE: You should always check the expiration date of the sterilization strip so you are assured that the strip will work as expected.
   Rationale. Placing a sterilization strip in the center of the pack indicates that the pack has been through the sterilization process if the strip has changed to the correct color according to the manufacturer.

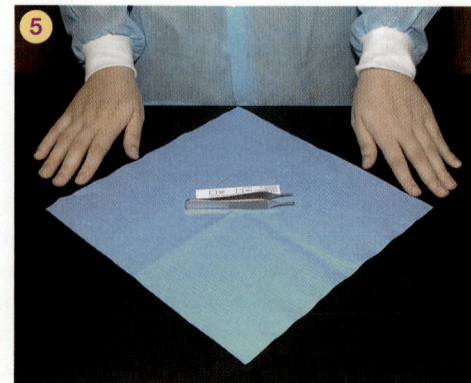

6. **Procedural Step.** Position the items in the pack just below the center of the wrap, with the longest part pointing toward the two side corners.

Continued

Infection Control and Asepsis **CHAPTER 31** 663

| PROCEDURE 31-8 | **Wrap Instruments for the Autoclave—cont'd** |

7. **Procedural Step. Wrap the instruments.**
   Starting with one piece of autoclave wrapping material, wrap the instrument pack as follows:
   a. Starting with the bottom flap, bring the wrapping material up snug against the instruments, then double-back 1 to 2 inches, leaving a flap. This "flap" will be used later to open the pack without touching and contaminating the instruments.

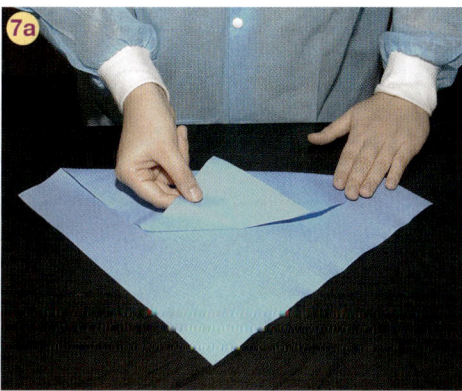

   b. Fold each corner in toward the center, one corner at a time, then double-back 1 to 2 inches, leaving a flap as you did with the bottom.

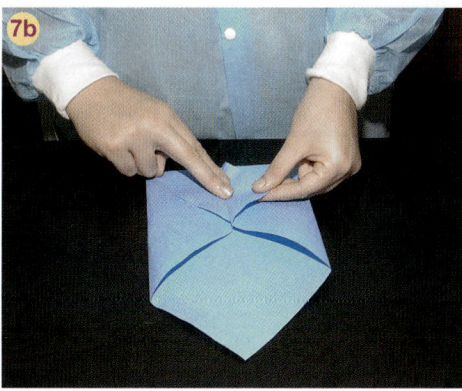

   c. Fold the remaining top edge of the pack in the same manner as the sides, doubling back 1 to 2 inches.
   d. Flip the now-squared pack forward so that only the remaining flap is visible. Fold the "flap" back. This completes the inside wrap.

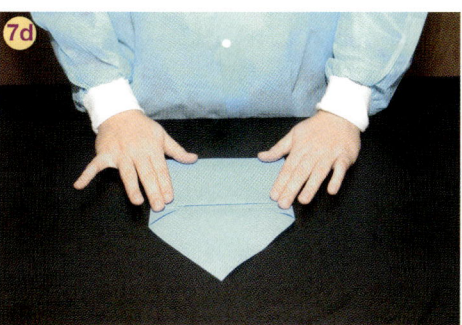

8. **Procedural Step. Repeat the wrapping process.**
   Repeat the process with a second piece of autoclave wrapping material in the same manner as the first layer, or wrap. This time, when you get to the last flap, fold it so it is on the outside of the pack; this flap will be used to tape the pack closed.
   Rationale. All instrument packs must be "double wrapped" to ensure sterility. The package should be wrapped firmly enough to allow for handling but loosely enough to allow for the penetration of steam.

9. **Procedural Step. Secure the package with autoclave tape.**
   Tear off a piece of tape from the roll that is long enough to secure the package. Fold a flap of tape on itself at one end to allow for easier removal of the tape once the package has been autoclaved.
   Rationale. Autoclave tape is like masking tape with stripes that change color when the package has been exposed to steam. This makes it possible to distinguish easily between packs that have been autoclaved and those that have not. Autoclave tape is not an indication of whether the pack is sterile, only that it has been through the sterilization process.

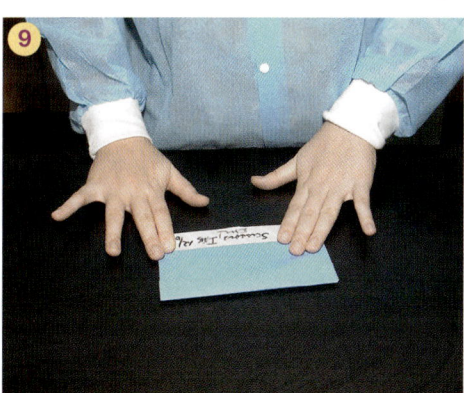

10. **Procedural Step. Label the autoclave tape.**
    With the waterproof pen, label the package with the following information:
    a. Instrument(s) enclosed or type of package (e.g., minor surgery).
    b. Date of autoclaving.
    Rationale. The date is important because wrapped sterile packs only maintain their sterility for 1 month. Any pack older than 1 month must be rewrapped and resterilized.
    c. Initials of the person who prepared the package.

11. **Procedural Step. Set the package aside until it is time to autoclave.**

INDIVIDUAL INSTRUMENT

12. **Procedural Step. Label the pouch.**
    With a waterproof pen, label the pouch with the name of the instrument, the date of sterilization, and the initials of the person wrapping the pack.
    Rationale. The package must be labeled before placing the instrument inside the pouch so that the pouch is not torn when labeling with the pen.

Continued

PROCEDURE 31-8 Wrap Instruments for the Autoclave—cont'd

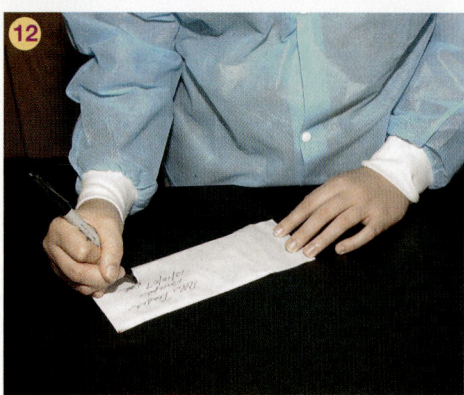

13. **Procedural Step.** Place the instrument carefully into the sterilization pack with the handles on the sealed edge or peel-apart side.
    a. Place the instrument in the pouch with the handle end first.
    Rationale. The handle end must be inserted into the pouch first because it is the opposite end of the pouch that will be opened after it is sterilized. This will allow the instrument to be appropriately grasped by its handle.
    b. Seal the pouch.
    Rationale. Depending on the style of the pouch, use the appropriate method of closure. Placing the handles on the edge that opens will allow the instrument to be handed in its functional position (the correct position for the physician to remove from the pack while maintaining sterility).
    - *Adhesive closure.* Peel the paper strip away to expose the adhesive. Fold the flap over, and press firmly to seal the paper to the plastic.
    - *Autoclave tape.* Fold the flap of the open end over to the plastic. With a piece of autoclave tape, seal the edge and around each corner.
    - *Thermal sealer.* Place the edges of the pouch under the heat bar, and apply pressure for 15 seconds.

    Rationale. Some pouches are packaged so that the peel-off paper end is inserted into the pack before sealing and serves as the sterilization indicator. If this is not available on the sterilization pack you use, you must insert a sterilization strip before sealing the pouch.

    NOTE: If the instrument package is opened and added to the sterile tray in a sterile manner, handle end–first insertion is not necessary. If the instrument package is being opened, however, and the instrument is presented to the physician to grasp from the package, the handle must be presented first. It is best to be in the habit of always inserting the handle end first into the sterilization pouch.

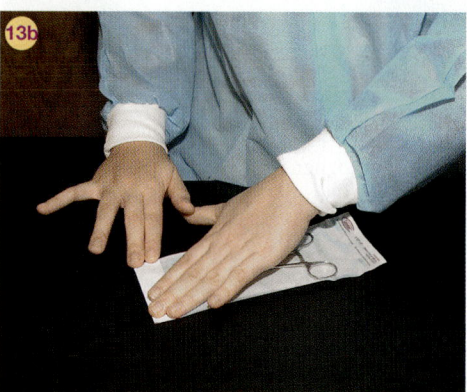

14. **Procedural Step.** Set the package aside until it is time to autoclave.

Infection Control and Asepsis **CHAPTER 31** **665**

PROCEDURE 31-9 — Sterilize Articles in the Autoclave

TASK: Properly sterilize supplies and medical equipment using an autoclave.

EQUIPMENT AND SUPPLIES
- Distilled water
- Heat-resistant gloves
- Wrapped packs (prepared in Procedure 31-8)
- Stainless steel canister containing 2 × 2–inch gauze squares, or items designated by instructor
- Autoclave with instruction manual
- Autoclave log
- Pen

SKILLS/RATIONALE

STANDARD PRECAUTIONS ARE TO BE FOLLOWED.

1. **Procedural Step.** Assemble previously wrapped autoclave packs, other items to sterilize, supplies, and equipment.
   Rationale. It is important to have all supplies and equipment ready and available before starting any procedure to ensure efficiency.

2. **Procedural Step. Fill the autoclave with distilled water.**
   Check the water level in the reservoir tank of the autoclave and fill it with distilled water as recommended by the manufacturer. Typically a "fill" line is marked on the inside of the reservoir.
   Rationale. Water used to fill the reservoir in the autoclave must be free of minerals, so distilled water is used. Minerals in tap water can corrode the stainless steel chamber of the autoclave and block the air exhaust valve. Water is used to build the steam necessary for sterilization.

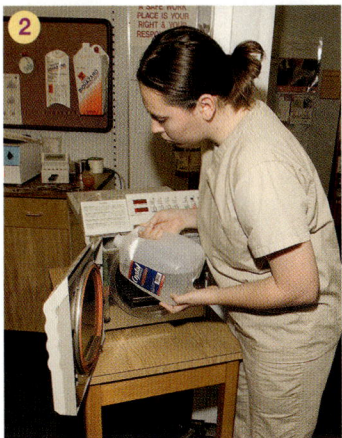

3. **Procedural Step.** Load the autoclave chamber with previously prepared items, leaving space for adequate circulation.
   a. Ensure that the items do not touch the chamber walls.
   b. Place wrapped packs on their side and stainless steel or glass items on their side with lids off so that the items inside (e.g., gauze) will be sterilized.
   c. If you are sterilizing dressing supplies and "hard" goods such as instruments together, place the dressing supplies on the top shelf and the hard goods on the bottom shelf.
   d. Place large packs 2 to 4 inches apart and small packs 1 to 2 inches apart.
   Rationale. The chamber must be loaded properly so that there is enough room for the steam to circulate. To sterilize the items effectively, steam needs to penetrate the middle portion of each item at its thickest point. Placing packs on their side maximizes steam circulation and effective drying.

4. **Procedural Step. Turn the autoclave control knob to "fill."**
   There is a "fill" line marked on the inside "floor" of the autoclave; allow the water to enter the inside chamber to this line. *Do not overfill the chamber.*
   Rationale. This allows water from the reservoir chamber to fill the inside chamber of the autoclave.

5. **Procedural Step. Close the door tightly.**
   Be sure to follow the manufacturer's instructions.
   Rationale. The door must be closed tightly so that the autoclave can properly heat the water to form steam and can operate with the amount of steam and temperature necessary for sterilization to occur. It is also important to lock the door properly because much pressure builds up during the autoclave cycle.

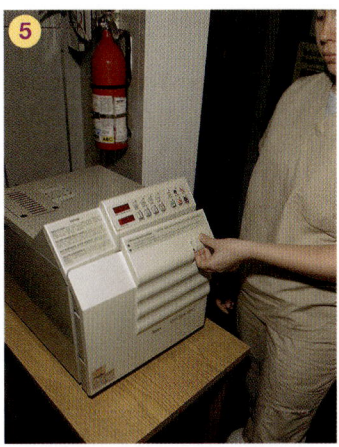

Continued

PROCEDURE 31-9 Sterilize Articles in the Autoclave—cont'd

6. **Procedural Step.** Turn the control knob to the "on" or "autoclave" setting to start the autoclave cycle.
   Rationale. The "on" control starts pressurization and increases the temperature of the autoclave.

7. **Procedural Step.** Check that the pressure gauge has reached 15 to 17 pounds of pressure and that the temperature has reached 250° F.
   If the gauge shows fluctuations in temperature or pressure, adjust them so they stay within the accepted range.
   Rationale. Adequate pressure must be achieved to reach the correct temperature of at least 250° to 270° F.

8. **Procedural Step.** Set the timer for the required time (typically 20 minutes).
   Rationale. For sterilization to occur, the autoclave must reach the required amount of pressure at the required temperature for the required length of time.

9. **Procedural Step.** After the time has expired, turn the control knob to "vent."
   NOTE: Remember to follow the manufacturer's recommendations for the autoclave you are using.
   Rationale. Venting the autoclave releases steam, which brings down the pressure. The pressure in the autoclave must drop to zero to be fully vented.

10. **Procedural Step.** When the pressure gauge returns to zero, open the door ½ to 1 inch.
    Never open the door until the pressure gauge is on zero.
    Rationale. Opening the door allows a more rapid escape of steam and drying of autoclave contents.
    NOTE: Opening the autoclave door before the pressure gauge has reached zero may result in steam burns or other injuries.

11. **Procedural Step.** Allow items to dry completely before removing them from the autoclave.
    Drying time is typically 15 to 60 minutes, depending on the articles being autoclaved.
    Rationale. Touching sterilized items before they are fully dry will allow microorganisms to penetrate the wrapping material and contaminate the articles that have just been sterilized, and sterilization will have to be repeated.

12. **Procedural Step.** Once the articles are completely dry, use heat-resistant gloves to remove items from the chamber.
    Rationale. The inner chamber of the autoclave should not be touched with bare hands. Heat is retained in the autoclave walls longer than in the articles being autoclaved, and injury could result.

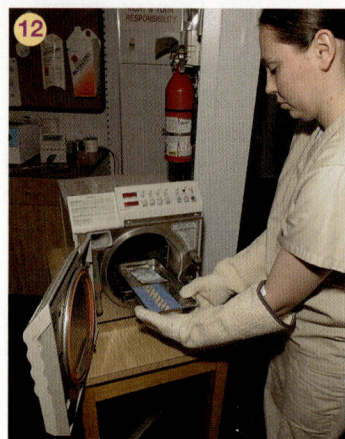

13. **Procedural Step.** Turn the autoclave control knob to the "off" position (unless the autoclave will be used again).

14. **Procedural Step.** Inspect each pack carefully.
    a. Make sure that the autoclave tape on the outside of a wrapped pack and the arrows on the back of the pouches changed color as expected.
    b. Ensure that no damage occurred to the sterilized packs during processing.
    NOTE: Autoclave tape changing colors only indicates the pack has been through the autoclaving process; it does not indicate that it is sterilized. Sterilization cannot be determined until the pack is opened at the time it is used, when the sterilization strip in the center of the pack can be checked.

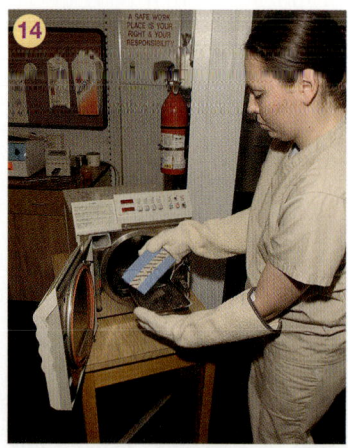

Continued

PROCEDURE 31-9 Sterilize Articles in the Autoclave—cont'd

15. **Procedural Step.** Store the autoclaved articles.
    Rationale. Make sure to store autoclaved articles in a clean, dust-proof area with the most recently sterilized items in the back so that those closest to the expiration date are used first.

16. **Procedural Step.** Record the date, the time the cycle was run, a description of the load, the duration of the cycle, chamber temperature, and your initials in the autoclave log.
    Comment on any change from the usual autoclave process.
    Rationale. Logging the articles autoclaved will provide quality assurance for all supplies in each autoclaved load in case any questions about adequate sterilization should arise.

    NOTE: The autoclave should be cleaned regularly according to the manufacturer's instructions to prevent buildup of minerals and other debris in the chamber and on the outside surface. Proper maintenance of the autoclave is necessary for proper sterilization of the materials.

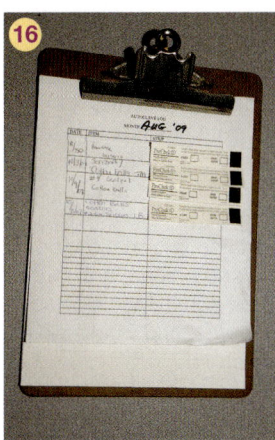

Chapter Summary

Reinforce your understanding of the material in this chapter by reviewing the curriculum objectives and key content points below.

1. **Define, appropriately use, and spell all the Key Terms for this chapter.**
   - Review the Key Terms if necessary.
2. **Explain why it is important for medical assistants to understand the basic principles of infection control.**
   - Understanding the principles of infection control helps medical assistants prevent the spread of disease in the medical office.
3. **Explain the difference between nonpathogenic and pathogenic microorganisms.**
   - Pathogenic microorganisms are disease producing; nonpathogenic microorganisms are not.
   - Nonpathogenic microorganisms help maintain homeostasis in the body, but can become disease producing if transported to an area outside their normal environment.
4. **List the six requirements that must be present for microorganisms to grow.**
   - Microorganisms need varying degrees and types of nutrients, darkness, temperature, pH, gases, and moisture to live and grow.
5. **List five classes of disease-causing microorganisms and give at least one example of a disease caused by each.**
   - Bacteria: gonorrhea, bacterial pneumonia, upper respiratory infection, syphilis, and diphtheria
   - Rickettsiae: Rocky Mountain spotted fever
   - Fungi: athlete's foot, vaginal yeast infection
   - Protozoa: dysentery
   - Viruses: HIV
6. **Describe the five parts of the "chain of infection," and give three examples of how this chain can be broken.**
   - The reservoir host, or carrier, is infected with the disease-causing microbes (or germs).
   - The germ leaves the body of an infected person by a route of exit (e.g., blood).
   - The infection is transmitted by direct or indirect contact (method of transmission such as touching, use of instruments).
   - Infection is transmitted to another person through a route of entry (e.g., broken skin).
   - The susceptible host becomes a reservoir host if infected, and the chain begins again.
     To break the chain, (a) practice frequent hand sanitization; (b) make good use of personal equipment, including gloves when handling biohazardous material; and (c) maintain Standard Precautions when working in the health care setting.
7. **Define the roles of the CDC and OSHA regarding Standard Precautions.**
   - CDC issues the Standard Precautions.
   - OSHA mandates and currently enforces these precautions.
8. **Demonstrate the correct procedure for practicing Standard Precautions.**
   - Review Procedure 31-1.
9. **Demonstrate the correct procedure for properly disposing of biohazardous materials.**
   - Review Procedure 31-2.

10. **List the five responsibilities of employers to protect employees against exposure to potentially biohazardous materials, according to the OSHA Bloodborne Pathogens Standard.**
    - Develop an exposure control plan.
    - Implement engineering controls and safe work practices.
    - Provide and train employees in the use of personal protective equipment (PPE).
    - Keep accurate records and follow mandated procedures for exposure incidents.
    - Communicate potential hazards to employees.
11. **List the six types of information found on a material safety data sheet (MSDS), and explain how an MSDS supports the "right-to-know" law.**
    - An MSDS contains information identifying a chemical, listing hazards and precautions for handling, identifying the chemical as carcinogenic (if applicable), providing first-aid procedures, and listing the contact information for the manufacturer.
    - There must be an MSDS on file for all chemicals in the medical office.
    - OSHA requires the manufacturers of these chemicals to make MSDSs available, usually as a package insert.
12. **Differentiate between medical asepsis and surgical asepsis.**
    - In medical asepsis, also called the "clean" technique, an object is clean and free from pathogens. Nonpathogenic microorganisms may still be present.
    - In surgical asepsis, also called "sterile" technique, *all* microorganisms have been removed.
13. **Explain the difference between normal flora and transient flora.**
    - Normal flora occurs naturally on the skin and helps the body fight infection.
    - Transient flora is picked up easily and can be pathogenic.
14. **List four methods of maintaining hand hygiene.**
    - Handwashing with soap and water or antiseptic hand cleanser, antiseptic hand rub, and surgical handwashing are all methods of maintaining hand hygiene.
15. **Demonstrate the correct procedure for handwashing for medical asepsis.**
    - Review Procedure 31-3.
16. **Demonstrate the correct procedure for hand sanitization using an alcohol-based hand rub.**
    - Review Procedure 31-4.
17. **Demonstrate the correct procedure for applying and removing nonsterile gloves.**
    - Review Procedure 31-5.
18. **Differentiate among sanitization, disinfection, and sterilization.**
    - Sanitization does not destroy all microorganisms or spores.
    - Disinfection destroys or inhibits the activity of pathogens but has no effect on spores.
    - Sterilization kills all microorganisms, including spores.
19. **Demonstrate the correct procedure for sanitizing instruments.**
    - Review Procedure 31-6.
20. **Demonstrate the correct procedure for performing chemical sterilization of items.**
    - Review Procedure 31-7.
21. **Explain the basic purpose and function of an autoclave.**
    - An autoclave is used to produce steam under pressure and is the primary method for sterilizing instruments in the medical office.
22. **Demonstrate the correct procedure for wrapping items for the autoclave.**
    - Review Procedure 31-8.
23. **Demonstrate the correct procedure for performing steam sterilization of items in an autoclave.**
    - Review Procedure 31-9.
24. **Describe how the autoclave is maintained on a daily and monthly basis.**
    - The inner chamber and door gaskets should be wiped with a damp, lint-free cloth daily.
    - A mild detergent should be used to clean the autoclave monthly, with careful rinsing to remove any residue.
25. **Explain the purpose of a chemical indicator, sterilization strip, and biological indicator.**
    - Chemical indicators alert the medical assistant after processing that conditions inside the autoclave (e.g., pressure, temperature) were right for sterilization.
    - Sterilization strips are embedded within the center of a dense pack to show that conditions for sterilization have occurred within the pack.
    - Biological indicators are used to determine the overall effectiveness of the autoclave.
26. **List three factors that influence the shelf-life of sterilized instruments.**
    - Instruments can be prepared, sterilized, and stored for 30 days up through several months (to 1 year), depending on the (a) type of packaging material, (b) environment in the storage area, and (c) how the package is sealed, among other factors.
27. **Analyze a realistic medical office situation and apply your understanding of infection control and asepsis to determine the best course of action.**
    - Medical assistants must be prepared to prevent cross-contamination and the spread of infection by practicing all safety precautions and procedures. Using PPE, remembering Standard Precautions on every patient at all times, and maintaining OSHA guidelines are essential practices that a medical assistant must perform daily.
28. **Describe the impact on patient care when medical assistants understand how to prevent the spread of disease and exposure to potentially biohazardous materials in the medical office.**
    - The role of the medical assistant is to control and prevent the spread of infection when performing patient care.
    - Common aseptic practices include proper handwashing, use of gloves to prevent transfer of pathogens, and proper preparation of items for sterilization.

PRACTICAL APPLICATIONS

If you have accomplished the objectives in this chapter, you will be able to make better choices as a medical assistant. Take another look at this situation and decide what you would do.

Janine is a new medical assistant in the office of Dr. McGee, a specialist in infectious diseases. Janine did her practical experience in a pediatric practice, often caring for children with viral and bacterial infections. As she begins her new employment, Janine asks to see the MSDSs and the current Exposure Control Plan. She also wants to know where the PPEs for her use are stored.

During patient care, medical workers often come in direct contact with many microorganisms, as Janine will in an office that specializes in infectious diseases. Janine's supervisor wants to be sure Janine is prepared to protect patients, other staff, and herself from infection. The supervisor reviews with Janine the importance of proper handwashing in infection control. Another important task for Janine will be performing both medical asepsis and surgical asepsis on a regular basis, so the supervisor assesses Janine's ability to perform these skills. The supervisor asks Janine what is done at the end of the day before leaving the office to break the cycle of infection. Janine responds that all medical workers should remove any garments that have been in direct contact with pathogens and nonpathogens and each person should carefully sanitize his or her hands.

Would you be prepared to take the necessary precautions to stop the spread of infection in the medical office?

1. What are "MSDSs"? What are "PPEs"? Why are both important to the health care worker?
2. What is "OSHA," and what are the requirements that a medical office must have to meet the OSHA standards?
3. What is included in the "Exposure Control Plan"?
4. What is the "chain of infection," and why is hand sanitization important in breaking this chain?
5. What is the difference between handwashing and hand sanitization in maintaining hand hygiene? Give two indications for the appropriate use of each.
6. What is the difference between medical asepsis and surgical asepsis?
7. What is the difference between sanitization and disinfection?
8. Is there a degree of sterilization in surgical asepsis? Defend your answer.
9. What is a non-pathogen? A pathogen?
10. How should Janine handle infectious waste from patients with a bacterial infection who are seen by Dr. McGee?

WEB SEARCH

1. **Research procedures that require the use of aseptic technique.** This exercise will enhance your knowledge concerning ways to break the chain of infection. The presence of microorganisms is not enough to promote infection. The chain of infection follows a designated pathway.

- **Keywords:** Use the following keywords in your search: aseptic technique, asepsis, bacteria, microorganisms, handwashing.

32 Preparing the Examination Room

evolve http://evolve.elsevier.com/klieger/medicalassisting

The medical assistant is responsible for preparing the examination room and the patient for the procedure that the physician will perform. How an examination room is stocked depends on the type of medical practice and the purpose for which the room will be used. Certain items, such as nonsterile disposable gloves and alcohol pads, are kept in all examination rooms because of the frequency of their use.

All examination rooms in the medical office should be stocked in the same manner with supplies stored in the same location in each room. This assists the physician and other health care team members by preventing delays in caring for the patient. When a specialty examination is planned, the medical assistant will set up the examination room to accommodate the needs and preferences of the practitioner (e.g., physician, nurse practitioner, or physician's assistant).

Preparing for a patient examination or procedure involves readying the examination room, sterilizing or cleaning the room, maintaining the room, and preparing the patient.

LEARNING OBJECTIVES

You will be able to do the following after completing this chapter:

Key Terms
1. Define, appropriately use, and spell all the Key Terms for this chapter.

Room Preparation
2. List four general considerations for examination room arrangement and preparation.
3. List and briefly describe the purpose of seven instruments typically stocked in an examination room.
4. List and briefly describe the purpose of six general supplies kept in an examination room.

Room Maintenance
5. Describe what should be done for maintenance to the examination table and work surfaces after a patient has left the examination room.
6. Describe what should be done to the instruments used during the examination after a patient has left the examination room.

Patient Preparation
7. Explain the medical assistant's role in preparing the patient to comply with the plan of care.

Patient-Centered Professionalism
8. Analyze a realistic medical office situation and apply your understanding of examination room preparation to determine the best course of action.
9. Describe the impact on patient care when medical assistants understand how to prepare the examination room for patients.

KEY TERMS

audiometer
lubricant
ophthalmoscope
otoscope
penlight
percussion hammer
specimens
speculum
tape measure
tongue depressor
tuning fork

PRACTICAL APPLICATIONS

Read the following scenario and keep it in mind as you learn about preparing the examination room for patients.

Julie, a medical assistant who was not educated in a medical assisting program, has been hired by a local family physician to assist with physical examinations. Today is her second day on the job. Her mentor has called in sick, so Julie is responsible for the clinical area by herself. Another physician, Dr. Johnson, will be performing the invasive procedures, and Julie is expected to have the room and patient ready for Dr. Johnson's examinations.

Julie finds the room too warm for her comfort, and she knows that it will be too warm for the physician in a lab coat, so she lowers the thermostat to 67° F. As Mrs. Sito is undressing, Julie barges into the room and leaves the door open. A male patient walks by and sees Mrs. Sito undressed.

During the examination, Dr. Johnson asks for the ophthalmoscope and otoscope. When he tries to use these, the necessary light will not work, so he asks for a penlight. Julie leaves the room to find the penlight and a tape measure. Dr. Johnson reaches for a cotton-tipped applicator and tongue depressors. Noticing that the supply is low, he asks Julie, "Would you please fill these containers?" Julie immediately departs to fill the jars, leaving Dr. Johnson alone with the patient, who needs a pelvic examination.

After Mrs. Sito leaves the room, Julie decides that the table paper does not look used. Thinking she will save the physician some money in supplies, she does not change the paper covering and brings in 5-year-old Joey Novelle, placing him on the table Mrs. Sito has just left. The sink still contains the dirty instruments used for the other patients. Joey's mother tells Dr. Johnson that she has never seen someone placed on dirty table paper, and she does not want her child to see dirty instruments in the sink.

At the end of Joey's physical examination, Dr. Johnson takes Julie to his office and explains that if she cannot properly prepare and clean the examination room in the future, he will have to find someone to replace her.

If you worked with Julie, what are some suggestions you would make to help her perform her duties more effectively?

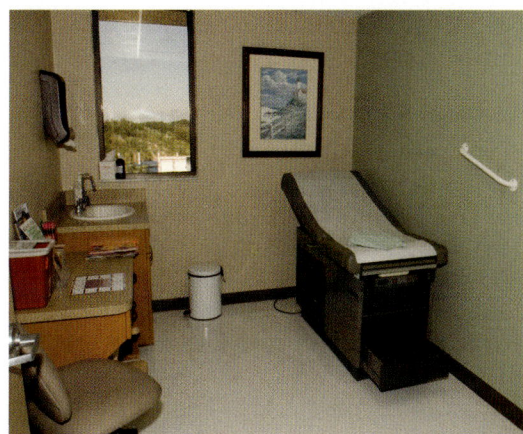

FIGURE 32-1 Patient examination rooms should provide privacy and accommodate those with disabilities.

ROOM PREPARATION

It is important for the examination room to be prepared before the patient arrives and the health care provider begins the examination or procedure. As shown in the scenario, an improperly prepared room, without the necessary equipment or supplies readily available, causes delays in caring for the patient. This is a failure to provide good service to the patient.

A helpful organizational tool for the medical assistant is to list all equipment and supplies needed for a particular procedure on an index card. Also, labeling the contents of the drawers helps when restocking items. Prescription pads should not be left on the counter in the examination room; pads should be safely stored away to prevent theft or misuse.

General Considerations

The examination room should provide privacy for patient interviews and examinations, should be appealing to the eye and comfortable, and should accommodate those with disabilities (Figure 32-1).

Privacy

Privacy is a key issue for patients. The patient may reveal sensitive information during the interview, so it is important that the door is closed and the medical assistant speaks in a voice that will not be overheard by others. This protects the patient's right to privacy and confidentiality as mandated by the Health Insurance Portability and Accountability Act (HIPAA).

If a patient is required to disrobe for the examination, the medical assistant should provide a gown and show the patient where to place removed clothing. Instructions should be given and even demonstrated to the patient on whether the gown should open in the front or back, which is usually based on the physician's preference. The assistant then should leave the room unless the patient requires assistance. Before reentering, the medical assistant should always knock to alert the patient that the door is opening and wait for a response from the patient.

Decor and Temperature

Room decor should be functional but should also promote a sense of warmth, friendliness, and tranquility. Lighting should not be overstimulating or too harsh. The room should not appear cluttered, and artwork may be placed on the walls and reading materials or pamphlets provided. The room should be comfortable for the patient.

Room temperature should not be too warm or too cold. The elderly patient may be more sensitive to a cool room because of loss of body fat and diminished circulation, and a blanket may need to be provided for comfort.

Accessibility and Safety

Appropriate accommodations need to be made in examination rooms to ensure that the room is accessible to all patients, including those in wheelchairs, as required by the Americans with Disabilities Act (ADA).

Safety measures should be taken to ensure patients do not injure themselves in the office. Such measures include slip-resistant flooring and a reception area free of obstacles that could cause a patient to trip (e.g., cords, throw rugs). In such cases, the office manager should be notified immediately and an incident report should be completed.

Equipment and Supplies

Equipment and supplies typically stocked in an examination room are those used during a general physical examination by the physician to evaluate the patient's health status. Medical assistants need to know some of the common instruments, equipment, and supplies needed and how each is used.

Equipment

In addition to blood pressure equipment (*sphygmomanometer* and *stethoscope*), other equipment typically kept in the examination room for physical examinations includes the following (Table 32-1 and Figure 32-2):

- **Ophthalmoscope:** Used to examine the retina and other internal structures of the eye. The head has a light, magnifying lenses, and an opening to look into the eye (Figure 32-3). Occasionally, the ophthalmoscope and the otoscope share a battery handle, and the heads of each are interchangeable.
- **Otoscope:** Used to examine the ear canal and eardrum (Figure 32-4). The head has a light and magnifying lens and is attached to a battery handle. Most ear speculums are disposable and are long and narrow. Replacing this type of **speculum** with a short and wide speculum allows the physician to examine the nasal area.
- **Penlight:** A small flashlight used to allow the physician to better examine the nose and the mouth; also used to check response of the pupils to light.

TABLE 32-1

Equipment in the Examination Room

Device or Item	Use
Ophthalmoscope	Inspect internal eye structure
Otoscope (with disposable speculum)	Inspect inner ear
Sphygmomanometer	Measure blood pressure
Stethoscope	Listen to heart, lung, and bowel sounds
Percussion hammer	Test reflex reactions
Tuning fork	Test for hearing loss
Thermometer	Measure body temperature
Sharps container	Hold used needles and other sharps for disposal
Tape measure	Measure length and diameter of surfaces
Gooseneck lamp	Allow for better inspection and viewing of body parts
Examination table (with footrest)	Allow for positioning of patient for examination
Penlight	Illuminate eyes to allow testing for dilation and constriction of pupils
Biohazard container	Hold biohazardous wastes (other than sharps)
Waste container with liner	Hold nonbiohazardous waste materials
Nasal speculum	View internal surfaces of nostrils

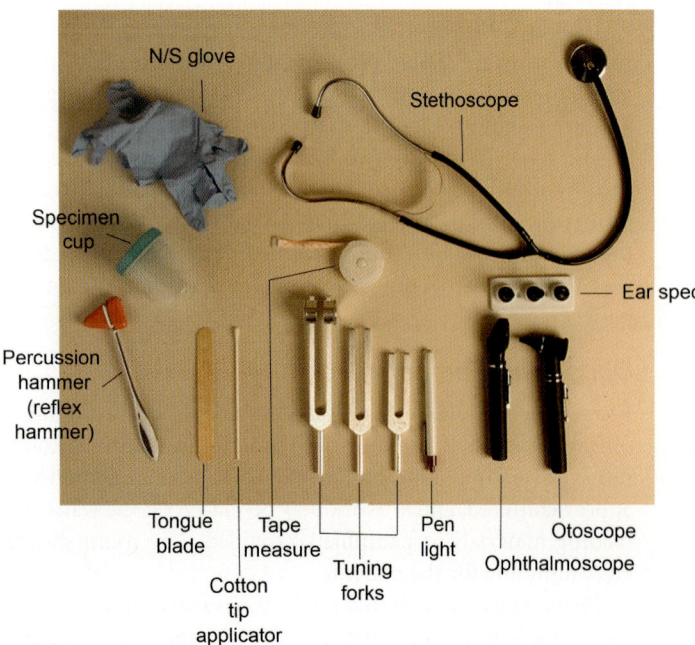

FIGURE 32-2 Instruments and supplies typically used for the physical examination.

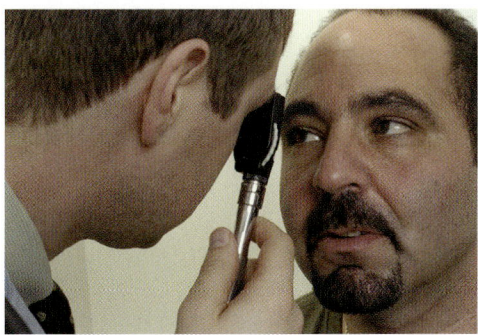

FIGURE 32-3 Physician using ophthalmoscope to view internal structure of the eye.

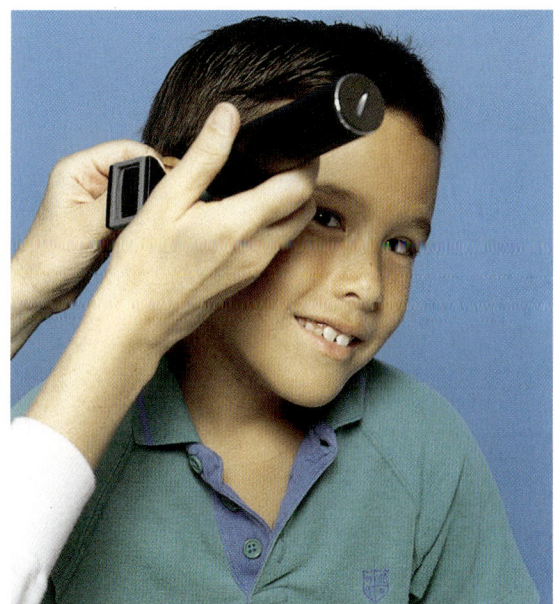

FIGURE 32-4 Physician using otoscope to examine the ear canal. (From Wong D, Hockenberry-Eaton M: *Wong's essentials of pediatric nursing*, ed 6, St Louis, 2001, Mosby.)

- **Tape measure:** Used to measure various body parts (e.g., head circumference of infant, body length) and the length of wounds.
- **Percussion hammer:** Instrument with a rubber triangular-shaped head used for tapping the tendon in the elbow, wrist, ankle, and knee to test for reflex action. The end of the stainless steel handle can be used on the sole of the foot to test for sensory perception. Figure 32-5 illustrates how the practitioner uses the hammer to test for various reflex actions.
- **Tuning fork:** Aluminum instrument with a handle (stem) and two prongs used to test hearing acuity (Figure 32-6). The physician strikes the prongs against the hand or knee, causing a vibration. The vibrating tuning fork stem is first placed behind the ear on the mastoid process to test hearing by bone conduction, then removed. The vibrating end is held near the ear canal to test hearing by air conduction. This is called the *Rinne test* and compares air conduction to bone conduction. The *Weber test* is used when the patient states hearing is better in one ear than the other. The vibrating tuning fork stem is placed in the center of the skull or on top of the head to see if the patient hears equally in both ears.
- **Audiometer:** Electronic device used to test hearing.

Part of the medical assistant's responsibilities is to make certain that all equipment is in good working order.

Supplies

Supplies in health care are typically disposable after one use. General supplies kept in the examination room include the following (Table 32-2):

- Disposable gloves: Gloves are always worn when coming in contact with body secretions. A gloved hand can be used to examine the mucous membranes of the mouth and other body parts.
- **Lubricant:** Water-soluble lubricant is used in conjunction with gloves to provide moisture when examining the rectal and vaginal areas.
- **Tongue depressor:** This disposable wooden device is used to hold the tongue down, allowing the physician to better see the mouth and throat (the oral cavity).
- Tissues: Used to wipe body secretions and excess lubricant (e.g., anal area after rectal examination).
- Cotton-tipped applicators: Used to collect specimens.
- Specimen containers: Used to hold and transport **specimens** to the laboratory.

Other common supplies include cotton-tipped applicators, disposable needles and syringes, microscope slides, thermometer covers, bandages, and alcohol wipes. These items typically depend on the the type of practice. The medical assistant must maintain the room with adequate supplies needed throughout the day for patient examinations and treatments, as well as to

TABLE 32-2

Supplies in the Examination Room

Item	Use
Alcohol wipes	Disinfect skin and equipment surfaces
Tongue depressors	Hold tongue during full-mouth or throat exam
Tissues	Wipe body secretions
Cotton-tipped applicators	Collect specimens; remove debris
Disposable gloves (nonsterile)	Provide protection against contact with body fluids
Lubricant (water soluble)	Assist in examination of rectal area by moistening to reduce friction
Patient gowns and capes	Cover body and allow easy access for examination
Drapes	Provide privacy and warmth
Hypoallergenic tape of various sizes	Secure dressings in place
Gauze squares (2 × 2, 4 × 4)	Wipe or cover an area
Sterile dressings	Cover wounds
Guaiac card and developer	Test for occult blood (usually fecal)

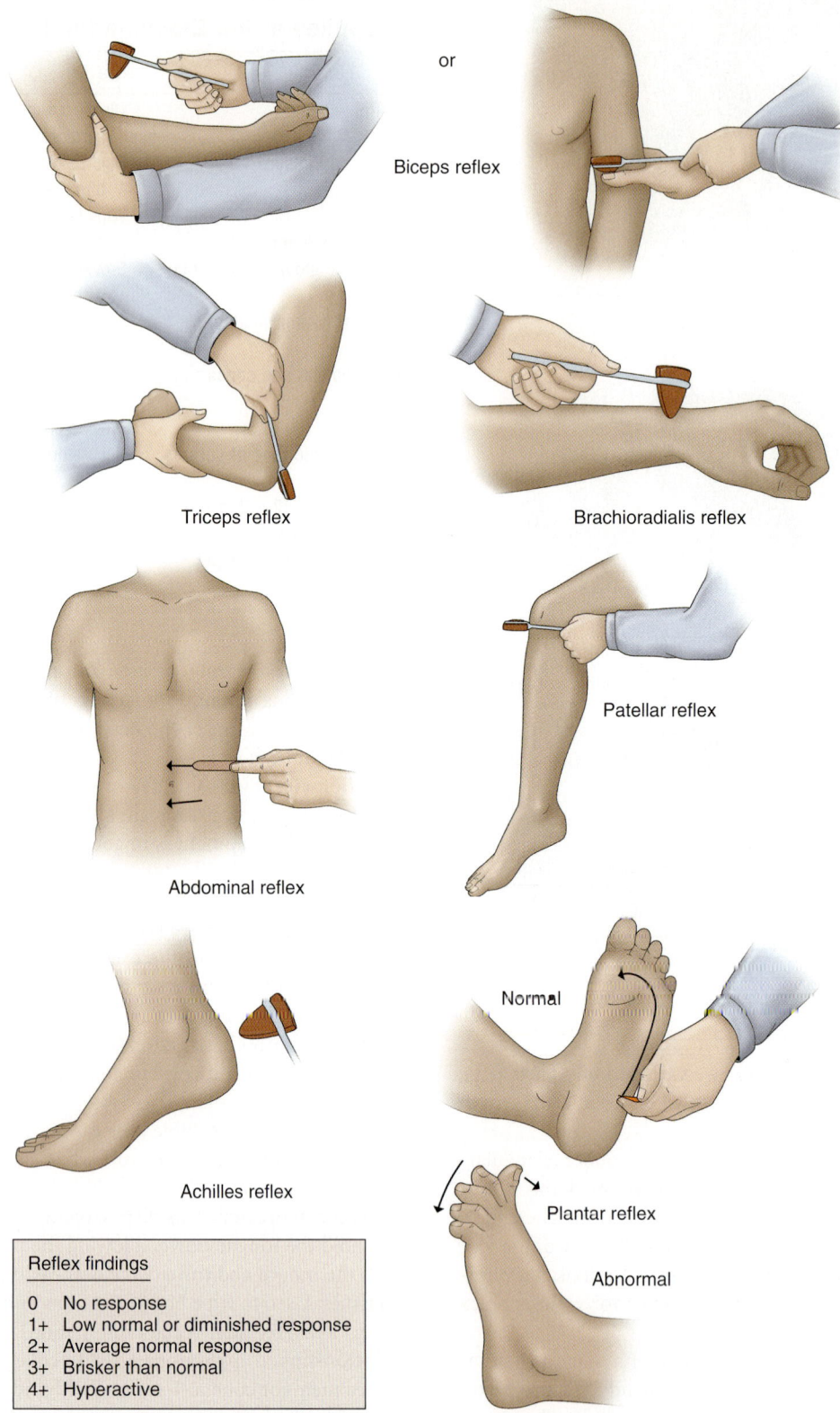

FIGURE 32-5 Testing reflexes with percussion hammer. *Inset,* Rating scale: 0 to 4+. (Modified from Leahy J, Kizilay P: *Foundations of nursing practice,* Philadelphia, 1998, Saunders.)

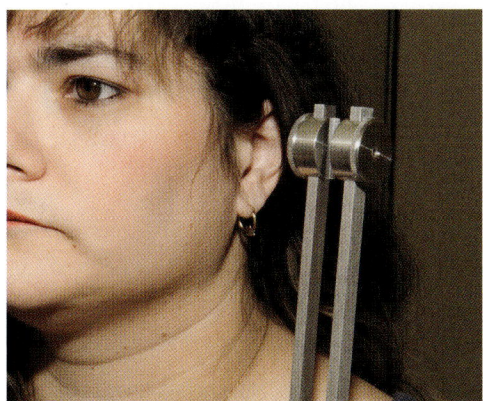

FIGURE 32-6 Tuning fork is used to test hearing acuity.

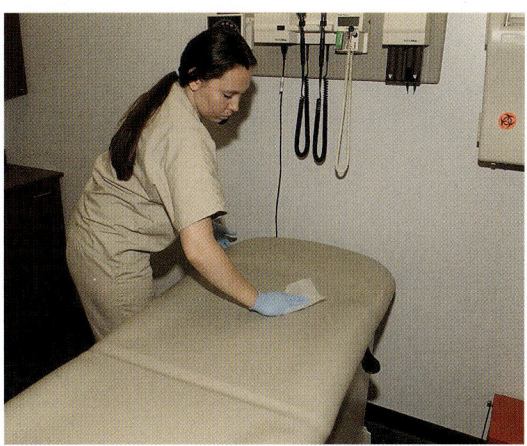

FIGURE 32-7 Examination table must be disinfected between patients.

anticipate the physician's needs based on the reason for the office visit.

Examination Table

The examination room will have an examination table, which can typically be raised or lowered by pushing or pulling a lever on the side of the table. The tables are usually covered with nonpermeable vinyl, which allows for easy cleaning with a disinfectant (e.g., 10% bleach solution, EPA-approved product) between patients (Figure 32-7).

To cover the table's surface, paper is often pulled from a roll underneath the head of the table and is secured at the bottom (Figure 32-8). A footrest or pullout platform at the end of the table should be available in the room for patients who may require assistance getting onto the examination table.

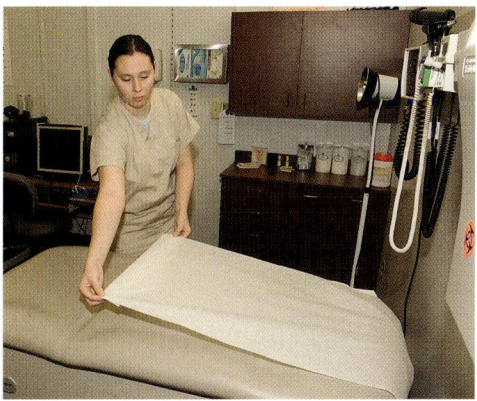

FIGURE 32-8 The medical assistant pulls clean paper covering down over the examination table.

> ### PATIENT-CENTERED PROFESSIONALISM
>
> - Why must the examination room promote privacy and offer appropriate accommodations for patient accessibility?
> - What is the medical assistant's role in room preparation?

ROOM MAINTENANCE

After a patient has left the room and has been escorted to the front of the office, the paper covering the examination table is removed, and the table is cleaned, dried, and re-covered with clean paper. Never bring a patient into a dirty examination room, and always ensure that the room is clean and odor free before bringing in the next patient.

Occupational Safety and Health Administration (OSHA) regulations state that all contaminated work surfaces must be decontaminated using an appropriate disinfectant as soon as possible after a procedure or immediately if potentially infectious contamination has occurred (e.g., contaminated body fluids). Medical assistants need to be especially careful to hold the dirty paper covering away from their clothing when removing it (Figure 32-9). Besides the table, all equipment and surfaces used must be sanitized and disinfected.

All instruments used during the examination need to be removed, cleaned, and sterilized if necessary. Instruments and equipment are then assembled and arranged to be neat and orderly. All supplies and equipment will be added to the room as required for the next patient. Any equipment for specialty examinations should be added to the examination tray as necessary (e.g., vaginal speculum, Pap smear supplies).

> ### PATIENT-CENTERED PROFESSIONALISM
>
> - What key element in infection control is the medical assistant providing by performing room sanitization?

PATIENT PREPARATION

The medical assistant has an important role in helping the patient comply with the physician-designed treatment plan. This involves preparing patients for procedures, as well as

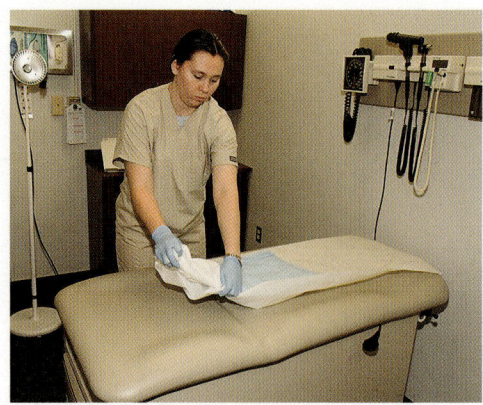

FIGURE 32-9 The medical assistant keeps the soiled paper table covering away from her clothing.

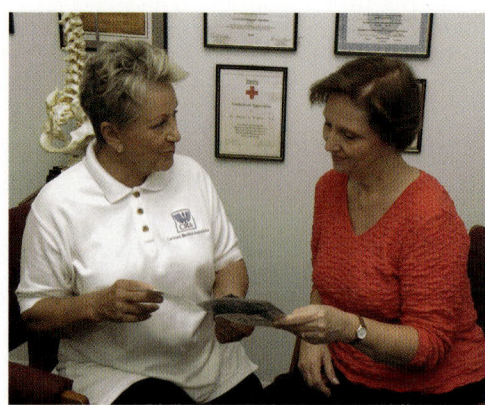

FIGURE 32-10 Patient teaching is made easier when written instructions are provided and the patient is allowed to ask questions. Keep in mind that some patients may not be able to read; therefore any teaching materials must be explained, not just given to the patient.

preparing them to comply with the plan of care after they leave the medical office. Once the physician has made the diagnosis, implementation of the plan of care requires patient cooperation. The medical assistant must be aware of barriers that would prevent the patient from following the plan, as discussed in Chapters 5 and 6.

To prepare the patient for carrying out the treatment plan, the medical assistant can address four major areas with the following questions:

1. *Does the patient understand the instructions?* Shaking the head "yes" does not mean the patient fully understands what is expected. Ask the patient to explain or demonstrate to you what is expected. Any additional teaching or clarification can take place during this "show and tell" time. Provide written instructions when available, and allow the patient to ask questions (Figure 32-10).
2. *Do the patient and family understand the time demands needed to follow the procedure preparation or treatment plan successfully?* For example, a patient scheduled for a sigmoidoscopy needs to follow a bowel evacuation procedure before the examination. The patient who needs to take medication with food in the morning must take enough time to eat breakfast.
3. *Will the patient's living environment allow the treatment plan to be followed?* For example, a patient newly diagnosed with diabetes has food concerns. Is the family supportive to help make certain the patient has a balanced diet or special foods?
4. *Is the patient hard of hearing or does the patient have other medical problems that could hinder understanding?* The medical assistant should always face the patient when speaking. Speak naturally and use nonverbal communication to send the message. To reinforce what is being said, have visual aids available.

PATIENT-CENTERED PROFESSIONALISM

- *In what ways can the medical assistant help the patient prepare for a procedure and comply with the treatment plan?*

CONCLUSION

An important part of the medical assistant's duties involves preparation for patient treatment. Before the patient arrives, the examination room must be prepared for the type of examination or procedure to be performed. In addition, the necessary supplies and equipment must be ready for the physician or other provider to use during the examination or procedure. Finally, medical assistants need to prepare patients for the procedure by educating them about anything they need to do before the procedure, as well as how they can comply with the treatment plan. Effective preparation saves time for the health care provider and the patient, ultimately providing for more effective patient care.

Chapter Summary

Reinforce your understanding of the material in this chapter by reviewing the curriculum objectives and key content points below.

1. **Define, appropriately use, and spell all the Key Terms for this chapter.**
   - Review the Key Terms if necessary.
2. **List four general considerations for examination room arrangement and preparation.**
   - Privacy, room decor, room temperature, and accessibility are four important considerations for examination rooms.
3. **List and briefly describe the purpose of seven instruments typically stocked in an examination room.**
   - An ophthalmoscope, otoscope, penlight, tape measure, reflex hammer, and tuning fork are kept in the examination room and used for physical examinations.
   - An audiometer is an electronic device used to test hearing.
   - Refer to Table 32-1.
4. **List and briefly describe the purpose of six general supplies kept in an examination room.**
   - Gloves, water-soluble lubricant, tongue depressors, tissues, cotton-tipped applicators, and specimen containers are usually kept in the examination room and used for physical examinations.
   - Refer to Table 32-2.
5. **Describe what should be done for maintenance to the examination table and work surfaces after a patient has left the examination room.**
   - The paper covering is removed and the examination table is cleaned and dried and re-covered with paper after the patient leaves the room.
   - All surfaces used must be disinfected.
6. **Describe what should be done to the instruments used during the examination after a patient has left the examination room.**
   - All instruments used during the examination must be removed, sanitized, and if necessary, sterilized.
7. **Explain the medical assistant's role in preparing the patient to comply with the plan of care.**
   - Medical assistants focus on the patient's understanding of instructions, time demands, living environment, and possible disabilities that may hinder understanding in helping patients comply with their treatment plans.
8. **Analyze a realistic medical office situation and apply your understanding of examination room preparation to determine the best course of action.**
   - The effective preparation of the examination room not only affects the functioning of the medical office, but also the care that patients receive.
   - Proper examination room preparation breaks the chain of infection.
9. **Describe the impact on patient care when medical assistants understand how to prepare the examination room for patients.**
   - The patient tends to have more confidence in the ability of the health care team (and the team's decision-making capability) when the equipment and supplies are readily available.
   - Infections may be prevented when proper room decontamination procedures are followed.

PRACTICAL APPLICATIONS

If you have accomplished the objectives in this chapter, you will be able to make better choices as a medical assistant. Take another look at this situation and decide what you would do.

Julie, a medical assistant who was not educated in a medical assisting program, has been hired by a local family physician to assist with physical examinations. Today is her second day on the job. Her mentor has called in sick, so Julie is responsible for the clinical area by herself. Another physician, Dr. Johnson, will be performing the invasive procedures, and Julie is expected to have the room and patient ready for Dr. Johnson's examinations.

Julie finds the room too warm for her comfort, and she knows that it will be too warm for the physician in a lab coat, so she lowers the thermostat to 67° F. As Mrs. Sito is undressing, Julie barges into the room and leaves the door open. A male patient walks by and sees Mrs. Sito undressed.

During the examination, Dr. Johnson asks for the ophthalmoscope and otoscope. When he tries to use these, the necessary light will not work, so he asks for a penlight. Julie leaves the room to find the penlight and a tape measure. Dr. Johnson reaches for a cotton-tipped applicator and tongue depressors. Noticing that the supply is low, he asks Julie, "Would you please fill these containers?" Julie immediately departs to fill the jars, leaving Dr. Johnson alone with the patient, who needs a pelvic examination.

After Mrs. Sito leaves the room, Julie decides that the table paper does not look used. Thinking she will save the physician some money in supplies, she does not change the paper covering and brings in 5-year-old Joey Novelle, placing him on the table Mrs. Sito has just left. The sink still contains the dirty instruments used for the other patients. Joey's mother tells Dr. Johnson that she has never seen someone placed on dirty table paper, and she does not want her child to see dirty instruments in the sink.

At the end of Joey's physical examination, Dr. Johnson takes Julie to his office and explains that if she cannot properly prepare and clean the examination room in the future, he will have to find someone to replace her.

If you worked with Julie, what are some suggestions you would make to help her perform her duties more effectively?

1. What part did the lack of education in the medical assisting field play in Julie making mistakes?
2. What temperature is appropriate for the patient examination room?
3. Why should Julie have been very careful to keep the door closed to the examination room in which a patient was placed?
4. What is the use of the ophthalmoscope and otoscope?
5. Should Julie have left the room to fill the containers of cotton-tipped applicators and tongue depressors? Explain your answer.
6. Why is changing the examination table's paper covering such an important task?
7. Do you think that Joey's mother and Dr. Johnson had a right to be upset?
8. What effect did the room's lack of preparation have on the appointments for that day?

WEB SEARCH

1. **Research different types of medical practices.** The equipment and supplies needed for the physical examination differ according to the type of examination and the physician's specialty.

- **Keywords:** Use the following keywords in your search: neurologist, orthopedist, pulmonologist, endocrinologist.

Body Measurements and Vital Signs

33

evolve http://evolve.elsevier.com/klieger/medicalassisting

Taking and recording body measurements and vital signs is an important part of providing effective care to patients. The health care team also must keep accurate records in these two areas to monitor their patients' health effectively. Monitoring body measurements and vital signs can provide early warning of diseases and other conditions that require treatment or intervention.

For these measurements to be useful, they must be *accurate.* Recording an inaccurate weight, height, temperature, pulse rate, respiratory rate, or blood pressure can prevent patients from receiving the best care possible. Therefore it is crucial that medical assistants understand these measurements, how to take them accurately, and how to document them correctly.

LEARNING OBJECTIVES

You will be able to do the following after completing this chapter:

Key Terms
1. Define, appropriately use, and spell all the Key Terms for this chapter.

Body Measurements
2. Explain the purpose of taking patients' weight and height measurements.
3. Accurately convert inches to centimeters and pounds to kilograms, and vice versa.
4. Demonstrate the correct procedure for measuring adult weight and height.
5. Demonstrate the correct procedure for measuring infant weight and length.
6. Demonstrate the correct procedure for measuring the head and chest circumference of an infant.
7. Explain how health care professionals use growth charts, and demonstrate how to plot weight and height (length) data on a growth chart.

Vital Signs
8. List the four vital signs and explain why they are taken at patient visits.

Temperature
9. List the five sites of the body that can be used to take a patient's temperature.
10. List five factors that can cause normal changes in body temperature.
11. List the normal body temperature range for oral, rectal, axillary, and tympanic temperatures.
12. Identify the four types of thermometers.
13. Demonstrate the correct procedure for accurately measuring and recording body temperature with a mercury-free glass thermometer.
14. Demonstrate the correct procedure for accurately measuring and recording oral, rectal, and axillary body temperature with an electronic or digital thermometer.
15. Demonstrate the correct procedure for accurately measuring and recording body temperature with a tympanic thermometer.
16. Demonstrate the correct procedure for accurately measuring and recording body temperature with a disposable oral thermometer.
17. Explain the considerations for using mercury-free glass thermometers in the medical office.

Pulse
18. Describe the body processes that create a pulse and explain why the pulse rate is measured.
19. Differentiate between *tachycardia* and *bradycardia,* and identify the normal pulse range for these age groups: birth to 1 year, 1 year to 6 years, 6 to 12 years, 12 years to adult, and elderly.
20. List eight pulse sites of the body.
21. List the three characteristics of the pulse that medical assistants should note in documentation.
22. Demonstrate the correct procedure for accurately measuring and recording radial pulse.

23. Demonstrate the correct procedure for accurately measuring and recording apical pulse.
24. Explain the purpose of a stethoscope and the need for sanitizing it between patients.

Respiratory Rate

25. Identify the normal respiratory rate for a child, an adult, and a geriatric adult.
26. Demonstrate the correct procedure for accurately measuring and recording respiratory rate.
27. List four abnormal breathing sounds that can be caused by respiratory problems.

Blood Pressure

28. Differentiate between *systolic* and *diastolic* blood pressure and state the normal range of each for an adult.
29. List six factors that influence a patient's blood pressure.
30. Demonstrate the correct procedure for accurately measuring and recording systolic blood pressure by palpation.
31. Demonstrate the correct procedure for accurately measuring and recording blood pressure by auscultation.

Patient-Centered Professionalism

32. Analyze a realistic medical office situation and apply your understanding of body measurements and vital signs to determine the best course of action.
33. Describe the impact on patient care when medical assistants understand how to accurately take and record body measurements and vital signs in the medical office.

KEY TERMS

afebrile	pulse
apical	pulse deficit
apical pulse	pulse pressure
axillary	pulse rate
baseline	radial artery
blood pressure	radial pulse
body temperature	rales
brachial artery	rate
bradycardia	rectal
carotid artery	respiration
Celsius (C)	respiratory rate
diastolic pressure	rhonchi
dorsalis pedis artery	rhythm
expiration	sphygmomanometers
Fahrenheit (F)	stethoscope
febrile	stridor
femoral artery	systolic pressure
hypertension	tachycardia
hypotension	temporal artery
inspiration	tympanic
mensuration	vital signs
oral	volume
popliteal artery	wheezes
posterior tibial artery	

PRACTICAL APPLICATIONS

Read the following scenario and keep it in mind as you learn about body measurements and vital signs and how they are taken and recorded in the medical office.

Stephanie works for a general practitioner who sees pediatric as well as adult and geriatric patients. Dr. Karas wants height and weight measurements for patients at each visit, regardless of the patient's age. Dr. Karas also wants head and chest circumference measurements taken for pediatric patients up to age 3 years.

Travis, a new patient, is a young teenager who does not want to have his weight and height measured because he is obese. He balks at having his temperature taken, stating that he knows he is not ill and "absolutely does not need to have that done." Stephanie tries explaining to Travis the differences in temperature, pulse, respiration, and blood pressure in different age groups. Finally, Travis agrees to have his temperature taken with a tympanic thermometer. When Stephanie starts to take Travis's blood pressure, he resists and tells her that he is scared and just knows that taking his blood pressure will hurt. Stephanie finally convinces Travis that she needs to take *all* his vital signs to prepare him for Dr. Karas's examination.

Would you be prepared to explain the importance of taking body measurements and vital signs to a new patient?

BODY MEASUREMENTS

Most medical assistants will be asked to take body measurements (**mensuration**) routinely in the medical office. Two important measurements are weight and height, which provide the physician with information about the patient's current health status. Comparing a child's height and weight progress to national growth charts can provide early warning of developmental problems.

Scales measure height in inches or in centimeters (cm). Scales measure weight in kilograms (kg) or in pounds (lb). Box 33-1 shows how to convert centimeters to inches and kilograms to pounds, and vice versa.

Adults

Most adults' weight is taken routinely at the time of the office visit, but height is taken on the first visit during a complete physical examination and thereafter only if a problem occurs, or at least every 3 to 5 years. These first measurements provide *baseline data* for future assessments and should be documented accurately in the patient's medical record. Comparisons are made based on past visits and current complaints. For example, a rapid weight gain or loss may be an indication that the body is in a diseased state. Older adults should be measured on at least a yearly basis or more frequently as indicated for signs of osteoporosis. All measurements can be compared to a standardized chart to determine if a patient's measurements are within acceptable limits.

BOX 33-1

English and Metric Conversions for Height and Weight Measurements

HEIGHT

To convert *inches* to centimeters (cm), **multiply** the number of inches by 2.5.
  Example
  60 inches = ? cm
  60 × 2.5 = 150 cm

To convert *centimeters* to inches, **divide** the number of centimeters by 2.5.
  Example
  200 cm = ? inches
  200 ÷ 2.5 = 80 inches

WEIGHT

To convert *pounds* (lb) to kilograms (kg), **divide** number of lb by 2.2.
  Example
  160 lb = ? kg
  160 lb ÷ 2.2 = 72.7 kg

To convert *kg* to *lb*, **multiply** the number of kg by 2.2.
  Example
  94 kg = ? lb
  94 × 2.2 = 207 lb

BOX 33-2

Documentation when Charting a Patient's Body Measurements

ADULT
1. Date
2. Time
3. Name of procedure:
   - Weight
   - Height
4. Results
5. Patient reaction, if any
6. Proper signature and credential

CHILD
1. Date
2. Time
3. Name of procedure:
   - Weight
   - Length
   - Head circumference
   - Chest circumference
   - Growth percentiles
4. Results
5. Patient reaction, if any
6. Proper signature and credential

CHARTING TIPS
1. Weight (Wt) is recorded in pounds (# or lb), fractions (¼, ½), and ounces (oz).
2. Weight can also be recorded in kilograms (kg).
3. Height (Ht) is recorded in inches (in or ″) or centimeters (cm), depending on office policy.

Certain diagnostic tests require a patient's weight and height. For example, when scheduling magnetic resonance imaging (MRI), the patient's weight is needed. Spirometry testing also requires a patient's weight and height. Procedure 33-1 explains the process of correctly obtaining the weight and height of an adult. Box 33-2 lists the necessary information when charting weight and height.

Weight

Measuring an adult's weight needs to be done in a private area. The patient can be fully clothed, and weight can be measured with or without shoes. Whether the patient is or is not wearing shoes should be documented, and an attempt should be made to weigh the patient the same way at each subsequent visit. Keep in mind that some medical offices specify that the patient should remove the shoes; check the policy of the office to be certain. A patient's weight is taken by having the patient step on the scale. The weight bars attached to the top of the balance-beam scale are moved to the correct calibration (Figure 33-1).

Height

The height of the patient is typically measured after completing the weight because the patient has already removed his or her shoes. Then, lift the measuring bar that is attached to the back of most scales to the top of the patient's head (Figure 33-2). It should rest on the patient's head, not the hair. Discuss each step with the patient before proceeding so the patient is not startled or hit with the extension bar. The measuring bar displays measurements from greater to lesser numbers. The

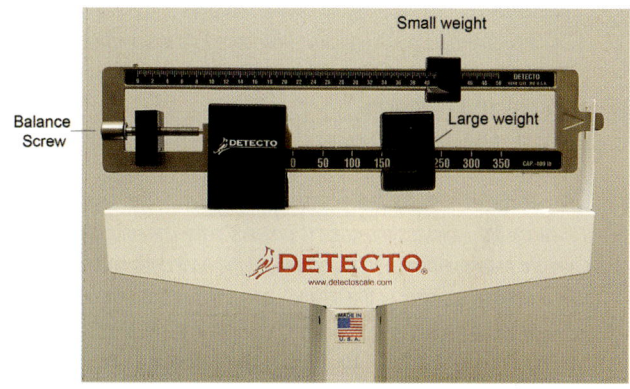

FIGURE 33-1 Balance-beam scale. Bottom bar has the large weight, and it is moved in 50-lb increments. The small weight is located on the top bar and can measure weight as little as ¼ pound. The height is measured by using the measuring bar.

bottom ruler displays measurements from lesser to greater and is typically used for children. The total reading is done in inches and is noted to the nearest quarter of an inch.

As a person ages, the bones become more brittle because the rate at which bones absorb calcium to replace bone decreases. Diets poor in calcium, lack of exercise, and decreased estrogen levels all affect bone strength. A patient with osteoporosis will lose height. Elderly persons also lose height because the discs between the vertebrae become thinner. Therefore, as adults age, their height should be monitored closely.

SECTION V Clinical Medical Assisting

PROCEDURE 33-1 Measure Weight and Height of an Adult

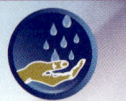

TASK: Correctly obtain accurate height and weight measurements of an adult patient.

EQUIPMENT AND SUPPLIES
- Paper towel
- Balance scale with bar measure for height
- Patient's medical record
- Pen

SKILLS/RATIONALE

STANDARD PRECAUTIONS ARE TO BE FOLLOWED.

WEIGHT

1. **Procedural Step.** Greet the patient, introduce yourself, and confirm the patient's identity.
   Rationale. Identifying the patient ensures the procedure is performed on the correct patient.

2. **Procedural Step.** Sanitize the hands.
   An alcohol-based hand rub may be used instead of washing hands with soap and water, unless hands are visibly soiled.
   Rationale. Hand sanitization promotes infection control.

3. **Procedural Step.** Assemble equipment and supplies.
   Rationale. It is important to have all supplies and equipment ready and available before starting any procedure to ensure efficiency.

4. **Procedural Step.** Check that the scale is properly calibrated and balanced.
   NOTE: The pointer should float in the middle of the balance bar when all weights are at zero.
   Rationale. Having the pointer float freely in the center of the balance bar indicates the scale is properly balanced and the patient's weight measurement will be accurate. If the float does not move freely or is not in the center of the balance bar, adjust the balance knob until it is properly aligned.

5. **Procedural Step.** Explain the procedure to the patient.
   Rationale. An explanation promotes patient cooperation and provides a means of obtaining implied consent.

6. **Procedural Step.** Place a clean paper towel on the scale platform.
   Rationale. The paper towel prevents transfer of microorganisms from patient to patient.

7. **Procedural Step.** Assist the patient onto the scale without shoes or heavy clothing. Be certain that both feet are totally on the scale
   NOTE: Ask the patient to empty pockets and remove any heavy outer clothing. If a patient is carrying a purse or other items, ask him or her to set them down during the procedure.
   Rationale. This provides for the most accurate measurement of body weight.

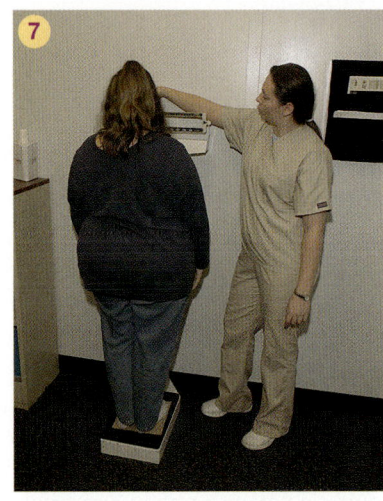

8. **Procedural Step.** Instruct the patient to stand still.
   Rationale. This promotes accuracy since movement will cause the scale balance to swing widely.

9. **Procedural Step.** Balance the scale by moving the large weight into the groove closest to the patient's estimated weight (e.g., 100, 150, 200, 250, or 300 lb.)
   NOTE: The grooves are calibrated in 50-lb increments. If the weight is moved too far, the pointer will tip to the bottom of the balance frame. You should then move the balance weight back one groove and move the smaller weight. Move the small weight by tapping it gently until it reaches a point at which the pointer floats in the center of the frame.
   Rationale. The pointer bar will float between the bottom and top frame when both the lower and upper weights balance with the patient's weight.

10. **Procedural Step.** Read the results by adding the large weight to the number behind the small weight (see Figure 33-1).

11. **Procedural Step.** Return the balance weights to the resting position.

Continued

Body Measurements and Vital Signs **CHAPTER 33** 683

PROCEDURE 33-1   **Measure Weight and Height of an Adult—cont'd**

12. **Procedural Step.** Record the weight in the patient's medical record (see the charting example).

HEIGHT

1. **Procedural Step.** Instruct the patient to stand erect and look straight ahead, with his or her back to the scale.
   The patient typically stands facing the scale during the weight measurement. Ask the patient either to step off the scale and turn around (so his or her back is to the scale), then step back on the scale, or to turn around carefully while staying on the scale, depending on the age and physical condition of the patient.
2. **Procedural Step. Raise the height of the bar.**
   Raise the bar in its collapsed position; lift the bar above the patient's head.
   Rationale. Keeping the bar collapsed during this step prevents injury to the patient.
3. **Procedural Step. Open the bar.**
   Open the bar out into a horizontal position, and move it down gently until it just touches the top of the patient's head. Leave this setting in place.

4. **Procedural Step.** Assist the patient in stepping off the scale.
5. **Procedural Step.** Read and record the measurement in the patient's medical record.
6. **Procedural Step.** Assist the patient in putting on shoes as required. Make certain that any items removed during the procedure are returned to the patient.
7. **Procedural Step.** Return the bar to the resting position.
8. **Procedural Step.** Sanitize the hands.
   Always sanitize the hands after a procedure or after wearing gloves.

CHARTING EXAMPLE	
Date	
7/31/xx	9:00 AM. Wt: 170 lb (shoes); Ht: 72"——————B. Larrson, CMA (AAMA)

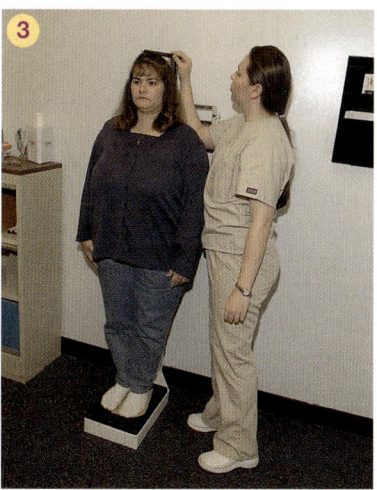

Infants and Children

Infants and children need to be weighed and measured at each visit. Procedure 33-2 explains the process of correctly obtaining the weight and length of an infant.

Weight

The birth weight of an infant should double within 6 months and triple within 1 year. The medical assistant should weigh the child and plot the gain or loss on the growth chart. Accurate body weight measurements are also important because medication dosages for children are calculated by body weight.

Height

Children will have their height recorded at each visit. This assists the physician in determining whether a proper growth rate is being maintained. Children from birth to 24 months should be measured lying down (see Procedure 33-2). After age 2 years, the child can stand (Figure 33-3). A child who is old enough may stand on the scale to be weighed, and after the weight is taken, the height can be measured.

Growth within a year from birth will average 10 to 12 inches. Table 33-1 shows the typical growth of a child from birth through age 18 years.

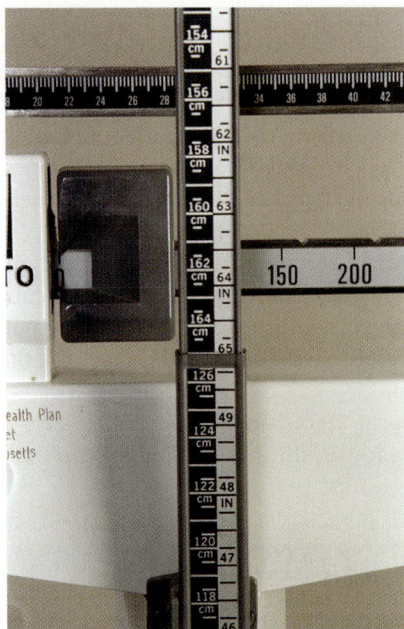

FIGURE 33-2 Patient measurement is done by using the movable ruler attached to the scale.

TABLE 33-1
Typical Growth Pattern: Birth to 18 Years

Age Group	Weight Increase	Height Increase
BIRTH TO TODDLER		
Birth to 1 year	Birth weight doubles by 6 months of age Birth weight triples by 1 year	10 to 12 inches per year
1 to 2 years	½ pound per month	3 to 5 inches per year
2 to 3 years	Average 3 to 5 pounds	2 to 2½ inches
PRESCHOOL		
3 to 6 years	3 to 5 pounds per year	1½ to 2½ inches per year By age 4, birth length doubles
SCHOOL AGE		
6 to 12 years	3 to 5 pounds per year	2 inches per year
ADOLESCENCE		
12 to 18 years	Gains half of adult weight *Girls:* 20 to 25 pounds *Boys:* 15 to 20 pounds	*Girls:* 4 to 5 inches *Boys:* 5 to 6 inches

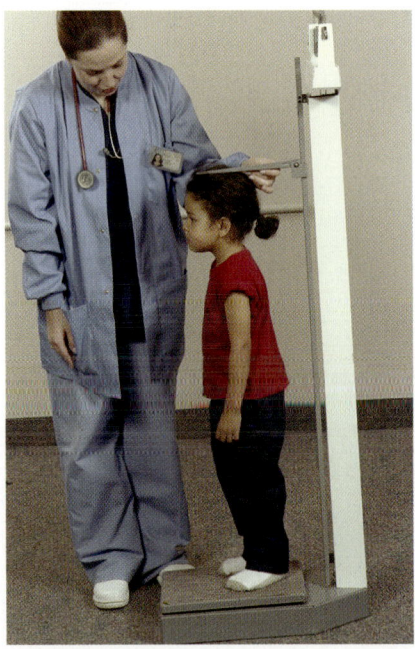

FIGURE 33-3 After age 2 years, a child can be measured standing up.

Chest Head and Circumference

An infant routinely has head and chest circumference measured. These measurements can be compared to the expected growth profile of other infants. Procedure 33-3 describes the process of measuring the head and chest circumference of an infant.

Head Circumference. An infant's head size is approximately 80% of an adult's by 1 year of age. Average head circumference at birth is 13.7 inches (35 cm), and this increases ½ inch (1.27 cm) a month for the first 6 months, and ¼ inch a month for the next 6 months. Knowing head circumference is important in making certain the growth plates in the head are growing. Two open "soft spots" (fontanels) allow for brain growth; the growth plates, or bony covering of the brain (the skull), gradually close, eliminating the soft spots. Evaluating the head size gives the physician information concerning growth plates and brain growth.

Chest Circumference. At birth, the infant's chest wall is underdeveloped. The chest circumference must be recorded to ensure that as the infant develops, the chest cavity is also developing.

Growth Charts

Growth charts provide documentation of a child's progress from infancy. A child's growth is compared to the statistical averages of children the same age. For example, if a child is in the 95th percentile for height, it means 95% of all children tend to be below his or her height, and 5% of all children tend to be above his or her height. The charts provide the physician with possible indications of nutritional deficiencies and growth abnormalities, including delayed growth patterns.

The medical assistant is responsible for correctly plotting the growth measurements on the chart. The information on these charts is only as good as the accuracy of the measurements (Figures 33-4 and 33-5). To plot the data collected, do the following:

1. Choose the correct chart according to gender and age.
2. Locate an infant's age in the bottom horizontal section and a child's age on the top horizontal section.

Text continued on p. 690

Body Measurements and Vital Signs CHAPTER 33

PROCEDURE 33-2 Measure Weight and Length of an Infant

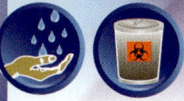

TASK: Correctly measure the weight and length of an infant to monitor development.

EQUIPMENT AND SUPPLIES
- Infant scale with disposable plastic-lined drape or pad cover
- Examination table paper
- Flexible tape measure
- Infant growth charts, male or female, as appropriate
- Patient's medical record
- Pen
- Ruler
- Waste container/biohazardous waste container

SKILLS/RATIONALE

STANDARD PRECAUTIONS ARE TO BE FOLLOWED.

WEIGHT

1. **Procedural Step.** Greet the parent or guardian, identify yourself, confirm the identity of the patient, and explain the procedure.
   Rationale. Identification of the infant is obtained through confirmation from the parent or guardian. This ensures the procedure is performed on the correct patient.

2. **Procedural Step.** Sanitize the hands.
   An alcohol-based hand rub may be used instead of washing hands with soap and water, unless hands are visibly soiled.
   Rationale. Hand sanitization promotes infection control.

3. **Procedural Step.** Assemble equipment and supplies and unlock the pediatric scale if necessary.
   Check the scale to ensure it is properly balanced. Follow the manufacturer's instructions. Typically, the scale is balanced in the same manner as an adult scale. The pointer should float in the middle of the balance bar when all weights are at zero.
   Rationale. It is important to have all supplies and equipment ready and available before starting any procedure to ensure efficiency. Having the pointer float freely indicates the scale is properly balanced. If the float does not move freely, adjust the balance knob until it is properly aligned.

4. **Procedural Step.** Place a plastic-lined disposable drape or pad cover on the scale.
   Rationale. This prevents cross-contamination from one infant to another.

5. **Procedural Step.** Undress the infant, including the diaper.
   You may ask the parent or guardian to undress the child.
   Rationale. The diaper must be removed when obtaining the infant's weight to prevent the diaper's weight from being included in the body weight.

6. **Procedural Step.** Gently place the infant in a recumbent position on the scale.
   The infant is weighed with one hand hovering closely over the body of the infant for safety and protection.
   Rationale. Do not place your hand directly on the infant, since this will cause an inaccurate weight measurement.

7. **Procedural Step.** Weigh the infant.
   First move the pound weight (large weight indicator). Be sure it is firmly placed in the notched groove. The appropriate pound will be the pound marker that does not cause the indicator point to drop to the bottom of the balance area. Next, move the ounce indicator (small weight) to the appropriate ounce. Adjust the weight by sliding the ounce indicator until the pointer floats in the center of the frame.
   Rationale. To obtain an accurate weight, the balance scale must be balanced. The child must be still for the scale to balance.

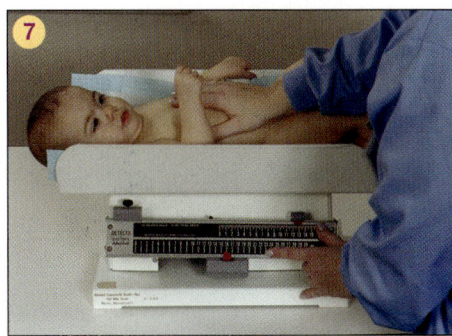

8. **Procedural Step.** Record the infant's weight in pounds and ounces in the medical record.

9. **Procedural Step.** Remove the infant from the scale.
   Hand the infant to the parent or guardian to place on his or her back on the examination table and replace the diaper.

10. **Procedural Step.** Return the balance weights to the resting position and lock. Discard the scale drape or pad.

Continued

PROCEDURE 33-2 Measure Weight and Length of an Infant—cont'd

LENGTH

1. **Procedural Step.** Position the infant in a recumbent position.
   If the scale or table is also equipped with a measuring device, place the crown (top) of the child's head against the headboard at the zero mark, asking the parent or guardian to hold the child's head in place.
   Rationale. If the scale or table is also used for measuring the child, this should be done before removing the child from the table.
2. **Procedural Step.** Exert mild pressure on the knees to straighten the child's legs and place the feet firmly against the upright footboard.
3. **Procedural Step.** Read the length in inches to the nearest fraction of an inch, according to office policy.
   Rationale. The length of the child is from the top of the head to the heel of the foot, and does not include the length of the foot. The length should be measured in inches to place on the growth chart.
4. **Procedural Step.** Record the results.
5. **Procedural Step.** Discard the drape or pad to prevent cross-contamination.
6. **Procedural Step.** Remove the infant from the scale.
   If the scale or table is not used for measuring, remove the child from the scale and place the infant on the examination table in a recumbent position with the table paper in place.
7. **Procedural Step.** Place a pen mark on the table paper to mark the top of the infant's head.

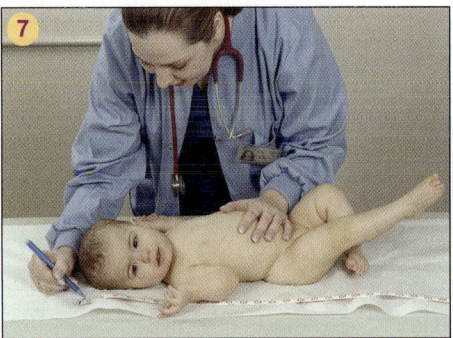

8. **Procedural Step.** Holding the infant, stretch the leg and foot down, and place a mark at the heel.
   This must be done without moving the infant on the table. Then, ask the parent or guardian to replace the diaper.
9. **Procedural Step.** Remove the infant from the table.
10. **Procedural Step.** Measure the length between the two pen marks using a tape measure.
    Rationale. The pen marks allow measuring the child without having to keep the tape measure straight under the child. Again, the legs must be straight and the heel at a right angle to the table to obtain the full length of the child. Removing the child allows you to measure between the pen marks, knowing that the tape measure is flat.
11. **Procedural Step.** Determine the infant's length.
    Read the length in inches to the nearest fraction of an inch, according to office policy. Record the length in the infant's medical record.
12. **Procedural Step.** Inform the parent or guardian of the measurements.
13. **Procedural Step.** Discard the protective paper on the examination table in the appropriate container. (If soiled with feces or urine, discard in a biohazardous waste container; otherwise discard in a regular waste container.)
14. **Procedural Step.** Sanitize the hands.
    Always sanitize the hands after a procedure or after wearing gloves.
15. **Procedural Step.** Plot the infant's weight and length on the growth chart (see Figures 33-4 and 33-5) and in the patient's medical record.
    NOTE: With an older and larger child (2 years of age), weight and height are obtained in the same manner as for an adult on a balance scale.

CHARTING EXAMPLE	
Date	
10/13/xx	11:00 a.m. Wt: 20 lb, 6 oz; Length: 33¼ in————K. Panatacos, CMA (AAMA)

Body Measurements and Vital Signs **CHAPTER 33** **687**

PROCEDURE 33-3 **Measure Head and Chest Circumference of an Infant**

TASK: Accurately measure the head circumference and chest circumference of an infant.

EQUIPMENT AND SUPPLIES
- Flexible tape measure
- Infant growth charts, male or female, as appropriate

SKILLS/RATIONALE

STANDARD PRECAUTIONS ARE TO BE FOLLOWED.

HEAD CIRCUMFERENCE

1. **Procedural Step.** Greet the parent or guardian, introduce yourself, and confirm the patient's identity.
   Rationale. Identifying the patient ensures the procedure is performed on the correct patient.
2. **Procedural Step.** Sanitize the hands.
   An alcohol-based hand rub may be used instead of washing hands with soap and water, unless hands are visibly soiled.
   Rationale. Hand sanitization promotes infection control.
3. **Procedural Step.** Assemble equipment and supplies.
   Rationale. It is important to have all supplies and equipment ready and available before starting any procedure to ensure efficiency.
4. **Procedural Step.** Explain the procedure to the parent or guardian.
   Rationale. Explaining the procedure promotes cooperation and provides a means of obtaining implied consent.
5. **Procedural Step.** Position the infant.
   Ask the parent or guardian to position the infant on his or her back on the examination table with the table paper in place.
6. **Procedural Step.** Position the tape measure around the infant's head slightly above the ears and top of the eyebrows and around the occipital prominence of the skull.
   Rationale. Placing the tape measure around the infant's head in this way helps to ensure accuracy when measuring the infant.

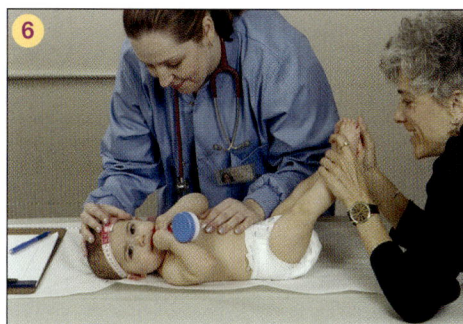

7. **Procedural Step.** Read the results to the nearest ¼ inch, or according to office policy.
8. **Procedural Step.** Write the results on the examination table paper.

Rationale. Results will be transferred to the patient's medical record and growth chart when the procedure is completed.

CHEST CIRCUMFERENCE

9. **Procedural Step.** Place the tape around the infant's chest at the nipple line.

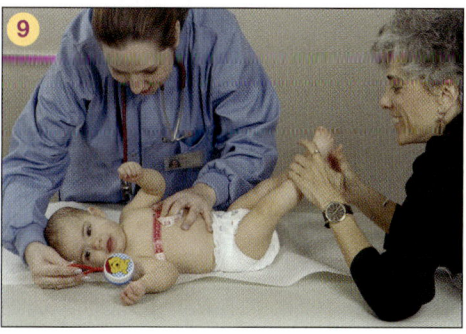

10. **Procedural Step.** Read the results to the nearest ¼ inch, or according to office policy.
11. **Procedural Step.** Write the results on the examination table paper.
12. **Procedural Step.** Hand the infant back to the parent or guardian.
13. **Procedural Step.** Inform the parent or guardian of the measurements.
14. **Procedural Step.** Discard the protective paper on the examination table in the appropriate container if the examination will not be done on the same table.
15. **Procedural Step.** Sanitize the hands.
    Always sanitize the hands after a procedure or after wearing gloves.
16. **Procedural Step.** Plot points on the growth chart and connect the dots using a ruler.
    Indicate the head and chest circumference measurement on the growth chart and in the patient's medical record.

CHARTING EXAMPLE	
Date	
1/13/xx	10:00 a.m. Head circumference: 37 in; Chest circumference: 36¼ in————————————L. Ramsey, CMA (AAMA)

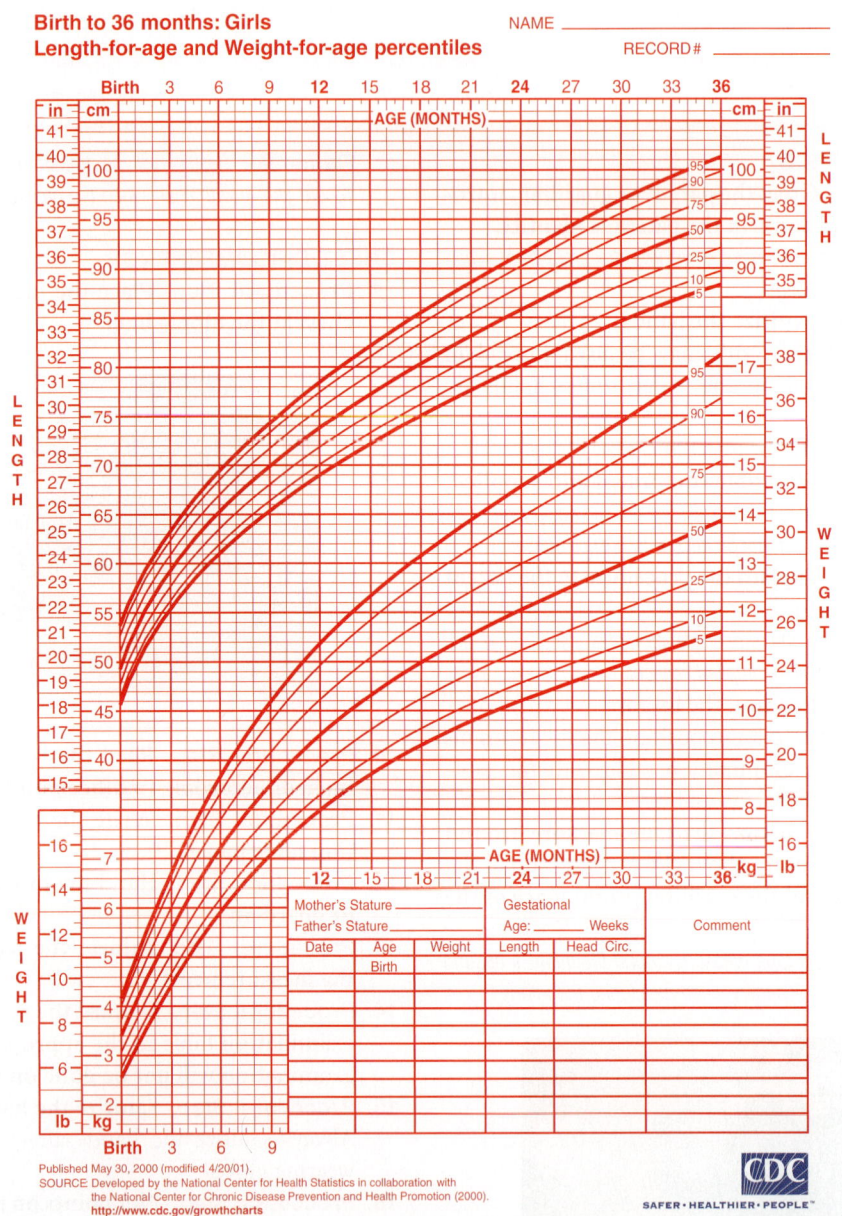

FIGURE 33-4 Use a growth chart to chart weight and length. This chart is for girls from birth to 36 months.

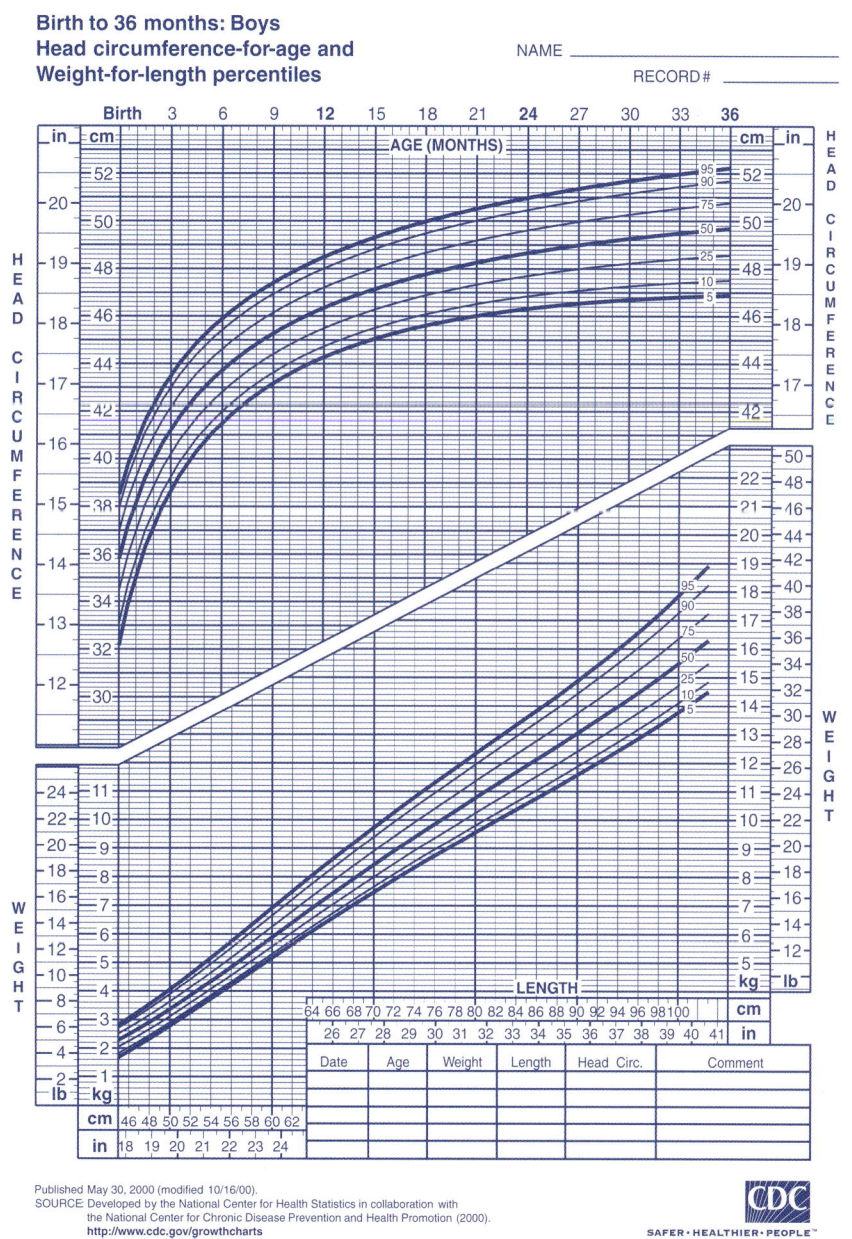

FIGURE 33-5 Use a growth chart to chart head circumference. This chart is for boys from birth to 36 months.

3. Locate the growth value in the vertical column under the correct category (e.g., length, weight).
4. Locate where the two lines meet (intersect).
5. Place a very small "x" on this location.
6. Follow the percentile line upward to read the value on the right side of the chart.

> **PATIENT-CENTERED PROFESSIONALISM**
>
> - Why would an elderly patient's weight and height be monitored more closely than a 28-year-old patient's?
> - What significance does knowing an infant's measurements have on the infant's overall health status?

VITAL SIGNS

A patient's temperature, pulse rate, respiratory rate, and blood pressure all provide *vital* (urgently needed, critical) information about the patient's present condition. This is why they are called **vital signs.** Vital signs provide the physician with important information about the patient's basic body systems. The medical assistant often takes the "vitals" of patients every time they visit the medical office and compares them to **baseline** measurements to detect changes in normal body functions. Vital signs are taken with the patient in a relaxed, comfortable position, either sitting or lying down. Once taken, the newly collected data are compared to data from prior visits to see even minor changes.

Accuracy is the number one priority when measuring, recording, and reporting vital signs. It is important to remember that vital signs must always be recorded in the order of temperature, pulse, respiration, and blood pressure. Documentation can be horizontal or vertical, but the order does not change because some of the results can be very similar numbers. Changes in vital signs can sometimes indicate health problems or disease conditions. If you are unsure of the accuracy of a measurement, notify the physician or ask a fellow health professional to verify your readings.

Temperature

Body temperature is the measurement of the amount of heat within a person's body. It reflects the balance between the heat produced and lost by the body. It is expressed in terms that describe an elevated temperature (**febrile,** or having a fever) or within normal range (**afebrile,** or not having a fever). A patient's temperature can be taken by the following methods:

- By mouth (**oral** temperature)
  - Should only be taken on alert and cooperative adults and children over age 5
  - Should not be used on patients who are mouth breathers, patients who are on oxygen, or patients who have recently eaten, smoked, or had something to drink, either hot or cold.
- Through the rectum (**rectal** temperature)
  - Taken in adults and children who cannot have their temperature taken orally
  - Should not be done on infants
  - Patient must be still to avoid breaking thermometer and perforating the rectum
  - Most accurate since few factors can alter the result
- Under the arm (**axillary** temperature)
  - Considered to be the least accurate measurement
  - Use when other methods cannot be used
  - Patient must hold arm tightly against side of the body
- Within the ear canal (**tympanic** [aural] temperature)
  - Reading within 1 to 3 seconds
  - Should not be used when ear drainage or heavy wax buildup is apparent
  - Tip must be pointed toward eardrum
- On the body surface
  - Plastic strip thermometers measure skin temperature, not body temperature

Temperature is a balance between the amount of heat produced in the body and the amount lost to the environment. As food is digested, energy is released and heat is produced. Body heat is lost through the skin, through breathing, and through elimination. A patient's body temperature remains fairly stable but can be affected by the following factors:

- *Time of day.* Body temperature is lower in the morning and higher in the afternoon and evening.
- *Health status.* Pregnancy and emotional status (including stress, depression, and anger) can raise body temperature, and mouth breathing can cause a lower temperature to register.
- *Medications.* Some medications can cause an increase or decrease in body temperature.
- *Recent activity.* Exercise can elevate body temperature, and food, drink, and gum chewing can either raise or lower body temperature.
- *Age.* As a person ages the regulatory mechanism for body temperature is not functioning as well as it once did because of changes in the body. This fact makes the temperature a less reliable indicator of the person's health. For example, an elderly patient usually has a lower body temperature; therefore 98.6° F may indicate a fever in an older patient. Always document temperature by rounding to the nearest tenth.

Temperature is measured in either **Fahrenheit (F)** or **Celsius (C).** Normal body temperature registers at 98.6° F, or 37° C. Table 33-2 lists the average body temperature ranges at different measurement sites. To convert Fahrenheit to Celsius, use the following formula:

$$C = (F - 32) \times \frac{5}{9}$$

To convert Celsius to Fahrenheit use the following formula:

$$F = \left(C \times \frac{9}{5}\right) + 32$$

The medical assistant can use several types of thermometers, including mercury-free glass, electronic or digital, tym-

TABLE 33-2
Average Body Temperature Ranges

Type	Site*	Range
Oral	Mouth	97.6° to 99.6° F
		36.5° to 37° C
Rectal	Rectum	98.6° to 100.6° F
		37° to 38.1° C
Axillary	Armpit	96.6° to 98.6° F
		35.9° to 37° C
Tympanic membrane	Ear	98.6° F to 99.4° F
		37° C to 38.1° C

*These sites have a rich blood supply near the surface; therefore, they can produce an accurate measurement.

BOX 33-3
Documentation when Charting Body Temperature in Children and Adults

1. Date
2. Time
3. Name of procedure:
   - Temperature
4. Assessment site (mouth, axilla, rectum, ear, skin)
5. Results (° F or C)
6. Patient reaction, if any
7. Proper signature and credential

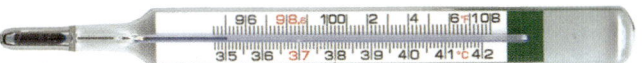

FIGURE 33-6 Mercury-free (alloy) oral thermometer (° F and C). (Courtesy RG Diagnostics, Wixom, MI.)

panic (aural), and plastic disposable thermometers. The type of thermometer used depends on what is available in the medical facility. The electronic or digital and tympanic thermometers are used most often. The rectal temperature normally registers 1° higher than an oral temperature, the tympanic temperature usually registers the same as the oral, whereas the axillary is 1° lower than the oral reading. When charting, remember to correctly chart the *type* of temperature taken. For example, indicate "A" for axillary and "R" for rectal so the physician does not mistake these temperatures for orally taken temperatures. Box 33-3 summarizes information needed when charting temperature.

Mercury-Free Glass Thermometer

Mercury thermometers are no longer used in the medical care setting because of environmental concerns, costs of mercury spills, and the availability of good mercury-free alternatives. The mercury-free glass thermometer is used less than the electronic or digital thermometer in the patient care setting but can be found in some medical offices (Figure 33-6).

A mercury-free glass thermometer may be used for oral and axillary temperatures. It is color-coded with a green end and has a long, narrow bulb filled with a nontoxic liquid alloy called Galinstan. When heated, the Galinstan alloy rises in the tube, and when cooled, it moves down the tube. The thermometer is marked with lines to indicate degrees. When reading Fahrenheit, the long lines indicate one degree and the short lines indicate two-tenths of a degree, whereas Celsius measures one degree with the long lines and one-tenth of a degree with the short lines. The medical assistant must hold the thermometer between the thumb and index finger at the stem (end away from the bulb) and read it at eye level. The lines must be visible, and the Galinstan alloy level must register. Find the silver line coming from the bulb and follow it until it ends. Procedure 33-4 provides step-by-step instructions for using the mercury-free thermometer.

The mercury-free rectal thermometer also has a long, narrow bulb end; is color-coded with a red end; and is marked in degrees the same way as the oral thermometer. To reduce the chance of spreading microorganisms, a disposable cover is used on both the oral and the rectal mercury-free thermometers.

As a general rule, the mercury-free thermometer is left in place 3 to 5 minutes for an oral or rectal temperature and 4 minutes for an axillary temperature.

Disadvantages of any type of glass thermometer include how easily it can break and the time it takes to obtain a temperature; however, glass thermometers are extremely accurate. When the disposable cover is removed, the thermometer is read according to the manufacturer's instructions and cleaned in soapy water and/or wiped clean with a cotton ball or gauze square saturated with alcohol. The thermometer is then briskly shaken, using a snapping motion of the wrist, until the silver contents are at or below 96 degrees and returned to its plastic case.

FOR YOUR INFORMATION

GLASS MERCURY THERMOMETER BREAKAGE IS A HEALTH RISK

Mercury thermometers are no longer used in the health care setting because of their dangers. Mercury is a toxic substance and can be harmful to humans and other animals. Mercury can damage the nervous system and is harmful to the environment. When a mercury thermometer breaks, mercury vapor is released into the air. The amount of mercury contained in a thermometer is small, but the mercury vapor in the air indoors poses the health risk. If a broken thermometer goes undetected or mercury seeps through the carpet, the quality of indoor air is affected. Some local governments (e.g., San Francisco) have banned the sale of mercury thermometers for home use, and the Department of Natural Resources in Broward County, Florida, offered a thermometer exchange in which nonmercury thermometers were traded for mercury thermometers.

Electronic or Digital Thermometer

Electronic thermometers are usually digital and are handheld, battery operated, and portable (Figure 33-7). The temperature is displayed quickly, within 4 to 60 seconds, on a small screen.

PROCEDURE 33-4

Measure Oral Body Temperature Using a Mercury-Free Glass Thermometer

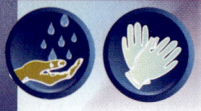

TASK: Accurately measure and record a patient's oral temperature.

EQUIPMENT AND SUPPLIES
- Mercury-free glass oral thermometer
- Thermometer sheath
- Disposable gloves
- Waste container
- Pen
- Patient's medical record

SKILLS/RATIONALE

STANDARD PRECAUTIONS ARE TO BE FOLLOWED.

1. **Procedural Step.** Sanitize the hands.
   An alcohol-based hand rub may be used instead of washing hands with soap and water, unless hands are visibly soiled.
   Rationale. Hand sanitization promotes infection control.

2. **Procedural Step.** Assemble equipment and supplies.
   Rationale. It is important to have all supplies and equipment ready and available before starting any procedure to ensure efficiency.

3. **Procedural Step.** Greet the patient, introduce yourself, and confirm the patient's identity.
   Rationale. Identifying the patient ensures the procedure is performed on the correct patient.

4. **Procedural Step.** Explain the procedure to the patient.
   Rationale. Explaining the procedure to the patient promotes cooperation and provides a means of obtaining implied consent.

5. **Procedural Step.** Determine if the patient has recently had a hot or cold beverage to drink, or has smoked.
   Rationale. Hot or cold substances in the mouth will prevent an accurate temperature measurement. You must wait a minimum of 10 minutes before measuring a patient's oral temperature if this is the case.

6. **Procedural Step.** Put gloves on and remove the thermometer from its plastic case.
   Do not touch the bulb end with your fingers.
   Rationale. The bulb end will be placed in the patient's mouth. Even though you will be placing a thermometer sheath on the thermometer before the procedure, there is less chance of contamination if the bulb is not touched.

7. **Procedural Step.** Inspect the thermometer for chips or cracks.
   Rationale. A chipped or cracked thermometer should be disposed of in a sharps container because it is unsafe for patient use and will provide inaccurate results.

8. **Procedural Step.** Read the thermometer to ensure that the temperature is 96° F or below.
   If the thermometer reads above 96° F, use a wrist snapping motion by holding the top of the thermometer until the silver content, Galinstan, is at or below 96° F.
   Rationale. Results will be inaccurate if the thermometer is registering a previously measured temperature.

9. **Procedural Step.** Cover the thermometer with a protective thermometer sheath.
   Rationale. This adds a layer of protection from cross-contamination.

10. **Procedural Step.** Ask the patient to open his or her mouth and place the probe tip under the tongue.
    Rationale. There is a rich blood supply under the tongue on either side of the frenulum linguae. The thermometer bulb should be placed in this area to receive the most accurate reading.

11. **Procedural Step.** Ask the patient to hold, not clasp, the thermometer between the teeth and to close the lips snugly around it to form an airtight seal.
    Rationale. Explain that the patient should not talk because the mouth must be closed, creating an airtight seal, for an accurate temperature reading.

12. **Procedural Step.** Leave the thermometer in place for a minimum of 3 minutes (average 3 to 5 minutes).
    The time should be monitored by a timer or watch.

13. **Procedural Step.** Remove the thermometer from the mouth and, holding the thermometer by the stem, remove the protective sheath and discard in a biohazardous waste container. Roll the thermometer back and forth in your hand until you can see the end of Galinstan that has risen up the interior column and corresponds with a number in degrees.
    Rationale. The thermometer can be read without a distorted view.

14. **Procedural Step.** Read the results.
    If the temperature is less than 97° F, reinsert the thermometer for an additional minute. Reread the thermometer as necessary.

Continued

PROCEDURE 33-4 Measure Oral Body Temperature Using a Mercury-Free Glass Thermometer—cont'd

15. **Procedural Step.** Sanitize the thermometer following the manufacturer's recommendations.
    This requires cleaning the thermometer with warm soapy water or an alcohol wipe.
16. **Procedural Step.** Remove gloves and discard in waste container.
17. **Procedural Step.** Return the thermometer to its storage container.
    Rationale. This ensures that the thermometer will be ready the next time it is needed.
18. **Procedural Step.** Sanitize the hands.
    Always sanitize the hands after a procedure or after wearing gloves.
19. **Procedural Step.** Document the results in the patient's medical record.

CHARTING EXAMPLE

Date	
9/17/xx	1:00 p.m. T: 101.2° F
	K. Lee, CMA (AAMA)

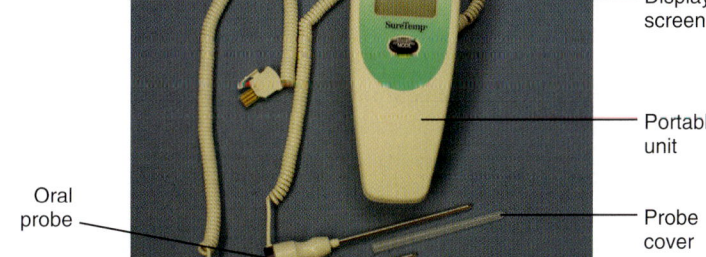

FIGURE 33-7 Electronic thermometer.

Temperature can be taken orally, axillary, or rectally with an electronic thermometer. Each machine has a color-coded oral and rectal probe. A disposable probe cover is placed over the probe to prevent cross-infection between patients. Depending on which one is used, the probe is inserted into the mouth, axilla, or rectum and left in place until a beep sounds from the thermometer. The temperature is displayed in degrees Fahrenheit. The medical assistant ejects the probe cover into a biohazardous waste receptacle.

Procedures 33-5, 33-6, and 33-7 provide information on correctly using the electronic or digital thermometer for measuring oral, rectal, and axillary temperatures, respectively.

Tympanic Thermometer

Tympanic thermometers are battery operated and digital and measure body temperature from the tympanic membrane of the ear (Figure 33-8). A disposable probe cover is used to prevent cross-contamination between patients. It registers the temperature within 1 to 2 seconds. For adults and children older than 3 years, the ear auricle is pulled back and up to straighten the ear canal before the tympanic probe is inserted into the ear. For children younger than 3 years, the ear pinna is pulled down and back. Procedure 33-8 explains the process of measuring temperature with a tympanic thermometer.

Disposable Oral Thermometer

Disposable oral thermometers can be paper or plastic and have chemically sensitive dots that change color when heated by the body. The temperature is visible within 60 seconds and is read by observing the highest reading among the dots that have changed color. Disposable oral thermometers are used primarily to determine if a patient is showing an elevation of temperature. Accuracy should be determined by using one of the other body temperature methods. Procedure 33-9 provides more information on taking temperature with a disposable oral thermometer.

Temperature-Sensitive Tape

Temperature-sensitive tape is usually applied to the forehead, but it can also be placed on the abdomen. The color of the tape changes according to body heat. The color range goes from "normal" to "above normal." When the color change ceases, the temperature is recorded. This is accomplished within 15 seconds (Figure 33-9). As with the disposable oral thermometer, temperature-sensitive tape is also used primarily to determine if someone has an elevation of temperature. Accuracy should be determined by using one of the other methods described.

Text continued on p. 702

SECTION V Clinical Medical Assisting

PROCEDURE 33-5

Measure Oral Body Temperature Using a Rechargeable Electronic or Digital Thermometer

TASK: Accurately measure and record a patient's oral temperature.

EQUIPMENT AND SUPPLIES
- Rechargeable electronic or digital thermometer
- Probe cover/thermometer sheath
- Waste container
- Disposable gloves
- Pen
- Patient's medical record

SKILLS/RATIONALE

STANDARD PRECAUTIONS ARE TO BE FOLLOWED.

1. **Procedural Step.** Sanitize the hands.
   An alcohol-based hand rub may be used instead of washing hands with soap and water, unless hands are visibly soiled.
   Rationale. Hand sanitization promotes infection control.

2. **Procedural Step.** Assemble equipment and supplies.
   Rationale. It is important to have all supplies and equipment ready and available before starting any procedure to ensure efficiency.

3. **Procedural Step.** Greet the patient, introduce yourself, and confirm the patient's identity.
   Rationale. Identifying the patient ensures the procedure is performed on the correct patient.

4. **Procedural Step.** Explain the procedure to the patient.
   Rationale. Explaining the procedure to the patient promotes cooperation and provides a means of obtaining implied consent.

5. **Procedural Step.** Determine if the patient has recently had a hot or cold beverage to drink or has smoked.
   Rationale. Hot or cold substances in the mouth will prevent an accurate temperature measurement. You must wait a minimum of 10 minutes before measuring a patient's oral temperature if this is the case.

6. **Procedural Step.** Remove the thermometer unit from its rechargeable base and attach the probe with the blue collar for measuring oral temperature.
   If using the digital thermometer cover the thermometer with a protective sheath, turn on the digital thermometer, and put on gloves.

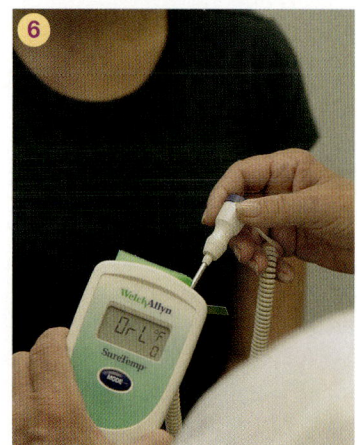

7. **Procedural Step.** Remove the thermometer probe from the probe holder.

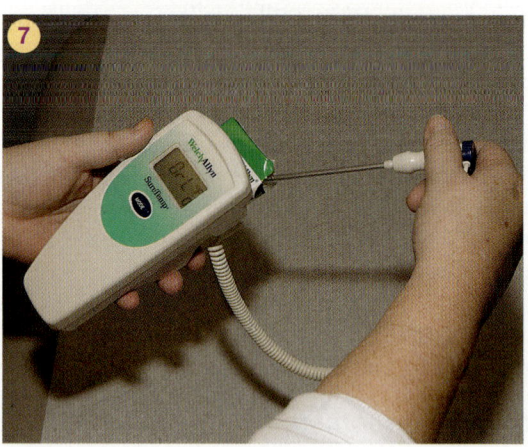

Continued

Body Measurements and Vital Signs **CHAPTER 33** 695

> **PROCEDURE 33-5** | **Measure Oral Body Temperature Using a Rechargeable Electronic or Digital Thermometer—cont'd**

8. **Procedural Step.** Assemble the thermometer probe and disposable probe cover.
   Secure the disposable probe cover over the thermometer probe by inserting the thermometer probe into a disposable probe cover while it is still in the box, which is usually placed near the charger. When the cover "snaps" onto the probe, withdraw the probe with the attached cover from the box.
   Rationale. If the probe cover is not attached, the thermometer will not measure the temperature and will not reset. Before taking the thermometer to the patient, be sure the digital reading shows "READY."

9. **Procedural Step.** Ask the patient to open his or her mouth. Place the thermometer probe with cover under the patient's tongue lateral to the center of the patient's jaw.
   Rationale. Heat from superficial blood vessels in the sublingual pockets produces the temperature readings.

10. **Procedural Step.** Ask the patient to close his or her mouth.
    Ask the patient to hold, not clasp, the thermometer between the teeth. Have the patient close the lips snugly around it to form an airtight seal.
    Rationale. Explain that the patient should not talk because the mouth must be closed, creating the airtight seal, for an accurate temperature reading.

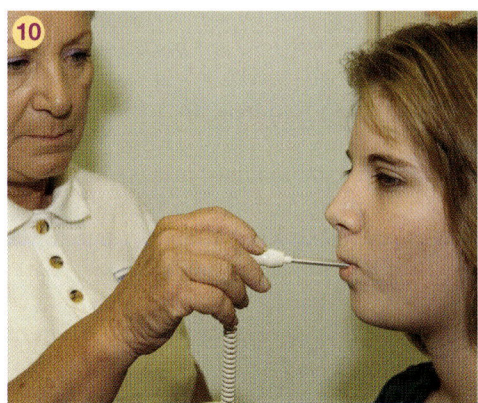

11. **Procedural Step.** When an alert signal is seen or heard, remove the thermometer from the patient's mouth.
12. **Procedural Step.** Read the results in the LED window of the unit or thermometer handle.
13. **Procedural Step.** Dispose of the thermometer probe cover or the disposable sheath.
    Immediately eject the probe cover into the waste container by firmly pressing the ejection button on the probe collar while holding the probe over the waste receptacle or peel the sheath away from digital thermometer. Do not allow the fingers to come in contact with the probe cover.

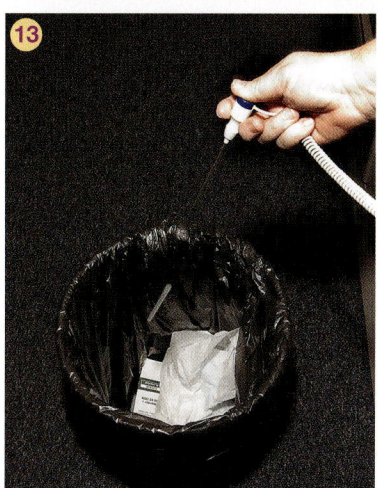

14. **Procedural Step.** Return the thermometer probe to the storage position of the thermometer unit or sanitize the tip of the digital thermometer with an alcohol wipe and store.

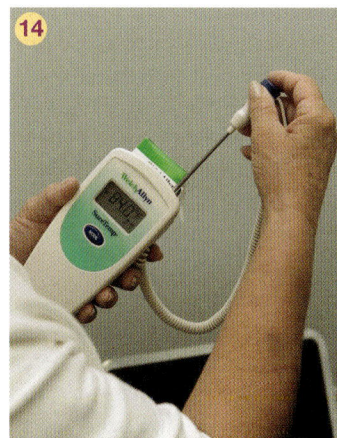

15. **Procedural Step.** Place the thermometer unit back on the rechargeable base.
    Rationale. This ensures that the thermometer will be ready the next time it is needed.
16. **Procedural Step.** Sanitize the hands.
    Always sanitize the hands after a procedure or after wearing gloves.
17. **Procedural Step.** Document the results in the patient's medical record.

CHARTING EXAMPLE

Date	
8/7/xx	11:00 a.m. T: 99.2° F———————
	——————T. Starling, CMA (AAMA)

PROCEDURE 33-6

Measure Rectal Body Temperature Using a Rechargeable Electronic or Digital Thermometer

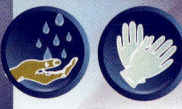

TASK: Accurately measure and record a patient's rectal temperature.

EQUIPMENT AND SUPPLIES
- Rechargeable electronic or digital thermometer
- Probe cover
- Disposable gloves
- Lubricant
- Biohazardous waste container
- Pen
- Patient's medical record
- Soft tissue
- Gauze squares

SKILLS/RATIONALE

STANDARD PRECAUTIONS ARE TO BE FOLLOWED.

NOTE: This procedure is performed in the same manner for children or adults with the obvious exceptions. This procedure addresses the steps required to perform the procedure on a child.

1. **Procedural Step.** Greet the patient, introduce yourself, and confirm the patient's identity.
   Identification of the child is obtained through confirmation from the parent or guardian.
   Rationale. Identifying the patient ensures the procedure is performed on the correct patient.

2. **Procedural Step.** Sanitize the hands.
   An alcohol-based hand rub may be used instead of washing hands with soap and water, unless hands are visibly soiled.
   Rationale. Hand sanitization promotes infection control.

3. **Procedural Step.** Assemble equipment and supplies.
   Rationale. It is important to have all supplies and equipment ready and available before starting any procedure to ensure efficiency.

4. **Procedural Step.** Explain the procedure to the patient's parent or guardian.
   Rationale. Explaining the procedure to the parent or guardian promotes cooperation and provides a means of obtaining implied consent.

5. **Procedural Step.** Remove the thermometer unit from its rechargeable base and attach the probe with the red collar for measuring rectal temperature.

6. **Procedural Step.** Remove the thermometer probe from the probe holder.

7. **Procedural Step.** Assemble the thermometer probe and disposable probe cover.
   Secure the disposable probe cover to the thermometer probe by inserting the thermometer probe into a disposable probe cover while it is still in the box, which is usually placed near the charger. When the probe cover "snaps" onto the probe, withdraw the probe with the attached tip from the box. Before taking the thermometer to the patient, be sure the digital reading shows "READY."
   Rationale. If the probe cover is not attached, the thermometer will not measure the temperature and will not reset.

8. **Procedural Step.** Place a plastic-lined disposable drape or pad cover on the table.
   Rationale. This prevents cross-contamination from one child to another. This also protects the tabletop from possible fecal contamination.

9. **Procedural Step.** Put on disposable gloves.
   Rationale. This protects you from possible contact with microorganisms in body secretions and feces from the child's anal area.

10. **Procedural Step.** Undress the child, including the diaper.
    The diaper must be removed just before obtaining the child's temperature. You may ask the parent or guardian to undress the child. Make sure the parent or guardian keeps the child from rolling from the examination table while you are preparing the thermometer.

11. **Procedural Step.** Squeeze a liberal portion of lubricant on gauze square.
    Lubricate the first 2 inches of the probe cover.
    Rationale. Lubricating 1½ to 2 inches of the tip helps with insertion of the thermometer.

12. **Procedural Step.** Have the parent or guardian hold the child firmly but comfortably so that the child lies still to avoid injury to the rectal wall.
    The child should be kept distracted so that you can insert the probe without resistance.

13. **Procedural Step.** Gently insert the tip of the thermometer probe about ½ inch for a child, or 1 to 2 inches for adults. Hold in place.
    NOTE: Do not force the thermometer. Do not use on infants.

Continued

PROCEDURE 33-6 Measure Rectal Body Temperature Using a Rechargeable Electronic or Digital Thermometer—cont'd

14. **Procedural Step.** When an alert signal is seen or heard, read the results in the LED window of the unit.
15. **Procedural Step.** Remove the thermometer probe.
    Remove and eject the probe cover into the waste container by firmly pressing the ejection button on the probe collar while holding the probe over the biohazardous waste receptacle. Do not allow the fingers to come in contact with the probe cover.
    Rationale. The plastic sheath on the tip has been exposed to microorganisms from the rectum that can transmit infection. Therefore the tip must be properly disposed of in a biohazardous waste container.
16. **Procedural Step.** Return the thermometer probe to the storage position on the thermometer unit.
17. **Procedural Step.** Place the thermometer unit back on the rechargeable base.
    Rationale. This ensures that the thermometer will be ready for use the next time it is needed.
18. **Procedural Step.** Wipe the child's anal area with tissue.
    Rationale. When the probe is removed from the rectum, the anal area on the child may become soiled.
19. **Procedural Step.** Remove soiled gloves and discard in a biohazardous waste container.
    Rationale. Gloves may have come in contact with microorganisms from the rectum.
20. **Procedural Step.** Sanitize the hands.
    Always sanitize the hands after a procedure or after wearing gloves.
21. **Procedural Step.** Document the results in the patient's medical record (Ⓡ indicates rectal).

CHARTING EXAMPLE	
Date	
8/7/xx	1:00 p.m. T: 101.2° F Ⓡ —————————
	b. Kioll, CMA (AAMA)

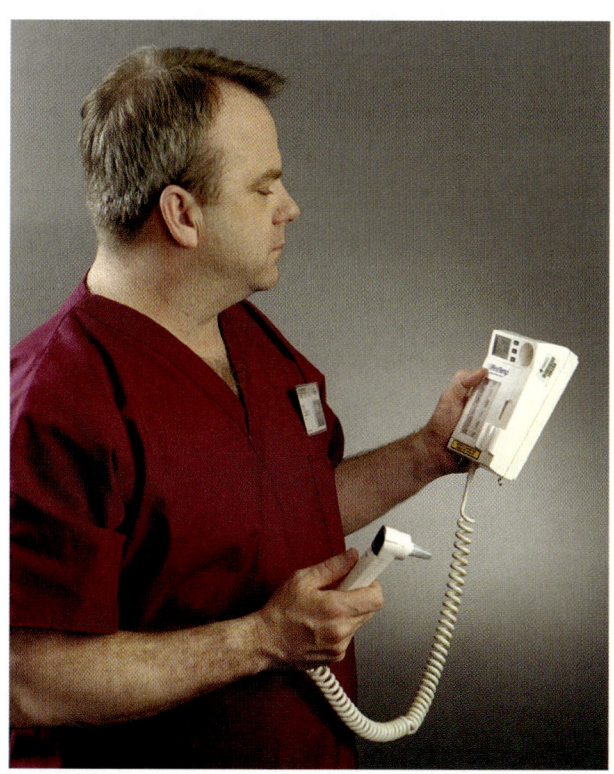

FIGURE 33-8 A medical assistant uses a tympanic thermometer that is battery operated, digital, and uses a disposable probe cover.

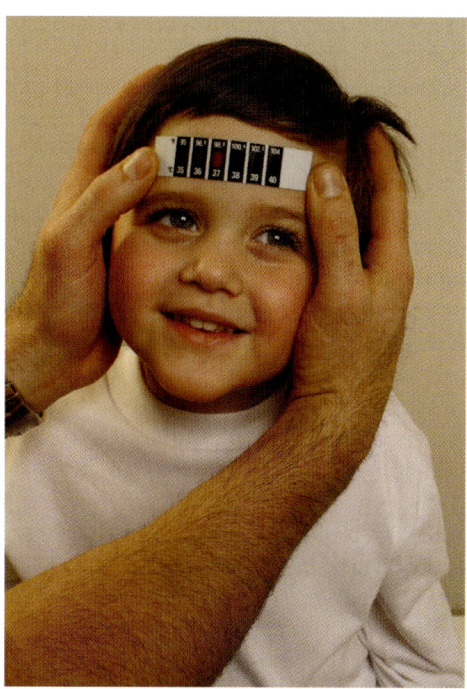

FIGURE 33-9 Temperature-sensitive tape is pressed onto the forehead and held in place until the color stops changing (generally 15 seconds). The results can be read by observing the color change and corresponding temperature indicated on the strip. (From Bonewit-West K: *Clinical procedures for medical assistants*, ed 7, St Louis, 2008, Saunders.)

PROCEDURE 33-7: Measure Axillary Body Temperature Using a Rechargeable Electronic or Digital Thermometer

TASK: Accurately measure and record a patient's axillary temperature.

EQUIPMENT AND SUPPLIES
- Rechargeable electronic or digital thermometer
- Probe cover
- Waste container
- Pen
- Patient's medical record

SKILLS/RATIONALE

STANDARD PRECAUTIONS ARE TO BE FOLLOWED.

1. **Procedural Step.** Greet the patient, introduce yourself, and confirm the patient's identity.
   Rationale. Identifying the patient ensures the procedure is performed on the correct patient.

2. **Procedural Step.** Sanitize the hands.
   An alcohol-based hand rub may be used instead of washing hands with soap and water, unless hands are visibly soiled.
   Rationale. Hand sanitization promotes infection control.

3. **Procedural Step.** Assemble equipment and supplies.
   Rationale. It is important to have all supplies and equipment ready and available before starting any procedure to ensure efficiency.

4. **Procedural Step.** Explain the procedure to the patient.
   Rationale. Explaining the procedure to the patient promotes cooperation and provides a means of obtaining implied consent.

5. **Procedural Step.** Remove the thermometer unit from its rechargeable base and attach the probe with the blue collar for measuring axillary temperature.

6. **Procedural Step.** Remove the thermometer probe from the probe holder.

7. **Procedural Step.** Assemble the thermometer probe and disposable probe cover.
   Secure the disposable cover to the thermometer probe by inserting the thermometer probe into a disposable probe cover while it is still in the box, which is usually placed near the charger. When the probe cover "snaps" onto the probe, withdraw the thermometer probe with the attached probe cover from the box. Before taking the thermometer to the patient, be sure the digital reading shows "READY."
   Rationale. If the probe cover is not attached, the thermometer will not measure the temperature and will not reset.

8. **Procedural Step.** Remove the patient's clothing as needed to access the axillary region.

9. **Procedural Step.** Pat the axilla and axillary area dry if needed.
   Rationale. Do not rub the area; friction may elevate the reading.

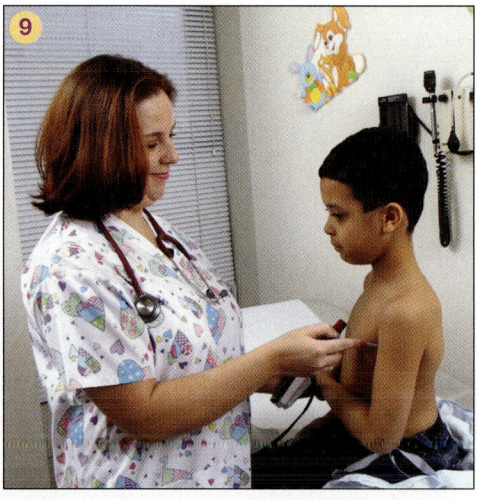

10. **Procedural Step.** Place the probe into the center of the patient's axilla (armpit).
    Make sure the probe touches only skin and not clothing.
    Rationale. If the probe touches clothing, it will produce an inaccurate reading.

11. **Procedural Step.** Instruct the patient to hold the arm snugly across the chest until the thermometer beeps.
    Rationale. Holding the arm snugly brings the body tissue into contact with the thermometer.

12. **Procedural Step.** When an alert signal is seen or heard, remove the probe from the patient's armpit.

13. **Procedural Step.** Read the results in the LED window of the unit.

Continued

PROCEDURE 33-7: Measure Axillary Body Temperature Using a Rechargeable Electronic or Digital Thermometer—cont'd

14. **Procedural Step. Dispose of the probe tip.**
    Immediately eject the probe tip into the waste container by firmly pressing the ejection button on the probe collar while holding the probe over the waste receptacle. Do not allow the fingers to come in contact with the probe cover.
15. **Procedural Step. Return the thermometer probe to the storage position on the thermometer unit.**
16. **Procedural Step. Place the thermometer unit back on its rechargeable base.**
    Rationale. This ensures that the thermometer will be ready for use the next time it is needed.
17. **Procedural Step. Sanitize the hands.**
    Always sanitize the hands after a procedure or after wearing gloves.
18. **Procedural Step. Document the results in the patient's medical record (Ⓐ indicates axillary).**

CHARTING EXAMPLE

Date	
7/1/xx	1:00 p.m. T: 97° FⒶ————L. Fisher, RMA

PROCEDURE 33-8: Measure Body Temperature Using a Tympanic Thermometer

TASK: Accurately measure and record a patient's temperature using a tympanic thermometer.

EQUIPMENT AND SUPPLIES
- Tympanic thermometer
- Disposable probe covers
- Patient's medical record
- Waste container/biohazardous waste container

SKILLS/RATIONALE
STANDARD PRECAUTIONS ARE TO BE FOLLOWED.

1. **Procedural Step. Sanitize the hands.**
   An alcohol-based hand rub may be used instead of washing hands with soap and water, unless hands are visibly soiled.
   Rationale. Hand sanitization promotes infection control.
2. **Procedural Step. Assemble equipment and supplies.**
   Rationale. It is important to have all supplies and equipment ready and available before starting any procedure to ensure efficiency.
3. **Procedural Step. Greet the patient, introduce yourself, and confirm the patient's identity.**
   Rationale. Identifying the patient ensures the procedure is performed on the correct patient.
4. **Procedural Step. Explain the procedure to the patient.**
   Rationale. Explaining the procedure to the patient promotes cooperation and provides a means of obtaining implied consent.

NOTE: To prevent an elevated reading, patients with hearing aids should remove them 15-20 minutes before taking the reading.

5. **Procedural Step. Remove the thermometer from the charger.**
6. **Procedural Step. Check to make sure the mode for interpretation of temperature is set to "oral" mode.**
7. **Procedural Step. Check the lens probe to be sure it is clean and not scratched.**
8. **Procedural Step. Turn on the thermometer.**
   If the thermometer is a model that turns on when the probe cover is attached, skip this step.
9. **Procedural Step. Insert the probe firmly into a disposable plastic probe cover.**
10. **Procedural Step. Wait for a digital "READY" display.**

Continued

PROCEDURE 33-8 Measure Body Temperature Using a Tympanic Thermometer—cont'd

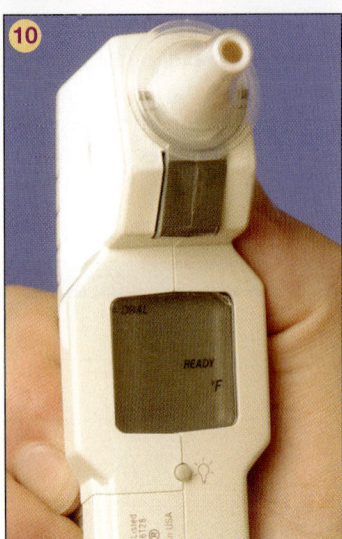

11. **Procedural Step.** Pull the patient's ear to straighten the auditory canal with the hand not holding the probe.

    For infants, pull the pinna down and then back; for children over 3 years and adults, pull the pinna up and back.

    Rationale. Correct positioning of probe allows for maximum exposure of tympanic membrane.

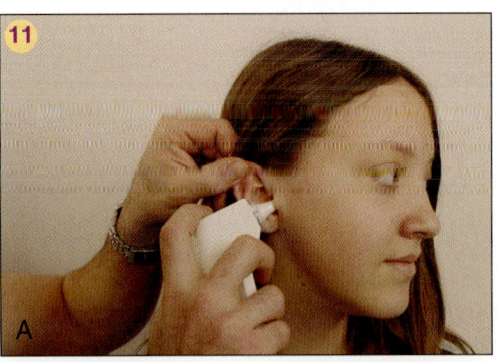

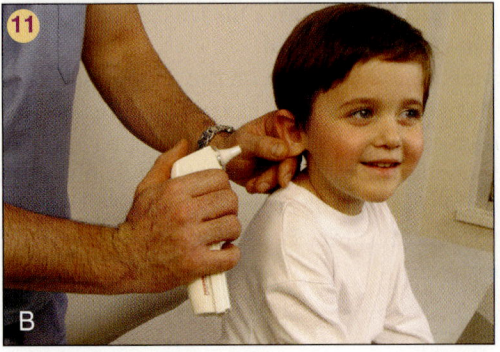

12. **Procedural Step.** Insert the probe into the patient's ear and tightly seal the auditory canal opening.

    Take care not to cause the patient any discomfort.

    Rationale. Sealing the opening of the auditory canal prevents air from altering readings.

13. **Procedural Step.** Position the probe.
14. **Procedural Step.** Depress the activation button.

    Hold the thermometer steady and depress the activation button for 2 seconds.
15. **Procedural Step.** Release the activation button.
16. **Procedural Step.** Remove the probe from the ear and read the temperature.
17. **Procedural Step.** Note the reading, making sure that the screen displays "oral" as the mode of interpretation.

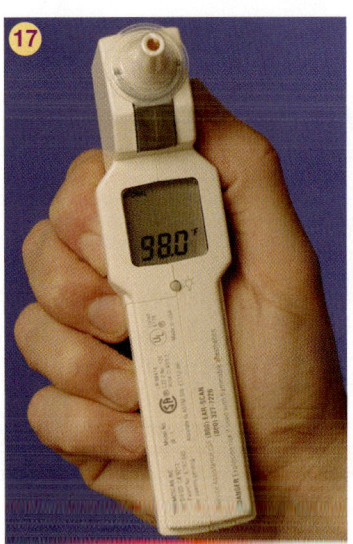

18. **Procedural Step.** Discard the probe cover in a biohazardous waste container if drainage.
19. **Procedural Step.** Replace the thermometer on the charger base.

    Rationale. This ensures that the thermometer will be ready the next time it is needed.
20. **Procedural Step.** Sanitize the hands.

    Always sanitize the hands after a procedure or after wearing gloves.
21. **Procedural Step.** Document the results in the patient's medical record (Ⓣ indicates tympanic).

CHARTING EXAMPLE	
Date	
3/31/xx	10:00 a.m. T: 99.8° F Ⓣ ———————
	——————— P. Konters, CMA (AAMA)

Photos from Bonewit-West K: Clinical procedures for medical assistants, ed 7, St Louis, 2008, Saunders.

Body Measurements and Vital Signs **CHAPTER 33** 701

| PROCEDURE 33-9 | **Measure Body Temperature Using a Disposable Oral Thermometer** | |

TASK: Accurately measure and record a patient's oral temperature using a disposable thermometer.

EQUIPMENT AND SUPPLIES
- Disposable thermometer
- Disposable gloves
- Waste container
- Patient's medical record

SKILLS/*RATIONALE*

STANDARD PRECAUTIONS ARE TO BE FOLLOWED.

1. **Procedural Step. Sanitize the hands.**
   An alcohol-based hand rub may be used instead of washing hands with soap and water, unless hands are visibly soiled.
   Rationale. Hand sanitization promotes infection control.

2. **Procedural Step. Assemble equipment and supplies.**
   Rationale. It is important to have all supplies and equipment ready and available before starting any procedure to ensure efficiency.

3. **Procedural Step. Greet the patient, introduce yourself, and confirm the patient's identity.**
   Rationale. Identifying the patient ensures the procedure is performed on the correct patient.

4. **Procedural Step. Explain the procedure to the patient.**
   Rationale. Explaining the procedure to the patient promotes cooperation and provides a means of obtaining implied consent.

5. **Procedural Step. Put on disposable gloves.**
   Rationale. This protects against possible contact with microorganisms in body secretions.

6. **Procedural Step. Open the thermometer packaging.** Typically, you "peel apart" the packaging.

7. **Procedural Step. Place the thermometer under the patient's tongue and wait 60 seconds.**

   Rationale. The thermometer must remain in the patient's mouth for the correct time or the results will be inaccurate. Disposable thermometers are also designed to be placed on the forehead.

8. **Procedural Step. Remove the thermometer and read the results by looking at the colored dots.**

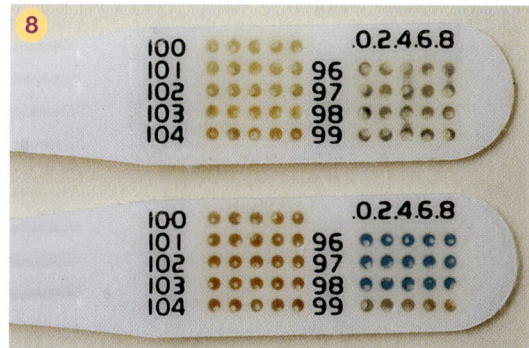

9. **Procedural Step. Discard the thermometer and gloves in a waste container.**

10. **Procedural Step. Sanitize the hands.**
    Always sanitize the hands after a procedure or after wearing gloves.

11. **Procedural Step. Document the results in the patient's medical record.**

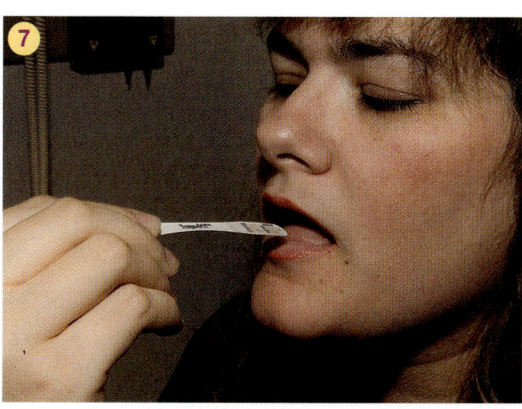

CHARTING EXAMPLE	
Date	
7/7/xx	9:00 a.m. T: 98.8° F ————————
	———————— D. DiMonda, CMA (AAMA)

Photo for step 8 from Sorrentino SA: Assisting with patient care, ed 2, St Louis, 2004, Mosby.

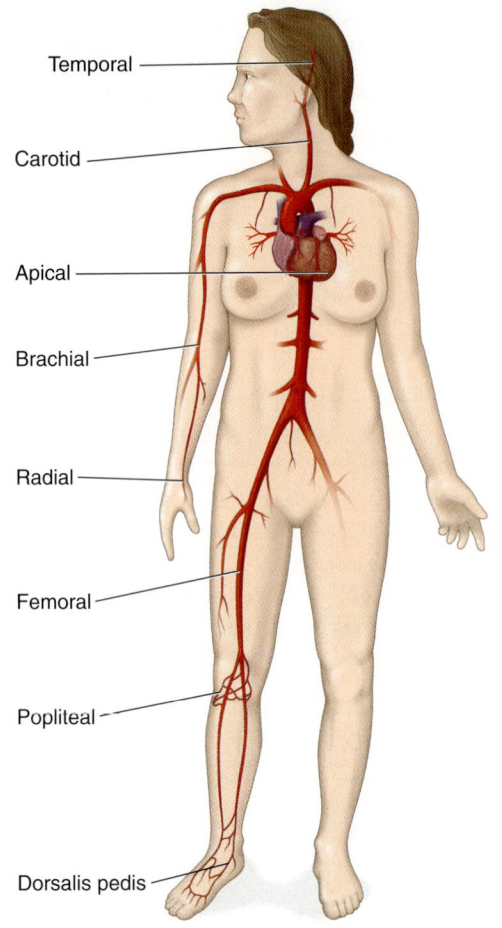

FIGURE 33-10 Pulse sites.

Pulse

The **pulse rate** is a measurement of the number of times the heart beats in a minute. The **pulse** is the vibration (pressure wave) felt when blood is forced from the aorta through the arteries and pressed against a bone. The vibration is caused by the contraction and expansion of an artery as blood passes through. Measuring the pulse provides information on how fast or how slow the heart is beating. The adult pulse rate is 60 to 100 beats per minute. If the rate is over 100 beats per minute, the patient is said to be experiencing **tachycardia**. Lower than 60 beats per minute is referred to as **bradycardia**.

Table 33-3 provides ranges for pulse rate in various age groups.

Pulse Characteristics

When taking the patient's pulse, the medical assistant must note the characteristics of (1) rate, (2) rhythm, and (3) volume. Any extreme variations in pulse rate, rhythm, and volume must be noted and recorded and the physician informed. *Never* make a patient return to the waiting room or wait in the examination room with a vital sign that is extremely abnormal. The physician should specify to the staff what elevation ranges require that the patient be seen immediately.

TABLE 33-3
Normal Pulse Rate Averages

Age Group	Range (beats/min)
Birth to 1 year	110 to 170
1 year to 6 years	80 to 120
12 years to adult	60 to 100
Elderly	55 to 70

Rate. Pulse rate and heartbeat are normally the same. When recording the **rate**, the number of beats felt per minute is recorded. It is acceptable to take a pulse for 30 seconds and multiply that number by 2 to obtain the rate, but it is better to take the pulse for a full 60 seconds. If the rate is irregular, the pulse rate must be counted for 1 full minute.

Many factors can affect the pulse rate. When taking a pulse you will notice that different age groups have different ranges of normal beats per minute (see Table 33-3). As a person ages, the normal number of beats per minute decreases. Differences can be caused by other factors as well. Females tend to have a faster pulse rate than males. A morning pulse will be slower than a pulse taken later in the day. A conditioned athlete's pulse will be slower than that of a patient who is the same age and gender but is not in the same physical condition. The heart rate will increase with physical exertion and emotional stress, but it will decrease with depression. These conditions, when apparent, should be charted. Medications, alcohol, and nicotine also can raise or lower a pulse rate, and the body's response to disease (e.g., infection) is to increase the pulse rate.

Rhythm. The **rhythm** is the time interval between each heartbeat. The medical assistant needs to pay close attention to the steadiness of the beat. A very steady, rhythmical beat is recorded as "regular." If a beat skips or if the rhythm speeds up, then slows down, or any variation from a steady rate occurs, the rhythm is recorded as "irregular" and the physician notified. The arterial walls of the older patient may become rigid, forcing a faster upstroke of blood, thereby causing a slightly irregular rhythm.

Volume. **Volume** refers to the strength or force of each heartbeat, as described by the following words:

- *Full* or "bounding" indicates an increase in blood volume; a *bounding pulse* feels strong and forceful.
- *Strong* indicates a normal blood volume.
- *Weak* or "thready" indicates a decrease in blood volume; a *thready pulse* feels like a small cord or thread under the finger.

Pulse Sites

There are several areas in the body where the pulse rate can be easily measured because the artery is near the surface of the body. The **apical** rate is taken over the apex of the heart with a stethoscope. Other pulse sites include the following arteries: **temporal, carotid, brachial, radial, femoral, popliteal, posterior tibial,** and **dorsalis pedis** (Figure 33-10). Table 33-4 provides information about common pulse sites. Remember the pulse site used should be the one closest to the area that is being checked for circulation. For example, you would not use the femoral artery to assess the circulation of the foot.

Pulse sites are used to measure the pulse and may be compressed to control bleeding. When counting a pulse, the fingers are placed over the artery, and gentle pressure is applied against a bone. This is often performed in conjunction with taking a blood pressure. Box 33-4 reviews information needed when charting a patient's pulse.

Pulse Measurement

Medical assistants need to be able to measure pulse at any of the pulse sites. Specific patient needs and conditions determine the site to be used.

Radial Pulse. The **radial pulse** is the most common site used to measure pulse rate. When taking routine vital signs, the pulse is found by placing two or three fingers over the radial artery about 1 inch above the wrist crease on the thumb side of the hand. If the pulse is regular and strong, count for 30 seconds and multiply the number by 2 to obtain the pulse rate. Medical assistants should wear a watch with a second hand to correctly time and document the pulse rate. If there are any variations, the pulse must be taken for 1 full minute. When charting, you must record the rate, rhythm, and volume (Procedure 33-10).

Apical Pulse. To take an **apical pulse**, a stethoscope must be used. The apex of the heart must be located by placing the fingertips on the left side of the chest, just below the left nipple in the intercostal space between the fifth and sixth ribs (Figure 33-11). The stethoscope is placed over the area, and the

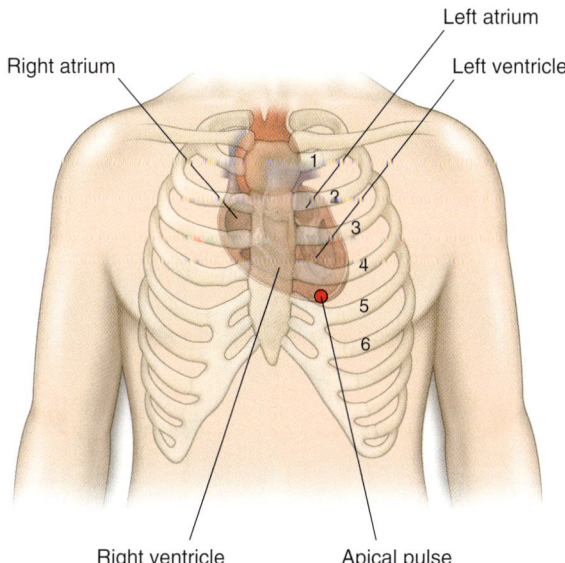

FIGURE 33-11 Apical pulse is found over the apex of the heart, which is located just below the left nipple between the fifth and sixth ribs. (Modified from Bonewit-West K: *Clinical procedures for medical assistants,* ed 7, St Louis, 2008, Saunders.)

BOX 33-4

Documentation when Charting a Patient's Pulse

ADULT
1. Date
2. Time
3. Name of procedure:
   - Pulse
4. Assessment site (typically radial or apical)
5. Results
   - Rate
   - Rhythm
   - Volume
6. Patient reaction, if any
7. Proper signature and credential

CHILD
1. Date
2. Time
3. Name of procedure:
   - Pulse
4. Assessment site (typically radial, apical, or brachial)
5. Results
   - Rate
   - Rhythm
   - Volume
6. Patient reaction, if any
7. Proper signature and credential

TABLE 33-4

Common Pulse Sites

Site	Location	When Used
Temporal	Just above ear	To control bleeding in patient with head injury
		When radial pulse not available
Carotid	Between larynx and sternocleidomastoid muscle	During CPR
Brachial	Inner aspect of elbow	When taking blood pressure
Radial	Thumb side of wrist	Most frequently, when recording pulse measurement
Femoral	Upper area of leg in middle groin region	To assess circulation to lower extremities and could be used during CPR
Popliteal	Behind knee	To assess circulation to lower extremities
Posterior tibial (pedal pulse)	Inside of the ankle	To assess circulation to feet
Dorsalis pedis	Top of foot	To assess circulation to feet
Apex of heart (apical pulse)	At base of heart in left fifth intercostal space	Infants and patients receiving medication (e.g., digitalis)
	Heard with stethoscope	Patients with irregular heartbeat

CPR, Cardiopulmonary resuscitation.

PROCEDURE 33-10 Measure Radial Pulse

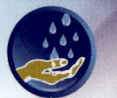

TASK: Accurately measure and record the rate, rhythm, and quality of a patient's pulse.

EQUIPMENT AND SUPPLIES
- Watch with a second hand
- Patient's medical record
- Pen

SKILLS/RATIONALE

STANDARD PRECAUTIONS ARE TO BE FOLLOWED.

1. **Procedural Step.** Greet the patient, introduce yourself, and confirm the patient's identity.
   Rationale. Identifying the patient ensures the procedure is performed on the correct patient.

2. **Procedural Step.** Sanitize the hands.
   An alcohol-based hand rub may be used instead of washing hands with soap and water, unless hands are visibly soiled.
   Rationale. Hand sanitization promotes infection control.

3. **Procedural Step.** Assemble equipment and supplies.
   Rationale. It is important to have all supplies and equipment ready and available before starting any procedure to ensure efficiency.

4. **Procedural Step.** Explain the procedure to the patient.
   Rationale. Explaining the procedure to the patient promotes cooperation and provides a means of obtaining implied consent.

5. **Procedural Step.** Observe the patient for any signs that may result in an increase or a decrease in the pulse rate.
   Rationale. Pulse rate can vary according to age, gender, physical activity, emotional state, metabolism, and medications.

6. **Procedural Step.** Position the patient.
   The sitting position allows easy access to pulse sites. The patient's lower arm should be in a comfortable position, with the forearm slightly flexed, and the hand palm down.
   Rationale. Position of the lower arm and extension of the wrist permits full exposure of the artery for palpation.

7. **Procedural Step.** Place the tips of the first two or middle three fingers of the hand over the groove along the radial artery of the patient's inner wrist.
   Rationale. The fingertips are the most sensitive parts of the hand, and the thumb has a pulse of its own.

8. **Procedural Step.** Apply light pressure against the radius, enough to allow the pulse to be felt.
   Rationale. A normal pulse can be felt with light pressure. Too much pressure occludes pulse and impairs blood flow.

9. **Procedural Step.** Count the pulse rate for 30 seconds and multiply by 2 if the pulse is regular.
   Determine strength, rhythm, and quality of the pulse. If the pulse rate is irregular, count the pulse for 1 full minute.
   Rationale. A 30-second count is accurate for a regular pulse rate. A longer time period is needed for any irregularities.

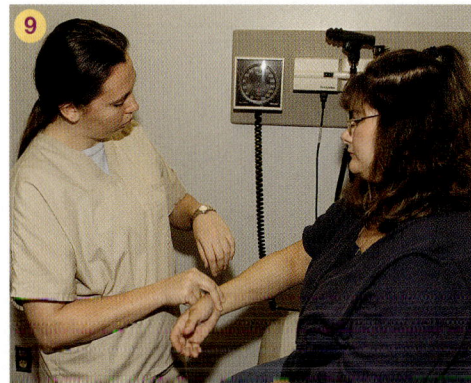

10. **Procedural Step.** Sanitize the hands.
    Always sanitize the hands after a procedure or after wearing gloves.

11. **Procedural Step.** Document the results in the patient's medical record; include the pulse rate, rhythm, and volume.
    NOTE: It is acceptable to chart just the pulse reading if the rate, volume, and rhythm are normal.

CHARTING EXAMPLE

Date	
7/30/xx	2:00 p.m. P: 72, Reg and strong —————— M. Crissip, CMA (AAMA)

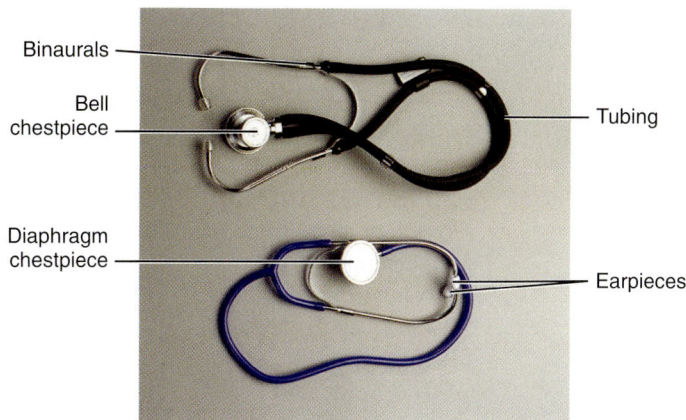

FIGURE 33-12 Parts of stethoscope.

medical assistant listens for the *lubb-dupp* sounds made by the heart. Each *lubb-dupp* is counted as one beat. Before some medications (e.g., digoxin) are administered, the patient's apical pulse must be taken. This is required when the radial pulse is less than 60. The difference between the apical pulse and the radial pulse is called a **pulse deficit**. Taking an apical pulse is often used with infants (Procedure 33-11).

Stethoscope

The **stethoscope** is an instrument used to listen to body sounds (e.g., heartbeat, bowel sounds, and lung sounds). Stethoscopes may be electronic or regular. Although it looks very similar to a regular stethoscope, the electronic stethoscope greatly amplifies the sounds of the heart, enabling the heart sounds to be heard better through clothing and faint sounds to be heard that may not be picked up with a regular stethoscope.

You need to know the parts of a stethoscope to understand its use and care (Figure 33-12). The *diaphragm* (larger, flat surface) is used to hear high-frequency sounds of the lungs (breath), bowel, and normal heart sounds. The *bell* (smaller, flat surface) is used to detect low-frequency sounds of the heart valves. General usage guidelines are as follows:

1. Clean the earpieces and diaphragm with alcohol before using.
2. Clean the tubing and check for cracks.
3. Place the earpieces forward in the ears so they point downward (toward the nose).
4. To be effective, ensure that the diaphragm does not touch clothing or the blood pressure cuff.
5. Place the diaphragm firmly and flatly against the patient's skin.
6. Hold the diaphragm in place with gentle pressure. Pressing too hard may decrease the ability to hear.

The potential for cross-contamination is very high because the stethoscope is used on many patients and is passed among health care workers. For these reasons, it is necessary to sanitize the diaphragm between patients (and the earpieces, if the stethoscope is used by more than one person).

Respiratory Rate

In addition to temperature and pulse, **respiratory rate** is another vital sign taken by the medical assistant. The number of cycles per minute is counted when taking a patient's respiratory rate. Breathing in (**inspiration**) and breathing out (**expiration**) is one cycle and is counted as "one." Adults have a respiratory rate of 16 to 20 cycles per minute. Children breathe faster—20 to 40 cycles in early childhood and 18 to 25 in later childhood—and older adults breathe slower—14 to 16 cycles. Because patients can voluntarily control **respiration,** it is best to measure respirations without the patient knowing. By continuing to hold the wrist after the pulse is taken, the patient may not know when the respirations are being counted and therefore will not adjust the breathing pattern.

Respirations are charted according to rate, rhythm, and depth with other patient documentation (Box 33-5).

Respiratory rate can be described as being normal, rapid, or slow. For every respiration, there are usually four pulse beats or heartbeats; this represents a 1:4 ratio of respirations to pulse beats. Both physical status and emotional state affect the rate of respirations. For example, a patient with an ele-

BOX 33-5

Documentation when Charting Respiration in Children and Adults

1. Date
2. Time
3. Name of procedure:
   - Respiration
4. Results
   - Rate
   - Rhythm
   - Depth
5. Patient reaction, if any
6. Proper signature and credential

PROCEDURE 33-11 Measure Apical Pulse

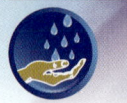

TASK: Accurately measure and record a patient's apical pulse.

EQUIPMENT AND SUPPLIES
- Watch (with a second hand)
- Stethoscope
- Alcohol wipe
- Patient's medical record
- Pen

SKILLS/RATIONALE

STANDARD PRECAUTIONS ARE TO BE FOLLOWED.

1. **Procedural Step.** Sanitize the hands.
   An alcohol-based hand rub may be used instead of washing hands with soap and water, unless hands are visibly soiled.
   Rationale. Hand sanitization promotes infection control.

2. **Procedural Step.** Assemble equipment and supplies.
   Rationale. It is important to have all supplies and equipment ready and available before starting any procedure to ensure efficiency.

3. **Procedural Step.** Greet the patient, introduce yourself, and confirm the patient's identity.
   Rationale. Identifying the patient ensures the procedure is performed on the correct patient.

4. **Procedural Step.** Explain the procedure to the patient.
   Rationale. Explaining the procedure to the patient promotes cooperation and provides a means of obtaining implied consent.

5. **Procedural Step.** Clean the earpieces and diaphragm of the stethoscope with an alcohol wipe.
   Rationale. Cleaning reduces the transmission of microorganisms.

6. **Procedural Step.** Position the patient in a supine (lying face up) or sitting position and carefully open the patient's shirt or blouse, taking care to protect the patient's modesty. Locate the fifth intercostal space at the midclavicular line (left nipple/under the breast).
   Rationale. Either position allows for access to the apex of the heart.

7. **Procedural Step.** Position the stethoscope.
   Warm the diaphragm of the stethoscope with your hand. Insert the earpieces of the stethoscope into your ears, with the earpieces directed toward the face, and place the chest piece (diaphragm) over the apex of the heart.
   Rationale. Warming the chest piece helps reduce the discomfort of having a cold object placed on the skin.

8. **Procedural Step.** Listen for the heartbeat (lubb-dupp) and count the number of beats for 1 full minute. Pay close attention to the rhythm and strength of the heartbeat.

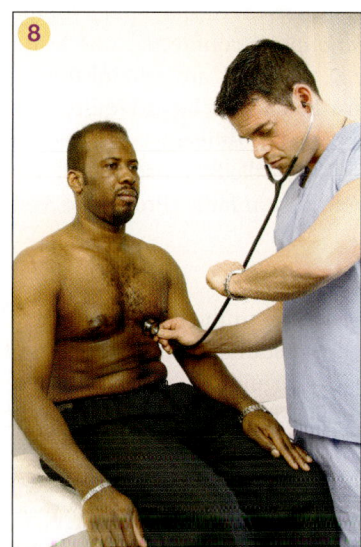

9. **Procedural Step.** Sanitize the hands.
   Always sanitize the hands after a procedure or after wearing gloves.

10. **Procedural Step.** Document the results in the patient's medical record; include the pulse rate, rhythm, and volume.
    Rationale. Good documentation techniques provide for a more complete patient record.

11. **Procedural Step.** Clean the stethoscope earpieces and diaphragm with an alcohol wipe.
    Regular disinfection can control nosocomial infections.

CHARTING EXAMPLE

Date		
2/15/xx	10:30 a.m. AP: 68	
		N. Stevens, CMA (AAMA)

Photo from Bonewit-West K: Clinical procedures for medical assistants, ed 7, St Louis, 2008, Saunders.

vated temperature will usually have an increase in pulse and respiratory rate. Procedure 33-12 explains the process of measuring respiratory rate.

Respiratory rhythm is concerned with breathing patterns. A regular rhythm will be even in rate and depth. The patient with irregular breathing patterns will inhale and exhale at different rates. For example, a patient with emphysema will be able to inhale without difficulty, but on exhalation the patient will struggle. When documenting a patient's breathing pattern, the use of specific terms to indicate difficult breathing (e.g., dyspnea, hyperpnea) alerts the physician to an apparent problem.

Recognition of *respiratory depth* includes an observation for shallow or deep respirations. Normal breathing is relaxed, effortless, and silent.

Patients with certain respiratory disease or conditions may have the following breath sounds:

- **Stridor** is a shrill sound heard on inspiration.
- **Rales** are caused by fluid or secretions in the bronchus and sound like tissue paper being crumpled.
- **Rhonchi** are low-pitched sounds created as air goes through mucus or narrowed bronchi.
- **Wheezes** are high-pitched sounds that occur when bronchial tubes are narrowed by disease (e.g., asthma).

The aging patient may experience a decrease in vital capacity and a decreased inspiratory reserve volume. Therefore inspirations may be shallower and the respiratory rate may increase.

Blood Pressure

Blood pressure is another vital sign taken in the medical office. As blood is being pumped through the circulatory system, pressure is exerted on the walls of arteries. How much pressure depends on the force of the heartbeat and the condition of the arteries. When the ventricles contract, the first measurable pressure is the **systolic pressure.** When the heart rests between contractions, the blood in the arteries exerts less pressure. This minimum pressure, or "resting" pressure, is the **diastolic pressure.**

Blood pressure is read in millimeters of mercury (mm Hg). The normal range for an adult systolic pressure is between 100 and 120 mm Hg, which means a blood pressure reading of 110/70 indicates the amount of force needed to raise a column of mercury to the 110 mm calibration during systole and to 70 mm during diastole. The normal diastolic pressure range is between 60 and 90 mm Hg. When recording a patient's blood pressure, write it as a fraction. The systolic is recorded first (on the top) and the diastolic is recorded second (on the bottom), for example, 130/82. **Pulse pressure** is the difference between the systolic and the diastolic reading. For example, the pulse pressure for a reading of 110/80 is 40 (110 − 70 = 40). The normal range for pulse pressure is 30 to 50 mm Hg.

The following factors influence a person's blood pressure:

1. *Gender.* Women usually have a lower blood pressure than men, but their blood pressure tends to rise after menopause.
2. *Age.* As a person ages, the arteries lose some of their elasticity. This increases as the person continues to age, thereby lowering blood pressure.
3. *Heredity.* Hypertension tends to run in families.
4. *Diet and exercise.* Diets high in sodium increase water retention in the body, thereby increasing blood pressure. Exercise increases heart rate and blood pressure. A person's blood pressure should not be taken immediately after exercise.
5. *Medications.* Some medications have side effects that will raise or lower a person's blood pressure.
6. *Emotional turmoil.* The body responds to stress with an increased heart rate and elevated blood pressure. "White coat syndrome" occurs when a patient who would not normally have elevated blood pressure reacts to being in the physician's office.
7. *Position.* Blood pressure tends to be lower when patients are sitting or lying down than when they are standing.
8. *Smoking and alcohol.* Blood vessels narrow as a result of alcohol use and smoking, which causes a rise in blood pressure.

Hypertension is high blood pressure, and **hypotension** is low blood pressure. *Orthostatic hypotension (postural hypotension)* occurs when the patient moves from a sitting or lying position to a standing position. Table 33-5 lists normal blood pressure ranges for children, as well as normal and some abnormal ranges in adults.

Blood pressure needs to be taken in a quiet area, away from distractions. Most often, this is done in the examination room. The patient can be sitting, standing, or lying down. The following styles of **sphygmomanometers** are available (Figures 33-13 and 33-14):

- The *aneroid mobile* sphygmomanometer has a large circular dial calibrated in pressure increments of 2 mm.
- The *aneroid* sphygmomanometer with cuff has a calibrated dial gauge with each line representing 2 mm Hg of pressure.

TABLE 33-5

Normal Blood Pressure Range (mm Hg)

CHILDREN

Age	Systolic/Diastolic
Birth to 1 year	95/70
Toddler to school age	100/70
6 to 13 years	110/74
14 to 18 years	120/76

ADULTS

Category	Systolic		Diastolic
Normal	<120	and	<80
Prehypertension	120 to 139	or	80 to 89
Hypertension, stage 1	140 to 159	or	90 to 99
Hypertension, stage 2	≥160	or	≥100

PROCEDURE 33-12 | **Measure Respiratory Rate**

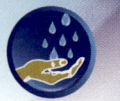

TASK: Accurately measure and record a patient's respiratory rate.

EQUIPMENT AND SUPPLIES
- Watch with a second hand
- Patient's medical record
- Pen

SKILLS/RATIONALE

STANDARD PRECAUTIONS ARE TO BE FOLLOWED.

NOTE: Assess the respirations after obtaining the pulse. Continue to place the fingers on the patient's wrist, or lightly place your hand on the patient's back, and count the respirations. This prevents the patient from altering rate and depth of breathing.

1. **Procedural Step.** Greet the patient, introduce yourself, and confirm the patient's identity.
   Rationale. Identifying the patient ensures the procedure is performed on the correct patient.

2. **Procedural Step.** Sanitize the hands.
   An alcohol-based hand rub may be used instead of washing hands with soap and water, unless hands are visibly soiled.
   Rationale. Hand sanitization promotes infection control.

3. **Procedural Step.** Assemble equipment and supplies.
   Rationale. It is important to have all supplies and equipment ready and available before starting any procedure to ensure efficiency.

4. **Procedural Step.** Explain the procedure to the patient.
   NOTE: This step should be eliminated if you feel the patient will consciously or unintentionally alter his or her breathing patterns.
   Rationale. Explaining the procedure to the patient promotes cooperation and provides a means of obtaining implied consent.

5. **Procedural Step.** Count each complete rise (inhalation) and fall (exhalation) of the chest as one respiration.
   Pay attention to the depth and rhythm of respirations.

6. **Procedural Step.** Count the respiratory rate for 30 seconds and multiply by 2.
   If the breathing pattern is irregular (<12 or >20), count for 1 full minute.

NOTE: Breathe with the patient to help you concentrate on the rise and fall of the patient's chest.

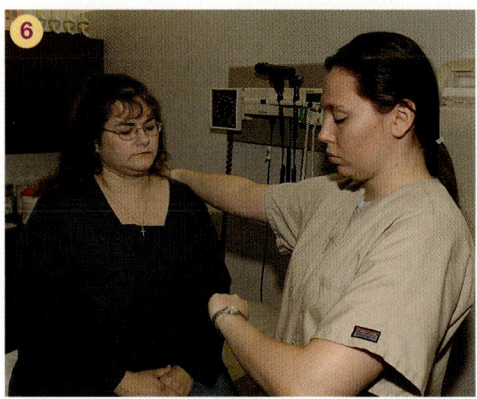

7. **Procedural Step.** Sanitize the hands.
   Always sanitize the hands after a procedure or after wearing gloves.

8. **Procedural Step.** Document the results in the patient's medical record; include rate, rhythm, and depth of the respirations.
   NOTE: It is acceptable to chart just the respiratory count if the rate, depth, and rhythm are normal.

CHARTING EXAMPLE	
Date	
4/19/xx	9:00 a.m. R: 16 ———— D. Bailey, RMA

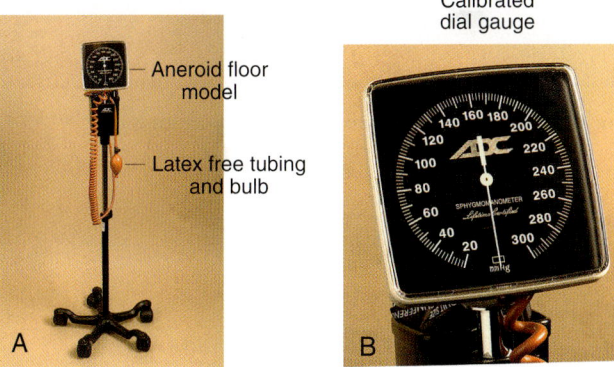

FIGURE 33-13 **A,** An aneroid floor model sphygmomanometer with latex-free tubing. **B,** Calibrated dial gauge.

BOX 33-6

Documentation when Charting Blood Pressure in Children and Adults

1. Date
2. Time
3. Name of procedure:
   - Blood pressure
4. Assessment site (typically brachial artery)
5. Results
   - Systolic pressure
   - Diastolic pressure
6. Patient reaction, if any
7. Proper signature and credential

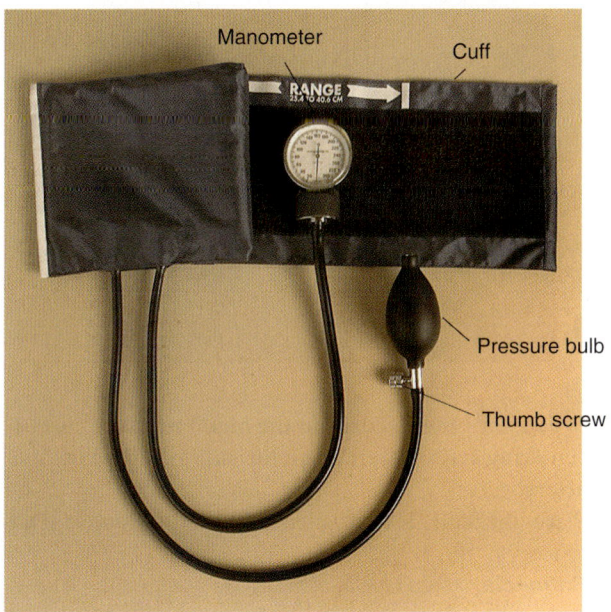

FIGURE 33-14 Parts of aneroid sphygmomanometer.

The proper blood pressure cuff size must be chosen. A cuff that is too wide or too narrow will produce an inaccurate reading up to 30 mm pressure. For example, a cuff that is too small will cause a false elevated reading and a cuff that is too large will produce an abnormally low blood pressure. Cuffs come in pediatric, standard or adult, obese or large, and thigh sizes (Figure 33-15). It is better to use a larger cuff when in doubt of which size to use. The cuff is never applied over clothing. Also, blood pressure should not be taken on arms that have shunts or intravenous (IV) lines or on the side where a mastectomy was done. Procedure 33-13 explains the process of accurately measuring and recording a patient's blood pressure and Box 33-6 lists the information necessary when charting blood pressure.

PATIENT-CENTERED PROFESSIONALISM

- *Why is accuracy so important when taking vital signs?*
- *What do vital signs tell the physician about the patient's current treatment plan?*

CONCLUSION

Body measurements and vital signs are true indications of the body's general state of health. These measurements need to be recorded and compared at regular intervals to help health care professionals recognize signs of possible disease or illness as well as determine a patient's general condition. When measured and recorded accurately, body measurements and vital signs provide essential objective (factual, measurable) information about a patient.

Accuracy is crucial; an incorrect reading or recording of information could lead to a misdiagnosis. This could contribute to delay or error in providing the care the patient needs. As you know, misdiagnosis could also lead to a lawsuit against the physician and medical assistant. The medical assistant has an ethical responsibility to use proper techniques when taking body measurements and performing procedures to measure vital signs.

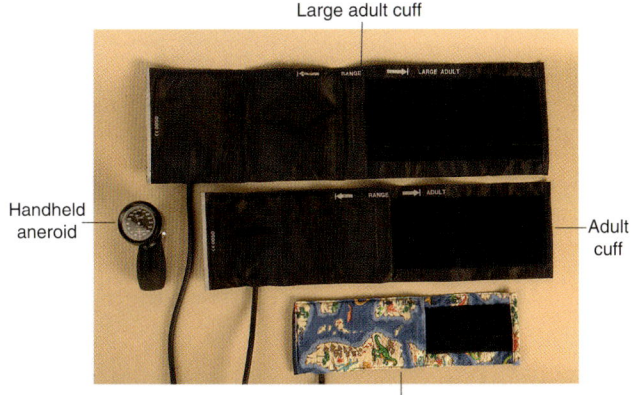

FIGURE 33-15 Blood pressure cuffs are available in different sizes. A different sized cuff can be attached to the handheld aneroid sphygmomanometer by way of a Luer connection.

SECTION V Clinical Medical Assisting

PROCEDURE 33-13 Measure Blood Pressure

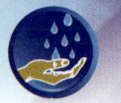

TASK: Accurately measure and record a patient's blood pressure by palpation and auscultation.

EQUIPMENT AND SUPPLIES
- Stethoscope
- Aneroid sphygmomanometer (proper size for patient)
- Alcohol wipe
- Patient's medical record
- Pen

SKILLS/RATIONALE

STANDARD PRECAUTIONS ARE TO BE FOLLOWED.

1. **Procedural Step. Greet the patient, introduce yourself, and confirm the patient's identity.**
   Rationale. Identifying the patient ensures the procedure is performed on the correct patient.

2. **Procedural Step. Sanitize the hands.**
   An alcohol-based hand rub may be used instead of washing hands with soap and water, unless hands are visibly soiled.
   Rationale. Hand sanitization promotes infection control.

3. **Procedural Step. Assemble equipment and supplies.**
   Assess the size of the patient's arm to determine the size of cuff needed.
   Rationale. It is important to have all supplies and equipment ready and available prior to starting any procedure, to ensure efficiency. Bladder of the blood pressure cuff should cover two thirds of the circumference of the upper arm.

4. **Procedural Step. Explain the procedure to the patient.**
   While explaining the procedure, observe the patient for any signs, such as anger, fear, pain, anxiety, or recent physical activity, that would influence the reading. Caffeine and smoking can also affect the blood pressure. If it is not possible to reduce or eliminate these influences, list them in the patient's record.
   Rationale. Explaining the procedure to the patient promotes cooperation and provides a means of obtaining implied consent.

5. **Procedural Step. Position the patient comfortably in a sitting or lying position.**
   Expose the upper arm by removing constrictive clothing. Position the patient's arm at heart level with the palm turned up. Always record the position of the patient when the blood pressure is taken.
   Rationale. Ensures proper cuff application and allows easy access to the brachial artery. The arm positioned above or below the level of the heart may cause inaccurate readings.

6. **Procedural Step. Palpate the brachial artery.**

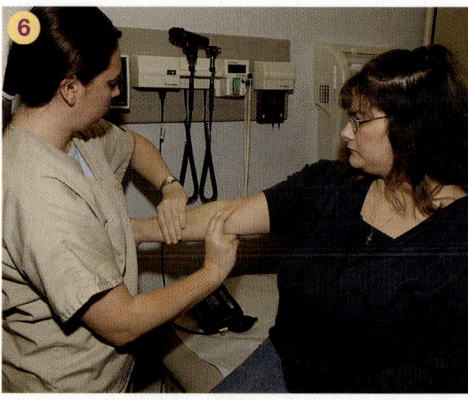

7. **Procedural Step. Position the blood pressure cuff by centering arrows marked on the cuff over the brachial artery.**
   Place the cuff 1 to 2 inches above the antecubital space.
   Rationale. Inflating the bladder over the brachial artery ensures proper pressure is applied during inflation.

8. **Procedural Step. Wrap the cuff firmly and smoothly around the arm and fasten.**
   The tubing, aneroid gauge, and pressure bulb must be pointed away from the patient's body.
   Rationale. An improperly fitting cuff causes false readings.

Continued

PROCEDURE 33-13 Measure Blood Pressure—cont'd

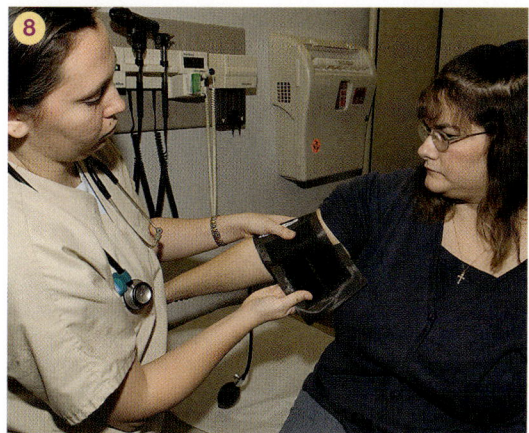

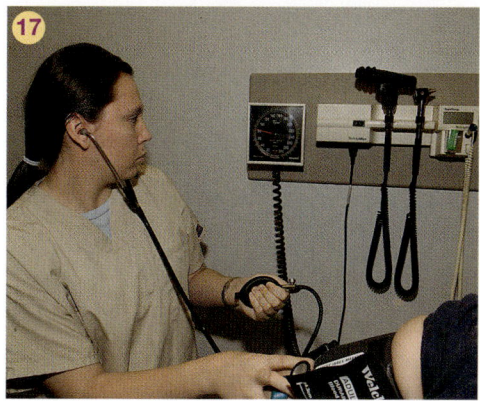

9. **Procedural Step.** Position the aneroid gauge so it can be easily seen.
   Rationale. Straining to see the lines on the gauge may cause inaccurate readings.
10. **Procedural Step.** Measure the systolic pressure by palpation first.
    Relocate the brachial pulse by palpating the artery while inflating the cuff.
11. **Procedural Step.** Close the valve on the pressure bulb by turning the screw valve clockwise until it is closed.
    Rationale. Closing the valve directs air flow into the cuff.
12. **Procedural Step.** Pump the cuff up by squeezing the bulb quickly and evenly until the artery is occluded; then slowly release the valve, deflating the cuff.
    Rationale. The inflated cuff compresses against the brachial artery, stopping blood flow through the artery. Deflating the cuff allows blood flow to resume and prevents venous congestion.
13. **Procedural Step.** Make note when the pulse disappears and when the pulse reappears. By locating where the pulse is strongest allows the best placement of the stethoscope.
    Rationale. NOTE: Blood pressure by palpation should be done on a patient's initial visit.
14. **Procedural Step.** Direct the earpieces of the cleaned stethoscope slightly forward and place them in your ears. Place the chest piece of the stethoscope over the brachial artery.
    Rationale. The earpieces should follow the angle of the auditory canal to facilitate hearing.
15. **Procedural Step.** Wait at least 30 seconds before reinflating the cuff.
16. **Procedural Step.** Close the valve of the pressure bulb by turning the screw valve in a clockwise direction until it is closed. Do not close it too tightly or it cannot be easily released.
17. **Procedural Step.** Reinflate the cuff at a smooth rate to at least 30 mm Hg above the palpated systolic pressure.
18. **Procedural Step.** Deflate the cuff at a constant rate of 2 to 3 mm Hg per second.
    Rationale. Deflating too rapidly or too slowly gives false readings.
19. **Procedural Step.** Listen for the first sharp sound.
    This is phase I of the Korotkoff sounds and indicates the systolic pressure.
20. **Procedural Step.** Continue to listen and steadily deflate the cuff until the last Korotkoff sound is heard, which indicates the diastolic pressure.

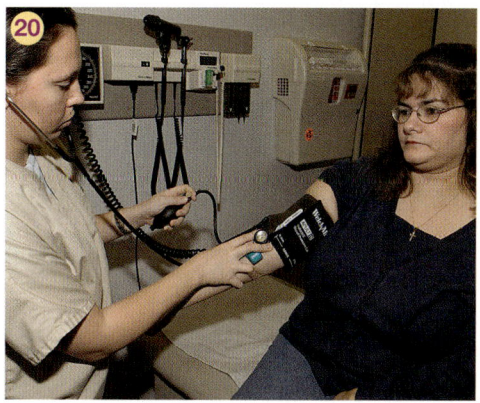

21. **Procedural Step.** If you could not obtain an accurate blood pressure reading, wait 1 to 2 minutes and repeat Steps 14 through 20.
    Rationale. Venous congestion results when blood pressure is taken and will alter a second reading if it is taken too soon.
22. **Procedural Step.** Remove the earpieces of the stethoscope from your ears and carefully remove the cuff from the patient's arm.

Continued

PROCEDURE 33-13 Measure Blood Pressure—cont'd

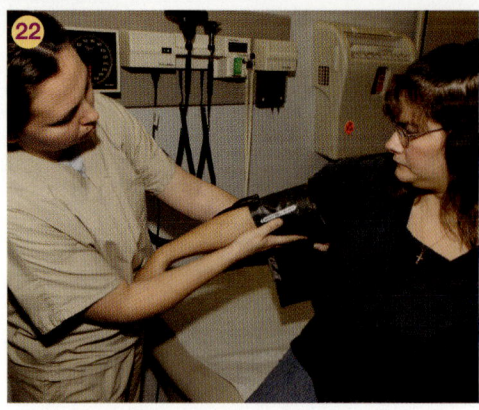

23. **Procedural Step.** Sanitize the hands.
    Always sanitize the hands after a procedure or after wearing gloves.

24. **Procedural Step.** Record the results in the patient's medical record; include which arm was used (right or left) and the patient's position (sitting, lying, or standing).

25. **Procedural Step.** Clean the earpieces and diaphragm with an alcohol wipe, and properly replace the equipment.

CHARTING EXAMPLE

Date	
9/11/xx	10:00 a.m. Ⓡ arm, blood pressure/sitting
	132/80 ——————————— J. Jonas, RMA

Chapter Summary

Reinforce your understanding of the material in this chapter by reviewing the curriculum objectives and key content points below.

1. **Define, appropriately use, and spell all the Key Terms for this chapter.**
   - Review the Key Terms if necessary.
2. **Explain the purpose of taking patients' weight and height measurements.**
   - Body measurements such as weight and height provide the physician with information about the patient's current health status by comparing it to previous visits.
3. **Accurately convert inches to centimeters and pounds to kilograms, and vice versa.**
   - To convert from centimeters to inches, divide by 2.5.
   - To convert from inches to centimeters, multiply by 2.5.
   - To convert from pounds to kilograms, divide by 2.2.
   - To convert from kilograms to pounds, multiply by 2.2.
4. **Demonstrate the correct procedure for measuring adult weight and height.**
   - Review Procedure 33-1.
5. **Demonstrate the correct procedure for measuring infant weight and length.**
   - Review Procedure 33-2.
6. **Demonstrate the correct procedure for measuring the head and chest circumference of an infant.**
   - Review Procedure 33-3.
7. **Explain how health care professionals use growth charts, and demonstrate how to plot weight and height (length) data on a growth chart.**
   - Children's weight and height are plotted on a growth chart and compared to national statistics.
   - Refer to Procedures 33-2 and 33-3 and Figures 33-4 and 33-5.
8. **List the four vital signs and explain why they are taken at patient visits.**
   - Body temperature, pulse rate, respiratory rate, and blood pressure are the four important vital signs.
   - Vital signs provide important information about a patient's present physical condition.
9. **List the five sites of the body that can be used to take a patient's temperature.**
   - Temperature can be taken orally, rectally, tympanically, on the skin, or under the arm (axillary).
10. **List five factors that can cause normal changes in body temperature.**
    - Time of day, health status, medications, recent activity, and age can all affect a person's body temperature.
11. **List the normal body temperature range for oral, rectal, axillary, and tympanic temperatures.**
    - Review Table 33-2.
12. **Identify the four types of thermometers.**
    - Mercury-free glass thermometers, electronic or digital thermometers, tympanic thermometers, and disposable oral thermometers (oral or temperature-sensitive tape) can be used to measure body temperature.
13. **Demonstrate the correct procedure for accurately measuring and recording body temperature with a mercury-free glass thermometer.**
    - Review Procedure 33-4.
14. **Demonstrate the correct procedure for accurately measuring and recording oral, rectal, and axillary**

body temperature with an electronic or digital thermometer.
- Review Procedures 33-5, 33-6, and 33-7.

15. **Demonstrate the correct procedure for accurately measuring and recording body temperature with a tympanic thermometer.**
    - Review Procedure 33-8.

16. **Demonstrate the correct procedure for accurately measuring and recording body temperature with a disposable oral thermometer.**
    - Review Procedure 33-9.

17. **Explain the considerations for using mercury-free glass thermometers in the medical office.**
    - Mercury-free glass thermometers can break easily, take a longer time to obtain a reading, and need to be cleaned between patients.

18. **Describe the body processes that create a pulse and explain why the pulse rate is measured.**
    - Pulse is the pressure felt when the wall of an artery is expanded and compressed.
    - The pulse rate provides information on how fast (or slow) the heart is beating.
    - Pulse sites can be used to measure pulse or to stop bleeding during an injury.

19. **Differentiate between tachycardia and bradycardia and identify the normal pulse range for these age groups: birth to 1 year, 1 year to 6 years, 6 to 12 years, 12 years to adult, and elderly.**
    - Tachycardia is a pulse rate over 100 beats per minute.
    - Bradycardia is a pulse rate lower than 60 beats per minute.
    - Review Table 33-3 for normal pulse rates by age group.

20. **List eight pulse sites of the body.**
    - Review Table 33-4.

21. **List the three characteristics of the pulse that medical assistants should note in documentation.**
    - Pulse rate, rhythm, and volume should be noted when the pulse is taken.
    - Any extreme variations in these characteristics must be recorded.

22. **Demonstrate the correct procedure for accurately measuring and recording radial pulse.**
    - Review Procedure 33-10.

23. **Demonstrate the correct procedure for accurately measuring and recording apical pulse.**
    - Review Procedure 33-11.

24. **Explain the purpose of a stethoscope and the need for sanitizing it between patients.**
    - A stethoscope is used to listen to body sounds; it amplifies the sounds so they can be heard clearly.
    - The potential for cross-contamination is very high with a stethoscope.

25. **Identify the normal respiratory rate for a child, an adult, and a geriatric adult.**

- Respirations are the "breathing in" of oxygen and "breathing out" of carbon dioxide.
- Children's normal respiratory rate is faster than adults' normal rate.
- Adults' normal respiratory rate is 16 to 20 cycles per minute.
- Older adults' normal respiratory rate is even slower than younger adults' normal rate.

26. **Demonstrate the correct procedure for accurately measuring and recording respiratory rate.**
    - Review Procedure 33-12.

27. **List four abnormal breathing sounds that can be caused by respiratory problems.**
    - Stridor, rales, rhonchi, and wheezes could indicate respiratory disease.

28. **Differentiate between systolic and diastolic blood pressure and state the normal range of each for an adult.**
    - Blood pressure is the measurement of pressure of the blood as it passes through an artery.
    - The systolic (contraction) and diastolic (resting) pressures are recorded as a fraction.
    - Review Table 33-5.

29. **List six factors that influence a patient's blood pressure.**
    - Gender, age, heredity, diet and exercise, medications, and emotional turmoil all influence a patient's blood pressure.

30. **Demonstrate the correct procedure for accurately measuring and recording systolic blood pressure by palpation.**
    - Review Procedure 33-13.

31. **Demonstrate the correct procedure for accurately measuring and recording blood pressure by auscultation.**
    - Review Procedure 33-13.

32. **Analyze a realistic medical office situation and apply your understanding of body measurements and vital signs to determine the best course of action.**
    - Medical assistants must be able to explain the need for each type of measurement and vital sign.
    - The physician uses the body measurements and vital signs to help provide a clear picture of the overall health of the patient.

33. **Describe the impact on patient care when medical assistants understand how to accurately take and record body measurements and vital signs in the medical office.**
    - Vital signs are measured to detect changes in normal body functions.
    - Taking vital signs is the first step in the assessment process.
    - Measurement of vital signs can provide information about the current treatment plan.

PRACTICAL APPLICATIONS

If you have accomplished the objectives in this chapter, you will be able to make better choices as a medical assistant. Take another look at this situation and decide what you would do.

Stephanie works for a general practitioner who sees pediatric, adult, and geriatric patients. Dr. Karas wants height and weight measurements for patients at each visit, regardless of the patient's age. Dr. Karas also wants head and chest circumference measurements taken for pediatric patients up to age 3 years.

Travis, a new patient, is a young teenager who does not want to have his weight and height measured because he is obese. He balks at having his temperature taken, stating that he knows he is not ill and "absolutely does not need to have that done." Stephanie tries explaining to Travis the differences in temperature, pulse, respiration, and blood pressure in different age groups. Finally, Travis agrees to have his temperature taken with a tympanic thermometer. When Stephanie starts to take Travis's blood pressure, he resists and tells her that he is scared and just knows that taking his blood pressure will hurt. Stephanie finally convinces Travis that she needs to take *all* his vital signs to prepare him for Dr. Karas's examination.

Would you be prepared to explain the importance of taking body measurements and vital signs to a new patient?

1. Why would Dr. Karas want height and weight measurements on each visit for patients in all age groups?
2. Why are growth charts important in treating pediatric patients?
3. Why are head and chest circumference measurements important in pediatric patients?
4. How can Stephanie convince Travis that it is important for his height and weight to be taken with each visit? How can she make the weight mensuration less upsetting to Travis?
5. What are the differences in temperature, pulse, respirations, and blood pressure in age groups?
6. How would a tympanic temperature reading differ from an oral temperature?
7. What does Stephanie need to explain to Travis about taking blood pressure?
8. Since Travis is upset, should Stephanie take his blood pressure immediately? Explain your answer.
9. What measurements are included in taking a patient's vital signs?

WEB SEARCH

1. **Research current information on detection, treatment, and prevention of hypertension.** All vital signs reflect the functions of the body necessary for life (e.g., body temperature regulation, respirations, heart rate, and blood pressure). Much research has been done on the causes and treatment of hypertension. Hypertension, referred to as the "silent killer," is a leading cause of death in the United States.
   - **Keywords:** Use the following keywords in your search: blood pressure, hypertension, American Heart Association.

Obtaining the Medical History

34

evolve http://evolve.elsevier.com/klieger/medicalassisting

A patient's medical and health history provides valuable information about the patient's present and past health and medical treatment. The physician uses this information to diagnose current illnesses or injuries and to monitor the patient's health as he or she ages. Because this information is so important, a complete medical history is taken for each new patient in the medical office.

The patient can provide some of the information needed for the health history in advance. The medical assistant or the physician must obtain other medical information during the office visit. In some cases the medical assistant takes much of this information in a patient interview. Taking a patient's medical history requires knowledge of the medical history form, good interviewing skills, and the ability to chart accurately.

LEARNING OBJECTIVES

You will be able to do the following after completing this chapter:

Key Terms
1. Define, appropriately use, and spell all the Key Terms for this chapter.

Sections of the Medical History
2. Demonstrate the correct procedure for completing a medical history form.
3. List seven sections of the medical history and briefly explain what type of information is collected in each.
4. Distinguish between *objective* and *subjective* data.

Interviewing Skills
5. State two positive outcomes of interviewing a patient effectively.
6. Explain the importance of maintaining the patient's privacy during and after the interview.
7. Explain the need for effective communication skills during a patient interview.
8. Demonstrate the correct procedure for recognizing and responding to nonverbal communication.

Charting
9. Explain the importance of charting patient statements and observations accurately.
10. Differentiate between "specific" and "general" patient statements and know when to obtain more detail.
11. Accurately record observations made during a patient interview.
12. Recognize judgmental statements in charting and explain the need for nonjudgmental documentation.
13. List seven guidelines for effective charting.

Patient-Centered Professionalism
14. Analyze a realistic medical office situation and apply your understanding of medical history taking to determine the best course of action.
15. Describe the impact on patient care when medical assistants understand how to take a patient's medical history appropriately and accurately.

KEY TERMS

charting
chief complaint (CC)
demographic
diagnosis (Dx)
familial
family history (FH)
Health Insurance Portability and Accountability Act (HIPAA)
hereditary
objective
open-ended questions
past history (PH)
present illness (PI)
"release of information" (ROI) form
review of systems (ROS)
signs
social history (SH)
subjective
symptoms

PRACTICAL APPLICATIONS

Read the following scenario and keep it in mind as you learn about taking a patient's medical history in the office.

Dr. Walker, an obstetrician/gynecologist and internal medicine physician, has hired Jenny to assist with taking medical histories for his patients. Dr. Walker sees many patients who have high-risk pregnancies because of an infectious disease. Sarah, a new patient who is 4 months' pregnant, has been referred to Dr. Walker because she is at risk for several infectious diseases.

Jenny goes to the waiting room and starts to ask Sarah questions about her pregnancy and her past medical history. Sarah tells Jenny that she does not want to discuss this with a medical assistant and would rather give the information to Dr. Walker. Jenny adamantly tells Sarah that if she does not want to cooperate, Dr. Walker will not see her as a patient. Sarah begins to cry but starts telling her history to Jenny. Trying to impress Sarah during the interview, Jenny uses medical terminology to ask questions and never looks at Sarah or makes any observations about Sarah's remarks.

After the history taking, Sarah is escorted to the examination room, where her vital signs are taken. After discussing her previous illnesses and family history, Dr. Walker examines Sarah and orders several laboratory tests, including tests for HIV and for syphilis. His tentative diagnosis is "possible HIV infection," and he confirms her pregnancy of 4 months. On leaving the office, Sarah makes an appointment for 2 weeks to discuss her test results and final diagnosis with Dr. Walker.

What should Jenny have done differently as a medical assistant initially taking Sarah's history?

SECTIONS OF THE MEDICAL HISTORY

A medical history form provides data or information about a patient that the physician can use to correlate the patient's symptoms and formulate a treatment plan. The medical history form is considered the foundation for understanding a patient's health status. These forms can be very comprehensive depending on the specialty (Figure 34-1), or they can be simple one- or two-page documents (Figure 34-2).

The sections of the medical history include personal data, chief complaint, present illness, past history, family history, social history, and review of systems. Procedure 34-1 describes the steps in completing a medical history form.

Personal Data

The personal data section requests basic information about the patient. This **demographic** material is completed by the patient and includes the patient's name, address, date of birth (DOB), social security number, gender, telephone number, insurance information, marital status, and occupation. The medical assistant should be ready to help patients who have difficulty completing this part of the medical history.

Chief Complaint

The **chief complaint** (**CC**) is the reason the patient wants to see the physician. The medical assistant should chart the CC concisely but with as much important information as possible and in the patient's own words. The CC is a brief statement of only one or two **signs** or **symptoms,** body location, character, severity of precipitating events (e.g., "what caused this problem?"), aggravating or relieving factors, and the duration (length of time) of the problem.

Symptoms that cannot be measured or seen are referred to as **subjective** information. If a patient states she has felt dizzy for the past 3 days, this symptom is subjective because dizziness cannot be measured or observed. **Objective** information can be measured or observed. For example, elevated blood pressure can be measured and reported (e.g., 160/100 mm Hg), thus this is an objective symptom. Box 34-1 provides more examples of objective and subjective data as listed in the sections of the medical health history.

When gathering information, the medical assistant should try and pinpoint the CC to a particular body system, time frame (onset, duration, frequency), degree of discomfort, and way in which it affects daily activities. Figure 34-3 provides examples of charting the CC based on the patient interview.

Present Illness

The **present illness** (**PI**) section provides an expansion of the CC, including when the problem began and any medications that have been taken to treat the problem. The PI contains more description about the current illness or injury, including the severity of the pain, whether symptoms have improved or worsened, and whether other minor symptoms are present. For example, a patient may state that he tripped on the stairs that morning and fell on his right arm, which is now swollen and painful; this is the CC. If he went on to explain in the interview that he applied ice to the right arm and took two Tylenol tablets with no relief, this information would go in the PI.

Sometimes the PI is based on a past medical problem. A patient's past illness may have been treated elsewhere. For example, if a patient with diabetes has moved from Ohio to Florida, the patient's new physician would want to see documentation of the patient's previous care. For this to occur, the patient or legal guardian must authorize the release of the patient's medical record by completing, signing, and dating a **"release of information" (ROI) form** (Figure 34-4) so that the release can be sent to the former physician to obtain the patient's medical records. The release form must specify which information is to be released, to whom, and for what purpose. The authorization typically expires 12 months after the date of signing, unless another date is indicated. Remember, not having a release form before sending any medical information is considered an invasion of privacy.

Text continued on p. 722

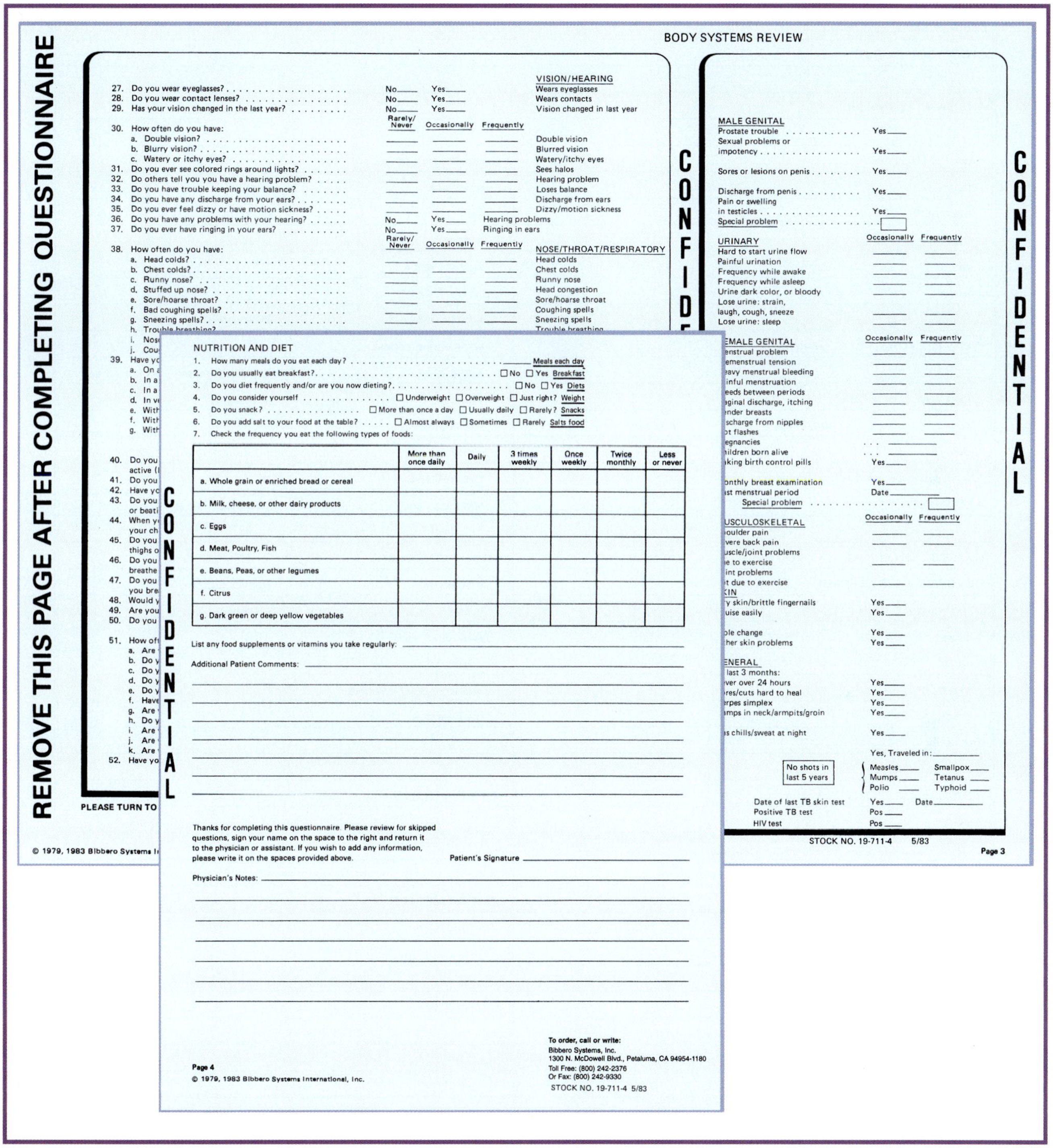

BODY SYSTEMS REVIEW

REMOVE THIS PAGE AFTER COMPLETING QUESTIONNAIRE

VISION/HEARING

27. Do you wear eyeglasses? . . . No___ Yes___ Wears eyeglasses
28. Do you wear contact lenses? . . . No___ Yes___ Wears contacts
29. Has your vision changed in the last year? . . . No___ Yes___ Vision changed in last year

	Rarely/Never	Occasionally	Frequently	
30. How often do you have:				
a. Double vision?	___	___	___	Double vision
b. Blurry vision?	___	___	___	Blurred vision
c. Watery or itchy eyes?	___	___	___	Watery/itchy eyes
31. Do you ever see colored rings around lights?	___	___	___	Sees halos
32. Do others tell you you have a hearing problem?	___	___	___	Hearing problem
33. Do you have trouble keeping your balance?	___	___	___	Loses balance
34. Do you have any discharge from your ears?	___	___	___	Discharge from ears
35. Do you ever feel dizzy or have motion sickness?	___	___	___	Dizzy/motion sickness

36. Do you have any problems with your hearing? . . . No___ Yes___ Hearing problems
37. Do you ever have ringing in your ears? . . . No___ Yes___ Ringing in ears

NOSE/THROAT/RESPIRATORY

	Rarely/Never	Occasionally	Frequently	
38. How often do you have:				
a. Head colds?	___	___	___	Head colds
b. Chest colds?	___	___	___	Chest colds
c. Runny nose?	___	___	___	Runny nose
d. Stuffed up nose?	___	___	___	Head congestion
e. Sore/hoarse throat?	___	___	___	Sore/hoarse throat
f. Bad coughing spells?	___	___	___	Coughing spells
g. Sneezing spells?	___	___	___	Sneezing spells
h. Trouble breathing?				Trouble breathing

i. Nos
j. Cou
39. Have yo
a. On
b. In a
c. In a
d. In v
e. With
f. With
g. With
40. Do you active (
41. Do you
42. Have yo
43. Do you or beati
44. When y your ch
45. Do you thighs o
46. Do you breathe
47. Do you you bre
48. Would y
49. Are you
50. Do you
51. How of
a. Are
b. Do y
c. Do y
d. Do y
e. Do y
f. Have
g. Are
h. Do y
i. Are
j. Are
k. Are
52. Have yo

PLEASE TURN TO

© 1979, 1983 Bibbero Systems I

CONFIDENTIAL

MALE GENITAL
Prostate trouble . . . Yes___
Sexual problems or impotency . . . Yes___
Sores or lesions on penis . . . Yes___
Discharge from penis . . . Yes___
Pain or swelling in testicles . . . Yes___
Special problem . . . ☐

URINARY	Occasionally	Frequently
Hard to start urine flow	___	___
Painful urination	___	___
Frequency while awake	___	___
Frequency while asleep	___	___
Urine dark color, or bloody	___	___
Lose urine: strain, laugh, cough, sneeze	___	___
Lose urine: sleep	___	___

EMALE GENITAL	Occasionally	Frequently
enstrual problem	___	___
emenstrual tension	___	___
avy menstrual bleeding	___	___
inful menstruation	___	___
eeds between periods	___	___
ginal discharge, itching	___	___
nder breasts	___	___
scharge from nipples	___	___
ot flashes	___	___

egnancies . . . ___
ildren born alive . . . ___
king birth control pills Yes___
onthly breast examination Yes___
st menstrual period Date___
Special problem . . . ☐

USCULOSKELETAL	Occasionally	Frequently
oulder pain	___	___
vere back pain	___	___
uscle/joint problems		
e to exercise	___	___
int problems		
t due to exercise	___	___

KIN
y skin/brittle fingernails Yes___
uise easily Yes___
ole change Yes___
her skin problems Yes___

ENERAL
last 3 months:
ver over 24 hours Yes___
res/cuts hard to heal Yes___
rpes simplex Yes___
mps in neck/armpits/groin Yes___
s chills/sweat at night Yes___
Yes, Traveled in:___

No shots in last 5 years { Measles___ Mumps___ Polio___ Smallpox___ Tetanus___ Typhoid___

Date of last TB skin test Yes___ Date___
Positive TB test Pos___
HIV test Pos___

STOCK NO. 19-711-4 5/83

Page 3

NUTRITION AND DIET

1. How many meals do you eat each day? . . . ___ Meals each day
2. Do you usually eat breakfast? . . . ☐ No ☐ Yes Breakfast
3. Do you diet frequently and/or are you now dieting? . . . ☐ No ☐ Yes Diets
4. Do you consider yourself . . . ☐ Underweight ☐ Overweight ☐ Just right? Weight
5. Do you snack? . . . ☐ More than once a day ☐ Usually daily ☐ Rarely? Snacks
6. Do you add salt to your food at the table? . . . ☐ Almost always ☐ Sometimes ☐ Rarely Salts food
7. Check the frequency you eat the following types of foods:

	More than once daily	Daily	3 times weekly	Once weekly	Twice monthly	Less or never
a. Whole grain or enriched bread or cereal						
b. Milk, cheese, or other dairy products						
c. Eggs						
d. Meat, Poultry, Fish						
e. Beans, Peas, or other legumes						
f. Citrus						
g. Dark green or deep yellow vegetables						

List any food supplements or vitamins you take regularly: ___

Additional Patient Comments: ___

Thanks for completing this questionnaire. Please review for skipped questions, sign your name on the space to the right and return it to the physician or assistant. If you wish to add any information, please write it on the spaces provided above.

Patient's Signature ___

Physician's Notes: ___

To order, call or write:
Bibbero Systems, Inc.
1300 N. McDowell Blvd., Petaluma, CA 94954-1180
Toll Free: (800) 242-2376
Or Fax: (800) 242-9330

Page 4
© 1979, 1983 Bibbero Systems International, Inc.

STOCK NO. 19-711-4 5/83

FIGURE 34-1 Comprehensive medical history form. (Courtesy Bibbero System, Inc., Petaluma, CA, (800) 242-2376, fax (800) 242-9330, www.bibbero.com.)

MEDICAL RECORD

NAME	AGE	SEX	S M D W
ADDRESS	PHONE	DATE	
E-MAIL	CELL PHONE		
SPONSOR	ADDRESS		
OCCUPATION	REF BY	ACKN	

CHIEF COMPLAINT

PRESENT ILLNESS

FAMILY HISTORY	URINARY TRACT
MOTHER FATHER	NOCTURIA FREQUENCY
BROTHERS	PAIN BURNING
SISTERS	BLEEDING INFECTION
TB DIAB MALIG	INCONTINENCE
HT DIS NEPH EPILIP	GENITAL TRACT
PSYCH	AGE AT MENST TYPE PERIOD
PAST HISTORY - GENL HEALTH	INTERMEN BLEEDING
	AMENORRHEA DYSMENORRHEA
CHILDHOOD DISEASES	VAG DISCH IRRITATION
SC FEV RHEUM FEV ALLERGY	PAINFUL PERIOD
OTHER USUAL WEIGHT	L M P
HAVE YOU EVER TAKEN FEN-PHEN/REDUX? YES NO	CHILDREN-L D S B
ACCIDENTS	MARRIED YRS. YOUNGEST CHILD
HABITS COFFEE TOBACCO ALCOHOL	NEURO-MUSCULAR
REVIEWS OF SYSTEMS	STRENGTH NERVOUSNESS
E E N T–EYES	SLEEP WORRY
EARS	MUSCULAR PAIN
NOSE	JOINT PAIN
THROAT	ABNORMAL SENSATIONS
NECK	DEFORMITIES
BREASTS	
HEART-LUNGS	OPERATIONS
PAIN	
DO YOU HAVE A PERSISTENT COUGH OR THROAT CLEARING NOT ASSOCIATED WITH A KNOWN ILLNESS (LASTING MORE THAN 3 WEEKS)? YES NO	
BLEEDING DYSPNEA	
IRREG EDEMA	TREATMENTS
GASTRO-INTESTINAL	
APPETITE DIET	
INDIGESTION PAIN	
NAUSEA VOMITING	COMMENTS
JAUNDICE BLEEDING	
BOWEL HABITS	
HEMORRHOIDS	
PAIN WITH STOOL ITCHING	
OTHER	

ITEM 060-1062/8184 PATTERSON OFFICE SUPPLIES 800-637-1140

FIGURE 34-2 General medical history form. (Courtesy Patterson Office Supplies, Champaign, Ill.)

PROCEDURE 34-1 Complete a Medical History Form

TASK: Obtain and record a patient's medical history using verbal and nonverbal communication skills and applying the principles of accurate documentation in the patient's medical record.

EQUIPMENT AND SUPPLIES
- Medical history form
- Patient's medical record
- Pens (red and black ink)
- Clipboard
- Quiet, private area

SKILLS/*RATIONALE*

1. **Procedural Step.** Assemble necessary supplies.
   Rationale. It is important to have all supplies ready and available before starting any procedure to ensure efficiency.

2. **Procedural Step.** Greet the patient, introduce yourself, and confirm the patient's identity.
   Rationale. Identifying the patient ensures the right patient is being interviewed.

3. **Procedural Step.** Escort the patient to a quiet, comfortable room that is well lit to conduct the interview.

4. **Procedural Step.** Explain why information is required and reassure the patient that the information gathered will be kept confidential.
   NOTE: It is important to explain to the patient that your purpose for reviewing the forms is to be sure that the physician has all relevant information about the patient's health history.
   Rationale. Patients are more comfortable and cooperative when they understand the reason for obtaining and recording their medical history.

5. **Procedural Step.** Seat the patient, then sit down next to the patient at eye level for questioning.
   Rationale. The patient feels less intimidated if the medical assistant is sitting rather than standing.

6. **Procedural Step.** Review the completed portion of the medical history form with the patient, looking for omissions or incomplete answers.
   Obtain any missing information from the patient by asking the appropriate questions.

7. **Procedural Step.** Speak clearly and distinctly and maintain eye contact (if appropriate) with the patient.
   Rationale. The patient should feel at ease to speak freely about the medical history; maintaining eye contact can assure the patient that you care and are listening. (However, keep in mind that some cultures consider eye contact to be inappropriate.)

8. **Procedural Step.** Once the medical history form has been reviewed, ask the patient to state the reason for today's visit.
   This is the patient's "chief complaint," or current medical problem. Ask open-ended questions requiring more than a "yes" or "no" answer to obtain the patient's chief complaint. The chief complaint should be limited to one or two symptoms and should refer to specific, rather than general or "vague," symptoms.

9. **Procedural Step.** Record the information briefly and concisely, using the patient's own words as much as possible.
   Use "c/o" for "complains of" and quotation marks when quoting the patient. Include the duration of the symptoms. Avoid using names of diseases or diagnostic terms. Use medical terminology to describe locations on the body but not disease processes.
   Rationale. This information is needed by the physician to make an accurate assessment and diagnosis. The physician usually completes the systems review during the pre-examination interview.

10. **Procedural Step.** Ask the patient about prescription, over-the-counter (OTC), and herbal medications; record all medications the patient is taking.
    If the patient is not taking any medications, write "none" in the medication section of the medical history form. Be sure to ask if the patient is taking vitamin supplements or nonprescription (OTC) medications such as pain relievers. Many patients will forget to mention such medications because they do not consider these to be drugs.
    Rationale. It is important that the physician have a complete list of medications because many medications have interactions with other medications.

11. **Procedural Step.** Inquire about allergies to medications, foods, and other substances, and record any allergies in red ink on every page of the history form.

Continued

PROCEDURE 34-1 Complete a Medical History Form—cont'd

If the patient does not have allergies, write "NKA" ("no known allergies") or "NKDA" ("no known drug allergies") in the record.

Rationale. This will alert the physician and all caregivers to the patient's allergies. The presence of an allergy may alter medication and treatment procedures as planned by the physician. Writing "NKA" or "NKDA" in the record informs the physician that you asked the question.

12. **Procedural Step.** Review and record information in all the following sections of the medical history form:
    - Family history
    - Social history
    - Past history
    - Hospitalizations
    - Surgeries
    - Injuries

13. **Procedural Step.** Record all information legibly and neatly in black ink.

    Rationale. Recording in ink maintains a medical record that is understandable and defensible in court and prevents alterations to documentation.

14. **Procedural Step.** Thank the patient for providing the information.

15. **Procedural Step.** Review the record for errors before giving it to the physician.

    Ask about any areas in which further clarification may be needed.

16. **Procedural Step.** Use the information to complete the patient's record as directed by office policy.

    All information about the patient must remain confidential and can only be discussed with the physician or health care member responsible for the patient's care.

BOX 34-1

Medical Health History: Objective and Subjective Data

SUBJECTIVE

Personal Data
Name, date of birth, marital status.

Chief Complaint
Patient symptoms and duration, self-medication (e.g., throbbing headache for 3 days with no relief from aspirin).

Past History
Past illnesses, past surgeries (e.g., gallbladder removed).

Family History
Causes of death, past or present diseases or illnesses (e.g., both parents died of heart disease; brother has high blood pressure).

Social History
Patient's lifestyle, including smoking, drinking, and occupation (e.g., worked in coal mine for 30 years).

OBJECTIVE

Systems Review
Physician records, past history, current findings.

Laboratory and Radiology Reports
Laboratory reports include complete blood count (CBC) and wound cultures.
Radiology reports include x-ray series and magnetic resonance imaging (MRI).

Diagnosis
Based on prior health history, signs and symptoms, and physical examination.

Treatment
Instructions for follow-up.

Progress Notes
Documentation of patient's care.

Patient Interview #1

Medical Assistant: What is the reason for your visit today?
Patient: My throat has been sore since Tuesday.
Medical Assistant: That's three days now isn't it? Have you had any fever?
Patient: I don't know. I don't think so.

Sample charting

6/12/XX	c/o sore throat x 3 days ——————— S. Williams, CMA (AAMA)

Patient Interview #2

Medical Assistant: Why have you come to see the doctor today?
Patient: I have had terrible stomach pain all morning.
Medical Assistant: Can you show me where it hurts?
Patient points to area 3 inches below belly button in the middle.
Medical Assistant: Have you taken anything to relieve the pain?
Patient: I took Maalox but it didn't help.
Medical Assistant: When did you take it?
Patient: At 9:30 this morning.

Sample charting

6/12/XX	Pt. c/o severe midline abdominal pain since this AM. Took Maalox at
	9:30 AM s̄ relief. ——————— S. Williams, CMA (AAMA)

Patient Interview #3

Medical Assistant: What is the reason for your visit today?
Patient: I have been having really bad headaches.
Medical Assistant: When did the headaches begin?
Patient: Well, I always have headaches occasionally, but lately I've had two or three a week, like for the last two weeks.
Medical Assistant: Are they in the front or back, can you show me?
Patient: They are all over. It feels like someone is hammering my head.
Medical Assistant: On both sides?
Patient: Yes.
Medical Assistant: What do you do when you have one?
Patient: I have to lie down. I've been taking ibuprofen but it doesn't help. When I have one I'm too sick to do anything.
Medical Assistant: Do you have any nausea or see flashing lights?
Patient: No.
Medical Assistant: Have you been sick or had any other problems?
Patient: Not really.

Sample charting

6/12/XX	Pt. c/o severe generalized headaches x 2 weeks, about 2-3 per week.
	Describes as "it feels like someone is hammering my head." Pain is not
	relieved by ibuprofen. Denies other symptoms or illness. ———————
	——————— S. Williams, CMA (AAMA)

FIGURE 34-3 Sample patient interview and charting of the chief complaint. (Modified from Hunt SA: *Saunders fundamentals of medical assisting—revised reprint,* St Louis, 2007, Saunders.)

RECORDS RELEASE Date ______________

To ____
DOCTOR

____
ADDRESS

I hereby authorize and request you to release

to ____
DOCTOR

____
ADDRESS

the complete medical records in your possession, concerning my illness and/or treatment during

the period from ______________ to ______________

Signed ______________
(PATIENT OR NEAREST RELATIVE)

______________ WITNESS Relationship ______________

FIGURE 34-4 "Release of information" request form ("records release" form).

Past History

Past history (PH) is a summary of the patient's prior and current health problems, major illnesses, or surgeries. This information is needed to assist the physician in treating the patient's current problem. Past diseases, conditions, or injuries can affect a person's present state of health. As part of a PH, information is gathered about the following:

- Childhood diseases
- Major or chronic illnesses
- Surgeries
- Hospitalizations
- Allergies
- Accidents or injuries
- Last examination date
- Current and past medications (prescription and nonprescription, over-the-counter, and herbal supplements)
- Immunizations

Family History

Family history (FH) includes a health inventory of the patient's immediate blood relatives. Health information is gathered about the patient's mother, father, brothers, sisters, and both maternal and paternal grandparents. The FH includes information about relatives' current state of health, significant health issues, and causes of death. The physician will reference the FH when studying a patient's current symptoms. Some diseases are **hereditary** (e.g., sickle cell anemia, hemophilia, or muscular dystrophy) or **familial,** meaning they are passed down from a parent. Diabetes mellitus is a common example of a familial disease, as are hypertension, heart disease, and allergies.

Social History

Social history (SH) presents an overview of the patient's lifestyle, including eating, drinking, smoking, education, exercise habits, past and present occupations, and when applicable, sexual habits. Although this information is sometimes awkward to obtain, it is important because it is helpful to the physician. The SH may provide insight as to the patient's ability to comply with the course of treatment. In addition, it may help the physician pinpoint the etiology of the disease. For example, a person's occupational history would include emotional or physical demands and environmental conditions such as chemical exposure and dust (e.g., coal, asbestos).

Review of Systems

The **review of systems (ROS),** also called the *systems review,* is a step-by-step review of each body system, past and present. The physician usually completes the ROS while doing a physical assessment of the patient. If these questions are included on a health history questionnaire completed by the patient, the medical assistant should go over these questions to ensure all the information is correct and was understood by the patient. One disease may impact another system without the patient's awareness. For example, a patient with severe back pain may think she has pulled a muscle, but the full ROS may detect a urinary tract infection (UTI).

An ROS starts at the head and moves downward. Table 34-1 provides typical information recorded by the physician. Using the patient's prior health history and reviewing symptoms related to the system, the physician can make a "tentative" (clinical) **diagnosis (Dx).** Box 34-2 describes the three

TABLE 34-1

Review of Systems (ROS): Examples of Patient Signs and Symptoms*

Body Part	Signs	Symptoms
Head	Fainting	Dizziness, headaches, pain
Eyes	Redness, discharge, swelling, excessive tearing	Pain, double vision, vision changes
Ears	Redness, discharge, hearing loss	Pain, ringing in ears, dizziness
Nose	Nosebleeds, discharge, obstruction	Altered smell, frequency of colds
Neck	Swelling, lumps	Tenderness, pain on movement
Mouth and throat	Swelling of gums, loose teeth, bleeding gums, yellow or white patches on mucous membranes, hoarseness, voice changes	Burning of tongue, sore throat
Chest	Cough, wheezing, shortness of breath, sputum production (color, quantity)	Pain with breathing, tightness
Cardiac	Palpitations, shortness of breath on exertion	Pain, tenderness of heart area
Abdomen	Swelling, bowel sounds	Pain, tenderness
Skin	Rashes, hives, itching, dryness, bruises, changes in skin color and texture of hair and nails	Burning, sensitive to touch, itching
General appearance	Fever, change in weight, night sweats, muscle weakness	Chills, fatigue

*Signs provide objective information, whereas symptoms are subjective complaints.

BOX 34-2

Types of Diagnoses

CLINICAL DIAGNOSIS
Physician uses patient's CC, PH, and PE.
Example: CC: joint pain, headache, irritability, weight loss. PH: unremarkable. PE: limited range of motion; other systems WNL.
Laboratory tests ordered: CBC with diff, sed rate, rheumatoid factor (RF)
Dx: Arthritis

FINAL DIAGNOSIS
Physician uses patient's CC, PH, PE, laboratory test results, and results of diagnostic procedures.
Test results: Moderate anemia, decreased WBC, increased sed rate, RF increased
Dx: Rheumatoid arthritis

DIFFERENTIAL DIAGNOSIS
Once treatment occurs, the patient is reevaluated to determine if the clinical diagnosis has changed. If it has changed, treatment is altered, and additional tests may be ordered.
Example: Patient is not responding to treatment. Developed skin lesions on the face, scalp, and neck. Rash appears on the face and the bridge of the nose. New symptoms and nonresponsiveness to treatment; additional tests ordered.
Dx: Lupus erythematosus

CBC, Complete blood count; *CC*, chief complaint; *diff*, differential; *Dx*, diagnosis; *PE*, physical examination; *PH*, past history; *RF*, rheumatoid factor; *sed rate*, sedimentation rate; *WBC*, white blood cells (count); *WNL*, within normal limits.

major types of diagnoses. Figure 34-5 is an example of a medical report completed by a physician.

PATIENT-CENTERED PROFESSIONALISM

- Why must the medical assistant be certain all information is completed in each section of the patient medical history form?
- Why must the medical assistant record the chief complaint concisely and in the patient's own words?

INTERVIEWING SKILLS

To encourage patients to describe their symptoms, different interview techniques have been developed by healthcare professionals. One group developed the PQRST interviewing technique to describe pain or other symptoms and assist the medical assistant in asking the appropriate questions for the condition:

P: Proactive—the medical assistant should be proactive (positive) when asking the patient to discuss the symptom or pain and what relieves it. The patient should be asked questions such as the following:

- When did the pain begin?
- Does any movement create pain? When does the pain occur?
- Are there any other items that exacerbate (make it worse) or alleviate the symptom (lying down, medications, breathing, etc.)?

Q: Quality—the quality of the symptom is a description of the severity or how the pain appears to the patient. The patient should be asked questions such as the following:

- Can you describe the pain (pricking, burning, or deep and aching)?

MEDICAL HISTORY AND REVIEW OF SYSTEMS

Ivan Shapiro
07/14/XX

HISTORY OF PRESENT ILLNESS
This 55-year-old white male presents with a history of chest tightness when exercising for the past month, which has increased in frequency during the last week. The tightness across the chest was first noticed when mowing the lawn. The episodes have been increasing in frequency until there are about one or two episodes per day, usually associated with exercise and all relieved by rest. Has taken antacids once or twice thinking that the pain might be due to indigestion without noticeable relief. Otherwise in good health.

MEDICATIONS
Not taking any prescription medications, but occasionally uses ibuprofen for relief of muscle pain; takes multivitamin daily.

ALLERGIES
Allergic to penicillin which results in urticaria. Has not taken penicillin for past 30 years.

PAST HISTORY
Had usual childhood diseases including mumps, measles, German measles, chicken pox. T&A when 6 years old. Fracture of left fibula at age 13; healed without problems. No other surgeries or medical problems.

FAMILY HISTORY
Father died at age 64 of MI. Mother living, has NIDDM, also being treated for hypertension. Siblings living and well. Has three children, all in good health. No other significant family history.

SOCIAL HISTORY
Smokes 20 cigarettes per day for the past 25 years. Social drinker. Drinks two cups of coffee daily.

OCCUPATIONAL HISTORY
Has been a carpenter for about 20 years. Worked on a farm for a few years after high school. No significant injuries due to occupation.

REVIEW OF SYSTEMS
Denies radiation of chest pain, has occasional indigestion, increasing in the past 6 months. Other than occasional muscle pain following physical exertion and recent chest pain, denies physical symptoms.

Joanne Hughes, MD

FIGURE 34-5 Sample medical report, including the patient history and review of systems. (From Hunt SA: *Saunders fundamentals of medical assisting—revised reprint,* St Louis, 2007, Saunders.)

- Rate the pain on a scale of 1 to 10.

R: Region/Radiation—the medical assistant should ask where the pain or symptom is located on the patient. Questions to ask the patient include the following:
- Where do you feel the pain?
- Does it travel to other parts of your body?

S: Severity/Signs and Symptoms—a rating scale is used in the assessment of the pain or any other side effects accompanying the pain (e.g., nausea, swelling, rash). Questions to ask the patient include the following:
- How does the pain compare to an earache, headache, or toothache?
- Are there any other issues accompanying the pain such as nausea?

T: Temporal Timing—exploring when the symptom started, how long it has lasted, if there are any patterns of the symptom, or if the pain is intermittent are critical questions while interviewing a patient. The medical assistant could ask questions such as the following:
- When did pain first occur?
- How long does the pain usually last?
- Is the pain constant or intermittent?

During the interview, it is critical for the medical assistant to maintain eye contact and make the patient feel as comfortable as possible while gathering the information. The medical assistant must present a feeling of genuine concern for the patient's well-being and show respect for the patient's concerns. All subjective and objective data should be accurately documented in the medical record appropriately and only Joint Commission–approved abbreviations should be noted in the chart. In addition, it is important to consider the patient's need for privacy and remember to use good communication skills.

Patient Privacy

The first step in interviewing any patient is to ensure the interview area is private and free from interruptions. A sense of confidentiality must be clearly demonstrated to the patient. This can be accomplished by going to a separate room and closing the door. When assured that the area is private, the patient will feel more comfortable being open about health details of a personal nature.

The **Health Insurance Portability and Accountability Act (HIPAA)** mandates, among other regulations, that appropriate measures must be taken to protect personal information. Besides being the law, the patient has a right to expect privacy. Only individuals directly involved in the patient's care are allowed access to the patient's medical record. All information provided by the patient (e.g., FH, SH) must be kept in strictest confidence.

Effective Communication

Effective communication enables the medical assistant to obtain the necessary information about the patient's medical history. As discussed in Chapters 7 and 8, remember to (1) make eye contact (unless this has cultural implications), (2) be a good listener (silent periods allow the patient time to express feelings), and (3) acknowledge the patient (positive facial expressions show you are listening).

Nonverbal cues may convey sensitivity toward the patient's needs and feelings. These include body language cues such as leaning toward the patient to show interest, nodding your head to encourage the patient to continue, and smiling at appropriate moments or showing signs of empathy to pain. This approach supports the patient and provides insight into the patient's attitudes about health and illness. Do not react to personal or "shocking" details the patient may reveal. It is important to be respectful and nonjudgmental, not reactive. Procedure 34-2 provides more information about recognizing and responding to nonverbal communication.

Explaining the reason for the health history form gives the patient confidence in the medical assistant's abilities because the patient can see that the assistant understands the need for the information. The patient feels more confident about providing information to a medical assistant who shows competence and professionalism.

> ### PATIENT-CENTERED PROFESSIONALISM
>
> - *Why must the medical assistant apply good communication skills when conducting the patient interview?*
> - *What are some advantages of the medical assistant interviewing the patient while obtaining the medical history versus the patient filling out a health questionnaire?*

CHARTING

Medical assistants are responsible for **charting** the information they obtain when taking the patient history. Charting must be clear, concise, objective (nonjudgmental), and correct.

Patient Statements

Charting patient statements that pertain to their health is key in providing a good database for the patient's physical examination. Having the patient pinpoint specific symptoms rather than make generalizations is most helpful. Always use quotation marks when charting the patient's words.

> **GENERAL STATEMENTS VERSUS SPECIFIC SYMPTOMS**
> *General:* "My hand seems to go numb all the time."
> *Specific:* "When I am working on the computer for more than 15 minutes, my right hand gets numb."

Allow patients to describe the reason for the visit or complaint in their own words. The medical assistant might have the tendency to make assumptions. Avoid using "yes" or "no" questions because patients tend to answer them with simply

PROCEDURE 34-2: Recognize and Respond to Verbal and Nonverbal Communication

TASK: Recognize and respond to basic verbal and nonverbal communication.

EQUIPMENT AND SUPPLIES
None.

SKILLS/*RATIONALE*

1. **Procedural Step.** Greet the patient, smile to welcome the patient, and introduce yourself.
2. **Procedural Step.** Verify the patient's name and use it with a courtesy title, such as Mr. or Mrs., unless otherwise instructed by the patient.
   Rationale. This ensures you are speaking to the correct patient, demonstrates a personal interest, and shows respect.
3. **Procedural Step.** Establish a comfortable physical environment.
   Establish an appropriate social distance, position yourself on the same level as the patient (not above or below), make eye contact (if culturally appropriate), reduce any physical noise (e.g., loud fans, sounds from nearby rooms), and provide privacy.
   Rationale. A comfortable environment free from distractions is required by the Health Insurance Portability and Accountability Act (HIPAA) of 1996.
4. **Procedural Step.** Verify that the patient feels comfortable.
5. **Procedural Step.** Establish the topic of discussion.
   If you need to introduce the topic, tell the patient what it is and why you will discuss it. If the patient will introduce the topic, ask the patient what he or she would like to discuss.
6. **Procedural Step.** Observe the patient for nonverbal communication cues.
   Nonverbal communication is communication without the use of words. It includes gestures, posture, facial expressions, eye contact, and physical touch. A medical assistant must be fully aware of any body language exhibited by the patient and report it, if necessary, according to the outcome of the response. The medical assistant must also be aware of his or her own body language when questioning a patient about sensitive material.
   Rationale. Observing the patient will help you become more sensitive to what the patient is saying without using words. This is especially important when discussing social habits like smoking, alcohol consumption, or drug usage. Eye contact is important to show confidence in asking the types of questions that may be required.
7. **Procedural Step.** Verify that the patient understands; ask open-ended questions that request the patient to explain his or her understanding.
   Rationale. An open-ended question can generate many different responses; it cannot be answered with a one-word response. Thus the information you receive from the patient will be more complete and accurate.
8. **Procedural Step.** Practice active listening; provide feedback.
   Active listening means focusing on the patient, what the patient is saying, how he or she is saying it, and what nonverbal messages he or she is sending. It also includes using the patient's verbal and nonverbal cues to ask follow-up questions. In active listening, it is important to verify your understanding of the message; a common approach is to "paraphrase" or repeat the message in a slightly different way. Another important part of active listening is eye contact.
   Rationale. This makes the patient feel that you are listening attentively and may help the patient to "open up."
9. **Procedural Step.** Near the end of the discussion, provide the patient with the opportunity to ask additional questions or to provide further clarification.
10. **Procedural Step.** Thank the patient for his or her comments and signal the end of the discussion.
    When possible, indicate what will happen next so that the patient knows what to expect.

"yes" or "no" without elaborating. This can result in the medical assistant forming an incorrect assumption because of oversimplification or misinterpretation of the patient's meaning. Using **open-ended questions** encourages patients to explain fully what they mean.

> **YES-NO QUESTIONS VERSUS OPEN-ENDED QUESTIONS**
> *Yes-no:* "Do you mean your foot is falling asleep?"
> *Open-ended:* "Tell me about the numbness in your foot."

Observations

In addition to what the patient says, the medical assistant must report what is seen, heard, felt, or smelled. Observations are based on the following areas:

- *Physical appearance* (e.g., patient's face is flushed, patient's clothes are loose fitting, patient is wearing long sleeves in hot weather)
- *Body structure* (e.g., poor posture, deformity)
- *Mobility* (e.g., gait slow, range of motion diminished)
- *Behavior* (e.g., answering questions inappropriately, disoriented, or unresponsive to questions)

Charting Tips

The medical assistant's notes should be concise. Only important information should be recorded.

Charting can be done in several forms, as discussed in Chapter 27. Box 34-3 reviews the necessary criteria for charting the patient's CC and information about the PI. Regardless of the form of charting used, the medical assistant should remember the following simple rules:

1. Always check the name on the chart and at the top of the page to be certain the correct patient is being charted.
2. Use black ink because it photocopies better than blue.
3. Ensure that writing is clear and legible.
4. Always begin charting with the date and time. Then make the entry and end with your first initial, last name, and credential (Figure 34-6).
5. Do not leave any space between the end of the entry and the signature.
6. Ensure accuracy with regard to information, spelling, abbreviations, and symbols. Credibility is ruined if words are misspelled or proper abbreviations are not used.
7. Use proper technique for correcting errors (Figure 34-7).

See Chapter 27 for common abbreviations in charting and correcting errors in medical records.

As mentioned previously, charting the patient's responses clearly and without judgment provides the physician with a foundation on which to build a treatment plan for the patient. Notes should never include judgmental statements. The medical assistant should not record his or her opinions, only observations and statements from the patient.

> **JUDGMENTAL VERSUS NONJUDGMENTAL CHARTING**
> *Judgmental:* Lack of good hygiene has caused the patient to have an infected toe.
> *Nonjudgmental:* Patient states foot has been sore for several days.
> *Judgmental:* The patient appears upset.
> *Nonjudgmental:* The patient is crying and wringing her hands.

BOX 34-3

Charting "Chief Complaint" and "Present Illness" Information

Before you chart the chief complaint (CC), the following information is needed:

1. Date
2. Time
3. CC (What brings you to the office today?)
   - **Signs and symptoms** (Patient's own words)
   - **Specific location of symptoms or pain**
   - **Onset** (When did it begin? or When did you first notice the symptoms?)
   - **Intensity** (How severe is it?)
   - **Precipitating factor** (What caused it to happen? What activities, situations, or positions make the pain worse or better?)
   - **Duration** (How long have you had these symptoms? Are they constant or intermittent? [Do they come and go?])
   - **Remedies** (What has the patient done before seeking medical attention?)
4. Proper signature and credential

DESCRIPTIVE TERMS
For Pain
Aching, sharp, throbbing, burning, cramplike, nagging

For Duration
Sudden, constant, intermittent, sporadic

For Intensity
Intense, moderate, mild; "On a scale of 0 to 10, with 0 being less severe and 10 most severe, describe your pain."

Charting Example

Date	
12/6/XX	9:00 a.m. Pt c/o sore throat x 3 days. T: 101.2° F.
	P. Smith, RMA

FIGURE 34-6 Charting example.

Date	error 2/14/XX	A. Weller, RMA
2/14/XX	1:15 p.m. Demerol 50 mg I.M. given Stat for pain in Ⓡ hip as ordered 25	A. Weller, RMA

FIGURE 34-7 The proper way to correct an error in the patient's record.

PATIENT-CENTERED PROFESSIONALISM

- Why must medical assistants chart only what they observe, hear, and see?

CONCLUSION

The medical history form is a key information tool used in treating the patient. It is a document that may be subpoenaed by the court, so accuracy and objective documentation are critical when writing in the medical record. Each section assists in answering questions about a patient's current state of health. The medical assistant can begin establishing rapport with the patient if the assistant is involved in the process of completing the health history. Charting should provide the physician with a "snapshot" explanation of why the patient is seeking treatment.

Effective listening and communication skills should be used when conducting a patient interview. Putting the patient at ease and demonstrating competence and professionalism give the patient confidence and a sense of security about sharing personal health information. Obtaining the necessary health and medical history information and documenting it accurately help establish a foundation for effective, quality patient care.

Chapter Summary

Reinforce your understanding of the material in this chapter by reviewing the curriculum objectives and key content points below.

1. **Define, appropriately use, and spell all the Key Terms for this chapter.**
   - Review the Key Terms if necessary.
2. **Demonstrate the correct procedure for completing a medical history form.**
   - Review Procedure 34-1.
3. **List seven sections of the medical history and briefly explain what type of information is collected in each.**
   - Demographic material: name, address, DOB, insurance information.
   - CC: main reason the patient wants to see the physician.
   - PI: expansion of the chief complaint.
   - PH: summary of the patient's prior health.
   - FH: inventory of the patient's immediate blood relatives.
   - SH: overview of the patient's lifestyle, including smoking, drinking, education, and exercise.
   - ROS: step-by-step review of each body system.
4. **Distinguish between *objective* and *subjective* data and provide an example of each.**
   - Objective data (signs) can be observed or measured.
   - Subjective data (symptoms) include patient complaints and feelings.
5. **State two positive outcomes of interviewing a patient effectively.**
   - The patient's alertness, level of orientation, grooming, and comfort level can be observed during an interview.
   - The interview is a good opportunity to establish a trusting relationship with the patient.
   - Describe the PQRST interview technique.
   - Proactive
   - Quality
   - Region
   - Severity/Sign/Symptom
   - Time
6. **Explain the importance of maintaining the patient's privacy during and after the interview.**
   - Patients are more likely to open up to the medical assistant when their privacy is assured.
   - HIPAA mandates that measures be taken to protect patient privacy.
   - Patients have a right to expect that their confidential information is being protected.
7. **Explain the need for effective communication skills during a patient interview.**
   - Effective communication encourages the patient to provide all the necessary information and allows the interviewer to receive and understand it.
   - Effective communication helps patients explain the situation completely without being influenced by the interviewer.

8. **Demonstrate the correct procedure for recognizing and responding to nonverbal communication.**
   - Review Procedure 34-2.
9. **Explain the importance of charting patient statements and observations accurately.**
   - The physician's treatment plan is based on the information gathered during history taking and the physician's examination of the patient.
   - Accurate documentation provides a thorough record of the office visit.
10. **Differentiate between "specific" and "general" patient statements and know when to obtain more detail.**
    - Encourage patients to provide detailed information with specific statements (e.g., "4 days" versus "a few days").
    - If patients do make general statements, ask questions to clarify the details.
11. **Accurately record observations made during a patient interview.**
    - Medical assistants should make note of what they see, hear, feel, and smell, in addition to what the patient says.
12. **Recognize judgmental statements in charting and explain the need for nonjudgmental documentation.**
    - Charting should be done using nonjudgmental statements (e.g., "the patient reports feeling sad much of the time and experiences constant fatigue" versus "the patient seems depressed").
    - Nonjudgmental statements provide the physician with a solid foundation on which to build a treatment plan for the patient.
13. **List seven guidelines for effective charting.**
    - First, the chart should be checked to make sure it is the correct patient's record.
    - Black ink should always be used.
    - Writing should be clear and legible.
    - Chart notes should include date and time and should be properly signed with first initial, last name, and credential.
    - No space should be left between the end of an entry and the signature.
    - No lines should be left between entries.
    - Charting should be done accurately, using correct information, spelling, abbreviations, and symbols.
    - Proper technique should be used for correcting errors.
14. **Analyze a realistic medical office situation and apply your understanding of medical history taking to determine the best course of action.**
    - Effective communication skills must be used to take the patient's history.
    - History taking is an opportunity for the medical assistant to build trust and rapport with the patient.
15. **Describe the impact on patient care when medical assistants understand how to take a patient's medical history appropriately and accurately.**
    - The medical history provides information about the patient's past and present, and proper collection of the data is necessary to formulate a diagnosis.
    - Properly collected data provide the physician with the necessary tools to make a diagnosis and treat the patient.

PRACTICAL APPLICATIONS

If you have accomplished the objectives in this chapter, you will be able to make better choices as a medical assistant. Take another look at this situation and decide what you would do.

Dr. Walker, an obstetrician/gynecologist and internal medicine physician, has hired Jenny to assist with taking medical histories for his patients. Dr. Walker sees many patients who have high-risk pregnancies because of an infectious disease. Sarah, a new patient who is 4 months' pregnant, has been referred to Dr. Walker because she is at risk for several infectious diseases.

Jenny goes to the waiting room and starts to ask Sarah questions about her pregnancy and her past medical history. Sarah tells Jenny that she does not want to discuss this with a medical assistant and would rather give the information to Dr. Walker. Jenny adamantly tells Sarah that if she does not want to cooperate, Dr. Walker will not see her as a patient. Sarah begins to cry but starts telling her history to Jenny. Trying to impress Sarah during the interview, Jenny uses medical terminology to ask questions, and she never looks at Sarah or makes any observations about Sarah's remarks.

After the history taking, Sarah is escorted to the examination room, where her vital signs are taken. After discussing her previous illnesses and family history, Dr. Walker examines Sarah and orders several laboratory tests, including tests for HIV and for syphilis. His tentative diagnosis is "possible HIV infection," and he confirms her pregnancy of 4 months. On leaving the office, Sarah makes an appointment for 2 weeks to discuss her test results and final diagnosis with Dr. Walker.

What should Jenny have done differently as a medical assistant initially taking Sarah's history?

1. Did Jenny handle the taking of the medical history correctly? Where should the history have been taken?
2. What actions would cause Sarah to think that Jenny is incompetent in taking a medical history?
3. Why is effective communication between the patient and the medical assistant so important when taking a medical history?
4. What is the "chief complaint" and how should it be documented?
5. What are signs? What are symptoms?
6. What is the correct name for the "tentative diagnosis"? What is the difference between this diagnosis and the "final diagnosis"?
7. Why would it be incorrect for the insurance coder to use the tentative diagnosis on the insurance claim form? What could be the repercussions if the laboratory tests are negative?
8. Why would it have been important for Jenny to observe Sarah during the taking of the medical history?

WEB SEARCH

1. **Research interviewing techniques.** When interviewing techniques are used effectively, time is saved and credibility with the patient is developed. The medical assistant can benefit from additional training to improve interviewing skills.

- **Keywords:** Use the following keywords in your search: interviewing techniques, communication skills, interviewing skills.

Assisting with the Physical Examination

35

evolve http://evolve.elsevier.com/klieger/medicalassisting

A patient may come to the medical office for many reasons. The person may be ill or injured, may be due for a general physical checkup, or may have been referred by another physician for a special procedure. The main purpose of a physical examination is for the physician to assess the status of the patient's health. Although the physician performs the examination and makes diagnoses, the medical assistant plays an important role in the physical examination.

The medical assistant's role is to prepare the examination room, prepare the patient for the examination, and then to assist the physician. Keep in mind that patients may be nervous or anxious. The manner in which the medical assistant handles the patient from the beginning of the office visit establishes the "mood" for the remainder of the visit. If the medical assistant makes the patient feel comfortable and at ease about the upcoming examination or procedure, the patient will be cooperative and comfortable with the physician.

Important aspects of assisting with the physical examination include giving the patient instructions, positioning the patient, knowing the methods of examination, and understanding what happens in vision and hearing examinations.

LEARNING OBJECTIVES

You will be able to do the following after completing this chapter:

Key Terms
1. Define, appropriately use, and spell all the Key Terms for this chapter.

Preparing the Patient
2. List the three main responsibilities of the medical assistant in preparing a patient for a physical examination.
3. List three responsibilities of the medical assistant in assisting the patient to disrobe for an examination.
4. Demonstrate the correct procedure for providing the physician and the patient with items needed to perform a complete physical examination.
5. Explain what a "consent-to-treat form" involves and when formal consent is needed for an examination.

Body Mechanics
6. Discuss why using proper body mechanics is essential when performing physical activities.

Positioning and Draping the Patient
7. Explain the importance of draping the patient appropriately for an examination or procedure.
8. List the three criteria for selecting the position to be used for an examination.
9. List nine examination positions and briefly explain what types of examinations are performed using each position.
10. Demonstrate the correct procedure for properly positioning and draping a patient in the sitting position.
11. Demonstrate the correct procedure for properly positioning and draping a patient in the recumbent position.
12. Demonstrate the correct procedure for properly positioning and draping a patient in the lithotomy position.
13. Demonstrate the correct procedure for properly positioning and draping a patient in the Sims' position.
14. Demonstrate the correct procedure for properly positioning and draping a patient in the prone position.
15. Demonstrate the correct procedure for properly positioning and draping a patient in the knee-chest position.

16. Demonstrate the correct procedure for properly positioning and draping a patient in the Fowler's and semi-Fowler's positions.

Examination Methods

17. List the four primary methods of examining used during a physical examination and briefly explain what occurs in each.

Vision Testing

18. State the purpose of a Snellen chart, and explain when each of the three types of Snellen charts should be used.
19. Demonstrate the correct procedure for accurately measuring and recording a patient's visual acuity with a Snellen chart.
20. List five types of common visual defects that are correctable by lenses or surgery.
21. Demonstrate the correct procedure for accurately measuring and recording a patient's color visual acuity with the Ishihara test.
22. Demonstrate the correct procedure for accurately measuring and recording a patient's near visual acuity with a Jaeger reading card.

Ear Examination

23. Differentiate between an ophthalmoscope and an otoscope and explain how each is used in the physical examination.

Patient-Centered Professionalism

24. Analyze a realistic medical office situation and apply your understanding of assisting with a physical examination to determine the best course of action.
25. Describe the impact on patient care when medical assistants understand how to assist the physician with the physical examination.

KEY TERMS

accommodation
auscultation
benign prostatic hypertrophy (BPH)
bruit
breast self-examination (BSE)
consent
crepitus
cyanosis
diaphoresis
distention
dorsal recumbent position
ecchymosis
erythema
Fowler's position
gingivitis
goniometer
HEENT
herpes simplex 1
horizontal recumbent position
inspection
jaundice
knee-chest position
lithotomy position
last menstrual period (LMP)
macrotia
microtia
murmur
ophthalmoscope
otoscope
pallor
palpation
patent
percussion
perforation
PERRLA
positioning
presbycusis
prone position
rales
rhonchi
Rinne test
range of motion (ROM)
Sims' position
sitting position
standing position
supine position
symmetry
thrill
tinnitus
Trendelenburg's position
testicular self-examination (TSE)
turgor
vertigo
visual acuity
vitiligo
Weber test

PRACTICAL APPLICATIONS

Read the following scenario and keep it in mind as you learn about assisting with the physical examination.

Beth is a medical assistant in the office of Dr. Havidiz, a family practitioner. Dr. Havidiz treats many low-income families, and many women in the community see him for gynecological visits. Holly, a new patient, comes to see Dr. Havidiz for a possible vaginal infection. Her demeanor shows her fear of the doctor's office, especially since this is the first time she has seen Dr. Havidiz. Dr. Havidiz was called to the hospital to see a critically ill patient earlier in the day, so appointments are delayed.

There is an available examination room when Holly arrives, so Beth takes her to the room and tells her to undress completely. Beth does not tell Holly how to put on the gown, but she stands in the room and watches Holly undress. While Holly is undressing, Beth asks the questions necessary to obtain the medical history. Beth then places Holly on the examination table in the lithotomy position and immediately leaves the room, giving the impression that she is in a great hurry. After 15 minutes, Holly has discomfort in her back but dares not move from the position because she does not want to delay the examination. After 30 minutes, Holly wonders just how much longer it will take for Dr. Havidiz to come and check her. Finally, Dr. Havidiz arrives and the examination begins.

During the examination, Beth leaves the room to answer a personal phone call, leaving Dr. Havidiz and Holly alone. As Holly leaves the office, she is in tears from back pain and appears to be very upset. Beth shows no sympathy or empathy for Holly. Two days later, Holly asks that her records be transferred to another physician and tells Dr. Havidiz that she has never been treated as rudely as she was in his office.

How might this situation have been avoided?

PREPARING THE PATIENT

Once the medical history has been completed and the patient's vital signs taken, the patient is ready for the examination. The medical assistant's major role in preparing a patient for the complete physical examination (CPX) is to have the patient gowned, appropriately positioned, and draped for the physician to perform the examination, and to assist the physician as necessary (Procedure 35-1). It is also important to consider

Assisting with the Physical Examination   CHAPTER 35   733

| PROCEDURE 35-1 | Assist with the Physical Examination |

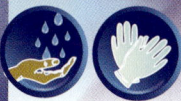

TASK: Prepare a patient and assist the physician or health care practitioner with a general physical examination.

EQUIPMENT AND SUPPLIES
- Examination table
- Table paper
- Patient gown
- Drape
- Urine specimen container
- Specimen collection system
- Snellen chart
- Patient's medical record
- Waste container
- Tongue depressor
- Gauze
- Clean surgical towel
- Stethoscope
- Sphygmomanometer
- Otoscope
- Ophthalmoscope
- Disposable gloves
- Waste container

SKILLS/RATIONALE

STANDARD PRECAUTIONS ARE TO BE FOLLOWED.

1. **Procedural Step. Sanitize the hands.**
   An alcohol based hand rub may be used instead of washing hands with soap and water, unless hands are visibly soiled.
   Rationale. Hand sanitization promotes infection control.

2. **Procedural Step. Assemble equipment and supplies.**
   Line the stainless steel instrument tray with a plastic-backed paper towel or clean surgical towel. Lay out the instruments and supplies for a general physical examination, making sure the items do not overlap. The instruments and supplies include:
   - Otoscope/ophthalmoscope (unless mounted on wall)

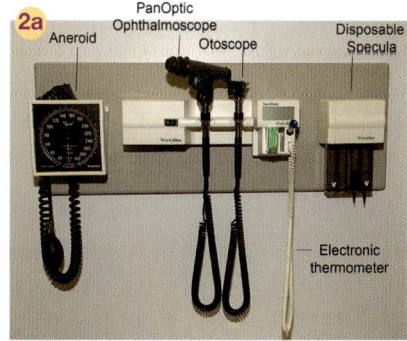

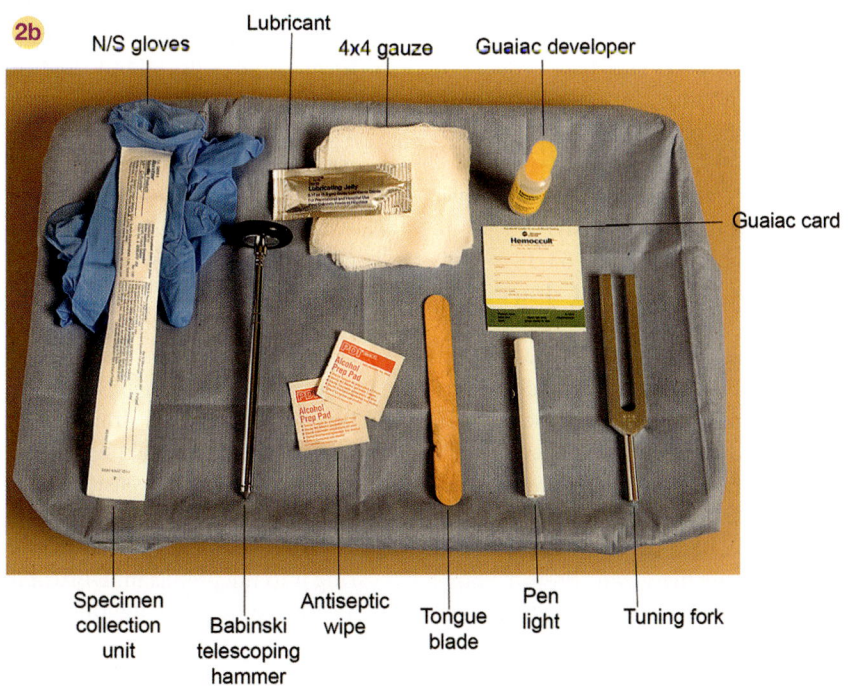

Continued

PROCEDURE 35-1 Assist with the Physical Examination—cont'd

- Penlight
- Percussion hammer
- Tuning forks
- Nonsterile disposable gloves
- Specimen collection system
- Antiseptic wipes

Other items that may be added to the tray include tongue depressor, gauze squares, water-based lubricant, and laboratory supplies (fecal occult blood testing supplies).

Rationale. It is important to have all supplies and equipment ready and available before starting any procedure to ensure efficiency.

3. **Procedural Step.** Obtain the patient's medical record.
4. **Procedural Step.** Greet the patient, introduce yourself, and confirm the patient's identity.
   Rationale. Identifying the patient ensures the procedure is performed on the correct patient.
5. **Procedural Step.** Explain the procedure to the patient.
   Rationale. Explaining the procedure to the patient promotes cooperation and provides a means of obtaining implied consent.
6. **Procedural Step.** Measure the patient's weight and height and chart the results.
   Refer to Procedure 33-1.
7. **Procedural Step.** Measure the patient's visual acuity and chart the results.
   See Procedure 35-9.
8. **Procedural Step.** Have the patient provide a urine sample (if required).
   Depending on the type or extent of the physical examination, a urine sample may be tested.
   Rationale. Having the patient void before the physical examination will ensure the patient is more comfortable during the examination.
9. **Procedural Step.** Escort the patient to the examination room.
10. **Procedural Step.** Measure the patient's vital signs and chart the results, if not done previously.
    Refer to Procedures 33-7, 33-9, 33-11, and 33-12.
11. **Procedural Step.** Provide a gown and drape the patient.
    Instruct the patient to change from street clothes into a patient gown. The gown should open in the back. Most male patients will not require a gown, but a drape should be provided to place over the patient's lap once seated on the examination table. Elderly patients may require assistance in changing into the gown and stepping up to sit on the examination table. Be sure to give the patient a few minutes to change into the gown. Protect your patient's right to privacy at all times. Knock on the door before entering once the patient has begun to change into the patient gown.

    Rationale. A drape provides for the patient's modesty and warmth.
12. **Procedural Step.** Allow the patient to change into the gown, inform the physician that the patient is ready, and make the patient's record available to the physician.
    Instruct the patient to have a seat on the end of the examination table when ready.
    NOTE: Never leave an elderly patient or a patient who has symptoms of dizziness sitting alone on an examination table because of the danger of falling or injury.
13. **Procedural Step.** Assist the physician with the examination of the body systems.
    The patient is generally placed in a sitting position for an examination of the upper body.
14. **Procedural Step.** Assist the physician with the eye examination.
    Hand the physician the ophthalmoscope. When instructed, dim the lights.
    Rationale. When the lights are dimmed the patient's eyes will dilate and the physician will be able to see the interior of the eye better.
15. **Procedural Step.** Assist the physician with the ear examination.
    Hand the physician the otoscope. A disposable otoscope speculum should be attached to the otoscope before it is passed to the physician in working position (handle first). Dispose of the otoscope speculum in a regular waste container on completion of this portion of the examination, unless there are obvious signs of contamination from blood (in which case you should dispose of it in a biohazardous waste container).
16. **Procedural Step.** Hand the tuning fork to the physician in working position (handle first).
    The physician will test the patient's ability to hear sound conducted first through the air, then through the bone of the skull.
17. **Procedural Step.** Assist the physician with the nose examination.
    Pass the nasal speculum and penlight or otoscope head and handle with wide speculum attached to the physician in working position (handle first). The physician will examine the patient's nasal cavities for nasal congestion, excessive nasal drainage from the sinuses, or the presence of abnormal growths.
18. **Procedural Step.** Assist the physician with the throat examination.
    Hold the tongue depressor at the center when transferring it to the physician. Discard the tongue depressor in a waste container when this portion of the examination has been completed, by either stepping on the foot pedal

Continued

PROCEDURE 35-1 Assist with the Physical Examination—cont'd

and allowing the physician to drop it directly into the container or by taking it from the physician by holding it at the center and throwing it away.

Rationale. The tongue depressor is passed by holding it in the middle so that the end inserted into the patient's mouth is not handled before or after use. This prevents contact with the patient's secretions, which may contain pathogens.

19. **Procedural Step.** Assist the physician with the lung and heart examination.

   Hand the physician a stethoscope if he or she does not already have one. (Most physicians will keep their own stethoscope in a pocket or around the neck.)

20. **Procedural Step.** Assist the physician with the examination of the upper extremity reflexes.

   Hand the physician the percussion hammer in working position (handle first).

21. **Procedural Step.** Position the patient as required for examination of the remaining body systems.

   This assessment includes palpation of the organs of the abdomen, strength and reflex testing of the lower extremities, auscultation of the abdomen for bowel sounds with a stethoscope, abnormalities that can be visualized, and observation of any abnormal smells.

   Positioning and draping procedures are described in Procedures 35-2 through 35-8.

   Rationale. Certain patient positions are required so that the physician can examine a particular part of the body.

22. **Procedural Step.** Assist the patient off the examination table as needed, to prevent the patient from falling.

   Rationale. Patients, especially the elderly, frequently become dizzy after being positioned on the examining table, and they often need assistance.

23. **Procedural Step.** Allow the patient time to change from the patient gown back into their street clothes.

   Provide assistance to the patient as needed. Tell the patient about the next steps of the examination. Allow adequate time for the patient to change clothes.

   Rationale. It is important to inform patients that they may change back into their clothes; otherwise, patients may remain in the patient gown.

24. **Procedural Step.** Allow time for further discussion between the physician and patient regarding prescriptions, medications, and a return visit. Ask the patient if he or she has any questions.

   Rationale. Answers and instructions given by the medical assistant involving medical care should be explained in terms the patient can understand. The medical assistant should answer questions within the scope of practice and refer other questions to the physician as necessary.

25. **Procedural Step.** Document any instructions given to the patient in the medical record.

26. **Procedural Step.** Clean the examination room according to Standard Precautions before the next patient arrives.

   Put on disposable gloves before cleaning the examination room. Cleaning the examination room includes:
   - Disposing of the patient gown and drape.
   - Changing the crumpled or soiled table paper.
   - Disposing of any waste materials in the appropriate container.
   - Removing soiled instruments.
   - Wiping down the examination table and counters.
   - Replenishing supplies as needed.

   Always clean the examination room immediately after the patient has left. Never bring a patient into a room with crumpled table paper and used instruments. Never clean a room in front of a patient. If the room has not been cleaned and you inadvertently bring the next patient into the examination room, apologize to the patient immediately. This is the only circumstance when cleaning a room in front of a patient would be acceptable. However, take steps to ensure this does not occur again.

27. **Procedural Step.** Sanitize the hands.

   Always sanitize the hands after every procedure or after using gloves.

---

whether informed consent is needed for an examination or procedure and to explain the examination or procedure completely to the patient. Answer questions and put the patient at ease before the examination begins.

Disrobing and Gowning the Patient

It is usually necessary for the patient to remove articles of clothing and put on a gown that can open to expose only the body part to be examined. The medical assistant must (1) choose the right type of gown for the procedure to be performed, (2) provide clear instructions for disrobing and gowning, and (3) assist patients who need help disrobing (e.g., elderly patient, patient with a disability). Remember, always respect the dignity of the patient by asking if he or she would like assistance.

The purpose or type of procedure will determine how much clothing the patient will need to remove. An upper respiratory complaint requires that only clothing from the waist up be removed, whereas a "well-woman visit" requires removal of all clothing except the socks. The physician's preference and need for accessibility will dictate whether the gown opening should be in the front or back. Gowns can be either *full length,* which covers the patient's body to the knees, or *half-length* (partial), which covers only the shoulders, chest, and back.

A medical assistant must respect the patient's right to privacy when the patient is to disrobe. Before leaving the room, make certain the patient understands what is to be done, how to wear the gown, how far to disrobe, and where to place their clothes. Assure the patient the physician will be arriving shortly. If the physician is delayed, be honest with the patient about the approximate waiting time.

Securing Consent

For a procedure that is beyond the basic wellness examination, it is necessary to obtain the patient's informed **consent**. A consent-to-treat form (procedure consent form) must be signed, dated, and witnessed (Figure 35-1). The physician must explain all details concerning the procedure, but the medical assistant can act as a witness. The consent-to-treat form must be included in the patient's chart before the procedure is performed. Remember that *implied* consent is only good for basic common procedures (e.g., electrocardiograms [ECGs], blood tests), whereas other procedures require written consent.

Failure to secure consent for procedures such as a colonoscopy or a stress test is considered assault and battery (see Chapter 4). Patients have the right to refuse treatments and procedures. In addition, patients can withdraw their consent at any time.

PATIENT-CENTERED PROFESSIONALISM

- Why must the medical assistant demonstrate competence when assisting the patient for a physical examination?

BODY MECHANICS

Body mechanics means using appropriate body movements to perform certain functions in a manner that protects the medical assistant's muscles and skeletal system from injury. Using correct techniques protects you from injury by aligning body segments to each other. By standing up straight, the main parts of the body (head, chest, and pelvis) are properly aligned one over the other to maintain good balance. Using good body mechanics reduces muscle fatigue and prevents strain on the spine by making the spine work with you to maximize body strength when lifting or moving objects. Using good body mechanics also provides balance and stability.

Remember your feet are your support base and the strongest and largest muscles in your body are those of the shoulders, upper arms, hips, and thighs. This is why we use these muscles to lift and move heavy objects. Before lifting, you must stand up straight with your feet slightly apart (about 18 inches) with one foot slightly ahead of the other (Figure 35-2). This position helps provide better stability and this stability prevents the medical assistant from becoming overbalanced, when assisting a patient out of a wheelchair, for example.

When lifting, get close to whatever is being lifted instead of reaching for it. Keep your back straight; bend at the hip and

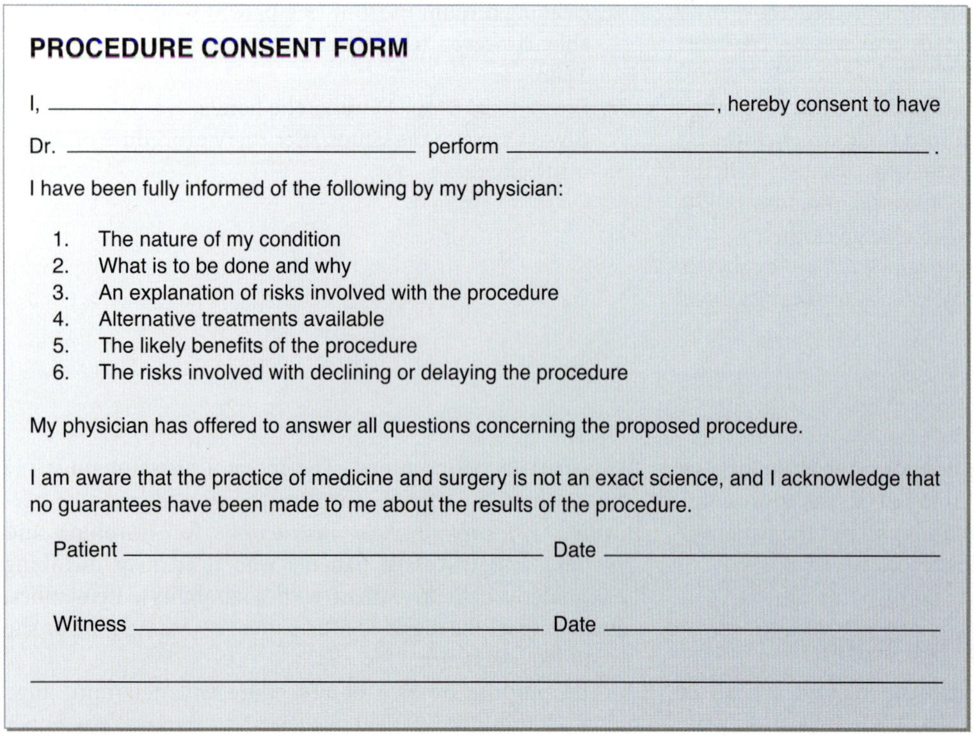

PROCEDURE CONSENT FORM

I, _____, hereby consent to have

Dr. _____ perform _____ .

I have been fully informed of the following by my physician:

1. The nature of my condition
2. What is to be done and why
3. An explanation of risks involved with the procedure
4. Alternative treatments available
5. The likely benefits of the procedure
6. The risks involved with declining or delaying the procedure

My physician has offered to answer all questions concerning the proposed procedure.

I am aware that the practice of medicine and surgery is not an exact science, and I acknowledge that no guarantees have been made to me about the results of the procedure.

Patient _____ Date _____

Witness _____ Date _____

FIGURE 35-1 Patient consent form to have procedure performed.

knees (Figure 35-3, *A*). Straighten your legs and use your upper arm and leg muscles to lift (Figure 35-3, *B*). When an activity requires a physical effort, use as many muscles as possible. For example, use both hands to pick up a heavy object, not just one hand. When picking something up off the floor, squat down rather than bending over at the waist, thus reducing the strain on the spine. Always carry objects close to the midline of the body, thus keeping the body in alignment.

PATIENT-CENTERED PROFESSIONALISM

- Why must the medical assistant use good body mechanics when lifting or moving objects?

POSITIONING AND DRAPING THE PATIENT

Another responsibility of the medical assistant is to position and drape patients appropriately for the procedures being performed. When **positioning** and draping, always consider the patient's comfort and minimize exposure of nonessential body parts.

Many types of positions are used for various procedures. Selection of a position depends on the examination or procedure to be performed. A patient's chief complaint and age are also important criteria to consider when choosing the best position. Medical assistants should be familiar with nine examination positions: sitting, standing, horizontal recumbent, dorsal recumbent, lithotomy, Sims', prone, knee-chest, and Fowler's positions.

Regardless of what position the patient will assume, it is the medical assistant's responsibility to explain to the patient the reason for the position and to provide clear instructions on assuming the position. Patient safety must be the prime consideration for the medical assistant during positioning (Box 35-1).

Sitting

The **sitting position** has the patient in an upright position at the end of the examination table without back support, using

---

BOX 35-1

Safety and Comfort in Patient Positioning

The medical assistant is responsible for patient safety. When positioning a patient, it is the responsibility of the medical assistant to make sure the patient is free from harm. For example, an elderly patient who is unsteady should never be left sitting on the examination table without someone in the room. If the medical assistant must leave the room, a family member or other caregiver must be present.

It takes time and practice to learn proper positioning techniques. A priority is to avoid causing additional discomfort or inflicting discomfort on the patient. When a male physician examines a female patient (or when a female physician examines a male patient), for the physician's legal protection, a medical assistant should be present. This provides support for the physician if the female (or male) patient complains of inappropriate touching, and it provides support for the female (or male) patient in an uncomfortable situation.

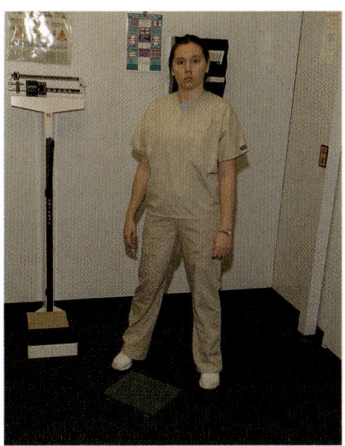

FIGURE 35-2 Good body position requires the medical assistant to stand up straight, feet slightly apart, with one foot slightly ahead of the other.

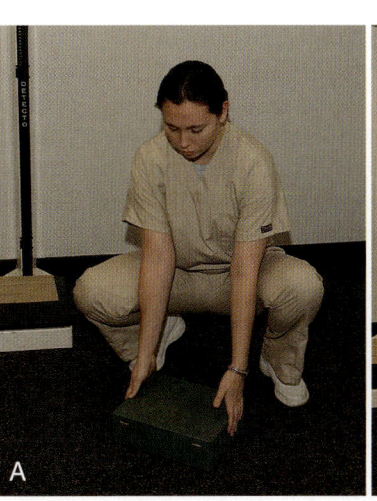 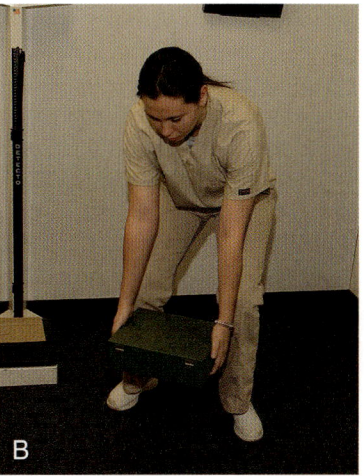

FIGURE 35-3 **A,** When lifting heavy objects, keep back straight, bend at the hip and knees, with feet apart. **B,** Use upper arms and leg muscles to lift.

the footrest for support (since the feet should not be left dangling for long periods). As needed, the drape extends from the waist and over the knees. Procedure 35-2 presents proper positioning and draping for the sitting position.

The sitting position is used most often to begin the physical examination because the upper extremities are clearly accessible (e.g., head, neck, and axillae). The neurological reflexes (knee, elbow, wrist, and ankle) can be tested in this position, and sitting provides the most comfort for the patient. Heart and lung sounds can be detected because sitting allows for maximum lung expansion, and sitting patients can easily answer questions for the physician concerning their state of health. The sitting position also provides better visualization of **symmetry** of upper body parts. If a patient is too weak to sit upright, the medical assistant should consider an alternative position, such as the supine position, for the examination.

Standing

The physician may need to evaluate coordination and balance by observing the patient in the **standing position** (erect) for seconds to minutes. No special draping is needed, but the gown must be able to cover the patient's whole body if this type of observation is performed.

Horizontal Recumbent (Supine)

In the **horizontal recumbent position,** or **supine position,** the patient is lying flat on his or her back with the arms to the sides and the head elevated with a pillow facing upward. The drape starts just under the arms and extends to the feet (Procedure 35-3).

Examination of the head, neck, anterior chest (lungs, heart, and breasts), abdomen, and lower extremities can be performed with the patient in the horizontal recumbent position. This position also provides easy access to pulse sites.

Dorsal Recumbent

In the **dorsal recumbent position,** the patient is in a supine position, but the knees are flexed (bent) sharply with the feet flat on the table. Bending the knees takes pressure away from the lower back and is more comfortable than the supine position for examining the abdomen. The drape is placed in a diamond shape, with the lower corner over the pubic area (see Procedure 35-3). When the physician wants to examine the pubic area, the corner is lifted up to expose the genitals.

The dorsal recumbent position allows for the examination of the vagina and rectal areas on the female and the rectal and genital areas on the male. It can also be used for examining the head, neck, axillae, and the anterior chest. This position may be used as an alternative to the lithotomy position for patients with severe arthritis or other disabilities or conditions.

Lithotomy

To place the patient in the **lithotomy position,** the dorsal recumbent position is assumed first. The buttocks are then moved to the edge of the table, and the feet are placed in stirrups. As with the dorsal recumbent position, the "diamond drape" is used. The medical assistant should help the patient into and out of this position (Procedure 35-4).

The patient is not placed in the lithotomy position until the physician is ready to examine the patient because it strains the back and it is difficult to maintain the position for a prolonged time. The lithotomy position is the best position for the Pap smear and pelvic examination.

Sims'

For the **Sims' position,** the patient first assumes the supine position and then moves to the left, side-lying position. The left arm is kept behind the body, and the right arm is up, flexed, and forward. Both legs are bent at the knee, with the right leg sharply bent to expose the anal area. The drape is positioned to cover the back from under the arms to the toes. Extra pillows may be needed for positioning purposes (Procedure 35-5). When the anal area is examined, the drape is adjusted.

The Sims' position can be used for both the rectal and vaginal examinations and enema administration.

Prone

In the **prone position,** the patient is lying on the abdomen with the head slightly turned to the side and the arms above the head or alongside the body. The drape starts just under the arms to the feet and is adjusted as needed during the examination (Procedure 35-6).

The back and lower extremities can be examined in the prone position. This position is most often used to assess the extension of the hip joints.

Knee-Chest

The **knee-chest position** begins with the patient in the prone position. The patient is assisted into a kneeling position, with the buttocks elevated and the head and chest lowered onto the table. The arms are above the head and bent at the elbow. For patient comfort, a pillow can be placed under the chest area (Procedure 35-7).

The patient is not placed in the knee-chest position until the physician is ready. The patient should never be left unattended in this position. The knee-chest position is most often used for sigmoidoscopy.

Fowler's

In the **Fowler's position,** the patient is lying in a supine position with the back of the table drawn up at either a 45-degree angle (*semi-Fowler's* position) or a 90-degree angle (*Fowler's* or *full Fowler's* position). The patient's legs are only slightly bent (Procedure 35-8).

Text continued on p. 747

Assisting with the Physical Examination **CHAPTER 35** 739

PROCEDURE 35-2 Sitting Position

TASK: Properly position and drape the patient for examination of the head, neck, chest, and upper extremities and measurement of vital signs.

EQUIPMENT AND SUPPLIES
- Examination table
- Table paper
- Patient gown
- Drape

SKILLS/*RATIONALE*

STANDARD PRECAUTIONS ARE TO BE FOLLOWED.

1. **Procedural Step. Sanitize the hands.**
   An alcohol-based hand rub may be used instead of washing hands with soap and water, unless hands are visibly soiled.
   Rationale. Hand sanitization promotes infection control.

2. **Procedural Step. Assemble equipment and supplies.**
   Rationale. It is important to have all supplies and equipment ready and available before starting any procedure to ensure efficiency.

3. **Procedural Step. Greet the patient, introduce yourself, and confirm the patient's identity.**
   Rationale. Identifying the patient ensures the procedure is performed on the correct patient.

4. **Procedural Step. Explain the procedure to the patient.**
   Rationale. Explaining the procedure to the patient promotes cooperation and provides a means of obtaining implied consent.

5. **Procedural Step. Provide a gown for the patient.**
   Prepare the patient for the particular type of examination being performed. Not all patients will require a gown, but if needed the opening is usually in the back.

6. **Procedural Step. Pull out the footrest of the table, and assist the patient to a sitting position.**

7. **Procedural Step. Drape the patient.**
   Draping will depend on the procedure being performed.
   Rationale. Draping provides warmth and prevents unnecessary exposure.

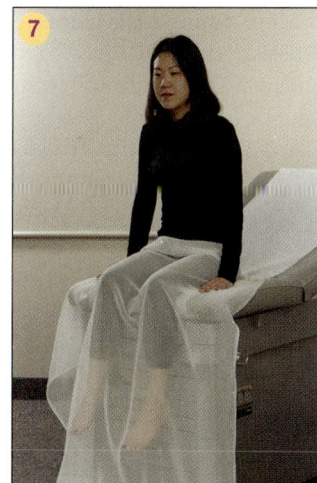

8. **Procedural Step. When the examination is complete, assist the patient from the table.**
   a. Return the footrest to its original position.
   b. Instruct the patient to dress; assist as needed.

9. **Procedural Step. Clean the examination room according to Standard Precautions.**
   Always clean the examination room immediately after the patient has left. Never bring the next patient into an unclean room.

10. **Procedural Step. Sanitize the hands.**
    Always sanitize the hands after every procedure or after using gloves.
    NOTE: Physically weak patients should not be placed in this position.

PROCEDURE 35-3 Recumbent Position

TASK: Properly position and drape the patient for catheter insertion, examinations of the abdomen, and general examination procedures.

EQUIPMENT AND SUPPLIES
- Examination table
- Table paper
- Patient gown
- Drape

SKILLS/RATIONALE

STANDARD PRECAUTIONS ARE TO BE FOLLOWED.

1. **Procedural Step. Sanitize the hands.**
   An alcohol-based hand rub may be used instead of washing hands with soap and water, unless hands are visibly soiled.
   Rationale. Hand sanitization promotes infection control.

2. **Procedural Step. Assemble equipment and supplies.**
   Rationale. It is important to have all supplies and equipment ready and available before starting any procedure to ensure efficiency.

3. **Procedural Step. Greet the patient, introduce yourself, and confirm the patient's identity.**
   Rationale. Identifying the patient ensures the procedure is performed on the correct patient.

4. **Procedural Step. Explain the procedure to the patient.**
   Rationale. Explaining the procedure to the patient promotes cooperation and provides a means of obtaining implied consent.

5. **Procedural Step. Provide a gown for the patient.**
   Prepare the patient for the particular type of examination being performed. Not all patients will require a gown, but if needed the opening is usually in the back.

6. **Procedural Step. Place the patient in the recumbent position.**
   a. Pull out the footrest of the table, and assist the patient to a sitting position.
   b. Have the patient move back on the table, and pull out the table extension supporting the patient's lower extremities.
   c. Assist the patient to lie down on his or her back with the head slightly elevated with a pillow. The arms can be placed above the head or alongside the body; this is the *horizontal recumbent* or *supine* position.

   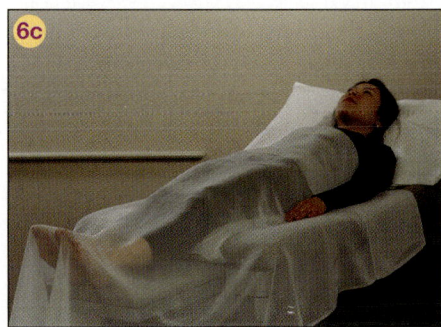

   d. To place the patient in a *dorsal recumbent* position, have the patient bend the knees and place each foot at the edge of the table.

   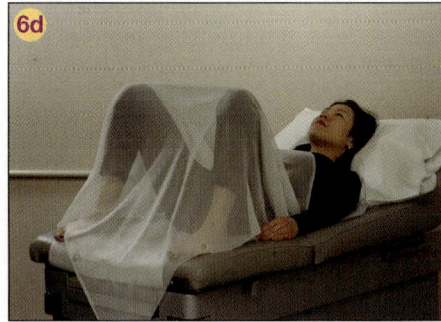

   e. Push in the table extension and footrest.

Continued

PROCEDURE 35-3 Recumbent Position—cont'd

7. **Procedural Step.** Drape the patient.
   a. The *horizontal* recumbent or supine drape is placed over the patient.
   b. The *dorsal* recumbent drape should be positioned diagonally.
   Rationale. Draping will depend on the procedure being performed.
8. **Procedural Step.** When the examination is complete, assist the patient from the recumbent position and into a sitting position.
9. **Procedural Step.** Assist the patient from the examination table.
   a. Return the footrest to its original position.
   b. Instruct the patient to dress; assist as needed.
10. **Procedural Step.** Clean the examination room according to Standard Precautions.
    Always clean the examination room immediately after the patient has left. Never bring the next patient into an unclean room.
11. **Procedural Step.** Sanitize the hands.
    Always sanitize the hands after every procedure or after using gloves.
    NOTE: Patients with respiratory and/or painful musculoskeletal disorders are more comfortable with the head of the table raised slightly for breathing difficulties and having the knees flexed to reduce tension on muscles of the back and abdomen.

PROCEDURE 35-4 Lithotomy Position

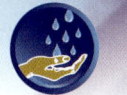

TASK: Properly position and drape the patient for a vaginal, pelvic, or rectal examination.

EQUIPMENT AND SUPPLIES
- Examination table
- Table paper
- Patient gown
- Drape

SKILLS/RATIONALE
STANDARD PRECAUTIONS ARE TO BE FOLLOWED.

1. **Procedural Step.** Sanitize the hands.
   An alcohol-based hand rub may be used instead of washing hands with soap and water, unless hands are visibly soiled.
   Rationale. Hand sanitization promotes infection control.
2. **Procedural Step.** Assemble equipment and supplies.
   Rationale. It is important to have all supplies and equipment ready and available before starting any procedure to ensure efficiency.
3. **Procedural Step.** Greet the patient, introduce yourself, and confirm the patient's identity.
   Rationale. Identifying the patient ensures the procedure is performed on the correct patient.
4. **Procedural Step.** Explain the procedure to the patient.
   Rationale. Explaining the procedure to the patient promotes cooperation and provides a means of obtaining implied consent.
5. **Procedural Step.** Provide a gown for the patient.
   Prepare the patient for the particular type of examination being performed. Not all patients will require a gown, but if needed the opening is in the front.
6. **Procedural Step.** Place the patient first in the supine position.
   a. Pull out the footrest of the table, and assist the patient to a sitting position.
   b. Have the patient move back on the table, and pull out the table extension supporting the patient's lower extremities.
   c. Assist the patient to lie down on his or her back with the head slightly elevated with a pillow. The arms can be placed above the head or alongside the body.
7. **Procedural Step.** Drape the patient.
   The drape should be placed diagonally.
   Rationale. Draping provides warmth and prevents unnecessary exposure.
8. **Procedural Step.** Pull out the stirrups.
   The stirrups should be level with the examination table and approximately 1 foot from each side of the table.

Continued

PROCEDURE 35-4 Lithotomy Position—cont'd

9. **Procedural Step.** Place the patient in the lithotomy position.
   a. Have the patient bend the knees, and place each foot into the stirrups.
   b. Push in the table extension and footrest.

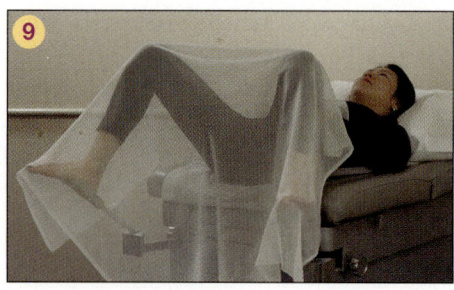

10. **Procedural Step.** Have the patient slide the buttocks to the edge of the table.
11. **Procedural Step.** Adjust the stirrups as needed.
    Rationale. Stirrups that are either too far apart or too close together will cause the patient discomfort. Stirrups too close to the table will not allow the patient's buttocks to reach the end of the table and will not permit enough knee flexibility.

12. **Procedural Step.** When the examination is complete, assist the patient from the lithotomy position.
    a. Have the patient slide the buttocks back from the edge of the table.
    b. Pull out the table extension and the footrest.
    c. Assist the patient out of the stirrups, supporting the legs.
    d. Place the legs on the table extension.
    e. Return the stirrups to their original position, and push in the table extension.
    f. Assist the patient to a sitting position.
13. **Procedural Step.** Assist the patient from the examination table.
    a. Instruct the patient to dress; assist as needed.
    b. Return the footrest to its original position.
14. **Procedural Step.** Clean the examination room according to Standard Precautions.
    Always clean the examination room immediately after the patient has left. Never bring the next patient into an unclean room.
15. **Procedural Step.** Sanitize the hands.
    Always sanitize the hands after every procedure or after using gloves.

PROCEDURE 35-5 Sims' Position

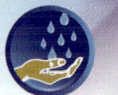

TASK: Properly position and drape the patient for a vaginal or rectal examination.

EQUIPMENT AND SUPPLIES
- Examination table
- Table paper
- Patient gown
- Drape

SKILLS/RATIONALE
STANDARD PRECAUTIONS ARE TO BE FOLLOWED.

1. **Procedural Step.** Sanitize the hands.
   An alcohol-based hand rub may be used instead of washing hands with soap and water, unless hands are visibly soiled.
   Rationale. Hand sanitization promotes infection control.
2. **Procedural Step.** Assemble equipment and supplies.
   Rationale. It is important to have all supplies and equipment ready and available before starting any procedure to ensure efficiency.
3. **Procedural Step.** Greet the patient, introduce yourself, and confirm the patient's identity.
   Rationale. Identifying the patient ensures the procedure is performed on the correct patient.

4. **Procedural Step.** Explain the procedure to the patient.
   Rationale. Explaining the procedure to the patient promotes cooperation and provides a means of obtaining implied consent.
5. **Procedural Step.** Provide a gown for the patient.
   Prepare the patient for the particular type of examination being performed. Not all patients will require a gown, but if needed the opening is usually in the back.
6. **Procedural Step.** Place the patient in the supine position.
   a. Pull out the footrest of the table, and assist the patient to a sitting position.

Continued

PROCEDURE 35-5 Sims' Position—cont'd

b. Have the patient move back on the table, and pull out the table extension supporting the patient's lower extremities.
c. Assist the patient to lie down on his or her back with the head slightly elevated with a pillow. The arms can be placed above the head or alongside the body.

7. **Procedural Step. Drape the patient.**
The drape should be placed diagonally, from under the arms to below the knees.
Rationale. Draping provides warmth and prevents unnecessary exposure.

8. **Procedural Step. Place the patient in the Sims' position.**
a. Have the patient turn to the left side.
b. Have the patient place the left arm behind the body and the right arm forward and bent at the elbow.
c. The right leg is sharply flexed upward and the left leg bent slightly.
d. Position the buttocks at the edge of the table.

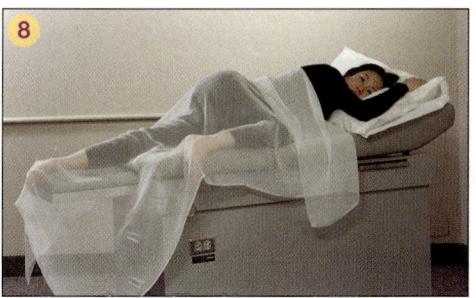

9. **Procedural Step. Adjust the drape as the physician examines the anal area.**

10. **Procedural Step. When the examination is complete, assist the patient to the supine position and then to the sitting position.**

11. **Procedural Step. Assist the patient from the examination table.**
a. Push in the table extension while supporting the lower extremities.
b. Pull out the footrest, and help the patient from the table as needed.
c. Return the footrest to its original position.
d. Instruct the patient to dress; assist as needed.

12. **Procedural Step. Clean the examination room according to Standard Precautions.**
Always clean the examination room immediately after the patient has left. Never bring the next patient into an unclean room.

13. **Procedural Step. Sanitize the hands.**
Always sanitize the hands after every procedure or after using gloves.
NOTE: Patients with joint deformities may not be able to bend the hip or knee.

PROCEDURE 35-6 Prone Position

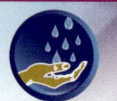

TASK: Properly position and drape the patient for examination of the back.

EQUIPMENT AND SUPPLIES
- Examination table
- Table paper
- Patient gown
- Drape

SKILLS/*RATIONALE*

STANDARD PRECAUTIONS ARE TO BE FOLLOWED.

1. **Procedural Step. Sanitize the hands.**
   An alcohol-based hand rub may be used instead of washing hands with soap and water, unless hands are visibly soiled.
   Rationale. Hand sanitization promotes infection control.

2. **Procedural Step. Assemble equipment and supplies.**
   Rationale. It is important to have all supplies and equipment ready and available before starting any procedure to ensure efficiency.

3. **Procedural Step. Greet the patient, introduce yourself, and confirm the patient's identity.**
   Rationale. Identifying the patient ensures the procedure is performed on the correct patient.

4. **Procedural Step. Explain the procedure to the patient.**
   Rationale. Explaining the procedure to the patient promotes cooperation and provides a means of obtaining implied consent.

5. **Procedural Step. Provide a gown for the patient.**
   Prepare the patient for the particular type of examination being performed. Not all patients will require a gown, but if needed the opening is usually in the back.

6. **Procedural Step. Place the patient on his or her back.**
   a. Pull out the footrest of the table, and assist the patient to a sitting position.
   b. Have the patient move back on the table, and pull out the table extension supporting the patient's lower extremities.
   c. Assist the patient to lie down on his or her back.

7. **Procedural Step. Drape the patient.**
   Draping will depend on the procedure being performed.
   a. The drape should be placed over any exposed area not being examined.
   b. For a female patient, the gown should extend high enough to cover the breasts, because she may be required to turn over and be positioned in the lithotomy or dorsal recumbent position later in the examination.
   Rationale. Draping provides warmth and prevents unnecessary exposure.

8. **Procedural Step. Place the patient in the prone position.**
   a. Have the patient turn onto his or her abdomen with the legs together by rolling toward you.
   b. Ask the patient to turn his or her head to one side.
   c. The patient's arms can be positioned above the head or alongside the body.

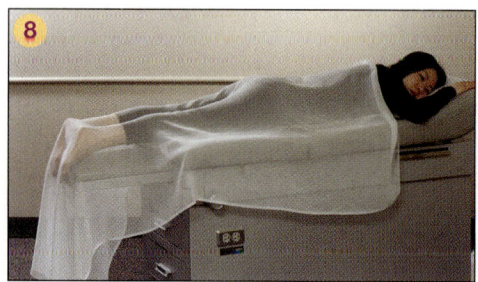

9. **Procedural Step. When the examination is complete, assist the patient to the supine position and then to the sitting position.**

10. **Procedural Step. Assist the patient from the examination table.**
    a. Push in the table extension while supporting the lower extremities.
    b. Pull out the footrest, and help the patient from the table as needed.
    c. Return the footrest to its original position.
    d. Instruct the patient to dress; assist as needed.

11. **Procedural Step. Clean the examination room according to Standard Precautions.**
    Always clean the examination room immediately after the patient has left. Never bring the next patient into an unclean room.

12. **Procedural Step. Sanitize the hands.**
    Always sanitize the hands after every procedure or after using gloves.
    NOTE: This position is poorly tolerated by patients with respiratory difficulties.

PROCEDURE 35-7 Knee-Chest Position

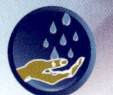

TASK: Properly position and drape the patient for a proctological examination.

EQUIPMENT AND SUPPLIES
- Examination table
- Table paper
- Patient gown
- Drape
- Tissue

SKILLS/*RATIONALE*

STANDARD PRECAUTIONS ARE TO BE FOLLOWED.

1. **Procedural Step. Sanitize the hands.**
   An alcohol-based hand rub may be used instead of washing hands with soap and water, unless hands are visibly soiled.
   Rationale. Hand sanitization promotes infection control.

2. **Procedural Step. Assemble equipment and supplies.**
   Rationale. It is important to have all supplies and equipment ready and available before starting any procedure to ensure efficiency.

3. **Procedural Step. Greet the patient, introduce yourself, and confirm the patient's identity.**
   Rationale. Identifying the patient ensures the procedure is performed on the correct patient.

4. **Procedural Step. Explain the procedure to the patient.**
   Rationale. Explaining the procedure to the patient promotes cooperation and provides a means of obtaining implied consent.

5. **Procedural Step. Provide a gown for the patient.**
   Prepare the patient for the particular type of examination being performed. Not all patients will require a gown, but if needed the opening is usually in the back.

6. **Procedural Step. Place the patient in the prone position.**
   a. Pull out the footrest of the table, and assist the patient to a sitting position.
   b. Have the patient move back on the table, and pull out the table extension supporting the patient's lower extremities.

7. **Procedural Step. Drape the patient.**
   The drape should be placed diagonally.
   Rationale. Draping provides warmth and prevents unnecessary exposure.

8. **Procedural Step. Assist the patient to lie down in the supine position, then the prone position.**

9. **Procedural Step. Have the patient bend the arms at the elbows and rest them alongside the head.**

10. **Procedural Step. Place the patient in the knee-chest position.**
    a. Ask the patient to raise the buttocks by moving up onto the knees while keeping the back straight.
    b. The patient may turn the head to either side.
    c. The patient should relax the upper body down onto the chest, supporting the majority of the body's weight and taking the strain off the knees.

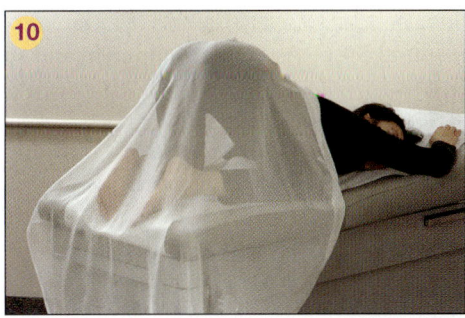

11. **Procedural Step. Adjust the drape as the physician examines the anal area.**

12. **Procedural Step. When the examination is complete, assist the patient to the prone then the supine position, and then to the sitting position.**

13. **Procedural Step. Push in the table extension while supporting the lower extremities and pull out the footrest.**

14. **Procedural Step. Allow the patient time to rest, then assist the patient from the examination table.**
    a. Hand the patient tissues and help the patient from the table, *or* assist the patient in cleaning up, then help the patient from the table.
    b. Return the footrest to its original position.
    c. Instruct the patient to dress; assist as needed.

15. **Procedural Step. Clean the examination room according to Standard Precautions.**
    Always clean the examination room immediately after the patient has left. Never bring the next patient into an unclean room.

16. **Procedural Step. Sanitize the hands.**
    Always sanitize the hands after every procedure or after using gloves.
    NOTE: Patient with joint deformities and/or arthritis may not be able to assume this position.

PROCEDURE 35-8 Fowler's Position

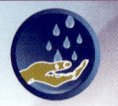

TASK: Properly position and drape the patient for examination of the head, chest, abdomen, and extremities.

EQUIPMENT AND SUPPLIES
- Examination table
- Table paper
- Patient gown
- Drape

SKILLS/RATIONALE

STANDARD PRECAUTIONS ARE TO BE FOLLOWED.

1. **Procedural Step. Sanitize the hands.**
   An alcohol-based hand rub may be used instead of washing hands with soap and water, unless hands are visibly soiled.
   Rationale. Hand sanitization promotes infection control.

2. **Procedural Step. Assemble equipment and supplies.**
   Rationale. It is important to have all supplies and equipment ready and available before starting any procedure to ensure efficiency.

3. **Procedural Step. Greet the patient, introduce yourself, and confirm the patient's identity.**
   Rationale. Identifying the patient ensures the procedure is performed on the correct patient.

4. **Procedural Step. Explain the procedure to the patient.**
   Rationale. Explaining the procedure to the patient promotes cooperation and provides a means of obtaining implied consent.

5. **Procedural Step. Provide a gown for the patient.**
   Prepare the patient for the particular type of examination being performed. Not all patients will require a gown, but if needed the opening is usually in the back.

6. **Procedural Step. Place the patient in Fowler's position.**
   a. Pull out the footrest of the table, and assist the patient to a sitting position.
   b. Have the patient move back on the table, and pull out the table extension supporting the patient's lower extremities.
   c. Have the patient lean back against the head of the table with a pillow under the head.
   d. For *Semi-Fowler's* position, the angle should be 45 degrees.
   e. For *full Fowler's* position, the angle is 90 degrees.

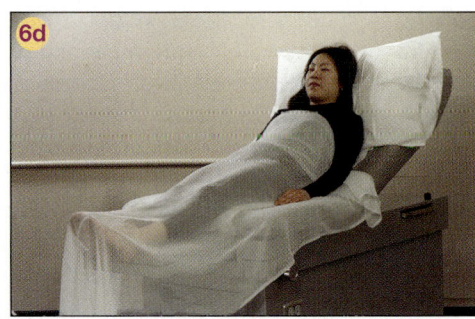

7. **Procedural Step. Drape the patient.**
   The drape should be placed over any exposed area not being examined.
   Rationale. Draping provides warmth and prevents unnecessary exposure.

8. **Procedural Step. When the examination is complete, assist the patient to the supine position and then to the sitting position.**

9. **Procedural Step. Assist the patient from the examination table.**
   a. Push in the table extension while supporting the lower extremities.
   b. Pull out the footrest and help the patient from the table as needed.
   c. Return the head of the table to its normal position.

Continued

PROCEDURE 35-8 Fowler's Position—cont'd

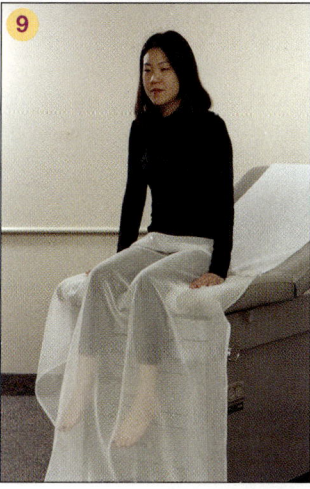

10. **Procedural Step.** Return the footrest to its original position. Allow the patient to get dressed (assist as needed).
11. **Procedural Step.** Clean the examination room according to Standard Precautions.
    Always clean the examination room immediately after the patient has left. Never bring the next patient into an unclean room.
12. **Procedural Step.** Sanitize the hands.
    Always sanitize the hands after every procedure or after using gloves.

Fowler's position helps the patient breathe easier and is used for examination of the upper extremities.

Trendelenburg's

In the **Trendelenburg's position**, the patient is supine on a tilted table with their head lower than their legs. The drape is positioned from the neck or underarms down to the knees. This position is used in some surgical procedures and emergency situations when a patient is experiencing shock or low blood pressure.

> **PATIENT-CENTERED PROFESSIONALISM**
>
> - Why is it important for the medical assistant to have the patient in the correct position and well supported during the physical examination?

EXAMINATION METHODS

The overall purpose of the physical examination is to examine the patient completely and to help the physician form a conclusion about the patient's health status. The medical assistant begins the assessment process by observing the patient (inspection) as soon as he or she greets the patient, and the physician carries the assessment through the physical examination. The patient's weight, height, and vital signs are taken before the physician begins the assessment. The physician uses the following assessment techniques to complete the physical examination:

- **Inspection** is a visual viewing of all body parts and surface areas for symmetry (equality of size and shape). The condition of the skin (e.g., turgor, Figure 35-4) and its color (Table 35-1), body movements (**range of motion [ROM]**), and body contours are observed (Figure 35-4, *A*).
- **Palpation** involves the physician using the hand to locate and touch major organs and lymph nodes and to detect tenderness, growths, and swelling in an area. Taking a patient's pulse is done by palpation (Figure 35-4, *B*).
- **Percussion** is used to check the nervous system and respiratory system. A percussion hammer is used to check for reflex action by tapping a tendon (Figure 35-5). The physician uses the fingertips to tap the patient's chest, back, and abdominal area while listening for distinctive sounds (Figure 35-4, *C*). Percussion is used to evaluate the size, borders, and consistency of body organs and to check for fluids in body cavities (e.g., lungs).
- **Auscultation** involves use of a stethoscope to detect the sounds of the heart, blood vessels, respiratory system, and intestines (bowels). Taking an apical pulse and recording blood pressure are other examples of this process (Figure 35-4, *D*).
- **Manipulation** involves the systematic movement of parts of the patient's body to determine the ROM of a joint. Physicians check for abnormalities affecting movement and may palpate an area during a manipulation.

These methods of assessment use the basic senses of sight, touch, smell, and hearing and require attention to detail.

> **PATIENT-CENTERED PROFESSIONALISM**
>
> - Why must the medical assistant understand the function of the various examination methods or assessment techniques?

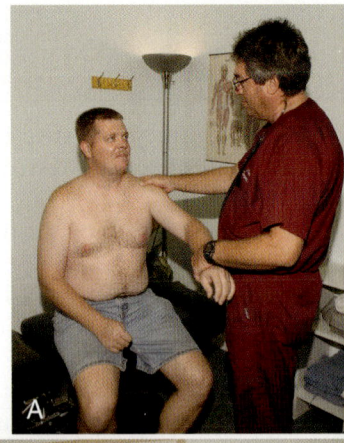
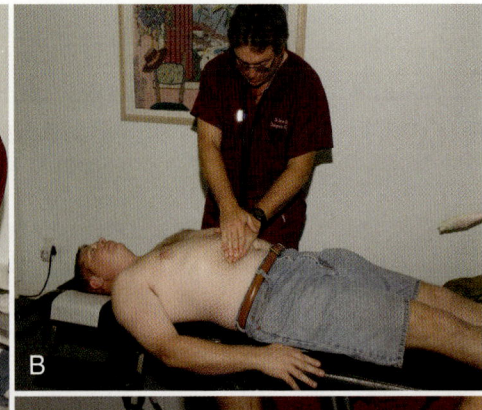
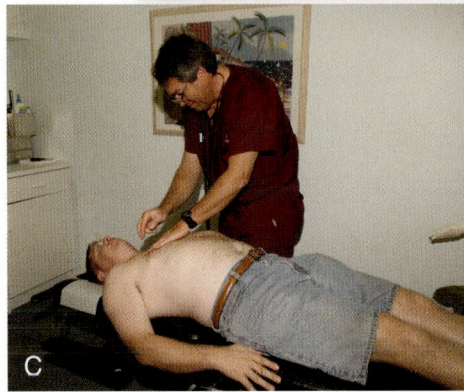
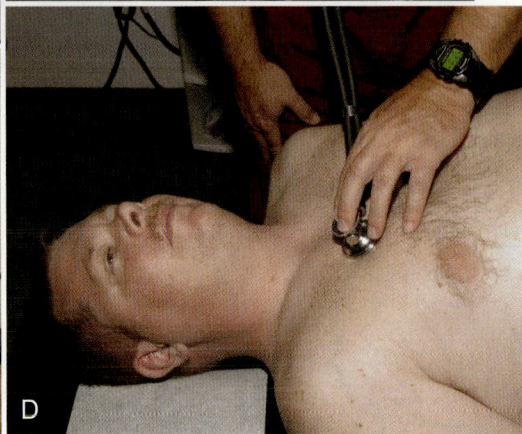

FIGURE 35-4 Methods of physical examination. **A,** Inspection. **B,** Palpation. **C,** Percussion. **D,** Auscultation.

TABLE 35-1

Elasticity and Color Variations of the Skin

Elasticity/Color	Condition	Indications	Sites
TURGOR			
Good or normal	Skin returns easily to its original place quickly	Adequate hydration	Patient's hand, sternum, forearm, and abdomen
Decreased	Skin remains suspended but slowly returns to its original place	Dehydration	Patient's hand, sternum, forearm, and abdomen
Increased	Unable to grasp skin	Edema	Patient's hand, sternum, forearm, and abdomen
COLOR CHANGES			
Cyanosis	Reduced amount of oxygen to tissue (hypoxia) causing a bluish discoloration	Cardiovascular and respiratory disorders and extreme cold environment	Nail beds, around lips, and base of tongue
Pallor	Decreased amount of oxyhemoglobin in the blood causing loss of color (pale)	Anemia	Conjunctivae, nail beds, palms of hands, and face
Vitiligo	Irregular patches of skin lacking pigment	Acquired skin disorder	Exposed areas of the skin (e.g., chest, arms, legs, etc.)
Jaundice	Increased deposits of bilirubins in tissues causing a yellow to orange skin discoloration	Liver disease and abnormal destruction of RBCs	Conjunctivae, sclera, and skin
Erythema	Redness of the skin or mucous membranes caused by vasodilatation and increased blood flow	Fever, blushing, alcohol consumption, and trauma	Face, trauma area, common sites for pressure sores (sacrum, shoulders)
Ecchymosis	Bluish-black discoloration to the skin or mucous membranes caused by blood being forced into the subcutaneous tissues (bruise)	Trauma and systemic skin disease	All areas of the body with subcutaneous tissue

RBCs, Red blood cells.

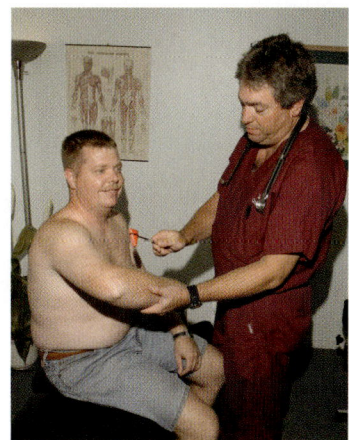

FIGURE 35-5 Checking tendon reflex with percussion hammer.

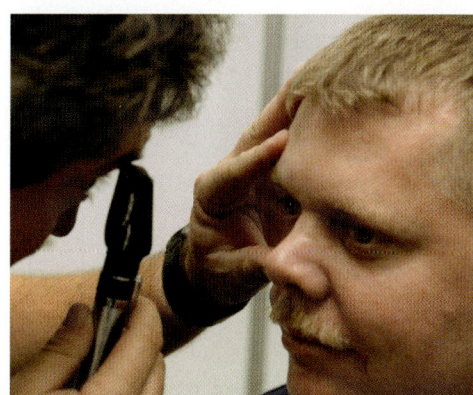

FIGURE 35-6 Using ophthalmoscope to view retina.

VISION TESTING

Vision tests are performed in the physician's office for a variety of reasons, including changes in visual acuity, blurred vision, and loss of vision. Vision tests may also be performed as part of a general physical examination. Most vision changes or visual defects are correctable with either eyeglasses or contact lenses (Table 35-2). The aging process causes the structure and function of the eyes to change, thus requiring some form of corrective lenses. When the lens loses its ability to adjust, it changes a person's field of vision (presbyopia). Vision testing assists in detecting both diabetes and hypertension.

The physician examines the interior of the eye with the **ophthalmoscope** (Figure 35-6). This instrument allows the physician to look at the condition of the retina, optic nerve, and the blood vessels of the eye. The medical assistant needs to make certain the light of the ophthalmoscope is working properly, and he or she may be asked to dim the lights when the physician is using this instrument. Extra bulbs and batteries should always be accessible in case of a malfunction.

The medical assistant is often responsible for testing the patient's **visual acuity** (ability to see) and color vision. Common tests include the Snellen eye chart, Ishihara color plates, and Jaeger reading card. Box 35-2 reviews the necessary criteria for charting visual testing procedures.

Snellen Eye Chart

The visual acuity test most often used in the medical office is performed with the use of a Snellen eye chart. The Snellen eye chart is a screening device and measures a patient's ability to view letters or images at a distance. Each row decreases in size to measure the patient's ability to see at a measured distance. Available visual acuity charts include the following:

- *Alphabet chart* is for English-speaking patients who know their alphabet (Figure 35-7, *A*).
- *Rotating "E" chart* is for non–English-speaking patients. The letter "E" is rotated in various positions (points in

TABLE 35-2
Correctable Visual Defects

Defect	Description
Hypermetropia or hyperopia (farsightedness)	Patient has trouble seeing objects clearly when they are close. Contour of crystalline lens is distorted.
Myopia (nearsightedness)	Patient has trouble seeing objects far away. Contour of crystalline lens is distorted.
Presbyopia ("old eye")	As people age, they are less able to see close objects clearly. Crystalline lens loses ability to adapt.
Astigmatism	Patient has trouble focusing; vision is blurred. Shape of cornea or lens prevents light from projecting on retina.
Strabismus (e.g., esotropia, or "cross-eye")	Eyes do not focus on an object at the same time. Main problem is muscle coordination. Eye exercises, surgery, and glasses can improve the various forms of strabismus.

BOX 35-2
Documentation when Charting Visual Testing Procedures

1. Date
2. Time
3. Name of visual test performed:
   - Snellen test
   - Jaeger test
   - Ishihara test
4. Results, indicating which eye was tested
5. Patient reaction, if any
6. Proper signature and credential

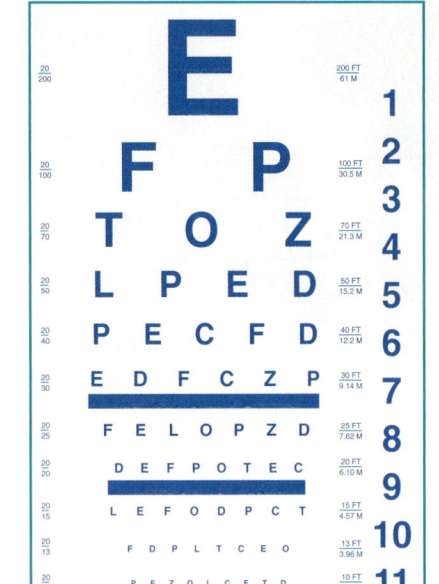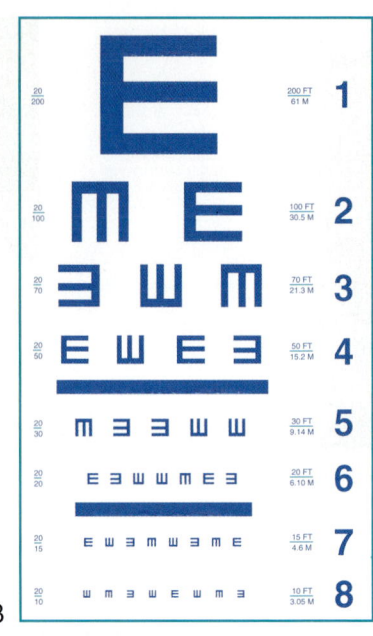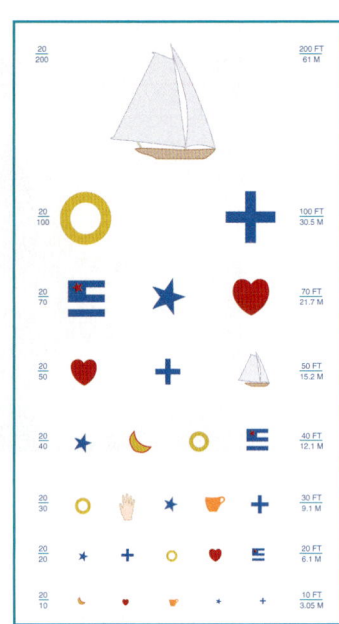

FIGURE 35-7 Snellen visual acuity charts. **A,** Alphabet eye chart. **B,** Snellen rotating "E" ("Big E") eye chart. **C,** Objects eye chart for testing preschoolers. (From Young AP, Kennedy DB: *Kinn's the medical assistant,* ed 10, St Louis, 2007, Saunders.)

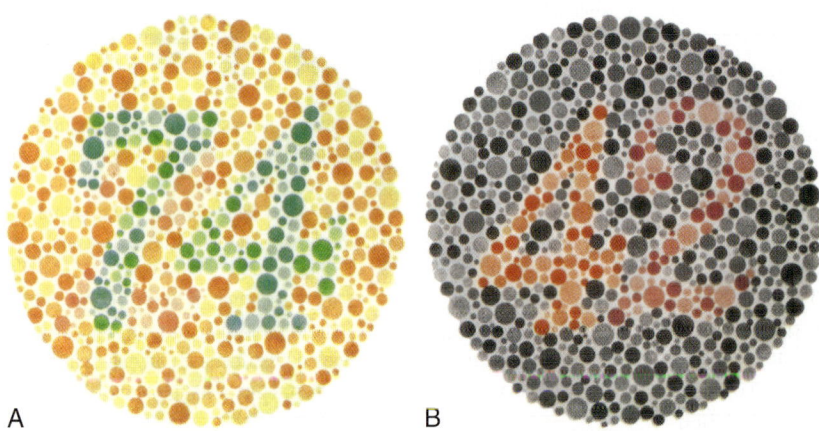

FIGURE 35-8 Ishihara color plates. **A,** Person with normal color vision reads 74, but red-green color-blind person reads 21. **B,** Red-blind person reads 2, but green-blind person reads 4. Normal-vision person reads 42. (From Ishihara J: *Tests for color blindness,* Tokyo, 1920, Kanehara.)

different directions) on the chart, and each row decreases in size (Figure 35-7, *B*).

- *Object chart* works well with preschoolers because it shows pictures of familiar objects that children can identify (Figure 35-7, *C*). Be sure the child understands what the picture depicts before you begin the examination.

The alphabet Snellen eye chart has rows of letters. Each row has a fraction listed on the left side. The top number of the fraction is always 20 feet. This means that the patient is standing 20 feet from the chart. The bottom number indicates the distance at which people with normal vision could read the row (e.g., 20/20 would mean the patient can read the 20 line at 20 feet for a given eye and 20/300 means that people with normal vision could see this line at 300 feet).

Each eye can be different with respect to its visual ability. Because of this, each eye must be tested independently and then both eyes together. Procedure 35-9 explains the process of accurately measuring and recording a patient's visual acuity using a Snellen chart.

Ishihara Color Vision Plates

Color vision is tested with Ishihara color vision plates (Figure 35-8). People with certain occupations, such as cosmetologists and airline pilots, are tested before schooling (Procedure 35-10).

Jaeger Reading Card

The Jaeger reading card (or chart) is used to test a person's ability to read at a prescribed distance. This test is conducted with a card containing sentences or phrases. The patient reads the card at varying distances, with each eye measured separately (Procedure 35-11).

Text continued on p. 755

Assisting with the Physical Examination **CHAPTER 35** 751

PROCEDURE 35-9 **Assess Distance Visual Acuity Using a Snellen Chart**

TASK: Accurately measure visual acuity using a Snellen eye chart, and document the procedure in the patient's medical record.

EQUIPMENT AND SUPPLIES
- Snellen eye chart
- Eye occluder (or index card, paper cup)
- Well-lit examination room
- Floor mark (20 feet from eye chart)
- Patient's medical record
- Pen

SKILLS/*RATIONALE*

STANDARD PRECAUTIONS ARE TO BE FOLLOWED.

1. **Procedural Step. Sanitize the hands.**
   An alcohol-based hand rub may be used instead of washing hands with soap and water, unless hands are visibly soiled.
   Rationale. Hand sanitization promotes infection control.

2. **Procedural Step. Assemble equipment and supplies.**
   Disinfect the occluder and allow it to dry completely.
   Rationale. It is important to have all supplies and equipment ready and available before starting any procedure to ensure efficiency. You should sanitize the occluder (if it is not disposable) between patients to prevent cross-contamination. It is important that the occluder dry completely before use; fumes from the antiseptic may burn the eyes, causing them to water and vision to blur.

3. **Procedural Step. Greet the patient, introduce yourself, and confirm the patient's identity.**
   Rationale. Identifying the patient ensures the procedure is performed on the correct patient.

4. **Procedural Step. Explain the procedure to the patient.**
   NOTE: For this procedure, the Snellen *alphabet* chart is used.
   The patient should be told that he or she will be asked to read several lines of letters. The patient should **not** have an opportunity to study or memorize the letters before beginning the test. The patient should be instructed not to squint during the test because squinting temporarily improves vision.
   Rationale. Explaining the procedure to the patient promotes cooperation and provides a means of obtaining implied consent. If the patient squints during the test, the results may be inaccurate.

5. **Procedural Step. Ask the patient if he or she is wearing contact lenses, and observe for eyeglasses.**
   The patient may be told to keep contacts in or glasses on during the test.
   Rationale. Most physicians prefer that corrective lenses be kept in place because this is a screening test.

6. **Procedural Step. Place the patient in a comfortable position 20 feet from the chart.**
   The patient may sit or stand.

7. **Procedural Step. Select the appropriate Snellen chart for the patient. (In this case the Snellen alphabet chart is used.)**
   Rationale. Selection of the chart is typically based on age and comprehension levels of the patient.

8. **Procedural Step. Position the center of the Snellen chart at the patient's eye level and stand next to the chart during the test to indicate to the patient the line to be identified.**

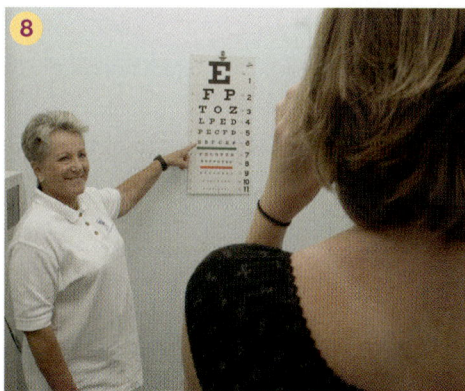

9. **Procedural Step. Ask the patient to cover the left eye with the eye occluder, but to keep the eye open.**
   Rationale. Keeping the left eye open prevents squinting of the right eye, which would increase visual acuity.

10. **Procedural Step. Measure the visual acuity of the right eye first.**
    NOTE: You should develop the routine of following the same steps with every patient, such as starting with the

Continued

PROCEDURE 35-9 Assess Distance Visual Acuity Using a Snellen Chart—cont'd

right eye first each time, because it reduces the opportunity for errors.

11. **Procedural Step. Ask the patient to identify verbally each letter (or picture or rotating "E" direction) in the row on the Snellen chart, starting with the 20/70 line.**
    Rationale. It is best to start at a line that is above the 20/20 line to give the patient a chance to gain confidence and to become familiar with the test procedure.

12. **Procedural Step. Proceed up or down the chart as necessary.**
    a. If the patient is able to read the 20/70 line, proceed down the chart until the patient can read the smallest line of letters with two errors or less.
    b. If the patient is unable to read the 20/70 line, proceed up the chart until the patient again can read the smallest line of letters with two errors or less.
    c. All errors are recorded in the patient's medical record with a minus sign (e.g., right eye 20/40–1).

13. **Procedural Step. Observe the patient for any unusual symptoms while he or she is reading the letters, such as squinting, tilting the head, or watering eyes.**
    Rationale. These symptoms may indicate that the patient is having difficulty identifying the letters.

14. **Procedural Step. Repeat the procedure to test the left eye by covering the right eye.**

15. **Procedural Step. Repeat the procedure without covering either eye.**

16. **Procedural Step. Chart the procedure.**
    a. Include the date and time, the name of the test (Snellen test), and the visual acuity results.
    b. The results must be charted as two numbers, or the number (fraction) on the left side of the chart next to the row read most accurately (e.g., right eye 20/20).
    c. Any unusual symptoms the patient may have exhibited during the test must be charted.
    d. Chart whether or not the patient was wearing corrective lenses during the test (e.g., left eye 20/40 w/contacts).

17. **Procedural Step. Sanitize the hands.**
    Always sanitize the hands after a procedure or after using gloves.

CHARTING EXAMPLE	
Date	
1/6/xx	9:30 a.m. Snellen test: right eye 20/20–1; left eye 20/40 ———— J. Biggs, SMA

PROCEDURE 35-10 Assess Color Vision Using the Ishihara Test

TASK: Measure color visual acuity accurately using the Ishihara color-blindness test.

EQUIPMENT AND SUPPLIES
- Ishihara color plate book
- Cotton swab
- Well-lit examination room (natural light preferred)
- Watch with second hand
- Patient's medical record
- Pen or pencil

SKILLS/RATIONALE   STANDARD PRECAUTIONS ARE TO BE FOLLOWED.

1. **Procedural Step. Sanitize the hands.**
   An alcohol-based hand rub may be used instead of washing hands with soap and water, unless hands are visibly soiled.
   Rationale. Hand sanitization promotes infection control.

2. **Procedural Step. Assemble equipment and supplies.**
   Rationale. It is important to have all supplies and equipment ready and available before starting any procedure to ensure efficiency.

3. **Procedural Step. Greet the patient, introduce yourself, and confirm the patient's identity.**

Continued

PROCEDURE 35-10 Assess Color Vision Using the Ishihara Test—cont'd

Rationale. *Identifying the patient ensures the procedure is performed on the correct patient.*

4. **Procedural Step.** Explain the procedure to the patient.
   Rationale. *Explaining the procedure to the patient promotes cooperation and provides a means of obtaining implied consent.*

5. **Procedural Step.** Identify the light source that will be used during the test.
   Rationale. *The Ishihara color-blindness test is most accurate when the test is given in a quiet room illuminated by natural daylight. Using artificial light may change the appearance of the shades of color on the plates, leading to inaccurate test results.*

6. **Procedural Step.** Use the first plate in the book as an example, and instruct the patient on how the examination will be conducted using this plate.
   Explain to the patient that he or she will have 3 seconds to identify numbers verbally or to trace a winding path formed by colored dots on each plate.
   Rationale. *The first plate is designed to be read correctly by all individuals and is used to explain the procedure to the patient.*

7. **Procedural Step.** Hold the color plates 30 inches from the patient.
   The plate should be held at a right angle to the patient's line of vision. Both eyes should be kept open during the test.

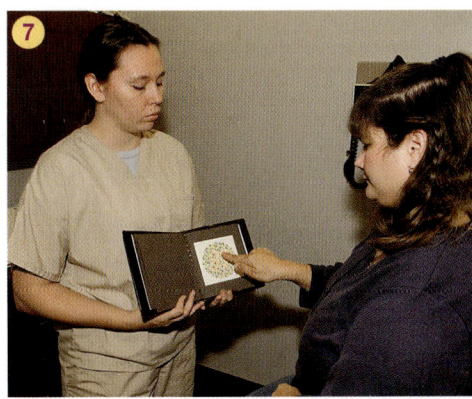

8. **Procedural Step.** Ask the patient to identify the number on the plate or, using a cotton-tipped swab, to trace the winding path.
   In some cases a patient may be asked to trace the numbers.
   Rationale. *Tracing ensures the number is read and not previously memorized. A swab is used because using the fingers would leave body oil on the paper and damage the plate.*

9. **Procedural Step.** Record the results after each plate, and continue until the patient has viewed and responded to all 11 plates.

10. **Procedural Step.** Record the results in the patient's medical record.
    Three methods are typically used to record the results in the patient's medical record:
    a. The first method is "pass/fail." The plate number is recorded, and if the patient was able to identify the number, "pass" is written next to it (e.g., Plate 2 = pass). If the patient cannot identify the number, an "X" is placed next to the plate number (e.g., Plate 4 = X).
    b. The second method of charting is similar to the first. Instead of "pass/fail," however, if the patient correctly identifies the number, the *number viewed* is placed next to the plate number (e.g., Plate 5 = 21). If the patient is unable to identify a number, an "X" is recorded to indicate that the patient could not read the plate in the same manner as the first example.
    c. The third method of charting requires that only the plate number with an "X" be recorded for the plates not read by the patient (e.g., Plate 4 = X, all other plates read correctly).

11. **Procedural Step.** Chart the results in the patient's medical record.
    a. Include the date and time, the name of the test (Ishihara test), and color vision results.
    b. Report any unusual symptoms that the patient may have exhibited during the test, such as squinting or rubbing the eyes.

12. **Procedural Step.** Return the Ishihara book to its proper place.
    Rationale. *The book of color plates must be stored in a closed position to protect it from light. Exposing the plates to excessive and unnecessary light results in fading of the color.*

13. **Procedural Step.** Sanitize the hands.
    Always sanitize the hands after every procedure or after using gloves.

CHARTING EXAMPLE

Date	
3/13/xx	2:30 p.m. Ishihara plates: all plates read correctly ———————— D. Teacher, SMA

PROCEDURE 35-11: Assess Near Vision Using a Jaeger Card

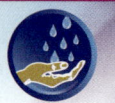

TASK: Measure near visual acuity accurately using the Jaeger near-vision acuity card. Document the procedure in the patient's medical record.

EQUIPMENT AND SUPPLIES
- Jaeger card
- Well-lit examination room
- Patient's medical record
- Pen
- 18-inch ruler or tape measure

SKILLS/RATIONALE

STANDARD PRECAUTIONS ARE TO BE FOLLOWED.

1. **Procedural Step. Sanitize the hands.**
   An alcohol-based hand rub may be used instead of washing hands with soap and water, unless hands are visibly soiled.
   Rationale. Hand sanitization promotes infection control.

2. **Procedural Step. Assemble equipment and supplies.**
   Rationale. It is important to have all supplies and equipment ready and available before starting any procedure to ensure efficiency.

3. **Procedural Step. Greet the patient, introduce yourself, and confirm the patient's identity.**
   Rationale. Identifying the patient ensures the procedure is performed on the correct patient.

4. **Procedural Step. Explain the procedure to the patient.**
   Rationale. Explaining the procedure to the patient promotes cooperation and provides a means of obtaining implied consent.

5. **Procedural Step. Have the patient sit in a comfortable position.**

6. **Procedural Step. Provide the patient with the Jaeger card.**

No. 1. .37M
In the second century of the Christian era, the empire of Rome comprehended the fairest part of the earth, and the most civilized portion of mankind. The frontiers of that extensive monarchy were guarded by ancient renown and disciplined valor. The gentle but powerful influence of laws and manners had gradually cemented the union of the provinces. Their peaceful inhabitants enjoyed and abused the advantages of wealth.

No. 2. .50M
fourscore years, the public administration was conducted by the virtue and abilities of Nerva, Trajan, Hadrian, and the two Antonines. It is the design of this, and of the two succeeding chapters, to describe the prosperous condition of their empire; and afterwards, from the death of Marcus Antoninus, to deduce the most important circumstances of its decline and fall; a revolution which will ever be remembered, and is still felt by

No. 3. .62M
the nations of the earth. The principal conquests of the Romans were achieved under the republic; and the emperors, for the most part, were satisfied with preserving those dominions which had been acquired by the policy of the senate, the active emulations of the consuls, and the martial enthusiasm of the people. The seven first centuries were filled with a rapid succession of triumphs; but it was

No. 4. .75M
reserved for Augustus to relinquish the ambitious design of subduing the whole earth, and to introduce a spirit of moderation into the public councils. Inclined to peace by his temper and situation, it was very easy for him to discover that Rome, in her present exalted situation, had much less to hope than to fear from the chance of arms; and that, in the prosecution of

No. 5. 1.00M
the undertaking became every day more difficult, the event more doubtful, and the possession more precarious, and less beneficial. The experience of Augustus added weight to these salutary reflections, and effectually convinced him that, by the prudent vigor of

No. 6. 1.25M
his counsels, it would be easy to secure every concession which the safety or the dignity of Rome might require from the most formidable barbarians. Instead of exposing his person or his legions to the arrows of the Parthians, he obtained, by an honor-

No. 7. 1.50M
able treaty, the restitution of the standards and prisoners which had been taken in the defeat of Crassus. His generals, in the early part of his reign, attempted the reduction of Ethiopia and Arabia Felix. They marched near a thou-

No. 8. 1.75M
sand miles to the south of the tropic; but the heat of the climate soon repelled the invaders, and protected the unwarlike natives of those sequestered regions

No. 9. 2.00M
The northern countries of Europe scarcely deserved the expense and labor of conquest. The forests and morasses of Germany were

No. 10. 2.25M
filled with a hardy race of barbarians who despised life when it was separated from freedom; and though, on the first

No. 11. 2.50M
attack, they seemed to yield to the weight of the Roman power, they soon, by a signal

Continued

| PROCEDURE 35-11 | Assess Near Vision Using a Jaeger Card—cont'd | |

7. **Procedural Step.** Instruct the patient to hold the card 14 to 16 inches away from the eyes. Measure the distance for accuracy.
8. **Procedural Step.** Ask the patient to read out loud the paragraphs on the card.
   The patient should read the card starting at the top and reading down to the smallest print the patient can read. As with the Snellen test, the near-vision acuity test is performed on each eye starting with the right eye.
9. **Procedural Step.** Document the number at which the patient stopped reading for each eye.
   Record the results and any problems experienced by the patient (e.g., squinting) in the medical record.
10. **Procedural Step.** Return the Jaeger card to its proper storage place.
11. **Procedural Step.** Sanitize the hands.
    Always sanitize the hands after every procedure or after using gloves.

CHARTING EXAMPLE

Date	
12/10/xx	10:15 a.m. Jaeger card: successfully read No. 7 (1.50M) c̄ contacts——————————————————— S. Lamb, SMA

PATIENT-CENTERED PROFESSIONALISM

- What are the responsibilities of the medical assistant in vision testing?

EAR EXAMINATION

The physician also examines the patient's ears in the CPX. Patient complaints involving the ear often include pain, discharge, hearing loss, ringing (**tinnitus**), or dizziness (**vertigo**). As a person ages, loss of hearing (**presbycusis**) occurs first as an inability to hear high-pitched sounds, then progresses to lower-pitched sounds. Auditory tests for hearing loss and equilibrium are discussed in Chapter 39.

The physician uses an **otoscope** to check the appearance of the ear canal and the eardrum or tympanic membrane (Figure 35-9). The otoscope uses a disposable *speculum* that fits the external ear canal of the patient. An adult's ear is examined by pulling the auricle upward and backward. A child's ear is examined by pulling the auricle downward and backward (up to age 3 years) to straighten the ear canal. Children are prone to ear infections because the eustachian tube is parallel with the pharynx. After visualizing the ear, the physician discards the speculum (most medical offices now use disposable specula).

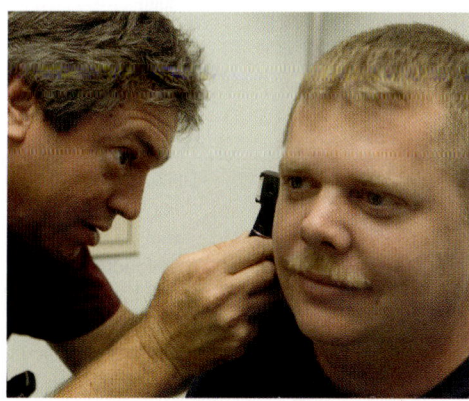

FIGURE 35-9 Otoscope to examine ear canal.

CONCLUSION

The medical assistant is responsible for having the patient ready for the physician and understanding the typical order in which a physician performs a physical examination and the instruments or supplies that are typically requested during the examination. This includes taking the vital signs and preparing the patient for an examination or a procedure. Having a patient in a gown and positioned properly allows the physician to begin the examination. The medical assistant should consider the patient's comfort level and safety at all times.

Understanding the proper methods for preparing the examination room and the patient and using proper techniques when assisting the physician will help the patient's appointment proceed smoothly and efficiently. This helps save both the physician's time and the patient's time. It also demonstrates professionalism and competence by conveying to the patient that he or she is in good hands.

Table 35-3 provides an overview of positions, body areas, assessment methods, abbreviations and medical terminology, and instruments and supplies needed for a physical examination.

PATIENT-CENTERED PROFESSIONALISM

- What are the responsibilities of the medical assistant in ear examinations?

TABLE 35-3

Physical Examination Overview

Position	Body Area	Assessment Technique	Common Terms and Abbreviations	Instruments Used
Sitting	Skin	**Inspection:** Color and pigmentation Change in surface texture **Palpation:** Temperature Edema, tenderness Moisture	**Pallor** **Erythema** **Cyanosis** **Jaundice** **Turgor** **Diaphoresis**	
	Head and neck	**Inspection:** Contour, shape, deformities Facial expression Scalp, hair **Palpation:** Swelling, tenderness (lymph node, thyroid) Temporal artery, temporomandibular joint	**HEENT** (head, eyes, ears, nose, and throat)	
		Auscultation: Carotid pulse	**Bruit**	Stethoscope with bell
	Eyes	**Inspection:** EOM function Pupillary light reflex Optic disc/retina/macula Color vision Visual acuity	**PERRLA** (pupils equal, round, react to light, and **accommodation**)	Penlight Ophthalmoscope Ishihara color plates, Snellen chart
	Ears	**Inspection:** Size, shape, color, redness, position, head alignment Eardrum (tympanic membrane): color, intact, position (flat, bulging) Hearing acuity	**Microtia** **Macrotia** **Perforation** **Weber test** **Rinne test**	Otoscope with ear speculum Tuning fork or audiometer
	Nose, mouth, and throat	**Inspection:** Symmetry, lesions Color and intact nasal mucosa Polyps, swelling **Palpation:** Sinus areas **Inspection:** *Lips:* color, cracking, lesions *Teeth, gums, tongue, mucosa:* color, lesions, breath odor, gag reflex **Palpation:** *Mouth:* tenderness, lumps	**Patent** **Herpes simplex 1** **Gingivitis**	Otoscope with short, wide-tipped nasal speculum *or* nasal speculum and penlight Penlight, tongue depressor, Disposable glove
	Breast	**Inspection:** Symmetry of size and shape	**BSE** (breast self-examination)	Small pillow, tape measure
Supine	Breast and axillae	**Palpation:** Lymph nodes Breast tissue		

TABLE 35-3
Physical Examination Overview—cont'd

Position	Body Area	Assessment Technique	Common Terms and Abbreviations	Instruments Used
Sitting	Chest	**Inspection:** Rib cage and vertebrae for deformities	"Barrel chest": protrusion of chest caused by hyperinflation of the lungs	
		Palpation: Lumps, tenderness Chest expansion		
		Percussion: Over lungs		
		Auscultation: Breath sounds	**Crepitus** **Rales**	Stethoscope
	Heart	**Auscultation:** Rate and rhythm	**Rhonchi** **Murmur** **Thrill**	Stethoscope with diaphragm and bell end pieces
Supine	Abdomen	**Inspection:** Contour; masses or bulges	**Distention** RLQ	Stethoscope
		Auscultation: Bowel sounds Vascular sounds (aorta, renal and femoral arteries)	LLQ	
		Palpation: All quadrants Liver, spleen, kidneys Tenderness		
		Percussion: All quadrants Liver and spleen		
	Arms and legs	**Inspection:** Color, size, lesions **Palpation:** *Pulses:* radial, brachial, femoral, popliteal, dorsalis pedis Inguinal nodes Temperature of feet and legs Muscle tone, tenderness, and masses ROM **Percussion:** Biceps, triceps, abdominal, patellar, Achilles, plantar reflexes	Reflex findings: 0: No response 1+: Low normal 2+: WNL 3+: Above normal 4+: Hyperactive	Goniometer Percussion hammer
Lithotomy position	Female genitalia	**Inspection:** External genitalia Vagina and cervix (obtain specimens) **Palpation:** Labia, Skene and Bartholin glands	**LMP** (last menstrual period)	Vaginal speculum, glove, slide, fixative or Thin Prep solution, cervical brush and spatula
	Anal canal	**Inspection:** Rectum **Palpation:** Rectum		Glove and lubricant
Standing position	Male genitalia	**Inspection:** Penis, scrotum, and testes	**TSE** (testicular self-examination) **BPH** (benign prostatic hypertrophy)	Glove Lubricant
	Anal canal	Anus **Palpation:** Penis, scrotum, and testes Inguinal hernia Prostate Rectum		

EOM, Extraocular; *LLQ*, left lower quadrant; *RLQ*, right lower quadrant; *ROM*, range of motion; *WNL*, within normal limits.

Chapter Summary

Reinforce your understanding of the material in this chapter by reviewing the curriculum objectives and key content points below.

1. **Define, appropriately use, and spell all of the Key Terms for this chapter.**
   - Review the Key Terms if necessary.
2. **List the three main responsibilities of the medical assistant in preparing a patient for a physical examination.**
   - The medical assistant is responsible for having the patient gowned, appropriately positioned, and draped for the physician to perform the physical examination.
3. **List three responsibilities of the medical assistant in assisting the patient to disrobe for an examination.**
   - The medical assistant must choose the right type of gown for the given procedure, provide clear instructions for disrobing and gowning, and assist patients who need help disrobing.
4. **Demonstrate the correct procedure for providing the physician and the patient with items needed to perform a complete physical examination.**
   - Review Procedure 35-1.
5. **Explain what a "consent-to-treat form" involves and when formal consent is needed for an examination.**
   - For invasive procedures beyond the basic examination, such as biopsies, the patient must sign a consent-to-treat form.
   - The form must be signed before the procedure is performed.
6. **Discuss why using proper body mechanics is essential when performing physical activities.**
   - Proper body mechanics allows the spine and large muscle groups to work with you to maximize body strength and to make lifting and moving objects easier.
7. **Explain the importance of draping the patient appropriately for an examination or procedure.**
   - Draping the patient provides warmth, comfort, and modesty.
8. **List the three criteria for selecting the position to be used for an examination.**
   - The position used depends on the procedure to be performed, the patient's chief complaint, and the patient's age.
9. **List ten examination positions and briefly explain what types of examinations are performed using each position.**
   - Sitting position is used to begin the physical examination because the upper extremities are easily accessible.
   - Standing position is used to evaluate coordination and balance.
   - Horizontal recumbent, or supine, position is used for examination of the chest, abdomen, and lower extremities.
   - Dorsal recumbent position is used for examination of the vaginal area for females and the rectal area for both males and females.
   - Lithotomy position is used for the pelvic examination in females.
   - Sims' position is used for rectal examinations, enema administration, and sigmoidoscopy.
   - Prone position is used to examine the back and lower extremities.
   - Knee-chest position is used for sigmoidoscopies.
   - Fowler's position helps the patient breathe easier and is used to examine the upper extremities.
   - Trendelenburg's position is used for emergencies and some surgical procedures.
10. **Demonstrate the correct procedure for properly positioning and draping a patient in the sitting position.**
    - Review Procedure 35-2.
11. **Demonstrate the correct procedure for properly positioning and draping a patient in the recumbent position.**
    - Review Procedure 35-3.
12. **Demonstrate the correct procedure for properly positioning and draping a patient in the lithotomy position.**
    - Review Procedure 35-4.
13. **Demonstrate the correct procedure for properly positioning and draping a patient in the Sims' position.**
    - Review Procedure 35-5.
14. **Demonstrate the correct procedure for properly positioning and draping a patient in the prone position.**
    - Review Procedure 35-6.
15. **Demonstrate the correct procedure for properly positioning and draping a patient in the knee-chest position.**
    - Review Procedure 35-7.
16. **Demonstrate the correct procedure for properly positioning and draping a patient in the Fowler's and semi-Fowler's positions.**
    - Review Procedure 35-8.
17. **List the four primary methods of examining used during a physical examination and briefly explain what occurs in each.**
    - Inspection is the visual viewing of all body surfaces for abnormalities and signs of disease.
    - Palpation uses touch to detect abnormalities.
    - Percussion uses the fingers to tap the body surfaces while listening for sounds.
    - Auscultation is accomplished by using a stethoscope to listen for body sounds.
18. **State the purpose of a Snellen chart and explain when each of the three types of Snellen charts should be used.**
    - Vision testing done in the medical office includes using the Snellen chart for distance viewing.
    - The alphabet chart can be used for English-speaking patients.

- The rotating "E" chart can be used for non–English-speaking patients.
- The object chart can be used for preschoolers.

19. **Demonstrate the correct procedure for accurately measuring and recording a patient's visual acuity with a Snellen chart.**
    - Review Procedure 35-9.
20. **List five types of common visual defects that are correctable by lenses or surgery.**
    - Hyperopia (farsightedness), myopia (nearsightedness), presbyopia ("old eyes"), astigmatism, and strabismus (e.g., "cross-eye") can be corrected.
21. **Demonstrate the correct procedure for accurately measuring and recording a patient's color visual acuity with the Ishihara test.**
    - Review Procedure 35-10.
22. **Demonstrate the correct procedure for accurately measuring and recording a patient's near visual acuity with a Jaeger reading card.**
    - Review Procedure 35-11.
23. **Differentiate between an ophthalmoscope and an otoscope and explain how each is used in the physical examination.**
    - An ophthalmoscope is used to look at the inner structures of the eye.
    - An otoscope is used to examine the external ear canal, tympanic membrane, and middle ear.
24. **Analyze a realistic medical office situation and apply your understanding of assisting with a physical examination to determine the best course of action.**
    - Care must be taken to treat the patient with dignity and respect during the physical examination.
    - The patient's safety and comfort are the primary concerns.
25. **Describe the impact on patient care when medical assistants understand how to assist the physician with the physical examination.**
    - Patient care is enhanced when the medical assistant is organized.
    - Patients have more confidence in their treatment plan when the medical assistant demonstrates competency and a caring attitude about their safety.

PRACTICAL APPLICATIONS

If you have accomplished the objectives in this chapter, you will be able to make better choices as a medical assistant. Take another look at this situation and decide what you would do.

Beth is a medical assistant in the office of Dr. Havidiz, a family practitioner. Dr. Havidiz treats many low-income families, and many women in the community see him for gynecological visits. Holly, a new patient, comes to see Dr. Havidiz for a possible vaginal infection. Her demeanor shows her fear of the doctor's office, especially since this is the first time she has seen Dr. Havidiz. Dr. Havidiz was called to the hospital to see a critically ill patient earlier in the day, so appointments are delayed.

There is an available examination room when Holly arrives, so Beth takes her to the room and tells her to undress completely. Beth does not tell Holly how to put on the gown, but she stands in the room and watches Holly undress. While Holly is undressing, Beth asks the questions necessary to obtain the medical history. Beth then places Holly on the examination table in the lithotomy position and immediately leaves the room, giving the impression that she is in a great hurry. After 15 minutes, Holly has discomfort in her back but dares not move from the position because she does not want to delay the examination. After 30 minutes, Holly wonders just how much longer it will take for Dr. Havidiz to come and check her. Finally, Dr. Havidiz arrives and the examination begins.

During the examination, Beth leaves the room to answer a personal phone call, leaving Dr. Havidiz and Holly alone. As Holly leaves the office, she is in tears from back pain and appears to be very upset. Beth shows no sympathy or empathy for Holly. Two days later, Holly asks that her records be transferred to another physician and tells Dr. Havidiz that she has never been treated as rudely as she was in his office. How might this situation have been avoided?

1. How did Beth invade Holly's privacy?
2. Under what conditions should Beth have taken Holly's history?
3. Why was it important to tell Holly how to put on the gown for the examination? How should the drape have been applied?
4. What examination methods would you expect the medical assistant to use while preparing Holly for an examination?
5. What methods of examination would you expect the physician to use during the examination?
6. What positions should have been used for Holly while she was waiting for the pelvic exam? What positions are inappropriate for a long wait? What explanation should Beth have given when placing Holly in the position?
7. How should Beth have handled the delay?
8. Why is it unethical for Beth to leave the room during the physical examination?
9. Do you think that Holly had a legitimate complaint to Dr. Havidiz about her treatment? Explain your answer.

WEB SEARCH

1. **Research the concept of *periodic* health examination versus the *annual* examination.** Replacing the annual examination with the periodic examination was done to promote the detection and prevention of specific diseases. Detecting a problem in its early stages can result in long-term benefits.

- **Keywords:** Use the following keywords in your search: preventive medicine, health examination, physical examination.

Electrocardiography

36

evolve   http://evolve.elsevier.com/klieger/medicalassisting

Electrocardiography is a method of measuring and graphically recording the electrical activity of the heart. It is the test used most frequently to diagnose heart disease. The **electrocardiograph** is the machine that records the heart's electrical activity that produces contraction and relaxation of the heart.

The **electrocardiogram** (ECG or EKG) provides a graphic picture of the heart's activity and indicates how long it takes (time) for an electrical impulse to travel through the heart during a heartbeat. This recording provides the physician with information to diagnose irregularities or changes in the electrical conduction of the patient's heart. Medical assistants performing ECGs should understand the purpose and use of electrocardiography, as well as how to obtain accurate tracings.

LEARNING OBJECTIVES

You will be able to do the following after completing this chapter:

Key Terms

1. Define, appropriately use, and spell all the Key Terms for this chapter.

Purpose of Electrocardiography

2. List two reasons why electrocardiography is performed.
3. List five common conditions that can be detected and evaluated using an ECG and explain how the ECG is able to provide this information.
4. List the five responsibilities of a medical assistant in obtaining a patient's ECG and also explain what the medical assistant should *never* do.

Electrical Impulses and ECG Patterns

5. Explain the sequence of events that creates the cardiac cycle.
6. Describe the role of the SA and AV nodes in generating and monitoring the electrical impulses in the heart.
7. Describe NSR and the four wave patterns that can occur within a normal time sequence.

Equipment and Supplies

8. List and describe the five basic components necessary for a good ECG tracing.
9. Describe ECG paper and explain the significance of "block" size.

10. Explain the need for standardization of an electrocardiograph.

Obtaining an ECG

11. Explain the considerations for clothing removal, proper positioning, and skin preparation when preparing a patient for an ECG.
12. Identify where electrodes are typically placed on the arms, legs, and chest.
13. Demonstrate the correct procedure for running a 12-lead ECG using a single-channel electrocardiograph with manual capacity.
14. Demonstrate the correct procedure for running a 12-lead ECG using a three-channel electrocardiograph with automatic capability, disposable electrodes, and a soft-touch keypad for entering patient data.
15. List three situations in which electrodes cannot be placed as usual and explain how the electrodes are to be placed in each of these situations.
16. Describe placement of the three standard limb (bipolar) leads and the tracings recorded with each.
17. Describe placement of the three augmented (unipolar) leads and the tracings recorded with each.
18. Describe placement of the six chest (precordial, or "V") leads.
19. Explain why a baseline ECG is needed.

Artifacts

20. Define and list the causes of the three main artifacts on ECGs.

Cardiac Arrhythmias

21. Differentiate between an artifact and an arrhythmia.
22. List and describe four types of sinus and atrial arrhythmias.
23. List and describe three types of ventricular arrhythmias.

Holter Monitor

24. Explain the purpose of a Holter monitor and describe how it is used with a patient activity diary.
25. Demonstrate the correct procedure for applying and removing a Holter monitor.

Cardiac Stress Testing

26. Explain the purpose of a cardiac stress (treadmill) test and describe the medical assistant's role in this procedure.

Patient-Centered Professionalism

27. Analyze a realistic medical office situation and apply your understanding of electrocardiography to determine the best course of action.
28. Describe the impact on patient care when medical assistants understand the purpose and use of electrocardiography in the medical office.

KEY TERMS

alternating current (AC) interference
amplifier
arrhythmia
artifact
atrioventricular (AV) node
augmented leads
baseline
bipolar leads
bundle branches
bundle of His
cardiac cycle
chest (precordial) leads
depolarization
electrocardiogram (ECG)
electrocardiograph
electrocardiography
electrodes
event monitor
galvanometer
Holter monitor
interval
ischemia
leads
myocardial infarction (MI)
normal sinus rhythm (NSR)
P wave
pacemaker
paroxysmal atrial tachycardia (PAT)
patency
polarization
PR interval
PR segment
premature atrial contraction (PAC)
premature ventricular contraction (PVC)
Purkinje fibers
QRS complex
QT interval
repolarization
rhythm strip
segment
sinoatrial (SA) node
sinus bradycardia
sinus tachycardia
somatic tremor
ST segment
standard limb leads
standardization
standardization mark
stylus
T wave
tracing
treadmill test
U wave
unipolar leads
"V" leads
ventricular fibrillation (V fib)
ventricular tachycardia (V tach)
wandering baseline
waves

PRACTICAL APPLICATIONS

Read the following scenario and keep it in mind as you learn about electrocardiography in this chapter.

Jim, a 55-year-old longtime smoker who is also overweight, has taken his grandchildren to the beach for the day. Mary, Jim's wife, notices that Jim is a little short of breath and seems to rub his chest often, so she asks if he is okay. Jim tells Mary that he thinks that he needs to get to a doctor because he has chest pain that is not subsiding. They drop off the children and immediately go to the medical office.

On arrival, Jim tells Gomez, the medical assistant, about his chest pain, which now seems to be in his left arm and left jaw. Gomez tells Jim that it is "probably just indigestion" and lets Jim sit in the waiting room. Finally, observing that Jim is very short of breath and is clasping his chest, Gomez asks the attending physician, Dr. Startz, if he can obtain an ECG.

Receiving approval for the ECG, Gomez quickly loads the paper into the electrocardiograph, not taking the necessary care to prevent markings on the ECG paper. Jim has suntan oil on his body and his chest is relatively hairy, so the electrodes do not attach with sufficient pressure to stay on the skin when the leads are placed on the tabs. Gomez places the electrodes in a haphazard manner, with no consideration of the way the tabs are facing. By this time, Jim is scared and experiencing a great deal of pain, which is causing diaphoresis, trembling, and twisting. Jim starts to sing and talk to relieve his tension, and the ECG has many artifacts. In a hurry to get the ECG to Dr. Startz because of Jim's declining condition, Gomez does not notice that the ECG also contains a wandering baseline. Even the rhythm strip is not readable.

On examination, Dr. Startz realizes the seriousness of Jim's condition and immediately sends him to the hospital, where another ECG and admission to the CICU are ordered. At the end of the day, Dr. Startz is upset and tells Gomez that if he cannot obtain a presentable ECG in an emergency situation, he might lose his job.

If you were the medical assistant in this situation, what would you have done?

PURPOSE OF ELECTROCARDIOGRAPHY

Electrocardiography is a painless, noninvasive procedure often done as part of a routine physical examination before surgery or as a baseline for cardiac testing. It is also used as a diagnostic tool to detect heart disease.

Electrocardiography can detect and evaluate the following conditions:

- A cardiac **arrhythmia** (abnormal cardiac rhythm; also called *dysrhythmia*).
- Heart damage caused by poor blood supply (**ischemia**).
- Presence of an electrolyte imbalance.
- Effects of cardiac medications.

- Damage caused by a heart attack, or **myocardial infarction (MI)**.

Medical Assistant's Role

The medical assistant who obtains a patient's ECG has the following responsibilities:

1. Properly preparing the patient.
2. Correctly operating the equipment.
3. Identifying and eliminating artifacts.
4. Properly labeling the ECG record.
5. Understanding and performing routine maintenance, proper care, and storage of the electrocardiograph.

The medical assistant is *never* to interpret the ECG or give any clue of the results of the ECG to the patient.

PATIENT-CENTERED PROFESSIONALISM

- Why must the medical assistant fully understand the ECG process and his or her responsibility?

ELECTRICAL IMPULSES AND ECG PATTERNS

Electrical impulses cause the heart to contract and relax; this is the "pumping" of the heart. The process of the heart pumping in a rhythmical cycle of contraction and relaxation is the **cardiac cycle,** considered to be one heartbeat. The recording of the ECG cycle provides a picture, or **tracing,** of the cardiac cycles.

Electrical impulses are generated and carried throughout the body. This electrical activity can be measured and recorded by using skin sensors called **electrodes.** Ten electrodes are attached to the skin and connected to an ECG machine by cables.

Box 36-1 reviews the conduction system of the heart as it relates to electrical impulses (Figure 36-1). See Chapter 12 for more information.

ECG Patterns

Each ECG tracing (Figure 36-2) shows how the heart is functioning and indicates the "ready" phase (polarization), the "action" phase (contraction, depolarization), and the "resting" phase (relaxation, repolarization) of the heart muscle (Figure 36-3). The tracing is described as letters or a combination of letters (e.g., P, QRS, and T). **NOTE:** Letters were chosen at random and are just used as an identifier to locate a certain point on the ECG tracing. Other characteristics of the ECG tracing are as follows:

- A flat line that separates the various waves is called a **baseline,** or *isoelectric line.* The baseline occurs when the entire heart is resting between beats and there is no electrical activity.

BOX 36-1

Conduction System Review

Together, the contraction and relaxation of the heart make up the cardiac cycle. The contraction phase is known as *systole,* and the relaxation phase of the heart cycle is known as *diastole.* The pumping action (muscle contraction) of the heart is a sequential chain of events. It begins when the *pacemaker of the heart,* the **sinoatrial (SA) node** (knot or group of specialized cells in upper right atrium), releases an electrical impulse that causes the heart muscle of the atria to contract, or depolarize. The SA node sends out electrical impulses at a rate of 60 to 100 beats per minute (beats/min). Blood is forced from the atria into the ventricles as the heart valves open.

The electrical impulse from the SA node travels to the **atrioventricular (AV) node,** which is located in the lower portion of the right atrium on the atrioventricular wall. The AV node monitors the heartbeat. If the heart rate drops below 50 beats/min, the AV node generates impulses to keep the heart beating at 40 to 60 beats/min. The impulse from the AV node is delayed momentarily to allow the ventricles to fill with blood from the atria. It then transmits the electrical impulse to the bundle of His, which further divides into right and left bundle branches.

Next, the impulse is transmitted to the Purkinje fibers. These fibers take the electrical impulse to both ventricles, causing them to contract. Blood is pumped from the right ventricle into the pulmonary artery and from the left ventricle to the aorta.

The heart muscle rests (repolarizes) when the impulse stops briefly. Then, the process starts over with the SA node sending out another electrical impulse.

- A **segment** is a small portion of the ECG between two **waves** showing heart activity or from the end of one wave to the beginning of the next.
- An **interval** indicates time and shows an entire wave with a segment.

The ECG cycle (single heartbeat) can be broken down into different components. The components include the P wave, the QRS complex, the T wave, and the U wave. Table 36-1 details cardiac events in the ECG cycle. Following the normal ECG tracing (one cardiac cycle), the heart is in a ready state, or **polarization** (no measurable activity). This appears as a flat line or baseline. **Normal sinus rhythm (NSR)** occurs with normal cardiac function. It appears when only one P wave, one QRS complex, one T wave, and occasionally a U wave occur. The rhythm measurement starts at the sinoatrial node and occurs within a normal time sequence (thus the name *normal sinus rhythm*).

P Wave and Related ECG Markings

The first electrical impulse shown on an ECG tracing is the **P wave.** It shows atrial contraction (impulse leaving the sinoatrial node), or atrial depolarization. **Depolarization** (activation) is a discharge of electrical energy that causes contraction.

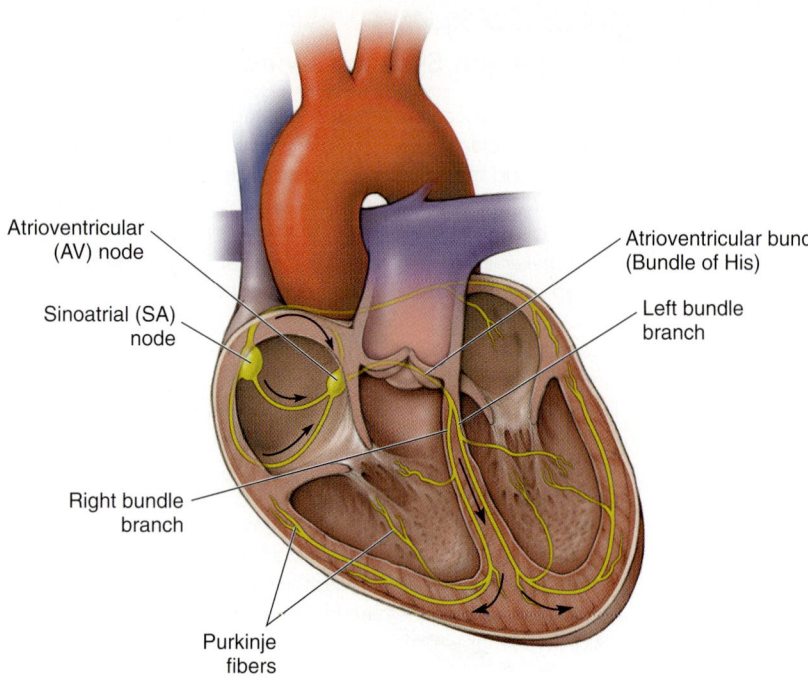

FIGURE 36-1 Conduction system of the heart.

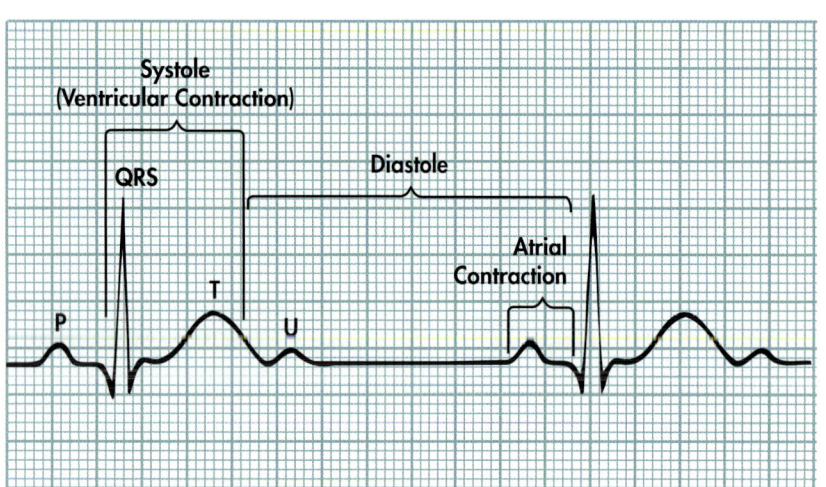

FIGURE 36-2 Normal electrocardiogram showing one cardiac cycle with events. (From Grauer K: *A practical guide to ECG interpretation*, ed 2, St Louis, 1998, Mosby.)

TABLE 36-1

Cardiac Events in the ECG Cycle

Event	Description	
P wave	Wave starts when SA node fires (discharges) and causes the atria to contract.	Atrial depolarization
PR segment	Transmission of the depolarization wave through the AV node, bundle of His, bundle branches, and Purkinje fibers.	
PR interval	Time it takes for an electrical impulse to be conducted through the atria and the AV node; measured from beginning of the P wave to the beginning of the QRS complex.	
QRS complex	Represents the depolarization (contraction) of the ventricles.	Ventricular depolarization
ST segment	Represents the ECG cycle from the end of the QRS complex to the beginning of the T wave. (Ventricles are between depolarization and repolarization.)	
T wave	Next deflection after ST segment.	Ventricular repolarization
QT interval	Represents the QRS complex, the ST segment, and the T wave (beginning of the Q to the end of the T).	

AV, Atrioventricular; *SA*, sinoatrial.

Polarization
"Ready phase"
(muscle ready to contract)

Think of a cat as it prepares itself for action.

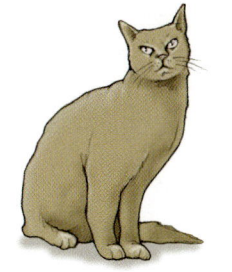

Depolarization
"Action phase"
(muscle contracting)

When the cat sees a mouse, it jumps into action.

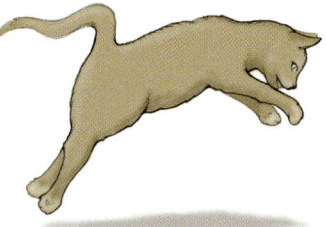

Repolarization
"Resting phase"
(muscle getting ready to contract again)

A cat rests after all the action to begin again.

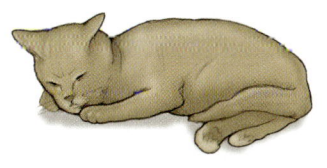

FIGURE 36-3 Phases of muscle contraction with polarizations.

The P wave is small, rounded, and upright and should not exceed 2 to 3 mm in height (Figure 36-4, A and B).

The **PR segment** shows how long it takes for the electrical impulse to go from the sinoatrial (SA) node to the atrioventricular (AV) node. It is measured from the end of the P wave to the start of the QRS complex.

The **PR interval** represents the time interval between the atrial contraction and the beginning of ventricular stimulation. In other words, the PR interval represents the time it takes for an electrical impulse to travel from the SA node through the atria and the AV node to the ventricles. The impulse continues through the **bundle of His** and down the **bundle branches** to the **Purkinje fibers.** The PR interval is measured from the beginning of the P wave and continues to the start of the QRS complex. Normal sequence time is between 0.12 to 0.2 second, depending on how rapidly the impulse is conducted.

QRS Complex and Related ECG Markings

The **QRS complex** shows when the electrical impulse reaches the Purkinje fibers. This is the ventricular depolarization (ventricular contraction) of both ventricles (Figure 36-4, C and D).
- The *Q wave* is represented by a downward (negative) deflection following the P wave.
- The *R wave* is an upward (positive) deflection or spike after the Q wave.
- The *S wave* completes the complex and is a downward and upward deflection that follows the R wave.

The normal duration of the QRS complex is 0.06 to 0.10 second.

The **ST segment** shows the time interval between the ventricular contraction and the beginning of ventricular relaxation.

T Wave and Related ECG Markings

The **T wave** indicates the resting phase, or **repolarization,** of the heart. In this part of the process, the cells are recharging for the next electrical impulse. The T wave is broad and rounded and usually larger than the P wave (Figure 36-4, E).

The **QT interval** shows the time needed for the ventricles to contract and recover.

U Wave

The **U wave** is a small, upward curve that may occasionally occur following a normal ECG tracing. A U wave could represent slow repolarization, low electrolytes, or a minor electrical discharge from the heart, but the exact representation is not known.

PATIENT-CENTERED PROFESSIONALISM

- Why is it the medical assistant's responsibility to know normal ECG patterns?

EQUIPMENT AND SUPPLIES

The **electrocardiograph** (ECG machine) interprets the electrical impulse of the heart and produces a graph tracing. Technological advances have reduced the size of the equipment while increasing the machine's capacity to interpret the ECG tracing. Medical assistants should understand the electrocardiograph and its parts, the type of paper used, and also how to standardize the ECG machine to ensure ECGs taken on different machines can be compared.

Electrocardiograph

There are two basic types of electrocardiographs (Figure 36-5). The *single-channel* 12-lead ECG machine monitors each lead separately. The *multichannel* (three-channel) machine records three leads at a time and switches automatically.

The basic components of the electrocardiograph are as follows:
- **Electrodes,** or sensors, are small devices made of a conductive material that are used to pick up the electrical activity of the heart generated by the myocardial cells. Remember there are only ten electrodes.
- **Leads** are covered wires that carry the electrical impulse from the sensors to the ECG machine. The 12-lead ECG provides a printout of the heart's electrical activity viewed from 12 different angles.

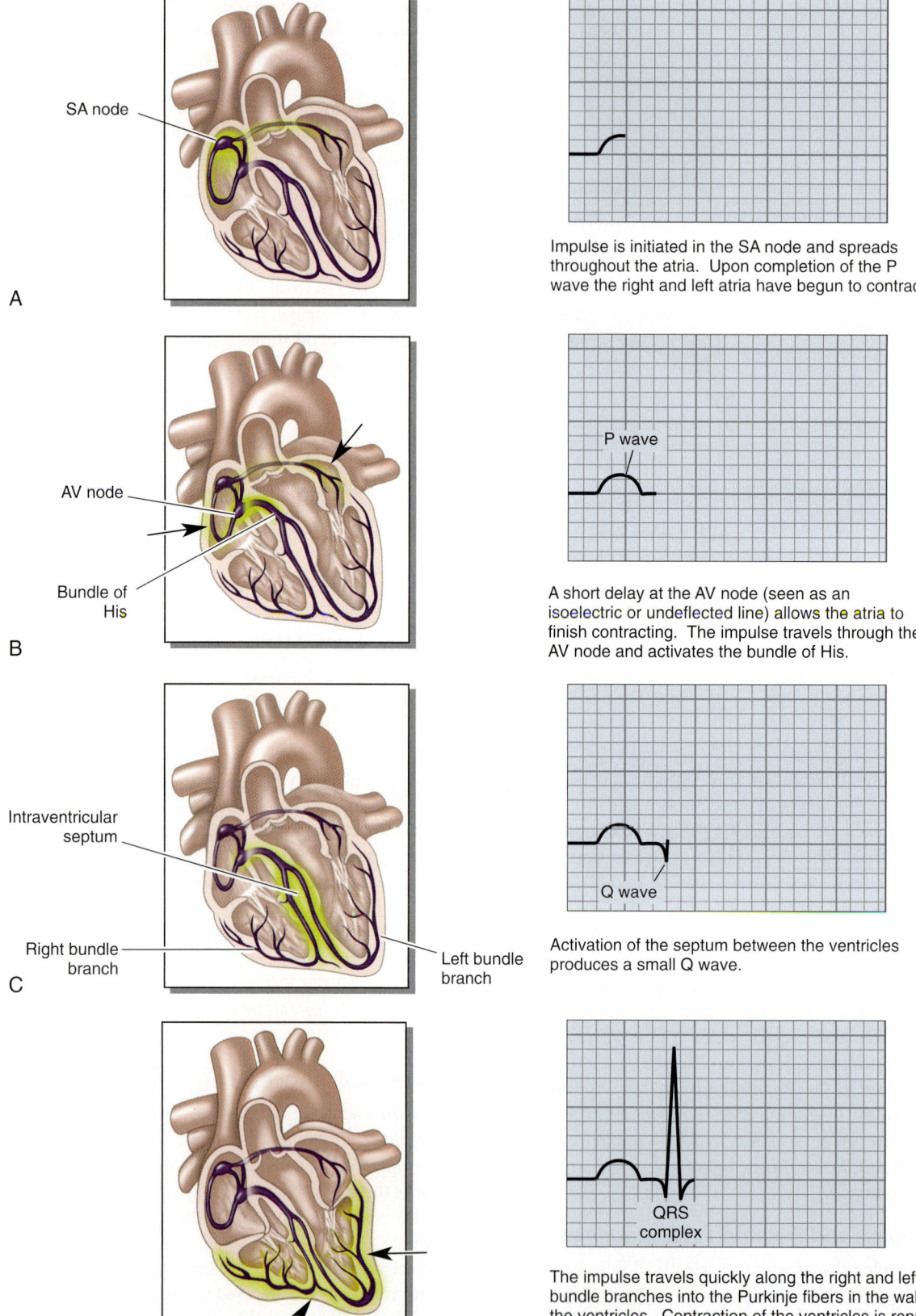

FIGURE 36-4 Cardiac activity related to the ECG tracing. (From Hunt SA: *Saunders fundamentals of medical assisting—revised reprint,* St Louis, 2007, Saunders.)

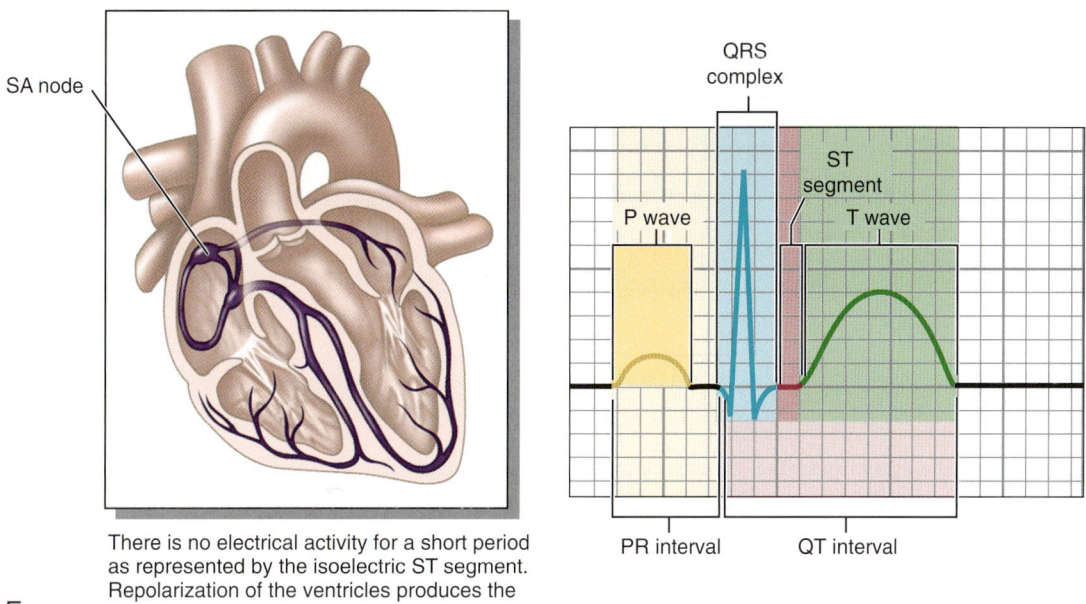

E   There is no electrical activity for a short period as represented by the isoelectric ST segment. Repolarization of the ventricles produces the T wave.

FIGURE 36-4, continued

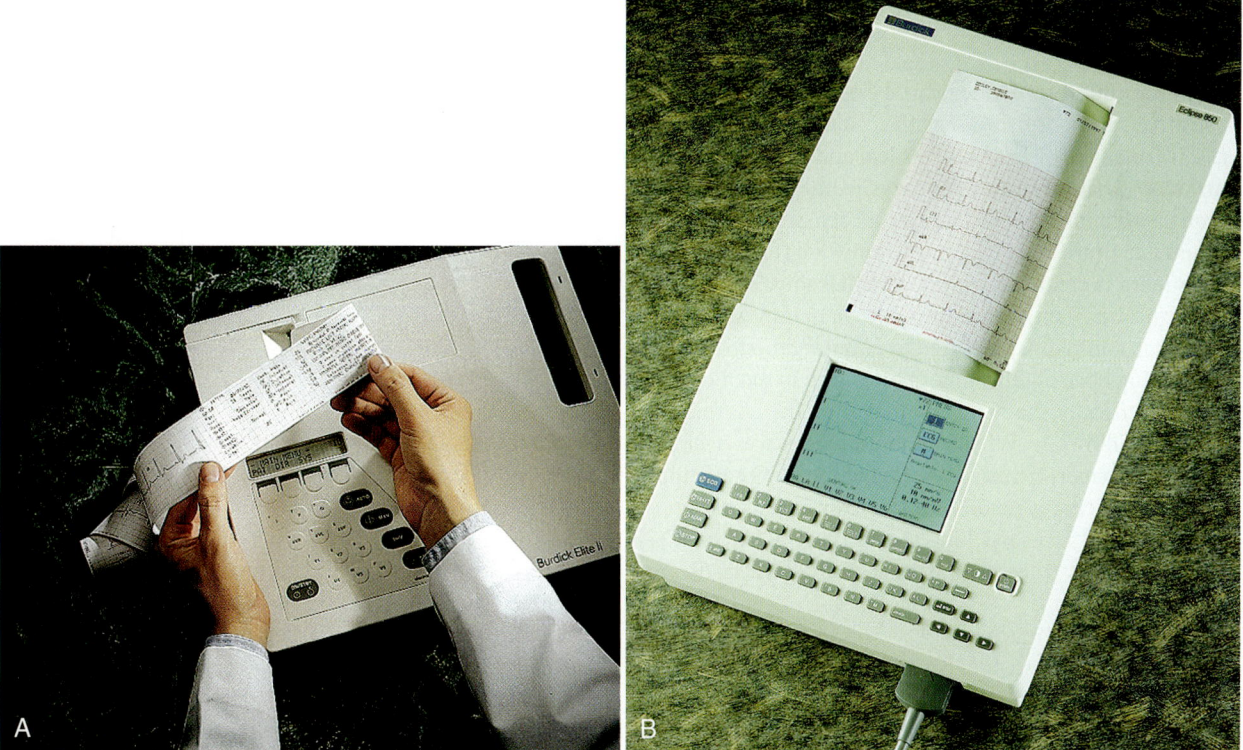

FIGURE 36-5 ECG machines. **A,** Simple one-step operation for 12-lead ECG in single-lead format. **B,** The Burdick Portable Eclipse 850 three-channel electrocardiograph with built-in computer program that interprets the tracing as it is being recorded. (Courtesy Quinton Cardiology, Inc., Bothell, Washington.)

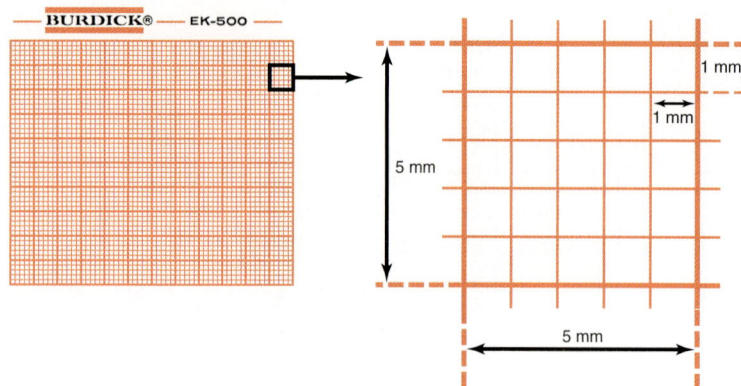

FIGURE 36-6 Example of ECG paper with an enlarged section indicating the size of the large and small squares. (Courtesy Burdick Corp., Deerfield, WI.)

- The **amplifier** magnifies (enlarges) the heart's electrical signal so that it can be recorded.
- The **galvanometer** detects and converts the amplified electrical signal into movement so a graph may be traced.
- A heated **stylus** records the motion on graph paper located in the machine by burning the impression on the heat-sensitive paper. In newer machines, the stylus uses ink to mark the ECG paper.

Electrodes are placed on the skin. Disposable electrodes are saturated with an electrolyte solution that conducts the electrical current from the body to the machine. Reusable electrodes require use of a gel, paste, or electrolyte-moistened flannel and must be cleaned after each use.

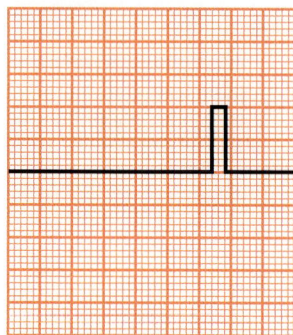

FIGURE 36-7 Normal standardization mark is 10 mm high. (Courtesy Burdick Corp., Deerfield, WI.)

ECG Paper

The ECG machine records the heart's electrical activity onto heat-sensitive and pressure-sensitive standardized graph paper. This ruled paper has both vertical and horizontal lines that make up small, thin-lined squares within a large, dark-lined square totaling 25 small squares. Each small square is one millimeter (mm) in height and 1 mm wide (Figure 36-6). A larger square is created from the 25 small squares (5 small squares high and 5 small squares wide, or 5 mm × 5 mm). Each wave and complex is measured by counting these squares. When counting horizontally, time is measured in seconds and when done vertically the height (voltage) of the complex is measured in millimeters. When a heated stylus moves over the plastic-covered paper, it burns a tracing of the ECG cycle into the paper or a tracing is made with ink from the stylus.

- A multichannel ECG machine uses an 8 × 11–inch ECG paper and prints 3 leads at a time until all 12 leads are recorded.
- The single-channel machine uses a roll of specially coated paper that is 3 inches wide. Each lead is recorded for 6 to 12 seconds.

Some physicians desire these ECGs to be mounted.

Standardization

Standardization is the process of making certain that an ECG taken on one machine will compare to a tracing taken on another machine. One milliwatt (mW) of electrical current

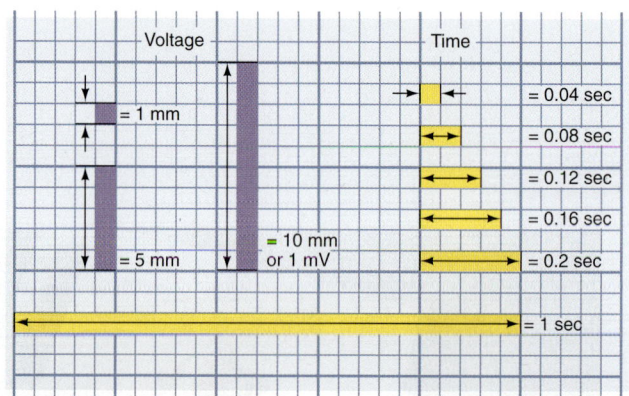

FIGURE 36-8 Representation of time and voltage on ECG paper. (Modified from Chester GA: *Modern medical assisting,* Philadelphia, 1998, Saunders.)

(strength of the heartbeat) causes the stylus to move 10 mm in height (10 small squares) (Figure 36-7). The ECG paper is usually set to run through the machine at a rate of 25 mm per second (mm/sec). Each small square passes the stylus every 0.04 second; therefore each large square represents 0.2 second (Figure 36-8). In 1 second, five large squares pass the stylus (Figure 36-9). When the speed is changed to 50 mm/sec, the width of the waves is doubled and complexes 50 mm/sec are used when the patient is tachycardic to allow ease of reading the rhythm strip. Remember, any change to the normal speed must be documented at the top of the ECG paper.

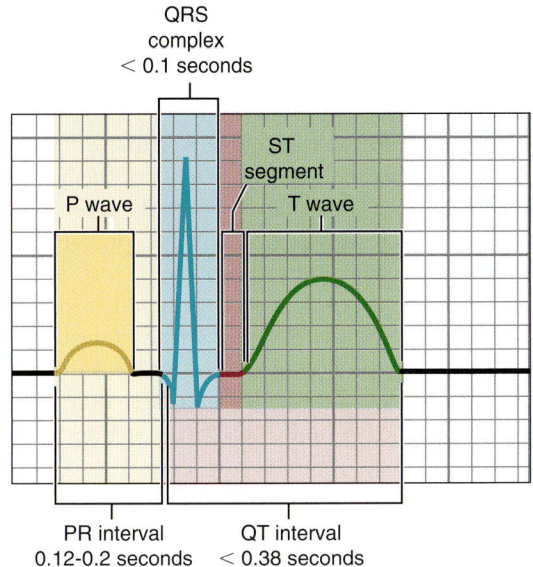

FIGURE 36-9 Normal ECG measurement. (From Hunt SA: *Saunders fundamentals of medical assisting—revised reprint*, St Louis, 2007, Saunders.)

Newer machines will automatically standardize before recording the first lead. However, older machines require the medical assistant to press a button and restandardize the machine when leads are changed. A **standardization mark** is printed each time this is done.

PATIENT-CENTERED PROFESSIONALISM

- *What is the significance of standardization, and how does it affect patient care?*

OBTAINING AN ELECTROCARDIOGRAM

When performing an ECG procedure, the medical assistant is often responsible for preparing the patient and placing electrodes and lead wires; the physician is responsible for its interpretation. Although the medical assistant should never discuss the results of the ECG with a patient (this is the physician's responsibility), it is helpful to understand how the ECG results will be used.

Preparing the Patient

The ECG procedure runs smoothly when the patient is properly prepared. The medical assistant needs to explain the procedure fully to the patient and reassure the patient that the procedure is simple and painless. The assistant (1) instructs the patient about what clothing must be removed, (2) places the patient in the proper position, (3) prepares the patient's skin for the electrodes, and (4) protects the patient's modesty.

Clothing

The patient will need to remove all clothing above the waist because any clothing could interfere with lead placement and tracing. Long pant legs must be rolled up, socks rolled down, and stockings and tights removed. The electrodes must come in complete contact with the skin. A gown or cape must be open in the front with a towel used for modesty, and care should be taken to have the patient remove jewelry that would interfere with electrode placement.

Positioning

The patient should be placed supine (lying on the back) with a small pillow under the head for comfort. The legs should be slightly separated and the arms at the patient's sides. The patient must be comfortable to prevent movement during the procedure. Incidental movement or discomfort from being cold causes muscle movement and results in an artifact. Elderly and obese patients may need extra care for comfort. Be alert to patients' feelings and protect their modesty by performing the procedure in a private area.

Skin Preparation

The skin where the electrodes will be applied must be clean and dry. Body lotions and oils and sweat are removed with an alcohol wipe. It is important to note that when alcohol is used on the skin it must be allowed to air dry or wiped off with a gauze square before applying the electrodes. Excessive hair may need to be shaved because the lead must be flat on the skin surface to receive the electrical impulse.

Placing the Electrodes

Electrodes are placed on the skin as follows:
- The *arm* electrodes are placed on the fleshy part of the upper arm with the tab facing toward the feet.
- The electrodes on the *legs* are placed on the fleshy part of the leg above the ankle with the tab facing toward the head. The right leg electrode is considered to be the grounding lead. Its purpose is to reduce electrical interference.
- The *chest* electrodes are placed with the tabs facing down. Make certain the chest hairs are separated, which is easily done with the fingers, to ensure complete skin contact. Chests that are overly hairy may require a small area to be

trimmed or shaved, or a gauze square can be used to abrade (roughen up) the skin to assist with good skin contact.

Procedure 36-1 describes single-channel ECG monitoring, and Procedure 36-2 outlines multichannel (three-channel) monitoring. Although most medical offices use a multichannel machine, some offices still use a single-channel system. Box 36-2 lists the information to be charted when obtaining an ECG.

Special Situations

Some patients have special requirements when electrodes cannot be placed as usual. To reduce muscle artifacts, some physicians request that the leg electrodes be placed on the abdomen or in the groin area.

Amputations, Casts, and Bandages. To accommodate a cast, bandage, or amputation of a leg or arm, the electrode must be placed as close to the usual site as possible. The electrode on the other limb should also be placed in the same location opposite the first. Sites may include the lower trunk or the shoulder. This variation should be documented in the patient's medical record.

Wounds. Electrodes cannot be placed on an open wound or on one that is recently healed. The site chosen should be as close to the preferred site as possible.

Large Breasts or Overweight. It is difficult to feel the intercostal spaces in large-breasted women and obese patients. The medical assistant can ask the patient to lift her breasts while the intercostal space is located. This provides accurate placement and is less embarrassing for the patient.

Placing the ECG Leads

Correct attachment of the electrodes and lead wires is critical to producing an accurate picture of the heart's electrical activity. There must be a *positive* lead, a *negative* lead, and a *ground* lead to provide a clear tracing. Electrical energy flows from the negative electrode toward the positive electrode. The *right arm* is always negative, and the *left leg* is always positive. The *right leg* is the ground lead. The position of the positive electrode on the body determines the portion of the heart viewed by each lead.

The heart can be viewed from the following four major surfaces (Figure 36-10):

- *Anterior surface:* front of the heart
- *Posterior surface:* back of the heart
- *Inferior surface:* bottom of the heart
- *Lateral surface:* side of the heart

A 12-lead ECG provides a complete picture of the heart's activity by measuring the electrical activity of the heart from 12 different angles. Why so many angles? The more angles or views that are represented increases the probability that abnormalities are recognized sooner.

The 12-lead ECG uses only 10 lead wires, which are attached to the chest, arms, and legs. Six leads attach to the chest electrodes, and the other four attach to the limb electrodes (arm and legs). The 12 leads are divided into three different types of leads: three standard limb leads, three augmented leads, and six chest leads.

FOR YOUR INFORMATION

ECG ANGLES

Imagine the heart in an upright position on a pedestal. Now, visualize walking around it and looking at it from all angles. The electrode placement will determine the portion of the heart being viewed. The different angles indicate how the electrical impulses travel through various parts of the heart. These angles are identified by a lead name or number.

Standard Limb Leads (Bipolar Leads)

Leads I, II, and III are called the **standard limb leads,** or **bipolar leads,** because they trace the electrical impulse of the heart from two different directions simultaneously. These leads record the *frontal plane* activity of the heart from top to bottom and from left to right. Each lead provides a different view of the heart.

BOX 36-2

Documentation when Charting 12-Lead ECG

1. Date
2. Time
3. Name of procedure: **electrocardiogram** (single channel or three channel)
4. Results
5. Patient reaction, if any
6. Proper signature and credential

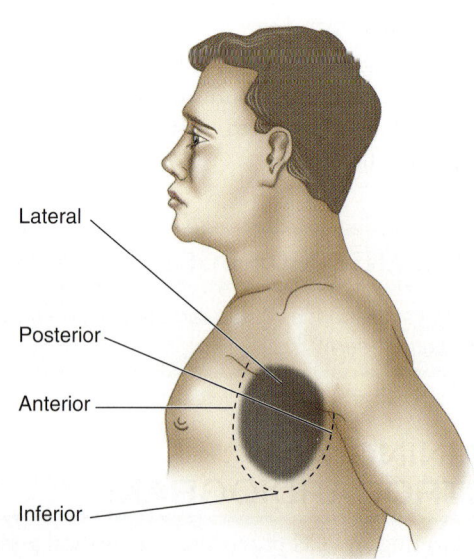

FIGURE 36-10 The 12-lead ECG can assess electrical activity from four major surfaces of the heart.

Text continued on p. 775

Electrocardiography CHAPTER 36   771

PROCEDURE 36-1   Obtain a 12-Lead ECG Using a Single-Channel Electrocardiograph

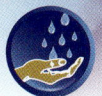

TASK: Obtain an accurate 12-lead ECG tracing by running a single-channel electrocardiograph with manual capacity.

EQUIPMENT AND SUPPLIES

- Single-channel electrocardiograph with lead wires
- ECG paper
- Disposable electrodes (self-adhesive)
- ECG mounting form and mounting supplies (such as an ECG paper cutter)
- Examination table
- Footstool
- Alcohol wipes (70% isopropyl)
- 4 × 4 gauze squares
- Disposable razor
- Patient gown
- Drape
- Blanket (optional)
- Small pillow
- Patient's medical record

SKILLS/RATIONALE

STANDARD PRECAUTIONS ARE TO BE FOLLOWED.

1. **Procedural Step. Sanitize the hands.**
   An alcohol-based hand rub may be used instead of washing hands with soap and water, unless hands are visibly soiled.
   Rationale. Hand sanitization promotes infection control.

2. **Procedural Step. Assemble equipment and supplies.**
   NOTE: Always have additional supplies within easy reach in case of malfunction or contamination.
   Rationale. It is important to have all supplies and equipment ready and available before starting any procedure to ensure efficiency.

3. **Procedural Step. Greet the patient, introduce yourself, and confirm the patient's identity.**
   Rationale. Identifying the patient ensures the procedure is performed on the correct patient.

4. **Procedural Step. Explain the procedure to the patient.**
   Rationale. Explaining the procedure to the patient promotes cooperation and provides a means of obtaining implied consent.

5. **Procedural Step. Ask the patient to remove all possible sources of electrical interference.**
   Such items include jewelry, watches, and tight clothing. Also have the patient empty pockets and remove any belts. Cell phones, laptop computers, and pagers should be turned off. All personal items should be kept in sight of the patient.
   Rationale. Metal items will interfere with the procedure and thus should be removed.

6. **Procedural Step. Establish a quiet, relaxing atmosphere.**
   The room temperature should be comfortable for the patient.
   Rationale. If the patient is cold, this may cause somatic interference.

7. **Procedural Step. Prepare the patient.**
   a. Ask the patient to remove clothing to the waist. Provide privacy and a gown.
   b. Ask the patient to leave the opening of the gown toward the front. The lower legs must also be uncovered (e.g., no pantyhose).
   c. Properly drape the patient over the uncovered body parts to prevent exposure and to provide warmth.

8. **Procedural Step. Position the patient.**
   a. Place the patient in a supine position on the table with the leg rest extended. The table should support the arms and legs so they do not dangle. A pillow can be placed under the patient's head and knees for comfort.
   b. If the patient must be elevated for comfort, document the approximate angle of elevation on the ECG. Keep the elevation as minimal as possible.
   Rationale. If the patient is lying on either side or the chest is elevated, the position of the heart in the chest cavity may be altered and thus produce inaccurate results. The chest, upper arms, and lower legs must be uncovered to allow for proper placement of the electrodes. The patient should be kept warm, and the arms and legs should not be allowed to dangle; otherwise, muscle artifacts could result.

9. **Procedural Step. Help the patient to relax.**
   Inform the patient that having an ECG recording is noninvasive and pain-free. Explain that he or she must lie still and not talk for an accurate recording to be obtained. Further explain that any movement will be picked up by the machine and recorded (as an artifact) or misinterpreted (as negative activity).
   Rationale. The patient should be mentally and physically relaxed for an accurate ECG recording because an apprehensive or moving patient produces muscle artifacts.

Continued

PROCEDURE 36-1 Obtain a 12-Lead ECG Using a Single-Channel Electrocardiograph—cont'd

10. **Procedural Step.** Position the ECG machine and turn it "on."
Place the ECG machine at the side of the patient, with the power cord pointing away from the patient; do not allow the cable to go underneath the table. Turn on the machine to allow the stylus to warm.
Rationale. Proper positioning of the ECG machine reduces alternating current (AC) interference.

11. **Procedural Step.** Label the beginning of the ECG paper with the patient's name, date, time, and current cardiovascular medications, or input the information directly into the machine.

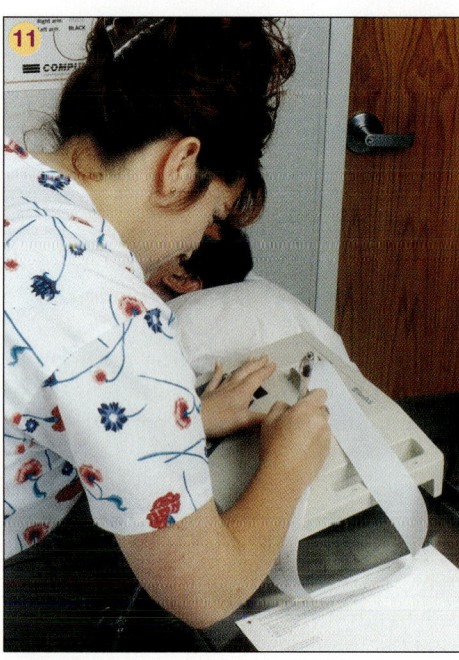

12. **Procedural Step.** Prepare the patient's skin for electrode placement.
Shave the skin as necessary. Remove excess oils or lotions by wiping the area where the electrode will be applied with an alcohol pad; allow to air-dry. A 4 × 4 gauze square can be used to rub the area to increase circulation and promote better contact for the electrodes.
Rationale. Excessive hair on the chest or legs may need to be trimmed or shaved. However, it may be possible to spread the hair with the fingers sufficiently to make good contact with the skin. The patient's skin must be dry and oil free to obtain good electrode adhesion to the skin.

13. **Procedural Step.** Apply the limb electrodes.
Apply the limb electrodes firmly to the freshly cleaned and dried fleshy areas of the arms and legs. The tabs on the arm electrodes should point downward toward the feet, and the tabs of the leg electrodes should point upward toward the head.

Rationale. Proper positioning of the tabs toward the cable (which will be plugged into the machine, connecting the machine to the patient) prevents the lead connectors from pulling and causing artifacts.

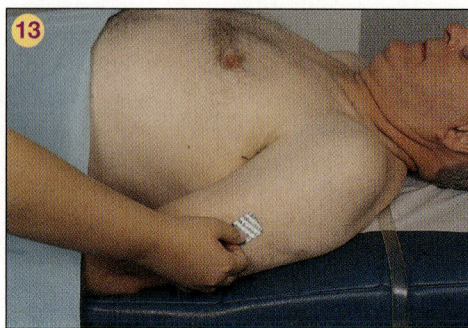

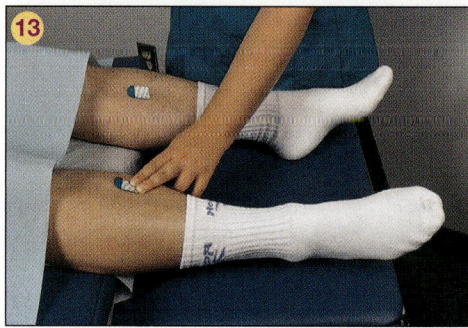

14. **Procedural Step.** Apply chest electrodes.
    a. Apply self-sticking chest electrodes on appropriate intercostal spaces with the tabs pointing down.
    b. Measure down to the fourth intercostal space on the right side of the chest for the V1 chest lead. Use the clavicle as a reference point to locate the fourth intercostal space. The *first* intercostal space is the area between the first and second ribs, the *second* intercostal space is the area between the second and third ribs, and so on. Apply the V1 electrode in the right *fourth* intercostal space close to the sternum.
    c. Place V2 directly across from V1 in the fourth intercostal space on the left side of the chest.
    d. V4 is positioned at the midclavicular line in the fifth intercostal space.
    e. V3 is positioned halfway between V2 and V4 in the fifth intercostal space.
    f. V5 and V6 are located laterally to V4, with V5 in the anterior axillary line and V6 in the midaxillary line.

Rationale. Careful placement of the electrodes promotes the chance of a reliable tracing. Placing the electrodes above a bone will cause artifacts on the ECG tracing.

Continued

PROCEDURE 36-1 Obtain a 12-Lead ECG Using a Single-Channel Electrocardiograph—cont'd

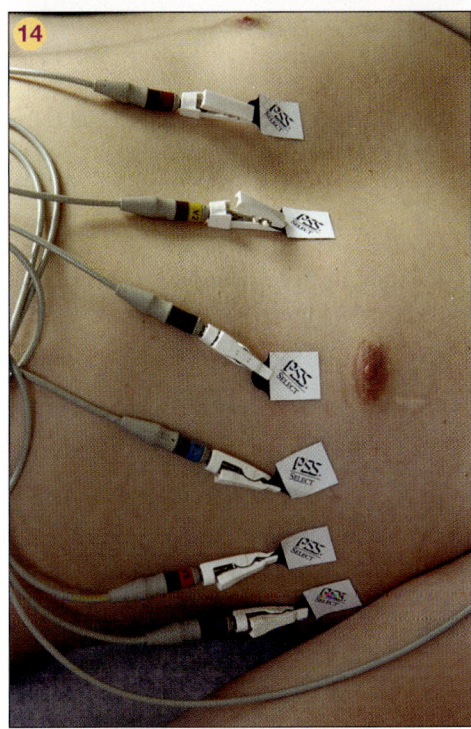

15. **Procedural Step. Connect the lead wires to the electrodes.**

    Insert an alligator clip (adapter) onto the metal tip of each lead (if not already placed). Attach the alligator clip to the tab of the proper electrode. The ends of these wires are usually color-coded and are identified with abbreviations—right arm (RA) = white, left arm (LA) = black, left leg (LL) = red, right leg (RL) = green, and chest (V) = brown—to help you connect the proper one to each electrode. The connection between the lead wire and the lead connector of the electrode should be tight, and the lead wires should be arranged to follow body contour.

    NOTE: When using plastic adapters, make certain the metal tip is in complete contact with the metal plate inside the adapter. Also, if using snap electrodes, turn the adapter sideways, open the jaws, and lock-snap it into the hole.

    Rationale. Following body contour prevents electrodes from being pulled off and reduces the possibility of artifacts.

16. **Procedural Step. Plug the cable into the machine.**

    The patient cable should be supported either on the table or on the patient's abdomen. This action prevents pulling or twisting of the lead wires or electrodes.

    Rationale. Twisting or pulling of the cable would reduce chest electrode contact with the patient's skin, as well as cause the patient discomfort.

17. **Procedural Step. Standardize the ECG machine.**

    Position the lead selector switch on "STD" and center the stylus. Set the "Record" switch to "RUN" (25 mm/sec) and check the standardization of the machine by momentarily pressing the "Standardization" button. The standardization mark should be 2 mm wide (two small squares); if the width of the standardization mark is less or more than 2 mm, the "Standardization" button should be depressed again for a longer or shorter time as required. Turn the machine to "AMP OFF" and determine the amplitude of the standardization mark by counting the small (1-mm) squares on the ECG graph paper. The standardization mark should be 10 mm (10 small squares) high. If it is more or less than this, adjust the machine until the proper standardization is reached (see Figure 36-6).

    Rationale. Standardizing the ECG machine ensures an accurate and reliable ECG for comparing to other ECGs.

18. **Procedural Step. Begin recording the ECG.**

    Center the stylus and run 8 to 10 inches or 6 to 12 seconds of leads I, II, and III by turning the "Record" switch to "RUN" (25 mm/sec) and turning the "Lead Selector" switch to the appropriate position. When recording, do the following:

    a. Make sure the recording stays near the center of the page. Use the "Position Control" knob if stylus adjustment is necessary. The entire ECG cycle must be recorded on the graph of the ECG paper. If any part of the cycle, such as the Q wave, is permitted to fall into the margin of the paper (which is not divided into a graph), it is difficult for the physician to interpret.

    b. Observe the amplitude of the R wave to determine whether a change in standard or stylus position is needed.

    c. Watch for artifacts appearing in the recording. If they occur, correct the problem and run the lead again.

    d. Mark each lead appropriately.

    e. Make certain the stylus is not burning a hole in the paper. Adjust the temperature if this occurs.

19. **Procedural Step. Record 5 to 6 inches of leads aVR, aVL, and aVF by turning the "Lead Selector" switch to the appropriate position.**

20. **Procedural Step. Record 5 to 6 inches of each chest lead (V1 to V6) by turning the "Lead Selector" switch to the appropriate position.**

    Most machines require that the machine be turned to "AMP OFF" when the chest leads are changed to prevent the stylus from thrashing. Remember to mark each lead.

Continued

PROCEDURE 36-1 Obtain a 12-Lead ECG Using a Single-Channel Electrocardiograph—cont'd

NOTE: Since the first chest lead (V1) is already positioned, most machines allow you to run the first seven leads (I, II, III, aVR, aVL, aVF, and V1) without having to turn the machine to "AMP ON." Some machines have an automatic selection process that runs the ECG.

21. **Procedural Step.** Ask the patient to lie as still as possible during the tracing, which will only take a few minutes, and correct artifacts as necessary while recording the tracing.
    If the ECG reading is not accurate, run the lead again.
    Rationale. Patient movement during recording of the tracing will cause artifacts on the ECG.

22. **Procedural Step.** If an arrhythmia occurs during the procedure, notify the nurse or physician immediately.

23. **Procedural Step.** Determine the accuracy of the ECG tracing and disconnect the patient from the electrocardiograph by removing all the lead wires and electrodes.
    Rationale. Providing an accurate tracing is extremely important to the physician in correctly diagnosing the patient. If the ECG tracing contains artifacts or interference, it may be difficult, if not impossible, for the physician to determine a diagnosis.

24. **Procedural Step.** Discard electrodes and any other waste material in the appropriate waste container.

25. **Procedural Step.** Thank the patient and allow the patient to dress.
    a. Assist the patient to a sitting position.
    b. Help the patient step down from the table, using a footstool if necessary.
    c. Provide the patient with privacy to redress and assist if necessary.

26. **Procedural Step.** Sanitize the hands.
    Always sanitize the hands after every procedure or after using gloves.

27. **Procedural Step.** Document any special information on the ECG tracing.

28. **Procedural Step.** Cut and mount the ECG as required.

29. **Procedural Step.** Handle the recording carefully and place the mounted recording in the appropriate place to be reviewed by the physician.
    Discard the excess ECG "scraps" in the waste container.
    Rationale. Careless handling of the recording can cause pressure marks, possibly leading to an inaccurate interpretation by the physician.

30. **Procedural Step.** Chart the procedure.
    Include the date, time, and the name of the procedure (12-lead ECG). Also, record any cardiac drugs that the patient is taking and any other information requested by the physician.

31. **Procedural Step.** Clean and return all equipment to its proper place.

CHARTING EXAMPLE

Date	
2/3/xx	3:30 p.m. 12-lead ECG completed. Patient tolerated procedure well. No complaints of chest pain during procedure. ECG mounted and given to Dr. Jones. ———————————————— D. Brenn, RMA

Step 11 and 14 photos from Young AP, Kennedy DB: Kinn's the medical assistant, ed 10, St Louis, 2007, Saunders; Step 13 photos from Bonewit-West K: Clinical procedures for medical assistants, ed 5, Philadelphia, 2000, Saunders.

PROCEDURE 36-2: Obtain a 12-Lead ECG Using a Three-Channel (Multichannel) Electrocardiograph

TASK: Obtain an accurate 12-lead ECG by running a multichannel (three-channel) ECG with automatic capability, disposable electrodes, and soft-touch keypad for entering patient data.

EQUIPMENT AND SUPPLIES
- Three-channel electrocardiograph
- ECG paper
- Disposable electrodes (self-adhesive)
- ECG mounting form and mounting supplies (such as an ECG paper cutter)
- Examination table
- Footstool
- Alcohol wipes (70% isopropyl)
- 4 × 4 gauze squares
- Disposable razor
- Patient gown
- Drape
- Blanket (optional)
- Small pillow
- Patient's medical record

SKILLS/RATIONALE

STANDARD PRECAUTIONS ARE TO BE FOLLOWED.

1. **Procedural Step.** Follow Steps 1 through 10 and Steps 12 through 16 of Procedure 36-1.
2. **Procedural Step.** Turn on the electrocardiograph, and enter the patient data using the soft-touch keypad.
   a. Always use your fingertips to enter the data; never use the fingernails, a pencil, or other sharp objects because these can damage the keyboard. As data are entered, the information will be displayed on the LCD screen. The patient data to be entered generally include the patient's name, identification number, age, gender, height, weight, and medications.
   b. The patient data are printed out at the top of the recording, along with the date and time of the recording.
   c. If the ECG machine is equipped with interpretive capabilities, this information is also used in the computer-assisted interpretation of the ECG.
3. **Procedural Step.** Press the "Start" or "Auto" button on the machine and run the ECG tracing.
   The machine will automatically insert a standardization mark at the beginning of each lead change, as well as identify the lead by placing lead markings at the top of the ECG paper.
4. **Procedural Step.** Follow Steps 21 through 30 of Procedure 36-1.

CHARTING EXAMPLE

Date	
1/2/xx	2:30 p.m. 12-lead ECG completed. Patient tolerated procedure well. No complaints of chest pain during the procedure. ECG given to Dr. Jones.———————————————— G. Coates, RMA

- *Lead I* records tracings from the right upper chest to the left upper chest. The electrodes are placed on the right arm (negative) and the left arm (positive), and they produce an upward deflection or positive wave (Figure 36-11, *A*). The lateral surface of the heart is viewed by Lead I.
- *Lead II* records tracings from the right upper chest to the left leg. Electrodes are placed on the right arm (negative) to the left leg (positive). Lead II also produces a positive upward deflection (Figure 36-11, *B*). Lead II shows the heart's rhythm better than the other leads, so it is considered the **rhythm strip**. The inferior surface of the heart is viewed by Lead II.
- *Lead III* records the electrical activity from the left upper chest to the left leg. The electrodes are placed on the left arm (negative) to the left leg (positive) (Figure 36-11, *C*). Lead III also views the inferior surface of the heart.

You may have noticed that by placing the electrodes on the right arm (RA), left arm (LA), and the left leg (LL), a triangle is formed. Each side of the triangle represents a lead (see Figure 36-11). Remember that the right leg (RL) is used as a ground or reference lead and is not considered.

Augmented Leads

The next set of leads is the **augmented leads,** or **unipolar leads.** Augmented leads measure the activity of one electrode on the body at a time. These tracings are increased in size (augmented) by the electrocardiograph so that they can be easily read and interpreted. Augmented leads have the same electrode placement as the standard limb leads and are referred to as the *aVR* (augmented Voltage right arm; also written aV_R), *aVL* (augmented Voltage left arm; also written aV_L), and *aVF* (augmented Voltage left foot; also written aV_F).

- The *aVR* lead records the activity from midway between the LA and LL to the RA, and this shows as a negative (downward) deflection. The *aVR* lead is not responsible for viewing any surface of the heart.

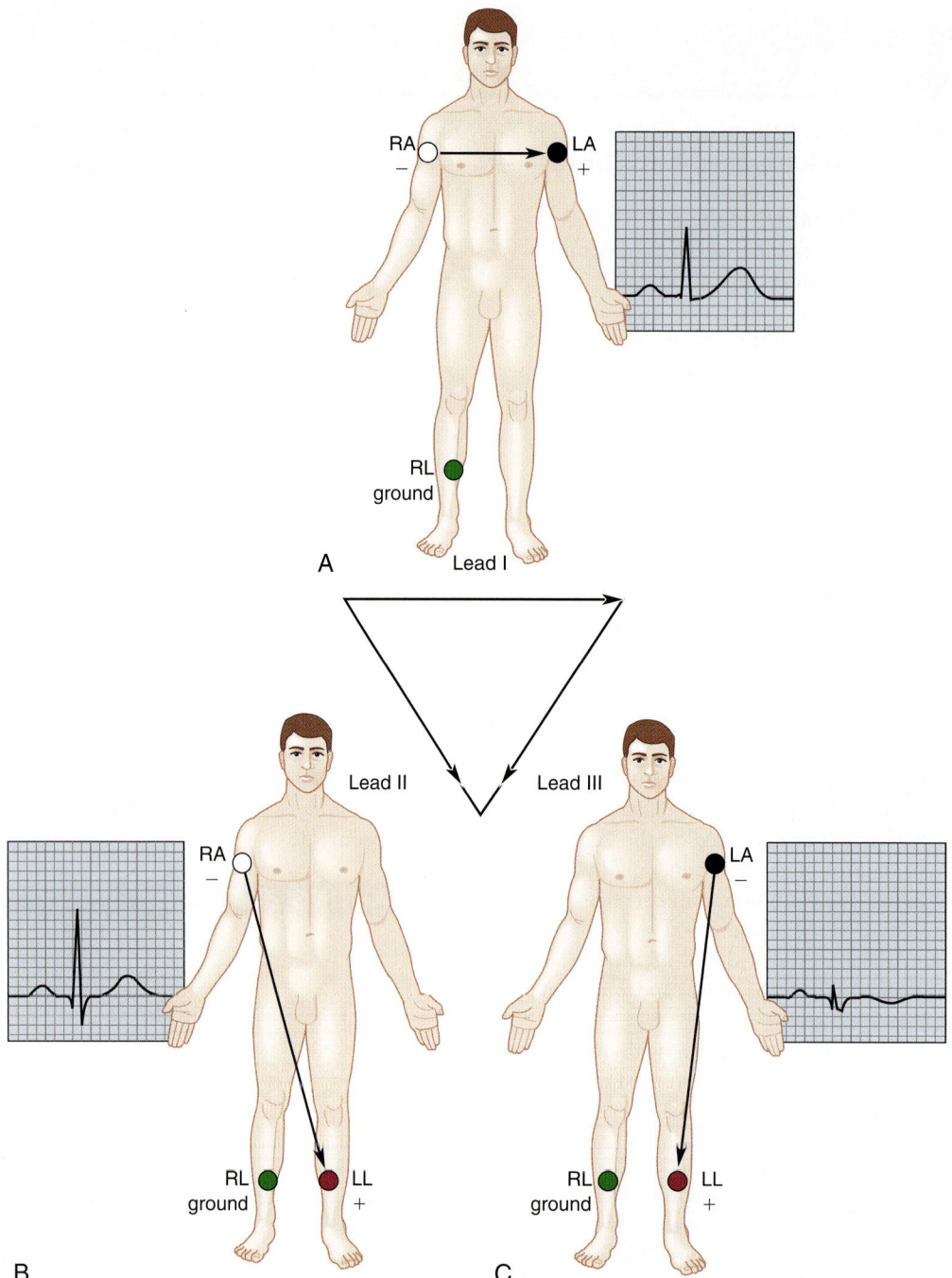

FIGURE 36-11 ECG lead wires and tracings. **A,** Lead I. **B,** Lead II. **C,** Lead III. (From Hunt SA: *Saunders fundamentals of medical assisting—revised reprint,* St Louis, 2007, Saunders.)

NOTE: Not having a negative deflection may indicate that either the electrodes or the lead wires are placed incorrectly (Figure 36-12, *A*).

- The *aVL* lead records the activity halfway between the RA and LL to the LA (Figure 36-12, *B*). This lead is responsible for viewing the lateral surface of the heart.
- The *aVF* lead records the activity halfway between the RA and LA to the LL (Figure 36-12, *C*). The *aVL* lead views the inferior surface of the heart.

Chest Leads

The **chest (precordial) leads,** or **"V" leads,** are the last six leads. These leads measure in only one direction. Precordial leads are located in front of the heart and view the heart in a *horizontal plane* from the anterior and left lateral surfaces of the heart. Each lead starts with the letter "V," and the leads are numbered V1 to V6 (also written V_1 to V_6; Figure 36-13). When placed, the leads go from the right side to the left side of the heart. Accurate placement of these leads is

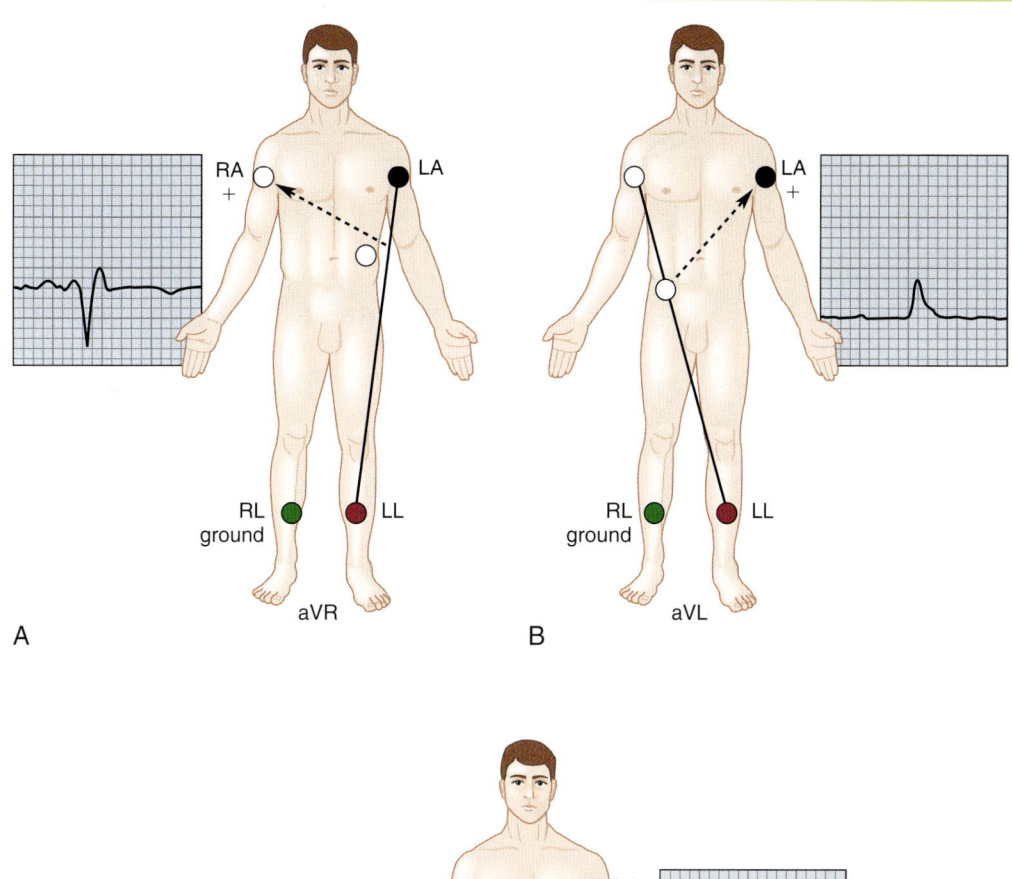
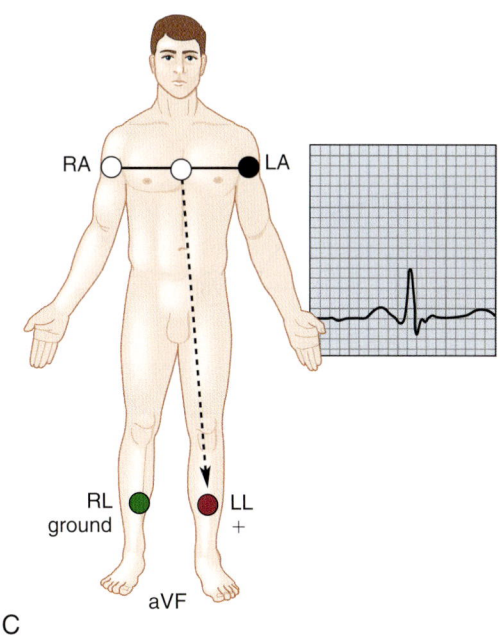

FIGURE 36-12 Augmented (unipolar) ECG leads and tracings. **A,** aVR. **B,** aVL. **C,** aVF. (From Hunt SA: *Saunders fundamentals of medical assisting—revised reprint,* St Louis, 2007, Saunders.)

extremely important to obtain a good tracing (Figure 36-14).

- *V1* is placed on the right sternal border in the fourth intercostal space. This is directly over the right atrium.
- *V2* is placed on the left sternal border in the fourth intercostal space. This is just anterior to the AV node.
- *V3* is placed midway between V2 and V4. This is over the ventricular septum.
- *V4* is placed on the left midclavicular line in the fifth intercostal space. This is over the ventricular septum but to the left of V3.
- *V5* is placed on the left anterior axillary line in the fifth intercostal space. This is over the lateral surface of the left ventricle.
- *V6* is placed on the left midaxillary line in the fifth intercostal space. This is also over the lateral surface of the left ventricle.

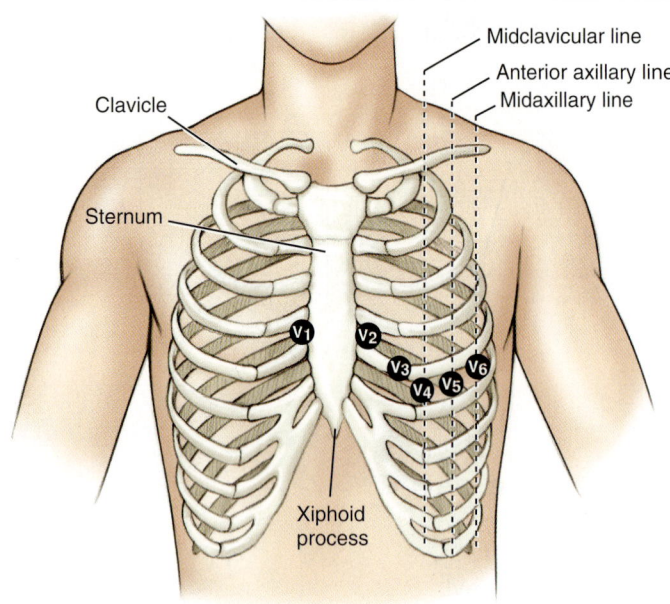

FIGURE 36-13 Precordial (chest) ECG leads: V_1 to V_6. (Modified from Hunt SA: *Saunders fundamentals of medical assisting—revised reprint,* St Louis, 2007, Saunders.)

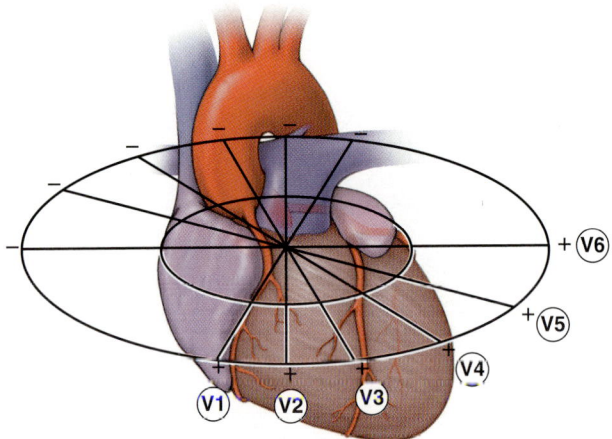

FIGURE 36-14 Precordial leads V1 to V6 are placed from the right side to the left side of the heart.

TABLE 36-2
Standard Marking Codes for ECG Leads

Electrodes Connected		Marking Code
STANDARD OR BIPOLAR LIMB LEADS		
Lead I	LL and RA	•
Lead II	LL and RA	••
Lead III	LL and LA	•••
AUGMENTED UNIPOLAR LIMB LEADS		
aVR	RA and (LA-LL)	–
aVL	LA and (RA-LL)	– –
aVF	LL and (RA-LL)	– – –
CHEST OR PRECORDIAL LEADS		
V	C and (LA-RA-LL)	V_1 – •
		V_2 – ••
		V_3 – •••
		V_4 – ••••
		V_5 – •••••
		V_6 – ••••••

LL, Left leg; *RA,* right arm; *LA,* left arm.

Lead Codes

A single-channel ECG machine with manual capacity does not automatically specify the lead names. Instead, a marker button is pushed on the machine, and corresponding dots and dashes are recorded (Table 36-2). The newer single-channel and multichannel ECG machines automatically specify the lead names (Figure 36-15).

ECG Results

The ECG tracing provides the physician with information about the current condition of the patient's heart. Comparing the patient's current ECG rhythm strip to a *baseline* ECG (an ECG done on a previous visit) provides a more accurate picture of the patient's condition and can help the physician identify changes in the patient's heart activity.

It is important to remember that each patient is to be treated as an individual. What is normal for one patient may not be normal for another. For example, if a patient normally has a heart rate of 100 beats per minute (beats/min) and the rate suddenly drops to 70 beats/min (without intervention), this "normal" heart rate may indicate a problem for the patient and the physician should be notified immediately.

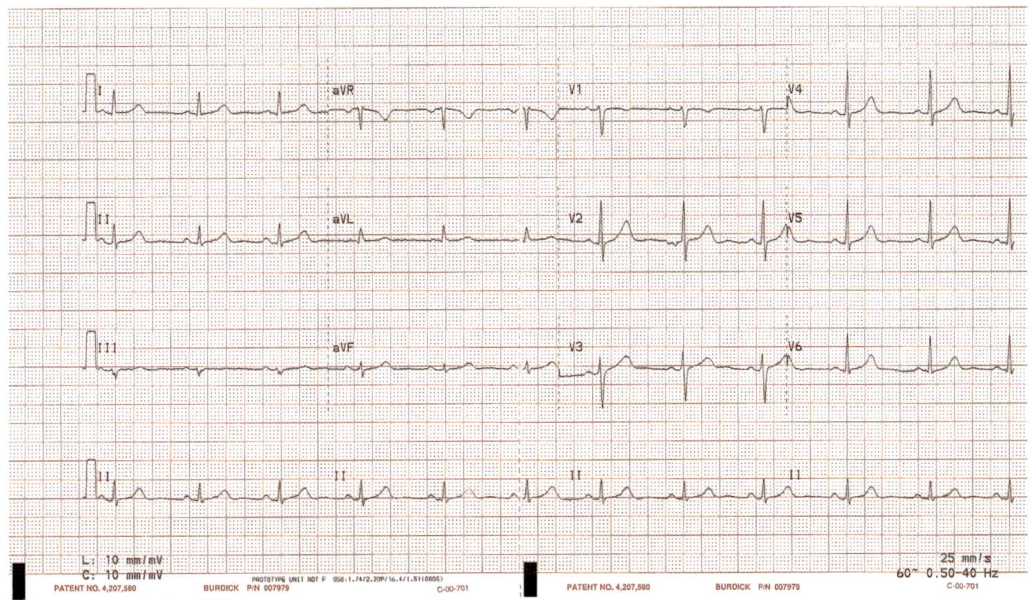

FIGURE 36-15 Three-channel ECG recording showing lead names. (Courtesy Burdick Corp, Deerfield, WI.)

FOR YOUR INFORMATION

LEGAL ASPECTS OF 12-LEAD ECG ACCURACY

In most ambulatory care settings, the medical assistant is responsible for performing the 12-lead ECG with accuracy. An inaccurate recording could result in a misdiagnosis. As a result, incorrect medications could be prescribed and legal actions could result.

The medical assistant must not react in an alarming manner when performing the ECG procedure. It is the medical assistant's responsibility to be aware of any possible legal implications that may cause potential problems for the physician and to try and avoid them.

Only the physician is to interpret the ECG. Even though some machines provide a computerized interpretation, this is not a substitute for the physician's interpretation. If a patient requests information about the results of an ECG, the patient must be referred to the physician.

PATIENT-CENTERED PROFESSIONALISM

- Why is it important for the medical assistant to attach the electrodes and lead wires correctly?

ARTIFACTS

The medical assistant is responsible for making certain an ECG tracing is free of unwanted markings, or artifacts (Figure 36-16). An **artifact** is a wave on an ECG caused by something other than the electrical activity of the heart. Artifacts interfere with the normal appearance of the ECG cycles and make it difficult for the physician to interpret the ECG tracing accurately.

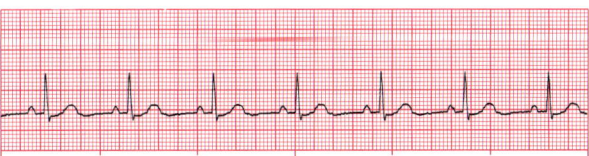

FIGURE 36-16 Example of normal sinus rhythm free of artifacts. (From Aehlert B: *Pocket reference for ECGs made easy*, ed 3, St Louis, 2006, Mosby.)

Since artifacts are caused by outside activity and not heart activity, these unwanted markings need to be eliminated. The first step in eliminating artifacts from the ECG recording is to recognize the type of artifact and to be aware of its cause. The three main artifacts are somatic tremor, wandering baseline, and electrical (AC) interference.

Somatic Tremor

A **somatic tremor** is a body tremor caused by voluntary or involuntary muscle movement of the patient. Muscle movements appear as small, jagged peaks of various heights and large, erratic spikes (Figure 36-17). Examples are shivering, talking, and involuntary movement caused by neuromuscular disorders. Remedies to prevent tremors include (1) providing the patient with a covering for warmth, (2) reassuring the patient if he or she appears anxious, (3) making the patient comfortable, and (4) requesting the patient not to talk during the procedure. If the patient has a nervous disorder, such as Parkinson disease, having the patient place the hands palms-down under the hips may help to control tremors. Always attempt to capture a readable tracing and write at the top of the best one "Best effort × (Times) [how many tracings were attempted]". For example "Best effort × 3" validates that an attempt was made to retrieve a readable tracing.

Wandering Baseline

Wandering baseline occurs when the tracing shifts from the baseline, or center of the paper, and moves over the ECG paper (Figure 36-18). Causes include electrodes not being applied properly to the patient's skin, tension on lead wires, dirty electrodes, hairy chests, and dried-out sensor pads. Eliminating this type of artifact involves (1) making certain the skin is cleaned properly and the tension on the electrodes is not too tight or too loose, (2) shaving the chest, and (3) using fresh, disposable electrodes or applying plenty of gel to clean reusable electrodes.

AC Interference

Alternating current (AC) interference results from electrical interference and appears as small, uniform spikes on the ECG tracing (Figure 36-19). AC interference can be caused by improper grounding of the ECG equipment, other electrical equipment leaking electricity, improper wall wiring, or lead wires not following body contour ("crossed" wires). Remember pagers, cell phones, and other electronic devices can cause this artifact to appear. This artifact can be fixed by making certain that the equipment is grounded and nearby equipment is unplugged. Repositioning lead wires to follow limbs and making certain the lead wires are pointed toward the hands and feet reduce the likelihood of AC interference.

> **PATIENT-CENTERED PROFESSIONALISM**
>
> - Why is it necessary for the medical assistant to understand how to prevent and eliminate artifacts from an ECG tracing?

CARDIAC ARRHYTHMIAS

When obtaining an ECG, the medical assistant needs to know the difference between an artifact and a cardiac arrhythmia. An arrhythmia, or *dysrhythmia,* can be an abnormality in heart rate, heart rhythm, or the conduction system. Remember, NSR begins in the SA node, which is located in the right atrium. The ability of the SA node to discharge properly is affected by changes in the nervous system, certain medications, hormones, and cardiac disease.

Cardiac arrhythmias are classified according to their effect on the anatomical structure of the heart. Common arrhythmias of the atria and ventricles include bradycardia, tachycardia, premature contraction, and fibrillation.

Sinus and Atrial Arrhythmias

Sinus and atrial arrhythmias are normally considered to be the least dangerous dysrhythmias. If the SA node fails to discharge, other tissues in the atria pick up the impulse and continue the conduction cycle.

Sinus Bradycardia

Sinus bradycardia occurs when the heart rate slows to less than 60 beats/min. The rhythm appears normal. The P wave appears as normal sinus rhythm. The PR interval is normal, and the QRS complex is not affected (Figure 36-20). Sinus bradycardia is often seen in well-conditioned athletes, but it can also result from myocardial infarction or medication (e.g., digoxin).

Sinus Tachycardia

Sinus tachycardia is an abnormally rapid heartbeat (100 to 180 beats/min) that results in decreased ventricular filling, thus causing a decrease in blood pressure. The P wave, PR interval, and QRS complex appear normal, but the QT inter-

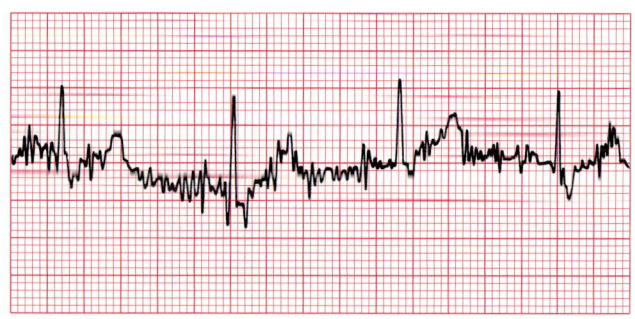

FIGURE 36-17 Somatic tremor. (From Aehlert B: *ECGs made easy*, ed 3, St Louis, 2006, Mosby.)

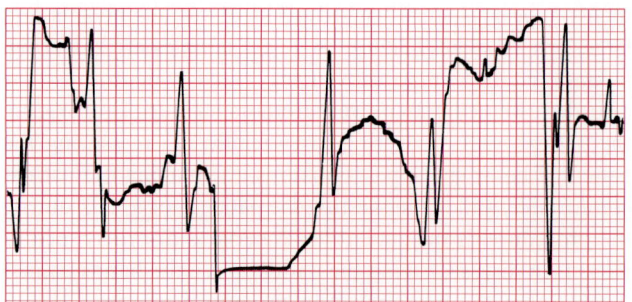

FIGURE 36-18 Wandering baseline. (From Aehlert B: *ECGs made easy*, ed 3, St Louis, 2006, Mosby.)

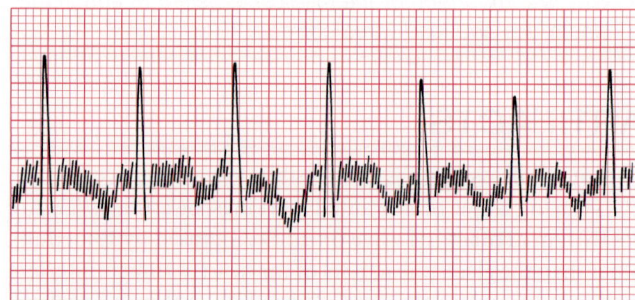

FIGURE 36-19 Alternating current (AC) interference. (From Aehlert B: *ECGs made easy*, ed 3, St Louis, 2006, Mosby.)

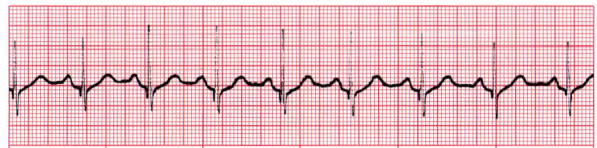

FIGURE 36-20 Example of sinus bradycardia. (From Aehlert B: *Pocket reference for ECGs made easy*, ed 3, St Louis, 2006, Mosby.)

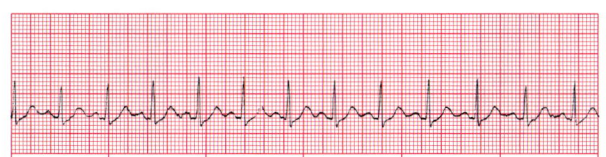

FIGURE 36-21 Example of sinus tachycardia. (From Aehlert B: *Pocket reference for ECGs made easy*, ed 3, St Louis, 2006, Mosby.)

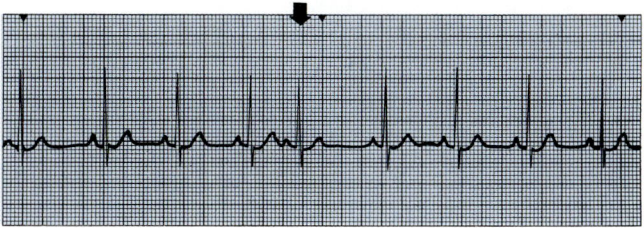

FIGURE 36-22 Example of premature atrial contractions (PACs). (From Huang S et al: *Coronary care nursing*, ed 2, Philadelphia, 1989, Saunders.)

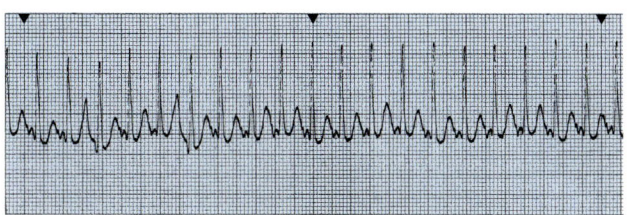

FIGURE 36-23 Example of paroxysmal atrial tachycardia (PAT). (From Huang S et al: *Coronary care nursing*, ed 2, Philadelphia, 1989, Saunders.)

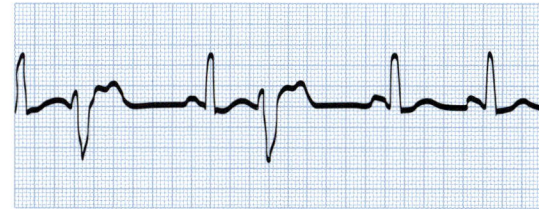

FIGURE 36-24 Example of premature ventricular contractions (PVCs).

val shortens (Figure 36-21). Sinus tachycardia is often seen in a patient after strenuous exercise, hemorrhage, dehydration, or heart failure and during times of anxiety.

Premature Atrial Contractions

A **premature atrial contraction (PAC)** occurs when an electrical impulse starts before the next expected beat. The P wave of the premature beat is abnormally shaped or may be inverted (Figure 36-22). The rate and the remainder of the ECG pattern are normal. A patient may complain of feeling a "skipped beat" or "extra beat," or the patient may be unaware of the PACs and may not report any symptoms. The problem begins when the atrial tissue becomes irritated from stimulation by caffeine, tobacco, stress, central nervous system (CNS) disturbances, thyroid disease, or heart disease. Treatment is aimed at eliminating the cause of the PACs.

Paroxysmal Atrial Tachycardia

Paroxysmal atrial tachycardia (PAT) is a sudden onset of tachycardia measuring 150 to 250 beats/min. The initial electrical impulse does not begin at the SA node; therefore the P wave is a different shape and is often inverted. The tachycardia stops spontaneously, as suddenly as it began. The heart rate then returns to a normal sinus rhythm. Each cardiac complex is very close together (Figure 36-23). A patient may complain of a sudden onset of pounding in the chest or a fluttering sensation. The patient may appear weak, may complain of breathlessness, and may experience periods of apprehension.

PAT may have no known cause or may be brought on by anxiety, stress, or excessive stimulants (e.g., alcohol, caffeine, or tobacco products). PAT may precede a ventricular arrhythmia, may occur when the heart muscle is experiencing hypoxia, or may be a sign of myocardial infarction. Because the ventricles will not fill completely, the patient experiences decreased cardiac output. Treatment is aimed at reducing the cause and therefore the increased heart rate.

Ventricular Arrhythmias

Ventricular arrhythmias are considered the most dangerous of all dysrhythmias. These arrhythmias usually cause incomplete ventricular contractions. This results in insufficient filling of the ventricles, which causes insufficient systemic circulation and oxygenation of tissues.

Premature Ventricular Contractions

A **premature ventricular contraction (PVC)** is usually seen with an injured or diseased heart. During PVCs the ventricles receive an impulse prematurely and contract early (before their time). The major problem is not only the frequency with which PVCs occur, but also the proximity of PVCs to the T wave of the preceding beat. The QRS complex will appear wider and have a bizarre shape because it does not follow the normal conduction pathway (Figure 36-24).

PVCs result from electrolyte imbalances, caffeine and other stimulants, emotions and stress, cardiac disease (including congestive heart failure and coronary artery disease), pulmonary disease, or a combination of factors. Intervention focuses on treating the cause of the PVC. PVCs are considered a

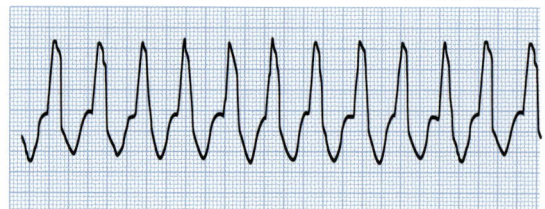

FIGURE 36-25 Example of ventricular tachycardia.

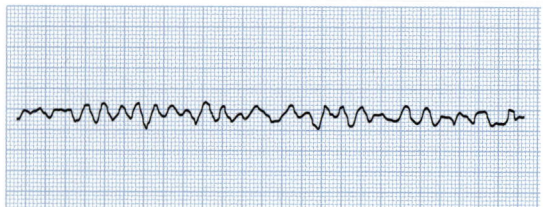

FIGURE 36-26 Example of ventricular fibrillation.

warning sign that a more serious ventricular dysrhythmia is possible.

Ventricular Tachycardia

Ventricular tachycardia (V tach) is defined by three or more consecutive PVCs and heart rate exceeding 100 beats/min. The QRS complex is wide and oddly shaped and usually there is a regular heart rhythm (Figure 36-25). Causes of V tach are similar to those for PVCs.

The longer and more sustained the V tach, the more serious it becomes. Since the heart rate is very fast, the ventricles do not have time to fill completely. This causes the cardiac output to decrease. As a result, the blood supply to the organs is decreased. The patient complains of chest pressure and a sense that the heart is "beating out of the chest." If not treated immediately, V tach can escalate into ventricular fibrillation and cardiac standstill.

Ventricular Fibrillation

Ventricular fibrillation (V fib) is the most life threatening of all arrhythmias (Figure 36-26). This is because the ventricles twitch, causing ineffective pumping action, and therefore, no circulation. Death will occur in 3 to 5 minutes if immediate medical care is not received. Immediate care may include starting cardiopulmonary resuscitation (CPR) within 1 to 2 minutes, use of a defibrillator, and/or administration of cardiac drugs.

Many medical offices include an *automated external defibrillator* (AED) as standard office equipment (Figure 36-27). A current trend is to provide lay volunteer training because defibrillators are now placed in public places such as schools and office buildings. Since quick response is important in saving a life, many community groups are supporting these efforts. It is important to remember that a patient with a pacemaker can be defibrillated as long as the paddles are not discharged directly over the battery pack.

Pacemaker Rhythm

Some patients experience conditions that will not allow the heart to function properly. When the SA node does not initiate or regulate the heartbeat correctly, an artificial **pacemaker** is implanted. The artificial pacemaker delivers electrical impulses to the heart muscle, causing depolarization and contraction.

The medical assistant needs to recognize the presence of a pacemaker rhythm on an ECG strip. A properly functioning

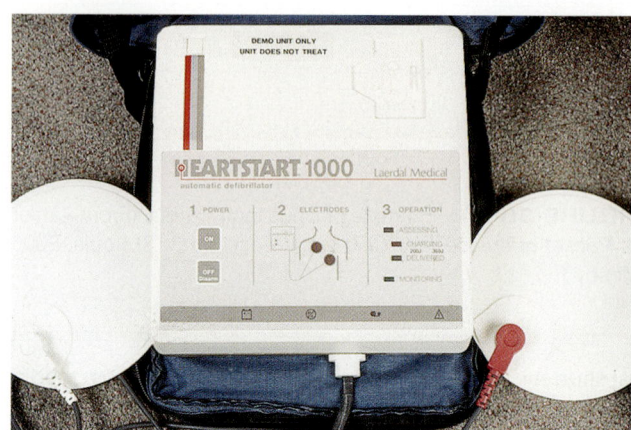

FIGURE 36-27 Automated external defibrillator (AED). (From Aehlert B: *ACLS quick review study guide,* ed 2, St Louis, 2001, Mosby.)

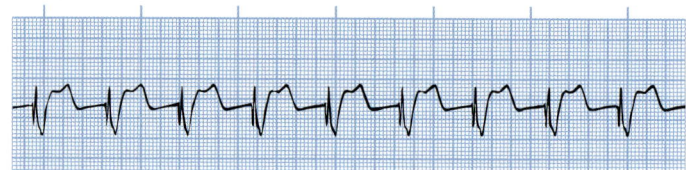

FIGURE 36-28 Pacemaker rhythm. (From Cohn EG, Gilroy-Doohan M: *Flip and see ECG,* ed 2, Philadelphia, 2002, Saunders.)

artificial pacemaker will produce rhythms with pacemaker spikes (Figure 36-28). The spike only indicates that the pacemaker mechanism is firing; it does not reveal ventricular contraction. Therefore the medical assistant must observe the patient for any clinical symptoms that would indicate problems.

PATIENT-CENTERED PROFESSIONALISM

- *Although medical assistants are not responsible for interpreting an ECG tracing or confirming the presence of an arrhythmia, why is it important for them to recognize various arrhythmias when obtaining an ECG?*

HOLTER MONITOR

Holter monitoring is an ECG-type test that monitors the heart rhythm of the ambulatory patient continuously for 24 to 48 hours. Because it is monitoring the patient for an extended

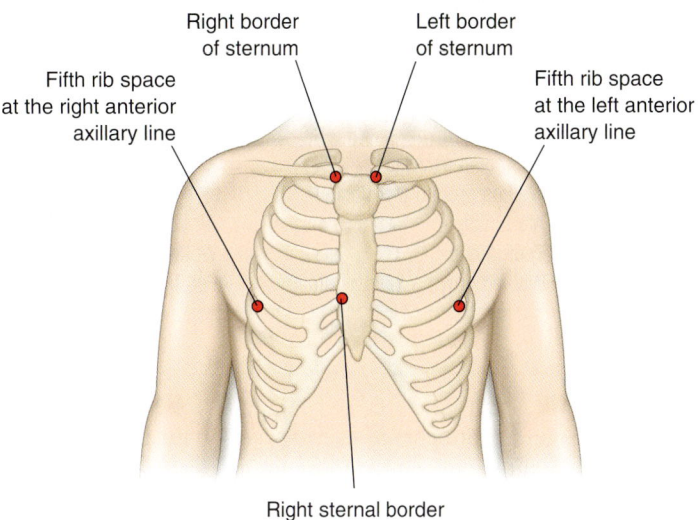

FIGURE 36-29 Positioning of electrodes for Holter monitoring.

time, the **Holter monitor** picks up intermittent problems (e.g., arrhythmias, cardiac ischemia) that may be missed during routine ECG or stress testing.

The Holter monitor consists of a small, battery-operated recorder box or a solid-state recorder that is strapped to the patient's shoulder or waist. The patient is asked to keep a diary of all activities, note any pain or discomfort, and record changes in emotional state during the monitoring. Also, patients may be asked to record medications and times taken. When the recording period is finished, a scanner or computer analyzes the tape. The physician reviews the recording and interprets it for any significant changes. The physician also correlates the recording with the patient's activity diary.

Only five leads are used to record a 12-lead tracing using the Holter monitor (Figure 36-29). Specific lead placement may differ for Holter monitors of different manufacturers.

Patient Preparation

As with the ECG, it is important to prepare patients effectively for Holter monitoring.
- Male patients with chest hair may need the sites shaved to allow the electrodes to adhere properly.
- Female patients need the electrodes placed firmly underneath the breasts. Proper skin preparation allows for good electrode adherence, and taping just below the electrode prevents accidental removal during regular activity.
- The patient is given instructions concerning the daily activities and the care of the monitor (Box 36-3). A diary or logbook is given to the patient with instructions to record all daily activities (Table 36-3).

Testing

The Holter monitor is worn and the diary used during the 24- to 48-hour testing period. When a patient experiences a symptom, the patient presses a "mark button" or "event

---

BOX 36-3

Patient "Do"s and "Don't"s When Wearing a Holter Monitor

DO:
- Keep the electrodes dry and in close contact with the skin.
- Maintain the diary accurately. Record all activities, including eating, sleeping, sexual activity, stress, exercise, stair climbing, and bowel movements.
- Press the event marker when significant symptoms (e.g., pain, dizziness) occur, and record the time, location, symptom, and activity in the diary.
- Call the physician's office if the recorder malfunctions or the electrodes loosen.
- Minimize use of electrical devices (e.g., electric toothbrushes or shavers).
- Maintain normal activities of daily living.

DON'T:
- Shower, bathe, or swim while wearing the monitor.
- Touch or move the electrodes. (This could cause artifacts.)
- Remove the monitor from its carrying case or handle the monitor.
- Use an electric blanket.

---

marker" on the recorder. This marks the point on the ECG where the symptoms are felt. The patient describes the symptom, activity, and time in the diary, and the monitor records the abnormality. For example, if the patient records that she felt chest pain at 6:00 AM and marked the ECG pattern at that time, the pattern may be significant for ischemia.

When the prescribed monitoring time has expired, the patient returns to the medical office. The physician places the tape for interpretation into a computerized analyzer. New models can transfer data directly to the computer.

TABLE 36-3

Activity Diary for the Holter Monitor

Time	Activity	Symptoms	Time	Activity	Symptoms
9 AM	**RECORDING STARTED**		1 PM	Resting in chair	Tightness relieved
10 AM	Walked around the block				
11 AM	Ate lunch				
Noon	Took a nap	Woke up and heart was pounding			
12:15 PM	Walked down a flight of stairs	Felt tightness in the chest			

Diagnoses and treatment are started based on the findings. The Holter monitor can be used to monitor the effectiveness of medication therapy and artificial pacemaker functioning.

Procedure 36-3 explains the process of applying and removing a Holter monitor, and Box 36-4 lists the necessary charting information.

PATIENT-CENTERED PROFESSIONALISM

- How important is it for the medical assistant to understand patient preparation, application, and removal of the Holter monitor?

BOX 36-4

Documentation when Charting Application of a Holter Monitor

1. Date
2. Time
3. Name of procedure: **applying Holter monitor**
   - Time started
   - Instructions provided
   - Return date and time given
4. Patient reaction, if any
5. Proper signature and credential

EVENT MONITOR

When monitoring is required over an extended period of time (a week to a month) an **event monitor** is prescribed for the patient. The event monitor is smaller than the Holter monitor and usually only has two electrodes that are placed on the chest area and connected to the monitor. The monitor is always on but will only store information when the *event marker* is pushed by the patient or picks up abnormalities it has been preprogrammed to identify. Transmissions can be done via telephone, when the electronic memory is full.

CARDIAC STRESS TESTING

The **treadmill test**, or *cardiac stress test*, is an exercise electrocardiography that is performed to determine if the heart is receiving enough blood during times of stress or exercise. It is an inexpensive (compared to invasive procedures), noninvasive procedure that provides valuable information about the heart's activity during physical activity. The test can show imbalances between myocardial oxygen demands and available supply. Before the test, the physician must provide the patient with information explaining the purpose of the test, proper preparation, and how the procedure will be done, and the patient must sign an informed consent form (Box 36-5).

The patient is attached to an ECG monitor while either riding a stationary bicycle or walking on the treadmill. During the test the speed of the treadmill is gradually increased, and the heart activity is recorded and analyzed for any electrical changes that may occur because of the increased stress placed on the heart. The stress test provides information on the **patency** (openness) of the patient's coronary arteries.

The medical assistant's role before the procedure is to attach the sensors and lead wires properly to the patient and record a baseline ECG, blood pressure, and heart rate. During the procedure the medical assistant can provide emotional support to the patient. The physician should always be present during the procedure.

The physician may order other types of cardiac stress tests for patients who are unable to tolerate increased activity levels. The heart can be exercised through the use of drugs that promote vasodilation (e.g., dipyridamole or adenosine). Cardiolite can also be used when the patient has an abnormal resting ECG to induce "artificial stress." The use of nuclear radioactive isotopes (e.g., Technetium Te99m Sestamibi) is another option that the physician may consider.

Box 36-6 lists additional types of cardiac procedures used to assess or treat cardiac disorders.

FOR YOUR INFORMATION

LEGAL ASPECTS OF CARDIAC STRESS TESTING

Informed consent is required for the cardiac stress test. The physician should explain the reason the test is being performed and any risk to the patient. An explanation of the consequences if the test is not *performed must also be provided, with alternative treatments and attendant risks.*

Electrocardiography **CHAPTER 36** 785

PROCEDURE 36-3 Apply and Remove a Holter Monitor

TASK: Demonstrate the correct procedure for applying and removing a Holter monitor.

EQUIPMENT AND SUPPLIES
- Holter monitor with battery
- Blank magnetic tape
- Patient activity diary
- Carrying case
- Disposable razor
- Belt or shoulder strap
- Disposable electrodes
- Nonallergenic tape
- Electrode cable with lead wires
- Gauze squares
- Alcohol wipes (70% isopropyl)
- Patient's medical record

SKILLS/RATIONALE

STANDARD PRECAUTIONS ARE TO BE FOLLOWED.

APPLYING THE MONITOR

1. **Procedural Step. Sanitize the hands.**
   An alcohol-based hand rub may be used instead of washing hands with soap and water, unless hands are visibly soiled.
   Rationale. Hand sanitization promotes infection control.

2. **Procedural Step. Assemble equipment and supplies.**
   NOTE: Always have additional supplies within easy reach in case of malfunction or contamination.
   Rationale. It is important to have all supplies and equipment ready and available prior to starting any procedure to ensure efficiency.

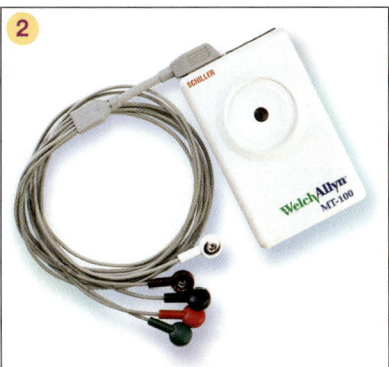

3. **Procedural Step. Greet the patient, introduce yourself, and confirm the patient's identity.**
   Rationale. Identifying the patient ensures the procedure is performed on the correct patient.

4. **Procedural Step. Explain the procedure to the patient.**
   Inform the patient that the Holter monitor will record the heart activity without interfering with his or her daily activities. Provide the patient with the guidelines for wearing a Holter monitor.
   Rationale. Explaining the procedure to the patient promotes cooperation and provides a means of obtaining implied consent. Also, the patient guidelines must be followed carefully to ensure an accurate recording.

5. **Procedural Step. Prepare the equipment.**
   Install a new alkaline battery and a blank magnetic tape following manufacturer's instructions.
   Rationale. Installing a new battery reduces the chance of the machine malfunctioning.

6. **Procedural Step. Prepare the patient.**
   Ask the patient to remove clothing to the waist. Provide a patient gown, if necessary, and instruct the patient to have the opening in the front.
   Rationale. Clothing must be removed for placement of the chest electrodes.

7. **Procedural Step. Have the patient sit on the examination table or have the patient lie down on the examination table.**

8. **Procedural Step. Locate and prepare the electrode placement sites.**
   Locate the electrode placement sites according to the diagram by the Holter monitor manufacturer. At each site, prepare an area of skin slightly larger than an electrode as follows:
   a. If necessary, shave the patient's chest at each position site.
   b. Cleanse the skin with an alcohol wipe and allow the area to dry completely.
   c. Lightly rub the skin with a gauze square until it is visibly reddened.
   Rationale. Preparing the skin helps the electrodes adhere better and assists with easier removal. Rubbing the skin with a gauze square prepares the site for better adherence.

9. **Procedural Step. Prepare the electrodes.**
   Peel the sticky backing from one of the electrodes. Avoid touching the adhesive as much as possible to prevent loss of stickiness from the adhesive. Check to make sure the electrode is moist. If it is dry, the electrode should not be used and a new electrode must be obtained.
   Rationale. The electrode should be moist to ensure good adherence and good conduction of electrical impulses.

Continued

PROCEDURE 36-3 Apply and Remove a Holter Monitor—cont'd

10. **Procedural Step. Apply the electrode.**
    a. Locate all electrode sites according to the diagram provided by the Holter monitor manufacturer.
    b. Apply the electrode with the snap fastener to the first position site with the adhesive side facing downward.
    c. Apply firm pressure at the center of the electrode and move outward toward the edges.
    d. Starting at the center of the electrode apply firm pressure and move outward.
    Rationale. Secure electrodes provide a quality tracing.
11. **Procedural Step.** Repeat Step 10 until all five electrodes have been applied.
12. **Procedural Step.** Attach the lead wires to the electrodes and place a strip of nonallergenic tape over the wires just below each electrode.
    Rationale. The tape relieves tension and pressure on the electrodes.
13. **Procedural Step.** Connect the lead wires to the electrode cable and tape the cable to the patient's chest.
    Rationale. The lead wires transmit the electrical impulses to the cardiac monitor.

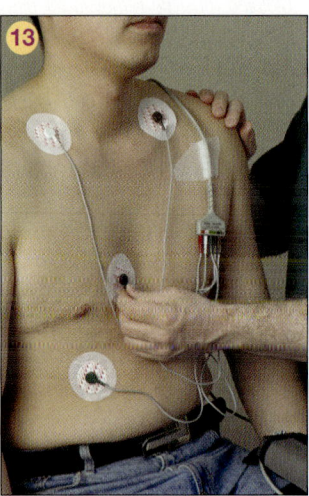

14. **Procedural Step.** Run a baseline tracing to check the recorder's effectiveness.
    Rationale. Checking the Holter monitor for proper functioning ensures a correct recording.
15. **Procedural Step.** Instruct the patient to redress and to be careful not to pull on the lead wires.
    The electrode cable should extend from under the patient's garment or between buttons.
16. **Procedural Step.** Place the recorder into its carrying case. Adjust the strap to avoid any pulling on lead wires.

Rationale. Straining or pulling on the lead wires may cause detachment of the electrodes.

17. **Procedural Step. Set the Holter monitor and record the start time.**
    a. Plug the electrode cable into the recorder.
    b. Verify the time and turn on the recorder according to the manufacturer's instructions.
    c. Record the start time in the patient activity diary.
    Rationale. The beginning time must be recorded for later correlation of the patient activity diary with cardiac activity.
18. **Procedural Step. Complete the patient information section of the patient activity diary.**
    Give the diary to the patient with verbal and written instructions on use of the monitor and proper documentation.
    Rationale. The patient diary is used to correlate patient symptoms with cardiac activity.
19. **Procedural Step.** Instruct the patient when to return for removal of the monitor.
    Be sure to remind the patient not to forget the diary.

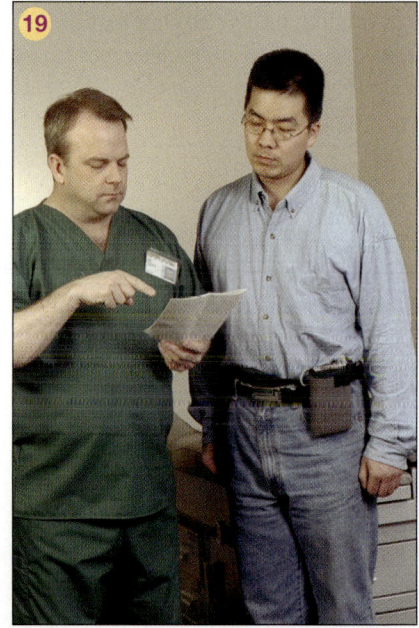

20. **Procedural Step. Sanitize the hands.**
    Always sanitize the hands after every procedure or after using gloves.
21. **Procedural Step. Chart the procedure.**
    Include the date and time, the name of the procedure (application of Holter monitor), and the start time. Also, chart instructions given to the patient.

Continued

PROCEDURE 36-3 Apply and Remove a Holter Monitor—cont'd

CHARTING EXAMPLE

Date	
3/28/xx	9:00 a.m. Holter monitor applied and started at 9:30 a.m. Patient given oral and written instructions for maintenance and care of Holter monitor. Instructions for diary completion given to patient. Patient was able to repeat all instructions. Patient to return 9:30 a.m. 3/29 to have the monitor removed.———————————————— M. DeMarce, RMA

REMOVING THE MONITOR

1. **Procedural Step.** Sanitize the hands.
2. **Procedural Step.** Assist the patient with removing clothing from the waist up.
3. **Procedural Step.** Turn off the monitor; remove the monitor strap and detach it from the lead wires.
4. **Procedural Step.** Remove the lead wires and electrodes from the patient.
5. **Procedural Step.** Clean the skin at the electrode sites.
6. **Procedural Step.** Allow the patient to redress and assist the patient if necessary.
7. **Procedural Step.** Obtain the activity diary from the patient.
8. **Procedural Step.** Sanitize the hands.
9. **Procedural Step.** Place the cassette in the computerized analyzer for recording.
10. **Procedural Step.** Attach the patient activity diary printout to the patient's medical record, chart the time that the monitor was returned, and give to the physician.

    NOTE: If the results are sent to an outside laboratory, the final analysis must be placed in the patient's medical record so that the physician can share the test results with the patient.

CHARTING EXAMPLE

Date	
3/29/xx	9:30 a.m. Removed Holter monitor from patient and activity diary retrieved. ECG printout, computer analysis, and diary given to Dr. Smith.———————————————— P. Konters, CMA (AAMA)

Step 2 photo courtesy Welch Allyn, Skaneateles Falls, NY.

BOX 36-5

Cardiac Stress Test Information for Patients

Cardiac stress testing (also known as an "exercise tolerance test" or "treadmill test") is a means of observing, evaluating, and recording your heart's response during a measured exercise test. This test determines your capacity to adapt to physical stress.

Various reasons that your physician may suggest this test for you include the following:
1. To aid in determining the presence of suspected coronary heart disease.
2. To aid in the selection of therapy.
    a. For angina pectoris (tightness or pain in the chest)
    b. After myocardial infarction (heart attack)
    c. After coronary bypass surgery (open heart surgery)
3. To determine your physical work capacity.
4. To authorize participation in a physical exercise program.

PREPARATION FOR THE TEST
1. Avoid eating a heavy meal within 2 hours of your appointment.
2. Take your medications as you usually do, unless your doctor advises you *not* to take them.
3. Wear a shirt or blouse that buttons down the front, with slacks, a skirt, jogging pants, or shorts.
4. Do not wear one-piece undergarments, jumpsuits, or dresses.
5. Tennis shoes are ideal if you have them. Otherwise, wear comfortable flat or low-heeled shoes. Do not wear clogs, sling-backs, crepe soles, boots, or high heels because they make walking on the treadmill more difficult.
6. Must sign a consent form for the procedure.

THE PROCEDURE
- When you arrive in the cardiology department, areas of your chest may be shaved to allow the electrodes to adhere tightly to your chest. A blood pressure cuff will be wrapped around your arm, and an electrocardiogram (ECG) is taken while you are at rest. The technician will then demonstrate how to walk on the treadmill and will answer any questions you may have.
- You will then perform a graded exercise test on a motor-driven treadmill. You will begin walking very gradually at a rate you can easily accomplish.
- Progressively throughout the test, the speed and grade of the treadmill will be increased, and you will be walking at a faster pace up a slight incline. At no time will you be asked to jog or run nor will you be asked to exercise beyond your capabilities.
- At all times during the test, trained personnel are in the room with you, monitoring your heart rate and blood pressure and observing you for signs of fatigue or discomfort. We do not want to exercise you to a level that is medically unsafe or physically distressing.
- An ECG is taken again when you finish walking. Your cardiologist will immediately interpret the results of the test and explain the findings to you. If necessary, medications or treatment will be discussed. A letter with the results of the stress test will be sent to your referring physician.
- The entire procedure will take 1 to $1\frac{1}{2}$ hours. If you have any questions regarding the cardiac stress test or any problems with your appointment, please contact us.

Modified from Young AP, Kennedy DB: *Kinn's the medical assistant,* ed 10, St Louis, 2007, Saunders.

BOX 36-6

Additional Cardiac Procedures

Ablation therapy: This nonsurgical technique destroys tissue in the heart along an abnormal electrical pathway of the heart conduction system. A catheter is inserted through a blood vessel near the neck or in the groin and advanced until it reaches the problem area in the heart. The tip of the catheter has electrodes that either cauterize the abnormal tissue or produce an intense cold that freezes this tissue.

Echocardiography: This procedure is also referred to as *ultrasonic cardiography* because it records pictures of the heart while at rest. A transducer held against the chest sends ultrasonic waves to the heart, and the echoes are converted into a moving image of the heart. Procedure is used to diagnose valve disorders, assess pumping function of the heart, and determine the severity of the cardiomyopathy.

Cardiac catheterization: This invasive procedure is used to diagnose or treat conditions affecting coronary artery circulation. A catheter is inserted into an artery or vein of the leg or arm. The catheter is advanced through the chambers of the heart and into the coronary arteries. Pumping ability of the heart is measured, and any occlusions are found.

Although none of these procedures is performed in a medical office setting, the medical assistant is usually responsible for scheduling the procedure at a hospital or outpatient facility.

PATIENT-CENTERED PROFESSIONALISM

- Why must the medical assistant be especially aware of his or her role when assisting during a stress test?

CONCLUSION

Electrocardiography is an important tool used by physicians to assess patients' current condition and identify changes that may have occurred. Accurate electrocardiography is a powerful tool and may show evidence of heart enlargement, insufficient blood flow to the heart, arrhythmias, and other changes in the heart's electrical activity. With an accurate ECG the physician is better able to assess, diagnose, and treat patients.

The medical assistant's role is to prepare the patient for the ECG procedure, place the electrodes and leads, and run the ECG recording. The medical assistant does not interpret the results of an ECG; this is the physician's role.

Chapter Summary

Reinforce your understanding of the material in this chapter by reviewing the curriculum objectives and key content points below.

1. **Define, appropriately use, and spell all the Key Terms for this chapter.**
   - Review the Key Terms if necessary.
2. **List two reasons why electrocardiography is performed.**
   - Electrocardiography is done as part of a routine physical examination or as a baseline for cardiac testing and is also used as a diagnostic tool to detect heart disease.
3. **List five common conditions that can be detected and evaluated using an electrocardiogram, and explain how the ECG is able to provide this information.**
   - An ECG can be used to detect and evaluate cardiac arrhythmia, ischemia, electrolyte imbalance, effects of cardiac medications, and damage caused by myocardial infarction.
   - An ECG provides information by measuring the time required for an electrical impulse to travel through the heart during a heartbeat.
4. **List the five responsibilities of a medical assistant in obtaining a patient's ECG and also explain what the medical assistant should never do.**
   - The medical assistant prepares the patient, correctly operates the equipment, identifies and eliminates artifacts, properly labels the ECG record, and understands the routine maintenance, care, and storage of the electrocardiograph.
   - The medical assistant should never discuss the results of the ECG with the patient; this is the physician's duty.
5. **Explain the sequence of events that creates the cardiac cycle.**
   - The contraction (systole) and relaxation (diastole) of the heart make up the cardiac cycle.
   - Review Figures 36-3 and 36-4.
6. **Describe the role of the sinoatrial (SA) and atrioventricular (AV) nodes in generating and monitoring the electrical impulses in the heart.**
   - The SA node (pacemaker) of the heart sends electrical impulses to both atria, causing them to contract and blood to be forced into the ventricles.
   - The AV node receives the electrical impulse from the SA node and transmits it to the bundle of His, both bundle branches, and finally to the Purkinje fibers, causing the ventricles to contract.
7. **Describe normal sinus rhythm (NSR) and the four wave patterns that can occur within a normal time sequence.**
   - NSR appears when only one P wave, one QRS complex, one T wave, and occasionally a U wave occur.
8. **List and describe the five basic components necessary for a good ECG tracing.**
   - Electrodes, leads, amplifier, galvanometer, and stylus are the basic ECG components.
   - ECG tracings show how well the heart is functioning.
   - The electrodes pick up electrical impulses generated by the myocardial cells. These impulses are carried to the electrocardiograph by the various lead wires. The amplifier enlarges the heart's signal so that it can be recorded, and the galvanometer converts this activity to movement that is recorded on heat-sensitive and pressure-sensitive ECG paper.
9. **Describe ECG paper and explain the significance of "block" size.**
   - Each wave in the ECG is measured by counting the squares on the ECG paper.
   - Each block represents a comparative height that the physician will use to count the rate and rhythm of the various leads.
10. **Explain the need for standardization of an electrocardiograph.**
    - An ECG taken on one machine should compare to a tracing taken on another machine.
11. **Explain the considerations for clothing removal, proper positioning, and skin preparation when preparing a patient for an ECG.**
    - The medical assistant must instruct the patient to remove any articles of clothing and jewelry that may interfere with testing.

- Medical assistants need to consider patient comfort, modesty, and safety when positioning the patient for the ECG.
- The patient's skin must be clean and dry where electrodes will be applied.
- The electrodes must lie flat on the skin surface; hair must be removed if necessary.

12. **Identify where electrodes are typically placed on the arms, legs, and chest.**
    - Correct placement of the electrodes and lead wires is critical to obtain an accurate reading.
    - The arm electrodes should be placed on the fleshy surface with the tab ends pointing toward the feet.
    - The leg electrodes should be placed on the calf with the tab ends pointing toward the head.
    - The chest electrodes are placed with the tabs facing down.

13. **Demonstrate the correct procedure for running a 12-lead ECG using a single-channel electrocardiograph with manual capacity.**
    - Review Procedure 36-1.

14. **Demonstrate the correct procedure for running a 12-lead ECG using a three-channel electrocardiograph with automatic capability, disposable electrodes, and a soft-touch keypad for entering patient data.**
    - Review Procedure 36-2.

15. **List three situations in which electrodes cannot be placed as usual and explain how the electrodes are to be placed in each of these situations.**
    - Amputations, casts, or bandages, wounds, and obesity or large breasts may prevent electrodes from being placed in their usual positions.
    - Electrodes must be placed close to the designated area such as on the trunk or shoulder. Notations should be made in the chart to document accommodated lead placement.

16. **Describe placement of the three standard limb (bipolar) leads and the tracings recorded with each.**
    - The limb leads are placed on both arms and both legs, with one electrode on each.
    - Standard limb leads record the frontal plane activity of the heart from top to bottom and from left to right.
    - Refer to Figure 36-11.

17. **Describe placement of the three augmented (unipolar) leads and the tracings recorded with each.**
    - The augmented leads are placed on both arms and both legs, with one electrode on each.
    - The augmented leads measure heart activity from a midway point.
    - Refer to Figure 36-12.

18. **Describe placement of the six chest (precordial, or "V") leads.**
    - The chest leads view the heart in a horizontal plane from the anterior and left lateral surfaces of the heart.
    - V1 is placed in the right sternal border in the fourth intercostal space.
    - V2 is placed in the left sternal border in the fourth intercostal space.
    - V3 is placed midway between V2 and V4.
    - V4 is placed in the left midclavicular line in the fifth intercostal space.
    - V5 is placed in the left anterior axillary line in the fifth intercostal space.
    - V6 is placed in the left midaxillary line in the fifth intercostal space.
    - Refer to Figures 36-13 and 36-14; also written V_1 to V_6.

19. **Explain why a baseline ECG is needed.**
    - A baseline ECG is done when the patient is in good health with no known cardiac problems. A current ECG may be compared with a baseline ECG to identify changes in the patient's heart activity.

20. **Define and list the causes of the three main artifacts on ECGs.**
    - Artifacts are unwanted markings on an ECG tracing caused by movement, improper electrode placement, and electrical interference.
    - Somatic tremors, wandering baseline, and AC interference are three major artifacts found on ECGs.

21. **Differentiate between an artifact and an arrhythmia.**
    - An arrhythmia results from abnormal electrical activity *within* the patient's heart, whereas an artifact is caused by movement or electrical interference *outside* the patient.
    - Cardiac arrhythmias are abnormalities in heart rate, heart rhythm, and the conduction system.

22. **List and describe four types of sinus and atrial arrhythmias.**
    - Sinus bradycardia occurs when the heart rate is less than 60 beats/min.
    - Sinus tachycardia occurs when the heart rate is 100 to 180 beats/min.
    - Premature atrial contraction (PAC) occurs when an electrical impulse starts before the next expected beat.
    - Paroxysmal atrial tachycardia (PAT) is a sudden onset of tachycardia measuring 150 to 250 beats/min.

23. **List and describe three types of ventricular arrhythmias.**
    - Ventricular arrhythmias are the most dangerous of all dysrhythmias.
    - Premature ventricular contraction (PVC) occurs when ventricles receive an impulse prematurely and contract early.
    - Ventricular tachycardia occurs with three or more consecutive PVCs and heart rate exceeding 100 beats/min.
    - Ventricular fibrillation occurs when the ventricles twitch, causing ineffective pumping action and resulting in no blood circulation.
    - Medical assistants need to recognize the presence of a pacemaker on an ECG strip and understand that the patient must be observed for clinical symptoms that would indicate ventricular problems.

24. **Explain the purpose of a Holter monitor and describe how it is used with a patient activity diary.**
    - The Holter monitor picks up intermittent problems that can be missed during a routine ECG.
    - The patient activity diary is used to record events that can later be linked by time to changes in the heart's electrical activity.
    - A Holter monitor is an ambulatory monitor that records heart activity for 24 to 48 hours.

25. **Demonstrate the correct procedure for applying and removing a Holter monitor.**
    - Review Procedure 36-3.
26. **Explain the purpose of a cardiac stress (treadmill) test and describe the medical assistant's role in this procedure.**
    - A cardiac stress test is an exercise electrocardiography test to determine if the heart is receiving adequate blood supply during physical activity.
    - The medical assistant is responsible for preparing the patient, properly attaching sensors and lead wires to the patient, and recording a baseline ECG, blood pressure, and heart rate.
    - The medical assistant also provides emotional support to the patient during the test.
27. **Analyze a realistic medical office situation and apply your understanding of electrocardiography to determine the best course of action.**
    - An accurate ECG tracing helps the physician diagnose and treat patients.
    - ECGs may be needed in emergency situations; the ability to obtain an accurate tracing is essential.
28. **Describe the impact on patient care when medical assistants understand the purpose and use of electrocardiography in the medical office.**
    - Patient care is enhanced when the medical assistant is knowledgeable about the operation and storage of the ECG equipment.
    - When the medical assistant understands the cardiac cycle and the importance of following the procedure for taking an ECG tracing, the patient benefits because the results are accurate.

PRACTICAL APPLICATIONS

If you have accomplished the objectives in this chapter, you will be able to make better choices as a medical assistant. Take another look at this situation and decide what you would do.

Jim, a 55-year-old longtime smoker who is also overweight, has taken his grandchildren to the beach for the day. Mary, Jim's wife, notices that Jim is a little short of breath and seems to rub his chest often, so she asks if he is okay. Jim tells Mary that he thinks that he needs to get to a doctor because he has chest pain that is not subsiding. They drop off the children and immediately go to the medical office.

On arrival, Jim tells Gomez, the medical assistant, about his chest pain, which now seems to be in his left arm and left jaw. Gomez tells Jim that it is "probably just indigestion" and lets Jim sit in the waiting room. Finally, observing that Jim is very short of breath and is clasping his chest, Gomez asks the attending physician, Dr. Startz, if he can obtain an ECG.

Receiving approval for the ECG, Gomez quickly loads the paper into the electrocardiograph, not taking the necessary care to prevent markings on the ECG paper. Jim has suntan oil on his body and his chest is relatively hairy, so the electrodes do not attach with sufficient pressure to stay on the skin when the leads are placed on the tabs. Gomez places the electrodes in a haphazard manner, with no consideration of the way the tabs are facing. By this time, Jim is scared and experiencing a great deal of pain, which is causing diaphoresis, trembling, and twisting. Jim starts to sing and talk to relieve his tension, and the ECG has many artifacts. In a hurry to get the ECG to Dr. Startz because of Jim's declining condition, Gomez does not notice that the ECG also contains a wandering baseline. Even the rhythm strip is not readable.

On examination, Dr. Startz realizes the seriousness of Jim's condition and immediately sends him to the hospital, where another ECG and admission to the CICU are ordered. At the end of the day, Dr. Startz is upset and tells Gomez that if he cannot get a presentable ECG in an emergency situation, he might lose his job.

If you were the medical assistant in this situation, what would you have done?

1. What are Jim's risk factors for coronary artery disease?
2. What symptoms did Jim have at the beach and later in the medical office?
3. Since Jim came to the office complaining of chest pain, what would have been the appropriate action for Gomez to take?
4. Why does ECG paper need to be handled carefully?
5. How should Gomez have prepared Jim's chest for the ECG and what effect did no preparation have on the ECG tracing?
6. What is an "artifact"? What actions by Jim caused the artifacts on the ECG?
7. What is a "wandering baseline" and what does this indicate?
8. How should the electrodes be turned when placed on the body?
9. How does a medical assistant obtain a rhythm strip on an ECG? What does the rhythm strip show?
10. What is the role of the medical assistant in obtaining an ECG tracing?

WEB SEARCH

1. **Research ablation techniques used to treat various tachycardia disorders.** Discuss how the procedure is done. How effective and safe is the procedure? What are the intended outcomes and advancements made in ablation treatment?

- **Keywords:** Use the following keywords in your search: ablation techniques, cardiac ablation, and radiofrequency ablation.

Radiography and Diagnostic Imaging

37

http://evolve.elsevier.com/klieger/medicalassisting

Radiography is the diagnostic technique of producing an image with radiation, usually x-rays. Sound waves and other types of energy can also be used to produce images of specific body areas. In radiography, a radioactive substance sends out radiation, or rays of energy, in different directions. Typical x-ray films use the radiation to create a picture of a specific body area. Diagnostic radiographic imaging provides valuable information; the physician can use the images and pictures to diagnose fractures or other disorders and diseases of the body.

Some states require additional training to take x-ray films, whereas other states allow the medical assistant to perform these tasks in the medical office under the physician's guidance. In addition, the medical assistant may be required to (1) schedule various procedures with outside **radiology** offices or departments, (2) order supplies, (3) assist with positioning, and (4) provide patient instructions before imaging. Therefore understanding the basics of all forms of diagnostic radiographic imaging is essential.

There are three basic types of diagnostic imaging: film-screen radiography, fluoroscopic imaging, and computer imaging. (In specialty areas of radiology, radiation is also used to treat cancer.) Medical assistants need to understand safety precautions when performing radiography, as well as the need to properly prepare patients for these procedures.

The duties of a basic or limited X-ray machine operator are outlined in each state's statute that covers regulation of professionals. Typically, the statute defines a basic x-ray machine operator as a person who is employed by a licensed practitioner (e.g., podiatric, chiropody, osteopathic, naturopathy, general practice, or chiropractic medicine) to perform certain radiographic functions under the direct supervision of that practitioner. Education of the limited radiographer includes either instruction or a clinical practicum, or both. This chapter covers basic principles of x-ray imaging and provides an overview of special imaging systems.

LEARNING OBJECTIVES

You will be able to do the following after completing this chapter:

Key Terms
1. Define, appropriately use, and spell all the Key Terms for this chapter.

Basics of Radiology
2. Use correct terminology when discussing radiology.
3. Discuss how an x-ray machine functions.
4. List the components of an x-ray room.

Film-Screen and Digital Radiography
5. Explain how electromagnetic energy is used to produce images on x-ray film.
6. List the advantages of digital radiography.
7. List the four views that can be taken in a chest radiograph ("x-ray") and describe the patient positioning for each.
8. Explain the patient preparation necessary for accurate mammography.

Fluoroscopic Imaging
9. Explain the difference between film-screen radiographic imaging and fluoroscopic imaging.
10. Explain the purpose of contrast media and state an important question to ask patients before contrast studies using iodine are performed.

Computer Imaging
11. Explain how ultrasonography uses sound waves to create images of soft tissue and internal organs.

12. Describe the patient preparation necessary for abdominal, gallbladder, kidney, and pelvic ultrasound tests.
13. Explain how magnetic resonance imaging (MRI) allows physicians to view detailed pictures from inside the body.
14. Describe the patient preparation necessary for MRI and list three important questions to ask the patient before the procedure.
15. Explain how computed tomography (CT) scans create a cross-sectional image of a target organ or body area.
16. Describe the patient preparation necessary for a CT scan.
17. Explain how positron emission tomography (PET) scans pinpoint cancer sites or other abnormally functioning areas in the body.
18. Describe the patient preparation necessary for a PET scan.

Employee Safety

19. List two safety precautions for employees working in areas where they could be exposed to radiation.

Medical Assistant's Role

20. Identify two topics the medical assistant must address with the patient when scheduling x-ray examinations.
21. State the most important task for the medical assistant after patient testing.

Patient-Centered Professionalism

22. Analyze a realistic medical office situation and apply your understanding of radiography and diagnostic imaging to determine the best course of action.
23. Describe the impact on patient care when medical assistants understand the concepts associated with radiography and diagnostic imaging and how patients are prepared for these procedures.

KEY TERMS

angiogram
caliper
cholecystogram
claustrophobia
collimator
computed tomography (CT)
computer imaging
contrast medium
diagnostic imaging
digital radiographic imaging
digital radiography
dosimeter
film-screen radiography
fluoroscopic imaging
fluoroscopy
intravenous pyelogram (IVP)
lower gastrointestinal series (lower GI)
magnetic resonance imaging (MRI)
mammogram
mammography
nuclear medicine
open MRI
positron emission tomography (PET)
radiograph
radiography
radiology
radiopaque
tomography
tracer
transducer
ultrasonography
ultrasound
upper gastrointestinal series (upper GI)
x-ray film
x-ray tube

PRACTICAL APPLICATIONS

Read the following scenario and keep it in mind as you learn about radiography and diagnostic imaging in this chapter.

Suzanne is a medical assistant who works for Dr. Sahara. Dr. Sahara has a medical office with the equipment for basic radiography. She sends her patients to specialized radiographic offices when more extensive testing is necessary. Dr. Sahara informs Suzanne that she has ordered these diagnostic imaging tests: (1) gallbladder ultrasound for middle-aged Mr. Donnolly; (2) baseline mammography for 40-year-old Mrs. Martens; (3) MRI for Mrs. Smith because of a possible brain lesion; and (4) chest radiograph for Mr. Charles, a patient with parkinsonism, because of possible pneumonia. Mr. Charles's chest x-ray film is inconclusive, so Dr. Sahara orders a CT scan. When the CT scan is suspicious, Dr. Sahara orders a PET scan for Mr. Charles 2 days later, and the results come back positive for cancer.

Would you be able to prepare patients for these procedures? Could you answer patient questions concerning these procedures?

BASICS OF RADIOGRAPHY

X-Ray Machine

The x-ray machine uses electromagnetic radiation to produce an image. The machine consists of an **x-ray tube** (generator source), a detection system (film or digital), and positioning hardware to align the x-ray tube and **x-ray film** with the object to be imaged. The x-ray beam is made up of electrons emitted from a heated cathode filament that is directed at a target (e.g., hand). X-ray machines work by generating a controlled voltage and current for a set period of time to the x-ray tube, which produces a beam of x-rays.

X-Ray Room

The x-ray room is a self-contained area (like a suite) that includes x-ray equipment, a control booth with a control panel, and a transformer cabinet. The walls are lined with lead to prevent x-rays from exiting outside the room. The x-ray equipment located in an x-ray room includes a tube support system, a radiographic table or an upright cassette holder, or both, as follows:

- A *tube support system* houses the x-ray tube, thereby controlling the size of the radiation field and allowing the body part being x-rayed to be in alignment with the x-ray beam and film. The tube support system can be mounted on the ceiling or on a tube stand.
  - A **collimator** is a device attached under the tube that is designed to restrict the size of the radiation field. The collimator provides a light field that outlines the exposure field and identifies the center of the field.

- A *radiographic table* is used to support the patient in a position that enhances the radiographic examination. Most tables are capable of motion (e.g., tilting), which allows for examination of the body at different angles. A radiographic table includes a space for film cassettes and a radiographic grid that minimizes *scatter radiation*.

- An *upright cassette holder* holds the x-ray film upright and can either have grids or not and is used when a cervical spine or chest film is needed.

The *control booth* is separated from the x-ray room by lead barriers that are contained within its walls and window. *Lead shields* are also used to protect the operator by minimizing scatter radiation that occurs during the exposure process. The *control panel* is located within the control booth and is designed to regulate x-ray exposure factors and to initiate x-ray exposure when a defined pattern of events occurs (Figure 37-1).

The *transformer cabinet* produces the high voltage needed for x-ray production. The cabinet is connected by cables to the x-ray tube and the control panel.

FILM-SCREEN RADIOGRAPHY

In **film-screen radiography,** the body part for which imaging is requested is placed between the x-ray tube and x-ray film (Figure 37-2). These procedures can be performed on patients in a standing, sitting, or supine position (Figure 37-3).

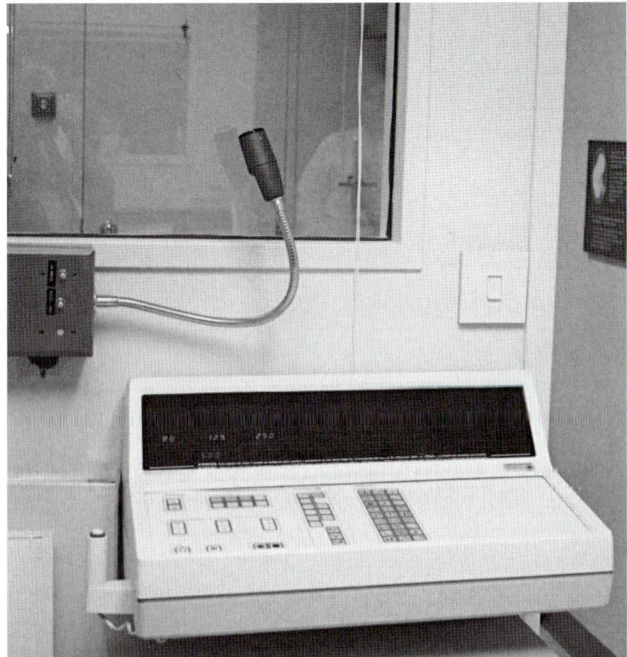

FIGURE 37-1 Control console. (From Long BW, Frank ED, Ehrlich RA: *Radiography essentials for limited practice,* ed 2, St Louis, 2006, Saunders.)

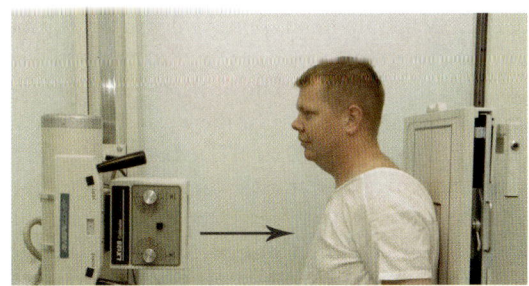

FIGURE 37-2 Patient is positioned between the film and the x-ray tube.

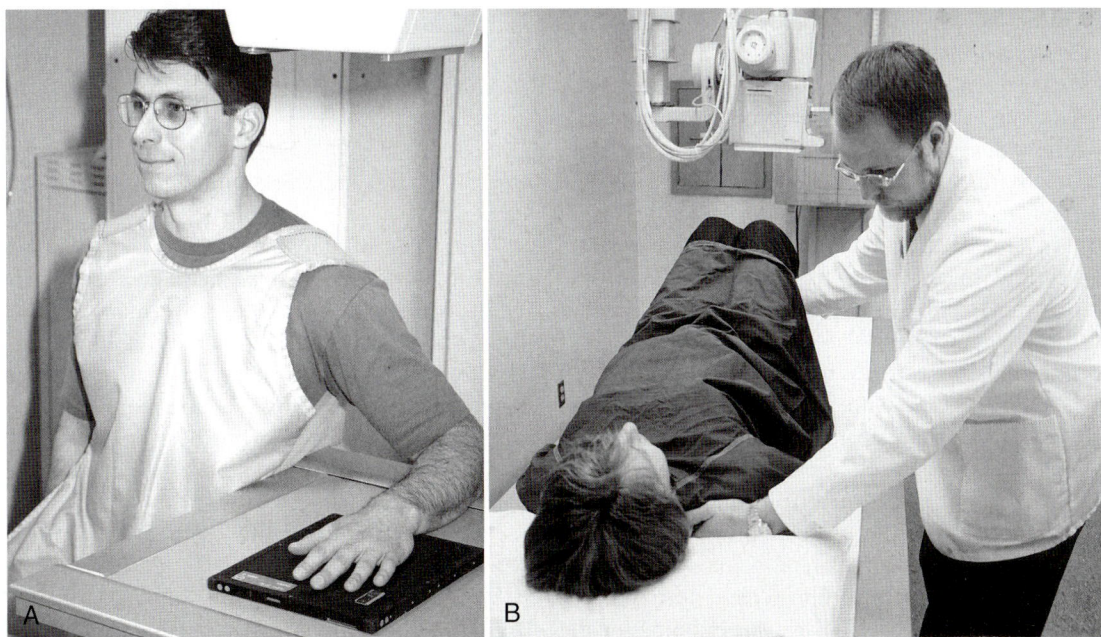

FIGURE 37-3 **A,** Patient seated at table for hand radiograph. **B,** Medical assistant assisting patient to lie on the radiographic table in a supine position. (From Long BW, Frank ED, Ehrlich RA: *Radiography essentials for limited practice,* ed 2, St Louis, 2006, Saunders.)

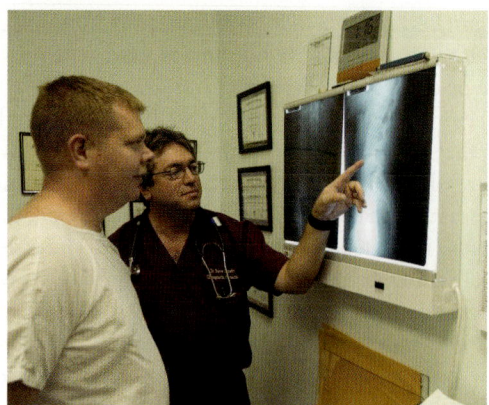

FIGURE 37-4 Physician explains x-ray results to a patient.

Electromagnetic energy from the x-radiation is directed at the film. The film is sensitive to the energy, and when developed, the picture or image (**radiograph**) that appears is the result of the x-ray energy. The recorded image looks like a photo negative, as follows (Figure 37-4):

- Maximum density areas are white because the x-ray beam could not penetrate them. Bone, a dense tissue, does not allow the radiation to pass through to the film, so bone appears on the film as a white or light-colored image.
- Minimal areas are gray because there was some penetration of energy or density. Muscle tissue does not absorb electromagnetic energy, so muscle tissue does not appear on the radiograph.
- Areas with no energy or little density are black because nothing stopped the radiation energy from reaching the film. Air, such as that within the lungs and intestines, does not absorb electromagnetic energy and appears black on the x-ray film.

The best images occur when the passage of energy is directed in a straight line through the desired area and onto a photographic cassette. Body structures do not lie at exact 90-degree angles to each other, so a body part may be rotated or positioned with sandbags or pillows to allow for clear projection of the x-ray beam.

The x-ray machine is designed to prevent x-ray leakage and confines the area of the x-rays to a small, specific part of the body. A lead shield (to protect the gonads), collar (to protect the thyroid), and glasses (to protect eyes) are used to protect sensitive organs when they are not being studied. The high-speed film used means less radiation is required, but protection is still necessary. Once the proper position is obtained, the x-ray machine operator (medical assistant) enters the shielded control booth. The patient is asked to hold his or her breath and remain still to avoid blurring on the film. See Box 37-1 for technical aspects of radiographic procedures.

Projection radiography using film-screen technology accounts for an estimated 65% of all diagnostic examinations. As with any procedure being performed in the medical office, the medical assistant responsible for basic x-ray operations will follow a predetermined protocol established by the medical facility and work within the confines of the state's statute.

Two types of film-screen radiography with which the medical assistant should be familiar are chest radiography (chest x-ray) and mammography (mammogram). If more diagnostic information is required, the physician may order tests from other departments, such as **nuclear medicine** or **diagnostic imaging.** Box 37-2 defines common diagnostic imaging tests. The type of medical imaging ordered by the physician depends on what part of the body is being examined and for what purpose.

Digital Radiography

Digital radiography, or *computed radiography (CR),* has the advantages of being compatible with existing x-ray equipment designed for film-screen imaging. Digital radiography uses the following four components:

BOX 37-1

Technical Aspects of Radiographic Procedures

- Selection of correct image receptor (IR) system (e.g., film cassette, image plate, or digital and computed radiography receptor). Purpose of the IR is to receive energy from the x-ray beam and to form an image of the body part.
- Align body part, IR, and central ray. Purpose is to control the size of the radiation field.
- Placement of the lead markers to signify right or left side of the radiograph.
- Perform quality control activities.
- Evaluate images produced for clarity.

BOX 37-2

Common Diagnostic Imaging Tests

- *Radiography (radiology) studies:* Radiation is used to show internal structures on x-ray films.
- *Ultrasonography:* High-frequency sound waves are used to create visual images of internal body structures.
- *Nuclear medicine:* Radionuclides are injected and travel throughout the body. Special equipment detects the material, and a computer creates an image.
- *Magnetic resonance imaging (MRI):* Specific parts of the body are exposed to an electromagnetic field. A scanner uses the information gathered to produce a three-dimensional image.
- *Computed tomography (CT) scan:* Internal structures are examined using a selected body plane. Rotating x-ray beam scans a cross-section and a computer reconstructs the image.
- *Fluoroscopy:* Internal organs are viewed in motion. Procedure is used for viewing the function of the stomach and intestinal structures and for cardiac catheterization.

- *Digital image receptor* intercepts the x-ray beam after it passes through the patient's body and produces a digital image (replaces film cassette).
- *Digital image processing unit* is a function performed by a computer system.
- *Image management system* controls the movement of images.
- *Information system* interfaces with a computer system to provide patient identification, scheduling, procedures performed, and so forth.

Major advantages of digital radiography are the ability to process images when recorded and rapid storage and retrieval. Digital images can be transferred from one location to another.

Chest Radiography

The chest radiograph, or "chest x-ray," provides an image of the lungs, heart, and large blood vessels (Figure 37-5). After the images are taken, a radiologist evaluates the results, and a report is sent to the primary physician. The following four views or projections are most often taken in an ambulatory care setting:

1. *Posteroanterior (PA) chest view* (posterior to anterior). The patient is facing the film holder and the x-ray tube is to the back. The hands are placed low on the hips with the palms facing outward, the shoulders are rolled forward with the scapulae moved forward, and the chin is elevated. The x-ray beam passes through the patient from the back to the front. Note that there are several ways to obtain a PA view (Figure 37-6, *A*).
2. *Anteroposterior (AP) chest view* (anterior to posterior). Two views: First, the patient is facing the x-ray machine, arms

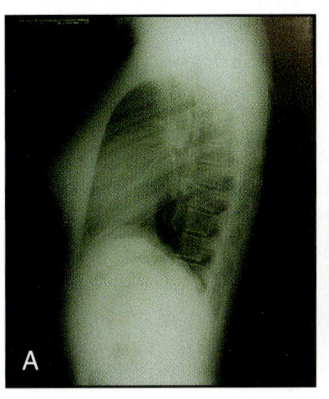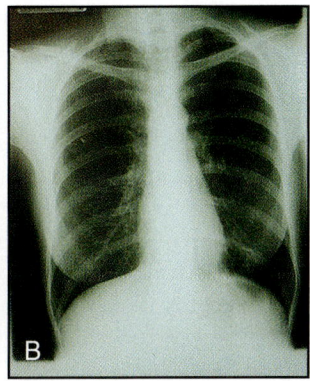

FIGURE 37-5 Chest radiographs. **A,** Lateral (side) view. **B,** AP (frontal) view (anterior to posterior). NOTE: Lead markers are not visible on radiograph. (From Young AP, Kennedy DB: *Kinn's the medical assistant,* ed 10, St Louis, 2007, Saunders.)

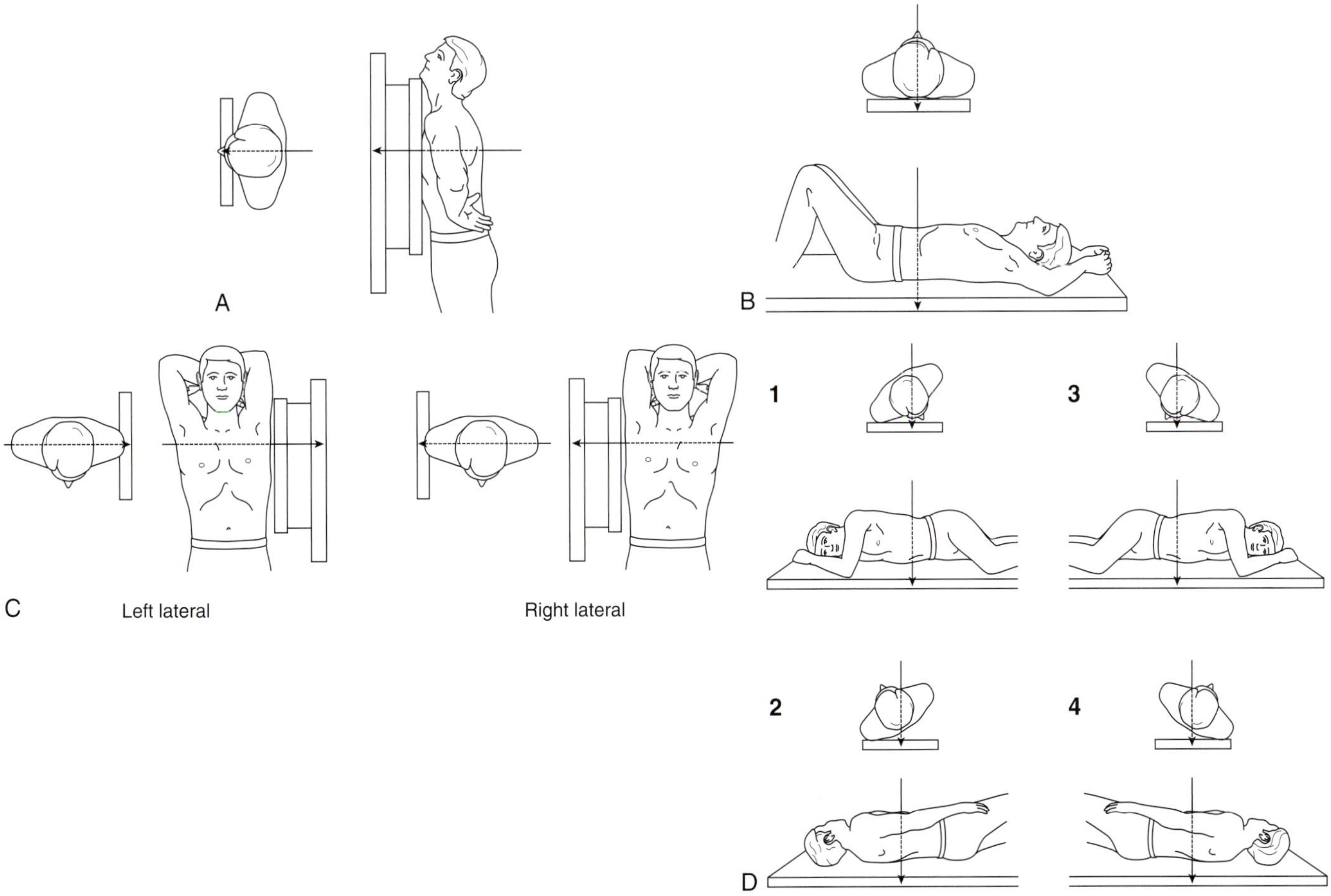

FIGURE 37-6 Projections used for x-ray studies. **A,** PA, posteroanterior. **B,** AP, anteroposterior. **C,** Lateral. **D,** PA, oblique projection. (From Long BW, Frank ED, Ehrlich RA: *Radiography essentials for limited practice,* ed 2, St Louis, 2006, Saunders.)

are at the patient's side, slightly abducted; with shoulders relaxed and slightly rotated forward (Figure 37-6, *B*). The x-ray beam passes through the patient from front to back. Second, the patient is in a dorsal recumbent position with knees slightly bent and the film holder is to the back.

3. *Lateral chest view.* The patient's feet, hips, and shoulders are in a lateral position to the film holder. The patient's arms are raised over the head with each hand grasping the opposite elbow and the chin elevated (Figure 37-6, *C*).
4. *Oblique chest view.* The x-ray beam is directed at an angle through the body part (Figure 37-6, *D*).

Patient Preparation

Before a chest x-ray film is taken, explain the procedure so that the patient knows what to expect (no advance preparation is necessary). Just before the procedure, remove all upper body jewelry. The patient is normally positioned in an upright position with the body weight equally distributed on both feet. The patient is asked to take a deep breath and hold it.

Mammography

Mammography is an x-ray examination of the breasts to detect abnormalities. It is considered to be one of the most effective methods for early detection of breast cancer. When scheduling a patient for a mammogram, keep in mind that the patient should make the appointment when her breasts are least tender (after her period). A **mammogram** is taken by positioning the patient's breast on a mammography machine and having a compression paddle apply pressure to the breast, flattening it (Figure 37-7). Mammography is usually performed bilaterally (on both breasts). Mammography may also be performed on males who have possible abnormalities of breast tissue.

Digital mammography, or full-field digital mammography (FFDM), is similar to standard mammography in that x-rays are used to produce an image of the breast. The differences are in the way the image is recorded, viewed by the physician, and stored. Standard mammography uses low energy x-rays, can only be viewed in one dimension, and is stored on large sheets of film. Digital mammography captures everything electronically and is viewed on a computer screen, thus allowing for a change in magnification, brightness, and contrast. In addition, digital mammography can be transmitted electronically from one location to another.

Patient Preparation

Patient preparation involves letting the patient know how to prepare for the mammography and what to expect during the procedure. The following areas should be addressed with the patient:

1. The patient should avoid caffeine for several days before the test.
2. No lotions, powders, or deodorant are to be used the morning of the examination.
3. The patient will be standing about 15 minutes for the procedures.
4. Explain that the x-ray machine will separately compress each breast, both superior to inferior and medial to lateral. There may be some discomfort, but full compression is necessary to achieve maximum results.
5. Advise patients to wear 2-piece outfits, so only clothing from the waist up needs to be removed.

Alternative methods used for detection of breast abnormalities are magnetic resonance imaging (MRI) and ultrasound. The MRI uses magnets and radiowaves instead of x-rays to produce very detailed, cross-sectional images of the body. A contrast medium (gadolinium DTPA) can be injected into the arm before the MRI, thus improving the ability of the MRI to show breast tissue detail. Women at high risk (e.g., family history) should get an MRI and a mammogram every year. Even though MRI is a more sensitive test in that it can detect cancer better than a mammogram, it may still miss some cancers that a mammogram would detect. A facility capable of doing an MRI-guided breast biopsy (if needed) is preferred to eliminate the need for another MRI. Women not at high risk should not have a breast MRI since the MRI has a higher false positive rate.

Breast ultrasound is sometimes used to evaluate breast problems that are found during a screening mammogram, especially with dense breast tissue. Research on breast imaging continues in order to increase the number of cancers found before being felt by the patient or the physician.

> ### PATIENT-CENTERED PROFESSIONALISM
>
> - *How would the medical assistant explain the purpose of radiography to a patient?*

FLUOROSCOPIC IMAGING

The film-screen radiographic imaging produces a view that is motionless, but in **fluoroscopic imaging,** or **fluoroscopy,** the image may include movement of contrast media (e.g., barium,

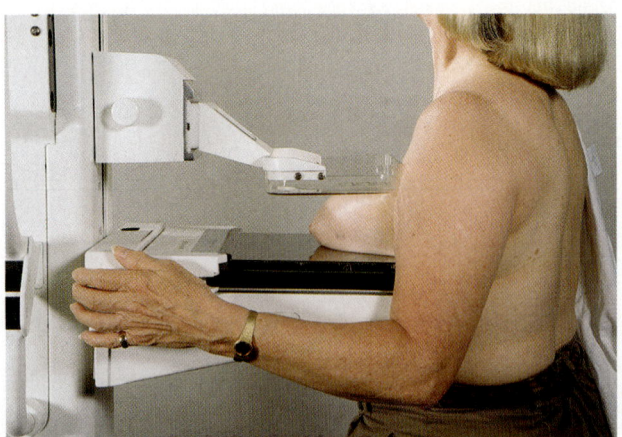

FIGURE 37-7 Patient positioning for mammography. (From Ballinger PW, Frank ED, editors: *Merrill's atlas of radiographic positions and radiologic procedures,* vol 2, ed 10, St Louis, 2003, Mosby.)

TABLE 37-1

Common Diagnostic Tests Requiring Contrast Media

Test	Purpose	Patient Preparation	Procedure
Upper gastrointestinal series (upper GI, barium swallow)	To examine esophagus, stomach, and small intestine for ulcers, obstructions, and inflammation.	Light evening meal. NPO after midnight.	Patient removes all clothing except shoes and socks; patient is gowned. Patient is positioned with the back against the film cassette. Patient drinks a barium solution through a straw while in front of a fluoroscope. Patient position is adjusted as needed for visualization. X-ray films are taken.
Lower gastrointestinal series (lower GI, barium enema)	To examine the colon for polyps, inflammation, diverticula, and other changes.	Low-residue diet for 2 days before examination; no dairy products. Use of a special bowel preparation kit as ordered. Light meal and NPO after meal except water. Enema and rectal suppositories the morning of examination; NPO.	Patient removes all clothing except shoes and socks; patient is gowned. Patient is positioned in Sims' position. Barium sulfate is inserted as an enema. Frequent side-to-side turning movement is needed to allow barium to move through intestines. X-ray films are taken.
Intravenous pyelogram (IVP)	To examine the renal pelvis, ureters, and bladder for cysts, stones, and tumors.	Light evening meal. Laxative taken the night before. NPO after midnight. Before the test, drink fluids. Empty bladder before procedure.	Dye is injected through IV catheter. As the kidneys excrete the dye, x-ray films are taken.
Cholecystogram	To study the gallbladder.	Low-fat evening meal. Take oral medication the evening before. NPO after medication.	Series of x-ray films is taken. Fatty meal given to stimulate gallbladder after preliminary films. Additional x-ray films are taken.
Angiogram	To detect tumors and obstructions, as well as lung, heart, and other organ problems.	NPO after midnight.	Sedative is given. Dye is injected into a vein using IV catheter. X-ray films are taken.

IV, Intravenous; *NPO*, Latin *nil per os*, nothing by mouth.

---

iodine) through a body part. Contrast medium outlines a specific area of the body on x-ray film. Fluoroscopy is used when real-time visualization is necessary. If you think of radiography as taking a snapshot or picture of a structure, think of fluoroscopic imaging as using a video camera.

Contrast Media

Fluoroscopic imaging requires the use of a **contrast medium** (plural *media*). A contrast medium is a **radiopaque** substance that enhances the imaging characteristic of the x-ray film by providing a difference in density. It provides a better visual effect because it allows organs to be outlined and tissues to absorb radiation better, thus allowing them to stand out on radiographs. Contrast media can be introduced into the body by swallowing, through injection, or with an enema. Typical contrast media are barium and iodine. Table 37-1 lists major tests using contrast media.

Patient Preparation

Patients scheduled for contrast studies using iodine should be asked about any possible allergy to any iodine compound or to shellfish. As with other procedures, tell the patient what will be done during the procedure and what to expect.

PATIENT-CENTERED PROFESSIONALISM

- How would the medical assistant explain the purpose of fluoroscopy to a patient?

COMPUTER IMAGING

Computer imaging, or **digital radiographic imaging,** is used in ultrasound, MRI, computed tomography, and nuclear medicine. Digital imaging reduces errors in processing because it does not rely on film, but instead it relies on computerized sensing and storage devices.

Ultrasonography

Instead of using ionizing radiation to diagnose, **ultrasonography** uses high-frequency sound waves to create an image

TABLE 37-2
Patient Preparation for Ultrasound Test

Ultrasound	Preparation
Abdominal*	NPO after midnight.
Gallbladder	NPO after midnight.
Kidney	NPO after midnight.
Pelvic	No dietary restrictions.
	Patient must drink four to six 8-ounce glasses of fluid (water, juice, coffee, or tea) 1 hour before the examination.
	Patient must not empty the bladder until after the test is done.
	NOTE: A full bladder provides the physician with a point of reference when visualizing the urinary bladder full.

NPO, Latin *nil per os*, nothing by mouth.
*Includes liver, gallbladder, kidneys, pancreas, spleen, and aorta.

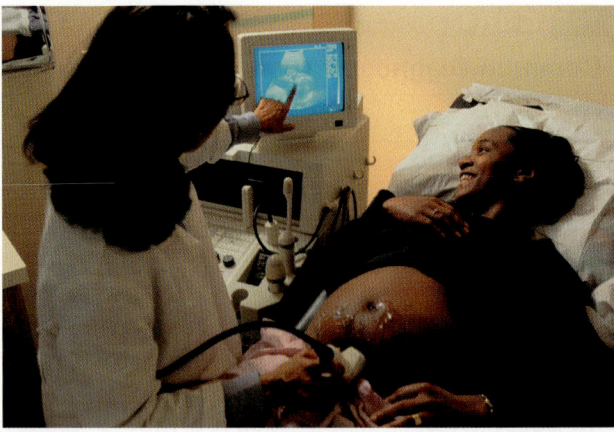

FIGURE 37-8 Fetal ultrasound. Technician moves a transducer across the patient's abdomen, and image appears on a television monitor. (From Hunt SA: *Saunders fundamentals of medical assisting—revised reprint,* St Louis, 2007, Saunders.)

(**ultrasound**) of soft tissue and internal organs. These sound waves are reflected by body tissues and recorded when a **transducer** (a computer mouse–like object) is moved over the skin, over the area to be examined.

Ultrasonography is a noninvasive and painless procedure that provides immediate feedback to the user. It can be used to visualize the abdominal area, the heart (echocardiogram), pelvic organs, and urinary organs. Table 37-2 lists patient preparations for various ultrasound studies. Newer uses include using a vaginal and rectal probe that can provide very clear images. A condom is typically used to cover the vaginal and rectal probe, making insertion easier.

Most people associate ultrasound examinations with pregnancy. Ultrasound is frequently used in the first trimester to confirm pregnancy and to view the gestational sac, fetal heart, and body movements, as well as to detect any uterine abnormalities. As the pregnancy progresses, ultrasonography is used to determine fetal size, position, and head circumference and to assess placental abnormalities and attachment (Figure 37-8).

Patient Preparation

Depending on the type of ultrasound procedure, the specific body area to be examined, and the reason the patient is having the test, the patient may need to take specific steps, such as fasting or drinking to have a full bladder, to prepare for ultrasonography. Regardless of the nature of the ultrasound, the medical assistant needs to let the patient know what to expect during the procedure.

Magnetic Resonance Imaging

Magnetic resonance imaging (MRI) allows the physician to see detailed cross-sectional images inside the body without the use of x-rays. A strong magnetic field and radiowaves are used to view anatomical structures. MRI is used to identify and evaluate blood clots, nerve damage, torn ligaments, and similar conditions.

MR images allow the physician to view anatomical structures more clearly than is possible with other forms of imaging because it basically creates a three-dimensional image of the body. MRI does not require the use of contrast media or radiation.

Patient Preparation

Patient preparation for MRI is simple. Patients can have a normal diet and continue to take their prescribed medications. Important questions to ask the patient include the following:

- Does the patient have any medical devices with metal (e.g., pacemaker, IUD [copper-7], surgical clips [e.g., aneurysm], metal prosthesis, hearing aids, dental bridges, glasses, or wig with metal clips)? Metal disturbs the signals needed to produce the image, which can cause blurring. Also, because the magnetic pull is so strong, a loose metal fragment could be pulled away from the patient's body, causing injury to the patient. Because clothing harbors metal, a gown will be provided for the patient. Even eye shadow and transdermal patches must be removed because they may be composed of metallic compounds (e.g., some patches have an aluminum backing).
- Is there any chance of pregnancy? MR scans are not recommended for pregnant women because the effects of strong magnetic fields on a fetus are not well-documented.
- Can the patient lie still for at least 30 minutes? Movement will blur the images.

The patient will be asked to lie flat (sometimes a small pillow is placed under the patient's knees for comfort), with arms at the side, on the scanning bed. Once the patient is comfortable, the bed is slid into the magnet tube (Figure 37-9). Since motion will affect the image, the patient must be still. A covering may be given to the patient to provide warmth. Some patients may be anxious, and others may experience **claustrophobia** in enclosed areas. In these situations, a mild sedative may be prescribed before the examination. The patient will hear a humming or thumping sound, which can

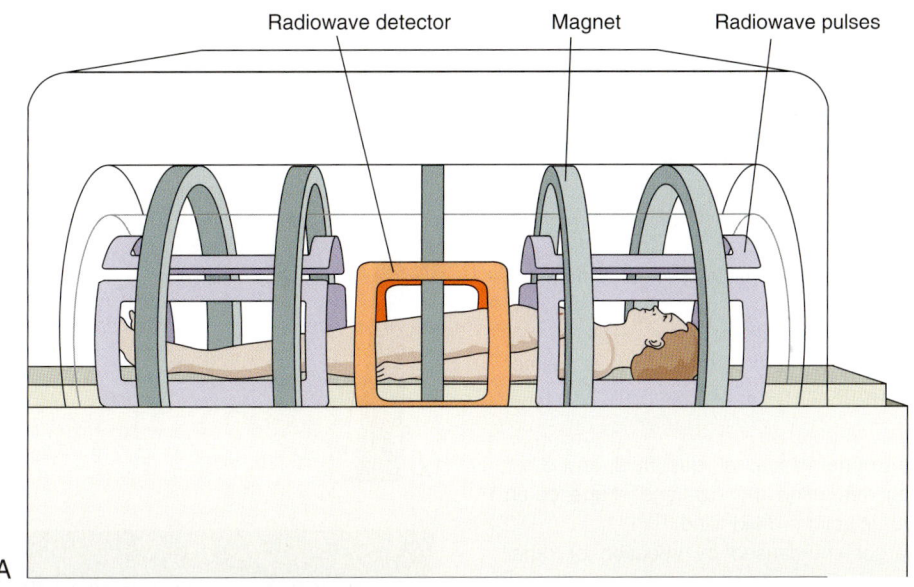
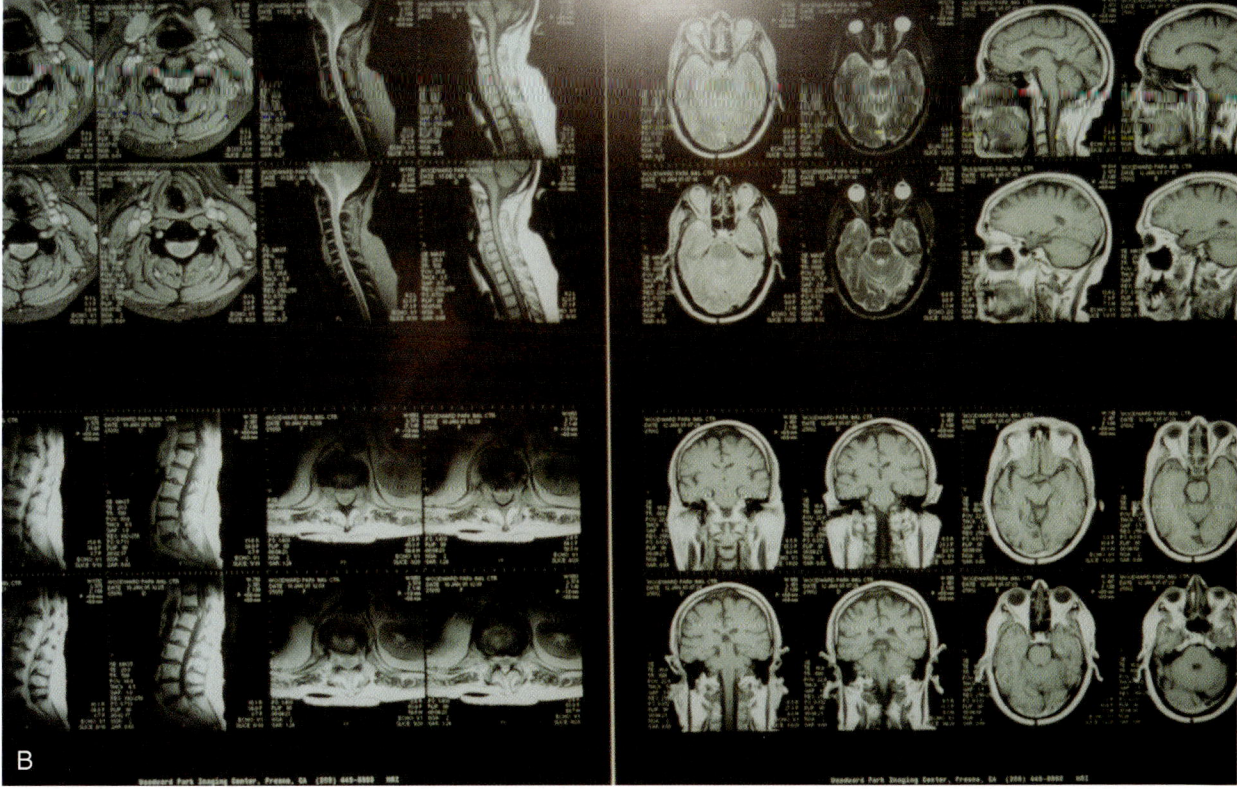

FIGURE 37-9 **A,** Magnetic resonance imaging (MRI) unit. **B,** MR images. (From Kinn ME, Woods MA: *The medical assistant,* ed 8, Philadelphia, 1999, Saunders.)

be lessened by wearing earplugs. After the examination, the patient can resume normal activities.

Technological advances have made **open MRI** a possibility for many patients. Instead of lying in the narrow magnet tube, the patient lies on an imaging table with more space around the body. Open MRI is often a good choice for children and for those who are claustrophobic or obese. Open MRI is now being used more frequently. The noise is less noticeable, and the feeling of being "closed in" is reduced.

Computed Tomography

Tomography is the use of radiography to see the body or an organ as a whole in a cross-sectional or "sliced" view. **Computed tomography (CT)** views the target organ or body area from different angles in a three-dimensional view; the CT scan is sometimes called a "CAT (computerized axial tomography) scan." Typical uses for CT scanning are the assessment of blood vessels (e.g., detecting aneurysms), the hepatic system,

BOX 37-3

Purpose and Diagnostic Uses of CT Scans

HEAD SCANS

To show brain structures and any abnormalities.
- Tumors growing in brain and spinal tissue.
- Blood clots forming because of a ruptured blood vessel in the brain.
- Enlarged ventricles resulting from cerebrospinal fluid not draining properly.
- Nerve and eye muscle abnormalities.
- Brain differences associated with mental illness, Alzheimer disease, and other disorders.

BODY SCANS

To distinguish among bone, tissue, fat, gas, fluid, and other body structures; can determine the size and shape of an organ and if a growth is solid or fluid filled.
- Lymph node enlargement caused by infection or other conditions.
- Pancreatic disease (can be diagnosed within 1 hour).
- Back problems, including ruptured vertebral discs.
- Lung cancer (growths can be viewed in areas not shown on regular x-ray films).

CARDIOVASCULAR SCANS

To show heart structures and blood vessels and any abnormalities.
- Abnormal blood flow within blood vessels can be detected through the use of high-frequency sound waves *(Doppler ultrasound)*.
- Structure and function of heart valves can be seen through the use of ultrasound *(echocardiogram)*.

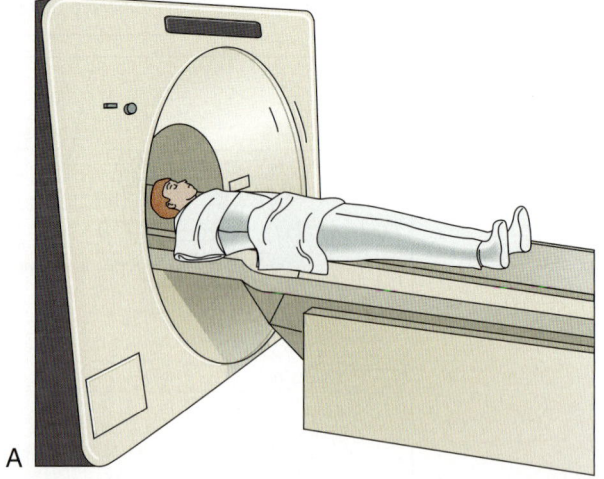
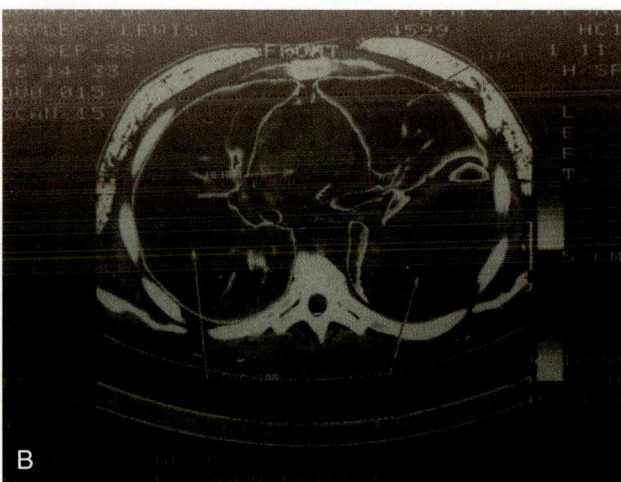

FIGURE 37-10 **A,** Computed tomography (CT) total scanner. **B,** Example of CT scan. (From Kinn ME, Woods MA: *The medical assistant,* ed 8, Philadelphia, 1999, Saunders.)

the kidney, and pulmonary systems. Box 37-3 lists other diagnostic uses of head, body, and cardiovascular CT scans.

The CT scanner x-ray tube focuses a narrow x ray beam across a layer, or "slice," of the body. Imagine a large donut that is upright. The patient lies on a platform and slowly moves through the donut hole. The x-ray tube is positioned on the edges of the hole. A motor rotates the ring around a section of the body, and after a complete revolution, the platform advances further into the hole so that the x-ray tube can scan the next section. The x-ray energy is absorbed differently by the body structures. Receptors detect the amount of radiation passing through the body. This information is relayed and stored in the computer. Numerous readings are stored in the computer. The computer analyzes the readings at the different angles and converts this information into a cross-sectional image. CT scans reveal more about the body and its structures than a typical x-ray. The radiologist interprets the resulting image and determines if further tests are needed.

Patient Preparation

If a contrast medium is used for a head and chest CT scan, the patient is advised to avoid food or fluids for 8 hours. The use of contrast media sharpens details better than the image produced by sound waves. It is important to ask the patient about any known allergies and to have the patient remove any metal objects. The patient lies in a supine position in a cylinder, with the head secured in a cradle if a CT head scan is ordered (Figure 37-10). Depending on what site is to be scanned, the average time needed for the scan is 1 hour.

An intravenous (IV) line is started to allow a site for the dye (contrast medium) to be injected, if needed. The patient must not move, since blurs could result.

FOR YOUR INFORMATION

CT SCANS
- *Radiation exposure for CT scans is reported to be two to three times as much as for a typical x-ray film.*
- *CT scans often detect the smallest abnormalities, allowing treatment to begin early.*

Positron Emission Tomography

Positron emission tomography (**PET**) is an imaging method that can evaluate the entire body with a single procedure. A patient is injected with a sugar **tracer,** which is taken up and concentrated in cancer cells or other cells such as the brain. These "sugar cells" (the cancer or other cells concentrated with sugar) send out signals that are picked up by a specialized camera. A computer in this camera converts these signals into pictures of the human body. Using this type of technology allows cancer and other sites to be pinpointed. CT scans and MRIs provide pictures of internal organs, but they do not identify abnormal functioning as the PET scan can.

Besides oncological purposes, PET scanning is also used in cardiology and neurology. For example, PET scanning is used to assess the potential benefits of coronary artery bypass surgery in high-risk patients and assists in the diagnosis of Alzheimer disease, Parkinson disease, and other neurological disorders.

Patient Preparation

The patient is asked to fast for at least 6 hours before the PET procedure. The patient is seated in a reclining chair and given an injection of the sugar tracer. After 45 minutes the patient is taken to an imaging table to lie down. The PET camera acquires information concerning the localization of the tracer in the body. These data are transmitted to a computer, and pictures of the body are formed. This part of the procedure takes another 45 minutes. A nuclear medicine physician reviews the PET scan in detail and sends a report to the primary physician.

> **PATIENT-CENTERED PROFESSIONALISM**
>
> - How would the medical assistant explain to a patient the need for tomography tests?

EMPLOYEE SAFETY

The medical assistant working in a medical office with an x-ray machine or any health care employee working in the radiology department can be exposed to particles of radiation if safety procedures are not followed.

All employees working in an area where the possibility of exposure to radiation exists should wear a personal monitoring device called a **dosimeter** (Figure 37-11). The dosimeter monitors the quantity of radiation exposure. It should be worn on the anterior surface, between chest and waist level. The device is usually referred to as a "film badge," and each employee is issued his or her own badge. To obtain an accurate exposure reading, the badge should not be shared among employees. It is usually worn clipped to the lab coat, uniform pocket, or collar. The two types of dosimeters are as follows:
- *Thermoluminescent dosimeter (TLD)* consists of a plastic badge containing lithium fluoride crystals that absorb x-

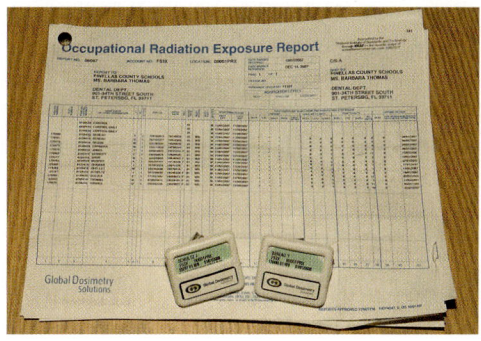

FIGURE 37-11 Optically stimulated luminescence (OSL) dosimeter with exposure report.

ray energy and give off energy in the form of light when heated.
- *Optically stimulated luminescence (OSL)* is a dosimeter that uses aluminum oxide as a radiation detector.

Both types of dosimeters are sent to a laboratory where they are analyzed for the amount of radiation exposure. This amount is compared to a control badge, and any amount of exposure measured on the control badge is subtracted from the amounts measured on the badge being analyzed.

The medical assistant should stand behind a lead barrier when performing radiography to ensure no exposure to radiation. Excessive exposure to radiation during pregnancy can result in birth defects and other problems in the child.

> **PATIENT-CENTERED PROFESSIONALISM**
>
> - Why must the medical assistant know safety measures when working with x-ray equipment?

MEDICAL ASSISTANT'S ROLE

Depending on the policies of the medical facility and state and local regulations, medical assistants may or may not be allowed to perform radiography. However, all medical assistants need to understand their role in patient care associated with radiography and diagnostic imaging.

Questions to Ask Patients

Before making arrangements for a patient to have an x-ray examination or diagnostic imaging done, the medical assistant should routinely ask the patient the following questions:

1. Has the patient had other x-rays or diagnostic tests done and for what?
2. If the patient is a female of childbearing age, is there a chance she could be pregnant? Asking the patient when her last menstrual period (LMP) occurred is a good indicator of pregnancy possibilities. Use the "10-day rule," which determines the patient is least susceptible to radiation to the gonads during the 10 days from the beginning of her

menses, since it is unlikely the woman will become pregnant during this time.
3. If the patient will have a contrast medium injected, is he or she aware of any allergies to the dye? For example, patients who have an allergy to shellfish, which have naturally occurring iodine content, should avoid media that contain inorganic iodine compounds.

Scheduling and Patient Preparation

The medical office will routinely schedule patients for x-ray examinations. The medical assistant should review any special procedures that will be required of the patient and provide written instructions for the patient to take home. The patient needs to be informed of the following:

- Approximate length of time the examination will take.
- Special preparations required (e.g., fasting, bowel prep, if contrast media is to be used).

If the medical assistant helps in taking the x-ray film in the office, patient preparation includes the following:

1. Ensuring proper identification of the patient.
2. Measuring the body part with a **caliper** and properly marking the area to be surveyed.
3. Positioning the patient and the central x-ray correctly. Film accuracy requires that the patient be placed in the correct position and the position be held without moving.
4. Ensuring that children and adults of childbearing age have the reproductive organs covered with a gonad shield to prevent damage to these organs (Figure 37-12). If the patient is pregnant, a release form must be signed stating that she understands the dangers from radiation to the fetus.
5. Providing reassurance as needed.
6. Developing the film properly, making certain the radiograph is free of artifacts. The film should be hung on the light box for the physician to view.

Postprocedural Duties

The medical assistant's most important task after patient testing is to be certain that a written report is received in the medical office for the physician to review. After review, the report must be filed in the patient's medical record. To make efficient use of the physician's and patient's time, the following can be done:

- Keep an x-ray log to monitor the return of diagnostic imaging reports.
- If a report is not received at the physician's office within a week, follow up with a call to the radiology department.
- The patient's medical record should be reviewed the day before the patient's visit to make certain all reports are available and the report has been signed off by the physician. Most physicians do not want to see patients without test results, and patients do not like to wait while results are being faxed.

> **PATIENT-CENTERED PROFESSIONALISM**
>
> - What is the medical assistant's role in preparing a patient for radiology studies?

CONCLUSION

Radiography has been a much-used diagnostic tool for nearly 100 years. In the last several decades, new technology has enabled digital computer imaging. These techniques enable physicians to diagnose illnesses and injuries quickly and efficiently. Diagnosing illness and injury in a timely manner allows the physician to determine the best course of treatment for patients and to implement the treatment plan more quickly.

Understanding the types of diagnostic imaging procedures, including film-screen radiography, fluoroscopy, and computer imaging, helps medical assistants provide better care to patients undergoing these tests, regardless of whether the assistant is directly involved in the procedure. Effectively preparing the patient allows the tests to run more smoothly and helps to produce better results.

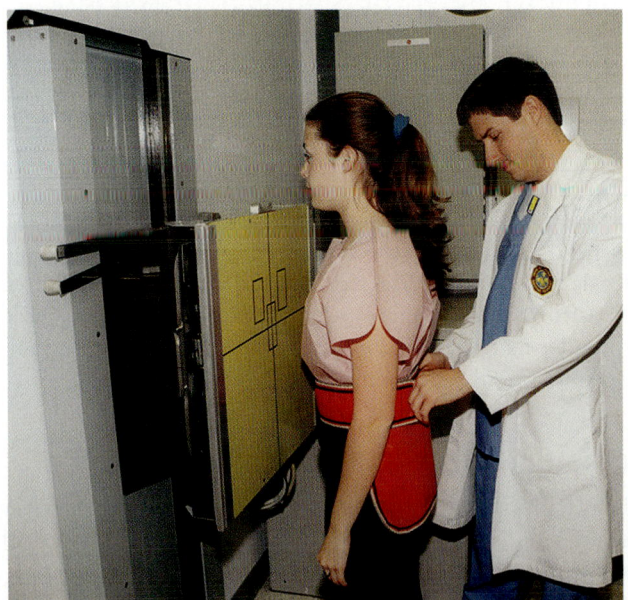

FIGURE 37-12 Patient wears lead apron to protect reproductive organs. (From Young AP, Kennedy DP: *Kinn's the medical assistant,* ed 10, St Louis, 2007, Saunders.)

Chapter Summary

Reinforce your understanding of the material in this chapter by reviewing the curriculum objectives and key content points below.

1. **Define, appropriately use, and spell all the Key Terms for this chapter.**
   - Review the Key Terms if necessary.
2. **Use correct terminology when discussing radiology.**
   - Review the terminology used in the various Boxes and Tables.
3. **Discuss how an x-ray machine functions.**
   - X-ray machine uses electromagnetic radiation to produce an image.
4. **List the components of an x-ray room.**
   - Tube support system houses the x-ray tube and controls the size of the radiation field.
   - Radiographic table supports patient and allows motion for examination at different angles.
5. **Explain how electromagnetic energy is used to produce images on x-ray film.**
   - Electromagnetic energy from the x-ray is directed at energy-sensitive film, with the body part between the energy source and the film.
   - White areas indicate no penetration of the energy (e.g., bones or total blockage) because of density, gray areas indicate some penetration of energy (some muscles and bones), and black areas indicate nothing blocking the penetration of radiation energy to the film (air) because of lack of density.
6. **List the advantages of digital radiography.**
   - Processes images when recorded.
   - Rapid storage and retrieval system.
   - Images can be transferred from one location to another.
7. **List the four views that can be taken in a chest radiograph ("x-ray") and describe the patient positioning for each.**
   - The posteroanterior (PA) view is a frontal view (posterior to anterior). The patient stands facing the film holder, and the x-ray tube is to the back; hands are low on the hips, palms face outward, shoulders and scapulae are moved forward, and the chin is elevated.
   - The anteroposterior (AP) view is a back view (anterior to posterior). The patient stands facing the x-ray tube, and the film holder is to the back; arms are slightly abducted at the sides, with the shoulders relaxed and slightly rotated forward.
   - The lateral view is a side view. The patient stands sideways to the film holder; the arms are raised over the head, with each hand grasping the opposite elbow, and the chin is elevated.
   - The oblique view is accomplished when the x-ray beam is directed at an angle through the body part.
8. **Explain the patient preparation necessary for accurate mammography.**
   - Patients should be told to avoid caffeine for several days before the test.
   - Patients should be told not to use lotions, powders, or deodorant the morning of the examination.
   - Patients should be informed how long they will stand and what will happen during the procedure.
   - Tell patients to wear 2-piece outfits so only clothing from the waist up needs to be removed.
9. **Explain the difference between film-screen radiographic imaging and fluoroscopic imaging.**
   - Film-screen imaging produces a still view; fluoroscopic imaging produces images in motion.
10. **Explain the purpose of contrast media and state an important question to ask patients before contrast studies using iodine are performed.**
    - Contrast media are radiopaque substances that enhance the imaging characteristics of the radiograph.
    - Before administering contrast media, always ask the patient if he or she is allergic to any iodine compound or shellfish.
11. **Explain how ultrasonography uses sound waves to create images of soft tissue and internal organs.**
    - Sound waves are reflected by body tissues and organs and recorded when a transducer is moved over the skin outside the area to be examined.
12. **Describe the patient preparation necessary for abdominal, gallbladder, kidney, and pelvic ultrasound tests.**
    - Review Table 37-2.
13. **Explain how magnetic resonance imaging (MRI) allows physicians to view detailed pictures from inside the body.**
    - A three-dimensional image of the body area is generated by a strong magnetic field and radio waves. Images are more clearly delineated with MRI than with other forms of imaging.
14. **Describe the patient preparation necessary for MRI, and list three important questions to ask the patient before the procedure.**
    - Patients can have a normal diet and take their prescribed medications before MRI is performed.
    - The medical assistant should ask the patient questions about (a) medical devices with metal, (b) chance for pregnancy, and (c) whether the patient can lie still for 30 minutes.
15. **Explain how computed tomography (CT) scans create a cross-sectional image of a target organ or body area.**
    - CT scans view a target organ or body area from different angles in a three-dimensional view.
    - The body or organ as a whole is viewed in a cross-sectional, or "sliced," view.
16. **Describe the patient preparation necessary for a CT scan.**
    - If contrast medium is used for a head and chest CT scan, the patient should avoid fluid and foods for 8 hours, and the patient should be asked about allergies

to iodine or shellfish. All metal objects should be removed from the patient.

17. **Explain how positron emission tomography (PET) scans pinpoint cancer sites or other abnormally functioning areas in the body.**
    - PET scans use tracers that are taken up by cancer or other cells. A specialized camera picks up the signals sent out by these cells, and a computer converts these signals into images.

18. **Describe the patient preparation necessary for a PET scan.**
    - Patients must fast for 6 hours before a PET scan.

19. **List two safety precautions for employees working in areas where they could be exposed to radiation.**
    - A dosimeter should be worn to monitor radiation exposure.
    - Employees should stand behind a lead barrier to block exposure to radiation.

20. **Identify two topics the medical assistant must address with the patient when scheduling x-ray examinations.**
    - Patients should be told (a) the approximate duration of the examination and (b) any special preparations required for the procedure.

21. **State the most important task for the medical assistant after patient testing.**
    - The medical assistant must be certain that a written report is received in the medical office for the physician to review.

22. **Analyze a realistic medical office situation and apply your understanding of radiography and diagnostic imaging to determine the best course of action.**
    - Medical assistants need to know about the types of imaging procedures that are performed and why and how each is used.

23. **Describe the impact on patient care when medical assistants understand the concepts associated with radiography and diagnostic imaging and how patients are prepared for these procedures.**
    - Continuity of patient care is maintained when the medical assistant is aware of the functions of various forms of radiography and can answer patients' questions.
    - Proper patient preparation is necessary to provide the best results from diagnostic imaging procedures.

PRACTICAL APPLICATIONS

If you have accomplished the objectives in this chapter, you will be able to make better choices as a medical assistant. Take another look at this situation and decide what you would do.

Suzanne is a medical assistant who works for Dr. Sahara. Dr. Sahara has a medical office with the equipment for basic radiography. She sends her patients to specialized radiographic offices when more extensive testing is necessary. Dr. Sahara informs Suzanne that she has ordered these diagnostic imaging tests: (1) gallbladder ultrasound for middle-aged Mr. Donnolly; (2) baseline mammography for 40-year-old Mrs. Martens; (3) MRI for Mrs. Smith because of a possible brain lesion; and (4) chest radiograph for Mr. Charles, a patient with parkinsonism, because of possible pneumonia. Mr. Charles's chest x-ray film is inconclusive, so Dr. Sahara orders a CT scan. When the CT scan is suspicious, Dr. Sahara orders a PET scan for Mr. Charles 2 days later, and the results come back positive for cancer.

Would you be able to prepare patients for these procedures? Could you answer patient questions concerning the procedures?

1. What protective equipment and safety features should Suzanne use when she is taking x-ray films in Dr. Sahara's office?
2. If Suzanne were asked to perform an "AP, PA, oblique, and lat" views of a forearm, in what positions would she place the arm?
3. What preparation would be needed for Mr. Donnolly's ultrasound of the gallbladder? Why would contrast media be used when the original x-ray films of the gallbladder were taken?
4. What does the white area on an x-ray film indicate? The gray area? The black area?
5. What preparation is necessary for Mrs. Martens's mammogram? What would happen if she were not prepared for the test?
6. Why was MRI used for diagnosing a possible brain lesion?
7. What patient preparation is necessary for a chest radiograph? Why did Dr. Sahara order a CT scan when the chest x-ray was inconclusive?
8. What does the PET scan show that is not in evidence with MRI? What is used as the tracer for cancer cells?
9. How would Mr. Charles's parkinsonism affect his x-ray films and MR images?
10. What role does the medical assistant play in scheduling patients for imaging tests?
11. What should Suzanne do if the x-ray report on the PET scan does not arrive within the week?

WEB SEARCH

1. Research qualifications for becoming certified in your state to take x-ray films in the medical office.

- **Keywords:** Use the following keywords in your search: office radiology, x-ray technician, radiologic technologist, limited radiography.

38 Therapeutic Procedures

evolve   http://evolve.elsevier.com/klieger/medicalassisting

Therapeutic procedures are performed to enhance the body's healing processes. These procedures also can assist patients with mobility. Physicians prescribe various therapeutic treatments and order therapeutic devices based on a patient's condition and the desired outcome. The medical assistant must understand and be able to use the proper techniques for eye and ear irrigation, bandaging, heat and cold therapy, ultrasound therapy, and measurement of patients for ambulatory devices. In addition, the assistant must provide instructions to patients on the use of these procedures. The medical assistant may also be asked to assist the physician with the application and removal of casts.

By performing these techniques effectively, the medical assistant can provide comfort and support to the patient while aiding in the healing process.

LEARNING OBJECTIVES

You will be able to do the following after completing this chapter:

Key Terms
1. Define, appropriately use, and spell all the Key Terms for this chapter.

Ear Treatments
2. Demonstrate the correct procedure for irrigating the external ear canal to remove cerumen or foreign objects.
3. Demonstrate the procedure for properly instilling prescribed medication in an affected ear.
4. Explain why extreme care must be taken when working with a patient's infected ear.

Eye Treatments
5. Demonstrate the correct procedure for irrigating a patient's eye to remove foreign particles.
6. Demonstrate the procedure for properly instilling prescribed medication in an affected eye.
7. Explain why the medical assistant should be careful not to touch the surface of the eye with the tip of the irrigating syringe, the tip of the eyedropper, or the finger.

Bandaging
8. List three common uses for bandages.
9. Differentiate between an elastic bandage and a Kling-type bandage.
10. List and briefly describe five basic bandage turns.
11. Demonstrate the procedure for properly applying a tubular gauze bandage to an affected area.

Cold Therapy
12. Explain the effects of local application of cold therapy on an injured body part.
13. Demonstrate the procedure for properly applying an ice bag.
14. Demonstrate the procedure for properly applying cold compresses.
15. Demonstrate the procedure for properly activating and applying a chemical cold pack.

Heat Therapy
16. Explain the effects of local application of heat therapy on an injured body part.
17. Demonstrate the procedure for properly applying a hot water bag.
18. Demonstrate the procedure for properly applying a heating pad.
19. Demonstrate the procedure for properly applying a hot compress to increase circulation.
20. Demonstrate the procedure for properly applying hot soaks for pain or swelling relief.

Ultrasound Therapy
21. List three therapeutic uses of ultrasound therapy.
22. Demonstrate the correct procedure for administering an ultrasound treatment.

Ambulation Devices

23. Explain the importance of ensuring that an ambulatory device properly fits the patient.
24. Demonstrate the procedure for properly measuring a patient for crutches.
25. Demonstrate the correct procedure for providing instructions to the patient for the appropriate crutch gait, depending on the patient's injury or condition.
26. Demonstrate the procedure for properly measuring and instructing the patient in the use of a walker.
27. Demonstrate the procedure for properly measuring and instructing the patient in the use of a cane.

Casts

28. Explain the purpose of a cast.
29. Demonstrate the correct procedure for providing supplies and assistance during plaster-of-Paris or fiberglass cast application and instructing the patient in cast care and nutritional requirements for healing.
30. Describe the process of cast removal and explain patient instructions that medical assistants may need to provide during the procedure.

Patient-Centered Professionalism

31. Analyze a realistic medical office situation and apply your understanding of therapeutic procedures to determine the best course of action.
32. Describe the impact on patient care when medical assistants understand the purpose and use of therapeutic procedures in the medical office.

KEY TERMS

air cast	heating pad
ambulation device	hot water bag
axillary crutches	ice bag
bandage turns	immobilization
cane	instillation
cast	irrigation
cast cutter	Kling-type bandage
cast padding	ointment
cast spreader	orthopedist
cerumen	patent
chemical hot/cold pack	plaster cast
circular turn	platform crutches
cold therapy	pressure ulcer
compress	recurrent turn
coupling agent	soak
crutches	spiral reverse turn
elastic bandage	spiral turn
fiberglass cast	stockinette
figure-eight turn	synthetic cast
forearm (Lofstrand) crutches	therapeutic procedures
gait pattern	tubular gauze
goniometer	ultrasound therapy
heat therapy	walker

PRACTICAL APPLICATIONS

Read the following scenario and keep it in mind as you learn about various therapeutic procedures performed in the medical office.

A multispecialty practice has medical assistants who work with each of the specialists. Allene, a medical assistant who has not had the benefit of training, works with Dr. Sumar, an ophthalmologist. Gerald, a graduate of a medical assisting program, works with Dr. Herzog, an orthopedist. The ophthalmologist and the otolaryngologist share the same examination room, but they use it on different days. Allene is not very busy one day, so she decides to clean the medicine cabinet and rearrange the drugs. She moves the ophthalmic medications to the spot where the otic medications are usually stored and vice versa.

When Dr. Sumar treats a patient with conjunctivitis the next day, Allene hands him an otic preparation for the eye instillation. Luckily, Dr. Sumar reads the label on the medication before instilling the drops into the patient's eye. Later in the day, Dr. Sumar reprimands Allene for handing him the otic drops.

Gerald is the person who communicates to the orthopedic patients the necessity of correct application of the bandaging, as well as the care of a cast after its application. For those who need cold or heat therapy, Gerald is responsible for the applications as ordered by Dr. Herzog and also performs the ultrasound treatments as indicated. During ultrasound treatments, Gerald is very careful to have sufficient coupling agent and to keep the head of the machine moving at all times.

Would you be able to step into the role of Allene or Gerald and perform their duties successfully?

EAR TREATMENTS

Ear treatments are performed in the medical office, often as a part of an ear examination. Ear irrigation and ear instillation are two procedures that medical assistants need to understand and be able to perform. You may want to review the structure and function of the ear in Chapter 17 before learning about ear irrigation and instillation. Box 38-1 reviews charting requirements when documenting ear treatments and other therapeutic procedures.

Ear Irrigation

Before examining the ear, the physician may request that ear **irrigation** be performed to remove an accumulation of impacted **cerumen** (earwax). This procedure may also be ordered to remove a foreign object. Procedure 38-1 explains how to perform ear irrigation.

When irrigating the ear, it is important to instill the solution toward the roof of the canal. Avoid using a solution that is cold or too warm, blowing air into the ear, or in any way touching the eardrum. When irrigating (flushing) the ear

PROCEDURE 38-1 Perform an Ear Irrigation

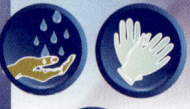

TASK: Irrigate the external ear canal to remove cerumen.

EQUIPMENT AND SUPPLIES
- Irrigating solution (may use warm tap water)
- Container to hold irrigating solution (sterile)
- Irrigating syringe or Reiner's ear syringe
- Ear basin for drainage
- Disposable barrier drape
- Disposable gloves
- Otoscope with disposable speculum
- Biohazardous waste container
- Gauze squares
- Patient's medical record

SKILLS/RATIONALE
STANDARD PRECAUTIONS ARE TO BE FOLLOWED.

1. **Procedural Step.** Sanitize the hands.
   An alcohol-based hand rub may be used instead of washing hands with soap and water, unless hands are visibly soiled.
   Rationale. Hand sanitization promotes infection control.

2. **Procedural Step.** Assemble equipment and supplies.
   Rationale. It is important to have all supplies and equipment ready and available before starting any procedure to ensure efficiency.

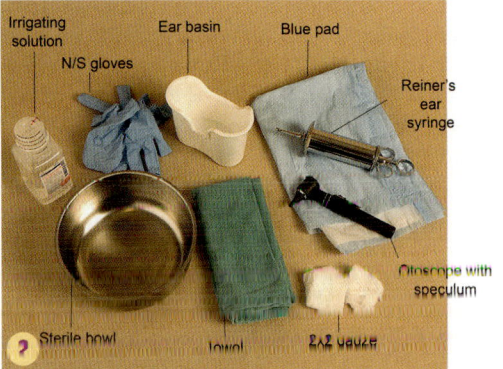

3. **Procedural Step.** Verify the physician's order.
   If a prepared irrigating solution is to be used, check the expiration date of the solution. As with all medications, ensure that the correct preparation is being used by reading the label three times: the first time when the irrigating solution is taken from the cupboard, the second time while the solution is poured into the basin, and the third time just before returning the solution to the cupboard. Also verify which ear is to be treated.
   NOTE: All medications must be returned to storage before patient use.

4. **Procedural Step.** Warm the irrigating solution to body temperature by running the container under warm tap water.
   The physician may order that warm tap water be used as the irrigating solution. For patient comfort, the water should be between 98.6° and 100° F.
   Rationale. The solution must be carefully compared with the physician's instructions. Outdated solutions must be discarded because they may cause adverse effects. If the solution is too cold or too warm, the patient may become dizzy or nauseated from overstimulation of the inner ear.

5. **Procedural Step.** Obtain the patient's medical record.

6. **Procedural Step.** Greet the patient, introduce yourself, and confirm the patient's identity. Ask the patient to have a seat on the end of the examination table.
   Rationale. Identifying the patient ensures the procedure is performed on the correct patient.

7. **Procedural Step.** Explain the procedure to the patient and ask the patient if they have an allergy to latex.
   Explain that the procedure usually is not painful but that the patient may feel some discomfort or a sense of pressure. Some patients may feel dizzy or nauseated. The patient may have a sensation of warmth or even burning as the solution comes in contact with the tympanic membrane.
   Rationale. Explaining the procedure to the patient promotes cooperation and provides a means of obtaining implied consent. Allergy to latex requires the use of nonlatex gloves. Although it is important to inform the patient of all outcomes of a procedure, it is equally as important not to alarm the patient. If patients are told that a procedure is going to feel a certain way or that they can expect to feel dizzy or nauseated, they may experience these discomforts simply because they were told they would.

8. **Procedural Step.** Put on disposable gloves.
   Rationale. This prevents the spread of infection.

9. **Procedural Step.** Examine the ear.
   Place a disposable ear speculum on the otoscope and gently pull the auricle upward and back (if an adult patient) to straighten the external auditory canal. Insert the otoscope and examine the external auditory canal and the tympanic membrane with the otoscope.
   Rationale. Viewing the external auditory canal and tympanic membrane before the irrigation provides a baseline for comparison on

Continued

PROCEDURE 38-1 Perform an Ear Irrigation—cont'd

completing the irrigation. You may also be able to visualize the placement of excessive cerumen or a foreign body that needs to be dislodged.

10. **Procedural Step. Position the patient.**
    a. Ask the patient to tilt the head slightly forward and toward the affected ear.
    b. Place a water-resistant disposable barrier on the patient's shoulder on the affected side.
    c. Provide an ear basin and ask the patient to hold the basin snugly against the head underneath the affected ear.

    Rationale. The water-resistant disposable barrier protects the patient's clothing and prevents water from running down the patient's neck, chest, and back. Proper positioning allows the solution to flow into the basin by gravity. The basin is used to catch the irrigating solution, any drainage, and cerumen. A gown may be offered to the patient before the procedure to protect the clothing from accidents.

11. **Procedural Step. Using the solution ordered to perform the irrigation, moisten 2 × 2 gauze squares and clean the outer ear (auricle, pinna).**

    Rationale. This will remove any discharge or other debris that may be present. Debris or foreign particles should not be introduced into the ear during the irrigation.

12. **Procedural Step. Pour the warmed solution into the sterile basin.**

13. **Procedural Step. Fill the ear-irrigating syringe with the ordered solution.**
    If air has been drawn into the syringe during this process, it must be expelled before the irrigation.

    Rationale. Introducing air into the auditory canal is painful for the patient, and, if introduced too forcefully, air can cause severe damage to the tympanic membrane.

14. **Procedural Step. Position the ear.**
    Straighten the external ear canal by gently pulling the ear upward and backward for adults and children over 3 years old or downward and backward for children age 3 years and younger.

    Rationale. Straightening the ear canal allows the irrigating solution to reach all areas of the auditory canal.

15. **Procedural Step. Irrigate the ear.**
    An ear irrigation may be ordered to remove a foreign body, soothe inflamed membranes, remove impacted cerumen, or clear discharge. The reason the irrigation was ordered will determine the length of irrigation.

    Insert the tip of the irrigating syringe into the ear canal and gently inject the irrigating solution toward the roof of the canal. It is important that the tip of the syringe not be inserted too deeply and that the solution is injected toward the roof of the canal to prevent damage to the tympanic membrane. The tip of the syringe must not obstruct the opening to the ear canal; the irrigating solution must be able to flow freely out of the canal.

Rationale. The irrigating solution should not be injected too forcefully and should not be directed at the tympanic membrane or damage to the tympanic membrane can occur. Directing the solution toward the roof of the external ear canal also helps when trying to dislodge foreign bodies; the stream of the solution will flow in over the top of the object, back behind it, and then out from the bottom, loosening the trapped particle. If the tip of the syringe is inserted too deeply, the patient will experience discomfort, and the tympanic membrane may be damaged. Patients often experience the most discomfort when the solution is injected directly at the tympanic membrane.

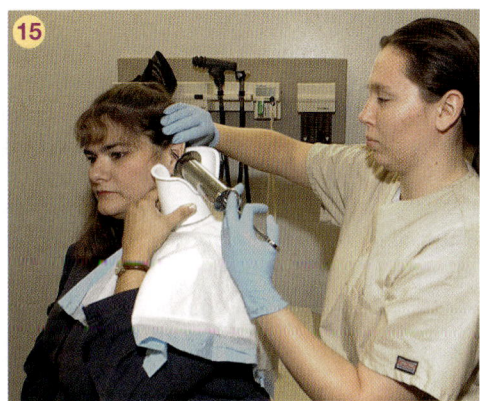

16. **Procedural Step. Continue irrigating until all the solution has been used or until the desired results have been achieved.**
    a. Refill the syringe as needed.
    b. If requested by the physician, periodically examine the ear canal with the otoscope to check the progress of the procedure, especially if the procedure has been ordered to remove cerumen or a foreign body.
    c. Observe the returning solution, and note the type of material present (e.g., cerumen, discharge, or foreign object) and the amount (small, moderate, or large).

    Rationale. All dislodged materials in the returning solution and the amount of the substance must be noted for the patient's medical record.

17. **Procedural Step. Conclude the irrigation.**
    a. Examine the ear canal with the otoscope at the end of the procedure.
    b. Gently dry the outside of the ear with a cotton ball or 2 × 2 gauze squares.
    c. Explain to the patient that the ear may feel sensitive for a few hours. Ask the patient to lie on the examination table with the affected ear down for approximately 15 minutes. A moistened cotton ball may be placed in the ear at the physician's request.

    Rationale. Lying on the examination table with the affected ear down allows any solution remaining in the ear to drain out. Placing a moist cotton ball in the ear canal provides a barrier and helps alleviate

Continued

PROCEDURE 38-1 Perform an Ear Irrigation—cont'd

discomfort or any sensitivity the patient may feel after the procedure.

18. **Procedural Step.** Remove gloves and sanitize the hands.

    Always sanitize the hands after every procedure or after using gloves.

19. **Procedural Step.** The physician will examine the ear and provide follow-up instructions to the patient.

    The physician may ask to examine the returned irrigating solution and will require the otoscope to examine the ear canal. Instructions are provided to the patient both verbally and in writing.

20. **Procedural Step.** Ask if the patient has any questions or would like clarification on any instructions. Thank the patient and escort the patient to the reception area for payment or scheduling follow-up appointment(s).

21. **Procedural Step.** Document the procedure.

    Include the date and time; which ear was irrigated; type, strength, and amount of solution used; amount and type of material returned in the irrigating solution; any significant observations; patient instructions; and patient reactions.

22. **Procedural Step.** Clean the equipment and examination room.

    Discard all used supplies in an appropriate waste container. If an item is contaminated with blood, it must be discarded in a biohazardous waste container.

    NOTE: Wear protective gloves when cleaning equipment and the examination room.

CHARTING EXAMPLE

Date	
12/3/xx	1:20 p.m. Irrigated right ear c̄ 250 cc sterile normal saline. Large amount of soft, brown, stringy cerumen removed. Patient tolerated procedure well. No complaints of dizziness, nausea, or pain.——————— E. Bryant, CMA (AAMA)

BOX 38-1
Documentation When Charting Therapeutic Procedures

1. Date
2. Time
3. Name or explanation of therapeutic procedure performed stating exact location on body
4. Results
5. Patient reaction, if any. If no reaction, can state, "Pt. tolerated procedure well."
6. Proper signature and credential

canal, the ear syringe must never block the canal because this will place pressure on the eardrum and could cause damage to the membrane. The medical assistant must be aware that the patient may experience dizziness after ear irrigation, and the assistant should assist the patient as needed.

Ear Instillation

Ear **instillation** is the process of administering medication to an affected ear. Before medication can be put into the ear, the ear canal must be **patent** (open). Procedure 38-2 explains the process of instilling prescribed medication to an affected ear. The medical assistant must take extreme care when working with a patient who has an infected ear. The inside of the ear is naturally sensitive, and it becomes very painful when infected.

EYE TREATMENTS

Eye treatments are also performed in the medical office. Eye irrigation and eye instillation are two procedures that medical assistants must be able to perform. You may want to review the structure and function of the eye in Chapter 17 before learning about eye irrigation and instillation.

FOR YOUR INFORMATION
KEEP EYE AND EAR MEDICATIONS SEPARATE

It is important to store eye medications and ear medications in separate places because their containers and packaging are similar. Also, ophthalmic preparations are sterile, whereas otic preparations are not sterile. Only sterile medications should be placed in the eye. These medications should be kept in the same location at all times to prevent the instillation of otic medication for ophthalmic uses.

Eye Irrigation

Eye irrigations are performed to rinse irritants or discharge away from affected eyes. Irritants and discharge can cause damage to the exterior eye. Rinsing them away minimizes tissue damage and soothes the irritated tissue. Procedure 38-3 describes the process of performing eye irrigation.

All irrigating solutions must be sterile. When performing eye irrigation, the medical assistant must be careful not to

Text continued on p. 817

Therapeutic Procedures CHAPTER 38 813

PROCEDURE 38-2 Perform an Ear Instillation

TASK: Properly instill prescribed medication to the affected ear.

EQUIPMENT AND SUPPLIES
- Otic drops with sterile dropper
- Cotton balls
- Disposable gloves
- Patient's medical record

SKILLS/RATIONALE

STANDARD PRECAUTIONS ARE TO BE FOLLOWED.

1. **Procedural Step.** Sanitize the hands.
   An alcohol-based hand rub may be used instead of washing hands with soap and water, unless hands are visibly soiled.
   Rationale. Hand sanitization promotes infection control.

2. **Procedural Step.** Assemble equipment and supplies.
   Rationale. It is important to have all supplies and equipment ready and available before starting any procedure to ensure efficiency.

3. **Procedural Step.** Verify the physician's order.
   Any medication that is instilled in the ear must be labeled with the word "otic." Check the expiration date of the solution. As with all medications, ensure that the correct preparation is being used by reading the label three times: (a) when the medication is taken from the cupboard, (b) while the medication is being drawn into the dropper, and (c) just before returning the solution to the cupboard. Verify the number of drops ordered and to which ear the medication is to be instilled.
   NOTE: All medications must be returned to storage before patient use.
   Rationale. The solution must be carefully compared with the physician's instructions to prevent an error. Outdated solutions must be discarded because they may produce adverse effects. Medications without the word "otic" must not be used in the ear because they could result in injury to the ear.

4. **Procedural Step.** Obtain the patient's medical record.

5. **Procedural Step.** Greet the patient, introduce yourself, and confirm the patient's identity.
   Rationale. Identifying the patient ensures the procedure is performed on the correct patient.

6. **Procedural Step.** Explain the procedure to the patient and ask the patient if they have an allergy to latex.
   Rationale. Explaining the procedure to the patient promotes cooperation and provides a means of obtaining implied consent. An allergy to latex requires the use of nonlatex gloves.

7. **Procedural Step.** Put on disposable gloves.
   Rationale. This prevents the spread of infection.

8. **Procedural Step.** Ask the patient to tilt the head in the direction of the unaffected ear.
   Rationale. In this position, gravity helps the medication to flow into the ear canal and to be retained for the required time.

9. **Procedural Step.** Warm and mix the medication, if necessary, and draw the medication into the dropper or, if using a soft-sided plastic container, remove the cap.
   If the medication bottle feels cold to the touch, gently roll it back and forth between your hands to warm and mix it.
   Rationale. If the medication bottle feels cold, the medication itself is probably cold. Cold medication may cause discomfort to the patient.

10. **Procedural Step.** Position the ear.
    Straighten the external ear canal by gently pulling the ear upward and backward for adults and children over 3 years old, or downward and backward for children age 3 years and younger.
    Rationale. The ear canal must be straightened to allow the medication to reach all areas of the auditory canal.

11. **Procedural Step.** Place the medication in the ear.
    Insert the tip of the dropper into the ear canal, making sure the dropper never touches the ear canal, or turn the

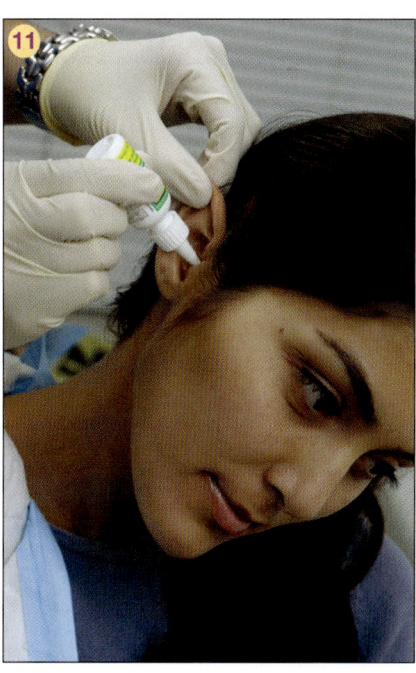

Continued

PROCEDURE 38-2 Perform an Ear Instillation—cont'd

soft-sided container downward. Instill the correct amount of medication (number of drops) ordered by the physician by squeezing the bulb of the dropper or squeezing the container gently. Medication should be instilled drop by drop along the side of the canal.

12. **Procedural Step. Discard any unused medication in the dropper or replace the cap.**
    Unused medication must be discarded before returning the dropper to the bottle. The dropper must never touch the patient or the outside of the bottle; if it does, the dropper must be discarded.
    Rationale. Unused solution must never be returned to the bottle because it would contaminate the remaining solution. Touching the dropper to the patient or the outside of the bottle contaminates the dropper.

13. **Procedural Step. Instruct the patient to rest on the unaffected side for approximately 5 minutes.**
    Rationale. Resting with the unaffected side down for 5 minutes allows the medication to distribute completely throughout the ear canal. If the patient sits up straight, the medication may run out and the patient will not receive the full benefit of the instillation.

14. **Procedural Step. If the physician orders it, loosely place a cotton ball moistened with the prescribed medication in the ear canal for 15 minutes.**
    Rationale. The moistened cotton ball prevents the medication from running out when the patient is upright. Moistening the cotton ball prevents the cotton ball from absorbing the medication.

15. **Procedural Step. Remove gloves and sanitize the hands.**
    Always sanitize the hands after every procedure or after using gloves.

16. **Procedural Step. Provide the patient with verbal and written follow-up instructions.**

17. **Procedural Step. Document the procedure.**
    Include the date and time, the name and strength of the medication, number of drops, which ear(s) received the instillation, any significant observations, and the patient's reaction.

18. **Procedural Step. Clean the equipment and examination room.**
    Discard all used supplies in an appropriate waste container.

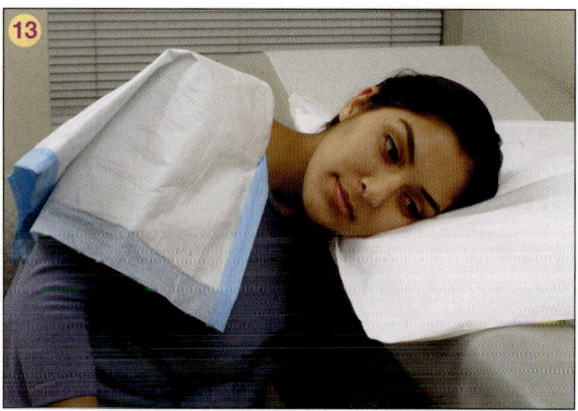

CHARTING EXAMPLE

Date	
12/4/xx	1:30 p.m. Ofloxacin, gtts v instilled, right ear. No discharge present. Pt tolerated the procedure well with no complaint of pain, dizziness, or nausea.————————————————L. Bradford, CMA (AAMA)

PROCEDURE 38-3

Perform an Eye Irrigation

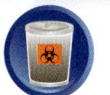

TASK: Irrigate the patient's eye(s) to remove foreign particles (by flushing irritants from the eye) and to soothe irritated tissue.

EQUIPMENT AND SUPPLIES
- Sterile irrigating solution
- Sterile container to hold the solution
- Sterile rubber bulb syringe or bottled solution
- Disposable gloves (powder free)
- Basin for the returned solution
- Sterile cotton balls or sterile gauze squares
- Disposable moisture-resistant towel
- Biohazardous waste container
- Patient's medical record
- Tissues

SKILLS/RATIONALE

STANDARD PRECAUTIONS ARE TO BE FOLLOWED.

1. **Procedural Step. Sanitize the hands.**
   An alcohol-based hand rub may be used instead of washing hands with soap and water, unless hands are visibly soiled.
   Rationale. Hand sanitization promotes infection control.

2. **Procedural Step. Assemble equipment and supplies.**
   Rationale. It is important to have all supplies and equipment ready and available before starting any procedure to ensure efficiency.

3. **Procedural Step. Verify the physician's order.**
   Typically, the physician will order normal saline as the irrigating solution. Check the expiration date of the solution. As with all medications, ensure that the correct preparation is being used by reading the label three times: the first time when the medication is taken from the cupboard, the second time while the medication is being prepared, and the third time just before returning the solution to the cupboard.
   NOTE: If both eyes are to be irrigated, two separate sets of supplies and equipment must be used to prevent cross-infection from one eye to the other.
   Rationale. The solution should be carefully compared with the physician's instructions to prevent an error. If the solution is outdated, consult the physician; it may produce undesirable effects.

4. **Procedural Step. Warm the irrigating solution to body temperature by running the container under warm running tap water (98.6° to 100° F).**
   Rationale. If the solution is too cold or too warm, it will be uncomfortable for the patient.

5. **Procedural Step. Obtain the patient's medical record.**

6. **Procedural Step. Greet the patient, introduce yourself, and confirm the patient's identity.**
   Rationale. Identifying the patient ensures the procedure is performed on the correct patient.

7. **Procedural Step. Explain the procedure to the patient and ask the patient if they have an allergy to latex.**
   Rationale. Explaining the procedure to the patient promotes cooperation and provides a means of obtaining implied consent. Allergy to latex requires the use of nonlatex gloves.

8. **Procedural Step. Position the patient.**
   Place the patient in a supine position. Ask the patient to tilt the head toward the affected eye. A moisture-resistant towel should be placed on the patient's shoulder to protect the patient's clothing. Position a basin tightly against the patient's cheek under the affected eye to catch the irrigating solution.
   Rationale. The patient is positioned to prevent solution from the affected eye from flowing into the unaffected eye and causing cross-contamination.

9. **Procedural Step. Put on disposable powder-free gloves.**
   Rationale. Using powdered gloves may irritate the patient's eyes if powder from the outside of the glove comes in contact with the eye.

10. **Procedural Step. Remove any debris or discharge from the patient's eyelid.**
    Moisten three or four cotton balls or gauze squares with the irrigating solution and wipe the eyelids and eyelashes from the inner canthus (next to the nose) to the outer canthus. Use each cotton ball or gauze square to wipe the eyelid only once and then discard.
    Rationale. Cleaning the eyelids prevents any foreign particles being driven into the eye during the irrigation. Cleansing from the inner to the outer canthus prevents cross-infection.

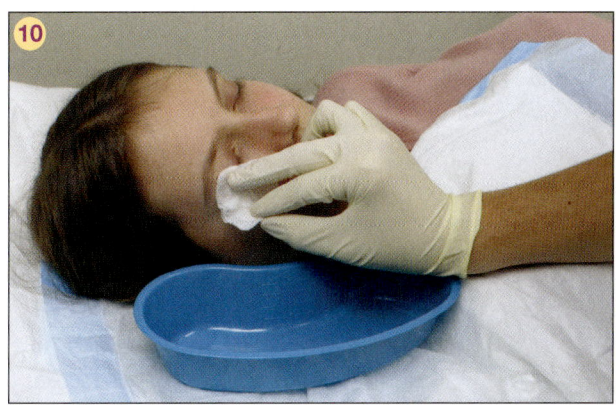

Continued

PROCEDURE 38-3 Perform an Eye Irrigation—cont'd

11. **Procedural Step.** **Prepare the irrigation syringe.**
    Remove the cap from the sterile irrigating solution bottle, being careful not to touch the tip of the bottle and keeping the inside of the cap up to prevent contamination. If you are using an irrigating syringe instead of using the solution directly from the sterile bottle, pour the warmed solution into the sterile basin. Fill the irrigating syringe by squeezing and releasing the bulb until the ordered amount of solution fills the syringe.

12. **Procedural Step.** **Expose the lower conjunctiva by separating the eyelids with the gloved index finger and thumb and ask the patient to stare at a fixed spot.**
    Rationale. Staring at a fixed spot limits the patient's eye movement during the irrigation. The patient will naturally want to close the eye during the irrigation, so it must be held open.

13. **Procedural Step.** **Irrigate the affected eye(s).**
    Rest the syringe or irrigating solution bottle on the bridge of the patient's nose, being extremely careful not to touch the eye or conjunctiva with the tip. Gently release the solution, at an even flow rate and directed at the lower conjunctiva, from the inner canthus toward the outer canthus.
    NOTE: If both eyes are being treated, two medical assistants may be required to perform the procedure or one eye may be irrigated at a time. Provide a gown and ask the patient to change clothes. Prepare two sets of supplies. Place the patient in a supine position and ask the patient to stare up at the ceiling. Place a towel under the patient's shoulders. A basin should be provided for both sides. Follow Steps 9 through 13, being certain that the irrigating solution runs from the inner to the outer canthus of both eyes.

    Rationale. Directing the solution away from the unaffected eye prevents cross-contamination. To avoid injury to the cornea, the irrigating solution must be directed at the lower conjunctiva.

14. **Procedural Step.** **Continue with the irrigation until the correct amount of solution has been used or as ordered by the physician.**
    You may be required to refill the irrigating syringe or to open a second bottle of sterile normal saline. The amount of the solution ordered will vary according to the purpose of the irrigation.

15. **Procedural Step.** **When the correct amount of irrigating solution has been used, dry the eyelids from the inner to the outer canthus (as in Step 10) using dry cotton balls or dry gauze squares.**

16. **Procedural Step.** **Provide the patient with tissue to wipe the face and neck as needed. Inform the patient that the eye(s) may be red and irritated.**

17. **Procedural Step.** **Remove gloves and sanitize the hands.**
    Always sanitize the hands after every procedure or after using gloves.

18. **Procedural Step.** **Provide follow-up instructions.**

19. **Procedural Step.** **Document the procedure.**
    Include the date and time; which eye was irrigated; type, strength, and amount of solution used; and any significant observations and patient reactions.

20. **Procedural Step.** **Clean the equipment and examination room.**
    Discard all used supplies in an appropriate waste container. If discharge or exudate was present, discard contaminated supplies in the biohazardous waste container.

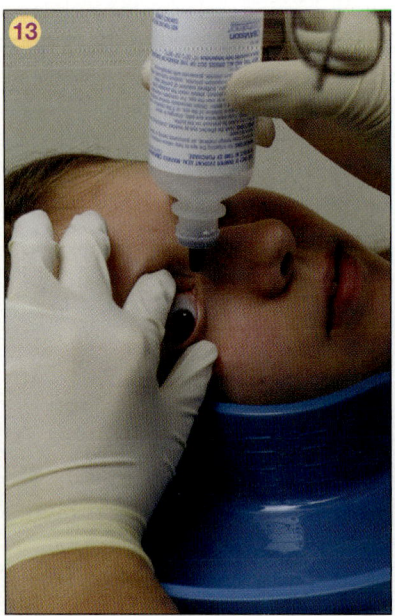

CHARTING EXAMPLE

Date	
12/3/xx	11:00 a.m. right eye irrigated c̄ 100 cc sterile normal saline to remove foreign particles. Several small brown flecks returned. Patient tolerated procedure well. No complaints of discomfort.————————— N. Collins, CMA (AAMA)

touch the surface of the eye or the finger with the tip of the irrigating syringe. Contact with either of these will contaminate the tip of the irrigating syringe and therefore anything else the tip contacts. Always irrigate with the patient's head tilted away from the unaffected eye to prevent cross-contamination.

Eye Instillation

Eye instillation is the application of prescribed medication to the eye. Eye medications are either a liquid or an **ointment.** Procedure 38-4 describes the process of performing eye instillation.

As with eye irrigation, be careful not to touch the surface of the eye with the tip of the eyedropper or the finger to prevent cross-contamination.

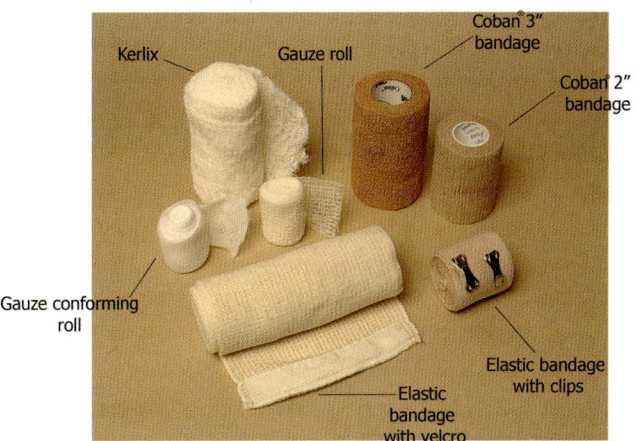

FIGURE 38-1 Various bandage types.

> ### PATIENT-CENTERED PROFESSIONALISM
> - Why is it important for the medical assistant to understand the purpose of and be knowledgeable about eye and ear treatments?

BANDAGING

Bandages have many uses, including the following:
- Support or **immobilization** of an injured body part.
- Securing a dressing (e.g., gauze) in place.
- Application of pressure to control bleeding.

Medical assistants need to be familiar with the types of bandages available and the basic bandage turns.

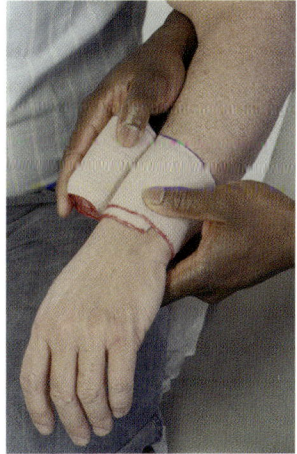

FIGURE 38-2 A circular bandage turn anchors a bandage.

Types of Bandages

The two types of bandages most often used by the medical assistant are elastic cloth bandages and wrinkled gauze–type roller bandages such as Kling bandages. Tubular gauze is also used in some medical offices. The type of bandage used depends on the type of injury or wound. These types of bandages work best on the elderly because of thin skin. Adhesive bandages may cause a skin tear if applied directly to the skin when removed.
- **Elastic bandages** can be stretched and molded around a body part. They can be removed and reused on the same patient as long as they are not soiled (Figure 38-1). Coban is a latex-free stretchable bandage that sticks to itself so fasteners are not needed.
- **Kling-type bandages** stretch but are not elastic. They are a soft woven material that molds around irregular areas and are most often used to hold dressings in place on the head or extremities (see Figure 38-1).
- **Tubular gauze** bandages consist of loose, elastic cotton fibers in a tubular roll and use a metal tube for application. Essentially, tubular gauze is used to cover rounded body parts such as fingers and toes. Tubular gauze can also be applied over a sterile dressing to keep the dressing in place. Procedure 38-5 explains the process of applying a tubular gauze bandage.

When applying a bandage, it is important to inspect the patient's skin for any break or swelling. In addition, be sure not to impair circulation when applying the bandage.

Bandage Turns

There are basically five **bandage turns** that are used either to support or to secure: the circular, spiral, spiral reverse, figure-eight, and recurrent turns. It is important to remember that all bandaging begins at the distal end and proceeds proximally.
1. The **circular turn** is used on areas that are uniform in width such as the fingers, toes, head, and wrist (Figure 38-2). Each turn overlaps the previous turn. A circular turn can also be used to anchor a bandage.

Text continued on p. 821

PROCEDURE 38-4 Perform an Eye Instillation

TASK: Properly instill prescribed medication in the affected eye(s).

EQUIPMENT AND SUPPLIES
- Ophthalmic drops with sterile eyedropper, or ophthalmic ointment ordered by physician
- Sterile cotton balls, or sterile gauze squares
- Tissues
- Disposable gloves (powder free)
- Patient's medical record

SKILLS/RATIONALE

STANDARD PRECAUTIONS ARE TO BE FOLLOWED.

1. **Procedural Step.** Sanitize the hands.
   An alcohol-based hand rub may be used instead of washing hands with soap and water, unless hands are visibly soiled.
   Rationale. Hand sanitization promotes infection control.

2. **Procedural Step.** Assemble equipment and supplies.
   Rationale. It is important to have all supplies and equipment ready and available before starting any procedure to ensure efficiency.

3. **Procedural Step.** Verify the physician's order.
   The medication should bear the word "ophthalmic." Check the expiration date. As with all medications, ensure that the correct preparation is being used by reading the label three times: (a) when the medication is taken from the cupboard, (b) while you are drawing the medication into the dropper, and (c) just before returning the solution to the cupboard. Verify the number of drops ordered (if a liquid) and to which eye the medication should be instilled.
   Rationale. The medication should be carefully compared with the physician's instructions to prevent a drug error. Any medication instilled into the eye should contain the word "ophthalmic." Medication without "ophthalmic" should never be placed in the eye because it could result in serious injury. If the medication is outdated, consult the physician; it may produce undesirable effects.

4. **Procedural Step.** Obtain the patient's medical record.

5. **Procedural Step.** Greet the patient, introduce yourself, and confirm the patient's identity. Ask the patient to have a seat on the end of the examination table.
   Rationale. Identifying the patient ensures the procedure is performed on the correct patient.

6. **Procedural Step.** Explain the procedure to the patient and ask the patient if they have an allergy to latex and to any eye medication.
   Rationale. Explaining the procedure to the patient promotes cooperation and provides a means of obtaining implied consent. This step protects the patient from an allergic response to the medication and to the latex.

7. **Procedural Step.** Place the patient in a sitting or supine position and ask the patient to stare at a fixed spot during the instillation.

8. **Procedural Step.** Put on disposable powder-free gloves and prepare the medication.
   If the medication bottle feels cold to the touch, gently roll it back and forth between your hands to warm the medication.
   Eyedrops: Withdraw the medication into the dropper.
   Eye ointment: Remove the cap from the tip of the tube.
   Rationale. If the medication bottle feels cold, the medication itself is probably cold. Cold medication may cause discomfort to the patient.

9. **Procedural Step.** Prepare the eye for instillation.
   a. Ask the patient to look up to the ceiling and keep both eyes open.
   b. Expose the lower conjunctival sac of the affected eye.
   c. Hold a gauze square or tissue in the fingers of your nondominant hand on the patient's cheekbone just below the affected eye.
   d. Gently pull the skin of the cheek downward.
   Rationale. Looking up with both eyes open helps keep the patient from blinking during the instillation and the dropper from touching the cornea. The gauze square or tissue placed on the cheek helps prevent the fingers from slipping.

10. **Procedural Step.** Instill the medication.
    Place the correct number of eyedrops in the center of the lower conjunctival sac of the affected eye or place a thin ribbon of ointment along the length of the lower conjunctival sac from inner to outer canthus. Use a twisting motion to end the ribbon of ointment to help keep the ointment in the eye. The tip of the dropper or ointment tube should be held approximately ½ inch above the eye sac and must never touch the eye.
    Rationale. Medication instilled into the eye must never be placed directly on the eye because it may cause damage to the cornea. Touching the dropper or tube to the eye results in contamination of these items.

Continued

PROCEDURE 38-4 Perform an Eye Instillation—cont'd

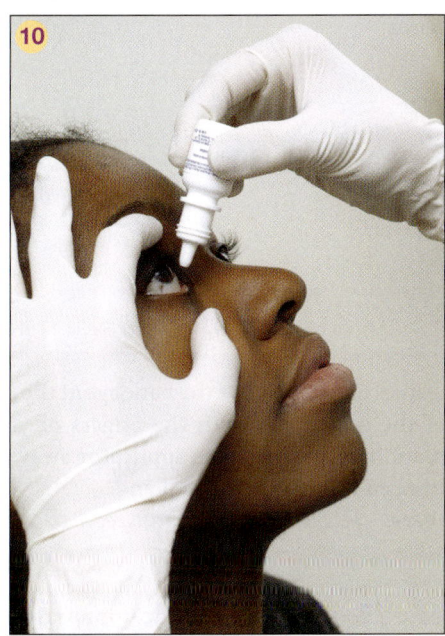

11. **Procedural Step.** Discard any unused solution from the eyedropper and replace the dropper into the bottle or replace the cap.

    Be careful not to let the dropper touch the outside of the bottle when replacing it. When using ointments, replace the cap on the tube.

    Rationale. Unused solution must not be returned to the bottle because it will contaminate the medication remaining in the bottle. Touching the dropper to the outside of the bottle contaminates the dropper; if this occurs, the entire bottle must be discarded.

12. **Procedural Step.** Instruct the patient about the instillation.
    a. Ask the patient to close the eyes gently and rotate the eyeballs.
    b. Advise the patient not to squeeze the eyelids because this will discharge the medicine.
    c. Explain that the patient's vision may be temporarily blurred.

    Rationale. Rotating the eyeballs provides even distribution of the medication across the entire eye. If the eyes are shut tightly, the drops or ointment may be pushed out. If the instillation blurs the patient's vision, arrangements must be made in advance for transportation because the patient must not be permitted to drive until vision is clear.

13. **Procedural Step.** Blot-dry the eyelid from the inner to the outer canthus with a dry gauze square to remove any excess medication.

    Provide the patient with a separate tissue for each eye. Apply gentle pressure to the inner canthus for 1 to 3 minutes.

    Rationale. Applying pressure to the inner canthus prevents eyedrops from going down the nasolacrimal sac. Advise the patient not to wipe the eyes with tissue but to blot any medication that may run out.

14. **Procedural Step.** Provide verbal and written follow-up instructions.

15. **Procedural Step.** Remove gloves and sanitize the hands.

    Always sanitize the hands after every procedure or after using gloves.

16. **Procedural Step.** Document the procedure.

    Include the date and time, name and strength of the medication, number of drops or amount of ointment, which eye(s) received the instillation, any observations noted, and the patient's reaction.

17. **Procedural Step.** Clean the equipment and examination room.

    Discard all used supplies in an appropriate waste container.

CHARTING EXAMPLE

Date	
12/5/xx	11:00 a.m. Chloromycetin 1%, gtts iii instilled both eyes. No discharge present. Patient tolerated procedure well with no c/o pain or discomfort.———————————————————— M. DeMarce, RMA

PROCEDURE 38-5: Apply a Tubular Gauze Bandage

TASK: Properly apply a gauze bandage to the affected area.

EQUIPMENT AND SUPPLIES
- Tube gauze applicator
- Roll of tubular gauze
- Nonallergic tape
- Patient's medical record

SKILLS/RATIONALE

STANDARD PRECAUTIONS ARE TO BE FOLLOWED.

1. **Procedural Step.** Sanitize the hands.
   An alcohol-based hand rub may be used instead of washing hands with soap and water, unless hands are visibly soiled.
   Rationale. Hand sanitization promotes infection control.

2. **Procedural Step.** Assemble equipment and supplies.
   Tube gauze applicators come in a variety of sizes. Select a size that is slightly larger than the appendage to be bandaged. Select a tube gauze that is wide enough to fit over the appendage but narrow enough to make a snug fit.
   Rationale. It is important to have all supplies and equipment ready and available before starting any procedure to ensure efficiency. The applicator should be larger than the body part to allow the gauze to slide easily over it.

3. **Procedural Step.** Obtain the patient's medical record.

4. **Procedural Step.** Greet the patient, introduce yourself, and confirm the patient's identity. Ask the patient to have a seat on the end of the examination table.
   Rationale. Identifying the patient ensures the procedure is performed on the correct patient.

5. **Procedural Step.** Explain the procedure to the patient.
   Rationale. Explaining the procedure to the patient promotes cooperation and provides a means of obtaining implied consent.

6. **Procedural Step.** Prepare the bandage.
   Pull an adequate length of gauze from the boxed roll, approximately 6 to 10 times the length of the appendage, depending on the desired thickness of the completed bandage. Cut the length of gauze from the roll. Spread one end of the tube gauze apart by inserting your fingers into the opening. Slide the now-open end of the tube gauze onto the applicator. Continue to push the tube gauze onto the applicator until the entire length of gauze has been loaded onto the applicator.

7. **Procedural Step.** Gently slide the applicator over the proximal end of the appendage.

8. **Procedural Step.** Anchor the bandage at the proximal end of the appendage with the fingers of your non-dominant hand and pull the applicator away from the proximal end toward the distal end.
   Rationale. The tube gauze must be secured in place to prevent it from sliding. If the bandage is not secured, the appendage will not be adequately covered.

9. **Procedural Step.** Pull the applicator approximately 1 inch past the distal end of the patient's appendage. Continue to hold the bandage in place with your fingers at the proximal end.
   Rationale. The bandage must extend beyond the length of the patient's appendage in order to secure it appropriately.

10. **Procedural Step.** Turn the applicator clockwise, one full turn to anchor the bandage.
    Rationale. Anchoring the bandage holds it securely in place.

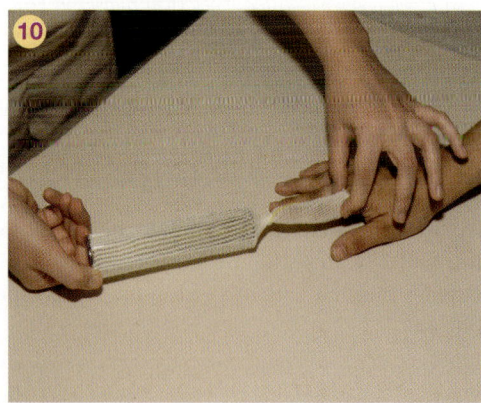

11. **Procedural Step.** Move the applicator back over the distal end of the appendage and gently push forward toward the proximal end of the patient's appendage.
    Rationale. Applying a second layer of bandaging material to the patient's appendage provides additional protective covering.

Continued

PROCEDURE 38-5 Apply a Tubular Gauze Bandage—cont'd

12. **Procedural Step.** Repeat Steps 9 to 11 to accomplish the number of layers needed.
13. **Procedural Step.** Complete the last layer at the proximal end, remove the applicator, and trim the excess gauze as needed.
14. **Procedural Step.** Apply nonallergic tape at the base of the appendage to secure the bandage.

    An alternative to adhesive tape is to secure the length of tube gauze remaining on the applicator around the patient's wrist or ankle. This is done by cutting the length of tube gauze down two sides, bringing it over the back of the hand or foot, and tying the two now-loose ends around the patient's wrist or ankle.

    NOTE: The tube gauze should never cross the patient's palm or sole.

15. **Procedural Step.** Sanitize the hands.

    Always sanitize the hands after every procedure or after using gloves.

16. **Procedural Step.** Document the procedure.

    Include the date, time, and location of the bandage application.

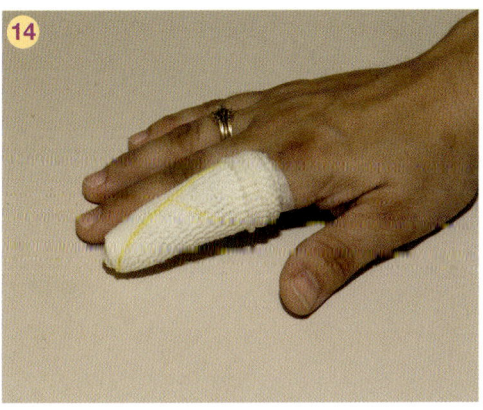

CHARTING EXAMPLE

Date	
3/10/xx	10:30 a.m. Tubular gauze bandage applied to the index finger of the Ⓡ hand. ——————— C. Cobb, CMA (AAMA)

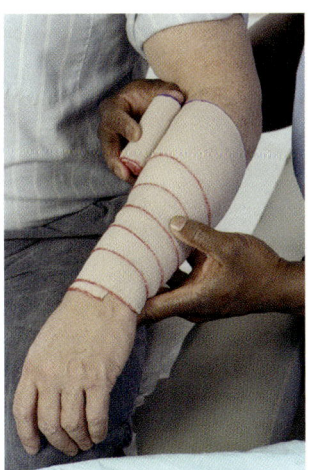

FIGURE 38-3 A spiral bandage turn is used to wrap the arm or leg. Always wrap from distal to proximal.

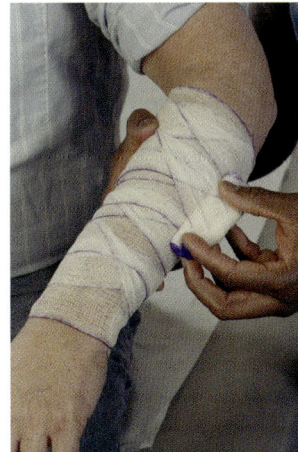

FIGURE 38-4 In a spiral reverse bandage turn, the direction of the spiral changes each time the bandage is brought around the limb.

2. A **spiral turn** is used where body parts are uniform in circumference, such as the arms and legs (Figure 38-3). The bandage progresses upward and each spiral turn overlaps the previous turn by ½ inch.
3. The **spiral reverse turn** is used when the area to be bandaged is a variety of widths such as the forearm and lower legs (calf area) (Figure 38-4). By reversing the turn, a smoother fit is accomplished, with less bulkiness. Each turn repositions the bandage downward and folds on itself, as in the spiral turn.
4. The **figure-eight turn** is most often used to hold a dressing in place or to support a jointed area such as the ankle or wrist. The bandage is applied on a slant and progresses upward, then downward, around the body part being wrapped (Figure 38-5).

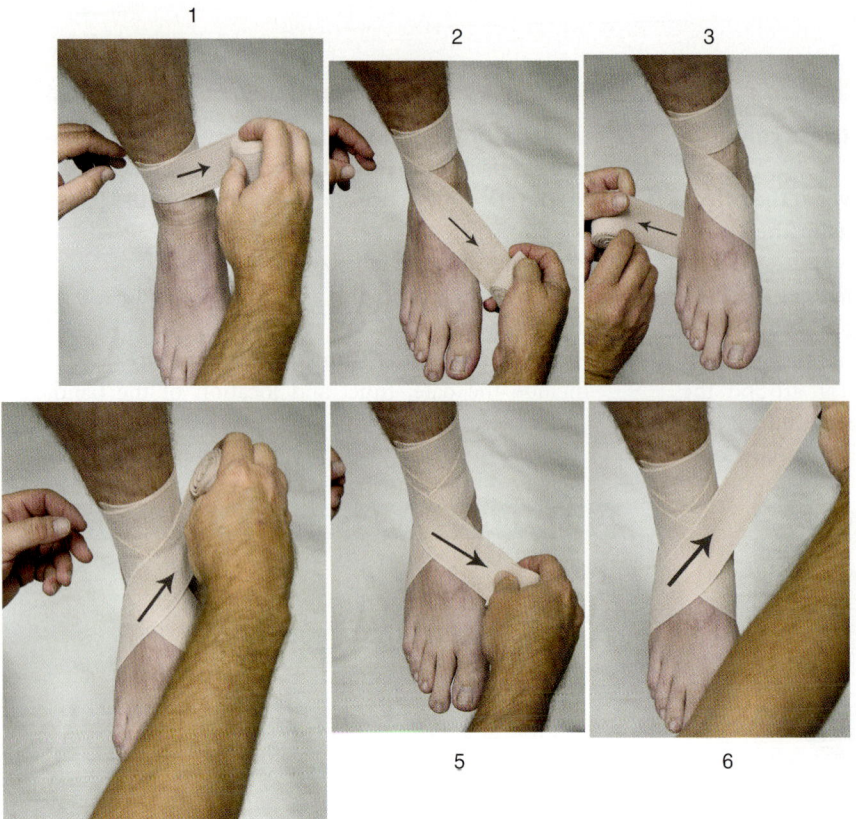

FIGURE 38-5 Use of figure-eight bandage turns for the ankle.

5. The **recurrent turn** is most frequently used for a stump area or for the head (Figure 38-6). The bandage is first anchored by using a circular turn and then moves back and forth over the end of the part to be bandaged. Each turn overlaps the next turn.

It is important to remember that once the bandage has been applied to the body part, the area below the bandage must be checked. Checking below the site for *capillary refill* (blood to fingers or toes) ensures that the application of the bandage is not too tight. Typical signs that circulation may be impaired include swelling, a pale or bluish color to the skin, coolness to the touch, and a complaint of pain, numbness, or tingling to the area.

Figure 38-7 illustrates various bandage-wrapping techniques for various body parts.

PATIENT-CENTERED PROFESSIONALISM

- Why must the medical assistant understand how the different types of bandages are to be used?
- What could happen if the medical assistant applied the wrong type of bandage turn?

COLD AND HEAT THERAPY

Hot and cold packs are effective tools for pain control. When applied alone or in combination, heat and cold therapy often provide relief not only from the pain itself but also from

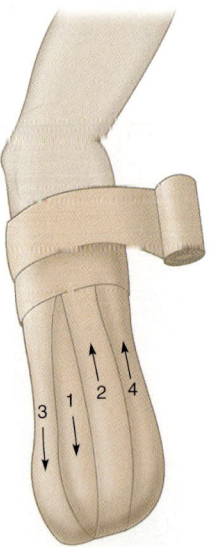

FIGURE 38-6 A recurrent bandage turn is used for a below-the-knee amputee. (Modified from Bonewit-West K: *Clinical procedures for medical assistants,* ed 7, St Louis, 2007, Saunders.)

accompanying swelling or infection. Each therapy causes physiological changes within the tissue.

Overuse of either hot or cold therapy may cause the opposite of the desired therapeutic effect (Box 38-2). Heat normally causes blood vessels to dilate, thus increasing blood supply to the surrounding tissues. Prolonged heat could cause the opposite: constriction and reduced blood supply. Cold normally

Therapeutic Procedures CHAPTER 38 823

Foot and ankle

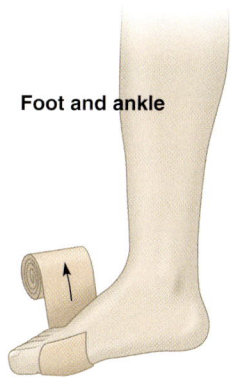

Use 3-inch width. Hold foot at right angle to leg. Start bandage on right of foot just back of the toes.

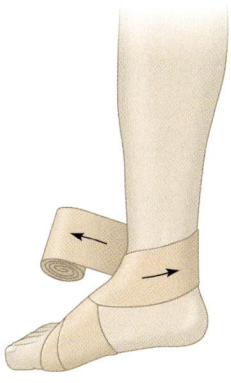

Pass bandage around foot from inside to outside. After two or three complete turns around foot, ascending toward the ankle on each turn, make a figure eight turn by bringing bandage up and over the arch –

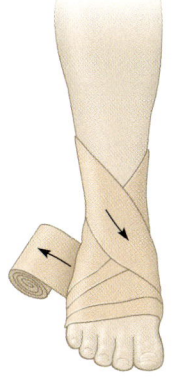

to the inside of the ankle – around the ankle – down over the arch – and under the foot.

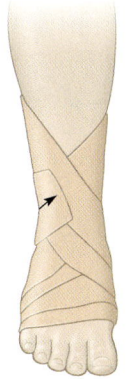

Repeat the figure eight wrapping two to three times. Fasten end by pressing the last 4 to 6 inches of unstretched bandage to the preceding layer.

Lower leg

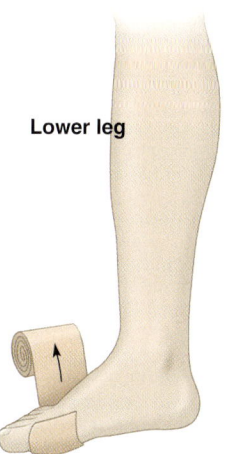

Use 3- to 4-inch width depending on the size of the leg. A leg wrap requires two rolls of bandage. Hold foot at right angle to leg. Start bandage on ridge of foot just back of the toes.

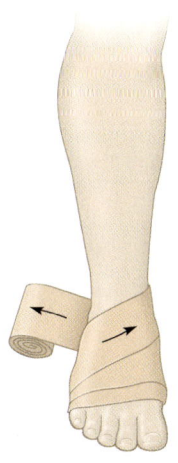

Pass bandage around foot from inside to outside. After two complete turns around foot, make a figure eight turn by bringing bandage up over the arch – to the inside of the ankle – around the ankle –

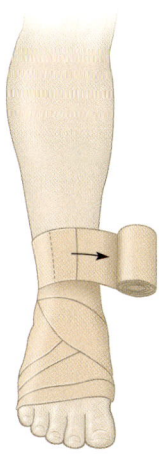

down over the arch – and under the foot. Start circular bandaging, making the first turn around the ankle. To begin the second roll of bandage, simply overlap the unstretched ends by 4 to 6 inches, press firmly, and continue wrapping.

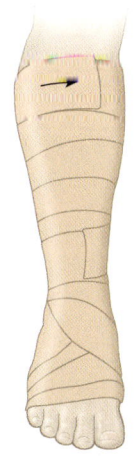

Wrap bandage in spiral turns to just below the kneecap. Fasten end by pressing the last 4 to 6 inches of unstretched bandage to the preceding layer.

Knee

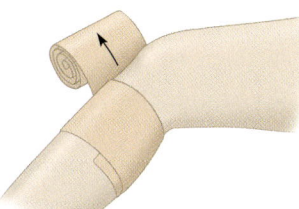

Use 4-inch width. Bend knee slightly. Start with one complete circular turn around the leg just below the knee.

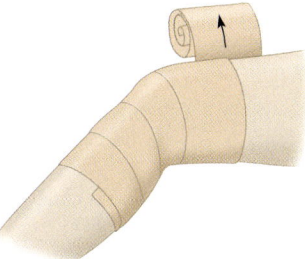

Start circular bandaging, applying only comfortable tension. Cover kneecap completely.

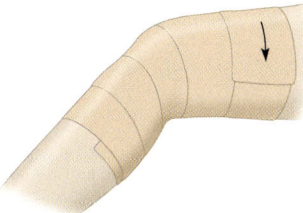

Continue wrapping to thigh just above the knee. Fasten end by pressing the last 4 to 6 inches of unstretched bandage to the preceding layer.

FIGURE 38-7 Bandage-wrapping techniques illustrating the circular, spiral, and figure-eight turns.

Wrist

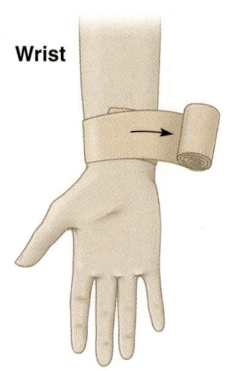 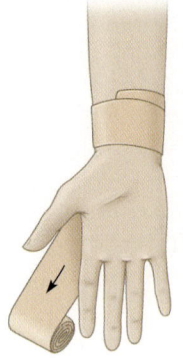 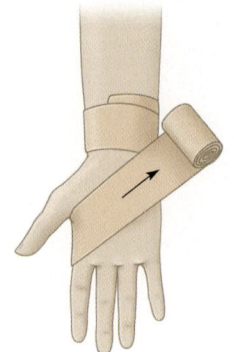 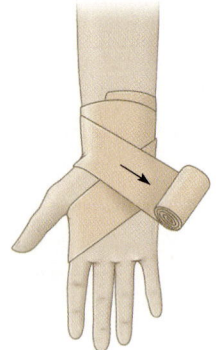 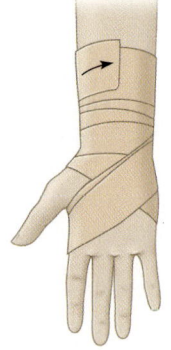

Use 2- or 3-inch width. Anchor bandage loosely at the wrist with one complete circular turn.

Carry the bandage across the back of the hand, through the web space between the thumb and index finger

and across palm to the wrist

Make a circular turn around the wrist and once more carry the bandage through the web space and back to the wrist.

Start circular bandaging, ascending the wrist. Fasten end by pressing last 4 to 6 inches of unstretched bandage to the preceding layer.

Elbow

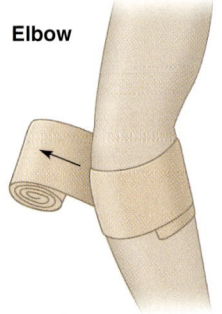 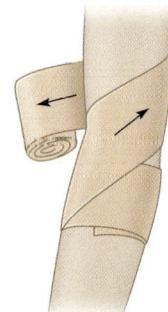 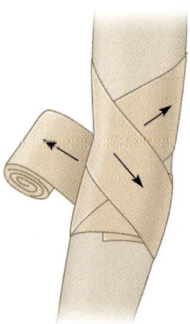 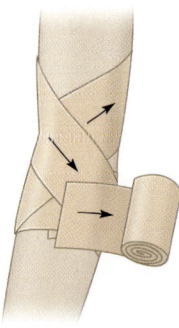 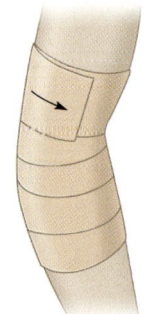

Use 3- or 4-inch width, depending on the size of the arm. Two rolls of bandage are required to complete the wrap. Start with a complete circular turn just below the elbow.

Wrap bandage in loose figure eights

to form a protective bridge across the front of the elbow joint.

Fasten end by pressing 4 to 6 inches of unstretched bandage to the preceding layer. Start second bandage with a circular turn below the elbow

over the first wrap. Continue spiral bandaging over the elbow, ascending to the lower portion of the arm. Fasten end with a circular turn.

Shoulder

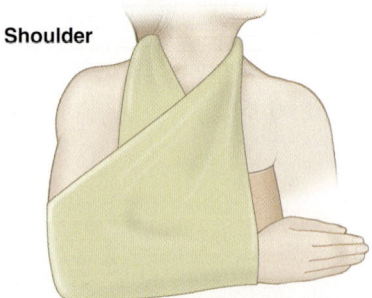 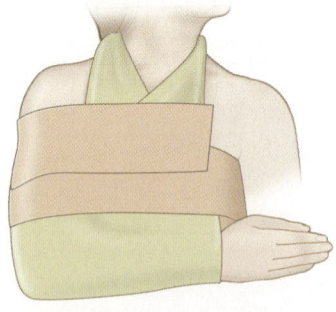 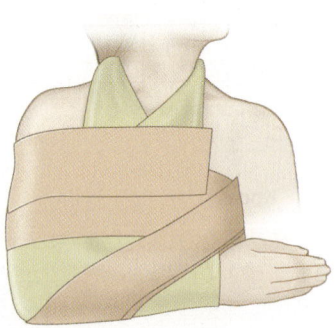

A shoulder wrap is used to provide additional support for an arm in a sling. Use 4- or 6-inch width. One or two rolls of bandage may be used. Start under the free arm.

Carry the bandage across the back, over the arm in the sling, across the chest and back under the free arm in complete circular, overlapping turns. Fasten the end by pressing 4 to 6 inches of unstretched bandage to underlying bandage.

Additional support can be obtained with a second bandage. Start at the back just behind the flexed elbow in the sling. Carry the bandage under the elbow, up over the forearm, around the chest and back, and repeat. Fasten end.

FIGURE 38-7, cont'd

> **BOX 38-2**
>
> **Injury Risk from Heat and Cold Applications**
>
> *Low body fat:* The elderly have reduced sensitivity to pain and young children have thinner skin layers, making them both susceptible to burns.
>
> *Broken skin:* Tissues of broken skin have fewer pain receptors and no temperature receptors, leaving the area susceptible to further injury.
>
> *New scar tissue:* New scar tissue has reduced sensation to temperature, leaving the tissue vulnerable to injury.
>
> *Peripheral vascular disease:* Patients with circulatory impairments (diabetes/arteriosclerosis) have a low sensitivity to pain and temperature and therefore are susceptible to tissue injury if hot or cold applications are not applied properly.

causes blood vessels to constrict and decreases the blood supply to the surrounding tissues. Prolonged cold could cause the opposite: dilation and increased blood supply. Timing of either therapy is essential to produce the desired effect.

Cold Therapy

Cold therapy is used to reduce or prevent swelling by temporarily decreasing circulatory flow to the injured body part. The use of cold applications causes the blood vessels to constrict, decreasing the blood supply to an area. The decrease in blood supply slows cellular growth and reduces bleeding.

Cold therapy is often prescribed after excessive muscle use, such as physical therapy; as a temporary anesthetic for burns; or it may be the initial treatment for an eye injury (e.g., black eye). Physicians may prescribe cold therapy to be followed by heat therapy 24 to 48 hours later or after swelling is brought under control. Methods of cold application include the ice bag, cold compress, and chemical cold pack.

Ice Bag

An **ice bag** is a device that holds ice cubes or ice chips so they can be applied to an area of the body to reduce swelling. Small cubes or ice chips are preferred because they allow the ice bag to mold easily. A protective covering must be applied to protect the patient's skin. Procedure 38-6 explains how to apply an ice bag to a swollen area.

Cold Compress

A **compress** is made of a soft, absorbent material (e.g., gauze squares, washcloth) and is moistened before being applied to a body part to penetrate the tissues more deeply. Cold compresses reduce pain caused by swelling, headaches, and injuries to an area. Procedure 38-7 describes the process of applying a cold compress to an affected area.

Chemical Hot/Cold Pack

A **chemical hot/cold pack** can also be used to relieve swelling in an area. A pack is activated when pressure is applied on the inner bag and it ruptures. Water is released into a larger bag, and the chemical reaction between the water and chemical crystals produces a warmth or coldness that lasts for 30 to 60 minutes. These bags are disposable and must be discarded when the effectiveness has worn off. Procedure 38-8 explains the process of applying a chemical cold pack.

Heat Therapy

Heat therapy, or the application of heat on the skin, is used to treat an infectious condition or a traumatized body area. Heat treatments are used to relieve discomfort from deep muscle tissue and muscle strains and spasms. Once swelling from an injury has been reduced (e.g., by cold therapy or 24 to 48 hours after injury), heat also provides comfort and aids the healing process by increasing blood flow to an area.

When heat is applied to a body surface, the blood vessels dilate. This increased blood supply to the area promotes growth of new cells and tissues by removing wastes faster and increasing nutrients to the site. The physician will specify the type of treatment, frequency, and duration.

To prevent injury to a patient, the medical assistant must carefully observe temperature and skin condition when applying any heat therapy to avoid burning or overheating. Heat therapy must *not* be applied if the following conditions exist:

- Major circulatory problems
- Pregnancy (heat could prematurely start uterine contractions)
- Damaged skin areas (e.g., blisters, burns, or scar tissue caused by poor circulation in the area or on existing reddened skin)

Methods of heat application include the hot water bag, heating pad, hot compress, and hot soak.

Hot Water Bag

A **hot water bag** is a device used to hold water warm enough to increase the blood supply to an area. The bag is filled one-third to one-half full of water, and the excess air is expelled from the bag (as air is a poor conductor of temperature). This allows the bag to mold more easily to the affected part. A protective covering placed over the bag helps absorb perspiration and reduces the risk of burns to the patient. Procedure 38-9 describes the process of applying a hot water bag.

Heating Pad

Although such pads are not frequently used in the medical office, the physician may recommend the patient use a **heating pad** at home. The medical assistant must be able to instruct the patient in its proper application.

The heating pad consists of a group of wires that take electrical energy and convert it to heat. The wires must never be bent because this would damage the pad and could result in overheating and a possible fire. No pins or wet dressings are used because they could result in an electrical shock to the patient. A heating pad should not be in place for longer than

Text continued on p. 831

PROCEDURE 38-6 Apply an Ice Bag

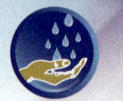

TASK: Properly apply an ice bag to a swollen area.

EQUIPMENT AND SUPPLIES
- Ice bag with protective covering
- Small pieces of ice (ice chips or crushed ice)
- Patient's medical record

SKILLS/RATIONALE

STANDARD PRECAUTIONS ARE TO BE FOLLOWED.

1. **Procedural Step.** Sanitize the hands.
   An alcohol-based hand rub may be used instead of washing hands with soap and water, unless hands are visibly soiled.
   Rationale. Hand sanitization promotes infection control.

2. **Procedural Step.** Assemble equipment and supplies. Check the ice bag for leaks.
   Rationale. It is important to have all supplies and equipment ready and available before starting any procedure to ensure efficiency. A leaking bag will get the patient wet.

3. **Procedural Step.** Obtain the patient's medical record.

4. **Procedural Step.** Greet the patient, introduce yourself, and confirm the patient's identity.
   Rationale. Identifying the patient ensures the procedure is performed on the correct patient.

5. **Procedural Step.** Explain the procedure to the patient.
   Rationale. Explaining the procedure to the patient promotes cooperation and provides a means of obtaining implied consent.

6. **Procedural Step.** Fill the bag one-half to two-thirds full with crushed or chipped ice.
   Rationale. Small pieces of ice allow the bag to mold better to the body area.

7. **Procedural Step.** Compress the empty top half of the bag to remove the air and replace the cap.

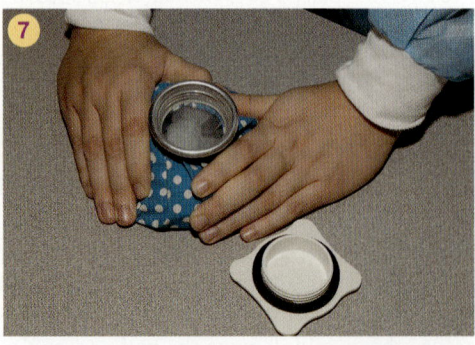

Rationale. The ice bag will mold to the affected area of the body more readily if the air has been removed from the bag, and removing the air keeps the bag colder for a longer period.

8. **Procedural Step.** Dry the outside of the bag, and place the bag inside a protective covering.
   The protective covering may be a disposable premade covering or simply a terrycloth towel.
   Rationale. The protective covering absorbs moisture.

9. **Procedural Step.** Apply the ice bag to the affected area, and ask the patient if the temperature is tolerable.
   Rationale. Application of cold is typically uncomfortable, but the patient will have more tolerance if you have explained the procedure and the patient understands the principle or reasoning behind the application.

10. **Procedural Step.** Leave the ice bag in place for the time prescribed by the physician.
    The duration is typically 20 to 30 minutes. Check the patient's skin every few minutes for any signs of increased redness or swelling, a mottled blue appearance, or extreme paleness. Ask the patient whether the area being treated is painful. If so, or if any of the conditions listed is apparent, remove the bag and notify the physician.

11. **Procedural Step.** Refill the bag with ice and change the protective covering as needed.

12. **Procedural Step.** Provide verbal and written follow-up instructions to the patient.

13. **Procedural Step.** Sanitize the hands.
    Always sanitize the hands after every procedure or after using gloves.

14. **Procedural Step.** Document the procedure.
    Include the date and time, method of cold application (ice bag), location and duration of the application, appearance of the application site, and the patient's reaction.

Continued

PROCEDURE 38-6 Apply an Ice Bag—cont'd

15. **Procedural Step. Properly care for the ice bag and covering, and return them to storage.**
    Drain the contents from the ice bag and dispose of or launder the protective covering as required. Clean the bag with detergent and warm water, rinse, and allow the bag to air-dry by hanging it upside down with the cap off. Allow the bag to fill with air and replace the cap before returning the bag to storage.
    Rationale. Allowing air to remain inside the bag with the cap on during storage prevents the sides from sticking together and the fabric from deteriorating.

CHARTING EXAMPLE

Date	
12/30/xx	9:30 a.m. Ice bag applied to Ⓡ wrist × 15 min. No complaints of discomfort, area is pink. Verbal & written instructions for home use provided. Pt. verbalized understanding of instructions. —— T. Franks, CMA (AAMA)

PROCEDURE 38-7 Apply a Cold Compress

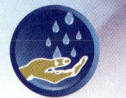

TASK: Properly apply a cold compress to an affected area.

EQUIPMENT AND SUPPLIES
- Ice cubes
- Washcloths or gauze squares (compress)
- Basin
- Towel
- Ice bag
- Patient's medical record

SKILLS/RATIONALE

STANDARD PRECAUTIONS ARE TO BE FOLLOWED.

1. **Procedural Step. Sanitize the hands.**
   An alcohol-based hand rub may be used instead of washing hands with soap and water, unless hands are visibly soiled.
   Rationale. Hand sanitization promotes infection control.
2. **Procedural Step. Assemble equipment and supplies.**
   Rationale. It is important to have all supplies and equipment ready and available before starting any procedure to ensure efficiency.
3. **Procedural Step. Prepare the water by placing a small amount of cold water in a basin and adding large ice cubes.**
   Rationale. Small ice cubes, ice chips, or crushed ice will stick to the compress. Using larger ice cubes also slows the rate at which the ice melts, keeping the water colder for a longer period.

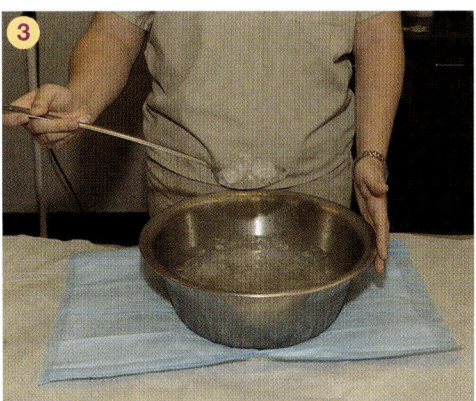

Continued

PROCEDURE 38-7 Apply a Cold Compress—cont'd

4. **Procedural Step.** Prepare an ice bag following the steps in Procedure 38-6.
5. **Procedural Step.** Obtain the patient's medical record.
6. **Procedural Step.** Greet the patient, introduce yourself, and confirm the patient's identity.
   Rationale. Identifying the patient ensures the procedure is performed on the correct patient.
7. **Procedural Step.** Explain the procedure to the patient.
   Rationale. Explaining the procedure to the patient promotes cooperation and provides a means of obtaining implied consent.
8. **Procedural Step.** Immerse the compress into the cold water, and wring the compress until it is moist but not dripping wet.
9. **Procedural Step.** Apply the compress gradually and gently to the affected area, allowing the patient to adjust progressively to the cold. Cover the compress with an ice bag.
   Rationale. Application of cold is typically uncomfortable, but the patient will have more tolerance if it is applied gradually and gently to the affected area. Covering the compress with an ice bag helps keep the compress colder for a longer time, reducing how frequently the compress needs to be changed.
10. **Procedural Step.** Ask the patient how the temperature feels.
11. **Procedural Step.** Place additional compresses in the cold water to be ready for use as needed.
12. **Procedural Step.** Repeat the application of the compress every 2 to 3 minutes for the duration specified by the physician.
    The duration is usually 15 to 20 minutes.
    NOTE: If an ice bag is used on top of the compress, the compress will not need to be replaced as frequently.
13. **Procedural Step.** Check the patient's skin periodically for signs of blueness or numbness, and ask the patient whether the site is painful.
    If any of these conditions is apparent, remove the bag and notify the physician.
14. **Procedural Step.** Add ice if needed to keep the water cold.
15. **Procedural Step.** Completely dry the affected area with a dry towel.
16. **Procedural Step.** Provide verbal and written follow-up instructions to the patient.
17. **Procedural Step.** Sanitize the hands.
    Always sanitize the hands after every procedure or after using gloves.
18. **Procedural Step.** Document the procedure.
    Include the date and time, method of cold application (cold compress), location and duration of the application, appearance of the application site, and the patient's reaction.
19. **Procedural Step.** Properly care for the equipment and return it to storage.
    Launder or dispose of compresses and towels. If an ice bag is used, see Procedure 38-6 for proper storage of the ice bag.

CHARTING EXAMPLE

Date	
11/10/xx	1:45 p.m. Cold compresses applied to ® cheek × 15 min. Area appears less swollen, and pt. states pain has lessened. Verbal and written instructions provided for patient follow-up care.————————————— ———————————— J. Jones, CMA (AAMA)

Therapeutic Procedures **CHAPTER 38** 829

PROCEDURE 38-8 Apply a Chemical Cold Pack

TASK: Properly activate and apply a chemical cold pack.

EQUIPMENT AND SUPPLIES
- Chemical cold pack
- Protective covering
- Patient's medical record

SKILLS/RATIONALE

STANDARD PRECAUTIONS ARE TO BE FOLLOWED.

1. **Procedural Step.** Sanitize the hands.
   An alcohol-based hand rub may be used instead of washing hands with soap and water, unless hands are visibly soiled.
   Rationale. Hand sanitization promotes infection control.

2. **Procedural Step.** Assemble equipment and supplies.
   Rationale. It is important to have all supplies and equipment ready and available before starting any procedure to ensure efficiency.

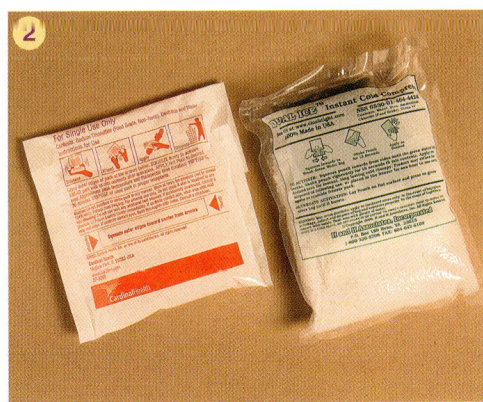

3. **Procedural Step.** Obtain the patient's medical record.

4. **Procedural Step.** Greet the patient, introduce yourself, and confirm the patient's identity.
   Rationale. Identifying the patient ensures the procedure is performed on the correct patient.

5. **Procedural Step.** Explain the procedure to the patient.
   Rationale. Explaining the procedure to the patient promotes cooperation and provides a means of obtaining implied consent.

6. **Procedural Step.** Follow the manufacturer's instructions to activate the chemical reaction creating the cold pack.
   The following steps are typical for most chemical cold packs:

   a. Shake the chemical crystals to the bottom of the bag.
   b. Apply firm pressure to the center of the bag to break the inner water bag.
   c. Shake the bag to mix the contents.

7. **Procedural Step.** Apply a cover to the bag and apply to the affected area.
   Rationale. Cold packs must never be placed directly on the patient's skin. A cover also protects the patient's skin from chemical burns if the bag leaks.

8. **Procedural Step.** Administer the treatment for the proper length of time, as ordered by the physician.
   Most chemical cold packs will remain cold for up to 60 minutes.

9. **Procedural Step.** Discard the bag in an appropriate container.

10. **Procedural Step.** Provide necessary verbal and written follow-up instructions to the patient.
    Rationale. The physician may provide a patient with a chemical ice pack to take home and use, so it is important that you provide the patient with thorough instructions.

11. **Procedural Step.** Sanitize the hands.
    Always sanitize the hands after every procedure or after using gloves.

12. **Procedural Step.** Document the procedure as you would for any cold application.

CHARTING EXAMPLE	
Date	
10/20/xx	3:30 p.m. Cold pack applied to Ⓡ forearm × 15 min. No complaints of discomfort, area is pink. Verbal & written instructions for home use provided. Pt. verbalized understanding of instructions.————————————————— T. Ponder, CMA (AAMA)

PROCEDURE 38-9 Apply a Hot Water Bag

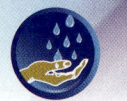

TASK: Properly fill and apply a hot water bag to an affected area.

EQUIPMENT AND SUPPLIES
- Hot water bag with protective covering
- Pitcher to hold water
- Bath thermometer
- Patient's medical record

SKILLS/*RATIONALE*

STANDARD PRECAUTIONS ARE TO BE FOLLOWED.

1. **Procedural Step.** Sanitize the hands.
   An alcohol-based hand rub may be used instead of washing hands with soap and water, unless hands are visibly soiled.
   Rationale. Hand sanitization promotes infection control.

2. **Procedural Step.** Assemble equipment and supplies.
   Rationale. It is important to have all supplies and equipment ready and available before starting any procedure to ensure efficiency.

3. **Procedural Step.** Obtain the patient's medical record.

4. **Procedural Step.** Greet the patient, introduce yourself, and confirm the patient's identity.
   Rationale. Identifying the patient ensures the procedure is performed on the correct patient.

5. **Procedural Step.** Explain the procedure to the patient.
   Rationale. Explaining the procedure to the patient promotes cooperation and provides a means of obtaining implied consent.

6. **Procedural Step.** Prepare the water to be used in the hot water bag.
   Fill a pitcher with hot tap water. Test the temperature of the water with a bath thermometer. It should range between 115° and 125° F (46° and 52° C) for adults and older children and between 105° and 115° F (41° and 46° C) for infants, children under 2 years of age, and elderly patients.
   NOTE: If the water temperature cannot be measured, the temperature should be adjusted to body comfort.
   Rationale. The temperature should never exceed 125° F (52° C) to avoid burning the patient.

7. **Procedural Step.** Fill the hot water bag one-third to one-half full of water.
   A hot water bag that is not completely full is lighter and easier to mold to the body area.

8. **Procedural Step.** Expel the excess air from the bag.
   Rest the bag on the table and flatten it while holding the neck upright until the water reaches the neck. Air can also be expelled by holding the bag upright and squeezing the unfilled part until the water reaches the neck screw in the stopper or fastening the top with special closure tabs.

Rationale. Air is a poor conductor of heat and also makes it difficult to mold the hot water bag to the body area.

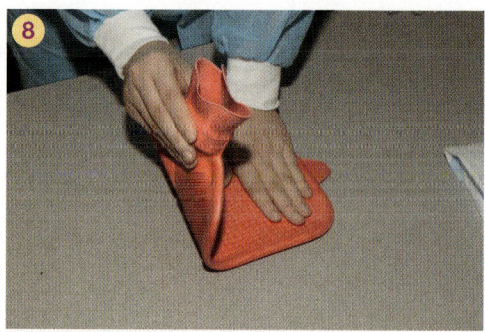

9. **Procedural Step.** Dry the outside of the bag and test for leakage by holding the bag upside down.
   Rationale. Leaking water will get the patient wet and may burn the patient.

10. **Procedural Step.** Place the bag in the protective covering.
    Rationale. The cover helps absorb perspiration and lessens the danger of burning the patient.

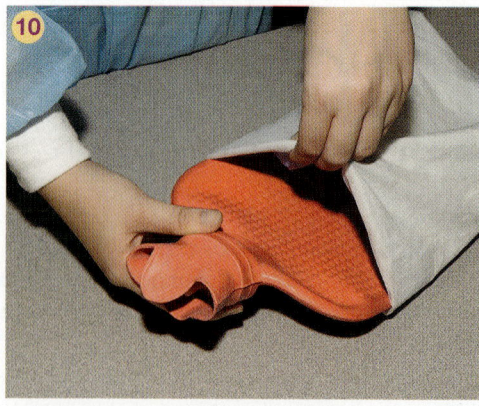

11. **Procedural Step.** Place the patient in a position of comfort, and place the bag on the patient's affected body area.

Continued

PROCEDURE 38-9 Apply a Hot Water Bag—cont'd

Ask the patient how the temperature feels. The hot water bag should feel warm but not uncomfortable.

Rationale. Individuals vary in their ability to tolerate heat.

12. **Procedural Step. Administer the treatment for the proper length of time, as designated by the physician.**
The duration is typically 10 to 20 minutes. Check the patient's skin periodically for signs of an increase or decrease in redness or swelling and ask the patient whether the site is painful.

13. **Procedural Step. Refill the bag with hot water as needed to maintain the proper temperature, making sure to remove an equal amount of the cooler water with each addition.**

14. **Procedural Step. Provide written follow-up instructions to the patient.**

15. **Procedural Step. Sanitize the hands.**
Always sanitize the hands after every procedure or after using gloves.

16. **Procedural Step. Document the procedure.**
Include the date and time, method of heat application (hot water bag), temperature of the hot water, location and duration of the application, appearance of the application site, and the patient's reaction.

17. **Procedural Step. Properly care for the hot water bag.**
Dispose of or launder the protective covering. Cleanse the hot water bag with a warm detergent solution, rinse thoroughly, and dry by hanging the bag upside down with the top removed. Store the bag by screwing on the stopper, leaving air inside to prevent the sides from sticking together.

CHARTING EXAMPLE

Date	
12/9/xx	10:00 a.m. Applied hot water bag, water temp @ 115° F, to ⓛ shoulder area for 20 minutes. Pt. states pain is relieved and skin is dry and intact. Provided verbal and written instructions for home use. Pt. verbalized understanding of instructions. ———————— P. Thomas, CMA (AAMA)

---

30 minutes and should never be placed on the high setting to avoid the potential for burns. The patient should be instructed not to use the pad when sleeping. Also, after 30 minutes, the therapeutic effect greatly diminishes and may even have the reverse effect. Procedure 38-10 explains the process of applying a heating pad.

Hot Compress

As with cold compresses, hot compresses are made of soft, absorbent materials and are moist when applied to penetrate the tissues more deeply. Hot compresses are used to increase circulation to an area for healing purposes. Procedure 38-11 explains how to apply a hot compress to increase circulation.

Hot Soak

A hot **soak** requires a body part to be submerged in a water bath with or without medication. Generally, a soak is applied to an extremity. A hot soak is used to clean an open wound and to increase blood supply to an area to aid in healing or reduce swelling. To use a hot soak on an open wound, sterile techniques must be used. Procedure 38-12 explains how to apply a hot soak to an affected area.

PATIENT-CENTERED PROFESSIONALISM

- Why must the medical assistant understand the proper uses of heat and cold?

ULTRASOUND THERAPY

Ultrasound therapy uses high-frequency sound waves. When used therapeutically, these sound waves produce heat and vibrations to affect soft tissues in the body. Low-intensity ultrasound is used for therapeutic purposes, including pain relief for muscle spasms, inflammation (e.g., tennis elbow), and arthritis. The therapeutic dose prescribed by the physician will produce the appropriate heat to facilitate the healing process.

As the sound waves are absorbed into body tissues, heat is produced. Also, because ultrasound therapy vibrates the soft tissues, a massage-like action takes place. A **coupling agent** must be used to make certain the energy given off by the ultrasound head (on the wand) is transmitted to the body tissues. This agent is a water-soluble lotion or gel that is spread over the area to be treated. The head of the wand must be in contact with the coupling agent to produce the desired effect. Never use ultrasound therapy over eyes or burn tissue.

The dosage is prescribed in watts (power) and in a time frame. The order will vary according to the site and severity of the condition. Areas of pain may respond better to low-to-moderate doses because less nerve activity is involved. The medical assistant must always ask how the patient is tolerating the treatment and must monitor the patient's condition throughout the ultrasound treatment. Procedure 38-13 explains how to administer ultrasound therapy.

Text continued on p. 838

PROCEDURE 38-10 — Apply a Heating Pad

TASK: Properly apply a heating pad to an affected area.

EQUIPMENT AND SUPPLIES
- Heating pad
- Protective cover
- Patient's medical record

SKILLS/RATIONALE

STANDARD PRECAUTIONS ARE TO BE FOLLOWED.

1. **Procedural Step.** Sanitize the hands.
   An alcohol-based hand rub may be used instead of washing hands with soap and water, unless hands are visibly soiled.
   Rationale. Hand sanitization promotes infection control.

2. **Procedural Step.** Assemble equipment and supplies.
   Rationale. It is important to have all supplies and equipment ready and available before starting any procedure to ensure efficiency.

3. **Procedural Step.** Obtain the patient's medical record.

4. **Procedural Step.** Greet the patient, introduce yourself, and confirm the patient's identity.
   Rationale. Identifying the patient ensures the procedure is performed on the correct patient.

5. **Procedural Step.** Explain the procedure to the patient.
   Instruct the patient not to lie directly on the heating pad.
   Rationale. Explaining the procedure to the patient promotes cooperation and provides a means of obtaining implied consent. Lying on the pad causes heat to accumulate and can burn the patient.

6. **Procedural Step.** Inspect the heating pad's electrical wires before each use to make sure they are intact.
   Rationale. Frayed or damaged wires can cause an electrical burn to the patient.

7. **Procedural Step.** Place the heating pad in the protective covering.
   Rationale. Covering the heating pad provides more comfort for the patient, functions to absorb perspiration, and also reduces the risk of a burn.

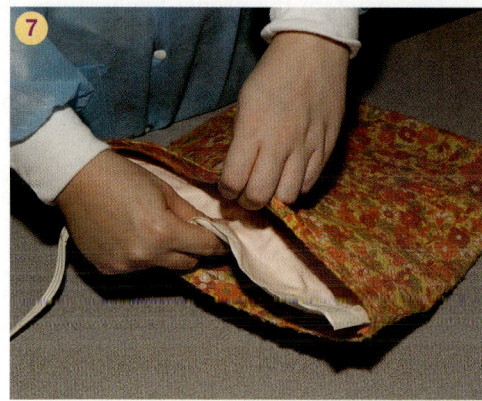

8. **Procedural Step.** Plug into an electrical outlet and set the selector switch at the setting, as designated by the physician (low or medium).

9. **Procedural Step.** Place the patient in a position of comfort and place the heating pad on the patient's affected body area.
   Ask the patient if the temperature is comfortable. The heating pad should feel warm but not hot. The patient should be cautioned not to turn the heating pad to a higher setting if it no longer feels hot enough after a time.
   Rationale. The patient's heat receptors eventually become adjusted to the temperature change, resulting in a decreased heat sensation, and the patient may be tempted to increase the temperature.

10. **Procedural Step.** Administer the treatment for the proper length of time, as ordered by the physician (usually 15 to 20 minutes).

Continued

PROCEDURE 38-10 Apply a Heating Pad—cont'd

Periodically check on the patient. Examine the site for signs of an increase or decrease in redness or swelling and ask the patient if the site is painful.

Rationale. Administering heat to an area of the body for a specified time increases circulation and promotes healing. After the specified period, typically 20 minutes, the treatment has the opposite effect. Leaving the heating pad on for longer than the specified time may also cause burns, redness, and swelling. If the site is painful, the treatment should be stopped and the physician notified.

11. **Procedural Step.** Provide verbal and written follow-up instructions to the patient.
12. **Procedural Step.** Sanitize the hands.
    Always sanitize the hands after every procedure or after using gloves.
13. **Procedural Step.** Document the procedure.
    Include the date and time, method of heat application (heating pad), temperature setting of the pad, location and duration of the application, appearance of the application site, and the patient's reaction.
14. **Procedural Step.** Replace the equipment to its appropriate storage area.

CHARTING EXAMPLE

Date	
12/20/xx	10:00 a.m. Heating pad temp set to low and applied to lower back area × 15 min. Pt. states relief. Area is dry and intact. Verbal & written instructions for home use provided. Pt. verbalized understanding of instructions. ——————— D. Goodwin, CMA (AAMA)

PROCEDURE 38-11 Apply a Hot Compress

TASK: Properly apply a hot compress to an affected area to increase circulation.

EQUIPMENT AND SUPPLIES
- Solution ordered by physician
- Bath thermometer
- Washcloths or gauze squares
- Basin
- Towel
- Patient's medical record
  Alternative: Commercially prepared hot moist heat packs

SKILLS/RATIONALE

STANDARD PRECAUTIONS ARE TO BE FOLLOWED.

1. **Procedural Step.** Sanitize the hands.
   An alcohol-based hand rub may be used instead of washing hands with soap and water, unless hands are visibly soiled.
   Rationale. Hand sanitization promotes infection control.
2. **Procedural Step.** Assemble equipment and supplies.
   Rationale. It is important to have all supplies and equipment ready and available before starting any procedure to ensure efficiency.
3. **Procedural Step.** Obtain the patient's medical record.
4. **Procedural Step.** Greet the patient, introduce yourself, and confirm the patient's identity.
   Rationale. Identifying the patient ensures the procedure is performed on the correct patient.
5. **Procedural Step.** Explain the procedure to the patient and the reason for applying the compress.

   Rationale. Explaining the procedure to the patient promotes cooperation and provides a means of obtaining implied consent. Moist heat improves vascular circulation, promotes relaxation, and increases mobility. Moist heat penetrates the tissues better than dry heat.
6. **Procedural Step.** Ask the patient to remove all jewelry in the area to be treated.
   Rationale. Applying any heat therapy, including a hot moist compress, over metal jewelry may burn the patient.
7. **Procedural Step.** Fill the basin one-half to three-fourths full of the solution ordered by the physician and check the temperature with a bath thermometer. The temperature for an adult should range between 105° and 115° F (41° and 44° C).
8. **Procedural Step.** Apply the compress.

Continued

PROCEDURE 38-11 Apply a Hot Compress—cont'd

a. Place the patient in a position of comfort.
b. Place the compress material (washcloth or gauze squares) into the hot water. Wring excess solution from the compress.
c. Cover the compress with a waterproof cover to help hold in the heat.
d. Gradually apply the compress to the affected site, allowing the patient to become accustomed to the heat.
e. Ask the patient if the temperature is comfortable. The compress should be applied as hot as the patient can comfortably tolerate within the acceptable temperature range.

Rationale. Covering the compress with a waterproof cover slows down the cooling process of the compress and reduces the number of times the compress will need to be rewarmed and reapplied.

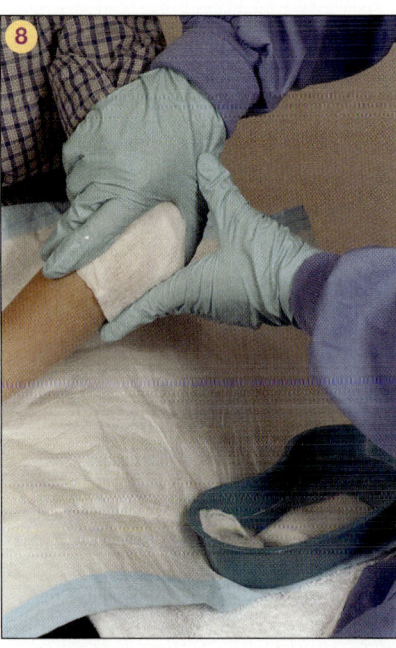

9. **Procedural Step.** Prepare additional compresses if needed during the application of the current compress so that they are ready for use when the current compress begins to cool.

10. **Procedural Step.** Reapply the compress as needed and periodically check the patient's progress.
Repeat the application of the compress every 2 to 3 minutes for the duration specified by the physician (usually 15 to 20 minutes). Periodically examine the site for signs of an increase or decrease in redness or swelling and ask the patient if the site is painful. Remove the compress immediately if either condition occurs and alert the physician.

11. **Procedural Step.** Periodically check the temperature of the water in the basin with the bath thermometer and replace the cooled water with hot water as needed.

12. **Procedural Step.** After the prescribed treatment time has elapsed, thoroughly and gently dry the affected part with a clean dry towel.

13. **Procedural Step.** Provide verbal and written follow-up instructions for the patient.

14. **Procedural Step.** Sanitize the hands.
Always sanitize the hands after every procedure or after using gloves.

15. **Procedural Step.** Document the procedure.
Include the date and time, method of heat application (hot compress), name and strength of the solution, temperature of the solution, location and duration of the application, appearance of the application site, and the patient's reaction.

16. **Procedural Step.** Properly care for the equipment and return it to its appropriate storage place.

CHARTING EXAMPLE

Date	
12/16/xx	1:30 p.m. Normal saline hot compresses at 110° F to Ⓛ forearm × 15 min. Site slightly reddened, warm to touch. No discomfort noted by the patient. Verbal and written instructions provided to pt. for home care. Pt. verbalized understanding of instructions. ———————————— A. Dickerson, CMA (AAMA)

Therapeutic Procedures **CHAPTER 38** 835

PROCEDURE 38-12 Apply a Hot Soak

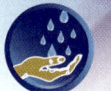

TASK: Properly apply a hot soak to an affected area for relief of pain or swelling.

EQUIPMENT AND SUPPLIES
- Soaking solution ordered by physician
- Bath thermometer
- Basin
- Bath towels
- Patient's medical record

SKILLS/*RATIONALE*

STANDARD PRECAUTIONS ARE TO BE FOLLOWED.

1. **Procedural Step. Sanitize the hands.**
   An alcohol-based hand rub may be used instead of washing hands with soap and water, unless hands are visibly soiled.
   Rationale. Hand sanitization promotes infection control.

2. **Procedural Step. Assemble equipment and supplies.**
   Rationale. It is important to have all supplies and equipment ready and available before starting any procedure to ensure efficiency.

3. **Procedural Step. Obtain the patient's medical record.**

4. **Procedural Step. Greet the patient, introduce yourself, and confirm the patient's identity.**
   Rationale. Identifying the patient ensures the procedure is performed on the correct patient.

5. **Procedural Step. Explain the procedure to the patient.**
   Rationale. Explaining the procedure to the patient promotes cooperation and provides a means of obtaining implied consent.

6. **Procedural Step. Fill the basin one-half to three-fourths full of the solution ordered by the physician and check the temperature with a bath thermometer.**
   The temperature for an adult should range between 105° and 115° F (41° and 44° C).

7. **Procedural Step. Place the patient in a position of comfort.**
   Pad the side of the basin with a towel, if needed.
   Rationale. The patient will be soaking for approximately 20 minutes and must be in a comfortable position to avoid fatigue and strain of the muscles. Padding the side of the basin may be done to provide comfort to the patient, if necessary.

8. **Procedural Step. Gently and slowly immerse the patient's affected body part into the solution.**
   Ask the patient if the temperature is comfortable.
   Rationale. The patient's affected body part should become accustomed to the change in temperature gradually.

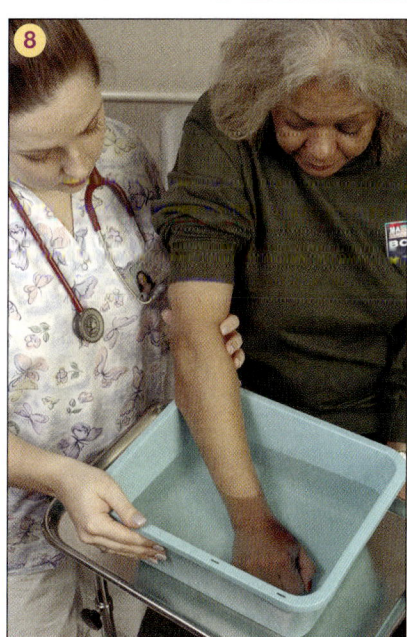

9. **Procedural Step. Periodically check the temperature of the water in the basin with the bath thermometer, and replace the cooled water with hot water as needed to keep the temperature constant.**
   Be very careful not to pour hot water directly onto the patient's skin. Add the water at the edge of the basin by pouring the hot water over your hand first, then stirring the hot water into the cooled water as you pour.
   Rationale. Water should be added away from the patient's body part to prevent splashing hot water on the patient. Stirring the water helps distribute the heat and keep the temperature constant.

PROCEDURE 38-12 Apply a Hot Soak—cont'd

10. **Procedural Step.** Apply the hot soak and periodically check on the patient.
    Continue applying the hot soak for the proper length of time, as ordered by the physician (usually 15 to 20 minutes). Periodically examine the site for signs of an increase or decrease in redness or swelling and ask the patient if the site is painful. Remove the patient from the hot soak immediately if either condition occurs and alert the physician.
11. **Procedural Step.** After the prescribed treatment time has elapsed, thoroughly and gently dry the affected part with a clean dry towel.
12. **Procedural Step.** Provide verbal and written follow-up instructions for the patient.
13. **Procedural Step.** Sanitize the hands.
    Always sanitize the hands after every procedure or after using gloves.
14. **Procedural Step.** Document the procedure.
    Include the date and time, method of heat application (hot soak), name and strength of the solution, temperature of the soak, location and duration of the application, appearance of the application site, and the patient's reaction.
15. **Procedural Step.** Properly care for the equipment and return it to its appropriate storage place.

CHARTING EXAMPLE

Date	
12/23/xx	3:00 p.m. Hot water soak @ 105° F applied to ® wrist × 15 min. Area pink and no discomfort noted by the patient. Verbal & written instructions provided to pt. for home care. Pt. verbalized understanding of instructions.————————————— M. Kohen, CMA (AAMA)

PROCEDURE 38-13 Administer an Ultrasound Treatment

TASK: Properly administer an ultrasound treatment.

EQUIPMENT AND SUPPLIES
- Ultrasound machine
- Coupling agent
- Paper towels or tissues
- Patient's medical record

SKILLS/RATIONALE

STANDARD PRECAUTIONS ARE TO BE FOLLOWED.

1. **Procedural Step.** Sanitize the hands.
   An alcohol-based hand rub may be used instead of washing hands with soap and water, unless hands are visibly soiled.
   Rationale. Hand sanitization promotes infection control.
2. **Procedural Step.** Assemble equipment and supplies.
   The coupling agent must be at room temperature.
   Rationale. It is important to have all supplies and equipment ready and available before starting any procedure to ensure efficiency. If the coupling agent is too cold or too warm, it will cause the patient discomfort. Some offices keep the coupling agent slightly warmed, as in a baby bottle warmer.
3. **Procedural Step.** Obtain the patient's medical record.
4. **Procedural Step.** Greet the patient, introduce yourself, and confirm the patient's identity.
   Rationale. Identifying the patient ensures the procedure is performed on the correct patient.
5. **Procedural Step.** Explain the procedure to the patient.
   Assure the patient that there should be minimal or no discomfort. If the patient experiences any discomfort or pain, the patient should tell you immediately, and the intensity of the treatment dosage should be decreased (per the physician's order) until the patient is comfortable.
   Rationale. Explaining the procedure to the patient promotes cooperation and provides a means of obtaining implied consent.
6. **Procedural Step.** Prepare the patient and treatment area.
   a. Place the patient in a position of comfort. Ask the patient to remove the appropriate clothing to expose the treatment area. Tell the patient that the coupling agent may feel cold.

Continued

PROCEDURE 38-13 Administer an Ultrasound Treatment—cont'd

b. Liberally apply the coupling agent to cover the treatment area completely. Never apply the coupling agent to the ultrasound machine wand.

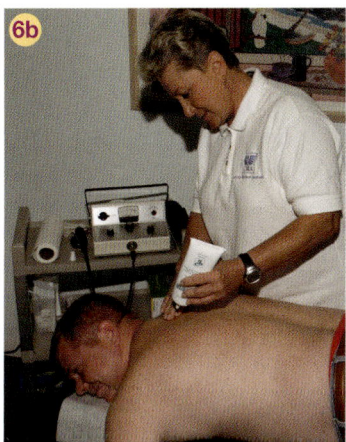

c. Use the ultrasound applicator head to spread the coupling agent evenly over the treatment area before turning on the machine.

Rationale. The treatment area should be adequately covered with the coupling agent but not to excess. The coupling agent is used to provide a better transmission of the ultrasound waves to the patient's tissues.

7. **Procedural Step. Set the ultrasound machine.**
   Turn the ultrasound machine "on" and place the intensity control knob at the minimum position. Set the timer to the required time ordered by the physician.
   Rationale. The timer activates the ultrasound machine, and the intensity must be at zero watts.

8. **Procedural Step.** Increase the intensity level (measured in watts) to the degree ordered by the physician.

9. **Procedural Step.** Place the applicator head at a right angle into the coupling agent on the patient's skin using firm pressure.
   Inform the patient that the applicator head may feel cold.

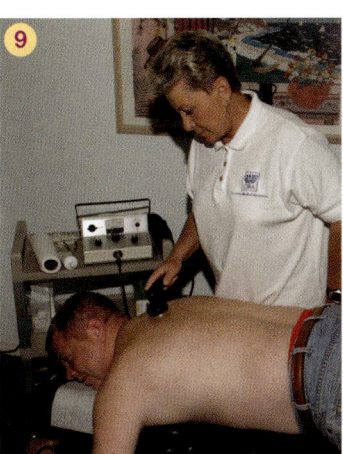

10. **Procedural Step.** Depending on the area of the body being treated, move the applicator in either a continuous back-and-forth sweeping motion or a circular motion.
    The back-and-forth sweeping motion is used for larger areas of the body (e.g., back, thigh). The circular motion is used for smaller areas and over bony prominences (e.g., wrist, ankle).
    Use short strokes, approximately 1 inch in length or diameter, continuously moving the applicator head at a rate of 1 to 2 inches per second. Gradually move the applicator head so that each stroke overlaps the previous stroke by ½ inch. Do not remove the applicator head from the patient's skin.
    Rationale. The applicator head must be in constant motion to prevent the tissues from overheating and creating a hot spot or burn. Removing the applicator head from the patient's skin and holding it in the air may cause the applicator head to overheat and may burn the patient when reapplied to the treatment area. The excessive heat may also damage the crystal in the applicator head.

11. **Procedural Step.** If the patient complains of any pain or discomfort, stop the treatment immediately and notify the physician.

12. **Procedural Step.** Continue the ultrasound treatment until the prescribed time has expired.
    The timer automatically shuts off the machine at the end of the prescribed time.

13. **Procedural Step.** Remove the applicator head from the patient's skin and turn the intensity control to the minimum position.

14. **Procedural Step.** Wipe the excess coupling agent from the patient's skin and applicator head with a paper towel or tissues.

15. **Procedural Step.** Instruct the patient to dress; assist as needed.

16. **Procedural Step.** Sanitize the hands.
    Always sanitize the hands after every procedure or after using gloves.

17. **Procedural Step.** Document the procedure.
    Include the date and time, location of the treatment, duration (in minutes), intensity used (in watts), and the patient's reaction.

CHARTING EXAMPLE

Date	
11/10/xx	10:45 a.m. Ultrasound treatment applied to Ⓡ lower back @ 2 watts for 15 min. Pt. states relief of discomfort. —————————————— C. Rabney, RMA

> **PATIENT-CENTERED PROFESSIONALISM**
>
> - Why must the medical assistant be knowledgeable about basic principles and proper procedure when performing ultrasound?

LASER THERAPY

Laser or light therapy is the use of specific wavelengths of light (red and near-infrared) to create therapeutic effects. The light can be provided by a cluster of low power laser diodes or light-emitting diodes (LED). The therapeutic effects of using low-level laser therapy have been documented to improve healing time and have shown reduction in pain and swelling in soft tissue. Chiropractic medicine appears to be the first to fully take advantage of this technology. Current research demonstrates that injuries treated with laser therapy heal faster and that laser therapy provides a positive effect on tissue repair. The main advantage of laser therapy over conventional forms of therapy is that no drugs or surgery are involved, there are fewer side effects or risks, and it is quick and convenient. The typical course of treatment lasts 5 to 10 minutes depending on what area is being treated. Currently, this procedure is performed by the doctor, but the medical assistant must be aware that it is an alternative therapy treatment of wounds and injuries.

AMBULATORY DEVICES

Many patients require assistance with walking after an injury (e.g., sprain, fracture) or surgery (e.g., joint replacement) and because of disease (e.g., gout, osteoarthritis, or polio) or congenital deformity. The type of **ambulation device** used depends on the patient's injury or condition.

The medical assistant must learn how to fit and adjust these assistive devices properly. Whether the ambulatory device is crutches, a cane, or a walker, improper fitting will likely cause decreased stability, increased use of the patient's energy, and decreased function, with the patient's safety at risk. Improper fit also may cause the patient to develop bad gait habits or unsafe gait patterns and may result in painful tissue trauma (e.g., under armpit if crutches are too high or low).

Crutches

Crutches allow a foot, ankle, leg, knee, or other area of the leg or hip to heal after an injury, surgery, or metabolic disease (e.g., gout). Crutches must be properly fitted, and a crutch-walking gait should be taught to promote ambulation. In addition, various gait (walking) patterns are used for stability, support, and mobility.

Types of Crutches

There are several types of crutches, including axillary, forearm, and platform crutches.

Axillary crutches are used when a patient needs less stability than provided by a walker or the patient cannot bear weight on an affected lower extremity. This type of crutch requires the patient to have good strength in the upper extremities and trunk muscles. Axillary crutches are usually made of wood or aluminum and most are easily adjustable for a proper fit. If improper gait patterns are used, damage to blood vessels and nerves in the axillary area may result.

When being measured for axillary crutches, the patient stands erect with the crutch tips about 6 inches away from the toes (using a **goniometer** at a 45-degree angle). Two fingers should fit between the axilla (armpit) and the top of the crutch pads. The handgrip is adjusted to the wrist crease with a 30-degree bend at the elbow. The weight is placed on the handgrips not the crutch pads. Procedure 38-14 explains the process of measuring a patient for axillary crutches.

Forearm (Lofstrand) crutches are used when more stability and support are needed than a cane can provide. Using the forearm crutch requires the patient to have superior standing balance and upper body strength (Figure 38-8).

Platform crutches are used by patients with poor arm strength. A shelf-like device with arm straps for supporting the forearm and a handgrip for grasping provides the patient with the needed stability (Figure 38-9).

Gait Patterns

The selection of the **gait pattern** depends on the patient's balance, coordination, strength, ability to bear weight, and energy level. Procedure 38-15 describes the process for providing instructions to a patient for the appropriate crutch gait, depending on the patient's injury or condition. The tripod

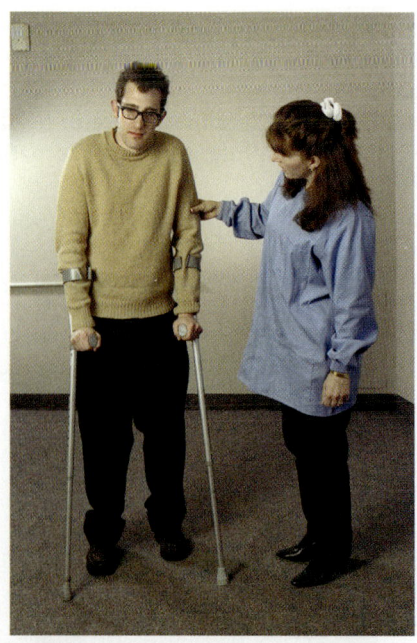

FIGURE 38-8 Medical assistant teaching a patient to use forearm crutches.

Therapeutic Procedures **CHAPTER 38** 839

PROCEDURE 38-14 — Measure for Axillary Crutches

TASK: Properly measure a patient for crutches.

EQUIPMENT AND SUPPLIES
- Crutches
- Goniometer
- Patient's medical record

SKILLS/*RATIONALE*

STANDARD PRECAUTIONS ARE TO BE FOLLOWED.

1. **Procedural Step. Sanitize the hands.**
   An alcohol-based hand rub may be used instead of washing hands with soap and water, unless hands are visibly soiled.
   Rationale. Hand sanitization promotes infection control.
2. **Procedural Step. Assemble equipment and supplies.**
   Rationale. It is important to have all supplies and equipment ready and available before starting any procedure to ensure efficiency.
3. **Procedural Step. Obtain the patient's medical record.**
4. **Procedural Step. Greet the patient, introduce yourself, and confirm the patient's identity.**
   The patient will most likely be in the examination room.
   Rationale. Identifying the patient ensures the procedure is performed on the correct patient.
5. **Procedural Step. Explain the procedure to the patient.**
   Rationale. Explaining the procedure to the patient promotes cooperation and provides a means of obtaining implied consent.

DETERMINING CRUTCH LENGTH

6. **Procedural Step. Position the patient.**
   Assist the patient as needed into a standing position. The measurement must be taken with the patient wearing at least one good walking shoe on the foot of the uninjured leg.
   Rationale. Measurement will not be accurate if the patient is sitting or is not wearing a shoe on the unaffected foot.
7. **Procedural Step. Position the crutch tips approximately 2 inches anterior and 4 to 6 inches lateral to the foot, creating a triangle.**
   The large dots in the accompanying figure represent the crutch tips.

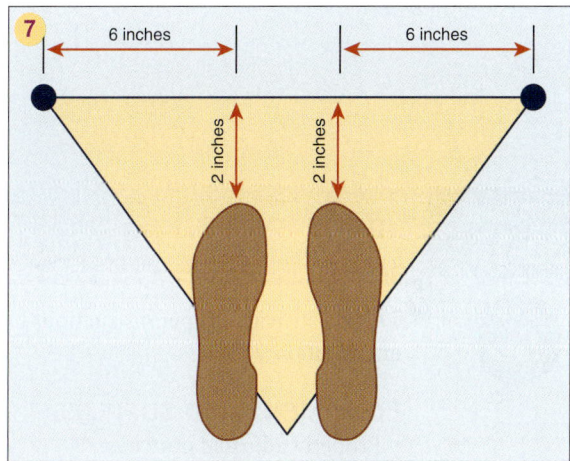

8. **Procedural Step. Adjust the crutches.**
   Remove the bolt and wing nut on the side of the crutch, and slide the support piece of the crutch either upward or downward to adjust the length of the crutch. The height of the crutch should be about 2 to 3 finger-widths below the patient's armpits. Replace the bolt and wing nut and tighten to secure the strut.

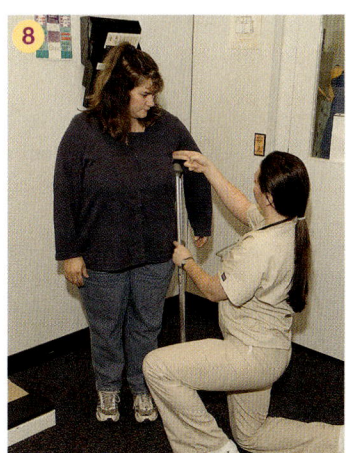

Continued

PROCEDURE 38-14 Measure for Axillary Crutches—cont'd

Rationale. Height adjustment is critical; without the gap of 2 or 3 finger-widths between the top of the crutch and the patient's armpit, nerve damage in the axillary region may result from the patient supporting body weight on the top of the crutch instead of on the handgrips.

HANDGRIP POSITIONS

9. **Procedural Step.** Once the height has been correctly adjusted, ask the patient to stand erect with a crutch beneath each axilla and to support his or her weight on the handgrips.

10. **Procedural Step.** Adjust the handgrips.
The handgrip level is adjusted in the same manner as the height was adjusted. Remove the bolt and wing nut and slide the handgrip upward or downward, as required. Secure the handgrip by replacing the bolt and tightening the wing nut. The handgrips should be adjusted so that the patient's elbows are flexed at an angle of 20 to 30 degrees. Verify the angle of the elbow using a goniometer.

11. **Procedural Step.** Perform a final check of the fit of the crutches.

PROCEDURE 38-15 Instruct the Patient in Crutch Gaits

TASK: Provide proper instructions to the patient for the appropriate crutch gait, depending on the injury or condition.

EQUIPMENT AND SUPPLIES
- Properly adjusted crutches
- Patient's medical record

SKILLS/RATIONALE   STANDARD PRECAUTIONS ARE TO BE FOLLOWED

NOTE: This procedure will most likely be performed immediately after adjusting the height and handgrip position of the crutches (see Procedure 38-14).

1. **Procedural Step.** Sanitize the hands.
An alcohol-based hand rub may be used instead of washing hands with soap and water, unless hands are visibly soiled.
Rationale. Hand sanitization promotes infection control.

2. **Procedural Step.** Assemble equipment and supplies.
Obtain the appropriate crutches previously fitted to the patient.
Rationale. It is important to have all supplies and equipment ready and available before starting any procedure to ensure efficiency.

3. **Procedural Step.** Obtain the patient's medical record.

4. **Procedural Step.** Greet the patient, introduce yourself, and identify the patient.
Rationale. Identifying the patient ensures the procedure is performed on the correct patient.

5. **Procedural Step.** Explain the procedure to the patient.

Rationale. Explaining the procedure to the patient promotes cooperation and provides a means of obtaining implied consent.

6. **Procedural Step.** Ask the patient to stand erect and face straight ahead.

7. **Procedural Step.** Position the crutches.
Place the tips of the crutches 4 to 6 inches anterior and 4 to 6 inches lateral to the side of each foot. This is referred to as the *tripod* position (see Figure 38-10).
Rationale. The tripod position provides the patient with a wide base of support and is the basic crutch stance used before crutch walking.

FOUR-POINT GAIT

8. **Procedural Step.** Instruct the patient in the four-point gait.
The four-point gait is a slower gait used for patients who are able to move each leg independently and bear weight on both legs. The patient moves one crutch forward, then the opposite foot forward. The other crutch is then moved forward, then the opposite leg. The four-point gait provides at least three points of contact at all times

Continued

PROCEDURE 38-15   Instruct the Patient in Crutch Gaits—cont'd

and is most often used for patients who have muscle weakness or poor muscular coordination (see Figure 38-11, D).

THREE-POINT GAIT

9. **Procedural Step. Instruct the patient in the three-point gait.**

   The three-point gait is used for the patient who can support full body weight on one leg and can touch the foot of the affected leg to the ground, but not bear weight on it. The patient moves forward by moving the crutches forward at the same time as the affected leg. The crutches bear the weight, and the affected foot touches the ground only for balance. The unaffected leg is then moved forward, and body weight is transferred to the unaffected leg. Patients who use this gait most often have musculoskeletal or soft tissue trauma to a lower extremity (e.g., fracture, sprain). This gait requires the patient to have good upper body strength and coordination (see Figure 38-11, C).

TWO-POINT GAIT

10. **Procedural Step. Instruct the patient in the two-point gait.**

    The two-point gait is used when a patient is capable of bearing partial weight on each leg. It is similar to the four-point gait but requires the patient to have greater coordination and balance. Two-point gait is an advanced gait and is typically used only after the four-point gait is mastered. The patient moves one crutch and the opposite leg forward while bearing partial weight on the opposite leg and crutch. The opposite crutch and opposite leg are then moved forward in the same manner (see Figure 38-11, B).

SWING GAITS

11. **Procedural Step. Instruct the patient in swing gaits.**

    The swing gaits include the *swing-to* gait and the *swing-through* gait. The gait is accomplished by moving both crutches forward and then swinging the legs up to meet the crutches (swing-to) or to stop slightly in front of the crutches (swing-through). Patients who use these gaits include those with severe lower extremity disabilities (e.g., paralysis) and those wearing supportive braces or prosthetic legs (see Figure 38-11, A).

12. **Procedural Step. Sanitize the hands.**

    Always sanitize the hands after every procedure or after using gloves.

13. **Procedural Step. Document the instruction.**

    Document in the patient's medical record that the patient was provided with verbal and written instructions, as well as a demonstration of the proper crutch use and gait, and that the patient understood the procedure and could return demonstrate the crutch gait to be used.

CHARTING EXAMPLE

Date	
8/16/xx	10:00 a.m. Patient instructed in basic 4-point gait after crutches adjusted appropriate for height. After several min of assisted gait, pt. demonstrated 4-point gait independently and appropriately. Questions answered and pt. discharged with crutches and telephone # to call for problem. Will rtn in 1 week for f/u. ———————————— S. Keill, CMA (AAMA)

position is the beginning position (Figure 38-10). Crutches can be used in four different gait patterns: four-point, two-point, three-point, and swing-through gaits.

Four-Point Gait. The four-point gait pattern requires the use of two ambulation aids (e.g., two crutches, two canes). The gait begins with the patient first placing one crutch or cane forward, followed by placing the *opposite* lower extremity forward (i.e., right crutch, left foot; left crutch, right foot). This gait is stable and slow but is the safest approach in crowded areas. The patient does not exert much energy because the patient must walk slowly to maintain balance (Figure 38-11, *D*).

Two-Point Gait. As with the four-point gait, the two-point gait requires two ambulation aids. Instead of using an alternating pattern, however, the crutch or cane is placed forward *at the same time* as the opposite lower extremity (Figure 38-11, *B*). This gait is quicker than the four-point gait and is closest to a person's normal gait. It requires more coordination because

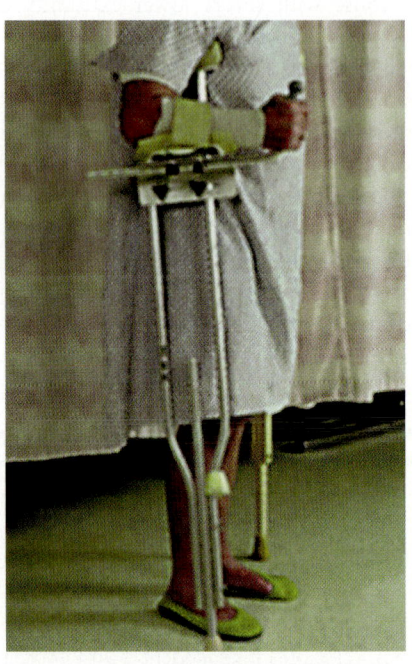

FIGURE 38-9 Patient with platform crutches. Patient uses forearms to lean on crutches. (From Zakus SM: *Mosby's clinical skills for medical assistants,* ed 4, St Louis, 2001, Mosby.)

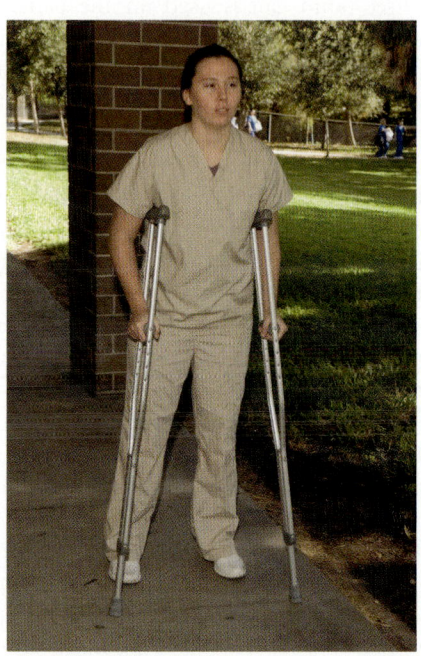

FIGURE 38-10 Basic crutch stance is the tripod position

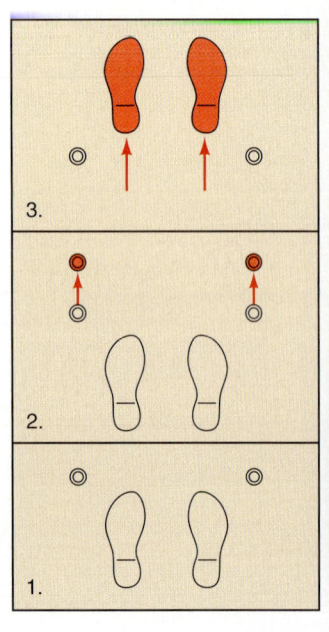
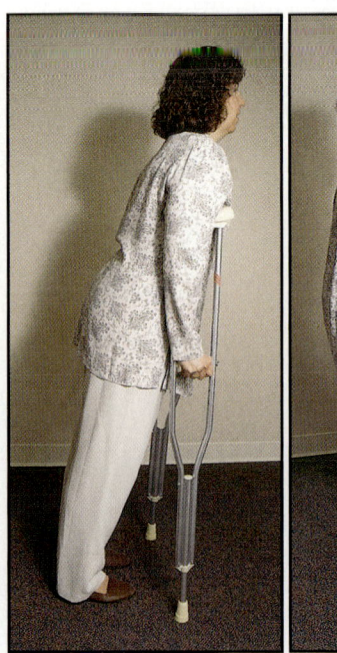
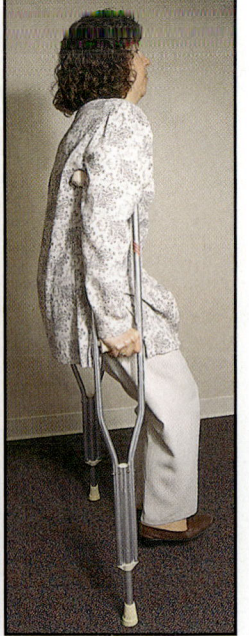

FIGURE 38-11 Crutch gait patterns. **A,** Swing-through gait. (Stand with both feet together; move both crutches; move both legs by swinging them forward.)

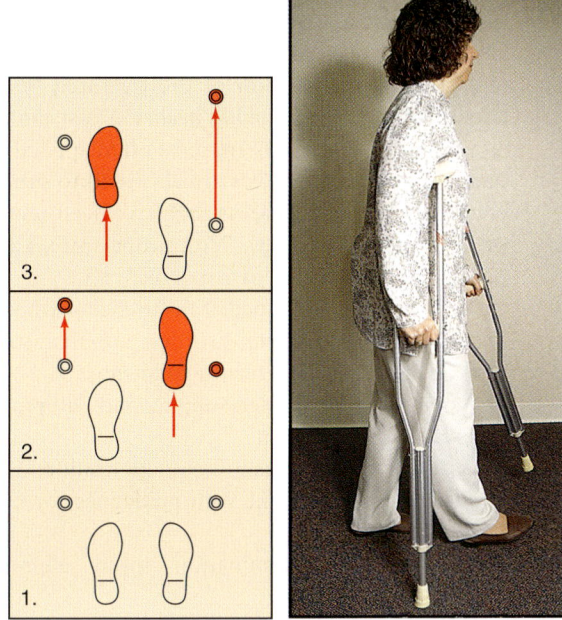
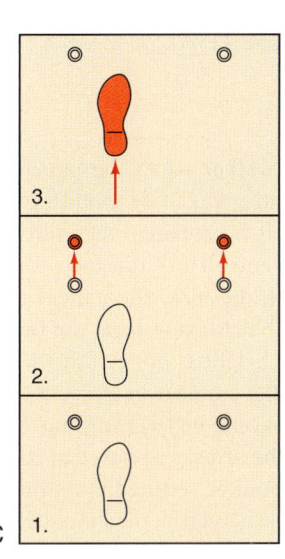
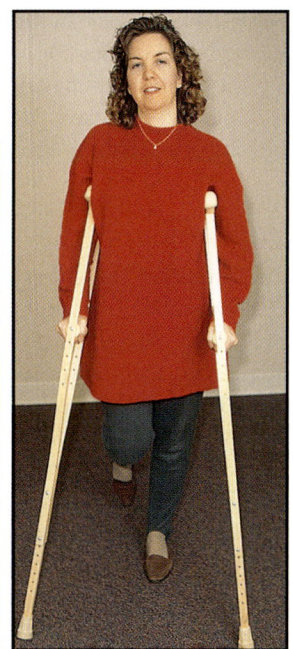
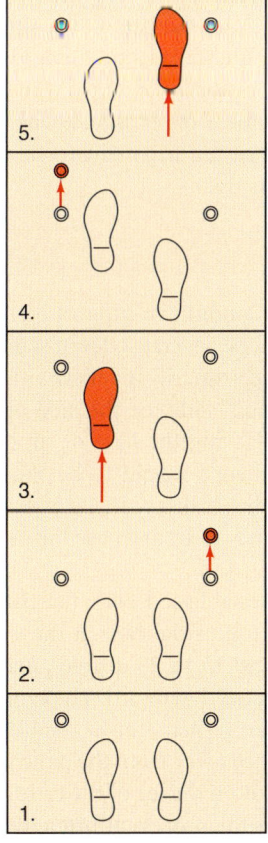
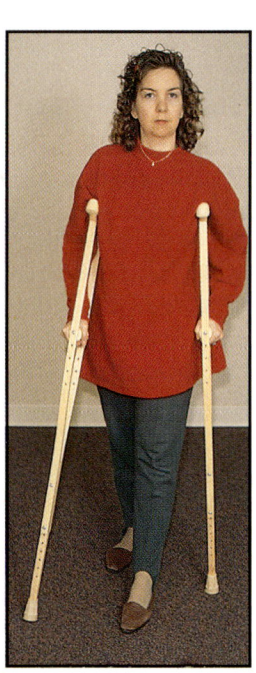

FIGURE 38-11, cont'd **B,** Two-point gait. (Stand with both feet together; move one leg together with one crutch on opposite side; move other leg with opposing crutch.) **C,** Three-point gait. (Stand with both feet together; move both crutches together with affected leg; move unaffected leg.) **D,** Four-point crutch gait. (Move right crutch; move left foot; move left crutch; move right foot.) (From Chester GA: *Modern medical assisting*, Philadelphia, 1998, Saunders.)

the upper extremity and the opposite lower extremity are moving at the same time. There is less stability with the two-point gait.

Three-Point Gait. The three-point gait, or *tripod* position, requires two crutches. The patient basically "steps through" the crutches. This gait is typically used when the patient can bear weight on one lower extremity but not the other (e.g., foot sprain). The non–weight-bearing extremity (leg not able to support weight) and crutches are moved forward, and the patient steps through the crutches (Figure 38-11, *C*). The three-point gait pattern is less stable than four-point gait but is quicker for the patient. The patient's upper body strength must be strong. The three-point gait also requires more energy from the patient.

Swing-Through Gait. In the swing-through gait, the patient moves both crutches forward. Both legs are swung through to a position ahead of the crutches. This gait is used with amputees, patients who have paralysis, or in cases where full weight-bearing is a problem (Figure 38-11, *A*).

Walkers

The physician prescribes a **walker** when the patient needs optimal stability, support, and a way to be mobile. It may be prescribed even when there is no apparent leg injury. There are various styles of walkers, and all are adjustable for proper fit. Walkers with wheels in front allow the patient to move more quickly but are less stable. Most walkers can be folded.

Measurement for proper height is done with the patient standing in the walker with the crossbar in front, as follows:
- The top of the handgrip should be level with the crease in the patient's wrist when the arms are relaxed at the sides.
- The feet of the walker should be resting flat on the floor.
- When the patient grasps the handgrip, the shoulders should be level and the elbows flexed 15 to 25 degrees.

The patient should move the walker forward 6 inches and then step into the walker. After the patient becomes stronger and more skilled at using the walker, the forward space may need to be adjusted. The medical assistant must observe the patient walking to determine if the fit is adequate. Procedure 38-16 explains how to measure a patient for a walker and provide instructions for its use.

Canes

A **cane** provides the least amount of support for the patient of all the ambulatory devices. Several styles of standard canes are available. A cane is used primarily to relieve weight bearing and is placed on the "good" side, or the side opposite the weaker lower extremity. Having the base of support on the strong side allows the patient's weight to be shifted toward this side and away from the weaker side. Be aware, however, that patients have a tendency to want to use the cane on their weak side.

Proper fitting can be established with the patient in an upright position and the top of the cane at the wrist crease. The elbow should be flexed 15 to 25 degrees, and the force of the cane should be directed downward. The cane should be alongside the patient's toes. When a *quad cane* (four-legged cane) is used, it is positioned away from the patient, reducing the risk of catching the foot on the leg of the cane and falling. Procedure 38-17 describes the process of properly measuring the patient for a cane and providing instructions for its use.

> **PATIENT-CENTERED PROFESSIONALISM**
>
> - Why does the medical assistant have to be knowledgeable about the proper fit and use of ambulatory devices?
> - Why must the medical assistant be able to instruct the patient in the use of ambulatory devices?

CASTS

The purpose of a **cast** is to immobilize a body part (e.g., arm, leg). The immobilization of the fractured bone allows for alignment until the bone has healed. A cast can be thought of as a rigid dressing. Casts are most often applied to bones that have been fractured. Casts are also used to promote postoperative healing and in areas that have been severely sprained or dislocated (Box 38-3). With proper care, a cast facilitates healing and speeds the patient's recovery.

Normally, an **orthopedist,** a physician whose specialty is to correct musculoskeletal disorders, applies casts. The medical assistant is responsible for the following:
- Assembling the needed supplies and equipment.
- Preparing the patient.
- Assisting the physician in cast application.
- Providing the patient with guidelines for cast care (Box 38-4).
- Cleaning the examination room after the patient leaves.

Cast Materials

Casts can be made of several types of materials: plaster-of-Paris, synthetic, fiberglass, and air. The type of material selected depends on the type of injury and its severity. Casts are applied to immobilize both the joint above and the joint below the fracture or injury.
- An **air cast** is a plastic cover filled with air that is used in emergency situations for stabilization.
- A **synthetic cast** is more of an *immobilizer* that can be removed when the limb is not being used; it is preferred for simple breaks (fractures) or sprains (Figure 38-12).
- Plaster and fiberglass casts are normally used for more complicated fractures.

Plaster Cast

A **plaster cast** is formed by wetting bandage rolls that contain calcium sulfate crystals and then molding the rolls to the injured body part. When the bandage roll comes in contact with water and is applied to the affected body part, the patient experiences a sense of warmth as the plaster hardens. As the bandage is being applied, it molds to the site. The medical assistant needs to instruct the patient not to lay the cast against anything until it dries; a dent in the cast will cause pressure on the underlying skin, which may result in pain and a **pressure ulcer** later. As the cast dries, usually within 72 hours, it forms a rigid protective dressing.

Fiberglass Cast

Using tapes in combination with a fiberglass or a plastic resin forms a **fiberglass cast.** The advantages of a fiberglass cast are that it is lighter, dries more quickly, and resists water better than a plaster cast (but cannot get soaking wet because the skin underneath may break down). Fiberglass also comes in various colors, which may appeal to adults (for stylistic reasons) as well as children.

PROCEDURE 38-16: Instruct the Patient in the Use of a Walker

TASK: Accurately measure and provide patient instructions for proper use of a walker.

EQUIPMENT AND SUPPLIES
- Walker
- Patient's medical record

SKILLS/RATIONALE

STANDARD PRECAUTIONS ARE TO BE FOLLOWED.

1. **Procedural Step.** Sanitize the hands.
   An alcohol-based hand rub may be used instead of washing hands with soap and water, unless hands are visibly soiled.
   Rationale. Hand sanitization promotes infection control.

2. **Procedural Step.** Assemble equipment and supplies.
   Rationale. It is important to have all supplies and equipment ready and available before starting any procedure to ensure efficiency.

3. **Procedural Step.** Obtain the patient's medical record.

4. **Procedural Step.** Greet the patient, introduce yourself, and confirm the patient's identity.
   Rationale. Identifying the patient ensures the procedure is performed on the correct patient.

5. **Procedural Step.** Explain the procedure to the patient.
   Rationale. Explaining the procedure to the patient promotes cooperation and provides a means of obtaining implied consent.

6. **Procedural Step.** Adjust the height of the walker.
   The top of the walker should be just below the patient's waist at the same height as the top of the hipbone. When properly adjusted, the patient's elbows will bend at approximately a 30-degree angle.

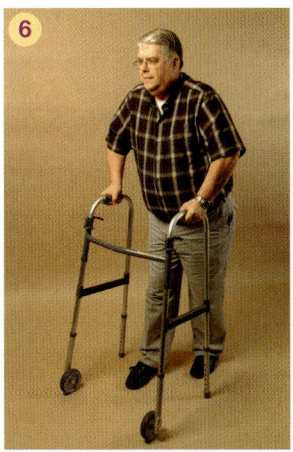

7. **Procedural Step.** Instruct the patient to stand in the center of the walker and grasp the hand grips. Now have the patient pick up the walker and move it forward approximately 6 to 8 inches.

8. **Procedural Step.** Have the patient move the dominant foot and then the nondominant foot into the "center" of the walker.

9. **Procedural Step.** Caution the patient to be sure he or she has good balance before moving the walker ahead again.
   NOTE: If the patient does not have enough strength to pick up the walker, obtain a walker that has wheels in the front, although they are not as stable.
   Rationale. Moving the walker forward requires that the patient have good balance before moving it. If not, the patient may fall and be injured.

10. **Procedural Step.** Repeat Steps 7 and 8 through the distance to be covered.

11. **Procedural Step.** Observe the patient for several repetitions to make sure the patient understands the process and can manage the walker.

12. **Procedural Step.** If the walker folds for storage or transport, provide the patient with instructions, demonstrate the process, and observe the patient performing this function. It may be necessary and desirable to involve a family member or other caregiver in this task as well.

13. **Procedural Step.** Sanitize the hands.
    Always sanitize the hands after every procedure or after using gloves.

14. **Procedural Step.** Document the instruction.
    Document in the patient's medical record that the patient was provided with verbal and written instructions as well as a demonstration of the proper use of the walker, and that the patient understood the procedure.

CHARTING EXAMPLE

Date	
9/12/xx	10:40 a.m. After properly adjusting the walker to patient, pt. demonstrated proper use of walker for stability. Wife present and both pt. and wife were shown how to fold walker for storage. Questions answered and pt. discharged with walker; rtn in 1 week for follow-up. — S. Patton, RMA

| PROCEDURE 38-17 | Instruct the Patient in the Use of a Cane | |

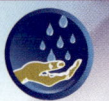

TASK: Accurately measure and provide patient instructions for proper use of a cane.

EQUIPMENT AND SUPPLIES
- Cane
- Patient's medical record

SKILLS/RATIONALE

STANDARD PRECAUTIONS ARE TO BE FOLLOWED.

1. **Procedural Step. Sanitize the hands.**
   An alcohol-based hand rub may be used instead of washing hands with soap and water, unless hands are visibly soiled.
   Rationale. Hand sanitization promotes infection control.

2. **Procedural Step. Assemble equipment and supplies.**
   Obtain the appropriate cane for the patient. Several styles of canes are available.
   Rationale. It is important to have all supplies and equipment ready and available before starting any procedure to ensure efficiency.

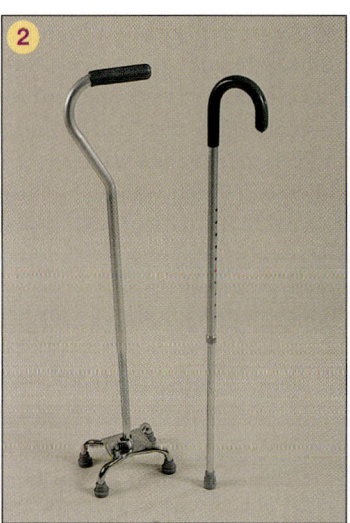

3. **Procedural Step. Obtain the patient's medical record.**

4. **Procedural Step. Greet the patient, introduce yourself, and confirm the patient's identity.**
   Rationale. Identifying the patient ensures the procedure is performed on the correct patient.

5. **Procedural Step. Explain the procedure to the patient.**
   Rationale. Explaining the procedure to the patient promotes cooperation and provides a means of obtaining implied consent.

6. **Procedural Step. Measure for the correct height of the cane.**
   For the cane to fit properly, the patient should stand straight. Measure from the crease at the patient's wrist to the floor. You may increase this measurement by 2 inches if it is more comfortable for the patient. The patient's elbow should bend at a 30-degree angle when the cane is adjusted correctly for the patient.

7. **Procedural Step. Position the cane.**
   Place the cane on the strong side of the patient's body (in the hand opposite the involved leg) 4 to 6 inches to the side of the foot. The top of the cane should be placed level with the greater trochanter of the hip, and the elbow should be flexed 30 degrees.
   Rationale. Provides added support for the weak or impaired side.

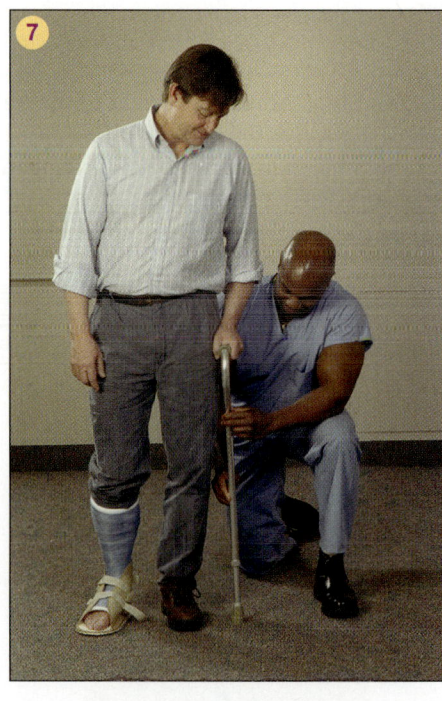

Continued

PROCEDURE 38-17: Instruct the Patient in the Use of a Cane—cont'd

8. **Procedural Step.** Instruct the patient to move the cane and affected leg forward at the same time (6 to 10 inches).
   Rationale. Body weight is supported by cane and uninvolved leg.
9. **Procedural Step.** Instruct the patient to move the unaffected leg forward just past the cane.
   Rationale. Body weight is supported by cane and uninvolved leg.
10. **Procedural Step.** Repeat Steps 8 and 9 through the distance to be covered.
11. **Procedural Step.** Document the instruction.
    Document in the patient's medical record that the patient was provided with verbal and written instructions, as well as a demonstration of the proper use of the cane, and that the patient understood the procedure.
12. **Procedural Step.** Sanitize the hands.
    Always sanitize the hands after every procedure or after using gloves.

CHARTING EXAMPLE

Date	
9/11/xx	11:50 a.m. Cane adjusted for patient use on left side for assisting c̄ with weakness in right ankle. Pt. was instructed and assisted in cane walking until comfortable, then demonstrated same independently. Questions answered; pt. discharged with cane and written instructions. Rtn in 1 wk for f/u.————— B. Larrson, CMA (AAMA)

BOX 38-3

Types of Casts

Short arm cast is used for a fracture or dislocation of the wrist. It extends from about mid-palm to just below the elbow.

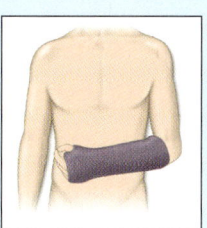

Long arm cast is used for a fracture of the forearm or upper arm (humerus). It extends from the axilla to mid-palm, with a 90-degree bend at the elbow.

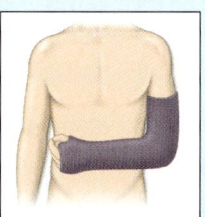

Short leg cast is used for fracture of the ankle. It extends from just below the knee to the toes. The foot extends naturally.

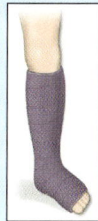

Long leg cast is used for fractures of the tibia, fibula, or femur. It extends from the upper thigh to the toes. The knee is slightly bent and the foot extends naturally.

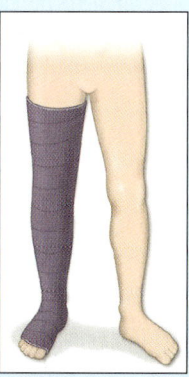

Walking cast is a cast with a walking heel.

Illustrations modified from Bonewit-West K: *Clinical procedures for medical assistants,* ed 6, Philadelphia, 2004, Saunders.

BOX 38-4

Patient Guidelines for Cast Care

1. A wet cast may be dried with a small fan. This allows air to circulate and assists in drying the cast.
2. Do not apply pressure to a wet or damp cast. This could create a pressure area under the cast and cause tissue damage.
3. Maintain elevation of the extremity with pillows to reduce swelling and discomfort.
4. Keep the cast uncovered until completely dry.
5. Frequently assess the fingers and toes for color, feeling, or temperature change (e.g., pain, bluish discoloration, tingling, or coldness to fingers or toes may be an indication that a cast is too tight because of swelling). The physician should be notified immediately if changes occur.
6. Do not insert any item between the cast and body part (e.g., coat hanger to scratch irritated skin). This prevents injury to and infection of the skin tissues.
7. Avoid getting the cast wet. Cover it with a protective covering when bathing. (A plastic bag that protects a newspaper works well.) The skin and tissue may break down if the cast becomes and remains wet.
8. Only use water-soluble marking pens to write on the cast. This allows the cast to "breathe."
9. Clean the cast with a damp cloth.

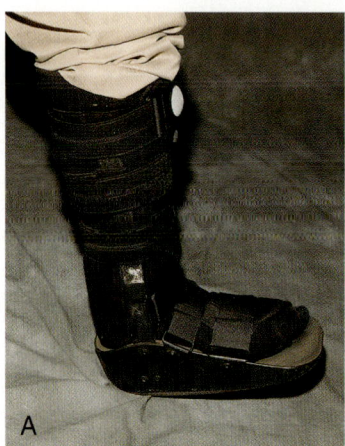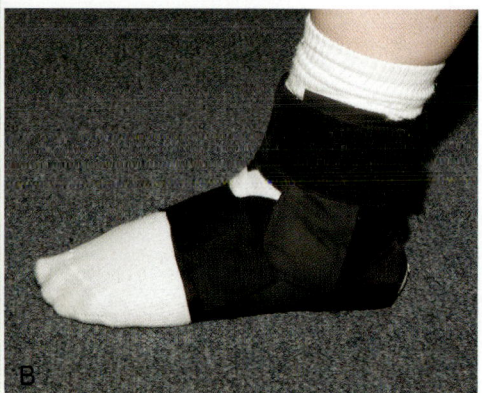

FIGURE 38-12 A, Synthetic boot cast. **B,** Synthetic foot immobilizer.

Cast Application

When the physician applies the cast, adequate space for blood circulation is needed for possible swelling and to allow healing. The medical assistant must check for capillary refill in fingers or toes (pressing the fingernails or toenails and watching the blood return). Application of the casting material involves the following stages:

1. *Inspecting the skin.* The area to be cast needs to be clean and dry. The location of all bruises, reddened areas, and skin breaks needs to be recorded in the patient's medical record.
2. *Applying the stockinette.* A **stockinette** is a knitted cotton material in tubular form. The diameter of the material stretches to accommodate a body part. A stockinette is used to protect the patient's skin at the edges of the cast. It is folded back over the casting material as it is molded. This keeps the hard casting material from rubbing the skin after the cast has been applied.
3. *Applying the cast padding.* The **cast padding** is a soft cotton material that comes in a roll of varying widths. The cast padding is applied over the stockinette. Its purpose is to protect the patient's skin when the cast is removed and to protect bony areas under the cast. Extra padding is applied to bony areas to prevent pressure ulcers and it is easily torn so the irregular bony areas can be padded more smoothly with fewer bumps.
4. *Applying cast bandage or tape.* Whichever type of cast is being applied, the material is applied over the cast padding. The number of layers of casting material used will depend on the desired strength needed. Gloves are required when applying the plaster or fiberglass material. Some physicians use a hand cream on their gloves to keep the fiberglass from sticking to the gloves.
5. *Allowing for drying time.* A cast must be allowed to dry adequately before weight bearing. To reduce strain on the body part and minimize swelling, the physician may prescribe an arm sling or crutches. The medical assistant must instruct the patient not to lean against anything with the cast until it is fully dry so the cast does not become damaged.

The patient needs to be reminded not to insert anything in the cast or use anything inside the cast to eliminate an itch (e.g., pen, pencil, or wire hanger). The object could injure the tissue and result in an infection.

Procedure 38-18 explains the process of providing supplies and assistance during the application of a plaster-of-Paris or

Therapeutic Procedures CHAPTER 38 849

PROCEDURE 38-18   Assist in Plaster-of-Paris or Fiberglass Cast Application

TASK: Provide supplies and assistance during cast application, and instruct the patient in cast care and nutritional requirements.

EQUIPMENT AND SUPPLIES
- Cast material to be used (plaster or fiberglass)
- Stockinette to fit extremity
- Sheet wadding (cast padding)
- Basin or bucket to hold warm water
- Scissors
- Disposable gloves
- Hand cream
- Patient's medical record

SKILLS/RATIONALE

STANDARD PRECAUTIONS ARE TO BE FOLLOWED.

1. **Procedural Step.** Sanitize the hands.
   An alcohol-based hand rub may be used instead of washing hands with soap and water, unless hands are visibly soiled.
   Rationale. Hand sanitization promotes infection control.

2. **Procedural Step.** Assemble equipment and supplies.
   Rationale. It is important to have all supplies and equipment ready and available before starting any procedure to ensure efficiency.

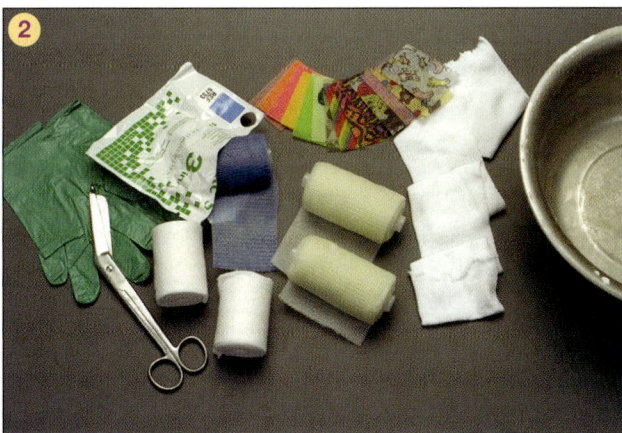

3. **Procedural Step.** Obtain the patient's medical record.
4. **Procedural Step.** Greet the patient, introduce yourself, and confirm the patient's identity.
   Rationale. Identifying the patient ensures the procedure is performed on the correct patient.
5. **Procedural Step.** Explain the procedure to the patient.
   Rationale. Explaining the procedure to the patient promotes cooperation and provides a means of obtaining implied consent.
6. **Procedural Step.** Place the patient in a position of comfort (sitting, lying down, or standing) for the type of cast to be applied.
   Body parts to be cast must be supported and in alignment for cast application.

7. **Procedural Step.** Clean and dry the area to be cast as directed by the physician and observe for areas of broken skin, redness, and bruising.
   Note observations in the patient's medical record.
   Rationale. Determining the condition of the skin before cast application provides information for later evaluation.

8. **Procedural Step.** Prepare the stockinette.
   Cut the appropriate size (width and length) of stockinette with 1 to 2 inches above and below the area being cast. The physician will apply and remove any creases. The physician will leave 1 to 2 inches of excess stockinette above and below the area to be cast.
   Rationale. Using stockinette that is too large could cause creases to form, thus causing tissue damage. Excess stockinette will be used later to finish the edges of the cast.

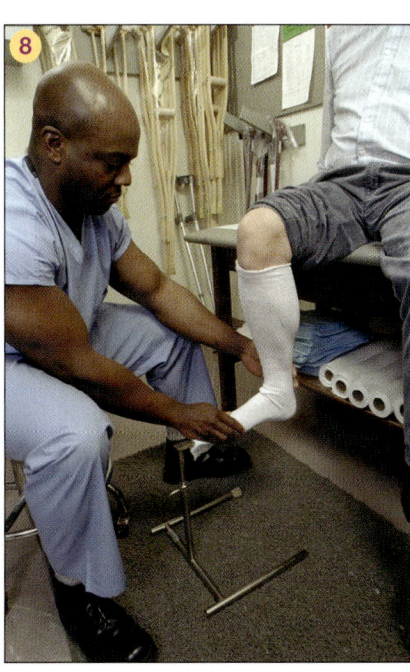

Continued

PROCEDURE 38-18 Assist in Plaster-of-Paris or Fiberglass Cast Application—cont'd

9. **Procedural Step.** Prepare the cast padding.

   Choose the appropriate size (width and length) of cast padding for the area being cast. The physician will apply the padding using a spiral bandage turn application. Extra padding will be added to areas of bony prominence (e.g., wrist, ankle bone).

   Rationale. Using cast padding that is too large could cause creases to form, resulting in pressure on skin tissue.

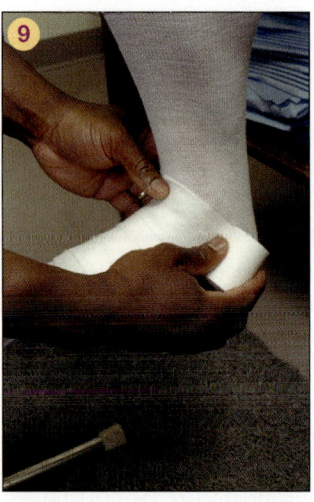

10. **Procedural Step.** When the physician is ready to apply the cast, put on disposable gloves.
11. **Procedural Step.** Prepare the plaster or fiberglass roll.

    Depending on the type of cast material used, do one of the following:
    a. Hold the plaster roll in the container of water until the bubbles stop (about 5 seconds). Remove it from the water and gently squeeze the excess water from the roll, and hand it to the physician.
    b. Hold the fiberglass roll under warm water for 10 to 15 seconds. Gently squeeze to remove excess water.

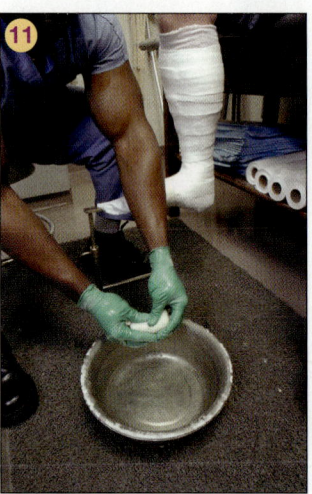

12. **Procedural Step.** Assist as needed by holding the body part in the position requested by the physician.
13. **Procedural Step.** Repeat Step 11 (a or b) until the cast is completed.
14. **Procedural Step.** Reassure the patient as needed.
15. **Procedural Step.** Assist with folding the stockinette or padding down over the outer edge of the cast to form a smooth edge.

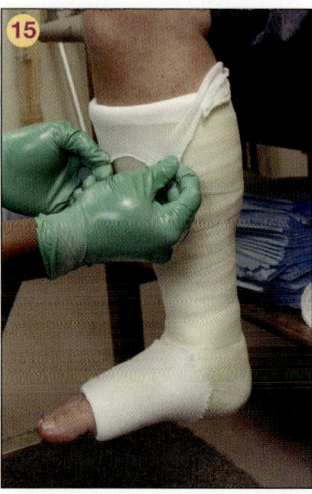

16. **Procedural Step.** Provide scissors or a plastic knife to the physician to trim areas around thumb, fingers, or toes as necessary.

    NOTE: Handle the casted extremity with palms only because fingers can cause indentations that could create pressure areas.
17. **Procedural Step.** Provide verbal and written cast instructions and isometric exercise instructions if prescribed by the physician.
18. **Procedural Step.** Clean the equipment and room.

    Discard water and excess materials.
19. **Procedural Step.** Remove gloves and sanitize the hands.

    Always sanitize the hands after every procedure or after using gloves.
20. **Procedural Step.** Document the procedure.

    Include the date and time, location, condition of underlying tissue and type of cast, and the patient's reaction. Document that the patient was provided with verbal and written instructions.

CHARTING EXAMPLE

Date	
12/14/xx	10:30 a.m. ® short leg fiberglass cast applied. Skin under cast is intact and clean, bruising over lateral ankle. Pt. tolerated procedure well. Pt. given verbal and written follow-up instructions and cast care.———P. Allen, CMA (AAMA)

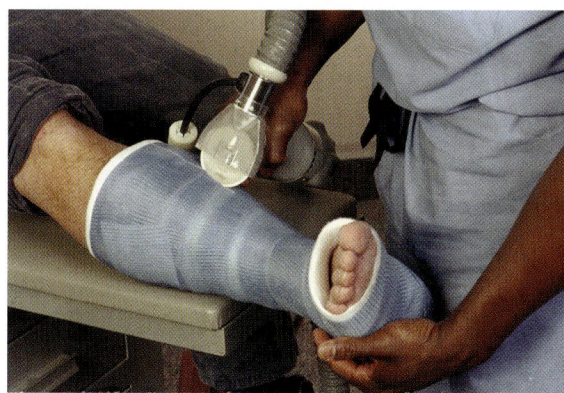

FIGURE 38-13 A cast cutter makes a separation in the cast without cutting through the wadding underneath.

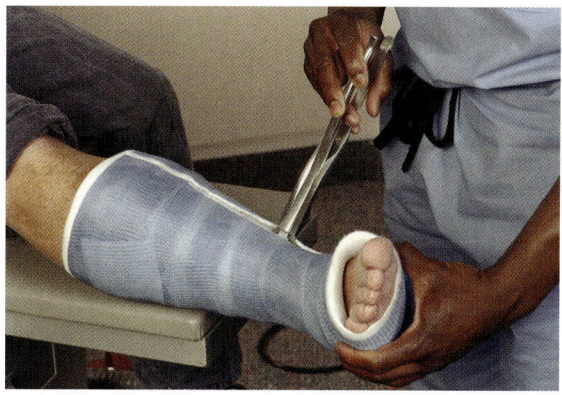

FIGURE 38-14 A cast spreader is used to increase the space between the two sections of the cast so that the wadding and stockinette can be cut with scissors.

fiberglass cast, as well as instructing the patient in cast care and nutritional requirements.

Cast Removal

To remove a cast, the physician uses a **cast cutter** to divide the cast in two parts (top and bottom). The cast cutter does not truly cut but instead vibrates back and forth to separate the casting material (Figure 38-13). A **cast spreader** is then used to open up the cast. Bandage scissors are used to cut through the cast padding and stockinette (Figure 38-14).

When the cast is removed, the normal appearance of the limb is pale (white to yellowish), and scaly, with old dried skin as well as a foul smell. The muscle tissue appears soft and flabby from lack of use. The medical assistant may need to provide instructions on skin care and exercises the physician has prescribed for regaining use of the limb. The physician will often prescribe physical therapy for the patient to regain the maximum range of motion of the affected limb. Some helpful hints for cast removal and aftercare are as follows:

1. Prove to the patient (especially children) that the cast saw will not hurt them. This can be done by touching the saw to their hand. This provides reassurance that the patient will not be cut.
2. If the cast is cut so that a top and bottom are available, the body part can be left in the bottom half until the physician checks the patient. This eliminates possible reinjury of the body part.
3. Explain to the patient that the condition of the skin under the cast will depend on the length of time the cast was in place and the integrity of the skin before the application of the cast.
4. Gently wash the body part with a warm, moist towel after the cast is removed. Avoid scrubbing the delicate skin because it will slough off within a few days, and hard scrubbing could cause the skin to break down.
5. The patient should be scheduled for exercises to increase mobility and muscle strength in the affected area.

PATIENT-CENTERED PROFESSIONALISM

- How would the medical assistant explain cast application and removal to a patient?

CONCLUSION

Many types of therapeutic procedures are prescribed by physicians and performed in the medical office. The physician must perform some of these procedures, but medical assistants can perform others or assist the physician with others. Therapeutic procedures reduce pain, help the body heal after injury or disease, and assist in patient mobility during recovery or when body parts are weak.

Understanding the correct techniques to perform these procedures is essential for medical assistants. Equally important is the ability to prepare for therapeutic procedures and provide the support and education that patients need before, during, and after the procedure. When these skills are mastered and performed with competence and professionalism, the patient's experience will be positive, and the patient will be more likely to follow the prescribed treatment plan.

Chapter Summary

Reinforce your understanding of the material in this chapter by reviewing the curriculum objectives and key content points below.

1. **Define, appropriately use, and spell all the Key Terms for this chapter.**
   - Review the Key Terms if necessary.
2. **Demonstrate the correct procedure for irrigating the external ear canal to remove cerumen or foreign objects.**
   - Review Procedure 38-1.
3. **Demonstrate the procedure for properly instilling prescribed medication in an affected ear.**
   - Review Procedure 38-2.
4. **Explain why extreme care must be taken when working with a patient's infected ear.**
   - When an ear is infected it becomes very painful and the tympanic membrane may be bulging and could rupture if care is not taken.
5. **Demonstrate the correct procedure for irrigating a patient's eye to remove foreign particles.**
   - Review Procedure 38-3.
6. **Demonstrate the procedure for properly instilling prescribed medication in an affected eye.**
   - Review Procedure 38-4.
7. **Explain why the medical assistant should be careful not to touch the surface of the eye with the tip of the irrigating syringe, the tip of the eyedropper, or the finger.**
   - Touching the surface of the affected eye could contaminate the syringe or eyedropper. This can result in cross-contamination if the contaminated items come into contact with other areas.
8. **List three common uses for bandages.**
   - Bandages can be used for support or immobilization, to hold dressings in place, and to apply pressure to control bleeding.
9. **Differentiate between an elastic bandage and a Kling-type bandage.**
   - An elastic bandage (Ace bandage) is made of cloth and contains elastic; it can be reused on the patient if not soiled.
   - A Kling-type bandage is made of stretchy loose fibers but contains no elastic.
10. **List and briefly describe five basic bandage turns.**
    - Circular bandage turn overlaps the previous turn.
    - Spiral bandage turn progresses upward, and each spiral overlaps the previous turn.
    - Spiral reverse bandage turn progresses downward and overlaps.
    - Figure-eight bandage turn is applied on a slant and progresses upward and then downward to support a dressing or joint.
    - Recurrent bandage turn is used for a stump or the head and begins with a circular turn and progresses back and forth, overlapping each turn.
11. **Demonstrate the procedure for properly applying a tubular gauze bandage to an affected area.**
    - Review Procedure 38-5.
12. **Explain the effects of local application of cold therapy on an injured body part.**
    - Cold therapy serves to temporarily decrease circulatory blood flow to an injured body part.
    - Decreased blood flow helps reduce or prevent swelling, slows cellular growth, and reduces bleeding.
13. **Demonstrate the procedure for properly applying an ice bag.**
    - Review Procedure 38-6.
14. **Demonstrate the procedure for properly applying cold compresses.**
    - Review Procedure 38-7.
15. **Demonstrate the procedure for properly activating and applying a chemical cold pack.**
    - Review Procedure 38-8.
16. **Explain the effects of local application of heat therapy on an injured body part.**
    - Heat therapy serves to increase blood flow to a traumatized body area.
    - Heat reduces pain and speeds up the inflammatory process, promoting cell and tissue growth by removing wastes faster and increasing nutrients to the area.
17. **Demonstrate the procedure for properly applying a hot water bag.**
    - Review Procedure 38-9.
18. **Demonstrate the procedure for properly applying a heating pad.**
    - Review Procedure 38-10.
19. **Demonstrate the procedure for properly applying a hot compress to increase circulation.**
    - Review Procedure 38-11.
20. **Demonstrate the procedure for properly applying hot soaks for pain or swelling relief.**
    - Review Procedure 38-12.
21. **List three therapeutic uses of ultrasound therapy.**
    - Ultrasound procedures are used for pain relief for muscle spasms, inflammation, and arthritis.
22. **Demonstrate the correct procedure for administering an ultrasound treatment.**
    - Review Procedure 38-13.
23. **Explain the importance of ensuring that an ambulatory device properly fits the patient.**
    - An ambulatory device that does not fit properly can decrease stability, increase use of energy, decrease function, and compromise patient safety.
    - Improper fit also may cause the patient to develop bad gait habits or unsafe gait patterns and may result in tissue trauma (e.g., armpit).
24. **Demonstrate the procedure for properly measuring a patient for crutches.**
    - Review Procedure 38-14.

25. **Demonstrate the correct procedure for providing instructions to the patient for the appropriate crutch gait depending on the patient's injury or condition.**
    - Review Procedure 38-15.
26. **Demonstrate the procedure for properly measuring and instructing the patient in the use of a walker.**
    - Review Procedure 38-16.
27. **Demonstrate the procedure for properly measuring and instructing the patient in the use of a cane.**
    - Review Procedure 38-17.
28. **Explain the purpose of a cast.**
    - Casts immobilize body parts to allow for proper alignment until bones or injured areas have healed.
29. **Demonstrate the correct procedure for providing supplies and assistance during plaster-of-Paris or fiberglass cast application and instructing the patient in cast care and nutritional requirements for healing.**
    - Review Procedure 38-18.
30. **Describe the process of cast removal and explain patient instructions that medical assistants may need to provide during the procedure.**
    - Patients must be instructed not to lean the cast on anything until it is dry and not to put anything in the cast or use anything inside the cast to scratch an itch.
    - A cast cutter, cast spreader, and bandage scissors are used to remove the cast, padding, and stockinette.
31. **Analyze a realistic medical office situation and apply your understanding of therapeutic procedures to determine the best course of action.**
    - When the medical assistant is knowledgeable about each procedure he or she performs, there is less chance for error when performing the procedure.
32. **Describe the impact on patient care when medical assistants understand the purpose and use of therapeutic procedures in the medical office.**
    - When the medical assistant understands the purpose and expected outcome of each therapeutic procedure, the patient benefits by having quality care.
    - Thoroughly understanding each procedure allows the medical assistant to answer all the patient's questions.

PRACTICAL APPLICATIONS

If you have accomplished the objectives in this chapter, you will be able to make better choices as a medical assistant. Take another look at this situation and decide what you would do.

A multispecialty practice has medical assistants who work with each of the specialists. Allene, a medical assistant who has not had the benefit of training, works with Dr. Sumar, an ophthalmologist. Gerald, a graduate of a medical-assisting program, works with Dr. Herzog, an orthopedist. The ophthalmologist and the otolaryngologist share the same examination room, but they use it on different days. Allene is not very busy one day, so she decides to clean the medicine cabinet and rearrange the drugs. She moves the ophthalmic medications to the spot where the otic medications are usually stored and vice versa.

When Dr. Sumar treats a patient with conjunctivitis the next day, Allene hands him an otic preparation for the eye instillation. Luckily, Dr. Sumar reads the label on the medication before instilling the drops into the patient's eye. Later in the day, Dr. Sumar reprimands Allene for handing him the otic drops.

Gerald is the person who communicates to the orthopedic patients the necessity of correct application of the bandaging, as well as the care of a cast after its application. For those who need cold or heat therapy, Gerald is responsible for the applications as ordered by Dr. Herzog, and Gerald also performs the ultrasound treatments as indicated. During ultrasound treatments, Gerald is very careful to have sufficient coupling agent and to keep the head of the machine moving at all times.

Would you be able to step into the role of Allene or Gerald and perform their duties successfully?

1. Why is it important for ophthalmic and otic preparations to remain in the same storage places?
2. What is the danger of placing otic medications into the patient's eye?
3. Would the ear patient have a problem if the ophthalmic preparation had been used for the ear instillation?
4. What reasons do you believe led to Allene's reprimand? What actions during the cleaning process could have caused the medication error?
5. Why is it important for Gerald to teach patients to apply bandages from distal to proximal?
6. What does Gerald need to teach a patient about caring for a plaster cast?
7. Why is it important for Gerald to keep the head of the ultrasound machine moving at all times?
8. Why should Gerald be concerned if the patient complains of heat during an ultrasound treatment?

WEB SEARCH

1. Research legal requirements regarding the performance of therapeutic procedures (e.g., ultrasound treatments) in your state.

- **Keywords:** Use the following keywords in your search: therapeutic procedures, medical procedures.

Specialty Diagnostic Testing

39

evolve http://evolve.elsevier.com/klieger/medicalassisting

To **diagnose**, or to identify a disease process, the physician must rely on the patient's signs, symptoms, history, and diagnostic test results. Diagnostic imaging techniques, electrocardiography, radiologic tests, and vision testing are discussed in previous chapters, and Chapter 42 discusses urinalysis and blood analysis. This chapter discusses other diagnostic tests performed in the medical office, including those associated with gynecological and obstetrical examinations, colon tests, pulmonary function, blood saturation, and hearing acuity.

LEARNING OBJECTIVES

You will be able to do the following after completing this chapter:

Key Terms
1. Define, appropriately use, and spell all the Key Terms for this chapter.

Gynecological Examination and Testing
2. Explain the importance of breast self-examination (BSE) and list five recommendations from the American Cancer Society regarding breast examination.
3. Demonstrate the correct procedure for instructing a patient in BSE.
4. List four purposes of a pelvic examination.
5. Describe the basic process used by the physician in a pelvic examination and describe how the speculum is used.
6. Explain the purpose of a Pap smear.
7. Explain the process used to label specimen slides and prepare them for transport to the laboratory.
8. Demonstrate the correct procedure for assisting the patient and physician during a pelvic examination and Pap smear.
9. List the three categories of the cytology report as described by the Bethesda System.
10. List three types of vaginitis and explain the etiology, signs and symptoms, and treatment for each.
11. Explain the education needs of a patient with a sexually transmitted disease (STD).
12. Briefly describe four commonly used types of contraception (birth control).

Obstetrical Examination and Testing
13. Explain the importance of prenatal care and describe how a serum pregnancy test confirms pregnancy.
14. Explain how the estimated date of delivery is established using Nägele's rule.
15. List seven types of tests performed at the initial prenatal visit.
16. Demonstrate the correct procedure for assisting the physician and patient during a follow-up prenatal examination.
17. List the five areas that are evaluated at a postpartum visit.

Colon Tests
18. Explain the purpose of fecal occult testing.
19. Demonstrate the procedure for providing the patient with accurate and complete instructions on the preparation and collection of a stool sample for fecal occult blood testing.
20. Demonstrate the procedure for accurately developing the fecal occult blood slide test.
21. Explain the purpose of sigmoidoscopy.
22. Demonstrate the correct procedure for assisting the physician and patient during sigmoidoscopy.

Pulmonary Function Tests
23. Explain the purpose of spirometry and list five indications for its use.
24. Demonstrate the procedure for accurately performing spirometry to measure lung volume.
25. Discuss the proper procedure for using a peak flow meter.

Pulse Oximetry
26. Explain the purpose of pulse oximetry and list five guidelines for its use.
27. Demonstrate the procedure for accurately determining a patient's blood oxygen saturation using pulse oximetry.

Hearing Acuity Tests
28. List the three types of hearing acuity tests and state the purpose of each.

Patient-Centered Professionalism

29. Analyze a realistic medical office situation and apply your understanding of diagnostic testing to determine the best course of action.
30. Describe the impact on patient care when medical assistants have a solid understanding of the purpose and procedures for diagnostic testing performed in the medical office.

KEY TERMS

abstinence
Apgar score
audiogram
audiologist
audiometry
barrier methods
Bethesda System
biopsy
blood chemistry
breast self-examination (BSE)
candidiasis
clinical information
colorectal
colposcopy
complete blood count (CBC)
conduction
contraception
corpus luteum
coverslip
culture and sensitivity (C&S)
cytology
cytology laboratory requisition
diagnose
diagnosis
dysplasia
dysuria
endocervical curettage (ECC)
estimated date of delivery/confinement (EDD/EDC)
fecal occult blood test (FOBT)
fixative
forced vital capacity (FVC)
Gardnerella
gestational diabetes
guaiac test
gynecologist
gynecology
hearing acuity tests
hormonal method
human chorionic gonadotropin (hCG)
intrauterine device (IUD)
lithotomy
"morning-after" pill
Nägele's rule
obstetrics
oximetry sensor
Pap smear
parturition
peak flow meter
pelvic examination
pelvimetry
photodetector
placenta
postpartum
prenatal care
protozoa
puerperium
pulmonary function tests (PFTs)
pulse oximetry
Rinne test
serum pregnancy test
sexually transmitted diseases (STDs)
sigmoidoscope
sigmoidoscopy
slide
specimen adequacy
specimens
spirometry
sterilization
test card
titer
trichomoniasis
tuning fork
tympanogram
vaginal irrigation
vaginal speculum
vaginitis
vital capacity (VC)
Weber test
wet mount

PRACTICAL APPLICATIONS

Read the following scenario and keep it in mind as you learn about diagnostic testing.

Kari, age 20, is a new patient in the office of Dr. Berg, a gynecologist. Francine is the medical assistant for Dr. Berg and has only been on the job for about 2 weeks. Arriving for her appointment, Kari is given the history and physical paperwork to fill out because she is a new patient. When Francine calls Kari to the back to question her further on some specifics regarding her menstrual periods and sexual activity, four other patients are sitting close to Kari in the lab/workup area. Later, Francine is overheard discussing Kari's history with co-workers by yet more patients in the waiting room.

After taking Kari to the examination room, Francine tells her to get undressed without providing instructions for putting on the gown and drape. When Francine returns to see if Kari is undressed, she then places her into the lithotomy position for what turns out to be a 30-minute wait.

When Dr. Berg starts to examine Kari, Francine leaves the room and tells Dr. Berg to call her when he is ready to do the pelvic examination. During the breast examination, Kari asks Dr. Berg about birth control and tells him that she has been sexually active with a partner who has been diagnosed with a sexually transmitted disease (STD). Dr. Berg completes the pelvic examination, obtaining a Pap smear, as well as cultures for STD and a wet prep. Dr. Berg takes the wet mount to the microscope for observation. He sees Francine in the hallway chatting with some co-workers and asks where she was when he needed her during the pelvic examination. She explains she never heard him call for assistance.

Dr. Berg returns to the examination room and begins discussing forms of birth control with Kari, asking if she would rather have a barrier method, an intrauterine device, or a hormonal method such as birth control pills. He also explains to her that she has trichomoniasis, an STD, as seen on the wet prep. Dr. Berg gives Kari a prescription to treat the trichomoniasis for herself and her sexual partner.

Would you be prepared to handle this situation better than Francine did?

GYNECOLOGICAL EXAMINATION AND TESTING

Gynecology is the branch of medicine that is concerned with maintaining women's health. This care includes sexual and reproductive functions, along with the diseases and conditions that affect these functions. A gynecological examination may be done by a **gynecologist** (a physician who specializes in the treatment of women, including diseases of the reproductive organs and breasts) or by a family physician as part of the wellness examination.

Examination and Prenatal Care

A gynecological examination includes the following:
- Breast examination
- Pelvic examination
- Pap smear (Papanicolaou test)
- Cultures for diagnosing vaginal infections and sexually transmitted diseases

Breast Examination

Breast self-examination (BSE), along with regular health checkups and mammograms, can play a vital role in the early detection of breast cancer. Therefore patients are encouraged to perform a BSE monthly and at least 1 week after the menstrual cycle when the breasts are less tender. Menopausal women or women who have had a hysterectomy should do a BSE on the same day of the month (e.g., the first of each month or the patient's birthday date). The medical assistant may be involved in educating patients about screening techniques for the identifying presence of masses or irregularities in breast tissue. Procedure 39-1 discusses how to instruct a patient in BSE. Because symptoms of breast cancer are not painful, close observation of any visual changes (e.g., inverted nipple, pitting or scaling of breast, discharge from the nipple, swelling, and lumps of any type) should be noted and reported immediately. See Box 39-1 for types of nipple discharge.

The American Cancer Society makes the following strong recommendations for BSE:

1. Monthly BSE should start at age 20.
2. BSE should be done the same time each month.
3. It is best if each breast is checked in the shower or bath, in front of a mirror, and while lying down. This allows for all breast tissue to be examined.
4. At age 30, besides the monthly BSE, it is recommended to have a clinical breast examination performed by a physician or other health care professional. The focus of this examination is to observe for changes in the size, texture, and shape of each breast and to locate any lumps in the breast tissue or under the arms.
5. At age 40, in addition to the BSE and clinical breast examination, an annual mammogram by a licensed technician is recommended.

NOTE: See Box-39-2 for guidelines for testicular self-examination.

Pelvic Examination

The **pelvic examination** is done to evaluate the shape, size, and location of the reproductive organs and to detect disease. The pelvic examination, in conjunction with the Pap smear, has proved to be an effective method for detecting changes in the cervical tissues that may be caused by cervical cancer or precancerous conditions. Cancer of the cervix is one of the most common cancers to affect women and the pelvic examination aids in early detection of this.

BOX 39-1

Types of Nipple Discharge

Most nipple discharge is benign and not related to an abnormality. Discharge can range in color from white to yellow to green and even bluish green. Discharge that is clear, thick, and mucus-like should be reported. Discharge that is bilateral (both breasts) is usually benign. A malignant condition is usually only on one side (unilateral).

DISCHARGE	CAUSE
Milky (cloudy, thin, nonsticky)	Lactation or increased mechanical stimulation (e.g., fondling, suckling, or irritation from clothing during exercise or activity). Drugs (birth control pills, methyldopa, and some tranquilizers and tricyclic antidepressants) or hormones that stimulate prolactin secretion. Smoking and hypertension can also stimulate prolactin. Pituitary tumor that causes excessive prolactin secretion.
Bloody or watery	Intraductal papilloma (benign growth), trauma, or infection (abscess).
Clear and mucus-like	Discharge that is spontaneous is suspicious and should be tested further.

BOX 39-2

Guidelines for Testicular Examination

Testicular cancer can be detected by a simple 3-minute examination performed easily in the shower. Doing the examination in the shower allows the fingers to glide over the skin making it easier to feel the texture underneath. Also, the heat causes the skin to relax, making the examination easier to perform.

1. Each testicle should be rolled between the thumb and fingers, applying slight pressure and checking for lumps (usually small and painless).
2. The epididymis, located behind each testicle, should be examined for lumps.
3. The vas deferens (tube that comes from the epididymis) should also be examined.

A lump, enlargement of one or both testicles, or a dull ache in the groin or testicles should be reported for follow-up.

Another woman should be in the room when a pelvic examination is being completed by a male physician. This often helps the patient feel more comfortable and provides a "chaperone" and assistant for the physician. The common position used for the pelvic examination is the **lithotomy** position. The procedure typically involves the following:

- The physician inspects the external genitalia for color, symmetry, and position of the urethra, vagina, and rectum. Any lesions, discharge, or odors are also noted.

PROCEDURE 39-1 Teach Breast Self-Examination

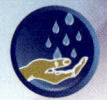

TASK: Instruct a patient in how to perform breast self-examination (BSE).

EQUIPMENT AND SUPPLIES
- Small pillow or rolled towel
- Model of breast with known irregularities
- BSE instruction sheet
- Patient's medical record

SKILLS/RATIONALE

STANDARD PRECAUTIONS ARE TO BE FOLLOWED.

1. **Procedural Step.** Sanitize the hands.
   An alcohol-based hand rub may be used instead of washing hands with soap and water, unless hands are visibly soiled.
   Rationale. Hand sanitization promotes infection control.

2. **Procedural Step.** Obtain the patient's medical record.

3. **Procedural Step.** Greet the patient, introduce yourself, and confirm the patient's identity.
   The most opportune time to instruct a female patient on how to perform BSE is after the yearly gynecological examination.
   Rationale. Identifying the patient ensures the procedure is performed on the correct patient.

4. **Procedural Step.** Place the breast model in the case on the counter and open the case but leave the model in the case.

5. **Procedural Step.** Explain the importance of performing the monthly BSE.
   BSE is important in the early detection of breast irregularities. The best time to perform BSE is 1 week after the beginning of the menstrual period, since this is when the breasts are least likely to be swollen or tender. Postmenopausal women should perform BSEs on the same day of each month; the patient's birthday date is an easy day to remember.
   Rationale. Explaining the importance of BSE promotes compliance.

6. **Procedural Step.** Ask the patient to take a look at the instruction card and explain the steps for BSE.
   Rationale. This shows that the patient has understood what needs to be done.

VISUAL INSPECTION

7. **Procedural Step.** Visually inspect both breasts in a mirror.
   Explain to the patient that she should remove clothing from the waist up and stand before the mirror with the arms relaxed at the sides, paying particular attention to the color and texture of the skin.
   Rationale. Regular examination of the breasts in a mirror will help the patient become accustomed to what looks normal.

8. **Procedural Step.** Explain to the patient that she should raise both arms at the same time and check to see if both breasts and nipples react to this movement in the same way.

9. **Procedural Step.** Explain to the patient she should rest her palms on the hips and press down firmly; flex the chest and tighten the chest muscles.
   Rationale. This allows any abnormalities to become more apparent.

10. **Procedural Step.** Bend forward at the waist with hands on the hips and check for dimpling of the skin or nipples.
    Rationale. Dimpling of the skin or nipples can be caused by the presence of a growing tumor and should be reported to the physician as soon as possible.

11. **Procedural Step.** Explain to the patient that she should stand up and gently squeeze the nipple of each breast with the fingertips to look for any discharge.

PALPATION

After the visual inspection, the patient is instructed to feel for lumps or thickening of breast tissue. Feeling for lumps or palpation of the breast is performed in two positions: lying down and standing.

12. **Procedural Step.** Before explaining to the patient how to palpate her own breasts, ask her to palpate the model, which will help her identify abnormalities.
    Rationale. Most models come with more than one lump or irregularity of varying depth and size, and these feel much like lumps found in the female breasts. If the patient can correctly locate all the irregularities, she has demonstrated that she can palpate the breast correctly.

13. **Procedural Step.** Instruct the patient how to use the pads of her index, middle, and ring fingers to palpate the model.
    Rationale. The pads of these fingers are the most sensitive.

14. **Procedural Step.** Ask the patient to use a small circular motion (the size of a dime) and apply continuous pressure while palpating the breast.

15. **Procedural Step.** Explain to the patient how to feel for lumps or thickening of breast tissue in a systematic pattern over all areas of the breast.

Continued

PROCEDURE 39-1 Teach Breast Self-Examination—cont'd

The pattern may be vertical lines about as wide as three fingers going up and then down or it may be a circular pattern, which begins at the outside top edge of the breast. A wedge pattern can also be used, which starts at the outside top edge of the breast.

16. **Procedural Step.** Explain to the patient how to palpate toward the nipple.

   After palpating the entire outer rim, instruct the patient to move an inch toward the nipple and make the same circling motion again and then move around the breast in smaller circles until the nipple is reached.

17. **Procedural Step.** Using the model, instruct the patient to palpate the same area using varying amounts of pressure to check the full thickness of the breast. First, palpate lightly, then a little deeper, and finally deeper still.

18. **Procedural Step.** When the patient moves her hand, instruct her to keep her fingers in contact with the skin and to keep the fingers on the breast to avoid missing a spot.

19. **Procedural Step.** Explain to the patient how to check the whole breast, from the armpit to the breastbone and from the collarbone to the bra line when doing the BSE at home.

20. **Procedural Step.** Explain to the patient why the supine is the best position for inspection of her own breasts.

   Once the patient has demonstrated how to palpate for lumps or thickening of breast tissue on the model, show her how to place a pillow or other support, such as a folded towel, under her shoulder and how to position her arm above her head.

   Rationale. It is easier for the patient to feel breast abnormalities if she is in the supine position. Placing the arm above the head allows the breast to flatten so that the patient can palpate her entire breast easily.

21. **Procedural Step.** Ask the patient if she has any questions about how to check her whole breast, from the armpit to the breastbone and from the collarbone to the bra line.

22. **Procedural Step.** Remind the patient of the importance of varying the amount of pressure while palpating and to cover the whole breast; remind her to keep the fingers in contact with the skin when moving her hand.

23. **Procedural Step.** Remind the patient to follow a pattern while palpating to ensure a thorough examination.

   The pattern can be vertical, circular, or a wedge.

24. **Procedural Step.** Remind the patient to repeat the process and examine her left breast with her right hand.

25. **Procedural Step.** Remind the patient to also palpate the breast in a standing position.

   Rationale. This makes it easier to feel the area of the breast near the underarm. Many women prefer to palpate their breasts for lumps while standing in the shower. Wet, soapy skin helps the fingers glide more smoothly over the breast and surrounding areas.

26. **Procedural Step.** Remind the patient to place her right hand on her right shoulder and palpate her right breast with her left hand, checking for any lumps, thickening, or hard knots.

   Rationale. This position makes it easier for examining the underarm area for lumps.

27. **Procedural Step.** Remind the patient that the process needs to be repeated for her left breast using her right hand.

28. **Procedural Step.** After a return demonstration by the patient, assist her with redressing, if needed.

FOLLOW-UP AND DOCUMENTATION

29. **Procedural Step.** Provide the patient with an instruction card, and ask the patient if she has any questions.

   Ask the patient to recall the steps necessary for successful completion of the examination to make sure she understands the process.

   Rationale. An instruction card to take home will help the patient remember what to do when she performs BSE by herself.

30. **Procedural Step.** Remind the patient that her health care provider will answer any questions she may have about any abnormalities she might find.

31. **Procedural Step.** Document the instruction in the patient's medical record.

   Include the date and time, a statement that the procedure was explained to the patient, a statement that the patient was able to locate irregularities in the breast model, confirmation of the patient's return demonstration of the procedure, a statement of the patient's receipt of education materials, a statement that the patient was asked if she had questions concerning the process, and the signature and credentials of the person recording the information.

CHARTING EXAMPLE

Date	
10/25/xx	2:30 p.m. Breast self-examination explained. Located lumps in breast model. Able to return information for breast examination by successfully demonstrating self-exam. Literature for breast self-examination provided. Had no further questions. ———— N. Collins, CMA (AAMA)

- Next, the physician inspects the internal genitalia by inserting a **vaginal speculum** into the vagina. Speculums come in small, medium, and large sizes. The physician determines speculum size based on the patient's physical and sexual maturity. Speculums may be disposable plastic or sterilized, reusable metal instruments. The speculum separates the walls of the vagina so that the vagina and cervix can be adequately visualized. The walls of the vagina and cervix are examined for lesions, color, discharge, and general condition.
- At this time, a Pap smear for **cytology** and various bacterial cultures can be obtained.
- On completion of the Pap smear, the physician palpates the internal genitalia and performs a bimanual examination, inserting two fingers (usually the index and middle finger) of a lubricated gloved hand into the vagina. The fingers of the opposite hand palpate the abdomen (Figure 39-1). By palpating the internal genitalia, the physician is able to evaluate the uterus and ovaries for size, shape, and position. Pain and tenderness can also be detected.
- The physician concludes the examination by inserting one gloved finger into the rectum (ages 40 to 50). This part of the procedure provides information about the size and position of the uterus, fallopian tubes, ovaries, and ligaments of the uterus. The physician also notes any bleeding, hemorrhoids, fissures, or fistulas of the rectum.

Papanicolaou Test

In 1883, George N. Papanicolaou, an American physician, developed a cytological screening test to detect atypical cell formation. The Papanicolaou test (**Pap smear**) is a screening tool that evaluates the squamous epithelial tissue covering the visible part of the cervix. Ideally, the medical assistant should schedule a patient so that the Pap test is about 1 week before the beginning of the menstrual period. The patient should be instructed not to douche, have sexual intercourse, or insert any vaginal medications 24 hours before the test, since this will wash away cellular deposits and change the acidity of the vaginal and cervical tissues.

Human Papillomavirus Test

A relatively new screening test, the human papillomavirus (HPV) test, also examines cells taken from the cervix but looks for the virus that causes cervical cancer instead of abnormal cells under the microscope as does the Pap test. This new technology for detecting cervical cancer has been found to be more accurate than the traditional Pap smear and is gaining approval in the United States. Currently, the Pap test and the HPV test are done together when women are known to be at high risk for cervical cancer (e.g., member of the family has been diagnosed). When the results of both tests are negative, it is a better indicator that the patient is free of cervical cancer.

The latest generations of preventive vaccines target the two most common high-risk HPVs known to cause cervical cancer. Both *Gardasil* and *Cervarix* target the two HPV types (16 and 18) that cause 70% of cervical cancers. Research continues to develop a vaccine against a broader range of HPVs.

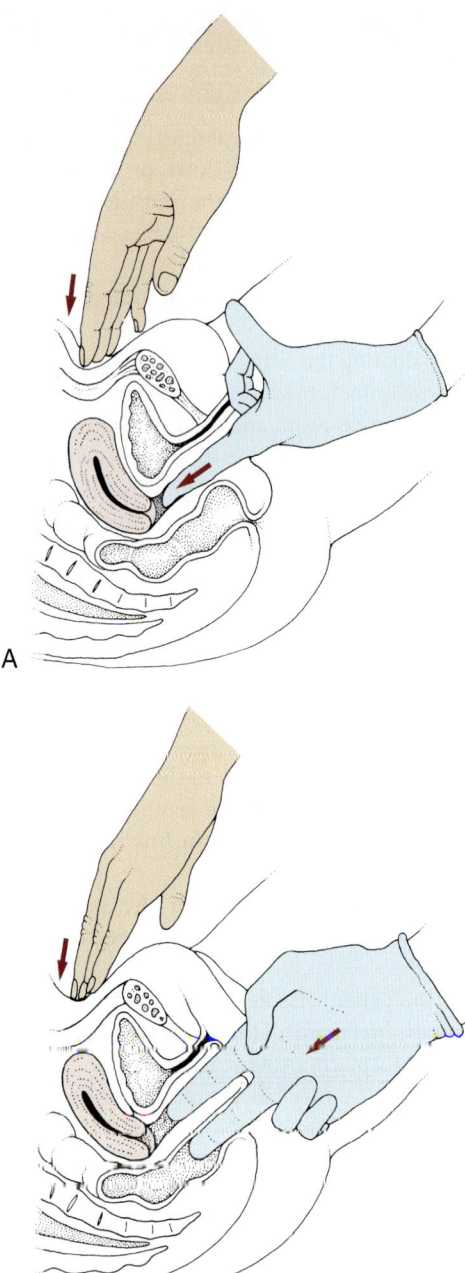

FIGURE 39-1 Bimanual (two-handed) pelvic examination. (From Ignatavicius DD, Workman ML, Mishler MA: *Medical-surgical nursing: a nursing process approach,* ed 2, Philadelphia, 1995, Saunders.)

Specimen Collection

As a part of the pelvic examination, **specimens** are collected. To obtain the specimens the physician inserts and opens a vaginal speculum. Depending on the physician's preference, the speculum may be rinsed and warmed with water before insertion. Once the speculum is opened, the cervical opening (or *os*) must be visualized and located for the cells to be

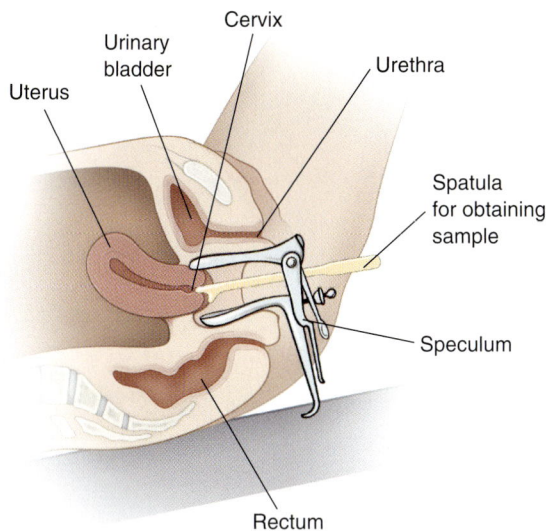

FIGURE 39-2 Method of obtaining sample for a Pap smear. (Modified from Chabner DE: *The language of medicine,* ed 7, Philadelphia, 2004, Saunders.)

obtained. The physician uses a plastic or wooden spatula, cotton applicator, or a cervical brush or broom to scrape cells gently from in and around the cervix (Figure 39-2). Cells can also be scraped from the vagina (Figure 39-3, *A*), the cervix (Figure 39-3, *B*), and the endocervical canal (Figure 39-3, *C*).

A patient's medical insurance plan may contain exclusions and limitations concerning certain preparations and types of readings (e.g., manual versus automatic).

"Liquid Prep" Method. The newest, most accurate way for obtaining cells for a Pap smear is done by a method called "liquid prep" (Thin Prep). A cervical brush or broom is used to obtain the cells from the cervix and endocervix. Once obtained, the cells are swished around in a liquid cytology transport medium. The container is labeled and sent to the laboratory. No fixative or other preparation is needed.

Slide Preparation. The cell samples are spread thinly on a glass **slide** with a frosted edge. The medical assistant labels each slide (on the frosted end with a marking pencil) with the patient's name and the location of each specimen, as follows:

V = vaginal (usually obtained only for women without a uterus such as after a hysterectomy)
C = cervical
E = endocervical

NOTE: Many slide containers are labeled underneath so the practitioner can see where to place the specimens.

The slide is either flooded with 95% ethyl alcohol or sprayed with a cytology **fixative** immediately after the smear is made. The spray fixative, if used, should not be sprayed too close to the sample to avoid damaging the specimen. The slides must be dry before being placed in a slide holder to be sent to a laboratory for inspection. Procedure 39-2 explains the process of assisting the patient and physician during a pelvic examination and Pap smear. Box 39-3 lists charting criteria necessary for sending specimens to the laboratory.

> **BOX 39-3**
>
> **Documentation When Charting for Transport of a Specimen to an Outside Laboratory**
>
> 1. Date
> 2. Time
> 3. Name of specimen being sent
> 4. Name of laboratory to which the specimen is sent
> 5. Test to be completed
> 6. Proper signature and credential

Laboratory Report. A **cytology laboratory requisition** must accompany all specimens to the laboratory for microscopic examination and evaluation (Figure 39-4). The cytologist looks for atypical or abnormal cells and signs of infection. If none are found, the Pap report will read *within normal limits* (WNL). Precancerous changes, or **dysplasia** (abnormal development of tissue), are reported when the cells are abnormal, but the surrounding tissue is not affected. Currently, Pap smear results are reported according to the **Bethesda System** (Table 39-1). This system divides the cytology report into the following three main categories (Figure 39-5):

1. **Clinical information:** Contains information concerning last menstrual period and previous cytology results.
2. **Specimen adequacy:** Concerns condition of the specimen (e.g., whether it is satisfactory for evaluation).
3. **Diagnosis:** Categorizes the specimen and indicates whether it is normal or abnormal. An unconfirmed diagnosis is given if abnormal findings are found (follow-up is recommended).

Follow-up. Because the Pap smear is a screening test, if findings are abnormal, further testing is indicated. These tests include **colposcopy, biopsy** of the cervix, and **endocervical curettage** (ECC). An abnormal Pap smear may be the result of inflammation of the tissue caused by a fungal or bacterial infection. An abnormal Pap smear is not a diagnosis; it is a result that leads to diagnosis by further testing and, if necessary, treatment.

Reproductive Disorders and Conditions

The pelvic examination and Pap smear may lead to a diagnosis of vaginitis. Sexually transmitted diseases can also be diagnosed using the results of the examination and Pap smear.

Vaginitis

Vaginitis is an inflammation of the vaginal tissue caused by fungus, bacteria, protozoa, or irritation from chemicals or foreign objects. The most common types of vaginitis are candidiasis and trichomoniasis. *Gardnerella* can also cause vaginitis. Many types of vaginitis can be treated with over-the-counter (OTC) vaginal preparations.

Text continued on p. 869

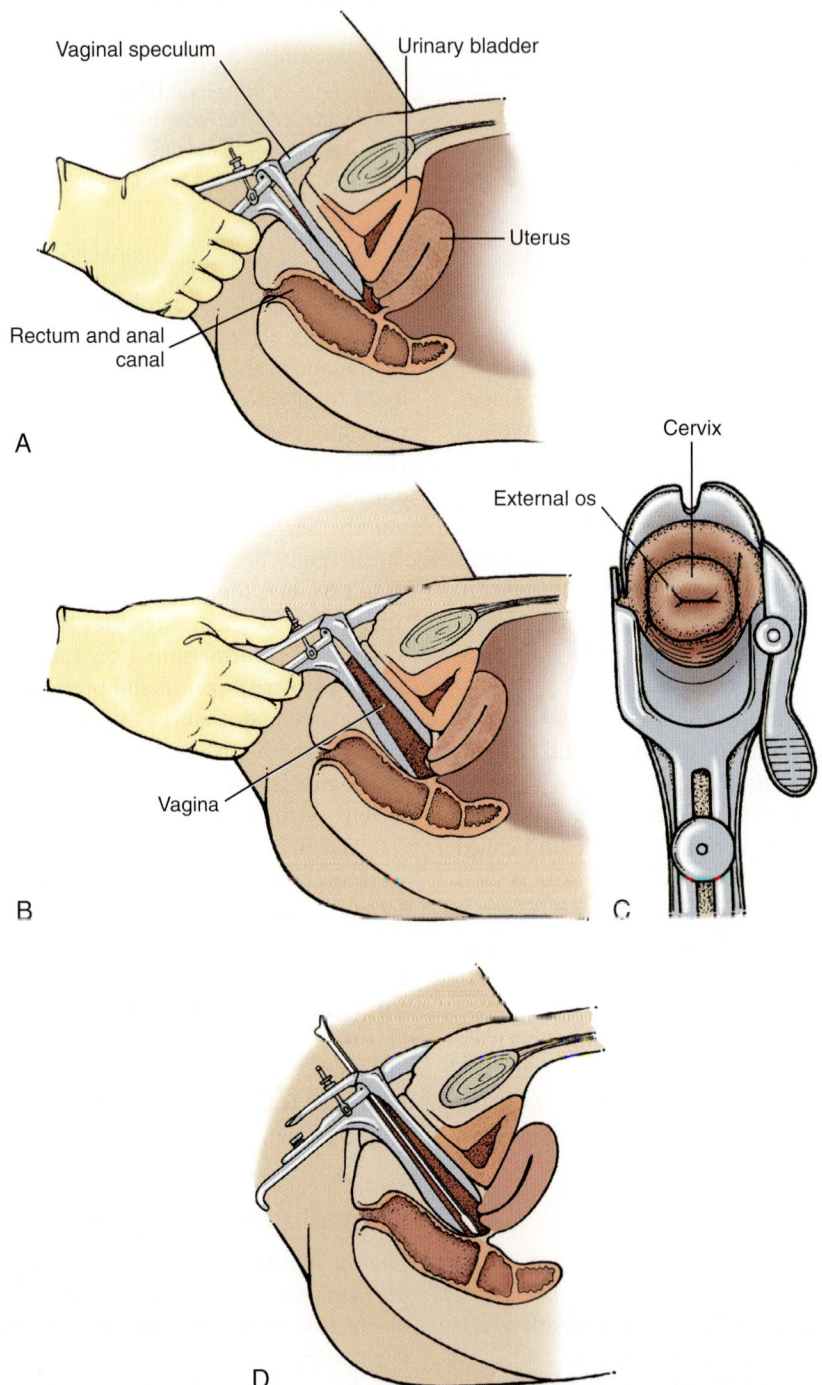

FIGURE 39-3 Obtaining a Pap smear. **A,** Insertion of speculum. **B,** Open speculum within the vagina. **C,** Examiner's view of the cervix through an open speculum. **D,** An instrument called an Ayre spatula is inserted through the speculum to obtain a cervical specimen for a Pap smear. (From Monahan FD, Neighbors M: *Medical-surgical nursing: foundations for clinical practice*, ed 2, Philadelphia, 1998, Saunders.)

Specialty Diagnostic Testing **CHAPTER 39** **863**

PROCEDURE 39-2

Assist with a Gynecological Examination

TASK: Prepare a patient for and assist the health care practitioner with a gynecological examination, including Pap smear (direct smear method and "liquid prep" method).

EQUIPMENT AND SUPPLIES

GENERAL
- Patient gown and drape
- Nonsterile disposable gloves
- Gauze squares
- Disposable vaginal speculum, or sterilized stainless steel speculum
- Light source
- Lubricant (water based)
- Tissues
- Cytology requisition
- Transport media
- Urine specimen container
- Fecal occult blood slide
- Fecal occult developer
- Biohazardous waste container
- Patient's medical record

"DRY PREP" (DIRECT SMEAR) METHOD
- Wooden spatula
- Endocervical brush; cotton-tipped applicator
- Microscope slides with frosted edge
- Slide holder
- Cytology fixative

"LIQUID-PREP" METHOD
- Cervical broom
- Plastic spatula
- Transport medium vial

SKILLS/RATIONALE

STANDARD PRECAUTIONS ARE TO BE FOLLOWED.

1. **Procedural Step. Sanitize the hands.**
   An alcohol-based hand rub may be used instead of washing hands with soap and water, unless hands are visibly soiled.
   Rationale. Hand sanitization promotes infection control.

2. **Procedural Step. Assemble equipment and supplies.**
   Rationale. It is important to have all supplies and equipment ready and available before starting any procedure to ensure efficiency.

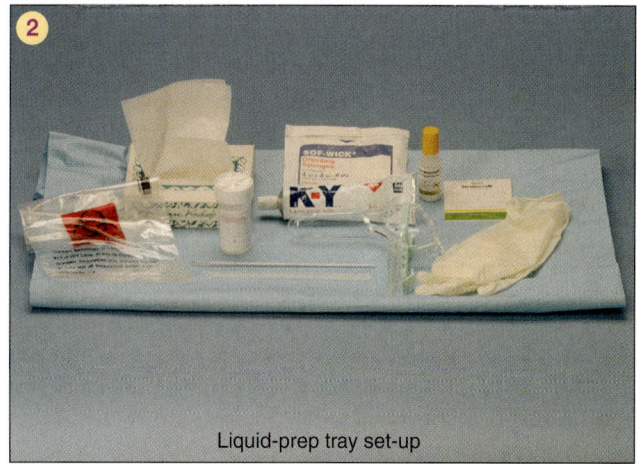
Liquid-prep tray set-up

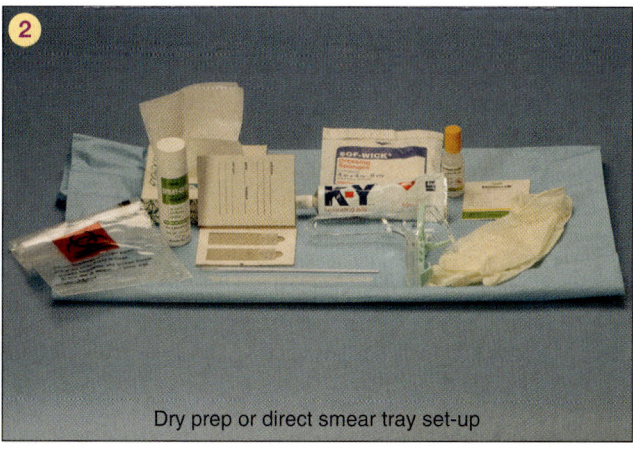
Dry prep or direct smear tray set-up

3. **Procedural Step.** Obtain the patient's medical record.

4. **Procedural Step. Complete the cytology requisition form.**
   Not all information may be available at this point and may need to be filled in later in the examination. Be as thorough as possible. The patient must provide some information such as the date of the first day of the last menstrual period (LMP).

Continued

PROCEDURE 39-2 Assist with a Gynecological Examination—cont'd

Rationale. Making sure to include all essential information required by the cytology laboratory lessens the risk of specimen rejection and provides information for a more accurate report.

5. **Procedural Step.** Greet the patient, introduce yourself, and confirm the patient's identity.
   Rationale. Identifying the patient ensures the procedure is performed on the correct patient.

6. **Procedural Step.** Ask the patient if she needs to empty her bladder before the examination.
   If the physician has ordered that a urine specimen be collected, provide the patient with a specimen container and directions for collection of a urine specimen.
   Rationale. An empty bladder makes it easier to palpate organs during the pelvic examination and is more comfortable for the patient.

7. **Procedural Step.** Escort the patient to the examination room and ask the patient to have a seat on the end of the examination table.

8. **Procedural Step.** Explain the procedure to the patient.
   Rationale. Explaining the procedure to the patient promotes cooperation and provides a means of obtaining implied consent.

9. **Procedural Step.** Obtain and record preliminary patient information.
   Measure the patient's vital signs and height and weight. Record the results in the patient's medical record. Ask the patient for any information you may need to complete the requisition form and ask if the patient has any particular complaints or concerns.
   Rationale. Vital signs and height and weight are routinely taken before an annual gynecological examination, usually before the patient is prepared.

10. **Procedural Step.** Prepare the patient.
    Instruct the patient to undress completely and put on the examining gown with the opening positioned in front. Ask the patient to have a seat at the end of the examination table with the drape across her lap.

11. **Procedural Step.** Position and drape the patient for the breast examination.
    When the physician is ready to begin the examination, help position the patient in a supine position, extending the end of the examination table with one hand while supporting the patient's legs with the other hand. Adjust the drape in preparation for a breast examination by positioning the top of the drape at the patient's waist. Tuck the patient gown beneath the drape. Adjust the gown opening for the breast examination.
    NOTE: If the patient has difficulty breathing in the supine position, the breast examination may be performed in a sitting or semi-Fowler's position.
    Rationale. The supine position is most appropriate for exposing the breasts for examination.

12. **Procedural Step.** Adjust the drape for the abdominal examination.
    After the breast examination is completed, with the patient still in the supine position, adjust the drape lower to cover the lower abdomen from the pubic area downward, then adjust the gown to expose the patient's abdomen for examination.

13. **Procedural Step.** Position and drape the patient into the lithotomy position for the pelvic examination.
    Ask the patient to bend both knees and place her feet on the corners of the examination table in a dorsal recumbent position, keeping the drape in place. Push in the table extension and pull out and adjust the stirrups approximately 1 foot from the end of the table. Assist the patient by raising both legs at the same time and positioning the patient's heels in the stirrups. Properly position the drape at an angle covering the patient's lower abdomen and legs with the corner of the drape hanging between the patient's legs. Once the patient's feet are securely positioned in the stirrups, ask the patient to slide down to the end of the table so that her buttocks are on the edge (it helps to tell them to slide until they hit your hand). Ask the patient to rotate her thighs outward as far as is comfortable.
    Rationale. Rotating the thighs relaxes the perineum so that the pelvic examination is more comfortable for the patient.

14. **Procedural Step.** Apply nonsterile disposable gloves (physician and assistant).
    Rationale. Since you may come in contact with body fluids from the vagina, disposable gloves should be worn.

15. **Procedural Step.** After the physician folds back the corner of the drape to expose the perineal area, adjust and focus the light on the perineum for the physician.
    Rationale. Direct light is needed to enable the physician to visualize the vagina and cervix.

16. **Procedural Step.** Warm the vaginal speculum under warm running water to prevent discomfort to the patient during insertion.
    The vaginal speculum may also have been stored in a warming drawer.
    Rationale. A cold speculum results in contraction of the vaginal muscles, making insertion difficult. Water should be the only lubricant used if a Pap smear is being performed; other lubricants can interfere with obtaining the cells needed for the examination.

17. **Procedural Step.** Encourage the patient to breathe deeply and evenly.
    Rationale. This also helps to relax the abdominal muscles. Focusing on breathing distracts the patient from the pelvic examination being performed. If the patient is relaxed, the examination proceeds more smoothly and is more comfortable for the patient.

Continued

PROCEDURE 39-2 Assist with a Gynecological Examination—cont'd

18. **Procedural Step.** Assist the physician with the pelvic examination (direct smear method).
    a. Using a lead pencil, mark the slides on the frosted edge with the patient's name, the date, and the source of the specimen. Use a "C" to identify the slide of the smear taken from the cervix, a "V" to identify the slide of the smear taken from the vagina, and an "E" to identify the slide of the smear taken from the endocervical canal.
    b. Pass the vaginal spatula to the physician by holding the spatula in the middle so that the physician grasps the rounded end. The physician will insert the S-shaped end of the spatula into the patient's cervix.
    Rationale. The instrument is held in the middle and is handed to the physician so that it can be grasped at the opposite end of the S.
    c. Hold the glass slide marked with a "C" by the frosted end for the physician to apply the specimen to the clear end. After the specimen has been applied to the slide, the applicator is discarded as biohazardous waste.
    d. Pass the endocervical brush handle-first to the physician by holding it in the middle.
    e. Hold out the slide marked with the "E" to receive the next specimen. The endocervical brush is then discarded as biohazardous waste.
    f. If a vaginal specimen is to be taken, hand the physician a cotton-tipped applicator handle-first for collection of a vaginal specimen. Hold out the glass slide marked with a "V" to receive this specimen. Discard the cotton-tipped applicator into the biohazardous waste container.
    g. Spray the Pap slides immediately (within 10 seconds) with a light coat of fixative. Hold the nozzle far enough away, about 6 inches, to coat the slides evenly with a light mist. The slide must be "fixed" before the samples dry, to preserve the shape of the cells. Place the slides in the microscope slide holder, leaving the lid open. The fixative must be dry before the lid can be closed.

    Rationale. Holding the spray nozzle too close may result in blowing the cells off the slides. The slides should be sprayed lightly with a continuous motion from left to right, then right to left, and allowed to dry thoroughly, usually for 5 to 10 minutes.

19. **Procedural Step.** Assist the physician with the pelvic examination ("liquid prep" method).
    a. Proceed with the procedure in the same manner as for the direct smear ("dry prep") method, except collect the cervical specimen with the plastic spatula and the endocervical specimen with the cervical brush or broom. The broom is typically used on pregnant women and the brush on nonpregnant women. The instruments are grasped in the middle and passed to the physician handle-first.
    b. Open the vial of liquid-prep transport medium. The physician will place the spatula and cervical brush or broom in the transport medium after the specimen has been collected.
    c. Rinse the broom in the liquid by pushing the end of it into the bottom of the vial 10 times and use the spatula to scrape the cells from the brush, swishing both around before removing them from the medium.
    Rationale. This ensures that the sample is adequately mixed with the liquid-prep transport medium.

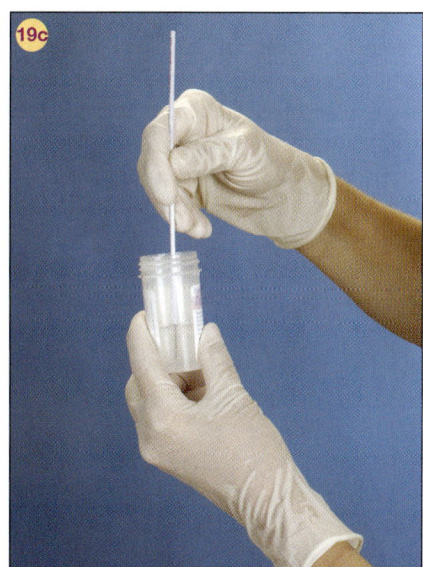

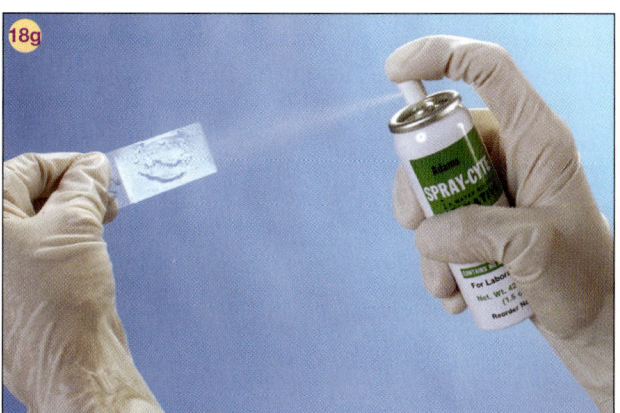

20. **Procedural Step.** Label the liquid-prep vial or slides as required by the laboratory.
    Include patient identification information and origin of the specimens. The vial may be labeled before or after the collection of the specimen, according to the provider's preference.
21. **Procedural Step.** Place the liquid prep vial or slides in a biohazard transport bag.

Continued

PROCEDURE 39-2 Assist with a Gynecological Examination—cont'd

22. **Procedural Step.** Assist the physician with the bimanual pelvic examination.
    a. Dispense some lubricant onto a 4 × 4 gauze square.
    b. After the physician passes the contaminated vaginal speculum to you, pass the gauze square with the lubricant to the physician. Some physicians will request that you apply the lubricant directly to their gloved hand. Do not allow the tube of lubricant to touch either the gauze square or the physician's glove.

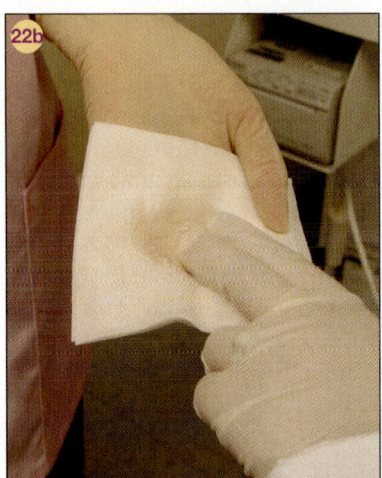

NOTE: If the vaginal speculum is disposable, discard it in the biohazardous waste container. If the speculum is metal, keep it separate from the clean equipment. Sanitize and prepare it for sterilization as soon as practical. To prevent body fluids from drying on the speculum, rinse the speculum under warm running water while wearing gloves.

Rationale. If the tube of lubricant touches the gauze square or the physician's gloved hand, the tube is considered contaminated and must be discarded.

   c. During the bimanual examination, support the patient by reminding her to relax and focus on breathing deeply.
   d. The physician may request an occult blood test on the fecal material adhering to the glove. Hold an occult blood slide out for the practitioner to apply fecal material (see Procedure 36-3 for the occult blood test).

23. **Procedural Step.** Remove and discard the gloves in a biohazardous waste container.

24. **Procedural Step.** Assist the patient from the lithotomy position and down from the examination table.
    On completion of the examination, assist the patient from the lithotomy position and into a sitting position by instructing the patient to push her feet against the stirrups and slide her buttocks back on the table. Pick up both legs at the knees at the same time to prevent strain on the lower back. Return the stirrups to their original position, pull out the end of the table, and place the feet onto it. Once the patient is comfortable, offer the patient tissues to remove excess lubricant. Assist the patient off the examination table as needed. Instruct the patient to dress. Leave the room to complete the cytology requisition form.
    Rationale. Patients may feel dizzy after the procedure and should be allowed to rest for a few minutes. Always assist patients as needed.

25. **Procedural Step.** Attach the completed cytology form to either the microscope slide holder or the transport medium vial and document the transport to the laboratory.

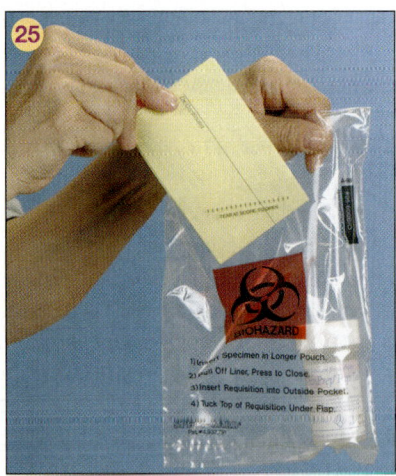

26. **Procedural Step.** Clean the examination room in preparation for the next patient.
    Discard all contaminated material in a biohazardous waste container. Wear nonsterile disposable gloves when cleaning the examination room. Never bring the next patient into an examination room that has items left from the last procedure (e.g., dirty speculum in sink).

27. **Procedural Step.** Sanitize the hands.
    Always sanitize the hands after every procedure or after using gloves.

28. **Procedural Step.** Document the procedure in the patient's medical record.

CHARTING EXAMPLE

Date	
8/07/xx	10:00 a.m. Pap smear collected and sent to Medical Center Laboratory for cytology. Pt. tolerated procedure well.— ———————— A. Policic, CMA (AAMA)

Step 2 photos from Bonewit-West K: Clinical procedures for medical assistants, ed 7, St Louis, 2008, Saunders.

CYTOLOGY REQUISITION Please Print Clearly

PATIENT INFORMATION

Name _____ Medical Record # _____ Sex M ____ F ____
         Last Name   First Name   Initial
Birthdate _____ Social Security # _____ Phone _____
Address _____
_____
_____
Physician ___Blackburn Primary Care Associates_____
             ___1990 Turquoise Drive, Blackburn WI 54937_____

SPECIMEN

____ Cervical   ____ Vaginal   ____ Vaginal with M.I.   ____ Endo Cervical   ____ Biopsy
____ Fluid/Washing/Brushing   ____ Fine Needle   ____ Buccal   ____ Other

Source _____
Pre-op DX _____

CLINICAL INFORMATION/REASON FOR PAP

Date collected _____ Date of LMP _____
Previous smear (Assession #/Date) _____

____ Screening for CA Cervix   ____ Hysterectomy   ____ Post Abortion   ____ Laser Rx   ____ PMB
____ Spotting   ____ Post menopausal   ____ Previous Abnormal   ____ Radiation Rx   ____ Cervicitis
____ Pregnant   ____ Hormone Rx   ____ Cervical Dysplasia   ____ Chemo Rx   ____ STD
____ Post partum   ____ BCPs   ____ Cryotherapy   ____ DES Exposure   ____ Smoker
____ Nursing   ____ IUD   ____ Conization   ____ Yeast Candida

FIGURE 39-4 Example of a laboratory slip that accompanies the Pap test. (From Hunt SA: *Saunders fundamentals of medical assisting—revised reprint,* St Louis, 2007, Saunders.)

GYN CYTOLOGY REPORT

RIVERVIEW MEDICAL LABORATORY
DEPARTMENT OF PATHOLOGY
2501 GRANT AVENUE
ST. LOUIS, MO 63146
(314) 555-3443

PATIENT: Heather Jones
PATIENT NO: 45876
DOB: 10/20/65
SUBMITTING: T. Woodside, MD

Date of Specimen: 7/01/05
Date Received: 7/02/05
Date Reported: 7/06/05
Performed By: Richard McVay, Cytotechnologist
Checked By: Melissa Wagner, Pathologist

SPECIMEN TYPE
☒ Thin Prep   ☐ Conventional Pap Smear

SPECIMEN ADEQUACY
☒ Satisfactory for Evaluation
☐ Unsatisfactory for Evaluation

GENERAL CATEGORIZATION
☐ Negative for Intraepithelial Lesion or Malignancy (see Interpretation/Result)
☒ Epithelial Cell Abnormality (see Interpretation/Result)
☐ Other (see Interpretation/Result)

INTERPRETATION/RESULT

A. BENIGN CELLULAR CHANGES
☐ Infection:
　☐ Trichomonas vaginalis
　☐ Fungal organisms morphologically compatible with Candida species
　☐ Cellular changes associated with herpes simplex virus
　☐ Bacterial infection morphologically compatible with gardnerella
　☐ Cytoplasmic inclusions suggestive of chlamydia

☐ Reactive changes
　☐ Without inflammation
　☐ With inflammation
　☐ Atrophy with inflammation (atrophic vaginitis)
　☐ Radiation effect
　☐ Repair
　☐ Hyperkeratosis
　☐ Parakeratosis

B. EPITHELIAL CELL ABNORMALITIES
☒ Squamous Cell
　☒ Atypical Squamous Cells of Undetermined Significance (ASC-US)
　☐ Atypical Squamous Cells of Higher Risk (ASC-H)
　☐ Low Grade Squamous Intraepithelial Lesion (LSIL)
　☐ High Grade Squamous Intraepithelial Lesion (HSIL)
　☐ Squamous Cell Carcinoma
☐ Glandular Cell
　☐ Atypical Glandular Cells of Undetermined Significance (AGUS)
　☐ Adenocarcinoma

FIGURE 39-5 Cytology report form (Bethesda System). (From Bonewit-West K: *Clinical procedures for medical assistants,* ed 7, St Louis, 2008, Saunders.)

TABLE 39-1

Bethesda System Classification for Pap Smear Results

Cells/Lesions	Cell Description	Follow-up	Class
Unsatisfactory specimen	Unsatisfactory for interpretation.	Repeat Pap smear.	0
WNL	Only normal cells on specimen; presence of some columnar cells increases specimen's reliability.	All women should begin Pap smear testing by age 18 or as soon as sexual activity commences; repeated yearly normal Pap tests may permit low-risk candidates to have routine screening every 1 to 3 years; by definition, over 90% of all women are now considered "high risk" and therefore benefit from yearly Pap tests.	1 Normal
Atypical squamous cell changes of nonspecific origin; consider infection or reactive or reparative changes	Many normal cells present, but within this normal group, some cells show irregular colors, shapes, and sizes.	Any known infection should be treated; if patient is suspected of having STD, additional testing should be done; in low-risk patients, test can be repeated in 2 to 4 months; in high-risk patients, further investigations, including colposcopy, are generally recommended.	2 Atypical
SILs **Low-grade lesions** (suspicious of cancer) HPV infections with changes in cells Mild dysplasia (CIN 1)	Some abnormal cells in smear; invasive cancer is not often found when only these types of cells are present.	Because Pap smear is a cancer *screening* tool, not a test that measures extent of disease, colposcopy or biopsy is the usual recommended follow-up for any patient in these last three class designations. HPV-introduced risk of cervical cancer may exist in infected cell for some time before cell begins to demonstrate microscopic physical changes in its appearance that can be appreciated by the Pap smear.	3 Suspicious
SILs **High-grade lesions** (possibly cancer) Moderate dysplasia (CIN 2) Severe dysplasia (CIN 3)	Even more bizarre and irregular cells; by appearance, most often found in advanced stages of dysplasia (CIN).		4 Suspicious
Squamous cells (probably cancer)	Represent classic appearance of cancer, usually indicating extensive, invasive disease.		5

CIN, Cervical intraepithelial neoplasia (grade); *HPV*, human papilloma virus; *SIL*, squamous intraepithelial lesions; *STD*, sexually transmitted disease; *WNL*, within normal limits.

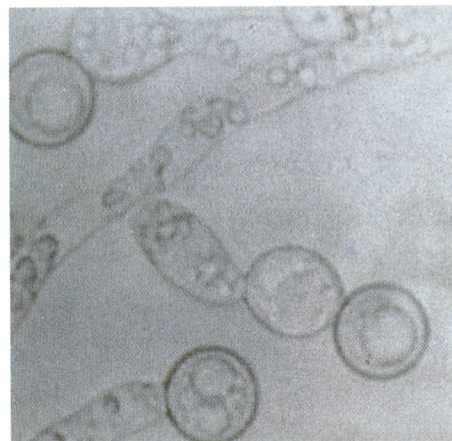

FIGURE 39-6 Candidiasis (moniliasis). (From Zitelli BJ, Davis HW: *Atlas of pediatric physical diagnosis*, ed 5, Philadelphia, 2007, Saunders.)

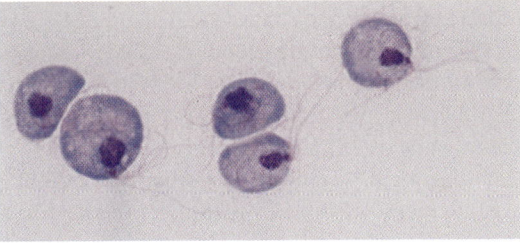

FIGURE 39-7 Trichomoniasis. (From Kumar V et al: *Robbins basic pathology*, ed 8, Philadelphia, 2007, Saunders.)

Candidiasis. **Candidiasis** is a fungal (yeast) infection of the vaginal tissue that may result from antibiotic use, oral contraceptives, diabetes, or pregnancy. These drugs or conditions change the pH of the vaginal mucosa, leading to an overgrowth of the fungus (Figure 39-6). Signs and symptoms include a thick, odorless, cottage cheese–like discharge. The patient complains of itching and possibly **dysuria**. A microscope slide (**wet mount**) is prepared by placing a small sample of the discharge on a slide. A drop of a 10% solution of potassium hydroxide (KOH) is added and covered with a **coverslip** to protect the specimen during microscopic examination. In some instances, two slides are prepared: one with KOH and the other with saline. Treatment varies from antifungal vaginal ointments, suppositories, or creams to oral medications.

Trichomoniasis. **Trichomoniasis** is an infection caused by **protozoa** and spread through sexual contact. Signs and symptoms include a yellowish green, frothy discharge; itching; and vaginal irritation with dysuria (Figure 39-7). Identifying this

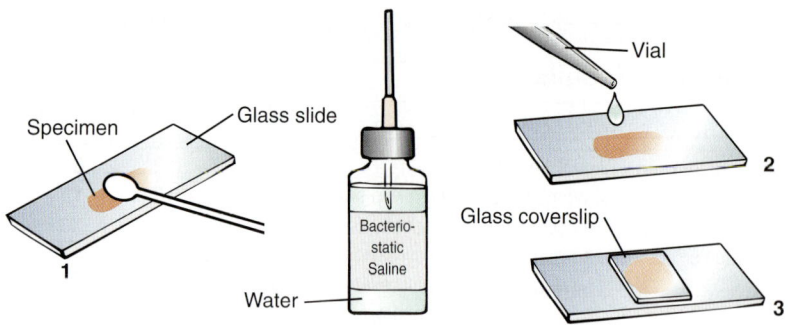

FIGURE 39-8 Preparation of a wet-mount slide for the identification of *Trichomonas vaginalis*. (From Stepp CA, Woods MA: *Laboratory procedures for medical office personnel*, Philadelphia, 1998, Saunders.)

Wet Mount (normal saline direct mount slide preparation)
1. Gently roll the specimen onto the slide.
2. Mix the specimen with one drop of saline.
3. Cover with coverslip and examine microscopically.

organism requires a microscope and a wet-mount slide prepared with normal saline (Figure 39-8). Treatment must include prescription medication, usually metronidazole (Flagyl), for both sex partners.

Gardnerella. *Gardnerella* is a genus of bacteria that normally lives in the vagina. When the normal pH of the vaginal tissues is disturbed, such as during **vaginal irrigation,** *Gardnerella* overtakes the environment and becomes problematic. A gray discharge with a "fishy" odor is the most frequent complaint from the patient. The use of an alkaline soap will increase the odor. The physician prepares a wet-mount slide using a 10% KOH solution. Treatment involves the use of metronidazole.

Sexually Transmitted Diseases

Sexually transmitted diseases (STDs) are passed between individuals through sexual contact (see Chapter 21). A patient with an STD must be educated about the need to notify sexual partners. All persons involved must be treated to correct the disease; otherwise, reinfection will occur, and all persons involved must be recultured before resuming sexual relations. STDs are diagnosed by **culture and sensitivity (C&S)** of the discharge. Remember, diseases that affect the health, safety, and welfare of the general public must be reported to the Department of Public Health.

Contraception (Birth Control)

The physician may discuss methods of birth control at the office visit. **Contraception,** or birth control, is an option that can be used to prevent pregnancy (conception). Religious beliefs and cultural attitudes can affect the patient's decision about the use of contraceptive methods. The medical assistant needs to be aware of various religious beliefs in the community and to be knowledgeable about the various birth control methods available. Common contraceptive options are as follows (Table 39-2):

- **Barrier methods** include the condom (both male and female), diaphragm, and cervical cap. Also in this category are contraceptive foams, jellies, and suppositories. These methods all place a physical or chemical barrier between the egg and sperm.
- An **intrauterine device (IUD)** is a small, T-shaped device positioned in the woman's uterus. It causes changes in the lining of the uterus, thus preventing the fertilized egg from implanting into the uterine wall, or it prevents the sperm from fertilizing the egg. IUDs contain copper or progestin and remain in the uterus for years.
- **Hormonal methods** include oral contraceptives (birth control pills), injections, patches, and vaginal rings. These items prevent ovulation by placing sex hormones into the woman's system gradually throughout the month.
- The **"morning-after" pill** relies on hormones being taken into the body shortly after unprotected intercourse. Instead of small daily doses, two large doses of female hormone are taken, one within 72 hours after intercourse and the second 12 hours after the first dose.

Each method disrupts the conception process at various points, and each has advantages and disadvantages. None of the methods can guarantee 100% accuracy; only **abstinence** and **sterilization** can provide this reassurance.

> ### PATIENT-CENTERED PROFESSIONALISM
>
> - Why is it important for the medical assistant to be knowledgeable about all aspects of gynecology?
> - Why is it beneficial for the medical assistant to be knowledgeable about reproductive disorders and conditions?

OBSTETRICAL EXAMINATION AND TESTING

Obstetrics is the branch of medicine that deals with the management of pregnancy, labor (childbirth), and the **puerperium** (postpartum period), which is the time after childbirth when the reproductive organs return to their prior state. To maintain the health of the mother and child, obstetrical examination and testing is necessary during these three stages.

TABLE 39-2 Common Methods of Contraception (Birth Control)*		
Method	Description	Mechanism
NONHORMONAL		
Condom (male)†	Latex sheath placed over erect penis.	Blocks entrance of sperm into uterus.
Condom (female)†	Plastic lining placed in vagina to cover the cervix.	Blocks entrance of sperm into uterus.
Cervical cap with spermicide	Plastic cap fits over cervical entrance.	Blocks entrance of sperm into uterus.
Diaphragm with spermicide	Soft rubber inserted into vagina to cover the cervix.	Blocks entrance of sperm into uterus.
IUD	Plastic T-shaped device containing copper placed inside uterus.	Causes changes to lining of uterus that prevent fertilized egg from implanting into uterine wall.
Surgical		
Vasectomy	Both vas deferens cut and tied.	No sperm in seminal fluid.
Tubal ligation	Fallopian tubes cut and tied.	No eggs reach fallopian tubes.
Chemical Barriers		
Creams, foams, jellies, suppositories, sponge	Contain spermicidal properties.	Kill sperm before they enter uterus.
HORMONAL		
Oral contraception ("the pill")	Hormone-containing pills taken daily (estrogen and progesterone).	Prevents ovulation.
Injection	Hormone-containing medication given once a month or every 3 months.	Prevents ovulation.
Patch	Hormone-containing patch is applied once a week for 3 weeks. Week 4: no patch.	Prevents ovulation.
IUD	Progestin-releasing plastic T-shaped device inserted into vagina.	Prevents ovulation.
Vaginal ring	Hormone-releasing ring inserted each month into vagina and left in place for 3 weeks, then removed during week 4.	Prevents ovulation.
"Morning-after" pill	Pill containing female hormones taken the morning after intercourse (within 72 hours). Take second pill 12 hours after the first dose.	Prevents implantation.
BEHAVIORAL		
Abstinence	No intercourse.	No sperm.
Rhythm (natural family planning, timed coitus)	Avoidance of intercourse for several days before and after ovulation.	No union of a sperm and egg.
Coitus interruptus (withdrawal)	Penis withdrawn before ejaculation.	Prevents sperm from entering vagina.

IUD, Intrauterine device.
*Some contraceptive methods (e.g., chemical barriers) are not adequate when used alone.
†When used correctly, latex condoms also can prevent spread of sexually transmitted diseases.

Pregnancy

Before learning about the examination and testing that occurs during pregnancy, it is helpful to review the prenatal developmental stages and the birth process in Chapter 21. An important aspect of obstetrics is the prenatal care given to the pregnant woman. The first examination is vital to establishing a care plan designed on baseline data. The medical assistant is involved in the preparation of the patient, which includes taking vital signs, measuring height and weight, and taking the patient history, and assisting the physician in various gynecological examinations.

Prenatal Care

Prenatal care promotes the health of the mother and baby. Prenatal care covers all conditions of the mother and fetus during pregnancy. This includes treatment of common problems associated with pregnancy such as urinary tract infections and anemia. Prenatal care also prevents or detects other conditions that could harm the mother and fetus during this time.

Examination

Prenatal care should begin when a woman suspects she may be pregnant after missing her first regular menstrual cycle and calls the medical office for an appointment. The physician determines if the woman is pregnant by requesting a **serum pregnancy test,** a blood test that confirms the presence of **human chorionic gonadotropin (hCG)** in the sample. The hCG stimulates the **corpus luteum** to secrete estrogen and progesterone. A positive (+) result is reported when the hCG reading is 100 units per milliliter (U/mL).

During the initial visit, a complete patient and family history (Figure 39-9) and physical examination are done to establish an **estimated date of delivery/confinement (EDD/EDC)** and the patient's general state of health. The medical assistant collects the patient's history and records the last menstrual period (LMP), which is used in **Nägele's rule** to calculate the due date (Box 39-4). If the LMP is not known, a date can be estimated by using the fundal height or by performing an ultrasound examination.

The physical examination includes vital signs, height and weight, and a full pelvic examination with initial bimanual **pelvimetry** and laboratory studies. The following tests are performed at the initial prenatal visit:
- Baseline Pap smear may also be performed.
- **Complete blood count (CBC)** to determine adequacy of cellular components of the blood.
- **Blood chemistry** to screen for random blood sugar, thyroid function, and electrolyte balance.
- Blood type and Rh factor to rule out maternal and fetal blood incompatibility.
- Syphilis testing to detect asymptomatic infections.
- Rubella **titer** to determine the presence or absence of antibodies to rubella.
- Urinalysis to detect infection, glucose, or protein.
- Vaginal cultures to rule out various viral, bacterial, fungal, and protozoal infections.

A pregnancy flow sheet is started and is used to record each subsequent visit (Figure 39-10). After the initial visit, the assessment of the patient's health continues on each subsequent visit. Weight, urinalysis (for glucose and protein), and blood pressure readings are performed at each visit. Periodic hemoglobin levels are also obtained to monitor for anemia. Glucose blood testing is done about the twenty-seventh week of pregnancy to check for **gestational diabetes.** Procedure 39-3 describes the procedure for assisting the physician and patient during a follow-up prenatal examination.

During each return prenatal visit, the medical assistant collects and records changes and new information. The return visits also allow the medical assistant to provide prenatal education, as well as emotional support to the patient when needed. The return physical examinations include measurement of the fundal height (Figure 39-11) and in the second trimester, measurement of the fetal heart tones (Figure 39-12).

Childbirth

Parturition (labor) is the physical process of the uterus expelling the fetus and the **placenta** and fetal membranes (afterbirth). The three stages of labor can be reviewed in Chapter 21. Within 1 minute after birth and again at 5 minutes after birth, the newborn is evaluated using a system called an **Apgar score.**

Postpartum Care

A patient is asked to return in 6 weeks after a vaginal delivery to evaluate her general state of health. After a cesarean birth, the patient is asked to return 2 weeks after surgery and then again 4 to 6 weeks after delivery. A **postpartum** visit includes the following:
- Vital signs: Any abnormal reading is reported, recorded, and evaluated.
- Weight: Nutritional counseling to help the patient lose weight if needed.
- Breast examination: Assessment for lumps and if breastfeeding, cracks in the nipples or other problems.
- Pelvic and rectal examination: Checking for muscle tone and size of uterus.
- Laboratory studies: CBC and urinalysis.

BOX 39-4

Estimated Date of Delivery/Confinement (EDD/EDC)

The estimated date of delivery (EDD) using Nägele's rule adds 7 days to the first day of the last menstrual period (LMP), subtracts 3 months, and adds 1 year (EDD = LMP + 7 days − 3 months + 1 year).

Examples:

LMP	December 1, 2004	12/01/04
+7 days	December 8, 2004	12/08/04
−3 months	September 8, 2004	09/08/04
+1 year	September 8, 2005	09/08/05

Question:
What happens if the LMP occurs in January, February, or March?
Answer:
Two adjustments must be made:
1. Think of January as month 13, February as month 14, and March as month 15.
2. Ignore +1 year.

For example:
Lisa Fisher's LMP was January 12, 2005.

LMP	January 12, 2005	01/12/05
+7 days	January 19, 2005	01/19/05
−3 months	October 19, 2005	10/19/05
+1 year		

Month	Day	Year
13	12	05
−3	+7	
10	19	05

PATIENT-CENTERED PROFESSIONALISM

- *How important is it for the medical assistant to understand the reason for all the prenatal and postpartum tests?*

Text continued on p. 877

GYNECOLOGICAL / OBSTETRICAL HISTORY

LAST NAME FIRST MIDDLE

PAT. HOSP. # ______

PRENATAL CLINIC / PHYSICIAN ______

PAT. CLINIC # ______

PATIENT - PLEASE COMPLETE SHADED AREAS

Birthplace	Age	Date of Birth	Race	Marital Status	Religion (Optional)
Your Occupation			Education Completed		
Baby's Father's Name	Father's Telephone	Father's Age	Father's Race	Father's Occupation	Father's Education Completed
Person To Contact In Emergency		Telepone	Alternate Telephone		Address

GENERAL HISTORY - SELF & FAMILY

Please check if you *or if* any of your relatives (such as children, brothers, sisters, grandparents, aunts, uncles) have had any of the conditions listed.
CIRCLE ANY CONDITIONS YOU ARE UNSURE OF.

FAMILY No	FAMILY Yes	SELF No	SELF Yes	CONDITION	PHYSICIAN NOTES
☐	☐	☐	☐	Cancer	
☐	☐	☐	☐	High Blood Pressure	
☐	☐	☐	☐	Heart / Valve Disease	
☐	☐	☐	☐	Rheumatic Fever	
☐	☐	☐	☐	Lung Disease	
☐	☐	☐	☐	Stomach / Bowel Problems	
☐	☐	☐	☐	Kidney Disease	
☐	☐	☐	☐	Urinary Problems, Infections or Malformations	
☐	☐	☐	☐	Diabetes Mellitus	
☐	☐	☐	☐	Anemia / Blood Disorders	
☐	☐	☐	☐	Other Endocrine / Hormone Disorders	
☐	☐	☐	☐	Nervous Mental Disorders	
☐	☐	☐	☐	Convulsive Disorders - Epilepsy	
☐	☐	☐	☐	Abnormal Babies	
☐	☐	☐	☐	Genetic Disease	
☐	☐	☐	☐	Twins	

FAMILY No	FAMILY Yes	SELF No	SELF Yes	CONDITION	PHYSICIAN NOTES
☐	☐	☐	☐	Infertility	
☐	☐	☐	☐	Blood Clots / Varicose Veins	
☐	☐	☐	☐	Blood Transfusions	
				Sexually Transmitted Diseases:	
		☐	☐	Genital Herpes	
		☐	☐	Condylomata (Warts)	
		☐	☐	Chlamydia	
				Infectious Diseases:	
		☐	☐	Hepatitis	
		☐	☐	Tuberculosis	
		☐	☐	PKU	
		☐	☐	DES Exposure	
		☐	☐	Other:	

Does the baby's father, or his family, have any history of abnormal babies or genetic disease? ☐ NO ☐ YES

HABITS / ENVIRONMENTAL FACTORS

TOBACCO & CAFFEINE

No	Yes	
☐	☐	Coffee / Tea____cups a day
☐	☐	Cola or other caffeinated drinks, ______ a day
☐	☐	Cigarettes - Now ____ a day ______ years
☐	☐	Cigarettes - Ever ____ a day ______ years
		When Stopped: ______

ALCOHOL

Alcohol No ☐ Yes ☐
______Drinks per day
______Drinks per week

MISC.

	No	Yes
1. Are you ever around cats?	☐	☐
2. Do you use a hot tub?	☐	☐
3. Do you have a regular exercise routine?	☐	☐
4. Do you, or have you, used drugs (marijuana, cocaine, uppers, downers)?	☐	☐

ALLERGIES / SENSITIVITIES (Detail)

ANTIBIOTICS ______
PAIN MEDICINE ______
ANESTHESIA ______
OTHER ______

Please list all times you have been hospitalized, operated on, or seriously injured.

Year	Operation, Illness, Injury	Hospital and City

LAST CONTRACEPTIVE

TYPE ______
DATE STOPPED ______

MENSTRUAL HISTORY

CYCLE ____DAYS ONSET ____AGE
LENGTH ____DAYS

LMP Mo. Day Year
EDC Mo. Day Year

Pregnancy History	Grav	Term	Preterm	Abortion S. E.	Living	C. Sections

No. of Preg.	Mo./Year	Baby's Sex	Wt.	Weeks Gestation	Hrs. Labor	Delivery Type	DETAIL COMPLICATIONS - MATERNAL / NEWBORN, ANESTHESIA IF C-SECTION, LIST INCISION TYPE
1							
2							
3							
4							
5							
6							

ORDER # 19-770 • BIBBERO SYSTEMS, INC. • PETALUMA, CA. © 1986
TO REORDER CALL TOLL FREE: (800) BIBBERO (800-242-2376) OR FAX (800) 242-9330 Mfd In U.S.A.

M.D. SIGNATURE DATE

FIGURE 39-9 Example of a pregnancy health history form. (Courtesy Bibbero Systems, Inc., Petaluma, CA (800) 242-2376; fax (800) 242-9330; www.bibbero.com)

PREGNANCY FLOW SHEET

LMP.________________
MO. DAY YEAR

☐ NORMAL ☐ ABNORMAL

EDC. ________________

PRE. PREG. WT. ________________

QUICKENING DATE________________

LAST NAME FIRST MIDDLE

PAT. HOSP. #________________

PRENATAL CLINIC / PHYSICIAN ________________

PAT. CLINIC # ________________

DATE	WEIGHT THIS VISIT	BLOOD PRESSURE	URINE PRO-TEIN	URINE SUG-AR	EST. WEEKS GEST. AGE (DATES/SIZE)	FUNDAL HEIGHT (CMS)	FETAL HEART TONES FHT	PRESENTATION	FETAL MOVE-MENTS	EDEMA		COMMENTS / COMPLAINTS / TREATMENT	NEXT VISIT	CHECK IF ADDIT. NOTES	INITIALS OF DR.

TELEPHONE CALLS

DATE / PERSON	QUEST.	ADVICE	DATE / PERSON	QUEST.	ADVICE

INITIAL LABORATORY RESULTS DATE:

BLOOD TYPE / RH: PATIENT: / FATHER: /

HEMOGLOBIN: HEMATOCRIT: WBC:

URINE: GLUCOSE: PROTEIN: MICRO: CULTURE:

ANTIBODY SCREEN: SICKLE CELL:

SEROLOGY: RUBELLA TITER:

PAP TEST: CERVICAL CULTURE:

TAY SACHS: GC:

CHLAMYDIA: ALPHA FETOPROTEIN:

ULTRASOUND: DATE: RESULTS:

ULTRASOUND: DATE: RESULTS:

GENETIC STUDY

______AMNIOCENTESIS DATE:__________RESULTS:__________

______CHORIONIC VILLI BIOPSY DATE:__________RESULTS:__________

POSTTERM (42 Wks.) MANAGEMENT

______NST (date) ________________

______CST (date) ________________

RhoGAM (28 - 32 Weeks)

☐ Indicated ☐ Given DATE:____________

GLUCOSE SCREEN (27 - 32 WEEKS)

DATE: ____________RESULT: ____________

HERPES CULTURE DATE / RESULT	HEPATITIS DATE / TEST / RESULT
/	/ /
/	/ /
/	/ /
/	/ /

ORDER # 19-773 • BIBBERO SYSTEMS, INC. • PETALUMA, CA. • © 1986 (REV. 3/95)
TO REORDER CALL TOLL FREE: (800) BIBBERO (800-242-2376) OR FAX (800) 242-9330 MFG IN U.S.A.

M.D. SIGNATURE DATE

FIGURE 39-10 Example of a pregnancy flow sheet. (Courtesy Bibbero Systems, Inc., Petaluma, CA (800) 242-2376; fax (800) 242-9330; www.bibbero.com)

PROCEDURE 39-3 Assist with a Follow-up Prenatal Examination

TASK: Assist the physician and patient during a follow-up prenatal visit.

EQUIPMENT AND SUPPLIES
- Flexible, nonstretchable centimeter tape measure
- Nonsterile disposable gloves
- Doppler fetal pulse detector
- Lubricant (water-based)
- Ultrasound coupling agent
- Vaginal speculum
- Examining gown and drape
- Biohazardous waste container
- Patient's medical record

SKILLS/RATIONALE

STANDARD PRECAUTIONS ARE TO BE FOLLOWED.

NOTE: For this procedure, all components of a follow-up prenatal examination will be included.

1. **Procedural Step. Sanitize the hands.**
   An alcohol-based hand rub may be used instead of washing hands with soap and water, unless hands are visibly soiled.
   Rationale. Hand sanitization promotes infection control.

2. **Procedural Step. Assemble equipment and supplies.**
   The prenatal examination tray setup may vary, depending on the extent of the examination. Not all prenatal follow-up examinations will include a Doppler fetal pulse or vaginal examination. Supplies for these procedures will not be included if they are not to be performed at this visit.
   Rationale. It is important to have all supplies and equipment ready and available before starting any procedure to ensure efficiency.

3. **Procedural Step. Obtain the patient's medical record.**

4. **Procedural Step. Greet the patient, introduce yourself, and confirm the patient's identity.**
   Rationale. Identifying the patient ensures the procedure is performed on the correct patient.

5. **Procedural Step. Collect the first morning urine specimen that the patient has brought from home.**
   Ask the patient if she has taken the necessary precautions to preserve the integrity of the specimen. Some physicians will request that a specimen be collected at the physician's office at the time of the appointment. If the physician has ordered that a urine specimen be collected on site, provide the patient with a specimen container and directions for collection of a urine specimen.
   Rationale. Specimens brought into the office must have been refrigerated if the specimen was collected more than 1 hour before the appointment; specimens that have been left standing out produce inaccurate test results. The specimen must also have been collected in a clean container. Often the office will provide patients with a specimen container at each visit to use for their next visit. Specimens should not be collected or transported to the office in empty medication bottles because there is a chance of residual contamination of the specimen by the medication.

6. **Procedural Step. Weigh the patient and document the results in the patient's medical record.**
   Most facilities have a central location for scales, and the patient should be weighed before being escorted to the examination room. If each examination room has its own scale, escort the patient to the examination room and then weigh the patient.
   Rationale. Weight loss or gain during pregnancy is vital in assessing fetal development and the health of the mother, and weight should be measured closely at every prenatal visit.

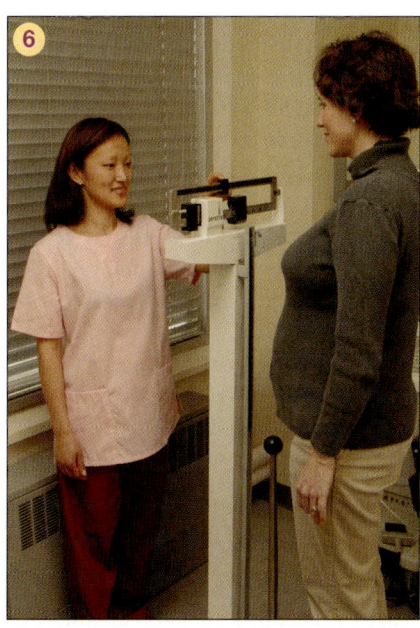

Continued

PROCEDURE 39-3 Assist with a Follow-up Prenatal Examination—cont'd

7. **Procedural Step.** Escort the patient to the examination room, and explain the procedure to the patient.
   Rationale. Explaining the procedure to the patient promotes cooperation and provides a means of obtaining implied consent.

8. **Procedural Step.** Document any patient problems, concerns, or chief complaint.
   Ask the patient to be seated. Ask the patient if she has experienced any problems or if she has any concerns or questions since her last visit. Document her responses in her medical record and answer her questions as appropriate. Direct the physician to answer any patient questions that are outside your scope of practice.
   Rationale. The physician uses this documentation to review and investigate any unusual or atypical signs or symptoms.

9. **Procedural Step.** Measure the patient's blood pressure and document the results in the patient's medical record.
   If the blood pressure is elevated, allow the patient a few minutes to relax, then measure again.
   Rationale. It is important to determine if blood pressure is elevated because of recent exertion, excitement, or stress, or if blood pressure is elevated because of a physiological condition.

10. **Procedural Step.** Prepare the patient for the examination.
    If the physician will be performing a vaginal examination, instruct the patient to remove *all* clothing (including undergarments), and provide her with a patient gown and drape. If no vaginal examination is to be performed, the patient may be required to remove only enough clothing to expose her abdomen.

11. **Procedural Step.** Test the urine specimen for glucose and protein using a reagent strip and document the results in the patient's medical record.
    Test the urine specimen while the patient is changing into a patient gown or any time before the physician examines the patient.
    Rationale. A urine specimen must be tested for protein and glucose at every prenatal visit for early detection of gestational diabetes or ketonuria.

12. **Procedural Step.** Inform the physician that the patient is ready to be examined and provide the physician with the patient's medical record for review.
    Rationale. The physician will review the measurements and test results before examining the patient as a means of comparison with the current examination findings.

13. **Procedural Step.** Position the patient.
    When the physician is ready to examine the patient, assist the patient onto the table and into a supine position. Drape the patient as required. Provide support and reassurance to the patient to help her relax during the examination. Provide for the safety of the patient and never leave a pregnant woman unattended on an examination table, especially if she is in her last trimester. Do not position the patient until the physician is ready for the examination.
    Rationale. Lying on the examination table in a supine position may be extremely uncomfortable for a pregnant patient. If the patient wants to lie down, suggest lying on the left side, with a pillow behind the back if in last trimester.

14. **Procedural Step.** Assist the physician as required for the prenatal examination.
    This typically includes handing the physician the tape measure for fundal measurement, preparing and handing the physician the Doppler fetal heart monitor and coupling agent, assisting the patient into the lithotomy position if a vaginal examination is performed, holding the glass slide and spraying the fixative if specimens are collected for determination of vaginal infection, and completing the requisition form if specimens are sent to the laboratory or transported outside the facility. If the specimens are examined on site, prepare the specimens for examination. Read and record the results in the patient's medical record. Follow all OSHA guidelines during the collection and processing of the specimen; follow Standard Precautions to prevent exposure to body fluids.

15. **Procedural Step.** After the examination, assist the patient from the examination table.
    Assist the patient into a sitting position and provide the patient with the opportunity to rest for a few minutes to prevent postural dizziness. Once the patient is comfortable, if a vaginal examination was performed, offer the patient tissues to remove excess lubricant. Assist the patient off the examination table as needed. Instruct the patient to dress and assist if needed. Leave the room to complete the cytology requisition form, if appropriate.
    Rationale. Patients may feel dizzy after the procedure and should be allowed to rest for a few minutes. Always assist patients as needed.

16. **Procedural Step.** Provide patient education and clarify any of the physician's instructions that the patient may question.

17. **Procedural Step.** Clean the examination room in preparation for the next patient.
    Discard all contaminated material in a biohazardous waste container. Prepare specimens and laboratory requisitions for transport as required. Wear nonsterile disposable gloves when cleaning the examination room. Never bring the next patient into an examination room that has items left from the last procedure (e.g., dirty speculum in sink).

18. **Procedural Step.** Sanitize the hands.
    Always sanitize the hands after every procedure or after using gloves.

Continued

PROCEDURE 39-3 Assist with a Follow-up Prenatal Examination—cont'd

EXAMPLE OF OB VISITS SUMMARY (FLOW SHEET)

Date	EGA	Wt	BP	UA-P	UA-G	FHT	FH	P
7-20-xx	11W2D	153	112/70	Neg	Trace	150	13	82
8-21-xx	15W3D	157	120/90	Neg	Trace	152	16	88

EGA, Estimated gestational age.

CHARTING EXAMPLE

Date	
8/21/xx	10:00 a.m. Pt states she is very anxious about pregnancy due to past history of miscarriage.——L. Kahl, CMA (AAMA)

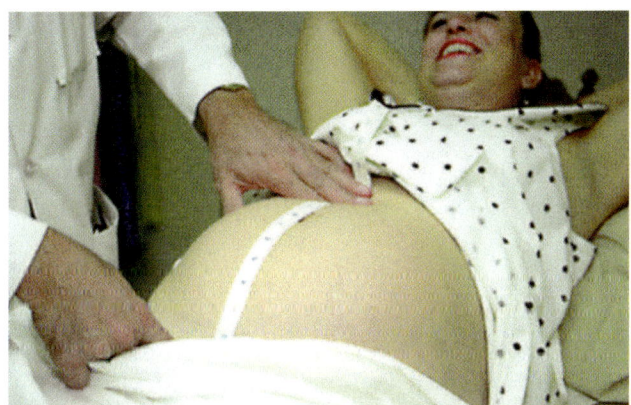

FIGURE 39-11 Measuring the height of the uterine fundus. (From Zakus SM: *Mosby's clinical skills for medical assistants,* ed 4, St Louis, 2001, Mosby.)

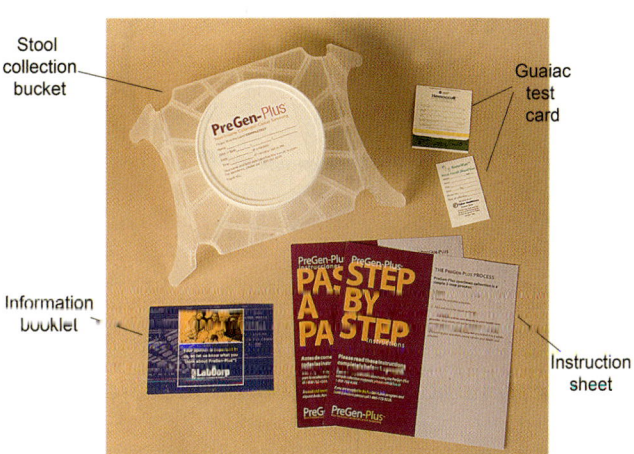

FIGURE 39-13 Testing kits for fecal occult blood.

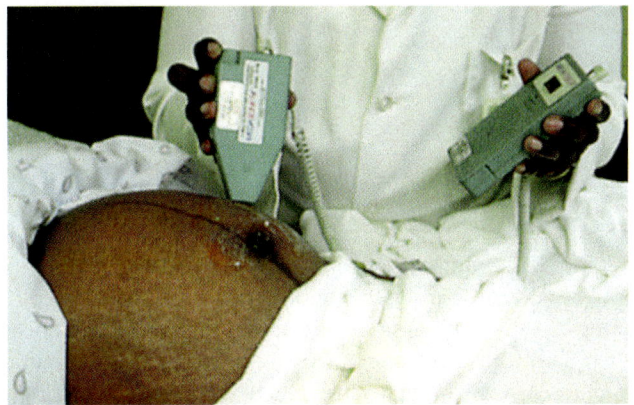

FIGURE 39-12 Listening to the fetal heart rate. (From Zakus SM: *Mosby's clinical skills for medical assistants,* ed 4, St Louis, 2001, Mosby.)

COLON TESTS

The most common colon procedures done in the medical office are tests for fecal occult blood and flexible sigmoidoscopy. In both of these colon procedures, the medical assistant provides the patient with diet and preparatory information and assists the physician during the procedures, making sure equipment and supplies are ready and available when needed. Colonoscopy is an extensive view of the entire colon that is usually scheduled as an outpatient procedure.

Fecal Occult Testing

A **fecal occult blood test (FOBT),** or **guaiac test** (e.g., Hemoccult, Seracult, or ColoScreen), is done to detect the presence of hidden blood in the stool. The FOBT cannot identify the *cause* of bleeding; it is performed to screen for **colorectal** bleeding. Positive test results require additional procedures to identify the location of the bleeding. A colonoscopy is normally recommended as a follow-up to a positive FOBT. Bleeding can occur in the stomach, intestines, and other digestive areas. A positive FOBT will lead to other tests to identify the cause (e.g., barium enema, sigmoidoscopy, colonoscopy, or a computed tomography [CT] scan).

Colorectal cancer is one possible cause of bleeding. Colorectal cancer is very prevalent in people over 40 years of age, and it is the second most common form of cancer in the United States. Symptoms tend to be general and are often ignored by the patient. Early screening can greatly reduce the risk of colon cancer. Figure 39-13 displays several types of screening tools used for detecting occult blood in stool.

Patient Preparation

During the FOBT, a stool specimen is placed on a **test card.** The medical assistant may provide the test card to the physician as part of the rectal examination or may provide three test cards to the patient to use at home and return to the office

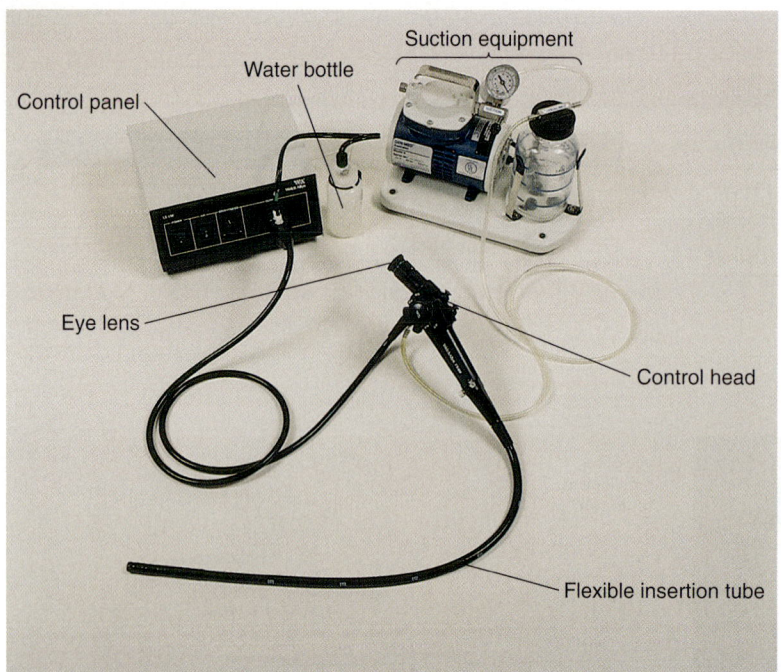

FIGURE 39-14 Flexible fiberoptic sigmoidoscope. (From Bonewit-West K: *Clinical procedures for medical assistants,* ed 7, St Louis, 2008, Saunders.)

BOX 39-5
Documentation When Charting for Patient Education

Before you chart instructions given to a patient, the following information is needed:
1. Date
2. Time
3. Supplies provided (if any)
4. Instructions provided for the procedure
5. Patient's understanding of the instructions
6. Proper signature and credential

BOX 39-6
Documentation When Charting Diagnostic Testing Procedures

1. Date
2. Time
3. Name of procedure
4. Results
5. Patient reaction, if any
6. Proper signature and credential

for testing. The medical assistant provides the patient with diet instructions before collection of a stool sample. Instructions are also given to the patient on properly collecting the stool sample. Procedure 39-4 explains how to provide a patient with accurate and complete instructions on the preparation and collection of a stool sample for testing. Box 39-5 lists charting information needed to document patient instructions.

Developing the Occult Blood Test

The medical assistant is also responsible for accurately developing the occult blood slide test. Regardless of the test card used, a chemical reagent called *guaiac* is impregnated on the testing paper. A developer (hydrogen peroxide) is placed on the guaiac paper directly over the smear. A color change (blue) indicates the presence of blood. Procedure 39-5 explains the process of accurately developing the occult blood slide test. Box 39-6 lists information necessary to chart diagnostic procedures.

Sigmoidoscopy

A *flexible* **sigmoidoscopy** is a procedure to examine the lower bowel to diagnose and treat conditions that affect this portion of the digestive system. A flexible fiberoptic **sigmoidoscope** is often used to visualize the mucosa of the rectum and sigmoid colon (Figure 39-14). This instrument magnifies the colon by 10 times and allows the physician to detect lesions, polyps, and other abnormalities. Further testing (e.g., proctoscopy) would be scheduled in a hospital area, such as an endoscopy unit, where more extensive equipment is used to evaluate what the sigmoidoscope cannot.

Patient Preparation

Normally, the physician has the patient eat a low-fiber diet the day before the scheduled examination. A mild laxative or an enema may be prescribed the evening before the test, with another enema the morning of the test. The procedure is done early in the morning, when the patient is usually fasting. On

Text continued on p. 883

Specialty Diagnostic Testing **CHAPTER 39** 879

| PROCEDURE 39-4 | **Instruct the Patient in Obtaining a Fecal Specimen** | |

TASK: Provide the patient with accurate and complete instructions on the preparation and collection of a stool sample for testing.

EQUIPMENT AND SUPPLIES
- Hemoccult slide testing kit:
  - 3 occult blood slides
  - 3 applicator sticks
  - Diet and collection instruction sheet
- Patient's medical record

SKILLS/RATIONALE

STANDARD PRECAUTIONS ARE TO BE FOLLOWED.

1. **Procedural Step. Sanitize the hands.**
   An alcohol-based hand rub may be used instead of washing hands with soap and water, unless hands are visibly soiled.
   Rationale. Hand sanitization promotes infection control.

2. **Procedural Step. Assemble equipment and supplies.**
   Obtain three fecal occult blood slides. Check the expiration date of each cardboard slide.
   Rationale. It is important to have all supplies and equipment ready and available before starting any procedure to ensure efficiency. Expired slides may render the test results inaccurate.

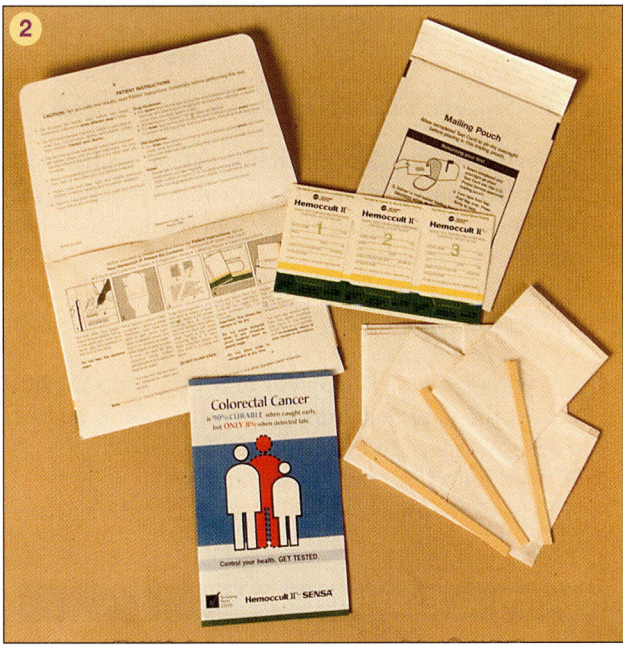

3. **Procedural Step.** Obtain the patient's medical record.

4. **Procedural Step.** Greet the patient, introduce yourself, and confirm the patient's identity.
   Rationale. Identifying the patient ensures the procedure is performed on the correct patient.

5. **Procedural Step. Explain the procedure to the patient.**
   Inform the patient that the test should not be conducted during a menstrual cycle or in the presence of hemorrhoidal bleeding.
   Rationale. Explaining the procedure to the patient promotes cooperation and provides a means of obtaining implied consent. Blood from sources other than fecal matter will provide inaccurate test results.

6. **Procedural Step. Provide the patient with verbal and written instructions.**
   Instructions should outline the correct dietary modifications to begin 48 hours before collection of the first stool sample and should explain that collection continues until all three slide specimens have been collected.
   a. Well-cooked fish and poultry are acceptable, but red or rare meat, processed meat, or liver should be avoided.
      Rationale. Red meat contains animal blood, which could cause a false-positive result.
   b. Vegetables in moderation are acceptable, but horseradish, turnips, and radishes should be avoided.
   c. Fruits in moderation are acceptable, but melons should be avoided.
   d. High-fiber foods, such as whole-wheat bread, bran cereal, and popcorn, are acceptable, but food high in roughage fiber should be avoided.
   e. Medications that contain aspirin, iron, or vitamin C should be avoided.
   Rationale. Following the outlined diet will provide more accurate test results. If the patient does not follow the diet modifications, inaccurate test results could occur.
   NOTE: Newer prep cards void the need to follow a special diet. Read the instructions that come with the guaiac cards being dispensed.

7. **Procedural Step. Provide the patient with the Hemoccult slide test kit.**
   The kit contains written instructions, three attached cardboard slides (numbered 1, 2, and 3), and three wooden applicator sticks (for three separate specimens).

Continued

PROCEDURE 39-4 Instruct the Patient in Obtaining a Fecal Specimen—cont'd

Each slide has two squares labeled "A" and "B" containing filter paper impregnated with guaiac.

8. **Procedural Step.** Instruct the patient to use a ballpoint pen to complete the required information on the front of the card.
   This information includes the patient's name, address, phone number, age, and the date of the specimen collection. This information should be completed before collection of specimens.

9. **Procedural Step.** Inform the patient of the requirements for proper care and storage of the slides.
   The slides must be stored at room temperature and protected from heat, sunlight, and strong fluorescent light.
   Rationale. Improper storage of the slides may result in deterioration of the guaiac impregnated on the filter paper, leading to inaccurate test results.

10. **Procedural Step.** Instruct the patient to collect a stool specimen from the first bowel movement after the 48-hour preparation period. The stool should not come in contact with the water in the toilet.

11. **Procedural Step.** Explain the stool collection procedure to the patient.

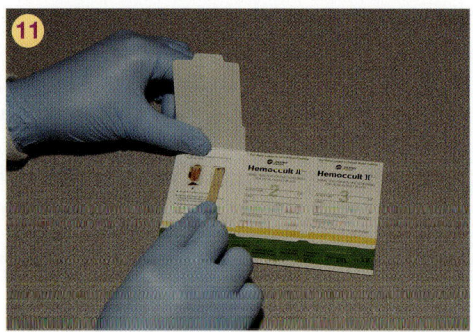

   a. The stool specimen may be collected directly from the stool in a container, on a disposable paper plate, or plastic wrap. Using one of the wooden applicators, obtain a small sample of the stool.
   b. Open the front flap of the first cardboard slide (located on the left in the series of three).
   c. Spread a very thin smear of the specimen over the filter paper in the square labeled "A."
   d. Using the opposite end of the same wooden applicator, obtain another small sample from a different area of the stool.
   e. Spread a very thin smear of the specimen over the filter paper in the square labeled "B."
   f. Close the front flap of the cardboard slide and indicate the date in the space provided.
   g. Discard the wooden applicator in a waste container.

   Rationale. Occult blood is not always distributed evenly throughout a specimen, so collecting two separate specimens from different areas of the sample provides a greater opportunity to find occult blood. The specimen must be spread thinly to provide adequate penetration through the filter paper.

12. **Procedural Step.** Instruct the patient to repeat the process on the next two bowel movements, repeating the collection steps.
    The specimen from the second bowel movement is placed on the middle slide, and the specimen from the third bowel movement is placed on the slide on the right.

13. **Procedural Step.** Instruct the patient to allow the slides to air-dry minimally overnight.

14. **Procedural Step.** Once all three specimens are collected and allowed to air-dry, instruct the patient to place the cardboard slides in the envelope, carefully seal it, and return it as soon as possible to the medical office.

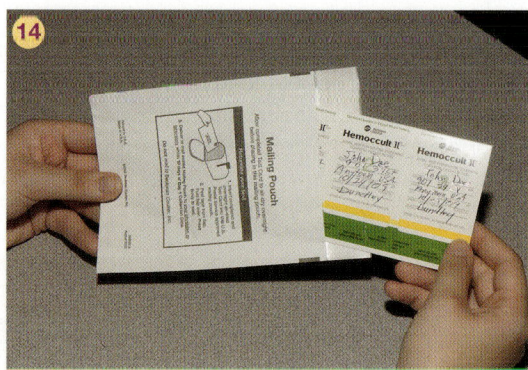

15. **Procedural Step.** Make sure the patient understands the instructions required for patient preparation, collection, and processing of the stool specimens and for storage of the slides.
    Allow time for patient questions.
    Rationale. Improper patient preparation and technique may lead to inaccurate test results.

16. **Procedural Step.** Document in the patient's medical record the date that the Hemoccult test and instructions were given to the patient.

17. **Procedural Step.** Sanitize the hands.
    Always sanitize the hands after every procedure or after using gloves.

CHARTING EXAMPLE

Date	
1/4/xx	9:30 a.m. Pt. given instructions for diet restrictions and stool collections. Written instructions provided. Pt. verbalizes understanding.————————————————— K. Key, CMA (AAMA)

Specialty Diagnostic Testing   **CHAPTER 39**   **881**

PROCEDURE 39-5

Test for Occult Blood

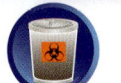

TASK: Accurately develop the occult blood slide test and document the results.

EQUIPMENT AND SUPPLIES
- Prepared cardboard slides
- Reference card
- Developing solution
- Nonsterile disposable gloves
- Biohazardous waste container
- Patient's medical record

SKILLS/RATIONALE

STANDARD PRECAUTIONS ARE TO BE FOLLOWED.

1. **Procedural Step. Sanitize the hands.**
   An alcohol-based hand rub may be used instead of washing hands with soap and water, unless hands are visibly soiled.
   Rationale. Hand sanitization promotes infection control.

2. **Procedural Step. Assemble equipment and supplies.**
   Rationale. It is important to have all supplies and equipment ready and available before starting any procedure to ensure efficiency.

3. **Procedural Step. Check the expiration date on the developing solution bottle.**
   Developing solution bottles must be stored with the cap tightly closed and must be kept from heat and light because the solution contains hydrogen peroxide.
   Rationale. Outdated solutions will cause inaccurate test results. The solution must be stored properly because the solution evaporates quickly and is flammable.

4. **Procedural Step. Obtain the patient's medical record.**

5. **Procedural Step. Prepare to develop the slides.**
   Obtain the specimens from the patient, and identify the specimens as belonging to the patient. The slides may be prepared and developed immediately, or they may be prepared and stored for up to 14 days (at room temperature) before developing.
   Rationale. Identifying that the specimens belong to the patient ensures the procedure is performed on the correct patient.

6. **Procedural Step. Apply nonsterile disposable gloves.**

7. **Procedural Step. Prepare the slides.**
   Open the back flaps of the cardboard slides (opposite side from where the specimens were applied). Apply two drops of the developing solution to the guaiac-impregnated test paper. The developing solution should not be added directly onto the stool specimen, but should be absorbed through the filter paper into the specimen.
   NOTE: The developing solution may cause irritation to the skin and eyes. If contact occurs, immediately flush the area with water.

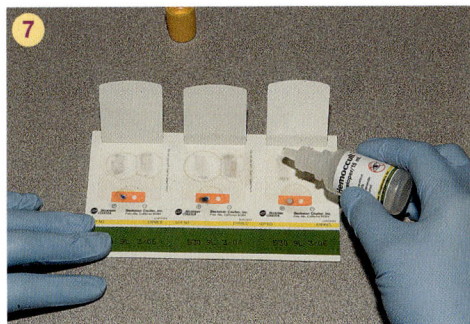

8. **Procedural Step. Obtain the test kit reference card.**
   A reference card is provided with each Hemoccult kit. The reference card provides an illustration of positive and negative results, which can be used as a guide for interpreting results.

Continued

PROCEDURE 39-5 Test for Occult Blood—cont'd

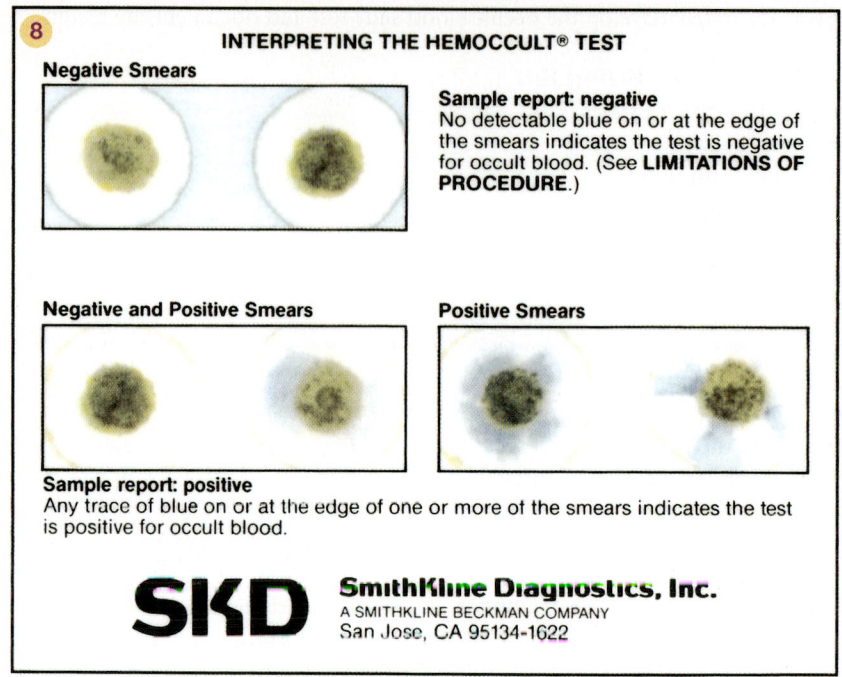

9. **Procedural Step. Read the test results within 60 seconds.**
   A positive result is indicated by any trace of blue color on the filter paper on or around the fecal matter. Occult fecal blood in excess of 5 mL per day will result in a positive reaction. If no detectable color change occurs, the result is considered negative.
   Rationale. Reading the results in the required time is important because the color reaction will fade after 2 to 4 minutes. The developer containing hydrogen peroxide causes the color reaction because heme, the compound in hemoglobin, oxidizes guaiac.

10. **Procedural Step. Perform the quality control procedure, and document the results in the quality control laboratory logbook.**
    Each Hemoccult kit is supplied with quality control slides.
    Rationale. Performing quality control procedures ensures that the test results are accurate and reliable.

11. **Procedural Step. Properly dispose of the Hemoccult slides in a biohazardous waste container.**
    Rationale. Fecal matter is considered a contaminant and should always be disposed of in the appropriate biohazardous waste container.

12. **Procedural Step. Remove gloves and sanitize the hands.**
    Always sanitize the hands after every procedure or after using gloves.

13. **Procedural Step. Document the results.**
    Include the date and time, brand name of the test (Hemoccult), and test results (recorded as positive or negative).

CHARTING EXAMPLE	
Date	
3/10/xx	Received by mail 3-10-xx. Occult testing done on stool specimens returned. Specimen 1 collected 3/6/xx pos; specimen 2 collected 3/8/xx neg; specimen 3 collected 3/9/xx neg. Dr. notified of results.————— B. Pizano, CMA (AAMA)

arrival, the patient is asked to empty the bladder. The patient is then provided with a gown and placed in the Sims' position.

Assisting with Sigmoidoscopy

During sigmoidoscopy, the end of the flexible tube is lubricated and inserted through the anal opening and slowly advanced to the sigmoid colon. Air is blown into the colon through a valve connected to the sigmoidoscope, which allows for better visualization. Suction can be performed to remove feces, mucus, and blood. The intestinal mucosa of the colon is examined while the sigmoidoscope is being inserted and also while it is being withdrawn. Procedure 39-6 explains the process of preparing the patient and assisting the physician and patient during sigmoidoscopy.

> ### PATIENT-CENTERED PROFESSIONALISM
> - How would the medical assistant explain the reason for colorectal testing to the patient?
> - What role does the medical assistant play before and during colon procedures?

PULMONARY FUNCTION TESTS

Pulmonary function tests (**PFTs**) are done to assess a patient's lung function (volume and capacity). The measurement of a patient's pulmonary function provides important information that can be used to assess the need for medications such as bronchodilators. Information from PFTs is also used to detect respiratory disease. Most tests require minimal equipment, are easy to perform, and are noninvasive.

Spirometry

In the medical office the most frequently performed PFT is **spirometry.** Spirometry is performed for the following reasons:

1. To detect the presence of lung dysfunction.
2. To screen the patient at risk because of the environment or smoking.
3. To assess changes in lung function over time.
4. To assess the patient's response to treatment.
5. To assess lung function before major surgery.

Spirometry is used to measure lung volume and lung capacity. To accomplish this, the patient is connected to the spirometer and instructed to perform actions that measure volume and airflow. The volume of air a patient inhales or exhales is measured over time.

The medical assistant should instruct the patient to loosen tight clothing and remove dentures to prevent interruption during the test. Nose clips may be provided to prevent air from escaping through the nose. Patient instructions depend on which PFT is ordered for routine screening, such as the following:

- **Vital capacity** (**VC**) is measured as the volume of air that can be expired when the patient exhales completely. The patient is asked to inhale as deeply as possible and to exhale completely into the mouthpiece.
- **Forced vital capacity** (**FVC**) is measured as the maximum volume of air that can be expired when the patient exhales forcefully. The patient is asked to inhale deeply until the lungs are full, then to blow all the air out of the lungs into the mouthpiece as fast and as hard as possible. This is done at least three times. The measurements are then averaged to obtain the best result.

Procedure 36-7 explains the procedure for accurately performing spirometry to measure lung volume.

Peak Flow Meter

A **peak flow meter** (**PFM**) is a handheld device that measures expiratory flow or the patient's ability to push air out of his or her lungs and is used to monitor respiratory conditions, for example asthma. Measurement results are used to access asthma severity, monitor response to prescribed medications, diagnose exercise-induced asthma, or detect asymptomatic decrease in lung function. When the patient blows into the PFM, his or her breath pushes the indicator marker (Figure 39-15). A high number usually indicates the air is moving easily through the lungs. Procedure 39-8 provides guidelines to assist a patient in learning to efficiently use a PFM.

A "normal" reading is recognized as each patient's own personal best. Once established, the patient can use established zones (green, yellow, and red) to assist him or her to recognize changes.

- *Green zone:* A reading within the green zone can be 80% to 100% of the patient's "normal" reading (personal best) and can be considered good management of asthma.
- *Yellow zone:* A reading within the yellow zone that is between 50% and 80% of the patient's "normal" reading requires some intervention. This may be in the form of taking medications or informing the physician of the results.
- *Red zone:* A reading within the red zone is below 50% of the patient's "normal" reading and signals a need for immediate medical care.

The physician and the patient should already have a plan that indicates what the patient should do in various situations. For example,

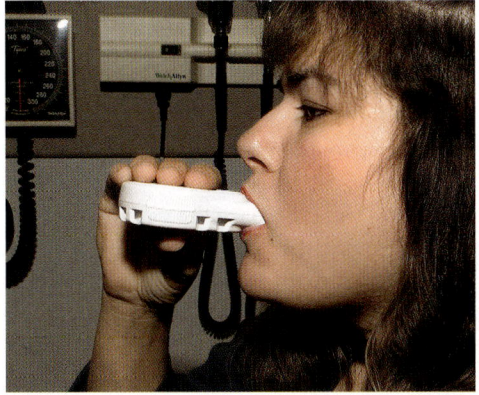

FIGURE 39-15 Patient using a peak flow meter.

Text continued on p. 888

PROCEDURE 39-6 Assist with Sigmoidoscopy

TASK: Assist the physician and the patient during sigmoidoscopy.

EQUIPMENT AND SUPPLIES
- Nonsterile disposable gloves
- Sterile specimen container with preservative
- Flexible sigmoidoscope
- 4 × 4 inch gauze squares
- Water-soluble lubricant
- Tissue wipes
- Drape
- Biopsy forceps
- Biohazardous waste container
- Patient's medical record

SKILLS/RATIONALE
STANDARD PRECAUTIONS ARE TO BE FOLLOWED.

1. **Procedural Step.** Sanitize the hands.
   An alcohol-based hand rub may be used instead of washing hands with soap and water, unless hands are visibly soiled.
   Rationale. Hand sanitization promotes infection control.

2. **Procedural Step.** Assemble equipment and supplies.
   Ensure the light source on the sigmoidoscope is working. Label the specimen container with the patient's name, the date, and the source of the specimen.
   Rationale. It is important to have all supplies and equipment ready and available before starting any procedure to ensure efficiency.

3. **Procedural Step.** Obtain the patient's medical record.

4. **Procedural Step.** Greet the patient, introduce yourself, and confirm the patient's identity.
   Rationale. Identifying the patient ensures the procedure is performed on the correct patient.

5. **Procedural Step.** Explain the procedure to the patient.
   Rationale. Explaining the procedure to the patient promotes cooperation and provides a means of obtaining implied consent.
   Ascertain that the patient's instructions for preparation have been followed.

6. **Procedural Step.** Ask the patient if he or she needs to empty the bladder before the examination.
   If the physician has ordered that a urine specimen be collected, provide the patient with a specimen container and directions for collection of a urine specimen.
   Rationale. An empty bladder allows the patient to tolerate the procedure more comfortably.

7. **Procedural Step.** Prepare the patient.
   Provide the patient with a patient gown and drape and ask the patient to remove all clothing from the waist down and put on the gown with the opening positioned in back. Ask the patient to have a seat on the examination table, assisting the patient as needed. Place a drape across the patient's lap.

8. **Procedural Step.** Position the patient.
   Once the physician has examined the patient and is ready to begin the procedure, place the patient in the Sims' or left lateral position.
   NOTE: If the medical office has a sigmoidoscopy table, the patient should first be aligned correctly on the table, then the table should be mechanically adjusted.

9. **Procedural Step.** Properly drape the patient so that the drape is placed at an angle and the corner of the drape can be lifted to expose the anus.
   A fenestrated drape (drape with one or more openings) can be used to cover the anus.
   Rationale. Draping the patient reduces exposure and provides warmth.

10. **Procedural Step.** Ensure the patient's comfort.
    Before starting the procedure, reassure the patient that even though the procedure may be uncomfortable, it will only last a short time. Ask the patient to breathe slowly and deeply through the mouth and encourage the patient to relax the muscles of the anus and rectum.

11. **Procedural Step.** Lubricate the physician's gloved index finger.
    The physician will begin with a digital examination.

12. **Procedural Step.** Lubricate the distal end of the sigmoidoscope before the physician inserts the sigmoidoscope into the anus.
    Rationale. The sigmoidoscope should be well lubricated for ease of insertion.

13. **Procedural Step.** Assist the physician with the suction equipment as required.

14. **Procedural Step.** Assist with the collection of a biopsy as needed.
    Hand the biopsy forceps to the physician and hold the specimen container to accept the biopsy. Because it is sterile, do not touch the inside of the container.

Continued

PROCEDURE 39-6 Assist with Sigmoidoscopy—cont'd

15. **Procedural Step.** On completion of the examination, apply clean gloves and clean the patient's anal area with tissues to remove any excess lubricant.
16. **Procedural Step.** Remove gloves and sanitize the hands.
    Always sanitize the hands after every procedure or after using gloves.
17. **Procedural Step.** Assist the patient from the examination table.
    Assist the patient to a sitting position and allow the patient to rest. Assist the patient off the examination table as needed. Instruct the patient to dress. Provide the patient a restroom to allow the patient to expel air that was used to inflate the colon during the procedure.
    Rationale. The patient should be allowed to rest after the procedure to prevent postural dizziness. Assisting the patient off the examination table as needed prevents falls and injuries.
18. **Procedural Step.** Prepare the laboratory requisition form and accompanying specimens.
    Complete the laboratory requisition form and attach it to the specimen, if a specimen was taken. Transport the requisition form and specimen to the laboratory pathology department in a sealed biohazard transport container.
19. **Procedural Step.** Clean the examination room in preparation for the next patient.
    Discard all contaminated material in a biohazardous waste container. The sigmoidoscope should be sanitized and disinfected according to the manufacturer's recommendations. The sigmoidoscope contains fiberoptics and should be handled with extreme care. Wear nonsterile disposable gloves when cleaning the examination room. Never bring the next patient into an examination room that has items left from the last procedure.
20. **Procedural Step.** Document the procedure in the patient's medical record.

CHARTING EXAMPLE

Date	
10/07/xx	9:00 a.m. Sigmoidoscopy c̄ 2 bx transported to Medical Center Laboratory for pathology. Pt. tolerated procedure well. Instructions for follow-up given and questions answered. —————— S. Bentley, CMA (AAMA)

PROCEDURE 39-7 Perform Spirometry (Pulmonary Function Testing)

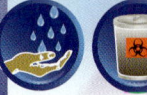

TASK: Prepare and operate a simple spirometer to measure lung volume.

EQUIPMENT AND SUPPLIES
- Spirometry machine
- Disposable mouthpiece
- Disposable tubing
- Nose clips
- Biohazardous waste container
- Patient's medical record

SKILLS/RATIONALE STANDARD PRECAUTIONS ARE TO BE FOLLOWED.

1. **Procedural Step.** Sanitize the hands.
   An alcohol-based hand rub may be used instead of washing hands with soap and water, unless hands are visibly soiled.
   Rationale. Hand sanitization promotes infection control.
2. **Procedural Step.** Assemble equipment and supplies.
   Calibrate the spirometer according to the manufacturer's instructions. Attach a disposable mouthpiece.
   Rationale. It is important to have all supplies and equipment ready and available before starting any procedure to ensure efficiency. Calibration of the spirometer ensures accurate test results.
3. **Procedural Step.** Obtain the patient's medical record.
4. **Procedural Step.** Greet the patient, introduce yourself, and confirm the patient's identity.
   Rationale. Identifying the patient ensures the procedure is performed on the correct patient.

Continued

PROCEDURE 39-7 Perform Spirometry (Pulmonary Function Testing)—cont'd

5. **Procedural Step. Explain the procedure to the patient.**
   Rationale. Explaining the procedure to the patient promotes cooperation and provides a means of obtaining implied consent.

6. **Procedural Step. Measure the patient's height and weight.**
   Rationale. Accurate height and weight measurements are important in calculating the patient's lung capacity.

7. **Procedural Step. Enter the patient's information into the spirometer.**
   The patient identification information is entered into the spirometer and should include gender, height, weight, and age and any other information requested on the machine. Some spirometer models have a bar code on the mouthpiece, which allows the machine to record multiple attempts for the same patient. For these models, the machine prompts the operator to "swipe the mouthpiece," and the operator moves the end of the mouthpiece with the bar code smoothly through a groove in the machine.
   Rationale. The computer database uses the patient's information along with the test results to calculate the patient's test values. If the patient is taking medications for breathing problems or smokes, the patient may be instructed to avoid taking the medication or smoking before the test.

8. **Procedural Step. Position the patient.**
   Instruct the patient to loosen any tight clothing to allow for deep breathing and forceful expiration. Have the patient sit with proper posture; legs should be uncrossed with both feet flat on the floor. If the patient is wearing dentures, they may need to be removed during the testing.
   Rationale. Proper posture and feet positioning help to obtain an accurate reading and to prevent injury from falling because the testing may cause lightheadedness.

9. **Procedural Step. Instruct the patient in the breathing maneuver.**
   a. If used, a nose clip is placed gently on the patient's nostrils to prevent the escape of air through the nose. All air must be exhaled through the mouthpiece and into the spirometer for the test to be valid. A nose clip may not be needed if the patient can exhale completely through the mouth.
   b. The patient relaxes, sits up straight, and takes the deepest breath possible until the lungs are completely full of air.
   c. The patient places the mouthpiece in the mouth and seals the lips tightly around it.
   d. The patient blows out through the mouth smoothly as hard and as long as possible until the lungs are completely empty, avoiding any coughing at the end. Instruct the patient that the mouthpiece should not be removed from the mouth until you tell the patient to do so.
   Rationale. Sitting up straight allows the chest to expand further and fill the lungs to a greater capacity. A tight seal around the mouthpiece must be created, as well as a tight seal of the nose when using nose clips. This ensures that all air is directed into the spirometer.

10. **Procedural Step. Perform the spirometry test.**
    Initiate the testing period by pressing a button on the spirometer. The machine will prompt you when to direct the patient to inhale and exhale.
    The most essential part of the spirometry test is the coaching you provide to the patient. For example, you could say "OK, now breathe in, and keep breathing in until you fill your lungs. Try to fill them some more ... keep inhaling ... don't stop until you can't take in any more air. Come on ... keep going! Now seal your lips around the mouthpiece and blow out! Keep blowing out until you don't have any more air in your lungs. Come on ... blow hard, keep blowing ... don't stop ... blow harder ... blow some more, you can do it ... keep going ... all the way ... you're doing great ... breathe smoothly! That was great! Now, if you can do that two more times, the test will be complete. The machine requires three good breaths to calculate the results. How do you feel?"
    Rationale. Studies have shown that coaching improves the patient's performance and results.

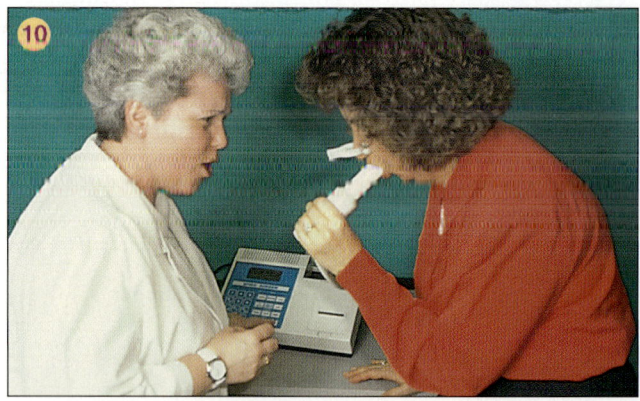

11. **Procedural Step. Allow rest periods for the patient, if needed.**
    If the patient becomes lightheaded or dizzy after exhaling, you should allow a rest period between attempts. If the patient does not exhale long enough or does not exhale with enough force, the spirometer will register the attempt as invalid. Usually, the best result of three attempts is printed as the result. If the patient is unable to produce three valid results, the machine will still print a test result, but you should document the type of diffi-

Continued

PROCEDURE 39-7 Perform Spirometry (Pulmonary Function Testing)—cont'd

culty the patient had with the test. If the patient cannot follow directions or if the patient becomes dizzy or tired, the test should be stopped. Most patients are unable to give a good effort after four or five attempts.

12. **Procedural Step.** Ensure the physician reviews the spirometry test results.
   A spirometry report is routed according to medical office policy. In general, it is important to make sure the physician sees and initials the report before it is filed in the medical record.

13. **Procedural Step.** Before documenting the procedure, make the patient comfortable and put the spirometer away.

14. **Procedural Step.** Discard the disposable components of the spirometry test in a biohazardous waste container.

15. **Procedural Step.** Sanitize the hands.
    Always sanitize the hands after every procedure or after using gloves.

16. **Procedural Step.** Document the test results.

CHARTING EXAMPLE

Date	
6/10/xx	Pt. performed three spirometry tests. Lightheadedness between efforts. See report. ———— M. Stewart, CMA (AAMA)

PROCEDURE 39-8 Instruct the Patient in the Use of a Peak Flow Meter

TASK: Properly provide instructions to a patient for the use of a peak flow meter.

EQUIPMENT AND SUPPLIES
- Peak flow meter (PFM)
- Patient's medical record

SKILLS/RATIONALE

STANDARD PRECAUTIONS ARE TO BE FOLLOWED.

1. **Procedural Step.** Sanitize the hands.
   An alcohol-based hand rub may be used instead of washing hands with soap and water, unless hands are visibly soiled.
   Rationale. Hand sanitization promotes infection control.

2. **Procedural Step.** Assemble equipment and supplies.
   Rationale. It is important to have all supplies and equipment ready and available before starting any procedure to ensure efficiency.

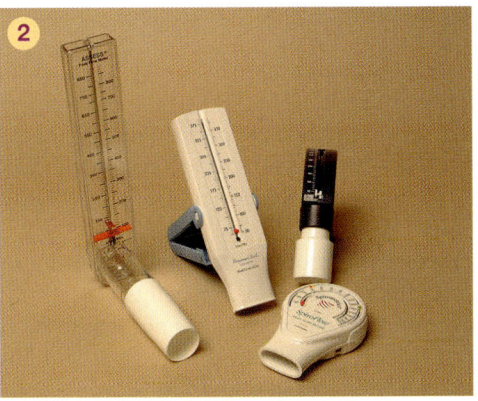

3. **Procedural Step.** Obtain the patient's medical record.

4. **Procedural Step.** Greet the patient, introduce yourself, and confirm the patient's identity.
   Rationale. Identifying the patient ensures the procedure is performed on the correct patient.

5. **Procedural Step.** Explain the procedure to the patient and family, if present. Place the sliding indicator marker (usually red) or arrow on the PFM at the bottom of the numbered scale (usually zero). Instruct the patient to remove any gum or food from his or her mouth.
   Rationale. Explaining the procedure to the patient and family promotes cooperation and provides a means of obtaining implied consent. Starting at zero each time provides accurate readings.

6. **Procedural Step.** Instruct the patient to stand up straight and hold the PFM upright, being careful not to block the opening in the back. If the patient is unable to stand up straight, have the patient sit in a chair.
   Rationale. Standing up straight increases lung expansion and promotes deep breathing.

Continued

PROCEDURE 39-8 Instruct the Patient in the Use of a Peak Flow Meter—cont'd

7. **Procedural Step.** Instruct the patient to take a deep breath (as deep as he or she can) and to put the mouthpiece of the PFM into his or her mouth with the lips tightly around the mouthpiece. Instruct the patient to keep his or her tongue away from the mouthpiece.
   Rationale: Maximal effort is needed for accurate reading and causes the indicator marker to move up the scale.

8. **Procedural Step.** Instruct the patient to blow out as hard and as quickly as possible with a "fast hard puff." Record the number on a piece of paper.
   Rationale. The force of the air coming out of the lungs causes the marker to move along the numbered scale.

9. **Procedural Step.** Instruct the patient to repeat the procedure two more times and to remember to slide the marker back to the bottom of the scale or zero.
   Rationale. The procedure has been done correctly when the numbers from all three tries are very close together.

10. **Procedural Step.** Document the highest of the three readings in the patient's medical record.
    Rationale: The patient cannot breathe out too much, but they can breathe out too little. Taking the highest reading indicates the patient's best effort and provides a baseline for evaluating future readings. When the patient knows the expected flow rate, he or she will be better prepared to recognize changes or trends.

11. **Procedural Step.** Provide the patient with a booklet to record daily readings and instruct the patient to measure readings close to the same time and same way each day.
    Rationale: Taking daily readings assists the physician to make important decisions concerning the patient's treatment.

12. **Procedural Step.** Sanitize the hands.
    Always sanitize the hands after every procedure or after using gloves.

CHARTING EXAMPLE

Date	
6/10/xx	Pt. performed three peak flow measurements with the highest reading 400. ———— J. Engleman, CMA (AAMA)

A "normal reading" for patient Suzy Patton is 500. Today, her reading is 350, which places her status in the *yellow zone*. She and her physician have established a plan in which she takes her relief medication, Albuterol (two puffs), and moves away from any triggers that cause her breathing problems, if known. After 15 minutes, she is to use her PFM again and see if her reading has returned to the *green zone*. If it has not, she is to call the office or seek emergency attention.

PATIENT-CENTERED PROFESSIONALISM

- How would the medical assistant explain to the patient the purpose of pulmonary function testing?

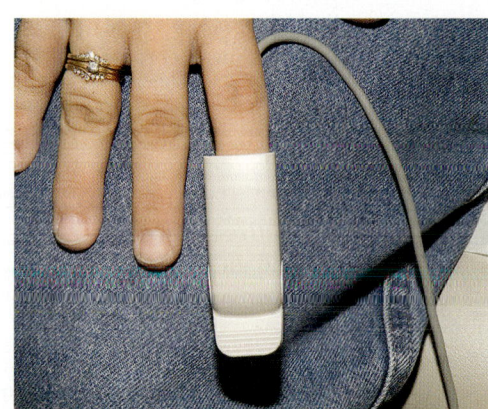

FIGURE 39-16 Pulse oximetry sensor.

PULSE OXIMETRY

Pulse oximetry is a noninvasive test that measures the amount of oxygen in a patient's blood. This test provides immediate results that can be used to detect changes in the oxygen saturation in arterial blood and determine how well the arterial blood is oxygenated (the efficiency of gas exchange within the lungs). In the medical office setting, an **oximetry sensor** is attached to a patient's finger (Figure 39-16). Light is sent through the capillary bed to a **photodetector** and a percentage measurement appears on a digital screen. Fingernail polish or a bandage on the finger where the probe is placed could cause errors in the readings.

Guidelines for performing pulse oximetry are as follows:

1. Always follow the manufacturer's recommendations.
2. Apply the sensor to the correct location (finger, toe, and earlobe).
3. Apply the sensor properly (not too tight or loose).
4. Disinfect the sensor between patients.
5. Make certain the site chosen has nothing to invalidate the reading (e.g., fingernail polish, bandage, cold fingers).
6. Report a reading of less than 95% immediately to the physician.

Procedure 39-9 explains how to apply the probe properly to obtain an accurate reading of the patient's blood oxygen saturation.

> **PATIENT-CENTERED PROFESSIONALISM**
>
> - Why must the medical assistant follow the guidelines established when using pulse oximetry for patient evaluation?

HEARING ACUITY TESTS

Hearing acuity tests are used to detect hearing loss and to look for **conduction** defects or nerve impairment. The Weber and Rinne tests both require a **tuning fork.** The Weber test checks that the loudness of the sound is heard the same in both ears, whereas the Rinne test compares air conduction with bone conduction. Audiometry is used to measure the degree of hearing. A **tympanogram** provides a graphic display of the results of *tympanometry.*

Weber Test

The **Weber test** assesses hearing loss in both ears at once. The tuning fork (256 or 512 Hz) is held by its base and struck against the palm of the opposite hand or the knee. The base of the vibrating fork is placed on the center of the patient's head—equal distance from the patient's ears (Figure 39-17). If hearing is normal, the patient will hear the sound equally in both ears.

The physician often performs the Weber and Rinne tests but can train and provide instructions for the medical assistant to perform these tests just as efficiently. If a patient has air conduction deafness, the patient will hear the sound better in the affected ear because bone will transmit sound directly to that ear. A person with presbycusis will have an apparent normal test result because he or she will hear the same in both ears.

Rinne Test

The **Rinne test** compares bone and air conduction by placing the base of the vibrating tuning fork to the patient's mastoid bone behind each ear (Figure 39-18). The patient is asked to report when the sound is no longer heard. The tuning fork is then held beside the ear, and the patient is asked if he or she can hear it. If the patient can, the hearing is normal. Normal results occur when air conduction hearing is greater than bone conduction hearing.

Audiometry

Audiometry is the measurement of hearing ability with an *audiometer* (Figure 39-19). The audiometer measures hearing

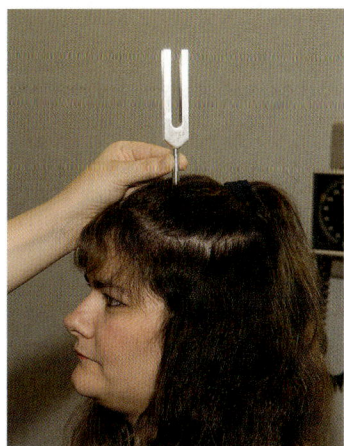

FIGURE 39-17 Weber test. With *normal hearing,* the patient hears the sound equally in both ears or in the center of the head. With *conductive hearing loss,* the patient hears the sound better in the problem ear. With *sensorineural hearing loss,* the patient does not hear the sound as well in the problem ear.

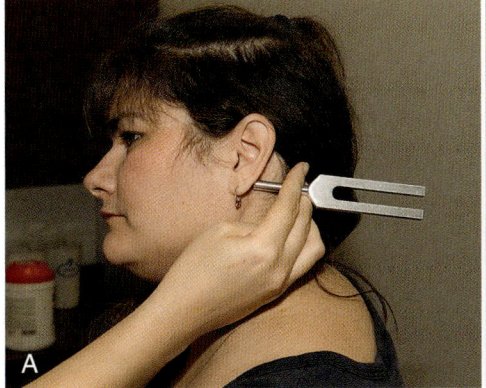 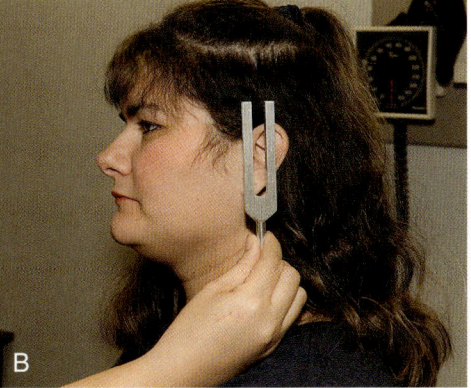

FIGURE 39-18 Rinne test. **A,** Bone conduction. **B,** Air conduction. With *normal hearing,* the patient hears the sound at least twice as long through air conduction as through bone conduction. With *conductive hearing loss,* the patient hears the sound longer by bone conduction than by air conduction. With *sensorineural hearing loss,* the sound is reduced, and the patient will also hear the sound longer through air conduction than through bone conduction but not twice as long.

PROCEDURE 39-9 Perform Pulse Oximetry

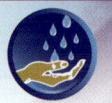

TASK: Accurately determine a patient's blood oxygen saturation using pulse oximetry.

EQUIPMENT AND SUPPLIES
- Pulse oximeter
- Probe
- Alcohol prep pads
- Patient's medical record

SKILLS/RATIONALE

STANDARD PRECAUTIONS ARE TO BE FOLLOWED.

1. **Procedural Step.** Sanitize the hands.
   An alcohol-based hand rub may be used instead of washing hands with soap and water, unless hands are visibly soiled.
   Rationale. Hand sanitization promotes infection control.

2. **Procedural Step.** Assemble equipment and supplies.
   Rationale. It is important to have all supplies and equipment ready and available before starting any procedure to ensure efficiency.

3. **Procedural Step.** Obtain the patient's medical record.

4. **Procedural Step.** Greet the patient, introduce yourself, and confirm the patient's identity.
   Rationale. Identifying the patient ensures the procedure is performed on the correct patient.

5. **Procedural Step.** Explain the procedure to the patient.
   Rationale. Explaining the procedure to the patient promotes cooperation and provides a means of obtaining implied consent.

6. **Procedural Step.** Ask the patient to have a seat in a comfortable position with the arms well supported.

7. **Procedural Step.** Connect the oximeter finger probe to the monitor.
   NOTE: Patients with long nails or with acrylic nails or dark nail polish, or patients who are missing fingers, may require the test to be performed on a toe or an ear.

8. **Procedural Step.** Turn on the power switch.

9. **Procedural Step.** Wipe the probe clean with the alcohol prep pad.
   Rationale. This prevents the possibility of cross-contamination.

10. **Procedural Step.** Apply the oximeter probe to the patient's finger.

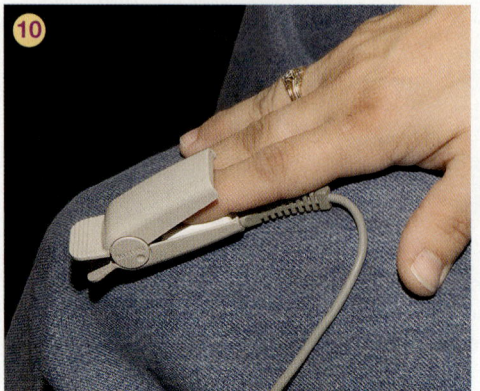

11. **Procedural Step.** Wait while the system stabilizes.

12. **Procedural Step.** Read the pulse rate and the arterial blood saturation on the digital display.

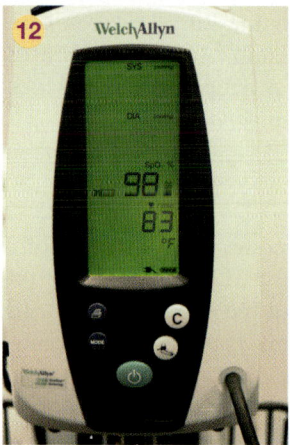

13. **Procedural Step.** Remove the sensor from the patient's finger.

14. **Procedural Step.** Sanitize the hands.
    Always sanitize the hands after every procedure or after using gloves.

15. **Procedural Step.** Document the pulse oximetry results in the patient's medical record.

CHARTING EXAMPLE	
Date	
1/13/xx	8:20 a.m. ® middle finger pulse oximetry results: P 80; SPO$_2$: 98. Pt. tolerated procedure well.———— D. Stewart, RMA

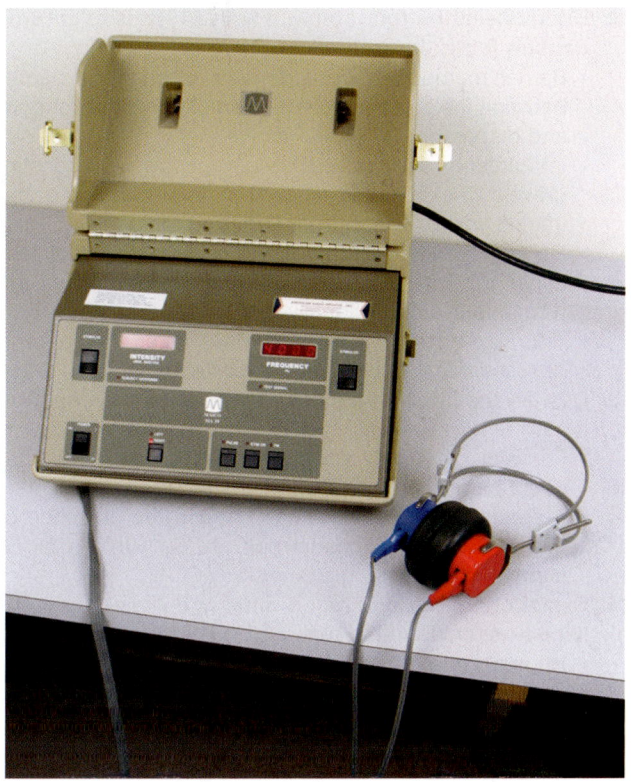

FIGURE 39-19 Audiometer.

sensitivity by producing an **audiogram,** which shows hearing loss as a function of tone frequency. The medical assistant can perform this test after receiving additional technical training, which is usually provided by the manufacturer or by an **audiologist.**

In audiometric testing, measurements are taken in decibels (dB). Most sounds that are associated with normal speech patterns fall in the range of 20 to 50 dB. An adult with normal hearing should be able to detect tones between 0 and 20 dB.

To perform audiometry, the room must be quiet to avoid outside interference. Headphones are provided to the patient, and when the audiometer sends a frequency, the patient is asked to signal when he or she hears the sound. The frequencies begin low and progress to high.

Tympanogram

Often babies will have fluid behind the eardrum, thus preventing the eardrum from vibrating. Therefore sounds are not carried forward and are not heard clearly. A *tympanometer* is used to provide information on the function of the structure and presence of fluid in the middle ear. Besides monitoring eardrum movement, it can also show any abnormalities in the middle ear.

Small soft, rubber probes are placed into each ear canal and air is moved into the ear canals to cause movement of the eardrum. The graphic result produced is referred to as a *tympanogram.* Remember the results only indicate if a problem exists not if there is a hearing loss. An abnormal reading requires further testing.

PATIENT-CENTERED PROFESSIONALISM

- What role does the medical assistant have in hearing acuity tests?

CONCLUSION

An accurate diagnosis must be made for a patient's treatment to be effective. Diagnostic testing provides objective information and gives the physician a clearer and more accurate picture of the patient's condition. Diagnostic testing and examination are important parts of gynecology and obstetrics. Diagnostic tests can also help physicians assess the state of a patient's colon, pulmonary functioning, blood oxygen saturation, and hearing acuity, depending on the needs of the individual patient.

Medical assistants need to have a good understanding of the purpose and use of each of these types of tests. In addition, they need to know their role in assisting the physician and patient to help ensure efficiency and accuracy in the testing procedures.

Chapter Summary

Reinforce your understanding of the material in this chapter by reviewing the curriculum objectives and key content points below.

1. **Define, appropriately use, and spell all the Key Terms for this chapter.**
   - Review the Key Terms if necessary.
2. **Explain the importance of breast self-examination (BSE) and list five recommendations from the American Cancer Society regarding breast examination.**

- BSE aids in the early detection of breast cancer.
- Monthly BSE should begin at age 20 and continue monthly.
- BSE should be done at the same time each month.
- At age 30, women should have a clinical breast examination performed by a health care professional.
- At age 40, women should have an annual mammogram in addition to monthly BSE and the clinical breast examination.

- Breast examinations should be done in the shower or bath, in front of a mirror, and while lying down.
3. **Demonstrate the correct procedure for instructing a patient in BSE.**
   - Review Procedure 39-1.
4. **List four purposes of a pelvic examination.**
   - Pelvic examination is done to evaluate the shape, size, and location of the reproductive organs and to detect disease.
5. **Describe the basic process used by the physician in a pelvic examination and how the speculum is used.**
   - External genitalia are inspected first.
   - Internal genitalia are inspected with the aid of a speculum by opening the speculum to reveal the cervical opening.
   - Pelvic examination in conjunction with the Pap smear is an effective method for detecting changes in cervical tissue.
6. **Explain the purpose of a Pap smear.**
   - The Pap smear evaluates the squamous epithelial tissue covering the visible part of the cervix.
7. **Explain the process used to label specimen slides and prepare them for transport to the laboratory.**
   - Each slide is labeled with the location of the specimen collection: V for vaginal, C for cervical, and E for endocervical. Usually, C and E are done on every woman but V only for posthysterectomy patients.
   - The slide must be fixed, allowed to dry, and placed in a slide holder to be sent to a laboratory for inspection.
   - For "liquid prep" specimens, the container is closed with the lid and labeled with patient identification.
8. **Demonstrate the correct procedure for assisting the patient and physician during a pelvic examination and Pap smear.**
   - Review Procedure 39-2.
9. **List the three categories of the cytology report as described by the Bethesda System.**
   - The Bethesda System divides the cytology report into three categories: clinical information, specimen adequacy, and diagnosis.
10. **List three types of vaginitis and explain the etiology, signs and symptoms, and treatment for each.**
    - Candidiasis is a fungal yeast overgrowth causing a cottage cheese–like discharge with itching and is treated with over-the-counter (OTC) vaginal preparations.
    - Trichomoniasis is a sexually transmitted protozoal infection causing a yellowish green, frothy discharge; both sex partners are given metronidazole (Flagyl).
    - *Gardnerella* is a genus of normal bacteria of the vagina that can become problematic when the normal pH of the vaginal tissues is disturbed, causing a fishy odor; metronidazole is prescribed for treatment.
11. **Explain the education needs of a patient with a sexually transmitted disease (STD).**
    - Patients with STDs must be educated about the need to notify sexual partners.
    - They should finish the treatment regimen completely and be recultured before assuming a cure and resuming sexual relations.
12. **Briefly describe four commonly used types of contraception (birth control).**
    - Barrier methods place a physical or chemical barrier between the egg and sperm. Examples include condom and diaphragm.
    - Intrauterine devices (IUDs; e.g., copper, progestin) prevent the fertilized egg from implanting into the uterine wall or sperm from fertilizing the egg.
    - Hormonal methods (e.g., oral contraceptives, injections) prevent ovulation by placing a hormone into the woman's system gradually throughout the month.
    - "Morning-after" pills are hormones taken in two large doses within 72 hours after unprotected sex.
13. **Explain the importance of prenatal care and describe how a serum pregnancy test confirms pregnancy.**
    - Prenatal care prevents and detects conditions that could harm the mother and fetus during pregnancy.
    - A serum pregnancy test can confirm the presence of human chorionic gonadotropin (hCG) within a blood sample, indicating pregnancy.
14. **Explain how the estimated date of delivery is established using Nägele's rule.**
    - Nägele's rule adds 7 days to the first day of the LMP, subtracts 3 months, and adds 1 year (as needed) to determine the estimated date of delivery.
15. **List seven types of tests performed at the initial prenatal visit.**
    - Besides a Pap smear, BSE, CBC, and blood chemistry, testing for blood type and Rh factor are done to rule out maternal and fetal blood incompatibility.
    - Tests are also performed to check for syphilis.
    - A rubella titer is drawn, and a urinalysis and vaginal cultures are done to rule out infection and STDs.
16. **Demonstrate the correct procedure for assisting the physician and patient during a follow-up prenatal examination.**
    - Review Procedure 39-3.
17. **List the five areas that are evaluated at a postpartum visit.**
    - Vital signs and weight are taken at a postpartum visit.
    - Breast, pelvic, and rectal examinations are performed.
    - Laboratory studies are performed, including CBC and urinalysis.
18. **Explain the purpose of fecal occult testing.**
    - Fecal occult testing detects the presence of blood in the stool (screens for colorectal bleeding).
19. **Demonstrate the procedure for providing the patient with accurate and complete instructions on the preparation and collection of a stool sample for fecal occult blood testing.**
    - Review Procedure 39-4.
20. **Demonstrate the procedure for accurately developing the fecal occult blood slide test.**
    - Review Procedure 39-5.
21. **Explain the purpose of sigmoidoscopy.**
    - Sigmoidoscopy examines the lower bowel to diagnose and treat conditions that affect this portion of the digestive system.
22. **Demonstrate the correct procedure for assisting the physician and patient during a sigmoidoscopy.**
    - Review Procedure 39-6.

23. **Explain the purpose of spirometry and list five indications for its use.**
    - Spirometry, the most frequently performed pulmonary function test, measures air entering and leaving the lungs.
    - Spirometry measures lung volume and lung capacity, detects the presence of lung dysfunction, screens the patient at risk from the environment or smoking, assesses changes in lung function over time, and assesses the response to treatment.
24. **Demonstrate the procedure for accurately performing spirometry to measure lung volume.**
    - Review Procedure 39-7.
25. **Discuss the proper procedure for using a peak flow meter.**
    - Review Procedure 39-8.
26. **Explain the purpose of pulse oximetry and list five guidelines for its use.**
    - Pulse oximetry measures the oxygen saturation of a patient's blood.
    - Always follow the manufacturer's recommendations.
    - Apply the sensor to the correct location (finger, toe, earlobe).
    - Apply the sensor properly (not too tight or loose).
    - Disinfect the sensor between patients.
    - Make certain the site chosen has nothing to invalidate the reading (e.g., fingernail polish).
    - Report a reading of less than 95% to the physician immediately.
27. **Demonstrate the procedure for accurately determining a patient's blood oxygen saturation using pulse oximetry.**
    - Review Procedure 39-9.
28. **List the three types of hearing acuity tests and state the purpose of each.**
    - The Weber test assesses hearing loss using a vibrating tuning fork on the center of the patient's head to determine if sound is heard equally in both ears.
    - The Rinne test compares bone and air conduction by placing the base of the vibrating tuning fork to the patient's mastoid bone behind each ear to determine when the sound is no longer heard.
    - Audiometry tests hearing ability with an audiometer by measuring hearing sensitivity with tones.
29. **Analyze a realistic medical office situation and apply your understanding of diagnostic testing to determine the best course of action.**
    - Medical assistants need to understand the legal and ethical principles that apply to assisting with all types of diagnostic testing.
30. **Describe the impact on patient care when medical assistants have a solid understanding of the purpose and procedures for diagnostic testing performed in the medical office.**
    - Patient care is enhanced when the medical assistant is knowledgeable about the purpose of each diagnostic test performed in the medical office.
    - The role of the medical assistant in diagnostic testing varies, but being able to answer the patient's questions concerning procedures is important to allow the patient to cooperate.

PRACTICAL APPLICATIONS

If you have accomplished the objectives in this chapter, you will be able to make better choices as a medical assistant. Take another look at this situation and decide what you would do.

Kari, age 20, is a new patient in the office of Dr. Berg, a gynecologist. Francine is the medical assistant for Dr. Berg and has only been on the job for about 2 weeks. Arriving for her appointment, Kari is given the history and physical paperwork to fill out because she is a new patient. When Francine calls Kari to the back to question her further on some specifics regarding her menstrual periods and sexual activity, four other patients are sitting close to Kari in the lab/workup area. Later, Francine is overheard discussing Kari's history with co-workers by yet more patients in the waiting room.

After taking Kari to the examination room, Francine tells her to get undressed without providing instructions for putting on the gown and drape. When Francine returns to see if Kari is undressed, she then places her into the lithotomy position for what turns out to be a 30-minute wait.

When Dr. Berg starts to examine Kari, Francine leaves the room and tells Dr. Berg to call her when he is ready to do the pelvic examination. During the breast examination, Kari asks Dr. Berg about birth control and tells him that she has been sexually active with a partner who has been diagnosed with an STD. Dr. Berg completes the pelvic examination, obtaining a Pap smear, as well as cultures for STD and a wet prep. Dr. Berg takes the wet mount to the microscope for observation. He sees Francine in the hallway chatting with some co-workers and asks where she was when he needed her during the pelvic examination. She explains she never heard him call for assistance.

Dr. Berg returns to the examination room and begins discussing forms of birth control with Kari, asking if she would rather have a barrier method, an intrauterine device, or a hormonal method such as birth control pills. He also explains to her that she has trichomoniasis, an STD, as seen on the wet prep. Dr. Berg gives Kari a prescription to treat the trichomoniasis for herself and her sexual partner.

Would you be prepared to handle this situation better than Francine did?

1. What was unethical about the way Francine took Kari's history? What HIPAA regulations did Francine not follow?
2. What are the issues concerning the privacy of Kari's medical record when Francine discussed the symptoms and patient history with co-workers?
3. How did Francine mishandle the preparation of the patient and the assistance with the physical examination?
4. Why do you think that Kari did not tell Francine about the sexual partner with an STD? Would you have told Francine if you had been in Kari's situation? Why?
5. What are the elements of a pelvic examination, and how should the medical assistant help with these?
6. Why would Dr. Berg do a gonorrhea and chlamydia culture? What other methods did Dr. Berg use to diagnose trichomoniasis?
7. What medication would you expect Dr. Berg to prescribe for both sexual partners, and why do both need to be treated?
8. What is included in barrier methods of birth control? What is included in hormonal methods? How is an IUD effective?

WEB SEARCH

1. Research the latest progress against cervical cancer. Discuss the history, controversy, and possible adverse reactions.

- **Keywords:** Use the following keywords in your search: HPV vaccine, cervical cancer, preventive vaccines.

Introduction to the Physician's Office Laboratory

40

evolve   http://evolve.elsevier.com/klieger/medicalassisting

One of the many duties of the medical assistant is to collect, prepare for transport, and process different types of specimens. Medical laboratories perform chemical, physical, and microscopic tests on blood, urine, and other body fluids. A medical laboratory's function is to collect and test specimens provided by the patient. The physician analyzes test results to assess the patient's general health, diagnose, and form a treatment plan as needed. A medical laboratory can be located in a variety of settings, including the physician office laboratory (POL), hospital, and outside (independent) reference laboratory. This chapter focuses on the POL.

When a specimen is collected and transported, the medical assistant must understand the importance of following federal and state protocols. Adherence to guidelines helps ensure the accuracy and usefulness of the results. In addition to understanding the laboratory regulations and safety guidelines, medical assistants must also be familiar with basic laboratory equipment; the process of carrying out laboratory tests; culture, urine, and blood collection; stool and sputum collection; and the range of normal test results.

LEARNING OBJECTIVES

You will be able to do the following after completing this chapter:

Key Terms
1. Define, appropriately use, and spell all the Key Terms for this chapter.

Laboratory Regulations and Safety
2. Explain the purpose of the Clinical Laboratory Improvement Amendments of 1988 (CLIA 88).
3. List three factors that determine whether a medical office will perform and process a specimen.
4. Briefly describe three CLIA-waived urine tests, six CLIA-waived blood tests, and seven CLIA-waived tests of other types.
5. Differentiate between quality assurance (QA) and quality control (QC) and briefly explain how each is accomplished in the medical office.
6. Demonstrate the correct procedure for using methods of QC.
7. Explain the need for safety precautions in the medical office laboratory and how they protect both staff and patients.

Basic Laboratory Equipment
8. Identify the parts of a compound microscope and explain its proper use and maintenance.
9. Demonstrate the procedure for successfully focusing a microscope from lower to higher power.
10. Explain the purpose and proper use of a centrifuge.

Laboratory Tests
11. List six categories of laboratory tests and briefly explain the purpose of each.
12. Explain the importance of effective patient preparation before laboratory tests are performed.
13. Explain the importance of completing a laboratory request form accurately.
14. Demonstrate the procedure for accurately completing a laboratory request form.
15. List three methods of specimen collection, and explain the need for collecting specimens accurately.
16. Demonstrate the procedure for accurately collecting a specimen for transport to an outside laboratory.
17. Explain the purpose of a laboratory report and why it must be accurate and transmitted to the physician in a timely manner.
18. Demonstrate the correct procedure for screening and following up on patient test results.

Culture Collection
19. Demonstrate the correct procedure for collecting an uncontaminated throat specimen to test for group A beta-hemolytic streptococci.

Urine Collection

20. Explain the purpose of a urinalysis and the need for avoiding sources of contamination and for processing urine specimens in the required time.
21. List four instructions the medical assistant should give to a patient who is to collect a random urine specimen and bring it to the medical office.
22. Demonstrate the correct procedure for obtaining a urine specimen from an infant using a pediatric urine collector.
23. Demonstrate the correct procedure for providing patient instructions on collecting a midstream clean-catch urine specimen to ensure validity of test results.
24. Demonstrate the correct procedure for providing patient instructions on collecting a 24-hour urine specimen to ensure validity of test results.
25. Explain the special considerations for handling drug screenings and specimens that may be used as evidence in a court of law.

Stool Collection

26. Explain the considerations for collecting stool specimens.
27. Demonstrate the correct procedure for the collection of stool specimens.

Sputum Collection

28. Explain the considerations for collecting sputum specimens.

Patient-Centered Professionalism

29. Analyze a realistic medical office situation and apply your understanding of the purpose and use of the physician office laboratory to determine the best course of action.
30. Describe the impact on patient care when medical assistants have a solid understanding of the processes and procedures used to collect specimens for testing in the medical office.

KEY TERMS

24-hour urine specimen
arm (microscope)
bacteriuria
base (microscope)
binocular
blood bank
Centers for Medicare and Medicaid Services (CMS)
centrifuge
certificate of provider-performed microscopy (PPM) procedures
certificate of waiver
chain of custody
chain of evidence
chemistry
Clinical Laboratory Improvement Amendments of 1988 (CLIA 88)
coagulation studies
coarse focus adjustment knob
compound
condenser
control samples
counterbalanced
crossmatching
cultures
drug screening
engineering controls
eyepiece
fine focus adjustment knob
first morning specimen
forensic
glucose tolerance test (GTT)
hematology
iris diaphragm
laboratory requisition
lens
light source
mechanical stage control knobs
microbiology
microhematocrit centrifuge
microscope
midstream clean-catch urine specimen
monocular
nosepiece
objectives
objective lens
ocular lens
oil-immersion lens
personal protective equipment (PPE)
physician office laboratory (POL)
plasma
postprandial specimen
quality assurance (QA)
quality control (QC)
random urine specimen
rapid screening test
reagents
serology
serum
solutes
sputum
stage
Standard Precautions
stool
swab-transport media system
timed specimen
urinalysis

PRACTICAL APPLICATIONS

Read the following scenario and keep it in mind as you learn about the POL.

The full-time laboratory technician at Dr. Macinto's office is on sick leave for a week. Dr. Macinto asks Sherri, a medical assistant, to fill in for the sick technician. Sherri has just been hired from another office, where she was trained by the physician. She has not done laboratory tests and has not prepared patients for laboratory work.

On the first day, Dr. Macinto asks Sherri to collect a midstream urine sample on a patient for a culture and sensitivity and to send some of the urine to an outside laboratory for a drug screen. Sherri hands the urine collection container to the patient without any instructions and allows the patient to go to the bathroom alone to collect the specimen. When the specimen is collected, Sherri leaves the drug screen on the counter to await the arrival of the laboratory courier for transport to the outside laboratory. Neither Sherri nor the courier signs for the specimen. Furthermore, the laboratory form is not complete, and no documentation was made of the collection of the specimen.

What things would you have done differently in this situation?

LABORATORY REGULATIONS AND SAFETY

Not all medical offices have a **physician office laboratory (POL).** Offices that do have a POL are regulated by government standards. Medical offices that do not have a POL are still required to take proper procedural steps in obtaining, labeling, and preparing any specimens to be sent to outside laboratories. Strict adherence to the Clinical Laboratory Improvement Act (CLIA) and Occupational Safety and Health Administration (OSHA) regulations is required.

CLIA Performance Standards

In 1988 the Federal Health Care Financing Administration (HCFA), now called the **Centers for Medicare and Medicaid Services (CMS),** developed the **Clinical Laboratory Improvement Amendments of 1988 (CLIA 88).** These regulations set minimum performance standards in the laboratory and mandated quality assurance and quality control standards. This act divided laboratory tests into three levels of complexity and established standards for personnel qualifications and quality control for testing at each of the three levels. The three levels are high complexity, moderate complexity, and waived tests (referred to as "CLIA-waived" tests). The more complex the test, the more training the laboratory personnel performing the test must have.

Whether a medical office performs and processes the specimen will depend on the type of practice, cost-effectiveness for performing the test "on site," and the level of complexity as defined by CLIA 88.

Laboratory Regulations

Medical laboratories are regulated by both state and federal agencies. CLIA 88 is monitored through CMS, the Centers for Disease Control and Prevention (CDC), and OSHA. CMS issues the certificate, and CDC and OSHA monitor compliance. The state health department is responsible for making certain their regulations meet or exceed the federal regulations. The amount of regulation to which a POL is subjected depends on the complexity of tests performed at the medical office.

CLIA-Waived Tests

Tests in the "waived" category are not held to the same personnel educational requirements as the other tests, but waived tests are still held to the same quality control and quality assurance standards. Waived tests do not require personnel to have specific training because the procedures are considered simple tests that can be performed with only a small amount of complexity. Table 40-1 lists typical CLIA-waived tests for urine and other body substances.

Moderate-Complexity Tests

A medical assistant with additional training in laboratory testing may qualify to perform some tests in the moderate-complexity range. Moderate-complexity testing involves proficiency testing, test management, quality control, quality assurance, and specialized training. These tests require that the medical assistant follow a certain protocol when performing each test. For example, hematology and blood chemistry tests performed on automated blood analyzers and microscopic analysis of urine sediment are moderate-complexity tests.

TABLE 40-1

Typical CLIA-Waived Tests

Waived Tests	Use
URINE	
Dipstick or tablet reagent: nonautomated tests for bilirubin, glucose, hemoglobin, ketones, leukocytes, nitrite, pH, protein, specific gravity, and urobilinogen	Screening of urine to monitor or diagnose various diseases (e.g., diabetes) and assess condition of kidneys and urinary tract
Urine pregnancy test (visual color comparison test)	Diagnosis of pregnancy
Urine chemistry analyzer	Screening of urine to detect abnormal values
OTHER	
Ovulation tests (visual color)	Detection of ovulation
Fecal and gastric occult blood	Detection of blood in feces or presence of blood in gastric contents
Tests for *Helicobacter pylori*	Detects antibodies specific for *H. pylori*
Streptococcus	Detects group A beta-hemolytic streptococci
Saliva alcohol tests	Detects alcohol in saliva

High-Complexity Tests

High-complexity tests require high levels of training and are not performed in the POL. They include cytology (Pap smear) and blood typing and crossmatching. Each state has its own regulations for laboratory personnel, and individual states' regulations may be more stringent than CLIA 88, which requires a facility to be appropriately certified for each test performed. For example, cytology testing and those laboratory tests requiring histopathology and manual cell counts are some of the tests included in high-complexity testing.

Certificates

A **certificate of waiver** is issued to a physician office laboratory qualified to perform only low-complexity tests.

A **certificate of provider-performed microscopy (PPM) procedures** is issued to a POL qualified to perform moderate-complexity and waived (low-complexity) tests and microscopic procedures. A medical assistant with additional training can perform moderate-complexity tests in the laboratory under the direct supervision of a medical technologist, medical laboratory technician, or physician (e.g., hematology and chemistry done with automated analyzers; wet-mount preparations being tested for bacteria, parasites, or fungi; and examinations of urine sediment and fecal material for the presence of leukocytes).

Quality Assurance

A **quality assurance (QA)** program for laboratory testing is designed to monitor and evaluate the quality and accuracy of the test results. It requires the medical office to ensure the reliability of test results by establishing a comprehensive set of written policies and procedures for performing the test and for patient education related to the testing. The facility must develop detailed instructions for specimen collection that include labeling, preservation, and transportation of specimens, as well as specific guidelines for training new personnel. A plan for the continuing education of employees and a program for the maintenance of equipment must also be included.

Quality Control

Quality control (QC) is a process that provides the medical assistant (or POL) the means to ensure that test results are accurate. This requires the following actions:

- Using **control samples** for each new batch of reagents or new supply of test kits daily.
- Using unexpired (fresh) **reagents** (Box 40-1).
- Conducting daily instrument calibration. All instruments must be calibrated according to the manufacturer's recommendations. This ensures that each patient's sample is measured under the same conditions.
- Properly documenting the samples and test results. Proper documentation should be used for every test. Document when a new test kit or reagent is tested. Include the date, time, expected results, actual results, and corrective action taken if results were not within known values.
- Performing preventive maintenance of equipment. Maintenance guidelines are provided with each piece of equipment. A regular schedule for routine maintenance should be established and documented by the user to maintain proper functioning of each piece of laboratory equipment.

BOX 40-1

Use of a Control Sample for Quality Control

1. A control sample having a known value is provided by the manufacturer.
2. This control sample is run as if it were a patient sample. This tests the technique of the operator, reagent effectiveness, and accuracy of the equipment.
3. The reagent is used to produce a chemical reaction. This chemical reaction provides a value.
4. This value is compared to a value range provided by the manufacturer.
5. Not all control samples use a reagent. For example, the HemoCue Photometer uses a control cuvette to check the machine's calibration. Each control cuvette has an assigned value (e.g., 12.1). Every morning before the machine is used, the control cuvette is placed into the machine and the registered value must match the assigned control value. Manufacturers will identify acceptable deviations (e.g., ±0.3 g/dL). Any reading not within the acceptable range means the machine must not be used until it has been serviced.

Procedure 40-1 outlines the process of using methods of QC.

Laboratory Safety

Attention to safety in the POL protects both the patient and the medical assistant. The ultimate goal of the medical assistant is to provide for quality patient care. Quality patient care depends on following safety guidelines established by government agencies (e.g., OSHA) that provide a safe working environment for employees. In turn, if the work setting is safe, the patient will benefit.

Chapter 31 contains information about the **Standard Precautions** developed by the CDC and enforced by OSHA, including information on the Bloodborne Pathogens Standard and its requirements concerning exposure control plans, **engineering controls, personal protective equipment** (**PPE**), exposure incidents, and the "right to know" law. Box 40-2 lists other OSHA safety guidelines for the POL. Box 40-3 lists general safety guidelines for the POL.

PATIENT-CENTERED PROFESSIONALISM

- Why must the medical assistant be aware of laboratory regulations and safety precautions in the POL?

BASIC LABORATORY EQUIPMENT

Because medical assistants perform several laboratory tests using technical equipment and supplies, they must be familiar with basic laboratory equipment. Medical assistants may be asked to order supplies, use automated equipment to process tests (e.g., HemoCue for hemoglobin, glucometer for glucose levels), maintain the equipment, and perform many tasks related to the care and maintenance of the equipment. As when using administrative office equipment, it is important to follow the manufacturer's instructions when performing tests with laboratory equipment.

The microscope and centrifuge are two basic pieces of equipment found in most POLs. Other automated pieces are advanced equipment (e.g., blood and urine analyzers) and may require additional training to operate. These types of equipment are fully computerized, and some automatically print out the test results.

Microscope

The **microscope** is one of the most important and frequently used pieces of equipment in the POL. The microscope magnifies objects too small to be seen with the naked eye. It is used when examining urine sediment, evaluating blood smears, performing cell counts, and identifying microorganisms.

Medical assistants who work in a facility with a POL may be required to use a microscope. Therefore it is necessary to

PROCEDURE 40-1: Use Methods of Quality Control (QC)

TASK: Practice QC procedures in the medical laboratory to ensure accuracy of test results through detection and elimination of errors.

EQUIPMENT AND SUPPLIES
- QC logbook
- QC samples (as provided in CLIA-waived prepackaged test kits)
- CLIA-waived prepackaged test kit
- Patient sample
- Copy of CLIA 88 guidelines
- Copy of state regulations and guidelines
- Patient's medical record

SKILLS/RATIONALE

STANDARD PRECAUTIONS ARE TO BE FOLLOWED.

NOTE: For this procedure, a CLIA-waived human chorionic gonadotropin (hCG) pregnancy test is performed.

1. **Procedural Step.** Sanitize the hands.
   An alcohol-based hand rub may be used instead of washing hands with soap and water, unless hands are visibly soiled.
   Rationale. Hand sanitization promotes infection control.

2. **Procedural Step.** Assemble equipment and supplies.
   Obtain the QC sample provided in a CLIA-waived prepackaged test kit.
   NOTE: Specially prepared QC samples are included with each CLIA-waived test kit. Manufacturer's directions must be followed and the QC samples tested along with patient samples. Each QC sample will specify how often the test must be performed to maintain the integrity of the test results. For example, a positive and a negative QC sample must be run each time that a patient sample pregnancy test is performed.
   Rationale. It is important to have all supplies and equipment ready and available before starting any procedure to ensure efficiency.

3. **Procedural Step.** Check the expiration date on the prepackaged test kit and on each QC specimen.
   Rationale. Outdated test kits and QC samples will cause inaccurate test results.

4. **Procedural Step.** Obtain the specimen from the patient and identify the specimen as belonging to the patient.
   Rationale. Identifying that the specimen belongs to the patient ensures the procedure is performed on the correct patient.

5. **Procedural Step.** Perform testing of the specimen following the specific protocols outlined for the sample by the manufacturer.

6. **Procedural Step.** Perform QC testing as outlined by the manufacturer's protocols for the specimen being tested.

7. **Procedural Step.** Determine the results for both the patient's specimen and the QC sample.
   Compare the test results with the standard reference values provided with the prepackaged CLIA-waived test kit.

8. **Procedural Step.** Document the results in the QC logbook and the patient's medical record.
   Rationale. When patient records are audited, the physician's office must be able to provide proof that a QC sample was completed for any CLIA-waived procedure that has been documented in a patient's medical record, as required by CLIA guidelines.

9. **Procedural Step.** Sanitize the hands.
   Always sanitize the hands after every procedure or after using gloves.

CHARTING EXAMPLE

Date	
8/2/xx	9:10 a.m. Pregnancy test performed on first morning urine specimen brought from home. Appropriate QC and patient tests performed. QC results documented in QC log. Negative test results for pregnancy. —————— F. Hamilton, CMA (AAMA)

BOX 40-2

OSHA Guidelines for Laboratory Safety*

PHYSICAL HAZARDS
If improperly used, any piece of laboratory equipment or its surroundings could promote hazardous work conditions. Proper training is therefore required.

Electricity
All equipment must be grounded according to established guidelines. Overloaded electrical circuits, frayed electrical cords, and use of extension cords must be avoided.

Fire
Fire extinguishers of the correct type to handle electrical or chemical fires must be present. All flammable chemicals must be stored in a fireproof cabinet.

Equipment
Laboratory equipment must be used according to the manufacturer's guidelines (e.g., autoclave, centrifuge).

CHEMICAL HAZARDS
Many chemical agents are used in the laboratory setting. If used improperly, chemicals can cause injury from toxic gas or can be caustic to skin.

Labeling
All chemicals must be identified with a label that contains hazard information, including name of the chemical, warnings, and name and manufacturer of the product.

Material Safety Data Sheet (MSDS)
An MSDS must be available for every potentially hazardous chemical in the laboratory (e.g., alcohol, bleach). The MSDS identifies the chemical, protective clothing needed when handling, which body systems could be affected by exposure to the chemical, and the first aid or medical treatment required. MSDSs must be available in all medical offices. An MSDS should come with each chemical product when ordered and should be stored in a yellow notebook in the work area (Figure 40-1).

Storage
Proper storage of flammable liquids and caustic chemicals is required.

OSHA, Occupational Safety and Health Administration.
*The employer must systematically evaluate the workplace and POL for any hazardous situation that could harm an employee.

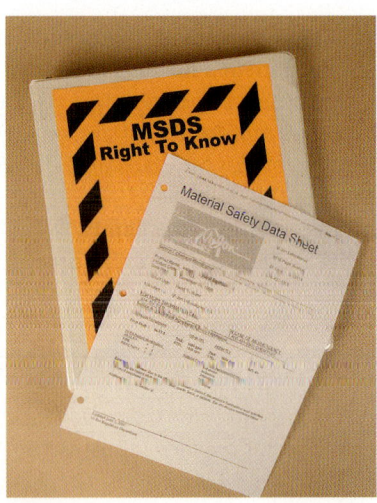

FIGURE 40-1 Laboratory MSDS notebook.

BOX 40-3

General Guidelines for Laboratory Safety

1. No shoes with open toes or heels.
2. Laboratory coats or protective outerwear must be worn while in the laboratory and removed when leaving the area.
3. Broken glass and sharps must be disposed of in a sharps container.
4. Long hair must be pulled back to prevent contamination and injury.
5. All work surfaces must be cleaned before and after procedures.
6. Hands must be sanitized before and after laboratory procedures.
7. Personal protective equipment (PPE) must be worn when a "splash" or aerosol contamination could occur.
8. No food or drink in the laboratory area.
9. Clean up all spills according to manufacturer's instructions if chemical, and if bodily fluids or bacterial in nature use a commercial cleanup kit if available.

be familiar with its parts and their function, be capable of operating it properly, and be able to maintain it.

Parts of a Microscope

Figure 40-2 shows the microscope and its various parts. Microscopes are either **monocular** (having one eyepiece, or **lens**) or **binocular** (**compound**, or having two eyepieces, or two sets of lenses). The parts of a microscope are mounted in a stand, which consists of an **arm** and a **base.** The stand supports the magnification system (objectives), accessories needed to operate it, and the stage, which holds the slide. The light or illumination source is situated in the base.

Operating the Microscope

To operate the microscope properly, the medical assistant needs to understand how magnification occurs, how the stage is used, how the light source functions, and how to focus the microscope.

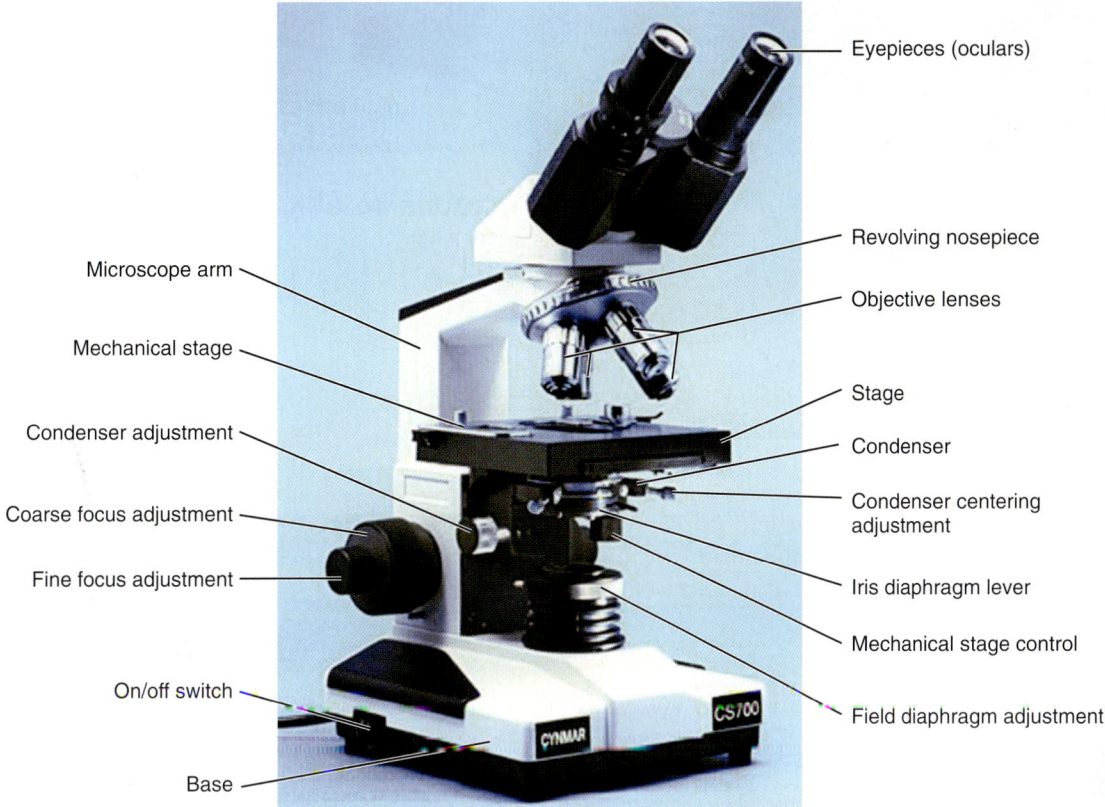

FIGURE 40-2 Parts of a binocular microscope.

Magnification. The compound microscope is the type most often used in the POL. It uses two sets of lenses to magnify an object. The first lens set is located in the **eyepiece**, or **ocular lens**, and the second lens set is the **objective lens**, commonly referred to as the **objectives**. The objectives are the set closest to the object being viewed. These two sets of lenses work together to magnify the specimen.

Magnification found in the ocular lens is 10 times (10×) the actual size of the object. Table 40-2 shows the total magnification. Most microscopes have three or four objectives: 4×, 10×, 40×, and 100× (oil immersion). The objectives are attached to the revolving **nosepiece**. Only one objective is used at a time. The lowest power is the shortest objective, and this is used first to scan the visual field and then focus on an object. To attain greater detail, the viewer advances to the next objective. The longest objective is the **oil-immersion lens** (100×), which allows for the most detail. This objective refracts light when a drop of immersion oil is placed between the lens and the specimen. Oil also allows the objective to move or slide without breakage. Differential of cells and Gram stain for bacteria are most often analyzed using this objective.

Stage. The **stage** is a platform that holds the slide for viewing and extends from the arm of the microscope. A hole located in the center of the stage allows light rays to enter from the light source (located below the stage) and reach the specimen. Movable clips are used to hold the slide securely on the stage. The **mechanical stage control knobs** allow the slide to be moved from right to left or front to back.

TABLE 40-2

Total Magnification = Ocular Lens × Objective Power

Ocular Lens	Objective Power	Total Magnification
10	4× (lowest power)	40×
10	10× (low power)	100×
10	40× (high power)	400×
10	100× (oil immersion)	1000×

Take extra care when placing the slide on the stage. Ease the slide gently between the clips, without releasing them too quickly, to avoid breaking the slide.

Light Source. The **light source** is usually located in the base of the microscope. Light passes upward to the specimen. The objective lens and the ocular lens of the eyepiece allow the viewer to have a magnified or enlarged image of the specimen. The **condenser** and the **iris diaphragm** are located between the stage and the light source, so the amount of light reaching the objective can be adjusted and controlled.

Focusing. Above the base, located on each side of the microscope, are the focusing knobs. The **coarse focus adjustment knob** (large knob) is used to bring the specimen into focus when the lower power objective is used. Once focused, the nosepiece can be rotated to increase the magnification by using higher power objectives. The **fine focus adjustment**

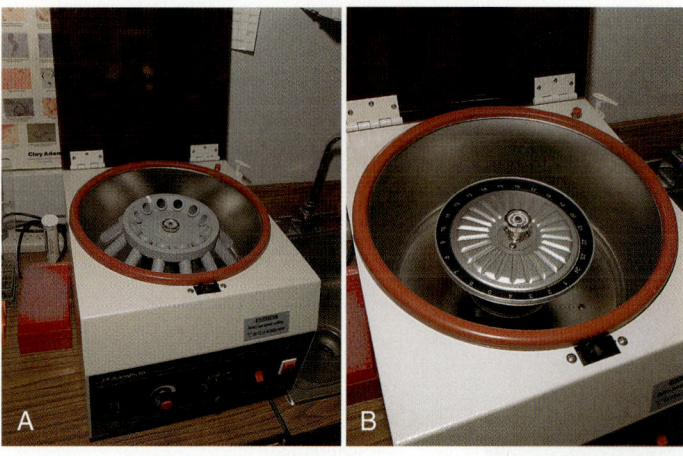

FIGURE 40-3 **A,** Regular centrifuge. **B,** Microhematocrit centrifuge.

knob is then used to bring the specimen into sharper focus. Procedure 40-2 describes how to focus the microscope from lower to higher power.

Care and Maintenance

To maintain optimal working order, microscopes must be properly maintained. They should have yearly maintenance performed by the manufacturer or a service representative. The microscope should be cleaned before and after each use. The following should be done to prevent damage to the microscope during cleaning, storage, and transportation:

- Clean all nonglass surfaces using a soft cloth.
- Use lens paper to clean all lenses. Wipe the ocular lens first, then the objectives. The oil-immersion objective should be cleaned last.
  NOTE: Use a new piece of lens tissue to clean the oculars, the objectives, and then the oil-immersion objective.
- Place the microscope in a protective covering or in a cabinet for storage.
- When transporting the microscope, firmly hold the arm of the microscope with one hand and support the base with the other.
  NOTE: Never slide the microscope on any surface, always lift and place it in the new location.
- Clean the oil-immersion lens with xylene or a special lens cleaner.

The microscope usually requires only minimal care to operate properly. Securing the microscope when transporting it by holding the arm and supporting the base, placing it gently on work surfaces, and cleaning it after use will help to avoid costly repairs.

Centrifuge

A **centrifuge** is a piece of laboratory equipment used to separate solid (or semisolid) material from a liquid by forced gravity. As the contents of the centrifuge tube are spun at a high speed, the solid or semisolid materials separate from the liquid portion and settle to the bottom of the tube. The centrifuge can separate **solutes** (materials suspended in a liquid) from urine and can separate **serum** or **plasma** from blood

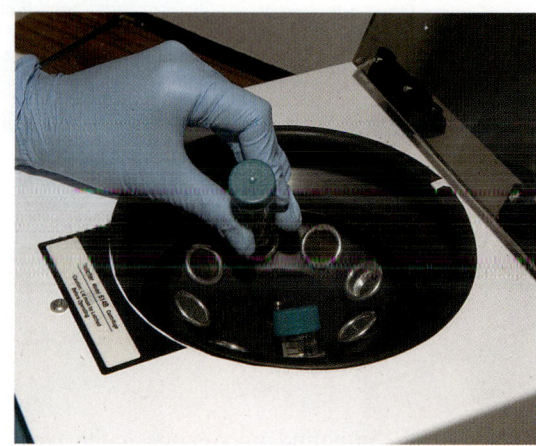

FIGURE 40-4 Placing specimen tubes in a centrifuge.

cells. This separation allows each part of the specimen to be studied.

Two types of centrifuge are typically used in the POL. A regular centrifuge uses large or small tubes to separate urine or blood components (Figure 40-3, *A*). The **microhematocrit centrifuge** processes blood in a capillary tube (Figure 40-3, *B*). Some centrifuges have both components in one machine.

Using the Centrifuge

Tubes placed in the centrifuge must always be **counterbalanced** (Figure 40-4). The area directly opposite the specimen tube must contain a tube of equal size and shape and must have an equal amount of fluid. Tubes with water are often used for this purpose when there are an unequal number of tubes to be centrifuged.

Centrifuges have a flat or domed safety cover. This cover must be closed before turning on the machine. This prevents glass and fluids from spraying into the air (aerosol droplet contamination). Some centrifuges have an additional safety feature that prevents the machine from working unless the cover is closed. A timer is set to process the specimen according to the manufacturer's instructions. A safety feature on

Introduction to the Physician's Office Laboratory   CHAPTER 40   903

PROCEDURE 40-2 Focus the Microscope

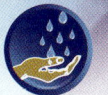

TASK: Focus the microscope on a prepared slide from low power to high power.

EQUIPMENT AND SUPPLIES
- Microscope with cover
- Lens paper
- Lens cleaner
- Specimen slide
- Soft cloth
- Tissue or gauze

SKILLS/RATIONALE

STANDARD PRECAUTIONS ARE TO BE FOLLOWED.

1. **Procedural Step.** Sanitize the hands.
   An alcohol-based hand rub may be used instead of washing hands with soap and water, unless hands are visibly soiled.
   Rationale. Hand sanitization promotes infection control.

2. **Procedural Step.** Assemble equipment and supplies and verify the order.
   Rationale. It is important to have all supplies and equipment ready and available before starting any procedure to ensure efficiency.

3. **Procedural Step.** Clean the ocular and objective lenses of the microscope with lens paper and lens cleaner.

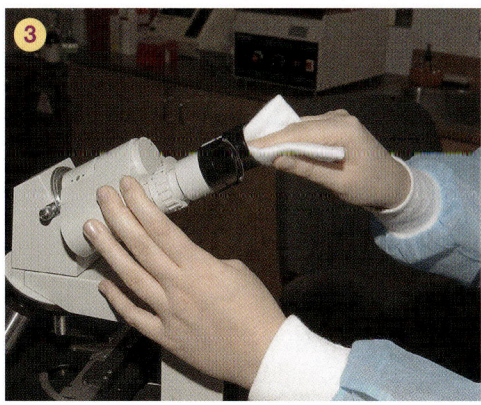

4. **Procedural Step.** Turn on the light source and adjust the ocular lenses to fit your eye span.

5. **Procedural Step.** Rotate the nosepiece to the scanning objective (4×) or to the low-power objective (10×) if the scanning objective is not attached to your microscope.
   Make sure the objective clicks securely into place.

6. **Procedural Step.** Place the slide on the stage and secure in the slide clip.
   The specimen side should be up.

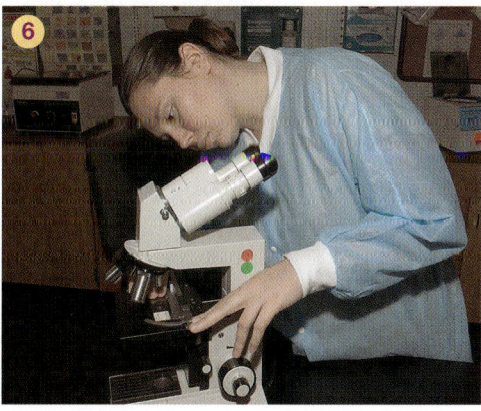

7. **Procedural Step.** Adjust the coarse focus adjustment knob.
   Viewing from the side, position the low-power objective until it almost touches the slide, either by raising the stage or by lowering the objective.
   Rationale. It is important to view from the side to prevent the objective from touching the slide.

8. **Procedural Step.** Open the diaphragm to allow in the maximum amount of light.

9. **Procedural Step.** Focus the specimen.
   Look through the ocular lens(es), and slowly turn the coarse focus adjustment knob to move the objective away from the specimen.

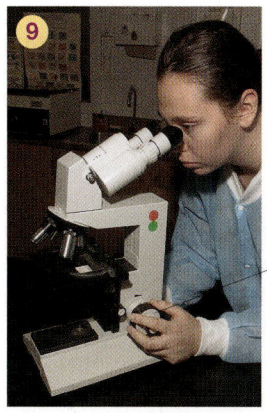

Coarse adjustment knob

Continued

> **PROCEDURE 40-2 Focus the Microscope—cont'd**
>
> 10. **Procedural Step.** Further focus the specimen into finest detail by using the fine focus adjustment knob.
> 11. **Procedural Step.** Adjust the diaphragm and condenser to regulate and adjust the amount of light focused on the specimen to obtain the sharpest image.
> 12. **Procedural Step.** Rotate the nosepiece.
>   Rotate the nosepiece to the low-power objective if the scanning objective was initially used or to the high-power objective if the low-power objective was initially used. Click securely into place. The specimen should still be in coarse focus. Using the fine focus adjustment knob, bring the specimen back into fine focus.
> 13. **Procedural Step.** Examine the specimen by scanning the slide using the stage controls to move it in four directions.
> 14. **Procedural Step.** Examine the specimen as required for the procedure or test and report the results.
> 15. **Procedural Step.** On completing your examination of the specimen, once again lower the stage or raise the objective, turn off the light, and remove the slide from the stage.
> 16. **Procedural Step.** Clean the stage with lens paper or gauze.
> 17. **Procedural Step.** Clean the objectives and ocular(s) with dry lens paper.
> 18. **Procedural Step.** Once clean, cover the microscope with a dust cover and return it to storage.
> 19. **Procedural Step.** Sanitize the hands.
>   Always sanitize the hands after every procedure or after using gloves.

most centrifuges is a safety lock that prevents the lid from being lifted during the spin cycle.

Centrifuge Tubes

Tubes used for centrifuging can have a cone-shaped or rounded bottom. The tubes can be made of glass or plastic and are disposable (glass tubes must be disposed of in a sharps container). Before placing a tube in the test tube compartment of the centrifuge, a rubber cushion should be placed in the bottom of the tube holder to minimize breakage.

> **PATIENT-CENTERED PROFESSIONALISM**
>
> - Why must the medical assistant understand the proper use and storage of laboratory equipment?

LABORATORY TESTS

Laboratory tests can be divided into several categories. Although the medical assistant will not perform some of these tests, it is important to be aware of their purpose in the POL. Categories and types of tests performed include the following:

- **Chemistry.** Chemistry test procedures are performed on a patient's serum (the liquid portion of the blood after a clot has formed and is then separated from the formed elements), plasma (from unclotted blood), urine, spinal fluid, and other body fluids. The tests are conducted to check for specific levels of chemicals, such as glucose, cholesterol, electrolytes (e.g., sodium, potassium), proteins, and drugs.
- **Hematology.** Hematology tests assess the formed elements of whole blood. This includes actual counting of the number of white cells (leukocytes), red cells (erythrocytes), and platelets in a blood sample. The cell shape, size, and level of maturity are also observed.
- **Coagulation studies** evaluate the clotting process of a patient's blood. These studies are often performed by the hematology department. Coagulation studies are performed to evaluate anticoagulant therapy and the blood's ability to clot.
- **Microbiology.** Microbiology tests are performed to study bacteria, fungi, viruses, and parasites found in body fluids. These tests aid in the identification of microorganisms and determination of their antibiotic sensitivity.
- **Serology.** Serology tests are performed to study the body's immune responses by detecting the antibodies in the serum. Serology includes testing for pregnancy, infectious mononucleosis, human immunodeficiency virus (HIV) infection, hepatitis, and some sexually transmitted diseases (STDs).
- **Blood bank.** The blood bank conducts studies for ABO blood groupings, Rh typing, and **crossmatching** blood for surgical patients.
- **Urinalysis.** Urinalysis testing studies the physical, chemical, and microscopic structure of urine. Tests are done on urine to screen for infection, drugs, glucose, human chorionic gonadotropin (hCG) for pregnancy, and other chemicals.

In addition to understanding the various types of testing, the medical assistant must understand the process of conducting laboratory tests, including patient preparation, use of the laboratory request form, specimen collection and transport, and the resulting laboratory reports.

Patient Preparation

The results of laboratory tests are only as good as the integrity (correctness) of the specimen collected. For example, if an ordered test required the patient to fast and the patient did not fast, the accuracy of the test would be in question. It is the medical assistant's responsibility to explain to the patient any special requirements, such as fasting or withholding medications, before collection of the needed specimen and to schedule the testing early enough that the patient can carry them out in time. Verbal and written instructions should be given to patients in a manner they understand.

- *Fasting* requires the patient to refrain from eating and drinking (except water in some cases) to prevent the results from being altered by certain foods, medications, and excess water or fluid. Fasting usually starts after midnight but can begin at 9 PM for some tests such as cholesterol testing. The specimen is collected in the early morning so that the patient can resume daily activities.
- *Medications* can sometimes interfere with test results. For example, insulin should not be taken until after the fasting blood specimen has been drawn to assess glucose tolerance. The physician will determine which medications the patient can take before testing.

A preprinted instruction sheet explaining the test to be done and its preparation is an ideal tool to help the patient be compliant. The medical assistant needs to make certain the patient understands the importance of preparing for the test properly. Allow the patient time to ask questions and provide any specific details as needed.

Laboratory Request Form

For laboratory tests to be processed correctly, a **laboratory requisition** must be completed correctly (Figure 40-5). All necessary information must be listed (e.g., diagnosis, collection site of specimen [such as forearm wound], whether patient was on antibiotics or fasting) for the specimen to be collected correctly. When incorrect paperwork accompanies a specimen to an outside laboratory, the test could be delayed or not performed at all, or the wrong test could be completed, or the test could be documented for the wrong patient. Patients do not like to come back for another specimen collection, and the physician does not expect a delay in testing, which in turn delays making a diagnosis and determining treatment plans. An incorrect form also suggests that the staff is unprofessional or incompetent. All outside laboratories have a requisition or request form; it may vary in style and format, but the information required is similar.

Procedure 40-3 explains the process of completing a laboratory requisition. Box 40-4 lists the necessary documentation for charting the transport of specimens to an outside laboratory. The completed requisition is attached to the specimen before transport. The laboratory requisition provides laboratory personnel with the physician's requested tests. Incomplete information delays the results and thus delays patient treatment.

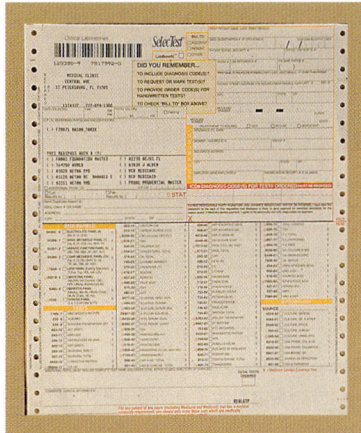

FIGURE 40-5 Laboratory requisition form.

BOX 40-4

Documentation when Charting for Transport of a Specimen to an Outside Laboratory

1. Date
2. Time
3. Name of specimen being sent
4. Name of laboratory to which the specimen is sent
5. Test to be completed
6. Proper signature and credential
7. Diagnosis code at time of examination
8. Name and patient demographics, including insurance information

Specimen Collection

QC measures should always be maintained during the collection process. The three different methods of specimen collection are as follows:

1. The specimen is collected and tested at the medical office.
2. The specimen is collected at the medical office, but it is transferred to an outside medical laboratory.
3. A physician with a written order refers the patient to an outside laboratory where specimen collection and testing take place.

Regardless of the method, the medical assistant is responsible for making certain the patient has received proper preparation instructions for the test to be done. For continued patient consideration, the medical assistant should ensure that the laboratory requisition is completed properly, then follow through to make certain the laboratory report is provided to the physician for analysis in a timely manner. If the report does not arrive in a timely manner, the medical assistant should follow up with the laboratory.

Specimen Containers

Before a laboratory test result can reflect the patient's true health status, the collection technique must be correct. Use of

PROCEDURE 40-3 Complete a Laboratory Requisition

TASK: Accurately complete a laboratory requisition form for specimen testing.

EQUIPMENT AND SUPPLIES
- Physician's written order for laboratory tests
- Laboratory requisition form
- Patient's medical record
- Pen

SKILLS/RATIONALE

STANDARD PRECAUTIONS ARE TO BE FOLLOWED.

1. **Procedural Step.** Obtain the patient's medical record and confirm the physician's orders for laboratory test(s).
   Rationale. Only tests that are ordered by the physician should be requested; confirming the order in the patient's record ensures accuracy.

2. **Procedural Step.** Obtain the laboratory requisition form for the laboratory where the test will be performed.
   Rationale. Requisition forms are typically provided by the laboratory. The physician's office may use several laboratories, thus it is important that the correct form and laboratory be used.

3. **Procedural Step.** Complete the section of the requisition requiring the physician's name and address.
   Rationale. If this section is left blank, the laboratory will not know where to send the test results, causing a delay in diagnosis and treatment for the patient.

4. **Procedural Step.** Complete the patient's demographic information.
   Some laboratory references require knowing a patient's age and gender.
   Rationale. Completing the patient demographic section ensures that the test results are reported for the correct patient.

5. **Procedural Step.** Complete the section of the requisition requiring the patient's insurance and billing information.
   Rationale. If this section is not completed, the physician and the laboratory may not receive a timely payment for services rendered.

6. **Procedural Step.** Complete the desired laboratory test(s) information.
   Indicate the ordered laboratory test(s) on the requisition and include the type of specimen collected and the source of the specimen (e.g., cytology, microbiology, fluid analysis, or other testing where analysis and reporting is site specific). All boxes must be clearly marked.
   Most laboratory requisition forms list all the tests that the laboratory routinely performs. Each test will have a box to check (or a bubble to fill in) or an area to circle to indicate which test is being ordered. A blank area toward the bottom of the form is usually provided to order tests not listed on the form.
   Rationale. It is important to indicate the specimen source, since many tests can be performed on several types of specimens (e.g., hCG pregnancy tests can be performed on urine and blood).

7. **Procedural Step.** Complete the section of the requisition requiring date and time of specimen collection.
   Rationale. Many laboratory tests are time sensitive, and the specimens must be processed within the time frame for the test results to be accurate.

8. **Procedural Step.** Enter the patient's diagnosis on the requisition as required.
   It may be necessary to code symptoms until the laboratory test rules in or rules out a diagnosis (e.g., nausea and vomiting—after test results, diagnosis becomes pregnancy).
   Rationale. Laboratory testing is performed to confirm or rule out a diagnosis. Diagnosis is required for billing the insurance company.

9. **Procedural Step.** Enter the type and amount of medication the patient is taking.
   Rationale. Some medications interfere with the accuracy of the test results.

10. **Procedural Step.** Complete the patient authorization to release, and assign the benefits portion as applicable.
    Rationale. This section must be completed for the laboratory to bill the patient's insurance company and release the test results to the physician's office.

11. **Procedural Step.** Attach the laboratory requisition securely to the specimen before sending it to the laboratory.
    Rationale. When specimens arrive at the laboratory without a requisition securely attached, the specimen is considered invalid and the ordered tests will not be performed, requiring the specimen to be recollected and reprocessed.

Continued

> **PROCEDURE 40-3 Complete a Laboratory Requisition—cont'd**
>
> 12. **Procedural Step.** Document in the patient's medical record and in the laboratory logbook that a specimen was sent for testing.
>
>   List type of specimen, special preparation that the patient may have performed, date, time, patient's name, where the specimen was sent, when the results are due to be returned (if known), and your initials.
>
>   *Rationale.* This step is important for follow-up.
>
> **CHARTING EXAMPLE**
>
> | Date | |
> |---|---|
> | 7/7/xx | 9:20 a.m. Urine 20 mL, clean-catch container, Vacutainer tube sent to Mullins Lab for urinalysis and C&S. Picked up at 10:05 a.m. ———— D. Scheble, RMA |
>
> **CHARTING EXAMPLE**
>
> | Date | |
> |---|---|
> | 8/4/xx | 9:00 a.m. Pt. presents to office fasting since 9:00 p.m. 8-3-xx. Blood sample drawn and spun for serum. Sent to Woodland Park Lab for Lipid Panel. Pt. tolerated procedure well. Juice and crackers provided after blood collection. Pt. instructed to schedule appt. in 5-7 days for test results. ———————— J. Lampley, RMA |

proper specimen containers is necessary to avoid contamination or deterioration of the specimen. Some specimens may require specific additives or preservatives to be added if the specimen will be sent to an outside laboratory or if it will involve a 24-hour urine collection. Remember, if you are not sure about the right test container for collection or proper times, call your laboratory personnel for clarification. They would rather answer questions before the test than after the test.

Timing

Proper collection times of a specimen are necessary to make the test values reliable, as follows:

- Glucose tolerance test (GTT) specimens must be carefully timed over a specified period to represent a patient's blood glucose level accurately.
- Most urine specimens need to be collected as the first specimen of the day because they provide more information about the patient's kidney function because of the concentration of the urine.

Transport

Outside laboratory testing requires the specimen be collected and taken to, or picked up by, the testing laboratory (Figure 40-6). Each laboratory service will supply the physician's office with transporting containers, special directions (if applicable) for obtaining the specimens and the amount needed, storage until picked up, and instructions for transporting the specimens. Most laboratory services have carriers trained to handle and deliver the specimens properly and on a timely basis. Outside laboratories have scheduled pickups, so when scheduling patients for specimen collection, remember to take this into consideration. Procedure 40-4 provides

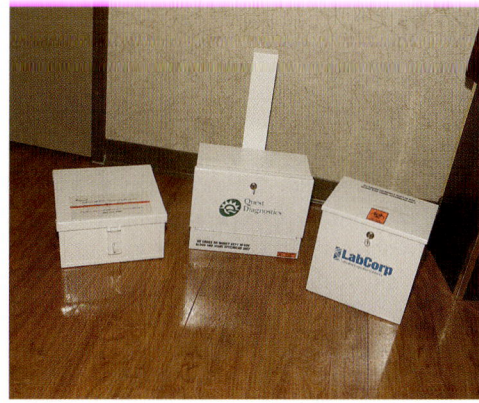

FIGURE 40-6 Outside laboratory pickup boxes.

instructions on proper collection techniques for specimens sent to an outside laboratory.

Laboratory Reports

The function of the laboratory report form is to provide the physician with the results of the laboratory test(s) performed. It contains necessary information to assist the physician with a diagnosis (Figure 40-7). Typical information for an outside laboratory includes the following:

1. Laboratory demographics (name, address, telephone number)
2. Ordering physician's name, phone number, and address
3. Patient's information (name, insurance, diagnosis, age, gender)
4. Date and time the laboratory received the specimen
5. Date and time results were reported to the physician's office
6. Tests to be performed

PROCEDURE 40-4

Collect a Specimen for Transport to an Outside Laboratory

TASK: Properly collect a specimen to be sent to an outside laboratory.

EQUIPMENT AND SUPPLIES
- Nonsterile disposable gloves
- Personal protective equipment (PPE)
- Specimen and container
- Laboratory request form
- Pen
- Patient's medical record
- Laboratory logbook
- Biohazardous waste container

SKILLS/RATIONALE

STANDARD PRECAUTIONS ARE TO BE FOLLOWED.

1. **Procedural Step.** Provide the patient with any advance preparation or special instructions.
   Such preparation may involve the following:
   a. Diet modification or specific dietary regimen
   b. Fasting
   c. Medication restrictions (either stopping or modifying dose)
   d. Collection of specimen at home

   Explain the process that the patient must follow for collections. Also provide the patient with written instructions to take home. If specimen collection is to be done in the physician's office, notify the patient of the time to report to the medical office.
   Rationale. The patient must prepare properly to provide a quality specimen; otherwise the test results will be invalid, causing a delay in treatment. The patient should not have to return to the office to have another specimen collected.

2. **Procedural Step.** Review the requirements in the laboratory directory for the collection and handling of the specimen ordered by the physician.
   These instructions may include the following:
   a. Proper supplies needed for collection
   b. Type of specimen to be collected (capillary, venous)
   c. Volume of specimen required for laboratory analysis
   d. Special preparation of the site
   e. Procedure to follow as the specimen is collected
   f. Proper handling and storage of the specimen after collection

   Telephone the laboratory with any questions regarding the collection or handling of the specimen to ensure specimen quality. Outside laboratories will provide a reference manual detailing their specimen collection requirements.
   Rationale. Reviewing the requirements beforehand prevents errors in collection and handling of the specimen and ensures quality that is acceptable for an accurate test.

3. **Procedural Step.** Complete the laboratory requisition form (see Procedure 40-3).
   If the tests results are needed by the physician as soon as possible, mark "STAT" on the request in bold letters.
   Rationale. The completed form provides the laboratory with the information necessary to perform the tests accurately.

4. **Procedural Step.** Sanitize the hands.
   An alcohol-based hand rub may be used instead of washing hands with soap and water, unless hands are visibly soiled.
   Rationale. Hand sanitization promotes infection control.

5. **Procedural Step.** Assemble equipment and supplies.
   Be sure to use the appropriate specimen container required by the outside laboratory. Inspect the container to make sure it is not broken, chipped, or cracked. If the specimen is to be collected in a sterile container, make certain the packaging material has not been broken.
   Rationale. It is important to have all supplies and equipment ready and available before starting any procedure to ensure efficiency. The appropriate specimen container must be used to ensure the collection of the proper type of specimen required by the laboratory. Damaged specimen containers are unsuitable for collection and should be discarded.

6. **Procedural Step.** Greet the patient, introduce yourself, and confirm the patient's identity. Escort the patient to the area where the specimen will be collected.
   If the patient was required to prepare for the test, determine whether the patient has prepared properly. Specimen collection is often an anxiety-producing experience for the patient, and reassurance should be offered to help reduce apprehension.
   Rationale. Identifying the patient ensures the specimen is collected from the correct patient.

Continued

PROCEDURE 40-4 Collect a Specimen for Transport to an Outside Laboratory—cont'd

7. **Procedural Step.** Collect the specimen.
   Use the following guidelines in specimen collection:
   a. Follow the OSHA standard (apply gloves or PPE as necessary).
   b. Collect the specimen using proper site preparation and technique.
   c. Collect the proper type and amount of the specimen required for the test.
   d. Process the specimen further as required by the outside laboratory (e.g., separating serum from whole blood).
   e. Place the lid tightly on the specimen container.
   f. Dispose of any materials used in the specimen collection in the appropriate waste container.
   Rationale. Proper collection of a specimen provides the laboratory with an acceptable sample for testing.

8. **Procedural Step.** Clearly label the tubes and specimen containers.
   Include the patient's name, date, physician's name, your initials, and any other information, such as the source of the specimen and time of collection, required by the laboratory.
   NOTE: QA procedures require labeling of blood specimen tubes *after* collection to ensure tubes have been drawn on the correct patient.
   Rationale. Properly labeled tubes and specimen containers prevent a mix-up of specimens.

9. **Procedural Step.** Record information about the collection in the patient's medical record and the laboratory logbook.
   Include the date and time of the collection, type and source of the specimen, laboratory tests ordered by the physician, and information indicating its transport to the outside laboratory, including the date the specimen will be sent.

10. **Procedural Step.** Properly handle and store (if necessary) the specimen, according to the laboratory's specifications.
    Rationale. The specimen must be handled and stored properly to maintain the integrity of the specimen.

11. **Procedural Step.** Prepare the specimen for transport to the outside laboratory.
    Be sure to include the completed laboratory request with the specimen, and double-check to make sure the name on the laboratory request and the specimen label is the same.

12. **Procedural Step.** Remove gloves and sanitize the hands.
    Always sanitize the hands after every procedure or after using gloves.

13. **Procedural Step.** When the laboratory report is returned to the physician's office, review the test results.
    a. Compare each test result with the normal range provided by the laboratory. If the test results are grossly abnormal, notify the physician immediately.
    b. Attach the laboratory report to the patient's record and submit it to the physician for review.
    c. Once the physician has reviewed and initialed the report, file the report in the patient's medical record and document on the flow chart as per office protocol.

CHARTING EXAMPLE

Date	
3/10/xx	8:00 a.m. Venous blood specimen collected for lipid profile from ® arm. Pt. was in a fasting state. Transported to Medical Laboratory Corp. on 3/10/xx.——————— E. Daly, CMA (AAMA)

---

7. Normal range or reference values for each test performed
8. Results of the tests performed

Most laboratory test results are meaningless unless standard values are available to compare the results. Since many factors can affect a person's results, such as gender, age, and race, a normal range is provided for each test. These values represent the range for the general population. Note that each laboratory's range may vary because of the equipment and reagents used to perform the tests. Therefore all tests should be compared to the range of the laboratory performing the test.

The medical assistant may be required to review the laboratory reports when received, immediately notifying the physician of abnormal findings. The physician must review and initial all laboratory reports before they are filed in the patient's medical record. If the patient does have an abnormal test result, the physician may want to see the patient. Laboratory reports can be mailed, delivered by the outside laboratory, or transmitted via the Internet, fax, or telephone. If receiving laboratory reports over the telephone, the medical assistant should repeat results recorded to verify correctness, obtain the identity of the phone reporter, and sign his or her initials to the report. Telephoned results should be followed by a hard copy or electronic copy.

Accuracy in recording results is important to avoid a misunderstanding and a possible misdiagnosis. A misdiagnosis could generate a lawsuit for misfeasance, so it is imperative to be accurate when documenting test results. Procedure 40-5 outlines the process of screening and following up on patient

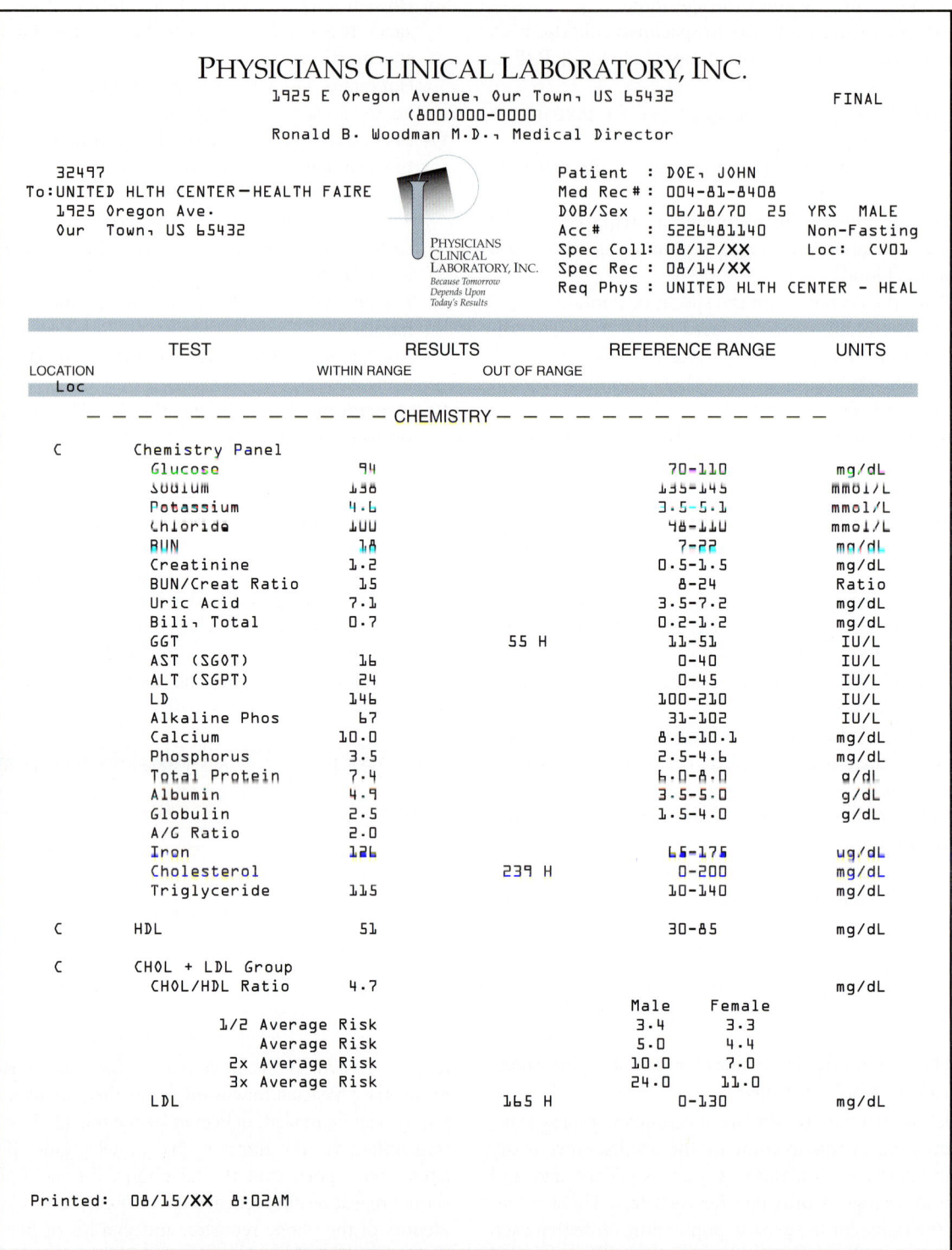

FIGURE 40-7 A test result form showing normal ranges and results. (From Stepp CA, Woods MA: *Laboratory procedures for medical office personnel*, Philadelphia, 1998, Saunders.)

Introduction to the Physician's Office Laboratory **CHAPTER 40** **911**

| PROCEDURE 40-5 | Screen and Follow-up on Patient Test Results | |

TASK: Follow-up with a patient who has abnormal test results.

EQUIPMENT AND SUPPLIES
- Laboratory test results
- Tickler file (3 × 5 cards or computer software program) or laboratory log of patient results
- Follow-up reminder cards
- Pen
- Patient's medical record

SKILLS/RATIONALE   STANDARD PRECAUTIONS ARE TO BE FOLLOWED.

NOTE: Follow office policy and procedures for contacting a patient with abnormal test results. Some physicians prefer to personally contact patients with abnormal results. Some test results should not be provided to the patient over the telephone, and the physician will require the patient to make an appointment and come to the office.

1. **Procedural Step. When the laboratory report is returned to the physician's office, review the test results.**
   Compare each test result with the normal range provided by the laboratory. Identify and highlight results outside the normal range. The laboratory will provide the reference ranges and may indicate on the report any results that fall outside the normal range. If abnormal results are not indicated by the laboratory, you should indicate them before submitting to the physician for review according to office protocol.

2. **Procedural Step. Attach the laboratory report to the patient's medical record and submit it to the physician for review.**
   After reviewing and initialing the report, the physician will determine what follow-up should occur.
   Rationale. Laboratory results that require immediate action must be handled in a timely fashion.

3. **Procedural Step. If the physician requests that you schedule the patient for a follow-up appointment, determine the most appropriate method of contact.**
   Remember to follow HIPAA guidelines.

4. **Procedural Step. Contact the patient and schedule an appointment.**
   NOTE: Do not discuss test results with a patient unless the physician has given you permission to do so and document your notification of the patient.

test results. Documentation of all patient communication concerning information on laboratory test results should include:
- Date test sent to laboratory
- Date results received and reviewed by the physician
- Date reported to patient (e.g., letter, follow up appointment scheduled)

Medical offices should have protocols in place regarding the reporting and documentation of laboratory tests.

PATIENT-CENTERED PROFESSIONALISM

- What professional components must a medical assistant have to make certain the patient is properly prepared, the correct collection method is used, and the specimen is transported to the laboratory within the proper time frame?

CULTURE COLLECTION

Cultures of a specific body area can be collected using a sterile polyester (Dacron) swab. Since delays in processing cannot be anticipated, a **swab-transport media system** should be used. Swabs in a transport media should be processed within 24 hours.

Wound

When wound cultures are collected, one or two sterile Dacron swabs should be used with transport media to ensure an adequate specimen has been collected (Figure 40-8). If the wound is deep, an *anaerobic* culture kit (which detects bacteria not needing oxygen to survive) may also be used to check for the presence of gangrene or other anaerobic bacteria.

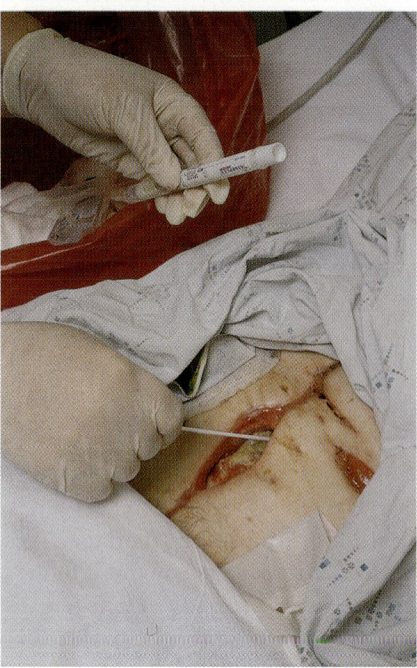

FIGURE 40-8 Sterile swabs are used to collect a specimen from a wound. (From deWit SC: *Fundamental concepts and skills for nursing*, ed 3, St Louis, 2009, Saunders.)

Throat

A throat culture is collected by using a sterile Dacron swab. The posterior pharyngeal and tonsillar areas are swabbed to perform a **rapid screening test** to detect the presence of group A beta-hemolytic streptococci. Avoid touching the tongue and the inside of the cheeks and teeth to prevent gathering of extraneous microorganisms. Immediately after the specimen is taken, the swab must be placed in the sterile collection tube containing the holding media. Procedure 40-6 outlines the process of throat culture collection.

> **PATIENT-CENTERED PROFESSIONALISM**
>
> - What collection criteria must be met for obtaining a swab culture?

URINE COLLECTION

The collection of a urine specimen from a patient is one of the most frequently performed procedures by a medical assistant. The process is simple, and the information provided about the patient's urinary system and body function is invaluable. A urinalysis can detect diseases of the kidney, other diseased states of body systems, and infections in the urinary tract. Proper collection of the specimen is imperative for the test results to be valid. QC practices require that all sources of contamination be avoided during the collection and while handling the specimen after the collection.

The medical assistant must process urine specimens within 1 hour of collection or refrigerate the specimen until processing can occur. Urine is an excellent culture medium, and any bacteria present in a urine specimen multiply rapidly at room temperature. Since one purpose of collecting a urine specimen is to screen for **bacteriuria** (bacteria in the urine) and, if necessary, to culture a urine specimen to identify the bacteria, timing is important. Box 40-5 provides information for charting laboratory procedures, such as urinalysis, done in the POL.

Medical assistants should be familiar with the various types of urine specimens that are collected; the collection of random, midstream clean-catch, 24-hour, timed, and specimens for drug-screening are covered in this chapter. Chapter 42 offers more information about performing urinalysis and analyzing urine specimens that have been collected.

Random Urine Specimen

A **random urine specimen** (collected any time during the day) is the type of urine most frequently collected from the patient. It is best collected after the patient has cleaned the urethral opening with an antiseptic wipe. This extra step removes any gross contamination. The ideal specimen is the **first morning specimen** because it is the most concentrated and has an acid pH, which preserves cells present. If the specimen is to be collected by the patient at home and then brought to the office for examination, it should be refrigerated until it can be transported. It should also be collected in a clean container or one provided by the office or laboratory. Instruct the patient not to touch the inside of the container if possible.

The medical assistant may be asked to collect an uncontaminated urine specimen from an infant. Special pediatric urine collection bags are available for obtaining this type of specimen. Procedure 40-7 outlines the steps in the process of collecting an uncontaminated urine specimen from an infant using a pediatric urine collector.

Midstream Clean-Catch Urine Specimen

A **midstream clean-catch urine specimen** requires the patient to follow a strict cleaning procedure. The medical assistant must explain to the patient the purpose for this type of specimen collection as well as the instructions for obtaining it. The patient should be told the importance of not touching the

Text continued on p. 918

> **BOX 40-5**
>
> **Documentation when Charting Laboratory Procedures Done in the POL**
>
> 1. Date
> 2. Time
> 3. Name of test performed
> 4. Results (using interpretation guide if provided by the manufacturer)
> 5. Patient reaction, if any
> 6. Proper signature and credential

Introduction to the Physician's Office Laboratory   **CHAPTER 40**   913

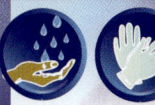

PROCEDURE 40-6   Collect a Specimen for CLIA-Waived Throat Culture and Strep A Test

TASKS: Collect an uncontaminated throat specimen to test for group A beta-hemolytic streptococci. Perform a strep A test.

EQUIPMENT AND SUPPLIES
- Nonsterile disposable gloves
- Personal protective equipment (PPE) as needed (goggles)
- Sterile polyester (Dacron) swab
- Culture transport system
- Test tube rack
- Tongue depressor
- Gooseneck lamp
- Timer
- Biohazardous waste container
- Patient's medical record
- Strep A kit

SKILLS/RATIONALE   STANDARD PRECAUTIONS ARE TO BE FOLLOWED.

SPECIMEN COLLECTION FOR THROAT CULTURE

1. **Procedural Step.** Sanitize the hands.
   An alcohol-based hand rub may be used instead of washing hands with soap and water, unless hands are visibly soiled.
   Rationale. Hand sanitization promotes infection control.

2. **Procedural Step.** Assemble equipment and supplies and verify the order.
   Rationale. It is important to have all supplies and equipment ready and available before starting any procedure to ensure efficiency.

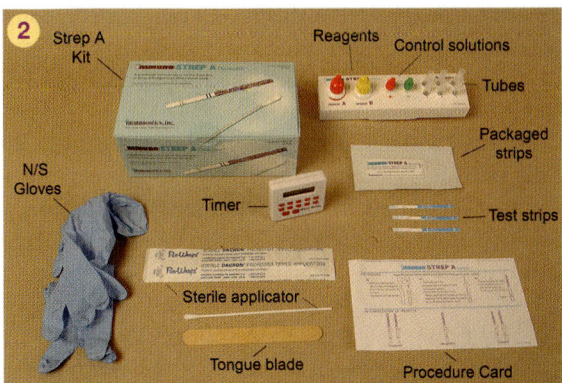

3. **Procedural Step.** Obtain the patient's medical record.

4. **Procedural Step.** Greet the patient, introduce yourself, and confirm the patient's identity.
   Rationale. Identifying the patient ensures the procedure is performed on the correct patient.

5. **Procedural Step.** Instruct the patient to have a seat on the end of the examination table and explain the procedure to the patient.
   Rationale. Explaining the procedure to the patient promotes cooperation and provides a means of obtaining implied consent.

6. **Procedural Step.** Visually inspect the patient's throat.
   If the patient is chewing gum or eating, ask the patient to dispose of the gum or food. Provide the patient with a tissue and throw the item in the waste container.
   Adjust lighting, such as a gooseneck lamp, as necessary to obtain proper visualization of the throat.
   Rationale. Visualization of the throat must be unobstructed to obtain an uncontaminated specimen.

7. **Procedural Step.** Apply gloves and PPE as required.

8. **Procedural Step.** Prepare the culture transport system.
   Peel open the wrapper containing the culture transport system. Stand the tube in the test tube rack.
   Rationale. The culture transport system will be used to send a specimen to the laboratory for confirmation of rapid strep test results.

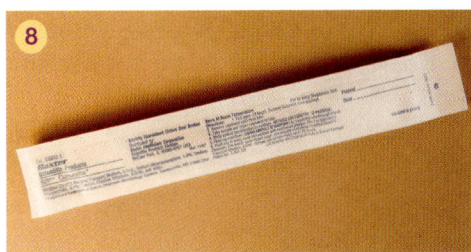

Continued

PROCEDURE 40-6 Collect a Specimen for CLIA-Waived Throat Culture and Strep A Test—cont'd

9. **Procedural Step.** Prepare the polyester (Dacron) swab.
   Open the sterile Dacron swab by peeling apart the paper wrapper halfway, leaving the tip of the swab inside the wrapper.
   Rationale. The Dacron swab will be used for collection of a specimen for the rapid strep test.

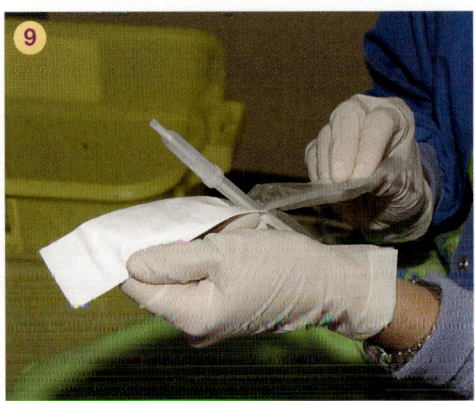

10. **Procedural Step.** Remove the culture transport system swab from the peel-apart package, being careful not to contaminate it by touching the tip to anything.
    Hold the swab in your dominant hand.
11. **Procedural Step.** Remove the Dacron swab from the paper wrapper, again being careful not to contaminate it by touching the tip.
12. **Procedural Step.** Place both swabs in your right hand with the tips close together, almost like one swab.
    The tips of the swabs may touch without becoming contaminated because both are sterile.
13. **Procedural Step.** Ask the patient to tilt the head back and open the mouth wide.
14. **Procedural Step.** Use a tongue depressor to hold down the anterior third of the tongue.
    Rationale. Using a tongue depressor to hold down the tongue provides visualization and access to the back of the throat.
15. **Procedural Step.** Carefully insert the swabs into the patient's mouth without touching the inside of the mouth, tongue, or teeth.
    Rationale. Touching the swabs to the inside of the patient's mouth, tongue, or teeth may contaminate the specimen, providing inaccurate test results.

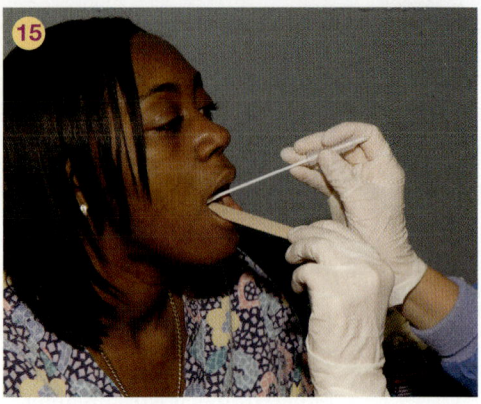

16. **Procedural Step.** Ask the patient to say "Ahh ..."
    Rationale. This reduces the tendency to gag.
17. **Procedural Step.** Firmly swab the back of the throat (posterior pharynx) with a figure-eight motion between the tonsillar areas.
    Make sure to touch any reddened areas, white patches, or areas where you see pus. Rotate the swabs to make sure each swab contacts as much of the tonsillar area as possible. To minimize gagging, swab quickly and firmly but without excess pressure.
    Rationale. The rotating motion is used to deposit as much of the material as possible onto the swabs. Most patients gag slightly, but excessive pressure on the back of the throat or moving the swab very slowly in the figure-eight pattern will increase discomfort for the patient.
18. **Procedural Step.** Continue to hold down the tongue with the depressor, and carefully remove the swabs from the patient's mouth without touching the tongue, teeth, or inside of the cheeks.
19. **Procedural Step.** Discard the tongue depressor in a biohazardous waste container.
20. **Procedural Step.** Immediately place the swab from the transport system firmly into the bottom of the tube so that it is dampened with the transport medium and secure tightly. Return the Dacron swab to the original wrapper.
    Avoid contamination of the swabs with anything from the environment. Some swab-transport systems require breaking an ampule after inserting the swab back into the collection device to release the transport medium.
21. **Procedural Step.** Label the transport tube and swab with the patient's name.
    Never label until the specimen has been collected.

Continued

PROCEDURE 40-6 Collect a Specimen for CLIA-Waived Throat Culture and Strep A Test—cont'd

If the transport tube is sent to the laboratory for confirmation, the label and a test requisition form must be completed.

22. **Procedural Step.** Once the specimens have been returned to their individual packaging, remove PPE and sanitize the hands.

Always sanitize the hands after every procedure or after using gloves.

STREP A TEST

NOTE: There are several manufacturers of strep tests. Follow the manufacturer's directions for testing. Directions below are specific to the QuickVue strep test but are relatively standard.

1. **Procedural Step.** Sanitize the hands.

   Sanitize the hands if you are not completing the strep test immediately after obtaining the specimen. An alcohol-based hand rub may be used instead of washing hands with soap and water, unless hands are visibly soiled.

   Rationale. Hand sanitization promotes infection control.

2. **Procedural Step.** Apply PPE (if not already applied).

3. **Procedural Step.** Assemble equipment and supplies.

   Obtain three of everything because a positive (+) and a negative (−) control must be run in addition to the patient's sample. Positive and negative controls must be run whenever a new kit is opened. The manufacturer supplies swabs that have been impregnated with different types of streptococcal bacteria. These swabs are treated the same as the patient swab. If they react as expected, then test has been performed correctly and everything is working properly. Before patient results can be reported, QC data must be satisfactory.

4. **Procedural Step.** Unwrap each of the three test strips that are wrapped in foil pouches.

5. **Procedural Step.** Record the lot number and expiration date of the kit on the log sheets.

   Rationale. Control and patient results are recorded after testing has been completed. The laboratory director reviews all log sheets.

6. **Procedural Step.** Label each tube for the controls positive (+) and negative (−) and patient.

7. **Procedural Step.** Add 4 drops of Reagent A, then 4 drops of Reagent B to the + tube. Tap bottom of tube to mix. Add swab from positive packet and rotate swab 10 times in tube. Let stand 1 minute. Remove swab from tube by pressing swab against the inside of the tube and squeeze tube while removing swab. (This allows as much of the liquid to stay in the tube as possible.)

   NOTE: There are two important things to remember:
   - Recheck the swab and tube label to make sure the correct swab goes into the correct tube.
   - Make sure the swab is inserted *completely* into the tube so that the reagent solution *covers* the swab.

8. **Procedural Step.** Place test strip in tube, making certain that the liquid reaches at least the "max" line. Read result at 5 minutes.

9. **Procedural Step.** Interpret the results according to manufacturer's instructions.

   Each test strip should have a pink line at the top mark. This is the internal control and is a measure of QA. If there is no pink line at the top mark, the results are invalid and the test must be repeated with a new specimen, a new test strip, tube, and fresh reagent solution. The positive strip will have two pink lines, one at the top and another one beneath. The negative strip will only have the top mark pink. A strip that has only a bottom marker or none at all is considered invalid.

   Rationale. QA is the procedural control confirming that the reaction between specimen and solutions took place as expected. Check for positive or negative test results.

   Two pink lines on the test strip mean the test is positive. Only a pink line at the top of the strip means the test is negative.

10. **Procedural Step.** Repeat steps 7 to 9 for the negative packet and then process the patient's specimen.

11. **Procedural Step.** Sanitize the hands.

    Always sanitize the hands after every procedure or after using gloves.

12. **Procedural Step.** Record the known controls on the QC log sheet.

13. **Procedural Step.** Document the test results from the patient's specimen.

CHARTING EXAMPLE

Date	
7/12/xx	11:15 a.m. Throat specimen collected from tonsillar area. QuickVue rapid strep test neg. Sent specimen to Medical Lab Corp. for confirmation test.————————————————————L. Patton, RMA

SECTION V Clinical Medical Assisting

PROCEDURE 40-7: Obtain a Urine Specimen from an Infant Using a Pediatric Urine Collector

TASK: Collect an uncontaminated urine specimen from an infant.

EQUIPMENT AND SUPPLIES
- Nonsterile disposable gloves
- Antiseptic wipes, or gauze squares, and antiseptic solution
- Sterile water and sterile gauze squares
- Pediatric urine collector bag
- Sterile urine specimen container and label
- Biohazardous waste container
- Patient's medical record

SKILLS/RATIONALE

STANDARD PRECAUTIONS ARE TO BE FOLLOWED.

1. **Procedural Step.** Sanitize the hands.
   An alcohol-based hand rub may be used instead of washing hands with soap and water, unless hands are visibly soiled.
   Rationale. Hand sanitization promotes infection control.

2. **Procedural Step.** Assemble equipment and supplies and verify the order.
   Rationale. It is important to have all supplies and equipment ready and available before starting any procedure to ensure efficiency.

3. **Procedural Step.** Obtain the patient's medical record.

4. **Procedural Step.** Greet the infant's parent or guardian, introduce yourself, and confirm the patient's identity.
   Rationale. Identifying the patient ensures the procedure is performed on the correct patient.

5. **Procedural Step.** Explain the procedure to the parent or guardian.
   Rationale. Explaining the procedure to the parent or guardian promotes cooperation and provides a means of obtaining implied consent.

6. **Procedural Step.** Apply gloves.

7. **Procedural Step.** Position the infant.
   Place the child in a supine position on the examination table. Remove the diaper and ask the parent or guardian to help spread the child's legs apart.
   Rationale. Placing the child in this position with the parent or guardian helping to spread the legs apart provides access to the genitalia and enables thorough cleansing of the area and application of the urine collection bag.

8. **Procedural Step.** Cleanse the child's genitalia thoroughly.
   Female infant: Using a separate antiseptic wipe for each side, cleanse the urinary meatus, wiping once from the pubis to the anus. Using a third wipe, cleanse directly over the urinary meatus. Rinse the area thoroughly with sterile water and sterile gauze squares, then wipe the area dry with a new sterile gauze square.
   Male infant: For uncircumcised males, retract the foreskin of the penis. Cleanse the area around the meatus and the urethral opening in the same manner used in the female patient. Use a separate antiseptic wipe for each area. Use a fresh antiseptic wipe to clean the scrotum. Rinse the area thoroughly with sterile water and sterile gauze squares, then wipe the area dry with a new sterile gauze square.
   Rationale. To prevent contamination of the specimen, the urinary meatus and surrounding area must be free from contaminants, which could affect the test results. Care must be taken to wipe only in a front-to-back motion, and each antiseptic wipe should be used only once to prevent contamination from the anal area. The cleansing agent must be rinsed off to prevent it from entering the urine specimen, which could affect the accuracy of the test results. The area must be wiped dry to ensure an airtight adhesion of the collection bag to prevent leakage of urine.

9. **Procedural Step.** Prepare the urine collection bag.
   Remove the urine collection bag from the peel apart packaging and remove the paper backing from the adhesive strip around the sponge ring of the bag, being careful not to touch the bag to any surface that could cause contamination.

10. **Procedural Step.** Firmly attach the urine collection bag.
    Female infant: The round opening of the bag should be placed so that it covers the upper half of the external genitalia. The opening of the bag should be directly over the urinary meatus with the bag directed toward the patient's feet.
    Male infant: The bag should be positioned so that the child's penis and scrotum are projected through the opening of the bag. The loose end of the bag should be directed toward the feet.
    Rationale. The urine collection bag must be attached securely to prevent leakage.

Continued

PROCEDURE 40-7 Obtain a Urine Specimen from an Infant Using a Pediatric Urine Collector—cont'd

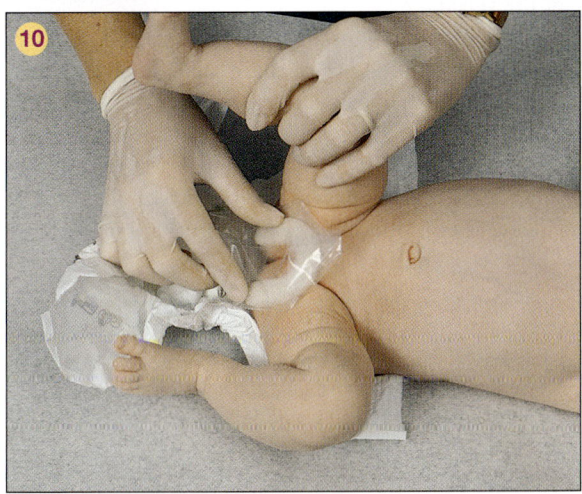

11. **Procedural Step.** Loosely diaper the child and check the urine collection bag every 15 minutes until a urine specimen is obtained. A parent or guardian should remain with the child during the collection.
    Rationale. The diaper helps hold the urine collection bag in place.
12. **Procedural Step.** Remove gloves and sanitize the hands.
    Always sanitize the hands after every procedure or after using gloves.
13. **Procedural Step.** When a sufficient volume of urine has been collected, apply new gloves and gently remove the urine collection bag.
    Rationale. Pulling the bag away from the child's skin too forcefully or too quickly may cause discomfort and irritation to the child's skin.
14. **Procedural Step.** Clean the genital area and re-diaper the child.
15. **Procedural Step.** Transfer the urine specimen into a sterile urine specimen container and tightly secure the lid.
    Dispose of the collection bag in a biohazardous waste container.
16. **Procedural Step.** Label the specimen container.
    Include the child's name, date, and time of collection, type of specimen, and the physician's name. Dispose of the collection bag in a biohazardous waste container.
17. **Procedural Step.** Process the specimen based on the physician office laboratory protocol.
    Either test the urine specimen per the physician's orders or prepare it for transfer to an outside laboratory. If the specimen is to be sent to an outside laboratory, complete a laboratory requisition form and securely attach it to the specimen before transport. If the specimen cannot be tested or transferred immediately, refrigerate it.
    Rationale. When a urine specimen cannot be tested immediately, a preservative must be added or the specimen must be refrigerated. When left sitting at room temperature, urine composition can change (e.g., a possible increase in bacteria and crystals).
18. **Procedural Step.** Remove gloves and sanitize the hands.
    Always sanitize the hands after every procedure or after using gloves.
19. **Procedural Step.** Document the procedure.
    Include the date, time of collection, and type of specimen. If the specimen is to be transported to an outside laboratory, document which tests were ordered and the name of the laboratory receiving the specimen.

CHARTING EXAMPLE

Date	
1/24/xx	10:00 a.m. Urine specimen collected for culture and sensitivity. Picked up by Lab Center on 1/24/xx.————————— —————————— T. Moore, CMA (AAMA)

Photo for Step 10 from Bonewit-West K: Clinical procedures for medical assistants, ed. 7, St Louis, 2008, Saunders.

inside of the sterile container and for wiping off the genital (urethral) area from front to back with the antiseptic wipes provided before urinating. The use of antiseptic wipes reduces bacterial contamination of the specimen, and although the specimen is not sterile, it is considered less contaminated than a random specimen.

Patients are instructed to start urinating in the toilet, stop, continue to urinate to collect a specimen, and then finish urinating in the toilet. By not collecting the first urine voided, the antiseptic residual and external bacteria from the urethral area are removed. This process also reduces the risk of contamination from the perineal area, which may contain anal contaminants. This procedure is usually done in the physician's office; the patient should be provided with detailed instructions and illustrations for collection. Procedure 40-8 provides patient instructions for collecting a midstream clean-catch urine specimen to ensure the validity of the test results.

24-Hour Urine Specimen

A **24-hour urine specimen** tests for kidney function. The patient collects urine over a 24-hour period. The specimen may need to be kept cool in an ice chest or other type of refrigeration. Some collection containers have a preservative that can be added to the specimen to maintain quality. This test is used to check for high levels of creatinine, uric acid, hormones, electrolytes, and medications. The medical assistant instructs the patient in proper collection technique. It is important to remind the patient that the first specimen is *not* collected. Instead, it is discarded, but the time is recorded. All urine is collected in this container through the first specimen the next morning. The specimen is processed in an outside laboratory. Procedure 40-9 provides instructions on preparing the patient to obtain an accurate 24-hour urine specimen.

Timed Specimen

A **timed specimen** collection is when a specimen is collected at certain intervals. This type of specimen is often used to aid in the diagnosis of diabetes. A **glucose tolerance test (GTT)** requires the fasting patient to provide a urine and blood sample before ingesting a measured amount of glucose solution, then at timed intervals thereafter (½ hour, 1 hour, 2 hours, and 3 hours). Deviation from this schedule invalidates the test results.

A 2-hour **postprandial** (after meal) **specimen** is collected to assess glucose metabolism. A patient may be asked to fast, have a blood and urine sample taken, then eat a high-carbohydrate meal. Two hours after the meal, the patient provides blood and urine samples, which are screened for elevated glucose levels. Some physicians only obtain a postprandial specimen, without the fasting specimen.

Drug Screen

Special handling is required for specimens that may be used as evidence in a court of law. For example, an industrial accident caused by drug or alcohol abuse will require the results of the urine or blood to be known. To be admissible, the collection, handling, processing, and testing of the specimen must maintain absolute quality and accuracy. A medical assistant may be involved in collecting a urine specimen for a **drug screening.** The **chain of custody** regulations describe how evidence—in this case the urine specimen—is to be collected and handled. These must be followed exactly to maintain the validity of the test results while protecting the donor's rights. The chain of custody provides strict guidelines for the collector of the specimen.

Forensic investigations are done in a methodical (step-by-step) manner and follow a **chain of evidence** (collection routine). The chain of evidence details each step and provides directions on handling every detail from beginning to end. Think of it as following a recipe: if you forget a step or an ingredient, the end result will not be very good. If the chain of evidence is not followed, the test results are suspect and are not usable in a court of law.

PATIENT-CENTERED PROFESSIONALISM

- *Why must the medical assistant know the criteria for the different types of urine collection and the processing procedures?*

STOOL COLLECTION

The way **stool** specimens are transported depends on what testing is to be performed. For tests requiring an unpreserved stool specimen, the collection of feces (stool) should be done with a clean container that is not contaminated by urine, menstrual blood, or water. One method is to insert a paper plate in the toilet bowl and then transfer the stool to a smaller container. The type of container supplied by the laboratory will depend on the test being performed. Unpreserved stool specimens should be placed in a sterile container. No special patient preparation is usually required. See Procedure 39-4 in Chapter 39 for instructing the patient on collection of a stool sample.

Ova and Parasites

A special kit with two or three collection tubes is needed for ova and parasite collection. Each container has a different type of fixative (Figure 40-9). Each container is filled to the fill line on the label with stool from the initial collection container. Once filled, the container is closed, mixed, labeled with the patient's name, and kept at room temperature or refrigerated until testing occurs.

PATIENT-CENTERED PROFESSIONALISM

- *Why would the medical assistant instruct the patient not to let the stool specimen become contaminated with urine, menstrual blood, or water?*

Introduction to the Physician's Office Laboratory   **CHAPTER 40**   919

PROCEDURE 40-8: Instruct a Patient in the Collection of a Midstream Clean-Catch Urine Specimen

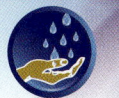

TASK: Instruct a patient in the correct method for obtaining a midstream clean-catch urine specimen.

EQUIPMENT AND SUPPLIES
- Midstream urine collection kit

or
- Sterile specimen container
- 3 antiseptic towelettes

SKILLS/RATIONALE

STANDARD PRECAUTIONS ARE TO BE FOLLOWED.

1. **Procedural Step. Sanitize the hands.**
   An alcohol-based hand rub may be used instead of washing hands with soap and water, unless hands are visibly soiled.
   Rationale. Hand sanitization promotes infection control.

2. **Procedural Step. Assemble equipment and supplies and verify the order.**
   Rationale. It is important to have all supplies and equipment ready and available before starting any procedure to ensure efficiency.

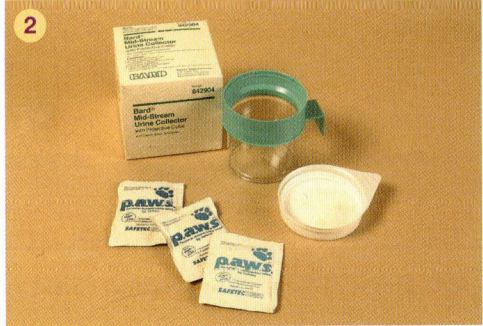

3. **Procedural Step. Greet the patient, introduce yourself, and confirm the patient's identity.**
   Rationale. Identifying the patient ensures the procedure is performed on the correct patient.

4. **Procedural Step. Explain the procedure to the patient.**
   Rationale. Explaining the procedure to the patient promotes cooperation and provides a means of obtaining implied consent.

5. **Procedural Step. Label the container with the patient's name and clinic identification number.**

6. **Procedural Step. Instruct the patient to wash and dry his or her hands.**

7. **Procedural Step. Instruct the patient to loosen the top of the collection container, being careful not to touch the inside of the container or lid and to place the sterile surface of the lid up.**
   Rationale. The container is sterile. Touching the inside of the container and lid will cause contamination and possibly produce inaccurate test results.

8. **Procedural Step. Provide the patient with written and verbal instructions.**

FEMALE PATIENT

a. Remove undergarments and be seated on the toilet.
b. Expose the urinary opening by spreading the folds of skin (labia) apart with one hand.
c. While holding the labia apart with one hand, use the other hand to cleanse the area around the opening by wiping each side once from front to back with a separate antiseptic wipe. The third wipe should be used to wipe directly across the opening from front to back.
   Rationale. The microorganisms from the genital area must be removed by cleansing with an antiseptic solution. Cleansing from front to back prevents microorganisms from the surrounding perineal and anal region from being drawn into the area that is clean.
d. Continue to hold the labia apart until the specimen has been collected.
e. Begin collection by voiding a small amount of urine into the toilet.
   Rationale. Voiding a small amount flushes microorganisms out of the distal urethra.
f. Instruct the patient to collect 1 ounce of urine by voiding into the sterile container (approximately two-thirds full), being careful not to touch the inside of the container.
   Rationale. Touching the inside of the container will contaminate it with microorganisms that normally reside on the skin.
g. Void the remaining urine into the toilet.
h. Wipe the area dry with a tissue.
i. Replace the sterile lid onto the container. Do not touch the inside of the lid.
   Rationale. Touching the inside of the lid may introduce contaminants into the urine specimen.
j. Wipe the outside of the cup as needed and leave the container on the counter, deliver it through the pass-through window into the laboratory, or hand it to the medical assistant, depending on office policy.
k. Discard the wipes, the kit, and everything else from the kit in a waste receptacle.

Continued

PROCEDURE 40-8 Instruct a Patient in the Collection of a Midstream Clean-Catch Urine Specimen—cont'd

l. Wash hands with soap and water. Return to the examination room.

MALE PATIENT
a. Expose the head of the penis. If the foreskin is in place, it should be retracted and held back until after the specimen has been collected.
b. Cleanse the area around the urethral opening by wiping each side once from top to bottom with a separate antiseptic wipe. The third wipe should be used to wipe directly across the opening from top to bottom. Cleansing from top to bottom prevents microorganisms from the surrounding region from being drawn into the area that is clean.
c. Begin collection by voiding a small amount of urine into the toilet.
   Rationale. Voiding a small amount flushes microorganisms out of the distal urethra.
d. Instruct the patient to then collect 1 ounce of urine by voiding into the sterile container (approximately two-thirds full), being careful not to touch the inside of the container.
   Rationale. Touching the inside of the container will contaminate it with microorganisms that normally reside on the skin.
e. Void the remaining urine into the toilet.
f. Replace the sterile lid onto the container. Do not touch the inside of the lid.
   Rationale. Touching the inside of the lid may introduce contaminants into the urine specimen.
g. Wipe the outside of the cup as needed and leave the container on the counter, deliver it through the pass-through window into the laboratory, or hand it to the medical assistant, depending on office policy.
h. Discard the wipes, the kit, and everything else from the kit in a waste receptacle.
i. Wash the hands with soap and water. Return to the examination room.

PROCEDURE 40-9 Instruct a Patient in the Collection of a 24-Hour Urine Specimen

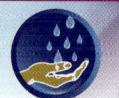

TASKS: Instruct a patient in the correct method for obtaining a 24-hour urine specimen. Send the urine specimen to the laboratory for processing.

EQUIPMENT AND SUPPLIES
- Large urine collection container
- Smaller container/toilet hat
- Written instruction sheet
- Laboratory requisition
- Patient's medical record

SKILLS/RATIONALE

STANDARD PRECAUTIONS ARE TO BE FOLLOWED.

COLLECTING THE SPECIMEN
1. **Procedural Step. Sanitize the hands.**
   An alcohol-based hand rub may be used instead of washing hands with soap and water, unless hands are visibly soiled.
   Rationale. Hand sanitization promotes infection control.

2. **Procedural Step. Assemble equipment and supplies and verify the order.**
   Rationale. It is important to have all supplies and equipment ready and available before starting any procedure to ensure efficiency.

Continued

PROCEDURE 40-9 Instruct a Patient in the Collection of a 24-Hour Urine Specimen—cont'd

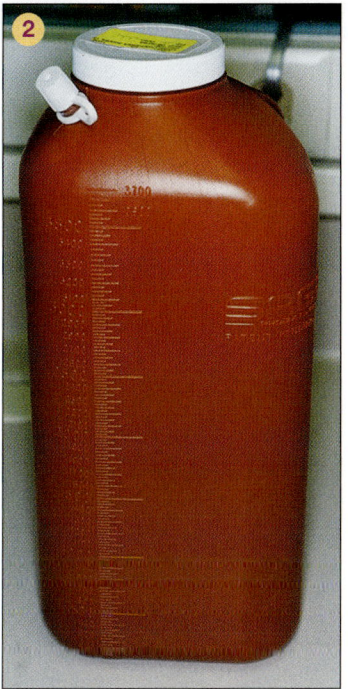

3. **Procedural Step.** Greet the patient, introduce yourself, and confirm the patient's identity.
   Rationale. Identifying the patient ensures the procedure is performed on the correct patient.
4. **Procedural Step.** Explain the procedure to the patient.
   Instruct the patient to consume their normal amounts of fluid for the duration of the procedure, except for the consumption of alcoholic beverages. Inform the patient there are no diet restrictions.
   Rationale. Explaining the procedure to the patient promotes cooperation and provides a means of obtaining implied consent. Intake of normal fluid amounts will provide more accurate information on the patient's normal output of urine.
5. **Procedural Step.** Provide the patient with the collection container and written instructions.
   Chart this information in the patient's medical record.
6. **Procedural Step.** Provide verbal and written instructions to the patient for collection of the specimen.
   a. On the first morning of the collection, empty the bladder as usual and note the time. Do not collect this first sample.
   b. Collect the next specimen either in a specified collection container (toilet hat or quart container) or directly into the large, plastic collection container.
   Some facilities will provide the patient with a "toilet hat" that can be placed over the toilet basin and under the seat, for ease of collection. The specimen is then transferred into the larger 24-hour collection container.
   Rationale. The specified collection container must be large enough to accommodate the entire amount of the specimen, since the goal is to collect all urine for a 24-hour period. If the patient forgets to collect a specimen or spills some of the urine, the collection must begin again the next morning.
   NOTE: Instruct patient to retrieve another container if the collection must be restarted.
   c. Instruct the patient to replace the lid on the large collection container and place the container in a refrigerator or cold ice chest. Some 24-hour urine collection containers are packaged with a urine preservative in the bottom of the collection container, so refrigeration of the specimen is not needed. If this is the case, instruct the patient not to remove the preservative. It must be left in the container.
   Rationale. The specimen must be kept cold or a preservative must be added to slow down the growth of bacteria and decomposition of the urine.
   d. Instruct the patient to repeat Steps b and c each time they urinate.
   e. Inform the patient that the urine specimen must only be collected in the specified container, and that all urine must be collected for the 24-hour period.
   Rationale. If the patient collects the specimen in nonspecified containers, there is a risk of contamination of the specimen. There is also the risk that the container will not be large enough to contain the entire specimen. It is important that every drop be collected.
   NOTE: If a 24-hour specimen collection has been ordered for a child, the parent or guardian must ensure that if the child wets the bed, the procedure is restarted the following morning.
   f. On the second morning, the patient should wake at the same time as the first morning and collect this last specimen in the container.
   Rationale. This provides an exact 24-hour specimen collection.
   g. Instruct the patient to secure the lid on the collection container and return the specimen to the physician's office the same morning of the last specimen collection.

PROCESSING THE SPECIMEN
7. **Procedural Step.** When the patient returns the specimen, ask the patient whether he or she encountered any difficulties during the 24-hour collection process.
   If problems were encountered that resulted in failure to collect the entire specimen, inform the patient that the procedure must be repeated starting the next morning. If this is the case, provide the patient with a second collection container and review the collection process with the patient again. Pay particular attention to any areas that created difficulties during the first collection process.

Continued

PROCEDURE 40-9 Instruct a Patient in the Collection of a 24-Hour Urine Specimen—cont'd

Rationale. *Because one component of the test requires measuring the quantity of urine, it must be stressed to the patient to follow the exact collection process and collect every specimen.*

8. **Procedural Step.** Prepare the specimen for transport to the laboratory.

   Complete a laboratory requisition form and label the specimen container. If the collection container does not already contain a preservative, one may be added to the specimen before transport to the laboratory. The laboratory will provide instructions if a preservative needs to be added.

9. **Procedural Step.** Document the results.

   Include the date and time, the type of specimen, and information on sending the specimen to the laboratory.

CHARTING EXAMPLES

Date	
1/26/xx	10:00 a.m. Container and verbal/written instructions provided to patient for 24-hour urine specimen collection. ————————— C. Miller, CMA (AAMA)
1/28/xx	10:00 a.m. 24-hour urine specimen sent to Medical Laboratory Corp. for creatinine clearance. ————————— C. Miller, CMA (AAMA)

Photo for Step 2 from Young AP, Proctor DB: Kinn's the medical assistant, ed 10, St Louis, 2007, Saunders

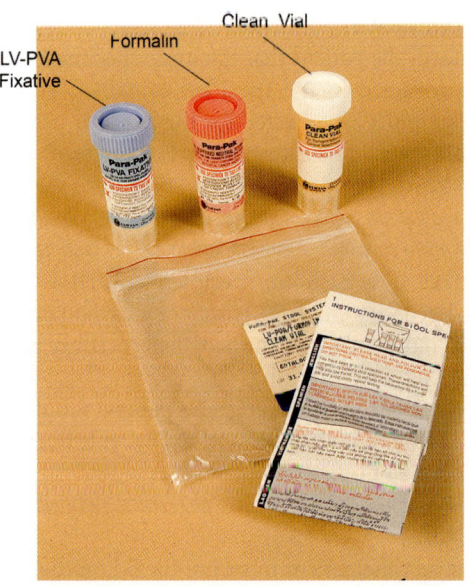

FIGURE 40-9 Ova and parasite collection containers.

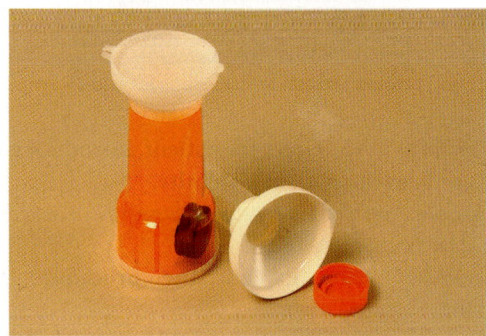

FIGURE 40-10 Sterile collection container for a sputum specimen.

PATIENT-CENTERED PROFESSIONALISM

- Why is it important for the medical assistant to understand proper collection technique for a sputum collection?

SPUTUM COLLECTION

Sputum is the secretion from the lungs produced in the bronchi and throat. To collect a sputum specimen, the patient is first asked to rinse the mouth to remove food particles. Then the patient is instructed to take three deep breaths and cough deeply "from the lungs." The specimen should be thick, colored, and sticky and is collected into a wide-mouthed container for culture and sensitivity testing (Figure 40-10). On awakening in the morning is an ideal time for collecting a specimen because the patient has not yet cleared the respiratory passages. Sputum testing is often done to rule out tuberculosis or determine the presence of blood (hemoptysis).

CONCLUSION

Medical assistants are often involved in the collection, preparation for transport, and processing of the many types of specimens collected at the POL. The physician can analyze specimens collected from a patient to assess the patient's general health, as well as to diagnose and determine treatment plans.

The medical assistant must understand and follow federal, state, and office protocols for collecting and transporting specimens. These protocols help ensure that accurate results are obtained from testing. Accurate test results are crucial.

Errors in specimen collection can cause delays in testing, diagnosis, and treatment or even lawsuits in some situations. The knowledgeable, skilled medical assistant helps protect the patient and the medical office by performing all procedures accurately, efficiently, and in accordance with all guidelines and protocols.

Chapter Summary

Reinforce your understanding of the material in this chapter by reviewing the curriculum objectives and key content points below.

1. **Define, appropriately use, and spell all the Key Terms for this chapter.**
   - Review the Key Terms if necessary.
2. **Explain the purpose of the Clinical Laboratory Improvement Amendments of 1988 (CLIA 88).**
   - CLIA 88 sets minimum performance standards for laboratories and defines three levels of complexity for performing laboratory testing.
3. **List three factors that determine whether a medical office will perform and process a specimen.**
   - The type of practice, the cost-effectiveness of the test, and the level of complexity of the test determine whether a medical office will perform and process a specimen or have the testing done elsewhere.
4. **Briefly describe three CLIA-waived urine tests, six CLIA-waived blood tests, and seven CLIA-waived tests of other types.**
   - Review Table 40-1.
5. **Differentiate between quality assurance (QA) and quality control (QC) and briefly explain how each is accomplished in the medical office.**
   - QA is designed to monitor and evaluate the quality of test results as processed by personnel.
   - QC is a process that provides the means to ensure that test results are accurate as processed by the equipment.
6. **Demonstrate the correct procedure for using methods of QC.**
   - Review Procedure 40-1.
7. **Explain the need for safety precautions in the medical office laboratory and how they protect both staff and patients.**
   - Safety precautions help prevent cross-contamination from worker to patient and from patient to patient, and help protect employees from exposure to potentially biohazardous materials from patients' body fluids.
8. **Identify the parts of a compound microscope, and explain its proper use and maintenance.**
   - A microscope consists of a stand (arm and base), magnification system (objectives), stage, and light source.
   - Understanding magnification, stage use, light source function, and how to focus the microscope allows the medical assistant to use it properly.
   - Microscopes must be properly maintained to keep them in optimal working order by cleaning all nonglass surfaces using a soft cloth, using lens paper to clean all lenses, placing the microscope in a protective covering or cabinet for storage, holding the arm firmly during transport, and cleaning the oil-immersion lens with a special cleaner.
9. **Demonstrate the procedure for successfully focusing a microscope from lower to higher power.**
   - Review Procedure 40-2.
10. **Explain the purpose and proper use of a centrifuge.**
    - A centrifuge separates solid material from liquid through forced gravity.
    - The separation of materials allows all parts of a specimen to be studied.
    - Always counterbalance the centrifuge with tubes on opposite sides with the same specimen or a tube of equal size and shape and amount of fluid.
    - Always follow the manufacturer's instructions for use and care of the centrifuge.
11. **List six categories of laboratory tests and briefly explain the purpose of each.**
    - Chemistry tests are performed on serum, plasma, urine, spinal fluid, and other body fluids to test levels of chemicals (e.g., glucose, cholesterol, electrolytes, proteins, or drugs).
    - Hematology (and coagulation) studies assess formed elements of whole blood (white and red blood cells, platelets) in a blood sample.
    - Microbiology tests are performed on various body fluids to study bacteria, fungi, viruses, and parasites.
    - Serology tests are performed on serum to study the body's immune responses by detecting antibody and antigen reactions.
    - Blood bank tests involve studies for ABO blood groupings, Rh typing, and crossmatching of blood for surgical patients.
    - Urinalysis studies the physical, chemical, and microscopic structure of urine.
    - Medical assistants perform some, but not all, of these laboratory tests.
12. **Explain the importance of effective patient preparation before laboratory tests are performed.**
    - Effective patient preparation helps ensure the accuracy of test results.
    - Patients should be given time to ask questions, and medical assistants should make certain that patients understand all instructions.
13. **Explain the importance of completing a laboratory request form accurately.**
    - Incorrect paperwork can cause a laboratory test to be delayed or not run at all.
    - An inaccurate laboratory request form may result in the wrong test being completed.
14. **Demonstrate the procedure for accurately completing a laboratory request form.**
    - Review Procedure 40-3.

15. **List three methods of specimen collection, and explain the need for collecting specimens accurately.**
    - Three ways to collect specimens include collection and testing at the office, collecting at the office and testing at an outside laboratory, and collecting and testing at an outside laboratory.
    - Accurate collection of the specimen helps ensure the sample will produce accurate test results.
16. **Demonstrate the procedure for accurately collecting a specimen for transport to an outside laboratory.**
    - Review Procedure 40-4.
17. **Explain the purpose of a laboratory report and why it must be accurate and transmitted to the physician in a timely manner.**
    - The laboratory report assists the physician in diagnosis.
    - When the laboratory report is accurate and on time, the physician can make a more accurate, timely diagnosis.
18. **Demonstrate the correct procedure for screening and following up on patient test results.**
    - Review Procedure 40-5.
19. **Demonstrate the correct procedure for collecting an uncontaminated throat specimen to test for group A beta-hemolytic streptococci.**
    - Review Procedure 40-6.
20. **Explain the purpose of a urinalysis and the need for avoiding sources of contamination and for processing urine specimens in the required time.**
    - Urinalysis can detect kidney disease, infections in the urinary tract, and other disease states of the body.
    - Contamination of a specimen makes test results less accurate.
    - Processing of urine specimens must be done in a timely manner as bacteria will multiply rapidly unless the specimen is refrigerated (or a preservative is used).
21. **List four instructions the medical assistant should give to a patient who is to collect a random urine specimen and bring it to the medical office.**
    - Purpose of the collection.
    - Importance of not touching the inside of the container.
    - First morning specimen is best.
    - Urine specimen should be refrigerated until it can be transported.
22. **Demonstrate the correct procedure for obtaining a urine specimen from an infant using a pediatric urine collector.**
    - Review Procedure 40-7.
23. **Demonstrate the correct procedure for providing patient instructions on collecting a midstream clean-catch urine specimen to ensure validity of test results.**
    - Review Procedure 40-8.
24. **Demonstrate the correct procedure for providing patient instructions on collecting a 24-hour urine specimen to ensure validity of test results.**
    - Review Procedure 40-9.
25. **Explain the special considerations for handling drug screenings and specimens that may be used as evidence in a court of law.**
    - Chain of custody regulations specify how evidence should be collected and handled.
    - Chain of evidence regulations specify how every detail of a forensic investigation should be handled from beginning to end.
26. **Explain the considerations for collecting stool specimens.**
    - A clean container (no urine, menstrual blood, or water) should be used to collect a stool sample.
    - No special patient preparation is necessary.
    - The type of container depends on the type of test being done.
27. **Demonstrate the correct procedure for the collection of stool specimens.**
    - Review Procedure 30-4 in Chapter 30.
28. **Explain the considerations for collecting sputum specimens.**
    - Sputum specimens are used for culture and sensitivity testing.
    - A good time for sputum collection is after awakening in the morning.
29. **Analyze a realistic medical office situation and apply your understanding of the purpose and use of the physician office laboratory to determine the best course of action.**
    - Medical assistants must understand and follow the procedures and policies associated with each laboratory procedure they perform.
    - Proper patient preparation is an important aspect of laboratory testing.
30. **Describe the impact on patient care when medical assistants have a solid understanding of the processes and procedures used to collect specimens for testing in the medical office.**
    - Accurate test results occur when the medical assistant properly collects or provides clear instructions to the patient for collection and follows proper processing procedures.
    - Patient care is enhanced when the medical assistant is knowledgeable about proper procedures for collecting and processing specimens.
    - Diagnosis and treatment of a patient begins sooner when test results are accurate.

PRACTICAL APPLICATIONS

If you have accomplished the objectives in this chapter, you will be able to make better choices as a medical assistant. Take another look at this situation and decide what you would do.

The full-time laboratory technician at Dr. Macinto's office is on sick leave for a week. Dr. Macinto asks Sherri, a medical assistant, to fill in for the sick technician. Sherri has just been hired from another office, where she was trained by the physician. She has not done laboratory tests and has not prepared patients for laboratory work.

On the first day, Dr. Macinto asks Sherri to collect a midstream urine sample on a patient for a culture and sensitivity and to send some of the urine to an outside laboratory for a drug screen. Sherri hands the urine collection container to the patient without any instructions and allows the patient to go to the bathroom alone to collect the specimen. When the specimen is collected, Sherri leaves the drug screen on the counter to await the arrival of the laboratory courier for transport to the outside laboratory. Neither Sherri nor the courier signs for the specimen. Furthermore, the laboratory form is not complete, and no documentation was made of the collection of the specimen.

What things would you have done differently in this situation?

1. What instructions should Sherri have given the patient for preparation for a midstream urine specimen?
2. How should urine for a drug screen be collected? What was the problem with leaving the specimen on the counter for the laboratory courier to collect?
3. Would the results of the test have been acceptable in a court case or to an employer who desired this information before hiring the person?
4. What is the difference between quality control and quality assurance? Is Dr. Macinto's office practicing quality assurance when Sherri is working in the laboratory?
5. Why is quality control so important when performing laboratory tests?
6. What is Dr. Macinto's responsibility in regard to Sherri's actions?

WEB SEARCH

1. **Research the history of the microscope.** The microscope is a valuable instrument in the physician office laboratory.

- **Keywords:** Use the following keywords in your search: microscope, electron microscope.

41 Phlebotomy

evolve http://evolve.elsevier.com/klieger/medicalassisting

The primary purpose of phlebotomy is to obtain blood specimens for diagnostic testing and it is performed by either venipuncture or capillary puncture. The medical assistant is often responsible for the collection of blood for laboratory analysis and point-of-care-testing (POCT). Manual dexterity, good communication and organizational skills, and a thorough knowledge of laboratory test requirements are expected of the medical assistant responsible for this function. The medical assistant must perform these tasks with confidence and expertise to ensure patient comfort, and it should be remembered that this skill requires patience and practice.

LEARNING OBJECTIVES

You will be able to do the following after completing this chapter:

Key Terms
1. Define, appropriately use, and spell all the Key Terms for this chapter.

Blood Collection
2. List methods of collecting blood and give the three factors that determine which method will be used.
3. Explain the purpose of a lancet in capillary blood collection.
4. Briefly describe five types of containers that can be used to collect capillary blood specimens.
5. Demonstrate the correct procedure for obtaining a capillary blood specimen acceptable for testing using the ring or middle finger.
6. Demonstrate the correct procedure for collecting a capillary specimen for phenylketonuria (PKU) screening using filter paper.
7. List four acceptable sites for performing venipuncture and the two factors in selecting the site.
8. State two reasons for failed venipuncture draws.
9. List the order of draw for the evacuated-tube (Vacutainer) system recommended by the Clinical and Laboratory Standards Institute (CLSI).
10. Demonstrate the correct procedure for obtaining a venous blood specimen acceptable for testing using the evacuated-tube system.
11. Demonstrate the correct procedure for obtaining a venous blood specimen acceptable for testing using the syringe method.
12. Demonstrate the correct procedure for obtaining a venous blood specimen acceptable for testing using the butterfly method.
13. Demonstrate the correct procedure for successfully separating serum from a blood specimen and transferring the serum from the collection tube to a transfer tube.

Patient-Centered Professionalism
14. Analyze a realistic medical office situation and apply your understanding of the purpose and use of the physician office laboratory to determine the best course of action.
15. Describe the impact on patient care when medical assistants have a solid understanding of the processes and procedures used to collect specimens for testing in the medical office.

KEY TERMS

bacteremia
blood bank
blood culture
butterfly method
capillary puncture
capillary collection tube
chemistry
Clinical Laboratory Improvement Amendments of 1988 (CLIA 88)
cultures
Cuvette
evacuated tube
evacuation blood collection system
filter paper
glass slides
hematology
hemoconcentration
heparin
lancet
microcontainers
multisample needles

Continued

order of draw
phlebotomy
pipette
pipetted
plasma
quantity not sufficient (QNS)
serology
serum
single-sample needles
syringe method
Vacutainer
vacuum tube
venipuncture
winged infusion set

TABLE 41-1
Typical CLIA-Waived Tests

Waived Tests	Use
BLOOD	
ESR (nonautomated)	Screening for inflammatory activity
Hemoglobin test: copper sulfate (nonautomated)	Monitors hemoglobin level in blood
Spun microhematocrit, blood count	Screening for anemia
Blood glucose level by monitoring device approved by FDA for home use	Monitors blood glucose level
Hemoglobin test by analytical instrument providing direct readout	Monitors hemoglobin level in blood; measures concentration of hemoglobin A_{1c} in blood, indicating glucose levels over a 3-month period
Hematocrit	Screening for anemia
OTHER	
Serum cholesterol and HDL	Total cholesterol monitoring
Prothrombin time	Evaluates anticoagulant effect

ESR, Erythrocyte sedimentation rate; *FDA*, Food and Drug Administration; *HDL*, high-density lipoprotein.

PRACTICAL APPLICATIONS

Read the following scenario and keep it in mind as you learn about the POL.

The full-time laboratory technician at Dr. Macinto's office is on sick leave for another week. Dr. Macinto asks Sherri, a medical assistant, to continue to fill in for the sick technician. Remember, Sherri had just been hired from another office, where she was trained by the physician. She has not done laboratory tests and has not prepared patients for laboratory work.

Mrs. Gorchetzki, a postmastectomy patient, is seen next. Dr. Macinto has ordered a fasting blood sugar and a fasting blood chemistry test. Without talking to Mrs. Gorchetzki about the preparation she has made for the test, Sherri gathers the supplies for the testing. Mrs. Gorchetzki mentions that she had bacon and eggs for breakfast. Sherri draws the blood sugar using a capillary puncture. Sherri performs the testing before doing quality control for the day. When the specimen is drawn for the blood chemistry, the laboratory request form asks for serum. Sherri starts the process of drawing the venipuncture specimen from the side of the mastectomy in a heparinized tube. Mrs. Gorchetzki tries to tell Sherri to collect the specimen from the other arm because it is easier to draw blood from that arm, but Sherri does not listen.

When Sherri places the specimen in the centrifuge, she spins only one tube. She pipettes off the liquid and sends it to the laboratory. As it turns out, the liquid sent to the laboratory is plasma, but the laboratory had requested serum.

What things would you have done differently in this situation?

BLOOD COLLECTION

Two methods of collecting a blood specimen performed in a medical office are capillary puncture and venipuncture. The method selected depends on the test to be performed (e.g., point-of-care testing [POCT], hemoglobin, or cholesterol) and the age and condition of the patient (e.g., infant, elderly adult with poor veins or weak veins). Table 41-1 provides those tests from blood specimens that are waived by the **Clinical Laboratory Improvement Amendments of 1988 (CLIA 88)**.

Capillary puncture is a skin (dermal) puncture to obtain a capillary blood sample. When a small sample of blood is required (e.g., for a self-monitoring glucose test), the capillary puncture is the method of choice. Capillary puncture also is often the preferred choice for infants and elderly patients, since drawing blood by venipuncture in these age groups may be difficult and could cause damage to veins and surrounding tissue.

Venipuncture is a puncture of a vein to obtain a venous blood sample. A larger quantity of blood can be drawn with a venipuncture, and this is the method of choice when several tests are ordered, or a larger amount of blood is needed.

Capillary Puncture

The most common sites for the collection of a capillary puncture are the lateral sides of the ring and middle fingers, and the outer borders of the heel (medial and lateral plantar) for infants (Figure 41-1). These sites are very vascular, and when punctured adequately, enough blood will be available to perform the ordered tests.

Poor collection techniques can alter the laboratory findings and therefore make the results useless.

- Avoid squeezing the area around the puncture site; this can also alter the results.
- To improve circulation before puncturing, the area can be warmed (e.g., moist heat, massaged or "milked," or warmed by having patients wash their hands in warm water).
- Callused and scarred areas should be avoided because they are difficult to puncture.
- Areas that are edematous (swollen) or cyanotic (bluish) should also be avoided because blood obtained from these areas usually does not produce accurate test results.

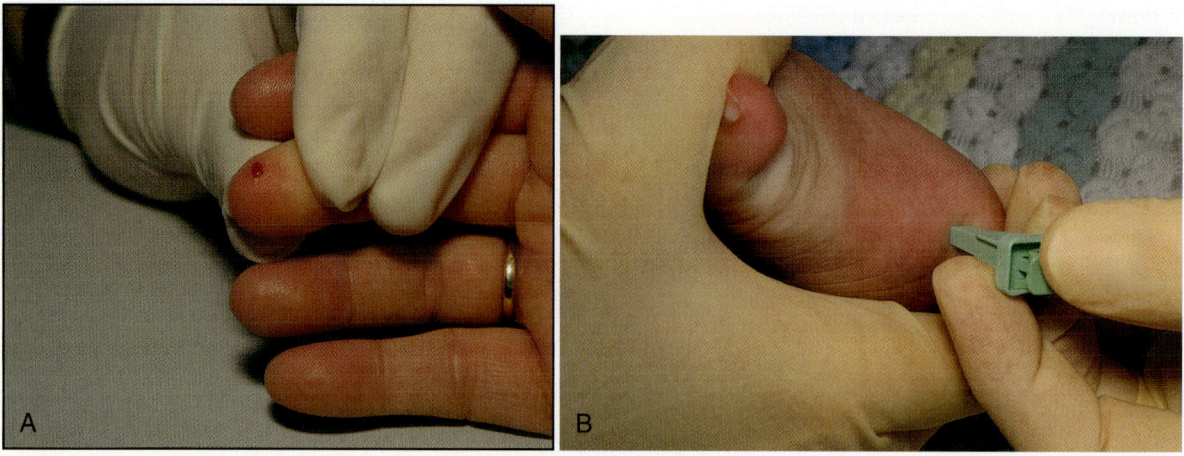

FIGURE 41-1 Capillary puncture sites. **A,** Fingertips. **B,** Infant's heel. (From Chester GA: *Modern medical assisting*, Philadelphia, 1998, Saunders.)

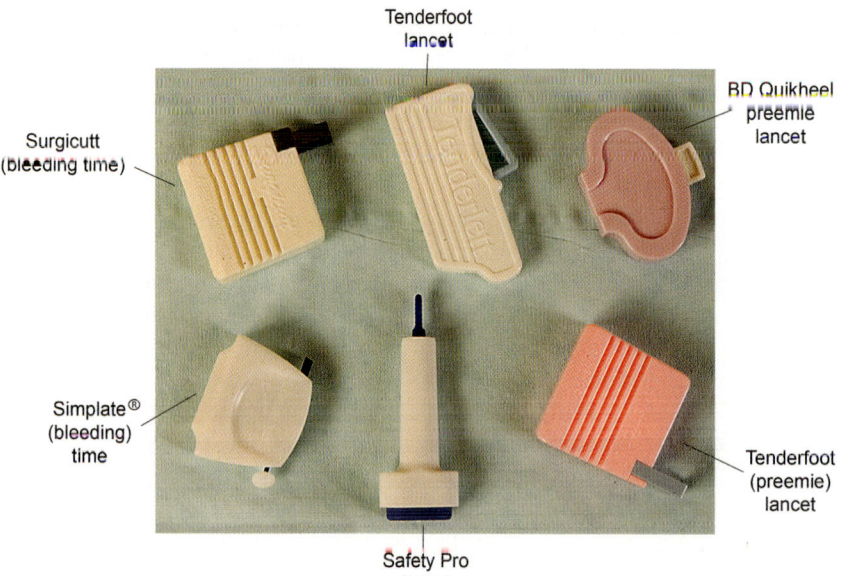

FIGURE 41-2 Adult and pediatric lancets.

Puncture Devices

A **lancet** is a small, sterile, needle-like piece of metal used to make a small puncture in the skin (dermis). Lancets are constructed to penetrate the skin at various depths depending on the type of patient (e.g., infant, child, or adult). For example, a lancet for an infant usually has an incision depth of 1 mm, whereas a lancet for an adult is larger and provides a deeper incision. The depth of a lancet should never be 3 mm or greater because this can cause inflammation in the site or accidental contact with the bone. Care must be taken to maintain the sterility of the lancet to prevent the accidental introduction of microorganisms into the puncture site. Skin punctures require a sterile device because the skin is broken.

Lancets are disposable and can be manual (pushing the point of a lancet into the skin), retractable or spring-loaded (depressing a plunger to force the blade into the skin and then retract it), or a reusable semiautomatic device. An example of a reusable semiautomatic lancet device is the Glucolet II (Bayer Corporation, Tarrytown, NY). A disposable lancet is placed in a spring-loaded holder, and a release button is depressed. The skin is penetrated to a depth that is determined by the lancet blade size. The lancet holder is reusable, whereas the lancet is used only one time. These devices are intended mostly for single users such as diabetic patients who perform their own skin punctures. Spring-loaded lancet devices in the medical office most often have a retractable blade, and some lock after use to prevent accidental reuse. Figure 41-2 illustrates varies types of adult and pediatric lancets. The type of lancet device used depends on the age of the patient and the amount of blood required. Immediately after use, lancets are discarded in the sharps container.

Collection Containers

Capillary blood specimens can be collected in and on a variety of microcollection devices, including microcontainers, capillary tubes, glass slides, cuvettes, or filter paper (used for phenylketonuria [PKU] testing), and other types of collection devices particular to a testing system (Figures 41-3 and 41-4).

- **Microcontainers** are small plastic tubes with a funnel-like top into which blood flows. These tubes use color-coded stoppers to identify the type of additive and laboratory use.
- **Capillary collection tubes** can be either plastic or glass-coated (although glass-coated tubes are not frequently used because of breakage) and are plain or contain **heparin** to prevent clotting.
- **Glass slides** can be used to collect a capillary blood sample for microscopic review.

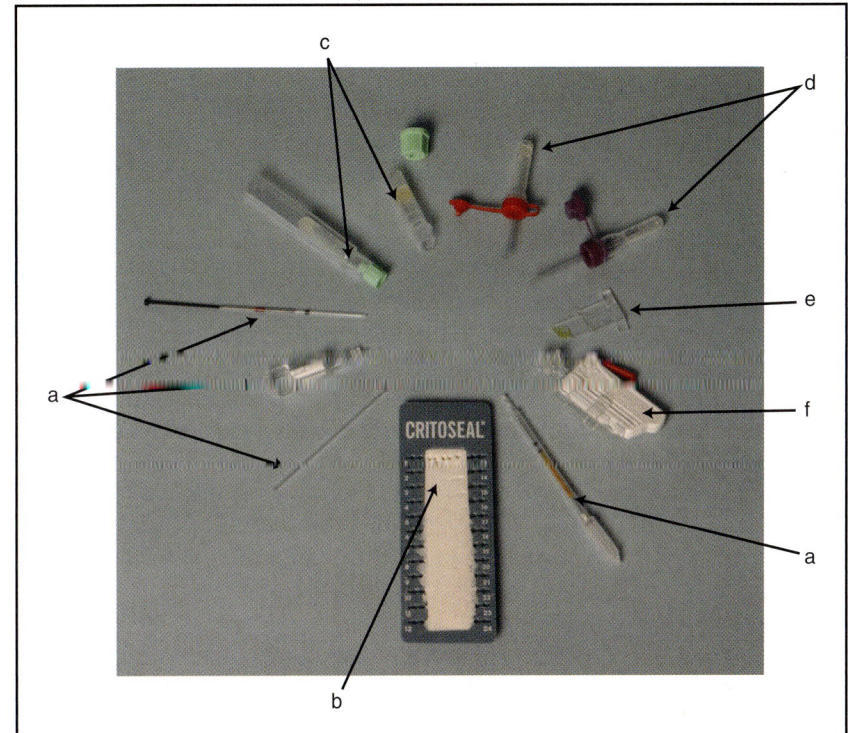

FIGURE 41-3 Collection devices used for capillary puncture specimens. *a*, Capillary collecting tubes; *b*, sealant for capillary tubes; *c*, Microtainers with color-coded lids; *d*, Microtainers with capillary tubes; *e*, cuvette; *f*, collection cup and lancet for protime testing. (From Garrels M, Oatis C: *Laboratory testing for ambulatory settings*, St Louis, 2006, Saunders.)

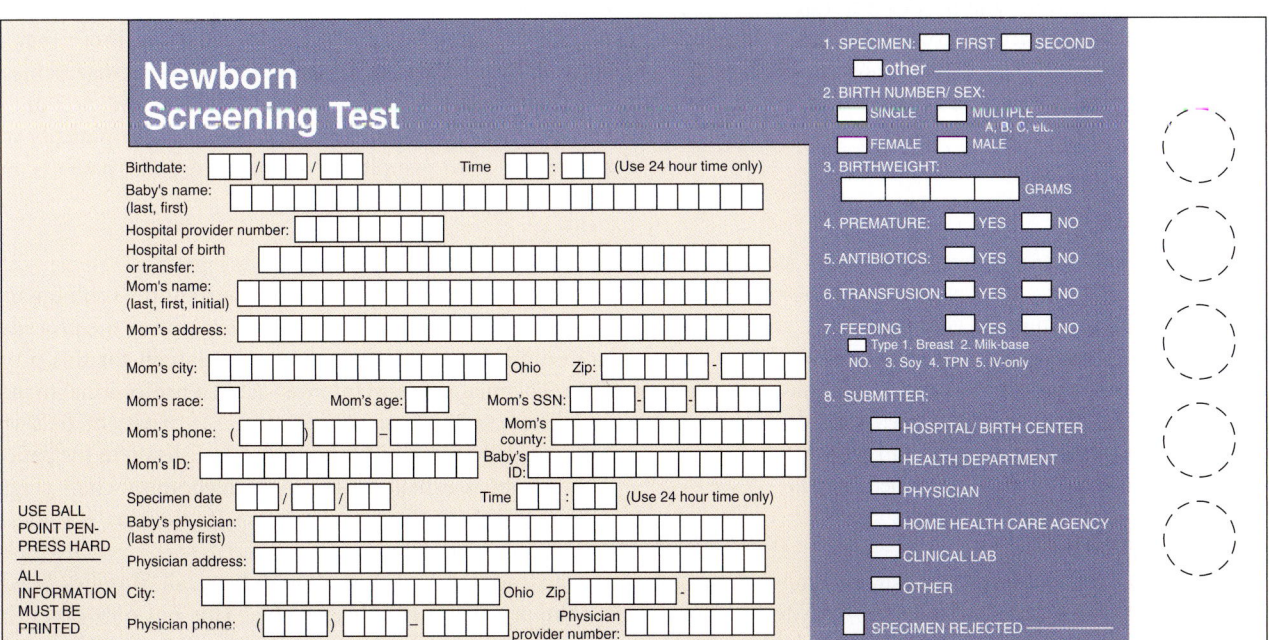

FIGURE 41-4 Example of filter paper used in PKU screening. (From Bonewit-West K: *Clinical procedures for medical assistants*, ed 7, St Louis, 2008, Saunders.)

- **Filter paper** can be used to blot an incised area to test for bleeding time or to collect a blood sample for PKU testing.
- **Cuvette** is a collection device used to hold specimens for spectroscopic readings (e.g., HemoCue).

Patient Preparation

Medical assistants need to know how to prepare the patient for a capillary puncture, as follows:

1. Gently massage the area to be punctured to increase blood circulation.
2. Cleanse the site with an alcohol wipe and allow to air-dry or wipe dry with a sterile gauze square.
3. When using the finger, puncture the skin at a slight angle and to the side of the fingerprint. This should be done on the middle or ring finger of the nondominant hand. **NOTE:** Never perform a capillary puncture on the fingers of an infant less than a year old or from the fingers on the side of the body where a mastectomy has been performed, since there is a lack of lymph fluid movement on that side of the body. If the blood does not flow freely, hold the finger in a downward position, allowing gravity to help with the blood flow.
4. Do not squeeze the finger; squeezing might cause the red blood cells to *hemolyze* (break up). The blood must be free flowing.
5. Wipe away the first drop of blood with sterile gauze. This first drop of blood will contain tissue fluid and alcohol from the skin prep, which dilutes the specimen, causing the clotting process to begin and distorting test results.
6. Fill the required collection devices, and give the patient a sterile gauze square to hold against the puncture site to stop the bleeding. Apply a latex-free bandage if needed.

Procedure 41-1 outlines the proper technique for using a disposable retractable microlancet to collect a specimen in a capillary tube. Procedure 41-2 explains how to collect a capillary specimen properly for PKU screening (filter paper method).

Venipuncture

Phlebotomy, another term for venipuncture, is accomplished by drawing blood directly from a vein. This process is considered an invasive procedure. In venipuncture, a sterile 18- to 22-gauge needle is inserted into a vein to remove a large specimen of blood for diagnostic testing. Venipuncture can be performed with a needle and syringe, winged infusion set ("butterfly"), or evacuated-tube system with a tube adapter (holder) and a multidraw (double-ended) needle.

Tourniquet Application

A tourniquet is used to disrupt the flow of venous blood to make the veins more visible and palpable (easy to feel) for a venipuncture site selection. The tourniquet should be 3 to 4 inches above the intended site because the vein may collapse as blood is drawn if the tourniquet is placed closer and the

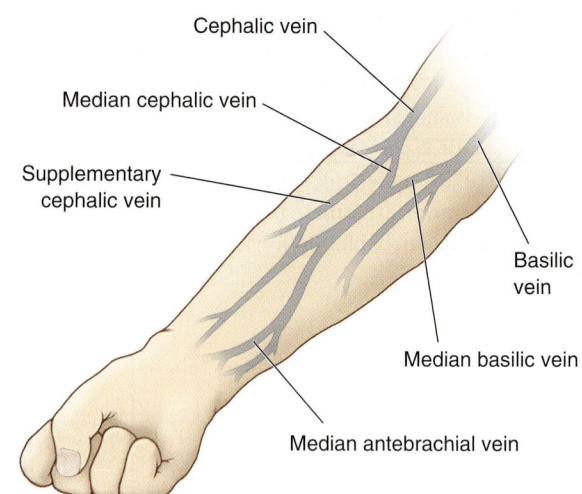

FIGURE 41-5 Veins of the arm. (From Stepp CA, Woods MA: *Laboratory procedures for medical office personnel,* Philadelphia, 1998, Saunders.)

tourniquet may become ineffective if placed farther away. The tourniquet should be positioned around the arm and should be kept flat. It should be applied tight enough to slow the venous flow without obstructing arterial flow. Applying the tourniquet too tightly or leaving it on longer than 1 minute causes blood pooling below the constricted area (see Procedure 41-3 for detailed instructions).

Venipuncture Sites

Venipuncture is usually performed at the antecubital fossa (space) of either arm. Vein selections include the median cubital, cephalic, or basilic veins of the forearm (Figure 41-5). The site depends on the age of the patient and condition of the patient's veins. The median cephalic vein is most often used for a venipuncture. Areas to avoid are those that are scarred, bruised, freckled, edematous, or otherwise damaged (e.g., tattooed). A venipuncture should never be done in an arm that has impaired circulation (e.g., in patients with stroke) or poor lymphatic drainage (e.g., in patients with mastectomy).

Patient Preparation

Patient preparation is extremely important for venipuncture. Properly identifying the patient and explaining the procedure to minimize anxiety help prepare the patient for this procedure. The medical assistant must act in a professional manner and listen to the patient's concerns. If a patient tells you, "They usually draw my blood from here," listen to the patient. The patient is usually seated in a phlebotomy chair (Figure 41-6). Ask the patient to lie down if previous episodes of fainting have occurred.

The medical assistant should have all supplies needed for the procedure readily available. This not only saves time but also projects an organized image. Having all supplies ready helps the patient feel relaxed and confident in the

Text continued on p. 940

Phlebotomy CHAPTER 41

PROCEDURE 41-1

Use a Sterile Disposable Microlancet for Skin Puncture

TASK: Obtain a capillary blood specimen acceptable for testing using the ring or middle finger.

EQUIPMENT AND SUPPLIES
- Nonsterile disposable gloves (latex-free)
- Alcohol wipe
- Sterile disposable retractable microlancet
- Sterile 2 × 2 gauze pads
- Sharps container
- Biohazardous waste container
- Bandage (latex-free)

SUPPLIES FOR ORDERED TESTS
Depending on the test ordered, the following supplies must be available (as appropriate):
- Unopette
- Microhematocrit capillary tubes
- Microcontainers
- Glass slides
- Glucometer or cholesterol device (as appropriate)
- Clay sealant tray

SKILLS/RATIONALE

STANDARD PRECAUTIONS ARE TO BE FOLLOWED.

1. **Procedural Step. Sanitize the hands.**
   Alcohol-based hand rub may be used instead of washing hands with soap and water, unless hands are visibly soiled.
   Rationale. Hand sanitization promotes infection control.

2. **Procedural Step. Assemble equipment and supplies and verify the order.**
   Depending on the test ordered and the age and size of the patient, select the lancet that will achieve the correct depth of puncture.
   Rationale. It is important to have all supplies and equipment ready and available before starting any procedure to ensure efficiency. Lancet systems come in a variety of depths; selecting the correct depth ensures that a specimen will be correctly obtained with minimal discomfort and minimal damage to the tissue or underlying bone.

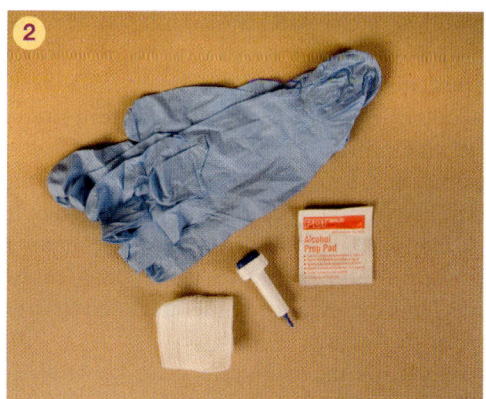

3. **Procedural Step. Greet the patient, introduce yourself, and confirm the patient's identity.**
   Rationale. Identifying the patient ensures the procedure is performed on the correct patient.

4. **Procedural Step. Explain the procedure to the patient.**
   If the test(s) ordered requires patient preparation, such as fasting or medication restrictions, confirm that the patient has followed the preparation orders. If the preparation has not been followed, inform the physician and document "noncompliance" in the patient's medical record. Reschedule the test as office policy or the physician dictates.
   Rationale. Explaining the procedure to the patient promotes cooperation and provides a means of obtaining implied consent. Test results will be inaccurate if the patient has not followed the required preparation orders.

5. **Procedural Step. Open the sterile gauze packet and place the gauze pad on the inside of its wrapper.**

6. **Procedural Step. Prepare the sterile lancet.**

7. **Procedural Step. Position the patient comfortably either sitting or lying down with the palmar surface of the hand facing up and the arm supported.**
   The patient must be positioned comfortably with the arm secure and supported. If the patient informs you that he or she faints "at the sight of blood," position the patient in a reclining position.

8. **Procedural Step. Select the appropriate puncture site.**
   The preferred site is usually the lateral tip of the ring or middle finger of the nondominant hand. Another puncture site is the medial or lateral surface of the heel of an infant.
   Rationale. The appropriate site selection will ensure adequate blood flow with minimal risk of injury to the patient.

9. **Procedural Step. Warm the site to increase blood flow.**
   If the patient's finger is cold, it can be warmed by gently massaging the finger five or six times from the base to the tip, or by placing the hand in warm water for a few minutes.
   Rationale. Blood flow will be greatly increased when the site is warm.

Continued

PROCEDURE 41-1 Use a Sterile Disposable Microlancet for Skin Puncture—cont'd

10. **Procedural Step.** Apply gloves.
11. **Procedural Step.** Cleanse the puncture site with an alcohol wipe and allow it to air-dry. Do not touch or fan the area after cleansing. Tell the patient to not touch the cleansed area.
    Rationale. Allowing the site to air-dry prevents hemolysis of the specimen from the alcohol and lessens the stinging sensation that accompanies the puncture when alcohol is introduced into the tissues. If not allowed to dry completely, alcohol residue may interfere with the accuracy of test results.

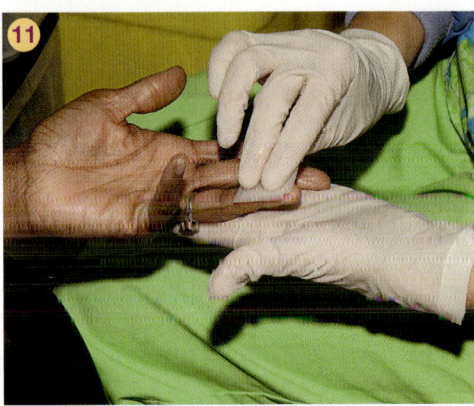

12. **Procedural Step.** While the puncture site is drying, prepare the lancet by removing the cover or tab from the end.
    Depending on the system used, the tab is either pulled straight out or twisted off.
13. **Procedural Step.** Position the lancet and perform the puncture.
    a. Hold the lancet between the first two fingers and position it firmly against the puncture site.
    b. Place the thumb on the activation button at the top of the device housing and firmly depress it to discharge the blade.
14. **Procedural Step.** Dispose of the lancet.
    When the blade is activated, it will puncture the skin and will retract automatically into the device housing. Immediately dispose of the lancet into the sharps container.
    Rationale. Proper disposal of contaminated sharps is required by the OSHA standard to prevent exposure to bloodborne pathogens.
15. **Procedural Step.** Wipe away the first drop of blood with the dry gauze.

    Rationale. The first drop of blood is not collected because it usually contains more tissue fluid than blood, which will result in an inaccurate test result.
16. **Procedural Step.** If necessary, massage the finger by applying gentle, continuous pressure from the knuckle to the puncture site to increase the blood flow.
    Do not squeeze the finger; tissue fluid will dilute the specimen. Lowering the puncture site will allow gravity to assist with the blood flow.
    NOTE: If the puncture is done correctly and at the right depth, the site will bleed properly. If not done properly, the procedure must be repeated at a new site with a new lancet. Performing the puncture correctly the first time is less traumatic to the patient.

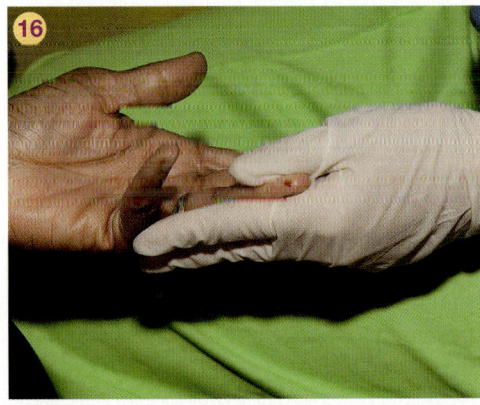

17. **Procedural Step.** Allow a second well-rounded drop of blood to form and quickly collect the specimen in the correct manner for the test(s) ordered.
    Rationale. Rapid collection is necessary to prevent coagulation.
18. **Procedural Step.** After the sample has been collected, apply pressure with a sterile gauze square directly over the puncture site.
19. **Procedural Step.** Bandage the puncture site.
    Check the puncture site to make sure it has stopped bleeding, and bandage it with a latex-free bandage to protect the wound. Discard any contaminated materials in the appropriate biohazardous waste container.
20. **Procedural Step.** Remove gloves and sanitize the hands before transporting the specimen to the laboratory for processing.
    Always sanitize the hands after every procedure or after using gloves.

Phlebotomy CHAPTER 41 933

PROCEDURE 41-2 Collect a Blood Specimen for a Phenylketonuria (PKU) Screening Test

TASK: Properly collect a capillary specimen to be used for PKU screening.

EQUIPMENT AND SUPPLIES
- Nonsterile disposable gloves (latex-free)
- Personal protective equipment (PPE)
- Sterile disposable retractable microlancet (lancet must be less than 2.4 mm in length)
- Infant heel warmer or warm compress
- PKU test card and mailing envelope
- Alcohol wipe
- Sharps container
- Biohazardous waste container
- Sterile 2 × 2 gauze pads
- Bandage (latex-free)
- Laboratory requisition form
- Patient's medical record

SKILLS/RATIONALE

STANDARD PRECAUTIONS ARE TO BE FOLLOWED.

1. **Procedural Step. Sanitize the hands.**
   An alcohol-based hand rub may be used instead of washing hands with soap and water, unless hands are visibly soiled.
   Rationale. Hand sanitization promotes infection control.

2. **Procedural Step. Assemble equipment and supplies and verify the order.**
   Select the lancet that will achieve the correct depth of puncture for the PKU screening test.
   Rationale. It is important to have all supplies and equipment ready and available before starting any procedure to ensure efficiency.

3. **Procedural Step. Greet the infant's parent or guardian, introduce yourself, and confirm the patient's identity.**
   Rationale. Identifying the infant and the infant's parent or guardian ensures the procedure is performed on the correct patient.

4. **Procedural Step. Explain the procedure to the child's parent or guardian.**
   Rationale. Explaining the procedure to the infant's parent or guardian promotes cooperation and provides a means of obtaining implied consent.

5. **Procedural Step. Open the sterile gauze packet and place the gauze pad on the inside of its wrapper.**

6. **Procedural Step. Prepare the sterile lancet.**

7. **Procedural Step. Position the infant.**
   Place the infant lying down in a supine position or lying across the parent's or guardian's lap. The child may also be positioned securely in the parent's or guardian's arms, leaving a foot exposed. The "burp" position is also very effective because the foot is in a downward position, allowing gravity to help with the flow of blood. The child should be placed in a comfortable position but must be securely supported.

8. **Procedural Step. Apply gloves.**

9. **Procedural Step. Select an appropriate puncture site.**
   The lateral and medial curves of the plantar surface of the heel (borders) can be used (see Figure 41-1).
   Rationale. These sites are used to prevent calcaneal (heel) damage.

10. **Procedural Step. Warm the puncture site with a commercially available infant heel warmer or a warm compress for approximately 5 minutes.**
    Rationale. Blood flow will be greatly increased when the site is warmed.

11. **Procedural Step. Position the puncture site.**
    Grasp the infant's heel firmly but gently. Hold the heel with your thumb below the puncture site and your index finger above the site in the arch of the child's foot. Cradle the foot in the palm of your hand and support it with your remaining fingers.
    Rationale. It is important that the foot be securely held because the child may try to kick or pull away.

12. **Procedural Step. Cleanse the puncture site with an alcohol wipe and allow it to air-dry.**
    Do not touch or fan the area after cleansing.
    Rationale. Allowing the site to air-dry prevents hemolysis of the specimen from the alcohol and lessens the stinging sensation that accompanies the puncture when alcohol is introduced into the tissues. If not allowed to completely dry, alcohol residue may interfere with the accuracy of test results.

13. **Procedural Step. Position the lancet and perform the puncture.**
    a. Hold the lancet between the first two fingers and position it firmly against the puncture site (bottom lateral surface of the newborn's heel).
    b. Place the thumb on the activation button at the top of the device housing and firmly depress it to discharge the blade.
    c. The puncture should be made at a right angle to the lines of the skin.

Continued

PROCEDURE 41-2   Collect a Blood Specimen for a Phenylketonuria (PKU) Screening Test—cont'd

14. **Procedural Step.** Dispose of the lancet.
    When the blade is activated, it will puncture the skin and will retract automatically into the device housing. Immediately dispose of the lancet into the sharps container.
    Rationale. Proper disposal of contaminated sharps is required by the OSHA standard to prevent exposure to bloodborne pathogens.

15. **Procedural Step.** Wipe away the first drop of blood with the dry sterile gauze.
    Rationale. The first drop of blood is not collected because it usually contains more tissue fluid than blood, which will result in an inaccurate test result.

16. **Procedural Step.** Allow a second well-rounded drop of blood to form, and quickly collect the specimen by gently touching the circle on the filter paper test card in the correct manner using filter paper test cards.
    Rationale. Rapid collection is necessary to prevent coagulation.
    Filter paper: Completely fill each of the circles on the PKU test card with a large drop of blood. The proper amount of specimen is obtained when the blood can be seen soaking completely through the filter paper from one side to the other.
    Rationale. The circles must be completely filled to ensure enough of a blood sample to perform the test. Most repeat tests are necessary because of an inadequate blood specimen.

17. **Procedural Step.** After the sample has been collected, apply pressure with a clean gauze square directly over the puncture site. Apply latex-free bandage over puncture site.
    Apply direct pressure until all bleeding has stopped. Never use a bandage on a child less than 2 years old; the child may choke on the bandage if it becomes loose.

18. **Procedural Step.** Discard any contaminated materials in the appropriate biohazardous waste container.

19. **Procedural Step.** Complete the information section of the PKU card.
    Rationale. Labeling the specimen after a successful collection and before leaving the examination room ensures that the correct specimen will be tested.

20. **Procedural Step.** Remove gloves and sanitize the hands.
    Always sanitize the hands after every procedure or after using gloves.

Continued

PROCEDURE 41-2: Collect a Blood Specimen for a Phenylketonuria (PKU) Screening Test—cont'd

21. **Procedural Step. Process and transport the specimen.**
    Filter test card: Allow the test card to dry for 2 hours at room temperature on a nonabsorbent surface. Cards should not be stacked together while drying. After the blood is completely dry, place the test card in its protective envelope and mail it to an outside laboratory for testing within 48 hours.
    Rationale. The test card should be mailed within 48 hours to ensure accurate test results.

22. **Procedural Step. Document the procedure.**
    Include the date and time, type of procedure, puncture site, and information regarding transfer to an outside laboratory.

    ### CHARTING EXAMPLE

Date	
2/10/xx	11:00 a.m. Blood specimen collected from Ⓛ medial aspect of heel. Sent to Medical Laboratory Corp on 2/10/xx for PKU test. ———————— K. Key, CMA (AAMA)

Photo from Sommer SR, Warekois RS: *Phlebotomy: worktext and procedures manual,* Philadelphia, 2002, Saunders.

PROCEDURE 41-3: Perform Venipuncture Using the Evacuated-Tube Method (Collection of Multiple Tubes)

TASK: Obtain a venous blood specimen acceptable for testing using an evacuated-tube system.

EQUIPMENT AND SUPPLIES

- Nonsterile disposable gloves (latex-free)
- Personal protective equipment (PPE) as required
- Tourniquet (latex-free)
- Evacuated-tube holder
- Evacuated-tube multidraw needle (21 or 22 gauge, 1 or 1½ inch) with safety guards
- Evacuated blood tubes for requested tests with labels (correct nonadditive or additive required for ordered test)
- Alcohol wipe
- Sterile 2 × 2 gauze pads
- Bandage (latex-free), CoFlex, or nonallergenic tape
- Sharps container
- Biohazardous waste container
- Laboratory requisition form
- Patient's medical record

SKILLS/RATIONALE

STANDARD PRECAUTIONS ARE TO BE FOLLOWED.

1. **Procedural Step. Sanitize the hands.**
   An alcohol-based hand rub may be used instead of washing hands with soap and water, unless hands are visibly soiled.
   Rationale. Hand sanitization promotes infection control.

2. **Procedural Step. Assemble equipment and supplies and verify the order.**
   Select the required evacuated tubes according to the tests to be performed. Check the expiration date of the tubes. Arrange the tubes in order of draw. Tap powdered additive tubes lightly below the stopper to dislodge any additive caught on the tube stopper. Phlebotomy supplies are often kept in a portable sturdy tray that keeps everything together in one place and is easy to transport from one examination room to another. When a phlebotomy supply tray is used, make sure that the tray is stocked with all the needed supplies and a variety of color-topped evacuated tubes.
   Rationale. It is important to have all supplies and equipment ready and available before starting any procedure to ensure efficiency. Checking for the tube expiration date is important because outdated tubes may no longer contain a vacuum, and as a result, they may not be able to draw blood into the tube. Outdated additives may cause inaccurate test results. If an additive remains trapped in the stopper, inaccurate test results may occur.

Continued

PROCEDURE 41-3 Perform Venipuncture Using the Evacuated-Tube Method (Collection of Multiple Tubes)—cont'd

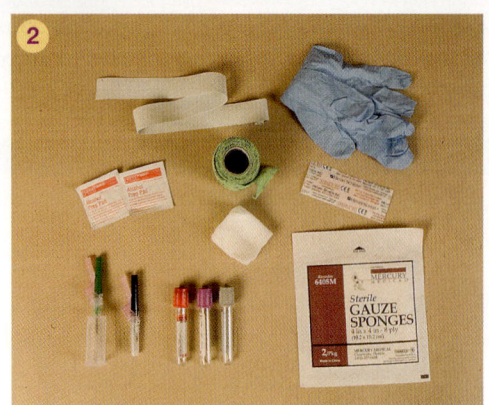

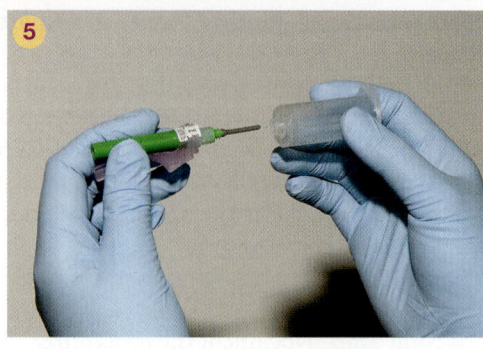

3. **Procedural Step.** Greet the patient, introduce yourself, and confirm the patient's identity. Ask the patient to have a seat in the phlebotomy chair. If the patient states that he or she "faints" when blood is taken, place the patient in a supine position on the examination table.

    Rationale. Identifying the patient ensures the procedure is performed on the correct patient. Placing the patient in the supine position makes it less likely that the patient will faint.

4. **Procedural Step.** Verify that any special diet instructions or restrictions have been followed (e.g., fasting) and explain the procedure to the patient.

    If the test(s) ordered requires patient preparation, such as fasting or medication restrictions, confirm that the patient has followed the preparation orders. When a patient is not properly prepared, the physician should be consulted for directions concerning how to proceed with the test.

    Rationale. Explaining the procedure to the patient promotes cooperation and provides a means of obtaining implied consent. Test results will be inaccurate if the patient has not followed the required preparation orders.

5. **Procedural Step.** Prepare the evacuated-tube system.

    Insert the rubber-tipped portion of the needle (posterior part of the needle) into the plastic holder. Screw the needle into the evacuated-tube holder or insert it into a quick-release holder and tighten securely. Keep the cover on the needle.

    Rationale. The needle must be tightened securely or it may fall out of the holder or be pushed farther than necessary into the patient's arm when the evacuated tube is pushed onto the needle.

6. **Procedural Step.** Prepare the gauze pad.

    Open the sterile gauze packet and place the gauze pad on the inside of its wrapper, or obtain sterile gauze pads from a bulk package.

7. **Procedural Step.** Position the remaining needed supplies.

    Place the first tube loosely in the plastic holder with the label facing downward. Place the remaining supplies within comfortable reach of your nondominant hand. Do not remove the needle cap.

    Rationale. Items used during the procedure should be positioned so that you do not have to reach over the patient, which may cause you to move the needle while it is still in the patient's arm. Puncturing the rubber stopper causes loss of the tube's vacuum.

8. **Procedural Step.** Position and examine the arm to be used in the venipuncture.

    a. Ask the patient to extend both arms in a slightly downward position. Examine the antecubital area. If the patient has a preference, examine it first but do not hesitate to select the other arm if it seems more acceptable. Select a suitable vein.

    b. The arm with the vein selected for the venipuncture should be in a downward position and not bent at the elbow. The arm should be supported on the armrest by a rolled towel or by having the patient place the fist of the other hand under the elbow.

    Rationale. Most adults have had previous venipunctures and know which veins are better for a successful draw. Asking a patient to state a preference gives the patient a sense of control over what is happening and increases patient comfort. By placing a rolled towel or having the patient place the fist under the elbow helps achieve proper positioning. Gravity helps to enlarge the veins.

Continued

PROCEDURE 41-3 Perform Venipuncture Using the Evacuated-Tube Method (Collection of Multiple Tubes)—cont'd

9. **Procedural Step.** Apply the tourniquet.
   a. Apply the tourniquet 3 to 4 inches above the bend in the elbow and stretch it slightly. Cross the ends in the front of the arm so that each hand is holding the opposite end of the tourniquet. The tourniquet should be tight enough to allow arterial blood to flow while preventing venous return. It should be "tight, but not *too* tight."
   b. Grasp the tourniquet's middle, where the ends cross, between your thumb and forefinger. With the left hand, loop the "underneath" flap on the left over the top, and tuck it under the tightened crisscross, but do not push it all the way through. Then let go of the tourniquet. The friction on the rubber will hold the end in place. You should see a loop just above the antecubital space, and the end "flap" should be easy to grab. (You will pull this end to release the tourniquet when you have completed the venipuncture.)

   NOTE: The tourniquet should not be left on for longer than 1 minute to prevent venous congestion, or excessive accumulation of blood in the vein (**hemoconcentration**). If you need to perform several assessments to locate the best vein, the tourniquet can be applied and reapplied as required.

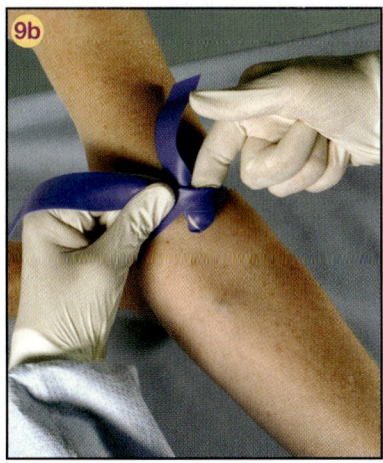

NOTE: Asking the patient to make a tight fist helps to locate deeper veins more easily. Do not leave the tourniquet on longer than 1 minute or have the patient pump (open and close) the fist, since these techniques cause hemoconcentration (blood pooling) and may lead to false test results. For example, the patient's potassium level could increase as much as 20%.

Rationale. The combined effect of the pressure of the tourniquet and the tightly clenched fist should cause the antecubital veins to stand out so that accurate selection of a puncture site can be made.

10. **Procedural Step.** Apply gloves and PPE.
    Rationale. Gloves and PPE are a precaution that provides a barrier against blood-borne pathogens.
11. **Procedural Step.** Thoroughly palpate the selected vein.
    Gently palpate the vein with the index finger to trace the direction of the vein and to estimate the size and depth of the vein. The vein feels like an elastic tube and gives under pressure while a tendon feels rigid and a sclerosed or thrombosed vein feels cordlike.
    Rationale. The index finger is most sensitive for palpating a vein.
12. **Procedural Step.** Release the tourniquet.
13. **Procedural Step.** Prepare the puncture site.
    Cleanse the site with the alcohol wipe using a circular motion from the center and working outward. Allow the site to air-dry. Once the site has been cleaned, do not palpate it again.
    Rationale. The site must be cleansed in a circular motion from the puncture site outward to help remove contaminants from the site. The site must be allowed to dry to prevent alcohol from entering the blood specimen and contaminating it, causing inaccurate test results. Touching or fanning the area causes contamination, and the cleansing process must be repeated. In addition, if the alcohol is not allowed to dry completely, it may cause the patient to experience a stinging sensation. Also the drying process helps to destroy microbes.
14. **Procedural Step.** Reapply the tourniquet.
    NOTE: According to CLSI, a tourniquet should not be reapplied for 2 minutes. If the site chosen needs to be palpated again, the site must be cleansed again.
15. **Procedural Step.** Position the holder.
    a. Grasp the holder with all five fingers: the forefinger under the top of the holder, the middle, ring, and fifth fingers supporting the underside of the tube, and the thumb holding the top of the holder just below the flange.
    b. Remove the needle cover and inspect for barbs and make sure the *bevel* of the needle is facing upward. Be sure the sheath on the safety device is flipped up and out of the way.
    c. Position the needle so that it follows the line of the vein. Twist the tube inside of the holder, without pushing onto the needle, so that the label is facing downward.
    Rationale. Positioning the needle with the bevel up allows for easier entry into the skin and the vein. With the label facing downward, you will be able to observe the blood as it fills the tube, which allows you to know when the tube is full.
16. **Procedural Step.** Perform the venipuncture.
    a. Warn that the patient will feel a little "stick."
    Rationale. Warning the patient before entering the vein prevents the element of surprise, which could cause the patient to pull away, causing the needle to be pulled out of the vein.

Continued

PROCEDURE 41-3 Perform Venipuncture Using the Evacuated-Tube Method (Collection of Multiple Tubes)—cont'd

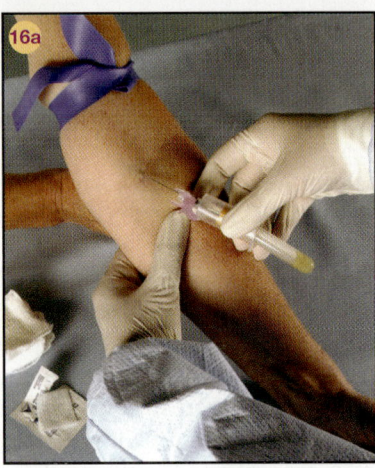

b. With the other hand, use your thumb to pull the skin taut below the intended puncture site to anchor the vein. Your thumb should be placed 1 to 2 inches below and to the side of the puncture site.
Rationale. Pulling the skin taut helps the needle glide in easily.

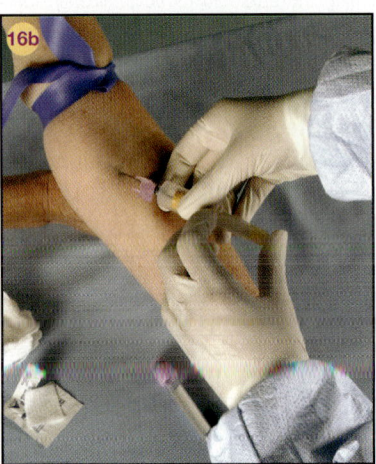

c. Following the direction of the vein, with one quick motion, smoothly pierce the skin and enter the vein at a small angle—about 15 degrees—and almost parallel to the skin.
Rationale. The angle of the needle is important because an angle of less than 15 degrees may cause the needle to enter above the vein, preventing puncture. An angle of more than 30 degrees may cause the needle to go through the vein, puncturing the posterior wall. This could result in a hematoma (blood in the tissues).

17. **Procedural Step. Secure the holder for blood collection.**
Support the holder on your middle finger by resting the middle finger against the patient's arm. Be careful to keep the holder steady in your dominant hand so that the needle does not move in the vein as you get ready to slide the tube "on." Then let go of the skin with the nondominant thumb and anchor the forefinger and middle finger of the nondominant hand on the flange of the holder.
Rationale. Firmly grasping the holder prevents the needle from moving deeper into the vein when inserting an evacuated tube. Moving the needle is painful for the patient.

18. **Procedural Step. Push the bottom of the tube with the thumb of your nondominant hand carefully while holding the holder and needle steady, so that the needle inside the holder pierces the rubber stopper of the tube.**
If everything is done correctly, blood will begin to fill the tube.

19. **Procedural Step. Change tubes as required by test orders by repeating Steps 17 and 18.**
When the tube has stopped filling, grasp the bottom of the tube with the left hand. Push against the flange with the thumb and pull the tube from the holder. This lets the rubber sleeve slide back over the end of the needle and prevents blood from dripping into the holder. Invert the purple-top tube about 8 to 10 times (do not shake the tube; this applies to any tube with additives), then place it upright in a rack so that it will not roll.
Rationale. Anchor the tube and tube holder firmly before changing tubes to prevent the needle from being pulled out of the vein or being inserted deeper. Inverting tubes with additives activates the anticoagulant. Shaking the tube hemolyzes the blood and damages blood cells.

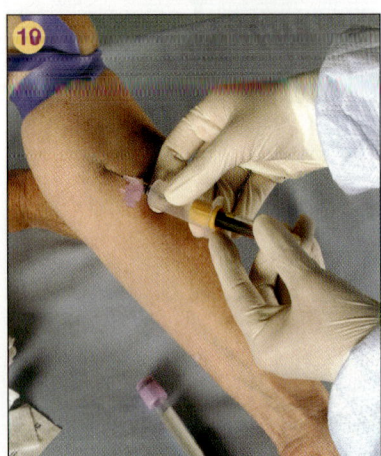

20. **Procedural Step. While the blood is filling the last tube, remove the tourniquet.**
With the dominant hand still holding the needle in place on the patient's arm, ask the patient to open the fist. Then release the tourniquet by pulling the loose left end upward with your other hand. This will allow blood to flow freely in the patient's arm again.

Continued

PROCEDURE 41-3 Perform Venipuncture Using the Evacuated-Tube Method (Collection of Multiple Tubes)—cont'd

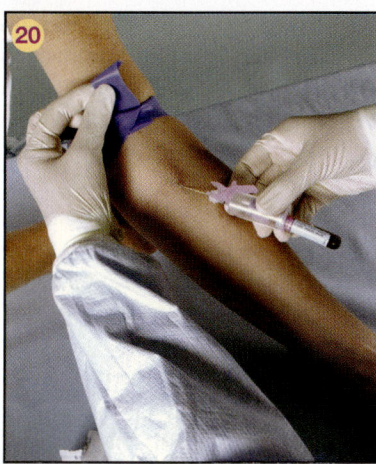

21. **Procedural Step.** Remove the needle and activate the safety needle device.

    After the last tube is removed and mixed, put it down, then pick up the sterile gauze with the nondominant hand and position the gauze over the needle. With one quick, smooth motion, remove the needle from the arm with the dominant hand and apply pressure with the gauze in the left hand immediately *after* you remove the needle. As you withdraw the needle, flip the safety shield over the needle tip with your right thumb and direct the needle down and away from yourself and the patient.

    NOTE: Do not place a gauze pad over the needle as it is being withdrawn, since this can scratch the patient's arm or dig the needle into the arm, causing pain. Always withdraw the needle completely first, then apply the gauze pad to the site.

    Rationale. Placing the gauze pad over the puncture site helps prevent tissue movement, absorbs small amounts of blood that ooze from the vein, and reduces patient discomfort. Careful withdrawal prevents further tissue damage. The needle sheath prevents needle sticks.

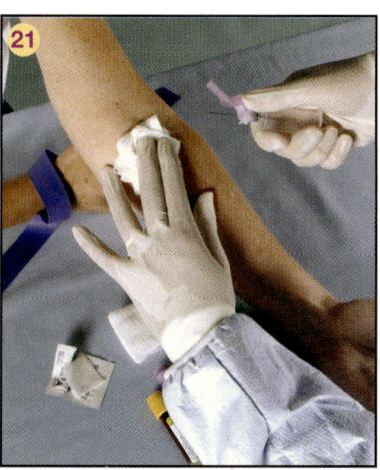

22. **Procedural Step.** Apply direct pressure on the venipuncture site to enhance the formation of a platelet plug. Secure the gauze dressing.

    Tell the patient to keep the arm straight to allow a good clot to begin forming over the puncture site.

    Rationale. Keeping the arm straight prevents dislodging the plug that has formed and prevents the formation of a hematoma.

23. **Procedural Step.** Instruct the patient to maintain pressure on the site for 1 to 2 minutes.

    NOTE: If any swelling or discoloration occurs, apply an ice pack to the site after bandaging it.

    Rationale. Do not allow the patient to bend the arm at the elbow, because this increases blood loss from the puncture site and causes bruising.

24. **Procedural Step.** Activate the safety device and discard the entire Vacutainer system in the biohazard sharps container.

25. **Procedural Step.** Label the tubes.

    Include the patient's name, the date, time of draw, test to be performed, and your initials.

    Rationale. It is important to label the tubes **after** collecting the specimen but **before** leaving the patient. If an unlabeled tube is sent to the reference laboratory, it will be rejected.

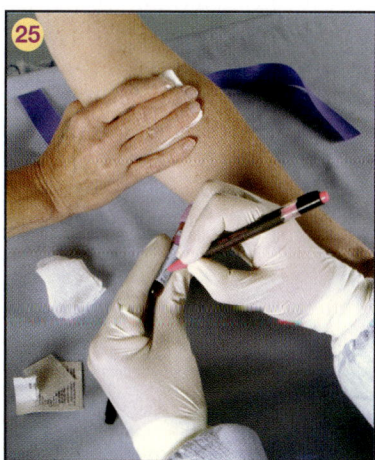

26. **Procedural Step.** After the tube(s) has been labeled, observe for any special handling procedures (e.g., frozen, chilled, warm); place the tube(s) into the biohazard transport bag with the laboratory requisition.

27. **Procedural Step.** Check to make sure the patient's arm has stopped bleeding, and then place a latex-free bandage or CoFlex over the gauze to create a pressure dressing. Caution the patient not to lift anything for an hour.

    Rationale. A slight pressure bandage will help to prevent further bleeding. Lifting could cause further bleeding leading to a hematoma.

Continued

PROCEDURE 41-3 Perform Venipuncture Using the Evacuated-Tube Method (Collection of Multiple Tubes)—cont'd

NOTE: Making certain that the bleeding has stopped is important for patients on anticoagulants. Continue with pressure until bleeding stops.

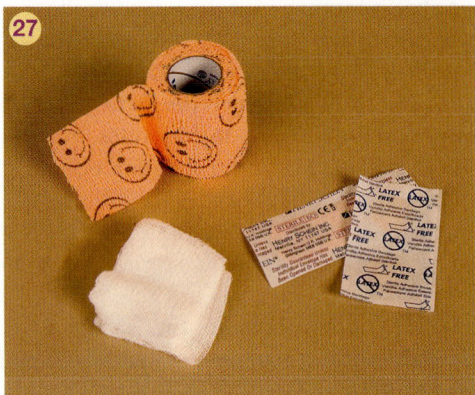

28. **Procedural Step.** Remove and discard the alcohol wipe and gloves.

    Before removing gloves, grasp the alcohol wipe in the palm of one gloved hand so that the wipe is enveloped in the gloves as you take them off. Remove the disposable gloves and discard them in the biohazardous waste container because they may have come in contact with blood.

29. **Procedural Step.** Sanitize the hands.

    Always sanitize the hands after every procedure or after using gloves.

30. **Procedural Step.** Complete the laboratory requisition form to include the collection date and time and place the requisition in the biohazard transport bag with the specimen(s).

31. **Procedural Step.** Ask and observe how the patient feels.

    Observe breathing, color, and skin moisture, looking for signs that the patient may feel faint. If the patient states he or she feels fine and there are no signs of fainting, prepare to document the procedure in the patient's medical record.

32. **Procedural Step.** Clean the work area using Standard Precautions.

33. **Procedural Step.** Document the procedure.

    Include the date and time, the test drawn, which arm and vein were used, and any unusual patient reaction.
    NOTE: Some physician's offices keep a laboratory log for all outside testing that includes patient name, date, test required, outside laboratory receiving the specimen, results, and the medical assistant's initials.

CHARTING EXAMPLE	
Date	
8/10/xx	10:00 a.m. Venous blood specimen collected from Ⓡ arm AC space for Lipid Profile; 2 SST tubes collected, centrifuged, and serum placed in transfer tube for pickup by Medical Laboratory Corp. ———— V. Koszarek, CMA (AAMA)

Photos for Steps 9b, 16b, 19, 20, 21, and 25 from Garrels M, Oatis C: *Laboratory testing for ambulatory settings,* St Louis, 2006, Saunders.

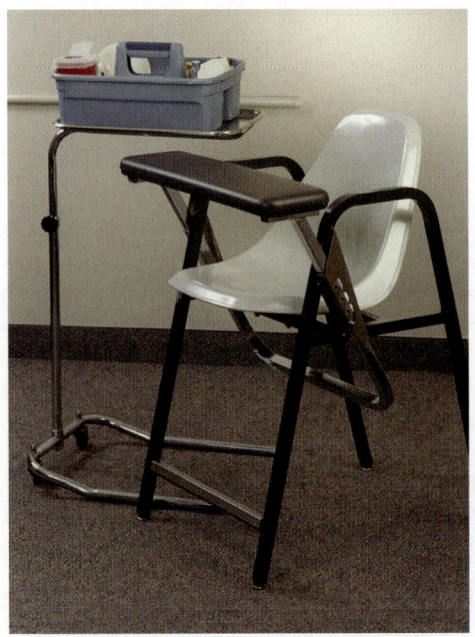

FIGURE 41-6 Phlebotomy chair.

medical assistant's ability to perform the venipuncture. Being relaxed and confident helps minimize the patient's discomfort, since the patient views these actions as professional behavior. Never tell the patient, "I've never done this before," or "It's my first time," or "I have trouble drawing blood," since all these statements will cause anxiety for both the patient and the medical assistant. Do a self-talk ("I can do it"), and be confident.

Evacuated Tubes

With the **vacuum tube** system, once the vacuum tube needle has pierced the vein and the selected tube's colored stopper (cap), a vacuum pulls the blood into the tube. Vacuum tubes allow for the blood specimen to enter directly into a collection tube (the **evacuated tube**) to be used for testing purposes. Tubes come in different sizes (e.g., pediatric and adult), with different colored stoppers, or tops. The color of the stopper identifies the type of test to be performed. The tubes are also marked with an expiration date and should be checked before use. Table 41-2 lists common stopper colors, additives, and laboratory uses.

TABLE 41-2
Common Stoppers, Additives, and Laboratory Uses

Vacutainer Colors*	Color	Hemogard Colors†	Additive and Function	Laboratory Use	Optimum Volume/Minimum Volume
ADULT TUBES					
Yellow		Yellow	SPS; prevents blood from clotting and stabilizes bacterial growth	Blood or body fluid **cultures**	5 mL/NA
Red		Red	None (Clot activator)	Serum testing, chemistry tests, **blood bank,** serology	10 mL/NA
Red/gray (marbled)		Gold	None, but contains silica particles to enhance clot formation	Serum testing	10 mL/NA
Light blue		Light blue	Sodium citrate; removes calcium to prevent blood from clotting	Coagulation testing (PT, PTT)	4.5 mL/4.5 mL
Green		Green	Heparin (sodium, lithium, ammonium); inhibits thrombin formation to prevent clotting	Chemistry tests	10 mL/3.5 mL
Green/gray (marbled)		Light green	Lithium heparin and gel for plasma separation	Plasma determinations	2 mL/2 mL
Lavender		Lavender	EDTA; removes calcium to prevent blood from clotting	Hematology testing (CBC)	7 mL/2 mL
Gray		Gray	Potassium oxalate, sodium fluoride; removes calcium to prevent blood from clotting; fluoride inhibits glycolysis	Chemistry tests, especially glucose/alcohol levels	10 mL/10 mL
Royal blue		Royal blue	Sodium heparin (also sodium EDTA); inhibits thrombin formation to prevent clotting	Chemistry trace elements	7 mL
PEDIATRIC TUBES‡					
Red		Red	—	—	2, 3, or 4 mL/NA
Lavender		Lavender	—	—	2 mL/0.6 mL, 3 mL/0.9 mL, 4 mL/1 mL
Green		Green	—	—	2 mL/2 mL
Light blue		Light blue	—	—	2.7 mL/2.7 mL

Modified from Rodak BF: *Diagnostic hematology*, Philadelphia, 1995, Saunders.
CBC, Complete blood count; *EDTA*, Ethylenediaminetetraacetic acid; *NA*, not applicable; *PT*, prothrombin time; *PTT*, partial thromboplastin time; *SPS*, sodium polyanethol sulfonate.
*Stopper colors are based on Vacutainer tubes (Becton Dickinson).
†Hemogard closures provide a protective plastic cover over the rubber stopper as an additional safety feature.
‡Additives and function, and laboratory uses are the same as for adult tubes.

Some tubes have an additive that in most cases acts as an anticoagulant. **Hematology** studies require tubes containing the anticoagulant ethylenediaminetetraacetic acid (EDTA). EDTA preserves the shape of the blood cells and prevents the platelets from clumping by removing calcium, thus preventing clotting. **Chemistry** and **serology** studies are drawn in a red or red-gray marbled stoppered tube or gold Hemogard tube that has no additives.

Order of Draw

When several evacuated tubes are to be collected for multiple studies, there is a recommended **order of draw** for the vacuum tubes (Figure 41-7). The Clinical and Laboratory Standards Institute (CLSI), formerly the National Committee for Clinical Laboratory Standards (NCCLS), established the order of draw for quality control purposes. Following the order of draw minimizes the chance of additives from a previous tube

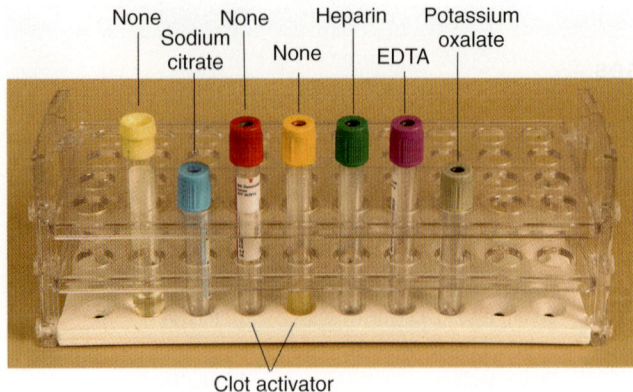

FIGURE 41-7 Hemogard tubes in order of draw.

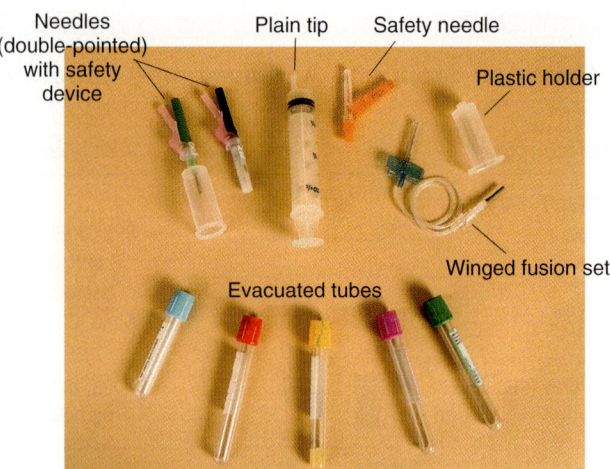

FIGURE 41-9 Equipment used for venipuncture.

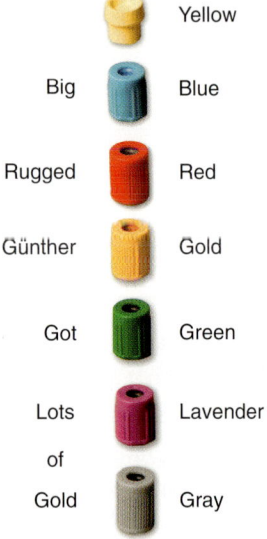

FIGURE 41-8 The order of drawing blood. Memorize "Big Rugged Günther Got Lots of Gold" to help remember the order, as shown.

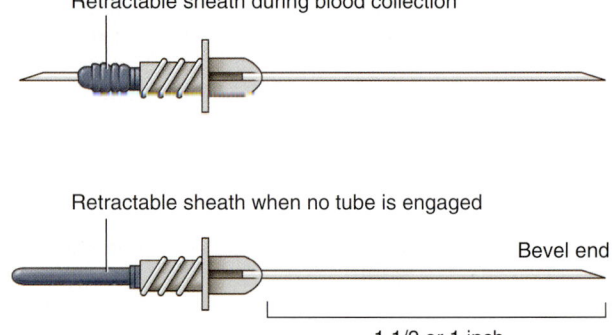

FIGURE 41-10 A multisample needle. (From Sommer SR, Warekois RS: *Phlebotomy: worktext and procedures manual,* Philadelphia, 2002, Saunders.)

getting into subsequent tubes when blood is drawn. The following color-topped tube order is recommended when the evacuated-tube (Vacutainer) system is used:

1. Yellow or blood culture tubes (sterile; special collection procedure required).
2. Light blue (sodium citrate): Forms calcium salts to remove calcium.
3. Red (no additives): Blood clots, and **serum** is separated when the specimen is centrifuged.
4. Red-gray or Hemogard gold (silicone clot activator): Gel at bottom of tube separated blood's formed elements from serum when centrifuged.
5. Light green (lithium heparin): **Plasma** is separated from gel at bottom of tube after being centrifuged.
6. Green (sodium heparin): Inactivates thrombin and thromboplastin.
7. Lavender (EDTA): Forms calcium salts to remove calcium.
8. Gray (potassium oxalate): Preserves glucose up to 5 days.

To assist in remembering the order of draw, memorize the sentence in Figure 41-8 or create one yourself.

Types of Equipment

Three types of equipment can be used in venipuncture: the evacuated-tube (Vacutainer) method, the syringe method, and the butterfly method (Figure 41-9).

Vacutainer Method. The **evacuation blood collection system,** or **Vacutainer,** has a holder, a double-ended sterile needle of various lengths and gauges, and a tube with a color-coded stopper and a premeasured space with or without an additive. The Vacutainer system allows for several tubes of blood to be drawn from a single venipuncture. This minimizes the chance of labeling errors and hemolysis.

Needles are available as **multisample needles** (retractable rubber sleeve) (Figure 41-10) or **single-sample needles.** When a multisample needle is used, the rubber sleeve retracts as the needle enters the stopper but then springs back to cover the needle when the tube is removed. Many manufacturers design needles with a recapping safety device to minimize the chance of an accidental needlestick (Figure 41-11). The holder is available in either an adult or pediatric size. The single-sample needle does not have a rubber sleeve, therefore allowing blood to exit through the needle when the tube is removed.

The holder has a flange at one end for the medical assistant's fingers and a grooved opening on the other end for the

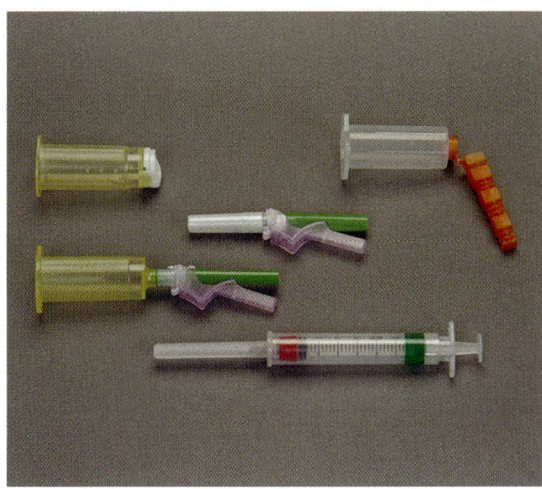

FIGURE 41-11 Safety venipuncture devices.

> **BOX 41-1**
>
> ### Reasons for Rejection of Specimen by Laboratory
>
> - Incorrect or incomplete labeling of specimen
> - No laboratory requisition
> - Insufficient filling of additive tubes
> - Insufficient quantity or **quantity not sufficient (QNS)** of specimen *(short draw)* for the test ordered
> - Collected in the wrong tube or container
> - Clotted specimen in an additive tube
> - Blood sample hemolyzed
> - Not refrigerated when required or thawed and refrozen
> - Patient not fasting when required

needle. The barrel of the holder is marked with a stopper guideline. It is only used one time and then disposed of in a biohazardous waste container, usually with the needle attached. The safety cap on the needle will be activated before disposal.

When the Vacutainer tube is pushed into the holder beyond the stopper guideline, the needle punctures the color-coded stopper, and the vacuum draws blood into the tube. Procedure 41-3 explains the process of venipuncture using the evacuated-tube method.

Syringe Method. The **syringe method** for venipuncture is used for patients with small or fragile veins (e.g., children, elderly persons). This method lessens the degree of pressure exerted on the vein to avoid the collapse of fragile veins. The medical assistant controls the vacuum created when the plunger of the syringe is pulled back slowly. When a blood sample is drawn with a needle and syringe, the blood sample must be transferred to the appropriate evacuated tube (e.g., sterile, light blue, lavender, green, gray, red, or red-gray). This is done by placing the syringe needle through the tube stopper. The vacuum exerted fills the tube automatically. Procedure 41-4 provides the steps for obtaining a blood specimen using the syringe method.

Butterfly Method. The **butterfly method** uses a **winged infusion set** attached to plastic tubing. The plastic tubing attaches to either a syringe tip or a Vacutainer holder. The butterfly method is used for infants, small children, or adults with small, difficult-to-find veins.

The "wings" make it easier to control and guide the needle. The medical assistant should make sure that he or she is actually holding the bottom, not just the top, of the wings for stability of draw. The forearm or hand is most often used in adults. A 23-gauge needle is typically used because this size will enter small veins easily and will not cause the vein to rupture. The most important step in a butterfly draw is to stabilize or anchor the vein before inserting the needle. The medical assistant then should "thread the vein" just under the skin to keep the needle inside the lumen of the vein while completing the draw. This is especially necessary when using the veins of the hand.

The butterfly method is often more comfortable for the patient, but it takes longer to perform the actual blood draw. Remember that using this method may cause an error in test results (e.g., potassium, serum iron) because a small-gauge needle can cause red blood cells (RBCs) to break up (hemolyze), thus releasing hemoglobin in the specimen. Procedure 41-5 explains how to obtain a venous blood specimen using the butterfly method.

Failed Draws

Regardless of the site or method chosen to perform the venipuncture, the patient must be prepared properly and the collection process done correctly. A partially filled tube, or *short draw,* is unacceptable because the ratio of additive to blood can produce inaccurate results. Box 41-1 lists other reasons that cause a laboratory to reject a collected specimen.

To become skilled and confident in venipuncture, the medical assistant must practice. Every venipuncture presents different challenges (e.g., an obese patient's veins will be deeper, an older patient's veins may collapse, or large veins may roll more easily). No more than two venipuncture attempts should be done on a patient. If unsuccessful after two attempts, notify the physician or ask a co-worker to examine the patient's veins and perform the procedure. Various factors affect a successful draw, so not every attempt will be successful (Box 41-2). Figure 41-12 illustrates various reasons for a failed draw.

Blood Culture Collection

When the body is in a diseased state, the blood may be invaded with microorganisms. When **bacteremia** (bacteria in the blood) is suspected, a blood sample is collected under sterile conditions. A venipuncture must be collected using a special aseptic technique to prevent possible contamination of the specimen from the skin. Figure 41-13 shows typical supplies used when collecting a specimen with this special technique.

Text continued on p. 952

PROCEDURE 41-4

Perform Venipuncture Using the Syringe Method

TASK: Obtain a blood specimen acceptable for testing using a syringe.

EQUIPMENT AND SUPPLIES
- Nonsterile disposable gloves (latex-free)
- Personal protective equipment (PPE) as required
- Tourniquet (latex-free)
- Test tube rack
- 10 cc (10 mL) syringe or 20 cc (20 mL) with 21- or 22-gauge needle with safety guards
- Evacuated blood tubes for requested tests with labels (correct evacuated tube required for designated test ordered)
- Transfer device
- Alcohol wipe
- Sterile 2 × 2 gauze pads
- Bandage (latex-free) or nonallergenic tape or CoFlex
- Sharps container
- Biohazardous waste container
- Laboratory requisition form
- Patient's medical record

SKILLS/RATIONALE

STANDARD PRECAUTIONS ARE TO BE FOLLOWED.

1. **Procedural Step. Sanitize the hands.**
   An alcohol-based hand rub may be used instead of washing hands with soap and water, unless hands are visibly soiled.
   Rationale. Hand sanitization promotes infection control.

2. **Procedural Step. Assemble equipment and supplies and verify the order.**
   Select the required evacuated tubes according to the tests to be performed. Check the expiration date of the tubes. Arrange the tubes in order of draw. Tap powdered additive tubes lightly below the stopper to dislodge any additive caught on the tube stopper. Phlebotomy supplies are often kept in a portable sturdy tray that keeps everything together in one place and is easy to transport from one examination room to another. When a phlebotomy supply tray is used, make sure that the tray is stocked with all the needed supplies and a variety of color-topped evacuated tubes.

   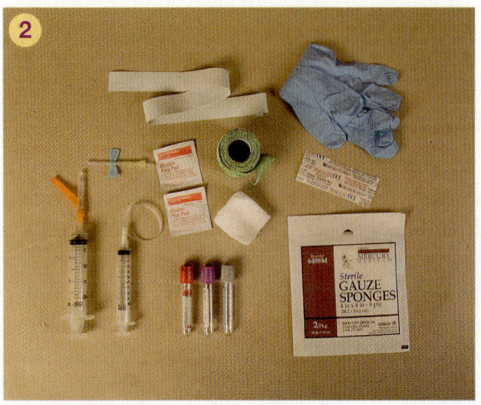

   Rationale. It is important to have all supplies and equipment ready and available before starting any procedure to ensure efficiency. Checking for the tube expiration date is important because outdated tubes may no longer contain a vacuum, and as a result, they may not be able to draw blood into the tube. Outdated additives may cause inaccurate test results. If an additive remains trapped in the stopper, inaccurate test results may occur.

3. **Procedural Step. Greet the patient, introduce yourself, and confirm the patient's identity.**
   Ask the patient to have a seat in the phlebotomy chair. If the patient states that he or she "faints" when they have blood taken, place the patient in a supine position on the examination table.
   Rationale. Identifying the patient ensures the procedure is performed on the correct patient. Placing the patient in the supine position makes it less likely that the patient will faint.

4. **Procedural Step. Explain the procedure to the patient. Verify that the special diet instructions or restrictions have been followed.**
   If the test(s) ordered requires patient preparation such as fasting or medication restrictions, confirm that the patient has followed the preparation orders. When a patient is not properly prepared, the physician should be consulted for directions concerning how to proceed with the test.
   Rationale. Explaining the procedure to the patient promotes cooperation and provides a means of obtaining implied consent. Test results will be inaccurate if the patient has not followed the required preparation orders.

5. **Procedural Step. Prepare the needle and syringe.**
   Make sure to keep the needle and the inside of the syringe sterile. Break the seal on the syringe by moving

Continued

PROCEDURE 41-4 Perform Venipuncture Using the Syringe Method—cont'd

the plunger back and forth several times, being careful to keep the plunger within the syringe. Loosen the cap on the needle, and check to make sure that the hub is screwed tightly into the syringe.

NOTE: Do not pull the cap straight off the needle, since this causes a "knee jerk" reaction and will cause you to stick yourself. Rock the cap gently back and forth at the hub of the needle, loosening it.

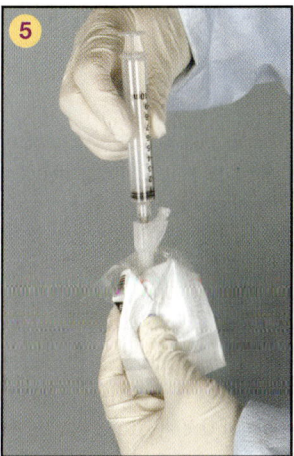

6. **Procedural Step.** Place the evacuated tubes to be filled in a test tube rack on a work surface.
   Make sure the tubes are placed in the correct order to be filled. If an evacuated tube contains a powdered additive, tap the tube just below the stopper to release any additive adhering to the stopper.
   Rationale. If an additive remains trapped in the stopper, inaccurate test results may occur.
7. **Procedural Step.** Open the sterile gauze packet and place the gauze pad on the inside of its wrapper, or obtain sterile gauze from a bulk package.
8. **Procedural Step.** Follow Steps 8 through 14 from Procedure 41-3.
9. **Procedural Step.** Position the syringe.
   Remove the cap from the needle. Hold the syringe by placing the thumb and index finger of the dominant hand near the needle hub while supporting the barrel of the syringe with the three remaining fingers. The bevel of the needle should be positioned facing up.
   Rationale. Positioning the needle with the bevel up allows for easier entry into the skin and the vein and allows the medical assistant to see when the needle enters the vein.
10. **Procedural Step.** Perform the venipuncture.
    a. Warn that the patient will feel a little "stick."
    Rationale. Warning the patient before entering the vein prevents the element of surprise, which could cause the patient to pull away, causing the needle to be pulled out of the vein.
    b. With the other hand, pull the skin taut beneath the intended puncture site to anchor the vein. Your thumb should be placed 1 to 2 inches below and to the side of the puncture site.
    Rationale. Pulling the skin taut helps the needle glide in easily.
    c. Following the direction of the vein, with one quick motion, smoothly pierce the skin and enter the vein at a small angle—about 15 degrees—and almost parallel to the vein.
    Rationale. The angle of the needle is important because an angle of less than 15 degrees may cause the needle to enter above the vein, preventing puncture. An angle of more than 30 degrees may cause the needle to go through the vein, puncturing the posterior wall. This could result in a hematoma (blood in the tissues).

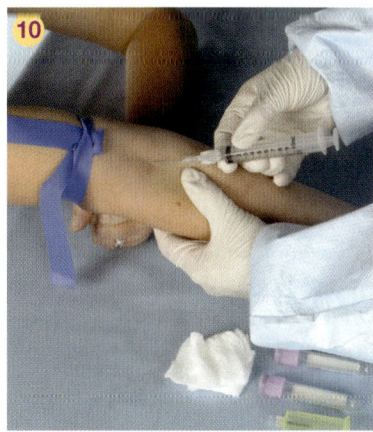

11. **Procedural Step.** Grasp the syringe firmly between the thumb and the underlying fingers.
    Blood may spontaneously enter the top of the syringe; this is called a *flash*. If a flash does not occur, gently pull back on the plunger of the syringe until blood begins to enter. Do not move the needle once the venipuncture has been made.
    NOTE: If no blood enters the syringe, slowly withdraw the needle, secure new supplies, and retry. The needle may not have threaded the vein, or it may have been resting on the vein wall.
    Rationale. Moving the needle is painful for the patient.

Continued

PROCEDURE 41-4 Perform Venipuncture Using the Syringe Method—cont'd

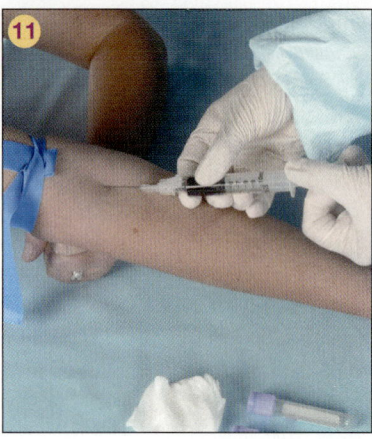

12. **Procedural Step.** Anchor the syringe and gently continue pulling back on the plunger until the required amount of blood is in the syringe.
    Be careful not to pull the needle out of the vein.
    Rationale. Pulling back on the plunger causes a vacuum, which draws the blood into the syringe. The blood should be withdrawn slowly from the vein to prevent hemolysis and to prevent the vein from collapsing.
13. **Procedural Step.** Release the tourniquet.
14. **Procedural Step.** Remove the needle.
    With one quick, smooth motion, remove the needle from the arm with the dominant hand and apply pressure with the gauze in the nondominant hand immediately *after* you remove the needle. As you withdraw the needle, flip the safety shield over the needle tip with your dominant thumb and direct the needle down and away from yourself and the patient.
    NOTE: Do not place a gauze pad over the needle as it is being withdrawn, since this can scratch the patient's arm or dig the needle into the arm, causing pain. Always withdraw the needle completely first, then apply the gauze pad to the site.

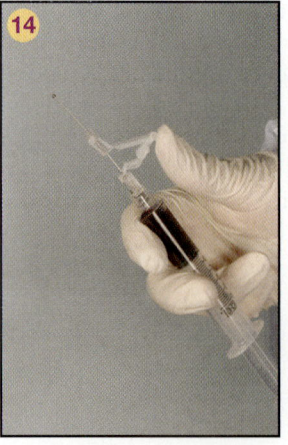

Rationale. Placing the gauze pad over the puncture site helps prevent tissue movement, absorbs small amounts of blood that ooze from the vein, and reduces patient discomfort. Careful withdrawal prevents further tissue damage. The needle sheath prevents needle sticks.

15. **Procedural Step.** Apply direct pressure on the venipuncture site to enhance the formation of a platelet plug.
    Tell the patient to keep the arm straight and not to bend at the elbow to allow a good clot to begin forming over the puncture site.
    Rationale. Keeping the arm straight prevents dislodging the clot that has formed.
16. **Procedural Step.** Instruct the patient to maintain pressure on the site for 1 to 2 minutes.
    NOTE: If any swelling or discoloration occurs, apply an ice pack to the site after bandaging it.
    Rationale. Maintaining pressure will help speed up the clotting process and prevent a hematoma. Do not allow the patient to bend the arm at the elbow because this increases blood loss from the puncture site and causes bruising.
17. **Procedural Step.** Attach the yellow safety transfer device to the tip of the syringe. Make sure the tubes are lined up in the correct order of fill in the tube rack.
    a. Remove the protected needle from the syringe and discard it into the sharps container.
    b. Attach the yellow safety transfer device to the tip of the syringe.
    c. Invert the syringe above the device and connect the correct vacuum tube for the test(s) requested.

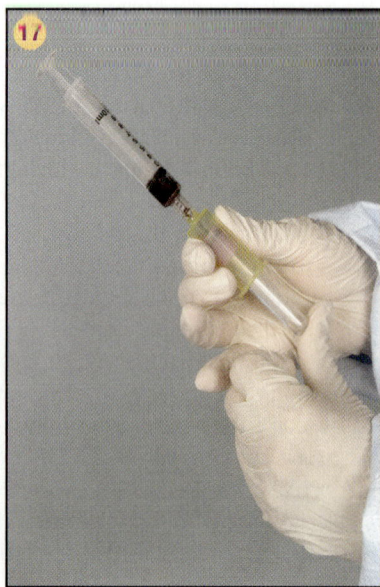

Continued

Phlebotomy CHAPTER 41 947

| PROCEDURE 41-4 | Perform Venipuncture Using the Syringe Method—cont'd | |

18. **Procedural Step.** Discard the entire system into the sharps container.
    Rationale. Proper disposal is required by the OSHA standard to prevent accidental needle stick injuries.
19. **Procedural Step.** Follow Steps 25 through 33 from Procedure 41-3.

CHARTING EXAMPLE

Date	
6/15/xx	12:00 p.m. Venous blood specimen collected from Ⓡ arm AC space. 1 EDTA tube for CBC to be picked up by Medical Laboratory Corp.——————————— ————————— S. Miller, CMA (AAMA)

Photos for Steps 5, 10, 11, 14, and 17 from Garrels M, Oatis C: Laboratory testing for ambulatory settings, St Louis, 2006, Saunders.

| PROCEDURE 41-5 | Perform Venipuncture Using the Butterfly Method (Collection of Multiple Evacuated Tubes) | |

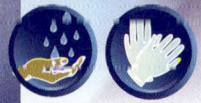

TASK: Obtain a venous blood specimen acceptable for testing using the butterfly method.

EQUIPMENT AND SUPPLIES

- Nonsterile disposable gloves (latex-free)
- Personal protective equipment (PPE) as required
- Tourniquet (latex-free)
- Test tube rack
- Winged-infusion set with Luer adapter and safety guard
- Multidraw needle (22 to 25 gauge) and tube holder or 10 cc (10 mL) or 20 cc (20 mL) syringe
- Evacuated blood tubes for requested tests with labels (correct evacuated tube required for designated test ordered)
- Alcohol wipe
- Sterile 2 × 2 gauze pads
- Bandage (latex-free) or nonallergenic tape or CoFlex
- Sharps container
- Biohazardous waste container
- Laboratory requisition form
- Patient's medical record

SKILLS/RATIONALE   STANDARD PRECAUTIONS ARE TO BE FOLLOWED.

1. **Procedural Step. Sanitize the hands.**
   An alcohol-based hand rub may be used instead of washing hands with soap and water, unless hands are visibly soiled.
   Rationale. Hand sanitization promotes infection control.
2. **Procedural Step. Assemble equipment and supplies and verify the order.**
   Select the required evacuated tubes according to the tests to be performed. Check the expiration date of the tubes. Arrange the tubes in order of draw. Tap powdered additive tubes lightly below the stopper to dislodge any additive caught on the tube stopper. Phlebotomy supplies are often kept in a portable sturdy tray that keeps everything together in one place and is

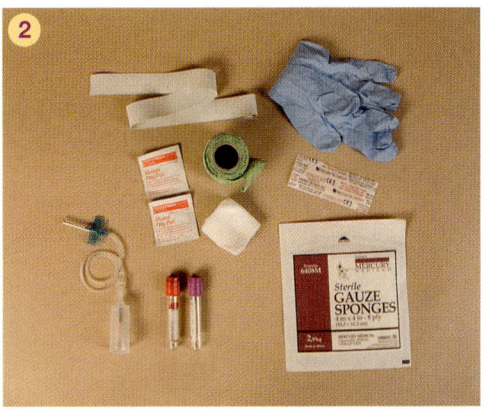

Continued

easy to transport from one examination room to another. When a phlebotomy supply tray is used, make sure that the tray is stocked with all the needed supplies and a variety of color-topped evacuated tubes.

Rationale. *It is important to have all supplies and equipment ready and available before starting any procedure to ensure efficiency. Checking for the tube expiration date is important because outdated tubes may no longer contain a vacuum, and as a result, they may not be able to draw blood into the tube. Outdated additives may cause inaccurate test results. If an additive remains trapped in the stopper, inaccurate test results may occur.*

3. **Procedural Step. Greet the patient, introduce yourself, and confirm the patient's identity.**
   Ask the patient to have a seat in the phlebotomy chair. If the patient states that he or she "faints" when blood is taken, place the patient in a supine position on the examination table.
   Rationale. *Identifying the patient ensures the procedure is performed on the correct patient. Placing the patient in the supine position makes it less likely that the patient will faint.*

4. **Procedural Step. Explain the procedure to the patient.**
   If the test(s) ordered requires patient preparation such as fasting or medication restrictions, confirm that the patient has followed the preparation orders. When a patient is not properly prepared, the physician should be consulted for directions concerning how to proceed with the test.
   Rationale. *Explaining the procedure to the patient promotes cooperation and provides a means of obtaining implied consent. Test results will be inaccurate if the patient has not followed the required preparation orders.*

5. **Procedural Step. Prepare the winged infusion set.**
   Remove the winged infusion set from its package. Extend the tubing to its full length and stretch it slightly to prevent it from coiling back up. Attach the winged infusion set to either a syringe or an evacuated-tube holder. If a holder is used, screw the adapter with the double-ended needle into the holder and tighten it securely. When using a syringe, tighten the Luer adapter onto the syringe.
   Rationale. *Extending the tubing straightens it to permit a free flow of blood in the tubing. An unsecured needle or syringe can come loose or pop off during the draw.*

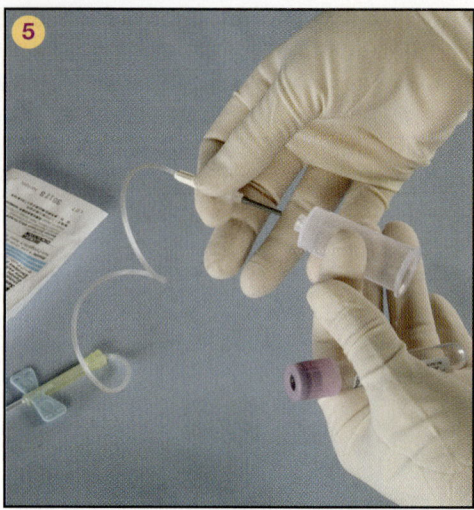

6. **Procedural Step. Open the sterile gauze packet and place the gauze pad on the inside of its wrapper or obtain sterile gauze pads from a bulk package.**

7. **Procedural Step. Position and examine the arm to be used in the venipuncture.**
   a. Ask the patient to extend both arms with the arms supported in a slightly downward position. Examine both arms. If the patient has a preference, examine the preferred arm first but do not hesitate to select the other arm if it seems more acceptable. Often a winged infusion set is selected because the patient's veins are very small or fragile in the antecubital space. If this is the case, inspect the back of the patient's hands for a suitable vein.
      Rationale *Most adults have had previous venipunctures and know which veins are better for a successful draw. Asking a patient to state a preference gives the patient a sense of control over what is happening and increases patient comfort.*
   b. The arm or hand with the vein selected for the venipuncture should be extended and placed in a straight line from the shoulder to the wrist with the antecubital veins facing anteriorly. The arm should be supported on the armrest by a rolled towel or by having the patient place the fist of the other hand under the elbow.
   c. If the back of the hand is used, extend the arm with the back of the hand facing up. The hand should be placed on a flat surface. Have the patient grasp a

Continued

PROCEDURE 41-5 Perform Venipuncture Using the Butterfly Method (Collection of Multiple Evacuated Tubes)—cont'd

hand roll with their hand and roll it toward you. This brings the veins closer to the surface. If using the forearm, position it over the towel in a similar fashion. The tourniquet is applied in the same manner but will be secured 3 to 4 inches above the venipuncture site (wrist or forearm).

8. **Procedural Step.** Follow Steps 9 through 14 from Procedure 41-3.

9. **Procedural Step.** If drawing from the hand, ask the patient to make a fist or bend the fingers downward. Pull the skin taut with your thumb over the top of the patient's knuckles.

10. **Procedural Step. Position the butterfly needle.**
    Grasp the "wings" and fold them together with the thumb and index finger of your dominant hand. Wrap the tubing from the medial aspect of your hand to the lateral aspect, allowing the tube holder or syringe to hang down loosely. Place evacuated tubes nearby if using the winged infusion set with a Luer adapter and tube holder.
    Rationale. Holding the winged infusion set in this manner allows more freedom of movement to insert the evacuated tube once the needle has been inserted into the vein.

11. **Procedural Step.** Remove the protective shield from the needle of the infusion set being sure the bevel is facing up.
    Rationale. Positioning the needle with the bevel up allows for easier entry into the skin and the vein.

12. **Procedural Step. Perform the venipuncture.**
    a. Warn that the patient will feel a little "stick."
       Rationale. Warning the patient before entering the vein prevents the element of surprise, which could cause the patient to pull away, causing the needle to be pulled out of the vein.
    b. With the other hand, pull the skin taut beneath the intended puncture site to anchor the vein. Your thumb should be placed 1 to 2 inches below and to the side of the puncture site.
       Rationale. Pulling the skin taut helps the needle glide in easily.
    c. Following the direction of the vein, with one quick motion, smoothly pierce the skin and enter the vein at a small angle—about 15 degrees—and almost parallel to the vein.
       Rationale. The angle of the needle is important because an angle of less than 15 degrees may cause the needle to enter above the vein, preventing puncture. An angle of more than 30 degrees may cause the needle to go through the vein by puncturing the posterior wall. This could result in a hematoma (blood in the tissues).

13. **Procedural Step.** After penetrating the vein, decrease the angle of the needle to 5 degrees until a "flash" of blood appears in the tubing.
    If no flash appears, thread the needle into the lumen of the vein a little farther. If still no flash, release the tourniquet, slowly remove the needle, reassemble supplies, and try again.

14. **Procedural Step. Secure the needle for blood collection.**
    Seat the needle by slightly threading it up the lumen (central area) of the vein. This helps to prevent the needle from twisting out of the vein during the remainder of the procedure. Do not let go of the needle or allow it to move. Securely rest the needle flat against the skin.
    Rationale. Seating the needle anchors the needle in the center of the vein. Moving the needle is painful for the patient.

15. **Procedural Step.** Insert the evacuated tube into the tube holder or gently pull back on the plunger of the syringe.
    If using an evacuated tube system, keep the tube and holder in a downward position so that the tube fills from the bottom up and not near the rubber stopper. Push the bottom of the tube with the thumb of your nondominant hand carefully so that the needle inside the holder pierces the rubber stopper of the tube. If everything is done correctly, blood will begin to fill the tube.
    Rationale. The tube must fill from the bottom up to prevent venous reflux.

16. **Procedural Step. Change tubes as required by the test ordered.**
    When the tube has stopped filling, grasp the bottom of the tube with your nondominant hand. Push against the flange with the thumb, and pull the tube from the holder. This lets the rubber sleeve slide back over the end of the needle and prevents blood from dripping into the holder. Invert additive-containing tubes approximately 8 to 10 times, then place them upright in a rack so they will not roll. (Do not shake the tubes.)

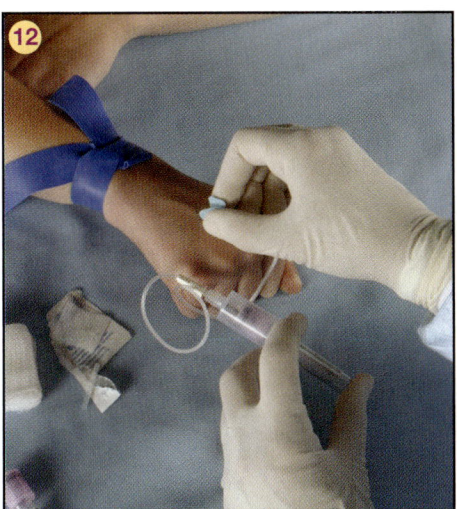

Continued

PROCEDURE 41-5 Perform Venipuncture Using the Butterfly Method (Collection of Multiple Evacuated Tubes)—cont'd

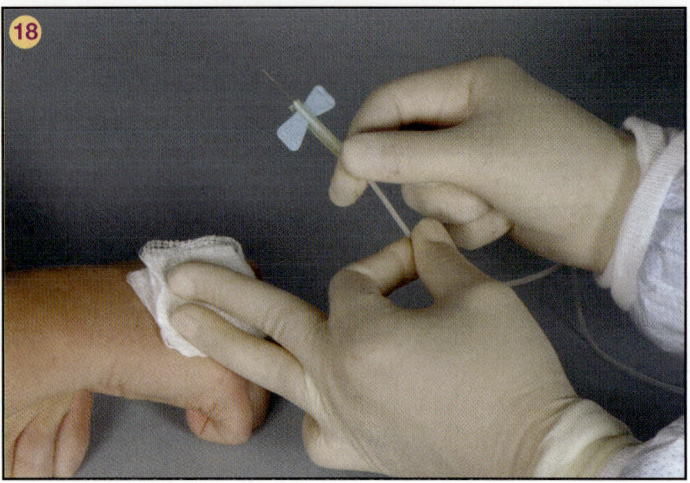

17. **Procedural Step.** Release the tourniquet.
18. **Procedural Step.** Remove the needle.
    With one quick, smooth motion, remove the needle from the arm with the dominant hand and apply pressure with the gauze in the left hand immediately *after* you remove the needle. As you withdraw the needle, flip the safety shield over the needle tip with your right thumb and direct the needle down and away from yourself and the patient.
    NOTE: Do not place a gauze pad over the needle as it is being withdrawn, since this can scratch the patient's arm or dig the needle into the arm, causing pain. Always withdraw the needle completely first, then apply the gauze pad to the site.
    Rationale. Placing the gauze pad over the puncture site helps prevent tissue movement, absorbs small amounts of blood that ooze from the vein, and reduces patient discomfort. Careful withdrawal prevents further tissue damage. The needle sheath prevents needle sticks.
19. **Procedural Step.** Apply direct pressure on the venipuncture site, and instruct the patient to raise the arm straight above the head.
    Tell the patient to keep the arm straight while raised to allow a good clot to begin forming over the puncture site.
    Rationale. Raising the arm straight above the head helps prevent a hematoma. Keeping the arm straight prevents dislodging the clot that has formed.
20. **Procedural Step.** Instruct the patient to maintain pressure on the site for 1 to 2 minutes, with the arm raised straight up above the head.
    NOTE: If any swelling or discoloration occurs, apply an ice pack to the site after bandaging it.
    Rationale. Maintaining pressure with the arm raised over the head will help speed up the clotting process and prevent a hematoma. Do not allow the patient to bend the arm at the elbow because this increases blood loss from the puncture site and causes bruising.
21. **Procedural Step.** If a syringe was used, transfer the blood to the evacuated tubes as soon as possible.
    See Step 17 in Procedure 41-4.
22. **Procedural Step.** Properly dispose of the winged infusion set.
    Always drop the butterfly set and holder in a sharps container. When using a quick-release holder, disconnect the multisample needle from the infusion set. If the quick-disconnect holder is contaminated with blood, it should be discarded.
    Rationale. Proper disposal of the needle is required by the OSHA standard to prevent accidental needle stick injuries.
23. **Procedural Step.** Follow Steps 25 through 33 from Procedure 41-3.

CHARTING EXAMPLE	
Date	
7/31/xx	10:30 a.m. Venous blood specimen collected for CBC from Ⓡ hand. Site without redness or edema.————————————————— R. Green, CMA (AAMA)

Photos for Steps 5, 12, and 18 from Garrels M, Oatis C: Laboratory testing for ambulatory settings, St Louis, 2006, Saunders.

BOX 41-2

Failed Blood Draws

Do not be discouraged. On certain days or with certain patients, a failed draw will occur. The best strategy for missing a blood draw is that strategy used for riding a horse: "When you fall off, get back on and try again." Never take it as a defeat; rather, look at a failed draw as a challenge. As mentioned, make two attempts, then ask someone else to do it.

The more you practice, the better you will be. The most important task in being able to perform venipuncture is "finding the vein." If you can locate, stabilize, and enter the vein's lumen (opening), you will be successful at drawing blood.

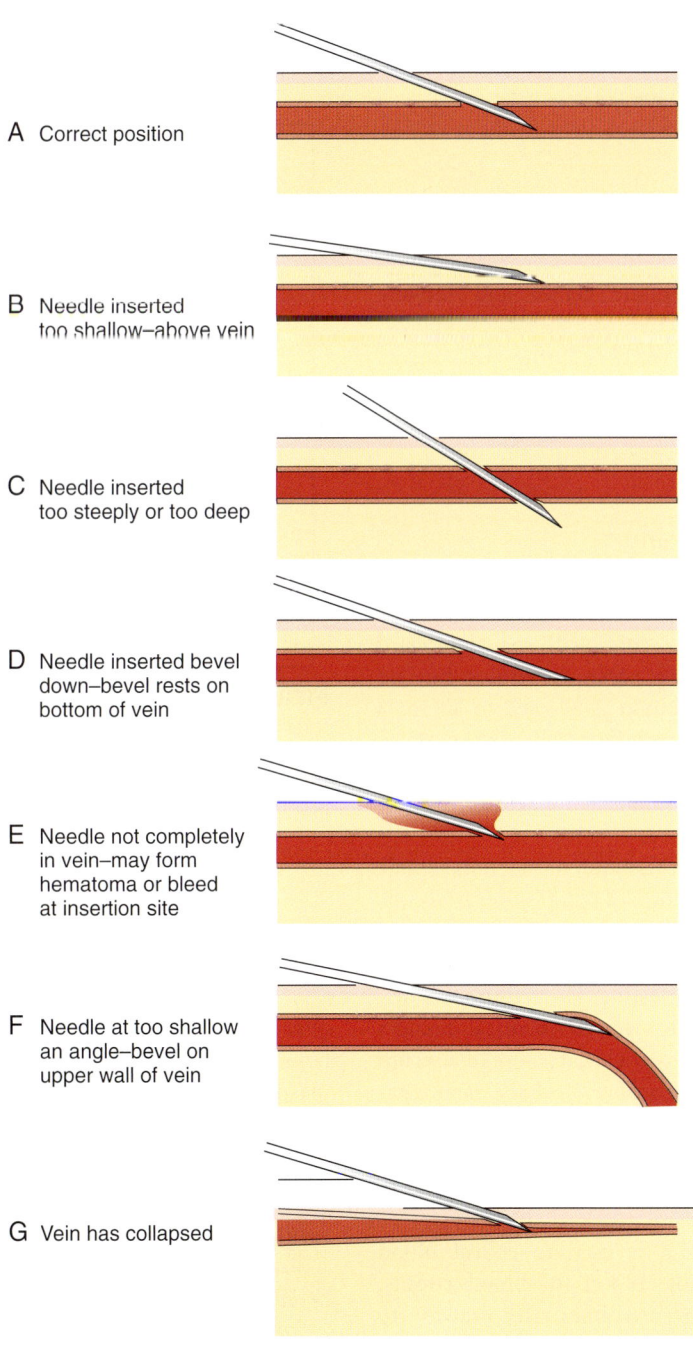

FIGURE 41-12 Causes of failed draws. (From Hunt SA: *Saunders fundamentals of medical assisting—revised reprint*, St Louis, 2007, Saunders.)

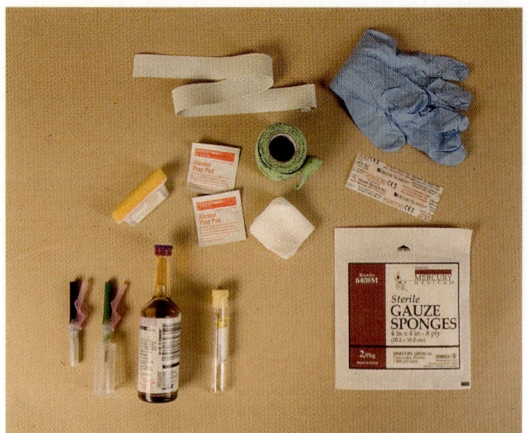

FIGURE 41-13 Blood cultures may be collected in sterile yellow tubes or bottles that fit into the plastic holder.

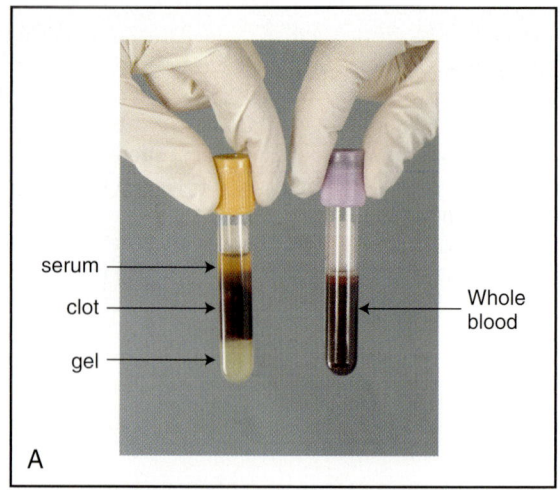

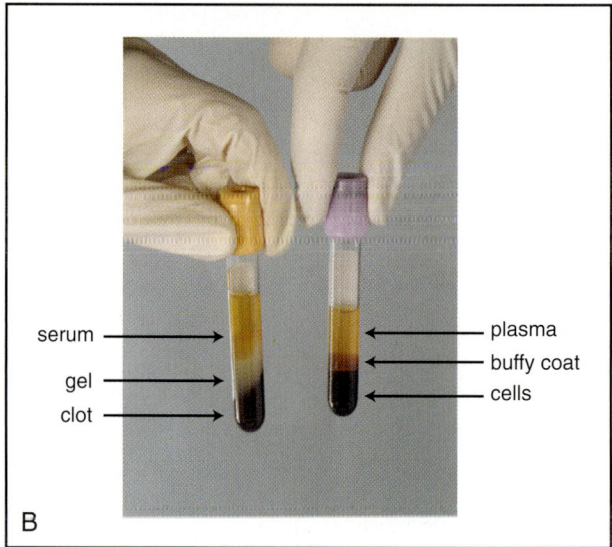

FIGURE 41-14 **A,** Gold tube with clotted blood and lavender tube with whole blood before centrifuging. **B,** Clotted and whole blood after centrifuging. Note the layers in each tube. (From Garrels M, Oatis C: *Laboratory testing for ambulatory settings,* St Louis, 2006, Saunders.)

For a **blood culture,** two blood samples are collected from different sites. Each site is cleaned with alcohol for 2 minutes using a "friction scrub" technique, followed by cleaning with povidone-iodine, starting from the center and moving outward. The blood sample is collected in either a yellow-stoppered tube or a special collection bottle with media designed to grow bacteria (Figure 41-14). Sometimes physicians request these samples be drawn at the outpatient or hospital laboratory to eliminate contamination factors.

Serum and Plasma Separation

If serum or plasma is required for a test, the blood specimen needs to be separated before transfer. The specimen is collected in a plain red, red/gray (marbled), or Hemogard gold Vacutainer tube containing serum separator but no additives. After collection, the blood is allowed to sit for a minimum of 30 minutes to allow a clot (jelly-like mass) to form. The tube is placed in the centrifuge and spun at the speed and time recommended by the manufacturer, usually 15 minutes.

The yellow liquid portion that is on top of the spun sample is serum. Serum is the liquid portion of blood minus the clotting factors (see Figure 41-14). The serum should be **pipetted** (usually using a **pipette**) from the tube and placed in a properly labeled transfer tube for later testing. The serum specimen is either refrigerated or frozen to prevent chemical changes unless the specimen can be tested quickly. The use of a serum separator tube provides a silicone gel barrier that aids in separation and allows for pouring the serum into the transfer tube instead of pipetting it. Procedure 41-6 describes the process of separating serum from whole blood and transferring it to a transfer tube.

A lavender tube with EDTA is used to collect blood specimens for plasma or whole blood for blood counts. This type of specimen is inverted 8 times after drawing to prevent clotting and platelet clumping. Blood collected in this type of tube is not required to sit and can be centrifuged immediately after collection (Figure 41-14, *B*). The plasma is pipetted off in the same manner as serum and stored until collection.

If either the serum or plasma becomes red or pink tinged after centrifuging, the specimen RBCs have ruptured, causing hemoglobin and cellular components to enter the serum or plasma. The specimen will have to be redrawn. Box 41-3 provides a list of reasons hemolysis occurs.

PATIENT-CENTERED PROFESSIONALISM

- Why is it important for the medical assistant to know proper patient preparation and collection methods for a capillary puncture?
- Why must the order of draw be followed?

Phlebotomy   CHAPTER 41   953

PROCEDURE
41-6

Separate Serum from a Blood Specimen

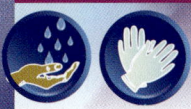

TASK: Transfer serum separated from blood by the process of centrifugation into a transfer tube.

EQUIPMENT AND SUPPLIES
- Nonsterile disposable gloves
- Personal protective equipment (PPE)
- Clotted blood specimen (centrifuged)
- Laboratory requisition form
- Biohazardous waste container
- Sharps container
- Transfer tube
- Transfer pipette
- Centrifuge

SKILLS/*RATIONALE*

STANDARD PRECAUTIONS ARE TO BE FOLLOWED.

1. **Procedural Step.** Sanitize the hands.
   An alcohol-based hand rub may be used instead of washing hands with soap and water, unless hands are visibly soiled.
   Rationale. Hand sanitization promotes infection control.

2. **Procedural Step.** Assemble equipment and supplies and verify the order.
   Rationale. It is important to have all supplies and equipment ready and available before starting any procedure to ensure efficiency.

3. **Procedural Step.** Apply gloves and other PPE.

4. **Procedural Step.** Verify orders against the laboratory requisition form and the specimen tube.
   Rationale. All identification must match for accuracy.

5. **Procedural Step.** Allow whole blood specimens, collected in a red-top evacuated tube, to clot at room temperature for a minimum of 30 minutes and no more than 45 minutes after collection.
   Rationale. Specimens require a minimum of 20 minutes sitting upright in a tube rack to form a sufficient clot removing all clotting factors. After 45 minutes the specimen starts to lose its integrity.

6. **Procedural Step.** Place two stoppered red-top tubes in the centrifuge to balance the centrifuge and close and latch the centrifuge lid securely.
   The centrifuge is balanced when tubes containing equal amounts of fluid are placed directly across from each other. If only one tube of blood is to be centrifuged, the second tube can be filled with an equal amount of water.
   Rationale. The tubes must remain stoppered during this process. If the centrifuge is not balanced, the blood tube could break, creating a biohazardous situation.

7. **Procedural Step.** Set the timer for 15 minutes.

8. **Procedural Step.** When the time has elapsed, allow the centrifuge to come to a complete stop before opening the lid and removing the tube.
   Rationale. This prevents the potential of aerosol spray contamination.

9. **Procedural Step.** Properly remove the stopper or apply a transfer device.

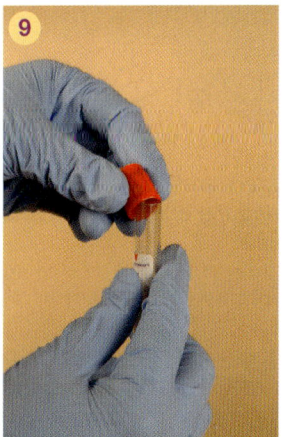

10. **Procedural Step.** Separate the serum from the top of the tube into a transfer tube using the transfer device or a disposable pipette.
    If a red/gray (marbled) or Hemogard gold tube is used, the serum may be poured into a transfer tube.

11. **Procedural Step.** Label the tubes and attach the laboratory requisition form.

12. **Procedural Step.** Properly dispose of all waste material in the appropriate waste receptacle.
    Any items contaminated with blood must be disposed of in a biohazardous waste container. Any items made of glass (tubes) must be disposed of in a sharps container. Items not contaminated with body fluids may be disposed of in regular waste containers.

13. **Procedural Step.** Package the specimen for transport to the laboratory.

14. **Procedural Step.** Remove gloves and sanitize the hands.
    Always sanitize the hands after every procedure or after using gloves.

BOX 41-3

Reasons Hemolysis Occurs

- Using a small-gauge (<23-gauge) needle
- When transferring blood from a syringe into a vacuum tube
- Improperly attaching a needle to a syringe (causes frothing of blood)
- Shaking a blood specimen to mix rather than invert
- Forcing blood into a vacuum tube when using a syringe

CONCLUSION

Medical assistants are often involved in the collection, preparation for transport, and processing of the many types of specimens collected at the POL. The physician can analyze specimens collected from a patient to assess the patient's general health, as well as to diagnose and determine treatment plans.

The medical assistant must understand and follow federal, state, and office protocols for collecting and transporting specimens. These protocols help ensure that accurate results are obtained from testing. Accurate test results are crucial. Errors in specimen collection can cause delays in testing, diagnosis, and treatment, or even lawsuits in some situations. The knowledgeable, skilled medical assistant helps protect the patient and the medical office by performing all procedures accurately, efficiently, and in accordance with all guidelines and protocols.

Chapter Summary

Reinforce your understanding of the material in this chapter by reviewing the curriculum objectives and key content points below.

1. **Define, appropriately use, and spell all the Key Terms for this chapter.**
   - Review the Key Terms if necessary.
2. **List methods of collecting blood and give the three factors that determine which method will be used.**
   - Venipuncture and capillary puncture are two methods of collecting blood
   - The test to be performed and the age and condition of the patient determine which method will be used
3. **Explain the purpose of a lancet in capillary blood collection.**
   - The sterile lancet makes a small puncture in the skin.
   - Lancets penetrate the skin at various depths depending on the patient and condition of the site.
4. **Briefly describe five types of containers that can be used to collect capillary blood specimens.**
   - Microcontainers, capillary tubes, glass slides, filter paper, and blood-diluting pipettes can be used to collect capillary blood specimens.
5. **Demonstrate the correct procedure for obtaining a capillary blood specimen acceptable for testing using the ring or middle finger.**
   - Review Procedure 41-1.
6. **Demonstrate the correct procedure for collecting a capillary specimen for phenylketonuria (PKU) screening using filter paper.**
   - Review Procedure 41-2.
7. **List four acceptable sites for performing venipuncture and the two factors in selecting the site.**
   - Venipuncture can be performed in the antecubital fossa of either arm, the cephalic veins, the basilic veins, or the forearm.
   - Site selection depends on the age of the patient and condition of the veins.
8. **State two reasons for failed venipuncture draws.**
   - Failed venipuncture draws can be caused by incorrectly positioning the needle or using the wrong angle.
9. **List the order of draw for the evacuated-tube (Vacutainer) system recommended by the Clinical and Laboratory Standards Institute (CLSI).**
   - Use the memory aid "Big Rugged Günther Got Lots of Gold" to help you remember the order of draw (see Figure 41-8).
10. **Demonstrate the correct procedure for obtaining a venous blood specimen acceptable for testing using the evacuated-tube system.**
    - Review Procedure 41-3.
11. **Demonstrate the correct procedure for obtaining a venous blood specimen acceptable for testing using the syringe method.**
    - Review Procedure 41-4.
12. **Demonstrate the correct procedure for obtaining a venous blood specimen acceptable for testing using the butterfly method.**
    - Review Procedure 41-5.
13. **Demonstrate the correct procedure for successfully separating serum from a blood specimen and transferring the serum from the collection tube to a transfer tube.**
    - Review Procedure 41-6.
14. **Analyze a realistic medical office situation and apply your understanding of the purpose and use of the physician office laboratory to determine the best course of action.**
    - Medical assistants must understand and follow the procedures and policies associated with each laboratory procedure they perform.

- Proper patient preparation is an important aspect of laboratory testing.
15. **Describe the impact on patient care when medical assistants have a solid understanding of the processes and procedures used to collect specimens for testing in the medical office.**
    - Accurate test results occur when the medical assistant properly collects or provides clear instructions to the patient for collection and follows proper processing procedures.
    - Patient care is enhanced when the medical assistant is knowledgeable about proper procedures for collecting and processing specimens.
    - Diagnosis and treatment of a patient begin sooner when test results are accurate.

PRACTICAL APPLICATIONS

If you have accomplished the objectives in this chapter, you will be able to make better choices as a medical assistant. Take another look at this situation and decide what you would do.

The full-time laboratory technician at Dr. Macinto's office is on sick leave for another week. Dr. Macinto asks Sherri, a medical assistant, to continue to fill in for the sick technician. Remember Sherri had just been hired from another office, where she was trained by the physician. She has not done laboratory tests and has not prepared patients for laboratory work.

Mrs. Gorchetzki, a postmastectomy patient, is seen next. Dr. Macinto has ordered a fasting blood sugar and a fasting blood chemistry test. Without talking to Mrs. Gorchetzki about the preparation she has made for the test, Sherri gathers the supplies for the testing. Mrs. Gorchetzki mentions that she had bacon and eggs for breakfast. Sherri draws the blood sugar using a capillary puncture. Sherri performs the testing before doing quality control for the day. When the specimen is drawn for the blood chemistry, the laboratory request form asks for serum. Sherri starts the process of drawing the venipuncture specimen from the side of the mastectomy in a heparinized tube. Mrs. Gorchetzki tries to tell Sherri to collect the specimen from the other arm because it is easier to draw blood from that arm, but Sherri does not listen.

When Sherri places the specimen in the centrifuge, she spins only one tube. She pipettes off the liquid and sends it to the laboratory. As it turns out, the liquid sent to the laboratory is plasma, but the laboratory had requested serum.

What things would you have done differently in this situation?

1. What color tube should have been used for the blood chemistry? What is the common tube used for whole blood and plasma?
2. Why should Sherri *not* have used the arm on the side of the mastectomy? What should she have done when Mrs. Gorchetzki told her that there was a vein that was usually used for venipuncture?
3. Why is it important to close the cover of a centrifuge when it is operating?
4. After Mrs. Gorchetzki stated that she had eaten breakfast, what should Sherri have done rather than collecting the blood specimens? What part of quality assurance was broken by Mrs. Gorchetzki's action of eating?
5. What is Dr. Macinto's responsibility in regard to Sherri's actions?

WEB SEARCH

1. **Research the current updates and history of the CLSI.** The organization is responsible for setting guidelines for the collection of diagnostic specimens by venipuncture, blood cultures collection, and the venipuncture in children.

- **Keywords:** Use the following keywords in your search: Clinical and Laboratory Standards Institute, CLSI.

42 Laboratory Testing in the Physician's Office

evolve   http://evolve.elsevier.com/klieger/medicalassisting

The purpose of the **Clinical Laboratory Improvement Amendments of 1988 (CLIA 88)** was to establish minimum quality standards for laboratory testing. Any facility wanting to become certified to perform certain laboratory tests and procedures must submit an application with a fee. The laboratory must also follow all regulations on using quality control testing, hiring knowledgeable personnel, using quality assurance measures, and submitting to periodic inspections. The standards established by CLIA 88 ensure the reliability of testing results. This protects the patient by ensuring that employees are not performing tests without the proper educational training.

As discussed in earlier chapters, some laboratory tests are **CLIA-waived tests.** This "waived" status means these tests are simple and have minimal risk for error. CLIA provides a certificate to perform waived tests to a facility when it agrees to follow proper laboratory practices. CLIA-waived tests can be performed in physician offices, clinical laboratories, and long-term care facilities; at the bedside in an acute care setting; by insurance companies; and in other settings by nonlaboratory health care workers.

CLIA-waived tests are simple to perform, but care must be taken to follow quality control measures to minimize inaccurate test results.

This chapter discusses CLIA-waived urinalysis and blood testing, as well as some non–CLIA-waived tests. Although some tests are not waived, the medical assistant should understand how they are done and their clinical significance (e.g., microscopic examination of urine sediment). Throat culture for group A beta-hemolytic streptococci, discussed in Chapter 40, is also a CLIA-waived test.

LEARNING OBJECTIVES

You will be able to do the following after completing this chapter:

Key Terms
1. Define, appropriately use, and spell all the Key Terms for this chapter.

Physical Properties of Urine
2. Explain what causes urine's color and what causes urine to have an abnormal color.
3. Describe the normal appearance of urine and explain what causes urine to have an abnormal appearance.
4. Explain why various odors occur in urine.
5. List two causes of low urinary output and three causes of high urinary output.

Chemical Properties of Urine
6. State two testing differences between a reagent strip and a reagent tablet.
7. Demonstrate the correct procedure for processing a urine specimen using a reagent technique.
8. List 10 tests performed during a routine urinalysis.
9. Explain how an automated urine analyzer processes reagent test strips.
10. List three brands of reagent tablets and their use in confirmatory tests.

Microscopic Examination of Urine

11. Explain why microscopic examination of urine sediment may be done.
12. Demonstrate the correct procedure for microscopic examination of urine.
13. List seven types of structures typically found in urine.

Urine Pregnancy Tests

14. Demonstrate the correct procedure for performing a urine pregnancy color-reaction test.

Blood Tests

15. Differentiate among hematology, serology, blood chemistry, and microbiology.

Hematology

16. State the purpose of a complete blood count (CBC) and list six types of information it provides.
17. State the purpose of measuring hemoglobin and list one automated device approved by CLIA for this use in the physician office laboratory (POL).
18. Demonstrate the correct procedure for obtaining a hemoglobin reading.
19. Explain the purpose of a hematocrit and what a low reading and a high reading may indicate.
20. Demonstrate the correct procedure for obtaining an accurate hematocrit value.
21. Explain the purpose of the erythrocyte sedimentation rate (ESR) and list two common methods used in the POL to perform ESR.
22. Demonstrate the correct procedure for performing ESR using the Westergren method.
23. Explain the purpose of a differential blood cell count and list five factors that affect the quality of a good blood smear.
24. Demonstrate the correct procedure for preparation of a blood smear slide.

Blood Chemistry

25. Explain how physicians use blood chemistry profiles.
26. Explain the purpose of cholesterol testing and list the desirable, borderline-high, and high cholesterol levels in test results.
27. Demonstrate the procedure for accurately collecting and processing a blood specimen for cholesterol testing.
28. Describe three tests performed to monitor a person's glucose level.
29. Demonstrate the procedure for accurately collecting and processing a blood specimen for glucose testing.

Serology and Immunology

30. Define serology and list seven types of serological or immunological testing.
31. List and describe four viewable reactions to additives that indicate positive results in serological testing.

Microbiology

32. Demonstrate the procedure for correctly obtaining a bacterial smear from a wound swab.
33. Explain the purpose of a Gram stain and briefly describe the staining process.
34. Explain why culture plates are inoculated, and briefly describe the process of streaking an agar plate.

Patient-Centered Professionalism

35. Analyze a realistic medical office situation and apply your understanding of laboratory testing in the physician office to determine the best course of action.
36. Describe the impact on patient care when medical assistants have a solid understanding of the purpose and procedures for laboratory tests performed in the medical office.

KEY TERMS

2-hour postprandial test
acetone
agar
agglutination
artifacts
automated urine analyzer
bacteria
bacterial smear
bacteriology
bacteriuria
bilirubin
bilirubinuria
casts
cellular casts
chemistry profile
CLIA-waived tests
Clinical Laboratory Improvement Amendments of 1988 (CLIA 88)
complete blood count (CBC)
confirmatory tests
crenated
crystals
culture and sensitivity (C&S)
culture plate
cystitis
diaphoresis
differential blood cell count
ethylenediaminetetraacetic acid (EDTA)
enzyme immunoassay (EIA)
erythrocyte sedimentation rate (ESR)
fasting blood sugar (FBS) test
fatty casts
first morning specimen
galactosemia
glucometer
glucose
glucose reagent strip
glucose tolerance test (GTT)
glycosuria
glycosylated hemoglobin (GHb) test
Gram stain
granular casts
high-density lipoprotein (HDL)
hematocrit (Hct)
hematology
hematuria
hemoglobin (Hb or Hgb)
hemoglobinuria
hemolyzed
high-power field (HPF)
human chorionic gonadotropin (hCG)
hyaline casts
immunoassays
immunological testing
immunology
ketones
ketonuria
low-density lipoprotein (LDL)
leukocyte esterase
low-power field (LPF)
lumen
lysis
media
mucous threads
myoglobinuria
nephron
nitrates
nitrites
parasites
plaque

Continued

platelet counts
point-of-care testing (POCT)
precipitates
proteinuria
qualitative
quantitative
random specimen
reagent strip
reagent tablet
red cell indices
renal epithelial cells
sediment
serological testing
serology
serum cholesterol
specific gravity
spermatozoa
squamous epithelial cells
streak
supernatant
timed specimen
total cholesterol
transitional epithelial cells
turbid
urinalysis
urobilinogen
urochrome
viscosity
waxy casts
Westergren method
Wintrobe method
yeasts

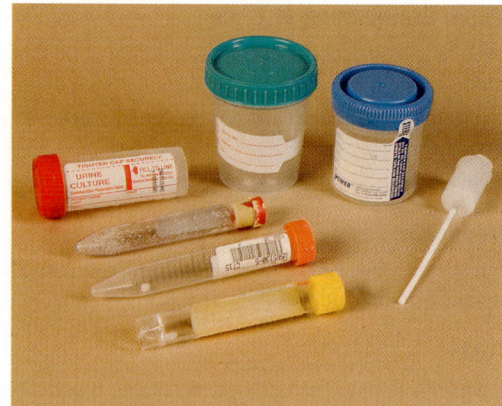

FIGURE 42-1 Containers for urine collection.

PRACTICAL APPLICATIONS

Read the following scenario and keep it in mind as you learn about laboratory testing in the physician office.

Dr. Carlson does not have a medical laboratory technician. Instead, she depends on the medical assistant to provide the test results of laboratory specimens that are ordered. Because of his training in a medical assisting program, Jerry is aware of the importance of quality control and quality assurance and that both should be done on a daily basis.

As part of the daily routine, Jerry, the medical assistant, is expected to perform physical and chemical testing of urine using reagent strips. Dr. Carlson also allows Jerry to examine specimens using a microscope to identify the urine sediment. Jerry completes hemoglobin testing using HemoCue and uses a centrifuge to spin hematocrits. As Jerry reads the hematocrit, he finds that the anticoagulated blood has separated into three layers, each of which has a specific characteristic.

Because CLIA-waived tests are often performed in a physician's office, Jerry and other medical assistants must be able to perform these tests on a daily basis. Would you be capable of performing these tasks?

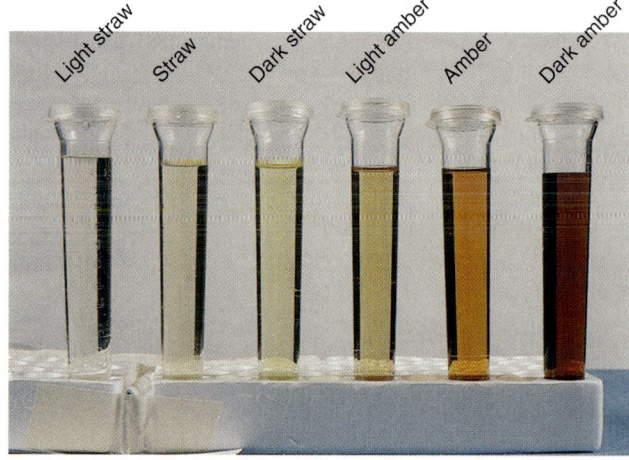

FIGURE 42-2 Color of urine. (From Bonewit-West K: *Clinical procedures for medical assistants*, ed. 7, St Louis, 2008, Saunders.)

URINALYSIS

Urinalysis is an examination of a urine specimen. It is one of the most common laboratory tests performed in the physician's office as part of a routine physical examination. Urinalysis involves the physical, chemical, and microscopic examination of the urine specimen. The medical assistant can perform the physical and chemical aspect of a urinalysis. However, a qualified member of the health care team must perform the microscopic portion because it is not a CLIA-waived procedure. (The microscopic aspect is only covered in this chapter to provide you with an overall understanding of the process.) Figure 42-1 is a display of various types of urine collection devices.

Physical Properties of Urine

A urinalysis can provide valuable diagnostic information concerning overall metabolic function of the kidneys and urinary tract. A visual inspection of the urine sample is made to assess its physical properties. This is the first step taken by the medical assistant when performing a urinalysis. Visual inspection includes observation of the color, appearance, and any distinctive odor from the specimen. A routine urinalysis does not require the medical assistant to record the amount or volume of the specimen, but the assistant needs to be aware if production amounts are within normal range (see Chapter 20).

Color

Normal urine color can vary from pale yellow or straw to amber (dark yellow) (Figure 42-2). **Urochrome** is the yellow pigment (derived from urobilin) left over when hemoglobin

TABLE 42-1
Urine Colors and Clinical Significance

Color	Clinical Significance
Pale yellow	High fluid consumption
	Diabetes mellitus
	Diabetes insipidus
	Diuretics
Straw	Normal
Amber	Concentrated specimen
	Dehydration
	Fever
	Excessive exercise
	Excessive fluid loss (diarrhea, vomiting)
Bright yellow	Excessive beta-carotene (carrots, high dose of vitamin A); vitamin supplements
Orange-yellow	Drugs (e.g., phenazopyridine [Pyridium]; warfarin [Coumadin])
Yellow-brown	Bilirubin
	Liver disease
	Excessive destruction of red blood cells
	Iron preparations
Greenish-yellow	Bilirubin
	Drugs (e.g., senna, cascara)
Blue-green	*Pseudomonas* infection
	High ingestion of asparagus
	Vitamin B
	Drugs (e.g., indomethacin [Indocin])
Red	Blood (menstrual)
	High ingestion of beets
	Red blood cells (hemoglobin)
	Drugs

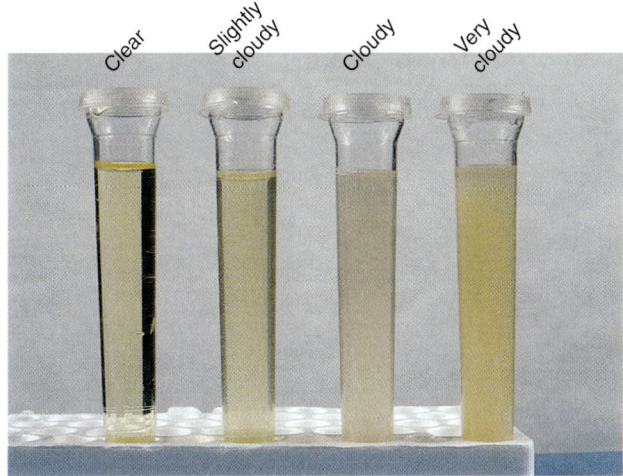

FIGURE 42-3 Appearance of urine. (From Bonewit-West K: *Clinical procedures for medical assistants*, ed. 7, St Louis, 2008, Saunders.)

breaks down during the destruction of red blood cells (RBCs). This is what gives urine its color.

Urine color is affected by food and fluid intake, medications, and waste products from a disease process. Usually a pale urine color indicates diluted urine, and a dark-yellow urine specimen indicates a concentrated specimen. In most cases, the more concentrated the specimen, the darker is the appearance.

Urine specimens may be collected at specific times of the day, which may affect the color, as follows:
- The **first morning specimen** is usually more concentrated because it has been in the bladder overnight.
- A **random specimen** (taken any time with no special preparation) may have less color because foods and fluids taken throughout the day affect its concentration.

Chapter 40 provides more information on specific methods for urine collection. Table 42-1 lists the clinical significance of various colors of urine.

Appearance

The appearance of urine can be described in terms such as *clear* or *transparent, hazy* (slightly cloudy), *cloudy,* **turbid** (particles floating within), and *milky* (very cloudy). A fresh urine specimen should appear clear or transparent. A fresh specimen that appears cloudy or turbid could be contaminated with bacteria, pus, mucus, or yeast. Since refrigeration or standing at room temperature for long periods causes a specimen to become cloudy, its appearance should be observed and recorded as soon as possible (Figure 42-3). Many factors can contribute to cloudiness, including crystals, the change of the specimen's pH from acid to alkaline as it sits and cools, blood cells, bacteria, and other substances. Further examination of the specimen with a microscope will help determine the cause of the cloudiness.

Besides abnormal color, the presence of *foam* that does not rapidly disperse from a fresh specimen is clinically significant. White foam that stays on top of a freshly voided specimen may indicate an increase in proteins (proteinuria), a clinical symptom for complications of diabetes, and heart and renal disease. Greenish yellow foam on an amber specimen may indicate the presence of bilirubin in the urine specimen (bilirubinuria); this is one of the clinical signs of hepatitis and other liver disorders.

Odor

Normal urine is described as being "aromatic," or not having a distinctive smell. It only develops an ammonia-like odor on standing. To prevent urine from developing the ammonia-like odor, a specimen must be tested within 1 hour of collection. The ammonia smell is caused by bacteria breaking down urea in the specimen. Several factors can affect the odor of a fresh specimen, as follows (Table 42-2):
- Foods, such as garlic and asparagus, can produce a strong odor in urine.
- A strong unpleasant (foul) odor is brought on by bacteria from a urinary tract infection (UTI).
- A "sweet-smelling" (fruity) scent is characteristic of a patient with uncontrolled diabetes because of ketones (a byproduct of fat metabolism) in the urine.

TABLE 42-2
Abnormal Urine Odors

Smell	Clinical Significance
Fruity	Starvation, anorexia
	Uncontrolled diabetes mellitus
Ammonia	Urinary tract infection (UTI)
	Long-standing specimen
Foul	Bacteria
"Musky"	Phenylketonuria (PKU) (metabolic disease)

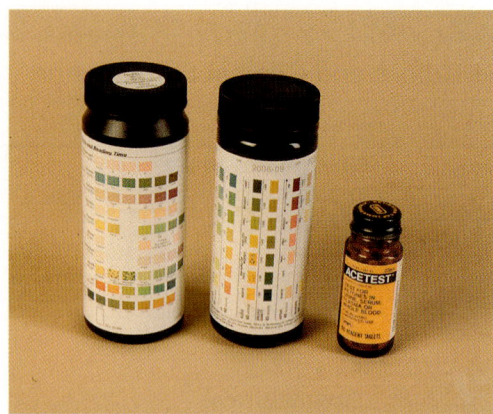

FIGURE 42-4 Examples of reagent strips and reagent tablets.

Volume

The normal volume of urine produced by an adult in a 24-hour period is 750 to 2000 mL (0.75 to 2 L). Smaller amounts are normal for infants and children. The major factor affecting urine output is fluid intake.

Factors affecting low output of urine include the following:
- Inadequate fluid intake
- Fluids lost during episodes of diarrhea, vomiting, and profuse sweating (**diaphoresis**) causing dehydration

High urine output may be caused by the following:
- Excessive fluid intake
- Diuretic medication for hypertension, congestive heart failure, and edema
- Reduction in antidiuretic hormone (ADH) secreted
- Uncontrolled diabetes insipidus or renal disease

During the patient screening process, a medical assistant must listen carefully when the patient describes fluid intake and output. For example, if a patient off-handedly remarks that she seems to be thirstier lately and is constantly urinating, this information must be charted so that the physician can further investigate possible causes. The physician may then order a **timed specimen,** in which urine is collected for 24 hours and a small sample is removed and analyzed.

Chemical Properties of Urine

When the filtering ability of the kidneys is damaged, substances not normally found in the urine (e.g., protein, blood) are present. The chemical composition of a urine specimen is measured in the physician office laboratory (POL) to detect these substances. This can be done by using a **reagent strip** (dipsticks) or a **reagent tablet** (Figure 42-4).

Differences between reagent strips and reagent tablets include the following:
- Reagent strips detect both the *presence* and approximate *amount* of these substances in the urine, whereas reagent tablet analysis only detects the *presence* of a particular substance (e.g., Acetest detects ketones) and not its quantity.
- Each chemical pad on the reagent strip tests for only one type of substance, whereas a reagent tablet can detect the presence of other related substances. For example, one chemical pad on the reagent strip only detects the presence of the sugar glucose in the urine, but a Clinitest (Ames) reagent tablet will detect the presence of other sugars (e.g., galactose, lactose, or fructose). When galactose fails to convert to glucose, for example, a congenital disorder called **galactosemia** is indicated. Reagent tablets can be used to confirm a particular substance in the urine (e.g., ketones, glucose).

Whether using a reagent strip or reagent tablet when performing laboratory tests, if the results do not fit with other test results or patient symptoms, the physician usually orders a retest. This can be done by (1) repeating the test on the same specimen or a new specimen, (2) performing a different test on the same specimen, or (3) running a test from a different type of specimen such as blood.

Reagent Strips

The Multistix 10 SG (Bayer, Tarrytown, NY) reagent strip tests for glucose, bilirubin, ketones, specific gravity, blood, pH, protein, urobilinogen, nitrites, and leukocytes. The Chemstrip 9 (Boehringer Mannheim, Norristown, PA) tests for all these substances but not for specific gravity. The type of reagent strip chosen by a medical practice depends on preference and the type of urine screening most often done in a particular medical office (e.g., an obstetric/gynecology office might use a reagent strip that tests for only glucose and protein).

Quality Control. Accurate results require medical assistants to use an appropriate technique and follow the quality control program established by the facility. Figure 42-5 shows reagents used to validate the quality of test materials. This includes (1) checking the expiration date on the bottle, (2) keeping the strips in their original container with the lid tight to prevent moisture and light from affecting the chemical pad, and (3) using a fresh specimen.

Using the Reagent Strip. The reagent strip is dipped into the fresh urine specimen, wetting all pads. It is removed immediately, and any excess urine is removed by dragging (or tapping) the strip edge gently against the rim of the container as it is removed. The strip is then held horizontally to prevent the chemicals on each pad from mixing with the others. When recording the results, the color of each chemical pad at time

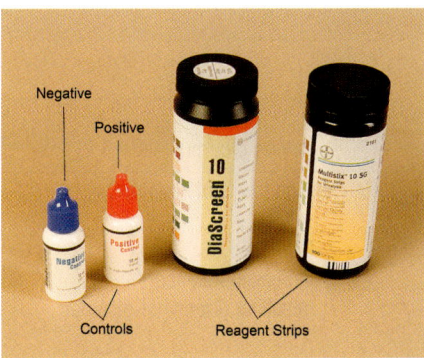

FIGURE 42-5 Reagent strips with controls for quality control purposes.

> **BOX 42-1**
>
> ### Documentation when Charting CLIA-Waived Tests
>
> 1. Date
> 2. Time
> 3. Name of test
> 4. Results
> 5. Patient reaction, if any
> 6. Proper signature and credential

intervals specified by the manufacturer is compared to a color scale located on the bottle. The medical assistant must be certain the specimen is fresh and must adhere to the times specified by the strip manufacturer because chemical reactions will continue to occur, resulting in elevated values.

Table 42-3 provides the normal values for each test, the clinical significance of each test, and possible reasons for false readings. Procedure 42-1 describes the proper technique for processing a urine specimen using a reagent technique. Box 42-1 reviews the necessary criteria for charting CLIA-waived tests.

Glucose. **Glucose** in the urine (**glycosuria**) may indicate the patient has diabetes. It also can be present after a heavy meal, emotional stress, or high doses of vitamin C. The presence of glucose in the urine is recorded as a trace, +1, +2, +3, or +4. Absence of glucose in the urine is recorded as negative. The test is usually read 30 seconds after the strip has been dipped into the urine.

Bilirubin. The presence of **bilirubin** in the urine is **bilirubinuria**. Bilirubin, a byproduct of hemoglobin breakdown, is normally processed into bile by the liver and excreted by the intestines. Bilirubin appearing in the urine is a clear sign of liver or biliary tract dysfunction or disease.

The test values are recorded as negative, +1 (small amount), +2 (moderate amount), or +3 (large amount). The test is read 30 seconds after the strip is dipped into the urine.

Ketones. **Ketonuria** is the presence of **ketones** in the urine. When the body does not have an adequate intake of protein, carbohydrates, or other energy-producing elements, the body will burn fatty acids. Ketones are a waste product of fat metabolism. Ketones will be excreted when the patient is diabetic, dieting, suffering from anorexia, starving, experiencing excessive diarrhea, and vomiting.

The values are recorded as negative, trace, small, moderate, or large. The results are read 40 seconds after the strip has been dipped into the urine.

Specific Gravity. The kidneys function to regulate the amount of urine that is produced and to maintain the concentration of various substances that provide homeostasis. Urine **specific gravity** shows the amount of dissolved substances in the urine. This test indicates the kidney's ability to concentrate urine. The specific gravity of urine depends on a person's fluid intake, various disease states (e.g., dehydration, renal or liver disease, congestive heart failure, or presence of protein or glucose in urine), and the ability of the kidneys to concentrate urine.

The specific gravity of urine is compared to that of distilled water (1). The normal range for specific gravity is 1.01 to 1.025 ± 5. Specific gravity of urine is highest in the morning. The higher the specific gravity of the urine, the darker is the specimen's color. An exception occurs when a specimen is obtained from a diabetic patient. The specimen may have a high specific gravity because of glucose in the urine but may appear light yellow. The results are read after 45 seconds.

Blood. The chemical pad for blood on the reagent strip will react to three different forms of blood: intact RBCs, hemoglobin from RBCs, and myoglobin from muscle tissue.

- **Hematuria** is the presence of intact RBCs in the urine caused by an infection (**cystitis**), injury, or trauma to the urinary tract, such as a kidney stone.
- **Hemoglobinuria** is the presence of hemolyzed RBCs in the urine. This can be caused by a hemolytic transfusion reaction, drug reaction, severe burns, and other conditions.
- **Myoglobinuria** is the result of severe muscle injury caused by trauma (e.g., automobile accidents, sports injuries).

In a physician's office, most positive blood reactions result from intact RBCs. Women who are menstruating (or in the days before or after menses) may have blood present in the specimen. Ask the patient the date of her last menses to determine if this may be a factor. The results are recorded as negative, trace, +1 (small amount), +2 (moderate amount), or +3 (large amount). The color strip is read after 50 seconds.

pH. The kidneys regulate the amount of acids produced by the metabolism of blood and fluids, and the lungs regulate metabolism by the amount of carbon dioxide excreted. These two processes regulate the body's acid-base balance. The pH value of urine ranges from 5 (acid) to 8 (alkaline) (Figure 42-6). An individual's urine is influenced by metabolic status, diet, medications, and any active disease process. For example, a diet high in proteins will produce acid urine, whereas a diet high in vegetables and dairy creates alkaline urine. Acid urine will become alkaline on standing because urea breaks down into ammonia. The chemical pad for pH is read after 60 seconds.

Protein. **Proteinuria** occurs when an increased amount of protein is excreted in the urine. It is an indicator of renal

Text continued on p. 966

TABLE 42-3

Reagent Strip Tests

Test	Normal Values	Clinical Significance (Abnormal Values Could Mean)	Test Error	Causes of Error
Glucose	Negative	Diabetes mellitus Pancreatitis	False positive	High levels of vitamin C
		Gestational diabetes Hyperthyroidism	False negative	Increased SG Increased ketones
Bilirubin	Negative	Cirrhosis Hepatitis	False positive	Intestinal disease or disorder
		Bile duct obstruction	False negative	Exposure to light Vitamin C Increased nitrites
Ketones	Negative	Excessive vomiting Diabetic acidosis Starvation Screening of proper insulin levels	False positive, false negative	Medications Red dyes Bacteria breakdown Incorrect timing
Specific gravity	1.01-1.025	Measures concentrating ability of kidneys	False positive False negative	Increased protein pH below 6.5
Blood	Negative	Glomerulonephritis Renal calculi Severe burns Trauma to kidney Strenuous exercise Muscle wasting Cystitis	False positive False negative	Menses Increased SG with crenated RBCs Increased nitrites Increased vitamin C
pH	5-8	Metabolic disorders Acid-base respiratory diseases Renal calculi Crystals UTI treatment/drugs	False readings	Run allowed from one test pad onto another
Protein	Negative	Renal disease (early) Muscle injury Severe infection or inflammation	False positive	Specimen contaminated with antiseptic solution Increased SG
		Glomerular problems High protein diet	False negative	Proteins other than albumin
Urobilinogen	2 mg/dL	Hemolytic diseases Hepatitis Cirrhosis	False positive	Metabolic disease Highly pigmented urine
		Liver cancer	False negative	Long-standing specimen Preservative (formalin)
Nitrites	Negative	Cystitis Pyelonephrosis	False positive	Long-standing specimen Preserved specimen done incorrectly
			False negative	Antibiotics Increased vitamin C Increased SG
Leukocytes	Negative	Cystitis Inflammation of urinary tract Organ transplant rejection	False positive	Increased pigment in urine Preservative (formalin)
			False negative	Increased glucose, protein, and vitamin C Antibiotics

SG, Serum glucose; *RBCs*, red blood cells; *UTI*, urinary tract infection.

PROCEDURE 42-1: Urinalysis Using Reagent Strips

TASK: Observe, record, and report the physical and chemical properties of a urine sample using Multistix 10 SG reagent strips.

EQUIPMENT AND SUPPLIES
- Nonsterile disposable gloves
- Personal protective equipment (PPE), as indicated
- Multistix 10 SG reagent strips
- Normal and abnormal quality control reagent strips
- Laboratory report form
- Quality control logsheet
- Urine specimen container
- Conical urine centrifuge tubes
- Digital timer or watch with second hand
- Paper towel
- Disinfectant solution
- Biohazardous waste container
- Patient's medical record
- Laboratory log

SKILLS/RATIONALE

STANDARD PRECAUTIONS ARE TO BE FOLLOWED.

1. **Procedural Step. Sanitize the hands.**
   An alcohol-based hand rub may be used instead of washing hands with soap and water, unless hands are visibly soiled.
   Rationale. Hand sanitization promotes infection control.

2. **Procedural Step. Assemble equipment and supplies and verify the order.**
   Check the expiration date of the reagent strips.
   Rationale. It is important to have all supplies and equipment ready and available before starting any procedure to ensure efficiency. Outdated reagent strips may lead to inaccurate test results.

3. **Procedural Step. Greet the patient, introduce yourself, and confirm the patient's identity. Escort the patient to the examination room or laboratory area.**
   Rationale. Identifying the patient ensures the procedure is performed on the correct patient.

4. **Procedural Step. Explain the procedure to the patient.**
   Rationale. Explaining the procedure to the patient promotes cooperation and provides a means of obtaining implied consent.

5. **Procedural Step. Ask the patient to provide a fresh clean-catch urine specimen.**
   Provide verbal and written instructions for the collection.
   NOTE: Chemical analysis of urine is best performed on a well-mixed, uncentrifuged specimen at room temperature. The reagent pads are temperature sensitive. Cold urine may produce false-negative results.
   Rationale. A freshly voided clean-catch specimen produces the most accurate results.

6. **Procedural Step. Apply gloves and other PPE as indicated.**

7. **Procedural Step. While waiting for the patient to collect the specimen, record the lot number and expiration date on the laboratory quality control log sheet.**
   The manufacturer displays this information on the outside of the bottle of reagent strips.
   Rationale. It is important to record the lot numbers and expiration dates of the reagent strips and controls. This gives the manufacturer and office a reference point in case the reagents or controls do not perform as expected.

8. **Procedural Step. Perform the Quality Control test as directed by the manufacturer.**
   NOTE: Quality control measures are only performed the first time a new bottle of reagent strips is used. Make certain the results are within the recommended parameters.
   If the controls do not fall within the acceptable ranges, the reagent strips cannot be used for patient samples until it is known why the controls are out of range and the problem has been fixed. Sometimes the reagent strips must be discarded.

9. **Procedural Step. Observe and record the physical properties of the patient's sample.**
   a. Assess that the quantity of the specimen provided is sufficient to perform the test.
   b. Identify the color of the urine specimen. Color is described as colorless, straw, yellow, or amber. The more concentrated the urine, the more the color intensifies.
   c. Identify the urine's clarity. Clarity is described as clear, slightly hazy, hazy, cloudy, or turbid (very cloudy) and is an indication of the amount of particulate matter in the sample. The cloudier the sample, the more particulate matter is present. The type of particulate matter is often identified on viewing urine sediment under the microscope.
   d. Urine odor is not reported in most cases unless it is particularly foul. The smell of a specimen may indicate a disease process.

Continued

PROCEDURE 42-1 Urinalysis Using Reagent Strips—cont'd

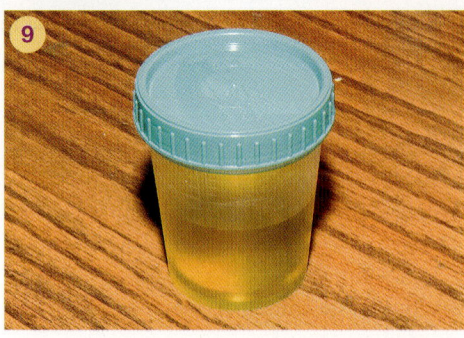

10. **Procedural Step.** Open the jar of reagent strips and remove one strip. Recap the bottle immediately.
    Rationale. Recapping the bottle prevents exposing the strips to environmental conditions (e.g., moisture, light, and heat), which can cause altered test results.

11. **Procedural Step.** Dip the strip in the specimen, and draw it out along the edge of the tube top to remove excess urine.
    Briefly blot it on a paper towel by tapping the lengthwise edge to remove any of the sample that may be clinging to the strip.
    Rationale. Excess urine can leach to other chemical pads on the strip causing inaccurate results.

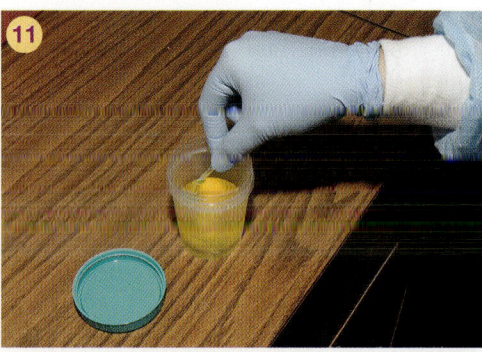

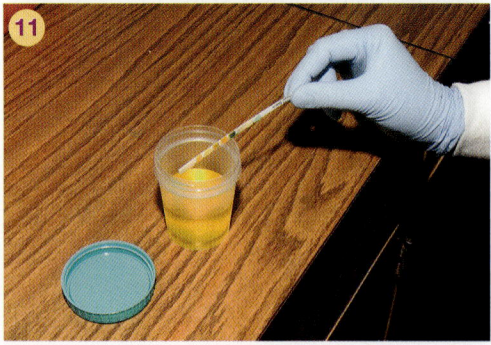

12. **Procedural Step.** Set the timer, or check the second hand on a watch to read the results after the recommended time has elapsed.

13. **Procedural Step.** After 30 seconds have elapsed, read the glucose and bilirubin results.
    Start by holding the reagent strip next to the color for the result of glucose and bilirubin. To avoid contaminating the chart, the strip should not touch the chart.

14. **Procedural Step.** After 40 seconds have elapsed, read the ketone results.

15. **Procedural Step.** After 45 seconds have elapsed, read the specific gravity results.
    NOTE: Specific gravity is defined as the concentration of dissolved substances in a specimen compared with distilled water, which is free of dissolved substances. Specific gravity may be measured with a urinometer, refractometer, or reagent strip.

16. **Procedural Step.** After 60 seconds have elapsed, read the blood, pH, protein, urobilinogen, and nitrite results.

17. **Procedural Step.** After 2 minutes have elapsed, read the leukocyte results.
    Compare the reagent strip color with the chart color that most closely matches it.

18. **Procedural Step.** After the reagent strip has been read, record the results and discard the reagent strip in the biohazardous waste container.
    NOTE: Visual interpretation of color on the reagent strip is likely to vary among individuals, so some laboratories use automated instruments for consistency in the readings. The strip is placed in the analyzer and is moved into the path of a light beam. The amount of light reflected is analyzed by a microprocessor and converted into a digital reading that is printed out.

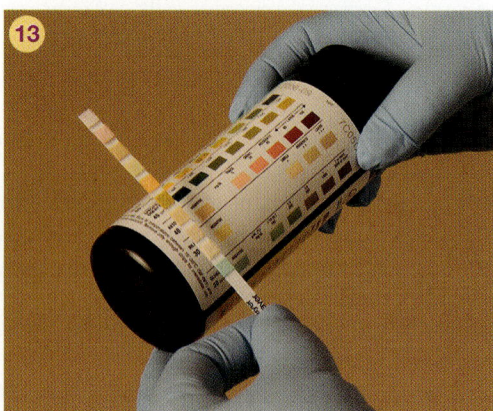

Continued

PROCEDURE 42-1 Urinalysis Using Reagent Strips—cont'd

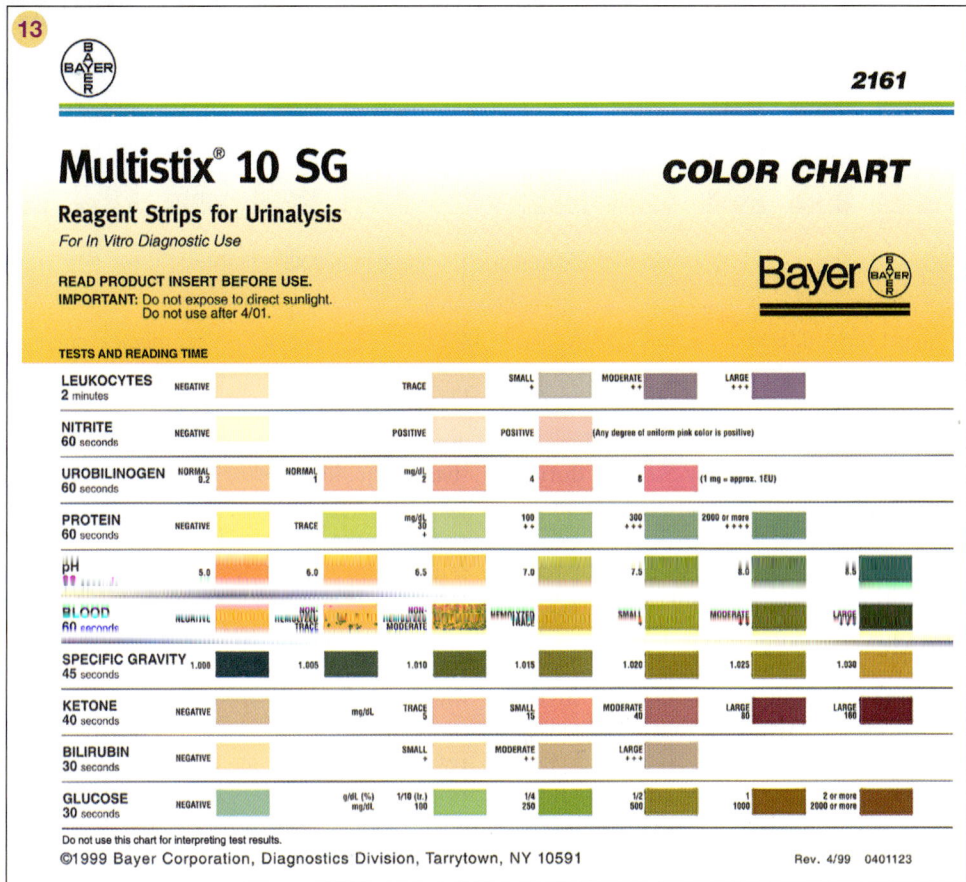

19. **Procedural Step.** Clean and disinfect the work area with a disinfectant solution.
20. **Procedural Step.** Remove gloves and dispose of in a biohazardous waste container.
21. **Procedural Step.** Sanitize the hands.
    Always sanitize the hands after every procedure or after using gloves.
22. **Procedural Step.** Report the result to the physician.
    Depending on the results of the physical and chemical properties of the patient's urine specimen, the physician may request that you prepare a urine sediment for microscopic examination.
23. **Procedural Step.** After the physician has reviewed the results, place the laboratory report form in the patient's medical record.

Color chart in Step 13 courtesy Bayer Corporation, a Siemens Healthcare Diagnostics company.

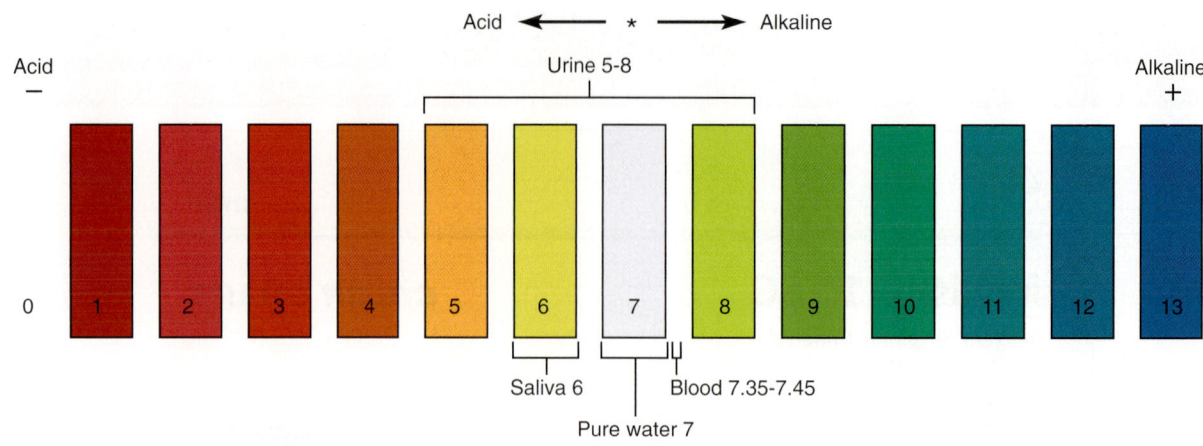

FIGURE 42-6 The pH scale. (Modified from Stepp CA, Woods MA: *Laboratory procedures for medical office personnel,* Philadelphia, 1998, Saunders.)

disease, complications of diabetes, congestive heart failure, or UTI. Proteinuria can also appear after heavy exercise, during pregnancy, and in newborns. The results are read after 60 seconds and recorded as negative, trace, +1, +2, +3, or +4.

Urobilinogen. Hemoglobin, when released from "worn out" RBCs, is converted to bilirubin in the liver. Intestinal bacteria break down bilirubin to form **urobilinogen.** Diseases of the liver (e.g., cirrhosis, hepatitis), bile duct obstruction, and antibiotic therapy increase the amount of urobilinogen in the urine. Since direct light breaks down bilirubin, the medical assistant must shield a specimen from light to avoid a false-negative reading. If the test does not detect a decrease in or absence of urobilinogen, the values are recorded as normal. An increase is recorded as positive. The strip is read 60 seconds after it has been dipped in urine.

NOTE: Urobilinogen is read in Erlich Units (EU), which is different from the readings of other chemicals.

Nitrites. Bacteria contain an enzyme that breaks down **nitrates** to **nitrites,** indicating **bacteriuria.** Common bacteria that infect the urinary tract are *Escherichia coli, Klebsiella, Proteus, Pseudomonas,* and *Staphylococcus.* The medical assistant should be aware that not all bacteria break down nitrates to nitrites, but that *E. coli* does and is the main cause of UTIs. Values are recorded as negative or positive. A color change of any degree is a positive sign for UTI. The reagent pad is read after 60 seconds.

Leukocytes. A reagent strip that tests positive for nitrites confirms the presence of **leukocyte esterase,** which is released from white blood cells (WBCs). Results are recorded as negative, trace, +1 (small), +2 (moderate), or +3 (large). A positive leukocyte reading without a positive nitrite reading may indicate a contaminated specimen. In this case, a fresh specimen should be obtained and the test redone. The results of the leukocyte reagent pad are not read for 2 minutes.

Automated Urine Analyzers. An **automated urine analyzer** uses the principle of light photometry to analyze a reagent test strip. The use of the analyzer eliminates the human error factor for color interpretation of a reagent strip. The Clinitek 50 Urine Chemistry Analyzer (Bayer, Tarrytown, NY), for example, is a benchtop, semiautomatic instrument. As with any automated equipment, it is important to make certain that the quality control and quality assurance program of the facility is followed.

When the analyzer is turned "on," the feed table moves out to a ready position. A self-test cycle begins, and when the cycle is completed, a reagent strip can then be used. A reagent strip is immersed in urine; the edge of the strip is touched to a paper towel to remove excess urine and then the strip is placed on the strip table, pad side up. It is automatically drawn into the instrument for analysis. Specimen results appear on a screen and are printed through a built-in printer (Figure 42-7). The reagent strip should be removed and discarded, and the strip table should be gently wiped with a damp, lint-free tissue. Quality control measures must be followed closely (e.g., correct use of positive and negative control strips) to ensure accurate reporting of test results (see Table 42-3).

Reagent Tablets

Reagent tablets, as mentioned, only test for one specific substance. The advantage is that some reagent tablets can be used with specimens other than urine (e.g., Acetest for serum, plasma, whole blood, and urine). Accurate results require that the medical assistant follow the prepackaged instructions exactly for each type of reagent tablet used. Care must be taken to not handle the tablets. They must be poured into the cap, and then into the test tube or placed on the mat. The Clinitest is used most often for pediatric patients, since sugars other than glucose can be detected. This test assists in the early detection of metabolic disorders in infants.

Confirmatory Tests. Reagent tablets are generally used for three **confirmatory tests:** Clinitest, used for glucose; Acetest, used for ketones; and Ictotest, used for bilirubin. As with reagent strips, reagent tablets must be kept in a dark bottle with the cap secure. Light or moisture can cause deterioration. The expiration date must be checked every time the tablets are used.

Glucose. The Clinitest 5-drop method can be used to confirm the presence of glucose and other types of sugars (e.g., fructose, lactose, galactose) in a urine specimen (Figure 42-8).

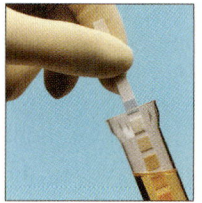
1. Dip reagent strip into sample and press the START button.

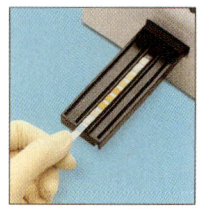
2. Blot side of reagent strip and place strip on test strip table.

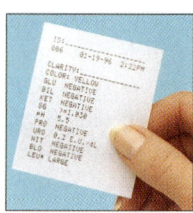
3. Instrument analyzes, displays, and prints results at the rate of one test per minute.

FIGURE 42-7 Clinitek 50 urine chemistry analyzer is a semiautomated instrument designed to read the reagent strip. Results appear on the display panel and are printed on a paper printout. (Courtesy Bayer Corporation, a Siemens Healthcare Diagnostics company.)

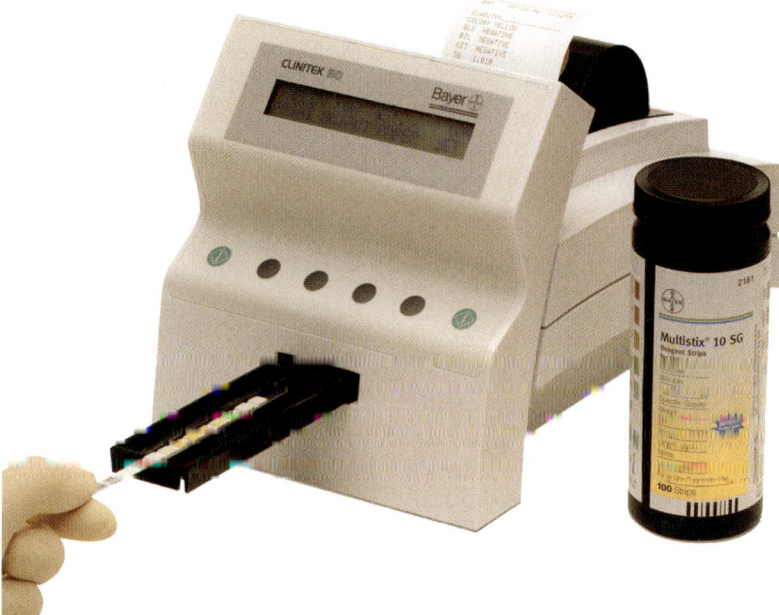

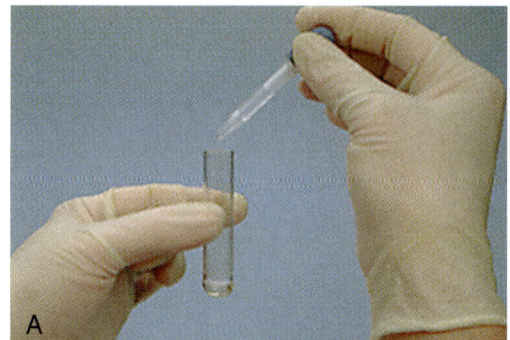
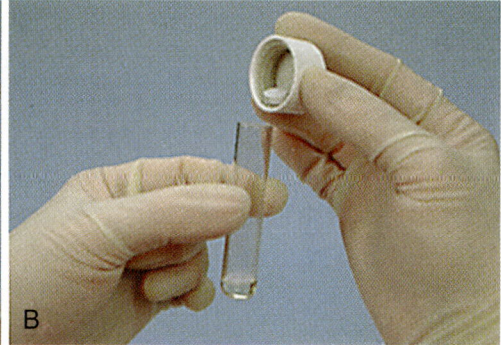
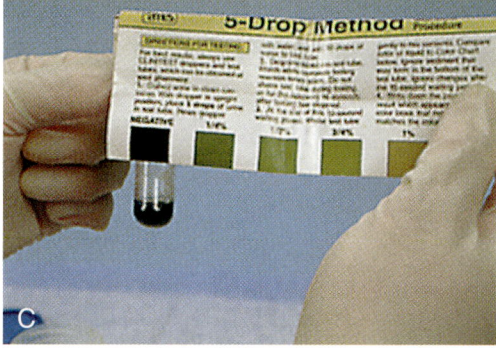

FIGURE 42-8 Clinitest procedure for urine testing. **A,** Place 10 drops of water into test tube containing 5 drops of urine. **B,** Add one Clinitest tablet to test tube. **C,** Compare contents in test tube with color chart. (From Zakus SM: *Mosby's clinical skills for medical assistants,* ed 4, St Louis, 2001, Mosby.)

Results are compared to a color chart at 15 seconds and recorded as negative, ¼%, ½%, ¾%, 1%, 2%, or more. Certain types of medication, such as cephalexin (Keflex) and probenecid (Benemid), as well as high doses of vitamin C, may cause a false-positive reading.

Ketones. The Acetest reagent tablet confirms the presence of **acetone** (ketones) in urine, serum, plasma, or whole blood (Figure 42-9). Results are determined after 30 seconds and recorded as negative, small, moderate, and large.

Bilirubin. The Ictotest confirms the presence of bilirubin in urine. Five drops of urine are placed on a small absorbent test mat. An Ictotest reagent tablet is placed in the center of the moistened mat. Two drops of distilled water are placed on the tablet. The results are negative if the mat shows no blue or purple color within 30 seconds. The results are positive for bilirubin if only these colors appear.

Microscopic Examination of Urine Sediment

Microscopic examination of urine sediment is not a CLIA-waived test. However, it is important for the medical assistant to understand the preparation of the specimen and the possible results. The purpose of microscopic examination of a urine sample is to identify cells and other formed elements present in urine. Casts, crystals, and other solids can be identified only by microscopic examination.

To perform this test, urinary **sediment** (solid material contained in the urine) is collected from a centrifuged urine specimen. The top liquid portion of the urine (the **supernatant**) is poured off, and the remaining sediment is examined under the microscope. A stain is often added to the sediment. This stain enables the health care professional to better visualize and identify structures.

The slide is first examined under **low-power field (LPF)** (10×) and low light for casts. The **high-power field (HPF)** (40×) is used to identify blood cells, crystals, bacteria, yeast, and parasites. Figure 42-10 illustrates various formed elements that can be found in a microscopic examination of urine sediment. Procedure 42-2 explains the process of microscopic examination of urine.

Blood Cells

RBCs can be found in small numbers in normal urine (0 to 5 RBCs/HPF). More than this amount is a sign of urinary tract injury (e.g., kidney stones), renal disease (e.g., pyelonephritis), or a systemic disease (e.g., hemophilia). In dilute urine, a *hypotonic* solution, the cells may appear swollen and may hemolyze. In concentrated urine, a *hypertonic* solution, the cells are shrunken (**crenated**). An RBC that has **hemolyzed** is colorless and cannot be seen under the microscope. RBCs are counted in several fields (5 to 10), totaled, and divided by the number of fields examined.

WBCs can be found in small numbers in normal urine (0 to 8 WBCs/HPF). Amounts greater than this are a clear indication of a contaminated specimen, UTI (e.g., cystitis, urethritis), kidney disease (e.g., pyelonephritis), or transplant rejection. WBCs are larger than RBCs and have a nucleus. WBCs are counted in several fields, totaled, and recorded as an average number per HPF.

Epithelial Cells

Epithelial cells line many structures in the body, including the urethra, bladder, and vagina. A few **squamous epithelial cells**

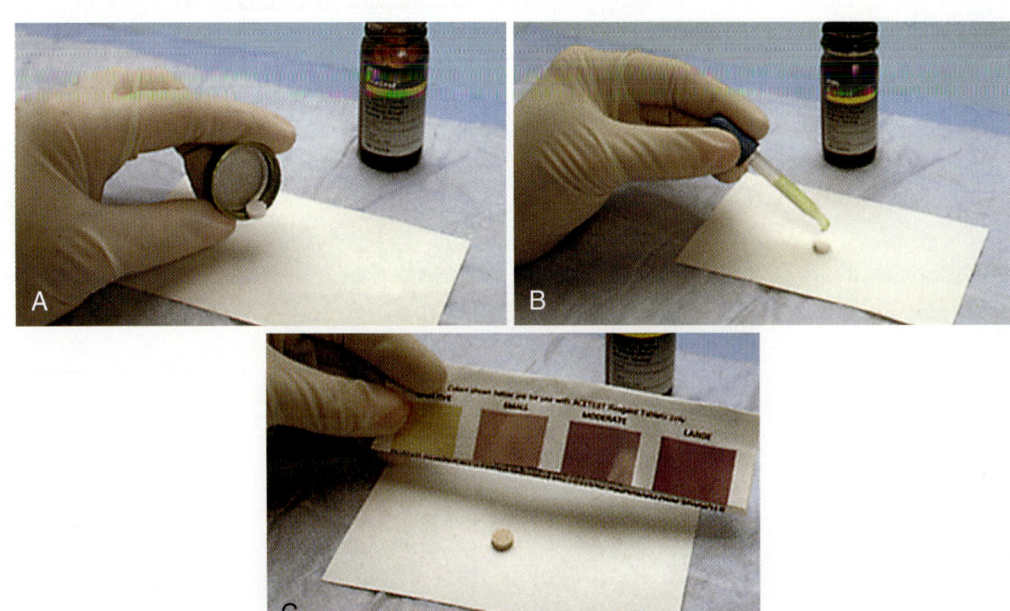

FIGURE 42-9 Acetest reagent tablet detects the presence of acetone and acetoacetic acid in the urine. **A,** Place the tablet on clean paper. **B,** Place 1 drop of urine on the tablet. **C,** Compare the tablet with the color chart. (From Zakus SM: *Mosby's clinical skills for medical assistants,* ed 4, St Louis, 2001, Mosby.)

CELLS IN URINE

Epithelial Cells Three types of epithelial cells may appear in urine sediment: renal tubular, transitional and/or squamous. Other types of cells may appear in urine but are difficult to identify due to morphologic changes caused by urine. Tubular cells are approximately 1/3 larger than white blood cells. Transitional epithelial cells may arise from the renal pelvis, ureters, bladder or urethra. They tend to be pear-shaped. Squamous cells are large and flat with a prominent nucleus. They originate in the urethra.

RENAL TUBULAR

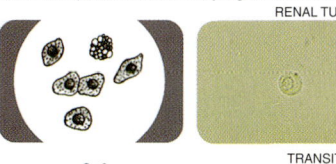

TRANSITIONAL

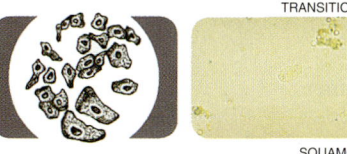

SQUAMOUS

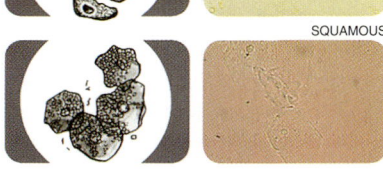

RBCs Red blood cells may originate from any part of the renal system. The presence of large numbers of RBCs in the urine suggests infection, trauma, tumors, renal calculi, etc. However, the presence of 1 or 2 RBC/(HPF) in the urine sediment, or blood in the urine from menstrual contamination, should not be considered abnormal.

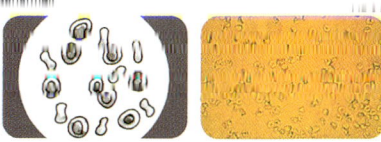

WBCs White blood cells in the urine (pyuria) may originate from any part of the renal system. The presence of more than 5 WBCs per HPF may suggest infection, cystitis, or pyelonephritis.

RENAL TUBULAR & WBC (SEDI-STAIN*)

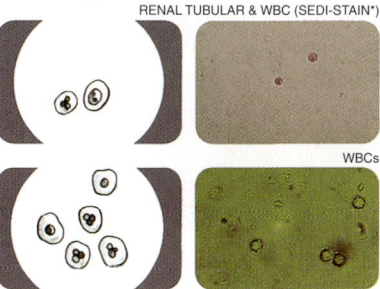

WBCs

CRYSTALS FOUND IN ACID, NEUTRAL AND ALKALINE URINE

Calcium Oxalate Calcium oxalate crystals most frequently have an "envelope" shape and appear in acid, neutral or slightly alkaline urine. They appear in the urine after the ingestion of certain foods, i.e., cabbage, asparagus.

CALCIUM OXALATE (BRIGHTFIELD)

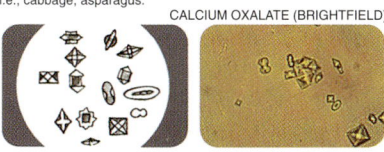

Hippuric Acid Hippuric acid crystals are colorless or pale yellow. They occur as needles, six-sided prisms, or star-shaped clusters. They appear in urine after the ingestion of certain vegetables and fruits with benzoic acid content. They have little clinical significance.

HIPPURIC ACID (BRIGHTFIELD)

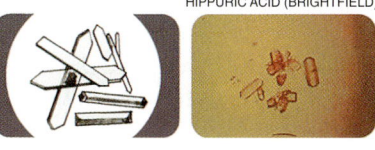

CASTS IN URINE

Hyaline Casts Hyaline casts are formed from a protein gel in the renal tubule. Hyaline casts may contain cellular inclusions. Hyaline casts will dissolve very rapidly in alkaline urine. Normal urine sediment may contain 1 to 2 hyaline casts per low power field (LPF).

HYALINE

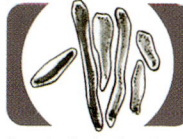 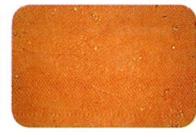

Granular Casts Granular casts are casts with granules present throughout the cast matrix. They are quite refractile. If the granules are small, the cast is defined as a finely granular cast. If granules are large, it is termed a coarsely granular cast. Granular casts can appear in urine in normal or abnormal states.

GRANULAR

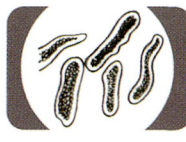 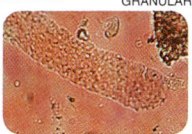

RBC Casts RBC casts are pathologic and their presence is usually indicative of severe injury to the glomerulus. Rarely, transtubular bleeding may occur, forming RBC casts. RBC casts are found in acute glomerulonephritis, lupus, bacterial endocarditis and septicemias. "Blood" casts are granular and contain hemo-globin from degenerated RBCs.

RBC CASTS

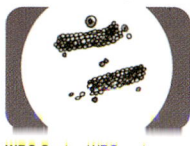 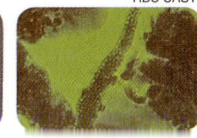

WBC Casts WBC casts occur when leukocytes are incorporated within the cast matrix. WBC casts will usually indicate an infection, most commonly pyelonephritis. They may also be seen in glomerular diseases. WBC casts may be the only clue to pyelonephritis.

WBC CASTS

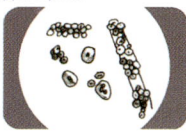 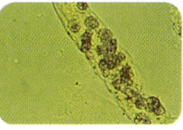

CRYSTALS FOUND IN ALKALINE URINE

Ammonium Blurate or Ammonium Urates Ammonium urates are yellow-brown in appearance and occur in urine as spheres or spheres with spicules ("thorny apples"). Both forms are frequently seen together. They appear in urine when there is ammonia formation in the urine present in the bladder. They are considered to have little clinical significance.

AMMONIUM URATES (BRIGHTFIELD)

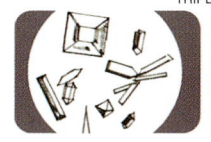 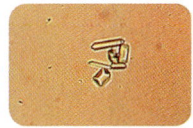

Triple Phosphate Triple phosphate crystals are common in urine sediment. They have a "coffin-lid" shape, are colorless and appear in alkaline urine. The ingestion of fruit may cause triple phosphate to appear in urine.

TRIPLE PHOSPHATE (BRIGHTFIELD)

CRYSTALS FOUND IN ACID URINE

Uric Acid Crystals Uric acid has birefringent characteristics; therefore, it polarizes light, giving multi-colors. Uric acid crystals are found in acid urine. Uric acid may assume various forms, e.g., rhombic, plates, rosettes, small crystals. The color may be red-brown, yellow or colorless. Although increased in 16% of patients with gout, and in patients with malignant lymphoma or leukemia, their presence does not usually indicate pathology or increased uric acid concentrations.

URIC ACID (BRIGHTFIELD)

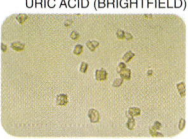

URIC ACID (POLARIZED)

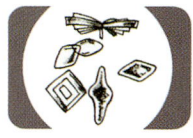 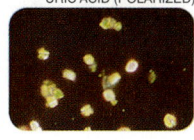

Leucine/Tyrosine Crystals Leucine and tyrosine are amino acids which crystallize and often appear together in the urine of patients with severe liver disease. Tyrosine usually appears as fine needles arranged as sheaves or rosettes and appear yellow. Leucine is usually yellow, oily-appearing spheres with radial and concentric striations.

TYROSINE (BRIGHTFIELD)

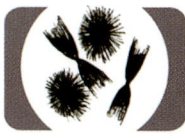 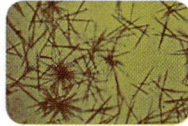

LEUCINE (BRIGHTFIELD)

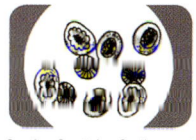 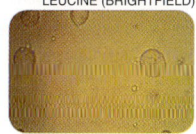

Cystine Crystals Cystine crystals are thin, hexagonal shaped (6 sided) structures. They appear in the urine as a result of a genetic defect. Cystine crystals and stones will appear in the urine in cystinuria and homocystinuria. Cystine crystals are frequently confused with uric acid crystals. Cystine crystals do not polarize light.

CYSTINE (BRIGHTFIELD)

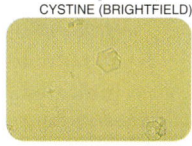

CYSTINE (POLARIZED)

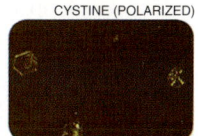

BACTERIA, FUNGI, PARASITES IN URINE

Bacteria Bacteria in the urine (bacteriuria) can result from contaminants in collection vessels, from periurethral tissues, the urethra, or from fecal or vaginal contamination as well as from true urinary infection.

BACTERIA

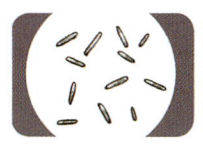 

Yeast Yeast cells vary in size, are colorless, ovoid, and are often budding. They are often confused with RBCs. *Candida albicans* is often seen in diabetes, pregnancy, obesity and other debilitating conditions.

YEAST

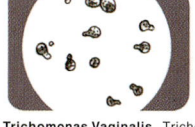 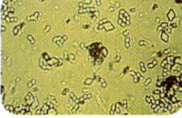

Trichomonas Vaginalis Trichomonas vaginalis is a flagellate protozoan which affects both males (urethritis) and females (vaginitis).

TRICHOMONAS VAGINALIS

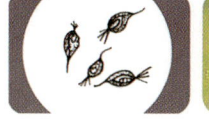 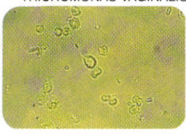

Selected Photomicrographs credited to Bowman Gray School of Medicine, Wake Forest University, N.C. and Rachel Lehman, MS, MT (ASCP).

FIGURE 42-10 Atlas of urine sediment. (Courtesy Bayer Corporation, a Siemens Healthcare Diagnostics company.)

SECTION V Clinical Medical Assisting

PROCEDURE 42-2 Prepare a Urine Specimen for Microscopic Examination

TASK: Prepare a urine sample for microscopic examination; mount a urine sediment sample on a microscope slide and position the slide on the microscope stage.

EQUIPMENT AND SUPPLIES
- Nonsterile disposable gloves
- Personal protective equipment (PPE), as indicated
- Midstream urine collection kit
- Conical urine centrifuge tubes with caps
- Disposable pipette
- Microscope slide and coverslip
- Centrifuge
- Paper towel
- Biohazardous waste container
- Laboratory logbook

SKILLS/RATIONALE

STANDARD PRECAUTIONS ARE TO BE FOLLOWED.

1. **Procedural Step.** Instruct the patient to provide a midstream clean-catch in preparation for a microscopic urinalysis.
2. **Procedural Step.** Sanitize the hands.
   An alcohol-based hand rub may be used instead of washing hands with soap and water, unless hands are visibly soiled.
   Rationale. Hand sanitization promotes infection control.
3. **Procedural Step.** Put on gloves and other PPE as indicated.
4. **Procedural Step.** If the physician orders a microscopic examination of the patient's urine, prepare a urine sediment sample.
   Prepare the patient's sample by gently rotating the specimen to mix the specimen. Pour 10 to 15 mL of the patient's specimen from the collection container into the urine centrifuge tube. When centrifuging specimens, the centrifuge must be balanced. Balance the specimen in the centrifuge by preparing a 10 mL tube of water to be placed opposite the urine tube. Visually compare the levels of urine and water in the tubes. If equal, the tubes will be balanced in the centrifuge. If not the same, adjust the levels by adding to or removing urine or water from one of the tubes.
   Rationale. If the centrifuge is not balanced, the specimen will not be processed correctly.

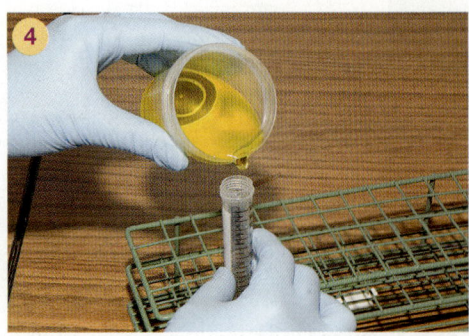

5. **Procedural Step.** Cap the tubes.
   Rationale. It is important to cap the tubes to prevent contamination of the centrifuge by aerosol or spray from the urine.
6. **Procedural Step.** Place the tubes in the centrifuge directly opposite each other for balance.
   If the centrifuge is not balanced, it will make a loud noise and bounce around after it is turned on.

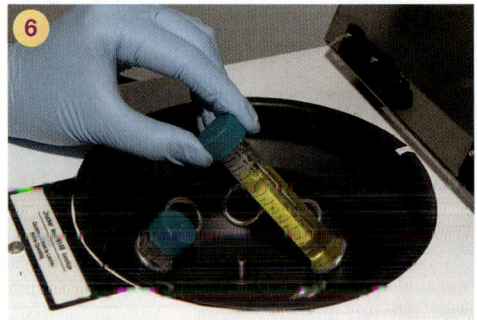

7. **Procedural Step.** Close the lid and set the timer on the centrifuge.
   The time and centrifuge speed vary according to laboratory policy and the specimen being spun. Typically, a urine sample is centrifuged for 5 minutes at a low speed. Some centrifuges start and stop automatically.
   Rationale. The lid must be closed before starting the centrifuge to prevent aerosol or droplet contamination.
8. **Procedural Step.** After the centrifuge stops, remove the cap from the specimen and discard it in the biohazardous waste container.
9. **Procedural Step.** Pour off the supernatant (clear upper fluid).
   Suction it off with a plastic transfer pipette and discard it until there is about 1 mL of urine left in the bottom of the tube.
   Or

PROCEDURE 42-2 Prepare a Urine Specimen for Microscopic Examination—cont'd

You may also pour off the supernatant from the top of the tube by inverting the tube over the sink. About 1 mL of sediment will remain in the bottom of the tube.

Be careful not to disturb the sediment while pouring off.

10. **Procedural Step.** Mix the sediment with the remaining urine in the bottom of the tube.

    Suction it up and down with the transfer pipette.

    You may also mix the sediment by gently tapping the side of the tube with your finger or on the countertop.

    Rationale. Failure to mix the sediment properly will cause errors in the report because the elements in the sediment centrifuge at different rates.

11. **Procedural Step.** Place a microscope slide on a paper towel and dispense a small drop of the mixed urine sediment in the center of the slide.

    Rationale. The slide should be placed on a paper towel in case of spills.

12. **Procedural Step.** Prepare the slide.

    Pick up a coverslip and hold it between the thumb and forefinger at two adjacent corners. Touch the opposite edge of the coverslip to the urine drop on the slide and the drop will spread across the edge of the coverslip. Carefully lower the coverslip over the drop so that no air bubbles are under it.

13. **Procedural Step.** Mount the slide on the microscope stage.

    Turn the coarse adjustment knob away from you to lower the stage, then place the slide between the spring-loaded clamps of the slide holder.

    Rationale. The slide holder positions the slide over the opening in the stage, which allows the light to pass through the specimen and into the objective lens.

14. **Procedural Step.** Remove gloves and dispose of in a biohazardous waste container.

15. **Procedural Step.** Sanitize the hands. Always sanitize the hands after every procedure or after using gloves.

16. **Procedural Step.** Inform the physician that the slide is ready for viewing.

17. **Procedural Step.** Record the results in the laboratory logbook as reported by the physician.

CHARTING EXAMPLE—LABORATORY LOGBOOK

Date	
1/17/xx	Microscopic examination of clean-catch urine specimen as reported by Dr. Carlson.
	WBC: 0-16/HPF
	RBC: 0-2/HPF
	Hyaline casts: 0-4/HPF
	Crystals: – Uric acid, moderate
	Bacteria: Few
	Mucus: Occasional
	— B. MacNeil, RMA

---

found in a urine specimen are normal. Abnormally large numbers in women indicate vaginal contamination. These squamous cells appear as large, clear, flat, irregularly shaped cells, and they have a small nucleus.

Renal epithelial cells or **transitional epithelial cells** appearing in large numbers indicate a kidney problem. Renal epithelial cells are round to oval in shape and contain a large nucleus. When present in large numbers, tubular damage (e.g., tubular necrosis, glomerulonephritis) is suspected. Transitional epithelial cells appear pear shaped and line the urinary tract from the renal pelvis to the top of the urethra. Large amounts indicate diseases of the bladder or renal pelvis.

Casts and Crystals

Casts are microscopic protein materials that harden and take on the shape of the **lumen** of the tubule, where they are formed within the **nephron**. These materials are flushed out of the tubule and appear in the urine as casts. The presence of casts in the urine usually signifies a disease process. Names of casts represent their cell and substance composition (Table 42-4).

Finding casts in urinary sediment is significant. The light should be low because casts are transparent. They tend to settle toward the edges of the coverslip. The average number of casts per LPF should be reported after 5 to 10 fields have been counted. Although casts are counted using low light and LPF, HPF must be used to classify them.

Crystals are often found in urine sediment. The type and number depend on the pH of the urine. Acid crystals include amorphous urates, uric acid, and calcium oxalate crystals. Crystals found in alkaline urine include amorphous phosphate, triple phosphate, calcium phosphate, and ammonium urate crystals. Crystals considered abnormal are leucine, tyrosine, cystine, and cholesterol and are found in the urine of patients with metabolic disease or on sulfa drugs.

When crystals form, they do so as the urine cools. They are observed under HPF. Crystals are counted using 5 to 10 fields and then dividing by the number of fields used.

Other Structures

Other structures found in urine include the following:
- **Bacteria** are rod-shaped or spherical organisms that appear in a urine specimen only if it becomes contaminated during collection or if the patient has a UTI.

TABLE 42-4
Types of Casts

Cast	Appearance	Indication
Hyaline casts	Colorless, cylinder-like structures with rounded ends	Occur in normal urine, after strenuous exercise, with unchecked hypertension, and with chronic renal disease
Granular casts	Hyaline casts that contain granules of disintegrated cells	Appear when patient has acute or chronic renal failure
Fatty casts	Cylinder-like structures that contain fat droplets	Appear in urine of diabetic patient or patient with nephrotic syndrome
Waxy casts	Appear glassy and smooth, and have sawtooth edges	Appear in urine during chronic renal disease and malignant hypertension
Cellular casts	Named according to what they contain (e.g., red blood cells, white blood cells, epithelial cells)	Appear in acute glomerulonephritis and other diseases

- **Yeasts** are oval shaped, vary in size, and have small buds. Yeast cells in the urine of a female patient are usually vaginal contaminants *(Candida albicans)*, such as found in diabetes mellitus, or may indicate UTI.
- **Mucous threads** from the urinary tract are normal in small amounts but indicate a urinary tract inflammation if found in large amounts. Microscopically, they appear as long, waxy, threadlike structures with pointed ends. Mucous threads are best observed under LPF.
- **Spermatozoa** are normal in small numbers in male urine and should be reported as "present" only if found in large numbers. Sperm, if seen in a female patient, is not an indicator of disease when seen on microscopic examination. It only indicates that the patient has had intercourse.
- **Parasites** (e.g., *Trichomonas*) are considered a contaminant.

Artifacts

Artifacts are contaminants sometimes found in urine. Powder, hair, fibers, and similar substances are typical contaminants if a specimen is improperly collected. Care should be taken to encourage the patient to provide an uncontaminated specimen.

Pregnancy Tests

Two types of pregnancy tests are performed in the POL: enzyme immunoassay and agglutination. These are both CLIA-waived tests. All pregnancy tests are based on the **qualitative** presence or absence of a hormone called **human chorionic gonadotropin (hCG)**. The hCG levels are detectable as early as 10 days after fertilization. Best results are obtained if the urine specimen is a first morning specimen, and is obtained before the fourth month of pregnancy.

Enzyme immunoassay (EIA) pregnancy tests are available in commercially prepared kits. The color-change tests are very reliable and have a high sensitivity to color reaction. Procedure 42-3 outlines the process of performing a urine pregnancy color-reaction test.

The slide or test tube **agglutination** tests are *inhibition* immunoassay tests. When a urine specimen containing hCG is mixed with either latex beads (on a slide) or antiserum (in a tube), no agglutination (clumping action) takes place. The absence of agglutination indicates a positive reaction for pregnancy. Therefore, when agglutination is visible, a negative reaction for pregnancy is recorded.

PATIENT-CENTERED PROFESSIONALISM

- What information is provided about a patient's state of health when a urinalysis is performed?
- Why must the medical assistant examine a urine specimen as soon as possible?

BLOOD TESTS

The processing of blood samples in a POL usually falls into one of three categories: hematology, blood chemistry, and serology. Hematology is the study of blood cells, blood cell–forming tissues, and coagulation factors. Blood chemistry is the complete (quantitative) analysis of the chemical composition of the blood, including electrolytes, hormones, and glucose. Serology identifies the antigen and antibody reactions in the serum of blood. Microbiology is another category for processing blood samples. A medical assistant can perform simple hemoglobin analyses, microhematocrits, and manual (nonautomated) sedimentation rates. Remember, reference ranges for various tests vary from infancy through adolescence as a result of growth cycles, hormone levels, and so forth. Specimens sent to an outside laboratory for processing will provide a test result with an accompanying reference range on the laboratory report. Remember, each laboratory uses different types of equipment, as well as different types of testing methods.

Hematology

Hematology is the study of all blood components, including erythrocytes (RBCs), leukocytes (WBCs), and thrombocytes (platelets). RBCs carry oxygen throughout the body and transport carbon dioxide from the body's tissues to the lungs to be exhaled. WBCs defend the body against allergens, bacteria, and viruses. Platelets assist in blood clot formation.

Laboratory Testing in the Physician's Office **CHAPTER 42** 973

| PROCEDURE 42-3 | **Perform a Urine Pregnancy Test** |

TASK: Perform a urine pregnancy test using a commercially prepared CLIA-waived kit (QuickVue).

EQUIPMENT AND SUPPLIES
- Nonsterile disposable gloves
- Personal protective equipment (PPE), as indicated
- Urine specimen (preferably first-voided morning specimen)
- Urine pregnancy testing kit (QuickVue)
- Biohazardous waste container
- Laboratory logbook
- Patient's medical record
- Disinfectant solution

SKILLS/RATIONALE

STANDARD PRECAUTIONS ARE TO BE FOLLOWED.

1. **Procedural Step.** Sanitize the hands.
   An alcohol-based hand rub may be used instead of washing hands with soap and water, unless hands are visibly soiled.
   Rationale. Hand sanitization promotes infection control.

2. **Procedural Step.** Assemble equipment and supplies and verify the order.
   Check the expiration date on the urine pregnancy test. It should not be used if the expiration date has passed.
   Rationale. It is important to have all supplies and equipment ready and available before starting any procedure to ensure efficiency. An expired pregnancy test may produce inaccurate test results.

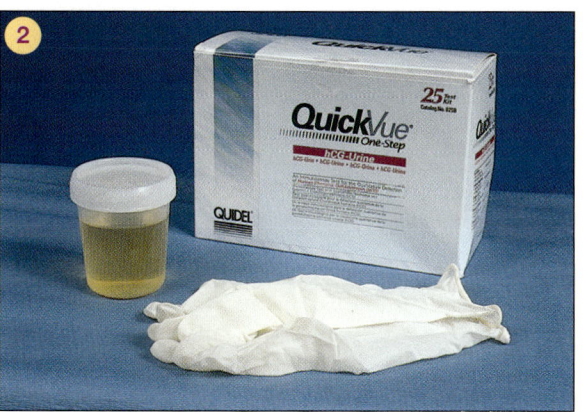

3. **Procedural Step.** Perform the quality control test as recommended by the manufacturer and document in the laboratory logbook.

4. **Procedural Step.** Greet and identify the patient and escort the patient to the examination room.

   (Only escort the patient to the examination room if the patient has not brought a urine specimen from home, and a specimen is to be collected in the office.)
   Rationale. Identifying the patient ensures the procedure is performed on the correct patient.

5. **Procedural Step.** If a urine specimen is to be collected in the office, explain the procedure to the patient.
   Rationale. Explaining the procedure to the patient promotes cooperation and provides a means of obtaining implied consent.

6. **Procedural Step.** Provide the patient with the collection container and instructions as needed.
   The patient may have brought the first morning specimen from home for analysis, and this step may not be necessary.

7. **Procedural Step.** Put on gloves and other PPE as indicated.

8. **Procedural Step.** Open the kit and remove one pregnancy test.
   Remove the test cassette from the foil pouch and place it on a clean, dry, and level surface.

9. **Procedural Step.** Begin the test by adding urine to the test cassette.
   Using the disposable pipette included with the kit, add 3 drops of urine to the sample well on the test cassette. Do not pick up or move the kit until you are ready to read the results. Dispose of the pipette in a biohazardous waste container.
   Rationale. Moving the test cassette after the urine has been added may produce inaccurate test results.

Continued

PROCEDURE 42-3 Perform a Urine Pregnancy Test—cont'd

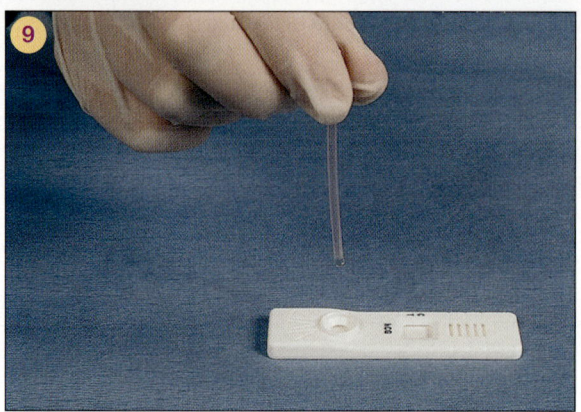

10. **Procedural Step.** Set the timer for 3 minutes and push start.
11. **Procedural Step.** Interpret the test results by observing color development and record the test results.
    Observe for the following changes through the result window.

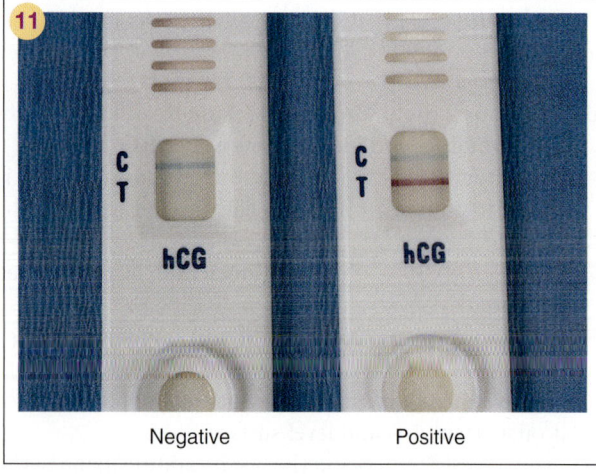

Negative: The appearance of the blue procedural control line only next to the letter "C" (indicates proper techniques) and no pink-to-purple test line next to the letter "T."
Positive: The appearance of any pink-to-purple line next to the letter "T" along with a blue procedural control line next to the letter "C."
No Result: If no blue procedural control line appears, the test result is invalid, and the specimen must be retested.

12. **Procedural Step.** Discard the test cassette in a biohazardous waste container.
13. **Procedural Step.** Disinfect the work area.
14. **Procedural Step.** Remove gloves and discard in a biohazardous waste container.
15. **Procedural Step.** Sanitize the hands.
    Always sanitize the hands after every procedure or after using gloves.
16. **Procedural Step.** Document the results in the patient's medical record and the laboratory logbook.
    Include date and time of the test, date of the patient's last menstrual period (LMP), name of the test, and results recorded (positive or negative).

CHARTING EXAMPLE	
Date	
2/11/xx	10:30 a.m. LMP: 1/02/xx. QuickVue preg test: Positive.————————B. Deal, RMA

Complete Blood Count

A **complete blood count (CBC)** is ordered to evaluate and monitor a patient's health and assist in the diagnosis of blood disorders (e.g., anemias, leukemias). The CBC is one of the most frequently performed laboratory tests on blood. It is not usually performed in the POL, but the medical assistant should be familiar with it and understand its importance. The CBC indicates the number of blood cells present in a volume of blood. Blood is composed of formed elements that float in plasma. The RBCs are the largest number of blood cells in the body and are made in the red bone marrow. The WBCs are formed in bone marrow and in lymphoid tissue and are larger than RBCs, but fewer in number. Platelets are the least numerous type of cells in the blood.

Besides blood cell counts, CBC measures the size and shape of the cells, hemoglobin, hematocrit, and reticulocytes (immature RBCs) and provides a differential of WBC types. Table 42-5 lists CBC ranges.

Additional hematology tests often run by laboratories are **red cell indices** and **platelet counts.** Red cell indices determine the size, content, and hemoglobin concentration of RBCs, and they also include a mean cell volume (MCV, average size of RBCs), mean cell hemoglobin (MCH, average cell hemoglobin), and mean cell hemoglobin concentration (MCHC, average concentration of hemoglobin in a given volume of RBCs). RBC count, hemoglobin, and hematocrit are necessary to calculate the RBC indices. Red cell indices are useful in determining types of anemias.

TABLE 42-5
Complete Blood Count (CBC)

Measurement	Range
Red blood cells	4.5-6 million/mm^3
Hemoglobin (adult)	12-18 g/dL
Hematocrit (adult)	37%-52%
Reticulocytes	0%-1.5%
White blood cells	5000-11,000/mm^3
Neutrophils	55%-70%
Eosinophils	1%-3%
Basophils	0.5%-1%
Lymphocytes	25%-30%
Monocytes	3%-8%
Platelets	150,000-400,000/mm^3

TABLE 42-6
Hemoglobin and Hematocrit Values

Group	Range (g/mL)
HEMOGLOBIN	
Men	14-18 g/dL
Women	12-16 g/dL
Child	10-14 g/dL
Infant	16-23 g/dL
HEMATOCRIT	
Men	42%-52%
Women	37%-47%
Child to 6 years	30%-40%
Child to 1 year	29%-43%
Infant to 6 months	35%-50%
Infant to 1 month	35%-49%
Newborn	51%-61%

Cell analyzers are used to perform all the tests required of the CBC and require advanced training for operation.

Hemoglobin

Hemoglobin (Hb or Hgb) is the component that gives RBCs their color. It carries oxygen to tissues and transports carbon dioxide to the lungs to be excreted. Hemoglobin measurement is used to detect blood loss and anemias. The test for hemoglobin can be performed on venous or capillary blood and can be measured as part of the CBC or as a separate test. Table 42-6 lists normal values. It is important to remember that values in children are age specific, therefore the values vary throughout the first 18 years. In contrast, the elderly will have slightly decreased values.

Several automated devices are available to measure hemoglobin's oxygen-carrying capacity. The HemoCue hemoglobin analyzer is approved by CLIA 88 for use in the POL. The analyzer uses a photometer to measure blood hemoglobin, with the results displayed on a digital screen. The HemoCue uses a microcuvette that automatically draws the right amount of blood from a capillary puncture. A dry reagent on the microcuvette starts a chemical reaction to determine the hemoglobin. Procedure 42-4 provides instructions on obtaining a hemoglobin reading using a HemoCue.

Hematocrit

A **hematocrit (Hct)** reading can be performed on venous or capillary blood. The Hct is a measurement of the percentage of packed RBCs in a volume of whole blood. For example, a Hct of 45% indicates that every 100 mL (deciliter [dL]) of blood contains 45 mL of packed RBCs and the remaining 55% is plasma (Table 42-6). Values, as with the hemoglobin, are age specific in children and show a slight decrease in the elderly.

To obtain a Hct reading, an anticoagulated blood specimen is collected in a capillary tube, sealed at one end, and spun in a microhematocrit centrifuge (or a centrifuge with Hct-reading potential). The specimen separates into the following three layers (Figure 42-11):

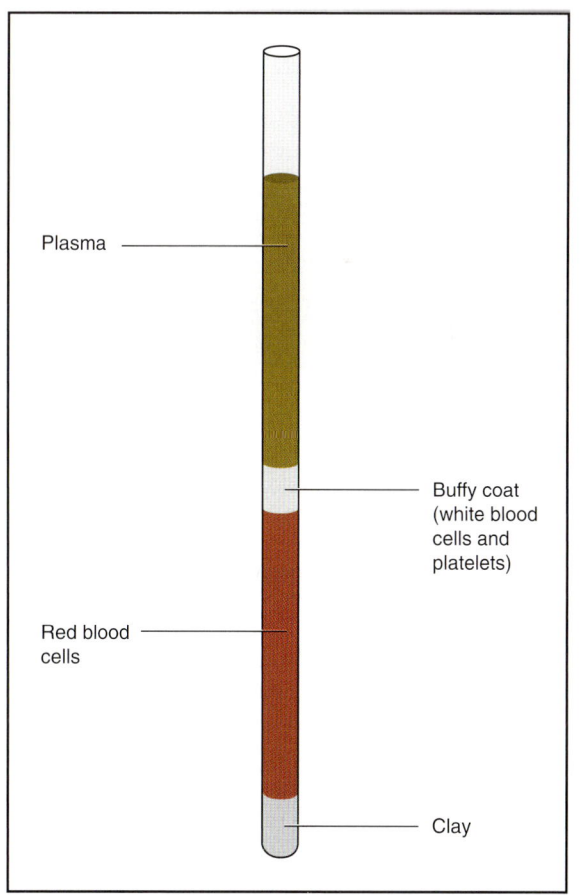

FIGURE 42-11 Hematocrit test results. The cellular elements are separated from the plasma by centrifuging an anticoagulated blood specimen, and the results are read at the top of the packed cell column. (From Rodak BF: *Hematology: clinical principles and applications*, ed 2, St Louis, 2002, Saunders.)

976 SECTION V Clinical Medical Assisting

PROCEDURE 42-4
Determine a Hemoglobin Measurement Using a HemoCue

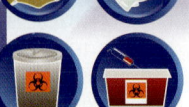

TASK: Accurately measure the hemoglobin of a blood specimen using a HemoCue.

EQUIPMENT AND SUPPLIES
- Nonsterile disposable gloves (latex-free)
- Personal protective equipment (PPE), as indicated
- Alcohol wipe
- Sterile disposable microlancet
- Sterile 2 × 2 gauze squares
- HemoCue
- Control cuvette
- Microcuvettes
- Disinfectant solution
- Sharps container
- Biohazardous waste container
- Patient's medical record
- Laboratory logbook
- Laboratory quality control logsheet

SKILLS/RATIONALE
STANDARD PRECAUTIONS ARE TO BE FOLLOWED.

1. **Procedural Step.** Sanitize the hands.
   An alcohol-based hand rub may be used instead of washing hands with soap and water, unless hands are visibly soiled.
   Rationale. Hand sanitization promotes infection control.

2. **Procedural Step.** Assemble equipment and supplies and verify the order.
   Rationale. It is important to have all supplies and equipment ready and available before starting any procedure to ensure efficiency.

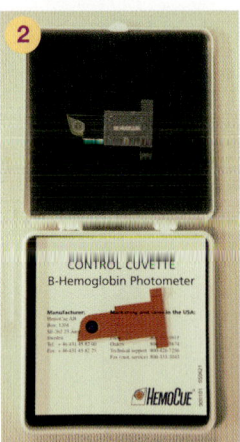

3. **Procedural Step.** Perform the quality control test as recommended by the manufacturer and document in the laboratory quality control logsheet.

4. **Procedural Step.** Prepare the HemoCue analyzer.
   a. Turn the power switch to the "on" position.
   b. Check that the meter reads zero.
   c. Place the control cuvette into the holder and push into the photometer.
   d. Validate the control values. If they are not within acceptable values, clean the test area and repeat the validation check.
   e. Fill a cuvette with a control solution.
   f. Place the cuvette into the holder and push into the photometer.
   g. Read the control result on the LED screen.
   h. Record the results.
   i. Dispose of the cuvette in a sharps container.

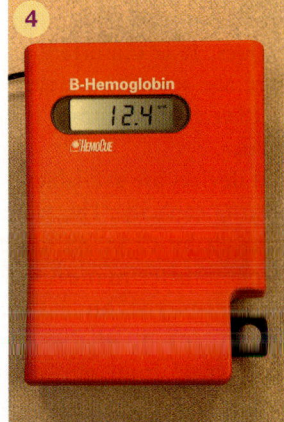

5. **Procedural Step.** Greet the patient, introduce yourself, and confirm the patient's identity. Escort the patient to the examination room or laboratory area.
   Rationale. Identifying the patient ensures the procedure is performed on the correct patient.

6. **Procedural Step.** Explain the procedure to the patient.
   Rationale. Explaining the procedure to the patient promotes cooperation and provides a means of obtaining implied consent.

7. **Procedural Step.** Again, sanitize the hands and apply gloves and PPE as indicated.

8. **Procedural Step.** Perform a capillary puncture and discard the lancet in a sharps container.
   Rationale. Proper disposal of the lancet is required by OSHA standards to prevent exposure to bloodborne pathogens.

Continued

PROCEDURE 42-4 Determine a Hemoglobin Measurement Using a HemoCue—cont'd

9. **Procedural Step.** Wipe away the first drop of blood with a gauze pad.
   Rationale. The first drop of blood is not collected because it usually contains more tissue fluid than blood, which could cause an inaccurate test result.

10. **Procedural Step.** Collect the specimen.
    Touch the pointed tip of the cuvette to the second well-rounded drop of blood. Allow the cuvette to fill on its own by capillary action.
    Rationale. Do not allow the patient's finger to touch the cuvette; the cuvette should touch only the drop of blood because the finger may break up or disintegrate the cells and render the test inaccurate.

11. **Procedural Step.** Wipe off any excess blood from the tip of the cuvette.

12. **Procedural Step.** Place the cuvette in its holder and push into the photometer.

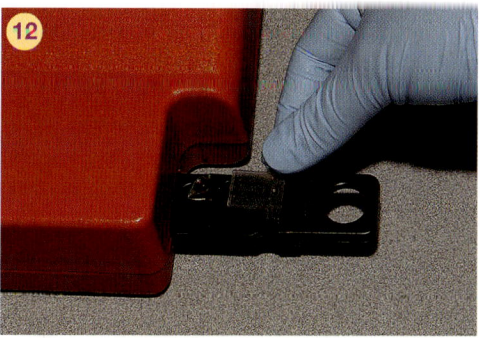

13. **Procedural Step.** Read and record the hemoglobin value.

14. **Procedural Step.** Discard the cuvette into the sharps container.

15. **Procedural Step.** Turn the equipment "off" as appropriate. Clean the equipment with a mild soap and water.

16. **Procedural Step.** Disinfect the work area with 10% bleach solution.

17. **Procedural Step.** Remove gloves and sanitize the hands.
    Always sanitize the hands after every procedure or after using gloves.

18. **Procedural Step.** Document the results in the patient's medical record and the laboratory logbook.
    Include date and time of the test, name of the test, and results.

CHARTING EXAMPLE

Date	
7/13/xx	9:00 a.m. Hb 16 g/dL per HemoCue.
	— O. Hodges, RMA

- Top layer = Plasma
- Middle layer = Buffy layer (coat) containing platelets and WBCs
- Bottom layer = Packed RBCs that have settled to the bottom because they are heavier than the other cells

The specimen is measured using a microhematocrit reader.

A patient's Hct should be approximately three times the value of the patient's Hb. For example, if a patient's Hb is 12 g/dL, multiply by 3 to obtain the patient's Hct (12 × 3 = 36%, ±3). Thus, if you know a patient's Hct, you can divide by 3 to obtain the Hb. A low reading may indicate anemia, and a high reading could be the result of polycythemia. Results other than the 1:3 ratio would require a retest. Procedure 42-5 explains the steps in performing a hematocrit.

Erythrocyte Sedimentation Rate

The **erythrocyte sedimentation rate (ESR),** or "sed rate," is a nonspecific screening test that confirms an inflammation is present somewhere in the body (e.g., respiratory infections, arthritis, pregnancy). ESR is a measurement of how fast RBCs settle to the bottom of a tube. The average rate is 1 mm every 5 minutes.

In a healthy person, ESR is slow and RBCs do not fall far. If inflammation is present, the test will show RBCs falling very quickly. The medical assistant will collect a venous blood specimen in a lavender tube, which contains the anticoagulant **ethylenediaminetetraacetic acid (EDTA).** Two common ESR methods used in the POL are the Westergren tube method and the Wintrobe tube method.

The **Westergren method** uses a disposable self-zeroing tube calibrated from 0 to 200. A blood sample from a blood tube containing EDTA is transferred to the tube, mixed with sodium citrate solution, and set upright in a sedimentation rack for 1 hour. Procedure 42-6 describes this process in detail using the Sed-Pac ESR system (Futura Medical Corp., Guildford, UK).

The **Wintrobe method** requires that an EDTA blood sample be transferred to a disposable tube. The Wintrobe tube is smaller than the Westergren tube and is calibrated from 0 to 100. The tube is placed in a sedimentation rack for 1 hour.

Text continued on p. 981

PROCEDURE 42-5

Perform a Microhematocrit Test

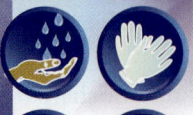

TASK: Accurately collect a capillary blood sample to spin and measure, and read a microhematocrit.

EQUIPMENT AND SUPPLIES
- Nonsterile disposable gloves (Latex-free)
- Personal protective equipment (PPE), as indicated
- Microhematocrit capillary tubes (heparinized)
- Sealing compound
- Alcohol wipe
- Sterile disposable microlancet
- Sterile 2 × 2 gauze squares
- Disinfectant solution
- Microhematocrit centrifuge
- Hematocrit reader
- Sharps container
- Biohazardous waste container
- Patient's medical record
- Laboratory logbook

SKILLS/RATIONALE

STANDARD PRECAUTIONS ARE TO BE FOLLOWED.

1. **Procedural Step.** Sanitize the hands.
   An alcohol-based hand rub may be used instead of washing hands with soap and water, unless hands are visibly soiled.
   Rationale. Hand sanitization promotes infection control.

2. **Procedural Step.** Assemble equipment and supplies and verify the order.
   Rationale. It is important to have all supplies and equipment ready and available before starting any procedure to ensure efficiency.

3. **Procedural Step.** Greet the patient, introduce yourself, and confirm the patient's identity. Escort the patient to the examination room or laboratory area.
   Rationale. Identifying the patient ensures the procedure is performed on the correct patient.

4. **Procedural Step.** Explain the procedure to the patient.
   Rationale. Explaining the procedure to the patient promotes cooperation and provides a means of obtaining implied consent.

5. **Procedural Step.** Apply gloves and PPE as indicated.

COLLECTING THE SPECIMEN

6. **Procedural Step.** Perform a capillary puncture and discard the lancet in a sharps container.
   Rationale. Proper disposal of the lancet is required by OSHA standards to prevent exposure to bloodborne pathogens.

7. **Procedural Step.** Wipe away the first drop of blood with a gauze pad.
   Rationale. The first drop of blood is not collected because it usually contains more tissue fluid than blood, which could cause an inaccurate test result.

8. **Procedural Step.** Collect the specimen by holding the tube at a slight downward angle.
   Allow another drop of blood to accumulate and touch the end of the capillary tube to the second drop of blood. Keep the tip of the capillary tube in the blood droplet. The blood will be drawn into the tube through capillary action. Continue filling the tube until it is about three-quarters full. Fill the second capillary tube in the same way. Wipe the outside of the filled capillary tube to remove excess blood.
   Rationale. Removing the capillary tube from the drop of blood may result in air bubbles within the tube, causing inaccurate test results. Allowing the capillary tube to press against the skin will close off the opening of the capillary tube and will not allow blood to enter the tube.

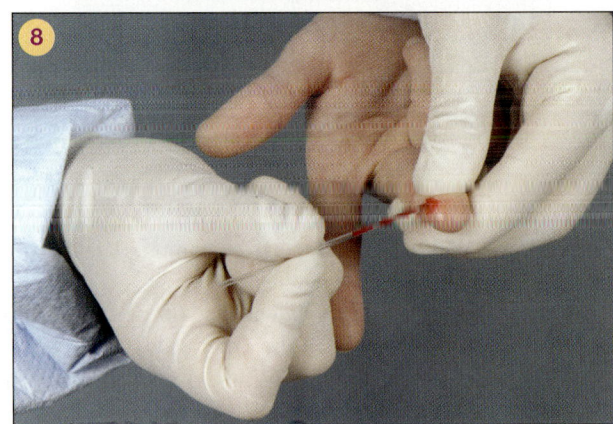

9. **Procedural Step.** After the sample has been collected, instruct the patient to hold a clean gauze square for direct pressure to the puncture site.

10. **Procedural Step.** Seal the dry end of the capillary tubes with clay (e.g., Critoseal, Hemato-Seal).
    To avoid splashing blood from the end used to collect the sample while sealing the tube, tilt the capillary tube slightly to allow air to enter the end of the tube used to fill it. When the dry end is sealed, air will be displaced instead of blood.
    Rationale. The capillary tubes must be properly sealed to prevent leakage of the blood specimen during centrifugation.

Continued

PROCEDURE 42-5 Perform a Microhematocrit Test—cont'd

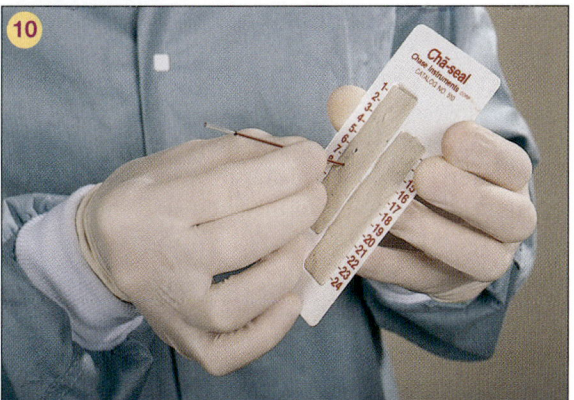

11. **Procedural Step.** Leave the capillary tubes embedded in the sealing clay to prevent damaging them.
    The clay board can be transported to the laboratory for the specimen to be processed.
12. **Procedural Step.** Check the puncture site.
    Make sure it has stopped bleeding and bandage it with a clean strip bandage to protect the wound. Discard any contaminated materials in the appropriate biohazardous waste container.
13. **Procedural Step.** Remove gloves and sanitize the hands.
    Always sanitize the hands after every procedure or after using gloves.

TESTING THE SPECIMEN
14. **Procedural Step.** Place the specimens in the centrifuge with the sealed ends securely against the gasket.
    Apply gloves and remove the patient samples from the clay. Place the capillary tubes opposite each other in the centrifuge for balance. Record the location of the patient samples in the centrifuge in the logbook.

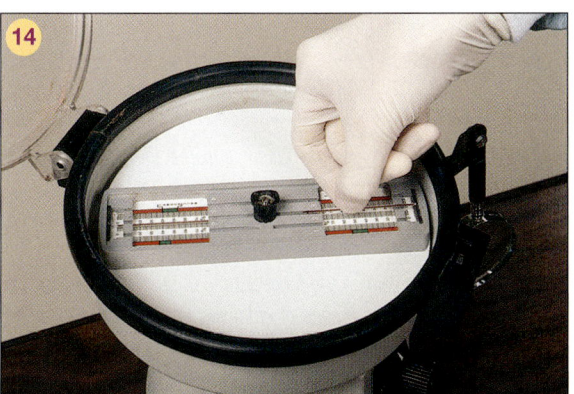

NOTE: For *quality assurance*, patient samples are run in duplicate, and the results of the two readings must agree within ±2%.
Rationale. When more than one patient's samples are being spun, recording the locations of the tubes is the only way to tell them apart after being placed in the centrifuge.

15. **Procedural Step.** Secure the locking top by placing it over the threaded bolt on the centrifuge head and turning the fastener until tight.
16. **Procedural Step.** Close and latch the lid of the centrifuge and spin for 5 minutes at 2500 rpm or the high setting.
    Most microhematocrit centrifuges are preset to the appropriate speed, so all that needs to be done is to set the timer for 5 minutes.
    Rationale. Spinning separates the blood into cells and plasma.
17. **Procedural Step.** Wait until the centrifuge comes to a complete stop before unlatching the lid, then remove the locking top.
    Rationale. The centrifuge must be stopped completely to prevent injury when removing the tubes.
18. **Procedural Step.** If the centrifuge does not have a built-in reader, place one of the tubes in the hematocrit reader. If the machine has a built-in reader, read the microhematocrit values on both tubes.
    Remove one of the tubes from its slot, taking care to note the number of the slot. Place the tube in the hematocrit reader with the junction of the clay and red blood cells against the zero line.

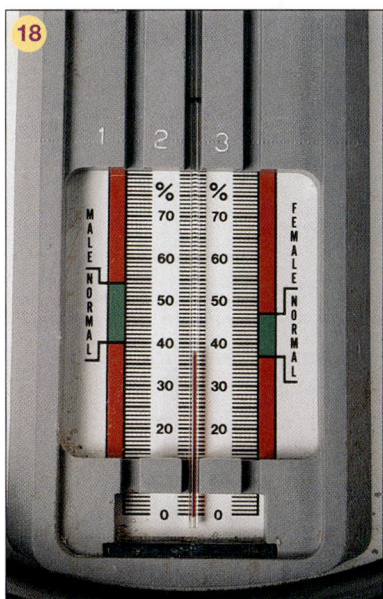

Continued

PROCEDURE 42-5 Perform a Microhematocrit Test—cont'd

19. **Procedural Step.** Read the first tube as the percentage of red blood cells or the hematocrit.
20. **Procedural Step.** Discard the capillary tube in a sharps container.
21. **Procedural Step.** Repeat the reading for the second capillary tube and discard.
22. **Procedural Step.** Average the two results and record the average value as the patient result.
    The two readings should not vary by more than ±2%. If they do, repeat the collection and run the test again.
23. **Procedural Step.** Disinfect the work area with a disinfectant solution.
24. **Procedural Step.** Remove gloves and sanitize the hands.
    Always sanitize the hands after every procedure or after using gloves.
25. **Procedural Step.** Document the results in the patient's medical record and the laboratory logbook.
    Include date and time of the test, name of the test, and results.

CHARTING EXAMPLE

Date	
6/12/xx	1:00 p.m. Hct: 42%. ——— A. Weller, RMA

Photos from Steps 10, 14, and 18 from Bonewit-West K: Clinical procedures for medical assistants, *ed 7, St Louis, 2008, Saunders; photo for Step 8 from Garrels M, Oatis C:* Laboratory testing for ambulatory settings, *St Louis, 2006, Saunders.*

PROCEDURE 42-6 Determine Erythrocyte Sedimentation Rate (ESR, Nonautomated) Using the Westergren Method

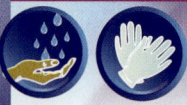

TASK: Properly fill a Westergren tube and observe and report ESR results accurately.

EQUIPMENT AND SUPPLIES
- Nonsterile disposable gloves
- Personal protective equipment (PPE), as indicated
- Supplies to perform venipuncture
- Ethylenediaminetetraacetic acid (EDTA)–anticoagulated blood specimen (lavender-top tube)
- Sed-Pac ESR system (reservoir, diluent, Dispette tube) with rack
- Transfer pipette
- Timer
- Disinfectant solution
- Biohazardous waste container
- Patient's medical record
- Laboratory logbook
- Sharps container

SKILLS/*RATIONALE*   STANDARD PRECAUTIONS ARE TO BE FOLLOWED.

1. **Procedural Step.** Sanitize the hands.
   An alcohol-based hand rub may be used instead of washing hands with soap and water, unless hands are visibly soiled.
   Rationale. Hand sanitization promotes infection control.
2. **Procedural Step.** Assemble equipment and supplies and verify the order.
   Rationale. It is important to have all supplies and equipment ready and available before starting any procedure to ensure efficiency.
3. **Procedural Step.** Greet the patient, introduce yourself, and confirm the patient's identity. Escort the patient to the laboratory area.
   Rationale. Identifying the patient ensures the procedure is performed on the correct patient.
4. **Procedural Step.** Explain the procedure to the patient.
   Rationale. Explaining the procedure to the patient promotes cooperation and provides a means of obtaining implied consent.
5. **Procedural Step.** Apply gloves and PPE as appropriate.
6. **Procedural Step.** Perform a venipuncture.
   Collect one EDTA tube (lavender top) of blood.
7. **Procedural Step.** Transport the specimen to the physician office laboratory.

Continued

PROCEDURE 42-6 Determine Erythrocyte Sedimentation Rate (ESR, Nonautomated) Using the Westergren Method—cont'd

8. **Procedural Step. Transfer the specimen.**
   Remove the stopper on the prefilled ESR vial and fill the reservoir to the indicated line with blood using a transfer pipette. Mix well.

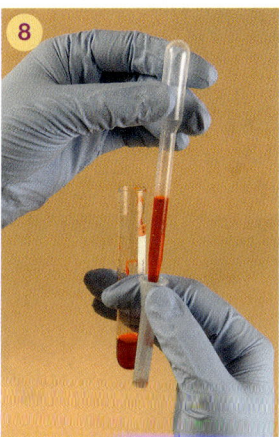

9. **Procedural Step. Insert the Dispette tube into the reservoir and push down until the tube touches the bottom of the reservoir.**
   The Dispette tube will auto-zero the blood, and any excess will flow into the closed reservoir compartment.

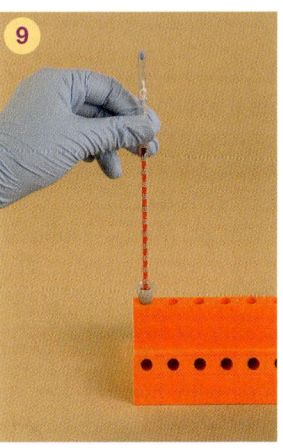

10. **Procedural Step. Place the ESR tube in a rack, making certain it remains vertical.**
    Rationale. Results will be inaccurate if the ESR tube is not kept vertical.

11. **Procedural Step. Set the timer for 1 hour.**

12. **Procedural Step. Read the results.**
    Observe the level of the meniscus of the blood in the tube after 1 hour. The scale is measured in millimeters; each line equals 1 mm.

13. **Procedural Step. Properly dispose of the ESR tube in a biohazardous waste container. Discard the lavender top tube in the sharps container.**

14. **Procedural Step. Disinfect the work area using 10% bleach solution.**

15. **Procedural Step. Remove gloves and sanitize the hands.**
    Always sanitize the hands after every procedure or after using gloves.

16. **Procedural Step. Document the results in the patient's medical record and the laboratory logbook.**
    Include date and time of the test, name of the test, and results.

CHARTING EXAMPLE

Date	
3/10/xx	2:15 p.m. ESR 9 mm/hr (Westergren).————————————— T. Bruno, CMA (AAMA)

The distance that the RBCs have fallen is recorded (Figure 42-12).

Table 42-7 compares the reference values of the Wintrobe and Westergren methods.

Blood Slide Differential

Another routine hematology procedure is the microscopic examination of blood. This involves the preparation, staining, and examination of a dried blood specimen on a glass slide. In most cases, only licensed laboratory technicians can perform these tests because they are not CLIA-waived. However, the medical assistant can prepare the blood smear in preparation for the procedure. Figure 42-13 shows slides ready for microscopic inspection.

A **differential blood cell count,** or "diff," is an important diagnostic test. An increase or decrease in one or several types of cells may occur in various disease conditions. The test differentiates WBCs (counts them by type) as a percentage per 100 cells. It also observes the shape of the RBCs and estimates the number of platelets.

When first learning this procedure, the medical assistant must remember that slide preparation takes time, patience,

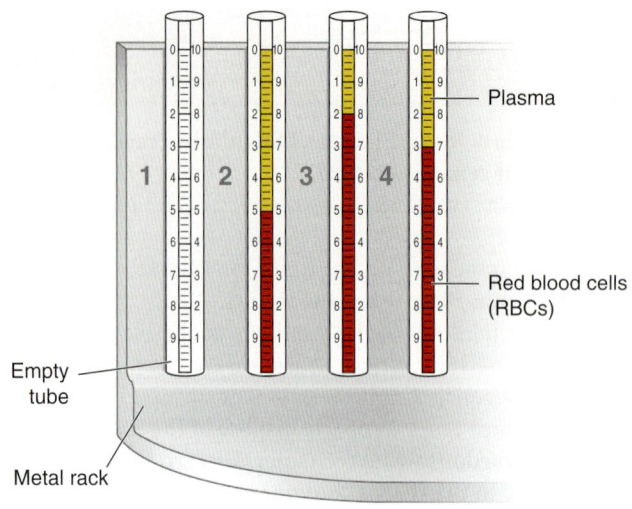

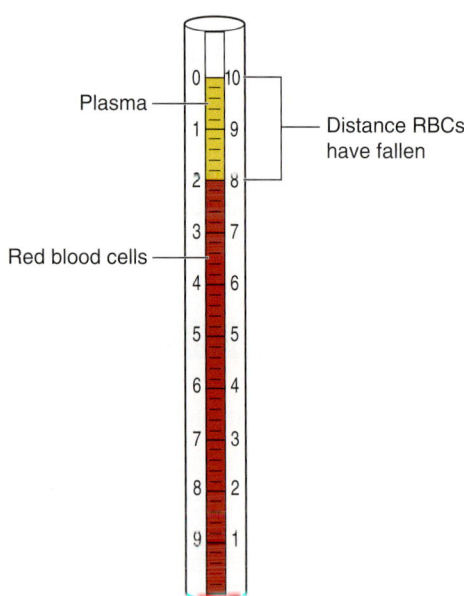

FIGURE 42-12 Wintrobe erythrocyte sedimentation rate (ESR) system. As with the Westergren method, the distance the red blood cells (RBCs) have dropped is determined in exactly 1 hour. (Modified from Stepp CA, Woods MA: *Laboratory procedures for medical office personnel,* Philadelphia, 1998, Saunders.)

TABLE 42-7
Erythrocyte Sedimentation Rate (ESR) Values

	Westergren Method	Wintrobe Method
MEN		
<50 years	0-15 mm/hr	0-7 mm/hr
>50 years	0-20 mm/hr	5-7 mm/hr
WOMEN		
<50 years	0-20 mm/hr	0-15 mm/hr
>50 years	0-30 mm/hr	25-30 mm/hr

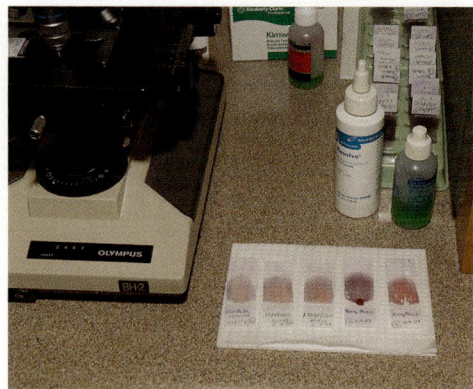

FIGURE 42-13 Slides prepared for a differential count.

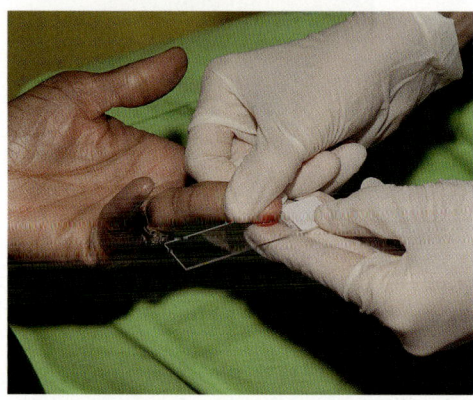

FIGURE 42-14 A drop of blood can be put directly onto the slide.

and practice. If the blood smear is too thick, the cells cannot be seen clearly, and it may not stain correctly. If it is too thin, the cells will be spread out, and the time needed to count increases. The medical assistant must be able to "feather" the blood smear to one cell layer thick.

The specimen can be from a capillary puncture (Figure 42-14), a freshly drawn specimen using a syringe, or an EDTA blood specimen. Basically, a drop of blood is pushed across a slide with another slide, as follows:

1. A medium-sized drop of blood is placed near the frosted edge of the slide, with the spreader slide at a 30-degree angle just in front of the drop of blood.
2. The spreader slide is pulled back until the edge comes in contact with the drop of blood.
3. The blood should spread evenly across the width of the spreader slide (Figure 42-15, *A*).
4. The spreader slide is then pushed toward the opposite end of the slide (Figure 42-15, *B*) and disposed of in a sharps container.
5. The slide should be placed on a flat surface immediately and allowed to air-dry. This prevents blood cell shrinkage.

The following factors can affect the quality of a good blood smear:

1. *Size* of the drop of blood. A small drop may produce a short, thick smear. A large drop can produce a longer, thinner specimen. A large drop can also produce too much

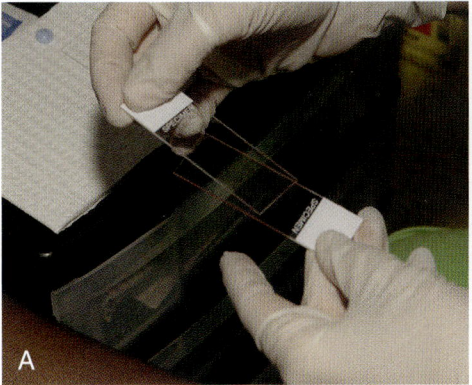
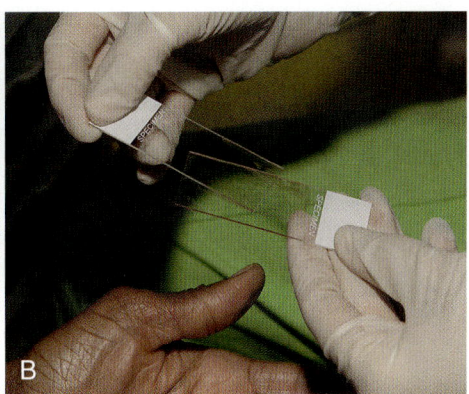

FIGURE 42-15 A, The spreader slide is placed directly in front of the blood at a 45-degree angle and spread evenly across the width of the slide. **B,** The smear will be heavier at the drop of blood end of the slide and thins out.

blood so that the smear has cells stacked on top of each other.
2. *Angle* of the spreader slide. An angle less than 30 degrees produces a long, thin slide. An angle greater than 30 degrees produces a shorter, thicker blood smear.
3. *Pressure* used. Pressure must be even during the process. The greater the pressure, the thinner is the smear. Uneven pressure creates ridges or gaps in the blood smear.
4. *Speed* of the spreading movement. Too much or too little speed can increase or decrease the thickness of the blood smear. The spreading movement must be smooth and continuous to achieve the desired thickness.
5. *Viscosity* (blood stickiness, or thickness). **Viscosity** can affect how evenly the smear can be done. If the blood is too thick or sticky, only masses of RBCs will be visible, and WBCs will not be seen.

Making a blood smear correctly depends on adjusting the technique according to the problem. Procedure 42-7 describes proper preparation of a blood smear.

Blood Chemistry

Blood chemistry is the **quantitative** (measurable, pertaining to amount) analysis of chemicals in the blood. Most blood chemistry tests are performed on serum. The test ordered will depend on the physician's diagnosis or the patient's present symptoms. The medical assistant must be conscious of the type of specimen required for each test ordered. Table 42-8 provides a reference range for various blood chemistry tests.

Specimens are frequently sent to an outside laboratory for processing so that qualified personnel and analyzers can perform the tests (Figure 42-16). A **chemistry profile** provides the physician with information about the patient's general state of health and includes lipid and carbohydrate metabolism and liver, thyroid, kidney, and cardiac function. Other profiles can be ordered to address a particular body system (e.g., liver, renal, cardiac, lipid).

Point-of-care testing (POCT) involves tests done in the physician's office for immediate feedback and can be performed by medical assistants. Such tests include cholesterol and glucose measurements. These tests require only a small sample of blood, so a capillary puncture is adequate. Blood

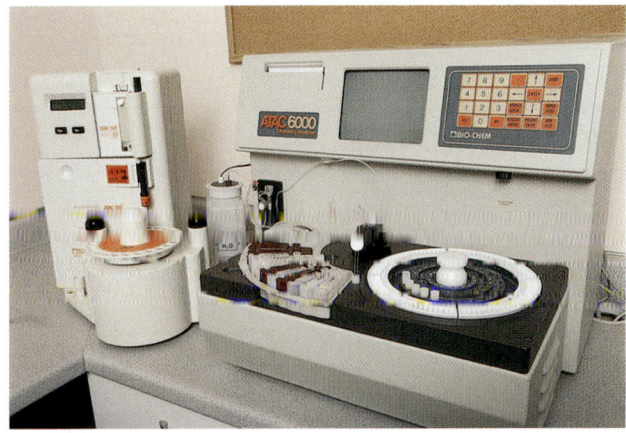

FIGURE 42-16 Blood chemistry analyzer. (ATAC Lab System, BioMed.)

glucose tests are performed for the diagnosis and control of diabetes mellitus. Cholesterol testing in the POL is used to monitor the patient's general health status and the effectiveness of cholesterol-lowering medications. "ProTimes" (coagulation and bleeding times or prothrombin times[PT] and partial thromboplastin times [PTT]) are also done on site to assist the physician with warfarin (Coumadin) adjustments. CLIA 88 requires that two levels of controls be performed daily: normal control and high level. This validates the accuracy of the equipment and reagents.

Cholesterol Testing

The body makes **serum cholesterol,** a white, fatlike substance, in the liver. Cholesterol is also metabolized from foods (e.g., organ meats, dairy products). It is contained within cell membranes. The body needs cholesterol for normal functioning and uses it to produce hormones and bile. Higher-than-normal levels of cholesterol in the blood cause narrowing of the blood vessels, leading to heart disease and stroke. The following three levels of cholesterol are measured:
- **Total cholesterol** is a combined measurement of the amount of LDL cholesterol and HDL cholesterol in the blood.

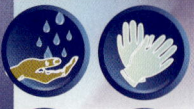
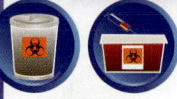

PROCEDURE 42-7

Prepare a Blood Smear

TASK: Prepare a blood smear for a differential count.

EQUIPMENT AND SUPPLIES
- Nonsterile disposable gloves
- Personal protective equipment (PPE), as indicated
- Supplies to perform capillary puncture or venipuncture
- Glass slides (frosted end)
- Pipette or DIFF-SAFE
- Slide holder
- Pencil
- Disinfectant solution
- Sharps container
- Biohazardous waste container

SKILLS/RATIONALE

STANDARD PRECAUTIONS ARE TO BE FOLLOWED.

1. **Procedural Step.** Sanitize the hands.
   An alcohol-based hand rub may be used instead of washing hands with soap and water, unless hands are visibly soiled.
   Rationale. Hand sanitization promotes infection control.

2. **Procedural Step.** Assemble equipment and supplies and verify the order.
   Slides must be clean and free from chips or cracks.
   Rationale. It is important to have all supplies and equipment ready and available before starting any procedure to ensure efficiency.

3. **Procedural Step.** Greet the patient, introduce yourself, and confirm the patient's identity. Escort the patient to the laboratory area.
   Rationale. Identifying the patient ensures the procedure is performed on the correct patient.

4. **Procedural Step.** Explain the procedure to the patient.
   Rationale. Explaining the procedure to the patient promotes cooperation and provides a means of obtaining implied consent.

5. **Procedural Step.** Apply gloves and PPE, as indicated.

6. **Procedural Step.** Label two slides on the frosted end, using a pencil, with the patient's name and the date.
   Rationale. Two slides will be smeared. Labeling the slides identifies the patient's specimen.

7. **Procedural Step.** Perform a venipuncture.
   Collect one EDTA tube (lavender top) of blood. Follow Procedure 41-3 or perform a capillary puncture following Procedure 41-1.

8. **Procedural Step.** Place a well-rounded, medium-sized drop (1 to 2 mm) of fresh whole blood on each slide as follows:

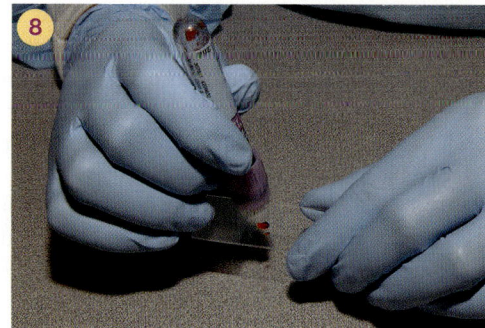

a. The cap from lavender-top tube is carefully removed, and a drop of blood is transferred to each glass slide using a disposable pipette. This is the least favorable method because it poses the greatest risk of aerosol and droplet contamination.

b. Blood is collected into an EDTA tube, and the specimen is transported to the POL, where a DIFF-SAFE is inserted into the top of the blood tube. The DIFF-SAFE with the attached tube is pushed down on top of each glass slide, releasing the drop of blood. This is the most accurate and safest method because it provides a measured drop of blood accurately and consistently and the risk is minimal.

From a *skin puncture:* Perform a capillary puncture and wipe away the first drop of blood. Place a drop of blood from the patient's finger onto each slide approximately $\frac{1}{4}$ inch from the frosted edge of the slide. Do not allow the patient's finger to touch the slide.

If only a differential and perhaps one other point-of-care test are ordered, a capillary puncture will provide a sufficient amount of blood. Again, this requires a great

Continued

PROCEDURE 42-7 Prepare a Blood Smear—cont'd

amount of skill and proficiency in smearing the slide. If a slide cannot be made from the first drops of blood, it may require a second puncture. With time and experience, however, this is an efficient method of collection and requires only a minimal amount of blood.

NOTE: The patient's finger must not touch the slide; it may cause hemolysis of the specimen and inaccurate test results. It may also cause the specimen to spread prematurely, and moisture and oils from the patient's skin can interfere with test results.

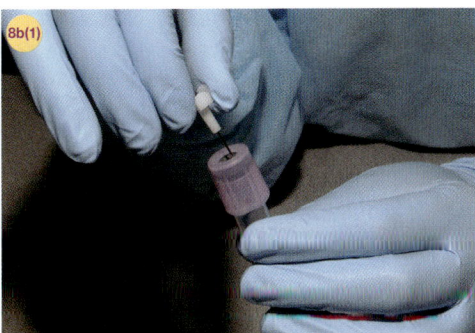

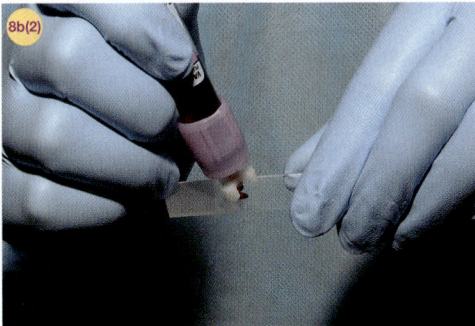

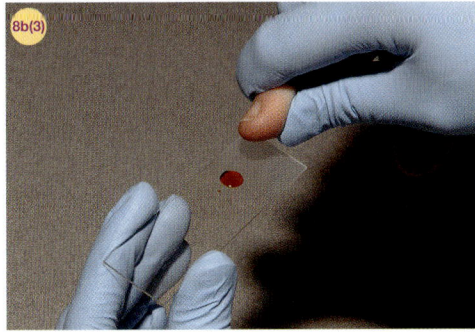

9. **Procedural Step. Spread the drop of blood back.**
Once the drop of blood is placed on the glass slide, take a second glass slide or "spreader" slide in your dominant hand. Place it directly in front of the drop of blood at a 45-degree angle. Slowly back the spreader slide into the drop of blood. Allow the drop of blood to spread evenly across the width of the slide.
Rationale. This ensures an even smear.

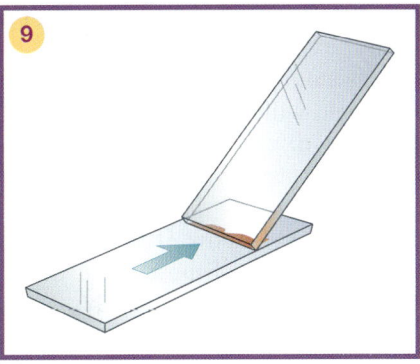

10. **Procedural Step. Spread the drop of blood forward.**
Lower the angle of the spreader slide to 30 degrees and quickly push the slide forward along the length of the stationary glass slide.
This movement is much like striking a match.
Rationale. If the angle is greater than 30 degrees, the smear will be too thick and will be difficult to read because the cells will be overlapping. If the angle is less than 30 degrees, the smear will be too thin, and the cells will be too spread out.

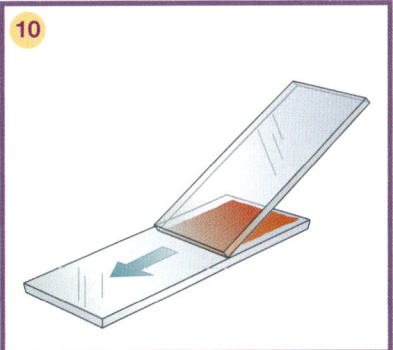

11. **Procedural Step. Evaluate the slide.**
The smear should be approximately one-half the slide's length. The blood smear will be heavier at the blood drop end of the slide, gradually thinning out to a feathered edge.
When held up to the light, a rainbow should be visible in the feathered end. The feathered end of the slide is only one cell thick and is the area where the physician will "read" the differential.
The smear should be free of holes, lines, clumps, or jagged edges. The feathered end should be free of streaks and spikes of blood extending from the feathered edge.

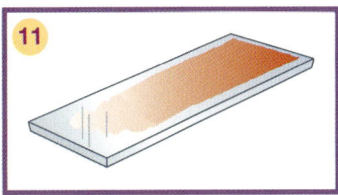

Continued

PROCEDURE 42-7: Prepare a Blood Smear—cont'd

12. **Procedural Step.** Repeat Steps 9 to 11 for the second glass slide.
13. **Procedural Step.** Allow both slides to air-dry standing at an angle, with the frosted end of the slide or the blood end down.
    Rationale. If the blood end of the slide is up, the blood may run down the slide and destroy the smear.
14. **Procedural Step.** Dispose of the spreader slide in a sharps container and dispose of all other contaminated or regular waste appropriately.
15. **Procedural Step.** Once the slides are completely dry (a minimum of 20 minutes), both slides can be placed in slide holders and transported to the laboratory.
16. **Procedural Step.** Disinfect the work area using a disinfectant solution.
17. **Procedural Step.** Remove gloves and sanitize the hands.
    Always sanitize the hands after every procedure or after using gloves.

Illustrations for Steps 9, 10, and 11 from Stepp CA, Woods MA: *Laboratory procedures for medical office personnel,* Philadelphia 1998, Saunders.

TABLE 42-8
Normal Blood Chemistry Values

Test	Reference Range for Adults	Test	Reference Range for Adults
Alanine aminotransferase (ALT)	4-36 U/L	Creatinine	Men: 0.5-1.2 mg/dL
Albumin	3.5-5.5 g/dL		Women: 0.5-1.1 mg/dL
Alkaline phosphatase (ALP)	30-120 U/L	Glucose, fasting (fasting blood sugar [FBS])	70-110 mg/dL
Amylase	95-290 U/L		
Anion gap (R factor) (AG)	10-18 mEq/L	Glucose, 2-hour postprandial (PPBS)	<140 mg/dL
Aspartate transaminase (AST)	0-35 U/L	Glucose tolerance test (GTT)	FBS: 70-110 mg/dL
Bilirubin, total	0.3-1 mg/dL		30 min: 110-170 mg/dL
Bilirubin, conjugated	0.1-0.3 mg/dL		1 hr: 120-170 mg/dL
Blood urea nitrogen (BUN)	10-20 mg/dL		2 hr: 70-120 mg/dL
Calcium (Ca)	9-10.5 mg/dL		3 hr: <120 mg/dL
Carbon dioxide (CO_2)	22-29 mEq/L	Iron (Fe)	60-180 µg/dL
Chloride (Cl)	98-106 mEq/L	Iron-binding capacity, total (TIBC)	250-400 µg/dL
Cholesterol, total (CH, Chol)	Desirable: <200 mg/dL	Lactate dehydrogenase (LD, LDH)	100-200 U/L
	Borderline: 200-240 mg/dL	Lipase	0-1 U/mL
	High: >240 mg/dL	Magnesium (Mg, Mag)	1.3-2.1 mEq/L
Cholesterol, low-density lipoprotein (LDL)	Desirable: <170 mg/dL	Phosphorus (P)	3-4.5 mg/dL
	Borderline: 170-200 mg/dL	Potassium (K)	3.5-5 mEq/L
	High: >200 mg/dL	Protein, total (TP)	6.2-8.2 g/dL
Cholesterol, high-density lipoprotein (HDL)	Men: 29-60 mg/dL	Sodium (Na)	136-145 mEq/L
	Women: 38-75 mg/dL	Triglycerides (TG, Trig)	40-160 mg/dL
Creatine kinase (CK)	Men: 15-160 U/L	Uric acid	Men: 3.5-7.2 mg/dL
	Women: 15-130 U/L		Women: 2.6-6 mg/dL

- **Low-density lipoprotein (LDL),** the "bad" cholesterol, picks up cholesterol from ingested fats and the liver and takes it to the blood vessels and muscles. When it builds up on the walls of blood vessels, LDL cholesterol causes heart disease.
- **High-density lipoprotein (HDL),** the "good" cholesterol, removes excess cholesterol from the body cells and takes it to the liver to be excreted.

Cholesterol test results are as follows:

Desirable cholesterol level:	<200 mg/dL
Borderline-high cholesterol level:	200-240 mg/dL
High cholesterol level:	>240 mg/dL

The primary use of cholesterol testing is to screen for high levels of blood cholesterol related to heart disease. The total amount of cholesterol, the amount of LDL and HDL cholesterol in the blood, and the ratios of each provide a good indicator of risk for artery disease. Cholesterol testing is often used to monitor liver and thyroid function. Procedure 42-8 explains the process of performing cholesterol testing.

Glucose Testing

The end result of carbohydrate metabolism is glucose, or sugar. Glucose is the main source of energy for the body. The body functions best if the blood glucose level remains constant. When not used for energy, glucose is stored in muscles and the liver as glycogen. When an overload of glucose is present, it can be stored as fat in the adipose tissue.

The hormone *insulin* allows glucose to enter the cells and be converted to energy. A person's blood glucose rises after an ingestion of glucose but should return to normal range after 2 hours.

Fasting Blood Sugar Test. The **fasting blood sugar (FBS)** test measures the glucose level in a blood sample. The patient is required to refrain from eating and drinking (except water) for at least 12 hours before testing. A blood sample is drawn, tested, and compared to the normal range of 70 to 110 mg/dL of glucose in the blood.

Two-Hour Postprandial Test. The **2-hour postprandial test** is used to screen for diabetes mellitus and to monitor the effects of a patient's insulin regimen. A patient is required to fast, then either eat a special meal or drink a glucose solution containing 100 g of glucose. Two hours after ingestion, a blood sample is drawn and compared to the normal range.

Glucose Tolerance Test. The **glucose tolerance test (GTT)** is more sensitive to the patient's ability to metabolize glucose. The patient fasts, blood and urine specimens are collected, and the patient ingests a special glucose drink. After this, blood and urine specimens are collected at 30 minutes, 1 hour, 2 hours, and 3 hours. Urine specimens are collected to measure the amount of glucose and ketones filtered out by the kidneys. The blood test determines if the glucose level has returned to within a normal range. The patient should be encouraged to drink water so the necessary specimens can be provided.

Glucometer. Measuring the amount of glucose in the blood is frequently performed in the medical office with a **glucometer.**

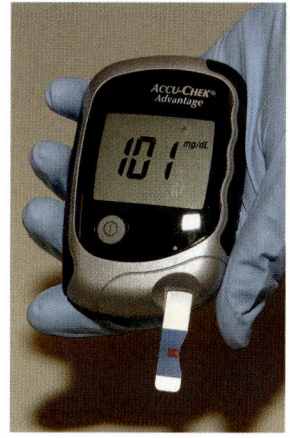

FIGURE 42-17 Glucometer.

BOX 42-2

Reasons for Errors in Glucose Readings

ERRORS IN PROCEDURE
- Not enough blood on test strip.
- Not wiping away the first drop of blood on the patient.
- Touching the finger to the test strip (allows substances from finger to be included in the reading).
- Using expired test strips.
- Touching the pad on the test strip while taking the strip from the bottle.
- If the test has a code, not checking that the code matches the strips.

OTHER REASONS FOR ERRORS
- Hematocrit readings that fall below or that exceed the normal range can cause an inaccurate low glucose reading.
- High levels of cholesterol and triglycerides may influence the blood glucose result.

On-site testing requires no special patient preparation and provides immediate feedback to the physician on the patient's status. This allows the physician to monitor the effectiveness of diabetic medications and diets.

Glucose Reagent Strip. Several manufacturers offer machines for home and clinical use that have a **glucose reagent strip** to test for glucose levels in blood. The medical assistant must follow the manufacturer's instructions for the specific device used in the medical office. Typically, a small drop of whole blood, usually obtained by capillary puncture, is applied to a reagent test strip. A glucometer uses a photometer to read the color change in the reagent paper. The result is automatically calculated and displayed in the window of the meter (Figure 42-17).

Box 42-2 lists reasons why a blood glucose reading could be inaccurate. Procedure 42-9 explains how to collect and process a blood specimen accurately for glucose testing.

PROCEDURE 42-8

Perform Cholesterol Testing

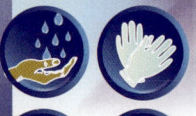
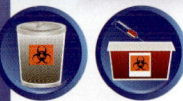

TASK: Collect and process a blood specimen accurately for cholesterol testing using the Cholestech LDX analyzer.

EQUIPMENT AND SUPPLIES

- Nonsterile disposable gloves (Latex-free)
- Personal protective equipment (PPE), as indicated
- Capillary puncture supplies
- Cholesterol testing device (Cholestech LDX)
- Cholesterol testing kit (capillary tube with plunger, test cassette)
- Disinfectant solution
- Sharps container
- Biohazardous waste container
- Quality control logsheet
- Sharps container
- Patient's medical record
- Laboratory logbook
- Disinfectant solution

SKILLS/RATIONALE

STANDARD PRECAUTIONS ARE TO BE FOLLOWED.

1. **Procedural Step.** Sanitize the hands.
   An alcohol-based hand rub may be used instead of washing hands with soap and water, unless hands are visibly soiled.
   Rationale. Hand sanitization promotes infection control.

2. **Procedural Step.** Assemble equipment and supplies and verify the order.
   Check the expiration dates of the test kits.
   Rationale. It is important to have all supplies and equipment ready and available before starting any procedure to ensure efficiency. Expired test kits may produce inaccurate test results.

3. **Procedural Step.** Prepare the test kit and analyzer.
   Remove the test kit from the refrigerator and warm to room temperature. Prepare the analyzer according to the manufacturer's instructions.

4. **Procedural Step.** Perform a quality control test as recommended by the manufacturer and document in the laboratory quality control logsheet.

5. **Procedural Step.** Greet the patient, introduce yourself, and confirm the patient's identity. Escort the patient to the laboratory area.
   Rationale. Identifying the patient ensures the procedure is performed on the correct patient.

6. **Procedural Step.** Explain the procedure to the patient.
   Rationale. Explaining the procedure to the patient promotes cooperation and provides a means of obtaining implied consent.

7. **Procedural Step.** Apply gloves and PPE as indicated.

8. **Procedural Step.** Perform a capillary puncture.

9. **Procedural Step.** Wipe away the first drop of blood.

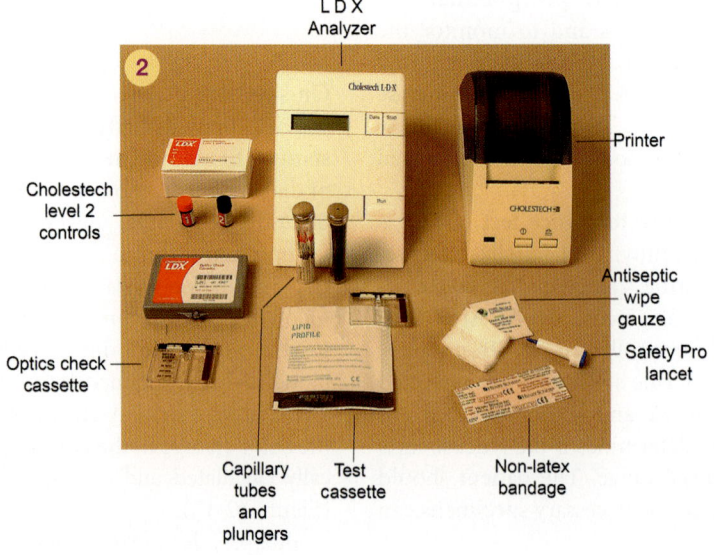

Continued

PROCEDURE 42-8 Perform Cholesterol Testing—cont'd

10. **Procedural Step.** Collect the blood specimen in a capillary tube.
    NOTE: The capillary specimen must be inserted into the cassette within 4 minutes of collection.
11. **Procedural Step.** Prepare the specimen.
    Place the end of the capillary tube in the sample well of the cassette and dispense the blood by pushing down on the plunger.
12. **Procedural Step.** Insert the cassette into the Cholestech LDX analyzer and activate the timer.
13. **Procedural Step.** When the timer stops, read the results.
14. **Procedural Step.** Discard the cassette, capillary tube, and plunger into a sharps container.
15. **Procedural Step.** Turn off the analyzer and wipe it with a damp cloth.
16. **Procedural Step.** Disinfect the work area using disinfectant solution.
17. **Procedural Step.** Remove gloves and sanitize the hands.
    Always sanitize the hands after every procedure or after using gloves.
18. **Procedural Step.** Document the results in the patient's medical record and the laboratory logbook.
    Include date and time of the test, name of the test, and results.

CHARTING EXAMPLE

Date	
4/30/xx	11:15 a.m. Cholesterol level 210 mg/dL using Cholestech LDX. ———————————————— M. Lenges, RMA

PROCEDURE 42-9 Perform Glucose Testing

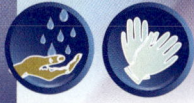
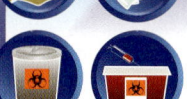

TASK: Accurately collect and process a blood specimen for glucose testing using Accu-Chek.

EQUIPMENT AND SUPPLIES
- Nonsterile disposable gloves (Latex-free)
- Personal protective equipment (PPE), as indicated
- Capillary puncture supplies
- Glucose testing device (Accu-Chek)
- Test strip
- Control solution
- Disinfectant solution
- Sharps container
- Biohazardous waste container
- Patient's medical record
- Laboratory quality control logsheet
- Laboratory logbook

SKILLS/RATIONALE
STANDARD PRECAUTIONS ARE TO BE FOLLOWED.

1. **Procedural Step.** Sanitize the hands.
   An alcohol-based hand rub may be used instead of washing hands with soap and water, unless hands are visibly soiled.
   Rationale. Hand sanitization promotes infection control.
2. **Procedural Step.** Assemble equipment and supplies and verify the order.
   Check the expiration dates of the test kits, and check the glucometer to make sure it is functioning properly.
   Rationale. It is important to have all supplies and equipment ready and available before starting any procedure to ensure efficiency. Expired test kits may produce inaccurate test results. The glucometer should be on a maintenance schedule for cleaning and battery replacement.

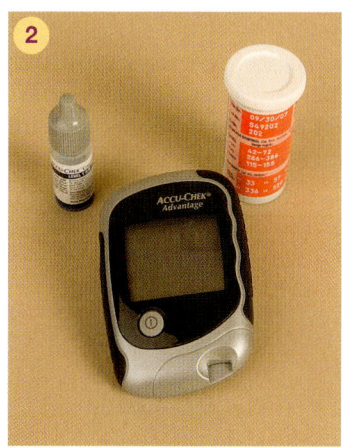

Continued

PROCEDURE 42-9 Perform Glucose Testing—cont'd

3. **Procedural Step.** Prepare the analyzer according to the manufacturer's instructions.

   Calibrate the glucometer by matching the glucometer code numbers to the code numbers on the vial of test strips. Adjust if necessary according to the manufacturer's instructions.

   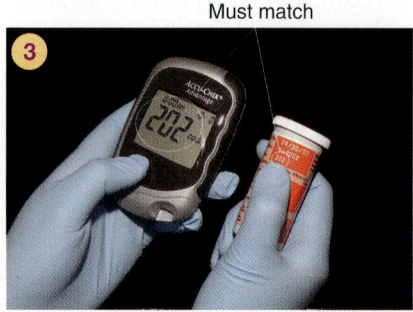

   Must match

4. **Procedural Step.** Perform a quality control test as recommended by the manufacturer and document in the laboratory quality control logsheet.

   The manufacturer displays the lot numbers and expiration dates on the outside of the bottle of test strips. Insert a control strip into the Accu-Chek glucometer. Apply a drop of control solution. Verify the accuracy of the control strip. Discard the control strip.

   Rationale. It is important to record the lot numbers and expiration dates of the test strips and controls. This provides a reference point in case the reagents or controls do not perform as expected. Recording the acceptable ranges of the controls lets you know immediately if the result obtained is acceptable.

5. **Procedural Step.** Greet and identify the patient and escort the patient to the examination room or laboratory area.

   Rationale. Identifying the patient ensures the procedure is performed on the correct patient.

6. **Procedural Step.** Explain the procedure to the patient.

   Rationale. Explaining the procedure to the patient promotes cooperation and provides a means of obtaining implied consent.

7. **Procedural Step.** Apply gloves and PPE as indicated.

8. **Procedural Step.** Insert a test strip into the test strip slot.

   After the monitor displays the code key number, it signals when to insert a test strip. Some models use a flashing icon of a test strip, others sound a beep, and still others use both a beep and a visual symbol. Within 30 seconds of the signal, insert a test strip in the slot.

   Some models have metal-colored bars at one end of the test strip. The test strip is inserted into the slot bars first, yellow pad facing up. When the flashing drop appears, the sample can be applied to the strip.

9. **Procedural Step.** Ask when the patient last had something to eat or drink (besides water).

   Rationale. The interval between the last consumption of food or beverage and the blood test for glucose may become a factor in the health care provider's evaluation of the result. If the last time the patient had anything to eat or drink was 12 hours or longer, the patient is considered to be fasting. The patient who has consumed food or a beverage within the last 12 hours is considered to be nonfasting.

10. **Procedural Step.** Perform a capillary puncture.
    Wipe away the first drop of blood.

11. **Procedural Step.** Apply a rounded drop of blood from the capillary puncture to the test strip.
    Make certain the test area is completely covered.

12. **Procedural Step.** When the glucometer timer stops, read the results.

13. **Procedural Step.** Discard the test strip into the biohazardous container.

14. **Procedural Step.** Turn off the glucometer and wipe it with a damp cloth.

15. **Procedural Step.** Disinfect the work area using 10% bleach solution.

16. **Procedural Step.** Remove gloves and sanitize the hands.
    Always sanitize the hands after every procedure or after using gloves.

17. **Procedural Step.** Document the results in the patient's medical record and the laboratory logbook.
    Include date and time of the test, name of the test, and results.

CHARTING EXAMPLE

Date	
11/22/xx	9:45 a.m. NON-FBS: 110 mg/dL.———————————— N. King, RMA

Glycosylated Hemoglobin Test. The **glycosylated hemoglobin (GHb) test** monitors diabetes treatment and control by measuring the amount of hemoglobin A_{1c} in the blood (Figure 42-18). When glucose is not used for energy and remains in the bloodstream, it attaches to the hemoglobin. Since the life span of an RBC is 120 days, GHb can be measured and an average glucose level obtained for the past 3 months.

Serology and Immunology

Serology is the laboratory study of blood serum for signs of antibodies produced by the antigen-antibody reaction. The body's immune system provides a defense against infection by producing antibodies against a disease-producing organism. When the body senses a foreign object or organism (antigen), it may produce antibodies to neutralize the offending organism. The body also produces antibodies against bacterial toxins, allergens, and blood allergens. **Immunology** is the study of how the immune system works to defend the body.

The testing of body fluids is referred to as **serological testing, immunological testing,** and **immunoassays.** Serological testing done in the POL involves the use of prepackaged test kits that analyze a reaction between an antigen and an antibody (Figure 42-19). Those performed in the medical office are for diseases seen most frequently by the physician (Box 42-3). Results are recorded as a reaction (positive) or lack of reaction (negative) to an additive. To be considered positive, the reaction must be viewable and measurable. Viewable reactions include the following:

- *Agglutination.* As discussed in Chapter 13 and earlier in this chapter, agglutination means "clumping." Think of the agglutination process as how a magnet attracts items. The antigen is the magnet, and it attracts antibodies to it. Figure

> **BOX 42-3**
>
> ### Serological Tests
>
> *Hepatitis test.* Detects viral hepatitis and determines what type of hepatitis.
>
> *Syphilis test.* Screening test for the syphilis antibodies (VDRL or RPR). Any active reaction results in a positive test result being recorded. Further tests are done to confirm a diagnosis of syphilis (e.g., FTA absorption test).
>
> *Mononucleosis test.* Aids in the diagnosis of infectious mononucleosis by testing for the presence of the heterophil antibody using serum, plasma, and sometimes whole blood (see Figure 42-20).
>
> *Rheumatoid test.* Detects rheumatoid factor (RF) in patients with rheumatoid arthritis.
>
> *Antistreptolysin O (ASO) test.* Detects ASO antibodies in the serum of a patient with a streptococcal infection or a disease occurring as a secondary infection (e.g., rheumatic fever, bacterial endocarditis).
>
> *C-reactive protein (CRP) test.* Detects an abnormal protein (CRP) in the blood during inflammation and tissue destruction. This screening test assists with the diagnosis of bacterial infections, malignancy, heart disease, and arthritis. Some research indicates that the buildup of **plaque** (fatty deposits) on the arterial walls is a result of an inflammatory response.
>
> *ABO and Rh blood typing.* Determines a patient's blood type and the presence or absence of the Rh factor.

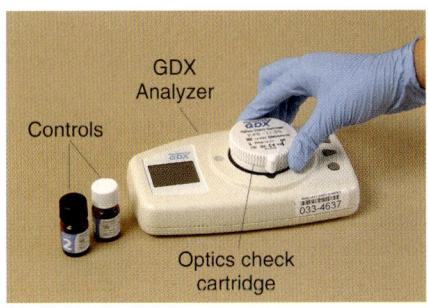

FIGURE 42-18 Cholestech GDX A1C used for point-of-care testing (POCT).

FIGURE 42-19 The Quick Vue Influenza Test is an immunoassay test.

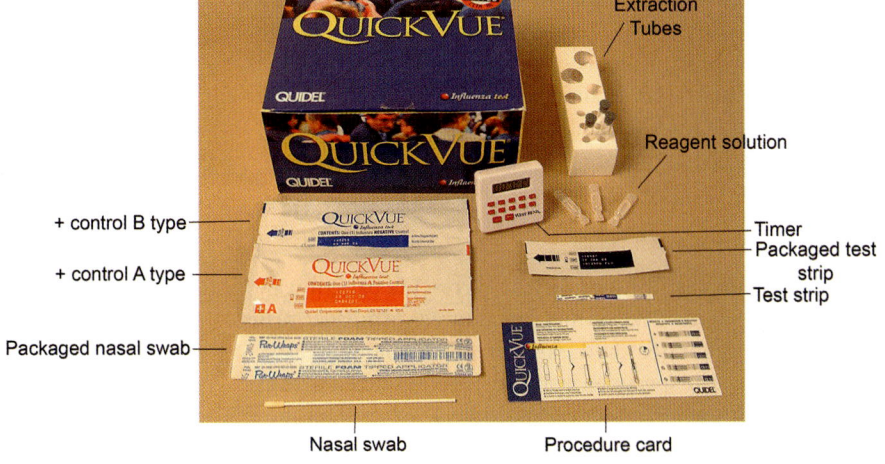

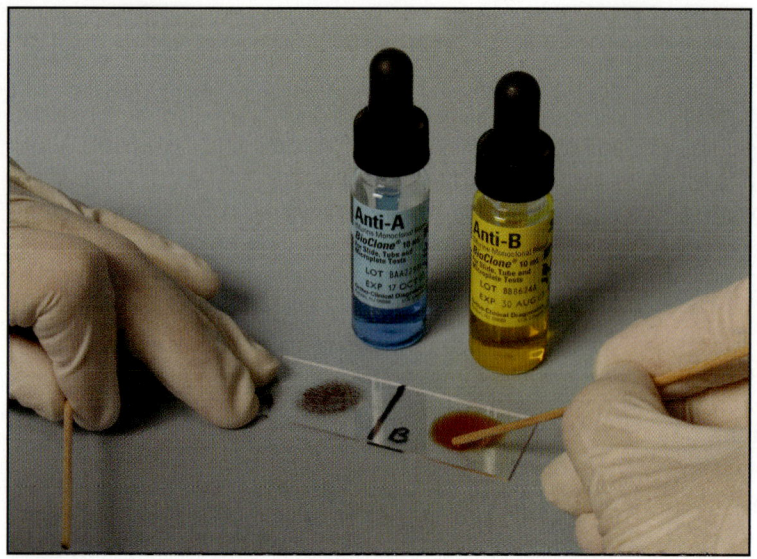

FIGURE 42-20 Blood can be tested for blood type by combining a drop of blood with anti-*A* and anti-*B* solutions. If antigens are present in the blood, agglutination will result. (From Garrels M, Oatis C: *Laboratory testing for ambulatory settings,* St Louis, 2006, Saunders.)

42-20 illustrates the agglutination process in blood typing.
- *Color change.* The color change technique is based on the use of an enzyme to test specifically for antigen-antibody sensitivity. Figure 42-21 provides an example of a product insert used to perform the mononucleosis test on whole blood using the color-change technique.
- *Precipitation* is a visible reaction between the antigen and antibody that produces a solid residue (**precipitates**).
- *Lysis* is the destruction of RBCs caused by an antibody-antigen response.

Microbiology

Bacteriology is the study of microorganisms, especially pathogenic (disease-producing) organisms. When a physician suspects a particular disease or infection or wants to identify a microorganism causing an infection, the physician may order a specimen be collected of a particular substance for microbiological review. The medical assistant or other health care professional may collect body fluids (e.g., urine, blood) or other specimens from the throat, wound, or lungs (sputum). The medical assistant may send these to an outside reference laboratory for processing or they may be processed in-house by a licensed laboratory technician. The preparation of bacterial smears and Gram staining may be done in the POL. Cultures may also be prepared.

Bacterial Smears

A direct bacterial smear may be taken from the patient using a sterile swab in the POL or may be cultured on an agar plate in an outside laboratory and transferred as a colony (cluster) to a glass slide. The specimen is then dried and stained to assist viewing under the microscope. Procedure 42-10 explains how to prepare a **bacterial smear** from a swab.

Gram Staining

The purpose of the **Gram stain** is to separate bacteria into two groups: gram-positive and gram-negative. The coloring of the cells of the bacteria allows for easier identification. Gram-positive microorganisms stain purple, and gram-negative microorganisms stain pink-red (Figure 42-22, *A* and *B*). Table 42-9 lists and illustrates staining properties of various bacteria. Figure 42-23 provides instructions for Gram staining.

If the specimen is sent to the laboratory for identification, it is often collected with a sterile swab. After collection, the swab is placed in a tube containing transport medium. This substance keeps the specimen moist until it can be processed.

Cultures

Inoculating a **culture plate** is done (when ordered) to identify which bacteria are causing the infection or which antibiotic to use for treatment. The successful growth of bacteria depends on the correct nutrients and environmental conditions. Most often, the cultures taken in the POL are for group A *Streptococcus* (throat), *E. coli* (urine), and *Staphylococcus* (wound).

Substances that support the growth of microorganisms are called **media**. Media selected could be a broth (liquid), a semi-solid, or a solid (**agar**) type. The agar could be either in a tube or on a Petri dish (culture plate). Some media are specific for particular organisms, whereas others support the growth of all bacteria. Throat cultures are usually cultured on a blood agar medium because this allows the *Streptococcus* bacteria to use the RBCs for growth. Urine cultures are either done on eosin–methylene blue agar or MacConkey agar specific for *E. coli.* Table 42-10 lists common culture media used to identify infectious bacteria.

Text continued on p. 998

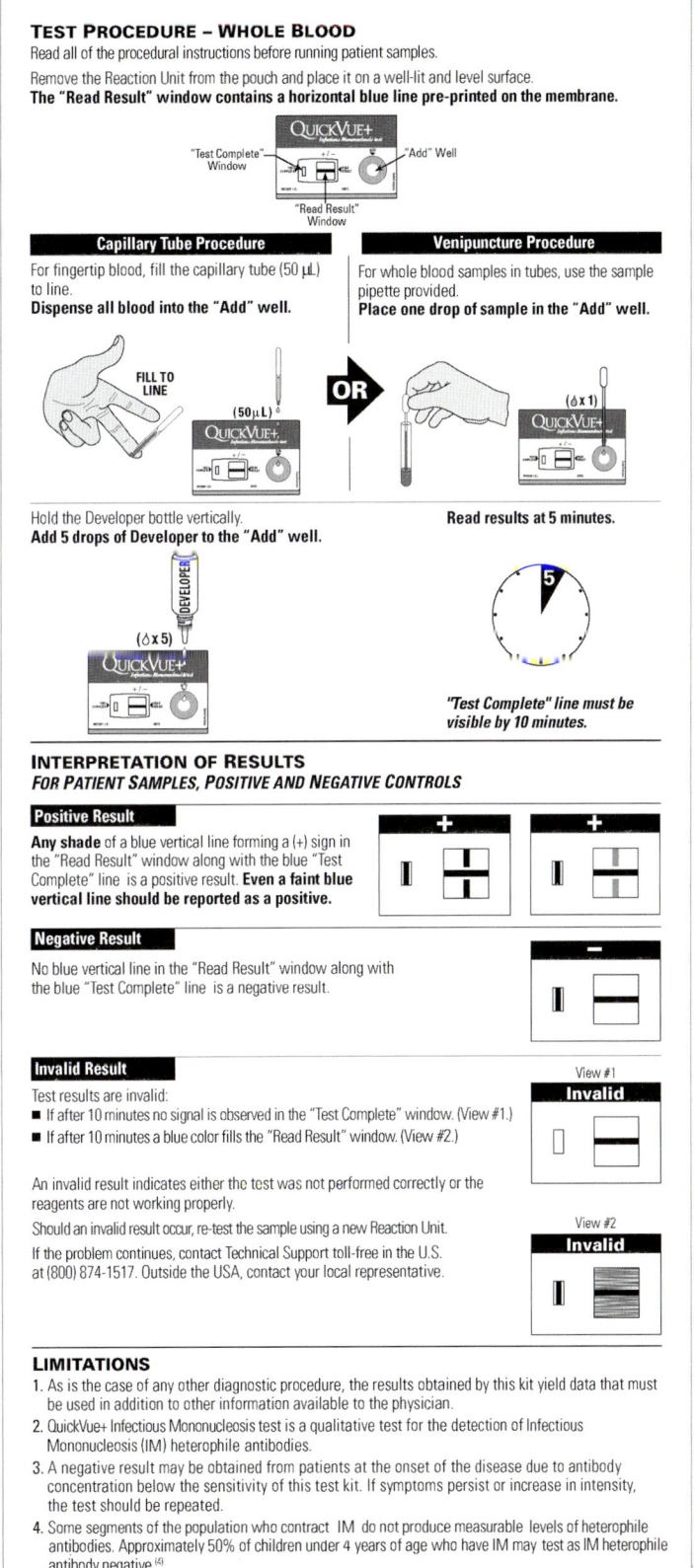

FIGURE 42-21 Procedure for performing the QuickVue + Infectious Mononucleosis Test. (Courtesy Quidel, San Diego).

PROCEDURE 42-10: Obtain a Bacterial Smear from a Wound Specimen

TASK: Collect a sample of wound exudates, using sterile collection supplies, without contaminating the specimen. Prepare the specimen for transport to the laboratory.

EQUIPMENT AND SUPPLIES
- Nonsterile disposable gloves (Latex-free)
- Personal protective equipment (PPE), as indicated
- Laboratory requisition form
- Plastic-backed paper towel
- Biohazard transport bag
- 4 × 4 sterile gauze
- Bottle of antiseptic solution
- Surgical tape
- Bandage roll
- Marking pen
- Agar-gel transport system (sterile tube with sterile swab and semisolid solution in the bottom)
- Disinfectant solution
- Biohazardous waste container
- Patient's medical record

SKILLS/RATIONALE

STANDARD PRECAUTIONS ARE TO BE FOLLOWED.

1. **Procedural Step.** Sanitize the hands.
   An alcohol-based hand rub may be used instead of washing hands with soap and water, unless hands are visibly soiled.
   Rationale. Hand sanitization promotes infection control.

2. **Procedural Step.** Assemble equipment and sterile supplies and verify the order.
   Check expiration date on the swab.
   Rationale. It is important to have all supplies and equipment ready and available before starting any procedure to ensure efficiency. Transport medium may dry up and lose its effectiveness past the expiration date.

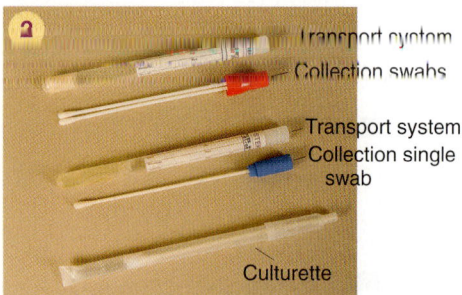

3. **Procedural Step.** Prepare a laboratory requisition form for submitting the specimen to the microbiology department.

4. **Procedural Step.** Greet the patient, introduce yourself, and confirm the patient's identity. Escort the patient to the examination room.
   Rationale. Identifying the patient ensures the procedure is performed on the correct patient.

5. **Procedural Step.** Explain the procedure to the patient.
   Rationale. Explaining the procedure to the patient promotes cooperation and provides a means of obtaining implied consent.

6. **Procedural Step.** Apply gloves and PPE as indicated.

7. **Procedural Step.** Position the patient for easiest access to the area from which the specimen will be collected.

8. **Procedural Step.** Remove the patient's old dressing and dispose of it in a biohazardous waste container.

9. **Procedural Step.** Change gloves.
   Rationale. Clean gloves are necessary when obtaining a specimen to prevent cross-contamination after the dressing is removed.

10. **Procedural Step.** Inspect the wound for odor, color, amount of drainage, and depth.
    Make a mental note of these characteristics for documentation later.

11. **Procedural Step.** Obtain the specimen.
    Carefully remove the sterile swab from the agar-gel tube so that it does not touch the sides of the tube as it is withdrawn. Being careful not to touch surrounding skin or anything other than the inside of the wound, insert the sterile swab into the wound where the drainage is most abundant.

12. **Procedural Step.** Move the swab around from side to side.
    Rationale. This ensures an adequate sample collection that will produce pathogens representative of any that may be causing the infection.

13. **Procedural Step.** Carefully return the swab to the tube.
    Make certain it does not touch the sides or the opening of the tube. Firmly slide the swab into the agar-gel so that the entire swab is suspended in the transport medium. If the transport medium is encapsulated, crush

Continued

PROCEDURE 42-10 Obtain a Bacterial Smear from a Wound Specimen—cont'd

the ampule to moisten the swab to keep it in optimum condition during transport.

14. **Procedural Step.** Label the specimen.
    Indicate the patient's name, identification number, date and time of collection, tests requested, site of collection, and physician's name. If you are using a computer system that generates a label, apply the label to the specimen instead.
15. **Procedural Step.** Place the agar-gel transport tube in a biohazard transport bag and seal the bag.
16. **Procedural Step.** Apply a clean bandage to the wound site.
17. **Procedural Step.** Dispose of all waste material appropriately and disinfect the work area.
18. **Procedural Step.** Remove gloves and sanitize the hands.

Always sanitize the hands after every procedure or after using gloves.

19. **Procedural Step. Complete the laboratory requisition form and transport the specimen as soon as possible to the laboratory.**
20. **Procedural Step. Document the procedure.**
    Include date and time of the procedure and condition of the wound.

CHARTING EXAMPLE

Date	
1/20/xx	11:45 a.m. Lesion Ⓛ ankle. Copious amounts of purulent discharge. Specimen obtained and sent to lab for culture.——————————— A. Reali, RMA

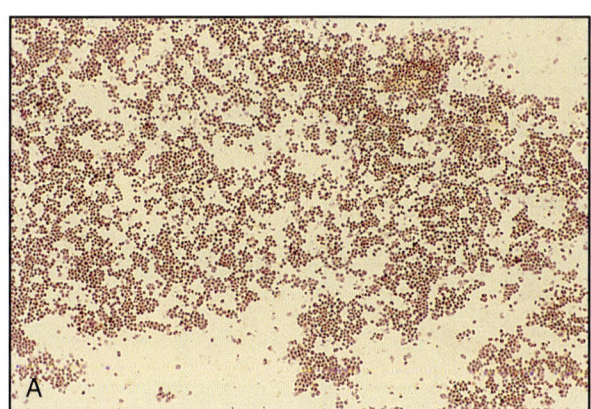
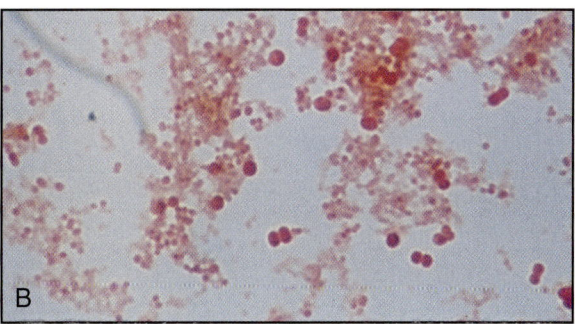

FIGURE 42-22 **A,** Gram-positive *Staphylococcus aureus*. **B,** *Neisseria gonorrhoeae* gram-negative bacteria. (From Mahon CR, Manusells G: *Textbook of diagnostic microbiology*, ed 2, Philadelphia, 2000, Saunders.)

TABLE 42-9
Identification of Bacteria Using Staining Techniques

Shape	Arrangement	Reaction	Appearance	Genus/Species
Sphere (diplococci)	Pairs and singles	Gram positive		Enterococcus species
		Gram negative		Neisseria gonorrhoeae
Sphere (streptococci)	Chains	Gram positive		Streptococcus pyogenes
Sphere (staphylococci)	Clusters	Gram positive		Staphylococcus aureus
Rod (bacilli)	Singles and chains	Gram positive		Bacillus anthracis Clostridium tetani
		Gram negative		Escherichia coli
		Acid fast		Haemophilus influenzae Pseudomonas aeruginosa Mycobacterium tuberculosis, M. leprae
Spiral (spirilla)		Gram negative		Treponema pallidum

From Hunt SA: *Saunders fundamentals of medical assisting—revised reprint*, St Louis, 2007, Saunders.

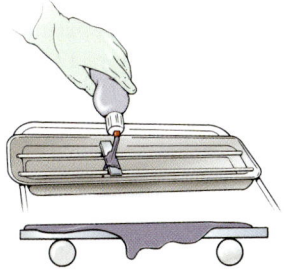
A Pour crystal violet stain onto one end of the slide until the slide is covered.

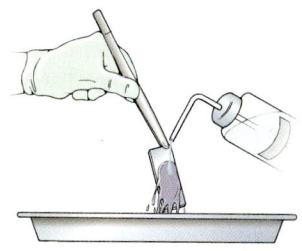
B Lift one end of the slide and rinse gently with distilled or deionized water.

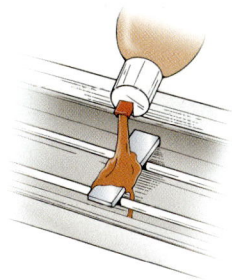
C Flood the slide with iodine solution.

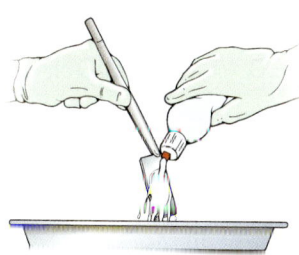
D Hold the slide at an angle and decolorize with an acetone/alcohol mixture.

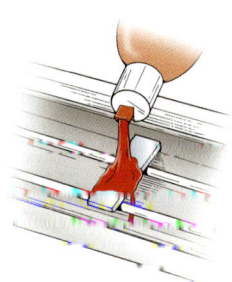
E Flood the slide with safranin.

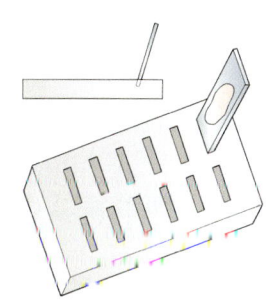
F Drain the slide and air-dry it in a slide dryer.

FIGURE 42-23 Gram stain technique. (From Stepp CA, Woods MA: *Laboratory procedures for medical office personnel,* Philadelphia, 1998, Saunders.)

TABLE 42-10
Primary Plating Media Typically Used in Culture Growths to Identify Infectious Bacteria

Medium	Form Used	Expected Isolates	Comments
Anaerobic CDC blood agar *(Brucella)* (BRUC, BRU)	Plate	All types of aerobic and anaerobic and gm (+) and gm (−) bacteria	Supports growth of all strict anaerobic and facultatively anaerobic bacteria.
Anaerobic colistin–nalidixic acid agar (ANA-CAN, CNA)	Plate and biplate	Growth of most gm (+) and gm (−) anaerobes; inhibits facultatively anaerobic gm (−) bacteria	
Anaerobic kanamycin–bile-esculin agar (KBE)	Plate and biplate	*Bacteroides fragilis* group	Provides presumptive identification of *B. fragilis* group.
Anaerobic kanamycin-vancomycin laked blood agar (KVLB, LKV)	Plate	*Bacteroides* species; pigmented anaerobic gm (−) rods, or *F. mortiferum*	Yeasts and kanamycin-resistant gm (−) bacilli may grow on this medium.
Chocolate/modified Thayer-Martin agar (CHOC/MTM)	Biplate	CHOC: *Haemophilus influenzae, Neisseria gonorrhoeae, N. meningitidis* MTM: *N. gonorrhoeae, N. meningitidis*	CHOC: see Chocolate agar. MTM: vancomycin inhibits gm (+) and colistin gm (−) bacteria; nystatin inhibits yeast.
Blood agar (BAP)	Plate	Both gm (+) and gm (−) organisms	
Chocolate agar (CHOC)	Plate	*H. influenzae, N. meningitidis*	Low agar content provides increased moisture.
Hektoen enteric agar (HE)	Plate	*Salmonella* and *Shigella* species	Has lactose, sucrose, and salicin, and most Enterobacteriaceae ferment one of these. Detects H_2S.
Löwenstein-Jensen agar (LJ)	Slant	Isolation of acid-fast bacilli	
MacConkey agar (MAC)	Plate	Gm (−) enteric bacilli	Bile salts inhibit gm (+) organisms.
Streptococcus selective agar (SXT)	Plate	Isolation of beta-hemolytic streptococci	Most gm (−) organisms are inhibited.

From Stepp CA, Woods MA: *Laboratory procedures for medical office personnel,* Philadelphia, 1998, Saunders.
NA, Not applicable; *gm* (+), gram-positive; *gm* (−), gram-negative; H_2S, hydrogen sulfide.

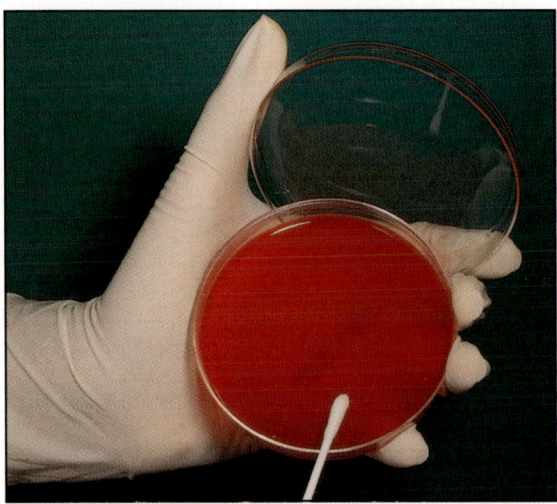

FIGURE 42-24 Method for streaking with culture swab. (From Chester GA: *Modern medical assisting*, Philadelphia, 1998, Saunders.)

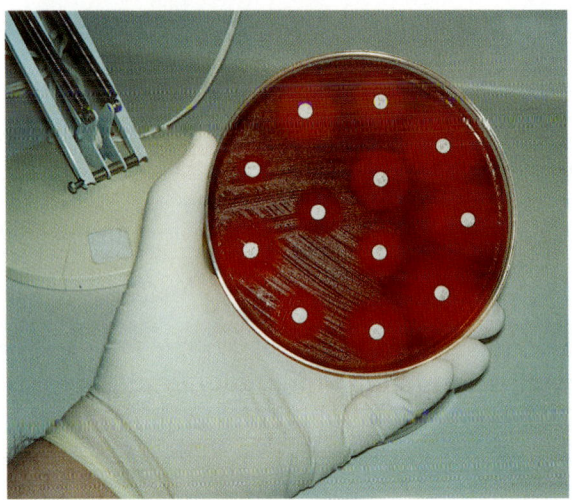

FIGURE 42-25 Zones of inhibition of bacterial growth around sensitivity disks. The greenish lines are bacterial colonies. (From Stepp CA, Woods MA: *Laboratory procedures for medical office personnel*, Philadelphia, 1998, Saunders.)

To inoculate, or **streak,** the culture medium (in an agar plate, swab, or other collection device), the specimen is passed over the medium in a zigzag pattern (Figure 42-24). After the inoculation is complete, the Petri dish is turned upside down (to discourage condensation) and placed in an incubator for 24 hours at 99° F (37° C). Sometimes, antibiotic disks are placed on the inoculated plate before incubation. With this test, the physician orders a **culture and sensitivity (C&S)** to determine the antibiotic to which the organism is most sensitive (Figure 42-25). *Culturing* is a laboratory technique that involves the growing of microorganisms on a special growth medium. The *sensitivity* test is a laboratory method that helps determine the effectiveness of many different antibiotics.

PATIENT-CENTERED PROFESSIONALISM

- *How would the medical assistant explain the function of hematology testing to a patient?*
- *How would the medical assistant explain liver and cardiac profiles to a patient?*
- *What are the advantages of point-of-care testing for the patient?*

CONCLUSION

The purpose of any laboratory testing is to aid the physician in diagnosis, treatment, or maintenance of the patient's current health status. All laboratory-testing procedures must follow established guidelines in order for the results to be considered valid. Medical assistants need to be aware of the types of CLIA-waived tests and procedures because these can be performed in physician offices. Even though these tests have a minimal risk for error, they must be performed carefully to produce results that will be helpful to the physician.

Chapter Summary

Reinforce your understanding of the material in this chapter by reviewing the curriculum objectives and key content points below.

1. **Define, appropriately use, and spell all the Key Terms for this chapter.**
   - Review the Key Terms if necessary.
2. **Explain what causes urine's color and what causes urine to have an abnormal color.**
   - Urochrome is the yellow pigment derived from urobilin in urine; it is left over when hemoglobin breaks down.
   - Fluid intake, medications, and waste products from a disease process can cause urine to have an abnormal color.
3. **Describe the normal appearance of urine, and explain what causes urine to have an abnormal appearance.**
   - Normal urine should appear clear or transparent.
   - Crystals, change of pH, blood cells, bacteria, and other substances can cause urine to have an abnormal appearance.
4. **Explain why various odors occur in urine.**
   - An ammonia smell is the result of bacteria breaking down urea in a specimen.

- Foods can also produce odor in urine.
- Odor can also be caused by bacteria, uncontrolled diabetes, and infection.

5. **List two causes of low urinary output and three causes of high urinary output.**
   - Low urinary output can be caused by low fluid intake or excessive fluid loss through diarrhea, vomiting, or sweating.
   - High urinary output can be caused by high fluid intake, reduced secretion of ADH, and uncontrolled diabetes.

6. **State two testing differences between a reagent strip and a reagent tablet.**
   - Reagent strips detect the presence and amount of substances; reagent tablets only detect the presence of substances, not the amount.
   - Reagent tablets test for only one substance; reagent strips detect the presence of one or several substances.

7. **Demonstrate the correct procedure for processing a urine specimen using a reagent technique.**
   - Review Procedure 42-1.

8. **List 10 tests performed during a routine urinalysis.**
   - Glucose, bilirubin, ketones, specific gravity, blood, pH, protein, urobilinogen, nitrites, and leukocytes are tested for during a routine urinalysis.

9. **Explain how an automated urine analyzer processes reagent test strips.**
   - The automated urine analyzer eliminates the human error factor by using light photometry to analyze a reagent test strip.

10. **List three brands of reagent tablets and their use in confirmatory tests.**
    - Clinitest reagent tablets confirm the presence of glucose.
    - Acetest tablets confirm ketones.
    - Ictotest tablets confirm bilirubin.

11. **Explain why microscopic examination of urine sediment may be done.**
    - Casts, crystals, and other solids can be identified only by microscopic examination.

12. **Demonstrate the correct procedure for microscopic examination of urine.**
    - Review Procedure 42-2.

13. **List seven types of structures typically found in urine.**
    - Red blood cells, white blood cells, epithelial cells, casts, crystals, artifacts, and other substances (e.g., bacteria, yeast, mucous threads, spermatozoa, parasites) can be found in urine.

14. **Demonstrate the correct procedure for performing a urine pregnancy color-reaction test.**
    - Review Procedure 42-3.

15. **Differentiate among hematology, serology, blood chemistry, and microbiology.**
    - Hematology is the study of blood cell–forming tissues and coagulation factors.
    - Serology is the study of antigen and antibody reactions in blood serum.
    - Blood chemistry is the complete quantitative analysis of the chemical composition of the blood.
    - Microbiology is the study of all microorganisms in the blood (bacteriology focuses on bacteria).

16. **State the purpose of a complete blood count (CBC) and list six types of information it provides.**
    - A CBC indicates the number of blood cells present in a volume of blood.
    - The CBC measures blood cell counts, hemoglobin, hematocrit, and reticulocytes; generates a differential of white blood cell types; and measures the size and shape of the cells.

17. **State the purpose of measuring hemoglobin and list one automated device approved by CLIA for this use in the physician office laboratory (POL).**
    - Hemoglobin measurement is used to detect blood loss and anemias.
    - HemoCue is an automated device approved by CLIA for use in the POL for analyzing hemoglobin.

18. **Demonstrate the correct procedure for obtaining a hemoglobin reading.**
    - Review Procedure 42-4.

19. **Explain the purpose of a hematocrit and what a low reading and a high reading may indicate.**
    - Hematocrit (Hct) is a measurement of the percentage of packed blood cells in a volume of whole blood.
    - A low Hct reading may indicate anemia; a high Hct reading could be the result of polycythemia.

20. **Demonstrate the correct procedure for obtaining an accurate hematocrit value.**
    - Review Procedure 42-5.

21. **Explain the purpose of the erythrocyte sedimentation rate (ESR) and list two common methods used in the POL to perform ESR.**
    - ESR confirms an inflammation is present somewhere in the body; it measures how quickly red blood cells settle in a tube.
    - The Westergren and Wintrobe tube methods are commonly used in the POL.

22. **Demonstrate the correct procedure for performing ESR using the Westergren method.**
    - Review Procedure 42-6.

23. **Explain the purpose of a differential blood cell count, and list five factors that affect the quality of a good blood smear.**
    - The differential blood cell count ("diff") is a test that differentiates white blood cells, observes the shape of red blood cells, and estimates the number of platelets.
    - Size of the drop of blood, angle of the pusher slide, pressure, speed, and viscosity affect the quality of the smear.

24. **Demonstrate the correct procedure for preparation of a blood smear slide.**
    - Review Procedure 42-7.

25. **Explain how physicians use blood chemistry profiles.**
    - Blood chemistry profiles give the physician information about the patient's general state of health.
    - Blood profiles can be ordered to address particular body systems.

26. **Explain the purpose of cholesterol testing and list the desirable, borderline-high, and high cholesterol levels in test results.**
    - Cholesterol is screened because high levels of blood cholesterol are related to heart disease.

- Cholesterol is also used to monitor liver and thyroid function.
- Desirable cholesterol level: less than 200 mg/dL; borderline-high level: 200 to 239 mg/dL; high level: greater than 240 mg/dL.

27. **Demonstrate the procedure for accurately collecting and processing a blood specimen for cholesterol testing.**
    - Review Procedure 42-8.

28. **Describe three tests performed to monitor a person's glucose level.**
    - A fasting blood sugar (FBS) test measures glucose level in a blood sample. The patient refrains from eating and drinking (except water) for at least 12 hours before testing. A blood sample is drawn, tested, and compared to normal range of 70 to 110 mg/dL of glucose.
    - The 2-hour postprandial test is used to screen for diabetes mellitus and to monitor the effects of a patient's insulin regimen. The patient is required to fast, then eat a meal or drink a glucose solution containing 100 g of glucose. Two hours after ingestion, a blood sample is drawn and compared to normal range.
    - Glucose tolerance test (GTT) is more sensitive to the patient's ability to metabolize glucose. The patient fasts, blood and urine specimens are collected, and the patient ingests a special glucose drink. Blood and urine specimens are collected at 30 minutes, 1 hour, 2 hours, and 3 hours to measure the amount of glucose and ketones filtered by the kidneys and to determine if the blood glucose level has returned to normal range.

29. **Demonstrate the procedure for accurately collecting and processing a blood specimen for glucose testing.**
    - Review Procedure 42-9.

30. **Define serology and list seven types of serological or immunological testing.**
    - Serology is the study of blood serum for signs of antibodies and the antigen/antibody response.
    - Refer to Box 42-3.

31. **List and describe four viewable reactions to additives that indicate positive results in serological testing.**
    - *Agglutination.* Antigen acts as a magnet and attracts antibodies to it causing "clumping."
    - *Color change.* Enzyme that causes color change in test results used to test specifically for antigen-antibody sensitivity.
    - *Precipitates.* Visible reaction between antigen and antibody producing a solid residue that settles out of liquid.
    - *Lysis.* Destruction of red blood cells caused by an antibody-antigen response.

32. **Demonstrate the procedure for correctly obtaining a bacterial smear from a wound swab.**
    - Review Procedure 42-10.

33. **Explain the purpose of a Gram stain and briefly describe the staining process.**
    - The purpose of Gram staining is to separate bacteria into two groups: gram positive and gram negative and to assist with the visualization of bacteria.
    - Review Figure 42-23.

34. **Explain why culture plates are inoculated and briefly describe the process of streaking an agar plate.**
    - Culture plates are inoculated to identify which bacteria are causing an infection or which antibiotic to use for treatment.
    - A zigzag pattern is used to inoculate the culture plate.

35. **Analyze a realistic medical office situation and apply your understanding of laboratory testing in the physician office to determine the best course of action.**
    - CLIA-waived tests permit a medical assistant to perform laboratory tests that provide the physician with immediate feedback.

36. **Describe the impact on patient care when medical assistants have a solid understanding of the purpose and procedures for laboratory tests performed in the medical office.**
    - When the medical assistant adheres to proper procedure when performing a urinalysis, valuable information is gained concerning kidney and liver function, acid-base balance, and the patient's ability to utilize carbohydrates.
    - Point-of-care testing (POCT) allows the physician to evaluate treatment.

PRACTICAL APPLICATIONS

If you have accomplished the objectives in this chapter, you will be able to make better choices as a medical assistant. Take another look at this situation and decide what you would do.

Dr. Carlson does not have a medical laboratory technician. Instead, she depends on the medical assistant to provide the test results of laboratory specimens that are ordered. Because of his training in a medical assisting program, Jerry is aware of the importance of quality control and quality assurance and that both should be done on a daily basis.

As part of the daily routine, Jerry, the medical assistant, is expected to perform physical and chemical testing of urine using reagent strips. Dr. Carlson also allows Jerry to examine specimens using a microscope to identify the urine sediment. Jerry completes hemoglobin testing using HemoCue and uses a centrifuge to spin hematocrits. As Jerry reads the hematocrit, he finds that the anticoagulated blood has separated into three layers, each of which has a specific characteristic.

Because CLIA-waived tests are often performed in a physician's office, Jerry and other medical assistants must be able to perform these tests on a daily basis. Would you be capable of performing these tasks?

1. What is meant by a "CLIA-waived" test?
2. What do reagent strips show? Are all reagent strips the same?
3. Why is it important for Jerry to wait for the designated amount of time before reading the results of a reagent strip?
4. When checking a urine specimen for physical properties, what is Jerry looking for?
5. What influences the physical properties of urine?
6. Can Jerry perform a microscopic examination of urine under CLIA standards? If not, what part of the microscopic examination can he perform?
7. What type of pregnancy tests can Jerry perform in the physician's office? What are the indications of a positive pregnancy result in each test?
8. When should a urine specimen be collected for a pregnancy test?
9. Can Jerry perform hemoglobin and hematocrit measurements? Why or why not?
10. What are the three layers found in centrifuged whole blood? How are these used to measure a microhematocrit?

WEB SEARCH

1. **Research the reliability of laboratory tests.** Investigate the criteria needed for clinical laboratory test reliability.

- **Keywords:** Use the following keywords in your search: CLIA, role of employees in laboratory testing, laboratory testing results.

43 Understanding Medications

evolve   http://evolve.elsevier.com/klieger/medicalassisting

Medications are chemicals used in the treatment, prevention, or diagnosis of disease. Patients may be given medication in the medical office, or the physician may give patients a prescription for a drug to be filled at a pharmacy. Medical assistants may be responsible for administering medication prescribed by the physician to patients during office visits.

Therefore it is important for medical assistants to understand the general types of drugs available, the regulations for administering drugs, the expected and unwanted effects of each drug administered, and the information contained in a prescription. This chapter helps you to understand these aspects of medications. Chapter 44 discusses the methods of administering medications, safety precautions, and patient education necessary to administer medications safely to all patients when prescribed.

LEARNING OBJECTIVES

You will be able to do the following after completing this chapter:

Key Terms
1. Define, appropriately use, and spell all the Key Terms for this chapter.

Pharmacology
2. Define pharmacology and differentiate between pharmacodynamics and pharmacokinetics.
3. List five reasons why drugs are prescribed by a health care professional.
4. Briefly describe the three ways drugs can be identified by name.
5. List three factors that determine the dosage prescribed by the health care practitioner for a patient.
6. Differentiate between average dose and cumulative dose and between lethal dose and toxic dose.

Drug Legislation
7. State the purpose of the Controlled Substances Act of 1970 and identify the organization established to set standards for drug products and its role in enforcement.
8. Describe the process for applying for and renewing DEA registration numbers and certificates.
9. List five rules that must be followed with controlled substances.
10. Describe the five drug schedules and list two examples of drugs from each.
11. Describe the inventory, ordering, and storage requirements for controlled substances.
12. List four drug references and explain their value for physicians and medical assistants.

Drug Administration
13. List the "seven rights" of drug administration and state the purpose of each.
14. Calculate the correct dose of a medication to be administered.
15. Convert dosage measurements to grains, grams, milligrams, pounds, and kilograms.
16. Explain how the body weight and body surface area (BSA) methods are used to determine pediatric doses.
17. Demonstrate the correct procedure for preparing an immunization record and filing it properly in the patient's record.
18. Discuss the immunization schedule for children and explain the time frame in which reactions can occur.

Drug Forms
19. List solid, liquid, and semisolid forms of drugs.

Drug Classifications
20. List five characteristics by which drugs can be classified.
21. Differentiate among side effects, adverse reactions, and toxic effects.

22. Explain what contraindications are and what the pharmacy does to alert patients to special instructions.

Prescriptions
23. List the nine pieces of information included in a prescription.
24. Explain the considerations for keeping a record of all medications a patient is taking.

Patient-Centered Professionalism
25. Analyze a realistic medical office situation and apply your understanding of medications to determine the best course of action.
26. Describe the impact on patient care when medical assistants understand the purpose and considerations for pharmacology and how medications are regulated and prescribed.

KEY TERMS

administer
adverse reactions
aerosols
average dose
booster dose
buccal tablets
caplets
capsules
contraindications
controlled substances
Controlled Substances Act
creams
cumulative dose
curative drug
DEA number
diagnostic drug
dispense
divided dose
drug
Drug Enforcement Administration (DEA)
Electronic prescribing (E-prescribing)
elixirs
emulsion
enteric-coated tablets
Food and Drug Administration (FDA)
gel caps
immunization
initial dose
inscription
layered tablets
lethal dose
liniments
local
lotions
lozenges
maintenance dose
maximum dose
minimum dose
nomogram
ointments
over-the-counter (OTC) drugs
parenteral
percutaneous
pharmacodynamics
pharmacokinetics
pharmacology
powders
prescribe
prescription
prophylactic drug
replacement drug
scored tablets
"seven rights"
side effects
sig, signature
solutes
solutions
solvent
spansules
sublingual tablets
subscription
superscription
suppositories
suspension
syrups
systemic
tablet
therapeutic drug
tinctures
topical
toxic dose
toxicity
transdermal patches
troches
unit dose
vaccine
Vaccine Information Statement (VIS)

PRACTICAL APPLICATIONS

Read the following scenario and keep it in mind as you learn about medications.

Glenn is a medical assistant in an office of a family physician. His employer, Dr. Carbello, sees patients of all ages. Because Glenn lives in a state where medical assistants are allowed to phone in prescriptions to the pharmacy, one of his regular duties is to call in prescriptions. Glenn is also responsible for performing the inventory on scheduled medications. Today, Dr. Carbello has asked Glenn to call a pharmacy with a prescription for meperidine for a patient who has a severe pain in her back.

After examining another patient, Mrs. Vouch, Dr. Carbello orders an antihistamine for itching, to be given by injection, and an antipyretic. Dr. Carbello tells Glenn to be sure that he tells Mrs. Vouch the side effects of the medications. Mrs. Vouch is also given a prescription for the antihistamine and antipyretic to take at home. The antihistamine is a capsule, and the antipyretic is a tablet. Both medications have systemic effects, and both can have indications of a toxic effect. As Mrs. Vouch leaves the office, Glenn asks her to call in the next week to tell him how the medications are helping with the itching.

If you were Glenn, would you be able to explain the side effects of the medications to Mrs. Vouch?

PHARMACOLOGY

A **drug**, or medication, is any substance that produces a physical or chemical change in the body. Drugs can be administered by mouth (oral); injected into a blood vessel (intravenous), fat (subcutaneous), muscle (intramuscular), or skin (intradermal); applied directly to the skin (**percutaneous** or **topical**); inhaled through nasal and oral passages (inhalation); or inserted into a body cavity (suppository).

Pharmacology is the study of drugs and how they affect the body. This includes drug sources, properties, and uses of a drug. Pharmacology may be further divided into the following areas of study:

- **Pharmacodynamics** is the study of the biochemical and the physiological effects of a drug within the body.
- **Pharmacokinetics** is the study of what happens to a drug from the time it enters the body until it leaves. This involves following a drug's absorption rate, the time it takes for the drug to act, and how the drug is distributed through and excreted from the body (Figure 43-1). Pharmacokinetics studies drug concentration in tissues over time.

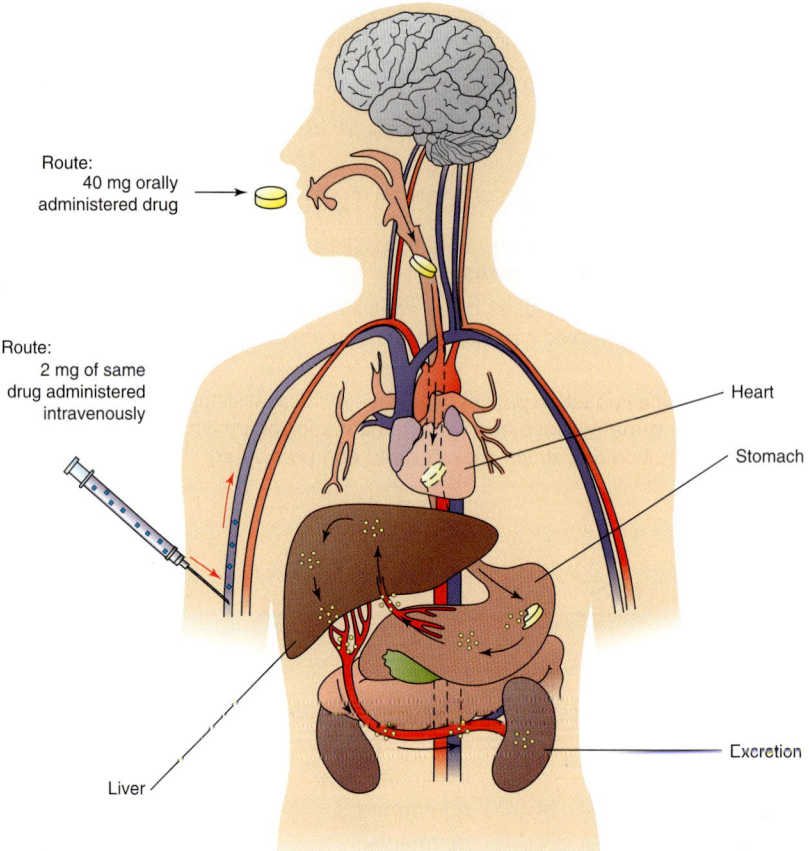

FIGURE 43-1 Pharmacokinetics studies what happens to a drug from the time it enters the body until it leaves. (Modified from Lilley L et al: *Pharmacology and the nursing process*, ed 4, St Louis, 2005, Mosby.)

Drugs are prescribed by a health care professional for their medical purposes, as follows:

- **Curative drug:** To heal disease or cure infection. For example, an antiinfective is a curative drug that can destroy or alter the cell metabolism of a disease-producing organism.
- **Diagnostic drug:** To assist with diagnosing disease during a procedure. For example, a radiopaque dye is a diagnostic drug injected to better view the function of the renal system during the radiograph of the kidney, ureter, and bladder (KUB).
- **Prophylactic drug:** To lessen or prevent the effects of a disease. For example, vaccines are prophylactic drugs used to prevent communicable diseases.
- **Replacement drug:** To replace substances normally found in the body. For example, replacement drugs are prescribed for hormone replacement therapy after menopause.
- **Therapeutic drug:** To restore the body to its presymptom state. For example, therapeutic medication for hypertension is used to lower blood pressure to a safe range. Therapeutic drugs are also used to treat symptoms (palliative); for example, medications for pain.

Drug Names

Most drugs can be identified in the following three ways (Figure 43-2):

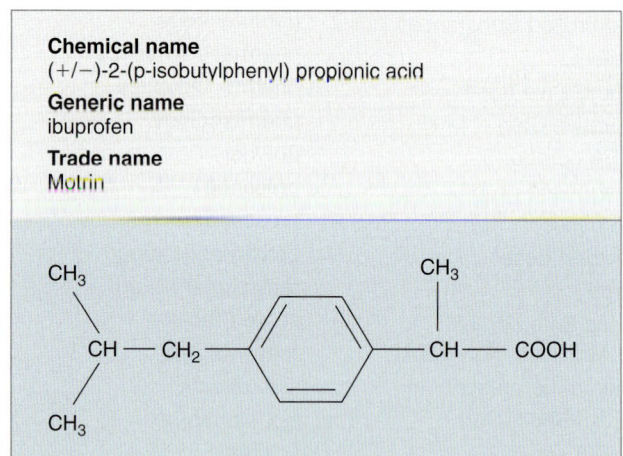

FIGURE 43-2 Chemical, generic, and trade names for the common analgesic ibuprofen are listed next to the chemical structure of the drug. (Modified from Lilley L et al: *Pharmacology and the nursing process*, ed 4, St Louis, 2005, Mosby.)

- *Chemical name:* The chemical name reflects the chemical composition or formula of the drug.
- *Generic name:* The generic name (*nonproprietary*) of a drug is its official (or legal) name and indicates its chemical structure or makeup. Generic names are given by the United States Adopted Name Council (USAN), and the official name is always written in lowercase letters. It

BOX 43-1

Factors Affecting Drug Actions

DIET
- Food may delay the absorption rate of medications and may be needed for the absorption of others.
- Alternative medications (e.g., herbs) and over-the-counter medications can alter the desired drug action.
- Certain foods may prevent the absorption of some medications, such as milk with tetracycline.

ENVIRONMENT
- Exposure to heat or cold. For example, patients living in warm weather normally would require lower doses of a vasodilator than those in colder climates.

PSYCHOLOGICAL
- Stress or high incidence of pain may require larger doses of an analgesic to increase the action of the prescribed medication.
- Different levels of depression will require adjusted amounts of medication for the patient to receive the expected action of the medication.

PHYSIOLOGICAL
- *Age:* Infants, young children, and elderly patients require different dosages to achieve the desired action.
- *Gender:* Women are normally prescribed lower maximum doses than men because women have less muscle mass and hormonal differences affect drug metabolism.
- *Body weight:* Drug's effect is determined by the relationship between the amount of medication prescribed and the patient's weight.
- *Disease status:* Decreased function of the organ responsible for breaking down the medication can influence the drug's action.

TABLE 43-1

Sources of Drugs

Source	Active Ingredient Example	Drug Example	Purpose
Plant	Belladonna	Atropine	Antispasmodic
Animal	Pancreas	Insulin	Hypoglycemic
Mineral	Calcium carbonate	Tums	Antacid
Synthetic	Mixing of chemical substances	Aspirin	Analgesic
Bioengineering	DNA technology	Humalog (insulin)	Hypoglycemic

is the generic name that is listed in official publications of standardized drugs (e.g., *United States Pharmacopeia*).

- *Trade name:* A trade name *(proprietary)*, or brand name, is the name used to market the drug by the pharmaceutical manufacturer and displays the symbol ®. A patent protects the rights of the original company that developed and marketed the drug for 17 years. The first letter of a trade name is capitalized, or the entire name may be written in all-capital letters (see Figure 43-8).

To prevent errors, the medical assistant must obtain the exact name and correct spelling of all ordered medications.

Drug Sources

The first attempts to treat disease in ancient times involved the use of herbs as medicine. Even today the healing properties of natural substances are accepted. Many of today's medications are derived from plant, animal, and mineral sources (Table 43-1). Synthetic and bioengineered (created with DNA) medications are also made in the laboratory. Modern technology has enabled many of these synthetic and bioengineered medications to be derived by converting natural sources to synthetic compounds (e.g., mold to penicillin).

Many physicians and researchers believe these synthetic compounds are far superior to the original sources because exact amounts can be calculated.

Drug Actions

Drugs work by combining with various parts of the cell either to block an action or to create a response.

> **EXAMPLE OF DRUG ACTION IN ANALGESICS**
> Analgesics are pain-killing drugs. Different analgesics cause different types of actions in the body. Some analgesics ease pain in or near the area of an injury and can also reduce inflammation. Other analgesics block pain signals from nerve endings to the brain. Analgesics can also reduce the electrical activity of neurons, thus reducing sensation to the affected area.
>
> To be effective or therapeutic, the medication must reach its intended site and have only a minimal effect on other tissues. Sometimes a drug produces a side effect or adverse reaction other than its intended purpose. Several factors influence how a drug reacts to a specific individual (Box 43-1). Age and weight are obvious considerations, but body surface area, allergies, tolerance, and interactions with other medications are other key factors.

Drug Dosage

The amount of drug prescribed by the health care practitioner is based on several factors, including age, weight, and gender (Box 43-2). The recommended adult dose is based on an age range between 20 and 60 years. Pediatric patients require smaller amounts based on their reduced kidney function, metabolism, and gastrointestinal (GI) motility. Weight is usually the determining factor. Geriatric patients also have a decrease in kidney, GI, and metabolic functions, but older patients may also have a disease process that could interfere with the absorption rate of the medication (Figure 43-3).

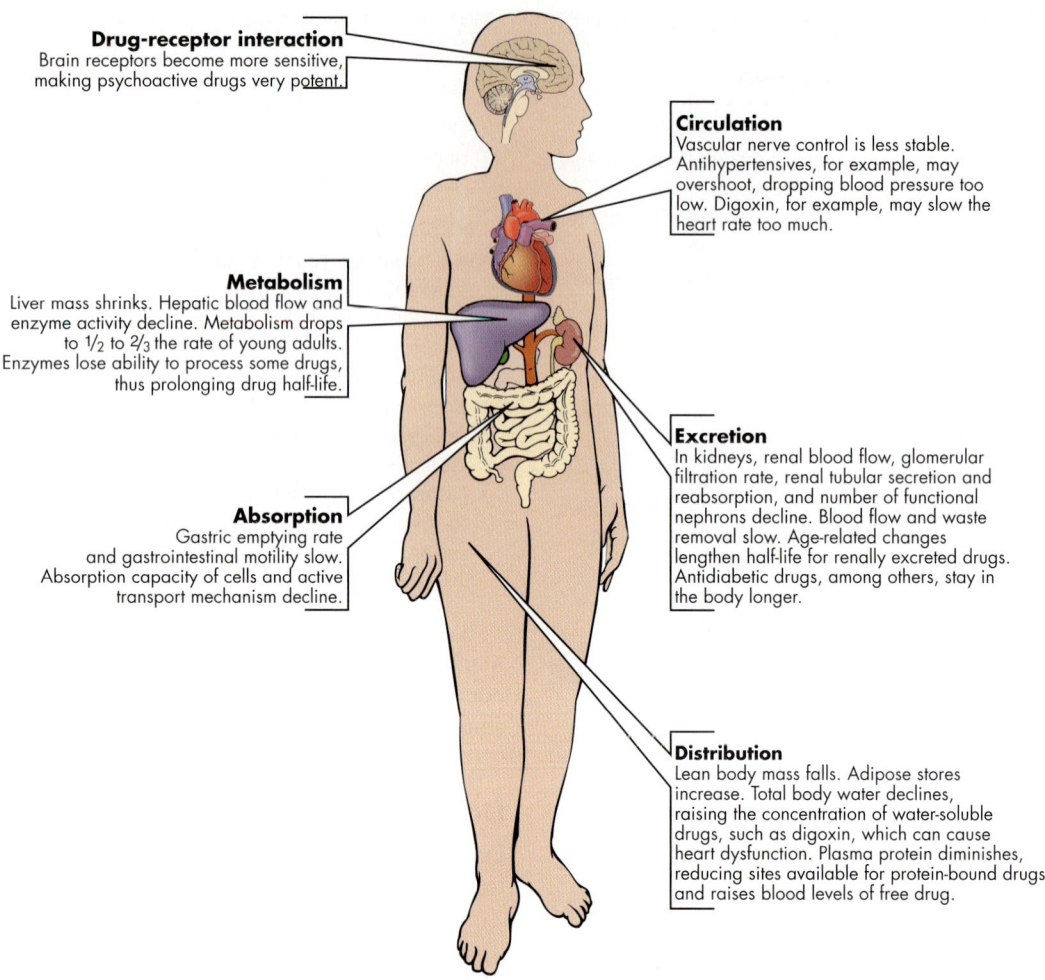

FIGURE 43-3 Effects of aging on drug metabolism. (From Lewis SM et al: *Medical-surgical nursing*, ed 6, St Louis, 2004, Mosby.)

BOX 43-2

Factors Affecting Amount of Drug Prescribed and Effectiveness

- *Weight and height* (body surface area) influence drug amount ordered and its effectiveness.
- *Age* involves consideration of the developmental conditions of the body's organs and tissues.
- *Gender* must be considered because of the difference in fat tissue, hormone balance, and other areas.
- *Electrolyte balance.* Knowing ratios is important because a drug may deplete existing electrolytes (e.g., diuretics can cause potassium imbalance). Replacement must occur with foods or supplements.
- *Disease processes.* Because the kidneys and liver are major areas for the excretion of drugs, these two systems must be able to break down and excrete the byproducts of drugs. Also, the cardiovascular system must be working properly to distribute the medication.
- *Tolerance* by the body tissue is important because some medications are given for long-term effects and the effects decrease over time.

As a medical assistant, you need to understand the meaning of important terms used to explain a drug dosage (Box 43-3).

PATIENT-CENTERED PROFESSIONALISM

- *Why is it important for medical assistants to be knowledgeable about the medications used in the office setting?*
- *What patient activities does the medical assistant perform that indirectly or directly relate to medications prescribed by the physician?*

DRUG LEGISLATION

The function of drug regulation (through legislation) is to protect the health and safety of the general public (Box 43-4). Table 43-2 follows the path of legislation beginning in 1906, when the Pure Food and Drug Act stated that only drugs listed in the *United States Pharmacopeia* and the *National Formulary (USP/NF)* could be prescribed and sold. Drug legislation was

BOX 43-3

Drug Dosage Terminology

- **Average dose:** Amount of medication proven to be effective with minimal side effects for an adult.
- **Cumulative dose:** Total amount of medication in the body after repeated doses or medication that accumulates in the body over time. Some medications must be taken for a time before the desired effect is reached, and others may have a toxic effect as the cumulative effect of a drug increases.
- **Divided dose:** Type of dosage when a total amount of medication is administered in separate doses.
- **Initial dose:** First dose of the medication administered.
- **Lethal dose:** Amount of medication that proves deadly to a patient.
- **Maintenance dose:** Amount of medication needed by the body to maintain its desired effect.
- **Maximum dose:** Largest amount of a medication that can be safely given to a patient at one time without causing adverse effects.
- **Minimum dose:** Smallest amount of medication that can be prescribed to be effective in treatment.
- **Toxic dose:** Amount of a medication that brings about signs and symptoms of toxicity or harmful side effects.
- **Unit dose:** Premeasured amount of medication individually packaged, usually in a single dose.

initiated to address issues on the clinical use of drugs and prevention of drug abuse. In 1938 the burden of proof shifted to the drug manufacturers by requiring that they provide documentation to prove a drug's safety. In 1970 the Controlled Substances Act was passed to control the use of dangerous drugs, tranquilizers, and stimulants.

By preventing the marketing of impure drugs, eliminating the practice of false labeling, and stopping the sale of worthless or dangerous drugs, the goals of legislative involvement are being met.

The **Food and Drug Administration (FDA)** was organized to set standards for the purity, strength, and composition

BOX 43-4

Drug Regulation Terminology

- **FDA:** Food and Drug Administration; tests and approves food, drug, and cosmetic products for the market.
- **DEA:** Drug Enforcement Administration; regulates the sale and use of controlled drugs.
- **Prescribe:** To indicate, by either written or verbal order, a medication to be given to the patient.
- **Dispense:** To deliver a medication into a patient's possession after it has been prepared.
- **Administer:** To give a medication to a patient.

TABLE 43-2

Federal Drug Legislation Addressing Clinical Use and Drug Abuse

Year	Federal Legislation	Purpose	Concerns
1906	Pure Food and Drug Act	Established written source for approved drugs: *U.S. Pharmacopeia* (USP) and *National Formulary* (NF). Began federal legislation to protect foods and drugs by requiring national standards for formula, strength, purity, and quality. Required preparations containing "dangerous" drugs be identified on the label.	Clinical use of drugs
1914	Harrison Narcotic Act	Established narcotic control for medications. Labeled habit-forming drugs as "narcotics." Established regulations for import, manufacture, sale, and use of opium, codeine, and related compounds. Later replaced by Controlled Substances Act of 1970.	Drug abuse prevention
1938	Federal Food, Drug, and Cosmetic Act (Revised)	Required Food and Drug Administration (FDA) review of drugs to determine safety by test results on toxicity. Required labeling of all drug contents. Required "habit forming" statement on container of drug.	Use of drugs
1951	Durham-Humphrey Amendment	Recognized over-the-counter drugs. Established procedures for prescription orders and refills. Required licensure to distribute or dispense medications. Required warning labels to identify potential for drowsiness, being a habit-forming drug, etc.	Drug abuse prevention
1962	Kefauver-Harris Amendment	Required registration and inspection of drug companies. Required truth in advertising. Required proof of drug safety before being approved by FDA for use.	Truth in advertising and drug safety
1970	Comprehensive Abuse Prevention and Control Act (Controlled Substances Act)	Identified five classes of habit-forming drugs and dropped the term "narcotic." Required detailed records of dispensing and established inventory requirements. Established the Drug Enforcement Administration (DEA) to enforce requirements of act. Required each prescriber, dispenser, or drug manufacturer to register with DEA.	Drug abuse prevention
1983	Orphan Drug Act	Provides incentives to drug manufacturers to produce medications for diseases involving only small populations.	Clinical use of drugs

of all food, cosmetic, and drug products, including prescription and **over-the-counter (OTC) drugs** (nonprescription drugs), during the manufacturing process. Using these standards, the FDA determines if a drug will be available with or without a prescription. By requiring a prescription, the FDA is saying that the patient must be monitored while taking the medication. A drug authorized by the FDA to be sold over the counter is considered safe and effective without the patient being monitored by a physician. The FDA requires that all health care practitioners who prescribe, dispense, or administer medications follow both state and federal laws. The FDA also has the authority to remove a drug from the market if it is found to produce effects that were not anticipated.

Controlled Substances Act of 1970

The purpose of the **Controlled Substances Act** of 1970 is to control the manufacture, free offering, and selling of drugs that have a potential for abuse. This legislation provides regulations for prescribing, refilling, dispensing, and use of these drugs.

The **Drug Enforcement Administration (DEA)** is the federal agency responsible for enforcing this act. All medical personnel who prescribe, administer, or dispense a controlled substance must register with the DEA. Form DEA-224 is used to apply for a **DEA number**. The DEA number must be written on any prescription for **controlled substances** (Figure 43-4). Controlled substances include opioid analgesics, stimulants, and depressants. The practitioner will receive a DEA registration number and a Controlled Substance Registration Certificate for a particular site. Each is valid for 3 years. If a physician has two offices, each site must have its own DEA number to dispense controlled substances. To renew, Form DEA-224a is completed and returned 60 days before the expiration date. It is the physician's responsibility to know when the renewal is due. Using a tickler file to remind the physician of the due date for the DEA renewal is an effective way to avoid lapse in coverage.

Box 43-5 outlines federal rules that must be followed when working with controlled substances. As a medical assistant, you need to become familiar with the regulations that apply to your state as well.

Drug Schedules

Drugs that have the potential for abuse and addiction included in the Controlled Substances Act of 1970 are classified into five groups, known as *schedules*. Within each schedule, regulations for drug use and rules for prescribing, refilling, and dispensing are listed (Table 43-3). Note that each schedule is indicated by the use of a Roman numeral, as follows:

- *Schedule I* drugs have no accepted medical use.
- *Schedule II* drugs have a use, but severe restrictions apply.
- *Schedule III* drugs do not have to be ordered on a special form, but records must be kept.
- *Schedule IV* and *Schedule V* drugs have a lower potential for abuse but could lead to dependency.

BOX 43-5

Rules for Dealing with Controlled Substances

1. Records concerning the dispensing and administration of controlled drugs must be kept for a minimum of 2 years.
2. A progress note must be in the patient's medical record concerning the dispensing or administration of controlled drugs, with a copy of the written prescription or order when administering.
3. A complete written inventory must be done every 2 years for all controlled drugs, and records must be kept for an additional 2 years.
4. Controlled drugs must be kept in a locked cabinet, separate from other drugs (e.g., samples).
5. Theft of controlled drugs must be reported to the local authorities and to the DEA. If an opioid analgesic is accidentally broken or spilled, its disposal must be witnessed by two people and logged in the controlled substance logbook.

The forms and reports required for each reportable incident will vary. The medical office staff must be familiar with what is required in their state of practice.

All controlled substance drug labels must clearly show the drug's assigned schedule. This is indicated by a capital "C" and the schedule number (Figure 43-5).

Inventory

If a medical facility stocks controlled substances, an initial inventory must be done to record the controlled substances on hand. If no controlled substances are kept at the site, a "zero" inventory is recorded. Thereafter, an inventory of all controlled substances must be conducted every 2 years.

It is best to log the administration of controlled substances each time one is given. This makes it easier to account for all inventoried drugs and to detect theft.

FOR YOUR INFORMATION

IMPORTANT INVENTORY NOTE

It is important that Schedule II drug inventories be kept separate from those of Schedule III, IV, or V. Schedule II inventories must include an exact count, whereas Schedules III, IV, and V inventories may use an estimated count or measure of the contents (unless the container holds more than 1000 tablets or capsules, in which case an exact count must be made).

Order Forms

For the physician to order Schedule II drugs, a DEA-222 (federal triplicate order form) is used. Other scheduled drugs (e.g., Schedule III, IV, and V drugs) do not require a triplicate order form. Instead, a logbook containing the invoice number from the drug supplier must be maintained for 2 years and kept another 2 years.

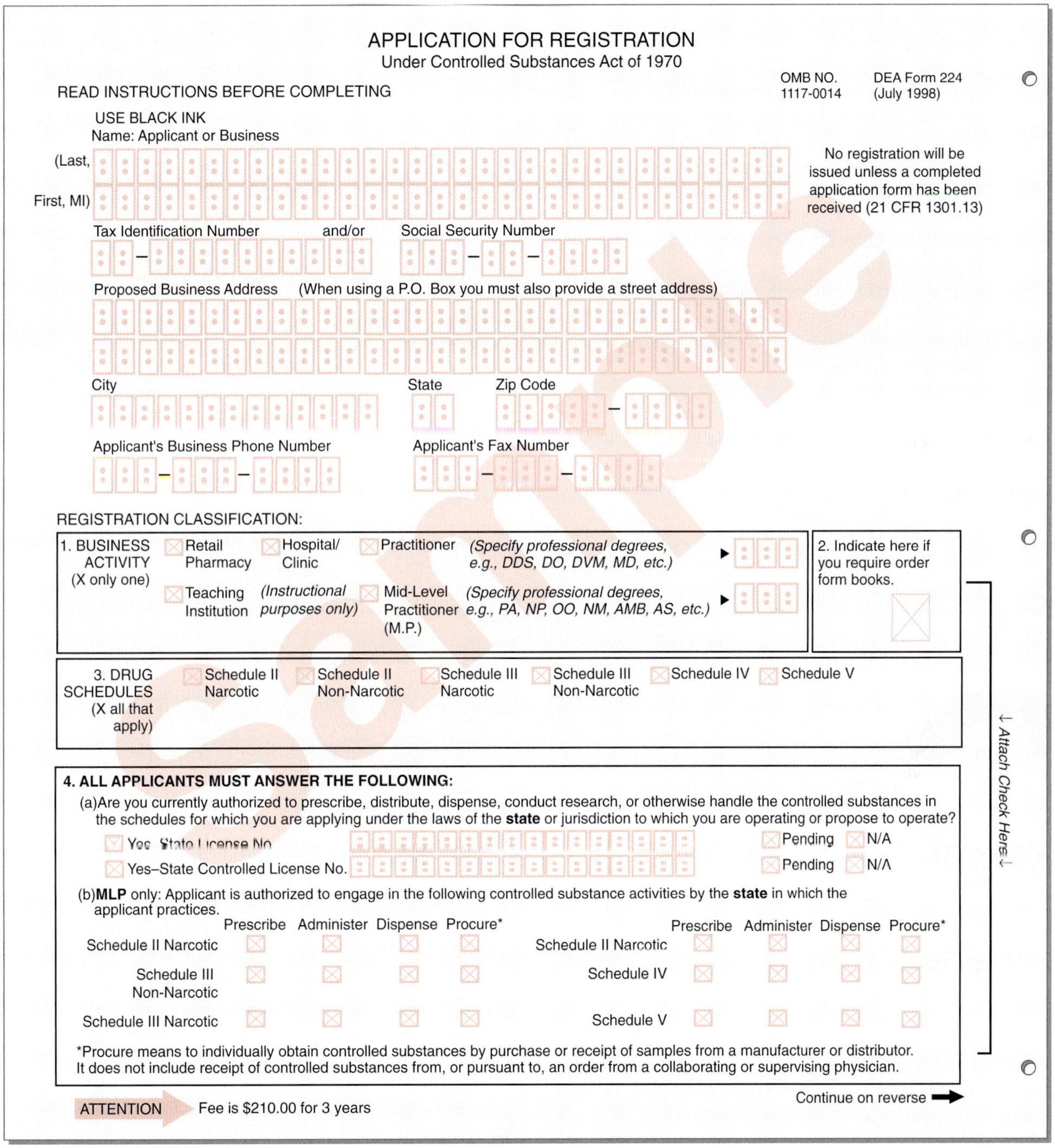

APPLICATION FOR REGISTRATION
Under Controlled Substances Act of 1970

READ INSTRUCTIONS BEFORE COMPLETING

OMB NO. 1117-0014 DEA Form 224 (July 1998)

USE BLACK INK

Name: Applicant or Business (Last, First, MI)

No registration will be issued unless a completed application form has been received (21 CFR 1301.13)

Tax Identification Number and/or Social Security Number

Proposed Business Address (When using a P.O. Box you must also provide a street address)

City State Zip Code

Applicant's Business Phone Number Applicant's Fax Number

REGISTRATION CLASSIFICATION:

1. BUSINESS ACTIVITY (X only one)
Retail Pharmacy
Hospital/ Clinic
Practitioner *(Specify professional degrees, e.g., DDS, DO, DVM, MD, etc.)*
Teaching Institution *(Instructional purposes only)*
Mid-Level Practitioner (M.P.) *(Specify professional degrees, e.g., PA, NP, OO, NM, AMB, AS, etc.)*

2. Indicate here if you require order form books.

3. DRUG SCHEDULES (X all that apply)
Schedule II Narcotic
Schedule II Non-Narcotic
Schedule III Narcotic
Schedule III Non-Narcotic
Schedule IV
Schedule V

4. ALL APPLICANTS MUST ANSWER THE FOLLOWING:

(a)Are you currently authorized to prescribe, distribute, dispense, conduct research, or otherwise handle the controlled substances in the schedules for which you are applying under the laws of the **state** or jurisdiction to which you are operating or propose to operate?

Yes–State License No. Pending N/A

Yes–State Controlled License No. Pending N/A

(b)**MLP** only: Applicant is authorized to engage in the following controlled substance activities by the **state** in which the applicant practices.

	Prescribe	Administer	Dispense	Procure*
Schedule II Narcotic				
Schedule III Non-Narcotic				
Schedule III Narcotic				
Schedule II Narcotic				
Schedule IV				
Schedule V				

*Procure means to individually obtain controlled substances by purchase or receipt of samples from a manufacturer or distributor. It does not include receipt of controlled substances from, or pursuant to, an order from a collaborating or supervising physician.

Attach Check Here

ATTENTION Fee is $210.00 for 3 years

Continue on reverse

FIGURE 43-4 Form DEA-224: Application for registration under the Controlled Substances Act of 1970. (Courtesy Drug Enforcement Administration, U.S. Department of Justice, Washington, DC.)

TABLE 43-3

Schedules of Controlled Substances

Schedule	Information	Examples
I	Abuse potential: High Medical use: Limited primarily to research with permission. Dependence: Severe	LSD, heroin, marijuana, mescaline, PCP, Ecstasy, Quaalude.
II	Abuse potential: High Dependence: High **NOTE:** Written prescription and physician must sign; no stamps. No refills. In emergency, phone order but written prescription to pharmacy within 7 days. If physician wants to administer in medical office, Form 222 is required for ordering medication from supplier, who sends a copy to DEA.	Methadone, meperidine, morphine, fentanyl, cocaine, codeine, amphetamines, methylphenidate (Ritalin), hydromorphone, hydrocodone, secobarbital, glutethimide, anabolic steroids.
III	Abuse potential: Moderate (less than I or II) (Opioid analgesics in combination with other nonopioid analgesic drugs or steroids with potential for abuse) Dependence: Low **NOTE:** Prescription by physician only, either written (to include faxed) or phone order accepted. Refillable up to five times in 6 months. Rx expires 6 months from issue date.	Barbiturate combinations, codeine preparations, testosterone.
IV	Abuse potential: Less than III Dependence: Low **NOTE:** Prescription can be written by health care professional but must be signed by physician. Also may be called in by health care professional after being ordered by physician. Refillable up to five times in 6 months. Rx expires 6 months from issue date.	Diazepam (Valium), chlordiazepoxide (Librium), alprazolam (Xanax), propoxyphene, phenobarbital, chloral hydrate, meprobamate.
V	Abuse potential: Less than IV Dependence: Limited **NOTE:** State statutes vary on prescription and dispensing guidelines. Rx expires 1 year from issue date.	Cough syrups with codeine, diphenoxylate and atropine (Lomotil), preparations containing paregoric.

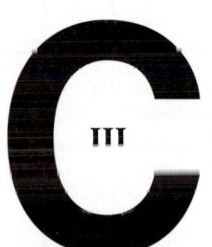

The large "C" indicates a controlled substance and the Roman numeral represents a schedule III (three) drug.

FIGURE 43-5 Controlled substance label.

Storage Requirements

Controlled substances must be kept separate from other drugs and must be kept in a locked cabinet. If theft occurs, Form DEA-116 must be completed and a police report filed. If a controlled substance must be discarded, the following rules apply:

- Discarding of a controlled substance must be witnessed by another individual (e.g., if only 25 mg of Demerol is needed and the prefilled syringe contains 50 mg, then 25 mg must be disposed of in front of a witness).
- Controlled substances can be sent to an appropriate state agency for destruction (when instructed to do so).
- A DEA agent may need to come to the facility and witness destruction.

Drug References

A *drug reference* is a publication listing drugs and information about each drug, or it can be an individual document about a specific drug (Figure 43-6). Pharmacists, physicians, and other health care professionals use drug references when prescribing medications. Four important drug references are the *USP/NF*, *Drug Facts and Comparisons* (both often used by registered pharmacists), package inserts, and the *Physicians' Desk Reference (PDR)*.

United States Pharmacopeia and National Formulary

The Federal Food, Drug, and Cosmetic Act recognizes a drug as official when it is listed in the *United States Pharmacopeia* and the *National Formulary* (USP/NF). This reference is published every 5 years by the Council on Pharmacology of the American Medical Association and only includes drugs that have been tested and certified as having met established standards of purity, quality, and potency. The NF supplies the formula for the medication.

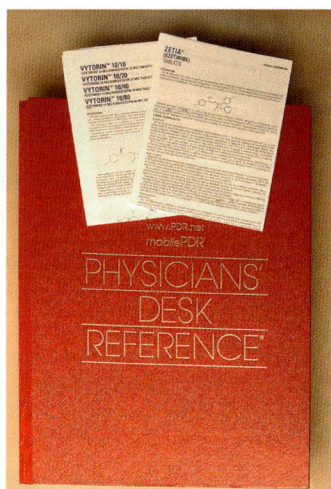

FIGURE 43-6 Reference materials: Package inserts and *Physicians' Desk Reference* (PDR).

Package Inserts

Package inserts are included with all prescription drugs sent to a pharmacy and included with samples distributed to the medical office. Information includes detailed specifics about the medication, such as chemical description, indications, precautions, recommended dosages, and adverse reactions. Inserts provide physicians and other health care professionals with a quick reference guide.

Physicians' Desk Reference

The PDR is published annually in conjunction with the pharmaceutical companies whose products are represented. During the year, supplements are created to keep the publication current. Most physicians use this publication as their source reference when needing information before prescribing medications. When using the PDR, it is important to understand how the book is organized. The PDR is divided into the following sections:

- *Section 1:* Manufacturer's Index (white pages). This index includes all participating drug companies, with full address, phone number, and emergency contact. Product names are listed with the page number.
- *Section 2:* Brand and Generic Name Index (pink pages). This index provides both generic and brand name products by page number.
- *Section 3:* Product Category Index (blue pages). This index lists categories with examples of product names.
- *Section 4:* Product Identification Guide (gray pages). This guide provides photos of various drug forms and products. The photos are arranged alphabetically by manufacturer.
- *Section 5:* Product Information (white pages). This is the main section of the book; each product is listed alphabetically within each manufacturer's section.
- *Section 6:* Diagnostic Product Information (white pages). This section provides usage guidelines for common diagnostic agents.

Figure 43-7 illustrates information and guidelines for using the PDR. The lists and indexes in the PDR make it easy for the medical assistant to identify a medication in several ways. If a patient brings in medication without a label on the container, the product identification section can be used for identifying trade name drugs. Knowing the brand or generic name of a drug allows a health care professional to locate information about the product easily.

Other information in the PDR includes the following:
- Key to Controlled Substance Categories
- Key to FDA use-in-pregnancy ratings
- Poison Control Centers
- FDA information, telephone numbers
- Vaccine Adverse Event Report Form
- Adverse Event Report Form (Med Watch)

The PDR is also available in an electronic version that can be accessed online or downloaded to a mobile computer.

PATIENT-CENTERED PROFESSIONALISM

- Why is it necessary for the medical assistant to understand the history behind legislative drug control?
- What was the main purpose of the Controlled Substances Act?
- Why must the medical assistant be knowledgeable about drug schedules, storage, and inventory methods in the medical setting?

DRUG ADMINISTRATION

Medications can be administered (given) in several ways (Table 43-4). The easiest and safest way is by mouth (PO). Medication can also be inserted into a cavity (e.g., rectal and vaginal suppositories), inhaled, placed directly on the skin (topical), or instilled, rubbed in, or injected into a blood vessel (intravenous [IV]), muscle (intramuscular [IM]), sterile cavity (e.g., knee), and under the skin (intradermal [ID]).

Drugs and immunizations must be administered correctly and at the correct dosage.

"Seven Rights" of Drug Administration

Medication errors can be avoided by following the **"seven rights"** of drug administration.

1. Right Patient

Errors in dispensing medications can occur when the patient is unfamiliar to the medical assistant. When patients have a decreased ability to identify themselves (e.g., non–English-speaking, pediatric, or confused patients), be absolutely certain the right person is receiving the medication. Use extra caution when two patients have similar names.

2. Right Drug

Many drug names are very similar. Therefore it is important to check the spelling and amount ordered carefully before

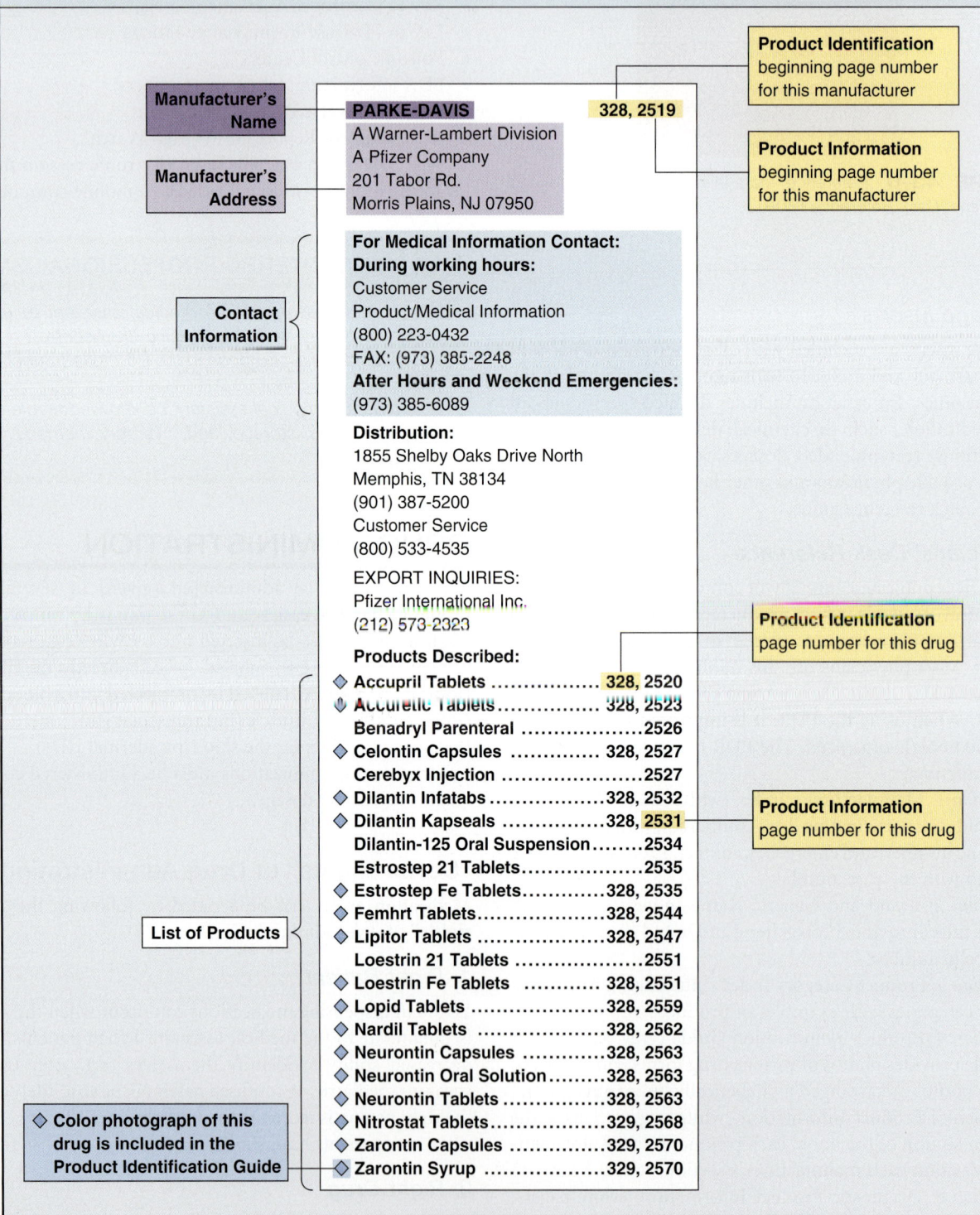

FIGURE 43-7 Guidelines for using the *Physicians' Desk Reference*. (From Bonewit-West K: *Clinical procedures for medical assistants,* ed 7, St Louis, 2008, Saunders.)

SECTION 4: PRODUCT IDENTIFICATION GUIDE
(Color Code: Gray)

This section provides a full-color (actual size) photograph of the tablets and capsules included in the PDR. The drugs are arranged alphabetically by manufacturer. A variety of other dosage forms are also illustrated, but are shown in less than actual size (e.g., inhalers, injectable drugs in vials). This section provides valuable assistance in identifying a drug.

SECTION 5: PRODUCT INFORMATION
(Color Code: White)

This index makes up the main section of the PDR and contains product information on approximately 3,000 drug products. The drugs are arranged alphabetically by manufacturer; under the manufacturer, the drugs are listed alphabetically by brand name. The information included in this section consists of the actual drug package inserts. The following information is included for each medication:

DESCRIPTION: This category consists of a general description of the drug and includes the following information: brand name (with pronunciation), generic name, drug category, dosage form (e.g., tablets, capsules), route of administration, chemical name and structural formula, and the inactive ingredients contained in the drug. This category also indicates if the product requires a prescription (Rx) or if it is available over-the-counter (OTC). The symbol C and a Roman numeral appearing next to the drug indicates that it is a scheduled drug and that a prescription written for this drug requires the physician's DEA number.

CLINICAL PHARMACOLOGY: This category describes how the drug functions in the body to produce its therapeutic effect. Also included is an analysis of the absorption, distribution, metabolism, and excretion of the drug after it enters the body.

INDICATIONS AND USAGE: This category presents a list of the conditions that the drug has been formally approved to treat by the Food and Drug Administration (FDA).

CONTRAINDICATIONS: This category includes situations in which the drug should not be used because the risk of using the drug in these situations outweighs any possible benefit. Contraindications include administration of the drug to patients known to have a hypersensitivity (allergy) to it and use of the drug in patients who have a substantial risk of being harmed by it because of their particular age, sex, concurrent use of another drug, disease state, or condition (e.g., pregnancy).

WARNINGS: This category describes serious adverse reactions and potential safety hazards that may occasionally occur with the use of the drug and what should be done if they occur.

PRECAUTIONS: This category includes information regarding any special care that needs to be taken by the physician for the safe and effective use of the drug. Information typically presented in this category includes:

- **General Precautions:** Lists any disease states or situations that may require special consideration when the drug is being taken.
- **Information for Patients:** Includes information that should be relayed to the patient to ensure safe and effective use of the drug.
- **Laboratory Tests:** Indicates the laboratory tests that may be helpful in following the patient's response to the drug or in identifying possible adverse reactions to the drug.
- **Drug Interactions:** Lists any known interactions of this drug with other drugs that can affect the proper functioning of the drug.
- **Laboratory Test Interactions:** Includes any laboratory tests that may be affected when taking the medication.
- **Pregnancy:** Indicates the pregnancy category of the drug.

ADVERSE REACTIONS: This category describes the unintended and undesirable effects that may occur with the use of the drug. Some adverse reactions are harmless and therefore are often tolerated by the patient in order to obtain the therapeutic effect of the drug. Other adverse reactions may be harmful to the patient and warrant discontinuing the medication.

OVERDOSAGE: This category describes symptoms associated with an overdosage of the drug as well as the complications that can occur and the treatment to institute for an overdosage.

DOSAGE AND ADMINISTRATION: This category lists the recommended adult dosage, the usual dosage range of the drug, and the route of administration (e.g., by mouth, sublingual, IM). Also included is information about the intervals recommended between doses, the usual duration of treatment, and any modification of dosage needed for special groups such as children, the elderly, and patients with renal or hepatic disease.

HOW SUPPLIED: This category indicates the dosage forms that are available (e.g., 20-mg tablets), the units in which the dosage form is available (e.g., bottles of 100; 5-ml multiple-dose vial), information to help identify the dosage form (shape and color), and the handling and storage conditions for the drug.

SECTION 6: DIAGNOSTIC PRODUCT INFORMATION

This section includes product information on diagnostic products. They are listed alphabetically by manufacturer and provide information on the use of these products. An example of diagnostic product included in this section is Tubersol, which is used to perform tuberculin testing.

Additional information included in the Physicians' Desk Reference is listed below:

- FDA Drug Information Centers
- Key to Controlled Substances Categories
- Key to FDA Use-In-Pregnancy Ratings

FIGURE 43-7, cont'd

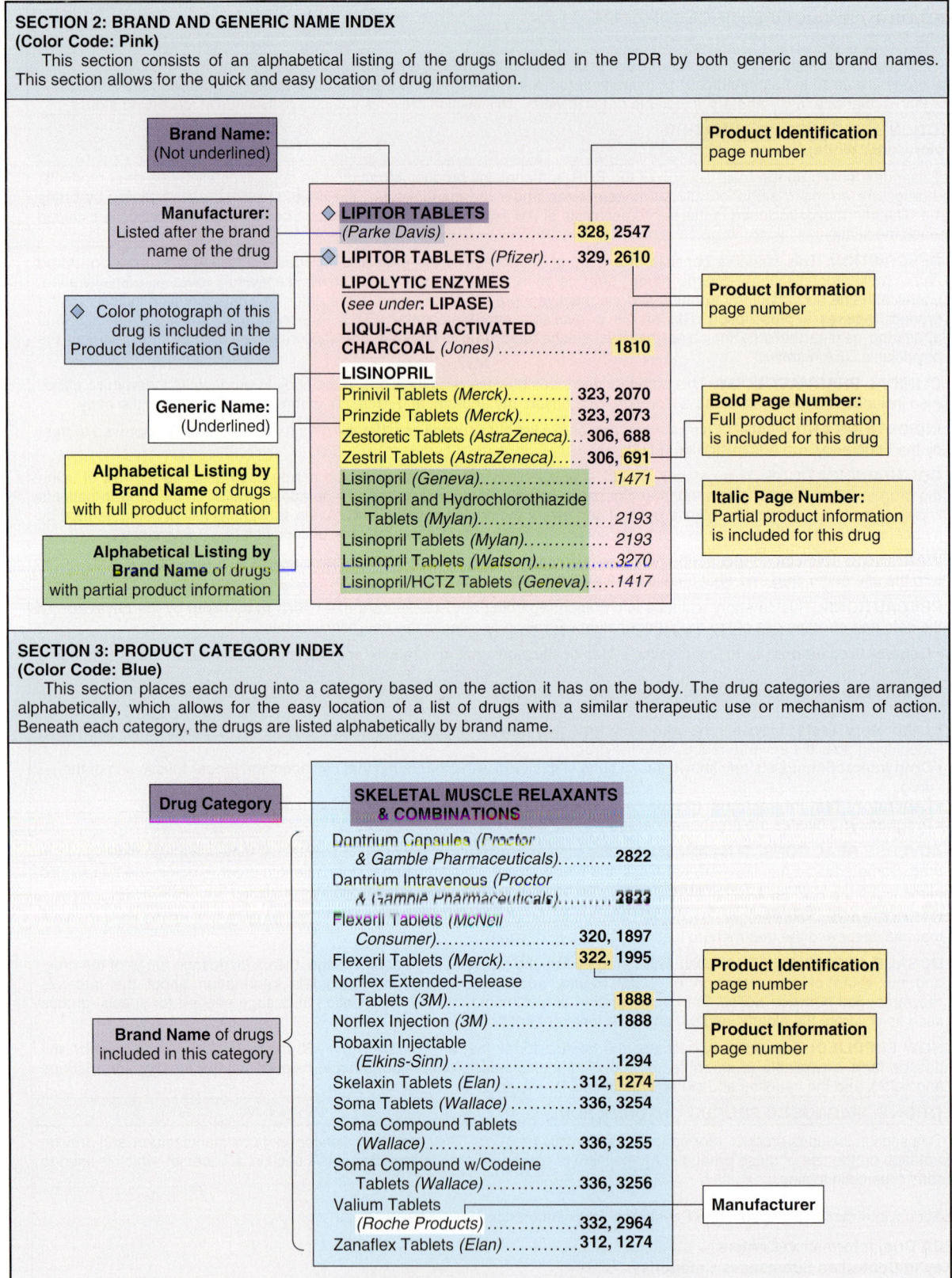

FIGURE 43-7, cont'd

TABLE 43-4
Methods of Drug Administration

Method	Form	Example	Procedure
Oral	Tablet capsule, liquids, caplets, spansules	Aspirin, Contac	Taken by mouth and swallowed.
Sublingual	Tablet, liquid, aerosol spray	Nitroglycerin	Placed under tongue.
Buccal	Tablet	Nitrogard, Tramadol	Placed between cheek and gum.
Rectal	Suppository	Anusol	Inserted into rectum for local effects, or if patient cannot take oral medications.
Intradermal	Sterile liquid	Allergy testing, TB testing, PPD	Small amount of medication injected under skin to test for reaction.
Subcutaneous (SubQ)	Sterile liquid	Insulin	Medication injected into subcutaneous tissue.
Intramuscular (IM)	Sterile liquid	Analgesics, antibiotics	Medication injected into muscle.
Topical	Liquid, semisolid, transdermal	Lotions, ointments	Applied to area directly and absorbed into skin.
Inhalation	Medicated aerosol droplets	Albuterol for local effects in respiratory tract	Liquid medications inhaled through nebulizer or metered-dose inhaler.
Intravenous (IV)	Solution	IV fluids for hydration	Enters into vein via needle.
Irrigation	Solution with medication	—	Solution washes cavity.
Instillation	Solution with medication	Visine, Debrox	Eyedrops, ear drops.

PPD, Purified protein derivative; *TB*, tuberculosis.

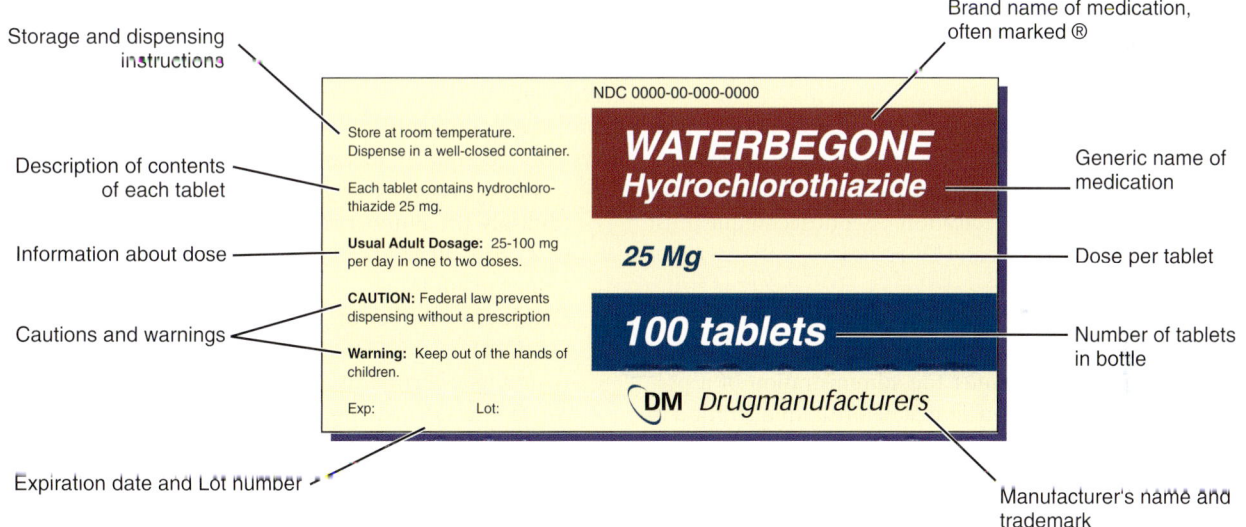

FIGURE 43-8 Information on a medication label. (From Hunt SA: *Saunders fundamentals of medical assisting—revised reprint,* St Louis, 2007, Saunders.)

administering any medication. For example, the drugs digoxin and digitoxin are both cardiotonic drugs, but the dosage and duration of action are very different for each. To ensure the patient is receiving the right drug, the medical assistant must read the label at least three times, as follows:
- Before removing the drug from storage
- Before pouring or preparing the medication
- Before returning the drug to storage

Figure 43-8 provides an example of a drug label showing various pieces of information.

3. Right Dose

A medication dosage is prescribed for a patient based on body weight, age, gender, and general state of health. For example, an emaciated (extremely underweight) patient or a pediatric patient would not receive the same dose as an average adult patient. Sometimes the amount of medication ordered by the physician is more than or less than the amount of the available drug form. In these situations, the amount administered to the patient must be calculated. Close attention is required so that the proper drug form (e.g., capsule, tablet, or suppository) is given for each dose of medication.

4. Right Route

The medical assistant must never vary from the route of drug administration prescribed. Since each drug route has a different rate of absorption, it is important to understand the significance of the route prescribed. Oral medications are considered to be the easiest to administer, but they absorb more slowly. If the absorption rate needs to be quicker, a medication would be best given through a **parenteral** route, such as IM or IV, or a route other than the digestive tract.

5. Right Time

Medications are to be taken when there is the best chance for maximum absorption and least chance for side effects. Some drugs must be taken on an empty stomach; others must be taken with food. Some drugs cannot be taken with certain foods or liquids.

> **FOR YOUR INFORMATION**
>
> FOOD-DRUG INTERACTION
>
> *Some drugs interact with certain foods or liquids. For example, grapefruit juice should not be taken with cholesterol-lowering drugs because an active ingredient in grapefruit reacts with these drugs and intensifies the action of the drug. If a patient takes 40 mg of simvastatin (Zocor) with grapefruit juice, the reaction produced may double the effects of the drug, overmedicating the patient.*

6. Right Technique

The right technique for medication administration must always be followed. If an injection is to be given subcutaneously (SubQ) and is given IM instead, the patient may not receive the benefits of the medication. Aseptic technique must always be used for injection and IV routes.

7. Right Documentation

The medical assistant must document the patient's medical record as soon as possible *after* the administration of a prescribed medication. Never document before administration in case you do not give the drug or other circumstances arise. When the medication is given by injection, the documentation must include the site used, what was given, and how the patient tolerated the procedure. The lot number, manufacturer, and expiration date of the drug may also be charted for certain medications, such as vaccinations (Box 43-6).

> **BOX 43-6**
>
> **Documentation when Charting Medications**
>
> 1. Date
> 2. Time
> 3. Name of medication
> 4. Dose administered
> 5. Injection site used, if applicable
> 6. Patient reaction, if any (record waiting time)
> 7. Patient education provided
> 8. Proper signature and credential
> 9. Expiration date, manufacturer, and lot number of drug, when applicable

Calculating Drug Dosage

The most important part of administering a drug is providing the correct amount. One method for calculating the proper dose is as follows:

$$\text{Dose order} \div \text{Dosage on hand} = \text{Dose amount}$$

> **EXAMPLE OF DOSAGE ORDER/DOSAGE ON HAND METHOD**
>
> If the physician orders 500 mg of a medication and the medication is supplied in 250 mg capsules, the dosage ordered (500 mg) is divided by the dosage on hand (250 mg). This provides the dosage amount of two capsules.
>
> $$500 \text{ mg} \div 250 \text{ mg} = 2 \text{ capsules}$$

Converting Measurements

Dosage must be calculated using the same measurements as the order. If a medication is ordered in grams and the dosage on hand is in milligrams, the medical assistant must convert the dosage ordered to what is available. Converting grams (g) to milligrams (mg) or grams to grains (gr) is easily done by learning that 0.06 g = 60 mg = 1 gr and 1 g = 15 gr. Table 43-5 lists other measurements and their equivalents. Figure 43-9 illustrates the basic units of the metric system. The following provides examples of converting different drug measurement systems (metric, apothecary).

Grams (g) to grains (gr):
- Multiply the number of grams by 15. For example: 2 g = (2 × 15) = 30 gr

Grains to grams:
- Divide the number of grains by 15. For example: 45 gr = (45 ÷ 15) = 3 g

Grams to milligrams (mg):
- Move the decimal point three places to the right. For example: 0.06 g = 060. = 60 mg

Milligrams to grams:
- Move the decimal point three places to the left. For example: 120 mg = 0.120 = 0.12 g

Milligrams to grains:
- Divide the number of milligrams by 60. For example: 60 mg = 60 ÷ 60 = 1 gr

Grains to milligrams:
- Multiply the number of grains by 60. For example: 15 gr = (15 × 60) = 900 mg

Calculating Infant or Child Dosage

Infant and child dosages are calculated according to body weight. An important conversion for the medical assistant to remember is that 2.2 lb = 1 kg.

Pounds (lb) to kilograms (kg):
- Divide the number of pounds by 2.2. For example: 100 lb = (100 ÷ 2.2) = 45.5 kg

Kilograms to pounds:
- Multiply the number of kilograms by 2.2. For example: 50 kg = (50 × 2.2) = 110 lb

TABLE 43-5

Approximate Apothecary, Household, and Metric Equivalents

Volume			Weight	
oz to mL	**m to gr**	**gr to mg**	**gr to mg**	
1 oz = 30 mL	45 m = 3 gr	gr xv = 1000 mg	15 gr = 1000 mg (1 g)	
½ oz = 15 mL	30 m = 2 gr	gr x = 600 mg	¼ gr = 15 mg	
	15 m = 1 gr	7½ gr = 500 mg	⅙ gr = 10 mg	
dr to mL	12 m = 0.75 gr	gr v = 300 mg	⅛ gr = 7.5 mg	
2½ dr = 10 mL	10 m = 0.6 gr	gr iv = 250 mg	1/10 gr = 6 mg	
2 dr = 8 mL	8 m = 0.5 gr	gr iii = 200 mg	1/15 gr = 4 mg	
1¼ dr = 5 mL	5 m = 0.3 gr	2½ gr = 150 mg	1/20 gr = 3 mg	
1 dr = 4 mL	4 m = 0.25 gr	gr ii = 120 mg	1/30 gr = 2 mg	
	3 m = 0.2 gr	1½ gr = 100 mg	1/40 gr = 1.5 mg	
1 m = 1 gtt	1½ m = 0.1 gr	gr i = 60 mg	1/60 gr = 1 mg	
1 t = 5 mL	1 m = 0.06 gr	¾ gr = 45 mg		
1 T = 15 mL	¾ m = 0.05 gr	½ gr = 30 mg	1 kg = 2.2 lb	
1 t = 60 gtt	½ m = 0.03 gr	⅓ gr = 20 mg	1 kg = 1000 g	
			1 mg = 1000 mcg	
HOUSEHOLD				
1 oz = 2 T				
8 oz = 1 cup = 240 mL	1 L = 1000 mL	1 lb = 16 oz		
2 pt = 1 qt = 1000 mL	1 mL = 16 gtt			
4 qt = 1 gallon = 4000 mL				

dr, Drams; *gr*, grains; *g*, gram; *gtt*, drop; *lb*, pounds; *m*, minims; *mg*, milligrams; *mL*, milliliters; *oz*, ounces; *T*, tablespoon; *t*, teaspoon.

Basic unit of weight: gram (g)

A candle used on a birthday cake weighs about one gram. We could also say that the candle weighs 1,000,000 μg or 1,000 mg or 0.001 kg.

Conversion equations for weight:

1,000 μg (micrograms) = 1 mg (milligram)
1000 mg (milligrams) = 1 g (gram)
1000 g (grams) = 1 kg (kilogram)

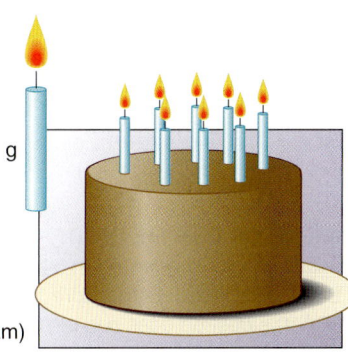

Basic unit of volume: liter (L)

A quart of milk contains a little less than a liter. We could say that the carton contains approximately 1000 mL.

Conversion equation for volume:

1000 mL (milliliters) = 1 L (liter)
1 cc (cubic centimeters) = 1 mL

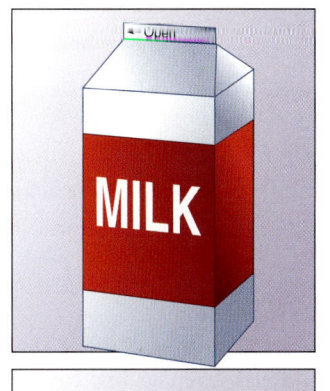

FIGURE 43-9 Basic units of the metric system. (From Hunt SA: *Saunders fundamentals of medical assisting—revised reprint*, St Louis, 2007, Saunders.)

Basic unit of distance: meter (m)

A yard is slightly less than a meter. A centimeter is slightly less than a half inch.

Conversion equation for distance:

1 cm = 10 mm
100 cm = 1 m

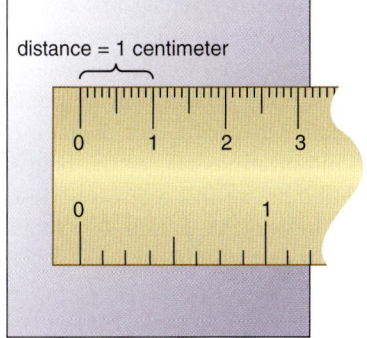

Two methods are currently used when calculating an infant's or a child's medication dose. The first involves using the child's body weight, and the second uses height and weight to determine body surface area.

Body Weight. The body weight method is the preferred method because it requires using the body weight in kilograms times the total amount in milligrams of medication desired per day.

> **EXAMPLE OF BODY WEIGHT METHOD**
> If a child weighs 60 lb, this weight is converted to kilograms:
>
> $$60 \text{ lb} \div 2.2 = 27 \text{ kg}$$
>
> If the physician wants the child to have 10 mg of medication per kilogram of weight per day, divided into two equal doses, the calculation proceeds as follows:
>
> $$\text{kg wt} \times \text{mg} = \text{dose}$$
> $$27 \text{ kg} \times 10 \text{ mg} = 270 \text{ mg per day}$$
> $$270 \div 2 = 135 \text{ mg per dose}$$

Body Surface Area Method. The body surface area (BSA) method uses a **nomogram** that shows a relationship between height and weight and body surface area. The height and weight are measured and charted on the nomogram (Figure 43-10). A straight line is drawn from the weight to the height, and then the place where the line crosses the BSA column is located.

> **EXAMPLE OF BSA METHOD**
> If a child's weight is recorded as 54 lb and height is 64 inches, the BSA scale reads 1; therefore the BSA is 1 m². Knowing the BSA, the desired dose can be calculated using the following formula:
>
> $$(\text{BSA}^2 \div 1.7) \times \text{Adult dose} = \text{Desired dose}$$
>
> (1.7 is BSA of an adult weighting 140 lb)
> If the adult dose of a medication is 500 mg, the dose for this child is 295 mg:
>
> $$(1[\text{BSA}] \div 1.7) \times 500 \text{ mg} = 295 \text{ mg}$$

Immunization

In the late eighteenth century, the first **vaccine** as an **immunization** was given against cowpox to prevent acquiring the dreaded disease smallpox. Since then, many vaccines have been developed to prevent polio, pneumonia, and other diseases. Infants begin their immunizations in the first few days because this is the age they are most vulnerable to disease. Immunizations trigger the body's immune system to build antibodies against a disease. Most childhood immunizations will be available in unit dose measurement; this makes medication preparation minimal.

Procedure 43-1 outlines the process of preparing an immunization record and filing it properly in the patient's medical record.

Immunization Timing

Timing of immunizations is important to obtain proper blood levels of needed antibodies. Figure 43-11 provides a chart with a recommended immunization schedule for ages 0 to 6 years and Figure 43-12 provides a schedule for persons 7 to 18 years. Side effects are usually minimal and limited to low-grade fever and tenderness where the injection was given (Table 43-6).

Besides administering the medication, the medical assistant is responsible for making certain a signature from the parent or legal guardian has been obtained on a consent form before giving the immunization. According to the *National Child Vaccine Injury Act (NCVIA)* of 1988, before administration of a vaccine, the parent or legal guardian must be given the **Vaccine Information Statement (VIS)** for the vaccine to be administered. The VIS provides updated information regarding the benefits and risks of the vaccine. Current VISs are available from local health departments and the Internet (www.cdc.gov/nip/publications/vis/). Any adverse reactions after the administration of any vaccine are reported to the *Vaccine Adverse Event Reporting System (VAERS)*. Assistance on how to obtain and complete VAERS forms can be obtained on the Internet (www.vaers.hhs.gov). The medical assistant also assists the parent or legal guardian with maintaining the immunization records and encourages them to follow the proposed schedule to obtain optimal results. A record of children's immunizations must be presented before they can enter school.

> **FOR YOUR INFORMATION**
>
> **RECOMMENDED IMMUNIZATION SCHEDULE**
>
> The Advisory Committee on Immunization Practices (ACIP) of the Center for Disease Control, American Academy of Pediatrics, and the American Academy of Family Physicians provide recommendations for immunization policies and procedures in the United States. Changes occur as a result of advances in immunology. Keeping current on the latest advances and changes in policy is possible by using the following Internet addresses:
> - www.cdc.gov/nip/acip
> - www.aap.org
> - www.aafp.org
>
> Vaccine-related updates are also available online at www.aapredbook.org.

Administering Immunizations

Some basic considerations when administering an immunization include the following:

1. *Selecting the correct site* (this allows for optimal distribution). An older child or adult receiving an IM injection will receive the injection in the deltoid or gluteus muscle,

PROCEDURE 43-1

Prepare and File an Immunization Record

TASK: Prepare an immunization record and properly document in the patient's medical record.

EQUIPMENT AND SUPPLIES
- Replicated medication container
- Replicated patient immunization form
- Physician's orders for immunization
- Patient's medical record

VACCINE ADMINISTRATION RECORD FOR CHILDREN AND TEENS

Patient Name: _____
Birthdate: _____
Chart number: _____

Vaccine	Type of Vaccine[1] (generic abbreviation)	Date given (mo/day/yr)	Source (F,S,P)[2]	Site[3]	Vaccine Lot #	Vaccine Mfr.	Vaccine Information Statement Date or VIS[4]	Vaccine Information Statement Date given[4]	Signature/ initials of vaccinator
Hepatitis B[5] (e.g., HepB, Hib-HepB, DTaP-HepB-IPV) Give IM.									
Diphtheria, Tetanus, Pertussis[5] (e.g., DTaP, DTaP-Hib DTaP-HepB IPV, DT Tdap, Td) Give IM.									
***Haemophilus influenzae* type b**[5] (e.g., Hib, Hib-HepB, DTaP-Hib) Give IM.									
Polio[5] (e.g., IPV, DTaP-HepB-IPV) Give IPV SC or IM. Give DTaP-HepB-IPV IM.									
Pneumococcal (e.g., PCV, conjugate; PPV, polysaccharide) Give PCV IM. Give PPV SC or IM.									
Rotavirus (Rv) Give oral (po).									
Measles, Mumps, Rubella[5] (e.g., MMR, MMRV) Give SC.									
Varicella[5] (e.g., Var, MMRV) Give SC.									
Hepatitis A (HepA) Give IM.									
Meningococcal (e.e., MCVS4; MPSV4) Give MCV4 IM and MPSV4 SC.									
Human papillomavirus (e.g., HPV) Give IM.									
Influenza[5] (e.g., TIV, inactivated; LAIV, live attenuated) Give TIV IM. Give LAIV IN.									
Other									

1. Record the generic abbreviation for the type of vaccine given (e.g., DTaP-Hib, PCV), *not* the trade name.
2. Record the source of the vaccine given as either F (Federally-supported), S (State-supported) or P (supported by Private insurance or other Private funds)
3. Record the site where vaccine was administered as either RA (Right Arm), LA (Left Arm), RT (Right Thigh), IN (Intranasal), or O (Oral).
4. Record the publication date of each VIS as well as the date it is given to the patient.
5. For combination vaccines, fill in a row for each seperate antigen in the combination.

From: Immunization Action Coalition • 1573 Selby Ave. • St. Paul, MN 55104 • (651) 647-9009 • www.immunize.org • www.vaccineinformation.org

Vaccine Administration Record courtesy Immunization Action Coalition, St. Paul, MN.

Continued

PROCEDURE 43-1   Prepare and File an Immunization Record—cont'd

SKILLS/RATIONALE

1. **Procedural Step.** Obtain the patient's medical record. Verify that the record and patient match.
   Rationale. This ensures the patient information is entered into the correct record.
2. **Procedural Step.** Confirm the date the previous immunization was ordered and administered.
3. **Procedural Step.** Verify that the immunization was given within the required time frame.
   Rationale. Some types of immunizations are not valid if not given within a specific time frame, and may require a series be repeated.
4. **Procedural Step.** Complete the "Vaccine Administration Record" and the patient's immunization record form.

IMMUNIZATION RECORD					
Name _____ Birthdate _____					
Immunization	DATE	DATE	DATE	DATE	DATE
Hep B (Hepatitis B)					
DTaP (Diphtheria, Tetanus, and Pertussis)					
Hib (Haemophilus influenzae Type b)					
IPV (Inactivated Polio Vaccine)					
PCV (Pneumococcal Conjugate Vaccine)					
Rv (Rotavirus)					
MMR (Measles, Mumps, and Rubella)					
Varicella (Chickenpox)					
Hep A (Hepatitis A)					
MPSV4 (Meningococcal)					
HPV (Human papillomavirus)					
Influenza (TIV or LAIV)					
Tetanus Booster					
Other					

5. **Procedural Step.** Chart the following information into the patient's medical record.
   a. Name of medication or immunization.
   b. Manufacturer, batch, and lot number.
   c. Date of expiration.
   d. Amount of medication or immunization given.
   e. Dose administered.
   f. Route of administration.
   g. Patient reaction. (Patient reactions vary depending on the type of immunization.)

   Some medical facilities will provide a patient with an immunization record that the patient retains for their records. This immunization record must be brought into the medical facility each time an immunization is given. The information recorded on the patient's immunization record must also be recorded in the patient's medical record.

6. **Procedural Step.** Sign the entry.
   Rationale. This is a legal document, and as such, it must have the signature and credentials of the person administering the immunization.
7. **Procedural Step.** Return the patient's record to the filing system.

CHARTING EXAMPLE

Date	
9/30/xx	10:00 a.m. MMR Lot #1234; Exp. 10/04/xx. 0.5 mL SubQ Ⓡ deltoid. No localized swelling or redness observed. No breathing difficulties noted. VIS (1/15/xx) given to mother. Instructed to call if temp greater than 103 degrees F or increased irritability occur. ——————————————— H. Buck, RMA

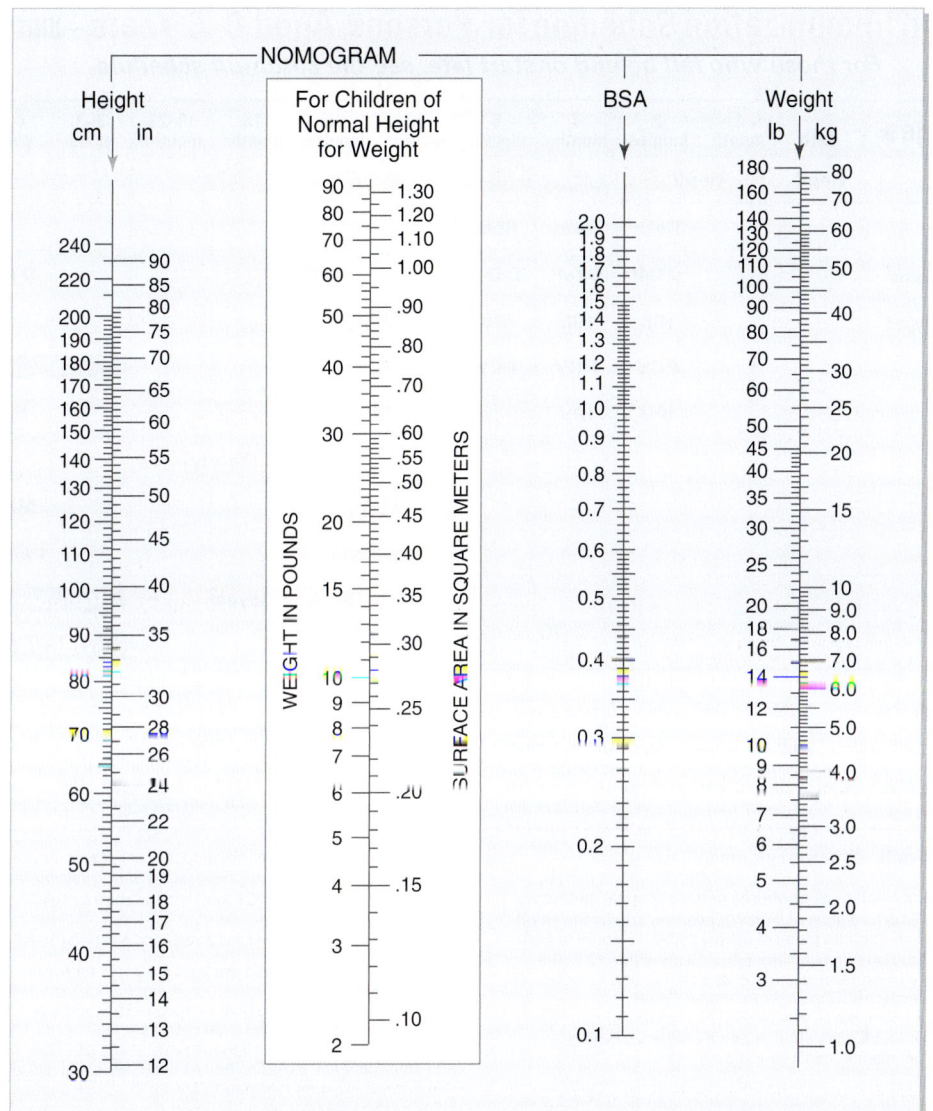

FIGURE 43-10 West body surface area (BSA) nomogram. (From Behrman RE et al: *Nelson textbook of pediatrics*, ed 16, Philadelphia, 2000, Saunders.)

TABLE 43-6
Possible Immunization Reactions

Immunization	Reaction*
Hepatitis B virus (HBV)	Localized tenderness where injection was given and mild-to-moderate fever
Polio (IPV)	Localized soreness and redness where injection was given
Haemophilus influenzae B (Hib)	Localized redness or warmth at site of injection
Diphtheria, tetanus (DTaP/Td)	Mild-to-moderate fever and tenderness at site of injection
Pneumococcal conjugate vaccine (PCV)	Mild-to-moderate fever and redness and tenderness at injection site
Measles, mumps, rubella (MMR)	Mild-to-moderate fever and redness and tenderness at injection site; 1 to 2 weeks after injection, mild rash may appear for 1 to 2 days
Chickenpox (VZV)	Mild-to-moderate fever and tenderness at injection site

*Reactions, if they occur, will usually begin 1 or 2 days after the vaccination and last 1 or 2 days.
IPV, Inactivated polio vaccine; *VZV*, varicella-zoster virus.

Recommended Immunization Schedule for Persons Aged 0–6 Years—UNITED STATES • 2008

For those who fall behind or start late, see the catch-up schedule

Vaccine ▼ Age ►	Birth	1 month	2 months	4 months	6 months	12 months	15 months	18 months	19–23 months	2–3 years	4–6 years
Hepatitis B[1]	HepB	HepB		see footnote 1		HepB					
Rotavirus[2]			Rota	Rota	Rota						
Diphtheria, Tetanus, Pertussis[3]			DTaP	DTaP	DTaP	see footnote 3	DTaP				DTaP
Haemophilus influenzae type b[4]			Hib	Hib	Hib[4]	Hib					
Pneumococcal[5]			PCV	PCV	PCV	PCV				PPV	
Inactivated Poliovirus			IPV	IPV		IPV					IPV
Influenza[6]						Influenza (Yearly)					
Measles, Mumps, Rubella[7]						MMR					MMR
Varicella[8]						Varicella					Varicella
Hepatitis A[9]						HepA (2 doses)				HepA Series	
Meningococcal[10]										MCV4	

Legend:
- ☐ (yellow) Range of recommended ages
- ☐ (purple) Certain high-risk groups

This schedule indicates the recommended ages for routine administration of currently licensed childhood vaccines, as of December 1, 2007, for children aged 0 through 6 years. Additional information is available at www.cdc.gov/vaccines/recs/schedules. Any dose not administered at the recommended age should be administered at any subsequent visit, when indicated and feasible. Additional vaccines may be licensed and recommended during the year. Licensed combination vaccines may be used whenever any components of the combination are indicated and other components of the vaccine are not contraindicated and if approved by the Food and Drug Administration for that dose of the series. Providers should consult the respective Advisory Committee on Immunization Practices statement for detailed recommendations, including for **high-risk conditions:** http://www.cdc.gov/vaccines/pubs/ACIP-list.htm. Clinically significant adverse events that follow immunization should be reported to the Vaccine Adverse Event Reporting System (VAERS). Guidance about how to obtain and complete a VAERS form is available at www.vaers.hhs.gov or by telephone, 800-822-7967.

1. **Hepatitis B vaccine (HepB).** *(Minimum age: birth)*
   At birth:
   - Administer monovalent HepB to all newborns prior to hospital discharge.
   - If mother is hepatitis B surface antigen (HBsAg) positive, administer HepB and 0.5 mL of hepatitis B immune globulin (HBIG) within 12 hours of birth.
   - If mother's HBsAg status is unknown, administer HepB within 12 hours of birth. Determine the HBsAg status as soon as possible and if HBsAg positive, administer HBIG (no later than age 1 week).
   - If mother is HBsAg negative, the birth dose can be delayed, in rare cases, with a provider's order and a copy of the mother's negative HBsAg laboratory report in the infant's medical record.

   After the birth dose:
   - The HepB series should be completed with either monovalent HepB or a combination vaccine containing HepB. The second dose should be administered at age 1–2 months. The final dose should be administered no earlier than age 24 weeks. Infants born to HBsAg positive mothers should be tested for HBsAg and antibody to HBsAg after completion of at least 3 doses of a licensed HepB series, at age 9–18 months (generally at the next well-child visit).

   4-month dose:
   - It is permissible to administer 4 doses of HepB when combination vaccines are administered after the birth dose. If monovalent HepB is used for doses after the birth dose, a dose at age 4 months is not needed.

2. **Rotavirus vaccine (Rota).** *(Minimum age: 6 weeks)*
   - Administer the first dose at age 6–12 weeks.
   - Do not start the series later than age 12 weeks.
   - Administer the final dose in the series by age 32 weeks. Do not administer any dose later than age 32 weeks.
   - Data on safety and efficacy outside of these age ranges are insufficient.

3. **Diphtheria and tetanus toxoids and acellular pertussis vaccine (DTaP).** *(Minimum age: 6 weeks)*
   - The fourth dose of DTaP may be administered as early as age 12 months, provided 6 months have elapsed since the third dose.
   - Administer the final dose in the series at age 4–6 years.

4. **Haemophilus influenzae type b conjugate vaccine (Hib).** *(Minimum age: 6 weeks)*
   - If PRP-OMP (PedvaxHIB® or ComVax® [Merck]) is administered at ages 2 and 4 months, a dose at age 6 months is not required.
   - TriHIBit® (DTaP/Hib) combination products should not be used for primary immunization but can be used as boosters following any Hib vaccine in children age 12 months or older.

5. **Pneumococcal vaccine.** *(Minimum age: 6 weeks for pneumococcal conjugate vaccine [PCV]; 2 years for pneumococcal polysaccharide vaccine [PPV])*
   - Administer one dose of PCV to all healthy children aged 24–59 months having any incomplete schedule.
   - Administer PPV to children aged 2 years and older with underlying medical conditions.

6. **Influenza vaccine.** *(Minimum age: 6 months for trivalent inactivated influenza vaccine [TIV]; 2 years for live, attenuated influenza vaccine [LAIV])*
   - Administer annually to children aged 6–59 months and to all eligible close contacts of children aged 0–59 months.
   - Administer annually to children 5 years of age and older with certain risk factors, to other persons (including household members) in close contact with persons in groups at higher risk, and to any child whose parents request vaccination.
   - For healthy persons (those who do not have underlying medical conditions that predispose them to influenza complications) ages 2–49 years, either LAIV or TIV may be used.
   - Children receiving TIV should receive 0.25 mL if age 6–35 months or 0.5 mL if age 3 years or older.
   - Administer 2 doses (separated by 4 weeks or longer) to children younger than 9 years who are receiving influenza vaccine for the first time or who were vaccinated for the first time last season but only received one dose.

7. **Measles, mumps, and rubella vaccine (MMR).** *(Minimum age: 12 months)*
   - Administer the second dose of MMR at age 4–6 years. MMR may be administered before age 4–6 years, provided 4 weeks or more have elapsed since the first dose.

8. **Varicella vaccine.** *(Minimum age: 12 months)*
   - Administer second dose at age 4–6 years; may be administered 3 months or more after first dose.
   - Do not repeat second dose if administered 28 days or more after first dose.

9. **Hepatitis A vaccine (HepA).** *(Minimum age: 12 months)*
   - Administer to all children aged 1 year (i.e., aged 12–23 months). Administer the 2 doses in the series at least 6 months apart.
   - Children not fully vaccinated by age 2 years can be vaccinated at subsequent visits.
   - HepA is recommended for certain other groups of children, including in areas where vaccination programs target older children.

10. **Meningococcal vaccine.** *(Minimum age: 2 years for meningococcal conjugate vaccine (MCV4) and for meningococcal polysaccharide vaccine (MPSV4))*
    - Administer MCV4 to children aged 2–10 years with terminal complement deficiencies or anatomic or functional asplenia and certain other high-risk groups. MPSV4 is also acceptable.
    - Administer MCV4 to persons who received MPSV4 3 or more years previously and remain at increased risk for meningococcal disease.

The Recommended Immunization Schedules for Persons Aged 0–18 Years are approved by the Advisory Committee on Immunization Practices (www.cdc.gov/vaccines/recs/acip), the American Academy of Pediatrics (http://www.aap.org), and the American Academy of Family Physicians (http://www.aafp.org).

DEPARTMENT OF HEALTH AND HUMAN SERVICES • CENTERS FOR DISEASE CONTROL AND PREVENTION • SAFER • HEATHIER • PEOPLE™

FIGURE 43-11 Recommended immunization schedule for persons aged 0-6 years.

Recommended Immunization Schedule for Persons Aged 7–18 Years—UNITED STATES • 2008

For those who fall behind or start late, see the green bars and the catch-up schedule

Vaccine ▼ Age ▶	7–10 years	11–12 years	13–18 years
Diphtheria, Tetanus, Pertussis[1]	see footnote 1	Tdap	Tdap
Human Papillomavirus[2]	see footnote 2	HPV (3 doses)	HPV Series
Meningococcal[3]	MCV4	MCV4	MCV4
Pneumococcal[4]	PPV	PPV	PPV
Influenza[5]	Influenza (Yearly)	Influenza (Yearly)	Influenza (Yearly)
Hepatitis A[6]	HepA Series	HepA Series	HepA Series
Hepatitis B[7]	HepB Series	HepB Series	HepB Series
Inactivated Poliovirus[8]	IPV Series	IPV Series	IPV Series
Measles, Mumps, Rubella[9]	MMR Series	MMR Series	MMR Series
Varicella[10]	Varicella Series	Varicella Series	Varicella Series

Legend:
- Range of recommended ages
- Catch-up immunization
- Certain high-risk groups

This schedule indicates the recommended ages for routine administration of currently licensed childhood vaccines, as of December 1, 2007, for children aged 7–18 years. Additional information is available at www.cdc.gov/vaccines/recs/schedules. Any dose not administered at the recommended age should be administered at any subsequent visit, when indicated and feasible. Additional vaccines may be licensed and recommended during the year. Licensed combination vaccines may be used whenever any components of the combination are indicated and other components of the vaccine are not contraindicated and if approved by the Food and Drug Administration for that dose of the series. Providers should consult the respective Advisory Committee on Immunization Practices statement for detailed recommendations, including for high risk conditions: http://www.cdc.gov/vaccines/pubs/ACIP-list.htm. Clinically significant adverse events that follow immunization should be reported to the Vaccine Adverse Event Reporting System (VAERS). Guidance about how to obtain and complete a VAERS form is available at www.vaers.hhs.gov or by telephone, 800-822-7967.

1. **Tetanus and diphtheria toxoids and acellular pertussis vaccine (Tdap).** *(Minimum age: 10 years for BOOSTRIX® and 11 years for ADACEL™)*
   - Administer at age 11–12 years for those who have completed the recommended childhood DTP/DTaP vaccination series and have not received a tetanus and diphtheria toxoids (Td) booster dose.
   - 13–18-year-olds who missed the 11–12 year Tdap or received Td only are encouraged to receive one dose of Tdap 5 years after the last Td/DTaP dose.

2. **Human papillomavirus vaccine (HPV).** *(Minimum age: 9 years)*
   - Administer the first dose of the HPV vaccine series to females at age 11–12 years.
   - Administer the second dose 2 months after the first dose and the third dose 6 months after the first dose.
   - Administer the HPV vaccine series to females at age 13–18 years if not previously vaccinated.

3. **Meningococcal vaccine.**
   - Administer MCV4 at age 11–12 years and at age 13–18 years if not previously vaccinated. MPSV4 is an acceptable alternative.
   - Administer MCV4 to previously unvaccinated college freshmen living in dormitories.
   - MCV4 is recommended for children aged 2–10 years with terminal complement deficiencies or anatomic or functional asplenia and certain other high-risk groups.
   - Persons who received MPSV4 3 or more years previously and remain at increased risk for meningococcal disease should be vaccinated with MCV4.

4. **Pneumococcal polysaccharide vaccine (PPV).**
   - Administer PPV to certain high-risk groups.

5. **Influenza vaccine.**
   - Administer annually to all close contacts of children aged 0–59 months.
   - Administer annually to persons with certain risk factors, health-care workers, and other persons (including household members) in close contact with persons in groups at higher risk.
   - Administer 2 doses (separated by 4 weeks or longer) to children younger than 9 years who are receiving influenza vaccine for the first time or who were vaccinated for the first time last season but only received one dose.
   - For healthy nonpregnant persons (those who do not have underlying medical conditions that predispose them to influenza complications) ages 2–49 years, either LAIV or TIV may be used.

6. **Hepatitis A vaccine (HepA).**
   - Administer the 2 doses in the series at least 6 months apart.
   - HepA is recommended for certain other groups of children, including in areas where vaccination programs target older children.

7. **Hepatitis B vaccine (HepB).**
   - Administer the 3-dose series to those who were not previously vaccinated.
   - A 2-dose series of Recombivax HB® is licensed for children aged 11–15 years.

8. **Inactivated poliovirus vaccine (IPV).**
   - For children who received an all-IPV or all-oral poliovirus (OPV) series, a fourth dose is not necessary if the third dose was administered at age 4 years or older.
   - If both OPV and IPV were administered as part of a series, a total of 4 doses should be administered, regardless of the child's current age.

9. **Measles, mumps, and rubella vaccine (MMR).**
   - If not previously vaccinated, administer 2 doses of MMR during any visit, with 4 or more weeks between the doses.

10. **Varicella vaccine.**
    - Administer 2 doses of varicella vaccine to persons younger than 13 years of age at least 3 months apart. Do not repeat the second dose if administered 28 or more days following the first dose.
    - Administer 2 doses of varicella vaccine to persons aged 13 years or older at least 4 weeks apart.

The Recommended Immunization Schedules for Persons Aged 0–18 Years are approved by the Advisory Committee on Immunization Practices (www.cdc.gov/vaccines/recs/acip), the American Academy of Pediatrics (http://www.aap.org), and the American Academy of Family Physicians (http://www.aafp.org).

DEPARTMENT OF HEALTH AND HUMAN SERVICES • CENTERS FOR DISEASE CONTROL AND PREVENTION
SAFER • HEALTHIER • PEOPLE™

FIGURE 43-12 Recommended immunization schedule for persons aged 7-18 years.

whereas an infant or small child receives it in the anterior lateral thigh. If multiple immunizations are given on the same day, different sites must be used for each.

2. *Choosing the correct route.* The route chosen by the physician for an immunization is as important as the site chosen. For example, the hepatitis B vaccine is best given IM in the deltoid because it loses optimal response if given in the gluteus. Measles, mumps, and rubella (MMR) vaccine is given SubQ.
3. *Providing the correct dose.* The size of the dose prescribed by the physician must be enough to receive the desired response. For example, a **booster dose,** one used to provide lifelong immunity, may be smaller than an initial dose(s) that begins the antibody response.

Medical assistants must be knowledgeable regarding proper dose and exact injection sites. Box 43-7 provides charting information required for vaccine administration.

BOX 43-7

Documentation when Charting Immunizations

1. Date
2. Time
3. Name of vaccine
4. Name of manufacturer
5. Expiration date
6. Lot number of vaccine
7. Dose administered
8. Route of administration
9. Injection site used
10. Patient reaction, if any (record waiting time)
11. Indication that permission has been signed
12. Provided Vaccine Information Statement (VIS) with print date
13. Proper signature and credential

FOR YOUR INFORMATION

NEEDLESTICKS

In June 2008 the federal advisory panel endorsed two new combination vaccines designed to reduce the number of needlesticks that young children must endure to receive the recommended immunizations.

- *Four-in-one vaccine that protects against diphtheria, tetanus, pertussis, and polio and is given once to pre-school aged children*
- *Five-in-one vaccine for diphtheria, tetanus, pertussis, polio and Hib. Toddlers get four doses by age 2.*

PATIENT-CENTERED PROFESIONALISM

- *Why must the medical assistant follow the "seven rights" of drug administration?*
- *When charting immunizations, why must the medical assistant be sure to include the information about the manufacturer, lot number, and expiration date?*

DRUG FORMS

Medications exist in three forms: liquid, solid, and semisolid.

Liquid Forms

Liquid forms include solutions, suspensions, emulsions, tinctures, lotions, liniments, elixirs, syrups, and aerosols.

- **Solutions** consist of one or more medications (**solutes**) dissolved in **solvent** (liquid). Water (both distilled and sterile), alcohol, and normal saline are typical solvents. True solutions are clear, and all forms of the solute are dissolved (e.g., hydrogen peroxide is very clear).
- **Suspension** occurs when the medication (solute) is evenly distributed within the solution, but is not dissolved. A suspension must be shaken to distribute the medication evenly before use (e.g., Maalox).
- **Emulsion** is a substance suspended in an oil based liquid into which it does not mix. It must be shaken before use (e.g., castor oil).
- **Tinctures** are medications mixed with an alcohol base (e.g., tincture of merthiolate).
- **Lotions** are water-based preparations with medications intended to soothe the skin (e.g., calamine lotion).
- **Liniments** are external preparations composed of a medication combined with a base of oil, water, alcohol, or soap. Liniments are rubbed into the skin (e.g., camphor liniment).
- **Elixirs** are solutions containing alcohol, water, sugar, and a drug or combination of drugs (e.g., Donnatal).
- **Syrups** are solutions of sugar and water containing dissolved drugs (e.g., cough syrups).
- **Aerosols** are drug suspensions that are administered in a mist. The suspension is packaged in a pressurized container, and when released, a spray of fine mist containing the medication is administered (e.g., metered-dose inhaler).

Solid Forms

Solid forms include tablets, capsules, caplets, gel caps, spansules, powders, and lozenges. Figure 43-13 shows various solid forms of drugs.

- **Tablets** are compressed powdered medication in the shape of a disk. Size, shape, and color vary. Sometimes a tablet is designed to dissolve in areas other than the stomach; these tablets are layered to alter the absorption rate (Figure 43-14). Other tablets may be scored to allow for halving the dose. A tablet may not be halved unless it comes prescored by the manufacturer. Box 43-8 lists and describes several types of tablets.

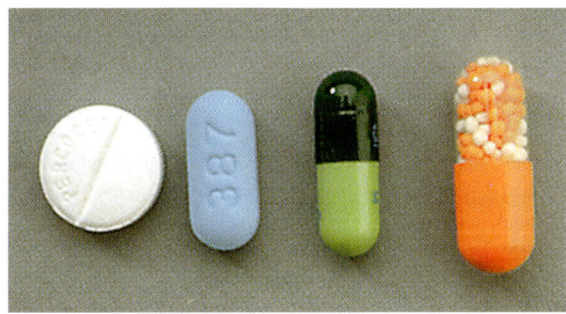

FIGURE 43-13 Solid forms of drugs. *Left to right,* Scored tablet, caplet, capsule, spansule.

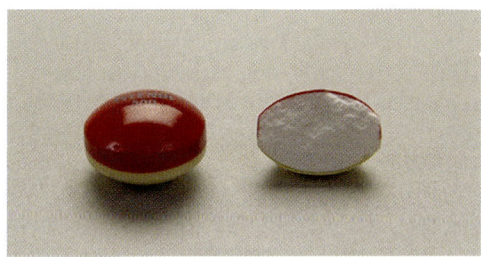

FIGURE 43-14 Thick outer covering of enteric-coated medication is visible in cross-section. The enteric coating is applied to tablets or capsules to prevent release and absorption of the contents until they reach the intestines.

BOX 43-8

Types of Tablets

- **Buccal tablets** are made to dissolve when placed between the cheek and gum.
- **Enteric-coated tablets** have a special coating that allows them to pass through the stomach and dissolve in the small intestine (see Figure 43-11).
- **Layered tablets** have two or more ingredients layered to dissolve and be absorbed at different times.
- **Scored tablets** have an indentation across the middle, which makes it easier to break in half.
- **Sublingual tablets** are made to dissolve when placed under the tongue.

- **Capsules** are rod-shaped, two-part containers made of a gelatinous substance. Capsules contain a powder (e.g., Prevacid).
- **Caplets** are rod shaped (like a capsule) or oval shaped, but they are solid like a tablet. Caplets have a special coating that allows them to be swallowed more easily (e.g., Aleve).
- **Gel caps** are made of a gelatinous substance, but they cannot be opened like a capsule. They contain an oil-based liquid (e.g., vitamin E).
- **Spansules** are capsules that contain small beads (granules) of medication that dissolve at various times (e.g., Contac).
- **Powders** are medications that are ground into a powder (e.g., Goody's Headache Powders).

- **Lozenges (troches)** are round, oval, or oblong-shaped sugar-based tablets that dissolve in the mouth, releasing medication (e.g., throat lozenges).

Semisolid Forms

Semisolid forms include transdermal patches, suppositories, ointments, and creams.

- **Transdermal patches** are medicated disks applied to the skin. The medication is absorbed through the skin over a set period.
- **Suppositories** are semisolid, cone-shaped medications combined with a base that dissolves when placed in a body cavity (e.g., Preparation H).
- **Ointments** are semisolid mixtures of medication mixed with an oil base such as lanolin or petroleum jelly (e.g., Neosporin).
- **Creams** are semisolid mixtures of medication in a water-soluble base (e.g., Monistat).

PATIENT CENTERED PROFESSIONALISM

- Why must the medical assistant know about the different drug forms?

DRUG CLASSIFICATIONS

A drug may be classified in various categories depending on different criteria. Medical assistants must understand the methods of classification, as well as the unwanted side effects that can occur with drugs.

Methods of Classification

Drugs can be classified in several ways, as follows:

1. *Drug's effect* (**local** or **systemic**). A drug that works locally acts on the site where it is applied such as eyedrops or topical medications. A drug that works systemically acts throughout the body (e.g., analgesics).
2. *Therapeutic effect.* Therapeutic effect refers to the intended effect of the drug. For example, an antidepressant is prescribed to elevate the person's mood by controlling the activation or inhibition of certain chemicals within the brain.
3. *Drug action.* A drug's action relates to the physiological effect on body tissues. Vasodilators, for example, work on different substances in the body to help widen (dilate) blood vessels.
4. *Body system affected.* Identifying medications that affect a certain body system can also be used to classify drugs. For example, by prescribing a diuretic, the urinary system is targeted to prevent water reabsorption.
5. *Chemical structure.* Classifying drugs by chemical structure is often done when replacing a substance produced in the body (e.g., hormones, vitamins, or minerals).

Table 43-7 lists drug classifications by action and use.

TABLE 43-7

Drug Classifications, Actions, and Uses

Class	Action	Treatment Uses	Examples
Adrenergics	Increase rate and strength of heartbeat Act as vasoconstrictor; dilate pupils and bronchi Relax muscular walls of GI and urinary tracts	Bronchitis, asthma, allergic condition, nasal congestion Treatment of shock to increase blood pressure	isoproterenol (Isuprel), pseudoephedrine (Sudafed), oxymetazoline (Visine), epinephrine
Adrenergic-blocking agents	Vasodilation to increase peripheral circulation, decrease blood pressure, and increase tone of muscle walls of GI tract	Hypertension, peripheral vascular disease	methyldopa (Aldomet), propranolol (Inderal), atenolol (Tenormin)
Analgesics	Opioid and opiate, nonopioid Block perception of pain in cortex	Relieve varying degrees of pain; lower blood pressure	*Opiates:* morphine, opioids, codeine, meperidine (Demerol), propoxyphene (Darvon) *Nonopioids:* aspirin, acetaminophen
Anesthetics	Block nerve impulses to brain to achieve loss of consciousness Dilate pupils; decrease respiration, pulses, and blood pressure	*Local anesthesia:* produces loss of pain or sensation without loss of consciousness *General anesthesia:* loss of consciousness results	*Local:* lidocaine (Xylocaine) *General:* thiopental (Pentothal)
Antacids	Neutralize hydrochloride in stomach or reduce its production	Hyperacidity, peptic ulcers	magaldrate (Riopan), calcium carbonate (Maalox)
Antianginals	Increased blood flow to the heart	Angina	nitroglycerine
Antiarrhythmics	Regulate rhythm of heartbeat	Cardiac arrhythmias	digoxin (Lanoxin), lidocaine
Anticholinergics	Increase heart rate Relax smooth muscle Reduce peristalsis Decrease secretions Dilate pupils	Reduce muscle spasm Treat bronchial asthma, peptic ulcers, and hypermobility of GI tract	atropine (Atropen), benztropine (Cogentin), ipratropium (Atrovent)
Anticoagulants	Inhibit blood clotting	Thrombophlebitis	warfarin sodium (Coumadin), heparin
Anticonvulsants	Prevent seizures or convulsions	Epilepsy, other neurological disorders	phenytoin (Dilantin), diazepam (Valium), phenobarbital
Antidepressants	Act as mood elevators	Psychotic or neurotic types of depression; anxiety	fluoxetine (Prozac), imipramine (Tofranil)
Oral hypoglycemics	Stimulate release of insulin from pancreas	Non–insulin-dependent (type 2) diabetes	metformin (Glucophage), pioglitazone (Actos), rosiglitazone (Avandia)
Antidiarrheals (antidiarrheics)	Inhibit diarrhea and hypermobility of GI tract	Diarrhea, flatulence, GI disorders	attapulgite (Kaopectate), diphenoxylate/atropine (Lomotil)
Antiemetics	Reduce vomiting and nausea Reduce vertigo	Treat or prevent nausea, vomiting, vertigo, and motion sickness	prochlorperazine (Compazine), trimethobenzamide (Tigan), meclizine (Antivert)
Antiflatulents	Relieve gastric or intestinal distention (usually used in combination with antacids)	Abdominal distention	simethicone (Phazyme)
Antihistamines	Reduce histamine produced in the body	Symptoms of allergies; treatment of ulcers	diphenhydramine (Benadryl), ranitidine (Zantac)
Antihypertensives	Reduce blood pressure by lessening resistance of blood flow, through relaxation of vasoconstricted peripheral vessels	Hypertension, migraine headache, arteriosclerosis	propranolol (Inderal), methyldopa (Aldomet), clonidine (Catapres)
Antiinfectives	Inhibit or kill growth of microorganisms	Disease caused by bacteria; used in viral infections to increase resistance to bacterial infection	penicillin, tetracycline, erythromycin, bacitracin (Polysporin), cephalexin (Keflex), ciprofloxacin (Cipro), sulfonamides (Bactrim, Septra)
Antiinflammatories	Steroidal or nonsteroidal; reduce inflammation	Arthritis, gout, and other inflammatory conditions	*Nonsteroidal:* naproxen (Naprosyn), ibuprofen, aspirin *Steroidal:* corticosteroids, prednisone

TABLE 43-7

Drug Classifications, Actions, and Uses—cont'd

Class	Action	Treatment Uses	Examples
Antineoplastics	Interfere with cell reproduction	Used in chemotherapy in treatment of cancer	L-asparaginase *Alkylating:* cyclophosphamide (Cytoxan), chlorambucil (Leukeran) *Antimetabolites:* 5-fluorouracil, cytarabine (Cytosar-U) *Antibiotic:* doxorubicin (Adriamycin)
Antiparkinsonians	Reduce nerve impulses causing tremors	Parkinsonian tremors	levodopa/carbidopa (Sinemet), levodopa (Larodopa)
Antipruritics	Relieve itching	Skin disorders; allergies that cause itching	calamine lotion, hydrocortisone ointment
Antipyretics	Reduce body temperature by febrile state; dilate peripheral vascular system	Pyrexia (fever)	aspirin, acetaminophen (Tylenol), ibuprofen (Motrin)
Antitussives	Decrease cough reflex	Cough suppressant in allergies or respiratory infections	dextromethorphan (Vicks 44)
Bronchodilators	Relax smooth muscle in bronchi	Asthma	albuterol (Proventil)
Diuretics	Increase removal of fluid from body tissues	Control edema in cardiac disease and hypertension	chlorothiazide (Diuril), furosemide (Lasix), spironolactone (Aldactone)
Expectorants	Help removal of mucus by liquefaction	Bronchitis and other respiratory conditions	guaifenesin (Robitussin)
Hematinics	Stimulate production of blood cells; increase amount of hemoglobin in blood	Anemias	ferrous sulfate (Feosol), ferrous fumarate (Femiron)
Hemostatics	Control bleeding or hemorrhage	Hemophilia; used in surgical procedures to stop or control bleeding	Gelfoam, fibrinogen, factor IX (Alpha Nine)
Hormones	Replace hormonal deficiencies in the body	Hypothyroidism, diabetes; other hormone replacement uses	levothyroxine (Synthroid), insulin, ovarian hormones, pituitary hormones, vasopressin (Pitressin)
Sedative-hypnotics	Act on CNS; interfere with nerve impulse transmission to brain Sedatives relax; hypnotics produce sleep, depress heart and respiration rates	Convulsions, insomnia	pentobarbital (Nembutal), secobarbital (Seconal), flurazepam (Dalmane)
Stimulants	Stimulate CNS; increase activity of vasomotor and respiratory centers of medulla Suppress fatigue and appetite	Exhaustion; specific abnormal patterns of behavior	caffeine, methylphenidate (Ritalin)
Tranquilizers	Reduce anxiety and tension; act as CNS depressants	Tension, anxiety; symptoms of neuroses and psychoses; muscle spasms	chlordiazepoxide (Librium), thioridazine (Mellaril), chlorpromazine (Thorazine)
Vaccines/toxoids	Antibodies provide passive immunity to disease; composed of certain "antigens," which are weakened disease-causing agents that cause body to manufacture its own antibodies	Prevent disease or lessen effect of disease	pneumococcal-7 valent conjugate (Prevnar), diphtheria and tetanus toxoids, diphtheria, pertussis, tetanus; measles, mumps; measles, mumps rubella; trivalent polio; tetanus toxoid; botulism antitoxin; diphtheria antitoxin
Vasodilators	Dilate blood vessels; usually used to increase peripheral circulation and blood flow to extremities	Specific drugs have specific actions; peripheral vascular disease, dysmenorrhea, angina, hypertension	nitroglycerin, verapamil (Calan), propranolol (Inderal)

CNS, Central nervous system; *GI,* gastrointestinal.

Unwanted Drug Effects

Along with the therapeutic effects, drugs may have unwanted effects as well. It is important to be aware of the side effects, adverse effects, and toxic effects of drugs, as well as contraindications to taking drugs.

Side Effects

Side effects are unwanted actions by a drug (e.g., dry mouth). All drugs have side effects, and some are more of a nuisance than harmful. Some side effects can even be beneficial. For example, diphenhydramine (Benadryl) is normally prescribed for allergies, but when ordered for bedtime, it is prescribed for sleep. Although side effects are unwanted, they are expected reactions.

Adverse Reactions

Adverse reactions are undesirable effects, and they may be harmful. For example, diarrhea or vomiting is an adverse effect of some antibiotics that may cause an electrolyte imbalance in the patient. Adverse reactions are both unwanted and unexpected.

Toxic Effects

Toxic effects, or **toxicity,** of a drug occurs when a drug accumulates in the body. For example, when giving the anticoagulant warfarin (Coumadin), levels need to be monitored to make certain the drug does not accumulate, exceeding the therapeutic levels and producing toxicity. In this case, excessive bleeding could occur.

Contraindications

Contraindications are factors (e.g., patient symptom or condition) indicating that a drug used under normal circumstances should not be prescribed because the risk of using the drug outweighs the benefit. For example, the rubella (measles) vaccine is safe, but it should not be given to women who are pregnant, people who are hypersensitive to neomycin or gelatin, and immunocompromised patients.

The pharmacy will attach warning labels to medications to alert the patient to special instructions or possible contraindications (Figure 43-15).

PATIENT-CENTERED PROFESSIONALISM

- How does the patient benefit when the medical assistant understands methods of drug classification?

PRESCRIPTIONS

A **prescription** is a legal document written by a licensed health care provider. It gives instructions to a pharmacist to provide a person with medication for a specific time in a specific amount (Figure 43-16). Table 43-8 lists the most common prescriptions that are filled and dispensed. A prescription is divided into the following sections:

TABLE 43-8

Common Prescriptions (New and Refill) Dispensed*

Brand Name (Manufacturer)	Generic Name
hydrocodone w/APAP (various)	hydrocodone w/APAP*
Lipitor (Pfizer)	atorvastatin
atenolol (various)	atenolol
Synthroid (Abbott)	levothyroxine
Premarin (Wyeth)	conjugated estrogens
Zithromax (Pfizer)	azithromycin
furosemide (various)	furosemide
amoxicillin (various)	amoxicillin
Norvasc (Pfizer)	amlodipine
hydrochlorothiazide (various)	hydrochlorothiazide
albuterol aerosol (various)	albuterol
Zoloft (Pfizer)	sertraline
Paxil (GlaxoSmithKline)	paroxetine
Zocor (MSD)	simvastatin
Prevacid (Tap Pharm)	lansoprazole
ibuprofen (various)	Ibuprofen
Toprol-XL (AstraZeneca)	metoprolol
Celebrex (Pharmacia Upjohn)	celecoxib
Zyrtec (Pfizer)	cetirizine
Levoxyl (Monarch Pharm)	levothyroxine
Allegra (Hoech Mar R)	fexofenadine
Ortho Tri-Cyclen (Ortho-McNeil)	norgestimate/ethinyl estradiol
Celexa (Forest Pharm)	citalopram
prednisone (various)	prednisone
Prilosec (AstraZeneca)	omeprazole
fluoxetine (various)	fluoxetine
acetaminophen/codeine (various)	acetaminophen/codeine
Ambien (Sanofi)	zolpidem
metoprolol tartrate (various)	metoprolol
lorazepam (various)	lorazepam
Fosamax (MSD)	alendronate
propoxyphene N-APAP (various)	propoxyphene N-APAP
Nexium (AstraZeneca)	esomeprazole
Singulair (MSD)	montelukast
Effexor XR (Wyeth)	venlafaxine

From www.rxlist.com/top200.htm.
APAP, Acetaminophen.
*Note that some popular drugs are prescribed in more than one strength or by specific brand name(s), as well as by generic name.

---

1. Physician demographics section is preprinted and provides the physician's name, address, and phone number.
2. Patient demographics section provides information about the patient (date, written name, address, age [if a child], and phone number).
3. **Superscription** section is where the symbol "Rx" appears; this means "to take" ("take thou") or "recipe."
4. **Inscription** line provides a place for the name of the medication ordered, its strength, and the drug's form.
5. **Subscription** section provides directions to the pharmacist for filling the prescription. This includes the number of doses and the quantity to be dispensed.
6. **Sig,** or **signature,** means "to write on label," and this section provides directions for the patient to include how much to

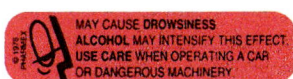
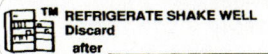
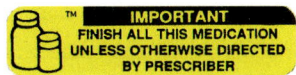
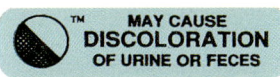
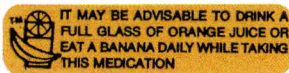
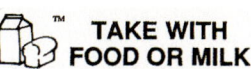

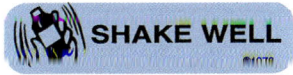
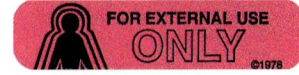
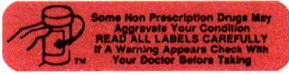
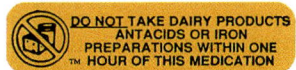
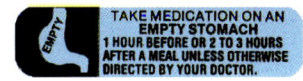

Swallow Whole. Do Not Chew Or Crush.

Do Not Take Aspirin Or Aspirin Containing Products Without Knowledge And Consent Of Your Physician.

Do Not Drink Alcoholic Beverages While Taking This Medicine.

Take This Medicine With A Snack Or Small Meal If Stomach Upset Occurs.

Do Not Use This Medicine If You Are Pregnant, Plan To Become Pregnant, Or Are Breastfeeding. Check With Your Doctor Or Pharmacist.

Read The Patient Information Leaflet That Came With This Medicine.

Take Or Use This Medicine Exactly As Directed. Do Not Skip Doses Or Discontinue Unless Directed By Your Doctor.

Obtain Medical Advice Before Taking Nonprescription Drugs. Some May Affect The Action Of This Medication.

Take Or Use This Medicine Exactly As Directed. Do Not Skip Doses Or Discontinue Unless Directed By Your Doctor.

Some Nonprescription Drugs May Aggravate Your Condition. If You Have Questions, Check With Your Doctor Or Pharmacist.

FIGURE 43-15 Warning labels attached to medication containers to alert the patient of special instructions. (From Zakus SM: *Mosby's clinical skills for medical assistants*, ed 4, St Louis, 2001, Mosby.)

take, how often to take, and in some cases, for how long and why. Table 43-9 lists common drug abbreviations.

7. Physician's signature line allows the physician to sign, thereby providing authorization for the drug to be dispensed by the pharmacist.
8. Refill line or box indicates how many times the prescription can be refilled and must be written on the label. Prescriptions cannot be refilled after 1 year, even if refills remain on the label.
9. DEA number line allows for the prescribing of controlled substances; it should be left blank for the physician to write in the number to prevent forgery of prescriptions for controlled substances.

The prescription form can vary in appearance. Some even have a box to indicate or to be checked for refills and labeling. Others have a preprinted line stating, "Dispense as written," which prevents the substitution of generic drugs. Some forms have a preprinted "yes/no" box that can be checked to indicate whether generic drugs are an acceptable substitute.

A survey published by *Med Track Alert* (http://www.mta.com/content/survey) found that 23% of Americans loan their prescription medications to someone else and 27% have borrowed prescription drugs. The drugs most frequently shared were allergy drugs (25%), painkillers (22%), and antibiotics (21%). Sharing medications can carry significant risks by producing unwanted drug effects. Remember, there are many factors affecting amount of drug prescribed and effectiveness (see Box 43-2).

In October 2008, all Medicaid prescriptions must be written on paper that is tamper-resistant. The CMS outlines that all prescription paper have the following three baseline characteristics:

Joan Smith, M.D.
456 Anywhere Lane
Right City USA 00020
Office (555-123-4567)
Fax (555-321-7654)

Patient Name Grace Wise **DOB** 07/30/43 **Date** 02/14/XX

Address 999 North Main St. Right City, USA 00020

℞ } **Superscription**

Inscription { Prevacid 30 mg

Subscription { Disp: #30 (thirty)

Signature { Sig: ṫ po QD

☒ **Dispense as written**

☐ **May substitute generic**

Refill None 1 2 3 4 ⑤

Signature: Joan Smith MD

DEA#:

FIGURE 43-16 Example of a prescription.

1. Prevent unauthorized copying of a completed or blank prescription form
2. Prevent the erasure or modification of information written on the prescription form by the prescriber
3. Prevent the use of counterfeit prescription forms

Each state is responsible for defining specific features that meet these criteria.

FOR YOUR INFORMATION

SUPERBUGS: ANTIBIOTIC RESISTANCE

In the 1940s, penicillin was first prescribed to treat an infectious disease. Since that time, over 150 antibiotics have been developed to halt the spread of infectious disease. Frequent use of antibiotics has given rise to bacteria that are resistant to many antibiotics. Superbugs emerge when an antibiotic fails to kill the bacteria it targets, and the surviving bacteria become resistant to that particular drug.

The consequences of this action are that as more bacteria become resistant to first-line treatments, illnesses last longer, side effects can be severe, and alternative medications usually cost significantly more. For example, the medications needed to treat multidrug-resistant forms of tuberculosis (TB) are 100 times more expensive than those needed to treat nonresistant TB.

ELECTRONIC PRESCRIBING

Electronic prescribing (E-prescribing) is thought to be a solution to the medical errors caused by the current paper-based prescriptions. Many of the same arguments used to encourage the use of Electronic Medical Records are used to encourage the use of E-prescribing. E-prescribing allows the sharing of prescription information among health care providers, thus improving the quality of patient care. The fact is medical errors can be reduced because the software used provides instant notification of drug interactions, drug allergy reactions, dosing errors, and therapeutic duplications. Efficiency would be improved since it would reduce the need for pharmacy callbacks caused by hard-to-read handwriting and the physician not prescribing the preferred drug for the patient's drug insurance plan. A prescription can be transmitted from the physician's office directly to the patient's pharmacy of choice.

A refill request would be entered into the pharmacy's system, and it is checked against availability of refills. If a refill is not available, the software system automatically routes a request to the physician's system that contains a patient's past medication history. The physician will also have available to them the number of refill requests and the number of different pharmacies at which a patient has tried to file a refill request.

TABLE 43-9
Commonly Used Drug Abbreviations

Abbreviation	Meaning	Abbreviation	Meaning
Ā	before	#	number (of tablets to disperse)
aa	of each	os	mouth
Ac	before meals	otic	ear
amt	amount	oz	ounce
Aq	water	p̄	after
Bid	twice a day	pc	after meals
c̄	with	per	by
Cap	capsule	po	by mouth
DAW	dispense as written	prn	when necessary
Dil	dilute	pulv	powder
disp	dispense	q	every
dr, d	dram	qam	every morning
Elix	elixir	q2h	every 2 hours
Et	and	qh	every hour
Fl	fluid	qid	four times a day
g, G, GM	gram	qs	quantity sufficient
GI	gastrointestinal	qns	quantity not sufficient
Gr	grain	®	right, or rectal
gtt, gtts	drop, drops	Rx	to take
GU	genitourinary	Tx	treatment or therapy
H₂O	water	s̄	without
ID	intradermal	SubQ	subcutaneously
IM	intramuscular	Sig	write or label
IV	intravenous	SL	sublingual
Kg	kilogram	sol	solution
L	liter	stat	immediately
Ⓛ	left	syr	syrup
mcg	microgram	tab	tablet
mEq	milliequivalent	tbsp	tablespoon
m, ♏	minim	tid	three times a day
ML	milliliter	tsp	teaspoon
NKA	no known allergy	ud	take as directed
Ns, NS, N/S	normal saline	X	times
Pt	pint or patient		

MEDICATION RECORD

The medical office must keep a record of all medications the patient takes, whether prescription or OTC drugs. The form is often preprinted and is always a part of the patient's medical record (Figure 43-17). The medication record is started when the patient is first seen and updated with each visit or refill request by telephone. The date, the name of the medication, and the frequency taken are recorded.

PATIENT-CENTERED PROFESSIONALISM

- Why must the medical assistant be aware of the purpose of the prescription form and the information required to complete it?

CONCLUSION

Advances in science and technology now give physicians many choices in finding the most appropriate medication to treat, prevent, or diagnose diseases. Medications may be part of the prescribed treatment plan, so it is important for medical assistants to understand what the drugs are and what they do. With this understanding, medical assistants can help educate patients and encourage them to follow their treatment plans. In addition, medical assistants may be responsible for administering some types of medications in the medical office.

To perform these tasks effectively, medical assistants need basic pharmacology knowledge, including understanding of the Controlled Substances Act, and must understand considerations associated with administration of drugs, calculation of drug dosages, immunizations, forms and classifications of drugs, prescriptions, and documentation.

MEDICATION RECORD

Patient Name Marilyn DeMarce   **DOB** 03/15/52
Primary Care Physician Dr. Spence

ALLERGY (Drug)	ALLERGY (Food)
Codeine	Eggs

IMMUNIZATION RECORD

Tetanus 7/06/09	Flu vaccine	
Pneumonia vaccine 9/20/09		
Hepatitis B		

OTC Drugs

ASA 81mg tab daily		

DATE	MEDICATION AND DOSAGE	FREQUENCY	REFILLS	STOP
2/09/09	Fluoxetine 40 mg	† QD po	8/10	
2/09/09	Premarin 0.3 mg	† HS po	8/10	
2/09/09	Medroxyprogesterone 2.5 mg	† HS po	8/10	
8/15/09	Zyrtec-D 5mg/120 mg	† tab 2x qd		
8/15/09	Cipro 250 mg	† po bid x 7 days		8/22/09

FIGURE 43-17 Example of a medication record.

Chapter Summary

Reinforce your understanding of the material in this chapter by reviewing the curriculum objectives and key content points below.

1. **Define, appropriately use, and spell all the Key Terms for this chapter.**
   - Review the Key Terms if necessary.
2. **Define pharmacology, and differentiate between pharmacodynamics and pharmacokinetics.**
   - Pharmacology is the study of drugs and their effect on the body.
   - Pharmacodynamics studies the biochemical and physiological effects of drugs within the body.
   - Pharmacokinetics studies the action of a drug from the time it enters the body until it leaves.
3. **List five reasons why drugs are prescribed by a health care professional.**
   - Drugs are prescribed for curative, diagnostic, prophylactic, replacement, and therapeutic purposes.
4. **Briefly describe the three ways drugs can be identified by name.**
   - The chemical name reflects the chemical composition or formula of the drug.
   - The generic (nonproprietary) name of a drug is its official (or legal) name and indicates its chemical structure or makeup.
   - The trade (proprietary) or brand name is used to market the drug by the pharmaceutical manufacturer and displays the symbol ®.
5. **List three factors that determine the dosage prescribed by the health care practitioner for a patient.**
   - Age, weight, and gender determine dosage; other factors include electrolyte balance, disease processes, and tolerance.

6. **Differentiate between average dose and cumulative dose and between lethal dose and toxic dose.**
   - The average dose is the amount of medication proven to be effective with minimal side effects for an adult. The cumulative dose is the total amount of medication in the body after repeated doses, or medication that accumulates in the body over time.
   - A lethal dose is the amount of medication that proves deadly to a patient. A toxic dose is the amount of medication that brings about signs and symptoms of toxicity or harmful side effects.
7. **State the purpose of the Controlled Substances Act of 1970, and identify the organization established to set standards for drug products and its role in enforcement.**
   - The Controlled Substances Act of 1970 was passed to control the use of opioid analgesics, tranquilizers, and stimulants.
   - The Drug Enforcement Administration (DEA) enforces the Controlled Substances Act.
8. **Describe the process for applying for and renewing DEA registration numbers and certificates.**
   - Form DEA-224 is used to apply for a DEA number.
   - Form DEA-224a is used to renew a DEA number.
9. **List five rules that must be followed with controlled substances.**
   Rules exist concerning the records and documentation that must be done when working with controlled substances, in addition to the type of storage needed and what should be done if controlled drugs are broken, spilled accidentally, or stolen.
   - Records concerning the dispensing and administration of controlled drugs must be kept for a minimum of 2 years.
   - A progress note must be in the patient's record concerning the prescribing or administration of controlled drugs.
   - A complete written inventory must be done every 2 years for all controlled drugs, and records must be kept an additional 2 years.
   - Controlled drugs must be in a locked cabinet, separate from other drugs (e.g., samples).
   - Theft of controlled drugs must be reported to the local authorities and to the DEA. If a controlled substance is accidentally broken or spilled, its disposal must be witnessed by two people and logged in the controlled substance logbook.
10. **Describe the five drug schedules and list two examples of drugs from each.**
    - Schedule I drugs have no accepted medical use.
    - Schedule II drugs must be kept separate from other drugs, must have separate inventory records, and require a written prescription.
    - Review Table 43-3.
11. **Describe the inventory, ordering, and storage requirements for controlled substances.**
    - Careful inventory records must be established and maintained if a medical facility stocks controlled substances.
    - Form DEA-222 must be used to order Schedule II drugs; Schedules III, IV, and V drugs only require a logbook with the invoice number from the supplier.
    - Controlled substances must be kept separate from other drugs and in a locked cabinet.
12. **List four drug references and explain their value for physicians and medical assistants.**
    - The *U.S. Pharmacopeia* and *National Formulary* (USP/NF), Drug Facts and Comparisons, package inserts, and *Physicians' Desk Reference* (PDR) are four important drug references.
    - Drug references allow physicians and medical assistants to identify medications and locate information about products easily.
13. **List the "seven rights" of drug administration and state the purpose of each.**
    - Right patient, right drug, right dose, right route, right time, right technique, and right documentation.
    - Following the "seven rights" of drug administration helps avoid medication errors.
14. **Calculate the correct dose of a medication to be administered.**
    - The most important part of administering a drug is providing the correct amount.
    - When calculating a dose, the same measurements must be used in the calculation as in the order.
15. **Convert dosage measurements to grains, grams, milligrams, pounds, and kilograms.**
    - Review Table 43-5 for measurement equivalents.
16. **Explain how the body weight and body surface area (BSA) methods are used to determine pediatric doses.**
    - The body weight method is preferred over the BSA method because it requires using the body weight in kilograms times the total amount of milligrams of medication desired per day.
    - The BSA method uses a nomogram chart.
17. **Demonstrate the correct procedure for preparing an immunization record and filing it properly in the patient's record.**
    - Review Procedure 43-1.
18. **Discuss the immunization schedule for children and explain the time frame in which reactions can occur.**
    - Timing of immunizations is important to obtain proper levels needed for production of antibodies.
    - Review Figure 43-11.
    - Review Figure 43-12.
19. **List solid, liquid, and semisolid forms of drugs.**
    - Liquid forms include solutions, suspensions, emulsions, tinctures, lotions, liniments, elixirs, syrups, and aerosols.
    - Solid forms include tablets, capsules, caplets, gel caps, spansules, powders, and lozenges.
    - Semisolid forms include patches, suppositories, ointments, and creams.
20. **List five characteristics by which drugs can be classified.**
    - Drugs can be classified by their area of effect (local or systemic), their therapeutic effect, how they work, the systems they affect, and their chemical structure.
21. **Differentiate among side effects, adverse reactions, and toxic effects.**
    - Side effects are unwanted actions that are not necessarily harmful and may be beneficial, but are expected.

- Adverse reactions are undesirable effects that may be harmful and are not expected.
- Toxic effects are unwanted actions that can produce toxicity.

22. **Explain what contraindications are and what the pharmacy does to alert patients to special instructions.**
    - Contraindications refer to circumstances when a drug should not be prescribed to a patient.
    - Pharmacies attach warning labels to medications to alert patients to special instructions.
23. **List the nine pieces of information included in a prescription.**
    - The physician's and the patient's demographics, superscription, inscription, subscription, signature, physician's signature line, refill line or box, and DEA number line are included in a prescription.
24. **Explain the considerations for keeping a record of all medications a patient is taking.**
    - The medical record must contain a record of all medications a patient is taking, whether prescription or OTC drugs, to prevent interactions.
25. **Analyze a realistic medical office situation and apply your understanding of medications to determine the best course of action.**
    - Medical assistants must understand and apply the legal and ethical aspects of working with medications.
26. **Describe the impact on patient care when medical assistants understand the purpose and considerations for pharmacology and how medications are regulated and prescribed.**
    - It is critical for medical assistants to understand the use and purpose of medications so that they can help educate patients and encourage them to follow their treatment plans.
    - In addition, medical assistants are responsible for administering some types of medications.

PRACTICAL APPLICATIONS

If you have accomplished the objectives in this chapter, you will be able to make better choices as a medical assistant. Take another look at this situation and decide what you would do.

Glenn is a medical assistant in an office of a family physician. His employer, Dr. Carbello, sees patients of all ages. Because Glenn lives in a state where medical assistants are allowed to phone in prescriptions to the pharmacy, one of his regular duties is to call in prescriptions. Glenn is also responsible for performing the inventory on scheduled medications. Today, Dr. Carbello has asked Glenn to call a pharmacy with a prescription for meperidine for a patient who has a severe pain in her back.

After examining another patient, Mrs. Vouch, Dr. Carbello orders an antihistamine for itching, to be given by injection, and an antipyretic. Dr. Carbello tells Glenn to be sure that he tells Mrs. Vouch the side effects of the medications. Mrs. Vouch is also given a prescription for the antihistamine and antipyretic to take at home. The antihistamine is a capsule, and the antipyretic is a tablet. Both these medications have systemic effects, and both can have indications of a toxic effect. As Mrs. Vouch leaves the office, Glenn asks her to call in the next week to tell him how the medications are helping with the itching.

If you were Glenn, would you be able to explain the side effects of the medications to Mrs. Vouch?

1. What is the importance of doing an inventory of Schedule II medications in the medical office?
2. Can Glenn call in a Schedule II medication? Why or why not?
3. What type of illness would you expect to be treated with an antihistamine?
4. What is the purpose of an antipyretic? What are some of the common antipyretics?
5. What are the "seven rights" that Glenn must follow when giving medications?
6. If Glenn does not know the interactions and the side effects of the antihistamine, what resource can he use to obtain this information?
7. What is the difference between a side effect and an adverse reaction?
8. What is the difference between a capsule and a tablet?
9. What is the difference between a "systemic effect" and a "local effect"? Give an example of each.
10. Why is it important for Glenn to explain "toxic effect" when the patient will be taking the medication at home on a regular basis?
11. What should Glenn document in the medical record at the office visit? What should he document when Mrs. Vouch calls in the next week?
12. Why is it important for Glenn to understand a drug's actions before giving the drug?
13. How are administering, prescribing, and dispensing a medication different?
14. How are the chemical name, generic name, and trade name of a medication different?

WEB SEARCH

1. **Research possible interactions when medications and herbal supplements are taken together.** Patients do not always provide information on herbal preparations that they are taking with their prescribed medications. The interaction between these drugs could be harmful to the patient. The medical assistant must be aware of this fact when asking patients for their list of "current medications."
    - **Keywords:** Use the following keywords in your search: herbal preparations, medication interactions, mixing medications.

44 Administering Medications

evolve http://evolve.elsevier.com/klieger/medicalassisting

As discussed in Chapter 43, medications can be administered by a variety of routes and in various forms, including oral, topical, vaginal and rectal, inhalation, and parenteral. This chapter discusses how each type of preparation is administered and what supplies and equipment are needed to administer these medications.

The selection of a drug route is based on the desired action on the body. For example, *systemic* action is chosen for general body aches, whereas application of a *topical* drug works well for localized pain. If the effects of a drug need to reach the body quickly, a *parenteral* route is selected (e.g., intravenous, intramuscular, or subcutaneous) because oral medications do not reach the bloodstream as fast and their onset of action is slower. A patient's physical and emotional state also must be taken into consideration when determining a route of administration. For example, an unconscious patient or someone unable to swallow will not be given medications orally.

The route chosen by the physician will be selected in terms of patient safety and the metabolism of the drug. All medications must be administered correctly. Injury or even death can result if medications are calculated or administered incorrectly. As a medical assistant, your goals when administering medications must provide patient safety. Be knowledgeable about the medications you are asked to administer. Use a drug reference if necessary. Never administer medications that you have not prepared yourself.

LEARNING OBJECTIVES

You will be able to do the following after completing this chapter:

Key Terms
1. Define, appropriately use, and spell all the Key Terms for this chapter.

Oral Administration
2. List the two forms of oral medication.
3. State three advantages of oral administration of medication.
4. Demonstrate the correct procedure for administering oral medications.

Topical Administration
5. List four forms of topical medication.
6. Demonstrate the correct procedure for applying a transdermal patch.

Vaginal and Rectal Administration
7. List three types of medications that can be inserted into the vaginal cavity.
8. Explain why medications for nausea and vomiting are often given rectally.

Inhalation
9. List three forms in which medications can be inhaled.
10. Explain how a nebulizer works.
11. Demonstrate the correct procedure for administering medication using a metered-dose inhaler with the closed-mouth technique.

Parenteral Administration
12. List one advantage and one disadvantage of parenteral administration of medication.
13. List five types of equipment used for parenteral administration of medication and explain the use of each.
14. Demonstrate the correct procedure for reconstituting a powdered medication to its proper dosage form.
15. Demonstrate the correct procedure for preparing a medication for injection by drawing it into a syringe from a vial.
16. Demonstrate the correct procedure for preparing a medication for injection by drawing it into a syringe from an ampule.

17. List four guidelines to help prevent accidental needlesticks.
18. List anatomical sites for administering intradermal, subcutaneous, and intramuscular injections.
19. Demonstrate the correct procedure for administering an intradermal injection.
20. Demonstrate the correct procedure for administering a subcutaneous injection.
21. Demonstrate the correct procedure for giving an infant an intramuscular injection, such as an immunization.
22. Demonstrate the correct procedure for administering an intramuscular injection to an adult.
23. Demonstrate the correct procedure for administering intramuscular medication using the Z-track injection technique.
24. List four categories of intravenous solutions.

Patient-Centered Professionalism

25. Analyze a realistic medical office situation and apply your understanding of medication administration to determine the best course of action.
26. Describe the impact on patient care when medical assistants understand the guidelines, safety requirements, and proper techniques for administering medications in the medical office.

PRACTICAL APPLICATIONS

Read the following scenario and keep it in mind as you learn about administering medications.

Sue, a medical assistant with no formal training, has been asked by her employer, Dr. Kenyon, to give Dylan, age 3 years, a single dose of acetaminophen, 250 mg. Dylan's record shows that he is allergic to penicillin and has had a severe rash in the past. Sue goes to the medicine cabinet and removes amoxicillin, 250-mg tablets, and takes a single tablet to Dylan. Sue does not bother to read the label except when taking the medication from the shelf. Dylan's mother tells Sue that her child is unable to swallow the tablet, but Sue continues to give the tablet, telling the mother that at age 3, Dylan should be able to swallow a tablet.

Sue leaves Dylan and his mother with the tablet. Margie, the other medical assistant in the office, asks Sue to prepare a medication for Mrs. Abbott, who needs a 1-mL estrogen injection. Margie tells Sue that this aqueous medication will be given intramuscularly and that she will be back to give the medication. In preparing the estrogen medication from a vial, Sue shakes the medicine and then draws it into a 5-ml syringe with a 25-gauge ⅝-inch needle. Margie returns and gives the medication that Sue prepared.

In the meantime, Dylan has choked on the tablet and is having difficulty breathing. Because Sue left the room, she is unaware of the situation. When Dr. Kenyon arrives in the room, he immediately recognizes a problem and calls in both Sue and Margie to help remove the tablet from Dylan's throat.

What would you have done differently as a medical assistant?

KEY TERMS

administration set	lumen
ampule	maintenance solutions
antipyretics	Mantoux test
aqueous	meniscus
aspiration	metered-dose inhaler (MDI)
beveled	nebulizer
bleb	ointment
buccal	oral
catheter	parenteral
cream	prefilled cartridge unit
deltoid muscle	shaft
dorsogluteal	spacer
drip rate	subcutaneous (SubQ) injection
enteral	sublingual
enteric-coated	suppository
gauge	syringe
heparin lock	topical
hub	transdermal patch
hydrating solutions	vastus lateralis muscle
hypertonic solutions	ventrogluteal
induration	vial
intradermal (ID) injection	wheal
intramuscular (IM) injection	winged infusion needles
intravenous (IV) therapy	Z-track method
isotonic solutions	
lotion	

ORAL ADMINISTRATION

The **oral** (or **enteral**) route of administering medication is the most frequently used method. Three advantages of the oral method of administration include the following:

1. Oral administration is considered the safest method because medications given can be retrieved easily if necessary.
2. Oral medications do not require special equipment.
3. Oral medications can usually be taken by the patient easily.

One disadvantage of the oral route is the possible aspiration of oral medications into the respiratory tract.

Oral medications are administered in either *solid* (e.g., tablet, capsule) or *liquid* (e.g., syrup, suspension) form. Oral drugs can be swallowed, or they can be absorbed through the mucous membranes into the bloodstream by placing the medication under the tongue (**sublingual**) or between the cheek and gum (**buccal**). Chapter 43 includes conversion techniques for calculating dosages ordered from drug labels for various types of administration. Completing the workbook exercises will help build your confidence in these calculations. Procedure 44-1 outlines the proper technique for dispensing solid

| PROCEDURE 44-1 | Administer Oral Medication | |

TASKS:
- Interpret the physician's orders for administering the oral medication.
- Calculate the required dose of the prescribed medication.
- Pour and measure an accurate dose of the prescribed medication.
- Document the medication administration in the patient's medical record.

EQUIPMENT AND SUPPLIES
- Medication ordered by physician (liquid or solid)
- Disposable medication cup (calibrated)
- Water, when appropriate
- Patient's medical record

SKILLS/RATIONALE

STANDARD PRECAUTIONS ARE TO BE FOLLOWED.

1. **Procedural Step. Sanitize the hands.**
   An alcohol-based hand rub may be used instead of washing hands with soap and water, unless hands are visibly soiled.
   Rationale. Hand sanitization promotes infection control.

2. **Procedural Step. Assemble equipment and supplies and verify the order.**
   Medications in the medical office should be organized for safety by placing them with the labels showing and grouping medications in alphabetical order according to their use and route or by action or class (as per office policy). Medications should always be stored in their original containers.
   Rationale. It is important to have all supplies and equipment ready and available before starting any procedure to ensure efficiency.

3. **Procedural Step. Check the expiration date of the medication.**
   NOTE: The expiration date on stored medications should be checked on a regular basis. Medications that have expired should be disposed of properly.
   Rationale. Medications used past expiration date may be inactive.

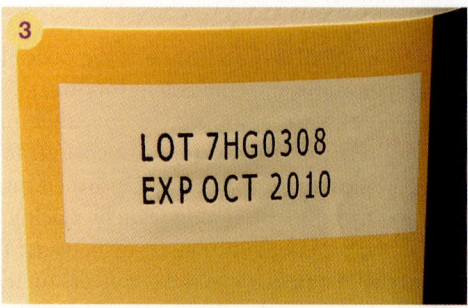

4. **Procedural Step. Follow the "seven rights" of medication administration:**
   Right drug—Check the label of the medication against the written order three times before administering the medication.
   Right dose—If the dose ordered does not match the dosage available, perform an accurate calculation to determine the correct dose.
   Right patient—Take the patient's medical record into the examination room and use it to verify the patient's identity before administering the medication.
   Right route—Check the written order to clarify the route of administration. If there are questions about the route, clarify the order with the health care provider.
   Right time—In the medical office, the time of day is usually less important than the interval between doses. Verify that the correct amount of time has passed since the last dose of the medication if the order is for a repeated dose.
   Right technique—Become familiar with the proper techniques for all routes of administration, and use the technique appropriate for the medication being administered.
   Right documentation—Immediately after giving the medication to the patient, document the details of the administration in the patient's medical record.

5. **Procedural Step. Select the right drug.**
   If the medication is unfamiliar, read the package insert or use a drug reference.

6. **Procedural Step. Perform the first of three checks of the medication.**
   Verify that the medication name on the label matches the medication name in the written orders.

Continued

PROCEDURE 44-1 Administer Oral Medication—cont'd

7. **Procedural Step.** Read the dosage information on the label and calculate the right dose using the following formula:

$$H \div D = Q$$

The components of this formula are as follows:

D is the *desired dose*, which is the amount of medication ordered.

H is the *available strength*, which is the amount of medication per dose as listed on the label.

Q is the *quantity*, which is the dose to be administered, or number of tablets, capsules, or other drug form, and contains the dose ordered.

NOTE: The dosage information is always on the medication label. It may be in small print and difficult to find, but it is always there.

8. **Procedural Step. Perform the second check of the medication against the written order.**

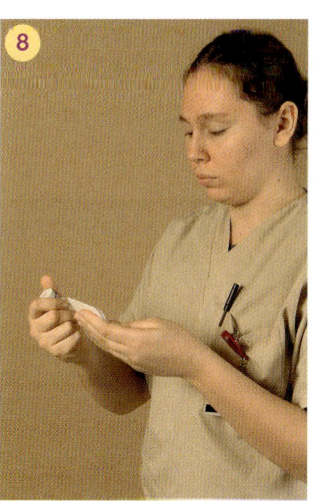

9. **Procedural Step.** Prepare the right dose and perform the third check before returning the medication to storage.

For *solid medication*, pour the required number of capsules, tablets, or other form into the bottle cap and transfer medication into a medication cup.

NOTE: Do not touch inside of the cup or lid of bottle.

For *liquid medication,* if it is a suspension, the medication must be gently shaken before pouring. Roll the medication between the palms of the hands to mix or rotate the bottle back and forth.

Rationale. Pouring solid medication into the lid prevents contamination of the medication and lid. Mixing liquid medication in this way prevents air bubbles. Continuing to check reduces the risk for error.

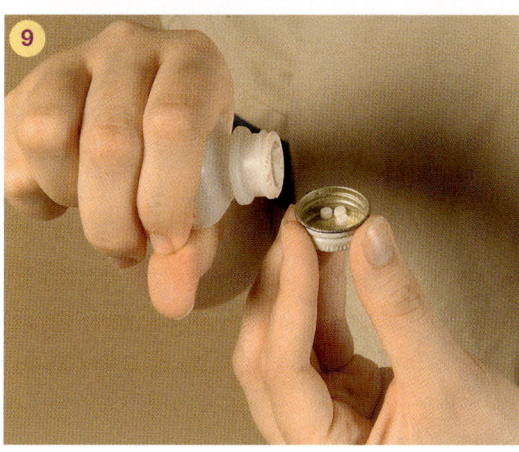

LIQUID MEDICATION

10. **Procedural Step. Remove the lid of the bottle and place it inside up on the counter.**

    Rationale. The contents of the medication container are sterile, as is the inside of the lid. Placing it inside up on the counter helps prevent contamination.

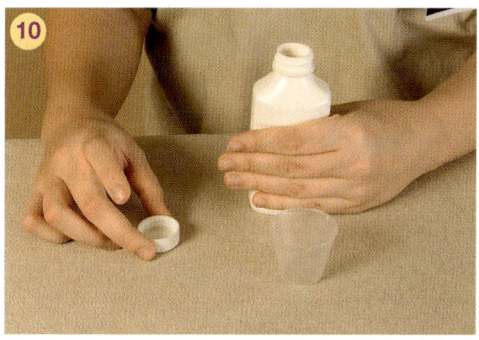

11. **Procedural Step.** When preparing to pour liquid medication, pick the bottle up so your palm covers the label, called "palming the label."

    Rationale. This keeps the label clean in case the liquid runs down the side of the bottle or spills.

12. **Procedural Step.** Determine how much liquid medication to pour.

    Locate the line on the medication cup that marks the volume representing the calculated dose. Place a thumbnail against the line to assist in measuring the correct amount when pouring.

13. **Procedural Step.** Pour the medication.

    Hold the medication cup at eye level when pouring to observe the level of the meniscus, which is the curved surface of the liquid. The *bottom* of the meniscus should touch the correct dose line on the medication cup.

Continued

PROCEDURE 44-1   Administer Oral Medication—cont'd

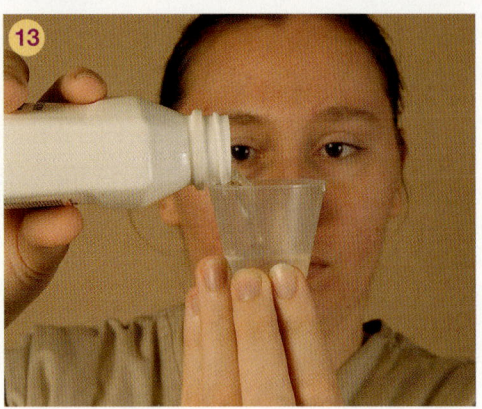

14. **Procedural Step.** Place the cup on a flat surface, and recheck the meniscus.
    Rationale. This ensures the medication has been poured accurately
15. **Procedural Step.** Before returning the bottle to the cabinet, perform the third check against the written order.
16. **Procedural Step.** Carry the medication cup carefully to avoid spilling.
    You may place it on a small tray if your office uses them.
17. **Procedural Step.** Administer the medication.
    Check to make sure that you have the *right patient* and that the patient is not allergic to the medication. Then use the *right technique* to administer the medication via the *right route* at the *right time*.
18. **Procedural Step.** Offer water to the patient, if appropriate.

Water is offered to patients who take solid oral medications such as tablets or capsules. Although not necessary with liquid medications, water may be offered as long as it will not dilute the medication. (Water should not be offered if the medication is a cough syrup, if indicated by the physician.)
NOTE: Liquid oral medications are ideal for children. A child who is able to hold a cup may take liquid medications in a medication cup. Children who are too young to hold a cup may be given liquid medications in an oral syringe, by dropper, or by a special medicine spoon.

19. **Procedural Step.** Remain with the patient until the medication has been swallowed.
    If the patient experiences any unusual reactions or serious or immediate side effects, notify the physician immediately.
20. **Procedural Step.** Sanitize the hands.
    Always sanitize the hands after every procedure or after using gloves.
21. **Procedural Step.** Document the administration of the medication.
    Use Box 44-1 as a guide.

CHARTING EXAMPLE

Date	
7/1/xx	9:30 a.m. Acetaminophen, 650 mg tabs, po. No reaction observed. ——————— ——————————— B. Thomas, RMA

and liquid oral medications. Box 44-1 reviews the necessary criteria for charting all medications administered.

Drug Action

Typically, the action of oral drugs takes 30 to 60 minutes. However, changes in the gastrointestinal (GI) tract brought on by food, physical activity, or emotions can accelerate or delay the absorption of oral medications. Some medications can be irritating to the stomach, causing nausea, gastric irritation, and heartburn. To minimize these effects, some medications have a special coating that allows them to pass through the stomach and enter the small intestine before being absorbed. These are referred to as **enteric-coated** medications.

Guidelines

General guidelines for preparing and administering oral medications are as follows:

BOX 44-1
Documentation when Charting Administered Medications

1. Date
2. Time
3. Name of medication
4. Dose administered
5. Injection site, if used
6. Patient reaction, if any (record waiting time)
7. Patient education provided
8. Proper signature and credential

1. Pour the required number of tablets, capsules, or other solid form of medication into the cap of the drug container, and then transfer them to a medication cup. If the medication is a unit dose (premeasured, individually packaged medication), place it directly into the medication cup.

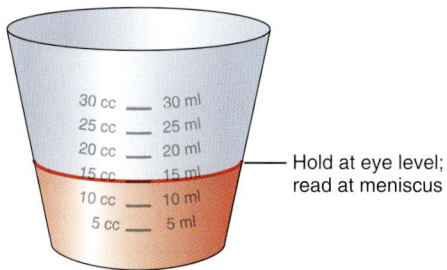

FIGURE 44-1 Medication cup containing 15 cc (mL) of medicine. (From Hunt SA: *Saunders fundamentals of medical assisting—revised reprint,* St Louis, 2007, Saunders.)

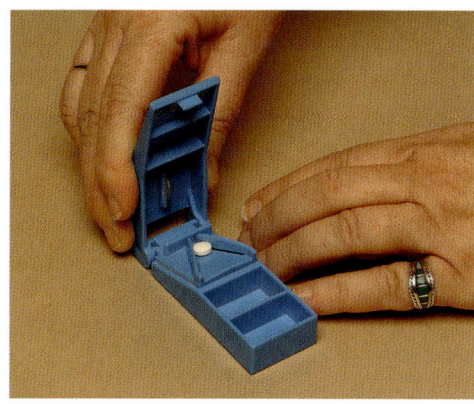

FIGURE 44-3 A "pill splitter" is used to halve scored pills.

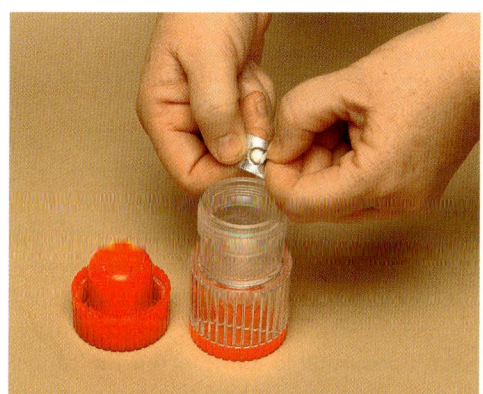

FIGURE 44-2 A pill is placed in the medication "crusher." The top is screwed onto the crusher and turned until the pill is crushed.

> **BOX 44-2**
>
> ### Examples of Tablets Not To Be Crushed*
>
> | | |
> |---|---|
> | Cardizem | Norflex |
> | Drixoral | OxyContin |
> | Entex | Phazyme |
> | Glucotrol | Procanbid |
> | Isordil | Respa |
> | Levbid | Sinemet |
> | Lithobid | Tiamate |
> | Niaspan | |
>
> *These examples are provided as illustration. This list is *not* a complete list of *all* tablets that should not be crushed. Always research any drug with which you are unfamiliar.

Do not touch the medication with the finger or hands, to avoid contamination.

2. When pouring liquid medication, shake well if it is a suspension. Hold the medicine cup at eye level and pour the required dose by observing the level of the **meniscus**. To recheck the poured amount, place the medication cup on a flat surface and read the level at the lowest point of the curve, called the meniscus (Figure 44-1). Always pour liquid medications into a marked (measured) container, never guess at the amount.
3. If a patient has difficulty swallowing, some pills can be ground in a medication "crusher" (Figure 44-2) and given in applesauce or pudding, but only if the manufacturer states this can be done. The amount of applesauce or pudding should be minimal so the patient will eat the entire amount and ingest all the medication.
   - Some medications should not be crushed because crushing alters their form and can minimize their intended action. For example, enteric-coated medications are not to be crushed because this eliminates the purpose of the coating. Box 44-2 provides examples of medications that should not be crushed.
   - Scored pills can also be cut by the use of a "pill splitter" (Figure 44-3). Pills that are not scored cannot be cut because the medication in each half would not be equal.
4. Check the medication against the physician's order at least *three times* before administering to the patient, as follows:
   a. Once when removing the medication from storage.
   b. A second time before preparing the medication.
   c. A third time when returning the medication to storage.

If the medication is dispensed per unit dosage, check this as well before administering.

PATIENT-CENTERED PROFESSIONALISM

- *Why is it important for the medical assistant to understand drug action of oral medications?*

TOPICAL ADMINISTRATION

Topical medications are applied to the epidermis (top layer of the skin) and mucous membranes (such as inside the mouth) and act either locally or systemically. Drug action

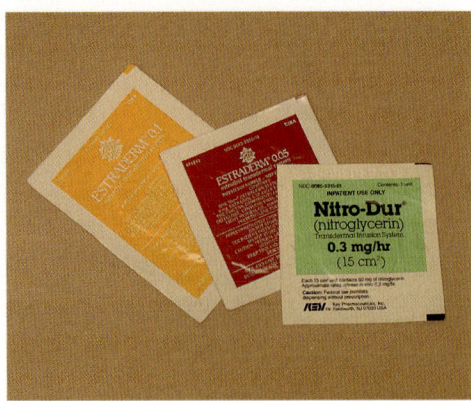

FIGURE 44-4 A variety of medications and doses are available as transdermal patches.

occurs within 1 hour of application. Topical applications include the use of creams, lotions, ointments, and transdermal patches.

Application

The administration of topical medications depends on the type of medicine.

Lotions and **creams** should be applied following the direction of hair growth of the area. This reduces entrance into the hair follicle and reduces the chance for infection.

The medication within an **ointment** is absorbed but not the greasy base. Therefore the ointment base should be removed before the next application.

A **transdermal patch** consists of a measured dose of medication. The medication is applied to the skin through the use of an adhesive-backed patch. When the patch is applied, the medication enters the bloodstream by absorption through the skin. The onset of drug action ranges from 30 to 60 minutes. Continuous absorption and systemic effects will occur over several hours, days, or even weeks. When reapplying a patch, the site of application must be rotated to avoid irritating the skin. Nitroglycerin, estrogen, and analgesics are medications often prescribed in patch form (Figure 44-4). Procedure 44-2 provides instructions for the application of a transdermal patch.

> **PATIENT-CENTERED PROFESSIONALISM**
>
> - Why is it important for the medical assistant to understand how topical medications should be applied?

VAGINAL AND RECTAL ADMINISTRATION

Medications can also be administered by inserting them into the vaginal or rectal cavity.

Vaginal

Medications inserted into the vaginal cavity can have a localized or a systemic effect. These drugs can be in the form of a cream, foam, or **suppository.** Patients may need specific instructions on proper insertion techniques. After a suppository is inserted into the vaginal cavity, the temperature of the body melts it and the drug is absorbed through the mucosa. The patient may need to remain in a recumbent position after inserting the medication. In this situation, insertion of the medication may be ordered at bedtime. Onset of action occurs in 15 to 30 minutes. Examples of vaginal medications include estrogen preparations and antifungal medications.

Rectal

Medications can also be inserted into the rectum for localized or systemic action. Medications for nausea and vomiting are often given rectally to avoid further upsetting the GI tract. Pain relievers and **antipyretics** (fever reducers) can also be given in suppository form.

Suppositories, both rectal and vaginal, are often packaged with a foil covering that must be removed before insertion. The patient is placed in the Sims' position and draped accordingly. The medical assistant applies gloves and places a small amount of a water-soluble lubricant on the suppository to allow for easy insertion. When the rectal suppository is inserted, it must be placed past the internal anal sphincter to allow for better absorption and to avoid being expelled before the drug is absorbed. Drug action occurs 15 to 30 minutes after insertion. Suppositories should be kept in a cool place and handled as little as possible to prevent the suppository from melting before insertion.

> **PATIENT-CENTERED PROFESSIONALISM**
>
> - What information must the medical assistant provide to the patient who is prescribed a medication in the form of a suppository?

INHALATION

Drugs can be inhaled as a gas, powder, or aerosol (fine mist). Inhaled medications are absorbed into the bloodstream through capillary action involving the mucous membranes of the nose and lungs. This route requires that specific instructions be provided to the patient. Both the nebulizer and the metered-dose inhaler are frequently prescribed for patients to use outside the medical office setting.

Nebulizer

A **nebulizer** provides a mist of medication (Figure 44-5). To inhale the medication, the patient closes the lips around a mouthpiece. An air compressor unit forces air into a

PROCEDURE 44-2   Apply a Transdermal Patch

TASK: Administer a transdermal patch and provide the patient with instructions for accurate application and safe removal.

EQUIPMENT AND SUPPLIES
- Medicated transdermal patch, as ordered by physician
- Nonsterile disposable gloves (Latex-free)
- Patient instruction sheet
- Patient's medical record

SKILLS/*RATIONALE*   STANDARD PRECAUTIONS ARE TO BE FOLLOWED.

1. **Procedural Step. Sanitize the hands.**
   An alcohol-based hand rub may be used instead of washing hands with soap and water, unless hands are visibly soiled.
   Rationale. Hand sanitization promotes infection control.

2. **Procedural Step. Assemble equipment and supplies and verify the order.**
   Medications in the medical office should be organized for safety by placing them with the labels showing and grouping medications in alphabetical order according to their use and route or by action or class (as per office policy). Medications should always be stored in their original containers.
   Rationale. It is important to have all supplies and equipment ready and available before starting any procedure to ensure efficiency.

3. **Procedural Step. Check the expiration date of the medication.**
   NOTE: The expiration date on stored medications should be checked on a regular basis. Medications that have expired should be disposed of properly.
   Rationale. Medications used past expiration date may be inactive.

4. **Procedural Step. Follow the "seven rights" of medication administration (see Procedure 44-1).**

5. **Procedural Step. Select the right drug.**
   If the medication is unfamiliar, read the package insert or use a drug reference.

6. **Procedural Step. Perform the first of three checks of the medication.**
   Verify that the medication name on the label matches the medication name in the written orders.

7. **Procedural Step. Read the dosage information on the label.**

8. **Procedural Step. Perform the second check of the medication against the written order.**

9. **Procedural Step. Return the package to storage, checking the medication for the third time.**
   NOTE: The physician may have ordered that the remainder of the doses (patches) in the package be given to the patient to take home, in which case the medication will not be returned to the cabinet.

10. **Procedural Step. Identify the right patient.**
    Determine that the patient is not allergic to the medication.
    Rationale. Identifying the patient ensures the procedure is performed on the correct patient.

11. **Procedural Step. Explain the procedure to the patient.**
    Discuss the side effects, contraindications, and reactions listed on the medication information sheet with the patient. Obtain a verbal acknowledgment of understanding from the patient.
    Rationale. Explaining the procedure to the patient promotes cooperation and provides a means of obtaining implied consent. When patients understand why taking a medication is important to their health and how the medication is to be taken and when, it increases the percentage of those who comply with their medication regimen.

12. **Procedural Step. Prepare to apply the transdermal patch.**
    The patient must expose an area that is relatively free from hair, such as the chest, upper back, or upper arm. The area must be clean and free from lotions and oils. Clean the area as needed. If the site needs to have hair removed, cut the hair close to the skin rather than shave, because shaving may cause nicks or cuts that will cause medication to absorb incorrectly.
    Rationale. The patch will not adhere to the skin properly if the area is covered with hair, lotions, or oils.

13. **Procedural Step. Instruct the patient that the location of the patch should be rotated to different sites at each application.**
    Rationale. Rotating sites at each application prevents skin irritation.

14. **Procedural Step. Apply the transdermal patch.**
    Apply gloves. Open the packaging and remove the patch. Peel away the protective covering from one half of the medication side of the patch. Firmly press down on the nonadhesive side of the patch to adhere it to the patient's

Continued

PROCEDURE 44-2 Apply a Transdermal Patch—cont'd

skin, while holding onto the still-protected half of the patch. Smooth down the edges.

Remove the backing from the other half of the protected patch, and adhere this half of the patch to the patient's skin. Smooth down the edges.

Rationale. It is important to wear gloves during this process to prevent absorption of the medication into your hands. Most transdermal patches are covered by two halves of protective backing, which allows you to apply the patch without touching the medication.

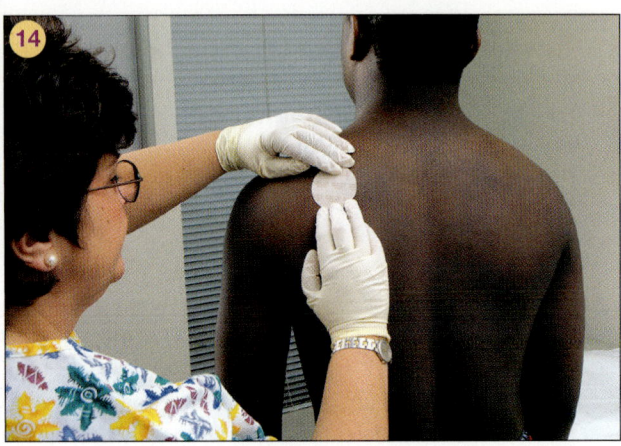

15. **Procedural Step.** Dispose of all waste material appropriately, and disinfect the work area.
16. **Procedural Step.** Remove gloves and sanitize the hands.
    Always sanitize the hands after every procedure or after using gloves.
17. **Procedural Step.** Instruct the patient on safe removal of the patch, its proper disposal, and applying a new patch at the same time each day.
    The patch should be disposed of in a lined container or flushed down the toilet, to prevent accidental exposure to the medication. Depending on the physician's orders and the type of medication, the patch may be left in place for a few hours to several days.
18. **Procedural Step.** Instruct the patient to wash and dry the hands after each application.
    Rationale. This prevents accidental exposure of the medication to others.
19. **Procedural Step.** Provide written care instructions to the patient.
    Rationale. Written instruction increases patient cooperation and compliance.
20. **Procedural Step.** Document the procedure.
    Include the date and time, name of the medication, dose given, site, and any significant observations or patient reactions.

CHARTING EXAMPLE

Date	
4/7/xx	2:15 p.m. Nitro-Dur, 5 mg/24-hour applied to Ⓡ chest area. No apparent reaction after 5 minutes. Patient instructed in removal and application. Pt given oral and written instructions and verbalized understanding. ——P. Rook, CMA (AAMA)

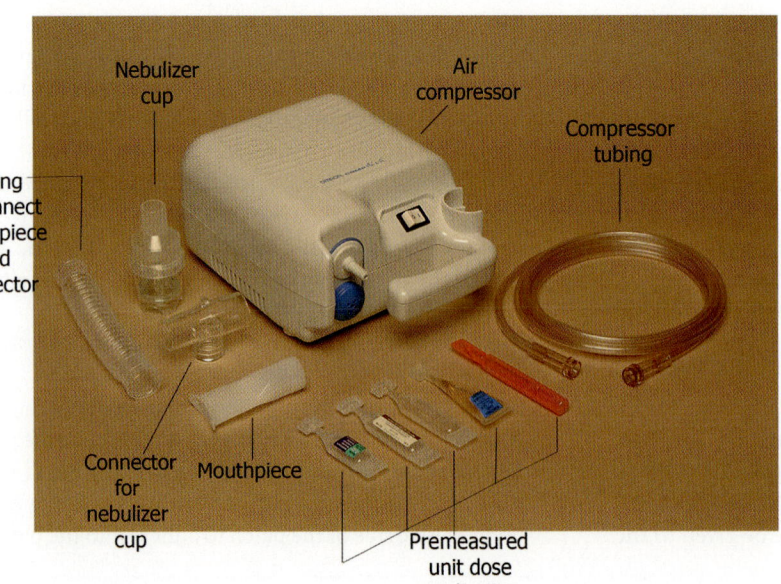

FIGURE 44-5 A nebulizer unit provides medications in a fine mist.

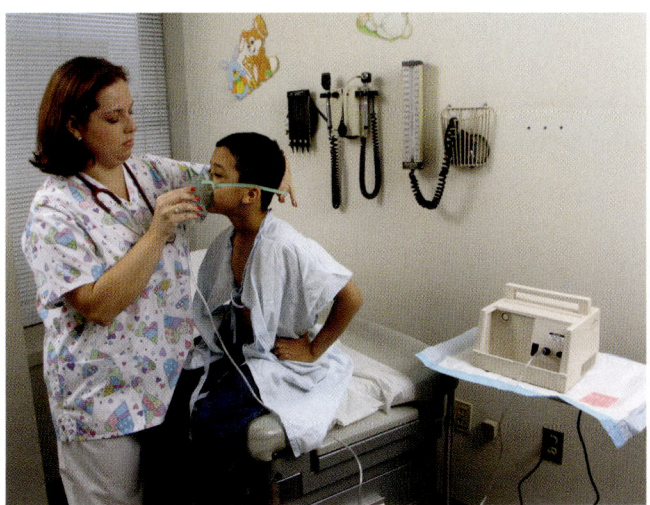

FIGURE 44-6 Child receiving a nebulizer treatment.

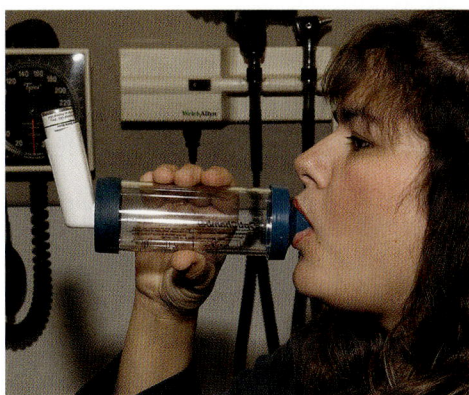

FIGURE 44-7 Metered-dose inhaler (MDI) with spacer attached.

medication compartment. The medication is rapidly absorbed because of the lungs' blood supply. As the patient exhales, a valve on the mouthpiece opens and allows the exhaled mist to escape. When all the medication is gone, the air compressor is turned off. A child can be fitted with a mask that covers the nose and mouth (Figure 44-6).

Metered-Dose Inhaler

A **metered-dose inhaler (MDI)** is a handheld device that dispenses medications into the airway and lungs. A **spacer** (added attachment) can be used to assist the patient who has difficulty coordinating between breathing and dispensing the medication (Figure 44-7). An elderly patient may have problems using an MDI because it requires coordination and strength to push the canister and breathe at the same time.

Since patients are responsible for self-administering their medications with the MDI, careful instructions are required to make certain the medication reaches the lungs. To reach the lungs, the inhaler must be depressed just as a person inhales. Usually, two "puffs" (doses) are ordered for medication distribution. The first puff opens the patient's airways and reduces inflammation, and the second dose, given approximately 1 minute later, enters deeper into the airway. Each dose is held for 10 seconds, and the patient is instructed to breathe out slowly through the nose. Procedure 44-3 provides instructions for administering medication using an MDI with the closed-mouth technique.

PATIENT-CENTERED PROFESSIONALISM

- How would the medical assistant explain to the patient the advantages of receiving medications through inhalation?

PARENTERAL ADMINISTRATION

Parenteral administration (taken into the body by injection) of medication involves injecting medication into the body by way of a needle. The advantage of parenteral administration is its quick action. Parenteral administration bypasses the GI tract, increasing the rate of absorption. The major disadvantages of parenteral administration are the occurrence of an adverse reaction that places the patient at immediate risk and the chance for infection because the skin has been broken.

To administer a medication by means of injection, an **aqueous** (water-based) solution is drawn from a vial, ampule, or a prefilled cartridge unit. The type of equipment needed to administer a parenteral medication is determined by the viscosity (thickness, stickiness) of the medication, body size of the patient, amount of medication, route of administration, and site of the injection. For example, penicillin G benzathine is very thick and the needle chosen must have a large lumen.

Equipment

After the physician determines that the parenteral route will be used for the medication, the medical assistant should select the proper equipment and supplies. All necessary equipment, including correct medication, syringe, and appropriately sized needle (to enter the required tissue type and allow for the appropriate flow rate), must be assembled. Box 44-3 lists key points on the selection of proper injection equipment.

Vial

A **vial** is a vacuum-sealed bottle that contains a sterile solution or a medication dissolved in a sterile aqueous solution or suspended in a sterile oil base (Figure 44-8).

Preparation. To make certain its contents are mixed, the vial should be gently rotated between the palms of the hands. Any medication that appears cloudy or has particles floating in the solution should be discarded (unless this is the medication's normal appearance). As with all medications, a vial should be checked for the expiration date and discarded if outdated. Remember, if the drug is a controlled substance, the

PROCEDURE 44-3

Instruct a Patient in Administering Medication Using a Metered-Dose Inhaler with the Closed-Mouth Technique

TASK: Properly provide instructions to a patient for the use of a metered-dose inhaler.

EQUIPMENT AND SUPPLIES
- Medication ordered by the physician
- Metered-dose inhaler (MDI)
- Spacer, if required
- Patient's medical record

SKILLS/RATIONALE

STANDARD PRECAUTIONS ARE TO BE FOLLOWED.

1. **Procedural Step.** Sanitize the hands.
   An alcohol-based hand rub may be used instead of washing hands with soap and water, unless hands are visibly soiled.
   Rationale. Hand sanitization promotes infection control.

2. **Procedural Step. Assemble equipment and supplies and verify the order.**
   Medications in the medical office should be organized for safety by placing them with the labels showing and grouping medications in alphabetical order according to their use and route or action or class (as per office policy). Medications should always be stored in their original containers.
   Rationale. It is important to have all supplies and equipment ready and available before starting any procedure to ensure efficiency.

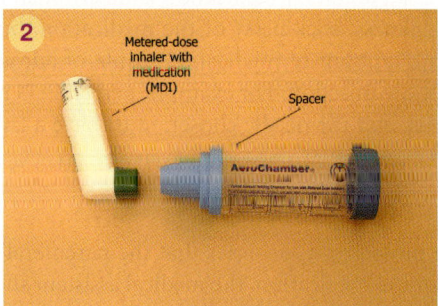

3. **Procedural Step. Check the expiration date of the medication.**
   NOTE: The expiration date on stored medications should be checked on a regular basis. Medications that have expired should be disposed of properly.
   Rationale. Medications used past expiration date may be inactive.

4. **Procedural Step. Follow the "seven rights" of medication administration (see Procedure 44-1).**

5. **Procedural Step. Select the right drug.**
   If the medication is unfamiliar, read the package insert or use a drug reference.

6. **Procedural Step. Perform the first of three checks of the medication.**
   Verify that the medication name on the label matches the medication name in the written orders.

7. **Procedural Step. Read the dosage information on the label.**

8. **Procedural Step. Perform the second check of the medication against the written order.**

9. **Procedural Step. Return the package to storage, checking the medication for the third time.**

10. **Procedural Step. Identify the right patient.**
    Determine that the patient is not allergic to the medication.
    Rationale. Identifying the patient ensures the procedure is performed on the correct patient.

11. **Procedural Step. Prepare the medication.**
    Instruct the patient to insert the correct medication canister into the mouthpiece, remove the cap from the MDI, and gently shake.
    Attach a spacer, if necessary by inserting MDI into end of spacer device (see Figure 44-5) or where indicated by the manufacturer.
    Rationale. Shaking the canister ensures the particles in the medication are aerosolized.

12. **Procedural Step. Instruct the patient to inhale deeply and then gently expel as much air as the patient comfortably can.**
    Rationale. This prepares the patient's airway for the medication.

13. **Procedural Step. Instruct the patient to place the mouthpiece in the mouth, holding the inhaler upright and closing the lips around it.**

Continued

PROCEDURE 44-3 Instruct a Patient in Administering Medication Using a Metered-Dose Inhaler with the Closed-Mouth Technique—cont'd

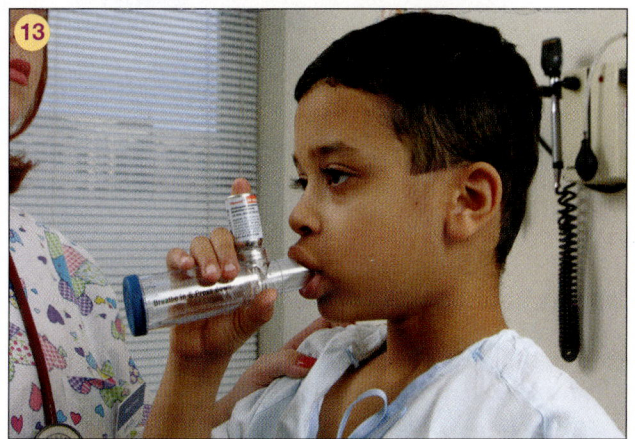

14. **Procedural Step.** Instruct the patient to inhale slowly through the mouth, depress the medication canister fully, breathe in slowly 2 to 3 seconds, and hold the breath for 10 seconds.
    Rationale. By holding the breath, the aerosol spray is able to reach deeper into areas within the airways.
15. **Procedural Step.** Have the patient remove the MDI from the mouth before exhaling, then exhale slowly, through the nose or pursed lips.
16. **Procedural Step.** Instruct the patient to exhale slowly.
    If a second dose of medication is ordered, the patient should wait at least 1 minute.
17. **Procedural Step.** Instruct the patient to keep the mouthpiece clean.
    Remove the canister, rinse the holder with warm water, and dry.
    Rationale. If medication accumulates around the mouthpiece, this may interfere with other doses of the medication reaching the patient's airways. It also promotes possible growth of bacteria.
18. **Procedural Step.** Instruct the patient to wash and dry the hands.
    The physician may recommend also rinsing the mouth after treatment to prevent a yeast infection from forming.
19. **Procedural Step.** Document the procedure.
    Include the date and time, name of the medication, dose given, instructions provided, and any apparent patient reactions.

CHARTING EXAMPLE

Date	
4/15/xx	10:00 a.m. Albuterol inhaler, 2 puffs as directed, with no apparent reaction. Verbal and written instructions provided. Pt verbalized understanding of instructions. —————— R. Williams, RMA

BOX 44-3

Key Points for Selection of Injection Equipment

1. Select needle length and gauge according to the following criteria:
   a. Patient safety and comfort.
      - This includes the patient's size and physical condition.
   b. Route and site chosen.
      - The needle length must be appropriate to reach the required depth to deliver the medication to the proper site.
   c. Viscosity of medication.
      - Aqueous medications require a smaller lumen.
      - Viscous-based medications require a larger lumen.
2. Select the syringe size based on the type of injection to be given and the amount of medication to be administered. The most common syringe sizes are 1, 3, and 5 cc (mL).
3. Select the correct cartridge holder for prefilled unit dose medications. The most common cartridge sizes are 1 and 2 cc (mL).

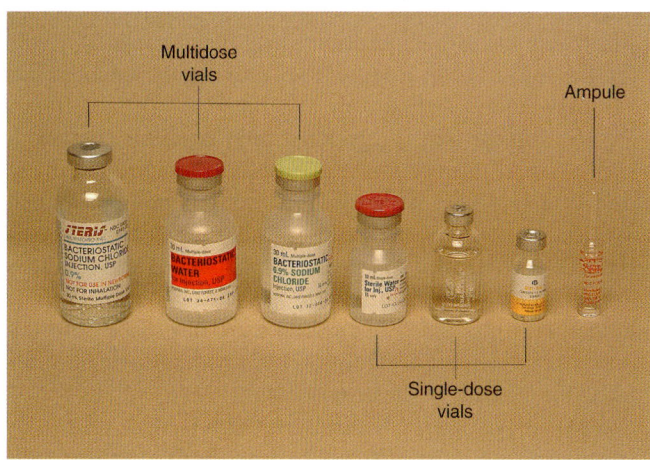

FIGURE 44-8 Vials can be multidose or single-dose containers, and an ampule is always single-dose.

discarding of it must be witnessed and documented. Some medications will be packaged in a vial as a powder, requiring reconstitution. Directions to reconstitute the medication must be followed according to the manufacturer's instructions. Procedure 44-4 provides a technique for reconstituting a powdered drug.

Administration. Medication is withdrawn from the vial by inserting a sterile needle through the rubber stopper on top of the vial. The rubber stopper is cleaned with an alcohol pad before inserting the sterile needle. To maintain the pressure in the vial, air equal to the amount of medication to be withdrawn from the vial is drawn into the syringe. If the vial is marked "single dose," one dose of medication is drawn from the vial, and the remainder of the vial is discarded. A multi-dose vial allows several doses of a drug to be drawn until the vial is empty. Procedure 44-5 provides instructions for withdrawing medications from a vial.

Ampule

An **ampule** is a specially shaped, single-dose glass container that has been hermetically sealed (see Figure 44-8). The neck is narrow, thin, and scored to allow for easy opening. Two other important characteristics of ampules follow:
- Air is never injected into the ampule. This would force medications out of the ampule.
- The container's shape will not allow medication to spill out, even when the ampule is inverted (upside down).

Preparation. Before opening an ampule, all medication must be removed from the stem by lightly tapping it. In addition, the neck must be cleaned with an alcohol pad to disinfect the container.

Administration. Even though the glass is designed not to splinter when snapped off, a special filtered needle is used to withdraw the medication to prevent glass contamination. The filtered straw or needle is replaced after the medication is withdrawn using the appropriate length and gauge of needle for the injection. Procedure 44-6 provides instructions for withdrawing medication from an ampule.

Prefilled Cartridge Unit. A **prefilled cartridge unit** contains a single-dose of medication (e.g., insulin, Demerol) for injection (Figure 44-9). If the prefilled unit contains too much medication, the unneeded portion is discarded. (If the medication is a controlled substance, the discarding must be witnessed and documented.) Cartridge units require a special holder with plunger. The cartridges are disposable, but the holders can be reused. Figure 44-10 provides instructions for using the TUBEX sterile cartridge unit.

Syringe. A **syringe** is a hollow tube (barrel) made of glass or plastic with a tip that attaches to a needle. The tube is calibrated and has a plunger that pulls or pushes medication into or out of it (Figure 44-11). Syringes are available in various sizes, such as 0.5, 1, 3, and 5 mL, but the 3-mL size is used most often and is calibrated in both tenths of a milliliter and minims. Figure 44-12 illustrates various types of syringes with safety devices, and Figure 44-13 shows the parts of a syringe that should not be touched because they are considered sterile. Only the barrel of the syringe can be safely handled.

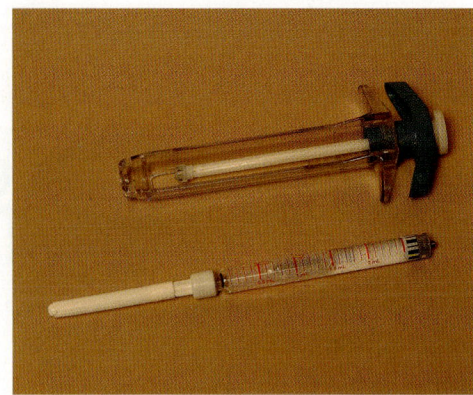

FIGURE 44-9 Parts of a prefilled cartridge used for a single-dose injection.

EXAMPLES OF SYRINGES

Tuberculin syringes are available in 1-mL capacity with calibrations in one-hundredths (1/100) of a milliliter and in minims. Insulin syringes are also 0.5- and 1-mL capacity and calibrated in units (e.g., 50 U [0.5 mL]). Insulin and tuberculin syringes may have permanently attached needles because the size of the needle is predetermined by site (e.g., under the skin), and "dead space" (medication remaining in the needle after injection) is eliminated.

When choosing a syringe, select the smallest syringe available that will hold the needed medication.

To eliminate cross-infection, disposable syringes are used in the health care setting. Only the outside of the barrel and the flared end of the plunger are touched. Touching other parts of the syringe contaminates the contents, and the syringe must be discarded.

In an effort to reduce needlestick injuries, the U.S. Occupational Safety and Health Administration (OSHA) requires that an employer, with the employees, evaluate the use of safer medical devices to reduce occupational exposure. Implementation of OSHA standards is expected to reduce the occurrence of needlestick injury. Figure 44-14 illustrates two safety-engineered syringes, and Figure 44-15 demonstrates the method to be used if recapping a syringe with needle is necessary before giving an injection. Box 44-4 provides more information about preventing needlesticks.

Needles

Needles are sterile metal objects constructed to fit on the tip of a syringe. Figure 44-16 illustrates various needles and their parts. Needles can be connected to the syringe by twisting the **hub** onto the tip and locking it in place (Luer-Lok) or by slipping it onto the tip of the syringe. The **shaft** of the needle determines the length of the needle. The point of the needle is slanted **(beveled).** The beveled point allows the needle to cut through the skin with minimal trauma. Needles come packaged in sterile peel-apart pouches or in sterile plastic

Text continued on p. 1059

Administering Medications CHAPTER 44 1049

PROCEDURE 44-4

Reconstitute a Powdered Drug

TASK: Properly reconstitute a powdered medication to its injectable dosage form.

EQUIPMENT AND SUPPLIES
- Vial of medication ordered by physician
- 70% isopropyl alcohol wipes
- Reconstituting liquid: sterile normal saline or manufacturer's indicated diluent
- Appropriate needle and syringe
- Sharps container

SKILLS/RATIONALE STANDARD PRECAUTIONS ARE TO BE FOLLOWED.

1. **Procedural Step. Sanitize the hands.**
   An alcohol-based hand rub may be used instead of washing hands with soap and water, unless hands are visibly soiled.
   Rationale. Hand sanitization promotes infection control.

2. **Procedural Step. Assemble equipment and supplies and verify the order.**
   Medications in the medical office should be organized for safety by placing them with the labels showing and grouping medications in alphabetical order according to their use and route or action or class (as per office policy). Medications should always be stored in their original containers.
   Rationale. It is important to have all supplies and equipment ready and available before starting any procedure to ensure efficiency.

3. **Procedural Step. Check the expiration date of the medication.**
   NOTE: The expiration date on stored medications should be checked on a regular basis. Medications that have expired should be disposed of properly.
   Rationale. Medications used past expiration date may be inactive.

4. **Procedural Step. Follow the "seven rights" of medication administration (see Procedure 44-1).**

5. **Procedural Step. Check the medication against the physician's order three times before it is administered:**
   a. Before removing the medication from storage.
   b. Before pouring or withdrawing the medication from the original container.
   c. Before returning the medication to storage.

6. **Procedural Step. Check the patient's medical record for drug allergies or conditions that may contraindicate the injection.**
   Rationale. This ensures that the medication is compatible with the patient, especially when administering antibiotics and analgesics.

7. **Procedural Step. Select the correct medication powder and diluent from the cabinet.**
   Most vaccines are stored in the refrigerator, and often the diluents to reconstitute them are stored there as well.

8. **Procedural Step. Read and follow the manufacturer's instructions for reconstituting the powder.**
   NOTE: Drugs that tend to be unstable when stored in liquid form are packaged as powders that need to be reconstituted before administration. Once the medication is reconstituted, the solution will be stable for a short time, as defined by the manufacturer. The manufacturer will specify the type and amount of diluent, or liquid, to be added to the powder. The manufacturer's directions must be followed exactly to ensure accuracy and patient safety.

9. **Procedural Step. Prepare the diluent vial.**
   If this is the first time the vial of diluent has been used, the hard metal or plastic cap protecting the rubber stopper of the vial must be removed before the first use. The vial may contain a single dose or multiple doses, depending on the medication. If the diluent vial being used is multidose and has been used previously, open the alcohol wipe and clean the top of the vial and allow to air-dry before withdrawing the dose.
   Rationale. Cleaning the top of the vial before inserting the needle to withdraw diluent prevents the needle from dragging contaminants into the vial, in turn contaminating the sterile diluent.

10. **Procedural Step. Prepare the needle and syringe.**
    Open the peel-apart sterile packaging surrounding the syringe and needle. Assemble the needle and syringe, if necessary. The syringe may come prepackaged with a needle attached, in which case you should tighten the needle to the hub. If the syringe and needle are packaged separately, once both packages have been sterilely opened, remove the small plastic cap covering the Luer-Lok on the syringe and attach the needle by twisting it securely onto the lock. Do not allow the hub of the needle to touch anything other than the Luer-Lok, or the needle may become contaminated. If this occurs,

Continued

PROCEDURE 44-4 Reconstitute a Powdered Drug—cont'd

discard both the syringe and the needle, and obtain a new one of each.

11. **Procedural Step. Remove the cover from the needle.**
Hold the barrel of the syringe with one hand while carefully removing the needle cover from the needle with the other hand. Place the needle cover on its side on the counter.

12. **Procedural Step. Insert the needle into the diluent vial.**
To minimize the risk of a needlestick injury, place the diluent vial on a flat surface without holding it. Hold the barrel of the syringe with one hand, guiding the needle as it pierces the rubber stopper of the vial. Once the needle is embedded in the rubber stopper, it is safe to grasp the vial with the other hand.

13. **Procedural Step. Fill the syringe.**
Invert the vial and syringe so that the tip of the needle is immersed in the diluent. If the manufacturer's instructions state that the entire contents of the diluent vial are to be used for reconstitution, pull the plunger of the syringe back until all the diluent has been removed from the vial. Otherwise, obtain the amount of diluent indicated by the manufacturer.

14. **Procedural Step. Carefully remove the needle from the vial stopper by pulling both hands away from each other.**
If air bubbles have entered the syringe, they may be injected along with the diluent into the vial containing the powder to be reconstituted; be sure and draw all diluent into the syringe.

15. **Procedural Step. Insert the needle into the medication vial.**
To minimize the risk of a needlestick injury, place the vial containing the powder to be reconstituted on a flat surface without holding it. Hold the barrel of the syringe with one hand, guiding the needle as it pierces the rubber stopper of the vial containing the powder. Once the needle is embedded in the rubber stopper, it is safe to grasp the vial with the other hand. Then inject the diluent into the vial containing the powder.

16. **Procedural Step. Carefully remove the needle from the vial stopper by pulling both hands away from each other.**
If the medication is to be withdrawn from the vial immediately after it has been reconstituted, recap the needle using a one-handed "scooping" technique.
Once the tip is no longer exposed, secure the needle cover to the needle hub with the other hand. If the medication will not be used until later, discard the needle and syringe as a single unit in a sharps container.

17. **Procedural Step. Mix the powder and diluent thoroughly by rolling the vial between your flattened palms until all the powder has been dissolved.**
The reconstituted solution vial must be labeled with the date and time it was reconstituted if (a) the medication is not to be withdrawn from the vial immediately after it has been reconstituted, or (b) it is a multidose vial. If it is a multidose vial, label it with date, time, reconstituted medication dosage, and your initials.
The reconstituted medication is stored according to the manufacturer's instructions until it is administered. If it has not been administered before the manufacturer's recommended expiration time after reconstitution, it must be discarded.

NOTE: When reconstituting pediatric medications, use only single-dose diluents because they do not contain preservatives. Bacteriostatic preservatives have been known to cause seizures in infants.

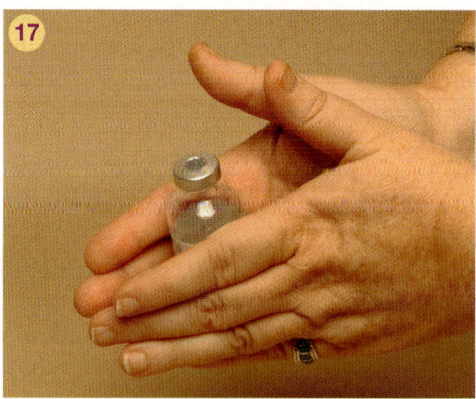

18. **Procedural Step. Sanitize the hands.**
Always sanitize the hands after every procedure or after using gloves.

Administering Medications **CHAPTER 44** 1051

PROCEDURE 44-5 **Prepare a Parenteral Medication from a Vial**

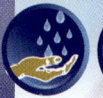

TASK: Measure the correct medication dosage in a 3-mL hypodermic syringe for injection from a vial.

EQUIPMENT AND SUPPLIES
- Vial of medication ordered by physician
- 70% isopropyl alcohol wipes
- Appropriate syringe for ordered dose
- Needle with safety device appropriate for site of injection
- 2 × 2 gauze squares
- Sharps container
- Patient's medical record

SKILLS/RATIONALE   STANDARD PRECAUTIONS ARE TO BE FOLLOWED.

1. **Procedural Step. Sanitize the hands.**
   An alcohol-based hand rub may be used instead of washing hands with soap and water, unless hands are visibly soiled.
   Rationale. Hand sanitization promotes infection control.

2. **Procedural Step. Assemble equipment and supplies and verify the order.**
   Medications in the medical office should be organized for safety by placing them with the labels showing and grouping medications in alphabetical order according to their use and route (as per office policy). Medications should always be stored in their original containers.
   Rationale. It is important to have all supplies and equipment ready and available before starting any procedure to ensure efficiency.

3. **Procedural Step. Check the expiration date of the medication.**
   NOTE: The expiration date on stored medications should be checked on a regular basis. Medications that have expired should be disposed of properly.
   Rationale. Medications used past expiration date may be inactive.

4. **Procedural Step. Follow the "seven rights" of medication administration (see Procedure 44-1).**

5. **Procedural Step. Check the medication against the physician's order three times before it is administered:**
   a. Before removing the medication from storage.
   b. Before pouring or withdrawing the medication from the original container.
   c. Before returning the medication to storage.

6. **Procedural Step. Check the patient's medical record for drug allergies or conditions that may contraindicate the injection.**
   Rationale. This ensures that the medication is compatible with the patient, especially when administering antibiotics and analgesics.

7. **Procedural Step. Calculate the correct dose to be given, if necessary.**

8. **Procedural Step. Prepare the vial.**
   If this is the first time the vial has been used, the hard metal or plastic cap protecting the rubber stopper of the vial must be removed before the first use. The vial may contain a single dose or multiple doses, depending on the medication. If the vial being used is multidose and has been used previously, open the alcohol wipe and clean the top of the vial and allow to air-dry before withdrawing the medication.
   Rotate the vial between the palms of the hands if medication needs to be mixed.
   Rationale. Cleaning the top of the vial before inserting the needle to withdraw medication prevents the needle from dragging contaminants into the vial, in turn contaminating the sterile medication. Allowing the alcohol to dry prevents alcohol from coating needle mixing with medication. Some liquid medications contain undissolved substances dispersed in a liquid and must be mixed before withdrawing for injection (e.g., insulin).

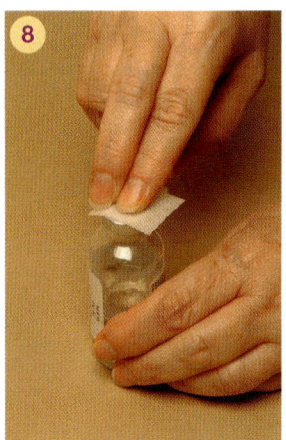

9. **Procedural Step. Prepare the needle and syringe.**
   Open the peel-apart sterile packaging surrounding the syringe and needle. Assemble the needle and syringe, if necessary. If the syringe comes prepackaged with a

Continued

PROCEDURE 44-5 Prepare a Parenteral Medication from a Vial—cont'd

needle attached, tighten the needle to the hub. If the syringe and needle are packaged separately, once both packages have been sterilely opened, remove the small plastic cap covering the Luer-Lok on the syringe and attach the needle by twisting it securely onto the Luer-Lok. Do not allow the hub of the needle to touch anything other than the Luer-Lok, or the needle may become contaminated. If this occurs, discard both the syringe and the needle, and obtain a new one of each.

The viscosity (thickness) of the medication, route, injection site, and patient size determine the needle length and gauge. The thicker the medication, the larger the lumen needed (e.g., 21 or 22 gauge).

10. **Procedural Step.** Draw air into the syringe.
    With the needle cover in place over the needle, draw an amount of air equal to the volume of medication that will be withdrawn from the vial up into the syringe.
    Rationale. This prevents a vacuum from forming inside the vial after the liquid is withdrawn.

11. **Procedural Step.** Remove the cover from the needle.
    Hold the barrel of the syringe with one hand while carefully removing the needle cover from the needle with the other hand. Place the needle cover on its side on the counter.

12. **Procedural Step.** Insert the needle into the vial.
    To minimize the risk of a needlestick injury, place the vial on a flat surface without holding it. Hold the barrel of the syringe with one hand, guiding the needle as it pierces the rubber stopper of the vial. Once the needle is embedded in the rubber stopper, it is safe to grasp the vial with the other hand. Then inject the air into the vial.

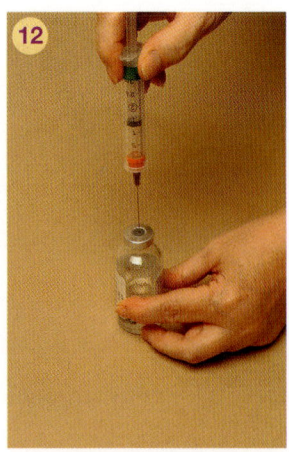

13. **Procedural Step.** Fill the syringe.
    Invert the vial and syringe so that the tip of the needle is immersed in the medication. Withdraw a little more than the required volume of medication from the vial.

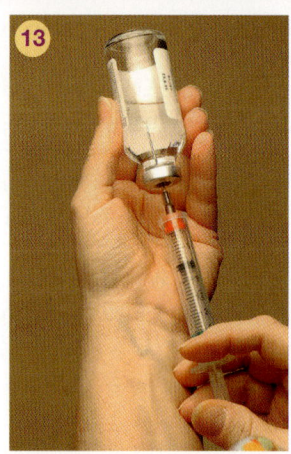

14. **Procedural Step.** Remove any air bubbles and measure the medication.
    If air bubbles have formed in the syringe, invert the syringe and tap the barrel with a finger or fingernail until the air bubbles rise to the surface of the liquid. Advance the plunger to expel the air; once you have removed the air from the syringe, measure the exact dose needed by advancing the plunger to the required mark on the barrel of the syringe.
    Rationale. The air must be inserted above the fluid level to avoid creating air bubbles in the medication. Too little air will make withdrawal difficult; too much air will increase the air pressure within the vial and cause the plunger to blow out. The needle must stay within the fluid to prevent pulling air up into the syringe, causing an inaccurate measurement of the medication.

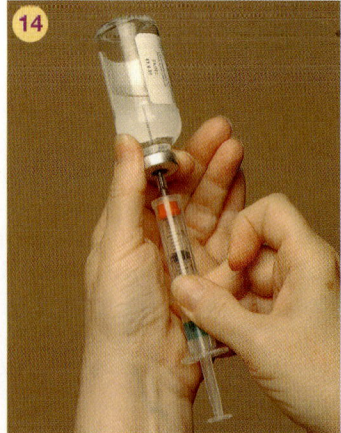

15. **Procedural Step.** Carefully remove the needle from the vial stopper by pulling both hands away from each other.

16. **Procedural Step.** Recap the needle if necessary.
    If a safety needle system is not being used, place the needle cover horizontally on a flat surface, hold the syringe with one hand, and carefully guide the exposed

Continued

PROCEDURE 44-5   Prepare a Parenteral Medication from a Vial—cont'd

needle into the cover and "scoop" the cover over the needle, being careful not to touch anything except the cover with the needle. Once the tip is no longer exposed, secure the needle cover to the needle hub with the other hand.

If the needle has been contaminated during the process, it must be exchanged for a clean needle before the medication is injected. The contaminated needle must be discarded in a sharps container.

17. **Procedural Step.** Compare the medication order to the vial label, and return the medication to its proper storage.
18. **Procedural Step.** Sanitize the hands.
    Always sanitize the hands after every procedure or after using gloves.

PROCEDURE 44-6   Prepare a Parenteral Medication from an Ampule

TASK: Measure the correct medication dosage in a 1-mL hypodermic syringe for injection from an ampule.

EQUIPMENT AND SUPPLIES
- Ampule of medication ordered by physician
- Ampule breaker or 2 × 2 gauze squares
- 70% isopropyl alcohol wipes
- Appropriate syringe for ordered dose
- Needle with safety device appropriate for site of injection
- Filter needle (used for ampule)
- Sharps container
- Patient's medical record

SKILLS/RATIONALE

STANDARD PRECAUTIONS ARE TO BE FOLLOWED.

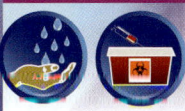

1. **Procedural Step. Sanitize the hands.**
   An alcohol-based hand rub may be used instead of washing hands with soap and water, unless hands are visibly soiled.
   Rationale. Hand sanitization promotes infection control.

2. **Procedural Step. Assemble equipment and supplies and verify the order.**
   Medications in the medical office should be organized for safety by placing them with the labels showing and grouping medications in alphabetical order according to their use and route (as per office policy). Medications should always be stored in their original containers.
   Rationale. It is important to have all supplies and equipment ready and available before starting any procedure to ensure efficiency.

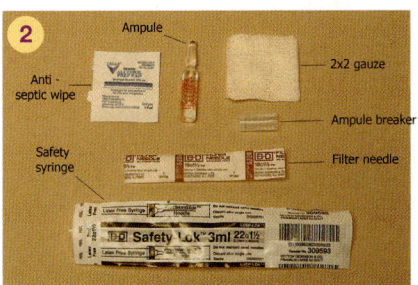

3. **Procedural Step. Check the expiration date of the medication.**
   NOTE: The expiration date on stored medications should be checked on a regular basis. Medications that have expired should be disposed of properly.
   Rationale. Medications used past expiration date may be inactive.

4. **Procedural Step. Follow the "seven rights" of medication administration (see Procedure 44-1).**

5. **Procedural Step. Check the medication against the physician's order three times before it is administered:**
   a. Before removing the medication from storage.
   b. Before pouring or withdrawing the medication from the original container.
   c. Before returning the medication to storage.

6. **Procedural Step. Check the patient's medical record for drug allergies or conditions that may contraindicate the injection.**
   Rationale. This ensures that the medication is compatible with the patient, especially when administering antibiotics and analgesics.

7. **Procedural Step. Calculate the correct dose to be given, if necessary.**

Continued

PROCEDURE 44-6 Prepare a Parenteral Medication from an Ampule—cont'd

8. Procedural Step. Clean the ampule.
Open an alcohol wipe, and clean the neck of the ampule and allow to air-dry before withdrawing the medication.

9. Procedural Step. Prepare the filter needle and syringe.
Open the peel-apart sterile packaging surrounding the syringe and filter needle. Assemble the needle and syringe. Avoid touching the ends of the hub of the needle or the tip of the syringe. As the medication is withdrawn, the filter in the hub of the needle will trap any glass fragments that may have fallen into the ampule.

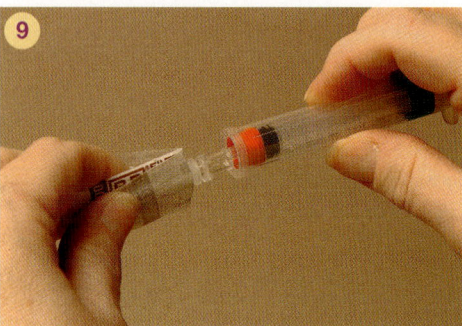

10. Procedural Step. Release liquid from the top of the ampule.
Examine the ampule to make sure there is no liquid trapped in the top section. To release any liquid from the top of the ampule, tap it lightly until the liquid runs down into the bottom of the ampule. The full volume of the ampule should be in the bottom section.

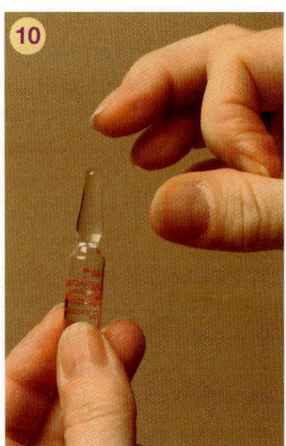

11. Procedural Step. Break the ampule.
Ease the ampule breaker over the top section of the ampule to the bottom of the neck. Grasp the ampule breaker and snap the neck away from the body to break open the ampule. Discard the top of the ampule and the ampule breaker into a sharps container and place the opened ampule on a flat surface.

If an ampule breaker is not available, the ampule may be opened by wrapping the neck of the ampule with an alcohol wipe or a 2 × 2 gauze square and snapping the top away from the body. Discard the top of the ampule and alcohol wipe or gauze in a sharps container, and place the opened ampule on a flat surface.

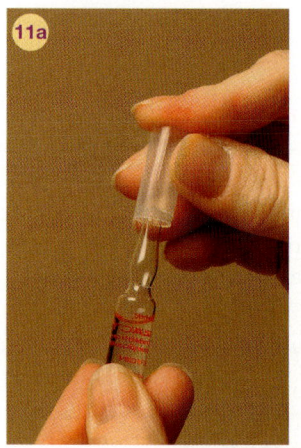 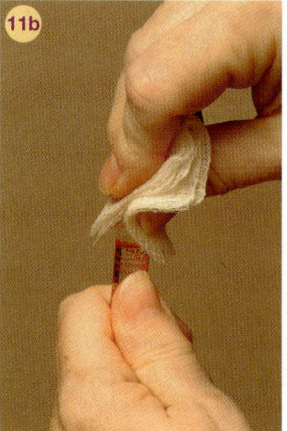

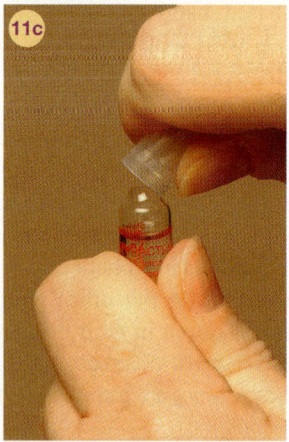

Continued

PROCEDURE 44-6 Prepare a Parenteral Medication from an Ampule—cont'd

12. **Procedural Step.** Remove the cover from the filter needle.
   Hold the barrel of the syringe with one hand and carefully remove the needle cover with the other hand. Place the needle cover on its side on the counter.

13. **Procedural Step.** Insert the filter needle into the ampule.
   To minimize the risk of a needlestick injury, place the ampule on a flat surface. Hold the barrel of the syringe with one hand, and carefully lower the needle into the ampule so that the bevel is below the surface of the liquid. Make sure the needle shaft does not touch the sides of the neck opening.
   Do not inject air into the ampule.
   Do not touch the broken edge of the ampule with the needle or fingers.
   After the tip of the needle is immersed in the liquid, the ampule may be picked up with the other hand and inverted. The needle shaft must not touch the sides of the neck opening as the ampule is inverted. The surface tension of the liquid will keep it in the ampule.

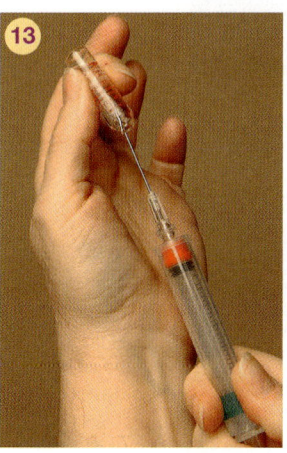

14. **Procedural Step.** Fill the syringe.
   Withdraw the entire amount of medication if appropriate, or a little more than the required volume of medication from the ampule. Avoid introducing excess air into the syringe in an attempt to draw up all the medication.

15. **Procedural Step.** Remove and recap the needle.
   Carefully remove the needle from the ampule. Once the tip is no longer exposed, place the needle cover over the needle using the one-handed "scoop" method.

16. **Procedural Step.** Replace the needle.
   Using sterile technique, exchange the filter needle for an injection needle with a safety device. Do not touch either the end of the hub of the needle or the tip of the barrel of the syringe.
   Rationale. The filter needle (or any needle that was used to withdraw a medication from an ampule) is never used to administer the medication to the patient. Changing needles eliminates the risk of administering glass fragments from the ampule along with the medication.

17. **Procedural Step.** Remove any air bubbles and measure the medication.
   Remove the cover of the new needle. If air bubbles have formed in the barrel, invert the syringe and tap the barrel with a finger or fingernail until the air bubbles rise to the surface of the liquid. Invert the syringe and advance the plunger to expel the air. After the air has been removed from the syringe, measure the exact dose needed by advancing the plunger to the required mark on the barrel of the syringe. Discard the excess medication into a receptacle.

18. **Procedural Step.** Recap the needle, if necessary.
   Recap the needle with a single-handed technique, as done previously, or by engaging the safety needle cover.

19. **Procedural Step.** Check the medication label, and discard the ampule in a sharps container.
   Keep the medication and syringe together until ready to administer.

20. **Procedural Step.** Sanitize the hands.
   Always sanitize the hands after every procedure or after using gloves.

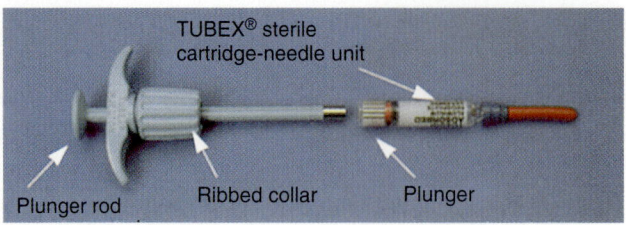

How To Load

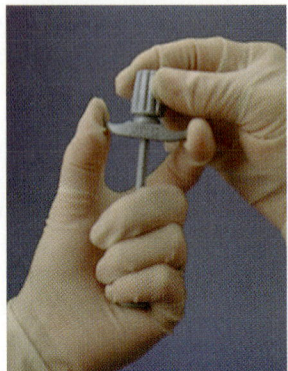

1. Turn the ribbed collar to the "OPEN" position until it stops.

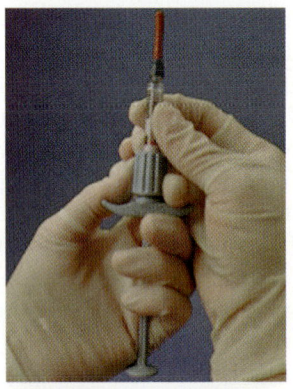

2. Hold injector with the open end up and fully insert the TUBEX sterile cartridge needle.

   Firmly tighten the ribbed collar in the direction of the "CLOSED" position.

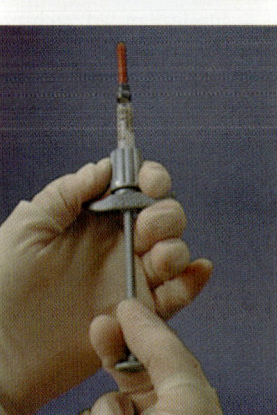

3. Thread the plunger rod into the plunger of the TUBEX sterile cartridge-needle until slight resistance is felt.

   The injector is now ready for use in the usual manner.

How To Unload And Discard Used Unit

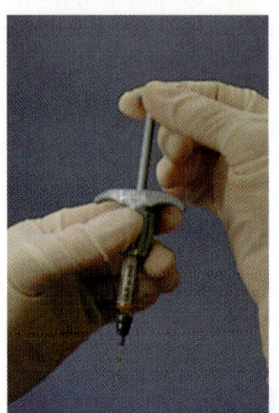

1. Do not recap the needle. Disengage the plunger rod.

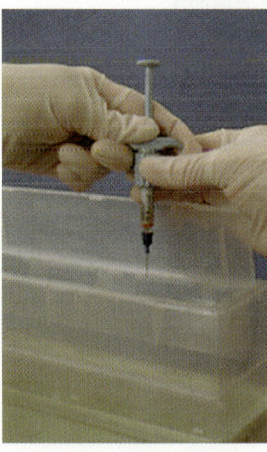

2. Hold the injector, needle down, over a needle disposal container and loosen the ribbed collar. TUBEX cartridge-needle unit will drop into the container. The TUBEX injector is reusable; do not discard.

FIGURE 44-10 Technique for using TUBEX injector (closed-injection system). The method of administration is the same as with a conventional system. Remove the needle cover by grasping it securely; then twist and pull. Introduce the needle into the patient, aspirate by pulling back slightly on the plunger, and inject. (From Zakus SM: *Mosby's clinical skills for medical assistants*, ed 4, St Louis, 2001, Mosby.)

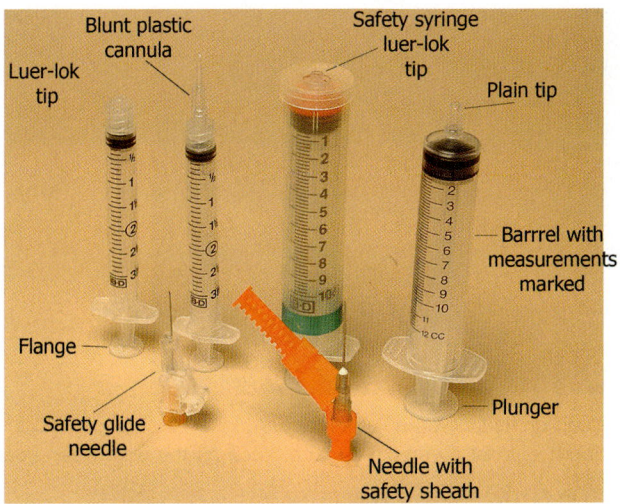

FIGURE 44-11 Parts of a syringe.

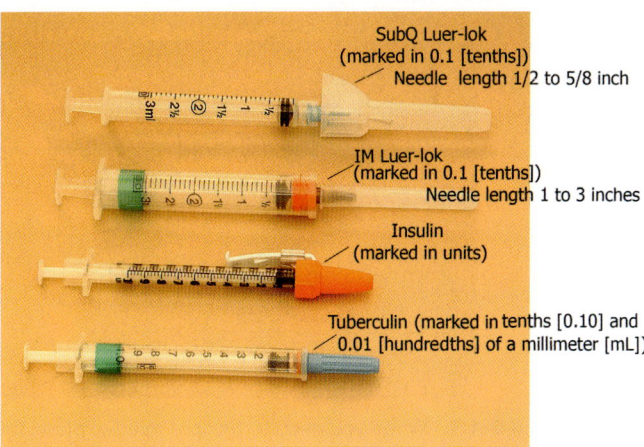

FIGURE 44-12 Various types of syringes used to administer injections.

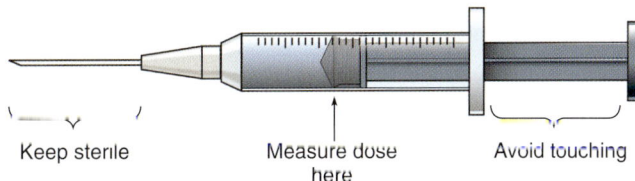

FIGURE 44-13 Parts of a syringe that should not be touched. (Modified from Potter PA, Perry AG: *Basic nursing*, ed 6, St Louis, 2007, Mosby.)

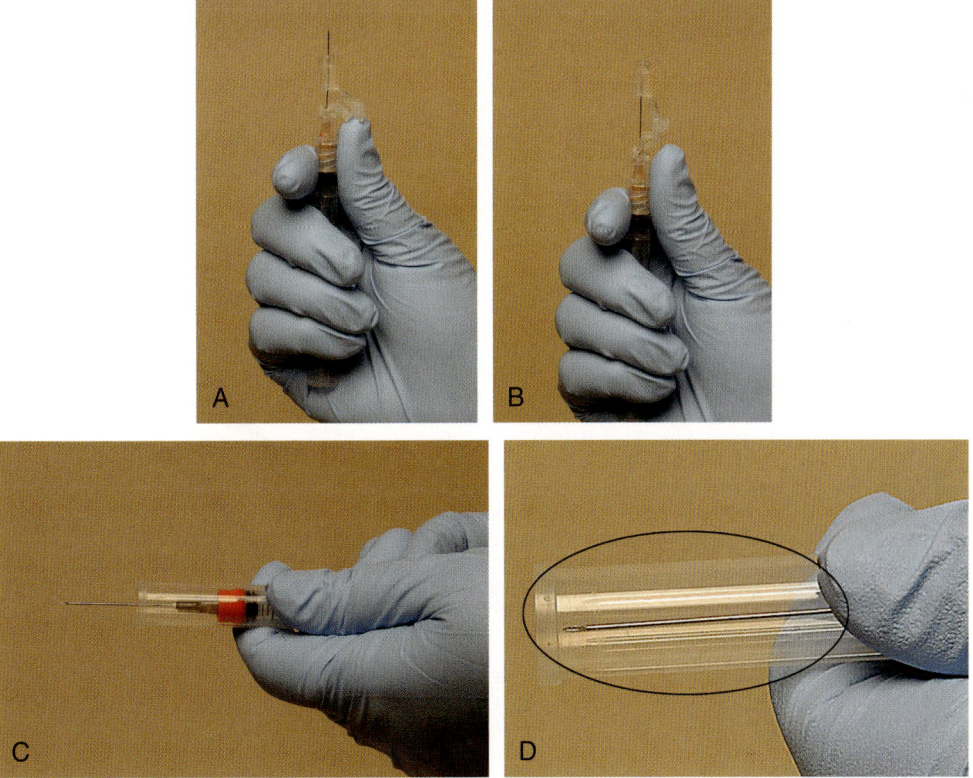

FIGURE 44-14 Safety-engineered syringes. **A** and **B,** Becton-Dickinson Safety Glide Syringe uses a hinged shield to cover the needle after it is used. **C** and **D,** Monoject Safety Syringe has a sliding shield that extends fully over the needle and is twisted and locked.

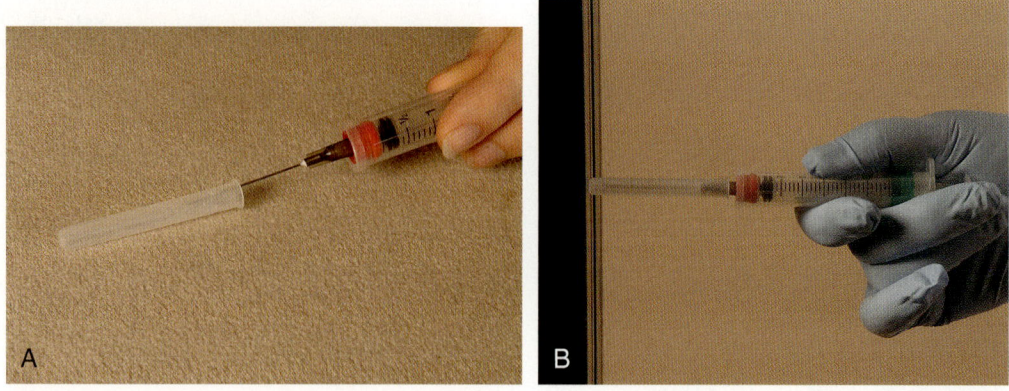

FIGURE 44-15 When you need to recap a needle, place the needle cap on its side on a flat surface. **A,** Insert the needle into the cap without holding the cap. **B,** Secure the cap on the needle by pushing it against a vertical surface, such as the wall. Keep your other hand behind your back during this procedure.

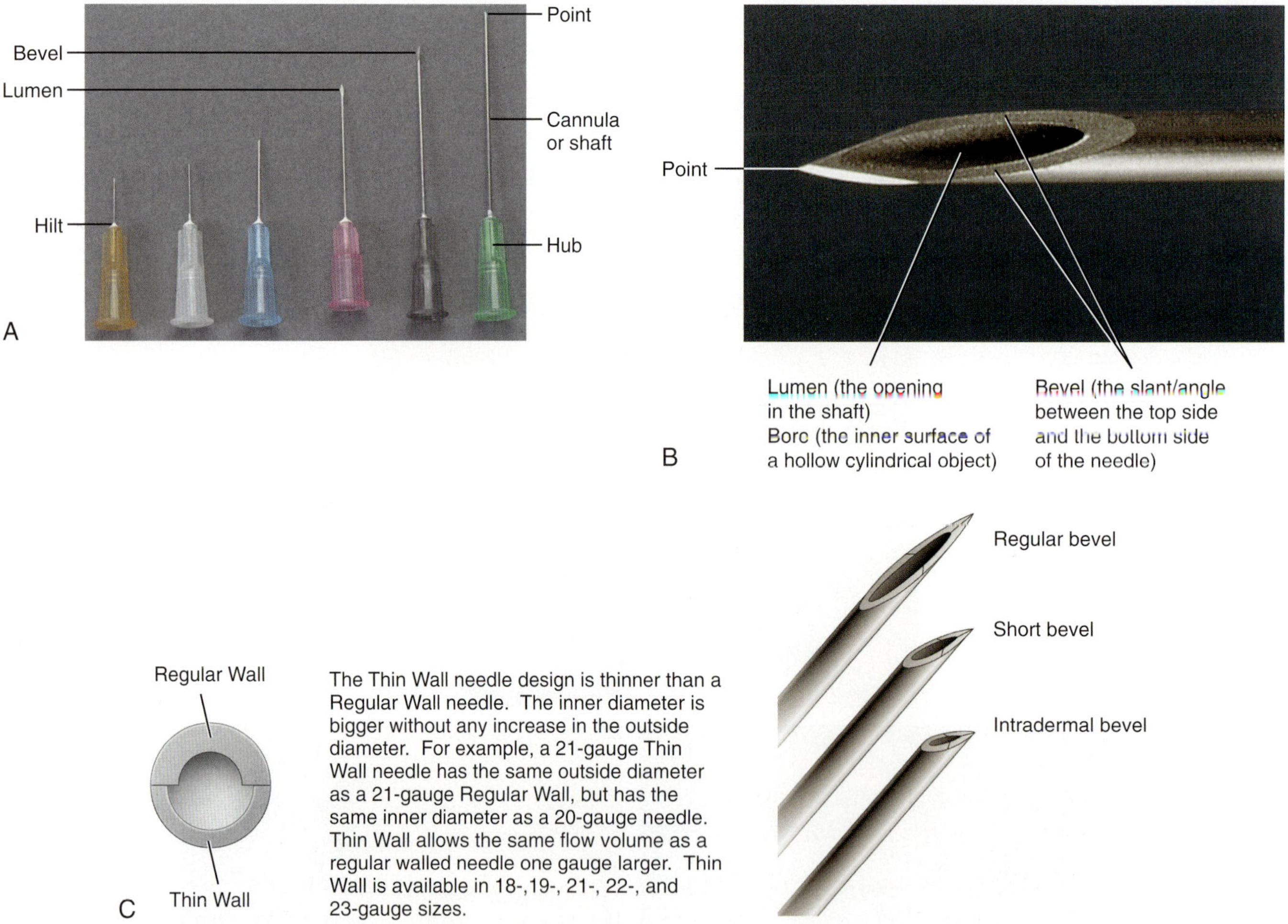

FIGURE 44-16 **A,** Various sizes and lengths of needles. The color of the hub identifies the gauge (diameter) of the needle for a particular manufacturer. **B,** Point, bevel, and lumen of needle. **C,** Types of needle walls and bevels. (From Zakus SM: *Mosby's clinical skills for medical assistants*, ed 4, St Louis, 2001, Mosby.)

BOX 44-4
Preventing Accidental Needlesticks

FEDERAL REGULATIONS

OSHA regulations protect the medical assistant from needlestick injury by requiring the following:
- Rigid, puncture-proof containers must be used to discard sharps.
- The needle and syringe must be discarded intact without recapping.
- The container must be tamper-proof, thus preventing accidental needlesticks to the medical assistant.
- Employers must have an exposure control and incident management plan in place and must educate employees in safety measures.

GENERAL GUIDELINES
1. Focus on the task at hand. Do not allow anything to cause a distraction. Immediately after the needle is removed from the patient, it must be discarded in the appropriate puncture-resistant container.
2. If absolutely necessary to recap a needle, use a single-handed "scoop" method (see Figure 44-15).
3. Properly use safety syringes and needles. Several styles of safety needles and syringes are available to reduce the risk of a stick from a contaminated needle.
4. Always dispose of needles and syringes as one unit in a puncture-resistant container. Never cut, bend, or remove a needle from the syringe before disposal.

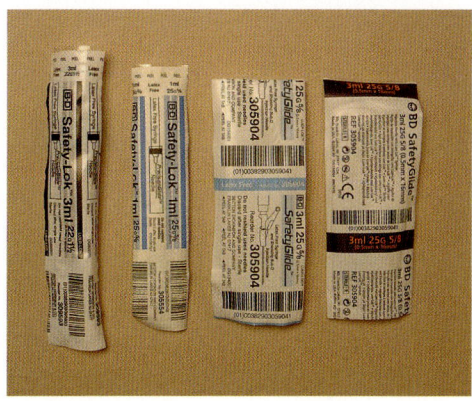

FIGURE 44-17 Syringe and needle packages labeled according to contents.

TABLE 44-1
Common Needle Length and Gauge Sizes

Method	Use	Length	Gauge
Intradermal (ID)	Allergy testing	⅜–½ inch	27-30
	Skin testing	⅜ inch	26, 27
	Tuberculin	½ inch	27
Subcutaneous (SubQ)	Immunizations	⅜ inch	25
	Insulin	½ or ⅜ inch	27, 28, 30
Intramuscular (IM)	Antibiotics	1-1½ inches	23
	Analgesics	1-1½ inches	22
	Corticosteroids	1-1½ inches	21, 22, 23
	Hormones	1-1½ inches	21, 23

TABLE 44-2
Injection Sites

Type	Amount	Site
Intradermal (ID)	0.05-0.1 mL	Forearm, upper chest, upper back
Subcutaneous (SubQ)	0.1-2 mL	Upper outer arm, thigh, abdomen
—Child	0.5 mL	Anterior vastus lateralis muscle, deltoid muscle
Intramuscular (IM)	1-2 mL	Deltoid (in adults with adequate muscle)
		Dorsogluteal, ventrogluteal, vastus lateralis
—Child	1-2 mL	Vastus lateralis, ventrogluteal
Z-track	1-3 mL	Dorsogluteal, ventrogluteal

tubes. Syringe and needle packages are color-coded to identify the gauge of the needle and syringe size (Figure 44-17).

Needle Selection. The various needle sizes allow for penetration of different depths of skin and tissue layers. The patient's size, the type of medication, and the injection site determine the length of the needle required. Table 44-1 shows the different needle lengths and gauges for parenteral methods. The **gauge** of the needle describes the opening, or **lumen,** of the needle. Selection of needle gauge is based on the thickness of the medication to be administered. Needle gauges range from 18 (thickest) to 30 (thinnest) and are color-coded. Each manufacturer identifies the gauge of its needles with a particular color on the hub and/or packaging.

Types of Injections

Several sites are used for administering medications by injection. Each site has a different tissue depth (Figure 44-18). When a medication is injected, the rate of absorption is rapid and cannot be altered. Once a medication has been injected, it cannot be returned. Therefore you must be very careful with injectable medications.

Proper skin preparation is necessary to minimize the chance of introducing bacteria into the body. The proper technique must be carefully followed to prevent trauma to the tissue. Box 44-5 provides some guidelines for administering parenteral medications. Table 44-2 lists various injection sites for parenteral methods.

Intradermal

An **intradermal (ID) injection** is placed just under the epidermis into the dermis. Only a small amount of medication can be administered through this route, usually 0.1 mL or less. The absorption rate is slow, and the drug reaction is localized. The sites used are the forearm, upper chest, and hairless area of the upper back (Figure 44-21). ID injections usually are not

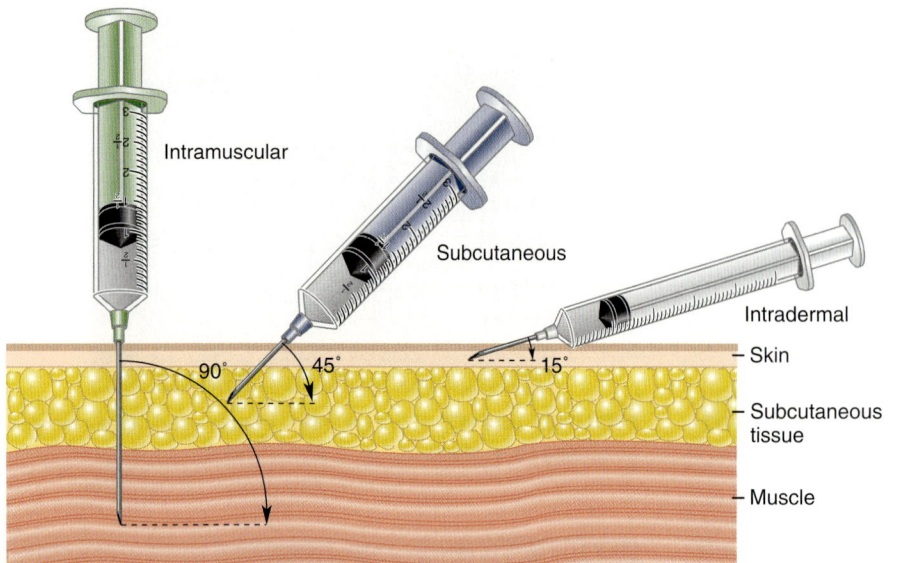

FIGURE 44-18 Intramuscular injections are given at a 90-degree angle, subcutaneous injections at a 45-degree angle, and intradermal injections at a 15-degree angle. (From Hunt SA: *Saunders fundamentals of medical assisting—revised reprint*, St Louis, 2007, Saunders.)

BOX 44-5

Guidelines for Administering Parenteral Medications

1. Selecting the proper site for intradermal, subcutaneous, or intramuscular injections will ensure that the medication is delivered to the right tissue type. Major blood vessels, nerves, and bones must be avoided.
2. Needles, syringes, and medication must remain sterile at all times.
3. The syringe, needle length, and gauge must be appropriate for the amount and type of medication to be given and the physical condition and body size of the patient.
4. The correct angle must be used for the type of injection given to ensure the medication reaches the correct tissues for absorption.
5. Aspirate, when appropriate, to make certain the needle has not entered a blood vessel. When injecting heparin or insulin and when giving an intradermal injection, ***do not aspirate.*** Keep in mind that you must document if you aspirate blood and that you must restart the procedure.
6. Entering a blood vessel requires the needle to be withdrawn and the process to be restarted with new medication and equipment, as well as proper documentation.
7. Rotate injection sites of frequently administered medications (Figure 44-19).
8. Aseptic technique must be maintained at all times.
9. Nonsterile gloves must be worn when administering an injection.
10. Dispose of used needles and syringes as a complete unit into a puncture-resistant container immediately after giving the injection (Figure 44-20). Do not recap needles, but activate the safety shield (if available) immediately after withdrawing from the injection site.
11. Warm refrigerated medications to room temperature. One method is to hold the medication securely in the palm of the hand.
12. Allow skin prep (alcohol) to air-dry before injecting medication. Do not blow on the site or wave your hand over it.
13. Inject the needle quickly.
14. Inject the medication slowly.
15. Remove the needle at the same angle it was inserted.
16. Massage the site when indicated.
17. Document the medication used, amount, time, site, patient reaction, and signature with credentials.

---

therapeutic but are administered for diagnostic purposes such as allergy testing or tuberculosis (TB) skin tests.

Administration. A tuberculin syringe with a ⅜- to ½-inch, 26- or 27-gauge needle is inserted at a 10- to 15-degree angle. When the medication is injected, a **bleb** or **wheal** (fluid-filled bump) appears (Figure 44-22). Since the medication is dispensed in an area with many nerves, the patient will experience a momentary burning or stinging sensation. Procedure 44-7 provides instructions for administering ID injections.

Allergy Testing. When testing for allergies, a small amount of an allergen is placed under the skin. Within 15 minutes, a patient who is sensitive to the allergen will develop an **induration** (area of hardened tissue). Positive results are determined by measuring the size of the induration and converting it to a numerical scale (Figure 44-23 and Box 44-6).

Tuberculin Testing. The tuberculin sensitivity test most often used is the **Mantoux test.** An ID injection of 0.1 mL of

Text continued on p. 1065

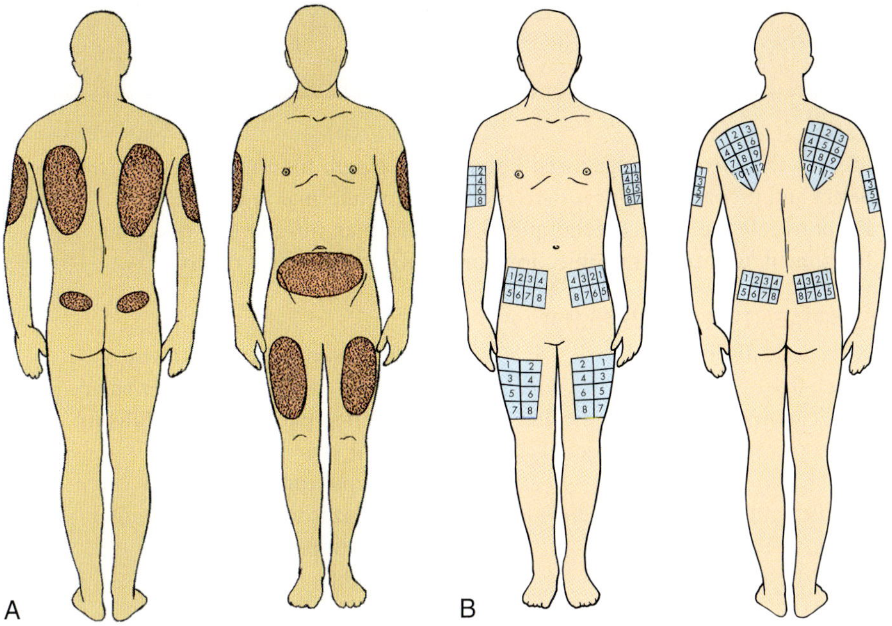

Administering Medications CHAPTER 44 1061

FIGURE 44-19 **A,** Rotation sites for insulin injections. **B,** Injection diagram to track rotation. (From Potter PA, Perry AG: *Basic nursing*, ed 5, St Louis, 2003, Mosby.)

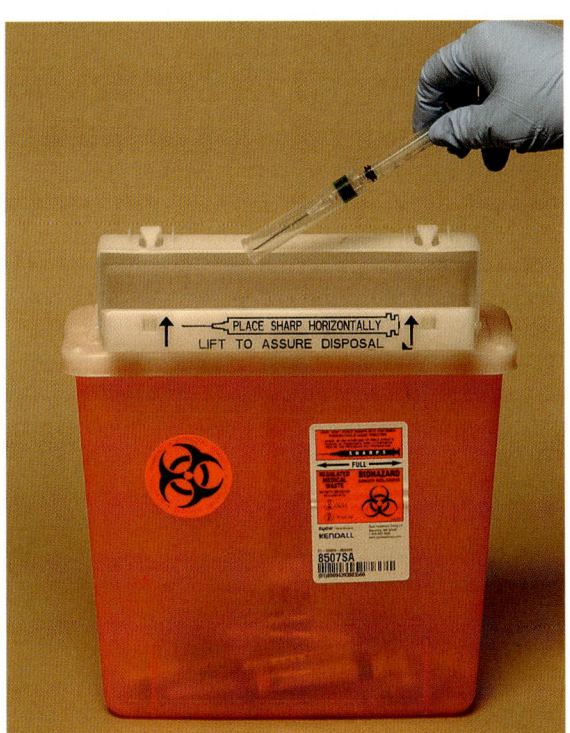

FIGURE 44-20 To prevent needlesticks, examination rooms have sharps containers.

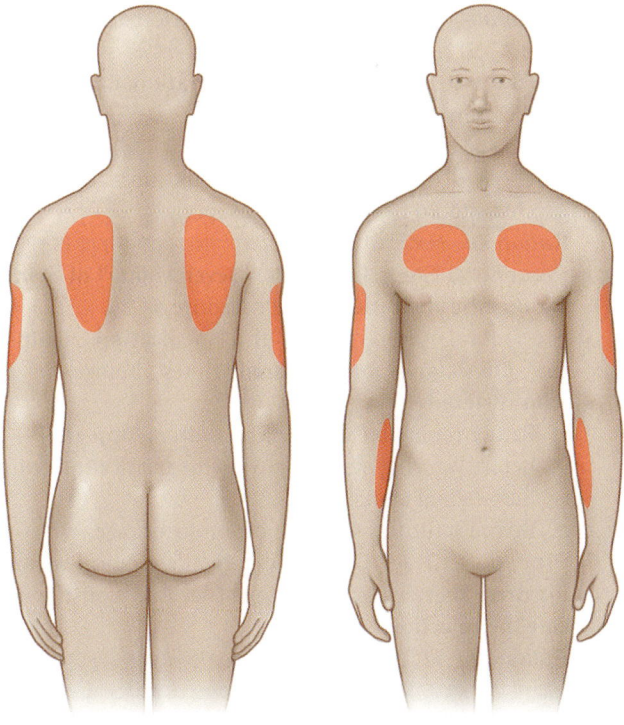

FIGURE 44-21 Sites recommended for intradermal injections.

PROCEDURE 44-7: Administer an Intradermal Injection

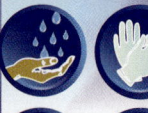
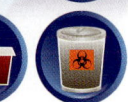

TASKS:
- Identify the correct syringe, needle gauge, and length for an intradermal injection.
- Select and prepare an appropriate site for an intradermal injection.
- Demonstrate the correct technique to administer an intradermal injection.
- Document an intradermal injection correctly in the medical record.

EQUIPMENT AND SUPPLIES
- Nonsterile disposable gloves (latex-free)
- Medication ordered by physician
- Appropriate syringe for ordered dose (tuberculin syringe)
- Needle with safety device (26- or 27-gauge, ⅜ inch to ½ inch)
- 2 × 2 sterile gauze
- 70% isopropyl alcohol wipes
- Small, flexible millimeter ruler
- Written patient instructions for post testing
- Light source
- Sharps container
- Biohazardous waste container
- Fine-tipped pen
- Patient's medical record

SKILLS/RATIONALE
STANDARD PRECAUTIONS ARE TO BE FOLLOWED.

1. **Procedural Step.** Sanitize the hands.
   An alcohol-based hand rub may be used instead of washing hands with soap and water, unless hands are visibly soiled.
   Rationale. Hand sanitization promotes infection control.

2. **Procedural Step.** Assemble equipment and supplies and verify the order.
   Rationale. It is important to have all supplies and equipment ready and available before starting any procedure to ensure efficiency.

3. **Procedural Step.** Check the expiration date of the medication.
   NOTE: The expiration date on stored medications should be checked on a regular basis. Medications that have expired should be disposed of properly.
   Rationale. Medications used past expiration date may be inactive.

4. **Procedural Step.** Follow the "seven rights" of medication administration (see Procedure 44-1).

5. **Procedural Step.** Check the medication against the physician's order three times before it is administered:
   a. Before removing the medication from storage.
   b. Before pouring or withdrawing the medication from the original container.
   c. Before returning the medication to storage.

6. **Procedural Step.** Check the patient's medical record for drug allergies or conditions that may contraindicate the injection.
   Rationale. This ensures that the medication is compatible with the patient, especially when administering antibiotics and analgesics.

7. **Procedural Step.** Calculate the correct dose to be given, if necessary.

8. **Procedural Step.** Follow the procedure for drawing the medication into the syringe (see Procedure 44-5 or 44-6).

9. **Procedural Step.** Greet the patient, introduce yourself, and confirm the patient's identity.
   The patient's medical record and the loaded syringe are brought into the examination room for the injection to be given.
   Rationale. Identifying the patient ensures the procedure is performed on the correct patient.

10. **Procedural Step.** Explain the procedure to the patient.
    Rationale. Explaining the procedure to the patient promotes cooperation and provides a means of obtaining implied consent.

11. **Procedural Step.** Select an appropriate injection site and properly position the patient as necessary to expose the site adequately.
    The sites most often used for intradermal injections are areas where the skin is thin, such as the anterior forearm, the upper back, or the upper chest. The upper arm may also be used to administer an intradermal injection if absolutely necessary. The area should not be scarred or inflamed and should be largely free of hair.

12. **Procedural Step.** Apply gloves.
    Rationale. Gloves provide a barrier precaution against bloodborne pathogens.

13. **Procedural Step.** Prepare the injection site.
    Clean the injection site with an alcohol wipe, working outward in a circular motion beginning at the center. Allow the site to air-dry. Do not touch the site after cleaning it.

Continued

PROCEDURE 44-7 Administer an Intradermal Injection—cont'd

14. **Procedural Step.** While the prepared site is drying, remove the cover from the needle.
Take care to pull the cover off without touching the needle. Check the site visually to be sure it has dried completely before the skin is pierced.
Rationale. Wet alcohol on the injection site causes the needle to sting when it is inserted. It may also interfere with test results.

15. **Procedural Step.** Secure the skin at the injection site.
Pull the skin at the injection site taut with the forefinger and thumb of the nondominant hand. The needle should be positioned almost parallel to the skin, at a very shallow 10- to 15-degree angle.
Rationale. Stretching the patient's skin taut will permit easier insertion of the needle.

16. **Procedural Step.** Puncture the skin.
Insert the needle, with the bevel facing upward, until the bevel barely penetrates the skin, to ensure penetration within the dermal layer of the skin.
The bevel should be visible beneath the transparency of the skin layer.
Rationale. Positioning the bevel up prevents the medication from being deposited into tissues below the dermis.

17. **Procedural Step.** Inject the medication.
Release the grasp on the forearm skin with the nondominant hand and use it to inject the medication slowly within the skin layer. *Do not aspirate* the injection site and keep both hands steady until all the liquid has been injected and forms a wheal of approximately 6 to 10 mm.
A certain amount of resistance should be felt as the medication is injected; this indicates that the needle is properly positioned in the superficial skin layer rather than in the deeper subcutaneous layer.
If the procedure is done correctly, a small raised area, known as a wheal, will form as the liquid accumulates within the dermis layer. If no wheal forms, the injection has been performed incorrectly and the physician should be notified.

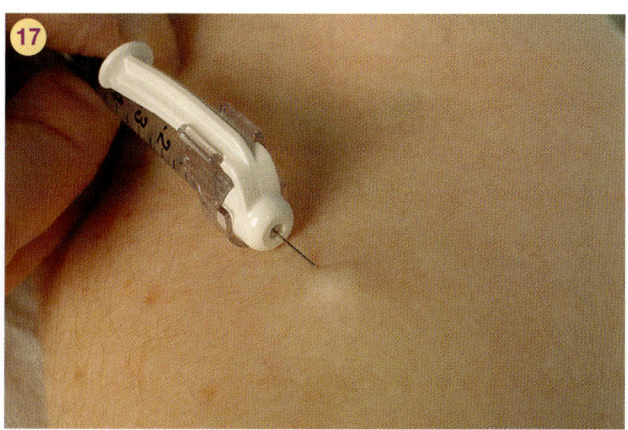

18. **Procedural Step.** Withdraw the needle from the injection site at the same angle it was inserted, and activate the safety device immediately.

19. **Procedural Step.** Dab the area with the gauze pad.
Do not apply pressure to the wheal. Discard the syringe and needle into a sharps container.
NOTE: *Do not* cover the site with a bandage.
Rationale. Massaging the wheal will disperse medication into tissue layers below the dermis and will interfere with the test results. Proper disposal of the needle and syringe is required by OSHA standards.

20. **Procedural Step.** Remove gloves and discard in a biohazardous waste container.

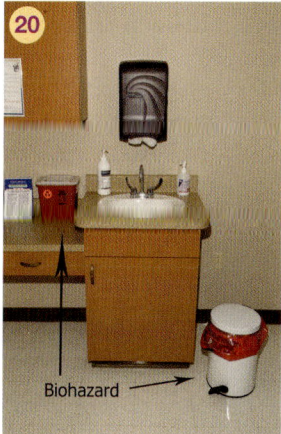

21. **Procedural Step.** Sanitize the hands.
Always sanitize the hands after every procedure or after using gloves.

22. **Procedural Step.** Check on the patient.
Ask the patient how he or she feels and observe once more for any signs of an immediate reaction, such as lightheadedness or fainting.
NOTE: The medical assistant should be especially careful and alert for any sign of a patient reaction when administering an allergy skin test. If the patient experiences an unusual reaction, notify the physician immediately.
Rationale. A reaction to an intradermal injection is usually lightheadedness or fainting resulting from fear of injections. If the medication is delivered correctly between the skin layers, a systemic reaction should not occur.

23. **Procedural Step.** Read or discuss with the patient the test results.
Perform one of the following, based on the type of skin test being administered, the length of time required for the body tissues to react to the test, and the medical office policy.
   a. Read the test results, using inspection and palpation at the site of the injection to assess the presence of and to determine the amount of induration.

Continued

PROCEDURE 44-7 Administer an Intradermal Injection—cont'd

b. Inform the patient of a date and time to return to the medical office to have the results read.
c. Instruct the patient in the proper procedure for reading and interpreting the results at home and reporting them to the medical office.

In all cases, the results must be read and interpreted according to the manufacturer's instructions that accompany the test.

24. **Procedural Step. Document the procedure.**

Include the date and time, name of the medication, dose given, lot number, expiration date, route of administration, injection site used, skin test results (as appropriate), and any significant observations or patient reactions.

NOTE: If the skin test results are to be recorded at a later date, the results will not be recorded at this time.

Rationale. The lot number and expiration date are documented so that should a problem arise with the batch of medication used, the drug can be recalled and individuals who received it identified. No procedure is completed until it has been documented.

CHARTING EXAMPLE

Date	
4/3/xx	1:00 p.m. Mantoux tuberculin test, 0.10 mL, ID, Lot # MG5768C Exp date 10-xx, given Ⓡ ant forearm. Instructed patient to return on 4/6 to have results read.— ————————— T. Isaacs, CMA (AAMA)

MANTOUX TEST

READING THE REACTION

1. **Procedural Step. Read the test results in 48 to 72 hours.**
2. **Procedural Step. After sanitizing the hands and applying nonsterile gloves, inspect the site, gently rub the test site with a finger, and lightly palpate for induration.**

Inspection requires a good light source. If induration is present, lightly rub the area from the area without induration to the indurated site to assess the entire size of the area of induration.

3. **Procedural Step. Mark the edges and measure the diameter of the area of induration from edge to edge (not the reddened area).**

If the area is only reddened but not indurated, do not take the measurement. The induration area is the area measured. A diameter of 10 mm or more indicates a positive test. Areas of redness without swelling should not be included in the measurement.

4. **Procedural Step. Record the diameter of induration that was measured, and notify the health care provider of the measurement.**

The medical assistant documents only what is observed and must not interpret the result.

5. **Procedural Step. Record the reading in millimeters.**

NOTE: Induration is the only criterion used in determining a positive reaction to a tuberculin test. It is a raised, hard, and reddened area at the injection site.

INTERPRETING THE REACTION

Induration 10 mm or more in diameter:
- Positive for possible past or present infection or exposure to infection with *Mycobacterium tuberculosis,* and further testing by x-ray or sputum examination is needed.
- Test does not have to be repeated, unless the validity of the test is in question.

Induration of 5 to 9 mm:
- Classified as doubtful, unless the patient has a close contact with an individual known to be positive for *M. tuberculosis.*
- In the presence of positive radiographic or clinical evidence of a disease resembling tuberculosis, the reaction should be read as "possibly positive."
- Repeat testing is indicated.

Induration of less than 5 mm:
- Negative reaction.
- No repeat test necessary, unless there is clinical suspicion of tuberculosis.

CHARTING EXAMPLE

Date	
4/5/xx	1:00 p.m. No reaction observed to Mantoux tuberculin test.— ————————— T. Isaacs, CMA (AAMA)

Step 17 photo from Potter PA, Perry AG: Basic nursing, ed 6, St Louis, 2007, Mosby.

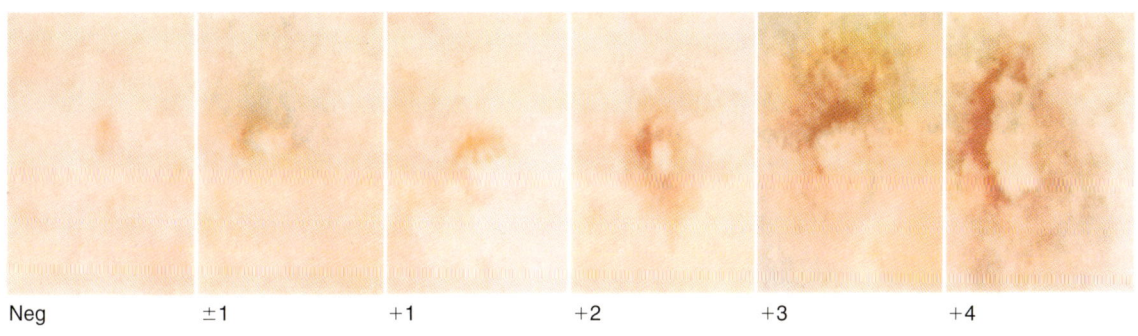

FIGURE 44-22 An intradermal injection deposits medication under the epidermis to form a wheal. (From Bonewit-West K: *Clinical procedures for medical assistants,* ed 7, St Louis, 2008, Saunders.)

FIGURE 44-23 Skin-prick and intradermal skin test results.

BOX 44-6	
Numerical Scale for Induration Reaction in Allergy Testing	
−	No reaction
±1	Induration of 1 mm or less
+1	Induration greater than 1 mm and up to 5 mm in diameter
+2	Induration greater than 5 mm and up to 10 mm in diameter
+3	Induration greater than 10 mm and up to 15 mm in diameter
+4	Induration greater than 15 mm in diameter

purified-protein derivative (PPD) is injected into the patient's forearm. If an induration of 10 mm or greater appears within 48 to 72 hours, the patient is said to be positive for exposure to the tuberculin bacteria *Mycobacterium tuberculosis*. Further tests (e.g., chest x-ray, sputum analysis) must be done to confirm a positive reaction that shows the person is infected with the bacteria.

Subcutaneous

A **subcutaneous (SubQ) injection** is placed into the fatty layer beneath the dermis. This method is used for small amounts of nonirritating medications. Because the blood supply in subcutaneous tissue is minimal, the absorption rate is slow. Sites chosen include the upper outer area of the arm, thigh, and abdomen (Figure 44-24). Medications given by SubQ injection must be water-soluble, nonirritating, less than 2 mL, and potent enough in small amounts to be effective. Vaccines (e.g., MMR), heparin, insulin, and influenza vaccines (flu shots) are all administered using the SubQ method. Because medications given by injection are sometimes irritating to soft tissue and nerve endings, it is recommended that repeated injections (e.g., insulin) be rotated to minimize tissue damage. Figure 44-25 provides recommended subcutaneous injection sites.

Administration. Typically, needles ⅝ to 1 inch with a gauge of 25 to 28 are attached to a 3-mL syringe. The needle is usually inserted at a 45-degree angle, but this can be increased to 90 degrees for obese patients or when insulin and heparin are injected with a short, fine needle. Before injecting the SubQ medication, the plunger is pulled back slightly to aspirate for blood to ensure the needle is not in a blood vessel. (**Aspiration** is *not* done for insulin or heparin doses.) When no blood appears and the needle is determined to be in the subcutaneous tissue, the medication is injected slowly and evenly. Procedure 44-8 provides instructions for the administration of a subcutaneous injection.

Intramuscular

An **intramuscular (IM) injection** is administered into a large muscle. The IM route of administration is used when rapid

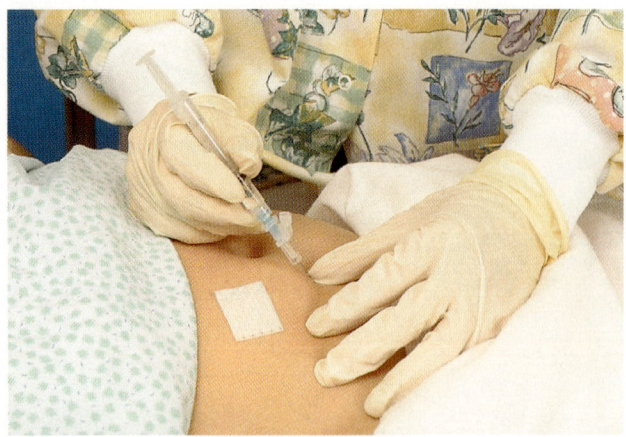

FIGURE 44-24 Administering subcutaneous heparin in the abdomen. (From Potter PA, Perry AG: *Basic nursing*, ed 5, St Louis, 2003, Mosby.)

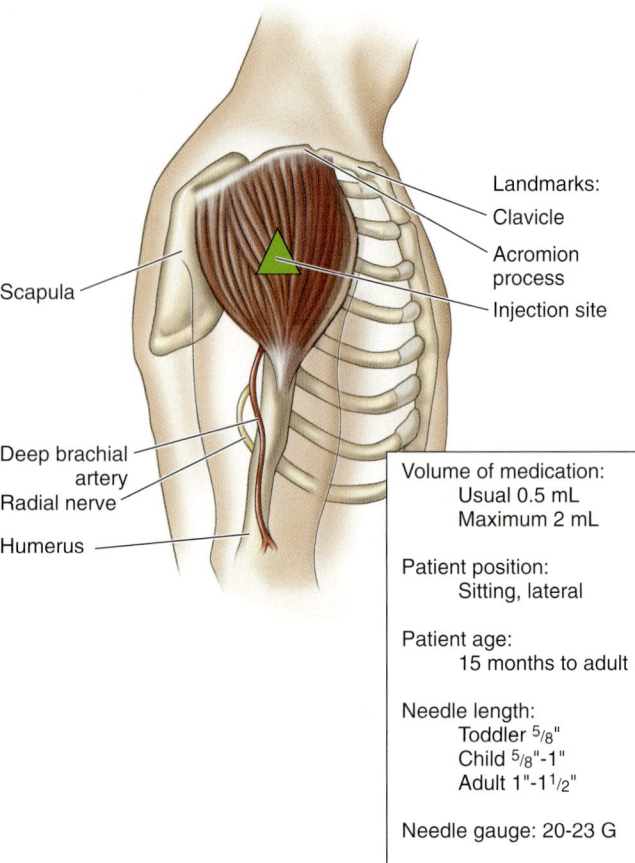

FIGURE 44-26 Deltoid muscle injection site. (From Hunt SA: *Saunders fundamentals of medical assisting—revised reprint*, St Louis, 2007, Saunders.)

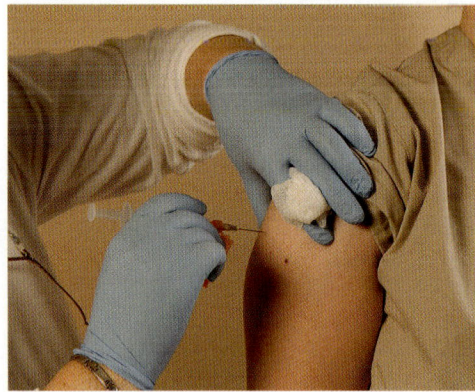

FIGURE 44-27 Intramuscular injection into the deltoid muscle.

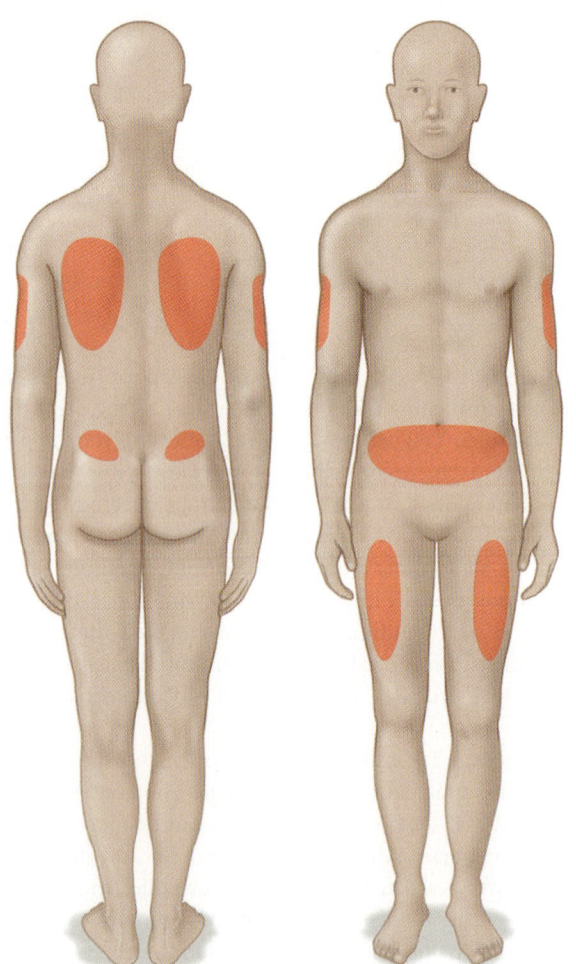

FIGURE 44-25 Sites recommended for subcutaneous injections.

absorption is needed. Sites frequently chosen for IM injection are the deltoid, vastus lateralis, and gluteus muscles.

Deltoid Muscle. The **deltoid muscle** is approved for both adults and older children. The injection should be given 1 to 2 inches (two fingerbreadths) below the acromion process and across from the axilla. No more than 2 mL for adults and 1 mL for children should be injected into this site. The medication should be aqueous. Figure 44-26 provides additional information on using the deltoid site, and Figure 44-27 illustrates an IM injection into the deltoid muscle. This site should only be used if the patient has well-developed muscle mass, since there is the potential for injury to the radial nerve and brachial artery.

PROCEDURE 44-8

Administer a Subcutaneous Injection

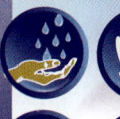
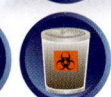

TASKS:
- Identify the correct syringe, needle gauge, and length for a subcutaneous injection.
- Select and prepare an appropriate site for a subcutaneous injection.
- Demonstrate the correct technique to administer a subcutaneous injection.
- Document a subcutaneous injection correctly in the medical record.

EQUIPMENT AND SUPPLIES
- Nonsterile disposable gloves (Latex-free)
- Medication ordered by physician
- Appropriate syringe for ordered dose (3-mL syringe, or tuberculin syringe if medication amount is less than 1 mL)
- Needle with safety device (25- or 27-gauge, ⅝ to 1 inch)
- 2 × 2 sterile gauze
- 70% isopropyl alcohol wipes
- Sharps container
- Biohazardous waste container
- Patient's medical record

SKILLS/RATIONALE

STANDARD PRECAUTIONS ARE TO BE FOLLOWED.

1. **Procedural Step.** Sanitize the hands.
   An alcohol-based hand rub may be used instead of washing hands with soap and water, unless hands are visibly soiled.
   Rationale. Hand sanitization promotes infection control.

2. **Procedural Step.** Assemble equipment and supplies and verify the order.
   Rationale. It is important to have all supplies and equipment ready and available before starting any procedure to ensure efficiency.

3. **Procedural Step.** Check the expiration date of the medication.
   NOTE: The expiration date on stored medications should be checked on a regular basis. Medications that have expired should be disposed of properly.
   Rationale. Medications used past expiration date may be inactive.

4. **Procedural Step.** Follow the "seven rights" of medication administration (see Procedure 44-1).

5. **Procedural Step.** Check the medication against the physician's order three times before it is administered:
   a. Before removing the medication from storage.
   b. Before pouring or withdrawing the medication from the original container.
   c. Before returning the medication to storage.

6. **Procedural Step.** Check the patient's medical record for drug allergies or conditions that may contraindicate the injection.
   Rationale. This ensures that the medication is compatible with the patient, especially when administering antibiotics and analgesics.

7. **Procedural Step.** Calculate the correct dose to be given, if necessary.

8. **Procedural Step.** Follow the procedure for drawing the medication into the syringe (see Procedure 44-5 or 44-6).

9. **Procedural Step.** Greet the patient, introduce yourself, and confirm the patient's identity.
   Recheck allergies with the patient. The patient's medical record and the loaded syringe are brought into the examination room for the injection to be given.
   Rationale. Identifying the patient ensures the procedure is performed on the correct patient.

10. **Procedural Step.** Explain the procedure to the patient.
    Rationale. Explaining the procedure to the patient promotes cooperation and provides a means of obtaining implied consent.

11. **Procedural Step.** Select an appropriate injection site and properly position the patient as necessary to expose the site adequately.
    Subcutaneous injections are given in areas where there is a substantial amount of connective tissue between the muscle and the skin to absorb the medication without damage to nerves, muscles, bones, or blood vessels. The upper outer aspect of the arm, the upper thighs, the lower abdomen, the upper back, and the flank region are all appropriate sites. If frequent injections are being given, the sites should be rotated.

12. **Procedural Step.** Apply gloves.
    Rationale. Gloves provide a barrier precaution against bloodborne pathogens.

Continued

PROCEDURE 44-8 Administer a Subcutaneous Injection—cont'd

13. **Procedural Step.** Prepare the injection site.

    Clean the injection site with an alcohol wipe, working outward in a circular motion beginning at the center. Allow the site to air-dry. Do not touch the site after cleaning it.

    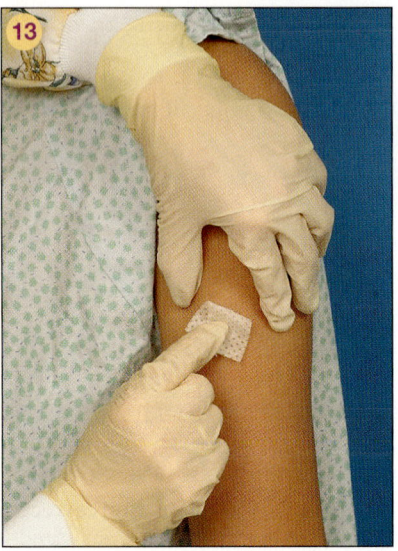

14. **Procedural Step.** While the prepared site is drying, remove the cover from the needle.

    Take care to pull the cover off without touching the needle. Check the site visually to be sure it has dried completely before the skin is pierced.

    Rationale. Wet alcohol on the injection site causes the needle to sting when it is inserted.

15. **Procedural Step.** Secure the skin at the injection site.

    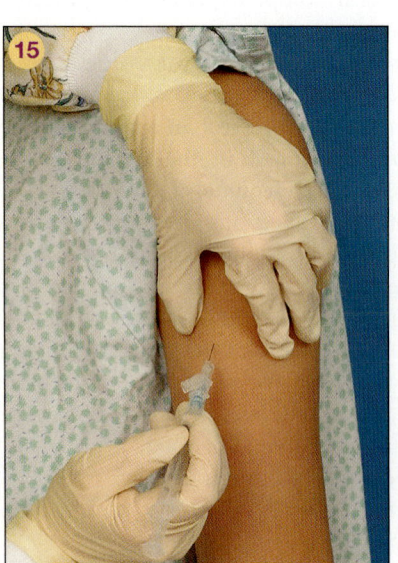

    Without touching the intended puncture location, grasp a generous portion of the skin around the injection site. Hold the syringe between the thumb and first two fingers with the ring and small fingers positioning the needle at a 45-degree upward angle. It is not necessary to position the bevel for a subcutaneous injection.

    Rationale. Grasping a portion of the patient's skin around the injection ensures that only subcutaneous tissue is injected.

16. **Procedural Step.** Puncture the skin quickly and smoothly.

    Make sure the needle is kept at a 45-degree angle.

17. **Procedural Step.** Check to see if blood aspirates into the syringe.

    Release the grasp on the tissue, and use the hand that was grasping around the injection site to pull back slightly on the plunger of the syringe (aspirate). *The needle should not be allowed to move during aspiration.* To avoid moving the needle, use the hand holding the barrel of the syringe to push inward to resist movement as the other hand pulls the plunger outward.

    NOTE: If blood is drawn into the syringe during aspiration, the needle has pierced a blood vessel and should be withdrawn from the site. In these situations, the loaded syringe and needle must be discarded and another dose with a new syringe and needle prepared.

    Rationale. Moving the needle in and out causes unnecessary pain to the patient and changes the needle's placement with the risk of entering a blood vessel.

18. **Procedural Step.** Inject the medication.

    If no blood is aspirated into the syringe when the plunger is pulled back, there is usually a sensation of pulling against pressure and it is safe to inject the medication. Push the plunger of the syringe slowly and steadily until

    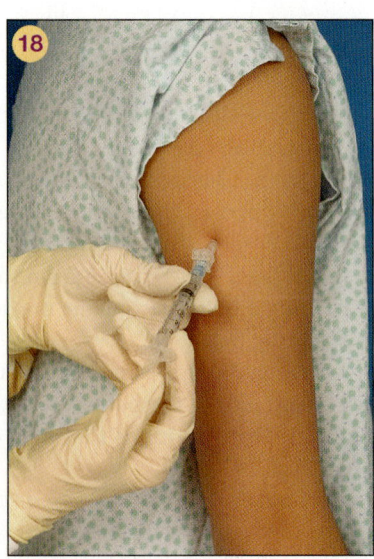

Continued

PROCEDURE 44-8 Administer a Subcutaneous Injection—cont'd

all the medication is delivered into the subcutaneous tissue. Take care to hold the syringe still while the medication is being injected.

19. **Procedural Step.** Place a gauze pad over the injection site and quickly withdraw the needle from the injection site at the same angle at which it was inserted.
Activate the safety device immediately.
Rationale. Withdrawing the needle quickly and at the same angle reduces discomfort. Using the gauze pad over the injection site prevents tissue movement and the stinging sensation that an alcohol wipe would cause.

20. **Procedural Step.** Massage the injection site.
Use the 2 × 2 gauze pad to massage the injection site gently but firmly. To avoid tissue damage after administering insulin or heparin, however, do *not* massage the injection site.
Rationale. Massaging the injection site helps to distribute the medication into the body tissue.

21. **Procedural Step.** Discard the syringe and needle into a sharps container.

22. **Procedural Step.** Remove gloves and discard in a biohazardous waste container.

23. **Procedural Step.** Sanitize the hands.
Always sanitize the hands after every procedure or after using gloves.

24. **Procedural Step.** Check on the patient.
Ask the patient how he or she feels, and observe the patient for any signs of an immediate reaction, such as dizziness, fainting, or severe pain at the injection site. Instruct the patient to remain in the office for another 15 to 30 minutes, since the most severe reactions (e.g., difficulty breathing, hives, and low blood pressure) are likely to begin within this time.

25. **Procedural Step.** Document the procedure.
Include the date and time, name of the medication, dose given, lot number, expiration date, route of administration, injection site used, and any significant observations or patient reactions.
Rationale. The lot number and expiration date are documented so that should a problem arise with the batch of medication used, the drug can be recalled and individuals who received it identified. No procedure is completed until it has been documented.

CHARTING EXAMPLE

Date	
4/1/xx	3:30 p.m. Ragweed allergy inj, 0.20 cc, Lot # JH4857B Exp date 7-xx, SubQ Ⓡ upper arm. Arm checked 15 minutes after administration. No reaction noted. Verbal and written follow-up instructions provided. ———————— J. Hammill, RMA

Steps 13, 15, and 18 photos from Potter PA, Perry AG: Basic nursing, ed 6, St Louis, 2007, Mosby.

Vastus Lateralis Muscle. The **vastus lateralis muscle** (thigh muscle) is located below the greater trochanter of the femur and the knee. The vastus lateralis muscle is the preferred site for infants and young children because it lacks major nerves and blood vessels and is one of the body's largest muscles. A child should be given the injection within the upper lateral quadrant of the thigh. An adult, however, receives the injection within the middle third of the muscle (Figure 44-28). This site provides for rapid drug absorption. Procedure 44-9 describes the procedure for giving an infant an IM injection and immunization.

Ventrogluteal Muscle. The **ventrogluteal** (*gluteus medius* and *gluteus minimus*) area is an injection site used from infancy to adulthood, since the area is free of major nerves and blood vessels and has a large muscle mass (Figure 44-29). All forms of injectable medication can be given in this site (e.g., aqueous, oil-based). The medical assistant places the patient in Sims' position with the palm of the patient's hand on the greater trochanter. The assistant places the index finger on the anterosuperior iliac spine and fans out the middle finger to touch the iliac crest. This forms a triangular injection area. The injection is made into the middle of the triangle formed by the assistant's index and middle fingers.

Dorsogluteal Area. The **dorsogluteal** area has been a traditional site for IM injections, but extreme care must be taken because of its proximity to major blood vessels and the sciatic nerve (Figure 44-30). Accidentally hitting the sciatic nerve would be extremely painful for the patient and could cause partial or permanent paralysis of the leg involved. Divide the gluteus area into quarters and give the injection in the upper outer quadrant.

To locate the correct injection site, the entire area must be visible and palpable. This is accomplished by marking off landmarks for proper positioning of the needle and clear visualization of the site. The patient should be in a comfortable position (e.g., leaning over examination table, lying down with the toes pointed inward) to relax muscle tension.

Administration. For most IM locations, no more than 3 mL of medication should be delivered at one time. If the dose is

Text continued on p. 1074

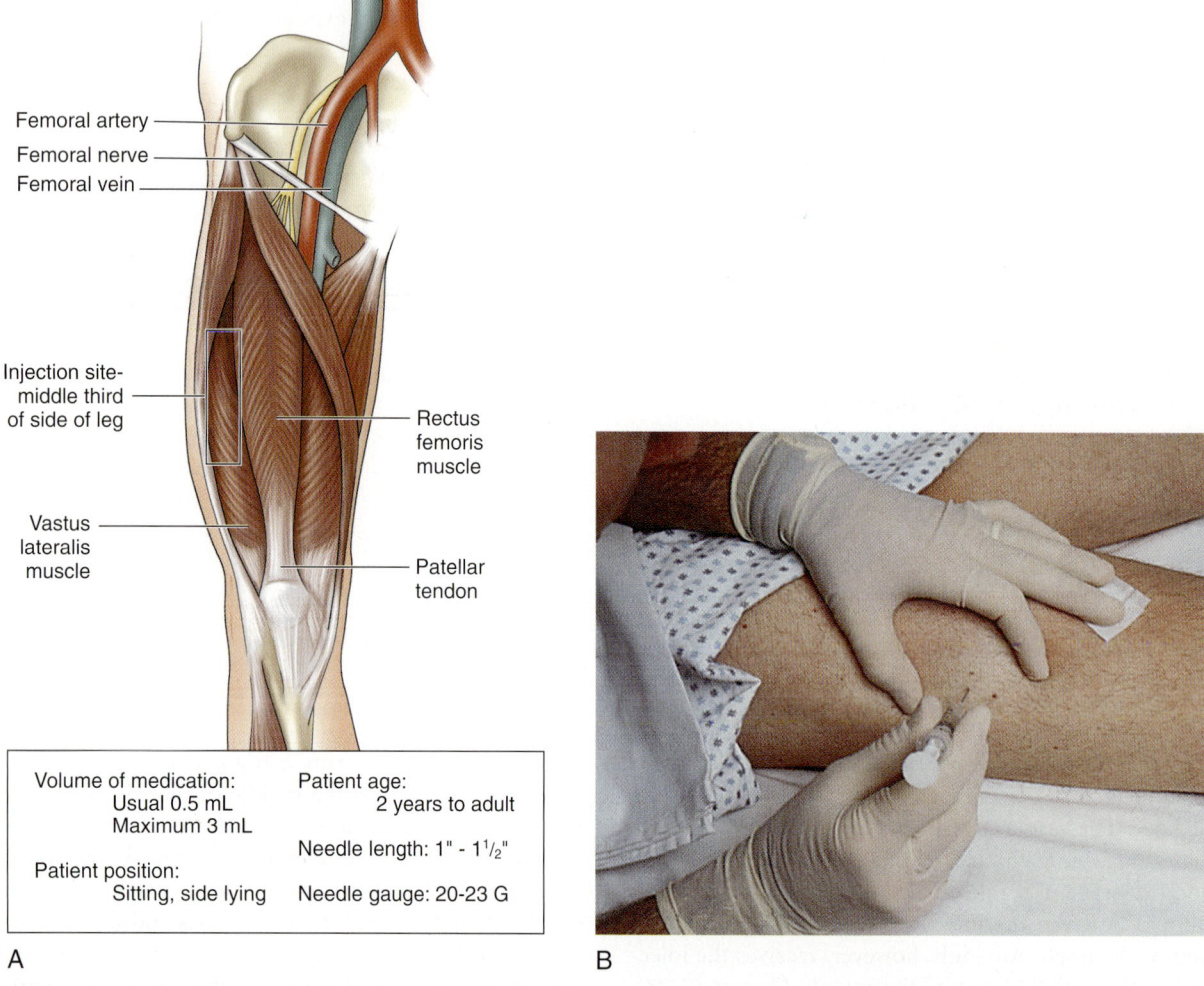

FIGURE 44-28 Vastus lateralis injection site (adults). (**A** from Hunt SA: *Saunders fundamentals of medical assisting—revised reprint*, St Louis, 2007, Saunders; **B** from Lilley L, Aucker R: *Pharmacology and the nursing process*, ed 3, St Louis, 2001, Mosby.)

PROCEDURE 44-9

Administer an Intramuscular Injection to a Pediatric Patient

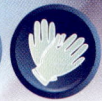
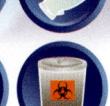

TASKS:
- Identify the correct syringe, needle gauge, and length for a pediatric intramuscular injection.
- Select and prepare an appropriate site for a pediatric intramuscular injection.
- Demonstrate the correct technique to administer an intramuscular injection.
- Document an intramuscular injection correctly in the medical record.

EQUIPMENT AND SUPPLIES
- Nonsterile disposable gloves
- Medication ordered by physician
- Appropriate syringe for ordered dose (3-mL syringe, or tuberculin syringe if medication amount is less than 1 mL)
- Needle with safety device (25- or 27-gauge, ⅝ to 1 inch)
- 2 × 2 sterile gauze
- 70% isopropyl alcohol wipes
- Sharps container
- Biohazardous waste container
- Patient's medical record

SKILLS/*RATIONALE*

STANDARD PRECAUTIONS ARE TO BE FOLLOWED.

1. **Procedural Step. Sanitize the hands.**
   An alcohol-based hand rub may be used instead of washing hands with soap and water, unless hands are visibly soiled.
   Rationale. Hand sanitization promotes infection control.

2. **Procedural Step. Assemble equipment and supplies and verify the order.**
   Rationale. It is important to have all supplies and equipment ready and available before starting any procedure to ensure efficiency.

3. **Procedural Step. Check the expiration date of the medication.**
   NOTE: The expiration date on stored medications should be checked on a regular basis. Medications that have expired should be disposed of properly.
   Rationale. Medications used past expiration date may be inactive.

4. **Procedural Step. Follow the "seven rights" of medication administration (see Procedure 44-1).**

5. **Procedural Step. Check the medication against the physician's order three times before it is administered:**
   a. Before removing the medication from storage.
   b. Before pouring or withdrawing the medication from the original container.
   c. Before returning the medication to storage.

6. **Procedural Step. Check the patient's medical record for drug allergies or conditions that may contraindicate the injection.**
   Rationale. This ensures that the medication is compatible with the patient, especially when administering antibiotics and analgesics.

7. **Procedural Step. Calculate the correct dose to be given, if necessary.**

8. **Procedural Step. Follow the procedure for drawing the medication into the syringe (see Procedure 44-5 or 44-6).**

9. **Procedural Step. Greet the patient's parent or guardian, introduce yourself, and confirm the patient's identity.**
   The patient's medical record and the loaded syringe are brought into the examination room for the injection to be given.
   Rationale. Identifying the patient ensures the procedure is performed on the correct patient.

10. **Procedural Step. Explain the procedure to the patient (depending on age) and the patient's parent or guardian as appropriate.**
    Rationale. Explaining the procedure to the patient and parent or guardian promotes cooperation and provides a means of obtaining implied consent.

11. **Procedural Step. Select an appropriate injection site and properly position the patient as necessary.**
    Remove the patient's clothing as necessary to make sure the entire area is exposed.
    The vastus lateralis muscle is the site of choice for pediatric patients up to age 12 months who are not walking. Once the child is walking, the deltoid region or ventral gluteus are usually used (stiffness and soreness of the vastus lateralis may occur when the child walks after injection to that site).
    Major nerves and blood vessels may lie close to the intramuscular injection site. The site must be free from conditions (e.g., bruise, scar tissue) that would contraindicate using the area.

Continued

PROCEDURE 44-9 Administer an Intramuscular Injection to a Pediatric Patient—cont'd

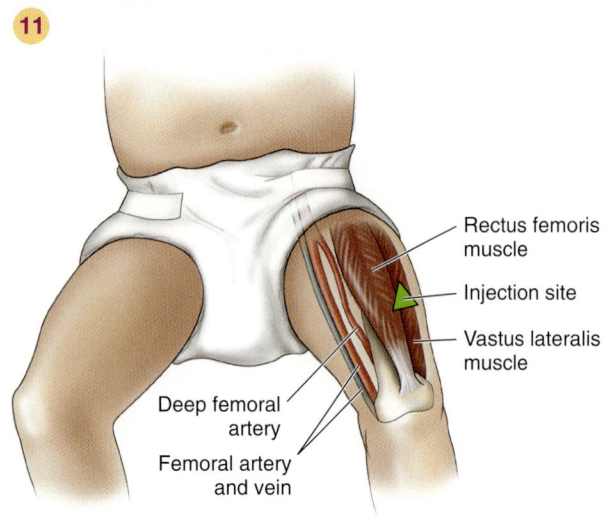

Volume of medication:	Patient age:
Infants 0.5 mL	Birth to 2 years
Pediatric 0.5-2 mL	
Patient position:	Needle length: ⅝"
Supine, sitting	Needle gauge: 22-25 G

12. **Procedural Step. Apply gloves.**
    Rationale. Gloves provide a barrier precaution against bloodborne pathogens.
13. **Procedural Step. Secure the patient.**
    Depending on the patient's age and the situation, the pediatric patient may need to be restrained by the parent or guardian. If the parent or guardian is unable to help restrain the child, a second health care professional should assume this task. Restraint should only be used as a very last resort. Gaining the child's cooperation is always less traumatic.
14. **Procedural Step. Prepare the injection site.**
    Clean the injection site with an alcohol wipe, working outward in a circular motion beginning at the center. Allow the site to air-dry. Do not touch the site after cleaning it.
15. **Procedural Step. While the prepared site is drying, remove the cover from the needle.**
    Take care to pull the cover off without touching the needle. Check the site visually to be sure it has dried completely before the skin is pierced.
    Rationale. Wet alcohol on the injection site causes the needle to sting when it is inserted.
16. **Procedural Step. Secure the skin at the injection site.**
    Without touching the intended puncture location, spread apart the skin around the injection site with the thumb and forefinger to compress the subcutaneous tissue. Hold the syringe between the thumb and first two fingers, with the ring and small fingers positioning the needle at a 90-degree angle to the injection site (perpendicular). It is not necessary to position the bevel for an intramuscular injection.
    Rationale. Compressing the subcutaneous tissue around the injection site ensures that muscle tissue is injected.
17. **Procedural Step. Puncture the skin quickly and smoothly, with the needle kept at a 90-degree angle.**
    The entire needle is inserted up to the hilt.
18. **Procedural Step. Check to see if blood aspirates into the syringe.**
    Release the grasp on the tissue and use the hand that was grasping around the injection site to pull back slightly on the plunger of the syringe (aspirate). *The needle should not be allowed to move during aspiration.* To avoid moving the needle, use the hand holding the barrel of the syringe to push inward to resist movement as the other hand pulls the plunger outward.
    NOTE: If blood is drawn into the syringe during aspiration, the needle has pierced a blood vessel and should be withdrawn from the site. In such situations, the loaded syringe and needle must be discarded and another dose with a new syringe and needle prepared.
    Rationale. Moving the needle in and out causes unnecessary pain to the patient and changes the needle's placement with the risk of entering a blood vessel.
19. **Procedural Step. Inject the medication.**
    If no blood is aspirated into the syringe when the plunger is pulled back, there is usually a sensation of pulling against pressure, and it is safe to inject the medication. Push the plunger of the syringe slowly and steadily until all the medication is delivered into the intramuscular tissue. Take care to hold the syringe still while the medication is being injected.
20. **Procedural Step. Place a gauze pad over the injection site and withdraw the needle from the injection site at the same angle at which it was inserted.**
    Activate the safety device immediately.
    Rationale. Withdrawing the needle quickly and at the same angle reduces discomfort. Using the gauze pad over the injection site prevents tissue movement and the stinging sensation an alcohol wipe would cause.
21. **Procedural Step. Massage the injection site.**
    Use the 2 × 2 gauze pad to massage the injection site gently but firmly. To avoid tissue damage after administering insulin or heparin, however, do *not* massage the injection site.
    Rationale. Massaging the injection site helps to distribute the medication into the body tissue.
22. **Procedural Step. Discard the syringe and needle into a sharps container.**
23. **Procedural Step. Remove gloves, and discard in a biohazardous waste container.**

Continued

PROCEDURE 44-9 Administer an Intramuscular Injection to a Pediatric Patient—cont'd

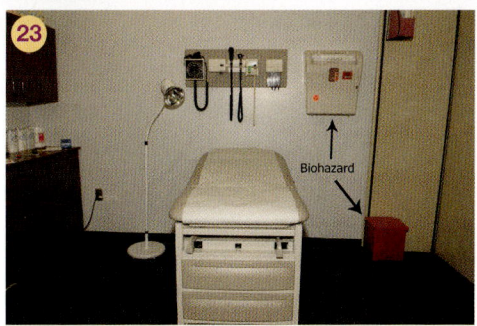

24. **Procedural Step.** Sanitize the hands.
    Always sanitize the hands after every procedure or after using gloves.

25. **Procedural Step.** Check on the patient.
    Observe the pediatric patient for any signs of an immediate reaction, such as dizziness, fainting, or severe pain at the injection site. If the injection is given in the dorsogluteal or ventrogluteal region, be sure the child can move the leg after the injection. The child should remain in the office for another 15 to 20 minutes, since the most severe reactions (e.g., difficulty breathing, hives, and low blood pressure) are likely to begin within this time.

26. **Procedural Step.** Document the procedure.
    Include the date and time, name of the medication, dose given, lot number, expiration date, route of administration, injection site used, and any significant observations or patient reactions.
    If the injection was an immunization, the immunization record must be completed as well. A VIS statement is provided and is also documented (see Procedure 43-1).
    Rationale. The lot number and expiration date are documented so that should a problem arise with the batch of medication used, the drug can be recalled and individuals who received it identified. No procedure is completed until it has been documented.

CHARTING EXAMPLE

Date	
8/13/xx	10:30 a.m. Td Lot # 27050, Exp date 2-xx IM (L) vastus lateralis. Verbal and VIS (6/10/xx) provided to parent. Tolerated injection well, no adverse effects noted. ———————————— T. Kremser, CMA (AAMA)

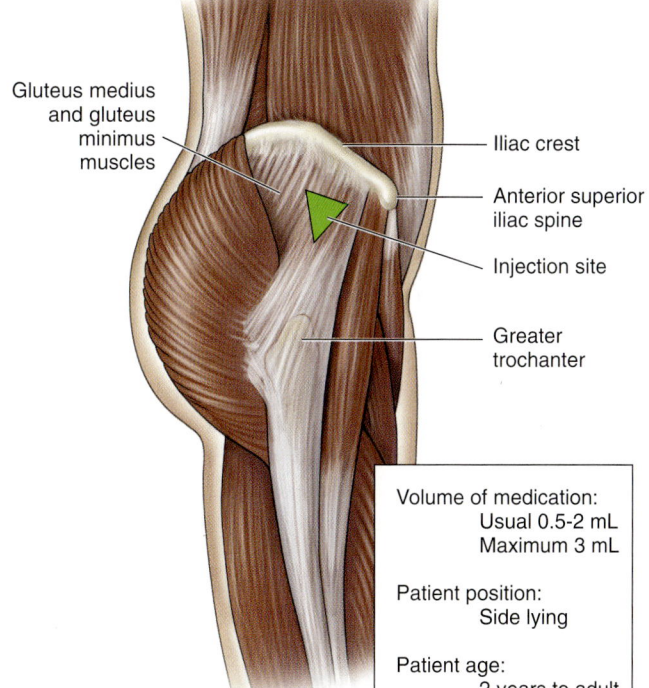

FIGURE 44-29 Ventrogluteal injection site. (From Hunt SA: *Saunders fundamentals of medical assisting—revised reprint,* St Louis, 2007, Saunders.)

Volume of medication:
 Usual 0.5-2 mL
 Maximum 3 mL

Patient position:
 Side lying

Patient age:
 2 years to adult

Needle length:
 Child 1"-1½"
 Adult 1½"- 2"

Needle gauge: 18-23 G

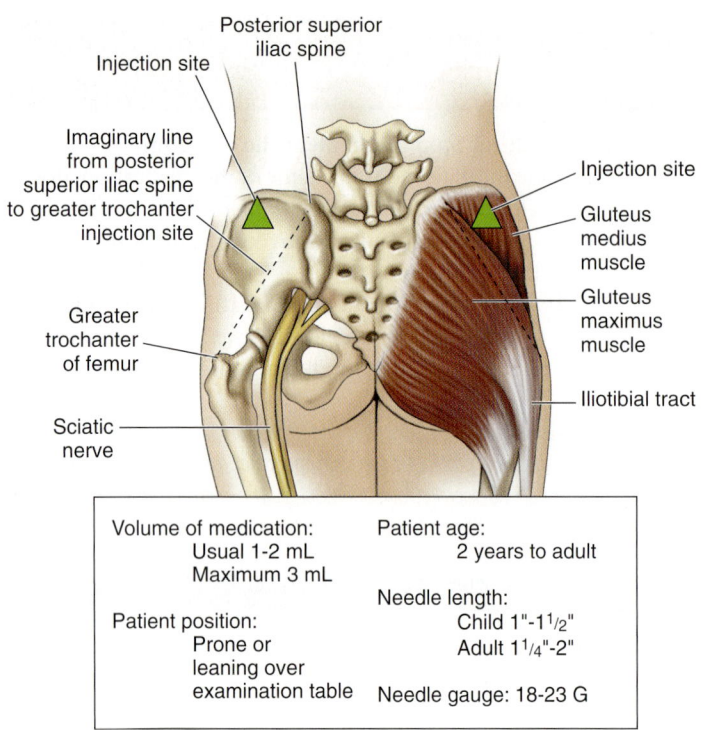

FIGURE 44-30 Dorsogluteal injection site. (From Hunt SA: *Saunders fundamentals of medical assisting—revised reprint,* St Louis, 2007, Saunders.)

larger, the medication should be divided into two smaller doses.

When giving an IM injection, the medical assistant should position the patient according to the site chosen. The site is wiped with alcohol. The needle should be inserted at a 90-degree angle and done quickly and smoothly to avoid tissue pulling. The syringe should be held steady while the needle is in the tissue. Caution must be taken to ensure the medication is deposited directly into a muscle and not into subcutaneous tissue or a blood vessel. Aspirate to determine if the needle has entered a blood vessel. If not, the medication is injected slowly and steadily. Once the needle is removed, the injection site should be gently massaged, unless contraindicated. Procedure 44-10 details the administration of an IM injection to an adult.

Z-Track Technique

The **Z-track method** is a special technique used for IM injections when a medication (e.g., iron) could cause skin discoloration or irritation to the subcutaneous tissue. The Z-track method stops medication from leaking back into the subcutaneous tissue. The preferred sites are the vastus lateralis and ventrogluteal muscles.

Administration. During the injection, the skin is pulled to one side and held. The needle is inserted at a 90-degree angle, the plunger is pulled back to aspirate, and the medication is delivered. There is a 10-second delay to allow the medication to disperse evenly, then the skin is released after the needle is withdrawn. This leaves a zigzag needle track that seals the needle path so the medication cannot leave the muscle tissue. The site is not massaged after injection. Procedure 44-11 provides Z-track instructions.

Intravenous Therapy

Administration of **intravenous (IV) therapy** (fluids and medications) allows for the fastest absorption, but it is also the most dangerous route because it enters directly into the bloodstream. The medical practice acts in each state, as well as medical office policy, will determine who can perform venipuncture, administer IV fluids, and give IV medications. Although the medical assistant may not currently have the responsibility to perform IV therapy, he or she may be required to set up supplies and equipment needed for IV therapy. Therefore it is important that the medical assistant have basic knowledge concerning fluid replacement, equipment and supply needs, scheduling requirements, and basic patient information.

Scheduling a patient for IV therapy at an outpatient facility requires that the medical assistant know the following information:

- Fluids the patient is to receive
- Medication(s) ordered
- Laboratory test(s) to be performed before and after treatment to monitor progress

Instructions given to the patient should include the date, time, and place where the IV therapy will occur. Any dietary restrictions, amount of time the infusion will take, and how to dress should also be provided. For example, a patient receiving IV fluids containing a chemotherapy medication will be at the facility 4 to 6 hours and should plan on wearing comfortable clothes. Often the facility will have a consultation setup with the patient to go over the procedure and meet the staff.

The next section provides a basic introduction to IV therapy guidelines.

Text continued on p. 1080

PROCEDURE 44-10 Administer an Intramuscular Injection to an Adult

TASKS:
- Identify the correct syringe, needle gauge, and length for an adult intramuscular injection.
- Select and prepare an appropriate site for an adult intramuscular injection.
- Demonstrate the correct technique to administer an intramuscular injection.
- Document an intramuscular injection correctly in the medical record.

EQUIPMENT AND SUPPLIES
- Nonsterile disposable gloves (Latex-free)
- Medication ordered by physician
- Appropriate syringe for ordered dose (3-mL syringe)
- Needle with safety device (21- to 25-gauge, 1 inch to 1½ inch)
- 2 × 2 sterile gauze
- 70% isopropyl alcohol wipes
- Sharps container
- Biohazardous waste container
- Patient's medical record

SKILLS/RATIONALE

STANDARD PRECAUTIONS ARE TO BE FOLLOWED.

1. **Procedural Step.** Sanitize the hands.
   An alcohol-based hand rub may be used instead of washing hands with soap and water, unless hands are visibly soiled.
   Rationale. Hand sanitization promotes infection control.

2. **Procedural Step.** Assemble equipment and supplies and verify the order.
   Rationale. It is important to have all supplies and equipment ready and available before starting any procedure to ensure efficiency.

3. **Procedural Step.** Check the expiration date of the medication.
   NOTE: The expiration date on stored medications should be checked on a regular basis. Medications that have expired should be disposed of properly.
   Rationale. Medications used past expiration date may be inactive.

4. **Procedural Step.** Follow the "seven rights" of medication administration (see Procedure 44-1).

5. **Procedural Step.** Check the medication against the physician's order three times before it is administered:
   a. Before removing the medication from storage.
   b. Before pouring or withdrawing the medication from the original container.
   c. Before returning the medication to storage.

6. **Procedural Step.** Check the patient's medical record for drug allergies or conditions that may contraindicate the injection.
   Rationale. This ensures that the medication is compatible with the patient, especially when administering antibiotics and analgesics.

7. **Procedural Step.** Calculate the correct dose to be given, if necessary.

8. **Procedural Step.** Follow the procedure for drawing the medication into the syringe (see Procedure 44-5 or 44-6).

9. **Procedural Step.** Greet the patient, introduce yourself, and confirm the patient's identity.
   The patient's medical record and the loaded syringe are brought into the examination room for the injection to be given.
   Rationale. Identifying the patient ensures the procedure is performed on the correct patient.

10. **Procedural Step.** Explain the procedure to the patient.
    Rationale. Explaining the procedure to the patient promotes cooperation and provides a means of obtaining implied consent.

11. **Procedural Step.** Select an appropriate injection site and properly position the patient as necessary.

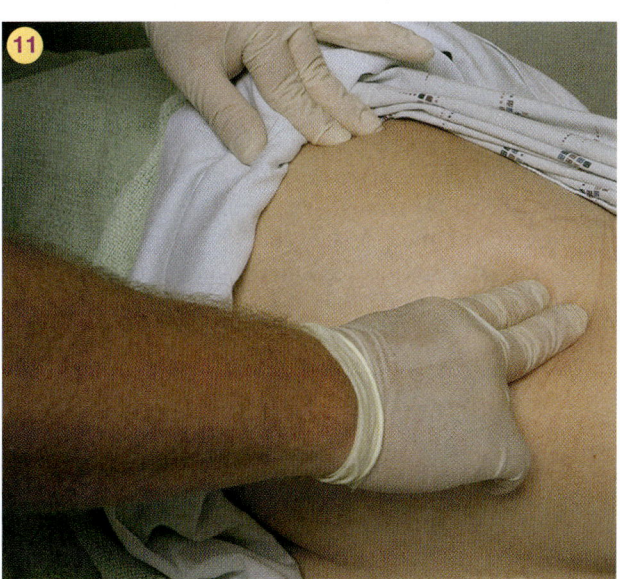

Continued

PROCEDURE 44-10 Administer an Intramuscular Injection to an Adult—cont'd

Remove the patient's clothing as necessary to make sure the entire area is exposed.

Intramuscular injections are given in muscle tissue areas beneath the subcutaneous tissue, where an abundance of blood vessels results in fast absorption of the medication. The most frequently used sites for an intramuscular injection are the deltoid region of the arm, the dorsogluteal region of the buttocks (upper outer quadrant), the ventrogluteal area of the thigh, or the vastus lateralis area of the upper leg.

The deltoid is used for injections of fluids up to 2 mL. Injections requiring larger volumes and injections of substances that are irritating or must be injected deep into a muscle should be made in the dorsogluteal or ventrogluteal area. Major nerves and blood vessels may lie close to the intramuscular injection sites. The site must be free from conditions (e.g., bruise, scar tissue) that would contraindicate using the area.

NOTE: For demonstration purposes the ventrogluteal injection site is being used.

12. **Procedural Step. Apply gloves.**
    Rationale. Gloves provide a barrier precaution against bloodborne pathogens.

13. **Procedural Step. Prepare the injection site.**
    Clean the injection site with an alcohol wipe, working outward in a circular motion beginning at the center. Allow the site to air-dry. Do not touch the site after cleaning it.

14. **Procedural Step. While the prepared site is drying, remove the cover from the needle.**
    Take care to pull the cover off without touching the needle. Check the site visually to be sure it has dried completely before the skin is pierced.
    Rationale. Wet alcohol on the injection site causes the needle to sting when it is inserted.

15. **Procedural Step. Secure the skin at the injection site.**
    Without touching the intended puncture location, spread apart the skin around the injection site with the thumb and forefinger to compress the subcutaneous tissue. Hold the syringe between the thumb and first two fingers, with the ring and small fingers positioning the needle at a 90-degree angle to the injection site (perpendicular). It is not necessary to position the bevel for an intramuscular injection.
    NOTE: If the patient has a small muscle mass (e.g., elderly), grasp the muscle with the thumb and forefinger.
    Rationale. Compressing the subcutaneous tissue around the injection site ensures that muscle tissue is injected. Grasping allows the medication to reach muscle mass rather than subcutaneous tissue.

16. **Procedural Step. Puncture the skin quickly and smoothly with the needle kept at a 90-degree angle.**
    The entire needle is inserted up to the hilt.

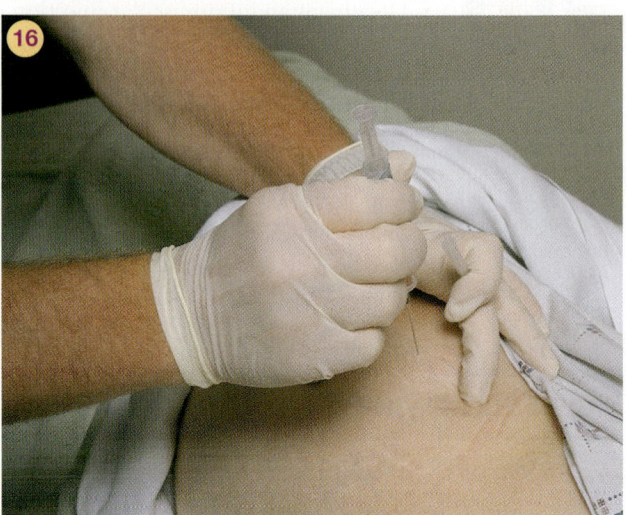

17. **Procedural Step. Check to see if blood aspirates into the syringe.**
    Release the grasp on the tissue, and use the hand that was grasping around the injection site to pull back slightly on the plunger of the syringe (aspirate). *The needle should not be allowed to move during aspiration.* To avoid moving the needle, use the hand holding the barrel of the syringe to push inward to resist movement as the other hand pulls the plunger outward.

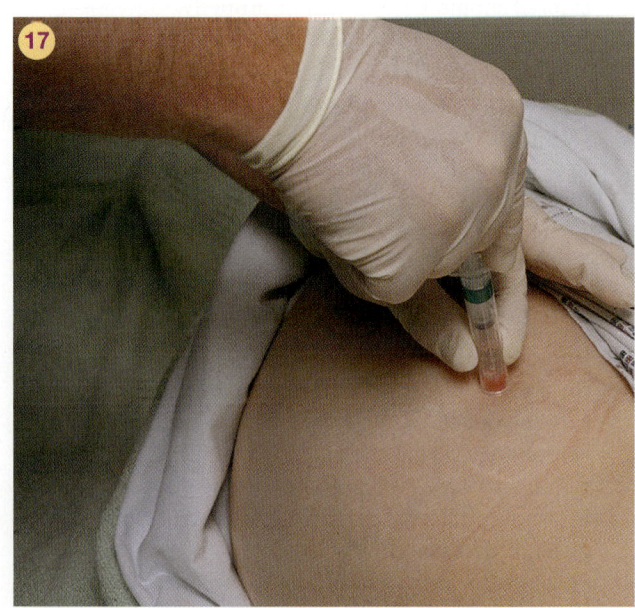

Continued

PROCEDURE 44-10	Administer an Intramuscular Injection to an Adult—cont'd

NOTE: If blood is drawn into the syringe during aspiration, the needle has pierced a blood vessel and should be withdrawn from the site. In such situations, the loaded syringe and needle must be discarded and another dose with a new syringe and needle prepared.

Rationale. Moving the needle in and out causes unnecessary pain to the patient and changes the needle's placement with the risk of entering a blood vessel.

18. **Procedural Step. Inject the medication.**
If no blood is aspirated into the syringe when the plunger is pulled back, there is usually a sensation of pulling against pressure and it is safe to inject the medication. Push the plunger of the syringe slowly and steadily until all the medication is delivered into the intramuscular tissue. Take care to hold the syringe still while the medication is being injected.

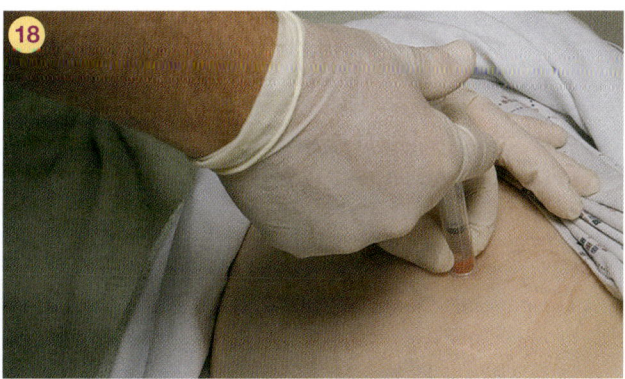

19. **Procedural Step.** Place a gauze pad over the injection site and quickly withdraw the needle from the injection site at the same angle at which it was inserted. Activate the safety device immediately.
Rationale. Withdrawing the needle quickly and at the same angle reduces discomfort. Using the gauze pad over the injection site prevents tissue movement and the stinging sensation an alcohol wipe would cause.

20. **Procedural Step. Massage the injection site.**
Use the 2 × 2 gauze pad to massage the injection site gently but firmly. To avoid tissue damage after administering insulin or heparin, however, do *not* massage the injection site.
Rationale. Massaging the injection site helps to distribute the medication into the body tissue.

21. **Procedural Step.** Discard the syringe and needle into a sharps container.

22. **Procedural Step.** Remove gloves and discard in a biohazardous waste container.

23. **Procedural Step. Sanitize the hands.**
Always sanitize the hands after every procedure or after using gloves.

24. **Procedural Step. Check on the patient.**
Ask the patient how he or she feels and observe the patient for any signs of an immediate reaction such as dizziness, fainting, or severe pain at the injection site. Instruct the patient to remain in the office for another 15 to 20 minutes, since the most severe reactions (e.g., difficulty breathing, hives, and low blood pressure) are likely to begin within this time.

25. **Procedural Step. Document the procedure.**
Include the date and time, name of the medication, dose given, lot number, expiration date, route of administration, injection site used, and any significant observations or patient reactions.
Rationale. The lot number and expiration date are documented so that should a problem arise with the batch of medication used, the drug can be recalled and individuals who received it identified. No procedure is completed until it has been documented.

CHARTING EXAMPLE	
Date	
4/4/xx	10:30 a.m. Penicillin G benzathine, 900,000 units, Lot # DC58767HG, Exp date 3-xx, IM, Ⓛ dorsogluteal. Verbal and written follow-up instructions provided. Tolerated injection well, no adverse effects noted.———————————————————— T. Kremser, CMA (AAMA)

Photos from deWit S: Fundamental concepts and skills for nursing, ed 3, St Louis, 2009, Saunders.

PROCEDURE 44-11: Administer an Intramuscular Injection Using the Z-Track Technique

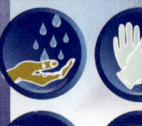

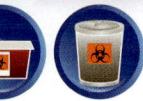

TASKS:
- Identify the correct syringe, needle gauge, and length for an intramuscular injection using the Z-track technique.
- Select and prepare an appropriate site for an intramuscular injection using the Z-track technique.
- Demonstrate the correct technique to administer an intramuscular injection using the Z-track technique.
- Document an intramuscular injection using the Z-track technique correctly in the medical record.

EQUIPMENT AND SUPPLIES
- Nonsterile disposable gloves (Latex-free)
- Medication ordered by physician
- Appropriate syringe for ordered dose (3-mL syringe)
- Needle with safety device (21- to 23-gauge, 1½ inch to 2 inch)
- 2 × 2 sterile gauze
- 70% isopropyl alcohol wipes
- Sharps container
- Biohazardous waste container
- Patient's medical record

SKILLS/RATIONALE

STANDARD PRECAUTIONS ARE TO BE FOLLOWED.

1. **Procedural Step.** Sanitize the hands.
   An alcohol-based hand rub may be used instead of washing hands with soap and water, unless hands are visibly soiled.
   Rationale. Hand sanitization promotes infection control.

2. **Procedural Step.** Assemble equipment and supplies and verify the order.
   Rationale. It is important to have all supplies and equipment ready and available before starting any procedure to ensure efficiency.

3. **Procedural Step.** Check the expiration date of the medication.
   NOTE: The expiration date on stored medications should be checked on a regular basis. Medications that have expired should be disposed of properly.
   Rationale. Medications used past expiration date may be inactive.

4. **Procedural Step.** Follow the "seven rights" of medication administration (see Procedure 44-1).

5. **Procedural Step.** Check the medication against the physician's order three times before it is administered:
   a. Before removing the medication from storage.
   b. Before pouring or withdrawing the medication from the original container.
   c. Before returning the medication to storage.

6. **Procedural Step.** Check the patient's medical record for drug allergies or conditions that may contraindicate the injection.
   Rationale. This ensures that the medication is compatible with the patient, especially when administering antibiotics and analgesics.

7. **Procedural Step.** Calculate the correct dose to be given, if necessary.

8. **Procedural Step.** Follow the procedure for drawing the medication into the syringe (see Procedure 44-5 or 44-6).

9. **Procedural Step.** Greet the patient, introduce yourself, and confirm the patient's identity.
   The patient's medical record and the loaded syringe are brought into the examination room for the injection to be given.
   Rationale. Identifying the patient ensures the procedure is performed on the correct patient.

10. **Procedural Step.** Explain the procedure to the patient.
    Rationale. Explaining the procedure to the patient promotes cooperation and provides a means of obtaining implied consent.

11. **Procedural Step.** Select an appropriate injection site and properly position the patient as necessary.
    Remove the patient's clothing as necessary to make sure the entire area is exposed.
    Intramuscular injections are given in muscle tissue areas beneath the subcutaneous tissue, where an abundance of blood vessels results in fast absorption of the medication. The most frequently used sites for an intramuscular injection using the Z-track technique are the dorsogluteal region of the buttocks, the ventrogluteal area of the thigh, or the vastus lateralis area of the upper leg. Major nerves and blood vessels may lie close to the intramuscular injection sites. The site must be free from conditions (e.g., bruise, scar tissue) that would contraindicate using the area.

12. **Procedural Step.** Apply gloves.
    Rationale. Gloves provide a barrier precaution against bloodborne pathogens.

Continued

PROCEDURE 44-11 Administer an Intramuscular Injection Using the Z-Track Technique—cont'd

13. **Procedural Step.** Prepare the injection site.
    Clean the injection site with an alcohol wipe, working outward in a circular motion beginning at the center. Allow the site to air-dry. Do not touch the site after cleaning it.

14. **Procedural Step.** While the prepared site is drying, remove the cover from the needle.
    Take care to pull the cover off without touching the needle. Check the site visually to be sure it has dried completely before the skin is pierced.
    Rationale. Wet alcohol on the injection site causes the needle to sting when it is inserted.

15. **Procedural Step.** Secure the skin at the injection site.
    Without touching the intended puncture location, use the nondominant hand to pull the skin around the injection site laterally, approximately 1 to 1½ inches. Hold the syringe between the thumb and first two fingers, with the ring and small fingers positioning the needle at a 90-degree angle to the injection site (perpendicular). It is not necessary to position the bevel for an intramuscular injection.

16. **Procedural Step.** Puncture the skin quickly and smoothly with the needle kept at a 90-degree angle.
    Insert the needle to ⅛ inch of the hilt.

17. **Procedural Step.** Continue to hold the tissue in place while aspirating and injecting the medication.
    The needle should not be allowed to move during aspiration.
    NOTE: If blood is drawn into the syringe during aspiration, the needle has pierced a blood vessel and should be withdrawn from the site. In such situations, the loaded syringe and needle must be discarded and another dose with a new syringe and needle prepared.
    Rationale. Moving the needle in and out causes unnecessary pain to the patient and changes the needle's placement with the risk of entering a blood vessel.

18. **Procedural Step.** Inject the medication.
    If no blood is aspirated into the syringe when the plunger is pulled back, there is usually a sensation of pulling against pressure and it is safe to inject the medication. Push the plunger of the syringe slowly and steadily until all the medication is delivered into the intramuscular tissue. Take care to hold the syringe still while the medication is being injected.

19. **Procedural Step.** Withdraw the needle.
    Wait 10 seconds, then withdraw the needle at the same angle at which it was inserted, and wipe the area with an alcohol wipe.

20. **Procedural Step.** Release the traction on the skin to seal the needle track as the needle is being removed.
    Activate the safety device immediately.
    Rationale. This prevents the medication from reaching the subcutaneous tissue and skin surface.

21. **Procedural Step.** Discard the syringe and needle into a sharps container.

22. **Procedural Step.** Remove gloves and discard in a biohazardous waste container.

23. **Procedural Step.** Sanitize the hands.
    Always sanitize the hands after every procedure or after using gloves.

24. **Procedural Step.** Check on the patient.
    Ask the patient how he or she feels, and observe the patient for any signs of an immediate reaction, such as dizziness, fainting, or severe pain at the injection site. Instruct the patient to remain in the office for another 15 to 20 minutes, since the most severe reactions (e.g., difficulty breathing, hives, and low blood pressure) are likely to begin within this time.

25. **Procedural Step.** Document the procedure.
    Include the date and time, name of the medication, dose given, lot number, expiration date, route of administration, injection site used, and any significant observations or patient reactions.
    Rationale. The lot number and expiration date are documented so that should a problem arise with the batch of medication used, the drug can be recalled and individuals who received it identified. No procedure is completed until it has been documented.

CHARTING EXAMPLE

Date	
4/2/xx	10:30 a.m. Iron dextran, 200 mg, Lot # 2379XZ, Exp date 10xx, IM, Z-track into Ⓡ dorsogluteal. No complaints of discomfort.——L. Hayes, CMA (AAMA)

BOX 44-7

Therapeutic Uses of Intravenous Solutions

1. Replace fluids and electrolytes.
2. Correct acid-base imbalance.
3. Administer medications (e.g., antiinfective, antiinflammatory).
4. Maintain ready access to the venous system.
5. Administer essential nutrients.
6. Administer blood products.

TABLE 44-3

Intravenous Solutions

Type	Examples
Hydrating solution	
Example: Dextrose in water	Dextrose 5% (D_5W, D5W)
	Dextrose 10% ($D_{10}W$, D10W)
Isotonic solution	
Examples: Saline solutions	0.9% sodium chloride (NaCl): normal saline (NS)
	Ringer's (sterile H_2O with NaCl, potassium chloride, and calcium chloride) used to replenish fluids lost due to vomiting and diarrhea
	Lactated Ringer's (sterile electrolyte solution with NaCl, calcium chloride, potassium chloride, and sodium lactate used for burns and infections)
Maintenance solutions	Plasmalyte
	Normosol
Hypertonic solutions	3% or 5% NaCl (saline)

Intravenous Fluids

To understand why IV fluids may be requested, it is necessary to know that the body can only function to optimum capacity when its physiological processes are in homeostasis. *Homeostasis* depends on the proper intake and output of fluids and electrolytes. Body fluids perform the following functions:

1. *Maintain* blood volume.
2. *Regulate* body temperature.
3. *Transport* nutrients to and from cells for cell metabolism.
4. *Aid* in digestion.

Box 44-7 lists therapeutic uses of IV fluids. The physician will select the appropriate fluid to meet the patient's needs. The most common IV solutions are specific combinations of water, sodium chloride (salt), dextrose (sugar), and other electrolytes. IV solutions are divided into the following four categories:

1. **Hydrating solutions** are used to hydrate the body or to prevent dehydration.
2. **Isotonic solutions** have the same *osmolality* (salt concentration) as a person's body fluids. They are used to replace cellular fluids lost through blood loss, vomiting, and other conditions. Isotonic solutions supply balanced amounts of water and sodium chloride.
3. **Maintenance solutions** are administered to replace electrolytes in severe cases of diarrhea and vomiting. Vitamins and minerals are often added to replenish amounts lost.
4. **Hypertonic solutions** are greater in osmolality than a person's body fluids and are used for overhydration.

Table 44-3 describes types of IV solutions.

Intravenous Fluid Administration

One of the goals of IV fluid administration is to correct or replace fluid volume and restore electrolyte imbalance. IV fluids must continuously be regulated because the patient's electrolyte levels will change as the fluids infuse. When IV administration is ordered, the medical assistant may be asked to initiate the IV therapy, or at least collect the needed equipment. The assistant begins by verifying the physician's solution order and collecting needed equipment and supplies. Understanding how to start an IV line, regulating the infusion rate, maintaining the system, and discontinuing the IV line when ordered are advanced medical assisting skills in some medical offices.

Basic Equipment and Supplies. Preparation for starting the IV infusion includes gathering needed supplies and equipment. Since the procedure requires entering directly into the bloodstream, sterile technique is required. Equipment includes sterile needles or catheters, skin-cleaning solution, gloves, tourniquet, dressing supplies, ordered solution, tubing, IV pole to suspend solution container, and possibly an IV pump. IV infusions in an ambulatory care setting are initiated with a winged infusion needle or a catheter (Figure 44-31), as follows:

- **Winged infusion needles,** often referred to as "butterfly" needles, are short needles with two plastic wings that are held during insertion. They are used when the veins of the patient are poor or small, for one-time therapy, and for short-duration therapy (less than 24 hours).
- A **catheter** is a small plastic tube that fits over or inside an IV needle. The size of the catheter selected depends on the type of solution and the condition of the patient's veins. A catheter is usually selected when the duration of fluid administration is longer than 24 hours.

Sometimes a patient may need IV medications at specific intervals (e.g., every 4 or 6 hours). When a patient does not require a continuous IV infusion, a resealable latex lock (**heparin lock**) can be used. The intermittent infusion device is a short needle with a catheter that has an attached injection port. It is taped into place, and the medication can be injected into the port when needed. The name "heparin lock" is often used because it is usually flushed with a dilute solution of heparin after each use to prevent clots from forming and blocking the catheter.

An **administration set** (delivery set) is used to deliver IV fluids from a sterile solution container to the patient. The set contains a spike for piercing the fluid container, tubing, and a drop (drip) device that determines the size and quantity of the fluid drop into the chamber (Figure 44-32). The tubing should be attached to the solution container before inserting the needle in the skin or the tubing to a heparin lock, and the fluid should flow through the tubing until the tubing is completely filled with fluid and no air bubbles are present.

Starting an Intravenous Line. The patient is assessed for a venipuncture site. The most common IV sites for adults are the arm and hand. For pediatric patients the foot is used (Figure 44-33). The site chosen should be the least restrictive to the patient. For example, if the patient is right-handed, it is best to start the IV line on the left side. In adults, hand veins have a lower risk of phlebitis than the upper arm.

After gathering equipment and supplies, sanitizing the hands, and applying gloves, the medical assistant explains the procedure to the patient. A tourniquet is applied 1 to 2 inches above the selected site. The site for the puncture is cleaned first with an alcohol wipe and then an antiseptic solution. The skin is punctured by a sharp, sterile, rigid needle (e.g., butterfly needle), or a needle with a partially covered plastic catheter, and is guided into the vein in the direction of the blood flow. When completed, the catheter should be taped securely without restricting circulation. The site can be dressed with a sterile gauze pad or a clear occlusive dressing that allows for inspection of the site.

Drip Rate. The physician will order the rate at which the IV fluid is to be given. The **drip rate** (infusion rate) can be calculated by knowing how much fluid is to be given per hour and how many drops equal 1 mL in the administration set (delivery set) that is used. Each administration set package states how many drops equal 1 mL using that set. Standard sets (macrodrip) can deliver 10, 15, or 20 drops per milliliter. Microdrip sets deliver 60 drops per milliliter and are used when small volumes of fluid are given. Usually, IV infusions in an outpatient setting are administered at a slow drip rate, so a microdrip chamber setup is used.

Discontinuing an Intravenous Line. To discontinue an IV line, the flow of the fluid must be stopped. The dressing and tape are loosened and removed. The catheter is gently removed, and pressure is applied to the puncture site with sterile gauze to prevent bleeding. A sterile dressing can be applied to the site.

Chart the appearance of the site and how the patient tolerated the procedure. Disconnect the catheter from the IV tubing and dispose of in the sharps container. Remove the IV solution container and tubing, and discard in the biohazardous waste container.

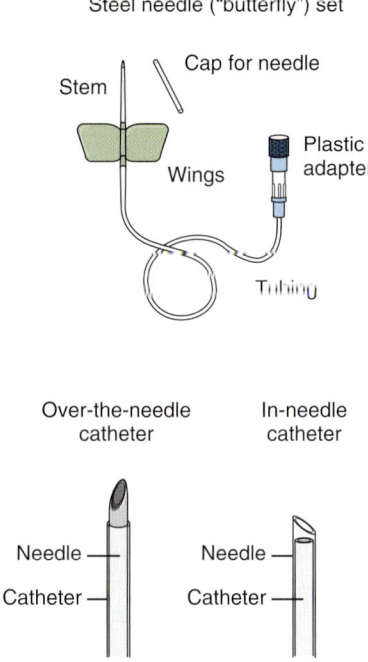

FIGURE 44-31 Intravenous cannulas: steel needle ("butterfly"), over-the-needle catheter, and in-the-needle catheter. (From Leahy JM, Kizilay PE: *Foundations of nursing practice*, Philadelphia, 1998, Saunders.)

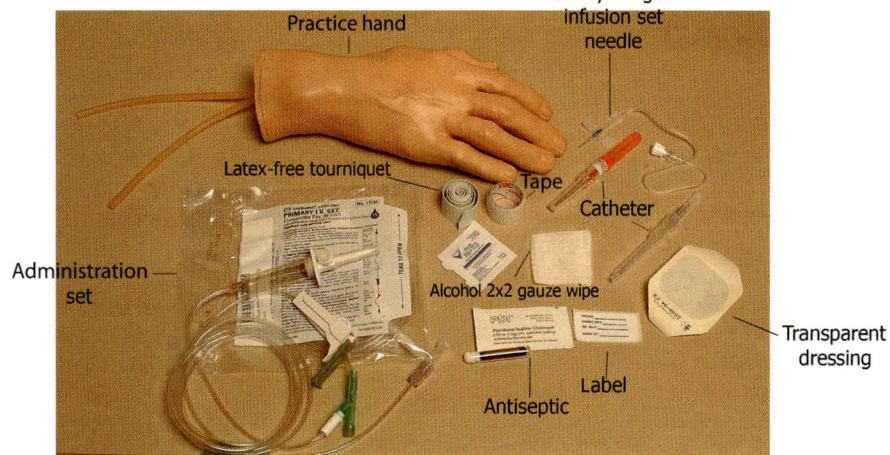

FIGURE 44-32 Intravenous administration set with supplies and practice hand.

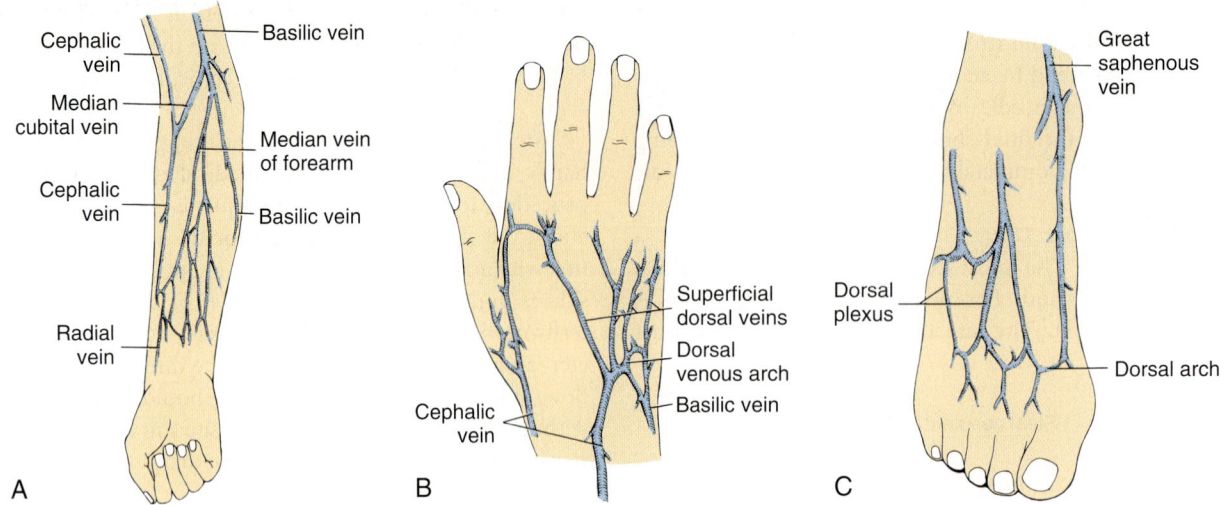

FIGURE 44-33 Common intravenous sites. **A,** Inner arm. **B,** Dorsal surface of hand. **C,** Dorsal surface of foot (used for children only). (Modified from Potter PA, Perry AG: *Basic nursing*, ed 6, St Louis, 2007, Mosby.)

PATIENT-CENTERED PROFESSIONALISM

- Why must the medical assistant be familiar with the equipment used for administering medications?
- Why must the medical assistant be knowledgeable about techniques for administering injections?

CONCLUSION

Medications can be administered in many ways, including orally, topically, vaginally, or rectally and through inhalation or parenteral methods. Medical assistants need to understand the purpose and use of each method in order to administer medications to patients accurately and efficiently.

When administering medications, as with any procedure, the medical assistant must be knowledgeable and focused and must use extreme care. By confirming the medication order, rechecking the medication three times, and observing the "seven rights" of medication administration, the medical assistant can greatly reduce the chance for error. It is the medical assistant's duty to be in compliance of all federal laws concerning controlled substances being administered.

Chapter Summary

Reinforce your understanding of the material in this chapter by reviewing the curriculum objectives and key content points below.

1. **Define, appropriately use, and spell all the Key Terms for this chapter.**
   - Review the Key Terms if necessary.
2. **List the two forms of oral medication.**
   - Oral medication comes in solid and liquid forms.
3. **State three advantages of oral administration of medication.**
   - Oral medications are considered the safest form of medication, no special equipment is required, and patients can take oral medications easily.
4. **Demonstrate the correct procedure for administering oral medications.**
   - Review Procedure 44-1.
5. **List four forms of topical medication.**
   - Creams, lotions, ointments, and transdermal patches are forms of topical medication.
6. **Demonstrate the correct procedure for applying a transdermal patch.**
   - Review Procedure 44-2.
7. **List three types of medications that can be inserted into the vaginal cavity.**
   - Creams, foams, and suppositories can be administered vaginally.
8. **Explain why medications for nausea and vomiting are often given rectally.**
   - Medications for nausea and vomiting are often given rectally to avoid further upsetting the gastrointestinal tract.
9. **List three forms in which medications can be inhaled.**

- Gases, powders, and aerosols (fine mist) are three forms in which medications can be inhaled.
10. **Explain how a nebulizer works.**
    - A nebulizer provides a mist of medication when the patient closes the lips around a mouthpiece, and an air compressor forces air rapidly into a medication compartment to be inhaled.
11. **Demonstrate the correct procedure for administering medication using a metered-dose inhaler with the closed-mouth technique.**
    - Review Procedure 44-3.
12. **List one advantage and one disadvantage of parenteral administration of medication.**
    - Parenteral administration allows quick drug action because it bypasses the GI tract, increasing the rate of absorption.
    - When adverse reactions occur, the patient is put at immediate risk.
13. **List five types of equipment used for parenteral administration of medication and explain the use of each.**
    - Vials, ampules, prefilled cartridge units, syringes, and needles are types of equipment used for parenteral administration of medication.
14. **Demonstrate the correct procedure for reconstituting a powdered medication to its proper dosage form.**
    - Review Procedure 44-4.
15. **Demonstrate the correct procedure for preparing a medication for injection by drawing it into a syringe from a vial.**
    - Review Procedure 44-5.
16. **Demonstrate the correct procedure for preparing a medication for injection by drawing it into a syringe from an ampule.**
    - Review Procedure 44-6.
17. **List four guidelines to help prevent accidental needlesticks.**
    - Review Box 44-4.
18. **List anatomical sites for administering intradermal, subcutaneous, and intramuscular injections.**
    - Review Table 44-2.
19. **Demonstrate the correct procedure for administering an intradermal injection.**
    - Review Procedure 44-7.
20. **Demonstrate the correct procedure for administering a subcutaneous injection.**
    - Review Procedure 44-8.
21. **Demonstrate the correct procedure for giving an infant an intramuscular injection, such as an immunization.**
    - Review Procedure 44-9.
22. **Demonstrate the correct procedure for administering an intramuscular injection to an adult.**
    - Review Procedure 44-10.
23. **Demonstrate the correct procedure for administering intramuscular medication using the Z-track injection technique.**
    - Review Procedure 44-11.
24. **List four categories of intravenous solutions.**
    - Hydrating, isotonic, maintenance, and hypertonic solutions are four categories of IV solutions.
25. **Analyze a realistic medical office situation and apply your understanding of medication administration to determine the best course of action.**
    - Always double-check to be sure you are administering the correct dosage.
    - Never administer a medication you did not prepare yourself.
26. **Describe the impact on patient care when medical assistants understand the guidelines, safety requirements, and proper techniques for administering medications in the medical office.**
    - To promote safety, the medical assistant must be knowledgeable about the medications he or she administers.
    - Following established guidelines and using proper technique when administering medications promote patient safety.

PRACTICAL APPLICATIONS

If you have accomplished the objectives in this chapter, you will be able to make better choices as a medical assistant. Take another look at this situation and decide what you would do.

Sue, a medical assistant with no formal training, has been asked by her employer, Dr. Kenyon, to give Dylan, age 3 years, a single dose of acetaminophen, 250 mg. Dylan's record shows that he is allergic to penicillin and has had a severe rash in the past. Sue goes to the medicine cabinet and removes amoxicillin, 250-mg tablets, and takes a single tablet to Dylan. Sue does not bother to read the label except when taking the medication from the shelf. Dylan's mother tells Sue that her child is unable to swallow the tablet, but Sue continues to give the tablet, telling the mother that at age 3, Dylan should be able to swallow a tablet.

Sue leaves Dylan and his mother with the tablet. Margie, the other medical assistant in the office, asks Sue to prepare a medication for Mrs. Abbott, who needs a 1-mL estrogen injection. Margie tells Sue that this aqueous medication will be given intramuscularly and that she will be back to give the medication. In preparing the estrogen medication from a vial, Sue shakes the medicine and then draws it into a 5-mL syringe with a 25-gauge $\frac{5}{8}$-inch needle. Margie returns and gives the medication that Sue prepared.

In the meantime, Dylan has choked on the tablet and is having difficulty breathing. Because Sue left the room, she is unaware of the situation. When Dr. Kenyon arrives in the room, he immediately recognizes a problem and calls in both Sue and Margie to help remove the tablet from Dylan's throat.

What would you have done differently as a medical assistant?

1. When should Sue have checked the medication to be sure she had the correct medication?
2. Does it make any difference that the medication ordered was acetaminophen and the medication given was amoxicillin? What are the specific dangers in this case?
3. Was the ordered dosage of the acetaminophen correct for a 3-year-old child? What should Sue have done to be sure the dosage was correct?
4. Why is it important for Sue to know the correct dosage of a medication rather than assuming that the physician is correct?
5. Why is oral administration of acetaminophen the correct route for a 3-year-old child?
6. If Dylan was unable to swallow a tablet, what form of medication could Sue have given him?
7. What are the dangers of giving a tablet to a child who is unable to swallow that form of solid medication?
8. If Dr. Kenyon had prescribed an injection of antibiotic for Dylan, where would the appropriate site have been for administration?
9. What mistake did Sue make while removing the medication from the vial? What mistake did she make in the selection of the syringe and the needle?
10. Because Sue prepared the medication for administration, and Margie administered the injection and documented the procedure, who is responsible if a mistake is made? Explain your answer.

WEB SEARCH

1. **Research current needlestick policies and locate data to verify if accidental injury from needlesticks is decreasing with the addition of safety-engineered needles.** According to a U.S. General Accounting Office report (GAO-01-60R), the annual needlestick injury rate in physician offices and clinics was equal to that of hospitals. This prompted the CDC to report that using safety-engineered needles and other medical devices could prevent 88% of needlestick injuries.
   - **Keywords:** Use the following keywords in your search: needlestick policy, safety-engineered medical devices, CDC.

Minor Office Surgery

45

evolve   http://evolve.elsevier.com/klieger/medicalassisting

Physicians can perform many minor surgical procedures in the office. Procedures done in the medical office have a low risk of postoperative complications. Common office procedures include cyst removal, removal of skin lesions, wound repair, biopsies, toenail removal, and incision and drainage of abscesses.

The medical assistant has an important role in preoperative and postoperative processes for minor office surgery, as well as in assisting the physician during surgical procedures. Medical assistants must understand the principles of surgical asepsis to prevent patient infection during a procedure. They must also be able to explain to patients the necessary preoperative and postoperative instructions as ordered by the physician.

LEARNING OBJECTIVES

You will be able to do the following after completing this chapter:

Key Terms
1. Define, appropriately use, and spell all the Key Terms for this chapter.

Before Surgery
2. List six areas in which medical assistants may need to provide preoperative instructions to patients and give an example for each area.
3. Explain the importance of obtaining informed consent.

Surgical Asepsis
4. Differentiate between medical asepsis and surgical asepsis.
5. List 12 guidelines that should be followed to maintain asepsis during a sterile procedure.
6. Demonstrate the correct procedure for performing a surgical scrub.
7. Demonstrate the correct procedure for putting on a sterile gown and sterile gloves.
8. Demonstrate the correct procedure for applying sterile gloves.
9. Demonstrate the correct procedure for removing contaminated gloves.
10. Demonstrate the correct procedure for opening a sterile package.

Surgical Instruments
11. List five classifications of surgical instruments and give an example of each.
12. List six commonly used surgical instruments and briefly describe each.
13. List four guidelines for the proper handling and maintenance of surgical instruments.

Assisting with Minor Office Surgery
14. Demonstrate the correct procedure for adding solutions to the sterile field without contaminating the setup.
15. Demonstrate the correct procedure for providing all equipment, supplies, and materials needed to assist the physician with a minor office procedure.
16. Differentiate among local, topical, and general anesthetics and explain the purpose and use of each.
17. Briefly describe four surgical procedures often performed in a medical office.
18. Briefly describe methods used for tissue removal.

Wound Care
19. Differentiate between an open wound and a closed wound.
20. Describe the healing process of a wound and list the three classifications of wound repair and healing.
21. Demonstrate the correct procedure for suture or staple removal and for changing a wound dressing.

22. Demonstrate the correct procedure for the application and removal of adhesive skin closures.
23. Explain the purpose of a sterile dressing.

Patient-Centered Professionalism

24. Analyze a realistic medical office situation and apply your understanding of minor office surgery to determine the best course of action.
25. Describe the impact on patient care when medical assistants have a solid understanding of the knowledge and skills necessary to assist in minor office surgery.

KEY TERMS

abscess incision and drainage	local anesthetics
ambulatory surgery setting	medical asepsis
anesthesia	needle holder
approximate	open technique
bandage scissors	open wound
box lock	operating scissors
catgut	pick-ups
cautery	preoperative instructions
chromic suture	probes
cicatrix	probing
clamping	purulent
closed technique	ratchet
closed wound	regional anesthesia
cryosurgery	retracting
curette	retractors
cutting	sanguineous
cyst removal	scalpel
debrided	second (secondary) intention healing
debridement	serosanguineous
decontaminates	serous
deep wound	shank
delayed primary (tertiary) intention healing	skin closures
dilating	skin lesion removal
dissecting	slough
dissecting scissors	splinter forceps
dressing forceps	sponge forceps
electrosurgery	staples
exudate	sterile dressing
first (primary) intention healing	superficial wounds
	surgical asepsis
forceps	surgical handwashing
general anesthetics	surgical glue
grasping	suture scissors
hemostatic forceps (hemostats)	sutures
	suturing
informed consent	thumb forceps
jaws	tissue forceps
laceration repair	topical anesthetics
laser	towel clamps
ligate	wound

PRACTICAL APPLICATIONS

Read the following scenario and keep it in mind as you learn about minor office surgery.

Shirley, a patient of Dr. Jones, has arrived at the office for removal of a cyst on her face that has been present for about 2 months. Anna is the medical assistant at the front desk, and Lori is the clinical medical assistant for Dr. Jones. Shirley has been asked to cleanse the area around the lesion with an antiseptic wash for the past 2 days. Shirley wants to know exactly what will be done and if she has to sign papers. Anna tells her that these papers can be signed at any time before the actual opening of the wound. Anna also tells Shirley that Lori will explain what will be done after Shirley is taken to the room where minor surgery is done.

As Lori sets up the surgical tray, she uses surgical asepsis. She uses a sterile tray and peel-back wrappers to set up the needed instruments. On the tray are a scalpel, several hemostat forceps, a probe, a needle holder, scissors, and two retractors.

After the surgery, Lori is in a hurry and piles the instruments in the basin before sanitizing them. When she documents the procedure for Dr. Jones, she only documents the date and the type of surgery.

Would you be prepared to step into Anna's or Lori's shoes and perform the needed tasks correctly?

BEFORE SURGERY

Before any surgery, patients must be given any necessary preoperative instructions and they must give their informed consent for the surgery.

Preoperative Instructions

The medical assistant plays a vital role in the success of any surgery by providing detailed **preoperative instructions.** These instructions may include specific preparation necessary (e.g., fasting laboratory tests, bowel prep). To be effective, the medical assistant should verbally review what the patient needs to do first, then provide written instructions to facilitate the patient's understanding of what needs to be done. This is also a good opportunity for patients to ask questions or clarify their understanding of what is expected. Box 45-1 lists typical areas that are addressed preoperatively.

Informed Consent

As described in Chapter 4, patients must thoroughly understand any planned surgical procedure, as well as its complications, contraindications, and risks, and must consent to the procedure before it is performed (**informed consent**). Although the medical assistant needs to ensure that the patient has signed the consent form, it is the physician's responsibility to explain the procedure, answer patient questions concerning the procedure, provide information about risks associated with the procedure, and indicate the probable outcome (Figure 45-1).

BOX 45-1

Areas and Examples Addressed by Preoperative Instructions

DIET MODIFICATION
- NPO (nothing to eat or drink) after midnight
- Fluid restrictions

MEDICATIONS
- Discontinue medications (e.g., aspirin products 3 days before surgery, anticoagulants 7 days before surgery)
- Taking antibiotics before surgery

PRETESTING REQUIREMENTS
- X-rays
- Laboratory tests (e.g., urine, complete blood count)

SUPPLIES NEEDED POSTOPERATIVELY
- Dressings
- Bandages

BOWEL PREPARATION
- Enema the night before surgery
- Enema the morning of surgery

ADJUSTMENT TO WORK OR SOCIAL SCHEDULE
- No driving for a certain amount of time, especially immediately after surgery

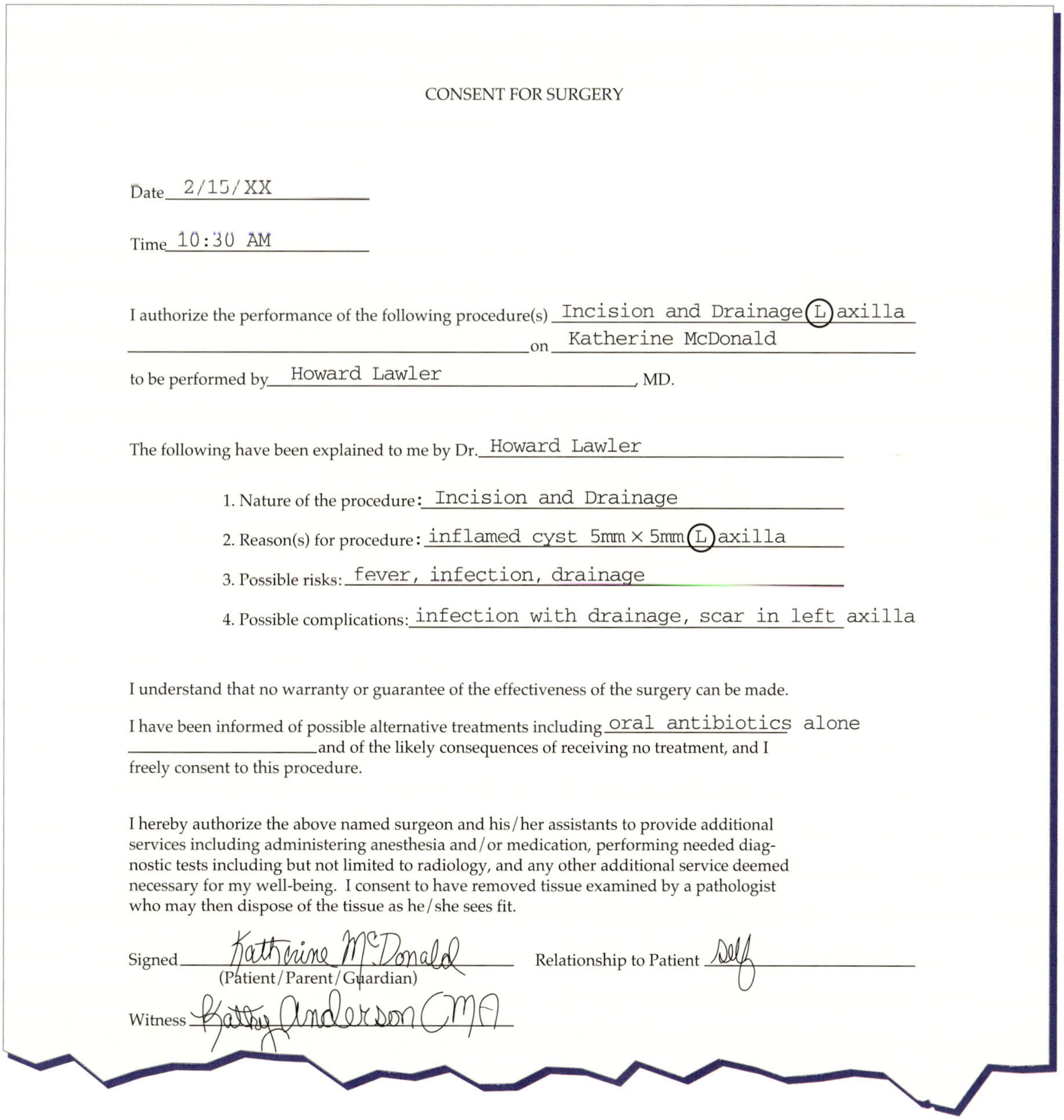

CONSENT FOR SURGERY

Date: 2/15/XX

Time: 10:30 AM

I authorize the performance of the following procedure(s) Incision and Drainage (L) axilla on Katherine McDonald to be performed by Howard Lawler, MD.

The following have been explained to me by Dr. Howard Lawler

1. Nature of the procedure: Incision and Drainage
2. Reason(s) for procedure: inflamed cyst 5mm × 5mm (L) axilla
3. Possible risks: fever, infection, drainage
4. Possible complications: infection with drainage, scar in left axilla

I understand that no warranty or guarantee of the effectiveness of the surgery can be made.

I have been informed of possible alternative treatments including oral antibiotics alone _____ and of the likely consequences of receiving no treatment, and I freely consent to this procedure.

I hereby authorize the above named surgeon and his/her assistants to provide additional services including administering anesthesia and/or medication, performing needed diagnostic tests including but not limited to radiology, and any other additional service deemed necessary for my well-being. I consent to have removed tissue examined by a pathologist who may then dispose of the tissue as he/she sees fit.

Signed: *Katherine McDonald* (Patient/Parent/Guardian)   Relationship to Patient: self

Witness: *Kathy Anderson CMA*

FIGURE 45-1 Example of a completed surgical consent form. (From Hunt SA: *Saunders fundamentals of medical assisting—revised reprint,* St Louis, 2007, Saunders.)

TABLE 45-1
Medical Asepsis versus Surgical Asepsis

	Medical Asepsis	Surgical Asepsis
Definition	Destruction of microorganisms, except bacterial spores (sanitizing and disinfecting)	Destruction of all microorganisms, including spores (sterilizing)
Purpose	To avoid cross-contamination from one person to another; to prevent reinfection of patient	Used in surgery when entering into any sterile cavity and when caring for large open wounds
Technique	Standard Precautions for isolation and for blood and body fluids	Invasive procedures, including surgery, biopsy, wound management, injection, and venipuncture
Procedure	All equipment and supplies clean and sanitized Wear clean gloves and any other necessary PPE Disinfect objects between patients	All equipment and supplies sterile Wear sterile gloves, gowns, and necessary PPE All objects must be sterilized between patients
Handwashing	Hands and wrists washed with soap, running water, and friction for 1 to 2 minutes Hands held downward so water drains off fingertips; hands dried with paper towel	Hands and forearms washed with antimicrobial soap, running water, and friction using a sterile brush and nail stick from 3 to 10 minutes Hands held up so water drains off elbows; hands dried with sterile towel

PPE, Personal protective equipment.

The patient must not be given any type of preoperative sedation before signing the consent-to-treat form. The medical assistant can only act as a witness to verify that the patient has signed his or her name to the form.

SURGICAL ASEPSIS

Medical asepsis, as you learned in Chapter 31, is also known as *clean aseptic technique.* The goal of medical asepsis is to decrease the number of microorganisms present. **Surgical asepsis,** or *sterile technique,* is used when the skin surface is broken, whether the break is intentional (e.g., surgical incision) or caused by trauma, and repair of the skin is essential. Because the skin acts as a barrier to microorganisms, a break in the skin provides a pathway for infection and disease. Surgical asepsis is the highest level of protection for patients. Table 45-1 compares medical and surgical asepsis. To prevent contamination of the surgical area from occurring during a surgical procedure, established guidelines must be followed (Box 45-2).

Before a surgical procedure, the medical assistant is responsible for preparing the room by providing sterile equipment, instruments, and supplies and taking steps to ensure the area does not become contaminated. The medical assistant may have an opportunity either to assist with minor surgery in the medical office environment or to participate in surgical procedures in an **ambulatory surgery setting.** The rules or guidelines established for hospital surgical suites also apply to the medical office and ambulatory surgery center. The prime function of all health care professionals caring for a patient during surgery is to prevent unnecessary harm to the patient (e.g., infection).

BOX 45-2
Guidelines for Preventing Contamination of Surgical Area

1. When performing surgical procedures, hands must be surgically scrubbed, properly gloved, and kept above the waist.
2. Once in sterile attire (e.g., wearing gown, gloves, mask), do not leave the sterile area. Surgical scrub, regowning, and regloving are required if you leave the surgical area.
3. Keep movement in the area to a minimum. Handle drapes gently using sterile technique.
4. Even though a mask is worn, minimize talking to reduce the risk of wound contamination from the mouth. Avoid sneezing and coughing. If sneezing or coughing is unavoidable, the face should be directed away from the sterile field and the mask replaced.
5. Place sterile items in the center of the field, with a 1-inch border maintained around the outside edge of the entire sterile field.
6. Reaching across the sterile field to distribute or retrieve supplies is not permitted.
7. Always face the sterile field.
8. All equipment and supplies used during a surgical procedure must be sterile.
9. If the sterility of an item is in doubt, the item is considered contaminated and must be replaced.
10. Worktables (e.g., Mayo stands) with sterile drapes are only sterile at table height. This includes only the surface working area.
11. Gowns are considered sterile in front from axillary line to the waist and in the sleeve 3 inches above the elbow.
12. The edge of a container holding sterile items is not sterile (e.g., the lip of a basin).

Surgical Handwashing

People are a major source of contamination to a surgical area. Therefore **surgical handwashing** and proper surgical attire are necessary for anyone coming in direct contact with the patient during a surgical procedure. Surgical handwashing goes beyond soap and water to reduce the number of pathogens present. The surgical scrub removes dead skin, oils, dirt, and pathogenic microorganisms. The soap used for a surgical scrub (e.g., Hibiclens, Betadine) has antimicrobial action and leaves a residue that is not entirely rinsed away. This residue acts as a barrier to prevent microorganisms from contaminating the skin again.

The sink used for a surgical scrub must be deep enough to prevent splashing that causes contamination. A knee control, foot pedal, or electronic sensor is ideal; if not available someone must be present to turn the water off, since hand-operated faucets do not allow the hands to remain clean once scrubbed. Procedure 45-1 explains how to perform a surgical scrub.

An alternative method being used in some surgical suites is the waterless surgical hand scrub such as Avagard and Triseptin. Both require that the area under the nails is cleaned before application of the waterless scrub and that the hands are clean and dry. The remaining steps are similar and as follows:
- Dispense one pump of the waterless surgical hand scrub into the palm of one hand.
- Dip the fingertips of the opposite hand into the waterless hand scrub and work it under the fingernails.
- Spread the remaining hand scrub over the opposite hand, wrist, and up to the elbow, paying particular attention to the nails, cuticles, and interdigital spaces.
- Repeat procedure with opposite hand with one pump of waterless scrub.
- Avagard requires that one additional pump is used and should be reapplied to both hands up to the wrists.
- Both require that the scrub be allowed to air-dry before putting on gloves.

Gowning and Gloving

After a physician has completed the surgical scrub, the medical assistant can assist the physician with moving the gown up over the shoulders and tying it. A **closed technique** for gloving ensures that the nonsterile hands never touch the outside of the gown or glove. Procedure 45-2 illustrates how to apply a sterile gown and gloves. When only the hands need to be covered for procedures (e.g., catheterization, skin preparation), an **open technique** for gloving can be used. Procedure 45-3 explains how to apply sterile gloves. Remember that the proper removal of sterile gloves is as important as the proper application. Procedure 45-4 outlines the process of removing sterile gloves to avoid spreading contaminants.

Sterile Supplies

Items in sterile packaging, whether from a manufacturer or sterilized by the medical assistant, must be able to be unwrapped without contamination. Chapter 31 reviews proper wrapping techniques.

Small packages (e.g., instrument tray) are wrapped so that the wrapping material can be opened either (1) by holding it in one hand, grasping the corners of the wrapper, and bringing them back over the hand (called a "peel-down" opening) or (2) by placing it on a flat surface and opening it there. Procedure 45-5 details how to open a sterile package. When a peel-back (or peel-down) wrapper is used, grasping the wrapper's edges and peeling the package apart (like peeling a banana) exposes the sterile item (Figure 45-2, A). One way to remove an item from a peel-back wrapper is by using sterile instruments (Figure 45-2, B). The other method is to reach for the object with sterile gloves (Figure 45-2, C).

PATIENT-CENTERED PROFESSIONALISM

- Why must the medical assistant understand the difference between medical asepsis and surgical asepsis?

SURGICAL INSTRUMENTS

Medical assistants must be familiar with the surgical instruments used for minor office surgery. Surgical instruments are normally made of stainless steel and either have a satin (dull) finish or a highly polished surface. The parts of an instrument are readily identifiable. This makes it easy to differentiate between one instrument and another. Instruments are classified according to their function, as follows:
- **Cutting** and **dissecting** instruments are used to cut tissues of the body. These include scissors, scalpels, biopsy punches, and curettes.
- **Grasping** and **clamping** instruments are used to hold body tissue. Grasping instruments pull back tissue for dissection (e.g., uterine tenaculum, thumb forceps) or hold surgical objects (e.g., needle holder). Clamping instruments clasp tissue or blood vessels between the jaws of the instrument. For example, a hemostatic clamp holds blood vessels. Figure 45-3 shows the identifiable parts of a clamp. The **jaws** hold, and the **box lock** is where the instrument is hinged. The **shank** is the area between the finger rings and the box lock. The **ratchet** interlocks to keep the instrument closed.
- **Retracting** instruments hold back the edges of a wound or hold tissue away from the work area during surgery. Examples are the Agricola lid retractor and the Volkmann finger retractor, which is used for holding tissue back.
- **Probing** and **dilating** instruments are used to probe or explore body cavities or wounds and to increase the diameter of an opening (e.g., urethra). Probes include the Williams lacrimal probe and the Pratt rectal probe. Dilators include the Walther female urethral dilator and the Hegar uterine dilator.
- **Suturing** instruments are used with suture materials to close a wound. Examples include the Mayo-Hegar needle holder, surgical needles, and Michel wound clips. Some

Text continued on p. 1101

PROCEDURE 45-1 Perform Handwashing for Surgical Asepsis

TASK: Prevent the spread of pathogens during a surgical procedure by performing a surgical scrub following standard precautions.

EQUIPMENT AND SUPPLIES
- Liquid antibacterial soap and nailbrush with nail cleaner, or prepackaged sterile scrub brush with antibacterial soap and nail cleaner
- Paper towels
- Warm running water (faucet with knee or foot control or electronic sensor)
- Sterile towel pack
- Regular waste container

SKILLS/RATIONALE

STANDARD PRECAUTIONS ARE TO BE FOLLOWED.

1. **Procedural Step.** Remove jewelry (rings, watch).
   Rationale. Jewelry traps microorganisms and dirt, which will not be washed away if jewelry is left on, preventing thorough handwashing.

2. **Procedural Step.** Open the sterile pack containing a scrub brush with a nail cleaner.
   Rationale. Sterile packs must be opened before washing hands to prevent contamination.

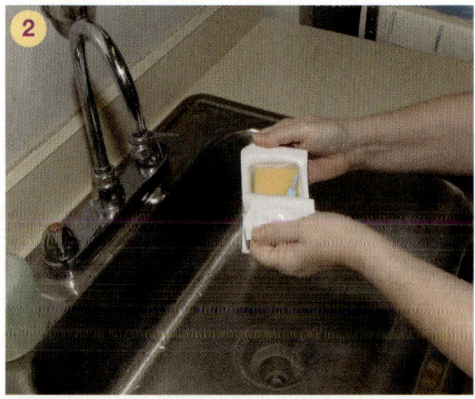

3. **Procedural Step.** Load the brush with liquid antibacterial soap.
   NOTE: Brushes can be purchased preloaded with antibacterial soap. If the brush is not preloaded with soap, antibacterial soap may be pumped onto the brush without touching the brush. Many facilities have a foot pump dispenser for this purpose or use a paper towel to pump the required amount of antibacterial soap.

4. **Procedural Step.** Turn on the faucets, using a paper towel if a knee or foot control or sensor is not available.

5. **Procedural Step.** Use a paper towel to adjust the water temperature if sensor or foot pedal is not available.

Discard the contaminated paper towel in a regular waste container. Water should be warm, not hot.
   Rationale. Water that is too hot can burn the skin. Water that is too cold does not promote the killing of microorganisms. Cold water also tends to dry the skin, which may cause the hands to chafe and crack, providing a means of entrance for microorganisms into the body.

6. **Procedural Step.** Wet the hands, wrists, and forearms.
   Stand away from the sink so that clothing is not touching the sink; wet hands, wrists, and forearms under the warm running water. The hands should be held upright at or above waist level at all times with the elbows bent, being careful not to touch the inside of the sink.
   NOTE: Some facilities have sinks equipped with knee controls rather than hand controls. The force of the water is controlled by moving the knee lever back and forth, and the temperature of the water is controlled by an up or down movement.
   Rationale. The sink is considered contaminated, and if clothing touches the sink, it may become contaminated by microorganisms. By holding the hands above waist level and bent at the elbows, bacteria and debris will be carried away from the tips of the fingers, the area deemed cleanest, down off the elbows and into the sink. Dropping the hands or fingers downward will contaminate the hands by allowing contaminated water and soap to run back down over the clean hands and fingers.

7. **Procedural Step.** Clean the fingernails with a nailbrush and or a nail cleaner.
   Rationale. Microorganisms collect underneath the fingernails, and using a nailbrush or nail cleaner removes the microorganisms without damaging the skin.

Continued

PROCEDURE 45-1   Perform Handwashing for Surgical Asepsis—cont'd

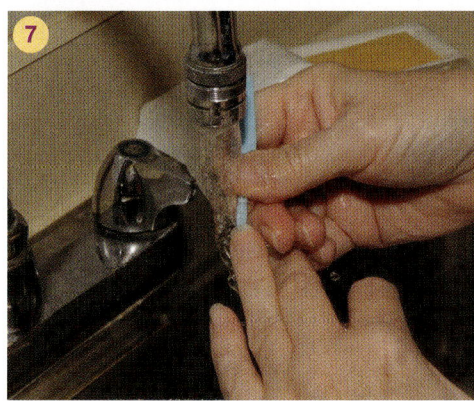

8. **Procedural Step.** Scrub the hands, wrists, and forearms.
   Work the scrub brush loaded with antibacterial soap into lather. Scrub the hands, wrists, and arms using a small circular motion in the following sequence for optimum asepsis.
   a. Anterior surface (palm side) of the fingers of the nondominant hand from tips down toward the palm. (Take special care to scrub between fingers.)

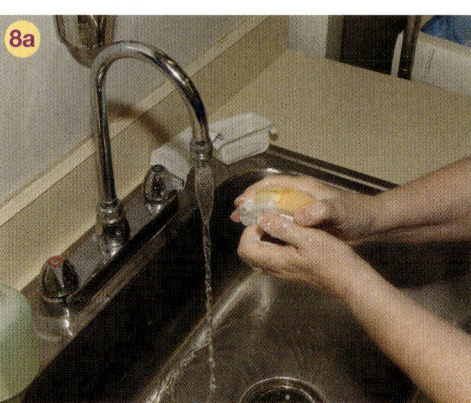

   b. Anterior surface of the fingers of the dominant hand.
   c. Palm of the nondominant hand.

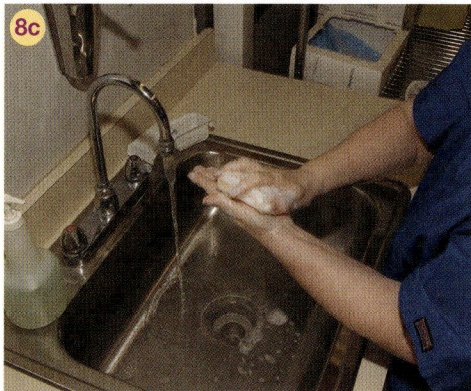

   d. Palm of the dominant hand.
   e. Posterior surface of the fingers of the nondominant hand.

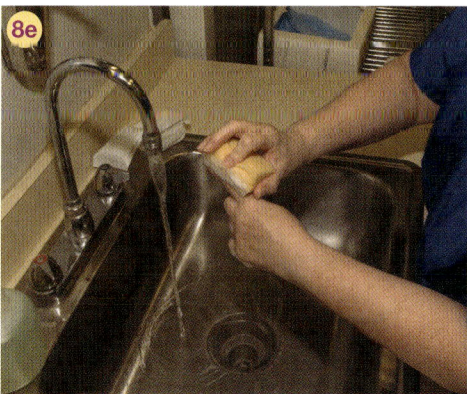

   f. Posterior surface of the fingers of the dominant hand.
   g. Back of the nondominant hand.
   h. Back of the dominant hand.
   i. Nondominant wrist all around.
   j. Dominant wrist all around.
   k. Nondominant arm scrub from the wrist down in a circular motion moving around the arm. (Do not return to an area once scrubbed.)

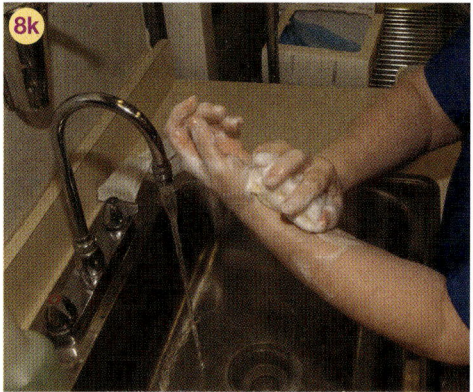

Continued

PROCEDURE 45-1 Perform Handwashing for Surgical Asepsis—cont'd

l. Dominant arm in a similar manner to the nondominant arm.

Rationale. Scrubbing in this manner causes friction, which dislodges microorganisms and other debris from the hands and arms.

9. **Procedural Step.** **Rinse the hands, wrists, and forearms.**

Drop the scrub brush in the sink, and rinse the hands thoroughly under the running water. Hold the hands in an upward position, allowing the soap and water to run from the fingertips, down the arms, and off the elbows. Run the arms under the water in one direction only. Remove them from the water and rinse them again. Use extreme caution not to touch the sink or faucet. If this occurs, the surgical scrub must be started again from the beginning. The brush is discarded after the procedure.

Rationale. Rinsing the hands in this manner allows microorganisms to run off the elbows and into the sink rather than running back down the hands. Removing the hands from the water after each rinse minimizes the risk of contamination from dragging microorganisms back and forth across the arms and hands.

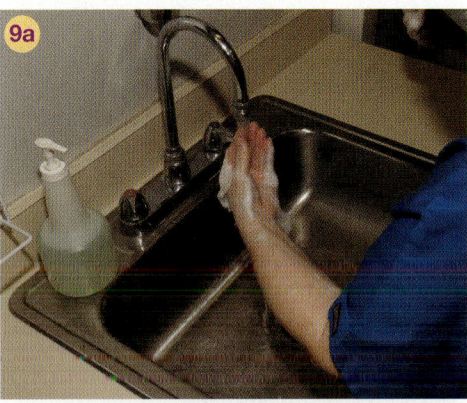

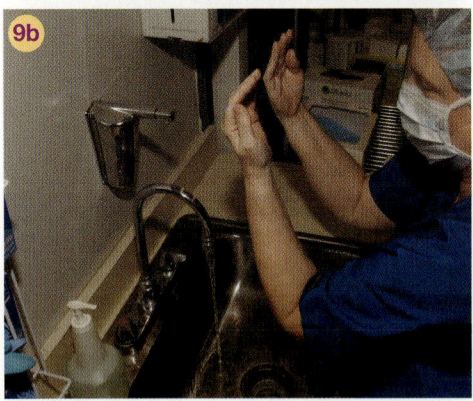

10. **Procedural Step.** **Turn off the water, using the knee or foot control or electronic sensor if available. If not available another staff member can turn off the water.**

11. **Procedural Step.** **Dry the hands and arms.**

Pick up a sterile towel by carefully grasping one corner. Pat the hands dry with one sterile towel. Use a second sterile towel to dry the arms.

NOTE: When drying the hands, be extremely careful not to allow sterile towels to touch the counters or your uniform or reach below waist level.

Rationale. Patting the hands and arms dry minimizes the risk of contamination and prevents the hands from becoming chapped. Make sure the hands are dried completely; damp skin may also cause chapping.

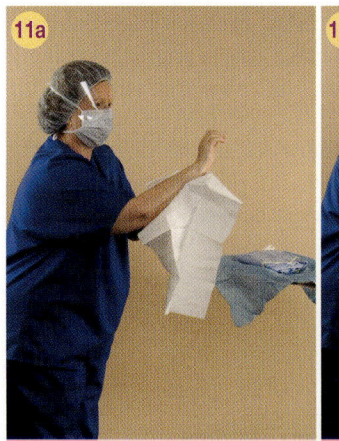 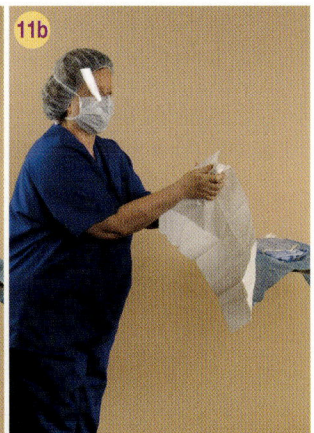

12. **Procedural Step.** **Discard used towels in a regular waste container or soiled-linen container.**

Be careful not to touch the container; keep the hands above waist level.

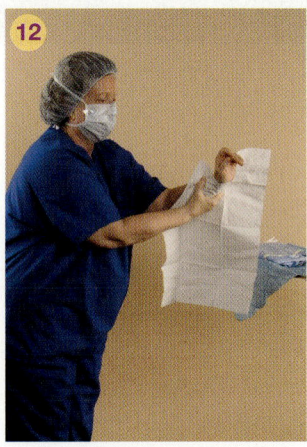

PROCEDURE 45-2 Apply a Sterile Gown and Gloves

TASK: Properly apply a sterile gown and gloves to maintain sterile technique.

EQUIPMENT AND SUPPLIES
- Supplies for surgical handwashing
- Sterile gown
- Sterile gloves
- Hair cover
- Mask
- Goggles (as needed for standard precautions)
- Regular waste container

SKILLS/RATIONALE
STANDARD PRECAUTIONS ARE TO BE FOLLOWED.

1. **Procedural Step. Remove jewelry (rings, watch).**
   Rationale. Jewelry traps microorganisms and dirt, which will not be washed away if jewelry is left on, preventing thorough handwashing. Jewelry must also be removed before sterile gloving because it may puncture the gloves.

2. **Procedural Step. Sanitize the hands.**
   An alcohol-based hand rub may be used instead of washing hands with soap and water, unless hands are visibly soiled. Hands must be sanitized before opening the glove package.
   Rationale. Hand sanitization promotes infection control.

3. **Procedural Step. Open the sterile package's outer wrapping.**
   On a clutter-free flat surface above waist level, peel apart the outer wrapper of the sterile gown package, sterile towel package, and sterile glove package. The outer portion of the inner wrapper may be touched if it is not lying on a sterile field. However, when the wrapper is completely open, only a 1-inch border of the inside may be touched with nonsterile hands. The remainder of the inside of the paper wrapper is considered sterile and should come in contact only with other sterile items.

4. **Procedural Step. Open the inner package.**
   Unfold the inner package containing gloves so that it lies flat on the surface. Turn it so that the labels for the right and left hands can be read. Open the inner package by grasping the side flaps and pulling them apart to expose the gloves. The flaps must *not* fold back against the gloves. The package is folded so that it automatically flattens the upper and lower flaps when the side flaps are pulled apart. The sterile gloves lie flat on the sterile inner wrap and should be oriented with left and right gloves positioned in front of the left and right hands. If the gloves are upside down, turn the package 180 degrees so the fold of the cuffs is at the front toward the person applying the gloves.

5. **Procedural Step. Apply the hair cover, mask, and goggles.**
   Rationale. Keeping the hair covered prevents hair from accidentally falling in a sterile field, causing contamination. Other personal protective equipment (PPE) prevents the spread of microorganisms and protects the medical assistant from exposure.

6. **Procedural Step. Perform a surgical scrub.**

7. **Procedural Step. Unfold the sterile gown.**
   Grasp the sterile gown, touching only within the 1-inch perimeter of the collar. Pull the gown up and away from the wrapper.
   Rationale. This prevents contamination of the gown.

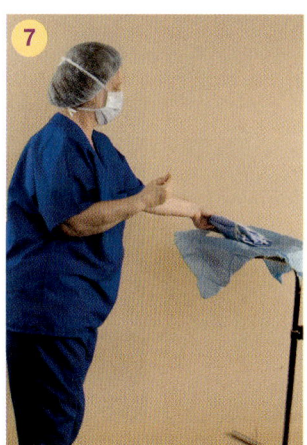

8. **Procedural Step. Apply the sterile gown.**
   Holding the gown away from the body, and touching only the inside of the gown, slide both hands into the sleeves. Do not "push" hands through the cuffs of the gown.
   Rationale. This keeps the gown sterile.

Continued

PROCEDURE 45-2   Apply a Sterile Gown and Gloves—cont'd

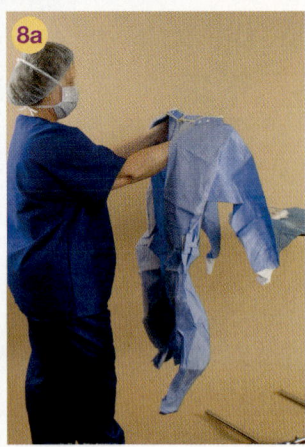
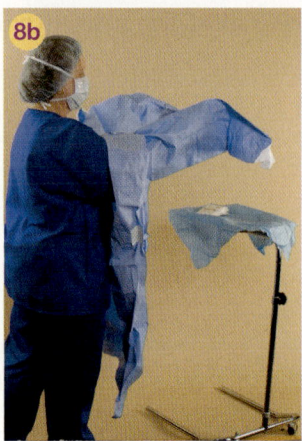

the cuff, gently push your hand through the end of the gown and into the glove at the same time you pull the glove over your hand.

NOTE: Be careful not to touch the front of the gown with nonsterile items when applying sterile gloves.

Rationale. This method ensures that your bare hand touches only the inside of the gown.

9. **Procedural Step.** Secure the sterile gown.
   A second assistant, touching only the inside of the gown, can pull the gown over your shoulders and secure the inside ties of the back of the gown.
   NOTE: Remember, surgically scrubbed hands must remain above the waist and in front of the body.
   Rationale. The gown must be fastened to prevent the flaps from contaminating the sterile field.

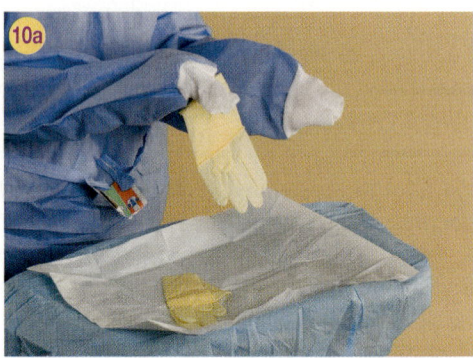
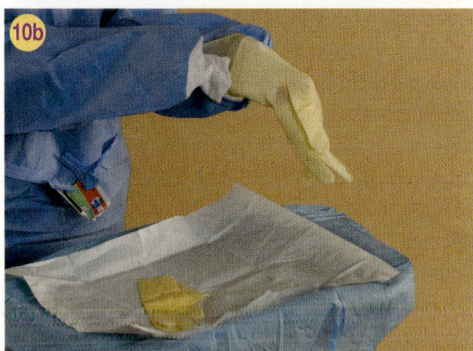
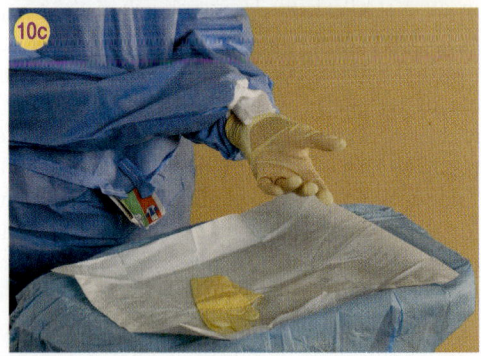

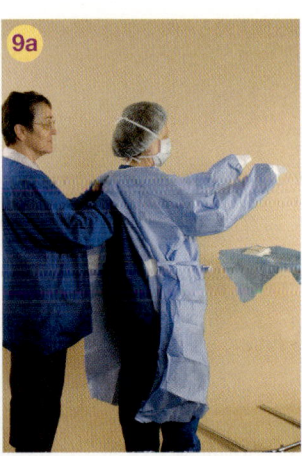
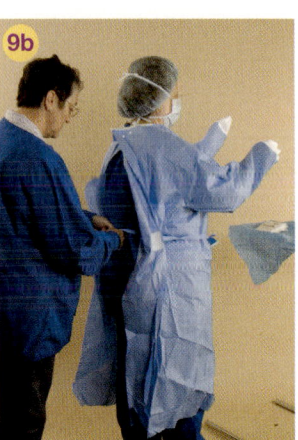

10. **Procedural Step.** Apply a sterile glove to the non-dominant hand.
    To apply gloves once the sterile gown is on, pick up the glove for your nondominant hand with your dominant hand, keeping your hand inside the sterile gown. Place the sterile glove in the palm of your nondominant hand, with the fingers of the glove running up your arm toward your elbow, thumb side touching the gown. Grasp the edge of the cuff with your fingers and by stretching out

11. **Procedural Step.** Apply a sterile glove to the dominant hand.
    With your gloved nondominant hand, slip your fingers under the cuff, pick up the glove for your dominant hand, and repeat Step 10.

Continued

PROCEDURE 45-2 Apply a Sterile Gown and Gloves—cont'd

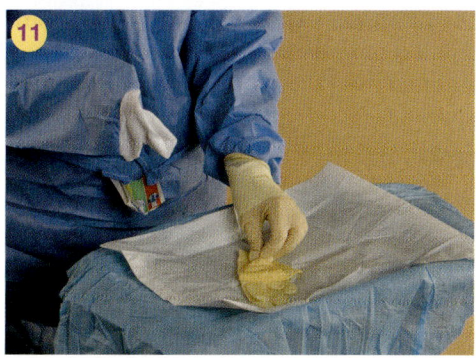
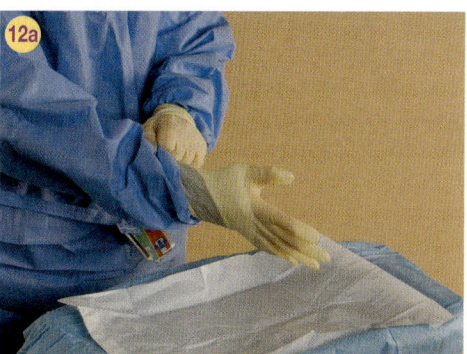
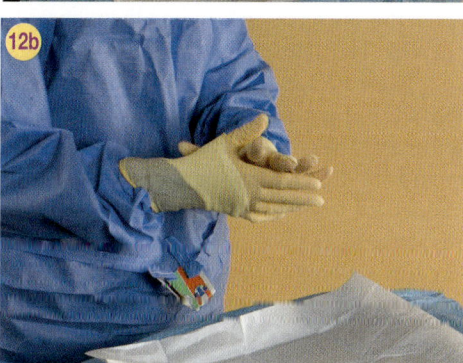

12. **Procedural Step.** Adjust the gloves and gown.
    Once both gloves are in place, the cuffs and fingers may be adjusted. The tie from the front of the gown may now be passed to the second assistant. The second assistant ties the gown in the back at the waist.
    NOTE: Be sure that the gloved hands stay above the waist and in front of the body and that the second assistant touches only the tips of the ties.

13. **Procedural Step.** Maintain sterile technique.
    Ensure that the hands never drop below waist level or touch nonsterile items. If either should occur, the entire process must be repeated from Step 1.

PROCEDURE 45-3 Apply Sterile Gloves

TASK: Properly apply sterile gloves to maintain sterile technique.

EQUIPMENT AND SUPPLIES
- Supplies for surgical handwashing
- Sterile gloves
- Regular waste container

SKILLS/RATIONALE

STANDARD PRECAUTIONS ARE TO BE FOLLOWED.

1. **Procedural Step. Remove jewelry (rings, watch).**
   Rationale. Jewelry traps microorganisms and dirt, which will not be washed away if jewelry is left on, preventing thorough handwashing. Jewelry must also be removed before sterile gloving because it may puncture the gloves.

2. **Procedural Step. Sanitize the hands.**
   An alcohol-based hand rub may be used instead of washing hands with soap and water, unless hands are visibly soiled. Hands must be sanitized before opening the glove package.
   Rationale. Hand sanitization promotes infection control.

3. **Procedural Step. Open the sterile package's outer wrapping.**
   On a clutter-free flat surface above waist level, peel apart the outer wrapper of the glove package. The inner package is sterile and should not be touched yet. The

Continued

PROCEDURE 45-3 Apply Sterile Gloves—cont'd

outer portion of the inner wrapper may be touched if it is not lying on a sterile field. However, when the wrapper is completely open, only a 1-inch border of the inside may be touched with nonsterile hands. The remainder of the inside of the paper wrapper is considered sterile and should come in contact only with other sterile items.

4. **Procedural Step.** Open the inner package.
   Unfold the inner package containing gloves so that it lies flat on the surface. Turn it so that the labels for the right and left hands can be read. Open the inner package by grasping the side flaps and pulling them apart to expose the gloves. The flaps must *not* fold back against the gloves. The package is folded so that it automatically flattens the upper and lower flaps when the side flaps are pulled apart. The sterile gloves lie flat on the sterile inner wrap and should be oriented with left and right gloves positioned in front of the left and right hands. If the gloves are upside down, turn the package 180 degrees so the fold of the cuffs is at the front toward the person applying the gloves.

5. **Procedural Step.** Aseptically sanitize the hands (see Procedure 45-1).
   When applying sterile gloves, handwashing for surgical asepsis (surgical scrub) is typically performed.
   Rationale. Handwashing promotes infection control.

6. **Procedural Step.** Pick up the sterile glove for the nondominant hand.
   Use the dominant hand to reach across the dominant glove and pick up the nondominant glove by pinching the bottom cuff fold between your thumb and forefinger. Only the inside of the glove, which is considered nonsterile, should be touched with bare hands or skin. To maintain sterility of the outside of the glove, do not touch the glove with bare hands or skin.

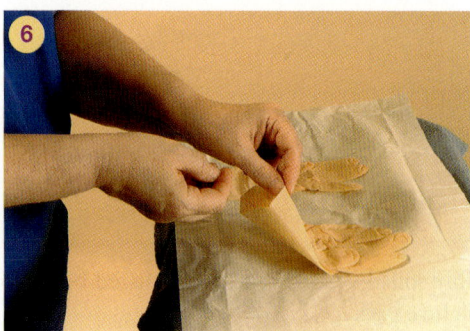

7. **Procedural Step.** Lift the entire glove from the paper and pull it onto the nondominant hand.
   Once lifted from the paper, the glove should not touch the paper again.

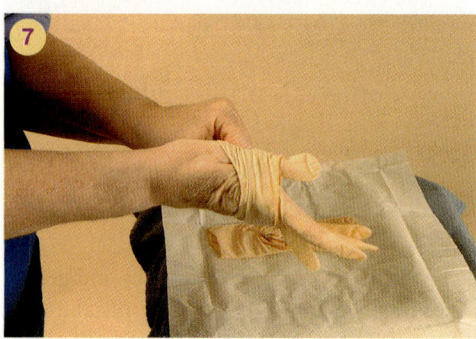

8. **Procedural Step.** Adjust the glove for the nondominant hand.
   Work the nondominant fingers into position while you pull the glove over the back of your nondominant hand and wrist while still holding the glove by the turned-down cuff. While you stretch the cuff of the glove away from the skin, pull the glove past the wrist as far as possible and release it when it will go no farther. A short cuff should remain and should not be turned over the skin because this increases the likelihood of contamination.
   With one glove in place, you must pay close attention to the sterile and nonsterile areas of the other glove. The outsides of both gloves are sterile and cannot touch your skin. The sterile outsides, however, can touch each other. Thus, once the second glove is on, you can touch the outside of each glove to the other.

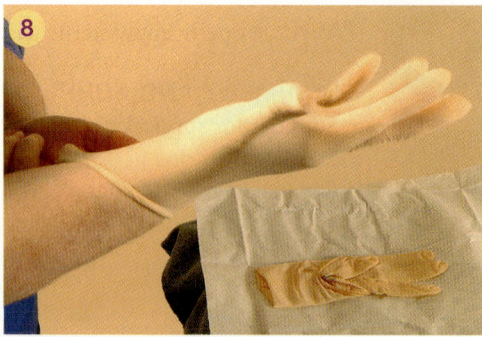

9. **Procedural Step.** Pick up the sterile glove for the dominant hand.
   With the gloved hand, pick up the second glove by placing your gloved fingers between the folded cuff and outside surface of the glove's fingers. The area under-

Continued

PROCEDURE 45-3   Apply Sterile Gloves—cont'd

neath the cuff will be on the outside, so it is considered sterile. No part of your gloved nondominant fingers or thumb may touch the inside of the dominant glove.

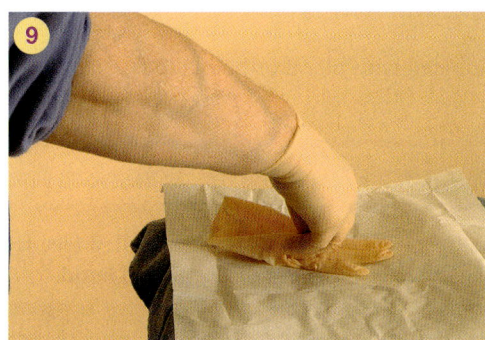

10. **Procedural Step.** Apply the sterile glove to the dominant hand.
Lift the glove completely off the paper and work your dominant hand into the glove, making sure that only the inner surface of the glove comes in contact with your skin. Your gloved nondominant hand must touch only the outer surface of the dominant glove and must not come in contact with the skin on your dominant hand or arm, or the inside surface of the cuff. It is helpful to pull the dominant hand away from the nondominant hand to stretch the glove slightly.

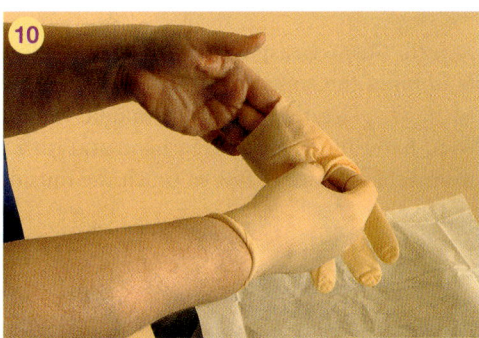

11. **Procedural Step.** Adjust the glove for the dominant hand.
Work your dominant fingers into position while you pull the glove over the back of your dominant hand and wrist while still holding the glove by the turned-down cuff. While stretching the cuff of the glove away from the skin, pull the glove past your wrist as far as possible and release it when it will go no farther. A short cuff should remain and should not be turned over the skin, because this increases the likelihood of contamination. You may adjust the gloves once the skin of the hands is covered, making sure that sterile surfaces touch only other sterile surfaces.

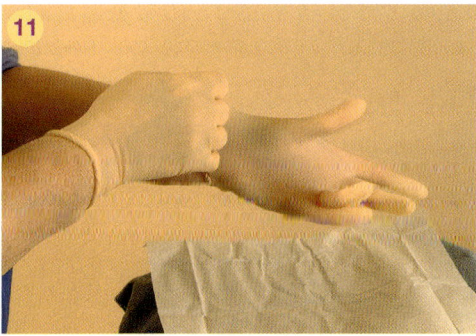

12. **Procedural Step.** Inspect the gloves for tears.
"Marry" your fingers by interlacing them and holding your hands away from your body above waist level, unless your hands are in use.
NOTE: If you touch any nonsterile area or tear a glove, one glove may be changed with the help of an assistant. The assistant removes the contaminated glove and opens a new package of sterile gloves. Still wearing one sterile glove, pick up the new sterile glove under the cuff and pull it onto your ungloved hand. Both gloves must be changed if no assistant is available.

PROCEDURE 45-4

Remove Contaminated Gloves

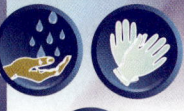

TASK: Properly remove contaminated gloves to avoid spreading contaminants.

EQUIPMENT AND SUPPLIES
- Gloves used in a procedure
- Regular waste container
- Biohazardous waste container (if gloves are contaminated with blood or body fluids)

SKILLS/RATIONALE

STANDARD PRECAUTIONS ARE TO BE FOLLOWED.

1. **Procedural Step.** Grasp the outside of one glove with the first three fingers of the other hand 1 to 2 inches below the cuff.
   Rationale. This avoids touching a soiled glove to a clean hand. Touching the skin with the dirty glove could contaminate the hand.

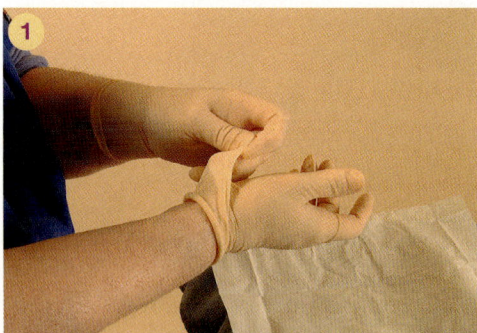

2. **Procedural Step. Remove the glove.**
   Stretch the soiled glove by pulling it away from the hand, and slowly pull the glove downward off the hand. As you pull the glove off, your arm should be extended away from your body, and your hands should be pointed downward. This will result in the glove coming off the hand inside out.
   Rationale. Pulling the outside of the glove with your fingers curled under the cuff will cause it to turn inside out as it is removed. This will confine the contaminants that were on the outside surface to the inside of the removed glove. If the glove has not been torn or damaged during your task, it can touch your skin once inside out.

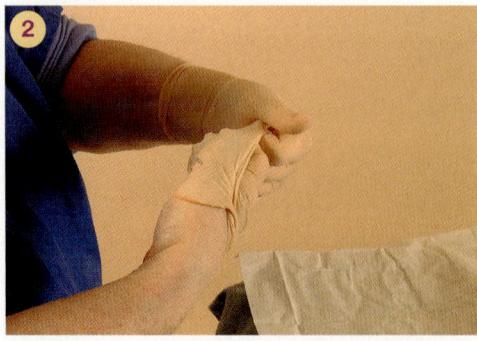

3. **Procedural Step.** As the glove is pulled free from the hand, ball it in the palm of the gloved hand.
   Rationale. Balling the glove into the still-gloved hand prevents loose fingers of the contaminated glove from accidentally touching a clean surface.

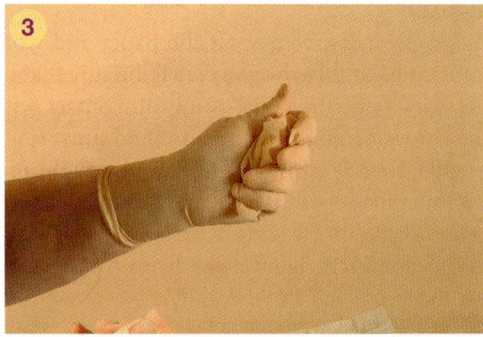

4. **Procedural Step. Grasp the second glove.**
   While holding the soiled glove in the palm of the still-gloved hand, place the index and middle fingers of the ungloved hand inside the gloved hand and turn the cuff downward, being careful not to touch the outside of the soiled glove.
   Rationale. This ensures that only clean skin touches clean skin.

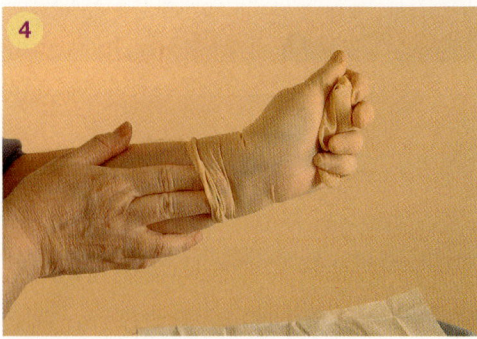

5. **Procedural Step. Remove the second glove.**
   Stretch the glove away from the hand and pull the cuff downward over the hand and over the balled-up glove, turning it inside out with the balled glove inside.

Continued

PROCEDURE 45-4 Remove Contaminated Gloves—cont'd

Rationale. By turning the glove inside out, all contaminated material is enclosed within the glove, reducing the chance of accidental contamination.

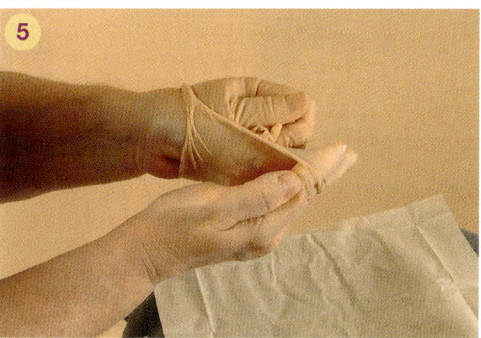

6. **Procedural Step.** Carefully dispose of the gloves in a biohazardous waste container (if gloves are contaminated with blood or body fluids).
   Rationale. Grossly contaminated gloves are considered hazardous even after the contamination has been turned to the inside. A red plastic biohazard bag is adequate for glove disposal because gloves do not have any sharp edges that could puncture the bag.
7. **Procedural Step.** Sanitize the hands.
   Always sanitize the hands after a procedure or after wearing gloves. Remember that gloving is not a substitute for thorough handwashing.

PROCEDURE 45-5 Open a Sterile Package

TASK: Maintain sterility while opening a prepackaged sterile item.

EQUIPMENT AND SUPPLIES
- Sterile prepackaged item
- Mayo stand, or other sturdy surface
- Regular waste container

SKILLS/RATIONALE

STANDARD PRECAUTIONS ARE TO BE FOLLOWED.

1. **Procedural Step.** Sanitize the hands.
   An alcohol-based hand rub may be used instead of washing hands with soap and water, unless hands are visibly soiled.
   Rationale. Hand sanitization promotes infection control.
2. **Procedural Step.** Assemble equipment and supplies and verify the procedure to be performed.
   Rationale. It is important to have all supplies and equipment ready and available before starting any procedure to ensure efficiency.
3. **Procedural Step.** Check the integrity of the outer covering of the sterile package.
   Observe the chemical indicator for a color change. Check the expiration date to make sure the wrapped package is still within the expiration date. Check the package for tears and moisture.
   Rationale. Packages should not be used if the color indicator has not changed, if the item is past the expiration date, and if the integrity of the package has been compromised.

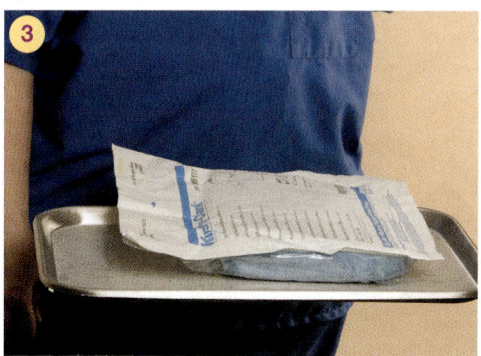

4. **Procedural Step.** Carefully peel back the outer protective wrapper.
   Rationale. The protective covering of disposable packages can become the sterile field when properly opened.

Continued

PROCEDURE 45-5 Open a Sterile Package—cont'd

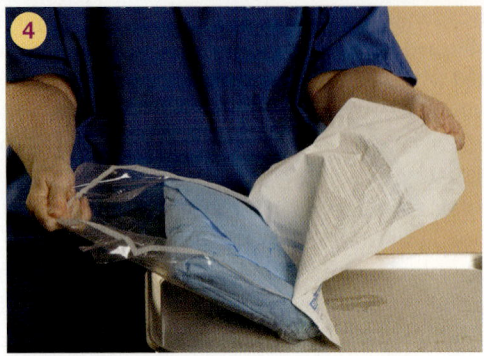

5. **Procedural Step.** Discard the outer wrap.
6. **Procedural Step.** Position the sterile package.
   Place the wrapped package on a clean Mayo stand or sturdy surface, with the top flap turned toward the body so that it can be opened away from your body.

   Small packages containing an article to be transferred to a sterile field may be opened in your hand; medium-sized to large packages should be placed on a sturdy surface or Mayo stand.

7. **Procedural Step.** Open the top flap.
   Open the top flap of the wrapper away from the body by grasping it in the 1-inch border that is considered nonsterile. Once the corner of the wrap has been touched, do not let it fall back onto the pack.
   NOTE: Never reach over the sterile contents since this contaminates the sterile field.

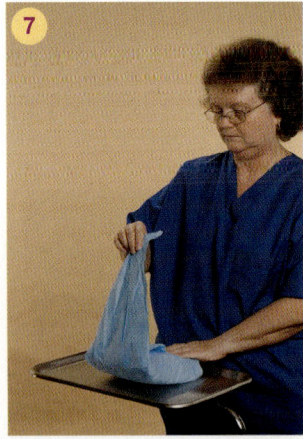

8. **Procedural Step.** Open the side flaps.
   Open the right then the left side flaps of the wrapper by grasping the corners within the 1-inch nonsterile border so that the final flap to be opened is the one that opens toward your body.

   The inside of the wrapper can now be used as a sterile field, or the contents can be transferred to a separate sterile field, according to office procedure.

   After the package is opened, it is critical to pay attention to sterile technique and to take every measure necessary to ensure that the field is not contaminated.
   Rationale. Grasping the corners only allows you to open the pack without passing your hands over the sterile area. Make sure to touch only the outside of the wrapper and only within the 1-inch border that is considered not sterile.

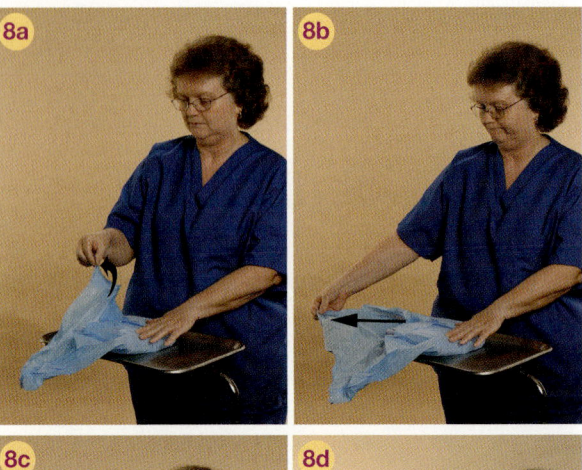

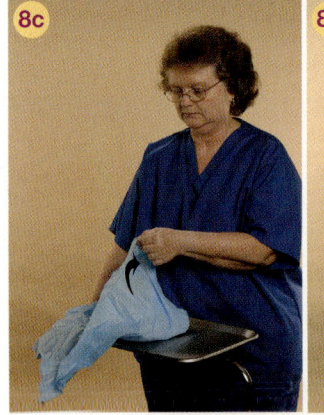 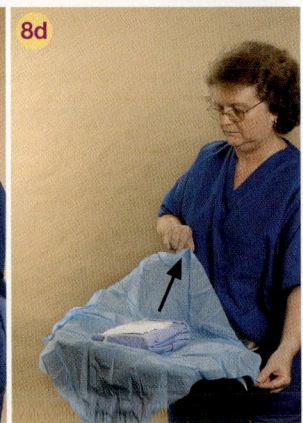

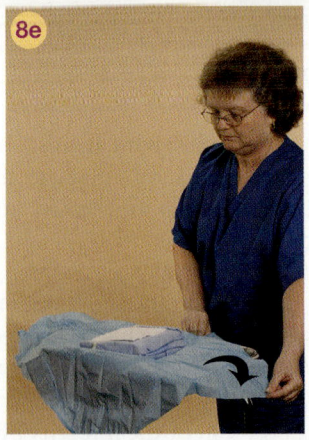

9. **Procedural Step.** Place a sterile towel over the tray and its contents.
   Without turning your back on the sterile field, open the sterile towel and lift it out of the package by the edges. Place the sterile towel over the sterile field, by working from your body out so your arms do not cross over the uncovered sterile field.
   Rationale: A sterile cover needs to be applied if the sterile tray will not be used immediately or the medical assistant leaves the tray unattended.

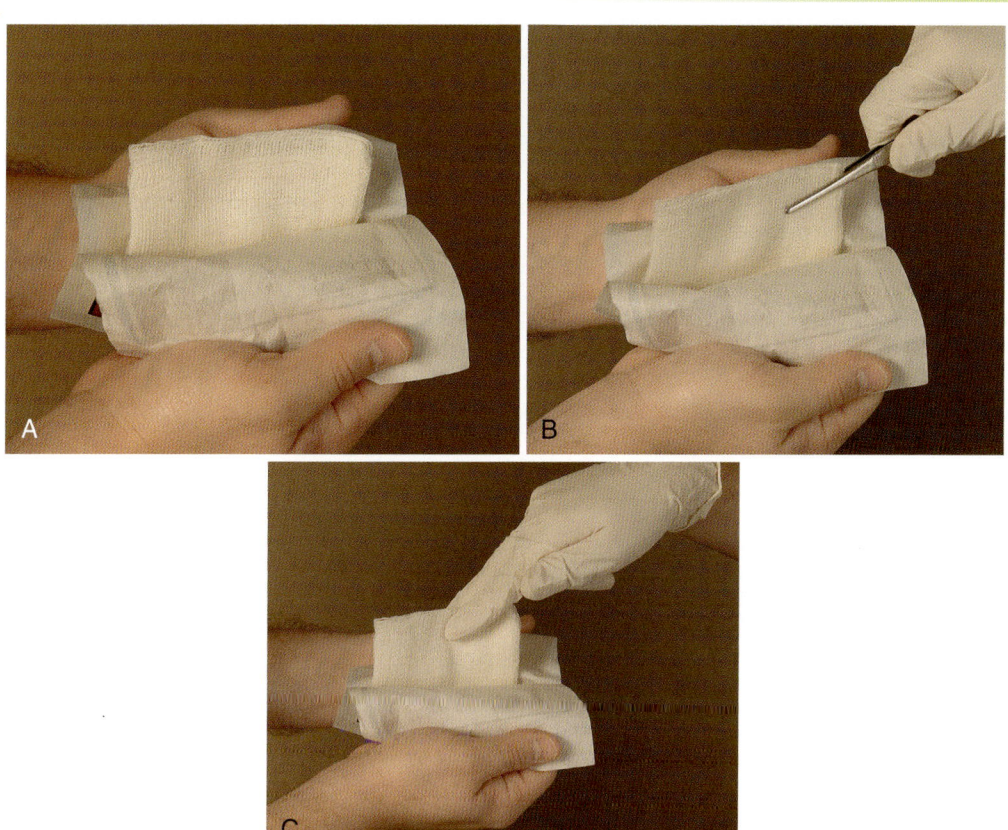

FIGURE 45-2 **A,** Opening peel-down (peel-back) package with sterile contents. **B,** Removing sterile dressing from a package using a sterile instrument. **C,** Removing sterile dressing from a package using sterile gloves.

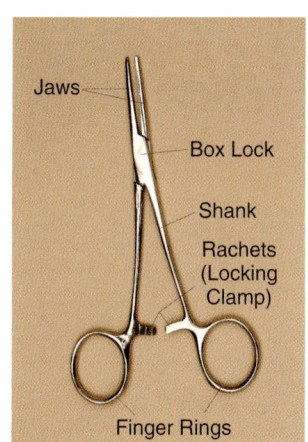

FIGURE 45-3 Parts of a clamp.

One of the medical assistant's greatest challenges is learning the names and functions of surgical instruments; Box 45-3 provides some guidelines.

Scalpels

A **scalpel** (knife handle) has a stainless steel surgical blade (Figure 45-4). Scalpel blades come in a variety of shapes and sizes; blade sizes range from 10 to 25. The tissue that needs to be cut determines the blade type needed. A straight, pointed blade is used for incision and drainage (I&D); a *convex* (curved outward) blade is used for growth removal (e.g., cysts); and a *concave* (pointed inward) blade is used for delicate tissue. Disposable scalpels are also available and are prepackaged with the blade attached. Disposable scalpels are discarded in a sharps container after use, as are the blades of nondisposable scalpels.

Forceps and Clamps

Forceps are two-pronged instruments for grasping or holding body tissue, foreign bodies, or surgical materials (Figure 45-5 and Figure 45-6).

- **Dressing forceps** have blunt ends with serrated tips (e.g., Adson) used for removing or applying dressing materials.

instruments may have a spring-type closure (e.g., thumb forceps). Others may have serrations that are crisscrossed (e.g., needle holder), horizontal, or longitudinal (e.g., Kelly forceps) or may even have teeth on the tips for grasping (e.g., Allis forceps). Medical assistants should be able to identify and care for minor surgical instruments used in the medical office.

BOX 45-3

Guidelines for Learning Surgical Instruments*

Associate the name of the instrument with something that is familiar to you. For example, a *thumb forceps* looks like a tweezers. You use your thumb and finger to close both the tweezers and the thumb forceps. A scalpel with a blade looks like a knife. You cut with both a knife and a scalpel.

Group like instruments together. For example, it is easier to learn the names of each type of retractor if all the retractors are together. Separate them further into those held by hand and those that use a mechanism to remain open.

Develop a goal as to how many instruments you will learn each day.

Review those instruments you have learned before taking on a new set.

Assemble an instrument tray where these instruments are used.

*With repeated use, the instruments' names and functions will make sense and will be easy to distinguish.

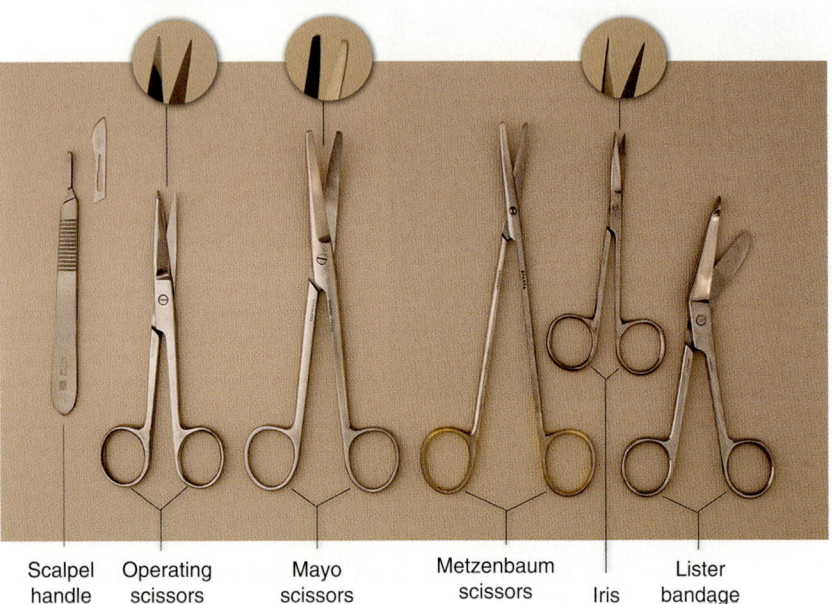

FIGURE 45-4 Cutting instruments.

Scalpel handle No. 3 with #10 blade | Operating scissors (S/S) | Mayo scissors (curved) | Metzenbaum scissors (curved) | Iris scissors | Lister bandage scissors

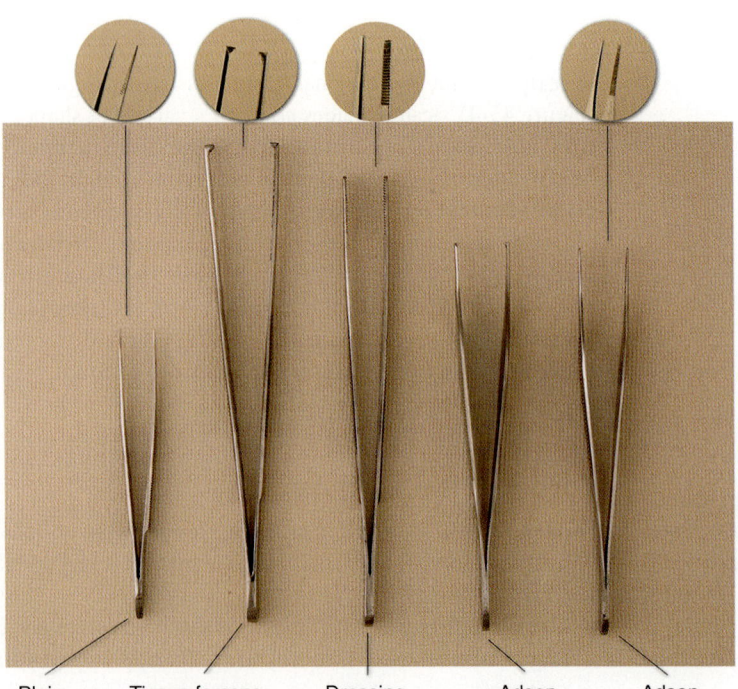

FIGURE 45-5 Dressing and tissue forceps.

Plain Splinter | Tissue forceps with teeth | Dressing forceps | Adson tissue | Adson dressing

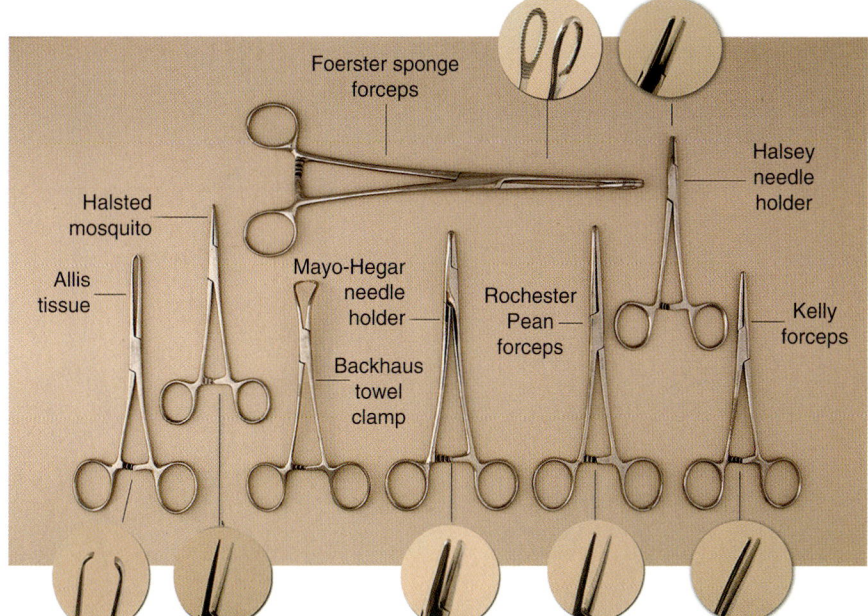

FIGURE 45-6 Grasping and clamping instruments.

- **Sponge forceps** have serrated rings at the tips to hold gauze sponges (absorbent material) to apply medications, cleanse areas, and absorb body fluids (e.g., blood).
- **Hemostatic forceps (hemostats)** are used to control bleeding. They have serrated tips, ratchets, and a box lock to grasp material or clamp off blood vessels and provide hemostasis until the blood vessel can be repaired (e.g., Kelly, Halsted mosquito forceps).
- **Thumb forceps,** or **pick-ups,** have serrated tips and a spring mechanism used to pick up or hold tissue.
- **Tissue forceps** have teeth that allow tissues or growths to be grasped (e.g., Allis tissue forceps).
- **Splinter forceps** have a sharp, pointed, and slender tip and a spring mechanism used to grasp fine objects or particles.
- A **needle holder** has serrated tips, box lock, and ratchets and is used to grasp a curved needle firmly and insert it through tissue. NOTE: A needle holder has the same mechanisms as clamps and forceps, but it is neither a clamp nor a forceps, having shorter and thicker blades.
- **Towel clamps** have two sharp points used to hold the edges of a sterile towel together to form a sterile fold or drape.

See Figure 45-6 for examples of different types of handles used for closing forceps.

Scissors

Scissors are instruments used for cutting (see Figure 45-4). The blades are either straight or curved, and the tips are sharp, blunt, or a combination (blunt-sharp).
- **Bandage scissors** have a bottom blade that is flat and dull on the end, allowing it to slide under a bandage to cut into the bandage before removing it. This blade prevents the skin from being cut or scratched.
- **Dissecting scissors** have thick blades with a fine cutting edge used to dissect and cut muscle tissue. Both ends are usually blunt/blunt (B/B) and have either straight or curved blades. For example, Lilly dissecting and Kahn dissecting scissors are used to divide tissue.
- **Operating scissors** have straight, delicate blades for cutting through tissue. The blade tips can be blunt/blunt (B/B); blunt-sharp (B/S), used when a sharp point is needed around delicate tissue; or sharp/sharp (S/S), with sharp tips on both blades (e.g., iris scissors).
- **Suture scissors,** or Littauer scissors, have a distinctive hook on one tip to get under the suture for cutting suture material and a blunt end to prevent cutting tissue.

Probes

Probes are used to feel inside a body cavity or wound, clear an obstruction, or drain fluids. They can be made of stainless steel, plastic, or rubber. Probes have a long, slender shaft with a rounded end, a grooved end, or an eyelet.

Retractors

Retractors are instruments used to hold back the edges of a wound or incision to expose the operative area (Figure 45-7). Retractors are placed in position, and tension is applied. This tension keeps the wound open.

Curettes

The **curette** is a long-handled instrument with a metal loop on one end (Figure 45-8). Curettes are used for scraping the inside of a cavity. The inner side of the loop is sharp to scrape mucous membranes, and the outer edge is dull to protect

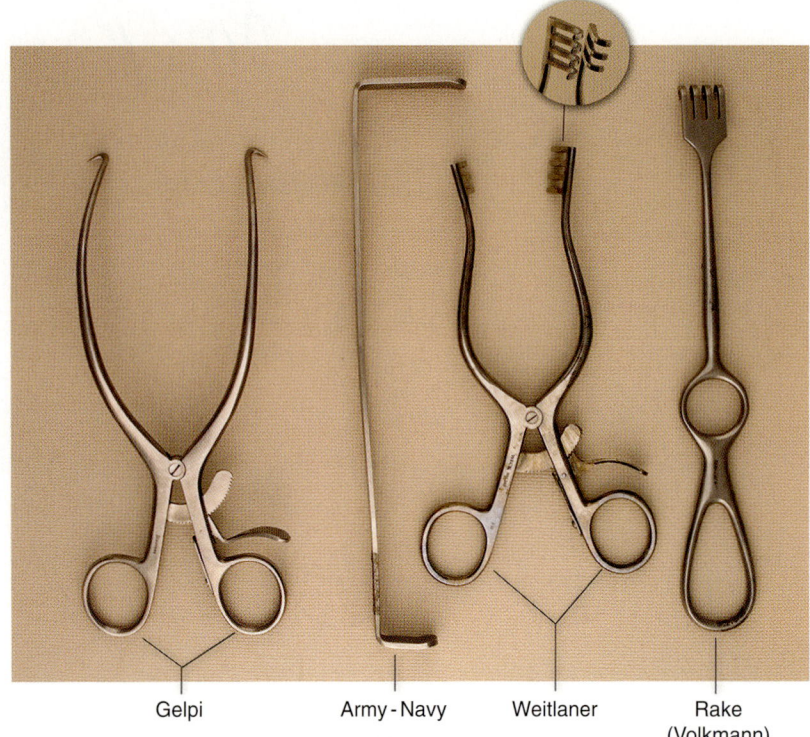

FIGURE 45-7 Retractors.

Gelpi   Army-Navy   Weitlaner   Rake (Volkmann)

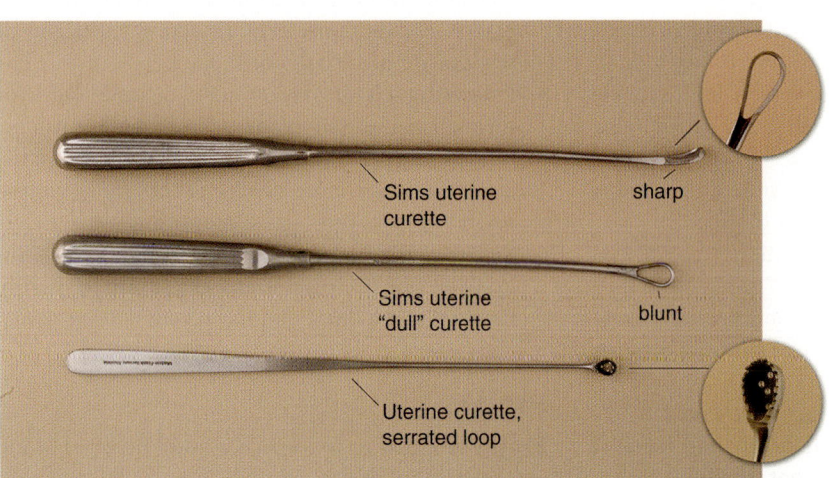

Sims uterine curette — sharp
Sims uterine "dull" curette — blunt
Uterine curette, serrated loop

FIGURE 45-8 Curettes.

against unwanted tissue damage. A curette can also be smooth on the inner and outer edges to allow scraping without cutting tissue.

Care of Instruments

Instruments can last for many years with proper handling and maintenance. Medical assistants should follow these simple guidelines:

1. Handle instruments gently.
2. Do not throw instruments into a basin, or pile them together. Instruments could be damaged in the attempt to untangle them. You also increase your risk of exposure to injury.
3. Keep sharp and cutting instruments separate from other instruments to avoid dulling them.
4. Rinse instruments as soon as possible to prevent blood from drying on them.
5. Use the instrument only for its intended purpose. For example, hemostats are used on delicate blood vessels; they are not made for prying open or pulling on objects.

PATIENT-CENTERED PROFESSIONALISM

- Why is it important for the medical assistant to be able to identify instruments by name and use?
- Why is proper care of instruments important?

ASSISTING WITH MINOR OFFICE SURGERY

The physician performs surgical procedures, but the medical assistant must provide assistance as needed and be alert to prevent breaks in technique such as accidental contamination (Box 45-4).

Before the surgical procedure, the medical assistant prepares the surgical room by disinfecting all surfaces, materials, and equipment in the room. The medical assistant can place the patient in the required position, prepare the incision site, and drape the area. The equipment, supplies, and instruments required by a physician for a minor office procedure depend on individual preference, as well as established standards. Often, an office will prepare an index card for each type of surgery performed. These index cards list all items needed for each type of surgery and aid the medical assistant in preparing the room and equipment according to the preferences of the physician.

Procedure 45-6 explains how to add a sterile solution to a sterile field without contaminating the setup. Box 45-5 reviews the necessary criteria for charting all minor office surgical procedures.

After the items for the surgery have been assembled on a sterile field using sterile gloves (Figure 45-9, A), they are covered with a sterile towel until they are ready to be used (Figure 45-9, B). (NOTE: Sterile forceps may also be used to prepare the necessary materials for a sterile field.) Some items to be used in the procedure are not sterile and will be placed on a side table until needed. For example, the outside wrapper on the sterile gloves is not sterile and must not be placed on the sterile field. The wrapper will be opened on the side table and the gloves applied. Procedure 45-7 details typical activities required of the medical assistant during a minor office procedure. Table 45-2 illustrates hand positions the physician can use to request instruments during surgery and techniques used for transferring them.

Other important aspects of minor office surgery include anesthesia, what common procedures are performed, and decontamination after surgery.

Anesthesia

Anesthesia is a lack of feeling or absence of normal feeling caused by a substance (e.g., medications), hypnosis, or trau-

---

BOX 45-4

Assistance Needed for Minor Surgery

BEFORE THE PROCEDURE
- Review preoperative and postoperative information and ensure that the patient can verbalize an understanding of the procedure
- Ensure a signed informed consent form has been obtained
- Locate equipment and supplies
- Assist in positioning the patient
- Prepare the area for treatment

DURING THE PROCEDURE
- Remove the cover from a sterile tray
- Adjust lighting (if not in sterile gown and gloves)
- Add instruments and supplies to the sterile field
- Add solutions to the sterile field without splashing (see Procedure 45-6)
- Use sterile gloves, and hand instruments and supplies to the physician
- Use sterile gloves, and retract tissue, sponge blood from the operative site, and cut sutures
- Hold the tissue specimen container

AFTER THE PROCEDURE
- Clean the surgical room after the procedure
- Prepare the proper laboratory forms for biopsy processing, label the container, and identify where results should be sent
- Chart the date, type of specimen sent, and name of the laboratory
- Discharge the patient to a responsible adult who also understands the discharge information
- Schedule a follow-up appointment for the patient

BOX 45-5

Documentation for Charting Minor Office Surgical Procedures

1. Date
2. Time
3. Name of procedure:
   - **Dressing change**
     - Location of dressing
     - Drainage type and amount
     - Condition of wound
     - Care of wound
     - Application of dressing
   - **Suture or staple removal**
     - Status of sutures or staples and incision line
     - Number of sutures or staples removed and location
     - Care of wound
     - Application of dressing
   - **Skin closure application**
     - Wound condition
     - Wound preparation
     - Number of skin closures applied and location
     - Application of dressing
   - **Skin closure removal**
     - Status of skin site
     - Number of skin closures removed and location
     - Wound care provided
     - Application of dressing
   - **Assisting with minor office surgery**
     - Action taken (e.g., dressing applied)
     - Type of specimen collected
     - Date, type of specimen sent, name of laboratory
4. Patient reaction, if any
5. Patient teaching and instructions provided (e.g., wound care, return date), time spent
6. Proper signature and credential

| PROCEDURE 45-6 | Pour a Sterile Solution | |

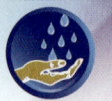

TASK: Add a sterile solution to a sterile field without contaminating the field.

EQUIPMENT AND SUPPLIES
- Sterile solution
- Sterile container
- Sterile towel
- Regular waste container

SKILLS/RATIONALE

STANDARD PRECAUTIONS ARE TO BE FOLLOWED.

1. **Procedural Step.** Sanitize the hands.
   An alcohol-based hand rub may be used instead of washing hands with soap and water, unless hands are visibly soiled.
   Rationale. Hand sanitization promotes infection control.

2. **Procedural Step.** Assemble equipment and supplies and verify the order.
   Rationale. It is important to have all supplies and equipment ready and available before starting any procedure to ensure efficiency.

3. **Procedural Step.** Read the label to make sure you have the correct solution and verify that the solution is not outdated.
   Treat solutions as you do medications and check the label two times before pouring—once when the solution is removed from storage and once when the bottle is opened—to make sure the correct solution is being poured and that the solution has not expired.

4. **Procedural Step.** Palm the label of the bottle.
   Rationale. This avoids drips that obscure the label information while pouring.

5. **Procedural Step.** Remove the cap.
   Touch only the outside of the cap and place the bottle cap with the opening facing up on a flat surface to prevent contamination. Cleanse the lip of the bottle opening by pouring some solution (to be discarded) from the bottle into a container not on the sterile field.

6. **Procedural Step.** Pour the solution.
   Holding the open bottle of solution 2 to 6 inches above the sterile container, pour the necessary amount of solution into the sterile container on the sterile field. Avoid splashing the solution on the sterile field.
   It is important to keep the bottle in the same position as when cleansing the lip of the bottle opening, so the solution poured into the sterile field will be poured over the cleansed area of the bottle opening.
   Rationale. It is important to avoid splashing the solution onto the sterile field because spillage would wet the sterile field and contaminate the entire surgical tray.

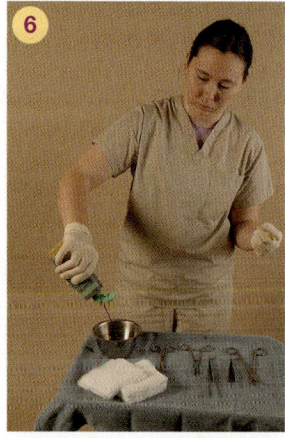

7. **Procedural Step.** Replace the cap on the bottle.
   Be careful not to touch the inside of the cap to anything except the bottle top. Perform a third check of the solution after you have poured the solution but before you return it to storage.

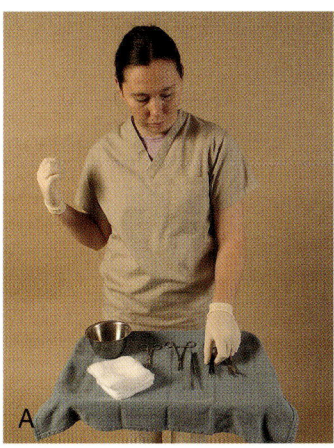 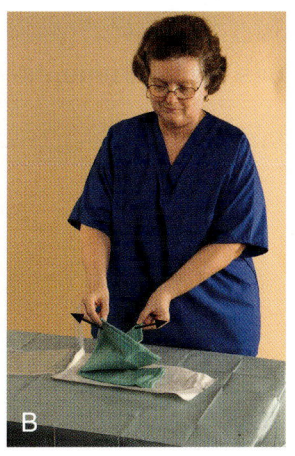 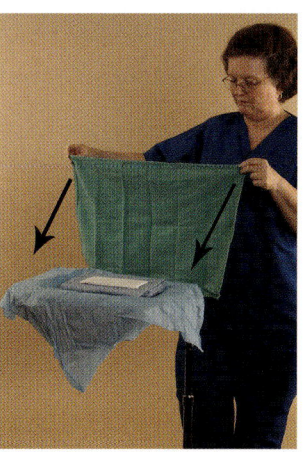

FIGURE 45-9 **A,** Sterile gloves are used to organize instruments for minor surgery. **B,** Sterile setups are covered with a sterile towel and when ready to use the towel is grasped at the top corners and pulled away from the sterile field.

TABLE 45-2
Hand Signals and Transfer Techniques for Instruments

Hand Positions	Instrument	Transfer Technique
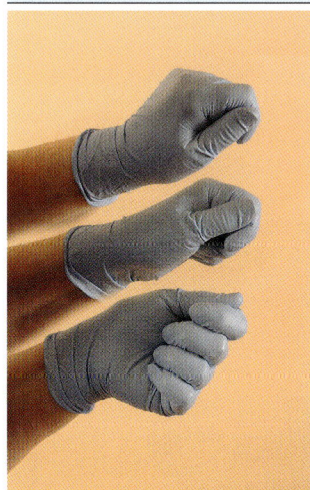	Needle holder	Pass with needle pointing up and suture material looped in other hand, hold by hinge
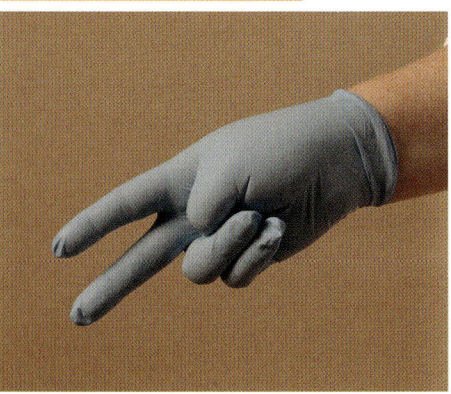	Scissors	Pass with handle first, hold at hinge

TABLE 45-2
Hand Signals and Transfer Techniques for Instruments—cont'd

Hand Positions	Instrument	Transfer Technique
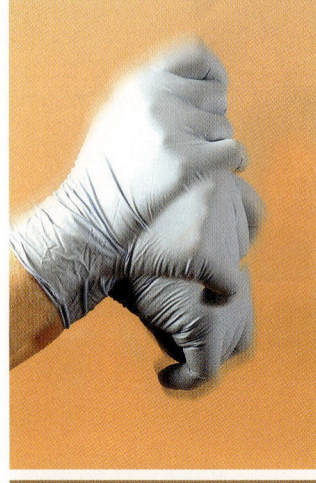	Scalpel	Pass with blade down and handle first, hold just below blade
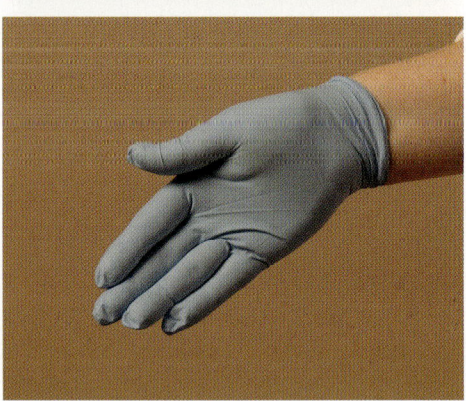	Tissue forceps	Pass the handle first, hold near the tip
	Hemostat	Pass handle first with ratchet disengaged, hold by the hinge

PROCEDURE 45-7: Assist with Minor Office Surgery

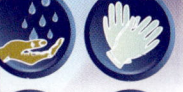

TASK: Provide all equipment, supplies, and materials needed to perform minor office surgery.
NOTE: For this procedure an Incision and Drainage (I&D) setup is being used.

EQUIPMENT AND SUPPLIES

STERILE "SKIN PREP" PACK
- Stainless steel bowl
- Stack of approximately 20 sterile 4 × 4 gauze squares
- 2 sterile towels

TYPICAL STERILE "INCISION AND DRAINAGE" PACK
- 1 Adson tissue forceps
- 1 Kelly hemostat
- 1 Dressing forceps
- 1 Mayo dissecting scissors
- 1 Sharp/sharp operating scissors
- 10 4 × 4 gauze squares

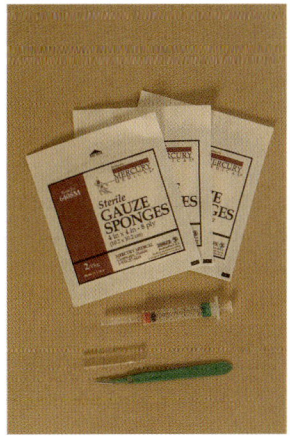

INDIVIDUAL STERILE ITEMS (AS NEEDED)
- Scalpel with blade appropriate for I&D
- 3-cc syringe (sterile)
- 25-gauge, ⅝-inch needle (sterile)
- Sterile dressing

ADDITIONAL SUPPLIES (SIDE TABLE)
- Fenestrated drape (sterile)
- Bottled sterile water
- Bottle chlorhexidine gluconate (Hibiclens)
- Povidone-iodine (Betadine) swabs, or other skin cleanser as preferred by physician
- 5-mL bottle lidocaine (Xylocaine) or other anesthesia, as ordered by physician
- Roll surgical tape
- Lister bandage scissors
- Conforming bandages (as required for type of surgery)
- 2 packages proper-sized sterile gloves (increase as required if others will scrub in)
- 2 packages sterile towels (increase as required if others will scrub in)
- Alcohol wipes
- Penrose drain
- Culture swab with transport system
- Disposable gloves

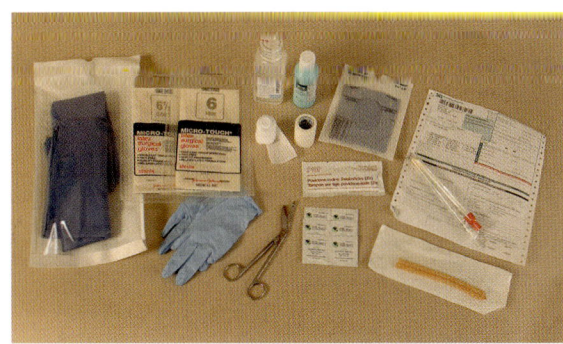

STAGING AREA FOR PHYSICIAN
- Sterile gown for physician (increase as required if others will scrub)
- Hair covers (depending on type of surgery)
- Masks (number required for everyone in surgical area)
- Goggles (as required)
- Shoe covers (as required)

OTHER ITEMS (DEPENDING ON MEDICAL OFFICE PROTOCOL)
- Urine specimen container (if urine sample needed)
- Patient gown and drapes
- Patient medical record with signed consent form
- Biohazardous waste container
- Sharps container
- Mayo stand
- Waterproof waste bag
- Laboratory request form
- Biohazard transport bag
- Disposable razor
- 2 plastic-backed underpads (Chux)

Continued

PROCEDURE 45-7 Assist with Minor Office Surgery—cont'd

SKILLS/RATIONALE

STANDARD PRECAUTIONS ARE TO BE FOLLOWED.

1. **Procedural Step.** Sanitize the hands.
   An alcohol-based hand rub may be used instead of washing hands with soap and water, unless hands are visibly soiled.
   Rationale. Hand sanitization promotes infection control.

2. **Procedural Step.** Assemble equipment and supplies and verify the order.
   Determine the type of surgery being performed and gather equipment and supplies accordingly.
   Some offices keep a card file on the types of supplies and equipment required or preferred by the physician for various surgeries. If this is the case, pull the card and assemble the equipment and supplies accordingly.
   Rationale. It is important to have all supplies and equipment ready and available before starting any procedure to ensure efficiency. It is also important to have back-up supplies of all sterile packs readily available in case of contamination.

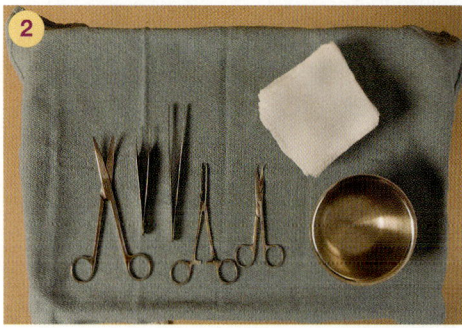

3. **Procedural Step.** Open sterile packs for surgical hand scrubs, physician's gown, and sterile towels in the staging area (not in the examination room). Cover with a sterile drape if items will not be used immediately.

4. **Procedural Step.** Prepare the examination room.
   Adjust temperature, room supplies (e.g., gloves), equipment (e.g., biohazard receptacles), and lighting.

5. **Procedural Step.** Greet the patient, introduce yourself, and confirm the patient's identity.
   Rationale. Identifying the patient ensures the procedure is performed on the correct patient.

6. **Procedural Step.** Explain the procedure to the patient.
   Rationale. Explaining the procedure to the patient promotes cooperation.

7. **Procedural Step.** Perform the following tasks:
   a. **Record** temperature, pulse, respiration, and blood pressure.
   b. **Verify** compliance of preoperative diet and medication instructions.
   c. **Verify** any allergies to medication (e.g., iodine).
   d. **Ask** the patient if they need to void.
   Rationale. The patient should be asked to empty the bladder before a surgical procedure, even if a specimen is not required, for the patient's comfort during the procedure.
   e. **Verify** that the patient has signed the informed consent form.
   Rationale. Written consent for the surgery must be obtained with the patient verbalizing a thorough understanding before signing the consent form and before beginning the procedure.
   f. **Ask** the patient to disrobe and put on a gown.

8. **Procedural Step.** Open a scrub pack in the examination room.
   Pour Hibiclens into a sterile bowl and put on clean disposable gloves.

9. **Procedural Step.** Position the patient.
   Rationale. The patient is positioned so that the surgical site is accessible and the patient is as comfortable as possible.

10. **Procedural Step.** Prepare the surgical site.
    Place an underpad (Chux) underneath the site to be cleaned. Unwrap the disposable razor and place it on the underpad. Use the disposable razor if needed to shave the area around the incision site. Shave against the direction of the hair growth. You must be careful not to nick the skin during shaving and to shave an area of about 4 inches around the surgical site. Scissors may be used to trim the hair down before shaving the area. Dispose of the razor in a sharps container.
    Rationale. Even the finest hair must be removed because hair can harbor microorganisms.

11. **Procedural Step.** Perform a surgical scrub of the incision site as follows:
    a. Starting at the point of incision and working outward in concentric circles, scrub the area for at least 5 minutes (time may vary according to office protocol).
    Rationale. Scrubbing from the point of incision outward in a circular motion carries contaminants away from the site.
    b. Discard gauze squares after one complete wipe. Never return to a previously scrubbed area with the same gauze square.

Continued

PROCEDURE 45-7 Assist with Minor Office Surgery—cont'd

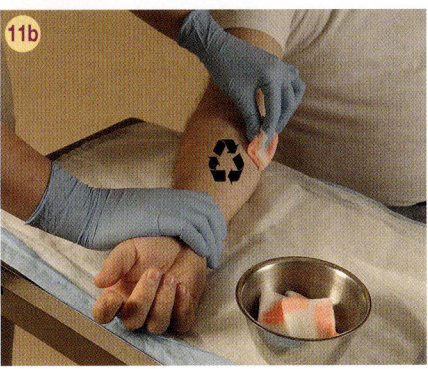

Rationale. Discarding the gauze square after each wipe prevents contaminants from being drawn back over the site.

  c. Rinse the site with sterile water.
  d. Pat dry with a sterile towel.
  e. Apply antiseptic skin cleaner if ordered by the physician (e.g., povidone-iodine).
  f. Remove the wet underpad and replace it with a clean, dry pad.

  NOTE: Be careful not to touch the incision site.

12. **Procedural Step. Drape the area with the fenestrated drape.**
    Caution the patient to remain still and not to touch the site or drape.
    Rationale. A fenestrated drape provides a cutout opening that is placed over the incision area.

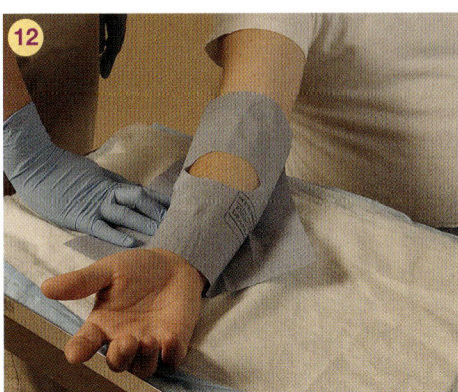

13. **Procedural Step.** Remove the surgical scrub pack and waste material from the room after completing the scrub and remove gloves.
14. **Procedural Step.** Sanitize the hands.
15. **Procedural Step.** Position the Mayo stand so that it is within easy reach of the procedure site.
16. **Procedural Step.** Open the sterile pack and set up the sterile field.
    Place medically aseptic articles on the side counter or table. Depending on the type of surgery, several actions can be taken at this point. If the physician is the only person "scrubbing in" to the surgery, only the outside wrapper of the sterile packages should be opened. If you are to scrub in, you must open only the outside wrap of the sterile packages. You would put on a mask, perform a surgical handwash, and apply a gown and gloves before returning to the room to set up the tray. For this procedure, however, you will not be scrubbing in.
    Rationale. Articles that are medically aseptic cannot be placed on the sterile field because they would contaminate it.
17. **Procedural Step. Tie the physician's surgical gown.**
18. **Procedural Step. Prepare the anesthetic as ordered by the physician.**
    a. Open the syringe and needle and add them to the sterile tray or hold them out for the physician to take from you. The physician will assemble the syringe and needle.
    b. As with any other medication, the label must be checked before the anesthetic is drawn up. Hold the label toward the physician for verification.
    c. Cleanse the stopper of the vial with alcohol and invert the vial so that the physician can insert the sterile needle into the stopper. The physician cannot touch the nonsterile bottle of anesthetic.
    d. After the physician injects air into the vial, pick up the vial and turn it upside down for the physician to withdraw the medication. It is important to hold the vial so that the syringe is at a height where the physician can read the calibration on the syringe.

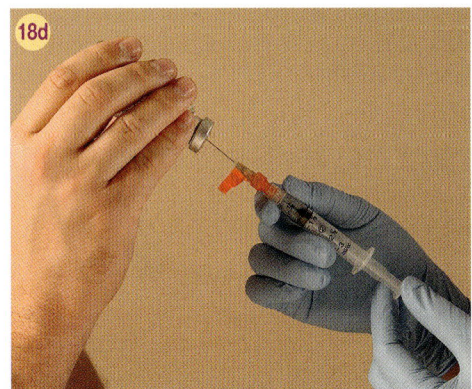

    e. After the physician withdraws the needle from the vial, hold the vial at eye level so that the physician can perform the final check before injecting the anesthetic at the surgical site.
19. **Procedural Step. Hand the physician the antiseptic skin cleanser (povidone-iodine swab), if not already done.**
    Be sure to prevent contaminating the sterile gloves.

Continued

PROCEDURE 45-7 Assist with Minor Office Surgery—cont'd

20. **Procedural Step.** Assist with sterile items.
    Hand the physician sterile items as requested or open sterile items and add them to the sterile tray, such as the individually wrapped scalpel and Penrose drain.

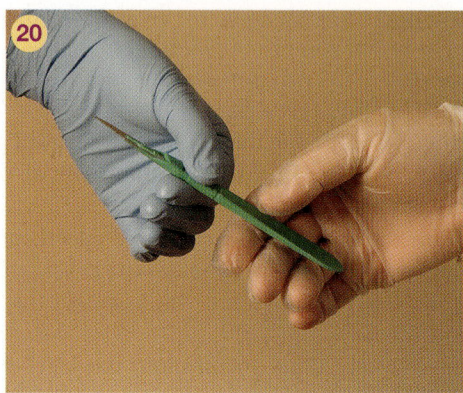

21. **Procedural Step.** Provide the physician with the wound collection system as needed.
    a. Label the specimen container and place it in a biohazard transport bag.
    b. Complete the laboratory requisition form.
    The specimen is labeled with the required patient demographics, date, and specimen type before being put into a biohazard transport bag. Then a laboratory requisition form is completed and inserted into the outside pocket of the specimen bag. The specimen will be taken later to the office laboratory or other designated site; it will await transport to the reference laboratory where it will be analyzed.

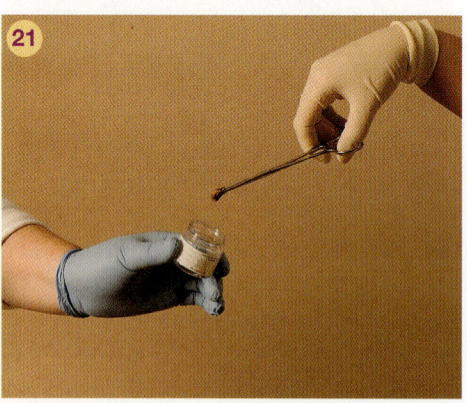

22. **Procedural Step.** Monitor the patient during the procedure.
    One of the most important roles of the medical assistant during a surgical procedure is to talk to patients and keep them occupied so they are not focusing on the surgical procedure.

23. **Procedural Step.** Apply sterile dressing.
    This may be done by the physician, or you may be asked to apply the dressing.

24. **Procedural Step.** Monitor the patient for the next 30 minutes.
    Make sure the patient is not lightheaded or dizzy after the procedure. During this time, do the following:
    a. **Monitor** vital signs.
    b. **Instruct** the patient on wound care, which includes keeping the surgical area elevated, dry, and clean.
    c. **Make** an appointment for follow-up.
    d. **Help** the patient relax.
    NOTE: A postsurgical patient should not be left unattended.

25. **Procedural Step.** Clean the examination room.
    Cleaning the room after a surgical procedure involves a few more tasks than after a nonsurgical patient visit, and always requires personal protection when handling anything that may have come in contact with body fluids. Gloves are adequate, and extra care should be taken to prevent accidental injury in disposing of sharps. The scalpel is disposable and is discarded in a sharps container. Collect surgical instruments carefully to prevent damage to the instruments and accidental sharps injury. After the patient has left, the instruments are brought to the utility room, where they will be rinsed and placed in a soaking solution until they can be sanitized, wrapped, and sterilized.
    a. Solutions are discarded, and the containers used for the solutions are gathered with the soiled instruments to be sanitized and sterilized.
    b. Any nonsharp, disposable item that may have come in contact with body fluids is discarded in biohazardous waste. The fenestrated drape, wraps, and barriers used for this procedure are disposable. After the patient leaves, sanitize the examination table and apply fresh paper.

26. **Procedural Step.** Follow up with the patient.
    a. After gloves have been disposed of and the hands sanitized, check the patient's vital signs and document in the medical record.

Continued

PROCEDURE 45-7 Assist with Minor Office Surgery—cont'd

b. Examine the dressing for excessive drainage; it should be dry. If the dressing has become wet or bloody or if the tape is discolored, notify the physician.

c. Patient instructions for wound care are an important element for postoperative care. The patient must know how to care for the site and when to return for the physician to evaluate the wound. This helps to prevent complications, but the patient should also know how to recognize complications and how to contact the office if complications occur. Instructions should be verbal and written.

27. **Procedural Step.** Document the procedure.

CHARTING EXAMPLE

Date	
4/30/xx	11:15 a.m. Nevus removed by Dr. Lopez on Ⓡ lower arm with the insertion of 3 sutures. Incision site covered with sterile dressing and taped. Dressing is dry. Pt alert with no complaints of dizziness or nausea following the procedure. BP 110/80, P-86 and regular. Verbal and written instructions on wound care given, and pt able to answer questions concerning the care. Appointment made for suture removal in 7 days. Specimen sent to Jones Lab. —— S. Spinks, RMA

---

matic injury. Anesthesia used for surgical or medical reasons could be local, topical, regional, or general.

Minor office surgery usually deals with **local anesthetics** because they produce a limited and brief loss of sensation in the area of injection, freezing, or application. A local injection is done in the area that will be cut, sutured, or probed. Epinephrine ("epi") is added to some local anesthetics because it causes the blood vessels to constrict, thereby holding the anesthetic in the tissues longer and minimizing bleeding. Examples of local anesthetics include lidocaine (Xylocaine), tetracaine (Pontocaine), and bupivacaine (Marcaine).

Topical anesthetics are applied to the skin and cause numbness to the nerve endings in just a few minutes. They can be sprayed (freezing the skin), swabbed, or applied in drops (e.g., eye procedures). The physician will test the patient's sensitivity in the area before proceeding with the procedure. Complications of local anesthesia include tissue damage and allergic reaction.

Regional anesthesia is accomplished when a local anesthetic is injected into and around a set of nerves. The patient remains awake but is unable to feel in a particular area (e.g., foot, leg, or lower back). As regional anesthesia wears off, the patient may be concerned that the area feels numb and heavy. The medical assistant can offer assurance that this is normal and that sensation and movement will gradually return.

General anesthetics produce unconsciousness by depressing the central nervous system. General anesthetics are used for major surgery performed in a hospital or ambulatory surgery center. Patients are usually required to have no food or water (NPO) after 9 PM or midnight the night before (or as ordered by the physician). After the procedure, operation of a vehicle is not recommended because this type of anesthesia is known to create psychomotor impairment for at least 24 hours after surgery. Patients must be made aware that they will need assistance getting home after the procedure.

Common Surgical Procedures

The most common surgical procedures done in a medical office are as follows:

- **Cyst removal.** Sebaceous cysts commonly occur on the face, scalp, ears, neck, and back. Because of irritation and pain, these benign capsules are frequently removed in the medical office under local anesthesia. An incision is made, the cyst removed, and the wound closed with suture material. A sterile dressing is applied. The specimen is often sent to the laboratory for an analysis.

- **Laceration repair.** A wound is cleaned and **debrided,** and a local anesthetic is used. Sutures bring the edges of the wound together. Adhesive skin closures (wound closure strips) can be used if the edges are smooth and the wound is fairly shallow with edges that can be easily brought together (this does not require the use of an anesthetic). A sterile dressing is applied.

- **Abscess incision and drainage.** An abscessed area is cleaned, and an incision is made to drain the area of exudate and infected matter. The wound is cleaned but not sutured because continued drainage of exudate is necessary. Sometimes a drainage tube is inserted and later removed. A thick sterile dressing is applied to monitor drainage.

- **Skin lesion removal.** Warts or other types of skin lesions are removed, often by the use of a freezing agent. Usually, liquid nitrogen is sprayed or applied by a large, cotton-tipped applicator on the area until it becomes white. Soon after, a blister forms. This blister scabs and eventually falls off (the patient should not try to forcefully remove the scab). A dressing is not applied, but the patient is told to keep the area clean.

Alternative Surgical Methods

Alternative methods to remove unwanted tissue are used when the patient's tissue does not need to be sent to the pathology laboratory for examination.

- **Electrosurgery** uses an electric current to cut or destroy tissue (e.g., skin tags, warts). Minimal blood is lost because blood vessels are cauterized during the process.
- A **laser** generates intense heat and energy creating a narrow beam of light that can be focused at unwanted tissue. A laser can be used to cut tissue, coagulate small blood vessels, and vaporize or remove tissues (e.g., warts, keloid, or tattoos) and body hair. Laser surgery causes less damage to surrounding tissue and promotes faster healing.
- **Cautery** uses chemicals (e.g., silver nitrate, sodium hydroxide) to destroy tissues (e.g., skin tags).
- **Cryosurgery** destroys tissues by using liquid nitrogen (extreme cold) (e.g., senile keratosis, planter's warts).

Decontamination after Surgery

After the patient has left the surgical room, the medical assistant **decontaminates** it. All instruments, both used and unused, are gathered and sanitized according to office policy. See Chapter 31 for information on sanitizing. Disposable linen is discarded in a trash receptacle; if contaminated with body fluids, linen is placed in the biohazardous waste container. Large pieces of equipment are wiped down with a disinfectant and allowed to dry. The examination table and any solid surfaces are wiped with a disinfectant.

> **PATIENT-CENTERED PROFESSIONALISM**
> - How does the medical assistant's role in minor office surgery promote patient health?

WOUND CARE

Wounds are often treated in medical offices. It is important for medical assistants to understand (1) types of wounds, (2) how wounds heal, (3) types of closures, (4) how to change a sterile dressing, and (5) how to instruct patients concerning the wound and its care. Remember the patient must understand the frequency of dressing changes and be instructed on how to identify the signs of infection. A handout on wound care is useful only if it is explained to the patient first.

Wound Types

A **wound** is a break in the soft tissue of the body. Figure 45-10 shows different types of wounds.

An **open wound** is a break in the skin or mucous membranes and can be classified as either superficial or deep. **Superficial wounds** do not extend beyond the subcutaneous layer (e.g., abrasions, lacerations). **Deep wounds** extend beyond the subcutaneous layer (e.g., puncture wounds).

A **closed wound** does not show a break in the skin. Instead, the tissues are bruised or bleed internally (e.g., contusion, hematoma). This type of wound is caused by trauma to the body.

Wound Healing

Effective wound healing is the goal after any surgery or wound repair. The healing process depends on the following factors:
- General state of the patient's health
- Good nutrition
- Adequate blood supply and normal clotting
- Use of proper aseptic technique during surgery and dressing changes

During wound healing, three tissues come together: epithelium, fibrous connective tissue, and blood cells. These tissues make up the scar tissue (**cicatrix**). The largest percentage of scar tissue is made up of fibrous tissue. Infection and necrotic tissue (dead tissue) increase the amount of scarring.

As soon as an injury or a surgical incision occurs, the inflammation process begins. The blood vessels constrict momentarily. The capillaries dilate, allowing plasma with its clotting factors to leave the capillaries to form a blood clot. As part of the inflammation process, neutrophils and macrophages (monocytes) clean up the injured area. As healing progresses, the clot becomes a scab. The space caused by the wound is replaced by granulation tissue, which has a rich blood supply. As new epithelial tissue grows from the granulation tissue at the wound edges, a scar forms. This scar tissue eventually fades to white as the blood supply decreases and blood vessels return to normal function.

Wounds are classified by the way they are repaired and how they heal. The three classifications of wounds are as follows:

1. **First (primary) intention healing** occurs when a clean surgical wound is closed and heals with minimal scarring and no infection (Figure 45-11, *A*).
2. **Second (secondary) intention healing** occurs when a large wound is not closed (e.g., pressure ulcer) and heals from the bottom up (granulation) (Figure 45-11, *B*). A large amount of scarring results.
3. **Delayed primary (tertiary) intention healing** occurs when the wound is left open because of infection or debris. Wounds with tertiary healing often require **debridement**, which is the removal of foreign or dead material such as necrotic tissue, dirt, glass, gravel, or metal fragments. When the infection or wound debris has been removed, the wound may be sutured. The amount of scarring and the rate of healing will vary for each individual (Figure 45-11, *C*).

Wound Closures

Sutures, staples, surgical glue, and skin closures may be used to close wounds. Both surgical glue and skin closures are examples of a noninvasive wound closure.

Sutures

Sutures are foreign materials used to **approximate** (bring together) skin edges or **ligate** (tie off) blood vessels until

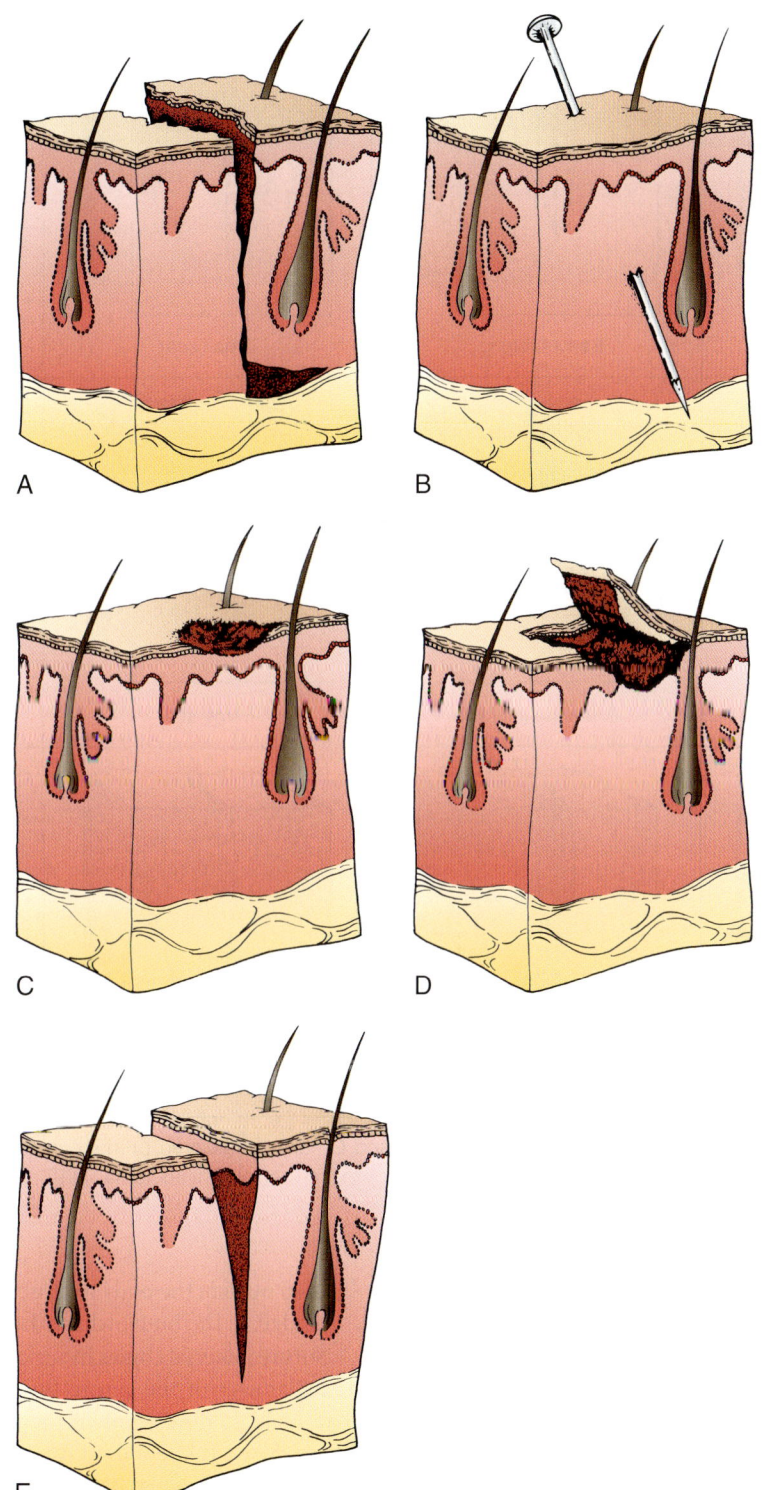

FIGURE 45-10 Types of wounds. **A,** *Laceration* is a jagged, irregular break or tear of tissue, usually caused by blunt trauma. **B,** *Puncture* is where the skin is pierced by a pointed object (e.g., pin, nail, splinter, and bullet). **C,** *Abrasion* is a superficial wound; skin scrape. **D,** *Avulsion* is where tissue is forcibly torn or separated, usually caused by accidents. **E,** *Incision* is a neat, clean cut from a sharp object (e.g., glass, knife, and metal). (From Buck CJ: *Step-by-step medical coding,* 2008 edition, St Louis, 2008, Saunders.)

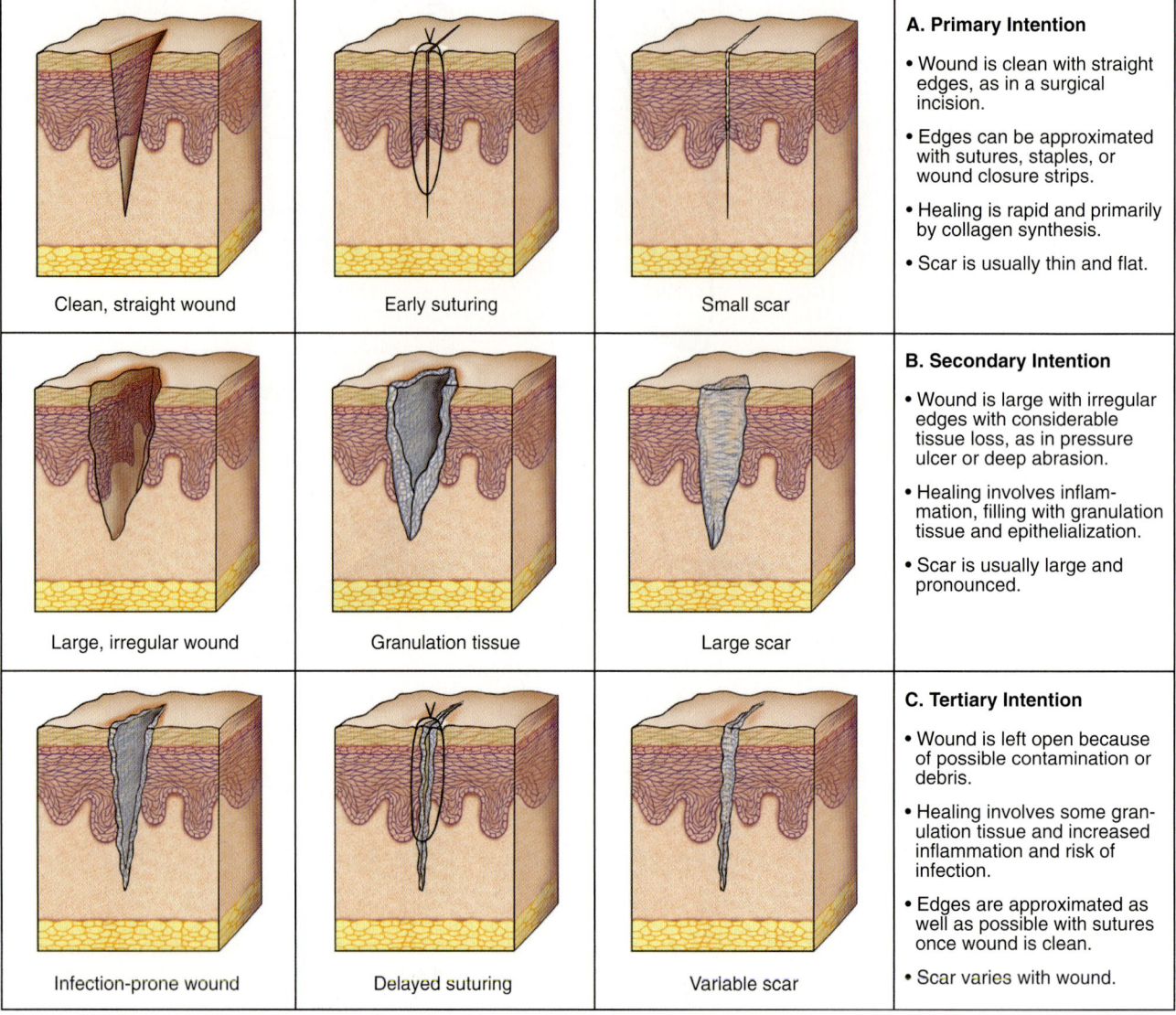

FIGURE 45-11 Wound healing by **A,** primary, **B,** secondary, and **C,** tertiary (delayed primary) intention. (Modified from Monahan FD, Neighbors M: *Medical-surgical nursing: foundations for clinical practice*, ed 2, Philadelphia, 1998, Saunders.)

healing is complete. A suture line may consist of a continuous line of suture material or a series of interrupted sutures individually tied (Figure 45-12). Sutures are made from different types of materials and are either absorbable or nonabsorbable.

- Some suture materials were once made of sheep intestines and referred to as "catgut," which dissolves (absorbs) inside the body over time. The term **catgut** is still used today, but today's catgut suture materials are usually made of a synthetic material. Catgut is used in tissues that heal rapidly and when absorption of suture material is desired.
- **Chromic suture** materials are specially treated and, as with catgut, dissolve after a time. Chromic sutures are used in areas that heal more slowly and when suture material needs to remain in place longer.
- Untreated materials, such as nylon, silk, stainless steel, and polypropylene, will not absorb. These suture materials are used outside the body to close wounds or incisions, or they are left in the body, where they embed in scar tissue.

Suture material comes in various sizes, as do suture needles. The diameter of the suture thread determines its size. Note that the higher the number, the smaller is the diameter of the suture. Size 1 is larger than size 0. Size 2-0 (00) is smaller than size 0. This "0" is also referred to or pronounced as "aught," as in "2-aught." The physician selects a suture size based on the amount of healing time required, the site of the wound, and the strength of the suture needed to close the wound. Figure 45-13 illustrates the different suture sizes and possible uses. Sutures also come in varying lengths. Figure 45-14 shows how packets of suture material are labeled.

Surgical needles can be straight or curved in various degrees (e.g., half-round, slight curve), and they have different types of pointed ends. A *sharp point* (cutting) needle cuts tissues, whereas a round pointed needle (tapered) separates tissues

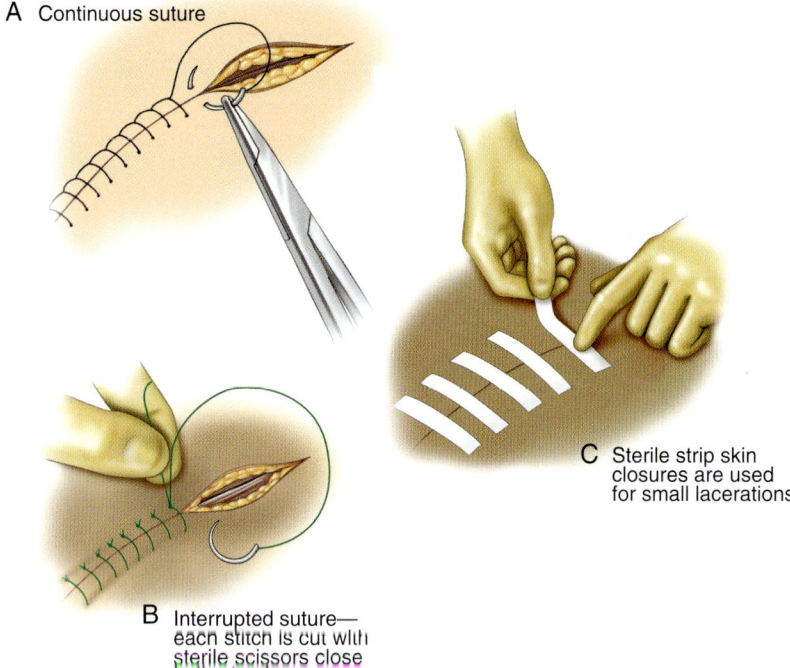

FIGURE 45-12 **A,** Continuous sutures. **B,** Interrupted sutures. **C,** Sterile strip skin closures. (From Hunt SA: *Saunders fundamentals of medical assisting—revised reprint,* St Louis, 2007, Saunders.)

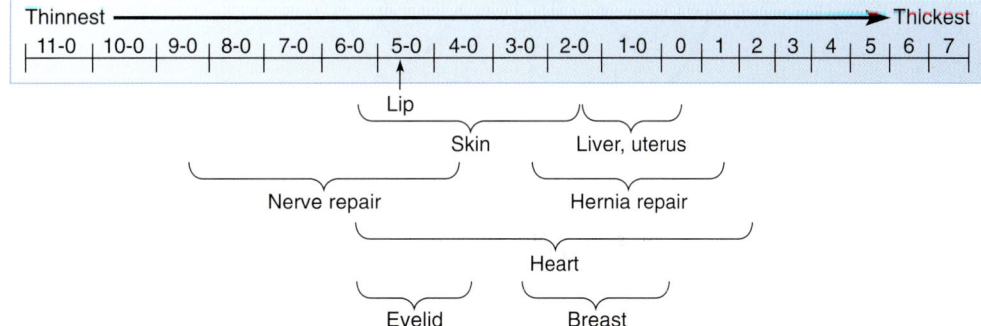

FIGURE 45-13 Suture material, thinnest to thickest.

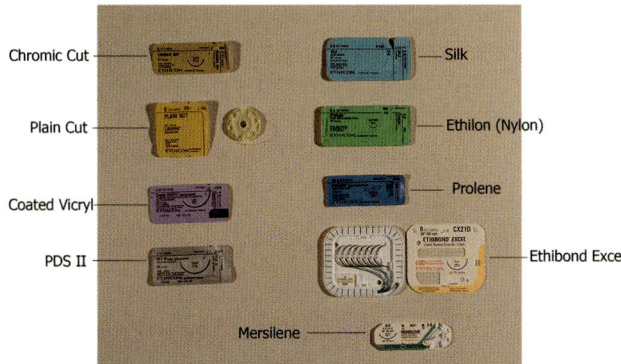

FIGURE 45-14 A variety of prepackaged suture materials with needles of various sizes and shapes.

(Figure 45-15). The suture material and type of needle that the physician requires for repair vary according to the area to be sutured and the physician's preference. Usually, a needle is already attached to the suture material; this is called a "swaged" needle. A needle holder must be used with a curved needle to penetrate tissue (Figure 45-16). Procedure 45-8 describes the process of suture removal.

Before removing sutures the wound margins should appear to be healing and closed. Typically, sutures are not left in place for more than 7 days because "suture marks" may be permanent. Often, skin closures are applied to strengthen the sutured area if under tension. Time for suture removal varies, but the following is typical:

- Face: 3 to 5 days
- Scalp: 7 days
- Chest and extremities: 8 to 10 days
- High tension (joints, hands): 10 to 14 days
- Back: 10 to 14 days

Staples

Staples can also bring tissue together (Figure 45-17). Staples are made of stainless steel and are sterile. They are used when greater stress will be placed on the suture line (e.g., scalp, trunk, and upper extremities). Staples are applied using a disposable skin stapler (Figure 45-18) and removed using a special staple-removing type forceps. One jaw of the staple

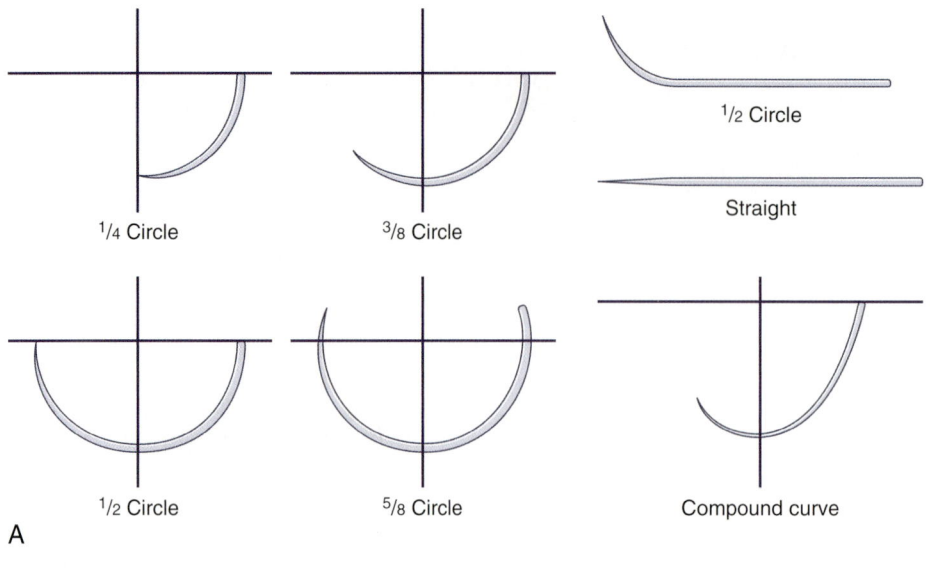

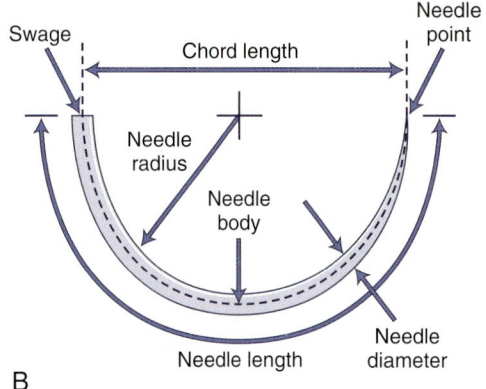

FIGURE 45-15 Surgical needle shapes. **A,** Needle shape and curvature. **B,** Characteristics of a needle. (From Fuller JK: *Surgical technology: principles and practice*, ed 4, St Louis, 2005, Saunders.)

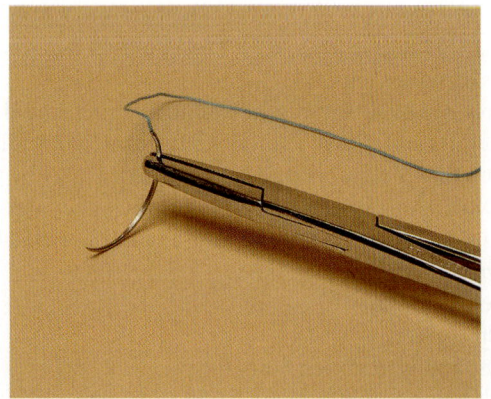

FIGURE 45-16 Curved needle positioned in needle holder.

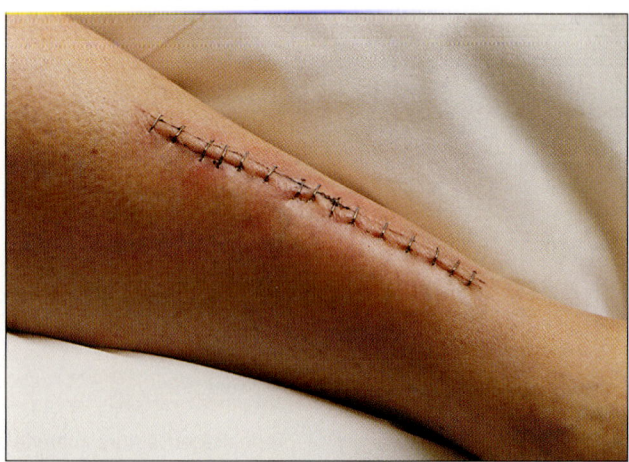

FIGURE 45-17 Suture line secured with staples. (From Potter PA, Perry AG: *Basic nursing*, ed 6, St Louis, 2007, Mosby.)

Minor Office Surgery **CHAPTER 45** 1119

PROCEDURE 45-8

Remove Sutures or Staples and Change a Wound Dressing Using a Spiral Bandage

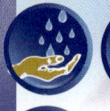

TASKS:
- Remove sutures from a healed wound as ordered by physician.
- Apply a sterile dressing to a wound.
- Apply a bandage over the sterile dressing, using a spiral turn.

EQUIPMENT AND SUPPLIES
- Nonsterile disposable gloves
- Sterile suture removal kit or staple removal kit
- Sterile gauze pads (size depends on size of wound to be covered)
- Antiseptic or sterile swabs
- Sterile gloves
- Waterproof waste bag
- Surgical tape
- Scissors
- Biohazardous waste container
- Patient's medical record

SKILLS/RATIONALE

STANDARD PRECAUTIONS ARE TO BE FOLLOWED.

1. **Procedural Step. Sanitize the hands.**
   An alcohol-based hand rub may be used instead of washing hands with soap and water, unless hands are visibly soiled.
   Rationale. Hand sanitization promotes infection control.

2. **Procedural Step. Assemble equipment and supplies and verify the order.**
   Determine whether the incision or wound has been sutured or stapled. Verify how many sutures or staples have been inserted.
   Rationale. It is important to have all supplies and equipment ready and available before starting any procedure to ensure efficiency. Verifying the correct number to be removed prevents accidentally not removing the correct number of sutures or staples.

3. **Procedural Step. Greet and identify the patient and escort the patient to the examination room.**
   Rationale. Identifying the patient ensures the procedure is performed on the correct patient.

4. **Procedural Step. Explain the procedure to the patient.**
   Ask the patient to describe any symptoms that should be reported to the physician such as drainage, pain, or an inability to move the extremities.
   Rationale. Explaining the procedure to the patient promotes cooperation and provides a means of obtaining implied consent.

5. **Procedural Step. Position the Mayo stand so that it is within easy reach of the procedure site.**

6. **Procedural Step. Create a sterile field, using a prepackaged sterile drape, and attach a temporary disposal bag (waterproof waste bag) to the edge of the Mayo stand.**

   Rationale. Contaminated items, such as the soiled dressing, may be discarded in the bag and the entire bag discarded later in biohazardous waste.

7. **Procedural Step. Open the suture removal kit or staple removal kit by peeling back the paper covering of the bubble pack.**

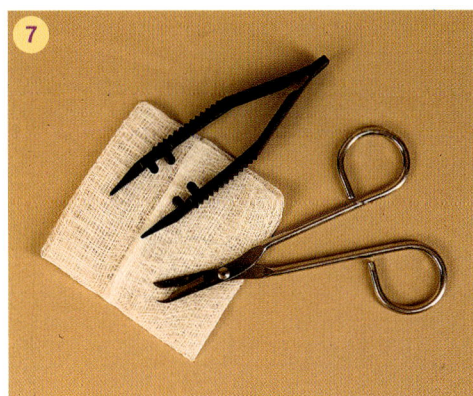

8. **Procedural Step. Apply nonsterile gloves.**
9. **Procedural Step. Remove the soiled dressing.**
   Examine for any signs of bleeding, excessive drainage, or infection before disposing of it in the plastic bag.
10. **Procedural Step. Check the incision line.**
    Be sure that the sutures are intact and that the laceration is not infected and has healed adequately. If excessive redness, swelling, or drainage is present, sutures or staples should not be removed, and the physician should be notified.

Continued

PROCEDURE 45-8 Remove Sutures or Staples and Change a Wound Dressing Using a Spiral Bandage—cont'd

Rationale. When a dressing is changed, the physician should view any incision or wound that is not healing normally before a new dressing is applied.

11. **Procedural Step.** Discard the contaminated dressing, sanitize the hands once again, and put on a clean pair of gloves to remove the sutures or staples.
12. **Procedural Step.** Cleanse the incision line.
    Before removing the sutures or staples, cleanse the incision line with an antiseptic swab from the center outward, so that potential skin contaminants are not drawn into the suture or staple holes.

TO REMOVE SUTURES

13. **Procedural Step.** Grasp the first suture to be removed.
    After the incision line has been cleansed and allowed to air dry, grasp the first suture to be removed with the dressing forceps by gently lifting upward until the thread is extended but not taut (this facilitates cutting).
14. **Procedural Step.** Cut the suture.
    Cut the suture next to the skin by slipping the curved end of the suture removal scissors under the knot and manipulating the straight edge of the scissors to cut the thread.
    Rationale. Cutting at skin level prevents the suture material, which has been exposed to contamination during the healing process, from being pulled through the skin.

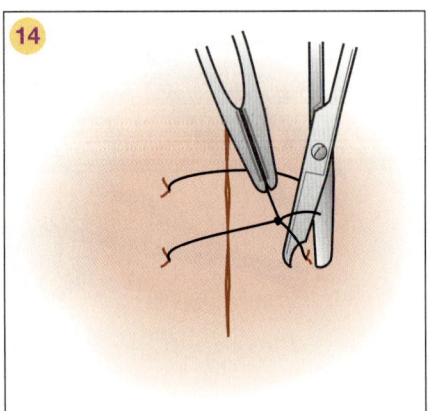

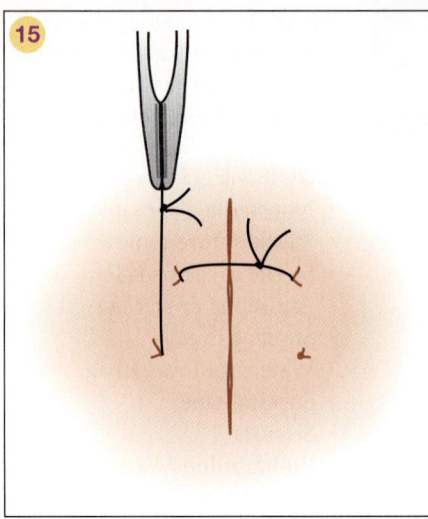

16. **Procedural Step.** Place each suture on the gauze square (included in the kit) after being removed.
    With attention to proper technique, the suture removal process is repeated for each suture that must be removed.
17. **Procedural Step.** Inspect and count the sutures on the gauze square before discarding them.
    Rationale. It is important to be certain that the number of sutures removed matches the number inserted and that the entire suture is present. This minimizes the potential for infection from a suture or any part of it being left in place.

TO REMOVE STAPLES

18. **Procedural Step.** Carefully place the bottom jaws of the staple remover under the staple to be removed.

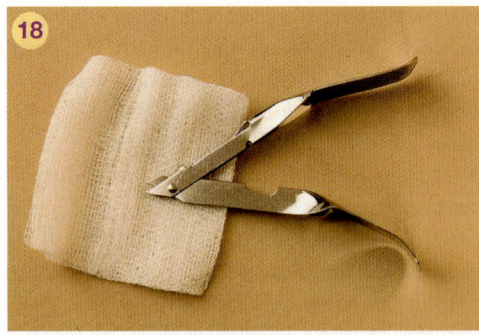

19. **Procedural Step.** Firmly squeeze the staple remover handles until they are fully closed.

15. **Procedural Step.** Use the dressing forceps to lift the suture straight upward, toward the suture line, and out of the skin.
    Rationale. Pulling straight upward and toward the suture line prevents tugging against the tissue and minimizes the possibility of reopening the suture line.

Continued

PROCEDURE 45-8 Remove Sutures or Staples and Change a Wound Dressing Using a Spiral Bandage—cont'd

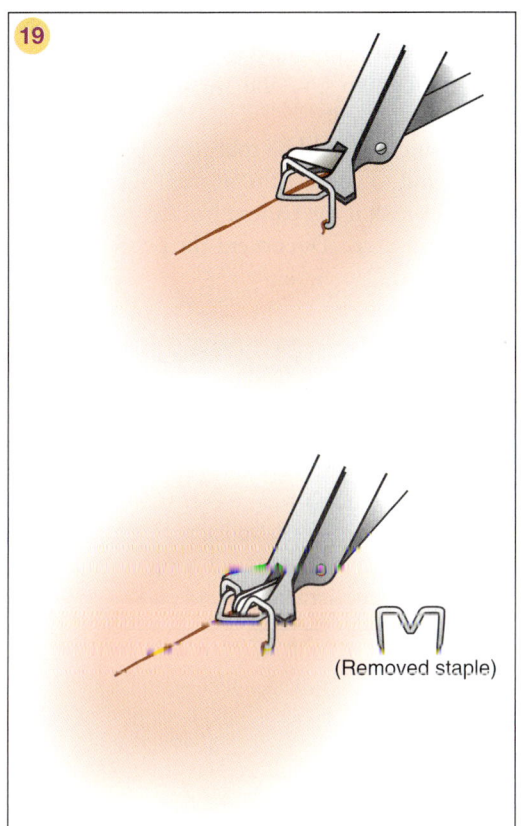

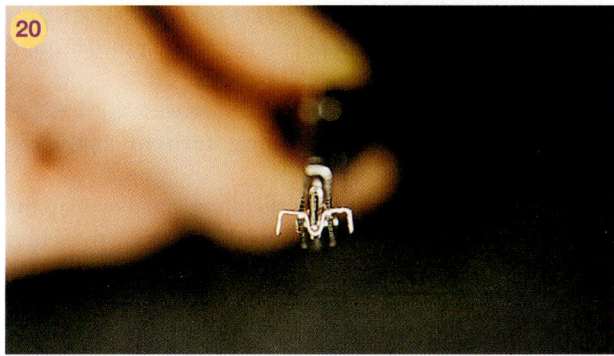

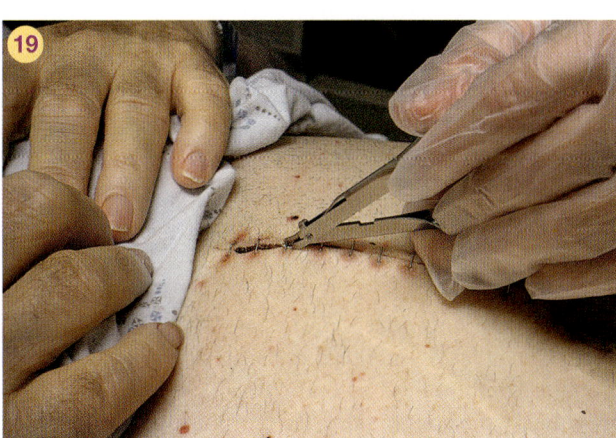

20. Procedural Step. Gently lift the staple remover upward to remove the staple from the incision line.

21. Procedural Step. Place the staple on the gauze square included in the staple kit.

22. Procedural Step. Continue in this manner until all the staples have been removed.

23. Procedural Step. Inspect and count the staples on the gauze square before discarding them.

CLEANING AND DRESSING A WOUND

24. Procedural Step. Clean the wound.

Clean any additional exudate from the healed portions of the wound after suture or staple removal and before applying a sterile dressing.

25. Procedural Step. After cleansing, use the sterile gauze squares to absorb excess antiseptic.

Do not touch the side of the gauze that contacts the wound.

26. Procedural Step. Apply a sterile dressing to cover the laceration and to protect the wound and any remaining sutures.

The dressing should cover the laceration site completely and extend 1 to 2 inches beyond it on all sides.

27. Procedural Step. Once the wound is covered, remove your gloves and discard the plastic waste bag in biohazardous waste.

28. Procedural Step. Sanitize the hands before bandaging the dressing.

Apply a bandage over a sterile dressing when the wound or laceration is on an appendage.

29. Procedural Step. Bandage the dressing.

Beginning at the distal portion of the wound beneath the dressing, place the end of the conforming gauze bandage on a slant. Encircle the appendage with the

Continued

PROCEDURE 45-8 Remove Sutures or Staples and Change a Wound Dressing Using a Spiral Bandage—cont'd

bandage while allowing the corner to extend. Then, turn the corner down and make another circular turn around the appendage to anchor the bandage.

Rationale. Bandaging is applied to hold the dressing in place.

30. **Procedural Step. Use a spiral turn to apply the bandage to an arm or leg.**

    Carry each turn upward at a slight angle and overlap the previous turn by about one-half to two-thirds the width of the bandage. Here, the spiral turn leaves about ¾ inch of the bandage showing with each turn.

31. **Procedural Step. Check the patient's fingers and hand or toes and foot for adequate circulation to be certain the bandage has not been applied too tightly.**

    Pallor or redness of the fingers or toes, swelling, pain, or a tingling sensation should alert the medical assistant to a problem and to reapply the bandage less tightly.

32. **Procedural Step. Assist the patient to a comfortable position.**

    Stand close by for a few seconds in case the patient becomes dizzy.

33. **Procedural Step. Instruct the patient when to return for removal of the remaining sutures if applicable.**

34. **Procedural Step. Disinfect the work area.**

35. **Procedural Step. Remove gloves and sanitize the hands.**

    Always sanitize the hands after every procedure or after using gloves.

36. **Procedural Step. Provide the patient with verbal and written wound care instructions.**

    Document in the patient's medical record that these instructions were provided to the patient. Remember, it is not enough to give the written instructions—they must be verbalized.

    The patient should be told to keep the wound clean and dry and to contact the office if signs of inflammation occur. Ask if the patient has any questions.

37. **Procedural Step. Document the procedure.**

CHARTING EXAMPLES

Date	
4/30/xx	11:15 a.m. Dry sterile 4 × 4 dressing applied on right forearm after removing 6 sutures. Well-healed suture line, wound edges well approximated. No signs of infection present. Pt provided verbal and written instructions for wound care.————————————— A. Reali, RMA

Date	
3/17/xx	10:30 a.m. Edges of wound well approximated with no signs of infection. Staples x6 removed from Ⓡ forearm. Dry sterile 4 × 4 dressing applied. Verbal and written instructions provided on wound care.————P. Konters, CMA (AAMA)

Steps 14 and 15 illustrations modified from Nealon TF: *Fundamental skills in surgery,* ed 4, Philadelphia, 1994, Saunders; Step 19 illustration courtesy Ethicon, Somerville, NJ; Step 19 photo from deWit S: *Fundamental concepts and skills for nursing,* ed 3, St Louis, 2009, Saunders; Step 20 photo from Potter PA, Perry AG: *Clinical nursing skills and techniques,* ed 6, St Louis, 2006, Mosby.

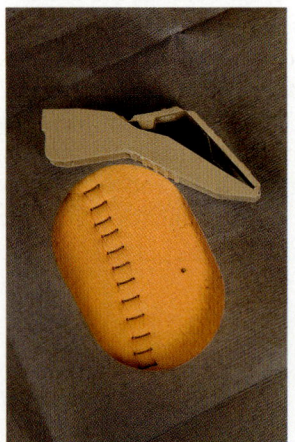

FIGURE 45-18 Disposable skin stapler and a fenestrated drape.

remover has prongs. These prongs are placed underneath the staple. The other jaw compresses the staple. As the handles are brought together, the staple uncrimps, causing the staple to be withdrawn from the skin. The process is repeated until all staples are removed. Procedure 45-8 describes the process of staple removal.

Surgical Glue

Surgical glue was approved by the FDA to be used in situations to close superficial incisions and lacerations. The glue is applied to the skin wound edges that have been brought together and bonds within 20 to 30 seconds. A second application can be applied after 45 seconds and dries completely in 60 seconds. A film forms over the wound and gradually falls off as the skin heals. Topical ointments are usually not prescribed for wound care since the glue may **slough,** and prolonged exposure to water should be avoided.

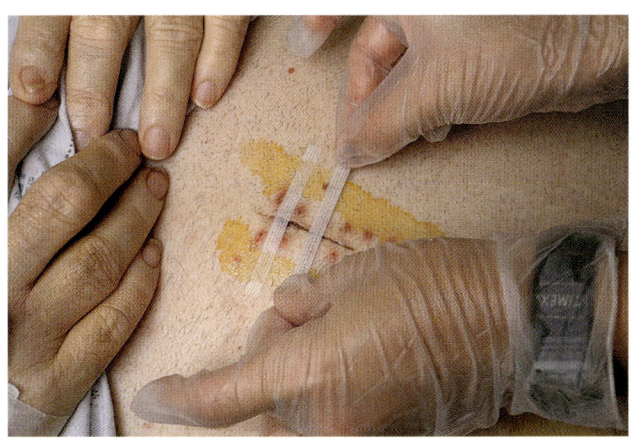

FIGURE 45-19 Skin closures are used to support the incision after suture removal. (From deWit S: *Fundamental concepts and skills for nursing*, ed 3, St Louis, 2009, Saunders.)

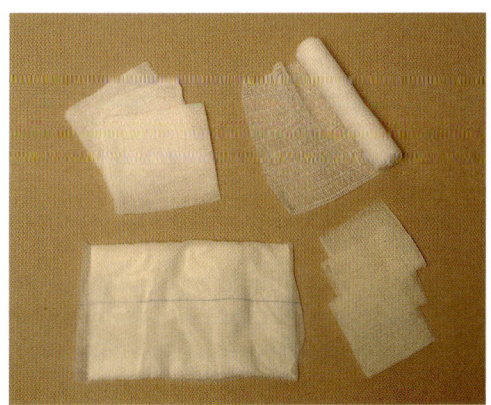

FIGURE 45-20 Various sizes of dressing materials.

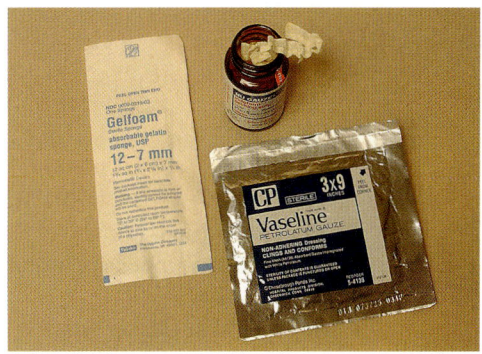

FIGURE 45-21 Alternative dressing materials (Gelfoam, Iodoform packing material, and Vaseline).

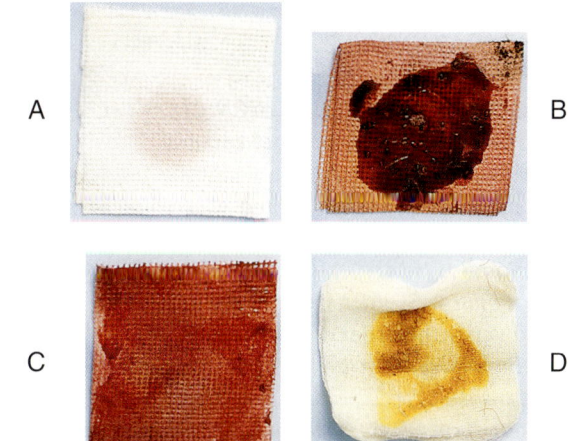

FIGURE 45-22 Wound drainage. **A,** Serous. **B,** Sanguineous. **C,** Serosanguineous. **D,** Purulent. (From Potter PA, Perry AG: *Fundamentals of nursing*, ed 6, St Louis, 2005, Mosby.)

Skin Closures

Skin closures are long, narrow adhesive strips that are used to close small wound areas instead of sutures (Figure 45-19). Closures can also be placed over an area where sutures or staples have been removed to keep the edges of the wound together. Skin closures do not control bleeding from the edges of a wound, and they cannot be used for deep tissue repair. The strips are applied at ⅛-inch intervals until the wound is approximated together (see Figure 45-12, *C*). To remove an adhesive strip, each tape is peeled off from the outside toward the wound. Procedure 45-9 describes the application and removal of skin closures.

Changing a Sterile Dressing

When a **sterile dressing** is applied to an open wound, sterile aseptic technique must be used. The purpose of the dressing is to protect the wound from infection. Figure 45-20 shows various types of dressing materials, and Figure 45-21 shows wound packing materials and alternative dressing materials.

Wound Drainage

When changing a dressing, a wound is evaluated for drainage or **exudate**. Exudate fluid or cellular debris seeps slowly from injured blood vessels through breaks in the skin. When charting the condition of the wound (degree of healing, condition of sutures), the amount of drainage (scant [small], moderate, or large [copious]), and the characteristics (appearance) of the drainage (color, odor, consistency) must be charted in the patient's record. Terms frequently used to describe wound drainage are as follows (Figure 45-22):

- **Serous** drainage consists of serum (clear or yellow fluid). For example, the fluid in a blister is serous drainage.
- **Sanguineous** drainage consists of blood from broken capillaries (blood tinged).
- **Serosanguineous** drainage consists of serum and blood.
- **Purulent** drainage consists of pus (white or yellow-green fluid). Pus contains leukocytes, tissue debris, and both live and dead bacteria.

Cleaning

Cleaning a wound rids the area of dead cells and bacteria. Using an antimicrobial cleaner (Figure 45-23), such as povi-

| PROCEDURE 45-9 | Apply and Remove Adhesive Skin Closures | |

TASK: Apply and remove skin closures using sterile technique.

EQUIPMENT AND SUPPLIES
- Nonsterile disposable gloves
- Sterile cotton-tipped applicator
- Sterile gloves
- Adhesive skin closure strips
- Antiseptic solution
- Sterile 4 × 4 gauze pads
- Sterile dressing forceps
- Sterile Iris scissors
- Surgical tape
- Antiseptic swabs (Betadine)
- Tincture of benzoin
- Biohazardous waste container
- Patient's medical record

SKILLS/RATIONALE

STANDARD PRECAUTIONS ARE TO BE FOLLOWED.

APPLICATION OF ADHESIVE SKIN CLOSURES

1. **Procedural Step. Sanitize the hands.**
   An alcohol-based hand rub may be used instead of washing hands with soap and water, unless hands are visibly soiled.
   Rationale. Hand sanitization promotes infection control.

2. **Procedural Step. Assemble equipment and supplies and verify the order.**
   Rationale. It is important to have all supplies and equipment ready and available before starting any procedure to ensure efficiency.

3. **Procedural Step. Greet and identify the patient and escort the patient to the examination room.**
   Rationale. Identifying the patient ensures the procedure is performed on the correct patient.

4. **Procedural Step. Explain the procedure to the patient and verify any known allergies (e.g., iodine).**
   Rationale. Explaining the procedure to the patient promotes cooperation and provides a means of obtaining implied consent. Verifying allergies prevents the patient from having an allergic reaction.

5. **Procedural Step. Position the Mayo stand so that it is within easy reach of the procedure site.**

6. **Procedural Step. Create a sterile field, using a prepackaged sterile drape, and attach a temporary disposal bag (waterproof waste bag) to the edge of the Mayo stand.**
   Rationale. Contaminated items, such as the soiled dressing, may be discarded in the bag and the entire bag discarded later in biohazardous waste.

7. **Procedural Step. Position the patient as required and inspect the wound.**
   Apply disposable nonsterile gloves. Inspect the wound for signs of infection (redness, swelling, or drainage) and notify the physician of any irregularities.
   NOTE: This information is documented in the patient's medical record at the end of the procedure.

8. **Procedural Step. Clean the wound using an antiseptic solution (e.g., Hibiclens).**
   Gently remove debris, skin oils, and exudates from at least 2 to 3 inches around the wound. Allow the area to air-dry.
   NOTE: Change gloves as needed to maintain cleanliness.
   Rationale. An antiseptic solution will help to disinfect the area from contaminants.

9. **Procedural Step. "Paint" the wound with a Betadine swab working from the center of the wound outward.**
   Use a new swab for each wipe. Again, allow the area to air-dry.
   Rationale. Allowing the area to air-dry gives the antiseptic time to work without introducing new contaminants.

10. **Procedural Step. Apply tincture of Benzoin.**
    Depending on office policy, a thin coat of tincture of benzoin may be applied with a sterile cotton-tipped swab on both sides of the wound. Do not allow the tincture of benzoin to touch the wound. Allow the skin to air-dry. Remove gloves and sanitize the hands.
    Rationale. Tincture of benzoin provides a "sticky" surface that assists with adherence of the strips to the skin.

11. **Procedural Step. Open the sterile adhesive strips.**

12. **Procedural Step. Apply sterile gloves.**

13. **Procedural Step. Prepare the adhesive strips.**
    Use a sterile dressing forceps to peel off one adhesive strip at a time.

14. **Procedural Step. Verify that the skin surface is dry and position the first strip over the center of the wound.**
    Firmly press one end of the adhesive strip to the patient's skin on one side of the wound. Stretch the adhesive strip across the incision line until the edges of the wound approximate.
    Rationale. Exact approximation of the wound promotes better healing and less scar formation.

Continued

PROCEDURE 45-9 Apply and Remove Adhesive Skin Closures—cont'd

15. **Procedural Step.** Continue applying adhesive strips.
    Place the next adhesive strip midway between the middle (first) strip and one end of the wound. Apply a third adhesive strip between the middle strip and the other end of the wound. Continue applying the strips at ⅛-inch intervals until the edges of the wound are approximated.
    NOTE: If at any time the skin surface becomes moist (e.g., perspiration, blood, or serum), dry the area with a sterile gauze pad before applying the next strip.
    Rationale. Applying the strips in this manner facilitates good approximation of the wound. Spacing the strips at ⅛-inch intervals allows for proper drainage of the wound while maintaining approximation.

16. **Procedural Step.** Apply the last adhesive strip(s).
    Once all adhesive strips are applied and the wound is in good approximation, apply adhesive strips parallel to the wound. (Some physicians prefer strips on both sides of the wound.)
    Rationale. This helps to lessen tension on the wound and holds the adhesive strips securely in place.

17. **Procedural Step.** Apply a dry sterile dressing over the strips, if indicated by the physician.

18. **Procedural Step.** Remove gloves and sanitize the hands.
    Always sanitize the hands after every procedure or after using gloves.

19. **Procedural Step.** Provide the patient with verbal and written wound care instructions as ordered by the physician.
    Document in the patient's medical record that these instructions were provided to the patient.
    The patient should be told to keep the wound clean and dry and to contact the office if signs of inflammation occur. Ask if the patient has any questions.

20. **Procedural Step.** Document the procedure.
    Include the date and time, location of the wound, appearance of the wound, wound preparation, number of strips applied, and care of the wound. Document instructions given to the patient about wound care.

CHARTING EXAMPLE

Date	
3/20/xx	10:30 a.m. Applied 6 skin strips to right shoulder wound after physician cleaned the wound with Betadine. Suture line in good approximation. No swelling or redness noted. Verbal and written wound care instructions provided to patient and wife. Patient to return in 4 days for removal of adhesive strips. ———— J. Shultz, RMA

REMOVAL OF ADHESIVE SKIN CLOSURES

1. **Procedural Step.** Sanitize the hands.
   An alcohol-based hand rub may be used instead of washing hands with soap and water, unless hands are visibly soiled.
   Rationale. Hand sanitization promotes infection control.

2. **Procedural Step.** Assemble equipment and supplies and verify the order.
   Rationale. It is important to have all supplies and equipment ready and available before starting any procedure to ensure efficiency.

3. **Procedural Step.** Greet and identify the patient and escort the patient to the examination room.
   Rationale. Identifying the patient ensures the procedure is performed on the correct patient.

4. **Procedural Step.** Explain the procedure to the patient.
   Rationale. Explaining the procedure to the patient promotes cooperation and provides a means of obtaining implied consent.

5. **Procedural Step.** Position the patient as required and remove the soiled dressing.
   Examine for any signs of bleeding, excessive drainage, or infection before disposing of it in the plastic bag.

6. **Procedural Step.** Check the incision line.
   Be sure that the adhesive strips are intact and that the laceration is not infected and has healed adequately. If excessive redness, swelling, or drainage is present, the physician should be notified before removing the strips.
   Rationale. When a dressing is changed, the physician should view any incision or wound that is not healing normally before adhesive strips are removed.

7. **Procedural Step.** Position a 4 × 4 gauze pad in close approximation with the wound and apply clean gloves.

8. **Procedural Step.** Remove the skin closures.
   Peel off the adhesive strips toward the incision line on one side of the incision site. *Never* pull strips away from or across an incision line. Start on the back end of the wound and work toward the center.
   Rationale. Pulling off adhesive strips away from or across a wound may pull the wound open. Working from the ends prevents excessive pressure in the center of the wound.

9. **Procedural Step.** Repeat Step 8 on the other side of the wound.
   Leave the strips adhered to the center of the wound. Gently lift the strip away from the wound surface. Place the strip on a 4 × 4 gauze square.

10. **Procedural Step.** Continue in this manner until all the skin closures have been removed.

11. **Procedural Step.** Cleanse the site with an antiseptic swab and apply a dry sterile dressing if indicated by the physician.

Continued

PROCEDURE 45-9 Apply and Remove Adhesive Skin Closures—cont'd

12. **Procedural Step.** Properly dispose of all contaminated supplies.
13. **Procedural Step.** Disinfect the work area.
14. **Procedural Step.** Remove gloves and sanitize the hands.

    Always sanitize the hands after every procedure or after using gloves.

15. **Procedural Step.** Provide the patient with verbal and written wound care instructions.

    You must document in the patient's medical record that these instructions were provided to the patient and that the patient verified his understanding by repeating the wound care instructions and was able to demonstrate how to change the dressing.

    The patient should be told to keep the wound clean and dry and to contact the office if signs of inflammation occur. Ask if the patient has any questions.

16. **Procedural Step.** Document the procedure.

    Include the date and time, status of the skin closures, number of skin closures removed, location of the site, and care of the wound. Document any instructions given to the patient.

CHARTING EXAMPLE

Date	
1/12/xx	2:00 a.m. Skin closures intact and in good approximation. No signs of infection. Strips x6 removed from Ⓡ shoulder. Incision line cleaned c̄ Betadine and sterile 4 x 4 dressing applied. Instructions provided on wound care. ————————— E. Gardner, RMA

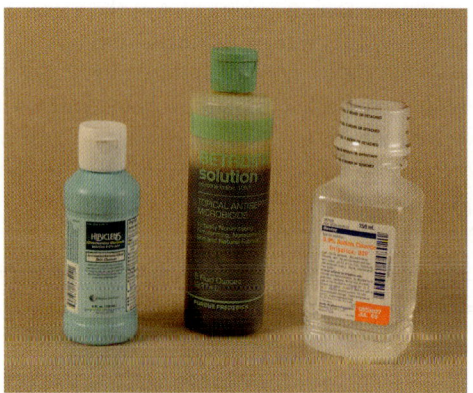

FIGURE 45-23 Cleansing solutions (Hibiclens, povidone-iodine, and sterile saline).

done-iodine (Betadine), chlorhexidine gluconate (Hibiclens), or sterile normal saline, as specified by the physician, along with sterile gauze, the wound is cleaned from the center of the wound outward. Be careful not to reopen the wound or break a forming clot or scab.

Dressing

The purpose of a wound dressing is to protect it from further injury, keep microorganisms out, and absorb drainage. Before applying a dressing, the skin is prepared to avoid damaging it when the dressing is removed later. A *primary* dressing provides the main layer of absorbency and protection for a wound. An *absorbent* dressing is placed over the wound site or over a nonadhering dressing. Surgical tape is best applied along one side of the dressing, repeating the application on the remaining sides to form a "picture frame."

The dressing material selected must be able to cover the wound, absorb any drainage, and prevent damage to newly formed tissue.

Dressing Change. Patients who have had minor surgery will return to the physician's office to have their dressing changed in approximately 5 to 10 days. See Procedure 45-8 for performing a sterile dressing change.

Patient Instructions

Patients need to know whether or not to change a dressing and when to change the dressing if needed. Often, the patient or a family member will change the dressing. Instructions should inform patients that each time a dressing is changed, the wound should be inspected for signs of infection, including swelling, hardness, redness, and warmth around the wound; any fever is noted as well. Patients should also be given wound care instructions regarding wetness and keeping the dressing dry.

As the wound heals, it should become smaller, and drainage should decrease. If no sign of healing is seen, patients should be instructed to contact the physician. The medical assistant must always document patient instructions, any literature provided, and patient feedback.

PATIENT-CENTERED PROFESSIONALISM

- Why is it important for the medical assistant to understand all aspects of wound care?

CONCLUSION

Cost-effective measures instituted by insurance providers are allowing many minor office procedures to be done in outpatient settings such as physician offices and outpatient surgery centers. The medical assistant plays a key role in ensuring that these surgical procedures are performed efficiently and effectively. Protecting the patient from harm is a responsibility of the medical assistant. By helping to maintain sterile technique, the medical assistant also helps to ensure that procedures performed in a surgical setting do not compromise the patient's health.

Chapter Summary

Reinforce your understanding of the material in this chapter by reviewing the curriculum objectives and key content points below.

1. **Define, appropriately use, and spell all the Key Terms for this chapter.**
   - Review the Key Terms if necessary.
2. **List six areas in which medical assistants may need to provide preoperative instructions to patients and give an example for each area.**
   - Patients may need preoperative instructions in diet modification, medications, pretesting requirements, supplies needed postoperatively, bowel preparation, and adjustment to work or social schedules.
   - Review Box 45-1.
3. **Explain the importance of obtaining informed consent.**
   - The patient needs to understand thoroughly what will happen and must consent to the procedure being performed.
   - Informed consent supports the legal and ethical right of the patient to make decisions about his or her health care.
4. **Differentiate between medical asepsis and surgical asepsis.**
   - Medical asepsis attempts to decrease the number of microorganisms present.
   - Surgical asepsis eliminates all organisms and spores.
5. **List 12 guidelines that should be followed to maintain asepsis during a sterile procedure.**
   - Review Box 45-2.
6. **Demonstrate the correct procedure for performing a surgical scrub.**
   - Review Procedure 45-1.
7. **Demonstrate the correct procedure for putting on a sterile gown and sterile gloves.**
   - Review Procedure 45-2.
8. **Demonstrate the correct procedure for applying sterile gloves.**
   - Review Procedure 45-3.
9. **Demonstrate the correct procedure for removing contaminated gloves.**
   - Review Procedure 45-4.
10. **Demonstrate the correct procedure for opening a sterile package.**
    - Review Procedure 45-5.
11. **List five classifications of surgical instruments and give an example of each.**
    - Surgical instruments may be categorized as cutting and dissecting instruments (e.g., scalpels), grasping and clamping instruments (e.g., hemostatic clamp), retracting instruments (e.g., Agricola lid retractor), probing and dilating instruments (e.g., Williams lacrimal probe, Walther female urethral dilator), and suturing instruments (e.g., Mayo-Hegar needle holder).
12. **List six commonly used surgical instruments and briefly describe each.**
    - Scalpels, forceps and clamps, scissors, probes, retractors, and curettes are often used for minor office surgery.
    - Scalpels are small, straight handles with a thin, sharp blade.
    - Forceps resemble tongs and are used for grasping; clamps are used to fasten or grip.
    - Scissors have curved or straight blades and sharp or blunt (or both) tips; they are used for cutting and dissecting.
    - Probes have a long, slender shaft with a rounded or grooved end or an eyelet; they are used to feel inside a body cavity or wound, clear an obstruction, or drain fluids.
    - Retractors are used to hold back edges of a wound or incision to expose the operative area.
    - Curettes are long-handled instruments with a metal loop on one end; they are used for scraping the inside of a cavity.
13. **List four guidelines for the proper handling and maintenance of surgical instruments.**
    - Instruments must be handled gently.
    - Instruments must not be thrown into a basin or piled with other instruments.
    - Sharp instruments should be kept separate and rinsed as soon as possible.
    - Instruments should be used for their intended purpose only.
14. **Demonstrate the correct procedure for adding solutions to the sterile field without contaminating the setup.**
    - Review Procedure 45-6.
15. **Demonstrate the correct procedure for providing all equipment, supplies, and materials needed to assist the physician with a minor office procedure.**
    - Review Procedure 45-7.
16. **Differentiate among local, topical, and general anesthetics and explain the purpose and use of each.**

- Minor office surgery usually involves local anesthetics because these produce a limited and brief loss of sensation in the area of injection, freezing, or application.
- Topical anesthetics are applied directly to the skin and cause numbness to the nerve endings.
- General anesthetics produce unconsciousness by depressing the central nervous system.

17. **Briefly describe four surgical procedures often performed in a medical office.**
    - In cyst removal the area is cleaned, an incision made, the cyst removed, and a sterile dressing applied.
    - For laceration repair the wound is cleaned and repaired (e.g., suturing, adhesive strips, staples) and the area covered with a sterile dressing.
    - For abscess drainage the area is cleaned, an incision made, and the area allowed to drain, and then covered with a sterile dressing.
    - For a skin lesion the area is cleaned and then frozen to destroy tissue.

18. **Briefly describe alternative methods used for tissue removal.**
    - Electrosurgery uses an electric current to cut or destroy tissue (e.g., skin tags, warts).
    - A laser generates intense heat and energy creating a narrow beam of light that can be focused at unwanted tissue.
    - Cautery uses chemicals (e.g., silver nitrate, sodium hydroxide) to destroy tissues (e.g., skin tags) to destroy unwanted tissue.
    - Cryosurgery destroys tissues by using liquid nitrogen (e.g., senile keratosis, planter's warts).

19. **Differentiate between an open wound and a closed wound.**
    - An open wound is a break in the skin or mucous membranes.
    - A closed wound does not show a break in the skin; only bruising and internal bleeding occur.

20. **Describe the healing process of a wound and list the three classifications of wound repair and healing.**
    - Injury or surgical incision begins the process of inflammation. A blood clot forms and becomes a scab, then scar tissue forms. The scar eventually fades to white as the blood supply decreases.
    - First (primary) intention healing, second (secondary) intention healing, and delayed primary (tertiary) intention healing are the three classifications of wound repair and healing.

21. **Demonstrate the correct procedure for suture or staple removal and for changing a wound dressing.**
    - Review Procedure 45-8.

22. **Demonstrate the correct procedure for the application and removal of adhesive skin closures.**
    - Review Procedure 45-9.

23. **Explain the purpose of a sterile dressing.**
    - Sterile dressings protect wounds from infection and capture drainage.

24. **Analyze a realistic medical office situation and apply your understanding of minor office surgery to determine the best course of action.**
    - All aspects of minor office surgery need to be documented fully and correctly.
    - It is important to instruct patients in the necessary preparation and follow-up for minor office surgery.

25. **Describe the impact on patient care when medical assistants have a solid understanding of the knowledge and skills necessary to assist in minor office surgery.**
    - The patient's healing process is enhanced when the medical assistant performs all aspects of asepsis properly.
    - Costs of health care depend on all procedures being performed efficiently.

PRACTICAL APPLICATIONS

If you have accomplished the objectives in this chapter, you will be able to make better choices as a medical assistant. Take another look at this situation and decide what you would do.

Shirley, a patient of Dr. Jones, has arrived at the office for removal of a cyst on her face that has been present for about 2 months. Anna is the medical assistant at the front desk, and Lori is the clinical medical assistant for Dr. Jones. Shirley has been asked to cleanse the area around the lesion with an antiseptic wash for the past 2 days. Shirley wants to know exactly what will be done and if she has to sign papers. Anna tells her that these papers can be signed at any time before the actual opening of the wound. Anna also tells Shirley that Lori will explain what will be done after Shirley is taken to the room where minor surgery is done.

As Lori sets up the surgical tray, she uses surgical asepsis. She uses a sterile tray and peel-back wrappers to set up the needed instruments. On the tray are a scalpel, several hemostat forceps, a probe, a needle holder, scissors, and two retractors.

After the surgery, Lori is in a hurry and piles the instruments in the basin before sanitizing them. When she documents the procedure for Dr. Jones, she only documents the date and the type of surgery.

Would you be prepared to step into Anna's or Lori's shoes and perform the needed tasks correctly?

1. What questions should Anna ask Shirley as she arrives at the office for the surgery?
2. Since Shirley is to receive a tranquilizer intravenously, what preparation should have been made for Shirley's safe return home?
3. Can Shirley wait to sign informed consent until after the incision has been made? Explain your answer.
4. Explain what role Lori can take in obtaining informed consent.
5. What is surgical asepsis? How does it differ from medical asepsis?
6. What is the difference between a sterile tray and peel-wrapped instruments? What is the indication for the use of each of these?
7. What is the use of a scalpel? Forceps? Probe? Needle holder? Retractors?
8. What did Lori miss in the correct documentation of the surgical procedure?
9. How did Lori mishandle the instruments after the procedure?
10. What instructions would you expect Lori to give to Shirley after the surgical procedure?
11. How will the lack of correct documentation affect the coding of this surgical procedure for insurance reimbursement?

WEB SEARCH

1. **Research hyperbaric medicine for people with wounds that resist healing.**

- **Keywords:** Use the following keywords in your search: wound care, hyperbaric medicine, wound healing.

46 Basic First Aid and Medical Office Emergencies

evolve http://evolve.elsevier.com/klieger/medicalassisting

Occasionally, medical emergencies occur in the medical office. Medical assistants are expected to respond according to the nature of the emergency. If the physician is present, the medical assistant alerts the physician and assists with the needs of the patient as directed. If the physician is not available, the medical assistant must assess the situation, call 911, and provide first aid as needed until help arrives.

Emergency situations can also occur outside the medical office; as a trained health care worker, you would be expected to manage the situation according to your scope of training until complete medical care can be obtained. The skills for handling medical office emergencies can be applied in "street" emergencies. Medical assistants need to understand the situations that require first aid, types of emergencies and what should be done for each, and how to perform basic life support procedures to be able to handle these situations.

LEARNING OBJECTIVES

You will be able to do the following after completing this chapter:

Key Terms
1. Define, appropriately use, and spell all the Key Terms for this chapter.

Incident Reporting
2. Explain the purpose of an incident report.
3. List the information needed to accurately complete an incident report.

Situations Requiring First Aid
4. Explain what a medical assistant should do first in an emergency situation.
5. Define first aid and list two guidelines that protect health care workers and victims from disease transmission.
6. List one situation requiring first-aid attention for each of the seven body systems.

Office Emergencies
7. Explain what causes fainting.
8. List seven guidelines for the emergency care of a patient who has fainted.
9. Describe the symptoms of a heart attack and explain the purpose of cardiopulmonary resuscitation (CPR).
10. List 10 guidelines for the emergency care of a patient who has heart attack symptoms.
11. Explain how a stroke differs from a heart attack and identify the signs of obstructed airway and cardiac arrest.
12. List six guidelines for the emergency care of a patient who has had a stroke.
13. List seven types of shock and explain what causes each.
14. List eight guidelines for the emergency care of a patient who has symptoms of shock.
15. Explain what a seizure is and what may cause one.
16. List eight guidelines for the emergency care of a patient who has had a seizure.
17. List and describe the two methods for controlling bleeding.
18. Explain the emergency care for patients with thermal, chemical, or electrical burns.
19. Differentiate between heat exhaustion and heat stroke.
20. Explain considerations for the emergency care of a patient with frostbite.
21. List the main goal for the emergency care of a fracture.
22. List four guidelines for assessing the degree of a dislocation.
23. List five guidelines for emergency care of a patient who has ingested poison.
24. List four guidelines for the emergency care of a patient who has inhaled poison.

25. Identify the symptoms of bites and stings.
26. Explain the difference between insulin shock and diabetic ketoacidosis (diabetic coma).
27. Explain "Hands-Only CPR" and its intended purpose.
28. Demonstrate the correct procedure for performing the Heimlich maneuver.
29. Explain what an AED is and explain how it is used.

Disaster Preparedness

30. Discuss the difference between natural and man-made disasters.
31. Discuss the advantages of registering with a disaster preparedness team.

Patient-Centered Professionalism

32. Analyze a realistic medical office situation and apply your understanding of handling office emergencies to determine the best course of action.
33. Describe the impact on patient care when medical assistants have a solid understanding of the knowledge and skills necessary to assist patients in office emergencies.

KEY TERMS

- anaphylactic shock
- automated external defibrillator (AED)
- bleeding
- burn
- cardiogenic shock
- cerebrovascular accident (CVA)
- cardiac arrest
- cardiopulmonary resuscitation (CPR)
- choking
- conscious
- defibrillation
- diabetic ketoacidosis
- direct pressure
- disaster
- dislocation
- epilepsy
- epistaxis
- first aid
- first-degree burn
- fracture
- frostbite
- full-thickness burn
- heat exhaustion
- heat stroke
- Heimlich maneuver
- hemorrhagic shock
- hyperglycemia
- hyperthermia
- hypoglycemia
- hypothermia
- incident
- incident report
- indirect pressure
- insulin shock
- Kussmaul breathing
- metabolic shock
- neurogenic shock
- partial-thickness burn
- poison
- psychogenic shock
- "rule of nines"
- respiratory arrest
- second-degree burn
- seizure
- septic shock
- shock
- splint
- sprain
- strain
- stroke
- syncope
- synergy
- third-degree burn
- unconscious
- within normal limits (WNL)

PRACTICAL APPLICATIONS

Read the following scenario and keep it in mind as you learn about first aid and office emergencies.

Mariah has type 1 diabetes mellitus and takes insulin on a regular basis. Dr. Naguchi is aware that Mariah does not follow her diet as she should and that her exercise habits are not consistent, so her diabetes is often not stable.

Mariah lives in the southern United States, where it is currently 100° F outside and very humid. Earlier today, Mariah was in the garden gathering vegetables. Later, she started canning the vegetables. Her house has minimal air conditioning. In her haste to complete what needed to be done in the garden, Mariah did not eat her lunch as she should have, although she took her entire dose of insulin.

During the afternoon, Mariah began to feel weak, experiencing dizziness and sweating, and her skin felt cool and clammy. Don, her husband, drove her the three blocks to Dr. Naguchi's office because she started complaining of chest pain and difficulty breathing. As soon as she arrives, Mariah appears to faint and falls, injuring her left ankle. As the medical assistant, Janis is the first health care professional to see what is happening to Mariah. After seeing Mariah, Dr. Naguchi orders an x-ray of her ankle to see whether she has a sprain, strain, or fracture.

If you were in Janis's place, would you know what to do in this situation?

SITUATIONS REQUIRING FIRST AID

Emergency situations require medical assistants to prioritize both the urgency of the situation and the status of the patient. Circulatory and respiratory symptoms are of primary concern and have first priority. Once the medical assistant begins providing emergency care, he or she must call 911 if appropriate, or have someone else place the call. If the emergency occurs in the medical office, first notify the physician if it is possible. Box 46-1 lists the information that will be requested when making a 911 call. Once emergency care is started, the medical assistant must stay with the victim until help arrives. For example:

PRIORITIZING URGENCY AND PATIENT STATUS

A car crashes outside the medical facility. The medical assistant reaches the car and sees the driver holding her chest, having difficulty breathing, and bleeding from a laceration on her forehead. The medical assistant must determine which illness or injury to attend to first. The circulatory and respiratory symptoms (holding chest, having difficulty breathing) take priority. The laceration is not life-threatening and can be attended to when the patient is stable.

First aid is the temporary care given to an injured or ill person until the victim can be provided complete emergency treatment. In the medical office, a medical assistant may be

BOX 46-1

911 Information

Be prepared to provide the following information when calling 911:

1. Name of caller and verification of address, to include floor level and room or suite number.
   - If using a cell phone, exact location including complete address, floor level, and room or suite number
2. Name and condition of the victim.
   - Patient's chief complaint and any known conditions
   - Observable signs and symptoms
   - Vital signs, if known
3. Care already given.

required to perform lifesaving first-aid measures (e.g., CPR), as well as basic first aid (e.g., applying a simple dressing to a skin break). Providing first aid should be done in ways that protect the health care worker and the victim from disease transmission. Therefore Standard Precautions should be followed when providing first aid, as follows:

- Wear protective gloves to avoid contact with blood and body fluids if possible.
- Do not touch areas that are soiled with blood, mucus, or other biohazardous materials without a barrier between you and the victim (Figure 46-1).

Box 46-2 provides general guidelines for providing emergency care, and Table 46-1 lists situations that may require first-aid attention.

PATIENT-CENTERED PROFESSIONALISM

- Why is it necessary to complete an incident report even if there is no apparent injury?

INCIDENT REPORTING

An **incident** is any unusual event that is not consistent with the routine activity within a health care facility. This includes a patient, visitor, or an employee of the health care facility. An incident can be a fall, an accidental needlestick injury, a medication error, or carelessness in performance of a procedure whether it leads to an injury of a patient or not. When an incident occurs, the health care professional involved or the person, often the medical assistant, who witnesses the incident completes an **incident report**. The incident report is a document that describes any unusual occurrence that happens while a person is on the premises of a health care facility. An incident report can be thought of as part of the medical facility's quality improvement plan or assessment tool for risk management.

Completing the Incident Report

It must be understood that completing an incident report is not an admission of negligence or placing blame on anyone

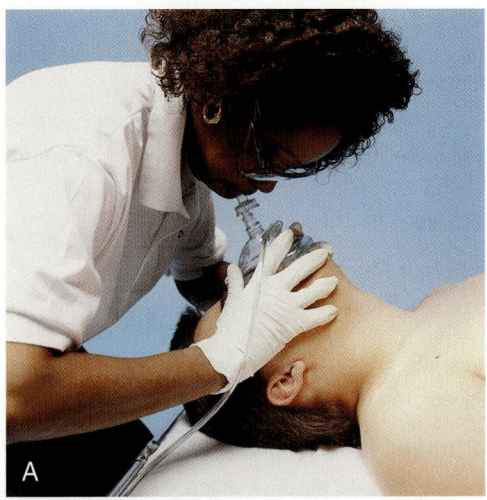
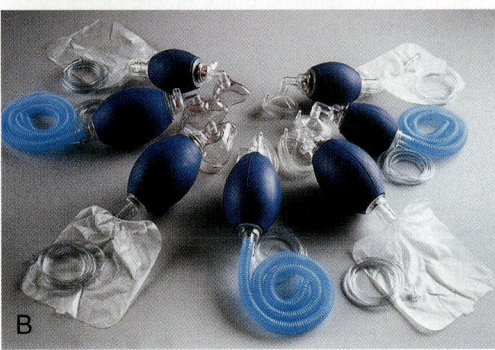

FIGURE 46-1 A, Mouth-to-mask ventilation technique. **B,** Disposable and reusable adult and pediatric bag-mask devices. (From Sanders MJ: *Mosby's paramedic textbook*, ed 3, St Louis, 2007, Mosby.)

TABLE 46-1

Situations Requiring First Aid

Body System Affected	Situation
Circulatory	Fainting
	Chest pain or heart attack
	Stroke
	Shock
	Bleeding
Respiratory	Obstructed airway (choking)
	Allergic reactions (anaphylaxis)
Digestive	Poisoning
Integumentary	Burns
	Wounds
	Heat or cold emergencies
Musculoskeletal	Sprains and strains
	Fractures and dislocations
Nervous	Seizures
Endocrine	Diabetic ketoacidosis
	Insulin shock

BOX 46-2

Guidelines for Providing Emergency Care

Important: Assess the emergency for your own safety first, to avoid creating another emergency.

1. Know your limits. Only do what is in your scope of training.
2. Stay calm and speak in a normal tone of voice. This assists in keeping the patient (if conscious), and other people around, calm. Explain what has happened and the extent of your training.
3. Practice Standard Precautions and follow the OSHA Bloodborne Pathogen Standards (see Chapter 31).
4. Assess the situation quickly and check for possibilities of life-threatening injuries. Use the "ABC" method to assess the patient:
   Airway
   Breathing
   Circulation
   This can be accomplished by (A) looking at the rise and fall of the patient's chest, (B) listening for air entering and leaving the patient, and (C) feeling for the patient's pulse.
5. Know how to acquire emergency medical response (e.g., call 911).
6. Do not move the patient unless he or she is in harm's way. Keep the person lying down.
7. Keep the patient warm (e.g., blanket, coats).
8. Look for a medical alert tag on the patient's wrist or neck.
9. Move bystanders away from the person. Do ask if anyone knows what happened.
10. Never leave the patient until emergency medical personnel have arrived and taken over. Provide information that you have observed.

person but a way to gather factual information of a problem that exists. A written report of the incident must be completed within 24 hours of the occurrence. The report must include observed, objective, and chronological information, which includes the following:
- Person's name
- Location and time of occurrence
- Factual description of what occurred and what was done
- Sequence of events leading up to the event (include victim's own words)
- Assessed extent of injury incurred (objective findings of health care professional reviewing)
- Observation of factors that may have contributed to the incident (e.g., "wet floor observed in bathroom where Amanda Packo fell")

The medical assistant must remember that the incident report is not a permanent part of the medical record and should not be referred to in the medical record. This action legally protects the health care facility and personnel involved.

Trend Analysis

A *trend analysis* is the ongoing review of data to detect significant patterns. Incident reports should indicate that an occurrence happens infrequently. After reviewing incident reports, if a different pattern begins to emerge, such as an unusual number of falls in a particular examination room, it can be the result of a dangerous condition. This adverse trend analysis identifies occurrences that need immediate attention.

PATIENT-CENTERED PROFESSIONALISM

- *Why must the medical assistant be able to recognize and quickly assess any situation that requires first aid or CPR?*

OFFICE EMERGENCIES

Despite efforts to prevent emergencies in the medical office with effective facilities management, Occupational Safety and Health Administration (OSHA) requirements, and Standard Precautions, office emergencies still occur. Medical assistants must be alert to unusual noises (screams, loud noises, or breaking glass), unusual sights (overturned chair, fire), unusual odors (smell of smoke, unrecognizable odors), and the unusual appearance or behavior of a patient (slurred speech, difficulty breathing, erratic behavior, or pale, moist skin). If the patient involved in an office emergency is **conscious,** the medical assistant can assess the patient's condition by asking questions. Also, stabilizing care can begin until help arrives. If the patient is **unconscious,** a 911 call should be made and care provided until help arrives. It is important to remember when providing emergency care to not put yourself in danger to help another. If you also become a victim, the crisis situation has now magnified.

Sudden illnesses that occur in the medical office often have similar symptoms. The medical assistant may not know the exact cause of the illness but can react to visual and auditory clues. For example, unusual breathing patterns may alert another individual that there is a problem. Chest pain should be treated as a heart attack, since it is better to err on the side of caution.

Some form of emergency equipment should be present in a medical office. Figure 46-2 shows a standard emergency cart, and Table 46-2 lists equipment, supplies, and medications often stored on an emergency cart. Medical assistants cannot prescribe medications, but they can administer prescribed medications, be responsible for checking the cart to make certain that medications are not outdated, and ensure that all supplies are present. The emergency cart should be inventoried on a regular basis, and it should be documented that the supplies have been checked. Figure 46-3 illustrates various items included on the cart that are used for airway management for a patient in respiratory distress.

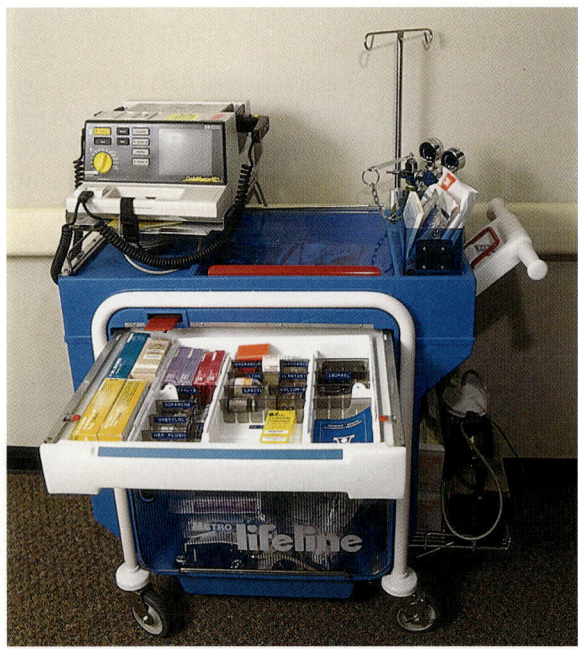

FIGURE 46-2 Standard emergency cart with defibrillator for use in emergencies. (From Chester GA: *Modern medical assisting*, Philadelphia, 1998, Saunders.)

Fainting

Fainting, or **syncope,** is a temporary loss of consciousness caused by an inadequate blood supply to the brain. Patients often describe the sensation before fainting as "everything is going dark." Following this sensation, they lose consciousness. Patients may complain of dizziness and nausea. They may appear pale, have cool skin, and be sweating. The body usually falls in a supine position, allowing the blood to flow back to the brain. Although fainting is not dangerous, the fall can cause injury. When patients regain consciousness, they sometimes experience confusion and anxiety.

If a patient indicates that he or she feels faint or lightheaded, it is best to have the patient sit down and lower the head to knee level (Figure 46-4, *A*). Alternately, have the patient lie down in a supine position on the floor or examination table with the feet slightly elevated (Figure 46-4, *B*). These positions increase the blood flow to the brain. Ask the patient if he or she has ever had this happen before, and if so, under what circumstances. Because fainting is a symptom of low blood sugar (hypoglycemia), heart attack (myocardial infarction), dehydration, and other conditions, this quick assessment assists you in determining what to do next. Patients have been known to become lightheaded when they see needles, such as during a blood drawing procedure, so be prepared.

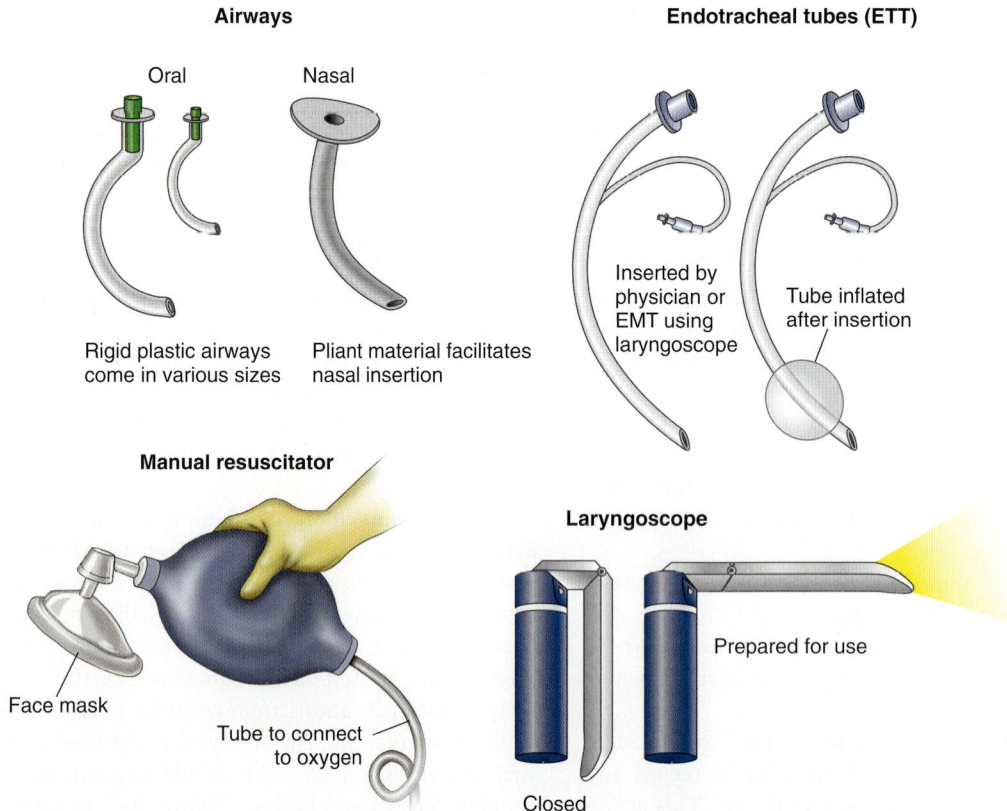

FIGURE 46-3 Equipment for emergency airway management. *EMT,* Emergency medical technician. (From Hunt SA: *Saunders fundamentals of medical assisting—revised reprint,* St Louis, 2007, Saunders.)

TABLE 46-2
Basic Medical Office Emergency Cart

Type of Equipment	Supplies Needed	Generic (Trade) Medications	Treatment
EQUIPMENT AND SUPPLIES			
Defibrillator with pads	ECG machine with cable/pads	adenosine (Adenocard)	Ventricular tachycardia
Oxygen tank and airway management	Flow meter, tubing, mask, nasal cannula	aminophylline	Acute bronchospasm (e.g., emphysema, bronchitis)
	Suction machine with tubing and catheters		
	Airways, both oral and nasal in assorted sizes	atropine	Bradycardia caused by hypotension
	Laryngoscope (handle and blades), assorted sizes	albuterol (Proventil)	Acute bronchospasm
		diazepam (Valium)	Seizures and acute anxiety attacks
	Endotracheal tubes	digoxin (Lanoxin)	Atrial tachycardia
	Ambu bag	diphenhydramine (Benadryl)	Hypersensitivity reactions
Intravenous (IV) supplies	Tourniquet	dopamine (Intropin)	Hypotension from cardiogenic shock
	Alcohol wipes	epinephrine (Adrenalin)	Restoring cardiac rhythm in cardiac arrest and acute allergic reactions
	Betadine swabs		
	Surgical tape	furosemide (Lasix)	Congestive heart failure and pulmonary edema
	Angiocaths and butterfly needles (assorted sizes)	isoproterenol (Isuprel)	Bradycardia that does not respond to atropine
	IV tubing		
	Arm board	lidocaine (Xylocaine)	Ventricular arrhythmias after MI
	IV fluids:	naloxone (Narcan)	Narcotic overdose
	Dextrose 5% (D5W)	nitroglycerin (Nitrostat)	Chest pain associated with angina and MI
	Normal saline (NS)		
	Lactated Ringer's solution	nitroprusside (Nitropress)	Elevated blood pressure in hypertensive crisis
	IV cutdown tray		
GENERAL SUPPLIES		norepinephrine	Hypotensive emergencies (Levophed)
	Gloves (sterile and nonsterile)	methylprednisolone (Solu-Medrol)	Acute allergic reactions when epinephrine is not effective
	Scissors (bandage, operative)		
	Hemostat	phenobarbital	Seizures, especially febrile seizures
	Syringes and needles (assorted sizes)	phenytoin (Dilantin)	Seizures, especially tonic-clonic
	Biohazard containers	procainamide (Pronestyl)	Ventricular arrhythmias when lidocaine is not effective
	Sterile gauze squares (2 × 2, 4 × 4)		
	Water-soluble lubricant	sodium bicarbonate	Acidosis after MI
	Penlight	verapamil (Calan)	Ventricular tachycardia that does not respond to adenosine
	Pen and paper		
	Pocket mask	activated charcoal	Ingested poisons
	Kling dressings	ammonia ampules	Fainting
	Blood pressure cuffs (all sizes)	glucagons or glucose	Hypoglycemia
	Stethoscope		

MI, Myocardial infarction.

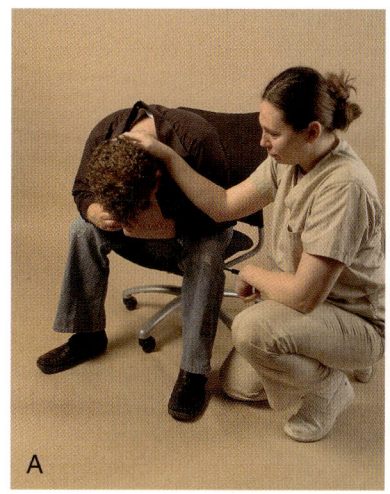
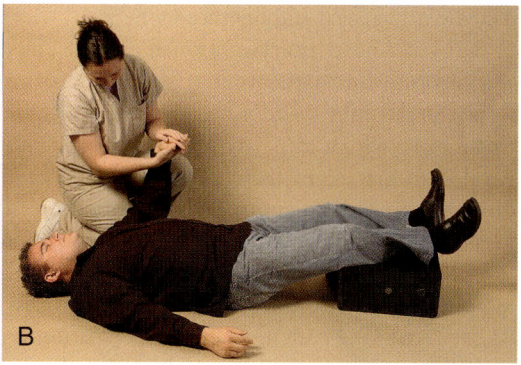

FIGURE 46-4 A, Prevention of fainting. **B,** Prevention and treatment of fainting.

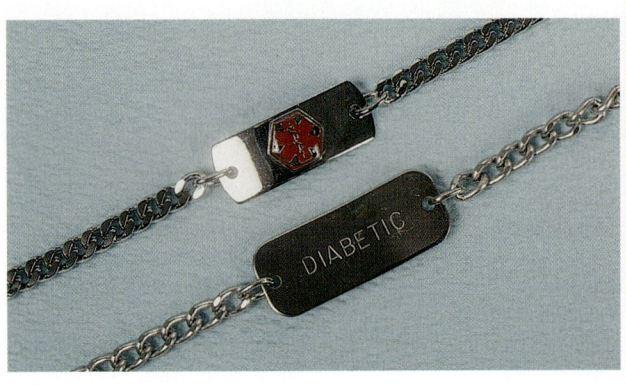 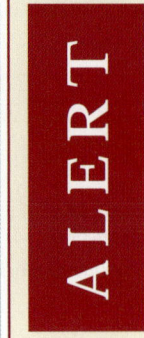

FIGURE 46-5 Diabetic medical identification. **A,** Diabetic medical alert bracelet. **B,** Diabetic wallet alert card. (From Bonewit-West K: *Clinical procedures for medical assistants,* ed 7, St Louis, 2008, Saunders.)

Guidelines for care of a patient who has fainted are as follows:
1. Quickly assess any life-threatening situation that may have caused the fainting.
2. Check for any medical alert tags or alert cards, since these provide information about certain medical conditions such as diabetes (Figure 46-5).
3. Move all furniture out of the way and keep the patient in a supine position. Slightly elevate the legs above the level of the heart (10 to 12 inches). If the patient vomits, turn the head to the side to prevent choking.
4. Check and clear the airway and determine if any injuries were sustained during the fall. Loosen any tight clothing.
5. Apply a damp, cool cloth to the patient's face.
6. Calm the patient as he or she awakens.
7. Ask if the patient has any known medical conditions. Do not allow the patient to sit upright immediately.

Chest Pain (Heart Attack)

Chest pain can be a sign of a heart attack and should be treated as an emergency until a medical diagnosis can be made. Symptoms include dusky skin color, diaphoresis, a bluish discoloration to the lips and nail beds, shortness of breath (SOB), and a rapid, weak pulse. Chest pain is described as "heavy" or "crushing" in the sternum area and may radiate down the left arm, jaw, and up into the shoulder area. Additional symptoms may include pain in one or both arms, back, neck, or stomach; cold sweat; nausea; and lightheadedness.

Signs of a heart attack in women and the elderly are often less obvious, and patients may describe an uncomfortable feeling in the chest as an ache, heartburn, or indigestion or a back, neck, jaw, or arm "ache." The medical assistant should remember that often these symptoms are vague and easily dismissed by the patient as a minor condition that does not need immediate attention. Remember, use open ended questions when interviewing the patient. This interviewing technique encourages the patient to describe the symptoms in detail, even if the patient feels the information is trivial.

Guidelines for the care of a patient who has symptoms of a heart attack are as follows:
1. Call for emergency assistance (911) and alert the physician.
2. Place the patient in a comfortable position, usually semireclining.
3. Assess the airway.
4. Loosen any tight clothing.
5. Ask if the patient is conscious; if he or she is, ask if he or she is taking any "heart" medication.
6. Administer any medications the patient may be taking (e.g., nitroglycerin, aspirin).
7. Administer oxygen with the physician's order.
8. Take the patient's vital signs.
9. Keep the patient warm.
10. Comfort and reassure the patient.

Stroke

A **stroke**, or **cerebrovascular accident (CVA),** occurs when the brain does not receive oxygen. This may result from a burst or blocked blood vessel leading to the brain or from pressure on the cerebral artery caused by a brain tumor. Stroke symptoms vary according to the severity and location of the blockage. A patient may complain of a severe headache with no known cause, sudden confusion, or vision changes that make it difficult to focus. A stroke is often painless and is usually the result of narrowed cerebral vessels caused by high blood pressure, heart disease, smoking, diabetes, and elevated cholesterol. It may also be caused by a hemorrhage or bleeding into the brain or an embolus or thrombus in the brain. Keep in mind that if a stroke occurs on the left side of the brain, the damage will be noticeable to the right side of the body, and vice versa.

Research studies have proved that women may have symptoms in addition to or instead of traditional stroke signs. These may include but are not limited to SOB, sudden hiccups, nausea, tiredness, and sudden pounding or racing heartbeat (palpitations).

FOR YOUR INFORMATION

RECOGNIZING STROKE WARNING SIGNS

The warning signs of stroke can be easily learned using the acronym **FAST**:

Facial weakness or numbness: Does one side of the face drop when asked to smile?

Arm weakness or numbness: When raising both arms, does one arm drift downwards?

Speech difficulty or difficulty understanding speech (aphasia): When trying to repeat a simple sentence, are the words slurred or incorrect?

Time to call 911: Emergency care is needed immediately in order to be evaluated and treated.

Additional symptoms: Blurred, double, or decreased vision; sudden dizziness; loss of balance or loss of coordination; sudden "out of the blue" headache; confusion or confused spacial orientation or perception.

GUIDELINES FOR THE CARE OF A PATIENT WHO HAS A STROKE ARE AS FOLLOWS

1. Call for emergency assistance (911) and alert the physician.
2. Assess the patient's airway. Turn the patient's head to the side to prevent the patient from choking on vomitus. A head tilt keeps the tongue from blocking the airway.
3. Elevate the head and shoulders slightly by placing a jacket or folded towel underneath. This relieves intracranial pressure.
4. Keep the patient quiet and warm. Maintain a confident attitude. Even though a patient may not be able to communicate, the person can hear what is being said. Anxiety can worsen the stroke.
5. If the patient develops difficulty with breathing, turn the patient on the side (paralyzed side down).
6. Take the patient's vital signs.

Shock

Shock is the progressive circulatory collapse of the body brought on by insufficient blood flow to all parts of the body. If left untreated, death can occur. Typical causes of shock include allergic reactions, exposure to extremes in heat or cold, heart attack, trauma, loss of blood, severe burns, and electrical shock. Symptoms include pale, cool skin; rapid pulse and breathing; disorientation; restlessness; and cyanosis around the lips and nail beds. Table 46-3 describes different types of shock and possible causes.

Guidelines for the care of a patient who has symptoms of shock are as follows:

1. Seek emergency assistance.
2. Maintain the patient's airway.
3. Place the patient in a supine position with the feet elevated above the heart (10 to 12 inches).
4. If bleeding is external, provide control by applying direct pressure.
5. Keep the patient warm and calm.
6. Do not give anything by mouth.

TABLE 46-3
Types of Shock

Type	Description
Anaphylactic shock	Severe allergic reaction (can become a sudden life-threatening situation) brought about by insect sting, drugs, foods, or any inhaled or ingested substance.
Cardiogenic shock	Cardiac muscles can no longer pump blood throughout the body; therefore the blood flow lessens, blood pressure drops, and the heart has difficulty pumping blood.
Hemorrhagic shock	Multiple trauma, severe burns, and internal bleeding all result in inadequate blood supply to tissues.
Metabolic shock	Diabetic coma, insulin shock, vomiting, and diarrhea result in loss of body fluids and metabolites, causing an imbalance in the body.
Neurogenic shock	Spinal or head injuries cause loss of nerve control over the circulatory system, causing decreased blood supply to an area.
Psychogenic shock	Psychological stress on the body causes shock (e.g., death in family, fear, or high anxiety).
Septic shock	Severe infection produces toxins that prevent the blood vessels from constricting; blood pools away from vital organs.

7. Never leave the patient alone.
8. Take the patient's vital signs.

Shock brought on by a severe allergic reaction (anaphylaxis) is caused by the following:

- Medication (e.g., penicillin, sulfa)
- Food (e.g., nuts [especially peanuts], shellfish, and eggs)
- Insect bite (e.g., fire ant, wasp, or honey bee)
- Plants (e.g., inhaled pollen)

The immediate treatment is a dose of epinephrine.

Common signs include difficult breathing, itching or burning sensation on the skin, and swollen tongue. Many patients that have severe allergies carry their own auto-injector epinephrine pen, and the medical assistant's role is to assist him or her to use it. Remember, many allergic reactions may appear mild but can become severe within minutes.

Seizures

A **seizure** is a sudden involuntary muscle activity leading to a change in level of consciousness and behavior. Seizures are normally brief and are brought about by a change in electrical activity in the brain. **Epilepsy,** a chronic brain disorder, accounts for many cases of seizure activity, but seizures can also be brought on by head trauma, heat stroke, electric shock, high fever, low blood sugar, and abuse or withdrawal of alcohol or drugs.

Guidelines for the care of a patient who has a seizure are as follows:

1. Quickly remove any objects from the area that could cause injury.

2. Maintain an open airway. ***Do not place anything between the patient's teeth.*** This could become an airway obstruction and cause vomiting.
3. Protect the patient's head by placing a folded towel, pillow, or clothing underneath the head.
4. Loosen any tight clothing that would interfere with breathing and remove eyeglasses.
5. Do not restrain the patient. Avoid overstimulation; this may cause further seizures.
6. Roll patient onto his or her side if vomiting occurs.
7. After seizure activity ceases, turn the victim to the side with the head extended and face slightly downward to help secretions drain and to allow the tongue to remain free of the airway.
8. Assess the patient's vital signs.
9. Allow the patient to rest after the seizure subsides. Reassure the patient and make him or her as comfortable as possible.

If a seizure occurs in the waiting room, move the patient to the examination room when fully conscious. When documenting the incident, the medical assistant should note the start and end time of the seizure and if any medications were administered because it is important for those who will provide advanced care to know what occurred. Moreover, the seizure victim may be incontinent during the activity and will need to be cared for accordingly. If a seizure or any other emergency occurs in the office or waiting room, the office staff/medical assistant is responsible for the other patients who are present. The waiting patients should not be permitted to remain in the area of the emergency. Remember, always protect the dignity of the patient.

Bleeding

Bleeding is the loss of blood from a ruptured, punctured, or cut blood vessel. The severity of bleeding depends on whether the bleeding is from an artery, vein, or capillary. The more blood vessel damage present, the more life-threatening the incident becomes. The average adult has a blood volume of 8 to 10 pints. A loss of 25% to 40% of the total volume can be fatal. Figure 46-6 shows the effects of blood loss from a patient and indicates how the body of the patient reacts to the blood loss.

- *Artery damage.* External arterial bleeding is easy to identify because the wound spurts bright-red blood. The blood is coming directly from the heart and is rich in oxygen (the reason for the bright-red appearance). If an artery is severed, the blood loss is rapid and severe. This type of injury requires direct pressure over the wound, as well as indirect pressure over the artery closest to the wound.
- *Vein damage.* When a vein is damaged, the blood flow is steady from the wound and is dark red. Since venous blood has less oxygen and contains more waste products than arterial blood, its color is darker. Injury to a vein is easier to control with direct pressure than injury to an artery.
- *Capillary damage.* A capillary injury does not flow freely but drips slowly or oozes. It forms a clot by itself or with the aid of a pressure dressing over the wound and seals off quickly.

Bleeding can be controlled by the use of direct or indirect pressure. **Direct pressure** is applied directly over the wound (Figure 46-7), whereas **indirect pressure** is applied over an arterial pressure point (Figure 46-8). When an extremity is injured, applying pressure and elevating the bleeding limb above the heart level slows the flow of blood and allows the wound to clot faster.

Epistaxis (nosebleed) can be caused by trauma, hypertension, high altitude, or an upper respiratory infection. The patient should be in a sitting position with the head tilted slightly forward (Figure 46-9, *A*). This prevents blood from going down the back of the throat and causing nausea. The nostrils should be pinched together to assist in clotting. An ice pack can be placed at the back of the neck or at the top of the nose area (Figure 46-9, *B*). The ice pack causes vasoconstriction of the blood vessels and is usually applied for 15 minutes. After the bleeding has stopped, the patient should be cautioned not to blow the nose because this would loosen the blood clot. Inability to stop the bleeding requires further emergency treatment, so the patient should be taken to a hospital.

Simple *wound care* for an abrasion or laceration is accomplished by cleaning the area with mild soap and water, rinsing, and blotting dry with a clean dressing. The purpose of wound care is to prevent infection, so cleaning and protecting the wound are important. After cleaning the site, a dressing is applied to protect the wound from further contamination and absorb any fluids. Tape is used to secure the dressing.

Burns

A **burn** is an injury to or destruction of body tissue caused by excessive physical heat (e.g., scalding water, hot iron), chemicals, electricity, or radiation. Box 46-3 reviews the depth and classification of burns, as well as the use of the "rule of nines" to evaluate surface area (see Chapter 23).

Proper treatment is started after both the depth and the total surface area of the burn have been determined. It is important to know what caused the burn (e.g., heat, chemical), the length of time the person was exposed (e.g., to the heat or chemical), and if the person has any medical conditions.

Call 911 in the following burn situations:
- Patient has breathing difficulty.
- Patient has burns to the head, neck, hands, feet, or genital area.
- Patient has chemical or electrical burns.
- Patient is very young or elderly.

Heat or Thermal Burns

Heat or thermal burns are best handled by taking the following actions:
1. Remove the person from the source of the burn (if this can be done without danger to yourself).

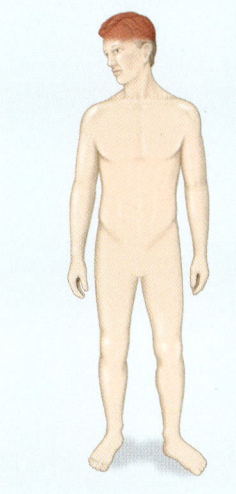
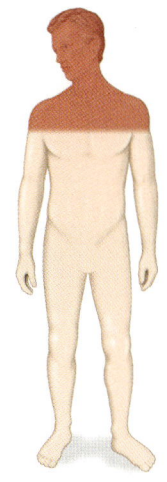
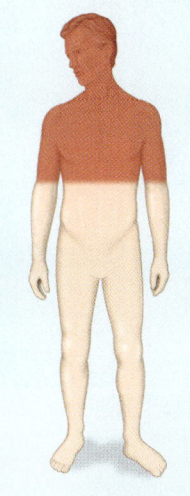
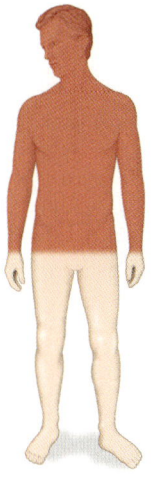

A
15% loss
Body Response:
- Vasoconstriction to maintain BP and homeostasis

Patient Response:
- Alert
- Vital signs
  - BP WNL
  - Pulse WNL
  - Respiration WNL
  - Temperature WNL
- Skin color WNL

B
30% loss
Body Response:
- Vasoconstriction
- Blood flow to some vital organs (i.e., heart) but decrease to kidneys, intestines and skin

Patient Response:
- Restless and confused
- Vital signs
  - BP — Decreased systolic/diastolic, only slight change
  - P increases, thready
  - R increases
  - T may decrease slightly
- Skin color pale, cool, and dry

C
40% loss
Body Response:
- BP falls since body cannot maintain vasoconstriction
- Blood flow to vital organs decreases

Patient Response:
- Confusion, restlessness, and anxiety increases
- Vital signs
  - BP decreases
  - P increases >100
  - R increases, rapid
  - T decreases
- Skin cool and extremities damp

D
>40% loss
Body Response:
- BP continues to drop, thus blood flow to organs and tissues is decreased further

Patient Response:
- Unresponsive or drowsy
- Vital signs
  - BP decreases
  - P increases >100
  - R increases, labored
  - T decreases
- Organ failure

FIGURE 46-6 The body's response to blood loss. *BP*, Blood pressure; *P*, pulse; *R*, respiration; *T*, temperature; *WNL*, within normal limits.

BOX 46-3

Depth and Classification of Burns

The depth of the burn and the extent of body surface area covered will determine its severity. Depth of burns is classified as either **partial-thickness burns** or **full-thickness burns**.
- Partial-thickness burns are divided into first-degree and second-degree burns.
  - **First-degree burns** are dry, red, painful, and slightly swollen and only involve the epidermis (e.g., sunburn).
  - **Second-degree burns** damage both the epidermis and the dermis. Symptoms include redness, swelling, and pain (because of nerve involvement), and the area is moist and blistered
- Full-thickness burns are **third-degree burns**. The epidermis and dermis are destroyed, and the underlying tissues are damaged. Patients with third-degree burns have little or no pain because the nerve endings are damaged. The damaged tissue appears white, tan, brown, black, or cherry red.

The surface area is evaluated according to the **"rule of nines."** The total body surface is divided into regions with assigned percentages related to the number 9 (e.g., arm to include shoulder to fingertip [front and back] 9%).

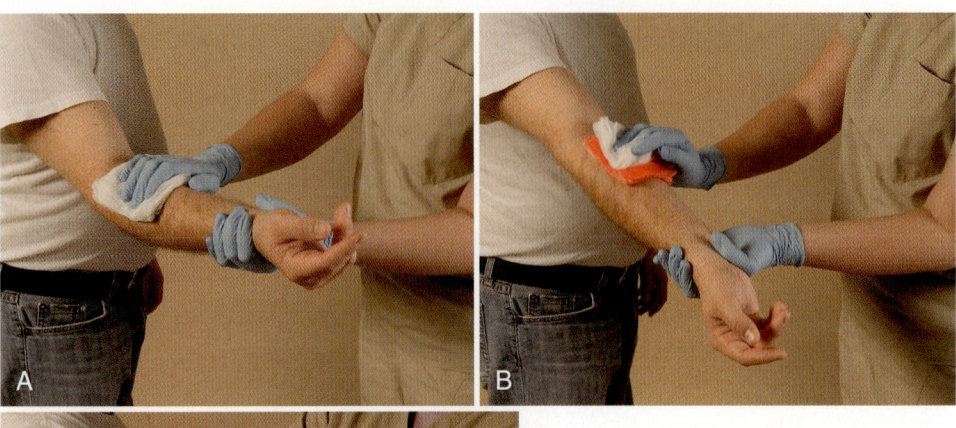
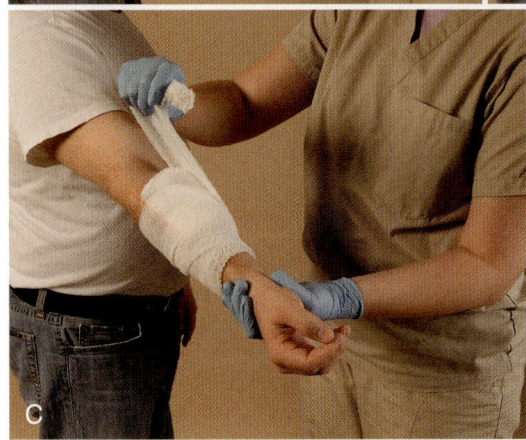

FIGURE 46-7 Control of bleeding. **A,** Apply direct pressure to wound with large, thick gauze dressing. **B,** If blood soaks through dressing, apply another dressing over the first one and continue to apply pressure. **C,** When bleeding has been controlled, apply a pressure bandage.

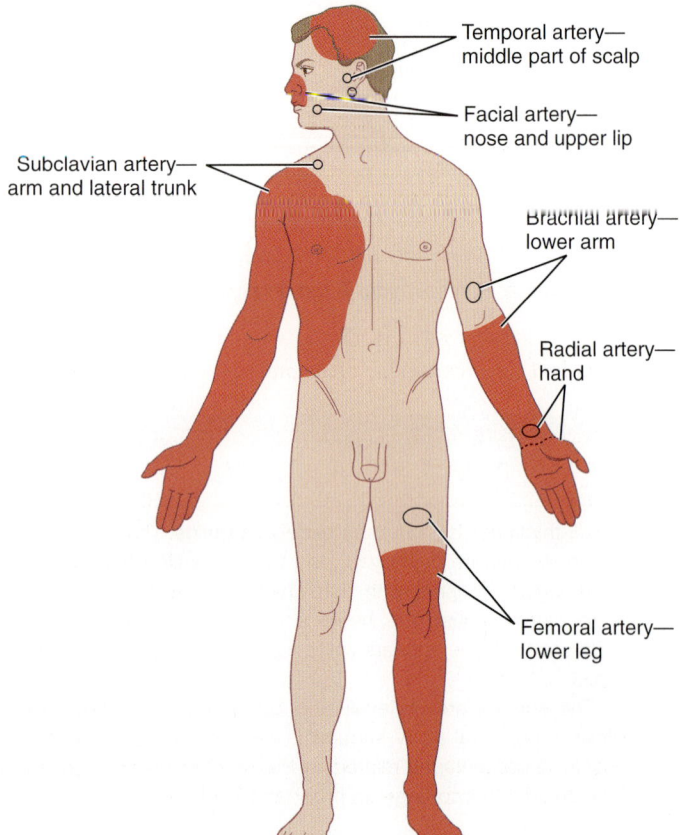

FIGURE 46-8 Pressure points to decrease arterial bleeding. (From Hunt SA: *Saunders fundamentals of medical assisting—revised reprint,* St Louis, 2007, Saunders.)

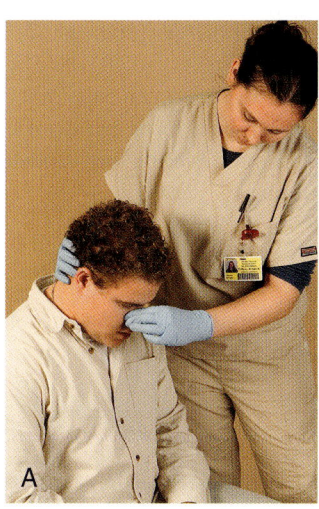
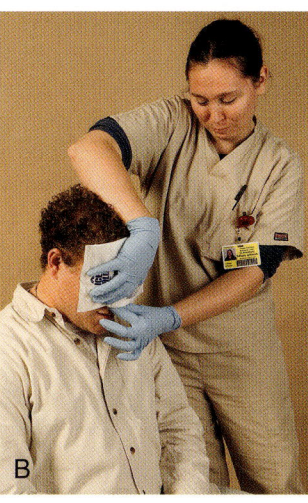

FIGURE 46-9 Care of a nosebleed. **A,** With the patient sitting and tilting the head slightly forward, apply direct pressure by pinching the nostrils together. **B,** An ice pack can be applied to the bridge of the nose to help control bleeding.

1. Cool the burned area by flushing with cool water or applying wet cloths.
3. Cover the burn with a dry sterile dressing or clean cloth.
4. In extreme cases, assess for respiratory and circulatory complications.
5. If necessary, start CPR and alert 911.

Chemical Burns

Chemical burns are best treated by removing the irritant from the skin as quickly as possible.

- Dry chemicals must be brushed off of the skin *before* flushing the area with water. Adding water to the chemical may activate it and cause greater damage.
- Liquid chemicals need to be flushed immediately with large amounts of water.
- Both dry and liquid chemical burns need to be covered with a dry sterile dressing after flushing.

Always remove clothing and jewelry that may trap chemicals against the skin or on which chemicals may have spilled.

Electrical Burns

Electrical burns occur when an electric current passes through the body (e.g., lightning, electricity). A victim who has apparently been affected by some form of electrical power must be approached carefully. Assess the situation and if a power line is down, wait for the power company to turn it off. Be certain the electrical source is off before administering first aid. At the scene, safety is a priority because you cannot provide assistance if you are injured by the electric current. Check the breathing and pulse of the victim and provide CPR if needed. Check for an entrance point and an exit point and treat accordingly.

Exposure

Exposure to excessive heat or cold causes localized tissue damage.

> **BOX 46-4**
>
> **Signs and Symptoms of Heat Emergencies**
>
> - Altered mental status (e.g., confusion, unresponsive to questions)
> - Complaints of dizziness or fainting
> - Weakness or feelings of exhaustion
> - Muscle cramps
> - Rapid, pounding heart rate

Hyperthermia

Hyperthermia (increased body temperature) can manifest itself as either heat stroke or heat exhaustion. Typical signs and symptoms of heat exposure emergencies are listed in Box 46-4. Treatments include removing the patient from the hot environment, gradually cooling the body by fanning, and comforting the patient until help arrives.

Heat exhaustion occurs when the body is subjected to excessive heat (e.g., furnace room at steel plant, lack of ventilation in room with excessive heat). Symptoms include excessive sweating and skin that appears pale and feels cool and clammy. The patient may appear confused or disoriented and may complain of headache, weakness, nausea, and being tired. People suffering heat exhaustion normally have increased shallow respirations, temperature of 101° to 102° F, and a weak, rapid pulse. They should be moved to a cooler environment, have restrictive clothing loosened, be provided large amounts of fluids, and have a cold compress applied to the forehead. If the patient feels faint, the treatment includes placing the patient in a supine position with the feet slightly elevated.

Heat stroke, or *sunstroke,* occurs when the body is subjected to high temperatures and humidity for long periods. The body becomes dehydrated, which causes a decrease in circulating blood. The patient's skin feels hot and is red and dry (not sweating). The patient acts confused, has a high body temperature (106° F or higher), and has increased pulse and respirations. The patient's pupils are equal but dilated, and the patient may complain of feeling weak and being dizzy. Treatment requires that the person be placed in a cool area. Clothes that retain body heat should be removed. Apply cool water to the patient's skin and ice packs to areas where heat is released in the body (e.g., armpits, back of neck, and groin). Slightly elevate the patient's head and shoulders. Take vital signs when equipment is available, and transport the patient for further medical attention as soon as possible.

> **FOR YOUR INFORMATION**
>
> *Elderly persons are more prone to heat-related emergencies because their circulatory systems are less able to compensate for the stresses brought on by the heat.*

Hypothermia

Hypothermia (decreased body temperature) can occur slowly when a person is exposed to extremely low temperatures for long periods or it can occur rapidly, as when someone falls through ice or into extremely cold water. The body loses its ability to generate heat when experiencing hypothermia. Signs and symptoms of hypothermia are listed in Box 46-5. Treatment includes removal of wet clothing and application of warm clothing. Provide a hot liquid to drink and place a hot water bottle on the neck, groin, and under each arm until help arrives.

Frostbite is the freezing of body tissue. Frostbite occurs when the tissues are subjected to extreme cold over time. The patient complains of numbness, which progresses to loss of feeling in the affected area. At first the skin appears red and has a sensation of burning and itching. The skin feels cold, is hard to the touch, and may appear white in the fingertips or toes. Pressure should not be applied, and the patient should not walk on frostbitten feet. The tissue should be protected, and immediate medical attention must be sought.

Treatment for frostbite requires the body part to be gradually rewarmed in water, which should not exceed 105° F. The area should not be rubbed, but it can be placed against another body part to rewarm. The person can be offered hot drinks, which will dilate the blood vessels, and should not smoke because this causes vasoconstriction.

Musculoskeletal Injuries

Medical assistants must also be prepared to give first aid for musculoskeletal injuries that may be brought to or occur in the medical office.

Fracture

A **fracture** is any break or crack in the bone caused by trauma or disease. The appearance of a deformity is a sign that a fracture has occurred. Swelling and pain often occur in the affected area. An *open* fracture pierces through the skin, a *closed* fracture does not pierce the skin, and a *greenstick* fracture bends but does not break the bone.

The main goal for the emergency care of a fracture is to immobilize the part above and below the fracture to prevent further damage. A **splint** immobilizes the affected body part and can be made from any firm material available (e.g., cardboard, rolled newspapers). A covering of soft material is placed over the splint and held in position with rolled bandage gauze. A sling can be made to elevate the extremity and help reduce swelling (Figure 46-10). Many devices are available to repair (reduce) a fracture, and the choice depends on the angle and severity of the break (Figure 46-11).

Dislocation

A **dislocation** occurs when one end of a bone is separated from its original position in a joint, usually by trauma. The

---

BOX 46-5

Signs and Symptoms of Hypothermia

- Decreased mental status (confusion, unresponsive to voice or touch)
- Abnormal skin temperature
- Decreased motor function (poor coordination, difficulty with speech)
- Slow pulse and respiration
- Shivering (and in late stages, lack of shivering)

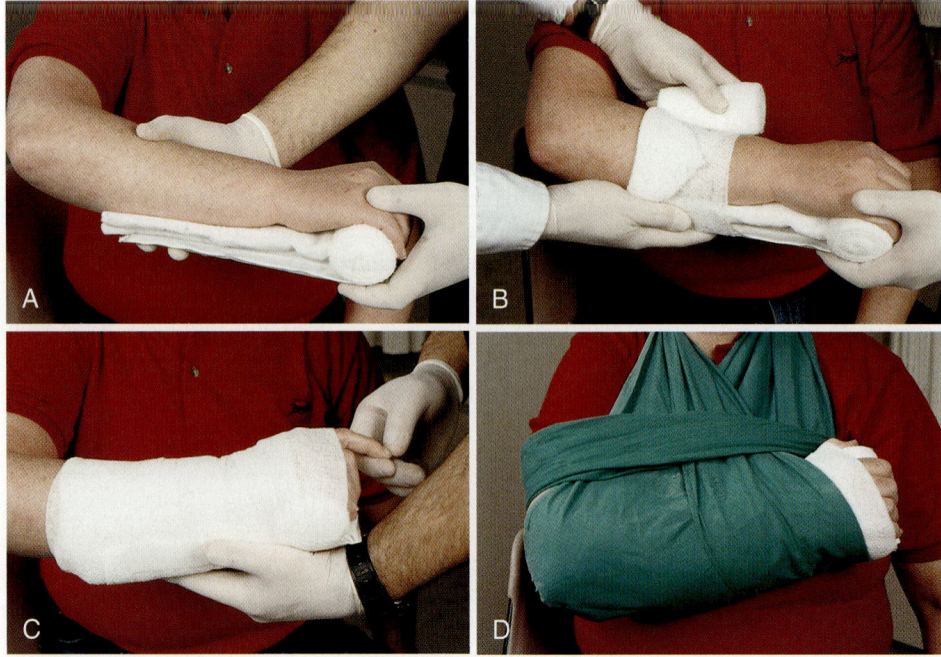

FIGURE 46-10 Emergency care of a fracture. **A,** A splint should immobilize the area above and below injury. **B,** A splint is held in place with a gauze roll bandage. **C,** After a splint is supplied, pulse below the splint should be checked to make sure the splint has not been applied too tightly. **D,** A sling can be used to elevate the extremity to reduce swelling. (From Henry M, Stapleton E: *EMT prehospital care*, ed 2, Philadelphia, 1997, Saunders.)

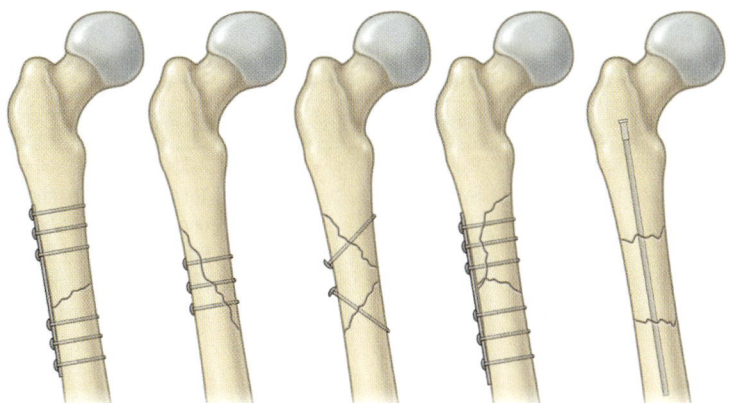

FIGURE 46-11 Devices used to reduce a fracture. (Modified from Beare PG, Myers JL: *Principles and practice of adult health nursing*, ed 3, St Louis, 1998, Mosby.)

patient experiences pain over the joint and loses motion. To assess the degree of dislocation, do the following:

1. Check the distal pulse to make certain the extremity below the dislocation is receiving a blood supply. For example, with a shoulder injury, check the radial pulse.
2. Splint above and below the dislocated joint.
3. Keep the patient warm and observe for shock.
4. Apply an ice pack to the area.

Sprain

A **sprain** is a full or partial tear of a ligament. Care should be taken to keep the injured area immobile. Based on the acronym RICE, begin treatment within 10 to 20 minutes of the injury, as follows:

- **R**est the injured area by splinting the area.
- **I**ce the area because cold reduces bleeding, swelling, and muscle spasms in injured muscles.
- **C**ompress the area by wrapping with an elastic bandage to minimize swelling.
- **E**levate the injured area to heart level if possible. This reduces circulation to the affected area.

Strain

A **strain** is a stretching or tearing of a muscle or tendon. As with a fracture, immobilize the area. Have the person assume a comfortable position to take pressure off the injured muscle. Apply heat to the area, and provide support if available.

Poisons

A **poison** is any substance that causes injury, illness, and even death in an individual. Signs and symptoms of having ingested a poison are listed in Box 46-6.

Ingested Poison

Ingested poisons are taken in by mouth and travel through the digestive system. When poison has been ingested, always call the nearest poison control center for advice. Inform the center of the type of poison ingested and if a medication is involved, the name of the medication, dosage, and the number of pills taken or missing from the bottle. If the person does not know how many pills were taken, the number remaining in the bottle can be subtracted from the number dispensed.

> **BOX 46-6**
>
> **Signs and Symptoms of Poison Ingestion**
>
> - Altered mental status (confusion)
> - Chemical burns around the mouth
> - Breath odor of chemical
> - Difficulty breathing
> - Nausea
> - Vomiting
> - Abdominal pain
> - Diarrhea

Emergency care for a person who has ingested poison is as follows:

1. Call 911.
2. Maintain the airway.
3. Position the patient to keep the airway clear.
4. Induce vomiting if the manufacturer or the poison control center provides this recommendation. Vomiting prevents absorption of the remainder of certain poisons if done within 1 to 2 hours of ingestion. Activated charcoal is the substance of choice for neutralizing poisons that have been swallowed. It should only be administered if the airway is clear and the patient's mental status is not impaired. *Do not induce vomiting* unless instructed to do so by the poison control center. If the patient has ingested corrosive or caustic (burning) materials or petroleum products (e.g., bleach, cleaners), rinse the mouth with cool water, without swallowing. The American Academy of Pediatrics no longer recommends the use of ipecac syrup.
5. Position the patient leaning forward to prevent aspiration of stomach contents.

Be prepared for poisoning and always have the poison control center's phone number posted at the receptionist's desk. Patients will often call the office first.

Inhaled Poison

Inhaled poison vapors and fumes usually result from a fire or chemical spill (e.g., carbon monoxide, cleaning solvents). Emergency care is as follows:

TABLE 46-4

Treatment Guidelines for Bites and Bee Stings

Bite or Sting	Symptoms or Signs	Treatment Guidelines
Snake bite, spider bite, scorpion bite	Pain Swelling Redness Bleeding	1. Ask victim to lie still with bitten area lower than the heart 2. Tie strip of cloth, shoestring, watchband, or belt about 3 inches above bite, making sure one finger can fit between strip and skin 3. Wash bitten area thoroughly with soap and water 4. Do not cut bite unless you have special training 5. Observe for signs of shock 6. Snake or spider: Try to identify markings on snake or type of spider; if dead, bring to emergency department (ED) 7. Transport victim to ED as soon as possible
Human and animal bites	Pain Swelling Redness Bleeding Human bites worst	1. Wash bite thoroughly with soap and water 2. Control bleeding by applying direct pressure; ice may be applied 3. Raise injured limb above level of the heart (helps control bleeding) 4. When bleeding stops, apply clean bandage (not too tight) 5. Wild animal: Try to capture or kill animal (without being bitten yourself) 6. Domestic animal: Obtain name and address of owner to report to health department 7. Seek medical attention for victim
Tick bites	Pain Tick may be attached	1. Remove tick if attached by cutting off its oxygen supply; cover tick with petroleum jelly or any oil, or gasoline; remove tick when it backs out of skin 2. Wash area thoroughly with soap and water 3. Seek medical attention if bite becomes infected or victim becomes sick, has joint pain, or develops rash on palms of hands (Lyme disease or Rocky Mountain spotted fever)
Bee stings	Pain Swelling Raised lump Stinger may be attached	1. If honeybee stinger attached, remove it carefully with tweezers, or scrape it with edge of knife or credit card 2. Avoid squeezing venom sac on tip of stinger 3. Wash area thoroughly with soap and water 4. Elevate stung area above the heart and apply ice to control swelling 5. Antihistamines may help localized swelling 6. Seek medical attention if site becomes infected or victim shows signs of severe allergic reaction (hives, itching, or wheezing)

1. Call 911.
2. Protect yourself and remove the patient from the source.
3. Loosen clothing that may affect breathing.
4. Assess breathing and perform rescue breathing or CPR if necessary.

Injected Poison

Injected poisons can be drugs or venom from spider, snake, and other insect bites. For insect stings, the area should be washed with soap and water after the stinger has been removed. Observe the patient for signs of an allergic reaction, such as redness, swelling, and difficulty breathing. Symptoms and treatments for bites and stings are listed in Table 46-4.

Diabetic Emergencies

Two types of emergencies can affect the diabetic patient: insulin shock (**hypoglycemia**) and diabetic ketoacidosis (**hyperglycemia**).

Insulin Shock

Insulin shock (low blood sugar level) occurs when the patient has taken too much insulin, has not eaten enough to use up the insulin taken, or has exercised heavily, using up available glucose in the body. The patient appears pale, and the skin feels cool and clammy. Patients usually complain of being lightheaded or hungry. They may appear restless or appear agitated. Vital signs are **within normal limits (WNL).**

To assess the situation, ask the patient if food was eaten after taking insulin. If the patient did not eat or only had time for minimal food, provide the patient with sugary nourishment (e.g., orange juice, white sugar dissolved in water, glucose gel or tablets) followed by proteins and fats, such as peanut butter, that will maintain the glucose level. The blood glucose level should be assessed with a glucose meter. If the condition does not improve, seek emergency assistance.

Diabetic Ketoacidosis

Diabetic ketoacidosis occurs when glucose builds up in the patient's blood without sufficient insulin, and ketones (acid waste byproducts) are produced. This situation requires a 911 call. A change in the patient's medical condition (e.g., infection, common cold) or glucose overload when eating without adequate insulin can lead to ketoacidosis. The patient tends to be confused and has diminished responsiveness. The skin feels hot and dry and is reddened. The patient's vital signs are

> **BOX 46-7**
>
> **Possible Food and Household Choking Hazards**
>
> Pieces of meat and uncooked vegetables
> Nuts
> Hard candy
> Marshmallows
> Chunks of peanut butter
> Balloons
> Coins
> Pen caps

severely affected. Respirations become very deep and gasping, then become rapid (**Kussmaul breathing**), and the pulse is thready and weak. A sweet or fruity odor caused by acetone buildup is detected. The physician will order a glucose level to assess the need for insulin to be given immediately (stat).

Choking

Choking is caused by a blockage in the trachea or from a swelling of the larynx caused by an injury. Box 46-7 lists possible food and household choking hazards, especially for children.

- A partial airway obstruction begins with a coughing episode and progresses to the patient not being able to breathe.
- With a complete airway obstruction, the patient cannot speak or breathe. The face will redden and will rapidly change to purple if the obstruction is not removed.

Patients who are conscious can usually indicate they are choking by clutching at their throat (Figure 46-12). This non-verbal communication is referred to as the "universal sign for choking." If the cough is forceful, allow the person to continue coughing, since this type of action indicates air is getting into the lungs. If the coughing fails to dislodge the obstruction, emergency action is needed to remove the cause of the obstruction. The type of action depends on whether the patient is conscious or unconscious.

Conscious Individuals

The **Heimlich maneuver,** or *abdominal thrust,* is an emergency procedure used to dislodge the cause of a blockage. Abdominal thrusts are only recommended for conscious patients with an airway obstruction.

The Heimlich maneuver is performed as follows:
1. The rescuer wraps his or her arms around the patient from behind.
2. The rescuer's fist, with thumb facing the abdomen of the victim, is placed just below the sternum and xiphoid process, and above the umbilicus. The other hand is placed over the fist.
3. An upward thrust is done in an attempt to dislodge the foreign body in the trachea. This pushes the diaphragm up, forcing air from the lungs and the obstruction from the trachea.

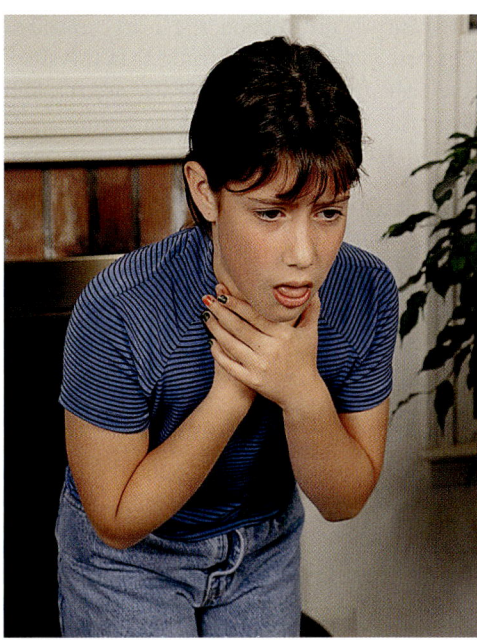

FIGURE 46-12 A choking person will usually clutch the throat. This is considered to be the universal distress signal. (From Sorrentino SA. *Assisting with patient care,* ed 2, St Louis, 2004, Mosby.)

Unconscious Individuals

For individuals who are unconscious, a combination of chest compressions and finger sweeps is used instead of the Heimlich maneuver. If the patient is unconscious, slightly blue, and no air movement is evident, do the following:
1. Check the airway by using a sweeping motion, then reposition the head and neck and have the patient attempt to breathe.
2. Reposition the patient if necessary and straddle the thighs or kneel beside the patient.
3. Give five abdomen thrusts with the heel of the hand. Always finger-sweep the mouth after each abdominal thrust, and repeat as needed.

An infant with a complete airway obstruction, as evidenced by the inability to cry or breathe, should have alternating blows to the back and chest thrusts to dislodge the foreign body forcibly from the airway.

> **PATIENT-CENTERED PROFESSIONALISM**
>
> - What are some general guidelines to help the medical assistant best handle an office emergency?
> - Why is knowledge of how to handle each specific type of office emergency critical to the safety of the patients who visit the office?

BASIC LIFE SUPPORT

Cardiac arrest is the sudden cessation of heart activity. It can occur at any time without warning. Unless the patient's heart activity is restored quickly, permanent brain damage or death will occur. If a patient stops breathing (**respiratory arrest**) because of an airway obstruction, the heart can still pump for several minutes. Starting rescue breathing in this situation can prevent the heart from stopping (cardiac arrest). Remember: always assess the situation before taking action.

Follow the basic "ABCs" before starting any type of resuscitation:
- *Airway* must be open.
- *Breathing* must be assessed.
- *Circulation* must be checked by feeling for a pulse.

Be especially aware of any head or neck trauma that could be associated with a spinal injury.

Cardiopulmonary Resuscitation

Cardiopulmonary resuscitation (CPR) is performed to restore breathing and cardiac activity to the heart. Most schools offering health care programs classes provide approved CPR training, therefore this chapter will highlight only current recommendations by the American Heart Association (AHA).

On March 31, 2008 an advisory statement from the AHA was published to clarify the 2005 AHA Guidelines for CPR and Emergency Cardiovascular Care (ECC), which states that bystanders should perform "Hands-Only CPR" if they are unable to provide rescue breaths. These recommendations emphasize that chest compressions are more important than mouth-to-mouth breathing for cardiac victims because the compressions are what actually keeps the heart pumping and the blood flowing. This action provides oxygen to the vital organs until more advanced breathing can be provided.

When someone suddenly collapses, the person nearest the victim should do the following:
- Call out to the victim and check the victim's pulse
- Call 911 or have someone else do it
- If unable to perform rescue breathing, compress the center of the chest with the heel of the hand
- Compressions must be done very fast, 30 compressions in 18 seconds using the heel of the hand and allowing the chest to compress after each compression
- Continue sequence until defibrillating equipment arrives, the victim responds, or paramedics take over

Data support that performing only "Hands-Only CPR" can be as effective as conventional CPR.

Automated External Defibrillator

The **automated external defibrillator (AED)** is a machine that analyzes the patient's cardiac rhythm and can deliver an electrical shock (**defibrillation**) to the heart to stop an erratic rhythm or restart the cardiac cycle. The chance of surviving sudden cardiac arrest decreases by 10% with every minute that passes without action. Technological advances allow these machines to be operated by almost everyone with minimal training.

There are two types of external defibrillators: fully automatic and semiautomatic. An AED should not be attached to a patient who is responsive or who has a pulse. Also, transdermal patches should be removed because they often have an aluminum backing, or the patch's paste medium is reactive to defibrillation.

Fully Automatic Defibrillator

The fully automatic external defibrillator requires the rescuer to place two defibrillator patches on the patient's chest, connect the lead wires, and turn on the AED. The machine will analyze and shock the victim with no action by the rescuer. After three shocks, check the pulse. The machine will state "clear the patient" before delivering the shocks, or "no shock indicated" if the AED does not detect a shockable rhythm. Once it is determined the patient has no pulse, CPR should begin. Even after successful resuscitation, the AED should not be disconnected because ventricular fibrillation could occur.

Semiautomatic Defibrillator

The semiautomatic defibrillator requires the rescuer to attach the patches and leads to the patient's chest, turn on the AED, and press a button. The computer analyzes the rhythm, and the computer-synthesized voice advises the rescuer what steps to take. This type of defibrillator requires more advanced training.

PATIENT-CENTERED PROFESSIONALISM

- *Why is it important for the medical assistant to be knowledgeable and skilled in cardiopulmonary resuscitation?*

DISASTER PREPAREDNESS

What were your first thoughts when you saw the word **disaster** (an event that creates destruction and or adverse consequences)? Terrorist attack! Since September 11, 2001, this has become an automatic response. That event also produced an even greater awareness of biological and chemical agents. What about Katrina? This hurricane devastated New Orleans not only because of its heavy rains and strong winds but also because of the flooding when the levees broke. Disaster preparedness is nothing more than making plans to prevent, if possible, an event that causes destruction and if unable to prevent it, respond and recover as quickly as possible.

Disasters can be divided into two major categories: natural and man-made. Box 46-8 provides a list of catastrophic events that require an immediate response from the community and various agencies (e.g., American Red Cross, the Salvation Army, and the Public Health Department) and health care professionals (e.g., licensed health care professionals [physicians, registered nurses] and soon to be added, allied health professionals [e.g., medical assistants, licensed practical nurses]). Effective emergency preparedness requires cooperation, communication, and coordination between all these groups. Collaboration (cooperation) strengthens coordination efforts, reduces overlap of assignments, and adds **synergy** to the disaster team. Working together optimizes resource use

> **BOX 46-8**
>
> ## Types of Disaster
>
> | NATURAL DISASTERS | MAN-MADE DISASTERS |
> |---|---|
> | Hurricanes | Terrorism |
> | Tornadoes | Bioterrorism |
> | Earthquakes | Chemical spills |
> | Floods | Nuclear accidents |
> | Wildfires | Transportation accidents |
> | Blizzards | Train, airplane, bridge collapse |
> | Heat waves | Infectious disease |
> | Tsunamis (tidal wave) | Severe acute respiratory syndrome (SARS) |
> | Landslides | West Nile virus |
> | Volcanic eruptions | Civil unrest |

and coordinates efforts to promote the health and safety of the community affected by the disaster.

Preparation

How can a community prepare for so many types of disasters? The answer to that question is "they can't." What can be done is to understand that each type of disaster is unique, but the planning and preparation are similar. Preparedness is the key to a successful disaster response. Preparing includes identifying resources that will be needed in the event of a disaster (e.g., communication equipment, supplies, and vehicles) and how these resources should be used.

Planning

The advantage of having a disaster preparedness plan is it provides a way to maximize the efforts of the team by providing a well-documented process that assists in the timely response and recovery of the area. Disaster planning requires the use of a management system approach. The plan will identify a designated "Chief" who is responsible for all functions of the plan unless they have been delegated. Typical duties include identification of priorities, coordination with outside agencies, and the approval of the team's action plan. The team can consist of but is not limited to the following:

Safety Officer, who monitors the safety of those affected and the response team's adherence to personal protective equipment (PPE) protocols.

Logistics Officer, who is responsible for supplies, equipment, food, and communication support.

Operations Officer, who directs activities and maintains discipline.

Some states support health care providers to increase their emergency (disaster) preparedness by enacting statutes that require disaster training as a requirement to renew their professional license. The Commission on Accreditation of Allied Health Education Programs (CAAHEP) proposes the inclusion of allied health care professionals to the disaster team. The rationale is that allied health professionals routinely provide those health care services needed in a disaster situation and therefore can reduce the shortage of providers in an emergency situation.

Practice

Drills, or practice sessions, provide team members with a clear understanding of their responsibilities during a disaster. Drills help evaluate the effectiveness and efficiency of the disaster plan and help coordinate resources and how they should be used. Practice in advance of an emergency allows everyone concerned to be better able to handle any situation.

Medical Assistant's Role

The medical assistant can supplement existing emergency and public health resources by contributing their vast knowledge and abilities during a crisis. This can be done by registering with an emergency preparedness unit before a disaster occurs. Registering has the following advantages for the medical assistant:

- Skills and competencies can be verified beforehand.
- Details of the unit's action plan will be known.
- Expectations will be understood.
- Advanced training will be given.
- Liability protection will be provided.

Failure to register in advance presents the following problems:

- Not enough time to verify credentials and competencies.
- Food and shelter accommodations are inadequate to provide for last minute personnel.
- You could get in the way because you do not know the plan.

Several agencies have formed to assist in organizing an emergency health care workforce that could help during a disaster situation to meet the increased patient/victim care and increased needs of the community. The *Emergency System for Advanced Registration of Volunteer Health Professionals (ESAR-VHP)* was initiated to provide a method for the supplemental health care workforce to respond immediately to a mass casualty event. An issue that arose in the aftermath of the World Trade Center destruction was the use of health care professional volunteers in an emergency or mass casualty event. Hospital administrators reported that they were unable to use medical volunteers because they were unable to verify the volunteers' basic identity, licensing, credentials (training, skills, and competencies), and employment.

The *Emergency Management Assistance Compact (EMAC)* is a congressionally ratified organization that provides aid from its list of health care volunteers in cases of an emergency. The *Medical Reserve Corps (MRC)* establishes teams of volunteer medical and public health professionals to contribute their skills in times of community need. A group that is composed of nonmedical volunteers is the *Community Emergency Response Team (CERT)*.

By becoming an active member of a disaster preparedness team, the medical assistant avoids getting in the way in the aftermath of a disaster since their role will be defined in advance of the emergency and within their scope of training.

The use of a medical assistant on a disaster preparedness team draws on their experience working with patients.

CONCLUSION

The purpose of performing first-aid measures is to provide emergency care within the scope of practice. When providing emergency care, the medical assistant must take care that the victim experiences no further injury. Detecting and responding to the situation in a competent manner is paramount. To do this, always assess the situation before beginning first aid. If a patient is conscious, permission to treat must be obtained. If the patient refuses, do not start any emergency care.

The Good Samaritan law was enacted to encourage people to assist others during an emergency situation. This law provides legal protection to those people who provide emergency care to ill or injured persons and minimizes the fear of legal consequences. The care provided can never exceed the scope of a person's training.

Medical assistants who are prepared to give first aid in office emergencies can make a difference in the lives of their patients. Because accidents can happen at any time, knowing what to do to assist the patient in each situation is essential. The knowledge and overall professional skills of the medical assistant are qualities that make the addition of the medical assistant to a disaster team a good decision.

Chapter Summary

Reinforce your understanding of the material in this chapter by reviewing the curriculum objectives and key content points below.

1. **Define, appropriately use, and spell all the Key Terms for this chapter.**
   - Review the Key Terms if necessary.
2. **Explain the purpose of an incident report.**
   - Documents the exact details of the occurrence while the facts are fresh in the minds of those who witnessed the event.
3. **List the information needed to accurately complete an incident report.**
   - Observed, objective, and chronological information is required. This includes the person's name, location and time of the incident, and any factual description of what occurred and what was done as a result of the incident.
4. **Explain what a medical assistant should do first in an emergency situation.**
   - Emergency situations require the medical assistant to prioritize both the urgency of the situation and the status of the patient.
5. **Define first aid and list two guidelines that protect health care workers and victims from disease transmission.**
   - First aid is the temporary care given to an injured or ill person until he or she can be provided with complete treatment.
   - Health care workers should wear protective gloves to avoid contact with blood and body fluids.
   - Areas that are soiled with blood, mucus, or other body fluids should not be touched without a barrier (e.g., CPR mouth barriers).
6. **List one situation requiring first-aid attention for each of the seven body systems.**
   - Review Table 46-1.
7. **Explain what causes fainting.**
   - Fainting is caused by an inadequate blood supply to the brain.

8. **List seven guidelines for the emergency care of a patient who has fainted.**
   - Assess for life-threatening cause; check for medical alerts; keep the patient supine and elevate the legs; check the airway and loosen clothing; apply a damp cloth to the face; calm the patient; and ask about medications.
9. **Describe the symptoms of a heart attack and explain the purpose of cardiopulmonary resuscitation (CPR).**
   - Dusky skin color, diaphoresis, bluish lips and nail beds, shortness of breath (SOB), and rapid, weak pulse are all symptoms of a heart attack.
   - Chest pain can be a sign of heart attack.
   - The purpose of CPR is to keep oxygen moving to the lungs and blood circulating throughout the body.
10. **List 10 guidelines for the emergency care of a patient who has heart attack symptoms.**
    - Always call for emergency assistance in a possible heart attack situation.
    - If a patient is exhibiting signs of a heart attack, follow these guidelines: call 911, position the patient comfortably, assess the airway, loosen clothing, determine if the patient is conscious and taking medication, administer the medication, administer oxygen, take vital signs, keep the patient warm, and comfort the patient.
11. **Explain how a stroke differs from a heart attack, and identify the signs of obstructed airway and cardiac arrest.**
    - A stroke occurs when the brain does not receive oxygen because of a burst or blocked blood vessel or pressure on the cerebral artery; a heart attack occurs because heart tissue is deprived of blood supply.
    - Stroke symptoms vary according to severity but can include facial and arm weakness or numbness, severe headache, sudden confusion, visual changes, and speech difficulty.
    - Heart attack victims may complain of chest pain, be diaphoretic, have SOB, be cyanotic, and have altered vital signs.

- A person with an obstructed airway will not be able to breathe or speak, whereas a heart attack victim may be able to breathe or have breath restored and the heart muscle is affected.

12. **List six guidelines for the emergency care of a patient who has had a stroke.**
    - Keep in mind that if stroke occurs on the left side of the brain, damage will be to the right side of the body, and vice versa.
    - If a patient has had a stroke, follow these guidelines: call 911, assess the airway, elevate the head, keep the patient warm, turn the patient on the side if there is difficulty breathing, and take vital signs.

13. **List seven types of shock and explain what causes each.**
    - Review Table 46-3.

14. **List eight guidelines for the emergency care of a patient who has symptoms of shock.**
    - Seek medical assistance, maintain the airway, place the patient supine with the feet elevated, apply direct pressure to external bleeding, keep the patient warm, do not give the patient anything orally, do not leave the patient alone, and take vital signs.

15. **Explain what a seizure is and what may cause one.**
    - A seizure is a sudden involuntary muscle activity with a change in behavior and level of consciousness.
    - Seizures are brought on by a change in the electrical activity of the brain.

16. **List eight guidelines for the emergency care of a patient who has had a seizure.**
    - Remove objects from the area, maintain the airway, protect the head, loosen clothing, do not restrain the patient and avoid overstimulation, turn the patient to the side after a seizure, assess vital signs, and allow the patient to rest.

17. **List and describe the two methods for controlling bleeding.**
    - Bleeding can be controlled by direct and indirect pressure.
    - Direct pressure is applied directly to the wound itself.
    - Indirect pressure is applied to the artery that supplies blood to the injured area.

18. **Explain the emergency care for patients with thermal, chemical, or electrical burns.**
    - The surface area of the burn is evaluated according to the "rule of nines."
    - Proper treatment is started after both depth and total surface area have been determined.
    - It is important to know the cause of the burn, length of exposure, and any medical condition.

19. **Differentiate between heat exhaustion and heat stroke.**
    - Heat exhaustion occurs when the body is subjected to excessive heat; symptoms include excessive sweating and pale, cool, clammy skin.
    - Heat stroke (sunstroke) occurs when the body is exposed to extreme heat and high humidity for long periods; symptoms include dry, hot, reddened skin and body temperature of 106° F or higher.

20. **Explain considerations for the emergency care of a patient with frostbite.**
    - Pressure should not be applied to frostbitten areas, and the patient should not walk on frostbitten feet.
    - The area should not be rubbed, and the body part needs to be gradually rewarmed.

21. **List the main goal for the emergency care of a fracture.**
    - Immobilization of the fractured area is the main goal of emergency care.

22. **List four guidelines for assessing the degree of a dislocation.**
    - Check the distal pulse, splint above and below the dislocated joint, keep the patient warm and observe for shock, and apply an ice pack to the injured area.

23. **List five guidelines for emergency care of a patient who has ingested poison.**
    - Call the poison control center for advice when a patient has ingested poison.
    - Call 911, maintain the airway, position the patient to keep the airway clear, induce vomiting if recommended, and position the patient leaning forward.

24. **List four guidelines for the emergency care of a patient who has inhaled poison.**
    - Call 911, protect yourself and remove the patient from the source of vapors and fumes, loosen clothing, and assess breathing and perform rescue breathing or CPR if necessary.

25. **Identify the symptoms of bites and stings.**
    - Review Table 46-4.

26. **Explain the difference between insulin shock and diabetic ketoacidosis (diabetic coma).**
    - Insulin shock occurs when the body has too much insulin and not enough glucose.
    - Diabetic ketoacidosis occurs when there is too much glucose and not enough insulin in the blood, and ketones are produced.

27. **Explain "Hands-Only CPR" and its intended purpose.**
    - "Hands-Only CPR" focuses on compressions to keep the heart pumping and the blood flowing.
    - This technique can be used by a bystander when a person collapses and the person is unresponsive and without a pulse.
    - Thirty (30) compressions are done very fast with the heel of the hand, within 18 seconds, and the compressions must continue until defibrillating equipment arrives, the victim responds, or paramedics take over.

28. **Demonstrate the correct procedure for performing the Heimlich maneuver.**
    - Rescuer wraps his or her arms around the patient from behind.
    - Rescuer's fist, with thumb facing the abdomen of the victim, is placed just below the sternum and xiphoid process and above the umbilicus. The other hand is placed over the fist.
    - An upward thrust is done in an attempt to dislodge the foreign body in the trachea.

29. **Explain what an automated external defibrillator (AED) is and how it is used.**
    - An AED analyzes cardiac rhythm and delivers an electric shock (defibrillation) to the heart to stop an erratic rhythm or restart the cardiac cycle.

30. **Discuss the difference between natural and man-made disasters.**

- Natural disasters are the result of the forces of nature, and man-made disasters result from human intervention causing an event of destruction.
31. **Discuss the advantages of registering with a disaster preparedness team.**
    - Skills and competencies can be verified.
    - Know details of the unit's action plan.
    - Understand expectations.
    - Receive advanced training.
    - Provided with liability protection.
32. **Analyze a realistic medical office situation and apply your understanding of handling office emergencies to determine the best course of action.**
    - Medical assistants must be prepared to act in emergency situations in the medical office; they must be aware of what is going on around them and must be prepared to act on the knowledge they have.
33. **Describe the impact on patient care when medical assistants have a solid understanding of the knowledge and skills necessary to assist patients in office emergencies.**
    - When the medical assistant is knowledgeable and skillful when emergencies arise in the medical office, the patient benefits.
    - Quick assessment by the medical assistant can prevent a delay in appropriate treatment.
    - When the medical assistant is prepared for medical emergencies, patient confidence is established in the medical practice.

PRACTICAL APPLICATIONS

If you have accomplished the objectives in this chapter, you will be able to make better choices as a medical assistant. Take another look at this situation and decide what you would do.

Mariah has type 1 diabetes mellitus and takes insulin on a regular basis. Dr. Naguchi is aware that Mariah does not follow her diet as she should and that her exercise habits are not consistent, so her diabetes is often not stable.

Mariah lives in the southern United States, where it is currently 100° F outside and very humid. Earlier today, Mariah was in the garden gathering vegetables. Later, she started canning the vegetables. Her house has minimal air conditioning. In her haste to complete what needed to be done in the garden, Mariah did not eat her lunch as she should have, although she took her entire dose of insulin.

During the afternoon, Mariah began to feel weak, experiencing dizziness and sweating, and her skin felt cool and clammy. Don, her husband, drove her the three blocks to Dr. Naguchi's office because she started complaining of chest pain and difficulty breathing. As soon as she arrives, Mariah appears to faint and falls, injuring her left ankle. As the medical assistant, Janis is the first health care professional to see what is happening to Mariah. After seeing Mariah, Dr. Naguchi orders an x-ray of her ankle to see whether she has a sprain, strain, or fracture.

If you were in Janis's place, would you know what to do in this situation?

1. What are the external factors that could have caused the symptoms that Mariah showed?
2. How should Janis handle this problem when several persons are in the waiting room with Don and Mariah?
3. What questions should Janis immediately ask Don?
4. What recent activities could have contributed to Mariah's problems?
5. If Mariah fainted and you were the medical assistant, what would you do for her immediately while someone was notifying the physician?
6. Knowing that Mariah has diabetes, what might you think happened, and what would you expect Dr. Naguchi to order for her?
7. Why would you be suspicious of hyperthermia? What should Janis do for these symptoms?
8. What symptoms does Mariah have that might indicate a heart attack?
9. How do a sprain, strain, and fracture differ and how is each treated? What treatment is common to all three conditions?

WEB SEARCH

1. **Research risk factors of a stroke.** Certain medical and hereditary conditions increase the risk of a stroke (e.g., diabetes, African American, family history of stroke).

- **Keywords:** Use the following keywords in your search: National Heart, Lung, and Blood Institute; National Stroke Association; American Heart Association, hypertension.

Beginning Your Job Search

47

evolve http://evolve.elsevier.com/klieger/medicalassisting

This text has taught you the qualities, skills, knowledge, and characteristics that will help make you a successful medical assistant. Everything you have learned in the previous chapters will prepare you for your first job. This final chapter shows you how to identify job opportunities, present yourself positively in writing a resumé and cover letter, prepare for an interview, and get that first job.

Before you begin actively looking for employment, take some time to consider the (1) type of setting in which you would like to work (e.g., hospital, ambulatory care, or private practice), (2) type of specialty in which you would like to work (e.g., pediatrics, cardiology), (3) type of schedule that would be best for you (e.g., part-time, full-time, evenings, or weekends), and (4) general location you would prefer (e.g., are you willing to move or commute or do you want something closer to home, accessible by car or public transportation?). Once you have a better idea of what type of position would be best for you, you will be more prepared to actively seek employment.

LEARNING OBJECTIVES

You will be able to do the following after completing this chapter:

Key Terms
1. Define, appropriately use, and spell all the Key Terms for this chapter.

Organizing Your Resources
2. List and briefly describe six methods of locating job positions.

Developing Your Materials
3. Explain the purpose of a resumé.
4. List two formats that can be used to create resumés and explain the focus of each.
5. List five sections that should always be included in a resumé.
6. Explain the purpose of a cover letter.
7. Describe the information that should be included in the first, second, and final paragraphs of a cover letter.

Contacting Potential Employers
8. Briefly describe four methods that medical assistants can use to contact prospective employers.

The Job Application
9. Explain the purpose of a job application.
10. List five guidelines for completing a job application.

The Job Interview
11. Explain the purpose of a job interview and list four issues the medical assistant should mention and five topics the employer should address during the interview.
12. Describe ways you can prepare for a job interview.
13. Provide clear, accurate, positive answers to six questions typically asked by employers during an interview.
14. Explain the importance of sending a follow-up note or "letter of thanks" after an interview.

Patient-Centered Professionalism
15. Analyze a realistic medical office situation and apply your understanding of the job-seeking process.
16. Describe the impact on patient care when medical assistants have a solid understanding of the knowledge and skills necessary to seek and obtain a job for which they are qualified and that they find fulfilling and rewarding.

KEY TERMS

chronological resumé
cover letter
employment agencies
functional resumé
heading
job application
job interview
networking
objective
placement services
references
resumé

PRACTICAL APPLICATIONS

Read the following scenario and keep it in mind as you learn about searching for a job in this chapter.

Dora has recently completed a medical assisting program and will be looking for new employment as a medical assistant in an ambulatory care setting. As she begins her search, she goes to the school placement office to see if the counselor knows of any jobs in the area. The counselor, Ms. Smith, states that she is unaware of any openings at present but will keep Dora in mind should someone call.

Next, Dora turns to the newspaper ads. She writes her resume and cover letter quickly because she is excited about a position she saw advertised in the classifieds. She is typically good at writing, so she doesn't bother to ask a friend to proofread her resumé and cover letter this time. (After all, it would only slow her down.) She is in such a hurry to apply for the job in the newspaper that she does not proofread or spell-check her materials. As a result, several words are misspelled, and the information that is supposed to be in chronological order is not.

Despite the errors on Dora's resumé and cover letter, she obtains an interview with a potential employer. When she arrives, she is surprised that the employer expects her to complete an application before the interview. After completing the application, she answers the employer's interview questions and asks a few of her own. Overall, she has a good feeling about this interview.

After the interview, Dora returns home and waits to hear from the potential employer, taking no further action and hoping that she has been chosen for the job.

Do you think Dora would be hired for this job? What would you have done differently?

ORGANIZING YOUR RESOURCES

When seeking employment in a medical setting as a medical assistant, getting organized is the first step. This process takes effort and careful planning, and you should make a list of the resources that you will use in your job search. The key to finding available positions is knowing where to look. Obvious places are the facility where your externship was completed, the school placement office, and the newspaper. Other valuable sources of employment information include employment agencies and the Internet.

Newspaper Classifieds

The classified advertising section of a newspaper can list medical assistant positions in several ways. Some newspapers list all health care positions under "Medical," whereas others break this section down using the particular job titles such as "medical assistant," "clinic office assistant," and "front/back office assistant." Some classifieds may be advertised for "either/or" types of respondents, so you should look in more than one section of the ads. For example, an ad that reads, "Clinical office assistant needed—LPN/MA may apply," might appear in both "licensed practical nurse" (LPN) and "medical assistant" (MA) sections, or it may appear in only one section of the newspaper.

Newspaper classified ads often give a brief description of the types of positions employers are trying to fill. The ad may describe duties, qualifications, and desired characteristics or qualities and may provide information on how to apply for the position. Some job classifieds also provide a salary range. Box 47-1 lists some abbreviations that are often used in employment classifieds.

Before responding to a newspaper classified ad, you should take the time to develop your contact materials (as discussed later) and carefully read the advertisement. Pay special attention to the type of contact requested by the employer (e.g., mail, phone, e-mail, or in person) and what information they request.

School Placement Services

Often, medical facilities call local schools to inform them of job vacancies. Many schools have **placement services** that help students obtain employment. Placement services may include help in writing or developing resumés and cover letters, interviewing tips, job search methods, and career planning in general. Check to see if your school or program offers placement services.

Employment Agencies

Private and public **employment agencies** exist to help individuals find employment. Employment agencies maintain lists of available jobs and help match employers to job seekers who have the skills and qualities needed. Private agencies charge a fee to either the employer or the person looking for a position for screening potential employees and placement, whereas public (state and local) employment agencies offer these services for free.

Direct Contact

If you are looking for employment in a particular area or specialty, contacting medical facilities directly is resourceful. Larger medical facilities may list employment opportunities on their website or may have a "hotline" that you can call to listen to a prerecorded listing of available jobs.

BOX 47-1

Abbreviations Used in Employment Classifieds

apps.	applicants, applications
ASAP	as soon as possible
avail.	available
B/F	back and front
ben.	benefits
co.	company
CV	Curriculum Vitae
emp.	employer, employee
EOE	equal opportunity employer
exp., exp'd	experience, experienced
flex.	flexible
FT, ft, f/t	full-time
hr.	hour
HS, hs	high school
immed.	immediate, immediately
K (as in $10K)	thousand
M-F	Monday through Friday
min.	minimum, minute
neg	negotiable
off.	office
pd.	paid
pos.	position
pref.	preferred
PT, pt, p/t	part-time
ref.	references
reimb.	reimbursement
req.	require, required
sal.	salary
tel.	telephone
w/	with
wk.	week, work
wpm, W.P.M.	words per minute
vac.	vacation
yr., yrs.	year, years
401K	type of retirement savings plan

You can also send a letter of inquiry to the employer to express your interest in working there. Always include a resumé with your letter of inquiry. Telephoning the medical facility's human resources department to ask if there are positions available is also appropriate. Whatever method you choose, always remember that the quality of your written and oral communication creates a first impression of you as a person. Make sure the first impression is a good one.

Another source of potential job opportunities is your local *medical society*, where physician members may advertise for staff. Check the medical society's website or call and inquire about employment opportunities.

Internet Job Search

Many websites are devoted to helping people search for jobs. Career search websites often allow users to search by position type, geographical location, specific company name, and any combination of these methods. Both browsing and keyword search functions are usually available.

Job search websites can be located by doing a keyword search on "jobs," "employment," and so on. Many newspapers also list their employment classified sections online. Also, as mentioned, larger medical facilities may have websites that list available positions online.

Networking

Networking is interacting with "contacts" or people you have met through various professional, educational, and social activities and asking for their help, advice, and suggestions when you are looking for a job. The people in your network may be able to give you job leads, offer you advice and information about a particular company or industry, and introduce you to others so you can expand your network. Many people hesitate to network because they feel awkward asking for help. However, networking is one of the best ways to find a job. Networking is a skill that improves with practice, so even if you are nervous at first, keep trying. People often enjoy talking about their jobs and career field and are willing to give career advice.

Assemble a list of potential contacts: your teachers, friends, your own physician(s), relatives, and so on. Even if your contact is not involved with health care or medical assisting, he or she may know someone who is involved or who knows of an opportunity in a health care setting (e.g., their family doctor may be looking for a medical assistant). Knowing someone already working in the health care field is an easy way to find out what is available. You can also join the local chapter of your professional organization and spread the word that you are seeking employment.

PATIENT-CENTERED PROFESSIONALISM

- *How do patients benefit when medical assistants perform an effective job search that matches them to positions they are qualified for and that interest them?*

DEVELOPING YOUR MATERIALS

Before you graduate and start looking for employment, begin developing materials that tell employers about who you are. Do not create a resumé the night before your interview; writing a resumé and good cover letters is a skill that takes time and practice. Create several versions of your resumé and ask teachers or someone you trust to critique them. Practice writing cover letters in answer to potential advertisements.

These two written documents act as an introduction to any potential employer. The cover letter introduces you to the employer, and the resumé highlights your qualifications. The resumé and cover letter should provide an overview of your education, employment history, and relevant experiences.

After reading these documents, the employer should want to learn more about you and your qualifications in an interview.

Unless specifically noted in an advertisement, resumés and cover letters should always be typed. Be sure neither document contains typographical errors or awkward grammar. Careful proofreading will help you find and correct errors before the documents are sent to a prospective employer. It is often difficult to see your own mistakes, so it is important to have a friend, teacher, or counselor review your job-seeking materials. Human nature suggests that we see what we want to see. For example, if you have been looking at your resume for hours, you might not see that you have typed "Registration of patience" instead of "Registration of patients." (The spell-check function on your computer will not catch this type of error because everything is spelled correctly; however, it does not make sense.) Any mistakes or "typos," even small ones, reduce your chances of getting an interview.

Resumé

The purpose of a **resumé** is to pique the interest of the prospective employer and schedule an interview. Although the cover letter may be read first, the resumé contains the information the employer most wants to see. Therefore your resumé must create a good first impression of you, your skills, and your experience. Computer software packages are available that provide guidelines, formatting styles, and suggestions for constructing a presentable resumé. If you do not have access to such software, or you want to individualize your resumé, consult the reference section of your library for "How To" books on resumé writing. As already emphasized, resumés should always be typed or printed on good-quality white or ivory paper, without any frills (e.g., borders, colored print).

Box 47-2 provides "do" and "don't" guidelines for resumé writing, and Box 47-3 describes two common resumé formats—chronological and functional (Figures 47-1 and 47-2). There is no one format that must be followed, but all resumés should include certain information needed by the employer, as follows:

- *Heading.* The **heading** is located at the top of the paper and includes your "demographics" (e.g., name, address, home telephone number, cellular phone number, and e-mail address, if available).
- *Objective.* Think of an **objective** as a career goal. Remember that your career goal must specifically match what the employer wants and needs. It is a good idea to adjust the objective of your resumé to match the position more closely each time you send out a resumé (Box 47-4).
- *Education and experience.* This section should contain a brief history of your work experience and a concise summary of your education. As a new medical assistant, you should begin with an educational summary. List your most significant education or training first. Then, list your present or most recent employment experience, and work back into the past. Include basic activities of each particular job, especially those that relate to the job you are seeking.

BOX 47-2

"Do"s and "Don't"s of Resumé Writing

DO:
- Be truthful and accurate.
- Keep sentences and paragraphs short.
- Use simple terms.
- Use correct spelling, punctuation, and grammar.
- Design to sell your strengths.
- Keep the resumé:
  (1) Neat
  (2) Brief
  (3) Concise
  (4) Easy to read
  (5) Relevant to the job objective

DON'T:
- Attach photographs.
- Include salary information.
- List gender, age or birthdate, weight, height, marital status, or health status.
- List education or experiences you never had.
- Inflate your previous job responsibilities.
- Use someone as a reference who will not give you a good recommendation.
- Use vague or elaborate jargon.

BOX 47-3

Common Resumé Formats

There is no "best" format for resumé writing. Select the format that is most appropriate for the type of position you are seeking, for your experience and education, and for the aspects of your resumé you want to highlight. The format chosen may be a combination of both the chronological and the functional resumé.

CHRONOLOGICAL RESUMÉ

A chronological resumé lists education and job experiences as they have occurred in order. This can be from the present to the past or the past to the present. However, the most common format is from the present to the past, or most recent experience first (Figure 47-1). Your current education level and current employment status would be listed first. Be prepared to explain any time gaps in your education or employment in an interview. Chronological resumés are the type used most often and are especially good for recent graduates and those with direct experience in the desired career field.

FUNCTIONAL RESUMÉ

A functional resumé relates your skills to the type of employment you seek (Figure 47-2). If you are looking for a job in an entirely new career and do not have direct experience, a functional resumé can be used to highlight the indirect experiences and transferable skills that will help you in the new career. Since functional resumés are organized by job skill rather than date, this type of resumé may deemphasize employment or education gaps.

```
                    Ruby Dunham
                9362 Caesar Creek Road
                   Mytown, OH 45458
                    (937) 555-1899
```

OBJECTIVE

- To obtain a position as a medical assistant

EDUCATION

- 2004: A.S. in Medical Assisting, Community College, Mytown, OH

EXPERIENCE

2001–present: Medical Transcriptionist, Community Hospital, Mytown, OH

- Transcribe 55 wpm
- Excellent attendance record
- Detail oriented
- Increased personal productivity each quarter

1999–2001: Secretary, State University School of Medicine, Mytown, OH

- Coordinated schedules of four full-time professors
- Maintained office supplies
- Created final examination scheduling guidelines for department
- Developed excellent written communication skills
- Operated a variety of office machines

1996-2000: Shift Manager, Burger World, Mytown, OH

- Managed 10 employees, including hiring, training, evaluating, and firing
- Developed excellent oral communication skills and team player concept
- Improved inventory control techniques, reducing losses by 10%
- Maintained cleanliness standards highest in chain
- Developed customer-focused service goals for store

FIGURE 47-1 Example of a chronological resumé. (From Chester GA: *Modern medical assisting*, Philadelphia, 1998, Saunders.)

BOX 47-4

Examples of Career Objective on Medical Assistant Resumé

- Entry-level position in the medical assisting field
- To secure a medical assistant position
- Seeking a position of challenge in a medical office environment
- To secure a medical assistant position within a medical office that will utilize my education and life experiences

NOTE: Avoid using "I."

```
                    Max Bryan, CMA
                1234 Rolling View Court
                   Mytown, OH 45431
                    (937) 555-3137
```

OBJECTIVE

- An entry-level position in medical assisting, with the opportunity to utilize and refine skills and training

EDUCATION

- 2004: A.S. in Medical Assisting, Community College, Mytown, OH. Dean's list senior year, cumulative GPA 3.5

STRENGTHS

- Possess excellent interpersonal and communication skills
- Demonstrate consistent positive attitude and high energy
- Caring and compassionate
- Responsible, self-motivated, precise in work
- Experienced in customer-focused service

ACCOMPLISHMENTS

- Tutored students in medical assisting and 12-lead ECG courses. Received excellent evaluations and positive results
- Certified Medical Assistant, active member of local AAMA
- Experienced in MS Office programs
- Consistent "excellent" ratings in clinical externships

COMMUNITY ACTIVITIES

- 1999–present: Organized, recruited, and trained 20 others for church hand bell choir, direct weekly practices and monthly performances
- 2000–present: Teach community CPR twice yearly to high school students
- Vice-President Student Government, Community College, Mytown, OH. Recruited members, organized fund raisers, campaigned successfully for policy changes

EMPLOYMENT

- 2002–present: Tutor, Community College, Mytown, OH
- Waiter, Scott's Place, Mytown, OH

FIGURE 47-2 Example of a functional resumé. (From Chester GA: *Modern medical assisting*, Philadelphia, 1998, Saunders.)

Use action words to describe job responsibilities or accentuate your strengths on a resumé (Box 47-5). Also, eliminate the use of "I." Instead of saying, "I supervised ten people," say, "Supervised ten people." List appropriate job-related skills.

- *Community activities.* Every medical practice draws on the community for its patients, and staff members often are involved in local community activities as a way to promote the practice. Always list your community or volunteer activities; for example, if you are the chairperson of a local blood drive, be sure to mention this. Such information shows you have organizational skills and that you are a well-rounded candidate.
- *References.* Do not list the actual **references** on your resumé but indicate they will be provided on request. Go to an interview with a properly typed list of references, including name, title, address, phone number, name of company, when you worked there, and which of your skills they are qualified to address. Always ask permission to use someone as a reference before putting the person on your list. Choose your references carefully. Use persons of responsibility: teachers, supervisors, former employers, and associates from professional organizations (Table 47-1).

FOR YOUR INFORMATION

There is no regulation that mandates that an employer conduct reference checks; however, employers can be held liable for negligent hiring when an employee performs an act that could have been foreseen by the employer had they completed a background check.

A good resumé is appealing to the eye, brief, and to the point. In addition, it is important to be truthful in your resumé. Do not exaggerate your employment history or skills because potential employers will always discover the truth when they speak with your references.

Cover Letter

A **cover letter** accompanies a resumé and basically introduces the medical assistant to the person in charge of screening job applicants. The letter should be brief, accurate, and concise. Ask yourself, "What do I expect this employer to understand about me from my letter?" and write the letter accordingly. It is best to revise your cover letter or create a new one every time you apply for a different job. This practice allows you to customize the cover letter to the individual company or business with the advertised position and prevents the appearance of a "form letter." Do not forget to change the date of the cover letter.

When typing your cover letter, use an appropriate format and writing style (see Chapter 22). Always proofread for spelling, grammar, keyboarding, or punctuation errors. Do not rely solely on your computer to catch errors. Ask at least two people to proofread your cover letter. Failure to do so may allow some errors to slip through, leaving the potential employer with the impression that you are careless.

Most cover letters contain the following paragraphs (Figure 47-3):

- The first paragraph identifies the position you are applying for and how you heard about it.
- The second paragraph should convince the employer that you would be an asset to the medical practice if hired. Always highlight the aspects of your educational and work experience that directly relate to the current job. Mention your enclosed resumé but do not summarize it in the cover letter.
- In the final paragraph, thank the employer for considering your resumé and ask for an interview.

BOX 47-5

Action Verbs to Use for Resumé Writing

accomplished	introduced
achieved	maintained
analyzed	managed
applied	measured
communicated	organized
conducted	planned
coordinated	prepared
created	presented
delegated	proposed
demonstrated	reviewed
developed	revised
established	supervised
generated	verified
increased	

PATIENT-CENTERED PROFESSIONALISM

- What is the impact on patients when prospective medical assistants are able to develop effective cover letters and resumés? How does the information in cover letters and resumés help physicians establish which applicants would be the most suitable for the available positions?

TABLE 47-1

Sample Reference List

Name, Title	Company Address and Phone Number	Time Period	Capacity
Mary Smith, Office Manager	Barkley Office Supply 1802 Allan Street Boon, PA 01010 215-555-4567	June to September 1990	Summer job taking inventory of office supplies. Ms. Smith was my supervisor.
Dean Allan, Volunteer Coordinator	Robert Barter Hospital 145 Rose Street Pember, PA 00022 871-555-9807	September 1990 to present	I volunteer at the hospital on weekends. Mr. Allan assigns duties for my shift.
Dr. Harry Klissel	Family Practice Associates 14322 George Pike Pember, PA 00022 871-555-7865	Current employer	Dr. Klissel is retiring and closing his practice. I have been his medical assistant for the past 5 years.

FIGURE 47-3 Example of a cover letter.

> 1555 High Street
> Stoyville, GA 00448
> November 1, 20XX
>
> Ms. J.C. Fagen
> Office Manager
> Medical Practice, Inc.
> 1000 S. Grant Street
> Stoyville, GA 00448
>
> Dear Ms. Fagen,
>
> Your ad for a medical assistant in *The Tribune* prompts this inquiry. I am a recent graduate of a medical assisting program in the area.
>
> My training at Medical Career College and work experience in the service industry appears to parallel the job description you provided in the ad. My medical assisting diploma includes an externship in a local medical office. My 12 months of training includes exposure to both an administrative and clinical setting. My 4.0 grade point average indicates my positive achievement record, which I have earned. The enclosed resume further details my qualifications.
>
> Please call me at your convenience at (898) 555-5555 to schedule an interview.
>
> Sincerely,
>
> *Charlene Wink*
> Charlene Wink
>
> Enclosure: 1

CONTACTING POTENTIAL EMPLOYERS

Once you have identified a job opportunity and prepared your resume, the next step is to contact the employer. The four primary ways to contact an employer are (1) fax, (2) electronic mail (e-mail), (3) telephone, and (4) standard mail (U.S. Postal Service). If a method of contact is specified, use the employer's preferred method (e.g., if e-mail is requested, use e-mail contact; if mailing a resume and cover letter is requested, use standard mail contact). If a method of contact is not specified, select the method most appropriate to the type of employer and position.

Regardless of the method you use, written documents will be needed. Any documents sent to employers, including your resume, cover letter, and supporting documents, should be free of errors. Keep a log of ads you have answered and employers you have contacted, to avoid sending your resume to the same place twice. This list can also serve as a follow-up reminder for future contact (Table 47-2).

Fax

Many medical offices place classified ads that describe the type of practice in the newspaper and request that a resume be forwarded to the fax number provided.

> *Example:*
> Wanted: Medical Assistant
> Busy Palm Harbor internal medicine office. Previous internal medicine experience preferred but will train right candidate. Certification expected within one year of hire. Duties include front and back office. Excellent benefits package, including tuition. Fax resume to 777-555-4567.

Websites and E-Mail

Often, a local medical society may have a website where physicians can post openings. Hospitals, large clinics, some private practices, and employment agencies also have websites where job opportunities are posted. The local chapter of your profes-

TABLE 47-2

Sample Job Log

Employer	Type of Ad and Contact	Response	Follow-Up
Hart Haven Hospital	Newspaper ad: the Tribune 1/12/XX Allen Arnold, Human Resources Fax: 806-555-2134	Cover letter and resumé sent by fax 1/14/XX	1/18/XX interview arranged
Ralston Clinic	Job hotline phone: 888-555-9090 Listed on 1/10/xx	Cover letter and resumé sent to e-mail address for clinic on 1/12/XX: graciea@ralston.xxx	Job still posted on hotline 1/16/XX

sional organization may also have a website with employment opportunities. The website will provide an e-mail address where the employer or agency may be contacted.

E-mail is increasingly becoming an acceptable form for responding to job postings. An e-mail address is often provided for sending cover letters and resumés. The e-mail may be used for a cover letter, and the resumé can be attached as a separate file and sent over the Internet.

Telephone

Some employment ads request that potential employees call a particular person to receive information. Medical office managers use the telephone call to screen job applicants. Because a medical assistant's office duties often involve communication skills, the telephone is a good way to screen job applicants. Remember, how you communicate is a major part of your overall image. What the office manager hears from you indicates the degree of professionalism you have attained.

If you telephone a prospective employer, keep the following guidelines in mind:

1. Call from a quiet area with no background noise or distractions (e.g., children, TV). If you are using a cellular phone, make sure it is fully charged.
2. Have a pencil and paper ready to take down important information.
3. Before answering a question, organize in your mind what you want to say and use proper grammar. Do not use slang and inappropriate language.
4. Speak clearly and keep your voice confident, pleasant, and not too loud or too soft.
5. When the telephone interview is completed, ask where you can send your resumé and thank the interviewer for his or her time.

Standard Mail

A job posting or position announcement may ask the job seeker to send his or her resumé, along with a cover letter, by standard mail. When preparing your materials for mailing, make sure they are neat. Again, print your resumé and cover letter on plain, good-quality white or ivory paper. Check carefully that you have correctly spelled the name and title of the person receiving your materials. Be sure to put your signature in the appropriate place on the cover letter. Make certain you have typed the correct address on the envelope and affixed the necessary amount of postage before mailing.

PATIENT-CENTERED PROFESSIONALISM

- How does the medical assistant's knowledge of the various methods of contacting prospective employers result in better care for patients?

THE JOB APPLICATION

A **job application** provides a potential employer with many details about you and your life. Even if you have sent in a resumé, most employers also require that you fill out a job application (Figure 47-4). As a potential employee, how you complete the application shows the employer how neat and organized you are. Many employers ask applicants to complete a job application at the interview so that they can see firsthand how the applicant spells, communicates in writing, and follows directions.

Typical information required on a job application includes the following:

- Complete name and address
- Social Security number (may be optional; when hired, must be provided)
- Telephone number where you can be reached during business hours and in the evening. Include your cell phone number, if you have one. You may need to record a new, professional-sounding voice message on your answering machine or voice mail if you are expecting prospective employers to call.
- Training or schools attended
- Past employment, salary, duties, responsibilities, and reason for leaving

When filling out a job application, neatness counts (Box 47-6). This is your chance to demonstrate your ability to complete paperwork in a neat, organized fashion. Always use a pen (or type, if possible) and print legibly. Use correct spelling and recheck for errors. Make an extra copy of your resumé to check exact dates.

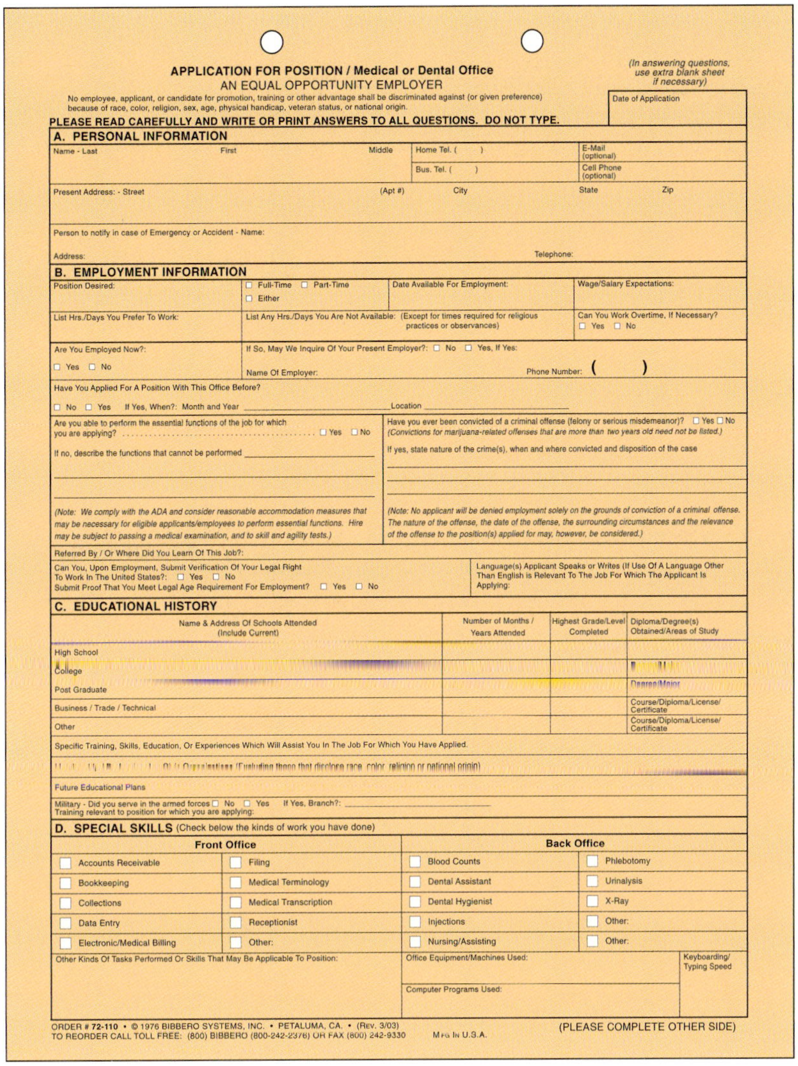

(In answering questions, use extra blank sheet if necessary)

APPLICATION FOR POSITION / Medical or Dental Office
AN EQUAL OPPORTUNITY EMPLOYER

No employee, applicant, or candidate for promotion, training or other advantage shall be discriminated against (or given preference) because of race, color, religion, sex, age, physical handicap, veteran status, or national origin.

Date of Application

PLEASE READ CAREFULLY AND WRITE OR PRINT ANSWERS TO ALL QUESTIONS. DO NOT TYPE.

A. PERSONAL INFORMATION

Name - Last | First | Middle | Home Tel. ( ) | Bus. Tel. ( ) | E-Mail (optional) | Cell Phone (optional)

Present Address: - Street | (Apt #) | City | State | Zip

Person to notify in case of Emergency or Accident - Name:
Address: | Telephone:

B. EMPLOYMENT INFORMATION

Position Desired: | ☐ Full-Time ☐ Part-Time ☐ Either | Date Available For Employment: | Wage/Salary Expectations:

List Hrs./Days You Prefer To Work: | List Any Hrs./Days You Are Not Available: (Except for times required for religious practices or observances) | Can You Work Overtime, If Necessary? ☐ Yes ☐ No

Are You Employed Now?: ☐ Yes ☐ No | If So, May We Inquire Of Your Present Employer?: ☐ No ☐ Yes, If Yes: Name Of Employer: | Phone Number: ( )

Have You Applied For A Position With This Office Before?
☐ No ☐ Yes If Yes, When?: Month and Year ________ Location ________

Are you able to perform the essential functions of the job for which you are applying? ☐ Yes ☐ No
If no, describe the functions that cannot be performed ________
(Note: We comply with the ADA and consider reasonable accommodation measures that may be necessary for eligible applicants/employees to perform essential functions. Hire may be subject to passing a medical examination, and to skill and agility tests.)

Have you ever been convicted of a criminal offense (felony or serious misdemeanor)? ☐ Yes ☐ No
(Convictions for marijuana-related offenses that are more than two years old need not be listed.)
If yes, state nature of the crime(s), when and where convicted and disposition of the case
(Note: No applicant will be denied employment solely on the grounds of conviction of a criminal offense. The nature of the offense, the date of the offense, the surrounding circumstances and the relevance of the offense to the position(s) applied for may, however, be considered.)

Referred By / Or Where Did You Learn Of This Job?:

Can You, Upon Employment, Submit Verification Of Your Legal Right To Work In The United States?: ☐ Yes ☐ No
Submit Proof That You Meet Legal Age Requirement For Employment? ☐ Yes ☐ No

Language(s) Applicant Speaks or Writes (If Use Of A Language Other Than English is Relevant To The Job For Which The Applicant Is Applying:

C. EDUCATIONAL HISTORY

	Name & Address Of Schools Attended (Include Current)	Number of Months / Years Attended	Highest Grade/Level Completed	Diploma/Degree(s) Obtained/Areas of Study
High School				
College				
Post Graduate				Degree/Major
Business / Trade / Technical				Course/Diploma/License/ Certificate
Other				Course/Diploma/License/ Certificate

Specific Training, Skills, Education, Or Experiences Which Will Assist You In The Job For Which You Have Applied.

[illegible] Organizations (Excluding those that disclose race, color, religion or national origin)

Future Educational Plans

Military - Did you serve in the armed forces ☐ No ☐ Yes If Yes, Branch?: ________
Training relevant to position for which you are applying:

D. SPECIAL SKILLS (Check below the kinds of work you have done)

Front Office		Back Office	
☐ Accounts Receivable	☐ Filing	☐ Blood Counts	☐ Phlebotomy
☐ Bookkeeping	☐ Medical Terminology	☐ Dental Assistant	☐ Urinalysis
☐ Collections	☐ Medical Transcription	☐ Dental Hygienist	☐ X-Ray
☐ Data Entry	☐ Receptionist	☐ Injections	☐ Other:
☐ Electronic/Medical Billing	☐ Other:	☐ Nursing/Assisting	☐ Other:

Other Kinds Of Tasks Performed Or Skills That May Be Applicable To Position: | Office Equipment/Machines Used: | Computer Programs Used: | Keyboarding/ Typing Speed

ORDER # 72-110 • © 1976 BIBBERO SYSTEMS, INC. • PETALUMA, CA. • (REV. 3/03)
TO REORDER CALL TOLL FREE: (800) BIBBERO (800-242-2376) OR FAX (800) 242-9330 MFG IN U.S.A.
(PLEASE COMPLETE OTHER SIDE)

A

FIGURE 47-4 Application for employment. **A,** Front, **B,** Back. (Courtesy Bibbero Systems, Inc., Petaluma, CA; (800) 242-2376; Fax (800) 242-9330; www.bibbero.com.)

BOX 47-6

Job Application Guidelines

1. Print all answers accurately and neatly.
2. Do not leave spaces blank. Use "N/A" (not applicable) or a dash to indicate the question was read but does not apply.
3. Account for periods of time not working in a positive manner. For example, "returned to school for graduate degree" or "volunteered at a clinic."
4. Account for reasons for leaving previous employment in an honest manner. For example, "reduction in workforce" or "unsafe working environment."
5. Answer potential salary questions as "open" if amount is not known. For example, "what salary would you expect for this position?"
6. Provide a phone number where a message can be left (both home and cell phone numbers).

NOTE: Bring an extra copy of your resumé so that you can easily reference dates, names, etc. Also, bring a separate list of references in case you are asked to provide them.

FIGURE 47-4, cont'd

> **PATIENT-CENTERED PROFESSIONALISM**
>
> - Job applications are an important part of the process of screening and gathering information from applicants. How does the patient benefit when prospective medical assistants complete job applications carefully and accurately?

THE JOB INTERVIEW

If your contact with the employer (whether through your resumé and cover letter, a phone screening, or other contact) was successful, you may be offered a **job interview.** The interview is your chance to make a good personal impression. It should be a "win-win" situation for both you and the interviewer. It is your opportunity to tell the interviewer about yourself and why you would like to work at the medical facility. It is also your chance to ask questions to make sure the position is right for you (Boxes 47-7 and 47-8).

Be aware that more than one person may talk with you at the interview. An office manager or clinical supervisor may interview you first and then present you to the physician(s) in the practice.

Before the Interview

You can prepare yourself for the interview by visualizing (1) what you want the interviewer to remember about you and (2) how you can leave these impressions. Follow these guidelines:

1. *Do your homework.* See if the potential employer has a website. If so, check it for current information. Are they adding beds to the hospital or physicians to the practice? The more you know about the employer in advance, the more confident you will be in asking intelligent questions.

2. *Make a list of questions* you need to ask for your own information. What are the benefits? Is there tuition assistance, on-site training, and opportunities for advancement? What is the vacation policy? Employers are impressed by organized, thoughtful questions that show you took the time to come prepared.

BOX 47-7

Interview Topics of the Employer and the Potential Employee

EMPLOYER
1. What will you bring to this medical office?
2. How much will it cost to hire you?
3. What is your motivation and work ethic?
4. Will you get along with the other employees and the patients?
5. Will you stay, or will you leave for a better offer?

POTENTIAL EMPLOYEE
1. Will the work environment be acceptable?
2. Will the salary and benefit package meet my needs?
3. Is there room to grow? Can I advance my skills and responsibilities?
4. How long will I find satisfaction with this job?

BOX 47-8

"Do"s and "Don't"s of Job Interviewing

DO:
- Find out as much as you can about the physician's office, especially the type of practice.
- Request directions to the interview.
- Practice answering possible interview questions before you go.
- Bring an extra copy of your resumé.
- Turn off your cellular phone when you enter the office.
- Be prepared with a typed list of several references, including names, addresses, and phone numbers.
- Arrive early.
- Dress appropriately (limit jewelry, cover tattoos).
- Go alone.
- Introduce yourself to the interviewer.
- Use a firm handshake and make eye contact.
- Wait to be asked to sit down.
- Place both feet on the ground and sit up straight.
- Show interest in what the interviewer has to say.
- Be enthusiastic, smile, and maintain eye contact.
- Sound professional. Avoid expressions such as, "Like, you know?"
- Ask questions.
- Keep answers to questions focused on the topic.
- Thank the interviewer at the end of the interview for his or her time and consideration.

DON'T:
- Arrive late.
- Wear inappropriate clothing (e.g., capris, sandals).
- Talk about personal problems.
- Complain about previous employers or fellow employees.
- Use slang or profanity.
- Chew gum, eat candy, or smoke before or during the interview.
- Wear heavy perfume, aftershave, or excessive makeup.
- Arrive with a cup of coffee in your hand.

3. *Be punctual.* A few days before the interview, do a "test run" to see how long it takes you to arrive at the location. This helps to ensure that you will not get lost or be late on the day of the interview.
4. *Dress professionally.* The day before the interview, select the clothes you will wear and be sure they are appropriate, clean, and pressed. If you are not wearing clinical attire, you should dress conservatively. Men should wear a jacket, shirt, and tie. Women should wear an appropriate-length skirt or slacks. Avoid tight-fitting, trendy, or flashy clothing. Decide how early you will need to shower, get dressed, and prepare for the interview the next day.
5. *Be enthusiastic.* Get plenty of sleep the night before the interview (it's hard to be enthusiastic when you're tired). Eat a good breakfast (or lunch if an afternoon interview).
6. *Make eye contact.* Practice answering interview questions and maintaining eye contact by role playing with a friend or relative.
7. *Review questions* you could be asked and plan how you will answer each. Role playing can help in this area as well.

When the time for your interview arrives, remember that first impressions are vital. Arriving early gives you time to gain your composure and not feel rushed. Wear appropriate clothing and be well groomed. Do not smoke (odor stays on clothes); do not chew gum; and do not wear heavy perfume, aftershave, or excessive makeup.

At the Interview

Greet your interviewer with a friendly smile, direct eye contact, and a firm handshake (Figure 47-5). Even if you have already sent a resumé to the office, always bring an extra copy with you. Make sure you bring your list of references. Remember, the resumé gets you the interview, but the interview gets you the job. The job interview is a professional situation, therefore do not use "street language" or slang terms. Always make direct eye contact with the interviewer (Figure 47-6).

Some interviewers start with small talk to "break the ice." Do not try to lead the conversation; the interviewer already

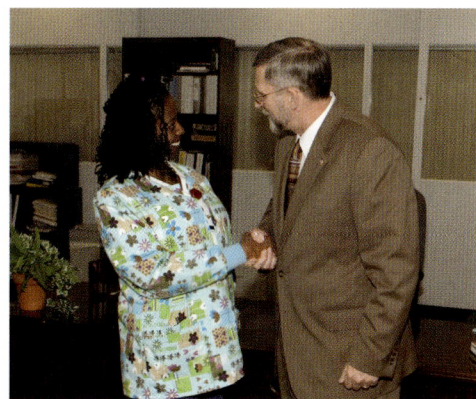

FIGURE 47-5 Greet your interviewer with a smile and a handshake.

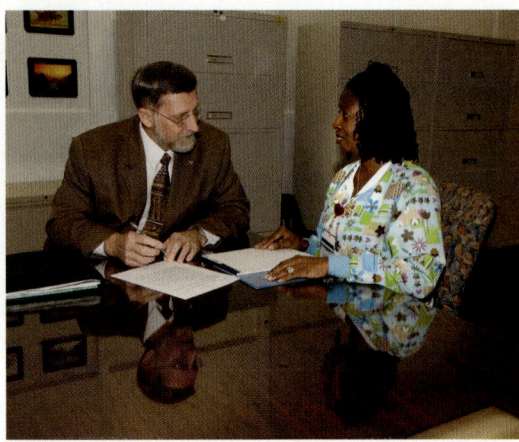

FIGURE 47-6 Make direct eye contact during the interview.

has decided what is to be asked and discussed. Box 47-9 lists questions commonly asked by employers at interviews.

Follow the lead of the interviewer; you can ask questions during lulls in the conversation, or you can ask them at the end of the interview. When asking questions, be sure to ask about the medical practice (e.g., patient load, growth plans, and other offices). Develop a clear idea of what you will be doing in the office; ask for a job description if one is available. Understand the expected hours of work and what orientation training is available. Do not be afraid to ask for a tour of the office or to meet the other staff, if possible.

When answering questions, have an understanding of how to respond. Be prepared for difficult questions if your resumé prompts them (e.g., "Why have you changed positions so often?"; "Why is there a lapse of 6 months when you were not employed nor in school?"; "Why have you not gone for certification?"). You should have honest answers to such questions ready because the employer has every reason to ask them.

> *Examples:*
> **Types of Interview Responses by Question**
> *"Do you think"* questions (e.g., "Do you think you will be able to work the hours specified?") require a *straightforward* and *logical* answer.
> *"How do you see"* questions (e.g., "How do you see yourself working with the different cultural groups who come to this office?") require a *thoughtful* answer.
> *"How do you feel"* questions (e.g., "How do you feel about referring someone to hospice?") require an *honest* answer.
> *"How would you handle"* questions (e.g., "How would you handle a patient who is always late for an appointment?") require an *action-oriented* answer.

Always answer questions completely and honestly. Use more than one-word answers to demonstrate your ability to communicate effectively. If an interviewer asks you something that you cannot answer, say so honestly. If the interviewer mentions a required skill in which you know you are weak, admit it immediately. Be prepared to say you are willing to learn and improve in that area. Always be a good listener.

Some topics are "off-limits" in interviews, meaning it is illegal for employers to ask job seekers certain questions (Box 47-10).

The interviewer should discuss at length exactly what the job entails, and outline salary, fringe benefits, and insurance. Do not argue about a salary that you feel is too low. Do inquire about the raise policy. At the end of the interview, you may

---

BOX 47-9

Typical Interview Questions or Statements

- *"Tell me about yourself."* This is a great opportunity to let the interviewer know why you are unique. This is a summary of who you are, what your achievements and skills are, and why you should be hired. For example, "Since graduating 2 years ago, I have been working at the hospital's eye clinic, where I was selected for advanced training in lens fitting."
- *"What did you like most about your former employer?"* The response to this will indicate qualities that you admire. For example, indicating that you liked the way your employer handled stressful situations will indicate that you too can "think on your feet."
- *"What did you like least about your former employer?"* Do not speak badly of your former employer, but refer to qualities that you find important. The response will provide an awareness of qualities you feel are important. For example, if your former employer was disorganized, the interviewer would expect you to be organized.
- *"What are your strengths?"* Choose from either your technical skills or personal traits. This should be answered to fit the job qualifications. For example, if the job requires multitasking (e.g., scheduling, answering phones), mentioning that you can perform several tasks at one time provides the interviewer with an idea of how you will fit into the busy practice. Assess your strengths honestly.
- *"What are your weaknesses?"* Do not answer "none," since this gives the impression that you are unrealistic. Use this question to show that you recognize you have weaknesses and are working on correcting them in a positive manner. For example, "I can't say 'no,' but I am learning that I must have time for myself and my family" shows your ability to assess a situation.
- *"What would you do if ... ?"* This type of question allows the employer to identify your ability to problem-solve, adapt to change, and work as a team member.
- *"Where would you expect to be professionally 5 years from now?"* Perhaps you are not yet certified, but you are preparing for the test. At some point, you may return to school for additional credits toward a bachelor's degree. Have a plan for professional development; employers know they reap the benefits.

BOX 47-10

Acceptable and Unacceptable Ways for Employers to Ask Interview Questions

AGE
Acceptable: "Are you over the age of 18?"
  Unacceptable: "How old are you?" "What is your date of birth?" "What year did you graduate from high school?"

RELIGION
Acceptable: "Can you work Saturdays and Sundays?"
  Unacceptable: "What church do you belong to?" Any question that inquires into a job applicant's religious background is illegal.

GENDER
Acceptable: No question regarding gender is acceptable.
  Unacceptable: "Do you wish to be addressed as Mrs., Miss, or Ms.?" "Do you have children?" "Do you plan to have more children?" "What arrangements have you made for child care?"

RACE
Acceptable: Stating that a photograph may be required after hiring is acceptable.
  Unacceptable: Stating that a photograph will be required with the application and asking about a person's ethnic origin are unacceptable.

SALARY
Acceptable: "What are your salary expectations?"
  Unacceptable: "What is the lowest salary you will accept?"

DISABILITY
Acceptable: "Is there any reason why you would not be able to perform the duties of this job?"
  Unacceptable: "Do you have any disabilities?" "What prescription drugs are you taking?"

RESIDENCE
Acceptable: "What is your place of residence?"
  Unacceptable: "Do you own or rent?"

MILITARY SERVICE
Acceptable: "Did you serve in the U.S. Armed Forces?"
  Unacceptable: "Are you currently in the military reserves?"

---

be offered a job on the spot or the interviewer may tell you he or she will get back to you in a day or so after all the applicants have been interviewed. If you are offered the job and you would like a day or two to think over the offer, let the interviewer know exactly when you will reply with your answer. Never accept an offer without knowing the entire package (preferably in writing): pay scale, benefits, vacation, education benefits, and so on. It is not unusual for an employer to follow up a job offer with a formal letter detailing the offer and benefits package.

At the end of the interview, always thank the interviewer for the opportunity to interview for the position and shake the person's hand. Ask when a decision on hiring will be made.

After the Interview

Always send a follow-up note or "letter of thanks" to the interviewer (Figure 47-7). This reaffirms that you are interested in the position and also leaves a good impression. Send a thank-you note whether you are hired or not. Being courteous is part of the job-seeking process, and the follow-up letter keeps your name in the employer's mind. Even if the employer decides you are not right for this position, he or she may keep your resumé on file for future positions.

If, despite your best efforts, you are not hired, do not become discouraged. Learn from each experience so that you can improve for your next interview. Immediately after each interview, jot down the questions you were asked, what went well, and what could have been done or answered differently. Work to improve any deficiencies, and keep looking for the position that best suits you.

PATIENT-CENTERED PROFESSIONALISM

- What is the benefit to patients when the medical assistant provides clear, informative information during an interview and has successful interviewing skills?
- Why might it be good for patients if a medical assistant decides that, based on the interview, he or she does not want to accept the job?

CONCLUSION

Completing your training to become a medical assistant is a great accomplishment. The reward for this accomplishment is securing a good job as a medical assistant. To get a job that is right for you, you must know where to look, how to develop materials that highlight your skills and training, and how to present yourself positively in an interview.

Once you are hired, you will have the opportunity to apply your administrative and clinical medical assisting skills with patients. Keeping the patient at the center of all your actions will help you provide the best care possible to patients and be a great asset to your employer. "Patient-centered professionalism" means being diligent, responsible, honest, and proactive; communicating clearly; following all procedures and guidelines; and practicing safety precautions to protect yourself, patients, and other staff members. Patient-centered professionalism helps ensure continued growth in both your skills as a medical assistant and your value to the practice. It will also help you make a positive difference in the lives of all the patients with whom you interact, which is one of the most rewarding aspects of the medical assisting profession.

> 411 Park Street
> Brooks, FL 33512
> December 1, 20XX
>
> Ms. Jane Delany
> Medical Lab Office
> 1807 Main Street
> Brooks, FL 33512
>
> Dear Ms. Delany,
>
> It was a pleasure to meet with you on Friday. Thank you for the opportunity to interview for the medical assistant position.
>
> I was pleased with what I learned about your office and your approach to patient service. Your attitude towards professionalism reflects my view.
>
> I am excited about the possibility of working with you and hope to be considered for one of the available positions.
>
> Sincerely,
>
> *Mary Marshall*
> Mary Marshall

FIGURE 47-7 Example of a follow-up (thank-you) letter.

Chapter Summary

Reinforce your understanding of the material in this chapter by reviewing the curriculum objectives and key content points below.

1. **Define, appropriately use, and spell all the Key Terms for this chapter.**
   - Review the Key Terms if necessary.
2. **List and briefly describe six methods of locating job positions.**
   - Classified ads in a newspaper list available positions with requirements.
   - School placement services assist the student in developing tools for the job search and often provide interview opportunities.
   - Employment agencies provide employment opportunities for a fee.
   - Direct contact of a medical practice can be done through their Internet site or in person.
   - Internet searches can be done by position and location.
   - Networking involves "contacts" made professionally, educationally, and socially.
3. **Explain the purpose of a resumé.**
   - A resumé provides information about an individual that will interest a prospective employer enough to arrange an interview.
4. **List two formats that can be used to create resumés and explain the focus of each.**
   - Chronological resumés are good for recent graduates or those with direct experience in the desired career field. Information can be organized from most recent to earliest or vice versa.
   - A functional resumé can be used to highlight indirect experiences and transferable skills that will help in a new career.
   - Review Box 47-3.
5. **List five sections that should always be included in a resumé.**
   - The resumé should contain a heading, a stated objective, a listing of the applicant's education and experience, any relevant community activities, and a notation that references will be provided on request.
6. **Explain the purpose of a cover letter.**
   - The cover letter's purpose is to introduce an applicant to the person in charge of screening applicants.

7. **Describe the information that should be included in the first, second, and final paragraphs of a cover letter.**
   - The first paragraph identifies the position you are applying for and how you heard about it.
   - The second paragraph convinces the employer that you would be an asset to the medical practice or facility.
   - The final paragraph asks for an interview.
8. **Briefly describe four methods that medical assistants can use to contact prospective employers.**
   - Faxing a cover letter and a resumé is often preferred by a medical practice.
   - Electronic mail is gaining use as a way to present a cover letter and resumé.
   - Telephone calls are often used to screen job applicants.
   - Standard mail is the traditional form of response in which a cover letter and the resumé are mailed to the medical facility.
9. **Explain the purpose of a job application.**
   - A job application provides the employer additional information about the job applicant.
   - Job applications also provide the employer insight into the applicant's ability to be organized and neat and to follow directions.
10. **List five guidelines for completing a job application.**
    - Review Box 47-6.
11. **Explain the purpose of a job interview, and list four issues the medical assistant should mention and five topics the employer should address during the interview.**
    - A job interview provides the job applicant a chance to meet the employer face-to-face, lets the employer know about the applicant, and allows for questions from both employer and applicant.
    - Review Box 47-7.
12. **Describe ways you can prepare for a job interview.**
    - Check if your prospective employer has a website, and review it for current information about the facility or practice.
    - Prepare a list of questions for the employer.
    - Visualize what you want the interviewer to remember about you and your interview.
    - Make arrangements to be on time.
    - Select the clothes that you will wear the day before the interview.
    - Get a good night's sleep and eat well before the interview.
    - Practice answering possible interview questions and making eye contact.
13. **Provide clear, accurate, positive answers to six questions typically asked by employers during an interview.**
    - Review Box 47-9.
14. **Explain the importance of sending a follow-up note or "letter of thanks" after an interview.**
    - A follow-up letter or note is courteous and lets the employer know of your continued interest in the position. It is also another way of putting your name in front of the employer again before an employment decision is made.
15. **Analyze a realistic medical office situation and apply your understanding of the job-seeking process.**
    - Creating professional, truthful, informative, error-free job-seeking materials can help you in obtaining a job.
    - Following the expected protocols of job seeking (e.g., having correctly formatted materials, communicating effectively in person and in writing, and following up with interviews) will make you more successful in your job search.
16. **Describe the impact on patient care when medical assistants have a solid understanding of the knowledge and skills necessary to seek and obtain a job for which they are qualified and that they find fulfilling and rewarding.**
    - When medical assistants have a job that is a good fit for their skills, beliefs, and lifestyle, they feel more fulfilled and are more likely to devote themselves to providing excellent patient care.

PRACTICAL APPLICATIONS

If you have accomplished the objectives in this chapter, you will be able to make better choices as a medical assistant. Take another look at this situation and decide what you would do.

Dora has recently completed a medical assisting program and will be looking for new employment as a medical assistant in an ambulatory care setting. As she begins her search, she goes to the school placement office to see if the counselor knows of any jobs in the area. The counselor, Ms. Smith, states that she is unaware of any openings at present but will keep Dora in mind should someone call.

Next, Dora turns to the newspaper ads. She writes her resumé and cover letter quickly because she is excited about a position she saw advertised in the classifieds. She is typically good at writing, so she doesn't bother to ask a friend to proofread her resumé and cover letter this time. (After all, it would only slow her down.) She is in such a hurry to apply for the job in the newspaper that she does not proofread or spell-check her materials. As a result, several words are misspelled, and the information that is supposed to be in chronological order is not.

Despite the errors on Dora's resumé and cover letter, she obtains an interview with a potential employer. When she arrives, she is surprised that the employer expects her to complete an application before the interview. After completing the application, she answers the employer's interview questions and asks a few of her own. Overall, she has a good feeling about this interview.

After the interview, Dora returns home and waits to hear from the potential employer, taking no further action and hoping that she has been chosen for the job.

Do you think Dora would be hired for this job? What would you have done differently?

1. What are the advantages of using a newspaper ad?
2. With whom would you network when seeking employment in your area?
3. If you were the employer, how would you feel about a resumé that had misspelled words? Would you still consider hiring this person?
4. Who should proofread a resumé? Why?
5. Why is the order of work experience on a resumé important?
6. If an ad requests that an applicant apply "in person" and you send a fax or e-mail, do you think the employer would consider your application? Explain your answer.
7. Why is a cover letter so important?
8. Why do you think that an employer may ask applicants to complete an application at the interview? What do you need to do to make a good impression on the application?
9. Why is a thank-you letter after an interview important?
10. Do you think you would have been chosen for the job if you had made the above mistakes? Explain your answer.

WEB SEARCH

1. **Research the website of the medical society in your area.** Many medical societies will assist their physician members in listing positions available at individual practices.

- **Keywords:** Use the following keywords in your search: Medical Society (use state and then find by county or parish).

Common Abbreviations, Acronyms, and Symbols

APPENDIX A

SYMBOLS

At	@
change	Δ
decrease; below	↓
degree	°
divide	÷
equal parts	aa
equals	=
female	♀
foot, minute	′
greater than	>
inch, second	″
increase	↑
infinity	∞
less than	<
male	♂
micro	μ
multiply, times	×
negative	−
none, without	Ø
number, pound	#
ounce	℥
percent	%
positive	+
ratio, "is to"	:
recipe, prescription, or take	℞
therefore	∴

ACRONYMS

AIDS	acquired immunodeficiency syndrome
APGAR	appearance, pulse, grimace, activity, respiration
BUN	blood urea nitrogen
CAT	computed axial tomography
CPAP	continuous positive airway pressure
DEXA, DXA	dual-energy x-ray absorptiometry
GERD	gastroesophageal reflux disease
HIPAA	Health Insurance Portability and Accountability Act of 1996
LASER	light amplification by stimulated emission of radiation
LASIK	laser-assisted in-situ keratomileusis
LEEP	loop electrocautery excision procedure
NSAID	nonsteroidal antiinflammatory drug
PET	positron emission tomography
SARS	severe acute respiratory syndrome
SIDS	sudden infant death syndrome
SOAP	subjective, objective, assessment, plan
TENS	transcutaneous electrical nerve stimulation
TURP	transurethral resection of the prostate

MEDICAL ABBREVIATIONS

A

a	before, artery
aa	of each
ABO	blood groups
ac, a.c.	before meals
AC	air conduction
Acc	accommodation
ACTH	adrenocorticotropic hormone
AD	admitting diagnosis, advance directive, Alzheimer disease
ad lib	freely, as needed, at pleasure
ADH	antidiuretic hormone
ADHD	attention-deficit hyperactivity disorder
ADL, ADLs	activities of daily living
AF	atrial fibrillation
AFB	acid-fast bacillus
AFP	alpha-fetoprotein test
AI	aortic insufficiency
AKA	above-knee amputation
ALS	amyotrophic lateral sclerosis
AMA	American Medical Association, against medical advice
ANA	antinuclear antibody
ANS	autonomic nervous system
AP	anteroposterior, apical pulse
aq	water (aqua), H$_2$O
ARDS	adult respiratory disease syndrome
ARF	acute renal failure
ARMD	age-related macular degeneration
AS	aortic stenosis
ASA	aspirin (acetylsalicylic acid)
ASAP	as soon as possible
ASD	atrial septal defect
ASHD	arteriosclerotic heart disease
astigm	astigmatism
AV	atrioventricular

B

BaE, BE	barium enema
BaS	barium swallow
baso	basophil

1167

BC	bone conduction		CPX	complete physical examination
BCP	birth control pill		CRF	chronic renal failure
BD	bipolar disorder		C-section, CS	cesarean section
BF	black female		CSF	cerebrospinal fluid
BID, bid	twice a day (*bis in die*)		CT, CAT	computed (axial) tomography
BKA	below-knee amputation		CTS	carpal tunnel syndrome
BM	black male, bowel movement		CV	cardiovascular
BMR	basal metabolic rate		CVA	cerebrovascular accident
BP, B/P	blood pressure		Cx	cervix
BPH	benign prostatic hypertrophy		CXR	chest x-ray film (radiograph)
bpm	beats per minute		cysto	cystoscopic examination
BSA	body surface area			
BSE	breast self-examination			
Bx	biopsy			

C

c	calorie
C	Celsius, centigrade
$\bar{c}$	with
C-1, C1	first cervical vertebra
C-2, C2	second cervical vertebra
C&S	culture and sensitivity
Ca^{++}	calcium
CA	cancer, chronological age
CA 125	tumor marker to monitor ovarian cancer
CA 15-3	tumor marker to monitor breast cancer
CA 19-9	tumor marker for pancreatic, stomach, and bile duct cancer
CA 27-29	tumor marker to check for recurrence of breast cancer
CAD	coronary artery disease
CAM	complementary and alternative medicine
Cap	capsule
cath	cardiac catheterization
CBC	complete blood count
CC	chief complaint
CCU	coronary care unit
CHD	coronary heart disease
CHF	congestive heart failure
CICU	cardiology intensive care unit, coronary intensive care unit
CK	creatine kinase
Cl^-	chloride
cm	centimeter
CMA (AAMA)	certified medical assistant
CNS	central nervous system
c/o	complains of
CO	carbon monoxide, cardiac output
CO_2	carbon dioxide
COLD	chronic obstructive lung disease
COPD	chronic obstructive pulmonary disease
CP	cerebral palsy
CPE	complete physical examination
CPK	creatine phosphokinase
CPR	cardiopulmonary resuscitation

D

d	day
D_5W, D5W	5% dextrose in water
D_5S, D5S	5% dextrose in saline
DAW	dispense as written
D&C	dilation and curettage
DDS	doctor of dental surgery
DEA	Drug Enforcement Administration
Decub	pressure ulcer
DI	diabetes insipidus
diff	differential WBC count
dil	dilute
DM	diabetes mellitus
DMD	doctor of medical dentistry
DNA	deoxyribonucleic acid
DNR	do not resuscitate
DOA	dead on arrival
DOB	date of birth
DOE	dyspnea on exertion
DPT	diphtheria, pertussis, tetanus
dr, ʒ	dram, drain
drsg, dsg	dressing
DSD	dry sterile dressing
d/t	due to
DTR	deep tendon reflex
DTs	delirium tremens
DVT	deep vein thrombosis
Dx	diagnosis

E

EBV	Epstein-Barr virus
ECG, EKG	electrocardiogram
ECHO	echocardiography
EDC	estimated date of confinement
EEG	electroencephalogram
EENT	eyes, ears, nose, throat
EGD	esophagogastroduodenoscopy
EMG	electromyography
elix	elixir
ENT	ear, nose, throat
EOM	extraocular movements
eos, eosins	eosinophil
ER	emergency room

ERT	estrogen replacement therapy		HGH	human growth hormone
ESR	erythrocyte sedimentation rate		HIV	human immunodeficiency virus
ESRD	end-stage renal disease		H/O	history of
ESWL	extracorporeal shock wave lithotripsy		HOH	hard of hearing
EST	exercise stress test		HPF	high-power field
et	and		HSV	herpes simplex virus
ETOH	alcohol		ht	height
			HTN	hypertension
			Hx	history
			hypo	under, hypodermic

F

F	Fahrenheit, female
FB	foreign body
FBS	fasting blood sugar
Fe	iron
FEV	forced expiratory volume
FH	family history
FHR	fetal heart rate
FHS	fetal heart sound
FHT	fetal heart tone
Fl	fluids
FOBT	fecal occult blood test
FSH	follicle stimulating hormone
FUO	fever of unknown origin
Fx	fracture

I

I&D	incision and drainage
IBS	irritable bowel syndrome
IC	irritable colon
ICU	intensive care unit
ID	interdermal
IDDM	insulin-dependent diabetes mellitus
IgA, IgD, IgG, IgM, IgE	immunoglobulins A, D, G, M, and E
IM	intramuscular
inf	infection
instill	instillation
I&O	intake and output
IOP	intraocular pressure
IUD	intrauterine device
IV	intravenous
IVC	intravenous cholangiogram
IVP	intravenous pyelogram

G

g, gm	gram
GA	gastric analysis; gestational age
Ga	gauge
GB	gallbladder
GC	gonococcus
GERD	gastroesophageal reflux disease
GI	gastrointestinal
GP	general practice, general practitioner
gr	grain
grad	gradually
gtt, gtts	drop, drops
GTT	glucose tolerance test
GU	genitourinary
GYN, gyn	gynecology

K

K^+	potassium
kg	kilogram
KJ	knee jerk
KUB	kidney, ureter, bladder

L

ⓛ, L, lt	left
L	liter
L-1, L1	first lumbar vertebra
L-2, L2	second lumbar vertebra
LA	left atrium
lab	laboratory
Lap	laparoscopy
lat	lateral
lb	pound
LE	lupus erythematosus
LH	luteinizing hormone
liq	liquid
LLL	left lower lobe
LLQ	left lower quadrant
LMP, lmp	last menstrual period
LP	lumbar puncture
LPF	lower power field

H

h, hr	hour
H&H	hemoglobin and hematocrit
H_2O	water
Hb, HGB, hgb	hemoglobin
HBV	hepatitis B virus
HCl	hydrochloric acid
hCG	human chorionic gonadotropin
HCT, Hct, hmct	hematocrit, packed-cell volume
HEENT	head, eye, ear, nose, throat
HgA, HgC, HgE, HgF, HgS	hemoglobins A, C, E, F, and S

LPN	licensed practical nurse	**O**	
LS	lumbosacral	O	oral, O₂, oxygen
LUL	left upper lobe	OB	obstetrics
LUQ	left upper quadrant	OB-GYN	obstetrics and gynecology
LV	left ventricle	OC	oral contraceptive
LVN	licensed vocational nurse	OD	overdose
L&W	living and well	OM	otitis media
lymphs	lymphocytes	OP	outpatient
		OPD	outpatient department
		OPS	outpatient service
M		OR	operating room
M, m	male, meter	os	mouth
m, ♏	minim	OT	occupational therapy
MA	mental age, medical assistant	OTC	over-the-counter (drug)
mcg, μg	microgram	oz	ounce
MCH	mean corpuscular hemoglobin (amount of Hgb in each RBC)		
MCHC	mean corpuscular hemoglobin concentration (amount of Hgb per unit of blood)	**P**	
		p̄	after
MCV	mean corpuscular volume (size of individual RBC)	P	pulse
		PA	posteroanterior, physician assistant
MD	muscular dystrophy	PAC	premature atrial contractions
mEq/L	milliequivalent per liter	Pap	Papanicolaou smear, stain, or test
mets	metastasis	PAT	paroxysmal atrial tachycardia
mg	milligram	path	pathology
MI	myocardial infarction	PBI	protein-bound iodine
mL	milliliter	pc, p.c.	after meals
mm	millimeter	PCN	penicillin
MMPI	Minnesota Multiphasic Personality Inventory	PCO₂	carbon dioxide pressure
		PE	physical examination, pulmonary embolism
MMR	measles, mumps, rubella (vaccine)	PERRLA	pupils equal, round, reactive to light and accommodation (normal)
MRI	magnetic resonance imaging		
MS	multiple sclerosis, mitral stenosis	PFS	pulmonary function studies
MSDS	material safety data sheet	PH	past history
MVP	mitral valve prolapse	pH	H⁺ concentration; denotes acidity and alkalinity
		PI	present history, previous illness
N		PID	pelvic inflammatory disease
Na⁺	sodium	PKU	phenylketonuria
N/A	not applicable	pm	afternoon, evening
NB	newborn	PMH	past medical history
NF	National Formulary	PMS	premenstrual syndrome
NGU	nongonococcal urethritis	PNS	peripheral nervous system
NIDDM	non–insulin-dependent diabetes mellitus	po, PO	by mouth (*per os*)
NKA	no known allergies	post	posterior
NKDA	no known drug allergy	pp	after meals (postprandial), after eating
noc, noct	night	PRL	prolactin
non rep	do not repeat	prn	as the occasion arises (*pro re nata*), as needed
NP	nurse practitioner		
NPO, npo	nothing by mouth	pro time	prothrombin time
NR	no refill	pt	patient, pint
NS	normal saline	PT	physical therapy; prothrombin time
NSR	normal sinus rhythm	PTA	percutaneous transluminal angioplasty
N&V	nausea and vomiting	PTH	parathormone
		PTT	partial thromboplastin time

PU	peptic ulcer		sol	solution
PVC	premature ventricular contraction		sp. gr.	specific gravity
PX	physical examination		S/S, S&Sx	signs and symptoms
			staph	staphylococcus
			stat, STAT	immediately
			STD	sexually transmitted disease
			strep	streptococcus
			subQ, Sub-Q	subcutaneous
			syr	syrup

Q

q	every
q2d	every 2 days
q3d	every 3 days
q2h	every 2 hours
q3h	every 3 hours
q4h	every 4 hours
qh	every hour
qid	four times a day
QNS	quantity not sufficient
QS, qs	quantity sufficient
qt	quart

T

T, temp	temperature
T-1, T1	first thoracic vertebra
T-2, T2	second thoracic vertebra
T_3	triiodothyronine
T_4	thyroxine
T&A	tonsillectomy and adenoidectomy
tab	tablet
TB	tuberculosis
TFS	thyroid function studies
TIA	transient ischemic attack
tid	three times a day (ter in die)
TLC	total lung capacity, tender loving care
top	topical
TPN	total parenteral nutrition
TPR	temperature, pulse, and respirations
tr	tincture
TSE	testicular self-examination
TSH	thyroid-stimulating hormone
TUR	transurethral resection
Tx	treatment

R

R	right, rectal
RA	rheumatoid arthritis, right atrium
rad	radiation absorbed dose
RAIU	radioactive iodine uptake
RBC	red blood cell, erythrocyte
RDS	respiratory distress syndrome
REM	rapid eye movement
RF	rheumatoid factor
Rh	rhesus factor in blood
RLL	right lower lobe
RLQ	right lower quadrant
RMA	registered medical assistant
RN	registered nurse
RNA	ribonucleic acid
R/O	rule out
ROM	range of motion
RUL	right upper lobe
RUQ	right upper quadrant
RV	right ventricle
Rx	prescription, treatment

U

U/A, UA	urinalysis
UGI	upper gastrointestinal
ung	ointment
URI	upper respiratory infection
USP	United States Pharmacopeia
UTI	urinary tract infection
UV	ultraviolet

V

v	vein
VA	visual acuity
VD	venereal disease
VDRL	Venereal Disease Research Laboratories (sometimes used loosely to mean a venereal disease report)
VF	visual field
vol	volume
VS	vital signs

S

s̄	without
SA	sinoatrial
segs	segmented neutrophils
SGOT (AST)*	serum glutamic-oxaloacetic transaminase (aspartate transaminase)
SGPT (ALT)*	serum glutamic-pyruvic transaminase (alanine transaminase)
SI	sacroiliac
Sig	instructions to patient
SL	sublingual
SLE	systemic lupus erythematosus
SLR	straight leg raising
SOB	shortness of breath

W

WBC	white blood cell, leukocyte
WDWN	well developed, well nourished

*Enzyme tests of liver function.

WF	white female	**Y**	
WM	white male	y	year
WNL	within normal limits	YOB	year of birth
wt, wgt	weight		

2004 National Patient Safety Goals: JCAHO "Do Not Use" List and ISMP Error-Prone Abbreviations, Symbols, and Dose Designations

Symbol or Abbreviation	Mistaken for	Should Write Instead
U (for unit)	Zero, four, or cc	"unit"
IU (for international unit)	IV (intravenous) or 10	"international unit"
Q.D., Q.O.D. (for "once daily" and "every other day")	Mistaken for each other: the period after the Q can be mistaken for an "I," and the "O" can be mistaken for "I."	"daily" and "every other day"
H.S. (for half-strength or for bedtime)	Half-strength or hour of sleep (at bedtime). q.H.S. mistaken for every hour	"half-strength" or "at bedtime"
S.C. or S.Q. (for subcutaneous)	SL for sublingual, or "5 every"	"Sub-Q," "subQ," or "subcutaneously"
D/C (for discharge)	Discontinue (and whatever medications follow)	"discharge"
c.c. (for cubic centimeter)	U (units) when poorly written	"mL" for "milliliters"
A.S., A.D., A.U. (for left, right, or both ears)	OS, OD, and OU	"left ear," "right ear," or "both ears"
O.D., O.S., O.U. for right, left, or both eyes	Mistaken for AD, AS, AU	"right eye," "left eye," or "both eyes"
Trailing zero (X.0) or lack of leading zero (.X mg)	Decimal point missed	Always write a zero before a decimal point (e.g., "0.6 mg").
MS (for morphine sulfate)	Magnesium sulfate	"morphine sulfate" or "magnesium sulfate"
SS	55	"sliding scale"; use "one-half" or ½
> and < for greater than and less than	Mistaken as opposite of intended; mistakenly use incorrect symbol; "<10" mistaken as "40"	"greater than" or "less than"
/ to separate two doses or indicate "per"	Mistaken as number 1 (e.g. "25 units/10 units" misread as "25 units and 110 units")	"per" to separate doses
@ for at	Mistaken as "2"	"at"
& for and	Mistaken as "2"	"and"
+ for plus or and	Mistaken as "4"	"and"
° for hour	Mistaken as "0" (e.g., "q2°" seen as "q20")	"hr," "h," or "hour"

From Joint Commission on Accreditation of Healthcare Organizations, 2004, and Institute for Safe Medication Practices, 2003.

Common Prefixes and Suffixes

APPENDIX B

Root word, prefix, or suffix	Meaning
A	
a-	no; not; without
ab-	away from
abdomin/o	abdomen
-abrasion	scraping
-ac	pertaining to
acid/o	acid
acous/o	hearing
acr/o	extremities; arms or legs
-ad; ad-	toward
aden/o	gland
adenoid/o	adenoids
adip/o	fat
adren/o, adrenal/o	adrenal glands
adrenalin/o	adrenalin
-aemia	blood
aer/o	air
agglutin/o	clumping
-al	pertaining to
alb/o, albin/o	white
albumin/o	protein
algesi/o	sensitivity to pain
-algia	pain
alkal/o	alkaline
all/o	other
alveol/o	alveolus; air sac
amb/i/o	both; around
amni/o; -amnios	amnion
amyl/o	starch
an-	not; without
-an	pertaining to
an/o	anus
andr/o	male; masculine
angi/o	vessel
ankyl/o	stiff; crooked; bent
ante-	before
anter/o	front
anthrac/o	coal
anti-, ant	against
apo	opposed; derived from
aort/o	aorta
append/o, appendic/o	appendix
-ar	pertaining to
arachn/o	arachnoid; spider
arteri/o, arter/o	artery
arteriol/o	arteriole
arthr/o	joint
articul/o	joint
-ary	pertaining to
-ase	enzyme
-asis	condition; pathological state
-asthenia	weakness
astr/o	star
ather/o	yellow, fatty plaque
atri/o	atrium
audi/o	hearing
aur/o	ear
aut/o; auto-	self
axill/o	armpit; axilla
az/o, azot/o	nitrogen
B	
bacter/i, bacteri/o	bacteria
bas/o	bottom; base
bi-	two
bi/o	life; living
-blast; blast/o	embryonic form
blephar/o	eyelid
brachy/o	short, small
brady-	slow
bronch/o, bronchi/o	bronchi (pl); bronchus (sing)
bronchiol/o	bronchiole
bucc/o	cheek
burs/o	bursa; sac
C	
calc/o, calcul/o	calcium; stone
calcane/o	calcaneus (heel bone)
cancer/o	cancer
-capnia	carbon dioxide
carcin/o	cancer of epithelial origin
-cardia	heart condition
cardi/o, card/o	heart
carp/o	carpus (wrist bones)
caud/o	tail
cec/o	cecum
-cele	hernia; tumor; swelling of
-centesis	surgical puncture; removal of fluid
cephal/o	head

1173

cerebell/o	cerebellum; little brain	dis-	negative; absence of
cerebr/o	cerebrum; brain	dist/o	distant; far
cervic/o	neck; cervix uteri	diverticul/o	diverticular
cheil/o	lip	dors/i/o	back; dorsal surface
chem/o	chemical	-drome	to run
chir/o	hand	duoden/o	duodenum
chlor/o	green	-dynia	pain
chol/e	gall; bile	dys-	bad; difficult; painful
cholecyst/o	gallbladder		
choledoch/o	common bile duct		
chondr/o	cartilage		
chori/o	chorion		
chrom/o	color	**E**	
-cidal	killing	ec-	outside; out of
circum-	around	-eal	pertaining to
-clasia; -clasis	break	ech/o: echo-	sound
-clast	to break	-ectasia, -ectasis	stretching; dilation
clavicul/o	clavicle (collarbone)	ecto-	situated on or outside
-cle, -cule	small, little	-ectomy	excision; surgical removal
cleid/o	clavicle	-edema	swelling
-clysis	irrigation; washing out	electr/o	electricity
coagul/o	coagulation; clot	-emesis	vomiting
coccyg/o	coccyx (tailbone)	-emia	blood condition
col/o	colon; large intestine	en-	inside, into
colp/o	vagina	encephal/o	brain
coni/o	dust; cone	end-, endo-	inside
contra-	against	enter/o	intestine; small intestine
cost/o	ribs	epi-	above; upon
crani/o	cranium; skull	epiglott/o	epiglottis
crin/o; -crine	secrete	episi/o	vulva
cry/o	cold	-er	one who
crypt/o	hidden	erythr/o	red
-cusis	hearing	es-	out of
cutane/o	skin	-esis	state of
cyan/o	blue	eso-	inward
-cyesis	pregnancy	esophag/o	esophagus
cyst/o	bladder; cyst; sac	esthesi/o, -esthesia	feeling, sensation of
cyt/o; -cyte	cell	etio-	cause of
-cytosis	abnormal increase of cells	eu-	good, normal
		ex-	out; without; away from
		exo-	outside; outward
		extra-	outside

D		**F**	
dacry/o	tear	femor/o	femur
dactyl/o	digits; fingers or toes	ferr/i/o	iron
de-	down; from; reversing; not	fet/o	fetus
demi-	half	fibr/o	fiber; fibrous
dendr/o	tree	fibrin/o	fibrin
dent/i, dent/o	teeth	fibul/o	fibula
derm/a, dermat/o	skin	-fida	split
-desis	binding; fusion	-flux	flow
dextro-	right	fore-	front
di-	twice; two; through	fruct/o	fruit
dia-	through; between; complete	fung/i	fungus
dipl/o	double; two	-fusion	pouring; to pour
dips/o; -dipsia	thirst		

G

galact/o	milk
gastro, gastero	stomach
gen/o; -genic; -genesis; -genous	beginning; origin
genit/o	organs of reproduction
ger/a; ger/o; geront/o	old; elderly
gigant/o	large
gingiv/o	gums
glomerul/o	glomerulus
gloss/o	tongue
glyc/o; glycos/o	sugar
gon/o	genitals; reproduction
gonad/o	gonads (ovaries or testes)
-grade	to go
-gram	a record; unit of metric system
gram/o	to record; a tracing or mark
-graph	instrument for recording
-graphy	process for recording
-gravida	pregnancy
gynec/o, gyn/o	female

H

heli/o	sun
hem/a, hem/o, hemat/o	blood
hemi-	half
hemoglobin/o	hemoglobin
hepat/o	liver
heter/o	different; other
hidr/o	sweat; perspiration
hist/o	tissue
hol/o	entire; complete
home/o, homo-	constant; sameness; like
humer/o	humerus (upper arm bone)
hydr/o, hydra	water
hyper-	excessive; more than normal
hypo-, hyph	beneath; below normal; less than
hypn/o	sleep
hyster/o	uterus

I

-ia; -iasis	condition
-iac	pertaining to
-iatrics; -iatry	medicine
-ic	pertaining to
ichthy/o	fish
idio-	individual
ile/o	ileum
ili/o	ilium; flank
immun/o	immune
in-	not; inside, within
infer/o	inferior; situated below
infra-	below
inguin/o	groin
inter-	between
interstit/o	space between
intra-	within
iod/o	iodine
-ion	process
irid/o	iris
is/o	equal
ischi/o	ischium
-ism	condition
-ist	one who specializes; specialist
-itis	inflammation
-ium	membrane; structure

J

jejun/o	jejunum
juxta-	close to; in proximity to

K

kal/i	potassium
kary/o	nucleus
kerat/o, ker/o	horny; hard, cornea
kilo-	thousand
kinesi/o, -kinesis, -kine	movement
kyph/o	humped

L

lacrim/o	tear
lact/o	milk
lapar/o	abdominal wall
-lapse	to sag: to fall
laryng/o	larynx (voice box)
later/o	side
lei/o	smooth
-lepsy	seizure
leuk/o	white
leut/o	yellow
lingu/o	tongue
lip/o	fat
lith/o; -lith, -lite	stone; calculus
-logist	one who studies; one who specializes in the study of
-logy	study or science of
lumb/o	lower back
lymph/o	lymph; lymphatics
lymphat/o	lymphatics
lys/o	destruction; separation; dissolving; breakdown
-lysin	that which destroys
-lysis	process of destroying; separating; breakdown
-lytic	capable of destroying; separating

M

macr/o, macro-	large
mal-	bad
malac/o, -malacia	soft; softening
mamm/o	breast
-mania	excessive preoccupation; excessive excitement
mast/o	breast
medi/o, med-, mid-	middle
mediastin/o	mediastinum
megal/o, -megaly	large; enlarged, enlargement
melan/o	black
men/o	month; menses
mening/o	meninges
ment/o	mind
meso-	middle
meta-	change; next (as in a series)
-meter	instrument used to measure
metr/o	measure; uterine tissue
-metry	process of measuring
micro-	small
mio-	smaller; less
-mission	sending
mon/o	one or single
morph/o	form; shape
muc/o	mucus
multi-	many
muscul/o	muscle
my/o	muscle
myc/o	fungus
myel/o	bone marrow; spinal cord
myocardi/o	heart muscle
myring/o	eardrum

N

narc/o	sleep, stupor
nas/o	nose
nat/o	birth
natr/o	sodium
necr/o	death
neo-	new
nephr/o	kidney
neur/o	nerve
non-	no; against
norm/o	normal
nos/o	disease; facility related
nucle/o	nucleus
nulli-	none

O

ob-	against
occipit/o	occiput
ocul/o	eye
odont/o	teeth
-odynia, adyn/o	pain
-oid, -ode	resembling; shape; form
-ole	small
olig/o	few
-oma	tumor
omphal/o	umbilicus (navel)
onc/o	tumor; mass
onych/o	nail
oo/o	egg
oophor/o	ovary
ophthalm/o	eye
-opia; opt/o, optic/o	vision; sight
-opsy	viewing
or/o	mouth
orchi/o; orchid/o	testis, testicle
orth/o	straight
os-	mouth; bone
-ose	sugar; carbohydrate
-osis	condition; disease; increase
oste/o	bone
-ostomy	creating an outlet
ot/o	ear
-ous	pertaining to; characterized by
ovi-, ovo-	egg
ox/o, oxy/o	oxygen

P

pach/y	thick
palat/o	palate
pan-	all of; entire
pancreat/o	pancreas
papul/o	pimple
par-, para-	near; beside; abnormal
-para	woman who has given birth
-paresis	slight, paralysis
par/o	to give birth
patell/o	patella (kneecap)
path/o; -pathy, -pathic	disease; emotion
ped/o	foot
pedi/o	child
pelv/i	pelvis
-penia	deficient; decreased
-pepsia	digestion
per-	throughout
peri-	around
periton/o	peritoneum
pes-	foot
pex/o; -pexy	surgical fixation
-phagia	swallowing
phag/o	eat; ingest
phalang/o	phalanges (finger and toe bones)
pharmac/o	drugs; medicine
pharyng/o	throat; pharynx
phas/o; -phasia	speech
phil/o; -pil, -philia	attraction
phleb/o	vein

-phobia	abnormal fear	-rrhagia, rrhage	hemorrhage; bursting forth of blood
phon/o	voice	-rrhaphy	suture; repair of
-phoresis	transmit	-rrhea	flow; discharge
phot/o	light	-rrhexis	rupture
phren/o	diaphragm; mind	rube-	red
-phylaxis	protection		
physi/o	nature		
-physis	growth		
pituitar/o	pituitary gland		

S

plas/o; -plasia	formation; development	sacchar/o	sugar
plast/o; -plasty	surgical repair	sacro-	sacrum
pleg/o; -plegia	paralysis	salping/o	uterine tubes; auditory tube; fallopian tube
pleur/o	pleura; rib area		
-pnea	breathing	-sarcoma	cancerous tumor of connective tissue
pneum/o	air; lung		
pneumon/o	lung	scapul/o	scapula (shoulder blade)
-pod; pod/o	foot	-schisis; schis/o, schiz/o, schisto-	split
-poiesis	production		
poikil/o	irregular	scler/o; -sclerosis	hard; hardening; white of eye
poly-	many	scop/o	examine; to view; to observe
post	after; behind	-scope	instrument used for viewing
poster/o	behind; toward the back	-scopic	pertaining to visual examination
-praxis	practice	-scopy	process of visually examining
pre-	before	seb/o	sebum
presby-, presby/o	elder; old age	semi-	half
primi-	first	semin/o	semen
pro-	before; for	seps/o	infection
proct/o	anus; rectum	sept/o	infection; septum
prostat/o	prostate gland	ser/o	serum
prote/o	protein	sial/o	saliva; salivary glands
proxim/o	near	-sis	state of
pseud/o	false	skelet/o	skeleton; skeletal system; bone
psych/o	mind	som/a, somat/o	body
-ptosis	sag; prolapse	son/o	sound
-ptysis	spitting	-spasm	cramp; twitching
pub/o	pubis	spermat/o	spermatozoa
pulm/o, pulmon/o	lungs	spher/o	round
py/o	pus	splen/o	spleen
pyel/o	renal pelvis	spondyl/o	vertebrae (spine)
pylor/o	pylorus	staphyl/o	cluster; uvula
pyr/o	fire; heat; fever	-stasis	stopping; controlling
		-stenosis, sten/o	stricture; narrowing
		stern/o	sternum (breastbone)

Q

quadri-	four	stert/o	fat
		steth/o	chest
		stomat/o	mouth
		-stomy	formation of an opening

R

rach/i, rachi/o	spine	strept/o	twisted
radi/o	radius; radiant energy	sub-	below; under
re-	back; repeat	super/o	situated above or uppermost
rect/o	rectum	super-	above; excess
ren/o	kidney	supra-	above; beyond
retro-	behind; backward	syn-	jointed; together
rheumat/o	rheumatism		
rhin/o	nose		

T

rhiz/o	root (spinal nerve root)	tachy-	fast; rapid
rhytid/o	wrinkle	tars/o	tarsals; edge of eyelid

tel/e	distant	ultra-	excess; more than; beyond
ten/o, tend/o	tendon	uni-	one
tendin/o, tenden/o	tendon	ur/o	urine; urinary tract
test/o	testes	ureter/o	ureter
tetra-	four	urethr/o	urethra
therm/o	heat	-uria	urine
thorac/i/o	chest	urin/o	urine; urination
thromb/i/o	clot or thrombus	uter/o	uterus
thym/o	thymus		
thyr/o, thyroid/o	thyroid gland		
tibi/o	tibia	**V**	
-tic	pertaining to	vag/o	vagus nerve
tom/o	to cut	vagin/o	vagina
-tome	instrument used in cutting	valv/o; valvul/o	valve
-tomy	incision; cutting	vas/o	vessel; duct; vas deferens
tonsill/o	tonsil	ven/o	vein
top/o	place; position	ventr/o	ventral; belly side
tox/o, toxic/o	poison	ventricul/o	ventricle of brain or heart
trache/o	trachea (windpipe)	venul/o	venule
trans-	through; across	vertebr/o	vertebrae
-tresia	opening	viscer/o	viscera; internal organ
tri-	three	vulv/o	vulva
trich/o	hair		
-tripsy	surgical crushing		
trop/o	to stimulate; to turn	**X**	
troph/o; -trophy	nutrition; development	xanth/o	yellow
-tropic	stimulate	xer/o	dry
-tropin	that which stimulates	xiph/i/o	xiphoid process
tympan/o	tympanic membrane		
		Y	
U		-y	condition or state
-ule	small		
uln/o	ulna		

Common Laboratory Test Values

APPENDIX C

NOTE: Common reference values may vary depending on the testing.

NORMAL URINE REFERENCE VALUES

Urine Volume

Age	Normal Reference Range (mL/24 hours)
Newborn	20-350
Child	300-1500
Adult	750-2000

Physical and Chemical Characteristics of Urine

Physical	Normal Reference Values	Average
Color	Straw (yellow) to amber, light to dark	Yellow
Turbidity	Clear to slightly hazy	Clear
Specific gravity	1.005-1.030	1.010-1.025
pH	5-8	6.5
Protein	Negative–trace	—
Glucose	Negative	—
Ketone	Negative	—
Bilirubin	Negative	—
Blood	Negative	—
Urobilinogen	0.1-1 EU/dL	0.1-1 EU/dL
Bacteria (nitrites)	Negative	—
Leukocyte esterase	Negative	—

Urine Sediment

Microscopic	Normal Reference Values
RBCs/HPF	Rare
WBCs/LPF	0-4
Epith/HPF	Occasional (may be higher in females)
Casts/LPF	Occasional hyaline
Bacteria	Negative
Mucus	Negative to 2+
Crystals	Only crystals, such as cystine, leucine, and tyrosine, are considered clinically significant.

NORMAL BLOOD CHEMISTRY REFERENCE VALUES

Test	Reference Range
Alanine transaminase (ALT) (SGPT)	4-36 U/L
Albumin	3.5-5.5 g/dL
Alkaline phosphatase (ALP)	30-120 U/L
Aspartate transaminase (AST) (SGOT)	0-35 U/L
Bicarbonate (HCO_3^-)	21-28 mEq/L
Bilirubin (total)	0.3-1 mg/dL
Blood urea nitrogen (BUN)	10-20 mg/dL
Calcium	9-10.5 mg/dL
Chloride	98-106 mEq/L
Cholesterol	<200 mg/dL
Creatinine	0.5-1.2 mg/dL
C-reactive protein	<1 mg/dL
Gamma-glutamyl transferase (GGT)	8-38 U/L
Glucose	70-110 mg/dL
Iron	60-180 mcg/dL
Phosphorus	3-4.5 mg/dL
Potassium	3.5-5 mEq/L
Sodium	136-145 mEq/L
T_3 (triiodothyronine)	75-220 mcg/dL
T_4 (thyroxine)	4-12 mcg/dL
Total protein (albumin/globulin)	6.4-8.3 g/dL
Triglycerides (TGs)	40-160 mg/dL
Uric acid	2.6-7.2 mg/dL

NORMAL HEMATOLOGY REFERENCE VALUES

Test	Reference Range
Hemoglobin	
Newborns	16-23 g/dL
One year	9.5-14 g/dL
Six years	10-15.5 g/dL
Adult males	14-18 g/dL
Adult females	12-16 g/dL
Microhematocrit	
Newborns	44%-64%
One year	30%-40%
Six years	32%-44%

Adult males	42%-52%	
Adult females	37%-47%	

Leukocyte Counts

Newborns	9-30 × 10⁹/L	9000-30,000/mm³
Children ≤2 years	6.2-17 × 10⁹/L	6200-17,000/mm³
Adults	5-11 × 10⁹/L	5000-11,000/mm³

Erythrocyte Counts

Newborn	4.8 × 7.1 × 10¹²/L	4.8-7.1 million/mm³
One year	4 × 5.5 × 10¹²/L	4.0-5.5 million/mm³
Six years	4 × 5.5 × 10¹²/L	4.0-5.5 million/mm³
Adult males	4.5 × 6 × 10¹²/L	4.5-6 million/mm³
Adult females	4.2 × 5.4 × 10¹²/L	4.2-5.4 million/mm³

Erythrocyte Indices

Mean corpuscular volume (MCV)	80-95 mm³/cell
Mean corpuscular hemoglobin (MCH)	27-31/RBC
Mean corpuscular hemoglobin concentration (MCHC)	32-36 g/dL

Platelet Count

Newborn	150,000-300,000/mm³
Children	150,000-400,000/mm³
Adult	150,000-400,000/mm³

Erythrocyte Sedimentation Rate (ESR)

Westergren method

Newborn	0-2 mm/hr
Children	0-10 mm/hr
Adult males	0-15 mm/hr
Adult females	0-20 mm/hr

One-Hour Sediplast ESR

Males	<50 years	0-15 mm
	>50 years	0-20 mm
Females	<50 years	0-20 mm
	>50 years	0-30 mm

Prothrombin Time

11-12.5 seconds

Partial Thromboplastin Time

60-70 seconds	Clotting times depend on the laboratory and the testing of that time for accurate clinical reference values for each test.

Bleeding Time

Ivy method	1-9 minutes

Differential Leukocyte Count

Leukocyte Type	Adult Reference Range
Neutrophil	55%-70%
Bands	3%-5%
Segs	54%-62%
Eosinophil	1%-3%
Basophil	0.5%-1%
Monocyte	3%-8%
Lymphocyte	25%-30%

Data from Pagana K, Pagana T: *Mosby's diagnostic and laboratory test reference,* ed 7, St Louis, 2005, Mosby; and *Illustrated guide to diagnostic tests*, Springhouse, PA, 1994, Springhouse. *Epith,* Epithelium; *HPF,* high-power field; *LPF,* lower power field; *RBCs,* red blood cells; *WBCs,* white blood cells.

NOTE: Results vary among laboratories.

English-to-Spanish Guide

APPENDIX D

BASIC TERMS

English	Spanish	Pronunciation
Yes	Sí	See
No	No	Noh
Please!	¡Por favor!	¡Pohr fah-bohr!
Thank you!	¡Gracias!	¡Grah-see-ahs!
You are welcome	De nada	Deh nah-dah
Health insurance	Seguro de salud	Seh-goo-roh deh sah-lood
Good morning!	¡Buenos días!	¡Boo-eh-nohs dee-ahs!
Good afternoon!	¡Buenos tardes!	¡Boo-eh-nohs tahr-dehs!
Very good!	¡Muy bien!	¡Moo-ee bee-ehn!
Hi! Hello!	¡Hola!	¡Oh-lah!
Goodbye	Adiós	Ah-dee-ohs
Who	¿Quién?	Kee-ehn
How	¿Cómo?	Koh-moh
Where	¿Dónde?	Dohn-deh
When	¿Cuándo?	Koo-ahn-doh
What	¿Qué?	Keh
Why	¿Por qué?	Pohr keh
Because	Porqué	Pohrkeh

NUMBERS

English	Spanish	Pronunciation
One	Uno	oo-noh
Two	Dos	dohs
Three	Tres	trehs
Four	Cuatro	koo-ah-troh
Five	Cinco	seen-koh
Six	Seis	seh-ees
Seven	Siete	see-eh-the
Eight	Ocho	oh-choh
Nine	Nueve	noo-eh-beh
Ten	Diez	dee-ehs
Fifteen	Quince	keen-seh
Twenty	Veinte	beh-een-the
Fifty	Cincuenta	seen-koo-ehn-tah
One hundred	Cien	see-ehn

PHRASES

English	Spanish	Pronunciation
May I help you?	¿En qué puedo servirle?	¿Ehn keh poo-eh-doh sehr-beer-leh?
Hello, my name is _____.	¡Hola! Me llamo _____.	Oh-lah mee yah-moh _____.
What is your name?	¿Cómo se llama usted?	¿Koh-moh seh yah-mah oos-tehd?
Please sit down in the waiting room.	Por favor siéntese en la sala de espera.	Pohr fah-bohr see-ehn-teh-seh ehn lah sah-lah deh ehs-peh-rah.
Do you understand?	¿Entiende?	¿Ehn-tee-ehn-deh?
I am going to ask some questions.	Voy a hacerle unas preguntas.	Voy ah ah-sehr-leh oo-nahs preh-goon-tahs.
How are you feeling?	¿Cómo se siente?	¿Koh-moh seh see-ehn-teh?
How are you?	¿Cómo está?	¿Koh-moh eh-stah?
Are you allergic to anything?	¿Tiene usted alergias?	¿Tee-eh-neh oos-tehd ah-lehr-hee-ahs?
Do you feel any pain?	¿Tiene dolor?	¿Tee-eh-neh doh-lohr?
What is the matter?	¿Qué le pasa/sucede?	¿Keh leh pah-sah/soo-seh-deh?
Is someone with you?	¿Hay alguien con usted?	¿Ah-ee ahl-gee-ehn kohn oos-tehd?
What medicines do you take?	¿Qué medicinas toma?	Keh meh-dee-see-nahs toh-mah?
Do you take any medications?	¿Toma usted algunas medicinas?	Toh-mah oos-tehd ahl-goo-nahs meh-dee-see-nahs?
Do you have any questions?	¿Tiene preguntas?	Tee-eh-neh preh-goon-tahs?
I am going to take your temperature.	Voy a tomar la temperatura.	Voy ah toh-mahr lah tem-pehr-ah-too-rah.

English	Spanish	Pronunciation	English	Spanish	Pronunciation
I am going to take your pulse.	Voy a tomar su pulso.	Voy ah toh-mahr soo pool-soh.	Speak slowly please.	Hable despacio por favor.	Ah-bleh dehs-pah-see-oh pohr fah-bohr.
I am going to take your blood pressure.	Voy a tomar su presión de sangre.	Voy ah toh-mahr soo preh-see-ohn deh sahn-greh.	I am going to give you an injection.	Voy a darte una inyección.	Voy ah dahr-teh oo-nah een-yehk-see-ohn.
			Repeat please.	Repitan por favor.	Reh-pee-than pohr fah-bohr.

Glossary

2-hour postprandial test Test measuring a patient's ability to metabolize food 2 hours after a meal.

24-hour urine specimen Collection of urine over a 24-hour period to test kidney function, checking for high levels of creatinine, uric acid, hormones, electrolytes, and medication.

A

A$_{1c}$ Hemoglobin A$_{1c}$; blood test measuring average blood glucose level over 3-month period.

AAMA American Association of Medical Assistants.

ABA number Number on all checks that identifies a payer's bank and location; assigned by American Bankers Association (ABA).

abandonment Failure to make arrangements for a patient's medical coverage.

abdominal (ab-DAHM-ih-nal) Referring or relating to the area of the abdomen.

abdominal reflex (ab-DAHM-ih-nal RE-flex) Abdominal wall draws inward on stimulation of abdominal skin.

abdominopelvic cavity (ab-DAHM-ih-no-PEL-vik KAV-ih-tee) Cavity between the diaphragm and pelvic floor.

abduction (ab-DUCK-shun) Motion that occurs when the extremity is moved away from the body.

abductors (ab-DUK-tors) Muscles that move a bone away from the midline.

ABHES Accrediting Bureau of Health Education Schools.

abnormalities Conditions that differ from the expected norm.

ABO blood groups Blood types (A, B, AB, or O).

abrasion (a-BRAY-shun) Epidermis is scraped off in an injury or through mechanical means.

abscess (AB-ses) Localized collection of pus that occurs on the skin or in body tissue.

abscess incision and drainage Process in which an incision is made into an abscessed area to promote drainage.

absorption (ab-SOARP-shun) Taking in of nutrients through the stomach and intestines (villi).

abstinence Contraceptive (birth control) method that prohibits sexual contact between partners.

abstract Brief summary of the contents of a manuscript or publication.

abuse Improper or harmful conduct by a health care business (e.g., insurance, medical office) in its fiscal or ethical practices.

acceptance Coming to terms with an issue (e.g., impending death or loss).

accommodation (ah-kom-oh-DAY-shun) Visual adjustment that allows for vision at various distances; ability of the eye to see objects in the distance and then adjust to a close object.

accounting Numerical language of business that describes its activities.

accounting equation Equation that expresses the relationship among assets, liabilities, and owner's equity.

accounts receivable (AR) Record of patient transactions showing an amount due.

acetabulum (as-ah-TAB-yoo-lum) Socket where the femur joins the pelvic girdle.

acetone Chemical formed when fats are metabolized rather than glucose.

acetylcholine (ah-see-till-KOH-leen) Neurotransmitter (chemical) used by nerve endings to send an impulse across a synapse to another nerve.

Achilles reflex (ah-KIL-eez RE-flex) Foot extends when Achilles tendon is tapped.

Achilles tendon (ah-KIL-eez TEN-don) Tendon that connects gastrocnemius muscle to heel bone.

acne (AK-nee) Disease of sebaceous gland associated with excessive sebum.

acquired immunity Immunity achieved through the body's production of antibodies either from disease process or through vaccination (active or passive immunity).

acromegaly (ack-roh-MEG-ah-lee) Overgrowth of bones and soft tissue of hands, feet, and face in adults when excessive growth hormone is secreted.

acromion process (ah-KRO-mee-on) Place where ridge of scapula and clavicle join; point of the shoulders.

acronym Word formed using the first letter of several words (e.g., SOAP).

actinic keratosis (AK-tin-ik kair-ah-TOH-sis) Precancerous skin growth caused by excessive exposure to the sun.

active files Current patient files.

active immunity Immunity provided by having the disease.

active listening Occurs when a listener maintains eye contact and provides responses to the speaker.

active transport Movement of materials across cell membrane using cellular energy.

acute (ah-KYOOT) Occurring now; of short-term duration.

acute renal failure (ARF) Renal failure occurring suddenly from trauma or any condition that impairs blood flow to kidneys.

Addison disease (ADD-ih-sun dih-ZEEZ) Deficiency of adrenocortical hormones.

adduction (ad-DUCK-shun) Motion that occurs when extremity is moved toward or added to the body.

adductors Muscles that move a bone toward the midline.

adenoids (AD-uh-noyds) Lymphoid tissues located in nasopharynx.

adenosine triphosphate (ATP) (ah-DEN-oh-seen try-FOS-fate) Nucleotide in all cells used to store energy and required for RNA synthesis; the energy of the cell.

adipose tissue (ADD-ih-pose) Fibrous tissue composed of fat cells.

adjective A word used to describe a noun or pronoun.

adjustment Addition or deduction of a designated amount to a balance owed.

administer To give medication to patient.

administration set Set for delivering intravenous fluids.

administrative Pertaining to general front office and financial activities.

administrative law Branch of law that functions to regulate business practices.

adolescence Developmental stage between childhood and early adulthood.

adrenal cortex (ah-DREE-nal KORE-tekz) Outer portion of adrenal gland that secretes steroids.

adrenal glands Glands located above kidney that secrete hormones to control metabolic rate and assist the body during stress.

adrenal medulla (ah-DREE-nal meh-DUL-ah) Portion of the adrenal gland that secretes epinephrine and norepinephrine.

adulthood Part of the human life span concerned with an individual during early, middle, and later years in life.

adverb A word used to describe a verb, adjective, or another adverb.

adverse reactions Undesirable and unexpected effects of medications that may be harmful.

advocate One that defends or maintains a cause.

aerobes (AIR-obes) Microorganisms that need oxygen to grow.

aerosols Drug suspensions administered in a mist.

afebrile (a-FEE-brill, a-FEH-brill) Without fever.

affective Type of learning based on feelings and emotions.

afferent nerves (AF-fer-ent) Nerves that carry impulses from the senses to the brain; conducting toward the brain.

agar Seaweed extract used to make certain media solid for bacterial cultures.

age of majority Person who is considered by law to have acquired all the rights and responsibilities of an adult (age 18 in most states).

agenda Document that includes length of meeting, topics covered, order of discussion, and person responsible for discussing each.

agent Representative of the facility (e.g., medical assistant acts as agent for physician).

agglutinate (ah-GLOO-ti-NAYTE), **agglutination** (ah-GLOO-tin-nay-shun) Process of blood cells clumping together when wrong blood type is transfused; result of an antigen-antibody reaction.

aging labels Labels on a chart that identify the year; also called *year labels*.

aging report Report that shows how long a debt has gone unpaid.

agranulocytes (a-GRAN-yoo-loh-sights) White blood cells without granules in the cytoplasm.

air cast Device that is inflated with air to immobilize an injured area.

akathisia (ack uh THEE zsa) Inability to remain calm and free of activity.

albinism (AL-bih-nizm) Genetic condition with total or partial loss of pigment because of inability to use melanin.

albuminuria (al-byou-mih-NEW-ree-ah) Presence of large amounts of serum albumin and other proteins in urine; usually a sign of renal disease or heart failure; also called *proteinuria*.

aldosterone (al-DOS-ter-own) Hormone responsible for increased sodium reabsorption; main mineralocorticoid.

alimentary canal (AL-ih-MEN-tah-ree kah-NAL) Digestive tract; extends from mouth to anus.

allowable charge Amount of a professional service fee that an insurance company is willing to accept.

alopecia (al-oh-PEE-shee-ah) Baldness; loss of hair.

alphabetic filing Filing method that uses the alphabet to determine how files are arranged.

alternating current (AC) interference Electrical interference; appears as small, uniform spikes on ECG tracing.

alveoli (al-VEE-oh-li) Tiny air sacs at the end of bronchioles through which gases are exchanged.

alveolus (al-VEE-oh-lus) Singular form of *alveoli*.

Alzheimer disease (ALTZ-hye-mer) A chronic progressive brain degeneration and dementia focusing on intellectual areas of the brain, causing loss of memory.

amblyopia (am blee OH pee ah) Dull or dim vision due to disease.

ambulation device Any device that assists a patient to walk.

ambulatory Having the ability to walk.

ambulatory surgery setting Nonhospital setting where surgery is performed and the patient is not hospitalized.

Americans with Disabilities Act (ADA) Federal act that provides equal accessibility to services by disabled persons.

amino acids Building blocks; byproducts of protein breakdown by enzymes.

amenorrhea Absence of menstruation.

amnesia (am-NEE-zsa) Inability to remember either isolated parts of the past or one's entire past.

amniocentesis (am-nee-oh-sen-TEE-sis) Sterile procedure to remove amniotic fluid to test for birth defects.

amniotic sac (AM-nee-AH-tik) Membrane (amnion) filled with fluid that surrounds and protects fetus.

amoebae (uh-ME-ba) Microscopic, single-celled parasitic organisms.

amphiarthrosis (am-fear-THRO-sis) Form of articulation (joint) with slight movement; connected by cartilage; plural *amphiarthroses*.

amplifier Device on electrocardiograph that magnifies or enlarges heart's electrical impulses so they can be recorded.

ampule Specially shaped single-dose glass container that contains a dose of medication and has been hermetically sealed.

Amsler grid Test to assess central vision that aids in the diagnosis of age-related macular degeneration.

AMT American Medical Technologists.

amyotrophic lateral sclerosis (ALS, Lou Gehrig disease) (ay-mye-oh-TROH-fic LAT-ur-ul sklih-ROH-sis) Motor neuron disease in which muscles of extremities atrophy and weaken with spasticity of extremities.

anabolism (ah-NAB-oh-lizm) Cellular activity of combining simple substances to form more complex substances.

anaerobes (an-AIR-obes) Microorganisms that do not require oxygen to grow.

anal canal Part of digestive tract between rectum and anus.

anal sphincter Muscle ring at end of digestive system that allows feces to exit from the body.

anaphylactic shock Severe allergic reaction caused by hypersensitivity to a substance (e.g., allergen, foreign protein).

anatomical position (an-ah-TOM-ih-kull poh-ZIH-shun) Position in which the body is upright and facing forward, with arms at the sides, palms and toes forward, feet slightly apart, and legs parallel.

anatomy (ah-NAT-O-mee) Study of an organism's structure.

androgen Any hormone that produces male sex characteristics; sex steroid.

anesthesia Absence of feeling; loss of sensation produced in a patient after administration of an anesthetic substance.

aneurysm (AN-yoo-rizm) Weakness in the wall of an artery.

anger Reaction caused by feeling of loss of control.

angiogram (AN-jee-o-gram) Diagnostic radiograph of the blood vessels using a contrast medium.

angiography (an-jee-OG-rah-fee) Series of x-ray films of blood vessels and lymphatics requiring radiopaque contrast medium.

ankylosis (ang-kih-LOH-sis) Bones fused together or crooked.

anorexia (an-oh-RECK-see-ah) Lack of appetite; psychological fear of gaining weight.

antagonistic (an-TAG-o-nis-tik) Referring to a muscle exerting an opposite action to that of another muscle.
anterior (an-TEER-ee-or) Referring to or in the front.
anterior cavity Space in front of lens between cornea and iris.
anterior descending artery Artery that supplies blood to the right and left ventricles.
antibody (AN-ti-BAH-dee) Protein produced in response to the presence of an antigen.
anticipation guide Pre-reading guide that presents questions and statements about what will be presented in the text; questions that guide the student to anticipate (guess) what will be learned.
antidiuretic hormone (ADH) (AN-ti-DI-u-re-tic HOR-mon) Hormone stored in posterior pituitary gland and needed to maintain fluid balance by reabsorption of fluids.
antigen (AN-ti-jen) Substance found in the body that marks cells as self or non-self and stimulates production of antibodies.
antioxidant Substance that acts against oxidizing agents.
antipyretics Medications that reduce fever.
antiseptic hand rub (an-tee-SEP-tik) Alcohol-containing substance used to clean the hands.
antiseptic handwash Antiseptic agent used to clean the hands.
antisocial Referring to personality exhibiting behavior that shows a disregard for the rights of others.
antonym Root word, prefix, or suffix that has the opposite meaning of another word.
anuresis (an-you-REE-sis) Condition of no urine production or urine output of less than 100 mL per day.
anus (AY-nus) End of digestive system.
anxiety Feeling of apprehension, unease, or uncertainty.
aorta (ay-OR-ta) Largest artery in the body.
aortic semilunar valve (ay-OR-tik seh-mee-LOO-nar) Heart valve that prevents blood from returning to left ventricle.
apex (AY-pex) Tip of the heart.
Apgar score System of measurement used to evaluate an infant at birth.
aphasia (ah-FAY-jhah) Inability to communicate through oral speech; often occurs after stroke.
aphonia (ah-FOH-nhah) Loss of ability to produce sounds.
apical Referring to the apex (or pointed area) of the heart.
apical pulse Heartbeat that is taken with a stethoscope over the apex of the heart.
apnea (AP-nee-ah) Absence of breathing.
aponeurosis (ah-pah-noo-ROE-sis) Wide, flat connective tissue that connects muscle to bone or other tissue.
appendices Additional information segments.
appendicitis (ah-pen-dih-SYE-tis) Inflammation of vermiform appendix.
appendicular area (ap-en-DIK-yoo-lar) Area of the body that includes upper (arms) and lower (legs) extremities.
appendicular skeleton Bones in upper and lower limbs and girdles that attach these to axial skeleton.
approximate To bring together skin edges.
aqueous Water-based.
aqueous humor (AK-wee-us HYOU-mor) Fluid portion of anterior chambers of the eye.
arachnoid (ah-RAK-noyd) Middle layer of meninges; resembles a spiderweb.
areola (ah-REE-o-lah, ah-ree-OH-lah) Dark-colored skin surrounding the nipple.
areolar tissue (ah-REE-oh-lar) Loose fibrous tissue between tissues and under mucous membranes.

arm (microscope) Part of the microscope that is held when moving the equipment; connects the objective and ocular lenses to the base.
arrhythmia Abnormal heart rate, rhythm, and conduction system; also called *dysrhythmia*.
arterial blood gases (ABG) Blood test that measures the amount of O_2 and CO_2 in the blood.
arterioles (ar-TEER-ee-ohls) Small arteries that carry blood to the capillaries.
artery (AR-tuh-ree) Blood vessel that transports blood high in oxygen from the heart.
arthritis (ahr-THRYE-tis) Inflammation of one or more joints; usually accompanied by pain, swelling, redness, and stiffness.
arthrography (ahr-THRO-grah-fee) X-ray of a joint.
arthroscopy (ahr-THROS-koh-pee) Visual examination of a joint with an arthroscope.
articular cartilage (ahr-TIK-yoo-lar KAR-ti-lij) Thin layer of cartilage that covers surface of bones at point where they come together.
articulate Join together, as with bones, by means of a joint.
articulation Point where bones are joined together; joint.
artifacts Unwanted changes in ECG tracing caused by movement, machine malfunction, or other factors; structures not normally present in a urine specimen.
artificially acquired immunity Process of providing immunity by vaccination.
ascending colon (ah-SEND-ing KOE-lon) Section of colon located on right side of the body next to small intestine.
ascites (as-SI-tez) Accumulation of fluid in peritoneal cavity caused by obstruction of portal circulation.
asphyxia (ass-FICK-see-ah) Pathological changes resulting from increased carbon dioxide in tissues and thus oxygen deficiency; insufficient intake of oxygen.
aspiration Pulling back, as in using suction to draw up blood in a syringe.
assault Threat or perceived threat of doing bodily harm to another person.
asset Anything of value owned by a business that can be used to acquire other items.
assimilation Taking in of nutrient material.
asthma (AZ-mah) Condition marked by recurrent attacks of labored breathing (dyspnea), with wheezing caused by spasmodic contraction of bronchi.
astigmatism (ah-STIG-mah-tizm) Refraction error caused by abnormal curvature of cornea and lens.
astrocytes (AS-troh-sites) Star-shaped nerve cells that hold blood vessels closer to nerve cells and serve as a barrier to transport water and salts between nerve cells and capillaries.
ataxia (uh-TACK-see-uh) Lack of muscle coordination.
atelectasis (at-ee-LEK-tah-sis) Incomplete lung expansion; lung collapse.
atlas First vertebra in the neck; supports the head.
atmospheric pressure Pressure of the outside air.
atom (AT-tum) Smallest division of an element.
atonic (ah-TON-ik) Absence of muscle tone.
atria (AY-tree-ah) Plural form of *atrium*.
atrioventricular bundle (ay-tree-oh-ven-TRIK-yoo-lar) Fibers of the atrioventricular node that send impulses to Purkinje fibers.
atrioventricular (AV) node (ay-tree-oh-ven-TRIK-yoo-lar) Specialized group of cardiac cells located in the lower left portion of the right atrium that produce the heart's electrical impulses.
atrium (AY-tree-uhm) Upper chamber of the heart (right or left).

atrophy (AT-roh-fee) Wasting away of muscle tissues caused by nonuse over long periods.

attention deficit hyperactivity disorder (ADHD) Inability to focus attention for short periods or to engage in quiet activities, or both; uncontrolled compulsive behavior.

attenuated Altered; weakened, as in a vaccine.

attitude Set of beliefs that is held about something (e.g., attitude toward test taking).

audiogram Record produced by an audiometer.

audiologist Specialist in audiology or hearing disorders.

audiometer (aw-dee-OH-meh-tehr) Electronic instrument used to test hearing.

audiometry (aw-dee-OH-met-tree) Test that measures sounds heard by the human ear; measurement of hearing ability.

auditory (AW-di-toe-ree) Hearing.

auditory meatus (AWL-di-toe-ree mee-AY-tus) Opening of ear in temporal bone.

augmented leads Leads that measure cardiac activity from one electrode on the body at a time; recordings are augmented (made larger) so they can be read.

auscultation (os-kull-TAY-shun) Listening for body sounds (e.g., heart, breathing, bowel), usually with a stethoscope.

autism (AW-tizm) Disorder characterized by a preoccupation with inner thoughts and marked unresponsiveness to social contact.

autoclave (AW-toe-KLAVE) Equipment that sterilizes objects through the use of steam under pressure or gas.

autoclave tape Special tape with marks that will change color when exposed to predetermined heat and/or pressure.

automated external defibrillator (AED) Machine that analyzes a patient's cardiac rhythm and delivers an electric shock if indicated.

automated urine analyzer Equipment that uses light photometry to analyze a reagent test strip.

autonomic nervous system (ANS) (aw-toe-NOM-ik) System controlled by CNS, mainly the cortex, hypothalamus, and medulla; responsible for involuntary actions of muscles and glands.

autopsy report Medical report that provides details about the cause of illness and death through both internal and external examination findings.

average dose Amount of medication proven to be effective with minimal side effects for an adult.

Avian influenza (H5N1) An infection caused by a virus spread when a wild bird infects a farm-raised bird.

axial skeleton (ACK-see-ul) Bones in central section of the body; skeleton of head, vertebrae, and bony thorax.

axial area Area of the body that includes the head, neck, and torso.

axillary (A) Underarm area; under the arm; armpit.

axillary crutches Devices that aid in walking and fit under the armpit.

axis (AK-sis) Second vertebra in neck; serves as a pivot when head turns from side to side.

axon (AK-sahn) Part of neuron attached to cell body that carries impulses to other neurons and body tissue; conduction portion of nerve.

azotemia (a-zoh-TEE-mee-ah) Nitrogenous waste, especially urea, accumulating in the blood.

B

B lymphocyte (LIM-foh-sight) Lymphocyte that matures in lymphoid tissue and produces antibodies that react against the toxins produced by bacteria.

Babinski reflex (ba-BIN-ske) Normal reflex when bottom of foot is stroked; great toe extends outward, and remaining toes curl.

bacilli (bah-SIL-i) Rod-shaped bacteria; singular *bacillus*.

backed up Copying data from a computer's hard drive to another storage device such as a floppy disk, CD, or "thumb drive" to protect against losing all data if the system fails or "crashes."

background knowledge What is already known before beginning a study; prior learning or understanding of a concept.

back-ordered Pertaining to out-of-stock items that will be shipped at a later date by a supplier.

bacteria (bak-TEE-ree-ah) Single-cell microorganisms; singular *bacterium*; may cause disease.

bacterial smear Placement of a bacterial specimen on glass slide for microscopic review.

bacteremia Bacteria in the blood; sepsis.

bacteriology Study of microorganisms.

bacteriuria Bacteria in the urine.

balance-billing Billing patients for the remaining balance after the insurance has paid its share of the charge.

balance sheet Report on the financial condition of a business on a certain date.

ball-and-socket joint One bone with ball-shaped head fits into socket of second bone.

bandage scissors Scissors with a flat bottom blade on the end that allows it to be placed under a bandage to be cut.

bandage turns Method of arranging a bandage on a body part.

bank statement Document that lists all the banking activities for a set period.

bargaining Process of making deals.

barrier method Birth control method that places a physical barrier between the egg and sperm.

Bartholin's gland One of two small mucus-secreting glands located on the posterior and lateral aspect of the vestibule of the vagina.

basal cell carcinoma (BAY-sal SELL kar-sih-NOH-mah) Malignant skin lesion that is raised, with blood vessels around the edges.

base (microscope) Bottom part of the microscope that contains the light source.

baseline Measurement of a vital sign that serves as a basis to which all subsequent measurements of that vital sign are compared; line that separates various cardiac waves; representative of the space between heartbeats while the heart is "resting"; called also *isoelectric line*.

basic benefits Insurance coverage for physician, hospital, and surgical fees.

basophils (BAY-soh-fills) White blood cells that respond to allergic reactions.

battery Intentional act of touching another person in a socially unacceptable manner without the person's consent.

beneficiary Person receiving insurance benefits.

benign (be-NINE) Not cancerous.

benign prostatic hyperplasia (BPH) (be-NINE PROS-tat-ik hi-per-PLA-ze-a) Enlargement of the prostate gland (nonmalignant).

benign prostatic hypertrophy Nonmalignant enlargement of the prostate.

beriberi Condition caused by a deficiency of thiamine (vitamin B_1).

Bethesda system Grading system used for a Pap smear.

beveled Slanted; the slant of a needle that makes piercing the skin easier.

biconcave Concave (depressed spheres) on both sides.

bicuspid valve See mitral valve.

bicuspids Teeth with two cusps on the grinding surface used for tearing food.

bile (byl) Fluid secreted by the liver, stored in the gallbladder, and discharged into the duodenum; aids in breakdown, digestion, and absorption of vitamins and fats.

bilirubin Byproduct of hemoglobin breakdown; orange-yellow pigment of bile.

bilirubinuria Appearance of bilirubin in the urine.

binocular Having two eyepieces or ocular lenses.

bioethics Ethical decisions and issues that deal with scientific situations.

biological indicator Preparation of live bacterial spores used to test the effectiveness of an autoclave.

biopsy Removal of tissue for a microscopic examination.

bipolar disorder Disorder marked by severe mood swings from hyperactivity (mania) to sadness (depression).

bipolar leads Standard limb leads.

birthday rule Insurance rule that states the policy of the parent whose birthday is first in the calendar year holds the primary insurance for any dependent.

bland diet Diet that uses foods that are not irritating to the digestive tract.

blank endorsement Type of endorsement in which only a signature is listed on the back of a check.

bleb Fluid-filled raised area under the skin.

bleeding Loss of blood from ruptured, punctured, or cut blood vessel.

blood antibody titer Test that shows if a person has had or been exposed to a particular antigen.

blood bank Organization that conducts studies for ABO blood grouping and Rh typing.

blood chemistry Laboratory test that reveals the levels of chemicals in the blood.

blood culture Sterile blood specimen drawn for use with a special medium to diagnose specific infectious diseases.

blood-diluting pipettes Thin glass tubes used to collect blood for manual blood counts.

blood pressure Pressure exerted on the walls of the arteries by blood during contraction and relaxation of the heart.

blood tissue Tissue composed of blood cells within plasma, with no fibers or ground substance.

blood urea nitrogen (BUN) (you-REE-ah) Blood test that measures amount of nitrogenous waste in circulatory system.

blood vessel Elastic tube-like channel through which the blood circulates.

body Main section of stomach; middle portion of sternum; middle of uterus.

body language Nonverbal signals using body motions.

body mass index (BMI) Formula that uses a chart to determine a person's predisposition for being overweight.

body plane Imaginary flat surface that divides the body into specific anatomical sections.

body temperature Measurement of the amount of heat produced by a patient's body.

bolus (BOE-lus) Food broken down by chewing and mixed with saliva ready to be swallowed.

bone density testing (BDT) Noninvasive test that determines the density of a bone.

bone marrow Organic material made of connective tissue and blood vessels that fills cavities of bones; two types are *red marrow*, responsible for manufacture of red and white blood cells, and *yellow marrow*, composed of fat cells and responsible for white blood cell production.

bone matrix (MAY-tricks) Fluids and collagen that make up bone tissue.

bone scanning Use of nuclear medicine to detect pathologies of bone.

bone tissue Tissue with hard fibers and calcium salts.

bookkeeping Systematic recording of business transactions, such as money owed and money paid.

booster dose Medication given to increase chances for long-term immunity, as with immunizations.

booted up Term used to indicate that the computer system has been activated and is ready for use.

Bowman's capsule C-shaped structure surrounding the glomerulus.

box lock Area where an instrument is hinged.

BPH Benign prostatic hypertrophy.

brachial artery (BRAY-kee-uhl) Artery located in the upper arm.

bradycardia (bray-dee-KAR-dee-ah) Pulse rate of less than 60 beats per minute.

brain Main functioning unit of CNS, located in skull and containing many neurons.

brainstem Area of brain located at top of spinal column including the medulla and pons, responsible for respiratory rhythm.

breach of confidentiality Break in right to privacy of personal information.

breach of contract The breaking of an established contract.

breast Mammary gland.

breast self-examination (BSE) Manual test performed by the patient over breast tissue that examines for abnormalities.

bronchi (BRAWN-kye) Main passageway in each lung leading from trachea to bronchioles for oxygen to enter the lungs.

bronchioles (BRAWN-kee-ols) Passageways between bronchi to alveoli for oxygen to reach alveoli.

bronchitis (brawn-KYE-tis) Inflammation of bronchial mucous membrane.

bronchodilators (brong-koh-dye-LAY-tors) Drugs that relax or dilate bronchi.

bronchoscopy (brong-KOS-skuh-pee) Endoscopic procedure used to examine the bronchial tubes visually.

browser Program for "surfing" the Internet.

bruit (BROO-ee) Blowing sound heard in narrowing arteries.

BSE Breast self-examination.

buccal (BUK-al) Pertaining to the cheek; between the cheek and gum.

buccal cavity Cavity containing the teeth and tongue.

buccal tablet Tablet that dissolves when placed between the cheek and gum.

bulbourethral gland (bul-boe-you-REE-thral) Gland on either side of the prostate that produces a fluid that provides a lubricant and becomes part of the semen; also called *Cowper's gland*.

bulimia Disorder characterized by compulsive overeating followed by self-induced vomiting or use of laxatives or diuretics.

bundle branches Branches of cardiac fibers that receive electrical impulses from the bundle of His.

bundle of His Atrioventricular (AV) bundle; small band of atypical cardiac muscle fibers that receive electrical impulses from the AV node.

burn Injury or destruction of tissue caused by excessive physical heat, chemicals, electricity, or radiation.

bursa (BUR-sah) Fibrous connective tissue filled with a synovial fluid; plural *bursae*.

bursae (BUR-SYE) Small sacs containing synovial-like fluid near the joints.
bursitis (burr-SYE-tis) Acute inflammation of bursae.
butterfly method Blood collection method using a winged-infusion set.

C

C&S Culture and sensitivity; test to determine which antibiotic is most effective against cultured organisms.
CAAHEP Commission on Accreditation of Allied Health Education Programs.
calcaneus (kal-KAY-nee-us) Heel bone.
calcium tetany (TET-uh-nee) Continuous muscle spasms caused by abnormal level of calcium in the blood.
caliper Hinged instrument that measures thickness or diameter.
caloric intake Amount of calories eaten.
calorie Unit of energy.
calorie-controlled diet Diet that minimizes or maximizes the amount of food intake based on caloric intake.
calyces (KAYL-ikz-cees) Cuplike edges of the renal pelvis that collect urine; also *calices*.
canals of Schlemm A tiny vein at the angle of the anterior chamber of the eye that drains the aqueous humor and funnels it into the bloodstream.
cancellous bone (KAN-seh-lus) Spongy, porous bone that contains red bone marrow; has lattice-like formation.
candidiasis (kan-dih-DYE-ah-sis) Fungal yeast infection affecting vaginal mucosa, skin, and other areas.
cane Handheld mobility device that provides minimal support for walking.
canines (KAY-nines) Teeth located to side of mouth; "eyeteeth."
canthus (KAN-thus) Angle at either side of slit between eyelids.
capillary (KAP-ih-lar-ee) Smallest blood vessel that moves oxygen into and removes waste products from body tissues.
capillary puncture Skin puncture to obtain a capillary blood sample.
capillary collection tube Small tube used to collect capillary blood.
capital goods Goods that are durable and are expected to last a few years; often expensive.
capitation Managed care plan that pays a predetermined amount to a provider over a set time regardless of the number of services rendered to their subscribers in that period.
caplet Rod-shaped, compressed powdered drug form.
capsule Rod-shaped gelatin container for drugs with two parts; something that holds; in urinary tract, Bowman's capsule.
caption Words that describe the contents, name, or subject matter on a label.
carbohydrates Substances that produce quick energy and are the body's primary source of energy.
carbon dioxide (CO_2) Gas waste released by the body cells.
carbuncles (KAR-bun-kulz) Large abscesses that involve connecting furuncles.
carcinoma (KAR-si-NO-ma) Cancerous or malignant tumor.
cardiac muscle (KAR-dee-ack) Involuntary muscle that is striated and found in the heart walls.
cardiac cycle Systole and diastole that reflect the contraction and relaxation of the heart or a heartbeat.
cardiac muscle Striated muscle that forms the heart wall.
cardiac region Area surrounding lower esophageal sphincter through which food enters stomach from esophagus.
cardiac sphincter See *lower esophageal sphincter*.
cardiac valves Tricuspid and bicuspid valves, which prevent blood in ventricles from backing up into atria when the ventricles contract.
cardiogenic shock Condition that occurs when the cardiac muscles can no longer pump blood throughout the body.
cardiologist (KAR-dee-AWL-oh-jist) Physician who specializes in the structure, function, and diseases of the heart.
cardiomegaly (KAR-dee-oh-MEG-ah-lee) Enlargement of the heart.
cardiopulmonary resuscitation (CPR) (kar-dee-oh-PUL-mah-ner-ee ri-sah-sah-TAY-shun) Emergency measure used to maintain cardiac and respiratory function when a person stops breathing and heart rate ceases; action performed to restore breathing and cardiac activity.
cardiovascular system (kar-dee-oh-VAS-kyoo-lar) Circulatory system; body system that consists of the heart and blood vessels.
caries (KAYR-eez) Tooth decay.
carotid artery (kuh-RAH-tid) Artery located on both sides of the neck.
carpal tunnel syndrome (KAR-puhl TUN-uhl SIN-drum) Compression of median nerve in wrist, causing pain and loss of movement.
carpals (KAR-puhls) Eight small bones of the wrist.
carrier Person who is the reservoir of a disease-producing organism but shows no signs or symptoms of the disease.
cartilage (KAR-tih-layj) Elastic substance attaching to the end of some bones.
cartilage tissue Dense, flexible tissue similar to bone tissue.
cast Plaster or fiberglass mold applied to immobilize a body part.
cast cutter Instrument used to divide a cast for removal.
cast padding Cotton material applied over a stockinette to protect the skin and to prevent pressure sores over bony areas.
cast spreader Instrument used to open the cast after it has been cut for removal.
casts Hardened protein material shaped like the lumen of a kidney tubule and washed out by urine.
catabolism (kah-TAB-oh-lizm) Cellular activity of breaking down complex substances into simple matter.
cataract (KAT-ah-rakt) Opacity of the lens.
catastrophic disability Loss of speech, loss of hearing in both ears, loss of sight in both eyes, or loss of use of two limbs.
catatonia (kat-tah-TOH-nee-ah) Paralysis or immobility from psychological or emotional rather than physical causes.
categorization scheduling See *cluster scheduling*.
catgut Suture material that dissolves inside the body over time.
catheter Small, sterile plastic tube that fits over or inside an intravenous needle.
cautery Uses chemicals (e.g., silver nitrate, sodium hydroxide) to destroy tissues
CBC Complete blood count; total count of each blood element.
CD-ROM Secondary storage device for computer data; holds more data than a floppy disk.
cecum (SE-kum) Large pouch forming first part of the large intestine.
celiac sprue Hereditary malabsorption disease coupled with mucosal damage to the small intestine caused by gluten (wheat) intolerance.
cell Fundamental unit of living tissue.
cell body Main part of the nerve cell.
cell membrane Wall that holds cytoplasm and gives the cell its shape and allows substances to enter and exit the cell.
cellular casts Hyaline casts that contain either white or red blood cells.

cellulitis (sell-yoo-LYE-tis) Infection of the skin and subcutaneous or connective tissue.
cellulose Chief part of the plant cell wall.
Celsius (C) Temperature scale that uses 0° as the freezing point and 100° as the boiling point of water.
Centers for Disease Control and Prevention (CDC) Federal agency established to protect the health and safety of people; responsible for establishing guidelines to prevent the spread of disease-producing microorganisms.
Centers for Medicare and Medicaid Services (CMS) Federal agency that oversees financial regulations of Medicare and Medicaid.
central nervous system (CNS) System of nerves that includes the brain and spinal cord.
central processing unit (CPU) Microprocessor; the "brain" of the computer.
centrifuge Laboratory equipment that separates solids or semi-solids from liquids by forced gravity.
centrioles (SEN-tree-ohlz) Organelles that coordinate cell division.
cerebellum (ser-eh-BEL-um) "Little brain" connected to brainstem that controls skeletal muscles for fine motor skills and coordination of voluntary muscle groups.
cerebral cortex (seh-REE-bruhl KORE-tekz) Area of the brain that controls conscious respiration.
cerebrospinal (seh-ree-broe-SPY-nal) fluid (CSF) Sterile, watery fluid formed within ventricles of the brain to cushion and protect CNS organs.
cerebrovascular accident (CVA) (suh-ree-broe-VAS-kyou-lahr) Stroke; blood vessel ruptures, or blood clot occludes a blood vessel in brain, decreasing blood flow to the area of the brain.
cerebrum (seh-REE-brum) Largest portion of the brain divided into two hemispheres, responsible for thinking, sensation, and voluntary actions.
certificate of provider-performed microscopy (PPM) procedures Certificate that allows a physician in the office laboratory to conduct both low-complexity and moderate-complexity tests.
certificate of waiver Certificate that allows physician office laboratory to perform low-complexity testing.
certified mail Special mail-handling method used to prove an item was mailed and received.
cerumen (see-ROO-men) Earwax; yellow or brown substance produced by sweat glands in external ear.
cervical (SER-vih-kal) Pertaining to the neck area of the spine ; also pertaining to the cervix (the neck of the uterus).
cervical vertebrae (SER-vih-kal VER-teh-brae) First seven vertebrae located in the neck; C1 to C7.
cervicography Technique similar to colposcopy for photographing part of or the entire uterine cervix.
cervix (SER-viks) Lower portion of the uterus; neck of uterus.
chain of custody Process by which evidence is handled.
chain of evidence Collection routine for a specimen used as evidence.
chalazion (ka-LA-ze-on) Small mass on eyelid caused by inflammation and blockage of a gland.
chamber Enclosed space in the body; a cavity.
CHAMPVA Civilian Health and Medical Program of the Department of Veterans Affairs; health benefits program that provides coverage to the spouse or widow(er) of a U.S. military veteran.
charting Process of documenting events and services concerning a patient's care; documenting what is observed or what is told by the patient.
chemical hot/cold pack Device that uses a chemical action to produce heat or cold.
chemical indicators Devices impregnated with a special dye that changes colors when exposed to the sterilization process.
chemistry Tests run on serum or other body fluids to identify specific chemicals and drugs.
chemistry profile Blood test that details the chemical composition of the blood.
chest (precordial) leads Leads that measure in only one direction.
chest x-ray Radiograph; radiological method used to visualize the lungs.
chief complaint (CC) Statement in the patient's own words that describes the reason for the office visit; should be documented in the patient's own words; reason why the patient wants to see the physician.
childhood Part of the human life span dealing with toddlers, preschoolers, school-age children, and adolescents.
chlamydia Member of genus *Chlamydia,* which can cause a sexually transmitted disease that produces a yellow, foul discharge.
choking Inability to breathe caused by a blockage in the trachea.
cholecystitis (kohl-ee-sis-TYE-tis) Inflammation of the gallbladder.
cholecystogram Radiograph of the gallbladder.
cholecystokinin Hormone that stimulates the gallbladder to release bile and the pancreas to release pancreatic juices in digestive enzymes.
cholelithiasis (kohl-oo-lith-EYE-ah-sis) Condition in which stones of calcium or cholesterol are in the gallbladder or lodged in the common bile duct; gallstones.
cholesterol Type of fat necessary for vitamin D and acid bile production.
cholinesterase (koe-lin-ES-ter-ayz) Enzyme that breaks down excess acetylcholine and stops its action at a synapse.
chordae tendineae (KOR-dee ten-DIN-EE) Fibrous cords that prevent the atrioventricular (tricuspid) valves from collapsing under pressure.
chorion (KO-re-on) Outer layer of embryonic sac that forms chorionic villi.
choroid (KOE-royd) Middle vascular part of eye; supplies oxygen and nutrients to the eye.
chromic suture Suture material that dissolves inside the body and is used in areas that are slow to heal.
chromosomes (KRO-mo-sohmz) Threadlike strands inside the cell nucleus that contain genetic information.
chronic (KRAH-nik) Occurring over the long term or recurring frequently.
chronic fatigue syndrome (CFS) Condition characterized by disabling fatigue, accompanied by many symptoms including muscle pain, joint pain, painful cervical or axillary adenopathy, impaired memory or concentration, and unrefreshing sleep.
chronic obstructive pulmonary disease (COPD) Combination of respiratory diseases, including chronic bronchitis, asthma, and emphysema, that have an etiology of destruction of the respiratory tract.
chronic renal failure (CRF) Renal failure resulting from long-term inability to excrete waste products.
chronological resumé Type of resumé that lists education and job experiences from most recent to earliest.
chyme (KYME) Semiliquid contents of the stomach and small intestines after becoming mixed with stomach acid.
cicatrix (sick-AY-tricks) Scar formation after a wound heals; scar tissue.
cilia (SIL-ee-uh) Hairlike projections derived from epithelial cells that sweep materials.

ciliary body (SIL-e-ar-e) Blood-rich ringed structure surrounding the lens and adjusting its shapes for near and far vision.
circular turn Bandage application in which each turn overlaps the previous turn.
circumcision (ser-kum-SIZH-un) Surgical removal of the prepuce.
circumduction (ser-kum-DUCK-shun) Combination of flexion, abduction, extension, and adduction; circular motion by a joint.
circumflex artery Artery that supplies oxygen to the left atrium and left ventricle.
clamping Compressing or gripping tissue or blood vessels with a surgical instrument, as with a clamp.
claudication (klah-dih-KAY-shun) Symptoms of pain and weakness in the legs that subside with rest.
claustrophobia (klos-troh-FOH-bee-ah) Fear of closed spaces.
clavicle (KLA-vih-kul) Collarbone.
clean claim Insurance claim that contains all the information required for processing with no errors or omissions.
clearinghouse Organization that receives electronic claim forms from medical providers and processes them for payment.
cleft palate, cleft lip Disorders that cause malformations of the lip, mouth, or upper jaw.
CLIA-waived tests Simple laboratory tests that can be performed in a licensed laboratory by non-laboratory health care workers.
clinical Pertaining to hands-on patient care.
clinical information Diagnostic information about the patient.
Clinical Laboratory Improvement Amendments of 1988 (CLIA 88) Legislation enacted to ensure the quality of laboratory results by setting performance standards.
closed reduction Repairing ("reducing") a fracture when the skin has not been surgically opened.
closed technique Method of applying a sterile gown and gloves that prevents nonsterile hands from touching the outside of a gown or glove.
closed wound Damage to tissues beneath skin without a visible break in the skin; tissues bruised but not cut.
clubbing Abnormal enlargement of ends of fingers caused by low oxygen level in the blood.
cluster scheduling Technique that groups several appointments for similar types of examination; also called *categorization scheduling*.
CMA (AAMA) Certified medical assistant through the American Association of Medical Assistants.
CMS-1500 Health insurance claim form, also known as the "universal" claim form, that can be filed with all insurance companies; formerly *HCFA-1500*.
CNS Central nervous system.
coagulation (koh-ag-yoo-LAY-shun) Clotting.
coagulation factors Substances in plasma that are released to form clots.
coagulation studies Studies that evaluate the clotting process of blood.
coarse focus adjustment knob Part of the microscope used to lower the stage for rapid focusing; used only with low-power objective.
cocci (KOK-sigh) Round or spherical-shaped bacteria; singular *coccus*.
coccygeal (kock-sih-JEE-ul) Referring to the tailbone (coccyx) area of the spine.
coccyx (KOCK-siks) Tailbone; below the sacrum.
cochlea (KOKE-lee-ah) Coiled portion of inner ear that contains the receptors for hearing.
coding Process of underlining a keyword to indicate how a document should be filed.
cognitive Type of learning based on what the patient already knows and has experienced.
co-insurance, coinsurance Fixed percentage of a medical cost that is paid by the patient after the insurance company has paid its portion of the charge.
cold boot Starting a computer when it has been in "off" mode.
cold therapy Therapy using ice or cold application to reduce or prevent swelling by decreasing circulatory flow to the injured body part.
collagen (KOL-a-jen) Hard protein substance formed when calcium and other minerals mix with osteoblasts and fibers to provide strength to tissue.
collagenous (KAHL-lah-jen-us) Strong and flexible; made up of collagen, a natural body protein that provides for tissue structure in connective tissues.
colon (KOH-luhn) Section of large intestine extending from cecum to rectum.
colostrum Milk substance without fat; first milk produced by the mother's mammary glands just before and after birth.
colorectal Pertaining to the colon and rectum.
colposcopy Examination of vaginal and cervical tissue with a colposcope.
columnar (ko-LUM-nar) Referring to cells that are tall and narrow.
combining form Root word with a vowel added (usually an *o*) to make pronunciation easier.
combining vowel Vowel added to a root word before any prefixes or suffixes.
comedo (KOM-eh-doh) Blackhead; pore that is blocked, usually with sebum and bacteria; may be pustular (whitehead) in closed form.
comminuted fracture Bone that has splintered or broken into many pieces.
common bile duct Duct that enters duodenum from gallbladder for release of bile into intestines.
communication The exchange of information between a sender and receiver.
compact bone Hard surface of all bone.
compassion Providing a sensitive emotional support.
compensation Defense mechanism in which a strength is emphasized to cover up a weakness in another area.
competence Proficiency in identified skills.
complete blood count (CBC) Laboratory test that provides information about red blood cells, white blood cells, and platelets; total count of each blood element.
complex carbohydrates Starches.
complex proteins Proteins that contain all the essential amino acids and are found in animal sources.
compound Substance composed of elements; having two sets of lenses on a microscope.
compound fracture Fracture in which bone protrudes through skin.
comprehensive plan Medical insurance plan that covers both basic and major medical costs.
compress Folded pad of soft absorbent material used for hot or cold therapy.
compromise To make a decision based on mutual agreement.
computed tomography (CT scan) (toh-MOG-rah-fee) Series of x-ray pictures taken at different angles and forming a composite, cross-sectional view of organ or area of interest.
computer imaging Techniques that display images with the use of contrast media.
concept map Drawing or map that uses words to describe and define a concept or main idea; relationships between items are shown by connecting them with lines or arrows.

concurrent condition Condition that occurs at same time as primary diagnosis and affects patient's treatment or recovery from the primary condition.

condenser Mechanism located between the stage and light source on a microscope that condenses the light for vision.

conditioning Process of removing staples and paper clips and mending a document before filing.

conduction Ability to move from one area to another, as in hearing with transmission of sound through nervous tissue.

conduction system Electrical signals through the heart causing a heartbeat.

condyles (KON-dials) Rounded projections at the end of a bone that anchor ligaments and articulates with adjacent bones to form a joint.

condyloid joint (KON-di-loid) Oval-shaped bone that fits into a concave bone.

cones Receptors of color.

confidential Private.

confidentiality Keeping something (e.g., information) private.

confirmatory test Test that confirms the presence of a specific substance in a specimen.

congenital (kon-JEN-ih-tahl) Referring to a condition or anomaly (abnormality) affecting an infant at birth, not necessarily inherited from the parents.

conization Removal of a cone-shaped sample of tissue, as in a cone biopsy.

conjunction A word used to join words or groups of words.

conjunctiva (kun-JUNK-tih-vah) Mucous membrane that lines the eyelids and anterior portion of the eyeball; keeps eye moist.

conjunctivitis (pink eye) (kun-JUNK-tih-VYE-tis) Inflamed conjunctiva.

connective tissue Tissue that supports and binds other body tissues.

Conn's syndrome Excessive production of aldosterone (hyperaldosteronism) that causes reabsorption of sodium chloride and water and excretion of potassium, leading to hypokalemia.

conscious Awake; aware of one's surroundings.

consensus A majority opinion.

consent Patient's permission for physician to proceed with an examination or procedure.

consideration Benefit or payment.

Consolidated Omnibus Reconciliation Act (COBRA) Federal legislation that requires employers with 20 or more employees to continue to offer health coverage to former employees for up to 18 months.

consonant Speech sound used to pronounce words that include all letters except *a, e, i, o, u,* and sometimes *y.*

constipation Difficulty in defecation caused by hard, compacted stool.

constitutional law Branch of public law concerned with relations between government and citizens.

constrict To make smaller; to decrease in size.

consultation Service provided by a health care provider at the request of another physician.

consultation report Medical report written by a specialist after seeing a patient for a primary physician.

continuity of care Care of the patient rendered by health care providers, with the medical record documenting all treatment by providers.

contraception Birth control.

contract Agreement between two or more persons resulting in a consideration.

contractility Ability of muscle to shorten and thicken when stimulated.

contraindications Factors (e.g., patient symptom or condition) that indicate a medication should not be prescribed because potential risks outweigh potential benefits.

contrast medium Radiopaque substance that enhances an image; plural *media.*

contributory factors Issues that affect a decision.

control samples Samples used for testing in which the values are known.

controlled substances Drugs that have a potential for abuse, misuse, and addiction.

Controlled Substances Act Legislation that controls the manufacture and sale of drugs with the potential for abuse and misuse.

contusion (kon-TOO-shun) Bruise.

conventions Ways of identifying special instructions through the use of abbreviations, symbols, and other short descriptions.

conversion Resolution of a psychological conflict through the loss of body function (e.g., paralysis, blindness).

coordination of benefits (COB) Insurance term stating that total reimbursement from primary and secondary insurance companies will not exceed the total cost of the charges.

coordination of care Approach to managing a patient's care when a provider asks other health care providers to assist.

co-payment, copayment Fixed fee that is paid by the patient at each office visit.

cornea (KOR-nee-ah) Anterior portion of the sclera; transparent (allows light through).

corneal reflex (KOR-nee-al RE-flex) Eye blinks when cornea is touched.

coronal plane (ko-ROH-nul) See frontal plane.

coronary arteries (KOR-oh-nair-ee) Blood vessels that branch from the aorta and supply the heart muscle with oxygen.

coronary circulation (KOR-oh-nair-ee SIR-kew-lah-shun) Movement of blood through the heart.

corporation Large business entity that has incorporated to avoid personal liability from the company's debts and taxes.

corpus luteum (KOR-pus LOO-tee-um) Small endocrine tissue located on the surface of the ovary following the release of an egg; secretes the progesterone required to maintain the endometrium during implantation and pregnancy.

cortex (KORE-tekz) Outer portion of the brain responsible for higher learning, perception, and initiation of voluntary movements; outer layer (e.g., of kidney).

corticoids (KOR-ti-coyds) Steroid hormones produced by the adrenal cortex; also called *corticosteroids.*

cortisol (KOR-ti-sol) Main glucocorticoid.

cost containment Term referring to methods used to control the rising costs of health care.

costal cartilage (KOS-tal KAR-til-lij) Cartilage that attaches the first seven pairs of ribs to the sternum.

counseling Discussion with the patient or family conducted by health care provider concerning the patient's diagnosis, test results, and other approaches to medical care.

counterbalanced Balanced on both sides.

coupling agent Water-soluble lotion or gel used to transmit energy provided by an ultrasound wand.

cover letter Job tool that serves to introduce an applicant to the person in charge of screening resumés for employment opportunities.

coverslip Thin piece of glass that fits over a specimen on a glass slide so the specimen can be examined under a microscope.

Cowper's gland See bulbourethral gland.

cramps Painful, involuntary skeletal muscle spasms or contractions.

cranial cavity (KRAY-nee-al) Cavity that holds the brain and is formed by the skull.
cranial nerves Twelve pairs of central nerves originating within the brain.
cranium (KRAY-nee-um) Skull; fusion of eight cranial bones with 14 facial bones that protects the brain.
cream Semi-solid mixture of medications in a water-soluble base for external use; applied to the skin.
creatinine clearance test (kree-AT-ih-nine) Test that measures the rate at which nitrogenous waste is removed from the blood by comparing its concentration in the blood and urine over a 24-hour period.
credit Amount representing a payment; recorded on the right side of an accounting sheet.
crenate (kre-NATE) To lose water and shrink up (e.g., when a cell shrinks up).
crenated Shrunken; formation of notches on the edges of red blood cells.
crepitation (krep-ih-TAY-shun) Joints rubbing against each other, making a grating sound.
crepitus Crackling sound heard in the lungs or joints.
cretinism (KREE-tin-izm) Underproduction of thyroid glands due to congenital reasons, causing a low metabolic rate, slow growth, and mental retardation.
criminal law Branch of public law that deals with the rights and responsibilities of the government to maintain public order.
Crohn disease Chronic inflammation of the ileum.
crossmatching Process of identifying blood compatibility by determining proteins on the red blood cells of the donor and recipient.
cross-reference Notification system showing a file stored in more than one place.
cross-sectional plane See transverse plane.
croup (kroop) Acute viral respiratory disorder in children characterized by a barking cough.
crust Scab; dried serum, blood, and pus.
crutches Devices that assist in walking when full weight cannot be placed on an injured lower extremity.
cryosurgery Destroys tissues by using liquid nitrogen (extreme cold) to destroy skin lesions
cryptorchidism (krip-TOR-kid-izm) Undescended or hidden testes.
crystals Translucent solids appearing in various shapes.
CSF Cerebrospinal fluid.
cuboid Large bone of the ankle; a tarsal.
cuboidal (kyoo-BOYD-al) Referring to cube-shaped cells that are one layer thick when forming tissues.
cultural diversity A mix of ethnicity, race, and religion in a given population.
cultures Growth of microorganisms in special media used to provide nutrition to the microbes.
culture and sensitivity (C&S) Laboratory test ordered to identify a microorganism and its susceptibility to antibiotics.
culture plate Covered container with nutritional substances that support growth of bacteria.
cumulative dose Total amount of medication in the body after repeated doses; medication that accumulates in the body over time.
cuneiforms Tarsal bones of the ankle.
curative drug Drug that heals from disease or cures from infection.
curette Long-handled instrument with a metal loop on one end to scrape inside a cavity.
curriculum vitae (CV) Type of physician's "resumé" that lists education, in-service training (internship, residency), hospital affiliations, professional organizations, and any publications written.
cursor Flashing line on a computer screen that indicates where the characters typed will appear.
Cushing syndrome Adrenal cortex oversecretes hormones, resulting in obesity, weakness, hypertension, and hyperglycemia; also results from ingesting corticosteroids.
cusps Flaps on a valve.
cuticle (KYOO-tih-kul) Narrow band of epidermis at the base and sides of the nail.
cutting Penetrating or dividing tissues of the body with a sharp-edged instrument.
cyanosis (SIGH-uh-NOH-sis) Bluish discoloration of nails or skin caused by lack of oxygen in the blood.
cyst (sist) Thick-walled sac that contains fluid or semi-solid material.
cyst removal Removal of a sebaceous cyst from body.
cystic duct Duct leading from the gallbladder into the common bile duct.
cystic fibrosis (SIS-tik fye-BROH-sis) Recessive genetic disorder of exocrine glands with defective chloride channels causing excretion of thick mucus into lungs.
cystitis (sis-TYE-tis) Inflammation of the urinary bladder.
cystoscopy (sis-TOS-koh-pee) Visual examination of the urinary bladder using a cystoscope.
cytology The study of the formation and structure of cells.
cytology laboratory requisition Laboratory form sent to the cytology laboratory that tells the laboratory what test is needed to examine the cells for abnormalities.
cytoplasm (SIGH-to-plazm) Fluid that bathes the organelles in the cell.

D

dacryoadenitis (dack-ree-oh-sis-TYE-tis) Inflammation of a lacrimal sac.
Daily Value (DV) Dietary standards that include a range of particular nutrients needed daily to optimize health.
damages Payment used to compensate for physical injury, damaged property, or loss of personal freedom or used as a punishment.
database Information source and storage.
database management Productivity software that allows the computer user to work with facts and figures.
day planner Organizational system (e.g., using a calendar, notebook, PDA) for planning and recording deadlines, tasks to be completed, events, and other activities.
daysheet Journal for recording the day's activities.
DEA number Number applied for and provided by the Drug Enforcement Administration that allows practitioners to prescribe scheduled drugs.
dead spaces Areas in the upper respiratory tract where air collects and never reaches the lungs.
deafness Interference with passage of sound waves from the outside to the inner ear; complete or partial inability to hear.
debit Amount representing a charge or debt owed; recorded on the left side of an accounting sheet.
debride To clean out a wound.
debrided Removed dead tissue.
debridement Removal of foreign or dead material from a wound.
debtor Person owing a debt.
decibels (dB) (DES-i-bels) Measurement of loud or soft sounds.

deciduous teeth (dee-SID-you-us) Teeth that will be lost; "baby teeth."
decontaminate To clean, sanitize, disinfect, and remove microorganisms or areas, such as after minor surgery.
decubitus ulcer (deh-KYOO-bih-tus) Pressure sore; bedsore.
deductible Yearly amount that the patient must pay "out of pocket" before the insurance will pay on any claims.
deep wound Wound that extends beyond the subcutaneous layer.
default A selection or option automatically chosen by most computer programs (when the user hits "enter") if not directed by the user to do otherwise.
defecation (def-eh-KAY-shun) Elimination of feces.
defense mechanism Filtering tactic used by the unconscious mind to avoid unpleasant situations.
defibrillation Electrical shock to the heart to maintain heart rhythm.
defined purpose Knowing what one is looking for before starting to read; having a clear idea of the goal or purpose of something written (e.g., the focus or main idea).
deglutition (dee-gloo-TISH-uhn) Act of swallowing.
delayed primary (tertiary) intention healing Healing that occurs when a wound is left open because of infection or debris or when a wound will not approximate correctly.
delirium (dih-LEER-ree-um) Condition of confused and irrational agitation.
deltoid muscle (DEL-toyd) Muscle of the shoulder shaped like an upside-down Greek delta (Δ).
delusion (dih-LOO-zhun) Persistent belief in an untruth.
delusional disorder Condition characterized by false beliefs, including grandiose and persecutory thoughts.
dementia (dee-MEN-shah) Irreversible impairment of intellectual capabilities.
demographics Biographical data; personal information.
dendrite (DEN-dryt) Part of neuron resembling tree branches that receives nerve impulses; toward the cell body.
denial Unconscious behavior that does not acknowledge unpleasant aspects of life.
dense tissue Fibrous tissue that is packed together.
deoxygenated blood (dee-AHK-see-GEN-a-ted) Blood that is low in oxygen.
deoxyribonucleic acid (DNA) (dee-ahk-see-rye-boh-noo-KLEE-ik) Substance that carries genetic information, considered the "blue print" of the cell.
dependent Person for whom another person is financially responsible.
depolarization Discharge of electrical energy that causes contraction, such as in heart muscle.
deposit Money placed in an account of a financial institution.
deposit slip Listing of all cash and checks to be deposited to a certain account of a business's financial institution.
depression Overall feeling of helplessness; feeling of persistent sadness accompanied by insomnia, loss of appetite, and inability to experience pleasure.
depressor Muscle that lowers a bone.
dermatitis Inflammation of the skin caused by irritation or riboflavin deficiency; may be infectious, contact (with a skin irritant), or atopic (allergic).
dermatologist (der-mah-TOL-oh-jist) Physician who specializes in the treatment of diseases and conditions of the skin.
dermatology (dur-mah-TOL-uh-jee) Study of the skin.
dermatome (DUR-mah-tohm) Surface area of the body (skin) where afferent fibers travel from a spinal root.
dermis (DER-mis) Layer of skin that lies beneath the epidermis.

descending colon Section of colon located on left side of the body.
development Progressive increase of body function throughout one's lifetime.
dexterity Ability to move with skill and ease.
diabetes insipidus (di-ah-BEE-teez in-SIP-ih-dus) Disease caused by release of insufficient antidiuretic hormone from posterior pituitary gland.
diabetes mellitus (di-ah-BEE-teez mell-EYE-tus) Primary disease of the insulin-producing pancreas.
diabetic diet Diet for patients who have difficulty with insulin secretion.
diabetic ketoacidosis State that occurs when there is too much glucose and not enough insulin in a patient's blood, and ketones are produced; acute insulin deficiency; also called diabetic coma.
diagnose To identify a disease process.
diagnosis (Dx) (dye-ag-NOH-sis) Determination of the nature of a disease based on signs, symptoms, and laboratory findings.
diagnostic Referring to the recognition or identification of diseases in the body.
diagnostic drug Drug that assists with diagnosing a disease during a procedure, such as radiopaque dye with x-rays.
diagnostic imaging Techniques used to produce a picture image that does not involve the use of radiation.
dialysis (dye-AL-ih-sis) Process used to clean the blood of toxins.
diameter The space across a vessel (from wall to wall).
diaphoresis (dye-ah-foh-REE-sis) Profuse or excessive sweating.
diaphragm (DYE-uh-fram) Main muscle of breathing that lies between the thoracic and abdominal cavities.
diaphysis (dye-AFF-ih-sis) Main shaft of long bones.
diarrhea (dye-ah-REE-ah) Frequent bowel movements of loose, watery stools.
diarthrosis (dye-ahr-THROE-sis) Joint with free movement; hinged or pivot joint; plural *diarthroses*.
diastole (dye-AS-toh-lee) Relaxation of the heart.
diastolic pressure (dye-AS-toh-lik) Minimum ("resting") blood pressure, occurring late in ventricular diastole (dilation, expansion) of the heart.
diencephalon (dye-en-SEF-a-lon) "Interbrain" located under the cerebrum that includes the thalamus and hypothalamus.
differential blood cell count (DIFF-er-EN-shul) Laboratory blood test that determines percentage of each type of white blood cell present in a blood sample.
diffusion (dif-YOO-zhun) Movement of a substance from an area of higher concentration to one of lower concentration.
digestion (di-JES-chun) Physical and chemical breakdown of food.
digital radiographic imaging Radiography using computerized imaging instead of conventional film or screen imaging.
digital radiography Computed radiography that uses the computer to produce images.
dilating Making wider or larger, as in a *dilating instrument* used to increase diameter of an opening.
dilation (dye-LAY-shun) Making larger; increasing in size.
dilation and curettage (D&C) Widening of the uterine cervix and scraping of the endometrium of the uterus.
diminutive Small; a small version of something.
diplococci (DIP-low-KOK-sigh) Spherical bacteria that appear in pairs; singular *diplococcus*.
diplomacy Ability to be tactful.
diplopia (dih-PLOH-pee-ah) Double vision.
direct contact Person-to-person contact; method by which most microorganisms are transmitted.

direct filing Filing system that requires knowing only the patient's name to initiate or locate the file.

direct pressure Pressure applied directly over a wound.

disability income insurance Insurance that pays benefits to the policyholder if he or she becomes unable to work because of an illness or injury that is not work related.

discharge summary Medical report that provides a comprehensive review of a patient's hospital stay.

discussion Process of talking with others about a concept or information for the purpose of understanding or clarification.

disinfection (dis-in-FEK-shun) Process of applying an antimicrobial agent to non-living objects to destroy pathogens and is considered an intermediate level of infection control since it does not destroy spores.

dislocation Displacement of a joint from its proper anatomical position.

dispense To deliver a medication into the patient's possession after it has been prepared.

displacement Defense mechanism in which aggressive behavior is placed onto something or someone else other than the source of frustration.

display panel Panel on a label that is used for marketing purposes.

disposable goods Expendable or consumable supplies that are used and then discarded.

dissecting Cutting apart or separating tissue, as in a *dissecting instrument* used to cut between tissues.

dissecting scissors Scissors that have thick straight or curved blades with a fine cutting edge used to cut through or between tissue layers.

distention (dis-TEN-shun) Swollen.

distracter Something that causes the sender or receiver not to give full attention to the message.

diuresis Increased urine production.

diuretics (dye-you-RET-iks) Medications that cause increased urine excretion.

diversity Having a variety of skills or types.

diverticulitis (dye-ver-tik-you-LYE-tis) Inflammation of small outpouches (diverticula) in the colon.

divided dose Total amount of medication that is administered in separate instances.

dominant Prominent trait or characteristic, as in a dominant gene.

donor Person who gives blood.

dorsal (DOR-sal) Back.

dorsal cavity (DOR-sal KAV-ih-tee) Cavity located in posterior (back) of the body made up of the cranial and spinal cavities.

dorsal recumbent position Patient is flat on the back with the knees and hips bent sharply and the feet flat on the table.

dorsalis pedis artery Artery located at the top of the foot.

dorsogluteal Area of the gluteus muscle in upper outer portion of the buttocks.

dosimeter Device that monitors the quantity of x-ray exposure to health care workers.

double booking Technique that schedules more than one patient during the same appointment time period.

Down syndrome Chromosomal disease that occurs because of a duplication of all or part of chromosome 21.

dressing forceps Instrument with blunt ends and serrated tips used for removing or applying dressing materials.

drip rate Infusion rate for intravenous fluids.

drug Medicine; any substance that produces a physical or chemical change in the body.

Drug Enforcement Administration (DEA) Agency responsible for enforcing the Controlled Substances Act; regulates the sale and use of controlled drugs.

drug screening Urine or blood collection to determine the presence or absence of specific substances.

duodenum (doo-oh-DEE-num) The first part of the small intestine.

dura mater (DOO-rah MAY-tuhr) Covering of the brain located closest to the skull and vertebral column.

dwarfism (DWAR-fizm) Undergrowth of bone and body tissue in children.

dysmenorrhea Pain associated with menstruation.

dyspepsia (dis-PEP-see-ah) Difficult digestion; uncomfortable feeling after eating; indigestion.

dysphagia (dis-FAY-jhah) Difficulty swallowing.

dysphonia (dis-FOH-nee-ah) Difficulty speaking; hoarseness.

dysplasia Abnormal development of tissue.

dyspnea (DISP-nee-ah) Difficulty in breathing; shortness of breath.

dysuria (dis-YOU-ree-ah) Painful or difficult urination.

E

E codes ICD-9-CM supplementary codes for external causes of injury and poisoning.

ecchymosis (eck-ih-MOH-sis) Hemorrhagic (bruised) area of skin caused by trauma to a blood vessel; collection of blood under skin causing skin to turn blue-black that changes to greenish brown.

ectopic pregnancy (eck-TOP-ik) Fertilized egg implants outside the uterus, usually in fallopian tube; formerly known as *tubal pregnancy*.

eczema (ECK-zeh-mah) Itchy, red rash with pustules, scales, crusts, or scabs caused by sensitivity to a substance; dermatitis.

edema (uh-DEE-muh) Abnormal tissue swelling.

editing Process of preparing a document or manuscript by correcting or revising its textual content.

EDTA Ethylenediaminetetraacetic acid; anticoagulant used for preserving blood for hematology studies.

efferent nerves (EF-er-ent) Nerves that carry impulses from the brain to the motor nerves; conducting away from the brain.

efficiency Performing tasks on time and accurately.

ego The part of the personality that is alert to reality and consequences of behavior.

ejaculation (ee-jak-yoo-LAY-shun) Forceful expulsion of seminal fluid.

ejaculatory duct (ee-JAK-yoo-lah-toe-ree) Duct where the ducts for seminal vesicles and vas deferens come together.

elastic (ee-lass-TIK) Easily stretched; recoiling after use.

elastic bandage Bandage containing elastic that stretches and molds to the body part to which it is applied.

elastic cartilage Most flexible cartilage, with elastic and collagenous fibers.

elasticity Ability of muscle to return to original length after stretching.

electrocardiogram (ECG) (EKG) (ee-lek-troh-KAR-dee-OH-gram) Recording of cardiac cycles; graphic picture of the heart's electrical activity.

electrocardiograph (ee-lek-troh-KAR-dee-OH-graf) Machine that records the electrical activity of the heart.

electrocardiography Noninvasive procedure used to detect the heart's electrical activity.

electrodes Devices made of a conductive material to pick up the electrical activity of the heart; sensors.

electroencephalogram (EEG) (ee-lek-troh-en-SEF-ah-loe-gram) Measurement of electrical activity of the brain.
electromyogram (EMG) Record of muscle activity that aids in diagnosing neuromuscular problems.
electromyography (ee-lek-troh-my-OG-rah-fee) Procedure that records the electrical activity of muscles.
electroneuromyography Tests and records neuromuscular activity by electrical stimulation; interpreting electromyograms.
electrosurgery Uses an electric current to cut or destroy tissue.
electronic medical record (EMR) Patient medical records kept in a computer file; also called "paperless chart."
element Basic chemical substance such as oxygen or carbon dioxide.
elimination Expelling of body wastes.
elixirs Solutions containing alcohol, water, sugar, and a drug or combination of drugs.
emancipated minor A minor who has legally been declared independent; held responsible for own debts.
embolus (EM-bo-lus) Clot that moves through the bloodstream.
embryo (EM-bree-oh) Developmental stage from second to eighth week of gestation.
emergency Situation in which a delay in treatment could be life threatening.
emesis (EM-eh-sis) Vomiting; forceful expulsion of stomach contents; "throwing up."
empathy Understanding how other people feel by placing oneself in their place.
emphysema (em-fih-SEE-mah) Pathological accumulation of air in the lungs resulting in abnormal distention and destruction of the alveoli; chronic pulmonary disease.
employee earnings record Document that shows individual employee earnings and deductions.
Employee's Withholding Allowance Certificate (Form W-4) Form that each new employee fills out to declare exemption from tax withholding for earnings.
employment agencies Agencies that charge a fee to an individual for finding employment or to an employer for finding an employee.
emulsification (ee-mul-si-fi-KAY-shun) Process of breaking down fat for digestion.
emulsion Substance suspended in an oil-based liquid that must be shaken before use.
encephalitis (en-sef-ah-LYE-tis) Infection of tissues of the brain and spinal cord.
encounter form Source document for billing purposes that contains patient account information and insurance codes for date of service; also known as *superbill*; form used in the medical office that identifies and records the patient's diagnosis and procedure performed on a specific date of service; office form attached to a patient's record where the physician records the diagnosis and the procedures and services performed for posting charges.
endocardium (en-doh-KAR-dee-um) Inner muscle layer of the heart.
endocervical curettage (ECC) Removal of endocervical tissue by scraping.
endocrine gland (EN-doh-krin) Gland that secretes a substance directly into the blood and lymph system; ductless glands that secrete hormones and other secretions into the blood or lymph for circulation throughout the body.
endocrinologist (EN-doh-krih-NOL-oh-jist) Specialist who treats diseases resulting from dysfunction of the endocrine system.
endometriosis (en-doh-mee-tree-OH-sis) Growth of endometrial tissue outside of the uterus in the pelvic cavity.

endometrium (en-doh-MEE-tree-um) Vascular inner lining of the uterus; holds the fertilized egg; sheds monthly as menses.
endoplasmic reticulum (ER) (end-oh-PLAZ-mik ree-TIK-yoo-lum) Tube-like structures that store and transport proteins within the cell.
endorse To sign or place (e.g., stamp) a signature on the back of a check that transfers the rights of ownership of funds to a financial institution.
endorsement Occurs when a state accepts the scores of a national examination.
engineering controls Equipment and facilities that minimize the possibility of exposure to microorganisms; promote safety in the laboratory.
enteral Taken through the digestive system.
enteric-coated Having a special coating that does not allow medication to dissolve until it reaches the small intestine.
enteric-coated tablet Tablet with a special coating that dissolves in the small intestine.
entity A particular type of business.
entry Written description of care provided to the patient.
enuresis (en-you-REE-sis) Involuntary discharge of urine at an age after bladder control should have been accomplished; bedwetting.
enzyme (EN-zyme) Complex protein produced by living organisms that causes biochemical changes; breaks down amino acids.
enzyme immunoassay (EIA) Pregnancy test that uses a color-change reaction.
eosinophils (EE-oh-SIN-oh-fills) White blood cells that react to the release of histamine in the body.
ependymal cells (ee-PEN-de-mal) Nerve cells that line the brain and central cavity of the spinal cord and serve as a barrier between CSF and tissue fluid.
epicardium (eh-pih-KAR-dee-uhm) Outermost layer of the heart wall.
epidermis (ep-i-DERM-is) Thin upper layer of the skin.
epididymis (ep-ih-DID-ih-mis) Place where sperm are stored on the posterior of the testes.
epididymitis (ep-ih-did-ih-MY-tis) Inflammation of the epididymis.
epidural space (ep-ih-DOO-ral) Space outside and between the dura mater and walls of the vertebral canal (vertebrae, skull).
epiglottis (ep-ih-GLOT-tis) Flap that prevents food from entering the larynx and trachea.
epilepsy (EP-ih-lep-see) Chronic brain disorder in which an individual has seizures.
epinephrine (EP-ih-NEFF-rihn) Adrenaline; hormone that converts stored sugar to energy, increases heart rate, and allows the body to respond to stress; secreted by the adrenal medulla.
epiphyseal plate (growth plate) (ep-ih-FEEZ-ee-ahl) Area at each end of a long bone responsible for bone growth; bone tissue replaces cartilage tissue, and the bone lengthens.
epiphysis (eh-PIF-ih-sis) Expanded ends of long bones filled with red bone marrow.
episiotomy (eh-piz-ee-OT-oh-mee) Surgical incision in the perineum to enlarge vaginal opening for passage of the infant at birth.
episode of care Term used to describe and measure the various health care services provided for a specific injury or period of illness.
epistaxis (ep-ih-STACK-sis) Nosebleed.
epithelial tissue (ep-ih-THEE-lee-al) Tissue that covers the body and internal cavities.
eponym The name of a specific person(s), place, or thing for whom or for which something (disease, procedure, instrument) is named (e.g., Alzheimer disease), or the name so derived (e.g., a simple urethropexy is known as the Marchal-Marchetti-Krantz procedure).

equilibrium Balance; sense of balance.
erect Upright.
erection (ee-REK-shun) Stiffening of the penis.
ergonomic (er-goh-NOM-ick) Pertaining to the study and analysis of human work devices that affect the anatomy.
erosion Destruction of the surface layer of skin.
erythema (er-ih-THEE-mah) Redness of the skin.
erythrocyte (ee-RITH-roh-sight) Red blood cell (RBC).
erythrocyte sedimentation rate (ESR) Screening test that confirms an inflammatory process in the body by measuring how quickly red blood cells settle to bottom of calibrated tube; "sed rate."
erythropoiesis (ee-RITH-roy-POY-e-sis) Process of red blood cell formation.
erythropoietin (ee-RITH-roy-POY-e-tin) Hormone that stimulates bone marrow to produce erythrocytes.
esophagitis (eh-SOF-ah-gi-tis) Inflammation of the esophagus.
esophagus (eh-SOF-ah-gus) Muscular tube that is a passageway for food between the pharynx and stomach.
esotropia (eh-soh-TROH-pee-ah) Turning inward of one or both eyes.
essential nutrients Nutrients that must be supplied to the body from a food source (vitamins, minerals, proteins, carbohydrates, fats, water).
established patient Patient who has been treated by a member of the health care team in the past 3 years.
estimated date of delivery/confinement (EDD/EDC) A mother's probable due date for birth based on her last menstrual period (LMP).
estrogen (ES-trow-jen) Hormone that prepares the uterus for the implantation of the fertilized egg and promotes female sex characteristics.
ethical standards Guidelines for professional decisions and conduct.
ethically In a way that distinguishes right from wrong.
ethics Moral principles.
ethmoid bone Bone located behind the nose and eye sockets.
etiology (ee-tee-OHL-ah-jee) Identification of the reason or cause for a disease.
eustachian tube (yoo-STAY-shun, u-STAY-kee-un) Tube that connects middle ear with nasopharynx and acts to equalize pressure between outer ear and middle ear.
euthanasia Intentional ending of the life of terminally ill persons.
evacuated tube Blood collection tube in which the internal atmosphere is a vacuum allowing blood to flow into the tube.
evacuation blood collection system System that includes a holder, double-ended sterile needle, color-coded stopper, and vacuum blood tube.
Event monitor Device worn by a patient to monitor cardiac activity for periods of one week to a month.
eversion (eh-VER-zhun) Turning outward.
examination Method by which a person is tested for knowledge; can be oral, written, or a combination of both; physical review of body system or systems.
excoriation (ecks-kore-ee-AYE-shun) Removal of surface epidermis by scratching, burn, or abrasion or through chemicals.
excretory system Urinary system; body system that separates and eliminates waste from blood, tissues, and organs.
exemption Amount of money earned that is not taxable.
exhalation (ex-hah-LAY-shun) Process of letting air out of the lungs; expiration.
exocrine gland (EKS-oh-krihn) Gland that secretes to the epithelial surface its substance through a duct (e.g., sweat glands, mammary glands).

exophthalmia (ek-sof-THAL-me-ah) Protrusion of the eyeballs from their orbits.
exophthalmometer Instrument used to measure the degree of forward displacement of the eye in exophthalmos.
exophthalmia (eck-soff-THAL-mee-ah) Abnormal condition characterized by a marked protrusion of the eyeballs.
exophthalmos (ek-sof-THAL-mus) Protrusion of the eyeballs; symptom of Graves disease.
exotropia (eck-so-TROH-pee-ah) Turning outward of one or both eyes.
expiration Process of air leaving the lungs; exhalation.
explanation of benefits (EOB) Form sent by the insurance carrier to the patient and the medical practice that explains the amount of reimbursement or reason for denial of a submitted claim.
exposure control plan Plan that identifies tasks that can expose employees to harmful risks and finds ways to decrease exposure.
exposure incident Contact with blood or other biohazardous and infectious material that occurs on the job.
expressed contract Written or oral contract agreeing to specific conditions.
extensibility Ability of muscle to stretch.
extension Motion that increases the angle of the bone between articulating bones.
extensor Muscle that straightens a joint.
external auditory canal Path that leads from the pinna to the middle ear.
external (lung) respiration Exchange of oxygen for carbon dioxide within the alveoli.
extracellular (eks-trah-SELL-yoo-lar) Occurring outside the cell, as in *extracellular fluid*.
extrinsic muscles (ek-STRIN-sik) Six skeletal muscles that allow the eye to move and that hold it to the orbit.
exudate Wound drainage, such as oozing pus or serum; fluid with cellular debris from inflammation.
eyepiece Part of the microscope through which the viewer looks to see an object; magnifies visual field by 10 times.

F

facilities management Maintaining the atmosphere and physical environment of an office.
facsimile Fax.
fad diet Diet that is structured to cause the quick loss of weight.
Fahrenheit (F) Temperature scale that uses 212° as the boiling point and 32° as the freezing point of water.
Fair Debt Collection Act of 1977 Act that governs how the collection of a consumer's debt must be handled.
Fair Labor Standards Act Legislation providing the standards for payment of hourly and salaried employees.
fallopian tubes (fah-LOW-pee-an) Tubes that connect ovary to uterus for passage of fertilized egg (bilateral); also known as *uterine tubes*.
false ribs Ribs that are indirectly connected to the sternum and are attached to vertebrae.
familial Occurring within a family; genetically acquired.
family history (FH) Health inventory of a patient's immediate family.
fantasy A daydream.
fascia (FAS-ee-a) Fibrous sheath that covers, supports, and separates muscles.
fasting blood sugar (FBS) test Blood test indicating the glucose level after a period of fasting (not eating).

fat-soluble vitamins Vitamins that are stored within the fatty tissues of the body (A, D, E, K).

fatty acids Organic acids produced by the breakdown of fats.

fatty casts Hyaline cast with fatty cells.

fax (facsimile) Method of communication in which written material is converted into electronic impulses transmitted by telephone lines.

fax machine Office equipment that scans a document, translates the information to electronic impulses, and transmits an exact copy of the original document from one location to another using a telephone line.

FDA Food and Drug Administration.

fear Appropriate reaction to genuine danger.

febrile (FEB-ril) With fever.

fecal Referring to or consisting of feces.

fecal occult test Test of stool specimen for the presence of minute amounts of blood.

feces (FEE-seez) Stool; body waste.

Federal Employees' Compensation Act (FECA) Legislation that covers nonmilitary employees of the federal government for work-related injuries.

Federal Insurance Contributions Act (FICA) Legislation that provides funds to support retirement benefits, dependents of retired workers, and disability benefits.

Federal Truth in Lending Act Legislation requiring a disclosure statement that informs a patient of a procedure's total cost, including finance charges; required when the patient will make more than four payments.

Federal Unemployment Tax Act (FUTA) Legislation that requires employers to pay tax based on employee's earnings to cover benefits if the employee becomes unemployed.

fee schedule Listing of a physician's charges for services.

feedback Evidence provided by instructors indicating a student's growth, progress, or mastery; verbal or nonverbal indication that a message was received; process that allows the body to stay in homeostasis in opposite response to a stimulus.

felony Serious crime against the public (e.g., practicing medicine without a license).

femoral artery (FEM-uh-rul) Artery located in the thigh.

femur Thighbone; long bone of upper leg.

fertilization (FUR-ti-ly-ZAY-shun) Joining of the egg and sperm.

fetus (FEE-tus) After 8 weeks of gestation, an embryo becomes a fetus until delivery.

fiberglass cast Cast made of fiberglass or plastic resin tapes.

fibers (FYE-burs) Long, threadlike structures in tissue that provide strength.

fibrin (FYE-brin) Protein that forms a clot.

fibrinogen (fye-BRIN-o-jen) Clotting factor.

fibrocartilage (FYE-broh-KAR-tih-layj) Combination of fibers and cartilage material.

fibrocystic disease of breasts (figh-broh-SIS-tik) Condition appearing as lumps in breast tissue, causing breast pain and tenderness.

fibromyalgia (FIGH-broh-my-AL-jee-ah) Syndrome that causes chronic pain in the muscles and soft tissue surrounding the joints.

fibromyositis (figh-bro-mi-O-si-tis) Muscle and tendon inflammation; same as *fibromyalgia*.

fibrous cartilage (FIGH-brus) Thick cartilage that connects bones to each other; found in vertebral disks.

fibrous tissue (FIGH-brus TISH-yoo) Tough durable tissue that connects and binds.

fibula (FIB-yoo-lah) Small bone of lower leg; lateral side of lower leg.

fiduciary (FI-due-SHE-a-re) A position of trusted responsibility.

fight, flight, or fright Body's response to threat.

"fight-or-flight" response Reaction by the sympathetic nervous system to respond quickly to stressful situations.

figure-eight turn Bandage turn that is applied on a slant and progresses upward and then downward to support a dressing or joint.

filing Process of putting documents in a folder.

film-screen radiography Radiography using special photographic film that blackens in response to the light from intensifying screens.

filter paper Special paper used to pass a liquid through or to collect a blood specimen.

filtration (fil-TRAY-shun) Process by which substances are taken out of a solution by passing through a partial barrier.

financial statements Reports that indicate the financial condition of a business.

fine focus adjustment knob Part of the microscope used for precise focusing of a specimen on a slide; used with both high power and oil immersion.

first aid Temporary care given to an injured or ill person until the victim can be provided complete treatment.

first-degree burn Burn that involves only the epidermis.

first morning specimen Urine specimen taken when patient first awakens; most concentrated specimen.

first (primary) intention healing Healing that occurs when a clean surgical wound is approximated or closed and heals with minimal scarring and no infection.

fiscal intermediary Agent; insurance company that processes Medicare claims.

fissure (FISH-yoor) Split or crack in the skin.

fissures Grooves or deep folds within the cortex.

fixative Substance that holds cells on a slide.

fixators (FICK-say-tors) Specialized synergistic muscles that stabilize the origin of a prime mover or immobilize a bone.

flaccid (FLAS-sid) Lacking muscle tone.

flat bones Thin, flattened bones found in the skull, ribs, and scapula.

flatulence Digestive bowel gas.

flashcards Learning aid used for memorization.

flexion Bending motion that brings two close bones together, decreasing the angle between articulating bones.

flexors Muscles that bend a joint or bring two bones closer together for flexion.

floating ribs Ribs attached to the vertebrae only and not the sternum.

floppy disk Secondary storage device for computer data.

fluorescein angiography Technique for examining the circulation within the blood vessels surrounding the retina.

fluorescein staining Test where fluorescein, an orange stain, is applied to the cornea to reveal corneal lesions.

fluoroscopic imaging, fluoroscopy Radiographic imaging in which the view allows the radiologist to view images in motion.

follicle (FAWL-ik-ul) Sac or tube that anchors and contains an individual hair.

follicle-stimulating hormone (FSH) Hormone that causes the egg to ripen in the graafian follicle.

font Character style (appearance) of typeface on a document.

fontanels (fon-tah-NELLS) Soft spots located between the cranial bones; also *fontanelles*.

Food and Drug Administration (FDA) Federal agency responsible for setting standards for the purity, strength, and composition of all drug, food, and cosmetic products.

food guide pyramid Tool developed by the U.S. Department of Agriculture (USDA) to provide a visual picture of the six food groups common to the American diet.
foramen (foe-RAY-men) Hole or opening for passage of nerves, blood vessels, and ligaments; plural *foramina*.
foramen magnum Large opening at base of the skull where the spinal cord joins the brain.
foramen ovale (foh-RAY-men oh-VAL-ee) Opening in septum between the atria before birth.
foramina Small openings in cranial bones for nerves and vessels; singular *foramen*.
forced vital capacity (FVC) Measurement of the maximum volume of air that can be expired when the patient exhales forcefully.
forceps Instrument used to grasp or hold body tissue, foreign bodies, and surgical materials.
forearm (Lofstrand) crutches Devices that provide contact with the hand and forearm.
forensics Collection of evidence (e.g., specimen) in a methodical manner for use in a court of law.
foreskin Skin folded over the end of the penis.
formed elements Blood components (blood cells; e.g., RBCs, WBCs, platelets).
fovea centralis (FOE-vee-ah) Depression in the retina; point of sharpest vision.
Fowler's position Patient is in a supine position with the head of the table either at a 45-degree (semi-Fowler's position) or a 90-degree (full-Fowler's position) angle.
fracture Break or crack in a bone caused by trauma or disease.
fraud Intentional misrepresentation of medical facts as they relate to a claim for health care services.
free edge Edge of nail extending beyond the nail body.
frenulum (FREN-yoo-lum) Structure that anchors the tongue to the floor of the mouth.
frequency Increase in number of times urination occurs over a short time.
frontal bone Bone that extends from top of the eye orbits to top of the head, forming the forehead.
frontal lobe Part of the brain that controls voluntary muscle action, speech, and judgment.
frontal (coronal) plane Vertical cut through the body that divides the body into anterior and posterior sections.
frontal sinuses Air-filled cavities located in area above the eye orbits.
frostbite Form of hypothermia that occurs when body tissues freeze.
full-block format Letter format that has all lines flush with the left margin.
full-thickness burn Burn that destroys the epidermis and dermis to include the nerve endings; third-degree burn.
functional resumé Type of resumé that relates the person's skills to the type of employment sought.
fundus (FUN-dus) Top portion of the stomach; upper part of the uterus above the fallopian tubes.
fungi (FUN-ji) Microorganisms that feed on organic material.
furuncle (FYOOR-ung-kul) Abscess that occurs around a hair follicle.

G

gait Way a person walks; style of walking; manner of walking.
gait patterns Patterns of walking used with crutches.
galactosemia Galactose in the blood.
gallbladder Small, muscular sac in which bile secreted by the liver is stored until needed by the body for digestion.
galvanometer Device that detects and converts the amplified electrical signal into a tracing on the ECG machine.
gametes (GAH-meets) Sex cells; reproductive cells; eggs and sperm.
ganglion (GANG-lee-ohn) Group of neuron cell bodies along the path of a nerve outside the CNS.
Gardnerella Genus of bacteria that exists in the vagina and can cause infection if pH is not balanced.
gastrin Controls gastric acid secretion.
gastritis (gas-TRY-tis) Inflammation of the stomach.
gastroenteritis (gas-troh-en-ter-EYE-tis) Inflammation and irritation of the stomach and intestines.
gastroesophageal reflux disease (GERD) (gas-troh-ee-sahf-ah-JEE-al REE-fluks) Backup of gastric juices into the esophagus.
gastrointestinal (GI) tract Digestive tract.
gatekeeper Primary care physician designated by an HMO to provide ongoing care to a patient and to authorize referrals to specialists when deemed necessary.
gauge Number that identifies the size of the inside opening, or lumen, of a needle.
gel cap Vessel made of a gelatinous substance to hold liquid medication.
general anesthetic Medication that produces unconsciousness by depressing the central nervous system.
general anxiety disorder General feeling of apprehension brought on by episodes of internal self-doubt.
gene Hereditary unit containing the coding sequence for protein synthesis found in chromosomes.
genetic counseling Counseling of individuals and prospective parents in the risks and treatment of inherited diseases.
genitourinary tract Male urinary and reproductive system.
genomics (je-NO-miks) The science of understanding the complete genetic inheritance of an organism.
gestation (jes-TAY-shun) Pregnancy.
gestational diabetes (jes-TA-shun-al dye-ah-BEE-teez) Condition that can occur during pregnancy when the effects of insulin are blocked by hormones produced in the placenta; pregnant woman is unable to metabolize carbohydrates; develops during latter part of pregnancy (24-28 weeks) and usually subsides with delivery.
gigantism (jye-GAN-tizm) Overgrowth of body tissue before puberty, including long bones.
gingivitis (jin-jih-VYE-tis) Inflammation of the gums in the mouth.
glands Specialized tissues that secrete or excrete a substance.
glans (glanz) penis Bulbous tissue at end of the penis.
glass slide Flat piece of glass used to hold a specimen for microscopic examination.
glaucoma (glaw-KOH-mah) Condition resulting when aqueous humor does not drain properly, increasing intraocular pressure, compressing choroid layer, and diminishing blood supply to retina.
glial cells (gly-al SELS) Cells that provide support for nervous tissue.
gliding joint Joint that allows flat surfaces to move across each other.
glomerulonephritis (glo-mair-yoo-low-neh-FRY-tis) Inflammation of glomeruli of nephron.
glomerulus (glo-MER-yoo-lus) Group of capillaries responsible for filtering blood in nephrons of kidney.
glossitis (GLOS-si-tis) Inflammation of the tongue.
glucagon (GLOO-ka-gon) Hormone that stimulates the conversion of glycogen to glucose.

glucocorticoids (gloo-koe-KOR-tih-koydz) Steroid hormones that promote release of glucose from glycogen and provide extra energy in stressful situations.
glucometer Device used to measure glucose in the blood.
glucose Sugar; end result of carbohydrate metabolism and the main producer of energy.
glucose reagent strip Chemical pad on a dipstick that tests for the presence of sugar.
glucose tolerance test (GTT) Blood test measuring the body's ability to break down glucose; urine and blood are collected at specified intervals after a special glucose solution is ingested; determines the body's ability to metabolize glucose over a specific time period.
glycemic index Scale that rates carbohydrate foods' effects on blood glucose levels from slowest to fastest.
glycerol Alcohol that is made up of fat.
glycosuria (glye-koh-SOO-ree-ah) Presence of glucose (sugar) in the urine.
glycosylated hemoglobin (GHb) test Hemoglobin A_{1c}; test that measures the amount of glucose attached to hemoglobin over a 3-month period.
goals Plans that are developed to reach one's mission in life; includes long-term goals (life goals) and the short-term goals that together help one to achieve long-term goals.
goiter (GOY-tuhr) Enlargement of the thyroid gland caused by underproduction or overproduction of thyroid hormones in adults; not caused by a tumor.
Golgi apparatus (GOAL-jee ap-ah-RA-tus) Organelles involved in packaging proteins and excreting materials from the cell.
gonads (GOH-nadz) Sex glands; ovaries and testes.
goniometer Device used to measure joint movements and angles.
gonioscopy Visualization of the angle of the anterior chamber of the eye.
gonorrhea Sexually transmitted disease caused by gonococci that produces no primary symptoms in females but dysuria in males.
Good Samaritan Act Legislation that provides protection from lawsuits for an individual who gives lifesaving or emergency treatment.
gouty arthritis (gout) (gowt-TE) Condition with swelling in the joints resulting from uric acid not being metabolized.
Gowers sign Manner in which a patient with muscular dystrophy stands from the supine or kneeling position.
graafian follicle Where the egg ripens in the ovary.
Gram stain Staining method used to identify the shape and pattern of microorganisms.
grammar Study of words and their relationship to other words in a sentence.
granular casts Casts appearing microscopically as short, plump, and coarse.
Granulation phase Phase 2 of healing process; flesh begins to form to later support tissue.
granulocytes (GRAN-yoo-loh-sights) White blood cells containing granules in the cytoplasm.
grasping Holding, as in a *grasping instrument* used to hold back tissue.
Graves disease Oversecretion of thyroid hormone in adults.
greatest specificity Coding to the highest level of documentation available; not using only a three-digit code when a four- or five-digit code exists to better describe the disease or procedure.
greenstick fracture Bone fractured and bent on one side but not on the other. Children are prone to this type of break because their bones have not completely ossified.
gross negligence Intentional omission or commission of an act.
gross wages Total amount of money earned before deductions are taken.
group policy Insurance policy purchased by a company for its employees.
group practice Practice owned by three or more people who are held legally responsible for the debts and taxes of the business.
group practice association Type of practice in which all the HMO's physicians and services are housed in the same location.
guaiac test (GWI-ak) Test for hidden (occult) blood in the stool or other body secretions.
guarantor Person who is responsible for paying the costs of a patient's treatment.
guidelines Rules that define items necessary to interpret and report procedures and services appropriately (e.g., for CPT codes).
guides Dividers used to separate file folders.
gustatory receptors (GUS-tah-toe-ree) Receptors in the taste buds that relay impulses of taste to the brain.
gynecologist Physician who specializes in the treatment of women, including diseases of the reproductive organs and breasts.
gynecology Branch of medicine that focuses on maintaining women's health.
gyri (JYE-re) Folds in the cortex, either fissures or sulci.

H

habit Established pattern of thinking or behaving.
hallucination Any unreal sensory perception that occurs with no external cause.
hamstrings Tendons behind knee responsible for extending hips and bending knees.
hand hygiene Maintaining the hands in a clean state by handwashing with soap and water, using an antiseptic solution, or using alcohol-based hand rubs.
handwashing Cleaning the hands with soap and water.
hard drive Main device in the computer used to store and retrieve information.
hard palate (PAL-at) Roof of the mouth.
hardware Mechanical devices and physical components of a computer system.
haversian system (hah-VER-shun) Structural unit of the bone that receives nutrition and removes wastes.
HCFA Common Procedure Coding System (HCPCS) Standardized coding system that uses CPT, national, and local codes to process Medicare claims. Used primarily for supplies, materials, injections, and for certain procedures and services not defined in CPT.
HDL High-density lipoprotein; "good" cholesterol.
head Rounded or necklike portion of a long bone.
headache A pain in the head from any cause.
heading Resumé section that includes the demographics (e.g., name, address, phone number) about the applicant.
Health Insurance Portability and Accountability Act (HIPAA) Exacted by U.S. Congress in 1996. Title I protects health insurance coverage for employees and their families when they change or lose their jobs. Title II requires national standards for electronic health care transactions and national identifiers. Title II also provides guidelines for maintaining confidentiality of patient information by health care providers and insurance carriers.
health maintenance organization (HMO) Organization that provides comprehensive health care services for plan participants at a fixed periodic payment.
hearing acuity tests Tests used to check for hearing loss.
heart Body pump that circulates the blood.

heartbeat Cardiac cycle; measurable contraction and relaxation of the heart.
heat exhaustion Form of hyperthermia marked by pale, cool, and clammy skin; shallow respirations; and weak pulse.
heat stroke Form of hyperthermia caused by dehydration causing a loss of consciousness.
heat therapy Therapy that uses application of heat to increase blood flow to a body area.
heating pad Electrical device that delivers a set temperature of heat for heat therapy.
HEENT Head, eyes, ears, nose, and throat.
Heimlich maneuver Abdominal thrust used in an emergency to dislodge the cause of a blockage.
hematemesis Vomiting of blood.
hematocrit (Hct) (hee-MAT-oh-krit) Measurement of the percentage of packed red blood cells in a volume of whole blood.
hematology Tests that assess the formed elements of blood, including red blood cells, white blood cells, and platelets.
hematopoiesis (HEE-mah-toe-poy-ES-siz) Production of blood cells; process of blood cell formation; also *hemopoiesis*.
hematuria (he-mah-TOOR-e-a) Presence of blood in the urine.
hemiparesis (heh-mee-puh-REE-sis) Muscle weakness of face or limb on one side of the body.
hemiplegia (heh-mee-PLEE-jee-ah) Paralysis of only one side of the body, often caused by stroke on opposite side of the brain.
hemoconcentration Blood pooling.
hemodialysis (hee-moh-dye-AL-ih-sis) Artificial kidney machine filters patient's blood and returns filtered blood back to patient.
hemoglobin (HEE-muh-GLOW-bin) Iron-containing pigment found in red blood cells used to transport oxygen; gives blood its color.
hemoglobinuria Hemolyzed red blood cells in the urine.
hemolysis (he-MAHL-ih-sis) Breaking down of the membranes of red blood cells.
hemolyze (he-MAHL-ez) To burst open red blood cells as a result of taking on too much liquid.
hemolyzed Damaged, burst cells; hemolyzed red blood cells are colorless and cannot be seen under magnification.
hemophilia (hee-moh-FILL-ee-ah) X-linked recessive bleeding disorder caused by a missing coagulation factor; most often seen in males.
hemoptysis (hee-MOP-tih-sis) Spitting of blood originating in the respiratory tract.
hemorrhagic shock Shock caused by inadequate blood supply to tissues as a result of trauma, burns, or internal bleeding.
hemorrhoids (HEM-oh-roids) Dilated veins in the rectum and anus.
hemostasis (HEE-moh-STAY-sis) Cessation of bleeding through a series of events: vasoconstriction, formation of a plug, and blood clotting.
hemostatic forceps (hemostats) Instrument with serrated tips, ratchets, and box lock used to clamp off blood vessels or to grasp material.
hemothorax (hee-moh-THOH-racks) Blood in the pleural cavity.
heparin Natural substance that prevents clotting; a vacuum tube additive that prevents the clotting of blood in the tube.
heparin lock Resealable latex lock to administer heparin directly into a vein.
hepatic duct (he-PAT-ik) Duct from the liver to the gallbladder.
hepatic portal system Blood vessels carrying blood from intestine to liver; drains intestinal capillaries and feeds hepatic capillaries.
hepatitis (hep-ah-TYE-tis) Inflammation of the liver caused by a viral infection.
hereditary Referring to a condition passed to a child by the parents; acquired through genetic makeup.
heredity Genetics.
hernia (HER-nee-ah) Protrusion (bulging) of an organ or part of an organ through a weakness in a muscle wall.
herpes simplex 1 (HER-peez SIM-plecks) Viral infection of the skin (lip-skin junction) at the site where skin and mucous membrane meet; "cold sores" or "fever blisters."
hiatal hernia (hi-A-tal HER-nee-ah) Protrusion of part of the stomach through the diaphragm into the chest cavity.
high-fiber diet Diet high in fiber to help with elimination.
high-power field (HPF) High magnification.
hilum (HYE-lum) Depression where blood vessels, nerves, and the ureter enter and exit the kidney; plural *hila*; located between the lungs; allows for the entrance and exit of blood vessels, nerves, bronchi, and lymphatic tissue.
hinge joint Joint that only moves in one direction.
Hirschsprung disease Chronic dilation of the colon; usually congenital.
hirsutism (HER-soo-tizm) Abnormal hairiness, especially in women.
history Information about past events.
history and physical (H&P) report Medical report that consists of a patient's subjective (medical history) and objective (physical examination) data.
history of present illness (HPI) Chronological description of the patient's present illness from the first sign or symptom to the present.
histrionic Showing excessive attention-seeking tendencies.
holistic Involving all health needs of the patient, including physical, emotional, social, economic, and spiritual needs (e.g., holistic patient care).
Holter monitor Ambulatory heart monitor that records heart activity during a 24- to 48-hour period.
homeostasis (hoh-mee-oh-STAY-sis) The body in balance.
homonym Word that has the same pronunciation, but a different spelling and meaning, than another word.
hordeolum (hor-DEE-oh-lum) (stye) Localized bacterial infection in the eyelid; stye.
horizontal recumbent position Patient lies flat on the back; supine position.
hormonal method Contraceptive method that prevents ovulation through the addition of hormones into the body.
hormone Internal secretion by a gland or an organ that moves through blood to another part of the body to regulate a body function.
hormone level test Blood test measuring amounts of antidiuretic, cortisol, growth, and parathyroid hormones.
hospice Bundle of services and team of people helping a family during the end stage of a patient's terminal illness.
host Computer that is the main computer in a system of connected terminals.
hot flashes Symptoms of an uncomfortable sense of warmth that occur during menopause because of a decrease in female hormones.
hot water bag Device that holds water warm enough to increase blood flow for heat therapy.
hub Part of the needle that fits or locks onto a syringe.
human chorionic gonadotropin (hCG) (ko-ree-ON-ik gon-ah-do-TROW-pin) Hormone produced during pregnancy that is responsible for the release of progesterone and estrogen to maintain the endometrium; maintains the corpus luteum; used to prove pregnancy on early testing.
humerus (HYOO-mur-us) Long bone of the upper arm.
Huntington chorea (disease) (HUN-ting-tuhn koh-REE-ah) Inherited condition with progressive muscular weakness and dementia.

hyaline cartilage (HIGH-ah-lin) Clear cartilage tissue.
hyaline casts Common casts found in urine that are pale and transparent; appear in unchecked hypertension.
hydrating solutions Solutions used to maintain adequate fluids in the body or to prevent dehydration.
hydrocele Scrotal swelling caused by an accumulation of fluid.
hydrogenated Polyunsaturated fats are made solid.
hyoid bone (HIGH-oyd) Bone located in the neck that anchors the tongue.
hypercalcemia (hye-per-kal-SEE-mee-ah) Increase of calcium in the blood.
hypercholesterolemia High level of cholesterol in the blood.
hyperglycemia (hye-per-glye-SEE-mee-ah) High blood sugar level; can cause diabetic coma.
hyperkalemia (hye-per-kuh-LEE-mee-ah) Increase of potassium in the blood.
hypernatremia (hye-per-nuh-TREE-mee-ah) Increase of sodium in the blood.
hyperopia (farsightedness) (hye-per-OH-pee-ah) Light rays entering the eye are brought into focus behind the retina.
hypersecretion Excessive secretion of a substance; oversecretion.
hypertension (hye-per-TEN-shun) Measurement of blood pressure that exceeds the acceptable range for the patient's age group.
hyperthermia Increased body temperature.
hypertonic (hye-per-TAH-nik) Pertaining to a solution that causes cells to shrink (excessively concentrated).
hypertonic solutions Solutions that have a higher salt concentration than a person's body fluids, thus causing the body to lose fluids.
hypertrophy (hye-PER-tro-fe) Enlargement of an organ.
hypocalcemia (hye-poh-kal-SEE-me-ah) Deficiency of calcium in the blood.
hypoglycemia (hye-poh-gly-SEE-me-ah) Low blood sugar level; can cause insulin shock.
hypokalemia (hye-poh-kuh-LEE-me-ah) Deficiency of potassium in the blood.
hyponatremia (hye-poh-nuh-TREE-me-ah) Deficiency of sodium in the blood.
hypophysis (hye-PAH-fih-sis) Pituitary gland.
hyposecretion Inadequate secretion of a substance; undersecretion.
hypotension (hye-poh-TEN-shun) Measurement of blood pressure that is below the expected range for the patient's age group.
hypothalamus (hye-poe-THAL-ah-mus) Gland that controls activities of pituitary gland; secretes oxytocin and ADH; regulates autonomic nervous system, body temperatures, release of hormones, and water balance.
hypothermia Decreased body temperature.
hypotonic (hye-poe-TON-ik) Pertaining to a solution that causes cells to swell (diluted or low concentration).
hypoxia (hye-POK-see-ah) Condition of low oxygen levels.
hysterosalpingography (his-tur-oh-sal-pin-GAH-gruh-fee) Method of producing radiographic images of the uterus and fallopian tubes.

I

ice bag Device that holds ice for cold therapy.
ichthyosis (ick-thee-OH-sis) Dry, scaly skin condition resembling fish scales.
id The unconscious part of the brain associated with biological drives, energy source, and needs gratification.
idiopathic Disease without an identifiable cause.
ileum (IL-ee-um) Last part of the small intestine.
ilium (IL-ee-um) Upper portion of the pelvic bones. (Not to be confused with *ileum,* which refers to the intestines.)
immobilization Prevention of movement; inability to move.
immunity (im-YOO-ni-tee) Defense against a specific disease.
immunization Protection against a disease by artificial active immunity.
immunoassay Laboratory technique that measures the reaction of an antigen to a specific antibody.
immunological testing Tests used to measure antigen-antibody reactions.
immunology The study of how the immune system works to defend the body.
impacted fracture Bone break in which one end of fractured bone is driven into itself.
impetigo (im-peh-TYE-go) Bacterial infection that forms pustules that rupture and form crusts; usually caused by streptococcal or staphylococcal infection.
implied contract Agreement that is created by a set of actions or behavior.
impotence (IM-poh-tens) Inability to have or sustain an erection during sexual intercourse.
inactive files Files of patients who have not been seen within a certain time span set by the medical practice (e.g., 3 years).
incident Any unusual event that is not consistent with the routine activity within a health care facility.
incident report Document that describes any unusual occurrence that happens while a person is on the property of a health care facility.
incision Smooth cut into the skin.
incisors Teeth located in the front of the mouth.
income statement Report showing the results of income and expenses over time.
incontinence (in-KON-tih-nents) Inability to retain urine or feces because of a loss of sphincter control.
incus (INK-us) (anvil) Part of middle ear that transmits sound vibrations from the malleus to the stapes.
indemnity (fee-for-service) plan Insurance plan in which patients pay the provider and submit a claim form for reimbursement from their insurance company.
independent practice association (IPA) Contractual agreement between private physicians, hospitals, and insurance companies to provide service to their members.
indexing Process of determining how a record will be filed.
indirect contact Method by which microorganisms are transmitted other than by person-to-person contact.
indirect filing Numeric filing system that requires a list containing cross-references of numbers and names to locate the file.
indirect pressure Pressure applied over an arterial pressure point.
individual policy Insurance policy purchased by individuals who are not members of any designated group.
induration Area of hardened tissue that occurs as a result of sensitivity to an allergen.
infancy Part of the human life span including birth through the first year.
infarction (in-FARK-shun) Death of tissue because of lack of blood to area.
infection control Established policies and procedures that must be followed to minimize the risk of spreading disease-producing microorganisms.
inferior (in-FEER-ee-or) That which is below.
inferior vena cava (in-FEER-ee-or VEE-nah KAY-vah) Vein that brings blood low in oxygen from the lower limbs and trunk.

infertility Inability or diminished ability to become pregnant.
Inflammatory phase Phase 1 of healing process; blood clot forms and stops blood from flowing.
influenza (in-flew-EN-zah) Flu; an acute viral infection of the upper respiratory tract.
informed consent Consent given after a patient has been informed in a manner the patient fully understands about complications, contraindications, and risks associated with a procedure, as well as alternatives and possibilities without treatment.
infraction Violation of a law resulting in a fine.
ingestion (in-JEST-shun) Process of taking nutrition into the body.
inhalation (in-hull-LAY-shun) Process of taking air into the lungs; inspiration.
initial dose First dose of medication administered.
initialized Formatted to hold data.
ink-jet printer Printer that produces characters and graphics by imprinting ink onto paper.
inner ear Part of the ear that contains receptors for sound waves and that maintains equilibrium.
inpatient Person who has been admitted to the hospital for continued care.
inscription Section of a prescription where the name of the medication is entered.
insemination Introduction of semen into the female.
insertion (in-SIR-shun) Part of a muscle anchored to a moving bone.
insidious Developing gradually (e.g., insidious disease or symptom); gradual, versus sudden, as in manifestation of disease.
inspection Visual viewing of body parts.
inspiration Process of taking air into the lungs; inhalation.
instillation Process of placing medication into an area as prescribed by a physician.
instructional terms Words or phrases that have a special meaning to provide needed information.
insulin (IN-soo-lihn) Hormone that functions to regulate metabolism of carbohydrates and fats, especially conversion of glucose to glycogen, which lowers blood glucose level; necessary for cells to be able to use glucose for energy.
insulin shock State that occurs when the body has too much insulin and not enough glucose (food) to use the insulin; severe hypoglycemia.
insurance claims register Log showing when insurance claims are filed.
integrative neurons (interneurons) (in-teh-GRAY-tiv) Neurons to the brain and spinal cord neurons that conduct nerve impulses between afferent (sensory) to efferent (motor) neurons.
integrity Quality of being honest and straightforward.
integumentary system (in-teg-yoo-MEN-tar-e) Body system made up of the skin, hair, nails, and sweat glands.
intercellular (in-ter-SEL-yoo-lar) The area between cells.
intercostal muscles (in-ter-KOS-tal) Muscles between the ribs used in breathing.
interface Connection between the user and the computer.
interferons (in-ter-FEER-ons) Proteins produced by T cells and cells infected with viruses that block the ability of a virus to reproduce.
interjection A word used to express strong feelings or emotion.
internal (cellular) respiration Exchange of oxygen for carbon dioxide at the cell level.
international law Laws that govern relations among nations.
Internet service provider (ISP) Company that provides a "host" access to the Internet (e.g., Earthlink, AOL).
internist Physician who specializes in the structure, function, and diseases of the internal organs.
interstitial fluid (in-ter-STISH-uhl) Fluid between the cells of tissue.
interstitial cystitis Inflammation of the bladder.
interval ECG pattern that shows the length of a wave with a segment.
interview Verbal format that allows the employer to form an impression about the job applicant.
intradermal (ID) injection Injection given just under the epidermis, or top layer of the skin.
intramuscular (IM) injection Injection given into muscle tissue.
intrauterine device (IUD) Birth control method that prevents a fertilized egg from implanting in the uterine wall.
intravenous pyelography (IVP) (in-truh-VEE-nus PYE-lo-gruh-fee) Imaging of the kidneys, ureters, and bladder using contrast dye injected intravenously.
intravenous (IV) therapy Administration of fluids and medications directly into a vein.
intrinsic muscles (in-TRIN-sik) Smooth muscles in the iris that control amount of light entering the eye.
intussusception (in-tus-sus-SEP-shun) Telescoping of one part of the intestine into another; usually occurs in the ileocecal area.
inventory records Documentation of physical assets and information that includes item description, date of purchase, price, and where purchased, as well as equipment serial numbers and service agreements.
inversion (in-VER-zhun) Turning inward.
invoice Form prepared by the vendor describing the products sold (by item number and quantity) and the price; used for paying vendor for purchased supplies and equipment.
involuntary Referring to muscles contracting independently; not under conscious control.
iris Colored portion of the eye between the lens and cornea that regulates amount of light entering the pupil; separates anterior and posterior chambers.
iris diaphragm Mechanism just below the microscope stage that adjusts the amount of light that enters the field of vision; connected to the condenser.
irregular bones Bones having no distinctive shape that make up spinal column, sphenoid and ethmoid of skull, sacrum, coccyx, and mandible.
irrigation Washing or rinsing out an area to remove foreign matter.
irritability Ability of muscle to respond to stimulation.
ischemia (iss-KEY-mee-ah) Deficiency of a blood supply to tissue because of obstruction; causes lack of oxygen to that tissue.
ischium (IS-kee-um) Lowest portion of the pelvic bones.
islets of Langerhans Pancreatic cells that produce insulin and cause secretion of glucagon.
isoelectric line See baseline.
isometric contraction Muscle tension increases, but the muscle does not shorten.
isotonic (eye-soh-TAHN-ik) The body's normal concentration of solutes in cells; pertaining to a solution that does not change cell volume.
isotonic contraction Muscle shortens, producing movement.
isotonic solutions Solutions that contain the same salt concentration as a person's body fluids.
itinerary Travel document that describes overall trip and indicates what is scheduled to happen each day.

J

jaundice (JAWN-dis) Yellowish discoloration of the skin and eye caused by breakdown of bilirubin.

jaws Holding part of a clamp.

JCAHO Originated as the "Joint Commission on Accreditation of Healthcare Organizations" and now called the "Joint Commission"; not-for-profit organization formed to promote specific improvements in patient safety.

jejunum (jeh-JOO-num) Second part of the small intestine responsible for absorption.

job application Form that, when completed, provides information about the person applying for employment.

job interview Verbal, face-to-face format that allows the employer to form an impression about the job applicant.

joint Place where two bones come together.

K

keloid (KEE-loid) Overgrowth of fibrous tissue at the site of scar tissue.

keratin (KER-ah-tin) Waterproof protein that toughens the skin.

Kernig sign Diagnostic sign for meningitis; patient seated or in supine position is unable to extend knee from flexed thigh position.

ketone Chemical formed when fats are metabolized.

ketonuria (kee-toh-NEW-ree-ah) Presence of ketones in the urine.

key components Three main factors (history, examination, and medical decision making) taken into account when selecting a level of E/M service in CPT coding.

key unit First unit to be filed.

keyboard Input device that includes letter and number keys and computer task keys.

kidney (KID-nee) Organ of the urinary system that produces urine.

kidney transplant Donor kidney replaces the kidney of a person with malfunctioning kidney to function as a kidney for the recipient.

kidneys, ureters, and bladder (KUB) Imaging of the kidneys, ureters, and bladder without a contrast medium.

Klinefelter syndrome Chromosomal disease that occurs in males when an extra X chromosome is present at birth.

Kling-type bandage Gauze bandaging material that stretches and molds to irregular-shaped areas.

knee-chest position Patient begins in the prone position, then moves into a kneeling position with the buttocks elevated and the chest on the table.

Kussmaul breathing Breathing pattern that begins with very deep, gasping respirations that become rapid and are associated with severe diabetic acidosis and coma.

KWL Reading comprehension strategy that uses a three-column approach and asks readers (1) what they *know* about what they are reading, (2) what they *want* to know, and (3) what they *learned* when finished.

kyphosis (ki-FO-sis) Curvature in thoracic area of the spine; hunchback.

L

labels Identifying names placed on an individual by others; stickers or other items that identify contents in a folder.

labia majora (LAY-bee-ah ma-JO-ra) Two large folds of skin that form the sides of the vulva.

labor Parturition; stages and process of expelling fetus and placenta at birth.

laboratory requisition Laboratory form showing the identification of a specimen and the laboratory test to be performed.

labyrinth (LAB-uh-rinth) Bones and membranes of inner ear that contain receptors for sound waves and maintain balance (equilibrium).

laceration Jagged cuts; wound tissue edges are irregular.

laceration repair Use of suture or adhesive strips to repair an open wound.

lacrimal bones (LAK-rih-mal) Bones that are part of the eye orbits situated alongside the nose.

lacrimal cavity Cavity containing the tear duct.

lacteals (LAK-tee-als) Structures that absorb nutrients for the lymph system.

lactic acid (LAK-tik) Waste product of muscle metabolism.

lactiferous ducts Ducts in the breast that transport milk to each nipple.

lactose intolerance (LACK-tose in-TAHL-er-ans) Deficiency of the enzyme lactase that prevents lactose from being digested properly.

lamellae (lah-MEL-ee) Thin layers of ground bone tissue arranged in patterns that determine bone type.

lancet Sterile needle-like piece of metal used to puncture the skin to collect a capillary blood specimen.

large intestine Portion of the intestine that extends from the small intestine to the anus.

laryngitis (lar-in-JIGH-tis) Inflammation of the larynx (vocal cords).

laryngopharynx (lah-ring-oh-FAR-inks) Area of the pharynx located above the larynx; extends from the epiglottis to the larynx.

larynx (LAR-inks) Musculocartilaginous structure serving as a passageway for air; guards entrance to the trachea and functions secondarily as the voice organ; commonly called the "voice box."

laser Generates intense heat and energy creating a narrow beam of light that can be focused at unwanted tissue

laser printer Printer that uses heat to fuse a fine dark powder (toner) onto paper to create graphics and text.

last menstrual period (LMP) Date that a woman had her last menstrual cycle.

lateral plane See sagittal plane.

laws General rules and standards to regulate conduct.

layered tablet Tablet containing two or more ingredients layered to dissolve and be absorbed at different times.

LDL Low-density lipoprotein; "bad" cholesterol.

lead time Time it takes to receive an order once placed.

leads Covered wires that carry electrical impulses from the sensors to the ECG machine.

learning log Writing study strategy where thoughts about learning are freely written in any format; a journal of information on what is being learned or has been learned.

ledger cards Records of debit and credit activity of a patient in the practice.

legislation Laws.

lens Transparent structure in anterior portion of the eye; focuses images on the eye; piece of glass with refracting capabilities.

lesions (LEE-shuns) Area of tissue that has pathologically changed.

lethal dose Amount of medication that proves deadly to a patient.

leukocyte (LOO-koh-sight) White blood cell (WBC).

leukocyte esterase Enzyme that is released from white blood cells.

leukopenia (loo-koh-PEE-nee-ah) Abnormal decrease in white blood cells.

levators Muscles that lift a bone.

liability Amount owed; debt.

libel Written form of defamation.

license Legal document that allows persons to offer their skills and knowledge to the public for compensation.

ligament (LIG-ah-ment) Tough fibrous band of fibers that connect bone to bone or support internal organs.
ligate To tie off.
light source Part of the microscope located in the base that allows for a better view of the specimen.
linear Referring to thought process that allows connections between thoughts; in a line.
lingual tonsils Lymphoid tissue near the root of the tongue.
liniments Oil, water, alcohol, or soap-based medications intended to be rubbed into the skin.
lipase Enzyme that breaks down fat.
liquid diet Diet consisting of all liquids.
lithotomy position Patient assumes the dorsal recumbent position first, then the buttocks are moved to the end of the table and the feet are placed in stirrups; used for the pelvic examination.
litigation Lawsuit.
liver Organ that secretes bile; active in formation of certain blood proteins and metabolism of carbohydrates, fats, and proteins.
LMP Last menstrual period.
local Primarily affecting the area where the medication is placed.
local anesthetic Medication applied to a small area to produce a limited loss of sensation to that area.
long bones Bones found in upper extremities and lower arms and legs; determine height.
longitudinal arch Skeletal structure that supports body weight and stretches from heel bone to phalanges (toes); formed by tarsals and metatarsals.
long-term memory Memory that is stored and can be retrieved throughout a person's lifetime.
loop of Henle Part of the tubular collection system in the nephron.
lordosis (lor-DOH-sis) Severe inward curvature in the lumbar area; swayback.
lotions Water-based preparations containing medications to soothe the skin; applied to the skin.
low-cholesterol, low-fat diet Diet low in saturated fats.
low-fiber diet Diet that contains low-residue foods that pass easily through the digestive system.
low-power field (LPF) Low magnification.
lower esophageal sphincter (LES) Sphincter located between the esophagus and the stomach; also called *cardiac sphincter*.
lower gastrointestinal series (lower GI) Radiographic examination of the lower intestinal tract during and after introduction of a contrast medium; also called *barium enema*.
lower respiratory tract Respiratory tract, including the trachea, lungs, bronchi, bronchioles, and alveoli.
lozenge Hard, candy-like tablet that dissolves in the mouth and releases medication.
lubricant Agent used to reduce friction by making a surface moist; used to facilitate anal and vaginal examinations.
lumbar (flank) (LUM-bar) Pertaining to the area between the chest (ribs) and pelvis (ilium) on the dorsal surface.
lumbar puncture (spinal tap) Withdrawal of spinal fluid for diagnostic purposes or for relief of pressure on the brain; also called *spinal tap*.
lumbar vertebrae Five vertebrae in lower portion of the back; L1 to L5.
lumen Opening in a vessel, intestines, or tube; opening of a needle.
lung cancer Malignant neoplasm of the lung.
lung scan Nuclear scanning test used to detect a blood clot.
lungs Organs responsible for respiration (oxygenation of blood and elimination of carbon dioxide).
lunula (LOON-yu-luh) White, moon-shaped base of the nail.
luteinizing hormone (LH) (LOO-tin-eye-zing) Hormone that starts ovulation in the female; develops interstitial cells in the male.
Lyme disease Bacterial skin disease that also affects the joints and connective tissue; carried by the tick as a vector.
lymph (LIMF) Fluid transported in the lymphatic vessels.
lymph nodes Small, oval-shaped bodies of lymphoid tissue that contain lymph and macrophages to fight infection.
lymphatic vessels (lim-FAH-tik) Vessels that transport lymph from the body toward the subclavian vein for return to the blood.
lymphatics (lim-FAH-tiks) Larger vessels formed by lymph capillaries.
lymphocyte (LIM-foh-sight) Type of leukocyte that is agranular; also a lymph cell.
lymphoid organs Spleen, tonsils, thymus, and lymph vessels.
lysis Destruction of red blood cells.
lysosomes (LYE-so-sohms) Organelles responsible for breaking down larger molecules; intracellular digestive system.

M

macrophage (MAK-roh-fahj) Cells responsible for destroying worn-out red blood cells and cellular debris; major phagocyte.
macrotia (mah-KROH-sha) Ears larger than 10 cm.
macula lutea (MACK-yoo-lah LOO-tee-uh) Yellowish spot in the retina that contains the fovea.
macule (MACK-youl) Flat, discolored area of the skin.
magnetic resonance imaging (MRI) Method of visualizing soft tissues of the body by applying an external magnetic field that causes hydrogen atoms in different body environments to release energy that is transformed into an image; procedure in which strong magnetic field and radio waves are used to produce images to view body structures.
main term Disease, condition, noun, synonym, or eponym that helps the coder find the correct code or range of codes in an index.
maintenance dose Amount of medication needed by the body to maintain its desired effect.
maintenance solutions Solutions administered to replace electrolytes lost and maintain electrolyte balance.
major medical benefits Insurance coverage beyond basic medical benefits used for expenses incurred by lengthy illness or serious injury.
major minerals Minerals used in significant amounts by the body (calcium, phosphorus, magnesium, sodium, iron, iodine, potassium).
malabsorption Inability of the digestive system to absorb required nutrients.
malaise (mah-LAYZ) Vague feelings of illness or discomfort.
malfeasance (mal-FEE-zunts) Performance of an unlawful act that causes harm.
malignant (mah-LIG-nant) Cancerous.
malignant melanoma (mel-ah-NOH-mah) Black, asymmetrical lesion with uneven borders that grows faster than normal moles.
malleus (MAL-ee-us) (hammer) One of the three bones of middle ear responsible for producing sound; connected to tympanic membrane and transmits vibrations to incus.
malnutrition Inadequate nutrition.
malpractice Specific type of negligence; liability.
mammary glands (MAM-a-ree) Glands located within the breasts that are responsible for producing milk.
mammogram X-ray of the breast.
mammography X-ray technique used to detect abnormalities (lesions and tumors) of the breast.

managed care Network of health care services and benefits designed for a group of individuals who pay premiums to join the insurance plan.

management service organization (MSO) Organization (e.g., hospital) that handles patient services for a medical practice (e.g., billing and payment services).

mandates Requirements.

mandible (MAN-dih-bul) Lower jawbone.

Mantoux test Tuberculin test.

manubrium (mah-NOO-bree-um) Upper portion of the sternum.

manuscript Document used for publication.

marginal artery Artery that supplies blood to the right atrium and right ventricle.

mastectomy (mass-TECK-tuh-mee) Removal of breast tissue. (Radical mastectomy refers to removal of breast with related lymph nodes.)

mastication (mass-tih-KAY-shun) Act of chewing.

mastoiditis (mas-toy-DYE-tis) Inflammation of the lining of mastoid cells.

material safety data sheet (MSDS) Forms that identify chemical structure and safety measures to be used in case of an accidental spill; fact sheet about chemicals that includes handling precautions and first aid procedures after a person has been exposed to a chemical.

matrix (MAY-tricks) Chart or table arranged in a rectangular grid of rows and columns and used to compare concepts or present information; substance within a cell from which it develops; method used to mark off or reserve time in a schedule.

maturation Growth and developmental process involving a person's physical, social, and emotional functioning.

maturation phase Phase 3 of healing process; scar tissue forms.

maxilla (MAX-ih-luh) Upper jawbone; plural *maxillae*.

maxillary sinus (MAX-ih-lahr-ee) Air-filled cavity within the maxilla.

maximum dose Largest amount of medication that can be prescribed to be effective without causing an adverse effect.

McBurney's point Landmark in right lower quadrant (RLQ) of abdomen over location of appendix.

meatus (mee-AY-tus) Opening to the outside of the body, as in the urethra.

mechanical stage control knobs Parts of the microscope that move a slide right to left or front to back.

media Nutritive substances used to grow bacteria and culture microorganisms; singular *medium*.

median plane See midsagittal plane.

mediastinum (ME-dee-ah-STYE-num) Area behind sternum and in front of lungs that separates lungs and includes trachea, esophagus, and large blood vessels.

Medicaid Federal- and state-funded assistance program that provides medical care for needy populations.

medical asepsis (ay-SEP-sis) Process of making an area clean and free of infectious materials; clean technique; reduces the number of microorganisms.

medical decision making How the physician looks at all the information gathered on examining and testing the patient and then factors this into a decision for a treatment plan.

medically necessary Pertaining to services deemed as needed for patients by the physician.

medical necessity Documentation that verifies a procedure is needed.

Medical Practice Acts Laws that govern the practice of medicine.

medical practice information booklet Booklet or brochure that provides nonmedical information for patients about standard office policies (e.g., billing, inclement weather) of a medical practice.

medical record Patient record that contains information about the patient's treatment history.

medical savings account (MSA) Special type of bank account set up to pay for medical care with pretax dollars.

Medicare Federal government health insurance program for people 65 years and older.

Medicare (as) secondary payer (MSP) Situation in which Medicare is not the primary payer but the secondary payer, because the Medicare recipient is covered by another policy considered to be the primary payer.

Medicare Part D Federally funded program that provides seniors and people living with disabilities with a prescription drug benefit.

Medicare tax Tax collected to support the federal health insurance program for people age 65 and older.

Medigap Medical supplemental (secondary) insurance for Medicare patients.

Medi-Medi Federal insurance program for patients receiving Medicare and Medicaid.

medulla (meh-DUH-lah) Part of the brain stem responsible for automatic control of respiration; inner portion of an organ, such as the kidney.

medulla oblongata (meh-DUH-lah ob-lon-GAH-tah) Lowest part of brainstem; connects to spinal cord and responsible for involuntary movements.

medullary cavity Central cavity of a bone.

meiosis (my-OH-sis) Cell division of sex cells.

melanin (MEL-ah-nin) Dark pigment that provides color to skin and protects against the sun's ultraviolet rays.

melatonin (mel-ah-TONE-ihn) Hormone that responds to natural light and plays a role in sleep.

melena (meh-LEE-nah) Black tarry feces caused by free blood in the intestines.

membrane (MEM-brayn) Specialized tissue that covers an organ surface, lines a body cavity, or is located between a space.

memo Informed written form of communication for interoffice use.

menarche (meh-NAR-kee) Beginning of the menstrual flow; first menses.

Ménière disease (may-nee-UR) Buildup of excess fluid in semicircular canals, which places excess pressure on the canals, vestibule, and cochlea, causing dizziness, ringing in ears, and sensation of fullness.

meninges (meh-NIHN-jeez) Tissues that provide a protective covering for the brain and spinal cord.

meningitis (meh-nihn-JYE-tis) Inflammation of the brain and spinal cord coverings.

meniscus Concave level where air and a liquid come together; the surface of fluid when placed in a column or container.

menopause Permanent cessation of the menstrual cycle.

menorrhagia Abnormal discharge of blood and tissue from the uterus.

menses (MEHN-sez) Monthly bloody discharge from endometrium of the uterus.

mensuration Taking body measurements.

mental growth An individual's cognitive development.

menus List of commands or options, typically found on the top of the computer screen, which can be selected by the user.

mesentery (MEZ-en-tair-ee) Connective tissue that covers the small intestines within the abdominal cavity.

metabolic shock Type of shock caused by excessive loss of body fluids and metabolites (body chemicals).

metabolism (muh-TAB-uh-lizm) Sum of all cellular activities and energy production after absorption of nutrients; all physical and chemical processes within the body, including anabolism and catabolism.

metacarpals (met-uh-KAR-puhls) Bones that form the hand.

metaphysis (meh-TAF-ih-sis) Growth center in children that lies between the epiphysis and diaphysis.

metastasis (meh-TAS-tah-sis) Process of a malignant tumor invading or spreading to other tissues in the body.

metastasized Cancer that has spread from its original (primary) site to a new (secondary) site.

metatarsals (met-uh-TAR-suhls) Long bones of the foot.

metered-dose inhaler (MDI) Handheld device that dispenses medication into the airway.

method of transmission Way microorganisms are passed on (spread) to other hosts or objects.

metrorrhagia (met-roh-RAH-zsa) Uterine bleeding other than that caused by menstruation.

microbiology Tests performed to study microorganisms.

microcontainer Small tubes for blood collection.

microglia cells Nerve cells that engulf cellular waste and destroy microorganisms in nerve tissue; special macrophages to protect CNS.

microhematocrit centrifuge Machine used to process a blood sample for a hematocrit reading by separating cells from plasma.

microorganism (mi-kro-OR-ga-ni-zem) Organism (e.g., bacterium) that can only be seen using a microscope; capable of reproducing; microorganisms include bacteria, fungi, viruses, and protozoa.

microprocessor Circuit found on the main board, that controls and coordinates many functions of the computer (e.g., speed of processing).

microscope Optical instrument used in a laboratory setting to view an organism too small to be seen with the naked eye.

microtia (mye-KROH-sha) Ears smaller than 4 cm.

micturition (mick-ter-RIH-shun) Urination; voiding.

micturition reflex Nerve stimulation that allows the expelling of urine from the bladder.

midbrain Part of brain connecting lower portion of cerebellum to pons; responsible for reflexes.

middle ear Cavity in the temporal bone filled with air that is connected to throat.

midline In the middle.

midsagittal (medial) plane (mid-SAJ-ih-tal) Vertical cut down the midline that divides the body into right and left halves.

midstream clean-catch specimen Urine specimen that requires a strict cleaning procedure collection during the middle of voiding.

mind map Drawing that depicts what an individual or group knows about a subject.

mineralocorticoids (min-er-al-oh-KOR-tih-koyds) Steroid hormones that control sodium, potassium, and water balance.

minerals Inorganic substances used in the formation of hard and soft body tissues.

minimum dose Smallest amount of medication that can be prescribed to be effective in treatment.

misdemeanor Crime that is punishable in jail for a year or less.

misfeasance Improper performance of an act resulting in harm.

mitochondria (my-tohe-KAHN-dree-ah) Organelles that are necessary for cell respiration to produce energy (ATP) within the cell.

mitosis (my-TOH-sis) Division of body cells.

mitral (bicuspid) valve (MY-tral) Heart valve located between the left atrium and left ventricle.

mnemonic device Creative device used to aid memory.

modem Device that transfers data from one computer to another over telephone or cable lines.

modified-block format Letter format that has all lines flush with left margin, except for first line of new paragraph (which is indented five spaces) and date, closing, and signature (which are centered).

modified-wave scheduling Appointment scheduling technique based on theory that each patient visit will not require the allotted time.

modifier Means by which the reporting physician can indicate that a service or procedure performed has been altered by some specific circumstance, but its definition or code has not changed.

molars Back teeth for grinding.

molecule (MAHL-eh-kyool) Two or more atoms.

monitor Display device that converts electrical signals from the computer into points of light that form an image.

monocular Having only one eyepiece.

monocytes (MAH-no-sights) Granular white blood cells that assist with phagocytosis.

monounsaturated fats Fats that are liquid at room temperature and help lower total cholesterol.

morbidity rate Rate of disease or illness or proportion of diseased persons in a given population or location.

"morning-after" pill Oral contraceptive that uses large doses of hormones to prevent conception following sexual intercourse.

mortality Death.

motherboard Circuit board that contains memory chips, power supply, and vital components for processing data in the computer.

motion sickness Excessive stimulation to the vestibular apparatus causing a feeling of nausea.

motor (efferent) neurons Neurons that transmit nerve impulses from the CNS to muscles and glands.

mouse Pointing device that directs activity on the computer screen.

mouth Oral cavity; body opening (orifice) through which humans take in food; also used for speech and, at times, breathing.

mucous threads Thin strands of mucus.

multiple sclerosis (skleh-ROH-sis) (MS) Chronic progressive autoimmune disease caused by irritation and degeneration of the myelin sheath, which is then replaced by scar tissue.

multisample needle Needle that can be used to take multiple blood samples because it has a retractable sleeve on one end of a double-ended needle; used with vacuum tubes.

mumps Viral infection of the parotid gland.

Munchausen syndrome Disorder characterized by the intentional presentation of false symptoms and self-mutilation.

murmur Abnormal heart sound; humming or low-pitched fluttering sound of the heart heard on auscultation.

muscle tissue Tissue composed of fibers that contract to cause movement.

muscle tone State of muscle in partial contraction.

muscular atrophy To lose muscle strength and decrease in size.

muscular dystrophy (DIS-troh-fee) Recessive muscle-wasting disease due to a defective muscle protein.

mutation Alteration of the genetic material of a cell.

myalgia Muscle pain.

myasthenia gravis (mye-as-THEE-nee-ah GRAY-vis) Disease with progressive weakness and atrophy of muscles.

myelin sheath (MY-eh-lin) Covering of an axon that has a whitish appearance.

myelinated Covered with myelin sheath, as over nerve fibers, and appearing as white matter.

myelogram (MYE-eh-loh-gram) X-ray film of spinal canal after injection of contrast medium.
myelography (mye-eh-LOG-rah-fee) X-ray films used to view structures of the spinal cord and surrounding areas using a dye.
myocardial infarction (MI) (my-oh-KAR-dee-ahl in-FARK-shun) Heart attack; death of heart tissue caused by blockage of the heart's blood vessels.
myocardium (my-oh-KAR-dee-um) Main muscle layer of the heart.
myoglobin Pigment responsible for red color of muscle and protein in muscle and that stores and transports oxygen.
myoglobinuria Globin from damaged muscle cells in the urine.
myometrium (mye-oh-MEE-tree-um) Thick muscular layer of the uterus.
myopia (nearsightedness) (mye-OHP-ee-ah) Light rays focus in front of the retina.
myositis Muscle inflammation.
myxedema (mick-se-DEE-mah) Undersecretion of thyroid hormone in adults that is acquired throughout life.

N

Nägele's rule (NAY-geh-lez) Method used to calculate a woman's due date by adding 7 days to the first day of the LMP, subtracting 3 months, and adding 1 year (as necessary).
nail body Fingernail that covers the nail bed.
nail root Part of the nail that lies under the cuticle.
nails Growths of hard keratin that protect the ends of the fingers and toes.
narcissistic (nahr-sih-SIS-tik) Exhibiting behavior that lacks empathy and sensitivity to the needs of others; concerned with self.
nasal bones Bones that form bridge of the nose.
nasal cavity (NAY-zul KAV-ih-tee) Cavity containing the nose.
nasal conchae (NAY-zul KONG-kee) Facial bones above roof of the mouth and walls of the nasal cavities.
nasal septum Partition dividing the nasal cavity into two parts.
nasopharynx (nay-zo-FAR-inks) Top of the pharynx; extends from posterior nares to soft palate.
National Provider Identifier (NPI) 10-digit lifetime identification number issued to health care providers by Medicare.
natural acquired immunity Process of immunity in which the body produces its own antibodies through disease.
nausea (NAH-see-ah) Inclination to vomit.
navicular Tarsal bone of the ankle.
nebulizer Air compressor unit that forces medication into the lungs.
necropsy Autopsy.
needle holder Instrument used to grasp a curved needle and insert it through tissue.
negative feedback Process that causes the body to respond to undersecretion or oversecretion of an element; reduces or stops a stimulus.
negligence Accidental omission or commission of an act that a prudent person would or would not do.
neoplasm (NEE-oh-plazm) Tumor; abnormal formation of new cells.
nephrologist Specialist who is concerned with kidneys and their structure and function.
nephron (NEF-ron) Functioning unit of the kidney.
nerve Bundle of fibers containing neurons and blood vessels (macroscopic).
nerve conduction studies Measurement of peripheral nerve stimulation using electrical impulses.
nerve fibers Bundle of axons.

nerve impulse Electrical signal that begins when a stimulus is received.
nerve tissue Tissue that carries electrical impulses to body structures.
net income Resulting figure when income is greater than expenditures.
net loss Resulting figure when expenditures exceed income.
net pay Total amount of money paid for work, minus deductions.
network Computers interconnected to exchange information; organized group of participating providers for an insurance plan; policies may have "in network" or "out of network" benefits.
networking Interacting with people met through various professional, educational, and social activities ("contacts") to assist in the job search.
neurogenic shock Loss of nerve control over the circulatory system causing decreased blood supply to an area.
neuroglia (noo-ROW-glee-ah) Supporting structures of nerve tissue, located in CNS, including phagocytic cells; do not transmit impulses.
neurolemma (noo-row-LEM-ma) Continuous plasma membrane around the myelin sheath.
neurologist (noo-ROL-oh-jist) Specialist in the medical treatment of nervous system disease.
neuromuscular junction Place where motor neuron comes in contact with a skeletal muscle cell.
neurons (NOO-rons) Nerve cells; functional unit of a nerve that sends and receives nerve impulses (microscopic).
neurotransmitters Chemical substances (e.g., adrenaline, acetylcholine) that cause a nerve impulse to cross synapses.
neutrophils (NEW-troh-fills) Granular white blood cells that are the body's first response to a bacterial infection.
nevus (NEE-vus) Mole or birthmark.
new patient Patient who has not received professional services from the physician, or another physician of the same practice, within the past 3 years.
night blindness Condition caused by a deficiency in vitamin A.
nipple Located at center of each breast; lactation ducts in breast lead to nipple and transport milk outside the body of a nursing mother.
nitrates Salts of nitric acid.
nitrites End products of nitrate metabolism from leukocyte metabolism.
nocturia (nock-TOO-ree-ah) Excessive urination at night.
nodes of Ranvier Spaces where myelin sheath does not touch itself.
nomogram Chart that shows the relationship of body surface area to height and weight in calculating drug dosage, usually for a child or an infant, but may be used with adults.
noncapital goods Equipment that is reusable but less expensive and less durable than capital equipment.
noncompliance Failure of a patient to comply with the physician's treatment plan; grounds for dismissal of a patient from a physician's medical care.
nonessential nutrients Nutrients provided in the body.
nonfeasance Failure to do what is expected.
nonessential Referring to nutrients provided by the body.
nonparticipating provider (non-PAR) Physician who has not signed a contract with an insurance company to participate in health care for the insured.
nonpathogens Non–disease-producing (nonpathogenic) microorganisms.
nonspecific immunity Process of immunity in which the body reacts to eliminate the effects of microorganisms.

nonstriated (non-STRY-aye-ted) Referring to muscle fibers that do not have bands or stripes.

nonsufficient funds (NSF) Indication that the payer did not have sufficient funds in the bank to cover the amount of a check written.

nonverbal Without using words (e.g., nonverbal communication).

norepinephrine (nor-ep-ih-NEF-rin) Hormone secreted by the adrenal medulla that allows the body to respond to stress by raising blood pressure.

normal flora Microorganism that naturally occurs within certain body systems; plural *floras, florae.*

normal sinus rhythm (NSR) Rhythm measurement that starts at the sinoatrial node, occurs within an established time frame, and follows an expected, established pattern.

nosepiece Part of the microscope that holds the objectives.

nostrils External openings of the nose; nares.

notebook computer Small, portable computer (size of a notebook).

noun A word used to name things, including people, places, objects, and ideas.

NPI National Provider Identifier; identification number issued to the provider by Medicare.

nuclear medicine Techniques that use radioactive material for patient diagnosis and treatment.

nucleolus (noo-KLEE-oh-lus) Organelle within the nucleus that forms ribosomes.

nucleus (NOO-klee-us) Organelle that functions as the control center of a cell and contains the chromosomes.

numbness A partial or total lack of feeling in a body part, resulting from an interruption of nerve impulses to a body part.

numeric filing Method of arranging files using numbers.

nutrients Chemical substances within food that are released during the digestive process.

nutrition Scientific study of how different food groups affect the body.

Nutrition Labeling and Education Act (NLEA) Federal act of 1990 to assist consumers in identifying nutritional content in food products.

nutritional fact panel Panel on a label that meets the requirements of federal regulatory boards.

nystagmus (nihs-TAG-muss) Rapid, involuntary, rhythmic movement of the eyeball.

O

obese Grossly overweight.

objective Concrete and factual; can be seen or measured; part of a resumé that states career goal(s) of person looking for employment; common name for objective lenses of a microscope that magnify by different powers or strengths.

objective lens Lens within the objective of the microscope that magnifies a specimen by a certain power.

oblique (oh-BLEEK) Angled.

obsessive-compulsive disorder (OCD) Disorder that interferes with ability to function on a daily basis and characterized by obsessive thoughts and compulsive actions.

obstetrics Branch of medicine concerned with the health management of women during pregnancy, childbirth, and the postpartum period.

occipital bone (OCK-sip-ih-tul) Bone that forms the back part of the cranial floor and covers the back part of the brain.

occipital lobe Lobe at the base of the posterior brain that controls vision.

occlusion (OH-clue-shun) Obstruction; something that blocks a blood vessel.

Occupational Safety and Health Administration (OSHA) Federal agency that enforces safe working conditions for all employees; enforces the use of safety measures in place under Standard Precautions.

ocular lens Eyepiece; magnifies the field by 10 times.

oil-immersion lens Microscope lens that uses a special oil to allow magnification of 100 times the size of the specimen.

ointment Petroleum-based or lanolin-based substance containing medications that is applied to external skin surfaces for healing or antiseptic reasons; semi-solid mixture.

olecranon process (oh-LECK-ruh-non) Extension of the ulna that forms the elbow.

olfaction (ohl-FACK-shun) Sense of smell.

oligodendroglia cells (ol-ih-GOO-DEN-dro-glee-ah) Nerve cells that produce and maintain myelin sheath.

oliguria (ol-ih-GOO-ree-ah) Diminished urine output.

omentum Structure that is part of the peritoneum attached to the stomach; folds over and protects the intestines.

oncology (ong-KOL-oh-jee) Study of cancerous tumors.

one-write system See *pegboard system.*

onychomycosis (on-ih-koh-mye-KOH-sis) Fungal infection of the nail.

opaque Not clear; cloudy.

open-ended questions Questions that require more than a "yes" or "no" answer.

open-hour scheduling Appointment scheduling technique that allows patients to be seen without an appointment.

open MRI Imaging table with more space used for MRI imaging versus the enclosed narrow magnet tube.

open reduction Repairing ("reducing") a fracture when the skin has been surgically opened.

open technique Application of only sterile gloves for performing a sterile procedure.

open wound Contusion where the skin is broken and the tissue below is exposed; break in the skin or mucous membranes.

operating scissors Scissors that have straight, delicate blades for cutting through tissue.

operative Pertaining to an action or surgical procedure.

operative report Medical report that lists surgical procedure done, pathological specimens, findings, and medical personnel involved.

ophthalmologist (ahf-thal-MOL-oh-jist) Specialist in treatment of eye disorders.

ophthalmoscope (ahf-THAL-moh-skope) Hand-held instrument used for viewing the internal structure of the eye, especially the retina, optic nerve, and blood vessels.

optic disc (OPP-tik) (blind spot) Area of no visual reception (no rods or cones) where optic nerve joins the retina.

optic nerve Nerve that carries visual impulses from the retina to the brain; second cranial nerve.

optical character recognition (OCR) Process by which electronic equipment scans printed documents and digitizes the information for computer processing.

oral By mouth.

orchitis Inflammation of one or both testes accompanied by pain and swelling.

orbital cavity (OR-bi-tul) Cavity containing the eye area.

order of draw Order or manner in which blood collection tubes are to be drawn.

order quantity Optimal quantity of a supply to be ordered at one time.

organ Structural unit of the body that has a unique function.
organ of Corti Receptor of hearing located in the cochlea.
organelle Structure contained within the cytoplasm of a cell; each organelle has a specific function.
organism An individual animal or plant that carries on life's function.
organize To bring order and form to a concept.
origin Term for a more fixed muscle anchored to nonmoving bone.
oropharynx (or-oh-FAR-inks) Area of pharynx located behind mouth; extends from soft palate to upper portion of epiglottis.
orthopedic (or-thoh-PEE-dik) Pertaining to treatment of the bones and joints.
orthopedist Physician whose specialty is to correct musculoskeletal disorders.
osmosis (os-MOH-sis) Diffusion of water through a membrane.
ossicles (OS-ih-kulz) Small bones of middle ear, including malleus, incus, and stapes.
ossification (os-ih-fih-KAY-shun) Formation of bone.
ostealgia (AHS-tee-AL-jee-ah) Pain within the bone.
osteitis (AHS-tee-EYE-tis) Inflammation of the bone.
osteoarthritis (AHS-tee-oh-ar-THRIGH-tis) Condition resulting from cartilage on the end of bones softening and the bones rubbing against each other; deterioration of joints.
osteoblast (AHS-tee-oh-BLAST) Bone-building cell.
osteoclast (AHS-tee-oh-KLAST) Bone-reabsorbing cell.
osteocyte (AHS-tee-oh-SITE) Mature bone cell made of organic and inorganic material, providing hardness to bone; maintains bone matrix.
osteoma (AHS-tee-oh-ma) Benign bone tumor that develops in the membrane of the skull.
osteomalacia (AHS-tee-oh-mah-LAY-shee-ah) Bone disease of adults characterized by deficiency of calcium and vitamin D and softening of bones.
osteomyelitis (AHS-tee-oh-my-eh-LYE-tis) Infection of the bone marrow and bone.
osteonecrosis (AHS-tee-oh-neh-KROH-sis) Death of bone tissue.
osteoporosis (AHS-tee-oh-por-OH-sis) Condition caused by more bone cells being destroyed than made; decrease in bone density leaves the bones porous and prone to fracture.
otitis externa (oh-TYE-tis eck-STER-nah) (swimmer's ear) Inflammation of the outer ear.
otitis media (oh-TYE-tis MEE-dee-ah) Inflammation of the middle ear.
otolaryngologist (oh-toh-lar-in-GOL-oh-jist) Specialist in treatment of ear, nose, and throat diseases.
otosclerosis (oh-toh-skleh-ROH-sis) Hardening of the ear bones.
otoscope (OH-toh-skope) Hand-held instrument used to examine the ear canal and eardrum.
otoscopy (OH-toh-sko-pee) Views the tympanic membrane and various parts of the outer ear.
out guides Separators that replace a file folder when it is removed from the file cabinet; contains a notation of the date and the name of who signed out the file.
out-of-town check Check drawn on a bank account that is not local.
outer ear External ear, including the pinna, external auditory canal, and tympanic membrane.
outpatient Person who is being treated in the hospital or medical center and who will be discharged within 24 hours.
out sourced Subcontracting work to a third party.
oval window Opening in inner ear that is in contact with the stapes.
ovarian cysts (oh-VAIR-ee-an) Fluid-filled sacs that form in the ovaries.
ovaries (OH-var-ees) Female sex glands (gonads); singular *ovary*.
over-the-counter (OTC) drugs Medications that are sold without a prescription.
overcompensation Defense mechanism in which exaggerated and inappropriate behavior is used to cover up an area of inadequacy.
ovulation (oh-vu-LAY-shun) Release of an egg from the ovary.
ovum (OH-vum) Gamete of reproductive cell; an egg; plural *ova*.
owner's equity Amount remaining after liabilities are subtracted from assets.
oximetry sensor Device attached to a patient's finger that detects oxygen content in arterial blood.
oxygen Gas necessary for cellular respiration and circulated to the tissues by the blood.
oxytocin (AHKS-ee-TOE-sin) Hormone stored in posterior pituitary gland and needed for uterine contractions during and after childbirth; allows for milk expulsion after delivery.

P

P wave ECG pattern that shows atrial contraction originating at the sinoatrial node.
pacemaker Sinoatrial (SA) node of heart; device that delivers electrical impulses to the heart muscle when the SA node is unable to do so.
packing slip Document received with an order that lists the items ordered and itemizes those sent and those to arrive at a later date.
Paget disease (PAJ-it) Slow, progressive disease of bone with excessive and abnormal resorption and formation of bone.
paid in full Endorsement qualifying that the balance of an account is zero after acceptance of a check.
pain Unpleasant sensation caused by a negative stimulation to the sensory nerve endings.
palatine bones (PAL-eh-tyne) Facial bones behind the hard palate that help to form walls of the nasal cavity and floor of the eye orbits.
palatine tonsils (PAL-eh-tyne TAHN-suls) Lymphoid tissue located in the oropharynx.
palliative (PAL-ee-ah-tiv) Relieving or soothing, but not curing; to be made comfortable by alleviating symptoms.
pallor (PAL-ur) Paleness; lack of color in skin.
palpation (pal-PAY-shun) Touching or feeling of body organs, lymph nodes, and tissue.
palpitation (pal-pih-TAY-shun) Subjective sensation of a rapid or irregular heartbeat.
pancreas (PAN-kree-ahs) Organ that secretes pancreatic juice into the duodenum (*exocrine*) and insulin and other substances into the bloodstream (*endocrine*); has both endocrine and exocrine functions; organ of the digestive system.
pancreatin (pan-kree-AH-tin) Medication that is a mixture of the enzymes of pancreatic juice, used as a digestive aid.
pancreatitis (pan-kree-ah-TYE-tis) Inflammation of the pancreas.
Pap smear Papanicolaou test; cells scraped from surface epithelium, usually from the cervix, are examined microscopically for malignancy.
papillae (pa-PIL-ahe) Small projections on the tongue that contain taste buds.
papule (PAP-youl) Small, solid, red raised area of the skin; a pimple.
paralysis Loss of muscle function, sensation, or both.
paranasal sinuses (par-ah-NA-sal) Cavities in skull connected to nasal cavities that lighten the weight of the skull.

paranoid Feeling of exploitation or of being harmed without a credible basis.

parasite (PAR-uh-sight) Infectious organism that needs a host to live or survive; living on or within a host.

parasympathetic nervous system (pahr-ah-sim-pah-THET-ik) System that returns the body back to balance after responding to a reactive state.

parathyroid glands (pahr-ah-THY-royd) Glands located in connective tissue surrounding the thyroid gland.

parathyroid hormone (PTH) Hormone that helps to maintain proper level of calcium in the body.

parenteral Route for medication given under the skin or other than the digestive tract.

paresthesia (pahr-es-THEE-zyuh) Abnormal touch sensation (e.g., prickling).

parietal bones (pah-RYE-eh-tal) Two bones that give shape to top of the skull and extend to the sides.

parietal lobe Lobe of the brain in mid-cerebrum that controls sensory functions (touch, pain, temperature interpretation).

parietal membrane Membrane that covers the wall of a cavity.

parietal pericardial membrane (pah-RYE-eh-tal pair-ih-KAR-dee-al) Outer layer of the heart sac.

Parkinson disease Slowly progressive degenerative disorder characterized by resting tremor, pill rolling of the fingers, and shuffling gait due to muscle weakness and rigidity.

parotid gland (pah-ROT-id) Salivary gland located at the side of the face in front of and below the external ear.

paroxysmal atrial tachycardia (PAT) (pah-rok-SIZ-mul tack-ee-KAR-dee-ah) Sudden onset and ending of atrial tachycardia, 150 to 250 beats per minute.

partial disability State in which a person can perform a portion of his or her job duties.

partial-thickness burn Burn depth that damages the epidermis or epidermis and dermis; second-degree burns.

participating provider (PAR) Physician who has signed a contract with an insurance company to provide services to the insured.

partnered reading Reading comprehension technique in which partners alternate reading passages and summarizing the meaning.

partnership Business owned by two people who are held legally responsible for the debts and taxes of the business.

parturition (par-tyou-RISH-un) Process of expulsion of the fetus; childbirth; labor.

passive immunity Immunity provided by antibodies being passed through the placenta or mother's milk or through gamma globulin.

passive listening Hearing what the speaker is saying, but not fully concentrating on the conversation.

passive transport Movement of materials across the cell membrane without using cellular energy.

password Special set of characters known only to the user and the person who assigned the password; designed to secure and protect unauthorized entry to a computer.

past history (PH) Summary of a patient's prior health.

patella (pah-TELL-ah) Kneecap.

patellar reflex (pah-TELL-ar) Knee-jerk response when patellar tendon is tapped.

patent Open; not obstructed.

pathogens (PATH-oh-jens) Disease-causing organism.

patency Describes the degree that an opening is unblocked.

patient Person who receives medical treatment; not necessarily the guarantor.

Patient Care Partnership Document produced by the American Hospital Association concerning communication between patients and hospitals.

patient education Teaching-learning process that takes place in a medical practice.

patient information brochure See medical practice information booklet.

Patient's Bill of Rights Document formulated by the American Hospital Association to define the rights of patients.

payable Representing liability; accounts payable are money and funds owed to someone else (e.g., vendor).

payee Person receiving payment of a debt.

payer Person paying a debt.

Payment Act Legislation requiring employers to withhold tax based on a scale and to pay it to the Internal Revenue Service.

payroll Employees' salaries, wages, bonuses, net pay, and deductions.

payroll register Document that shows information about earnings and deductions for each employee.

pectoral girdle (pek-TOR-uhl) Shoulder; attaches arms to axial skeleton.

pediculosis (pee-dik-you-LOH-sis) Parasitic skin disorder caused by lice.

pegboard Device used to write the same information on several forms at one time.

pegboard system Recording system using a pegboard designed to increase the efficiency of recording daily transactions; also called *one-write system.*

pellagra Disease caused by a deficiency of niacin in the body.

pelvic (PEL-vik) Pertaining to the area of the pelvis or lower abdomen.

pelvic examination Internal examination to evaluate the size, shape, and location of the reproductive organs and to detect disease.

pelvic girdle Bones that connect the legs to the axial skeleton.

pelvic inflammatory disease (PID) Infection that involves the uterus, uterine tubes, and surrounding tissue.

pelvimetry Measurement of the pelvis by estimating bimanually or by x-ray.

penis Male organ for copulation that is suspended from the front and sides of the pubic arch and contains the urethra.

penlight Instrument used to enhance examination in a cavity and to check for pupillary response to light.

pepsin (PEP-sin) Digestive enzyme found in gastric juice that catalyzes the breakdown of protein.

perception An individual's view of a situation based on the environment.

percutaneous Route for medication given through the skin.

percussion Tapping to check for reflexes or sounds of body cavities.

percussion hammer (per-KUSH-un) Instrument used to measure tendon reflexes.

perforation Tear or hole in an organ or body part (e.g., eardrum rupture, perforated bowel).

pericardial membrane (per-ih-KAR-dee-al) Membrane that surrounds the heart.

pericardium (pair-ih-KAR-dee-um) Sac that surrounds the heart.

perimetrium (per-ih-MEE-tree-um) Serous layer of the uterus.

perineum (per-ih-NEE-um) Area between vagina and anus in females; area between scrotum and anus in males.

periosteum (per-ee-OS-tee-um) Outer covering of bone that provides support of blood vessels that nourish the bone and provides attachment of muscles, tendons, and ligaments.

peripheral nervous system (PNS) (pur-RIFF-uh-ruhl) System of nerves that connect the CNS to body tissue; nervous system outside the brain and spinal cord.

peripherals External components attached to the computer, such as the speakers.

peristalsis (per-ih-STAL-sis) Wavelike motions that propel food through the digestive tract.

peritoneal dialysis (pehr-ih-toh-NEE-al dye-AL-ih-sis) Solution is passed through the patient's peritoneal cavity and drained to remove waste products that the kidney cannot excrete.

peritoneum (per-ih-tow-NEE-um) Abdominal membrane that divides into the parietal and visceral membranes.

permanent teeth Adult teeth.

pernicious anemia Condition caused by the body's inability to absorb vitamin B_{12}.

PERRLA Pupils equal, round, and react to light and accommodation.

personal digital assistant (PDA) Pocket-sized computer used for appointments, phone numbers, notes, and other information (e.g., Palm Pilots, Blackberries).

personal mission statement Sentence that describes a person's purpose in life.

personal protective equipment (PPE) Protective items used to prevent exposure to blood and body fluids, required by CDC Standard Precautions to minimize exposure.

pertinent past, family, and social history (PFSH) Pertinent background information about a patient's family and the patient's social habits, as directly related to the patient's current problem.

pertussis (per-TUS-is) Whooping cough; bacterial infection of the pharynx, larynx, and trachea.

petechiae (pee-TEE-kee-ee) Small purple or red spots appearing on the skin as a result of hemorrhages within the dermis.

petty cash Amount of cash kept on hand to be used for making payments for incidental supplies.

phagocytes (FAJ-oh-sights) White blood cells that engulf foreign material.

phagocytosis (FAJ-oh-sigh-TOH-sis) Process of engulfing or digesting foreign material.

phalanges (fay-LAN-jez) Bones that form the fingers (or toes).

pharmacodynamics The study of the biochemical and physiological effects of a drug within the body.

pharmacokinetics The study of what happens to a drug from the time it enters the body until it leaves.

pharmacology The study of drugs and how they affect the body.

pharyngeal tonsils Lymphatic tissue located on the posterior wall of the nasopharynx.

pharyngitis (far-in-JIGH-tis) Inflammation of the throat; sore throat.

pharynx (FAR-inks) (throat) Passageway that transports air into the lungs and food and liquids into the esophagus.

phenylketonuria (PKU) (fen-il-kee-toh-NEW-ree-ah) Recessive trait causing the abnormal presence of phenylketones in the urine.

phlebitis (fle-BY-tis) Inflammation of the walls of the veins.

phlebotomy Process of drawing blood from a vein; venipuncture.

phobias Irrational fears of objects, activities, or situations.

photodetector Device that records the percentage of oxygen in the blood after a light source passes through arterial blood.

phrenic nerve Nerve responsible for stimulating the diaphragm in breathing.

physical growth An individual's growth and development in physical size and in motor and sensory skills.

physician office laboratory (POL) Laboratory within the medical office setting.

physiological Relating to the body's responses to its internal and external environment.

physiology (fiz-ee-AHL-oh-jee) Study of an organism's function.

pia mater (PEE-ah MAY-ter) Covering of the brain closest to the brain and spinal column that is delicate tissue rich with small blood vessels.

pick-ups Common name for thumb forceps; also used by some physicians as another name for transfer forceps or sponge forceps.

pineal gland (PIHN-ee-ahl) Small, cone-shaped organ in the brain that secretes melatonin.

pinna (PIN-ah) (auricle) External portion of the ear (flap).

pinocytosis (pin-oh-sye-TOH-sis) Process where cells ingest or absorb fluids or nutrients.

pipette Narrow tube used for transferring liquids by suction.

pipetting Taking a small sample from a larger sample using a pipette.

pitch Pertains to high or low sound created by sound waves.

pituitary gland (pih-TOO-ih-terr-ee) Master gland; under control of the hypothalamus.

pivot joint Joint that allows for rotation.

placement services Agencies that assist job seekers in finding employment.

placenta (pluh-SEN-tah) Organ that provides nourishment and oxygen to the fetus during pregnancy; special tissue that attaches to the uterus.

placenta abruptio Premature separation of placenta from uterine wall, either partially or completely; hemorrhage may result; obstetrical emergency during which mother needs immediate medical attention.

placenta previa Attachment of the placenta implants in lower portion of uterus and partially or completely covers cervix.

plan Action created to solve a problem, as in a patient treatment plan.

plantar reflex Bottom of foot is stroked and toes flex.

plaque (plack) Food debris and saliva debris that accumulate on the teeth and trap bacteria; fat deposits on the inside wall of an artery.

plasma (PLAZ-mah) Liquid matrix (portion) of blood.

plaster cast Mold made by wetting bandages that contain plaster that hardens when it dries to immobilize a body part.

platelet (PLAYT-let) Cell fragment responsible for clotting; thrombocyte.

platelet counts Total number of platelets in a blood sample.

platform crutches Devices used for walking that provide a shelf-like device to support the forearms and a handgrip.

pleura (PLOO-rah) Serous membrane around the lungs that provides moisture to prevent friction during respiration.

pleural cavity (PLOO-rahl KAV-ih-tee) Cavity containing the lungs.

pleurisy (PLOOR-ih-see) Inflamed pleural surfaces of the lungs.

plexus Network of nerves.

plural Noun that refers to two or more things.

pneumonia (new-MOW-nee-ah) Inflammation of the lung tissues.

pneumothorax (new-mow-THOH-racks) Accumulation of air or gas in the space between visceral pleura and parietal pleura (pleural space).

PNS Peripheral nervous system.

point Size of typeface; number of characters per inch.

point-of-care testing (POCT) Tests done in the physician office laboratory for immediate feedback.

point-of-service (POS) plan Open-ended HMO option that allows members to visit physicians outside the plan (out of network) but offers better reimbursement and lower payments to use physicians within the plan (in network).

poison Substance that causes injury, illness, and even death; toxin.

polarization Phase when the heart is in a ready state to contract.

policy manual Manual that explains the policies used in the day-to-day operations of the medical office and provides general information that affects all employees.

polycystic kidney (pah-lee-SIS-tik) Replacement of kidney tissue with marble-like cysts.

polydipsia (pol-ee-DIP-see-ah) Excessive thirst.

polyp (POL-ip) Stalk-like growth extending out from the mucous membrane; usually benign growth that can be attached to mucosal lining of colon.

polyphagia (pah-lee-FAY-jee-ah) Excessive appetite.

polyunsaturated fats Fats that are liquid at room temperature and found in vegetable oil.

polyuria (pah-lee-YOOR-ee-ah) Excretion of abnormally large amounts of urine; excessive urination.

pons (PONZ) Part of the brainstem responsible for automatic control of respiration; middle section of the brain stem that acts as a bridge between the brain and spinal cord, controlling the face, hearing, balance, blood pressure, and heart rate.

popliteal artery Artery located behind the knee.

pore Opening on the surface of the skin that provides a pathway for fluid to leave the body.

portion Actual amount of food consumed at any one time, which may be more or less than a serving.

positioning Placing a patient in a particular posture.

positive feedback Process that increases secretion of hormone when needed; increases a stimulus.

positron emission tomography (PET scan) (POZ-ih-tron ee-MIH-shun toh-MAH-gruh-fee) Imaging technique that evaluates physiological and biochemical processes using a glucose molecule with radioactive material attached; sugar tracer is injected into the body and picked up by cancer cells that send out signals that can be picked up by a camera that forms pictures of various body parts. Also used with cerebral and arteriovascular diseases.

postage meter Automated stamp machine.

postdated Written using a future date, as in postdated check.

posterior (pos-TEER-ee-or) Referring to or in the back; behind.

posterior cavity Space between the iris and lens.

posterior descending artery Artery that supplies blood to the left and right ventricles.

posterior tibial artery Artery located on the inside of the ankle.

postpartum Time from immediately after birth to 6 weeks after birth.

postprandial specimen Urine or blood specimen taken after a meal.

posttraumatic stress disorder (PTSD) Severe anxiety resulting from past trauma; mental impairment that affects daily living.

powders Medications that have been ground into powder form.

power notes Note-taking strategy in which main concepts and subconcepts are identified and recorded in a simple format.

PR interval Time interval between atrial contraction and the beginning of ventricular contraction.

PR segment Time interval necessary for an electrical impulse to cause contraction of the atria and begin contraction of the ventricles.

practice management Sum total of managing all the facets (financial, personnel, patient) of running a medical practice.

preauthorization Authorization for payment sought in advance from the insurance company for a patient's specific procedure or treatment.

precertification Method used for determining in advance how much the patient's insurance policy will reimburse for a particular service or procedure.

precipitates Particles in a solution brought on by a chemical reaction.

predisposing factor Reason or group of reasons that influences a person's chance for contracting a disease.

preexisting condition Documented medical condition that is present in the patient before the insurance policy goes into effect.

preferred provider organization (PPO) Health care system that provides a list of providers who have signed a contract with the insurance carrier to provide services to the insured.

prefilled cartridge unit Container with a single dose of medication for injection.

prefix Word part placed at the beginning of a root word to change its meaning.

pregnancy (PREG-non-see) Time from fertilization of the egg to birth of offspring.

pregnancy-induced hypertension Elevated blood pressure that occurs during pregnancy caused by cardiovascular changes in the body.

prejudice Negative opinion(s) toward an individual because of the individual's affiliation with a specific group.

premature atrial contraction (PAC) Condition in which an electrical impulse in the atria starts before the next expected heartbeat.

premature ventricular contraction (PVC) Condition in which the ventricles receive an impulse prematurely and contract before their time.

premenstrual syndrome (PMS) Combination of physical and emotional symptoms (tension, irritability, headache, fatigue, restlessness, depression, breast tenderness) appearing before the start of menstrual flow and stopping with its onset.

premium Monthly, quarterly, or annual payment for insurance coverage.

prenatal Before birth.

prenatal care Care provided before birth that promotes health for both mother and child.

preoperative instructions Detailed instructions given to the patient before surgery.

preposition A word used to begin a prepositional phrase.

prepuce (PRE-pyoos) Foreskin of the penis.

presbycusis (pres-beh-KOO-sis) Progressive hearing loss occurring in old age.

presbyopia (pres-bee-OH-pee-ah) Lens loses its ability to change shape during accommodation for close objects. Also known as "old eyes."

preschool 3 to 5 years.

prescribe To indicate a medication to be given to a patient verbally or in writing.

prescription Legal document written by a licensed health care provider to a pharmacist for the dispensing of a drug.

present illness (PI) Expansion of a patient's chief complaint.

presenting problem Symptom, disease, or condition that is currently causing a problem and that is the reason for the patient visiting a health care provider.

pressure ulcer Ulcer created when the skin over a bony area has contact and pressure with an irritating source for long periods causing ulceration or breakdown of the skin.

preventive maintenance Regular servicing to prevent the breakdown of equipment.

primary care physician (PCP) Physician responsible for most of the ongoing care of a patient.

primary diagnosis Condition considered as the patient's major health problem; used in outpatient coding.

prime mover Muscle responsible for movement when a group of muscles is contracting at the same time; muscle that provides major energy to movement.

principal diagnosis Diagnosis, determined after study, which was the cause for a patient's hospital admission; used only for inpatient coding.

printer Output device that reproduces information from a computer onto paper.

prioritize To decide which situation requires the most attention; to organize tasks or activities by their level of importance.

private law Branch of law concerned with rights and duties of private individuals.

probes Instruments used to feel inside a body cavity.

probing Exploring, as in a *probing instrument* used to explore body cavities or wounds.

problem list List of a patient's medical complaints.

problem-oriented medical record (POMR) Chart format that is arranged according to a patient's health complaint.

procedures manual Manual containing specific instructions on how procedures are to be performed.

process Projection on or outgrowth of a bone.

professional Person who conforms to the technical and ethical standards of a profession.

professional discounts Discount given to other professionals working in the same field as a provider.

progesterone (pro-JES-ter-own) Hormone produced by the corpus luteum that maintains the uterus during pregnancy.

progress notes Written findings of a patient's condition; data concerning a patient's medical care and its results.

projection Defense mechanism in which there is an unconscious rejection of an unacceptable thought, desire, or impulse, placing blame on something or someone else.

prolactin (pro-LAK-tin) Hormone that stimulates milk production.

prolapse of uterus (PRO-laps) Displacement of the uterus into the vagina.

prompt Message displayed by the computer to request information or help the user proceed.

pronation (pro-NAY-shun) Turning downward.

prone position Position in which the body is lying on the belly with the face down.

pronoun A word used to take the place of a noun.

proofreading Reviewing a written work for errors; process of reading and correcting a document or manuscript for technical errors (e.g., spelling, punctuation).

prophylactic Preventive, as in measures taken to prevent disease.

prophylactic drug Medication that lessens or prevents the effects of a disease.

proprioception Awareness of body position of a body part in reference to another.

prostaglandins (pros-tah-GLAN-dins) Large group of hormone-like substances responsible for regulation of blood pressure, pain threshold, inflammation, and blood clotting.

prostate gland (PRAH-stayt) Gland at the base of the penis that produces an alkaline fluid that neutralizes acidity of the urethra and of vaginal secretions.

prostatic cancer (PRAH-sta-tik) Cancer of the prostate.

prostatitis (pros-tah-TYE-tis) Infection of the prostate.

protein Substance that builds and repairs body tissue and breaks down enzymes so they can be absorbed by the small intestine.

proteinuria (proh-teen-YOU-ree-ah) Presence of excess serum protein in the urine; also called *albuminuria*.

prothrombin (proh-THROM-bin) Substance needed for clot formation.

protozoa (proh-tuh-ZOH-ah) Single-cell animals; singular *protozoan, protozoon*; parasitic organisms that have the ability to move.

provider Health care facility (e.g., medical office) or the personnel (e.g., physician, medical assistant) rendering medical treatment to a patient.

pruritus (proo-RYE-tus) Severe itching.

psoriasis (soh-RYE-uh-sis) Idiopathic, hereditary dermatitis with dry, scaly, silver patches with definite borders, usually on both arms, legs, and the scalp.

psychiatry (sye-KYE-ah-tree) Medical specialty that deals with the treatment and prevention of mental illness; medical science that deals with the origin, diagnosis, prevention, and treatment of developmental and emotional components of mental disorders.

psychogenic shock Psychological stress on the body.

psychology (sye-KAHL-uh-jee) Scientific study of the mind and the behavioral patterns of humans and animals.

psychomotor Type of learning based on motor skills needed to perform tasks.

psychosis (sye-KOH-sis) Impaired perception of reality.

psychosocial Pertaining to some form of social action and how it affects an individual.

psychosocial growth An individual's emotional and social development.

psychosomatic Physical illness brought about by psychological problems.

ptosis (TOE-sis) Drooping (e.g., upper eyelid unable to remain open).

pubis (PYOO-bis) Area that joins the hipbones together anteriorly.

public law Branch of law that deals with offenses or crimes against the welfare or safety of the public.

puerperium The time period after childbirth; postpartum.

pulmonary artery (PULL-mon-air-ee) Artery that carries oxygen-poor blood from the right ventricle to the lungs.

pulmonary circulation Movement of blood from the heart to the lungs and back.

pulmonary edema Fluid in the lungs.

pulmonary embolism (EM-boh-lizm) Closure of the pulmonary artery or one of its branches when a clot dislodges and obstructs the vessel either partially or completely.

pulmonary function tests (PFTs) Tests (e.g., spirometry) that measure how well the lungs take in and exhale air and how efficiently the lungs transfer oxygen into the blood; measure lung volume and capacity; assess lung function.

pulmonary semilunar valve (seh-mee-LOO-nar) Valve that prevents backflow into the right ventricle.

pulmonary vein Vein that carries oxygenated blood from the lungs back to the left atrium.

pulse Rhythmical throbbing of an artery felt when the artery is pressed against a bone.

pulse deficit Condition in which the radial pulse rate is less than the apical pulse rate.

pulse oximetry Method to measure the amount of oxygen in a patient's blood.

pulse pressure Difference between the systolic and diastolic blood pressure.

pulse rate Number of heartbeats per minute.

punctuality Ability to be on time.

punctuation Marks within and between sentences that separate, emphasize, and clarify the different ideas within a sentence or group of sentences.

puncture Piercing of the skin by a sharp object.

pupil Opening at center of the iris that regulates the entrance of light.

purchase order Document used to order supplies; contains the name, address, and telephone number of a vendor and the quantity, price, and description of the items ordered.

purge To clean out, as with excessive data in patient files.

Purkinje fibers (per-KIN-jee) Fibers that form right and left branches of bundle of His and extend along outer walls of ventricles, causing them to contract; receive impulses from the bundle branches and take them throughout the heart muscle.

purpura (PUR-pew-rah) Small hemorrhages into the skin and tissues.

purulent Wound drainage that consists of pus.

pustule (PUS-tyoul) Small, raised area of the skin containing pus.

pyelonephritis (pye-uh-loh-neh-FRY-tis) Inflammation of the renal pelvis and nephron, including connective tissue of kidneys.

pyloric sphincter (pie-LOR-ik) Sphincter that allows chyme to exit from stomach into small intestine; opening between stomach and small intestine.

pyloric stenosis Narrowing of pyloric sphincter between stomach and duodenum.

pylorus (pye-LORE-us) Area of stomach closest to duodenum.

pyramids (PIR-a-midz) Triangular shapes; sections within the kidneys that contain the tubules.

pyuria (pye-YOU-ree-ah) Presence of pus in the urine.

Q

QRS complex ECG pattern that shows when the impulse moves through ventricles and reaches the Purkinje fibers, depicting contraction of both ventricles.

QT interval Time interval that shows the time needed for the ventricles to contract and recover.

quadrants (KWOD-rants) Clinical division of the abdominal area into four parts.

qualified endorsement Type of endorsement that qualifies the acceptance of a check received; done when one person accepts payment for another.

qualitative Presence of a substance (e.g., hCG in a pregnant woman's urine or blood); positive or negative results.

quality assurance (QA) Process designed to monitor and evaluate the quality and accuracy of test results.

quality control (QC) Process that provides for accuracy of laboratory tests performed by using a known value for a precheck.

quantitative Amount of a substance able to be measured; actual amounts.

quantity not sufficient (QNS) Insufficient amount of a specimen for performing the desired test.

quid pro quo (kwid-pro-kwo) Latin phrase meaning "something for something"; equal exchange, similar to give and take.

R

radial artery (RAY-dee-al) Artery in the wrist area.

radial pulse Pulse felt at the radial artery when palpated at the wrist over the radius.

radioactive iodine (RAI) uptake scan Test that detects the thyroid's ability to concentrate and retain iodine.

radiograph Picture or image created on film when exposed to x-rays; x-ray film.

radiography (ra-de-O-gra-fee) Imaging technique using x-rays or gamma rays to make a film record (radiograph, x-ray film) of internal structures based on changes in tissue density, especially skeletal system's soft tissue.

radioimmunoassay (RIA) Test using nuclear medicine that detects hormone levels in the blood using radionuclides.

radiology Branch of medicine dealing with radioactive substances (x-rays, isotopes).

radiology report Medical report that describes the findings and interpretation of a radiologist.

radiopaque (ra-de-o-PAKE) Able to be seen using an x-ray technique.

radius Bone of the lower arm located on the thumb (medial) side.

rales (rayls) Crackling sounds heard on auscultation during inspiration; breathing sounds of "tissue paper being crumpled" caused by fluid or secretions in the bronchus.

random access memory (RAM) Read and write memory that the CPU uses for storage.

random specimen Urine specimen collected at any time; any specimen taken anytime without special preparation.

range of motion Extent of movement of a joint.

rapid screening test Test used to detect disease using various methods; can be used to detect group A beta hemolytic streptococci.

rapport Harmonious relationship that considers both the physical and the emotional needs of those involved.

ratchet Part of an instrument used to keep it closed by interlocking both sides.

rate Numerical measurement of heartbeats or respirations per minute; a characteristic of measuring the pulse or respiration.

rationalization Inventing acceptable reasons for one's behavior.

read-only memory (ROM) Stored data that can be read but not changed (e.g., instructions to the CPU on how to set itself up).

reagent strip Dipstick containing several chemical pads that detect a specific substance in a body fluid.

reagent tablet Tablet that reacts to a substance, confirming its presence.

reagents Solutions used when testing specimens in the laboratory.

receipt-charge slip Charge form with two parts: right side lists previous balance, treatments, and patient's name; left side lists charge for treatments, payments received, and current balance; also called *statement-receipt*.

receptor (re-SEP-tor) Sensory nerve ending.

recessive Not prominent trait or characteristic, as in a recessive gene.

recipient Person who receives blood.

reciprocity Exchange that occurs when one state accepts another state's licensing requirements.

recommended dietary allowances (RDAs) Established amounts of essential nutrients in a diet that help decrease the risk of chronic disease.

reconciled State of a checkbook and a bank statement being in balance.

rectal (℞) By means of the rectum.

rectum (REK-tum) Portion of digestive tract that extends from sigmoid colon to anal canal.

rectus Straight.

recurrent turn Bandage turn used for a stump or the head that begins with a circular turn and progresses back and forth overlapping each turn, until the area is covered.

red blood cells (RBCs) Cells in the blood that transport oxygen and carbon dioxide to and from the tissues.

red cell indices Tests that determine the size, content, and hemoglobin concentration of red blood cells.

reduction Returning the bones to their original position.

references List of people who can vouch for the job seeker's character and work habits; can be provided to a potential employer on request.

referral Transfer of a patient's care to another health care provider at the request of a member of the health care team.

reflex Involuntary reaction that results from a stimulus.

refraction (ree-FRAK-shun) Bending of light rays as they pass from one medium to another.

regional anesthesia Type of anesthesia produced when a local anesthetic is injected into and around a set of nerves.

regions Clinical division of the abdominopelvic area into nine sections.

registered mail Special handling method used when the contents have a declared monetary value.

regular diet Diet that contains all foods from the food guide pyramid according to recommended proportions.

regurgitation (ree-gur-jih-TAY-shun) Backward flow of blood.

relative value scale (RVS) Scale that compares the relative value of medical procedures.

relative value unit (RVU) Component of the resource-based relative value scale; three RVUs considered are for work done, practice overhead, and cost of malpractice insurance.

release of information (ROI) Authorization signed by the patient that gives the provider permission to disclose certain health information to the insurance carrier or other health care providers or pertinent parties (e.g., attorney) as deemed appropriate.

release of information form Legal form signed by a patient that indicates who can see the patient's health records.

releasing Marking or placing initials on a document to indicate it can be filed.

reliability Dependability; the quality of being able to be counted on to do one's job well.

renal artery (REE-nul) Artery that takes blood into the kidney.

renal calculi (KAL-ku-lye) Kidney stones made of mineral salts.

renal computed tomography Imaging that shows a transverse view of the kidney.

renal epithelial cells Epithelial cells released by the kidney indicating disease.

renal failure Progressive loss of nephrons, resulting in loss of renal function.

renal failure diet Diet is ordered when a patient's kidneys are not able to get rid of all the wastes in their blood.

renal pelvis Collecting area for urine at the proximal end of the ureter.

renin (REH-nin) Hormone responsible for blood pressure control.

reorder point Minimum quantity of a supply to be available before a new order is placed.

reorganization Changing the order or format of a concept in a logical way to aid in understanding or learning; putting information into a different format.

replacement drug Medication that replaces substances normally found in the body.

repolarization Rest phase of the ECG cycle.

res ipsa loquitur (ras ep-sa lo-kwi-tur) Latin phrase meaning "the thing speaks for itself"; legal principle that applies when the situation itself shows negligence.

reservoir host Infected person; one who is carrying the disease-causing germs but may not have symptoms of disease.

resident flora Bacteria that normally reside in a particular area.

residual disability State in which a person is recovering from total disability but is not capable of performing former duties.

resistance Ability of the body to fight off infection or disease.

resource-based relative value scale (RBRVS) Scale that uses a complex formula to determine Medicare fees based on geographical area expenses (e.g., overhead, cost of malpractice insurance).

respiration (RES-pih-RAY-shun) Process of inhaling oxygen to the lungs and exhaling carbon dioxide; inspiration and expiration.

respiratory rate Cycle of breathing to include inspirations and expirations in a minute.

respondeat superior (ra-spon-de-aht su-per-e-or) Latin phrase meaning "let the master answer"; legal doctrine that places responsibility on physicians for actions by their employees.

restrictive endorsement Type of endorsement in which payee indicates sole purpose for funds; ex. endorsement "for deposit only" on the back of a check for deposit with signature indicates that check is to be used for that purpose only (deposited to that particular account) and therefore cannot be exchanged for cash.

resumé Document that provides an employer with the work history and personal information about a potential employee.

retention (of urine) Abnormal accumulation of urine in the bladder due to loss of muscle tone in the bladder.

reticular (reh-tik-yoo-lur) Occurring in networks to support small structures such as capillaries and nerve fibers.

reticular tissue Fibrous tissue that forms a network for the spleen, lymph, bone marrow, muscular tissue, liver, lungs, kidneys, and mucous membranes of the GI tract, as well as walls of blood vessels.

reticulocyte (re-TIK-yoo-loh-sight) Immature red blood cell.

retina (RET-ih-na) Innermost layer of eye containing the cones, rods, and blood vessels.

retracting Pulling back tissue, as in a *retracting instrument* used to hold tissue away from a surgical area.

retractors Instruments used to hold back the edges of a wound.

retroperitoneal (reh-trow-per-ih-tow-NEE-al) Located behind the peritoneum.

revalidation Recertification.

review of systems (ROS) An inventory of body systems obtained through a series of questions seeking to identify signs and symptoms that the patient may be experiencing or has experienced; step-by-step review of each body system.

Rh factor Rhesus factor, an antigen factor in blood.

rheumatoid arthritis (RA) (roo-MA-toyd) Chronic joint disease that affects the connective tissue and joints.

rheumatoid factor test Test to detect presence of rheumatoid factor (RF) in the blood; a test for rheumatoid arthritis.

rhinitis (rye-NIGH-tis) Inflammation of nasal mucosa from either viral, bacterial, or allergic origin.

rhonchi (RONG-kye) Wheezes heard on auscultation during inspiration and/or expiration; low-pitched sounds created as air goes through narrowed bronchi.

rhythm Interval between each heartbeat or respiration.

rhythm strip Lead II recording on ECG that shows the heart's rhythm.

ribonucleic acid (RNA) Substance responsible for transmitting genetic information from the nucleus to the cytoplasm and controls proteins in cells.

ribosomes (RYE-bo-sowmz) Organelles that manufacture proteins within the cell by translating the codes in messenger RNA.

ribs Flat bones that protect the lungs and heart; 12 pairs articulate to the thoracic vertebrae.
rickets (RICK-ehts) Bone disease (condition) caused by a lack of vitamin D in children.
rickettsiae Microorganisms that live in a particular species of insect and are transmitted (spread) through its bite; singular *rickettsia*.
"right to know" law Hazard communication standard that allows each employee to know of potential exposure problems.
Rinne test Test that uses a tuning fork to compare bone conduction and air conduction of sound; compares air conduction to bone conduction in the hearing response.
risk management Proactive management of potential risks that could result in a lawsuit.
RMA Registered medical assistant.
rods Receptors for black and white and peripheral vision.
ROM Range of motion.
root Part of the hair that lies beneath the surface of the skin or scalp.
root word Main meaning of a word.
rotation Motion that occurs when one bone moves or turns on its own axis.
rotators Muscles that move a joint on its axis.
round window Area below the oval window that separates middle ear and inner ear.
route of entry Way in which a microorganism enters the body.
route of exit Method by which a microorganism leaves the body.
rugae (ROO-gay) Muscular folds of stomach that aid in digestion; also allow bladder to expand.
"rule of nines" Method of evaluating a surface area of a burn; the surface is divided into regions with percentages assigned.

S

sacral (SAY-kral) Referring to the sacrum area of the spine.
sacrum (SA-kyrum) Five vertebrae after lumbar vertebrae that fuse into one; S1 to S5; located between hipbones.
saddle joint Joint shaped like a saddle that fits into a concave-convex socket.
safety stock Items kept on hand to avoid running out of supplies until a reorder is obtained; backup supply.
sagittal (lateral) plane (SADJ-ih-tul) Vertical cut that divides the body into right and left portions.
salary Predetermined amount of pay for a designated period.
saliva (sa-LI-va) Watery mixture of secretions from the salivary glands.
sanguineous Wound drainage that consists of blood.
sanitization (SAN-uh-tuh-zay-shun) Process that reduces the number of microorganisms on an item.
sarcoma (sar-KOH-mah) Malignant bone tumor of the bone marrow and cartilage cells.
SARS Severe acute respiratory syndrome; highly contagious respiratory illness.
saturated fats Animal fats and tropical oils; solid at room temperature.
scabies (SKAY-beez) Parasitic skin disorder caused by an itch mite.
scanner Device that converts texts or graphics on paper into an electrical format that a computer can display, print, and store.
scalpel Instrument with a knife blade used to make an incision.
scapulae (SKAP-yoo-lay) Shoulder blades.
schizoid Showing indifference to social relationships.
schizophrenia (skit-soh-FREE-nee-ah) Condition characterized by disturbances in thought content, perception, sense of self, and both personal and interpersonal relationships.
school age 6 to 11 years.
sclera (SKLEH-rah) White of the eye; tough outer layer.
scleroderma (sklehr-oh-DER-mah) Chronic idiopathic progressive systemic disease of the skin.
scoliosis (skoh-lee-OH-sis) Lateral curvature of the spine.
scored tablet Tablet with indentations across the middle that allow it to be broken in half.
scrotum (SKROW-tum) Sac that holds the testes outside the body.
scurvy Condition caused by a lack of vitamin C in the diet.
search engine Specialized program designed to find specific information on the Internet.
sebaceous glands (she-BAY-shus) Oil glands; release oil that lubricates the skin and hair.
sebum (SEE-bum) Oil that lubricates the skin and hair.
second-degree burn Burn that damages both the epidermis and dermis; partial-thickness burn.
second (secondary) intention healing Healing that occurs when a wound is not totally approximated, but rather heals with granulation and causes scarring.
secondary condition (diagnosis) Condition (or diagnosis) that the patient experiences at the same time as the primary diagnosis.
secretin Hormone that stimulates pancreas to secrete bicarbonate ions to neutralize acid chyme.
sediment Solid material that settles to the bottom of a urine specimen.
segment ECG pattern between two waves.
seizure Sudden involuntary muscle activity leading to a change in level of consciousness and behavior.
self-esteem Feelings of self-worth.
sella turcica (SEL-ah TUR-sih-kah) Bony projection in the sphenoid bone that holds the pituitary gland.
semen (SEE-men) Fluid of male reproductive system that contains spermatozoa; mixture of prostate and bulbourethral fluids and sperm cells.
semicircular canals Inner ear structures that control equilibrium and detect motion.
seminal vesicles (SEM-ih-nul VESS-ih-kuls) Saclike production site of fluid that mixes with sperm and provides nutrition and energy to sperm.
seminiferous tubules (sem-ih-NIF-ur-us) Place where sperm are formed within the testes.
semipermeable Quality of a membrane that allows some materials to pass through but not others.
sensory (afferent) neurons Neurons that transmit nerve impulses to the CNS from within and outside the body.
sentence Group of words that express a complete thought.
septa (SEP-tah) Plural form of *septum*.
septic shock Severe infection with toxins that prevent blood vessels from constricting, causing blood to pool away from vital organs.
septum (SEP-tum) Partition between two sides, as in the heart.
sequela Secondary result of another disease; aftereffect.
serological testing Testing of body fluids to analyze a reaction between antigen and antibody.
serology Tests that study the body's immune response by detecting antibodies in the serum; study of blood serum for antigen-antibody reactions.
serosanguineous Wound drainage that consists of serum and blood.

serous (SEER-us) Wound drainage that consists of serum or clear fluid.
serous membrane Membrane that lines closed cavities.
serum (SEER-um) Liquid portion of blood after blood cells and clotting elements form a clot; used for testing chemicals found in blood.
serum calcium (Ca) Laboratory test to measure amount of calcium in the blood.
serum cholesterol White, fatlike substance made in the liver.
serum pregnancy test Blood test to detect the presence of human chorionic gonadotropin (hCG).
serving Individual quantity of food or drink taken as part of a meal.
"seven rights" Guidelines for drug administration: right patient, drug, dose, route, time, technique, and documentation.
sexually transmitted disease (STD) Disease spread through sexual contact.
shaft Part of the hair that is seen extending above the skin or scalp; part of the needle that determines its length.
shank Area of an instrument between the finger rings and the box lock.
sheath Covering.
shingles (herpes zoster) Acute viral inflammation of dorsal root ganglia.
shock Progressive circulatory collapse brought on by insufficient blood flow to all parts of the body.
short bones Cube-shaped bones that appear in wrists and ankles.
short-term memory Memory that holds a small amount of information for a short time.
sickle cell anemia Recessive disease resulting in crescent-shaped red blood cells.
side effects Unwanted actions of drugs that may be expected.
sig, signature Section of a prescription that provides directions for the patient.
sigmoid colon (SIG-moyd KOE-lon) S-shaped section of the colon between the descending section and the rectum.
sigmoidoscope Instrument used to view the sigmoid region of the colon.
sigmoidoscopy Technique of viewing the sigmoid region of the colon with a sigmoidoscope.
sign(s) Something that can be seen or measured (objective finding); observable evidence that can be seen or measured; objective data.
simple fracture Bone break in which bone does not break through skin.
simple carbohydrates Sugars that have a high caloric value but no nutritional value.
simple proteins Proteins found in whole grains, beans, nuts, and seeds.
Sims' position Patient is first in the supine position, then turns onto the left side with the right leg sharply bent upward.
single-sample needle Double-ended blood collection needle without a retractable sleeve.
sinoatrial (SA) node (sye-noh-AY-tree-al) Specialized group of cardiac cells (tissue) that functions as natural "pacemaker" of the heart; located in upper portion of the right atrium and responsible for the electrical impulse that "fires" the heart.
sinus (SIGH-nus) Air-filled cavity in a bone that reduces the weight of bone.
sinus bradycardia Slow heart rate, less than 60 beats per minute.
sinus tachycardia Rapid heart rate, 100 to 180 beats per minute.
sinuses (SIGH-nus-uz) Cavities in the skull connected to the nasal cavities.

sinusitis (sigh-nuh-SYE-tis) Inflammation of the paranasal sinuses.
sitting (position) Patient's body is at a 90-degree angle.
skeletal (SKEL-eh-tal) Voluntary muscles attached to bones of the skeleton that allow body movement.
skeletal muscle Striated, voluntary muscle used for movement.
skeletal system Bony framework of the body.
skin biopsy Removal of skin tissue for examination.
skin closures Long, narrow adhesive strips used to close small wounds; also called "wound closure strips."
skin lesion removal Removal of warts or other skin lesions through the use of a freezing agent or surgery.
skin test Test to observe the reaction of the skin to a certain substance.
slander Spoken form of defamation.
slide Flat glass plate used to hold specimens for examination under the microscope.
slit-lamp examination Examination of various layers of the eye.
slough Fall off.
small intestine Smaller, upper part of the intestines where digestion is completed and nutrients are absorbed by the blood.
smooth muscle A nonstriated involuntary muscle found in most hollow organs (e.g., digestive tract, blood vessels).
soak Procedure that requires a body part to be immersed in water warm enough to increase blood flow to an area or cold enough to slow blood flow to an area.
SOAP Type of chart format that divides each patient problem into subjective data, objective data, assessment, and plan for treatment.
social history (SH) Overview of a patient's lifestyle, including smoking, education, exercise, occupation, and other environment factors.
Social Security Disability Income Insurance (SSDI) Federal program for individuals who become disabled as a result of injury or illness not related to their employment.
sodium-restricted diet Diet low in sodium-rich foods and seasonings.
soft diet Diet containing foods that are low in residue and easy to digest.
software "Intelligence" of a computer; tells the computer what to do; computer program.
sole proprietorship Business owned by one person who is legally responsible for the debts and taxes of the business; also known as *private practice*.
solute (SOL-yoott) Substance dissolved in a liquid or semi-solid.
solutes Materials suspended in liquid that are not dissolvable; particles of medications in a liquid base.
solution Liquid with dissolved substances.
solvent Liquid that dissolves or holds solid substances.
soma Body cells.
somatic cells Body cells other than reproductive cells.
somatic nervous system (soh-MAT-ik) System of nerves that transmits impulses to skeletal muscles and is responsible for reflex action.
somatic tremor Body tremor caused by voluntary or involuntary muscle movement.
somatoform disorder Disorder characterized by complaints of symptoms with no organic cause or physiological dysfunction.
sorting Arranging documents in a particular order for filing ease.
sound card Internal component in a computer for multimedia that functions for sound and animation.
source-oriented format Chart format that has dividers that separate the different types of patient information.
spacer Attachment added to metered-dose inhaler that acts as a reservoir and changes the characteristics of the medication.

spansule Capsule that contains time-released beads of medication.

spasms Involuntary muscle twitches.

spatial Referring to the feeling of space; sense of where one "is."

special endorsement Type of endorsement in which a payee signs a check made out to the payee over to another payee.

specialization Focus on a particular work specialty that occurs when additional training and educational requirements have been met.

specific gravity Measurement of the weight of dissolved substances in the urine compared with distilled water.

specific immunity Selective immune response of the body against a particular microorganism.

specimen Sample of a larger part, such as body tissue or cells.

specimen adequacy Term that refers to the condition of a specimen.

speculum (SPEK-u-lum) Instrument for viewing a cavity (e.g., ear, nose).

spermatozoa (spur-mat-ah-ZOH-ah) Sperm; reproductive cells of the male.

sphenoid bone (SFEE-noyd) Middle portion of cranial floor that holds cranial bones in place.

sphincters (SFINK-terz) Ringlike muscles that allow openings to open and close.

sphygmomanometer (sfig-moh-muh-NOM-uh-tur) Instrument used to measure blood pressure.

spina bifida (SPY-nah BIFF-ih-dah) Condition in which the spinal column in the lumbar and sacral areas does not close completely at birth.

spinal cavity (SPY-nal KAV-ih-tee) Cavity along the dorsal surface that holds the spinal cord.

spinal column Bony structure (vertebrae) that surrounds and protects the spinal cord.

spinal cord Nerve tissue surrounded by the spinal column; long bundle of nerves that conduct impulses to and from the brain.

spinal nerves Nerve fibers extending from the spinal cord; 31 pairs carry motor impulses from the spinal cord toward muscles or glands and organs.

spinal tap See lumbar puncture.

spinous process (SPI-nus) Projection extending from vertebral bone to serve as attachment for the ribs.

spiral fracture Bone break in which bone is twisted; abuse cases have shown this type of injury.

spiral reverse turn Bandage turn that progresses upward and reverses on itself at intervals to assist in making the bandage fit.

spiral turn Bandage turn in which the bandage progresses upward and each spiral overlaps the previous turn.

spirilla Spiral or corkscrew-shaped bacteria; singular *spirillum*.

spirometer (spy-ROM-u-ter) Instrument used to measure breathing volumes.

spirometry Type of test that measures lung volume and capacity over time.

spleen Organ that stores and destroys red blood cells and produces lymphocytes and monocytes.

splint Firm material used to immobilize above and below a fracture to prevent further damage.

splinter forceps Spring-type instrument with sharp, pointed, slender tips used to grasp fine objects or particles.

sponge forceps Instrument with serrated rings at the tips used to hold gauze sponges.

sponsor One who assumes responsibility for another person or group; the person who carries the insurance.

spores Bacteria with a hard wall capsule that is resistant to heat.

sprain Injury in which ligaments around a joint are torn or ruptured.

spreadsheet Productivity software application that helps the user do calculations by entering numbers and formulas in a grid of rows and columns (e.g., Excel).

sputum (SPYOU-tum) Mucus coughed up from the lungs; lung secretion produced by the bronchi.

SQ3R Reading comprehension strategy: *s*urvey; *q*uestion; *r*ead, *r*ecite, *r*eview.

squamous (SKWAH-mus) Referring to cells with a flat, patchlike shape.

squamous cell carcinoma (SKWAH-mus kar-sih-NOH-mah) Skin cancer that appears as a firm papule with ulcerations.

squamous epithelial cells Cells that appear flat and irregularly shaped under magnification.

SSDI Social Security Disability Income Insurance.

SSI Supplemental Security Income.

ST segment Time interval between the ventricular contraction and the beginning of ventricular relaxation.

stage Part of microscope that holds the slide.

standard limb lead Bipolar lead; insulated device that carries the electrical impulses to the ECG and traces the electrical impulse of the heart in two different directions simultaneously.

Standard Precautions Guidelines established by the CDC to reduce the spread of infection.

standardization Process of ensuring that an ECG taken on one machine will compare to a tracing taken on another machine.

standardization mark Mark made on the ECG paper that indicates the ECG is standardized.

standing (position) Erect; a position where the body is in an upright position.

stapes (STAY-peez) (stirrup) Stirrup; part of middle ear that transmits sound vibrations from the incus to internal ear; smallest bone in the body.

staphylococci (staff-eh-low-KOK-sigh) Bacteria that appear in clusters; of the genus *Staphylococcus*; singular *staphylococcus*.

staples Skin closures made of stainless steel.

State Unemployment Tax Act (SUTA) Legislation mandating that the state collect tax money for benefits to be used by workers who become unemployed.

statement Document indicating the activity in an account.

statement of owner's equity Report that shows changes in the owner's financial interest over time.

statement-receipt See receipt-charge slip.

statute of limitations Time limits to bring forth a lawsuit.

statutes Laws.

stem cells Main cells from which all other cells develop.

stenosis (ste-NOH-sis) Condition in which blood cannot flow through valves into the next chamber; caused by hardening of flaps or scar tissue on flaps.

stereotyping Holding the belief that all members of a culture or group are the same.

sterile Free from all microorganisms, including spores.

sterile dressing Sterile material, such as gauze, used to cover a wound.

sterility Inability to produce sperm in the male or to become pregnant in the female.

sterilization (STIR-uh-luh-zay-shun) Process that destroys all microorganisms including spores; contraceptive method that does not allow the egg or sperm to travel the normal pathway in the body.

sterilization strip Chemical indicator embedded within the center of a wrapped, dense pack that shows conditions for sterilization within the pack.
sternum (STER-num) Breastbone.
steroid Organic compound derived from fats and formed in the adrenal cortex.
stethoscope Instrument used to listen to body sounds from the heart, bowel, and lungs.
stimulus Change in the environment of a nerve cell; causes action.
stockinette Knitted cotton material used over extremities to cover an area before application of cast material.
stomach Muscular saclike portion of the alimentary canal between the esophagus and small intestines; one of main organs where food is broken down for digestion.
stomatitis Inflammation of mucous lining of mouth.
stool Feces; end product of the digestive system expelled from rectum.
strabismus (strah-BIHZ-muss) (cross eye) Condition in which movements of the eyeball are not coordinated because of congenital weakness of external eye muscles (esotropia is a medial strabismus whereas exotropia is a lateral strabismus).
strain Stretching or tearing of a muscle or tendon caused by trauma.
streak To inoculate or put a specimen onto a culture plate in an established pattern.
stream scheduling Appointment scheduling technique that accounts for the actual time a patient needs to be seen.
streptococci (STREP-toh-KOK-sigh) Bacteria that appear in chains; of the genus *Streptococcus*; singular *streptococcus*.
stress Body's response to any demand put on it, whether positive or negative.
striated (STRY-ate-ed) Referring to muscle fibers that are divided by bands or stripes.
stridor (STRYE-dor) High-pitched breathing associated with obstructed airway; shrill sound heard on inspiration.
stroke Cerebrovascular accident (CVA); condition caused by narrowed cerebral vessels, hemorrhage into the brain, and formation of an embolus or thrombus, resulting in a lack of blood supply to a portion of the brain.
stylus Heated device that records the heart's activity on heat-sensitive graph paper.
subarachnoid space (sub-ah-RAK-noyd) Space between the pia mater and arachnoid membrane; contains CSF.
subconscious The part of the consciousness that is not fully aware.
subcutaneous (subQ) injection Injection given into the fatty layers of the skin beneath the dermis.
subcutaneous layer Skin layer that lies beneath the dermis and consists mainly of adipose tissue and loose connective tissue.
subdural space (sub-DOO-ral) Space between the dura mater and arachnoid membrane.
subject Part of a sentence that identifies who or what is being discussed.
subjective Information provided by the patient that cannot be proven.
subjective findings Information provided by the patient (symptoms) and generally not measurable by health professionals.
sublingual (sub-LING-gwal) Under the tongue.
sublingual gland Salivary gland located in the front of the mouth, under the tongue.
sublingual tablet Tablet that dissolves when placed under the tongue.
subluxation (sub-luck-SAY-shun) Partial dislocation of a joint.

submandibular gland (sub-man-DIB-yoo-lar) Salivary gland located below the lower jaw.
subpoena (su-PE-na) Legal document that requires a person to appear in court or to be available for a deposition.
subpoena duces tecum (su-pe-na du-ces ta-cum) Legal document that requires a person to appear in court and bring the records.
subscriber Person who carries the insurance.
subscription Section of a prescription that provides directions to the pharmacist for filling the prescription.
sudden infant death syndrome (SIDS) Sudden, unexpected death of apparently healthy infant; commonly called "crib death."
sudoriferous glands (soo-doe-RIF-uh-rus) Sweat glands; maintain body temperature.
suffix Word part or series of word parts added to the end of a root word to change the meaning.
sulci Shallow grooves in the brain; singular *sulcus*.
super glue A substance used to close superficial wounds.
superbill See *encounter form*.
superego The part of the personality that includes the values and standards designed to promote proper behavior.
superficial wounds Surface wounds that do not go beyond the subcutaneous layer.
superior That which is above.
superior vena cava (soo-PEER-ee-your VEE-nah KAY-vah) Vein that brings blood low in oxygen from the head and upper limbs.
supernatant Top, liquid portion of a specimen that has been centrifuged to remove solid particles.
superscription Section of a prescription with instructions to the patient about how to take the medicine.
supination (soo-pih-NAY-shun) Turning upward.
supine position Position in which the body is lying on the back with the face up.
Supplemental Security Income (SSI) Federal program that offers disability income at a fixed rate and qualification for Medicare insurance; person receiving SSI is limited in amount of outside income he or she can earn.
suppository Semisolid, cone-shaped medication that melts within a body cavity.
surfactant Substance that decreases surface tension within the alveoli.
surgical asepsis Removal of all microorganisms from an object, including spores; sterile technique used to prevent the spread of microorganisms when skin or mucous membranes have been broken.
surgical handwash Cleaning the hands with an antiseptic solution using a prescribed time and action.
surgical handwashing Special handwashing technique that decreases the total number of pathogens present; surgical scrub.
susceptible host Person, insect, or animal that can be infected easily by a particular microorganism.
suspension Solution that has undissolved particles and must be shaken to distribute evenly before administration.
suspensory ligament Ligament that holds the lens in place.
suture scissors Scissors that have a distinctive hook on one tip to get under a suture for cutting the suture material.
sutures (SOO-churs) Sterile material, such as silk or nylon, used to close a wound; immovable joints found in the head.
suturing Closing or pulling together tissue using suture material.
swab-transport media system Device used to keep a swab with a specimen moist until it can be processed for testing.
symmetry Pertains to being equal in size and/or shape.

sympathetic nervous system (sim-pah-THET-ik) System responsible for the body's response to stress or any perceived emergency situations; "fight or flight."

sympathy Having concern for another person's situation.

symptom (SIMP-tum) Something that a patient can describe but that cannot be measured or seen (subjective); subjective data reported by the patient.

symptomatic Pertaining to the characteristics of body function or changes that indicate a particular disease.

synapse (SIN-aps) Space between end of one neuron and beginning of next neuron; place where nerve impulses are transmitted.

synarthrosis Joint with no movement such as the sutures of the head; plural *synarthroses*.

syncope (SIN-koh-pee) Fainting.

synergistic (SIN-er-jis-tik) Referring to muscles acting or working together.

synonym Root word, prefix, or suffix that has the same or nearly the same meaning as a given word, prefix, or suffix.

synovial cavity (sih-NO-vee-al) Joint cavity filled with a fluid.

synovial fluid Fluid that reduces friction caused by joint movement.

synthesize To make or take in; the body synthesizes substances.

synthetic cast Limb immobilizer of fiberglass used for simple fractures and sprains.

syringe Hollow tube made of glass or plastic marked with specific measurements and with a tip that attaches to a needle.

syringe method Blood collection method using a syringe and sterile needle.

syrup Solution of sugar, water, and dissolved drugs.

system, body system Combination of structures that perform organized functions to sustain life.

systemic Absorption of medication with its effects working throughout the body.

systemic circulation (sis-TEM-ik SIR-kew-lah-shun) Movement of blood from the heart throughout the entire body and back.

systole (SIS-toh-lee) Contraction of the heart.

systolic pressure (sis-TOHL-ik) First measurable sound of blood pressure when the heart contracts.

T

T-account Tool used to analyze the effect of a transaction on an account.

T lymphocyte Lymphocyte that matures in the thymus gland and directly attacks foreign substances (e.g., viruses).

T wave ECG pattern that shows resting of the heart; repolarization.

tablet Compressed powdered medication.

tachycardia (tack-ee-KAR-dee-ah) Pulse rate above 100 beats per minute.

tactful Acting with sensitivity when dealing with people.

tactile (TAK-tile) Pertaining to the sense of touch.

talipes (TAL-ih-peez) Foot deformity of one or both feet; clubfoot.

talus (TAL-us) Tarsal bone of the ankle joint.

tape backup External storage unit.

tape measure Device used to measure body parts and wound length.

target organ Organ containing receptors that cause it to react to certain hormones.

tarsals (TAR-sals) Seven bones that form hind part of the foot; ankle bones.

taste buds Minute terminal sensory organs of the gustatory nerve located in various areas on the tongue to differentiate sweet, sour, salty, and bitter.

Tay-Sachs disease Recessive disease affecting the nervous system of persons with Eastern European Jewish heritage, causing mental and physical retardation.

temperature Measurement of the amount of heat produced.

temporal artery (TEM-puh-ruhl) Artery located on each side of the head.

temporal bone Bone located at side of the skull.

temporal lobe Lobe at side of the brain over the ear that controls hearing, smell, and taste.

tendon Connective tissue that connects muscles to bones.

terminal-digit filing Method of filing that organizes records by their final digits.

test card Specimen card for stool collection.

testes (TEHS-teez) Male gonads, singular *testis*; also known as *testicles*.

testicular cancer (tehs-TICK-yoo-lar) Cancer in one or both testicles.

testicular self-examination (TSE) Procedure done by the male to detect tumors or other abnormalities in the testes.

testosterone (tehs-TOS-teh-rohn) Male hormone responsible for male sex characteristics.

tetany (TE-tah-nee) Twitching and cramping of a muscle caused by low serum (blood) calcium level; continuous muscle spasms.

thalamus (THAL-uh-mus) Area of the brain responsible for relaying messages from parts of the body; monitors sensory stimuli.

thalassemia (thal-ah-SEE-mee-ah) Group of hereditary anemias that causes changes in hemoglobin of red blood cells; *Cooley anemia*.

therapeutic diet Diet required for health maintenance, special testing, or disorders.

therapeutic drug Medication that restores the body to its presymptomatic state.

therapeutic procedures Procedures done to enhance the body's healing processes and assist in patient mobility.

third-degree burn Burn that destroys the epidermis and dermis to include the nerve endings; full-thickness burn.

third party Person or company involved in the physician-patient relationship but not part of implied contract.

third-party check Check signed over to another party, who is not the original payee.

thoracic (tho-RAS-ik) Pertaining to the chest area of the spine.

thoracic cavity The chest area.

thoracic vertebrae Part of spinal column that joins with the 12 pairs of ribs in thoracic cavity.

thorax Chest area.

thrill Palpable vibration.

thrombin (THROM-bin) Substance formed by the combination of prothrombin and calcium.

thrombocyte (THROM-boh-sight) Platelet.

thrombus (THROM-bus) Stationary clot.

thrush Fungal infection of the mouth.

thumb forceps Spring-type instrument with serrated tips used to pick up or hold tissue; also called pickups.

thymosin (THYE-moh-sin) Hormone secreted by the thymus that helps to develop the T cells; needed for the immune system to function properly.

thymus gland (THIGH-mus) Lymphatic organ located in the mediastinum and a primary site for T cell formation; endocrine gland and lymphatic organ important to the immune system.

thyroid function tests (TFTs) Blood test assessing T_3, T_4, and calcitonin.

thyroid gland (THY-royd) Gland located in anterior neck on both sides of trachea and larynx.

tibia (TIB-ee-uh) Large bone of lower leg; shinbone.

tic douloureux (TIK doo-loo-ROO) (trigeminal neuralgia) Neuralgia of fifth cranial nerve producing excruciating pain of the face.
tickler file Reminder aid that organizes events by date.
tidal volume Amount of air taken into and out of the lungs during respiration.
time management Organization of time to accomplish goals; choices that are made about how time is used.
timed specimen Urine or blood specimen collected at specified intervals for a set time.
time-specified scheduling Appointment scheduling technique that provides a definite time for the patient to be seen.
tinctures Liquid medications mixed with an alcohol base.
tinea (TIN-ee-ah) Fungal infection of the skin.
tinnitus (tih-NIGH-tus) Ringing in the ears.
tissue (TI-shu, TISH-yoo) Body structure composed of groups of cells with similar structure that network together to carry out a specific task.
tissue forceps Instrument with teeth that allow tissues or growths to be grasped.
tissue scrapings Process of removing superficial tissue for examination.
titer Measurement of the amount of a substance in a specimen.
to-do list List of tasks to be completed in a given period; items are crossed off as they are completed.
tomography Radiography that views the body or organ as a whole in a cross-sectional view.
tongue Organ in the mouth used for taste, chewing, swallowing, and speech.
tongue depressor Instrument is used to hold the tongue down or move it from side to side when examining the mouth.
tonometry Measurement of intraocular pressure (glaucoma).
tonsils (TAHN-sills) Lymphoid tissue located in pharynx and base of the tongue.
tonus Slight tension in the muscle, which is always present, even at rest.
toddler 13 months to 3 years.
tophus Chalky deposit (calculus) containing sodium urate that develops in fibrous tissue; plural *tophi*.
topical For use on the surface of the skin; route for medication applied to the skin or mucous membranes.
topical anesthetic Medication applied to the skin to cause numbness to the area.
torso (TOR-so) Trunk of the body, including the chest, abdomen, and pelvis.
tort Negligent, wrongful act that causes harm, committed by a person against another person or property.
torticollis (wry neck) Contracted (shortened) state of cervical muscles or sternocleidomastoid muscle, causing twisting of neck and tilting of head to one side.
total calcium Blood test measuring calcium.
total cholesterol Combined measurement of LDL and HDL cholesterol.
total disability State in which an individual is unable to perform the requirements of any employment.
touch screen Monitor that displays options that can be selected by touching them on the screen.
towel clamps Instrument with sharp points to hold the edges of a sterile towel together, usually to form a drape.
toxemia Toxic condition in pregnancy that produces high blood pressure and decreased kidney function.
toxic dose Amount of medication that brings about the signs and symptoms of toxicity.

toxic shock syndrome (TSS) Septic infection caused by strains of staphylococcal bacteria.
toxicity Harmful effects of drugs on the body.
trace minerals Minerals used by the body in small amounts (copper, cobalt, manganese, fluorine, zinc).
tracer Special radiographic medium that tags body cells, such as cancer cells.
trachea (TRAY-kee-ah) Passageway that conducts air to and from the lungs; commonly called the "windpipe."
tracing Recording of the ECG cycle.
trackball Pointing device that has a ball that is rolled to position the pointer on the screen; serves the same function as a mouse.
trans-fatty acids Substances formed when polyunsaturated fats are made solid.
transaction Financial activity of a business.
transcriptionist (trans-KRIP-shun-ist) Person who listens to recorded dictation and converts it to a written document.
transdermal patch Medicated disk applied to and absorbed from the skin; adhesive-backed patch that contains a premeasured dose of medication that is absorbed through the skin.
transducer Device that is moved over the skin to record sound waves.
transfusion (trans-FU-shun) Process of taking blood from a donor and infusing it into a recipient.
transient flora Microorganism that easily transfers to hosts because of its location.
transient ischemic attack (TIA) (iss-KEE-mik) Temporary stoppage of blood to the brain; "mini stroke."
transitional epithelial cells Renal epithelial cells appearing in kidney disease.
transverse arch Skeletal structure that supports body weight and extends from one side of foot to other side; formed by tarsals and metatarsals.
transverse colon Section of the colon located across the abdomen.
transverse (cross-sectional) plane Horizontal cut that separates the body into superior and inferior parts.
treadmill test Exercise electrocardiography that is done to determine if the heart is receiving enough blood during exercise; called also *cardiac stress test*.
Trendelenburg's position Position where the head is low and the body and legs are on an incline.
TRICARE Comprehensive federal health care program for active-duty and retired U.S. military personnel and eligible family members; formerly known as CHAMPUS.
trichomoniasis Infection with *Trichomonas* protozoa spread through sexual contact, making it an STD.
tricuspid valve (trye-KUS-pid) Heart valve located between the right atrium and right ventricle.
triglycerides Dietary fats that have been broken down into fatty acids and glycerol.
trigone (TRY-gohn) Triangular area in the bladder formed by entrance of ureters and exit of urethra.
trochanter (troh-KAN-tur) Bony prominence of the femur that provides a place for muscle attachment.
troches Lozenges.
true ribs Ribs that attach directly to the sternum.
trunk The body, except for the head and limbs.
TSE Testicular self-examination.
tuberculosis (pulmonary) (too-ber-kyoo-LOH-sis) Bacterial infection of the lungs caused by mycobacteria, although bacteria can affect other areas of the body.

tubular gauze Gauze bandage made in a tubular shape that can be used to cover rounded body parts.
tumor Mass caused by uncontrolled cell and tissue growth; can be malignant or benign.
tuning fork Instrument used to test hearing acuity by air or bone conduction.
turbid Not clear or transparent; particles floating within; cloudy.
turgor (turbidity) Normal tension in the skin; skin resiliency.
Turner syndrome Chromosomal disease affecting females that occurs when an X chromosome is missing at birth.
tutorial Self-guided, step-by-step learning process that teaches generic skills needed to use software.
tympanic (tim-PAN-ik) Area of the eardrum.
tympanic membrane (eardrum) Structure that transmits sound waves to ossicles of the middle ear.
type and crossmatch Process of determining a person's blood type and establishing compatibility of another's blood type for transfusions.
Tzanck test Microscopic examination of cellular tissue from skin lesions.

U

U wave Normal, small upward curve that occasionally follows a complete ECG cycle after the PQRST; has unknown indication.
ulcer (UL-ser) Area of open skin caused by loss of superficial tissue, usually accompanied by sloughing of inflamed and dead tissue.
ulcerative colitis (UL-sur-a-tiv koh-LYE-tis) Inflammation of mucosa of the colon.
ulna (UL-nah) Bone of the lower arm located on the (lateral) side (little finger).
ultrasonography Visualization of deep structures of the body using sound waves to produce an image of the interior structure of a hollow organ.
ultrasound Imaging of soft tissue and internal organs using high-frequency sound waves.
ultrasound therapy Therapy that uses high-frequency sound waves to produce heat and vibrations to aid in the healing of inflammation in soft tissue.
umbilical cord (um-BIL-ih-kul) Structure that connects the fetus to the placenta.
umbilicus (um-BIL-i-kus) The navel.
unconscious Not responding to stimuli.
unipolar leads See augmented leads.
unit dose Premeasured amount of medication individually packaged, usually in a single dose.
universal donor Blood type with neither type A nor type B antigens; type O blood.
universal recipient Blood type with A and B antigens; type AB.
unsaturated fats Fats that are liquid at room temperature.
Unique Personal Identification Number (UPIN) Number assigned to a physician by Medicare to track physician activity and payments.
upper gastrointestinal series (upper GI) Radiographic examination of the esophagus, stomach, and upper small intestines during and after the introduction of a contrast medium; also called *barium swallow*.
upper respiratory infection (URI) Inflammation and edema of mucous membranes of the upper respiratory tract.
upper respiratory tract Respiratory tract, including the nose, sinuses, pharynx, and larynx.
urea (you-REE-ah) Nitrogen waste product excreted in the urine.

uremia (you-REE-mee-ah) Azotemia; accumulation of toxins, such as urea, in the blood.
ureters (you-REE-terz) Pair of muscular tubes that carry urine from the kidneys to the bladder.
urethra (you-REE-thrah) Membranous canal that transports urine from bladder to outside the body; tube from bladder and through penis by which semen and urine are released.
urgency Feeling of the need to urinate immediately.
urinalysis (you-rih-NAL-ih-sis) Physical, chemical, and microscopic examination of the urine; analysis of urine specimen.
urinary bladder (YOUR-ih-nair-ee) Hollow muscular organ that holds urine before it is excreted from the body.
urinary reflux Backflow of urine from the bladder into the ureters during urination.
urinary system Body system that eliminates waste in the body and maintains water and chemical balance.
urination Process of excreting urine; micturition; voiding.
urine Liquid and dissolved substances excreted by the kidneys.
urine glucose Urine test for the presence of glucose.
urine ketones Urine test for the presence of ketones.
URL Uniform (or universal) resource locator; Internet address.
urobilinogen Breakdown of bilirubin by intestinal bacteria.
urochrome Yellow pigment derived from urobilin that is left over when hemoglobin breaks down during red blood cell destruction.
urologist Specialist in the treatment of diseases of the kidneys, urinary tract, and male reproductive organs.
urticaria (er-tih-KARE-ee-ah) Hives; raised areas that are smooth and cause itching.
User ID Combination of letters and numbers that serves as identification of the person using the computer.
usual, customary, and reasonable (UCR) Referring to typically charged or prevailing fees for health services in a geographical area.
uteri-body Middle of the uterus.
uterine fibroids (YOU-tur-in FYE-broyds) Smooth muscle tumors within the uterus, usually benign.
uterine tubes See fallopian tubes.
uterus (YOU-tur-us) Organ that functions to receive the fertilized egg.
uvula (YOU-vue-lah) Small mass of tissue hanging from soft palate at back of mouth.

V

V codes ICD-9-CM supplementary codes for factors influencing health status and reasons for contact with health services when a diagnosis needs further explanation or when the patient has no disease process for coding.
V leads Chest (precordial) leads.
vaccination (vak-suh-NAY-shun) Process of injecting antigens of a disease into the body to produce artificially acquired immunity.
vaccine Medication used to prevent disease.
Vaccine Information Statements (VIS) Information sheets produced by the CDC that explain to vaccine recipients, their parents, or their legal guardian both the benefits and risks of a vaccine; required by federal law to be supplied whenever (before each dose) certain vaccinations are given.
Vacutainer Blood collection tube with a colored stopper; used with the evacuation blood collection system.
vacuum tube Blood collection tube with a vacuum; evacuated tube.

vagina (vah-JYE-nuh) Muscular area located between cervix and vulva.
vaginal irrigation Irrigation of large amounts of solution into the vagina as a method of cleansing.
vaginal speculum Instrument used in a pelvic examination to view the cervix.
vaginitis Inflammation of vaginal tissue caused by fungus, bacteria, protozoa, or irritation of tissue.
vagus nerve (VAY-gus) Nerve that controls secretions of hydrochloric acid, among many other functions.
valve Structure that controls fluid direction, as in blood through the heart.
valvular insufficiency Condition in which the heart valves lose their ability to close tightly.
varices Plural of varix.
varix Twisted and swollen vein; *varicose* (VAR-ih-kose) veins.
vas deferens (vas DEF-her-henz) Tube by which sperm leave the epididymis and travel to the urethra for ejaculation.
vasoconstrict (VAY-zoh-kon-STRIKT) To make a blood vessel narrower.
vasodilate (VAY-zoh-dye-LATE) To make a blood vessel wider.
vastus lateralis muscle Thigh muscle located between the greater trochanter of the femur and the knee.
vein Blood vessel that carries blood low in oxygen toward the heart.
venae cavae (VEE-nay KA-vay) Largest veins in the body; bring oxygen-poor blood from the body to the right atrium.
vendor Entity that sells supplies, equipment, and services (e.g., office cleaning).
venipuncture Puncture of a vein to obtain a venous blood sample.
Venn diagram Diagram using circles to represent concepts; overlapping areas of the circles represent similarities between concepts, and the other areas represent differences.
ventilation Movement of air in and out of the lungs; breathing.
ventral (VEN-tral) Front.
ventral cavity Anterior (front) cavity that includes the chest area, abdomen, and pelvic area.
ventricle (VEN-tri-kuhl) Lower chamber of the heart (right or left); larger than atrium; small cavities within the brain responsible for production of CSF.
ventricular fibrillation (V fib) Life-threatening condition of ventricular twitching that causes ineffective pumping action, stopping blood circulation.
ventricular tachycardia (V tach) Three or more consecutive PVCs with heart rate exceeding 100 beats per minute.
ventrogluteal Muscle area formed by the gluteus medius and gluteus minimus.
venule (VEN-yool) Small vein that carries blood from capillary to the vein.
verb A word in a sentence that expresses action or a state of being.
vermiform appendix (VER-mih-form) Wormlike appendage attached to the cecum that is lymphoid tissue.
verrucae (veh-ROO-kay) Warts; contagious raised epithelial growths caused by papillomavirus.
vertebra (VER-tuh-bruh) Bones of the spinal column; one of a series of bones that protect the spinal cord.
vertebrae (VER-tuh-bray) Bones of the spinal column.
vertebral arteries Pair of arteries branching from the subclavian arteries and dividing into two cervical and five cranial branches.
vertebral column (VER-tuh-brul) Flexible, curved, segmented structure composed of vertebrae that are stacked on one another.

vertigo (VER-tih-goh) Dizziness.
vesicle (VES-ih-kul) Blister; collection of clear fluid under the skin.
vestibular apparatus Portion of inner ear that handles equilibrium; consists of vestibule and semicircular canals.
vestibule (VES-tih-byool) Inner ear structure behind the cochlea that controls the sense of position in space.
veteran Retired member of the U.S. military services.
viable Alive, living.
vial Vacuum-sealed bottle that contains a sterile solution with or without medication or a sterile oil-based substance.
vicarious liability Liability of an employer for the wrongdoing of an employee while on the job.
villi (VIL-i) Vascular projections of the small intestine that aid in absorption.
Vincent infection Painful ulcerations of the mucous lining of the mouth; "trench mouth."
viruses (VI-rus-ez) Smallest of all microorganisms; visible only under electron microscopy.
viscera (VIS-er-ah) Organs of any cavity; internal organs.
visceral layer (VIS-er-ul) Serous membrane that covers the outside of an organ.
visceral membrane Membrane that covers the organs.
visceral pleura (VIS-er-ul PLOO-rah) Membrane that covers an organ in the thoracic cavity.
viscosity Stickiness, or thickness, as of the blood; state of being viscous (sticky).
visual acuity Ability to see at different distances.
vital capacity (VC) Measurement of the volume of air that can be expired when the patient exhales completely.
vital signs Systematic measurement of a patient's temperature, pulse rate, respirations, and blood pressure.
vitamin Organic compound needed by the body to function.
vitiligo (vit-ih-LYE-goh) Loss of pigment in the skin; milk-white patches.
vitreous humor (VIT-ree-us HYOO-mor) Jelly-like substance in the posterior chamber that gives the eyeball its shape.
voiding Urination or micturition.
volume Strength or force of each heartbeat.
voluntary Referring to muscles contracting by effort; controlled by choice.
volvulus (VOL-view-lus) Colon twisting on itself.
vomer Bone that forms lower wall between the nostrils; nasal septum.
voucher Paper showing the date, amount of transaction, what was purchased, and who purchased the item.
vowel Speech sound used to pronounce words (e.g., *a, e, i, o, u,* and sometimes *y*).
vulva (VUL-vah) Female external genital area between mons pubis and vagina.

W

wages Money paid for work done by an employee and calculated by multiplying the hourly wage rate times the number of hours worked.
waiver A release form.
walker Lightweight mobility device providing a stable platform that is used when a patient needs optimal stability and support.
wandering baseline Shift on the ECG tracing from the baseline or center of the paper.
warm boot Term used when the system has been on and must be restarted because it "freezes up."

warranty card Card accompanying a purchased item that protects the buyer against defective parts for a certain time.

warts See verrucae.

water-soluble vitamins Vitamins not stored in the body (C, B complex, thiamine, riboflavin, niacin, pantothenic acid, pyridoxine, folic acid, B_{12}).

wave ECG pattern that represents specific electrical heart activity.

wave scheduling Appointment scheduling technique that divides an hour block into average-appointment time slots.

waxy casts Urinary casts that appear glassy and smooth with saw-tooth edges under microscopic view.

Weber test Test to determine whether hearing loss is conductive or sensorineural; used to evaluate hearing quality in both ears by placing a vibrating tuning fork stem on the center of the skull and determining if sound is equal in both ears; also determines air conduction deafness.

Westergren method Method measure ESR using a self-zeroing tube calibrated from 0 to 200.

wet mount Slide preparation used to observe for fungal or bacterial growth.

wheal (wheel) Slightly elevated area on the skin; bump resembling a hive (e.g., insect bite) or seen after a properly placed intradermal injection; fluid-filled bump.

wheezes High-pitched musical sounds caused by narrowing of the respiratory passage; heard mainly during expiration; heard when bronchial tubes are narrowed by disease.

white blood cells (WBCs) Cells in the blood that help provide protection against infection and disease.

whorls Ridges that fit snugly over the papillae on top of the dermis; coils or spirals that form fingerprints.

winged infusion needles "Butterfly needles"; special needles with tabs that resemble butterfly wings used to grasp during insertion.

winged infusion set Blood collection needle set with "wings" to aid in guiding the needle.

Wintrobe method Method to measure ESR using a disposable tube calibrated from 0 to 100.

within normal limits (WNL) Values found within established guidelines.

wizards Sequence of screens that direct the user through a multistep software task.

Wood's light examination (ultraviolet lamp) Device used to detect certain pathogens on the skin.

word map Drawing or map that uses words to describe and define a word.

word processing Computer-based application used to produce text-based documents.

work practice controls Work practices that minimize the possibility of infectious exposure to employees.

work-related injury Injury that has occurred to an employee when performing the duties of his or her job.

workers' compensation System that provides insurance to the employer for a worker injured on the job; insurance program that requires employers to pay the medical expenses and lost wages for workers who are injured on the job or who have job-related illness.

wound Break in the skin or soft tissue.

wrist Area between lower arm and hand.

write-off Amount of money not able to be collected.

X

x-ray film Special photographic film that blackens in response to light; also called a radiograph.

x-ray tube Vacuum tube that creates x-radiation.

xerophthalmia Condition of dry and dull corneas and conjunctival areas.

xiphoid process (ZIH-foyd) Lower tip of the sternum.

Y

year labels See aging labels.

yeasts Oval-shaped fungi with small buds.

Z

Z-track method Intramuscular technique for administering medication that requires the pulling back or displacement of tissues during the injection to prevent discoloration of the skin.

zip drive External disk storage device that holds large amounts of data.

zygomatic bones (zye-goh-MAH-tik) Cheekbones.

zygote (ZYE-goat) Fertilized egg; contains all the genetic material.

Index

A

A$_{1c}$. *See* Glycosylated hemoglobin A$_{1c}$
AAMA. *See* American Association of Medical Assistants
ABA number, 559–560
Abandonment, 50, 69
ABCDE rule, 427, 427t
ABCs. *See* Airway, Breathing, Circulation
Abdomen muscles, 359t–360t, 362
Abdominal cavity, 171–172
Abdominal reflex, 294
Abdominal thrust. *See* Heimlich maneuver
Abdominal wall muscles, 359t–360t
Abdominal x-ray, 272b
Abdominopelvic cavity, 171–172, 194
Abduction, 337, 348
ABGs. *See* Arterial blood gases
ABHES. *See* Accrediting Bureau of Health Education Schools
Ablation therapy, 788b
ABMS. *See* American Board of Medical Specialists
Abnormalities
 chromosomal disease and, 180–181, 194
ABO blood group, 226. *See also* Blood
Abortion, 66
Abrasion, 428
Abscess, 430b
Abscess incision, 1113, 1128
Absence, 23
Absorption, 263, 266, 269f, 270t
Abstinence, 870
Abstract, 504
Abuse, health insurance and, 604
AC. *See* Alternating current (AC) interference
Acceptance, stages of grief and, 82, 84
Accessory gland (male), 385
Accessory organs, 261, 263, 263f, 268–271, 270t, 277–278
Accommodation, of eyes, 311, 756t–757t
Account management, computerized, 551–557
Accounting, principles of, 544–548
Accounting equation, 545, 545f, 578
Accounts receivable (AR), 547–548
Accrediting Bureau of Health Education Schools (ABHES), 29, 30f
Acetabulum, 333–334
Acetone, 968
Acetylcholine, 354
Achilles reflex, 294
Achilles tendon, 341t–343t, 354
Acne, 422–423
Acquired immunity, 237, 238f
Acquired immunodeficiency syndrome (AIDS), 144, 238t, 239f, 240
 record retention and, 539
 special considerations for, 237–239, 239b

Page numbers followed by f indicate figure(s); t, table(s); b, box(es).

Acromegaly, 412t–414t, 415f
Acromion process, 332
Acronym, 11
 indexing of, 534–535, 535t
ACTH. *See* Adrenocorticotropic hormone
Actinic keratosis, 425, 426f, 435
Active file, 542
Active immunity, 237
Active learning, 14–16
Active listening, 108, 109b, 109t, 115
Active reading, 11, 14–15
Active transport method, 178, 194
Active writing, 15
Activities of daily living (ADL's), 302
Acute
 coding guidelines and, 589b
 definition of, 271
Acute needs scheduling, 492, 511
Acute renal failure (ARF), 374t–375t
Adam's apple, 246f, 247
Addison disease, 407–408, 412t–414t
Adduction, 337, 348
Adductors, 357
Adenoids, 247. *See also* Tonsils
Adenosine triphosphate (ATP), 178, 354
ADH. *See* Antidiuretic hormone
ADHD. *See* Attention deficit hyperactivity disorder
Adipose tissue, 188t–189t, 189
Adjective, 153
 correct use of, 110t
Adjustment, 568, 579
ADL. *See* Activities of daily living
Administer, 1007b
Administration set, 1080–1081, 1081f
Administrative law, 48
Administrative Simplification Provision, HIPAA and, 60
Administrative skills, 25, 27b–29b
Adolescence, 91
 12 to 18 yrs of, 91b–92b, 92f
 nutrition and, 144
Adrenal cortex, 405t, 407–408
Adrenal gland, 405t, 407–408
Adrenal medulla, 405t, 408
Adrenocorticotropic hormone (ACTH), 405t, 406
Adult, body measurements of, 680–681, 681b–683b
Adulthood
 19-45 yrs of, 93, 93b, 93f
 45 to 59 yrs of, 93, 93f
 60 to 69 yrs of, 94, 94f
 70+ yrs of, 94, 94b, 95f
Adults, body measurements of, 680–681
Adverb, correct use of, 110t
Adverse reactions, 1028, 1033–1034
Advocate, 456
AED. *See* Automated external defibrillator (AED)
Aerobes, 638b

Aerobic, 354
Aerosols, 1024
Afebrile, 690
Affective learning, 125–126
Afferent nerve, 190
Afferent neuron. *See* Sensory neuron
Agar, 992
Age
 pulse rate and, 702t
 special needs patients and, 123, 124b, 124f
Age of majority, 47b, 50
Agenda, 454, 458
Agent, 51
Agglutination, 972, 991–992, 992f, 1000
Aggression, 81t
Aging individuals
 endocrine system and, 411b
 nervous system and, 302b
 nutrition and, 144
 reproductive system and, 391b
 skeletal muscles and, 362, 362b
 skin and, 430b
 urinary system and, 378b
Aging labels, 521b–522b, 532
Aging report, 547–548, 578
Agranulocytes, 225, 227t
Agricola lid retractor, 1089–1101
AHA. *See* American Heart Association; American Hospital Association
Aha moment, 2–3
AIDS. *See* Acquired immunodeficiency syndrome
Air cast, 844
Airway, Breathing, Circulation (ABCs), 1133b, 1146
Akathisia, 303b
Albinism, 421
Albuminuria, 222b
Aldosterone, 370, 408
Alimentary canal, 263. *See also* Digestive tract
Allergens, 237
Allied health professionals, 41, 41f
Allis forceps, 1089–1101
Allowable charges, 606
Alopecia, 430b
Alphabet chart, 749–750, 750f, 758
Alphabetic Index, 598–599
 CPT manual and, 592–593
 ICD-9-CM and, 585
Alphabetic Index of Diseases, 586b, 589, 589b
 ICD-9-CM Volume 2 and, 586
Alphabetic Index to External Causes of Injury and Poisoning. *See* E codes
Alphabetical filing method, 533–536
Alphabetical filing system, 528, 538b
 advantages of, 534, 541
 disadvantages of, 534, 541
 rules for, 534–536, 541
Alphanumerical, 532
ALS. *See* Amyotrophic lateral sclerosis
Alternating current (AC) interface, 780, 780f

1225

Alveoli, 248, 258
Amblyopia, 314b
Ambulation device, 838
Ambulatory, 25, 37
Ambulatory devices, 838–844
Ambulatory surgery setting, 42, 1088
Amenorrhea, 390b
American Academy of Pediatrics, ingested poison and, 1143
American Association of Medical Assistants (AAMA), 30
  code of ethics of, 62b, 70
  credentialing and, 27b, 30–31, 30f, 32t–33t
American Board of Medical Specialists (ABMS), 37–38, 39f
American Cancer Society, breast self examination and, 857
American Heart Association (AHA), cardiopulmonary resuscitation and, 1146
American Hospital Association (AHA), 66, 67b, 70, 604
American Medical Association (AMA), 539, 609–610
  code of ethics of, 62b
  CPT-4 manual and, 591
American Medical Technologists (AMT), 30, 30f
  recertification by, 31b
  RMA credential and, 31
American Registered Nurse Practitioner (ARNP), 40, 41f
Americans with Disabilities Act (ADA), 60
  examination room accessibility and, 672
  facilities management requirements of, 458
Amino acids, 142, 269f, 270t
  eight essentials of, 142b
Amnesia, 303b
Amniocentesis, Down syndrome and, 180–181
Amniotic sac, 393
Amoebae, 298t–299t
Amphiarthroses, 336
Amplifier, 765–768
Ampule, 1047f, 1048
  administration of, 1048, 1053b–1055b
  pre-filled cartridge unit and, 1048f, 1053, 1056f
  preparation of, 1048
  syringes and, 1053
Ampulla, 384
Amsler grid, 314b, 315t–316t
AMT. See American Medical Technologists
Amylase, 264, 269f
Amyotrophic lateral sclerosis (ALS), 298t–299t
Anabolism, 177t, 271
  definition of, 278
Anaerobes, 638b
Anaerobic, 354
Anaerobic culture kit, 911
Anal canal, 267–268
  diseases of, 273t–276t
Anal sphincter, 267
  digestive role of, 277
Analgesics, 1005b
Anaphylactic shock, 237, 1137t
Anastomose, 205–206
Anatomical directions, 168, 170t

Anatomical position, 166t, 168, 169f, 195
Anatomy, body structure and, 166, 168
Androgen, 383–384, 408
Anemia, 231t–232t
Anesthesia, 1105–1113
Aneurysm, 215t–216t
Anger, 82, 84
  response to illness and, 99
Angiogram, 799t
Angiography, 296b
Ankle, 334, 359t–360t
Ankylosis, 341t–343t
Anorexia, 144, 272b, 411b
ANS. See Autonomic nervous system
Answering machine, 446
Answering service, 446
Answering systems, 446
Antagonist, prime mover muscle, 356
Antagonistic, 353
  ANS and, 203–204
Anterior body plane, 168–169
Anterior cavity, 311–312, 312f
Anterior descending artery, 205, 207f
Anterior lobe, 405t, 406, 406f
Anterior pituitary gland, 389
Anti-benign prostatic hyperplasia, 385t
Antibiotic resistance, 1030b
Antibodies, 222
Anticipation guide, 11, 12f
Antidiuretic hormone (ADH), 287–289, 370, 406
Antigen, 226
Antioxidant, 138t
Antipyretics, 1042
Antiseptic hand rub, 648
Antiseptic handwash, 648
Antisocial, 304b
Antonym, 163–164
Anuresis, 373b
Anus, 267
Anvil. See Incus
Anxiety, 78
  medical conditions and, 78b, 83
Anxiety disorder, general, 304b
Aorta, 200–201, 202f–203f, 204–205, 205f–206f
Aortic semilunar valve, 200–203, 205f, 217
Apex, 201f
  of the heart, 200
Apgar score, 394, 396b, 872
Aphasia, 296b
Aphonia, 253b
Apical pulse, 702f, 706b
  measurement of, 703–705, 703f
Apical rate, 702–703
Apnea, 253b
Aponeurosis, 354
Appeal, lawsuit process and, 55t
Appendices
  CPT manual and, 592, 592t, 599
  for Volume 1, ICD-9-CM manual, 588, 588b
Appendicitis, 273t–276t
Appendicular area, 173, 175f
Appendicular skeleton, 328–335, 328b, 329f, 348
Appointment book, 485–489, 485f, 486b–488b, 510
  abbreviations for, 488b

Appointments
  cancellation of, 492, 511
  for special circumstance, 492–493
  late arrival and, 492
  reminders and, 493, 493f, 511
  techniques of, 489–493, 491f
Approximate
  sutures and, 1114–1116
Aqueous
  water-based solution and, 1045
Aqueous humor, 311
AR. See Accounts receivable
Arachnoid membrane, 285, 287f
Arbitration, lawsuit process and, 55t
Areola, 389
Areolar tissue, 188t–189t, 189
ARF. See Acute renal failure
Arm, muscles of, 359t–360t
Arm (microscope), 900
ARMA. See Association of Records Managers and Administrators
ARNP. See American Registered Nurse Practitioner
Arrhythmia, 762–763
  conduction system disorders and, 204
Arterial blood gases (ABGs), 254b
Arterioles, 211
Artery, 211–213, 212t
  damage to, 1138
Arthritis, 341t–343t, 349
  gouty (gout), 341t–343t
Arthrography, 340b
Arthroscopy, 340b
Articular cartilage, 336–337, 348
Articulate, 328–331
Articulations, 335–338
Artifacts, 779–780, 972
Artificial insemination, 66
Artificially acquired immunity, 237
Ascending colon, 261, 267
Ascites, 272b
Asphyxia, 253b
Aspiration, 1065
Assault, 51
Assessing, teaching process and, 126
Assessment, 525–527, 588
Asset, 545, 578
  types of, 546–548, 578
Assimilation, 138
Assisted living facility, 42
Association of Records Managers and Administrators (ARMA), 534
Asthma, 254t–256t
Astigmatism, 315t–316t, 317f
Astrocytes, 284
Ataxia, 296b
Atelectasis, 253b
Athlete's foot. See Tinea pedis
Atlas, 332
Atmospheric pressure, 249, 250f
Atom, 174, 194
Atonic, 353–354
ATP. See Adenosine triphosphate
Atria. See Atrium
Atrial arrhythmia, 780–781
Atrial depolarization, 764t
Atrial flutter, conduction system disorders and, 204b

Atrioventricular (AV) node, 203, 203f–204f, 217, 763b, 764f
Atrioventricular bundle, 203, 764f. See also Bundle of His
Atrium, 200, 202f–205f, 217
Atrophy
  menopause and, 389
  of muscles, 364t
Attention deficit hyperactivity disorder (ADHD), 304b
Attenuated, 237
Attitude, 2, 12f, 16
  positive, 23–24, 24b
Audiogram, 889–891
Audiologist, 889–891
Audiometrist, 318
Audiometry, 318, 318b, 889–891, 891f
  audiometer and, 672–673, 677
Auditory, 314
Auditory canal, external, 314
Auditory meatus, 329–331
Augmented leads, 770–776, 777f
Aural temperature. See Tympanic temperature
Auricle. See Pinna
Auscultation, 717, 718b, 756t, 757t, 758
Autism, 304b
Autoclave, 657, 657b, 660f, 665b–667b, 668
  maintenance of, 657, 662b–664b, 668
Autoclave tape, 648, 661f
Automated external defibrillator (AED), 782, 782f, 1146, 1149
  types of, 1146
Automated file, 529–532
Automated urine analyzer, 962t, 966, 967f, 999
Autonomic nervous system, 290, 294f
Autonomic nervous system (ANS), 203–204, 217, 292, 292t, 294f
Autopsy report, 508, 512
Auxiliary input devices, 464–465
AV. See Atrioventricular node
Average dose, 1007b, 1033
Axial area, 173
Axial skeleton, 328–332, 328b, 329f, 348
Axilla. See Underarms
Axillary temperature, 690, 691t
Axis, 332
Axon, 283
Azotemia, 369

B

B lymphocytes, 237
Babinski reflex, 294
Bacilli, 638
Back-ordered, 451
Back-up, 470, 471f, 472
Background knowledge, 2, 11
Backup, 470, 471f, 472
Bacteremia, 943
Bacteria, 638, 639f, 639t, 667, 971–972
Bacterial infection, 432t–433t
Bacterial smear, 992, 994b–995b
Bacteriology, 992
Bacteriuria, 373b, 912, 966
Balance, nutritional principles and, 137, 148
Balance billing, 611–612
Balance sheet, 548, 578
Balanced Budget Act of 1997, 615

Ball-and-socket joints, 337
Bandage scissors, 1103
Bandage turns, types of, 817–822
Bandages, types of, 817, 817f
Bandaging, 817–822
  techniques of, 823f–824f
  turns for, 817–822
Bank statement, 560, 563f
  reconciliation of, 560
Banking, procedures of, 557–560
Bankruptcy Act, 58
Bargaining, 82–84
Barium enema, 272b
Barium swallow, 272b
Barrier methods, 870, 892
Bartholin's glands, 389
Base (microscope), 900
Baseline, 690
  ECG patterns and, 763
  ECG results and, 778
Basic benefits, 606
Basophils, 227t
Battery, 51
BDT. See Bone density testing
Bee sting. See Poison, injected
Beginning of life issues, right to die and, 66
Behavior, change of, 77t
Being on time. See Punctuality
Beliefs, personal, cultural differences and, 122
Beneficiary, 612
Benign mole, 425–427, 427f, 427t
Benign prostatic hyperplasia (BPH), 387t, 756t–757t
Benign tumors, 179b
Beriberi, 139t
Bethesda System, 861, 868f, 869t, 892
Beveled needle, 1048–1059
Biconcave
  erythrocytes and
  red blood cells and, 223
Bicuspid, 264
Bicuspid valve, 205f
Bifurcate, 205–206
Bile, 138, 266, 269f, 270
Bilirubin, 270, 961
  reagent tablets and, 968
Bilirubinuria, 961
Billing cycle, 568
  types of, 568
Billing statement, 566–567
Binocular microscope, 900
Bioethics, 66
Biohazard symbol, 641f, 646b, 648f
Biological indicator, 648, 657b, 661f, 668
Biopsy, 861
Bipolar disorder, 304b
Bipolar leads. See Standard limb leads
Birth, process of, 394, 395f, 400
Birth control. See Contraception
Birthday rule, 605, 632
Bit, 461
Bites. See Poison, injected
Blackhead. See Comedo
Bladder, urinary system and, 367
Bland diet, 147
Blank endorsement, 559, 579
Bleb, 1060. See also Wheal
Bleeding, 1138, 1139f, 1149

Blind spot. See Optic disc
Blood
  calcium levels of, 407f, 410
  circulation of, 218
  composition of, 222–229
  diseases of, 228–229, 231t–232t, 240
  functions of, 222
  pH of, 222
  supply of, 204–205
  terms for, 227b
  types of, 226–228, 230t, 240
Blood antibody titer, 420t, 872, 892
Blood bank, 904, 923
Blood cartilage, 188t–189t
Blood cells, 239. See also Formed elements
  urine and, 968
Blood chemistry, 872, 983–991, 986t, 999
  analyzer of, 983, 983f
Blood collection, 927–954
Blood culture, 952, 952f
  collection of, 943–952, 952f
Blood pressure, 707–709
  documentation of, 709b
  factors of, 707
  measuring of, 710b, 711b, 713
  ranges of, 707, 707t
Blood recipient, 227
Blood slide differential, 981–983, 982f
  preparation of, 982, 982f–983f
Blood smear, 984b–986b
  qualities of, 982–983
Blood system, 191t–193t
Blood tests, 972
Blood tissue, 187–190
Blood types, 226–228
Blood urea nitrogen (BUN), 374b
Blood vessels, 200–201, 218
Bloodborne Pathogens Standard, 58, 668
  regulations of, 58–60
Blue Cross/Blue Shield, 603, 610, 633
BMI. See Body mass index
Body
  areas of, 175f
  measurements of, 679
  mechanics of, 736f, 737f, 758
  organizational levels of, 174–193
  sensations of, 421
  skin protection of, 420
  systems of, 174–193, 191t–193t, 196–197
  temperature regulation of, 421, 422f, 435
Body cavity, 169–173, 170f, 171t
Body cells, 409–410
Body fluids, 1080
Body language, 106–107, 106f
Body mass index (BMI), 136f, 137b, 137t
  nutritional principles and, 136–137, 148
Body measurements, 679, 712
  accuracy in, 679
  conversion tables for, 681b, 712
Body movements, nonverbal communication and, 107
Body plane, 168–169, 170f
Body surface area (BSA), 1033
  drug dosage and, 1018, 1018b, 1021f
Body temperature
Body tissue, 181–190
Body weight method, drug dosage and, 1018, 1018b

Boldface type, 586
Bolus, 264, 269f
Bone
　deficiencies of, 341t–343t
　development of, 325
　diseases of, 341t–343t
　growth of, 347–348
　repair of, 328
　shapes of, 348
　structure of, 325–327, 348
　surface markings of, 326–327, 326f, 327t
　types of, 327–328, 327f
Bone cells, 325
Bone density testing (BDT), 340b
Bone marrow, 326
Bone matrix, 325–326
Bone neoplasm, 341t–343t
Bone scan, 340b
Bone tissue, 187–190, 188t–189t
　formation of, 347
Bookkeeping, 28b–29b, 543, 579
　procedures of, 549–557
Booster dose, 1018–1024
Booted up, 462–463
Bowman's capsule, 371–372
Box lock, 1089–1101, 1101f
BPH. *See* Benign prostatic hyperplasia
Brachial artery, 702–703, 702f
Bradycardia, 702, 713
Brain, 281, 285–289, 286b, 288f, 305
　blood circulation and, 205–211, 218
Brain freeze, 290b
Brain stem, 251, 288f, 291f
　parts of, 289
Breach of confidentiality, 440b
Breach of contract, 50
Breakfast, importance of, 136b
Breast, 389
　fibrocystic disease of, 392t–393t
Breast self examination (BSE), 390–391, 756t–757t, 857, 857b–859b
　recommendations for, 857, 891
Breastbone. *See* Sternum
Breathing, 248–252, 258, 260. *See also* Respiratory rate
Bronchi, 248, 249f, 258
Bronchioles, 248
Bronchitis, 249b, 254t–256t
Bronchodilators, 253t
Bronchoscopy, 254b, 257f
Browser, 465–466
Bruise. *See* Contusion
Bruit, 756t–757t
BSE. *See* Breast self examination
Buccal, 1037–1040
Buccal cavity, 172, 173f, 264
Buccal tablets, 1025b
Bulbourethral gland, 385. *See also* Cowper's gland
Bulimia, 144
BUN. *See* Blood urea nitrogen
Bundle branches, 764f, 765
Bundle of His, 203, 203f–204f, 764f, 765
Burns, 428–429, 429f, 1138–1141, 1139b
　classification of, 428–429
Bursa, 336–337, 348
Bursitis, 341t–343t, 349

Business letters, 499–504, 499b, 501b, 501f–502f, 503b, 512
　closing of, 499b
　elements of, 499–501
　format of, 501f–502f
Business names, indexing of, 534, 534t
Butterfly method, 943, 947b–950b
Byte, 461

C

C. *See* Celsius
C&S. *See* Culture and sensitivity
Ca. *See* Serum calcium
Calcaneus, 334
Calcitonin, 406–407
Calcium, 328
Calls. *See* Incoming calls; Outgoing calls
Caloric intake, 134
Calorie-controlled diet, 146
Calories, 136b
Calyces, 371, 372f
Canals of Schlemm, 311, 312f
Cancellous bone, 328
Cancer
　cell growth and, 179b
　cervical, 392t–393t
　lung, 254t–256t
　nutrition and, 144–145, 148–149
　prostatic, 387t
　testicular, 387t
Candidiasis, 392t–393t, 869, 869f, 892
Cane, 844
　measuring for, 846b–847b
Canines, 264
Canthus, 312–313
Capillary, 213
　damage to, 1138
Capillary collection tube, 929–930
Capillary puncture, 927–930, 928f, 931b–935b
　blood collection and, 927–930
　collection containers for, 929–930, 929f
Capital goods, 450, 453
Capitation, 607, 609, 632–633
Caplets, 1024–1025
Capsule, 1024–1025
　kidneys and, 371
Caption, 532, 533f
Carbohydrates, 136b, 140–141, 148, 269f
　sources of, 141b
Carbon dioxide (CO_2), 204, 243, 245
Carbuncles, 430b
Carcinoma, 341t–343t
　basal cell, 425, 426f, 435
　squamous cell, 427, 427f, 435
Cardiac arrest
　life support and, 1145–1146
Cardiac arrhythmia, 780–782
Cardiac catheterization, 788b
Cardiac cycle, 202–203, 203f, 763
Cardiac muscle, 186, 186t, 355–356
Cardiac output, 203
Cardiac region, 265
Cardiac stress test, 784, 788b
　legal aspects of, 784b
Cardiac valves, 200–201, 217. *See also* Heart valves; Valve

Cardiogenic shock, 1137t
Cardiologist, 206
Cardiomegaly, 200–201
Cardiopulmonary resuscitation (CPR), 251–252, 1146
　emergency care for, 1146
Cardiovascular system. *See* Circulatory system
Career planning, 33–34
Caries, 273t–276t
Carotid artery, 702–703, 702f
Carpal tunnel syndrome (CTS), 341t–343t, 349, 447b
Carpals, 333
Carrier, 642
Cartilage, 324–328
Cartilage tissue, 187–190
Cash, asset types and, 546
Cast
　application of, 848–851
　care of, 848b
　materials for, 844
　removal of, 851
　types of, 844–851, 847b
Cast cutter, 851, 851f
Cast padding, 848
Cast spreader, 851, 851f
Casts
　types of, 972t
　urine sediment and, 971
Catabolism, 177t, 271
　definition of, 278
Cataract, 315t–316t
Catastrophic disability, 614
Catatonia, 303b
Catecholamines, 408
Category III codes, CPT manual and, 594
Catgut, 1116
Catheter, 1080, 1081f
Cautery, 1114, 1128
CBC. *See* Complete blood count
CC. *See* Chief complaint
CD-ROM, 462f, 463
CDC. *See* Centers for Disease Control and Prevention
Cecum, 266
Celiac sprue, 273t–276t
Cell, 175–181, 194, 196
　structure of, 175–176, 177t
Cell body, 283, 284f
Cell division, 178–179
Cell growth, 196
　cancer and, 179b
Cell membrane, 175, 177t, 194
Cellular casts, 972t
Cellulitis, 432t–433t, 433f
Cellulose, 140
　sources of, 141b
Celsius (C), 690
Centers for Disease Control (CDC), and Infection control, 640
Centers for Disease Control and Prevention (CDC), 58, 640, 667
　Standard Precautions and, 640
Centers for Medicare and Medicaid Services (CMS), 583–584, 611, 897
　fee structures and, 610
Central nervous system (CNS), 285–290, 287f, 354

Central processing unit, 462–463
Central processing unit (CPU), 462–463
Centrifuge, 902–904, 902f, 923
Centrifuge tubes, 904
Centrioles, 177t, 178f
Cerebellum, 288f, 289
Cerebral cortex, 251, 258
Cerebral hemispheres, 287
    lobes of, 290f
Cerebrospinal fluid (CSF), 286, 287f, 291f
    purpose of, 305
Cerebrovascular accident (CVA), 298t–299t, 301f
Cerebrum, 287, 288f, 305
CERT. See Community Emergency Response Team
Certificate of provider-performed microscopy (PPM) procedures, 897
Certificate of waiver, 897
Certified mail, 496b
Certified Medical Assistant (CMA), 41
    credentials of, 31, 31f
    occupational analysis of, 27b
    requirements of, 32t–33t
    testing for, 31
Certified Nursing Assistant (CNA), 41
Cerumen, 318, 809
Cervical
    spinal cavity and, 172–173
    spinal column divisions, 173f
Cervical vertebrae, 332, 333f
Cervicography, 391b
Cervix, 386–387
CEU. See Continuing education unit
CF. See Conversion factor
Chain of custody, 918
Chain of evidence, 918
Chain of infection, 639–640, 640f, 667
    and infection control, 639–640, 667
Chalazion, 315t–316t
Chambers, heart, 200, 202f
CHAMPVA, 604, 614, 633
Change, adapting to, 76–77, 77t
Charge form, 551
Chart documentation, 514, 529b
Charting, 527, 541, 721f, 725–727
    guidelines for, 527–529
    medical record and, 527–528
    tips for, 727, 727b, 727f–728f
Checks, 557–559
    requirements for, 557–559
    returned, 568
    types of, 558, 579
    writing of, 558–559, 558f, 579
Cheekbones. See Zygomatic bones
Chemical burns, 1141, 1149
Chemical hot/cold pack, 825, 829b
Chemical indicator, 657, 668
Chemicals
    cell formation and, 174
Chemistry, 904, 941
Chemistry profile, 983
Chemistry tests, 904, 923
Chemotherapy, topical, 428
Chest. See Thorax
Chest leads, 776–777, 778f
Chest muscles, 357, 359t–360t

Chest pain, 1136
    guidelines for, 1136
Chest radiography, 797–798, 797f
Chest x-ray, 254b, 258f
Chief complaint (CC), 588, 716, 720b, 721f, 728
    E/M coding and, 596
Child abuse, 56b
Childbirth, 872
    nutrition and, 143
Childhood, 86, 88–91
Children
    blood pressure ranges and, 707t
    body measurements, 685b–686b
    communicating with, 124b
    communication and, 124b
    drug dosage calculation for, 1016–1018
    nutrition and, 143
Choking, 1145, 1145b, 1145f
Cholecystitis, 273t–276t
Cholecystogram, 799t
Cholecystography, 272b
Cholecystokinin, 268
Cholelithiasis, 273t–276t
Cholesterol, 142, 142b
Cholesterol testing, 983–987, 988b–989b, 999–1000
    heart disease and, 987
Cholinesterase, 354
Chordae tendineae, 200–201
Chorion, 393
Choroid, 311
Chromic suture, 1116
Chromosomal disease, abnormalities and, 180–181
Chromosomes, 176
Chronic, coding guidelines and, 589b
Chronic disease
    definition of, 271
    nutrition and, 144–145
Chronic fatigue syndrome, 298t–299t
Chronic obstructive pulmonary disease (COPD), 254t–256t
Chronic renal failure (CRF), 374t–375t
Chronological resumé, 1154b, 1155f, 1164
Chyme, 264–265, 269f
Cicatrix, 430b, 1114
Cilia, 177t, 178f, 246
Ciliary body, 311
Circle of Willis, 205–206
Circular E: Employer's Tax Guide, 575
Circular turn, 817–822, 817f
Circulatory system, 191t–193t, 196, 243
    functions of, 199–200, 217
Circumcision, 385
Circumduction, 338, 348
Circumflex artery, 205, 207f
Civil law. See Private law
Claims. See also Electronic claims
    billing/coding requirements of, 622
    CMS-1500 form and, 622
    follow-up of, 630, 631f
    insurance carrier guidelines and, 622
    methods of, 625
    preventing rejection and delay of, 629–630, 634
    processing of, 625
    proper documentation and, 621–622, 634
    submitting of, 620–629
    tracking of, 625–629

Clamping instruments, surgery and, 1089–1101, 1101f
Clamps, 1127
Clarification, communication evaluation and, 105
Clarifying, positive communication techniques and, 120t
Classroom activities, 15
Claudication, 207b, 215t–216t
Claustrophobia, 800–801
Clavicle (collarbone), 332
Clean aseptic technique. See Medical asepsis
Clean claim, 620, 629, 634
Clear-liquid diet, 145
Clearinghouse, medical claims, 625, 634
Cleft lip, 182t–183t, 185f
Cleft palate, 182t–183t, 185f
CLIA 88. See Clinical Laboratory Improvement Amendments of 1988
CLIA-waived tests, 897, 956
    blood collection and, 941t
Clinical and Laboratory Standards Institute (CLSI), 941–942, 956
Clinical diagnosis, 723b
Clinical duties, 25, 27b, 31b
Clinical information, 601
Clinical Laboratory Improvement Amendments of 1988 (CLIA 88), 896–897, 923, 983
    blood tests and, 927
Clinical medical assisting, 28b–29b
Clinical skills, 27b
Clitoris, 389
Clone, 68
Closed reduction, 345
Closed technique, gloving and, 1089
Closed wound, 428, 435–436, 1114, 1128
Clothing, cultural differences and, 96–98
CLSI. See Clinical and Laboratory Standards Institute
Clubbing, 253b, 257f
Cluster scheduling, 492, 511
CMA. See Certified Medical Assistant
CME. See Continuing medical education
CMS. See Centers for Medicare and Medicaid Services
CMS-1500 claim form, 588, 599, 622–625, 623f–624f, 626b–628b
    third party liability and, 611, 611f
CNA. See Certified Nursing Assistant
CNS. See Central nervous system
Co-insurance, 567, 606, 608f
Co-payment, 567, 606
CO_2. See Carbon dioxide
Coagulation factor, 226, 229f
Coagulation studies, 904
Coarse focus adjustment knob, 901–902
COB. See Coordination of benefits
COBRA. See Consolidated Omnibus Reconciliation Act
Cocci, 638
Coccygeal, spinal column divisions and, 172–173, 173f
Coccyx, 332
Cochlea, 318
Code format, 593–594
Coding, 523b, 582, 589b
    filing and, 538

Cognitive learning, 125
Cold boot, 462–463
Cold therapy, 825
Colic, 272b
Colitis, ulcerative, 273t–276t
Collagen, 325
Collagenous, matrix tissue fibers, 187–190
Collarbone. See Clavicle
Collection process, 570, 572b–574b, 579
  payment plans and, 569, 569f, 570b–571b
Collimator, 794
Colon, 266, 277. See also Large intestine
  parts of, 261
Colon tests, 877–883
  sigmoidoscopy and, 878–883
Colonoscopy, 272b
Color coding, 537
Color coding filing methods, 537
Color-coding/A-Z guides, 532
Colorectal, 877
Colposcopy, 391b, 861
Columnar
  cell classification and, 184t
Combining form, 154t–155t, 172
Combining vowel, word parts and, 153
Comedo, pustular (whitehead), 422–423
Comedo (blackhead), 422–423
Comments, stereotyped, 121t
Comminuted fracture, 345, 346t–347t
Commission on Accreditation of Allied Health Education Programs (CAAHEP), 29, 30f, 32t–33t
  emergency planning and, 1147
Common bile duct, 271
Communication. See also Effective communication
  medical office, 474
  positive techniques of, 119, 119f, 120b, 120t
  process of, 103, 103f, 115
  written, 109–111, 512
Community Emergency Response Team (CERT), 1147
Community resources, 455–456, 457b
Compact bone, 328
Comparative negligence, 53
Compassion, 24–25
Compensation, 81t, 83–84
  lawsuit damages and, 54t
Compensatory damages, lawsuit damages and, 54t
Competence, 23–24
Complete blood count (CBC), 872, 892, 974–975, 975t, 999
Complete physical examination (CPX), 732–735
Complex carbohydrates, 140
Complex proteins, 142, 148
Compound binocular, 900. See also Binocular microscope
Compound fracture, 345, 346t–347t
Comprehensive plans, 606
Compress, cold, 825, 827b–828b
Compression fracture, 346t–347t
Compromise, 24
Computed radiography (CR). See Digital radiography
Computed tomography, 801–802

Computed tomography (CT) scan, 254b, 300f, 340b, 411b, 801–802, 802f
  patient preparation for, 802, 802f
Computer, 446–447
  components of, 461f–462f, 462–465
  functions of, 461–462
  health issues and, 447b
  HIPPA and, 447b
Computer imaging, 799–803
Computer security, 465, 466b
Computer skills, 460
Computer systems
  components of, 471
  functions of, 471
  medical practice management and, 468–471
Computer use
  basics of, 465–468
  HIPAA regulations and, 465, 466b
Computer vision syndrome (CVS), 447b
Concept map, 11–14, 13f
Conception. See Fertilization
Concurrent condition, 588–589, 599
Condenser, 901
Conditioning, 541
  filing and, 538
Conduction, 889
Conduction system, 201–203, 217, 764f
Condyle, 327t, 330f, 334
Condyloid joint, 337
Cones, 311
Confidence, 24
Confidential, 24
Confidentiality, 532b, 620
  breach of, 61–62, 62b, 70, 440b
  HIPAA requirements and, 54, 63b
Confidentiality agreement, example of, 440b
Confirmatory tests, 966–968
Congenital, genetic disorders and, 180
Conization, 391b
Conjunction
  correct use of, 110t
  indexing of, 534
Conjunctiva, 311, 312
Conjunctivitis (pinkeye), 315t, 316t, 316f
Conn's syndrome, 412t–414t
Connective tissue, 181, 187–190, 188t–189t, 194
  disorders of, 190b
Conscious, patient condition and, 1133
Consensus, 24
Consent, 736
  informed, 51
Consent to treat form, 516–518, 524, 541
Consent to use and disclose form, 516–518
Considerate. See Tactful
Consideration, 49–50
Consolidated Omnibus Reconciliation Act (COBRA), 604, 632
Consonant, 157–161, 161t
Constipation, 272b
Constitutional law, 48
Constrict, 215t–216t
Consultation, E/M coding and, 596
Consultation report, 505, 512
Consumer protection, 58
Continuing education, 22
Continuing education units (CEU), 31, 31b, 47
Continuing medical education (CME), 47
Continuity of care, 515

Contraception, 892
  methods of, 871t
Contract
  definition of, 49–50
  types of, 50–51
Contract law, 45
Contractility, 356
Contraction
  isometric, 354, 355f
  isotonic, 354, 355f
Contraindications, 1028, 1034
Contrast medium, 799, 799t
  patient preparation for, 799
Contributing factor, E/M service and, 599–600
Contributory factor, E/M service and, 597
Contributory negligence, 53
Control booth, x-ray room and, 795
Control panel, x-ray room and, 795, 795f
Control samples, 898
Controlled substance, 1008, 1008b, 1009f, 1033
  inventory of, 1008, 1008b, 1033
Controlled Substances Act of 1970, 1006–1008, 1033
Contusion, 363b, 428
Conventions, 588
  ICD-9-CM manual and, 585–586, 585b
Conversion, 304b
  of measurements, 681b, 1016, 1017f, 1017t
Conversion factor (CF), 610
Conversion reaction, 81t
Coordination of benefits (COB), 605, 632
Coordination of care, 597
COPD. See Chronic obstructive pulmonary disease
Coping, 80–83
Cornea, 311
Corneal reflex, 294
Coronary arteries, 205
Coronary circulation, 205, 218
Corporation, 37
Corpus callosum, 287
Corpus luteum, 389, 871–872
Correspondence, written
  guidelines for, 498
  letter and memo preparation for, 499–504, 512
  management of, 498–510
  manuscript preparation for, 504–508
  medical transcription and, 509–510
  proofreading of, 498–499, 503b
  report preparation for, 504–508
Cortex, 287, 371
Corticoids, 407
Cortisol, 407–408
Cost containment, 610, 633
Costal cartilage, 332
Council on Ethical and Judicial Affairs (CEJA), 61b
Counseling, E/M coding and, 596, 600
Counterbalanced, 902, 902f, 923
Coupling agent, 831
Course focus adjustment knob, 901–902
Cover letter, 1156, 1157f, 1164
Cover sheets, fax machine and, 443f
Coverslip, 869
Cowper's gland, 385. See also Bulbourethral gland

CPR. *See* Cardiopulmonary resuscitation
CPT codes, 551, 591
CPT manual, 591–592
    organization of, 592, 592b
    sections of, 599
CPT system, purpose of, 591
CPT-4 manual. *See* CPT manual
CPU. *See* Central processing unit
CPX. *See* Complete physical examination
Cramps (muscle), 363b
Cranial bones, 286b
Cranial cavity, 172, 173f, 194
Cranial nerve, 286, 286t, 288f
Cranium, 328–331
Creams, 1025, 1042
Creatinine clearance test, 374b
Credentialing, 47
Credentialing examinations, 32
    comparisons of, 32t–33t
Credentials, 30–32, 30b, 30f
Credit, 545, 578
Crenate
    concentrated urine and, 968
    hypertonic IV solutions and, 177
Crepitation, 341t–343t
Crepitus, 756t–757t
Cretinism, 412t–414t
CRF. *See* Chronic renal failure
Criminal law, 49b
Crohn disease, 273t–276t
Cross-eye. *See* Strabismus
Cross-reference, 534, 534t
Crossmatching, 904
Croup, 254t–256t
Crust, 430b
Crutches, 838–844
Cryosurgery, 428, 435, 1114, 1128
Cryptorchidism, 383, 385f
Crystals, 971
CSF. *See* Cerebrospinal fluid
CT. *See* Computed tomography (CT) scan
CT scan. *See* Computed tomography (CT) scan
CTS. *See* Carpal tunnel syndrome
Cuboid, 334
Cuboidal cell classification, 184t
Cultural diversity, 36, 95–98, 95b, 97t, 122
Cultural influences, 76, 83
Culture and sensitivity (C&S), 870, 998, 998f
Culture collection, 911–912, 912f
Culture plate, 992, 1000
Cultures, 941t, 992–998, 997t
Culturing, 998
Cumulative dose, 1007b, 1033
Cuneiform, 334
Curative drug, 1004
Curette, 1103–1104, 1104f, 1127
Current Procedural Terminology (CPT), 591, 609–610. *See also* CPT codes
Curriculum vitae (CV), 605
Cursor, 463
Cushing syndrome, 412t–414t, 415f
Cusps, 200–201
Cuticle, 423
Cutis anserina. *See* Goose flesh
Cutting instruments, 1089–1101
Cuvette, 929–930
CVA. *See* Cerebrovascular accident

CVS. *See* Computer vision syndrome
Cyanosis, 208t–209t, 756t–757t
Cyst, 424–425, 435
Cyst removal, 1113, 1128
Cystic duct, 271
Cystic fibrosis, 182t–183t
Cystitis, 961
Cystoscopy, 374b
Cytology, 857–860, 897
Cytology laboratory requisition, 861, 867f
Cytoplasm, 175–176, 177t, 178f, 194
Cytoscopy, 377f

D

D&C. *See* Dilation and curettage
Dacryoadenitis, 314b
Daily value (DV), 131–132
Damages
    lawsuits and, 53
    types of, 54t
Data records, 516–524, 517b–518b, 519f
Database
    information sources and, 524–527
    management of, 468, 472, 524
Date of birth (DOB), 521b, 522b
Day planner, 6, 7f
Daysheet, 550f, 551
dB. *See* Decibels
DEA. *See* Drug Enforcement Administration; U.S. Drug Enforcement Agency
DEA number, 1008, 1033
Dead spaces, 251–252
Deafness, 319t
Death, 81–83
Debit, 545, 578
Debrided, 341t–343t, 1113
Debridement, 1114
Debtor, 570
Decibels (dB), 318, 891
Deciduous teeth, 264
Decision-making process, 24
Decontaminates, 1114
Decubitus ulcer, 430b
Deductible, 606, 608t
Deep wound, 1114
Defamation, intentional torts and, 52–53
Default, 469–470
Defecation, 267
Defending, as communication barrier, 121t
Defense mechanism, 80–81, 81t, 83–84
Defibrillation, 1146
Defibrillator
    fully automatic, 1146
    semiautomatic, 1146
Defined purpose, 10
Deglutition, 264
Delayed primary (tertiary) intention healing, 1116f, 1128
Delegate, 6
Delirium, 303b
Delivery, of message, 104, 115
Deltoid muscle, 357
    intramuscular injection and, 1066, 1066f
Delusion, 303b
Delusional disorder, 304b
Dementia, 304b
Demographic, 716, 728
Dendrites, 283

Denial, 81t, 82–84
Dense tissue, 188t–189t, 189
Deoxygenated blood, 204
Deoxyribonucleic acid (DNA), 427
    cell nucleus and, 176
Dependability, 23
Dependent, 575, 604
Depolarization, 763–765, 765f
Deposit, 559–560, 559f, 561b, 579
    methods of, 562f
Deposit slip, 559–560, 560f
Deposition, lawsuit information and, 55t
Depreciation, 447–448
Depression, 82, 84, 304b
Depression fracture, 346t–347t
Depressors, 357
Dermatitis, 139t, 432t–433t
Dermatologist, 430
Dermatology, 419
Dermatome, 290, 302f
Dermis, 421
Descending colon, 261, 267, 277
Detoxification, 270
Development, human life span and, 86–94
Developmentally delayed, 125–128
Dexterity, 24–25
Diabetes, gestational, 397t
Diabetes insipidus, 415t
Diabetes mellitus, 412t–414t, 416f
    signs of, 417b
Diabetic diet, 145
Diabetic emergency, 1144–1145
    types of, 1144
Diabetic ketoacidosis, 1144–1145, 1149
Diagnose, 855
Diagnosis (Dx), 583, 588, 598, 720b
    Bethesda System and, 861
    types of, 722–723, 723b
Diagnostic coding, 583–590, 588b–590b, 598
Diagnostic drug, 1004
Diagnostic imaging, 796, 796b
    types of, 793
Diagnostic procedures, 27b
Diagnostic suffix, 153–156, 160t, 161f
Dialysis, 376b, 377b
Diameter, 211
Diaphoresis, 208t–209t, 430b, 756t–757t, 960
Diaphragm, 171, 200, 201f, 206f, 248
Diaphysis, 326f, 328
Diarrhea, 272b
Diarthroses, 336
Diastole (S_2), 202
Diastolic pressure, 707, 713
Diencephalon, 287–289, 291f, 305
Diet therapy, 145–147
Dietary guidelines, 131–134, 148
    updates to, 132b
Diff. *See* Differential count
Differential blood cell count, 981, 982f, 999
Differential count (diff), 225
Differential diagnosis, 723b
Diffusion
    passive transport systems and, 176–177, 179f–180f, 194
Digestion, 263, 269f
Digestive diseases and disorders, 271t, 272b, 273t–276t

Digestive organs, 261, 264–268
Digestive process, 269f
   stages of, 277
Digestive system, 191t–193t, 196, 261, 263–264, 263b, 263f, 277
   diseases and disorders of, 271–276
Digestive tract. *See also* Alimentary canal
   areas of, 277
Digital radiographic imaging. *See* Computer imaging
Digital radiography, 796–797
Digital subscriber lines (DSL), 464
Digital thermometer, 691–693, 693f, 694b–699b, 712
Dilating instruments, 1089–1101
Dilation, 215t–216t
Dilation and curettage (D&C), 391b
Diminutive endings, 158t
Diplococci, 638
Diplomacy, 24
Diplopia, 296b, 314b
Direct cause, lawsuits and, 53
Direct contact, 642, 667, 1152–1153, 1164
Direct filing system, 533–534
Direct pressure
   bleeding and, 1138, 1140f
Directory, 467b, 471
Disabilities, 123, 128
Disability income insurance, 614–615, 633
   types of disabilities and, 614–615
Disaster
   planning for, 1147
   practice for, 1147
   preparation for, 1147
   types of, 1146, 1147b
Disaster preparedness, 1146–1148, 1150
   medical assistant's role and, 1147–1148
Discharge summary, 508, 512
Disclaimer, facsimile cover sheets and, 442–443
Discussion, in classroom, 15–16
Disinfection, 654, 668
Dislocation, 345, 346, 1142–1143, 1149
Dispense, 1007b
Displaced fracture, 346t–347t
Displacement, 81t, 83–84
Display panel, 134
Disposable goods, 450
Disrobing, 735–736, 758
Dissecting instruments, 1089–1101
Dissecting scissors, 1103
Distance, nonverbal communication and, 107
Distention, of abdomen, 756t–757t
Distracter, message and, 104–105, 115
Diuresis, 373b
Diuretics, 373t–375t
Diverticulitis, 273t–276t
Divided dose, 1007b
DO. *See* Doctor of Osteopathy
DOB. *See* Date of birth
Doctor of Medicine (MD), 39, 39t
Doctor of Osteopathy (DO), 39, 39t
Domain name, 466, 466b
Domestic Violence Law, 58b
Dominant genes, 179
Donor, universal, 227
Dorsal, posterior body plane and, 168–169, 193–194

Dorsal cavity, 170f, 171t, 172–173, 194
Dorsal recumbent position, 738, 740b–741b, 758
Dorsalis pedis artery, 702–703, 702f
Dorsogluteal area, 1069, 1074f
Dosage
   calculation of, 1016–1018, 1016b, 1033
   child calculation of, 1016–1018
Dose, drug administration and, 1015
Dosimeter, 803, 803f
Double booking scheduling, 492, 511
Down syndrome, 180–181, 182t–183t, 185f
Dressing forceps, 1101–1103
Drip rate, 1081
Drug, 1003, 1029f
   labels and, 1011–1015, 1015f
Drug administration, 1011–1024, 1015t
   documentation of, 1016, 1016b
Drug classifications, 1025, 1026t–1027t, 1033
   methods of, 1025
Drug Enforcement Administration (DEA), 1007b, 1008, 1033
Drug legislation, 1006, 1007b, 1007t
Drug reference, 1010–1011, 1011f, 1033
   package inserts and, 1011
Drug route, 1015–1016, 1036
Drug schedules, 1008, 1010f, 1010t, 1033
Drug screening, 918, 924
Drugs. *See also* Medication administration
   actions of, 1005, 1005b
   dosage of, 1005–1006, 1006b–1007b, 1006f
   forms of, 1024–1025
   identification of, 1004–1005, 1004f
   names of, 1004–1005, 1004f, 1015f, 1032
   sources of, 1005, 1005t
   unwanted effects of, 1028
DSL. *See* Digital subscriber lines
Ductus arteriosus, 206
Ductus venosus, 206
Duodenum, 266, 268, 269f, 277
Dura mater, 285
Durable power of attorney for health care, 56, 58, 59t
Duty
   dereliction of, 53
   lawsuits and, 53
DV. *See* Daily value
Dwarfism, 412t–414t
Dx. *See* Diagnosis
Dying. *See* Death
Dysmenorrhea, 390b
Dyspepsia, 272b
Dysphagia, 272b
Dysphonia, 253b
Dysplasia, 861
Dyspnea, 253b
   sickle cell anemia and, 182t–183t
Dysrhythmia. *See* Arrhythmia
Dysuria, 373b, 869

E

E codes, 588, 588b
E-prescribing. *See* Electronic prescribing
E/M. *See* Evaluation and Management (E/M)
Ear, 318, 318b
   diseases and disorders of, 319t
   documentation of, 813f–814f
   drug classifications of, 318t

Ear *(Continued)*
   inner, 314–318
   instillation of, 812, 813b–814b
   irrigation of, 809–812, 810b–812b
   structure and function of, 314–318, 317f
   tests and procedures for, 318b
   treatment of, 809–812
Ear examination, 755
Eardrum. *See* Tympanic membrane
Earnings, 575–576
ECC. *See* Endocervical curettage
   See also Emergency Cardiovascular Care
Ecchymosis, 231t–232t, 430b
ECG. *See* Electrocardiogram
ECG cycle, cardiac events in, 764t
ECG lead, legal aspects of, 779b
ECG leads. *See also* Electrocardiogram (ECG)
   placement of, 770–777
ECG paper, 768, 768f
ECG patterns, 763–765, 764f
Echocardiography, 788b
Echoing, feedback clarification and, 105
Eczema, 430b
EDD/EDC. *See* Estimated date of delivery/confinement
Edema, 233
EDTA. *See* Ethylenediaminetetraacetic acid
EEG. *See* Electroencephalography
Effective communication, 25
   and interviewing skills, 725, 726b, 728
   barriers to, 121t
   english skills and, 25
   facial expressions and, 25
   medical assistant and, 474
   patient teaching and, 121b, 121f
Efferent nerve, 190
Efficiency, 23
Ego, 73, 83
EHR. *See* Electronic health record
EIA. *See* Enzyme immunoassay
Ejaculation, 385
Ejaculatory duct, 384
Elastic, matrix tissue fibers and, 187–190
Elastic bandage, 817
Elastic cartilage, 188t–189t, 190, 326
Elasticity, muscle tissue and, 356
Elder abuse, signs of, 56b
Elderly person
   communication with, 128
   heat stroke and, 1141b
Electrical burns, 1141, 1149
Electrical impulses, 763–765, 763b, 764f
Electrocardiogram (ECG), 204f, 217, 761, 770b, 778, 779b
   angles of, 770b
   placing electrodes for, 769–770
   placing leads for, 770–777
Electrocardiograph, 761, 765–768, 768f
   types of, 765
Electrocardiography, 28b–29b, 761
   equipment and supplies, 765–769
Electrodes, 763, 765–768
   placement of, 769–770
Electroencephalography (EEG), 296b, 300f
Electromyography (EMG), 296b, 363b
Electroneuromyography, 296b
Electronic claims, 625, 634
   clearinghouses for, 625

Electronic health record (EHR), 486. *See also* Electronic medical record
Electronic mail (e-mail), 114–116, 114b
Electronic medical record (EMR), 468, 516, 540
Electronic Patient Records (EPR). *See* Electronic medical record
Electronic prescribing (E-prescribing), 1030
Electronic technology, 112–116
Electrosurgery, 1114, 1128
Elephantiasis, 235f, 235t
Elimination, 263
Elixirs, 1024
EMAC. *See* Emergency Management Assistance Compact
Email. *See also* Electronic mail
　employer contact and, 1158, 1165
Emancipated minor, 50
Embolus, 215t–216t
Embryo, 393, 400
Emergency
Emergency Cardiovascular Care (ECC), AHA Guidelines for, 1146
Emergency care, 1133b, 1148. *See also* First aid
Emergency equipment, 1133, 1134f, 1135t
Emergency Management Assistance Compact (EMAC), 1147
Emergency preparedness unit, medical assistant and, 1147
Emergency scheduling, 492
Emergency System for Advanced Registration of Volunteer Health (ESAR-VHP), 1147
Emesis, 272b
EMG. *See* Electromyography
Emotional abuse, 56b
Emotional support. *See* Compassion
Empathy, 24, 82
Emphysema, 249b, 254t–256t
Employee earnings record, 577, 578f, 580
Employee safety, 803, 803f
Employee's Withholding Allowance Certificate (Form W-4), 575
Employer contact, 1157–1158, 1158t, 1165
　fax machine and, 1157
Employer-sponsored group plans, 604
Employment, law and, 58, 58t
Employment agency, 1152, 1164
EMR. *See* Electronic medical record
Emulsification, 265–266
Emulsion, 1024
Encephalitis, 298t–299t
Encounter form, 469–470, 551, 552f, 621f, 622
End-of-life issues, right to die and, 66, 70
Endocardium, 200, 202f
Endocervical curettage (ECC), 861
Endocrine disorders
　drug classification for, 410t
　signs and symptoms of, 411b
　tests and procedures for, 411b
Endocrine gland, 186, 403, 404f, 405t, 417
Endocrine hormone, disorders of, 415t
Endocrine system
　activity in cells and organs, 408–410
　aging and, 411b
　body systems and, 191t–193t
　diseases and disorders of, 402, 410, 412t–414t
　function of, 403–404, 417

Endocrinologist, 410
Endocrinology, 402
Endometriosis, 392t–393t
Endometrium, 387
Endoplasmic reticulum (ER), 177t, 178f
Endorse, 559
Endorsement
　checks and, 559, 559f
　licensure and, 46
Endoscopy, 272b, 272f
Engineering controls, 643, 646b, 898
Enteral. *See* Oral drug administration
Enteric-coated tablets, 1025b, 1040
Entity, 37
Entry
　progress notes and, 516–518
Enuresis, 373b
Envelope preparation. *See also* Outgoing mail
　for outgoing mail, 497–498, 497b, 498f, 503b, 511
Environment, distracters and, 104–105
Enzyme immunoassay (EIA), 972, 973b–974b
Enzymes, 142, 264, 269f, 270t
EOB. *See* Explanation of benefits
Eosinophils, 225, 227t
Ependymal cells, 284
Epicardium, 200, 202f
Epidermis, 421
Epididymis, 384, 384f
Epididymitis, 387t
Epidural space, 285–286
Epigastric, 264
Epiglottis, 247–248, 264
Epilepsy, 298t–299t, 301b, 1137
　guidelines for, 1137–1138
Epinephrine, 408
Epiphyseal plate (growth plate), 328
Epiphysis, 326f, 328
Episiotomy, 389
Episode of care, 609, 632–633
Epistaxis, 254t–256t, 1138, 1141f
Epithelial cells, 968–971
Epithelial tissue, 181–186, 184t, 194
　disorders of, 186b, 186f
Eponym, 152, 152b, 163
Equal Employment Opportunity Commission (EEOC), 60
Equilibrium, 289, 314, 318
Equipment
　buying of, 458
　in examination room, 672–673, 672f, 672t, 677
　leasing of, 448, 458
Equipment inventory, records of, 447–448
Equipment maintenance, 448
　preventive actions for, 448
　procedure for, 449b–450b, 458
Erect, 333–334
Erectile dysfunction, 385. *See also* Impotence
Erection, 385
Ergonomic, 341t–343t, 446
Erlich Units (EU), urobilinogen and, 966
Erosion, 430b
Erythema, 432t–433t, 756t–757t
Erythroblastosis fetalis, 230f, 231t–232t
Erythrocyte sedimentation rate (ESR), 341t–343t, 977–981, 999

Erythrocytes, 222–224, 224f
Erythropoiesis, 223–224, 226f
Erythropoietin, 223–224, 368
ESAR-VHP. *See Emergency System for Advanced Registration of Volunteer Health (ESAR-VHP)*
Esophagitis, 273t–276t
Esophagus, 247, 264, 266f, 269f
　digestive role of, 277
Esotropia, 314b
ESR. *See* Erythrocyte sedimentation rate
Essential nutrients, 138, 148
Established patient
　appointments for, 489
　E/M coding and, 595–596
　greeting of, 475–476
　medical records of, 540
　work-related injury and, 518
Estimated date of deliver/confinement (EDD/EDC), 872, 872b, 892
Estrogen, 386, 389, 408
　function of, 399
Ethical standards, 23
Ethics
　code of, 62b, 69
　health care and, 61–68
　medical, 28b–29b
　standards of, 23, 61–66
Ethmoid bone, 329–331
Ethylenediaminetetraacetic acid (EDTA), 941, 977
Etiology, 181
EU. *See* Erlich Units
Eustachian tube, 314
Euthanasia, 66
Evacuated tube method, 935b–940b, 940–941, 941t
Evacuation blood collection system, 942–943
Evaluation
　teaching process and, 126
　verbal communication and, 105
Evaluation and Management (E/M) coding
　code determination for, 595–598, 600
　CPT coding and, 595
　factors of, 596, 599
　guidelines for, 598
　vocabulary of, 595–596
Evaluation and Management (E/M) service
　CPT manual organization and, 592
　levels of, 599
Event monitor, 784
Eversion, 338
Examination
　E/M service types of, 596–597, 599
　licensure and, 46
　methods of, 747
Examination room
　accessibility and safety in, 672
　decor and temperature in, 671–672
　maintenance of, 675, 676f, 677
　patient preparation and, 675–677, 676f
　privacy in, 671
Examination room preparation
　equipment, 672–673, 677
　examination table and, 675, 675f, 677
　general considerations of, 671–672, 671f
　supplies for, 673–675, 677

Excision, 428
Excoriation, 430b
Excretion, 368
Excretory duct, 384
Excretory system, 368. See also Urinary system
Exemption, 575
Exhalation, 249, 251f
Exocrine gland, 186, 403, 417
Exophthalmia, 314b, 411b
Exophthalmos, 412t–414t
Exotropia, 314b
Expiration, 245, 250f, 705
Explanation of benefits (EOB), 611, 634
Exposure, medical emergencies and, 1141–1142
Exposure control plan, 643, 646b, 668
Exposure incident, 643, 646b
Expressed contract, 50–51, 69
Extensibility, muscle tissue and, 356
Extension, 337, 348
Extensors, 357
External carotid arteries, 205–206, 218
External respiration, 249, 258
External storage devices, 463
Extracellular, fibrous structure and, 187–190
Extrinsic eye muscle, 312–313, 313t
Extrinsic muscle, 312
Exudate, wound drainage and, 1123
Eye
  structure and function of, 311–313, 320
  treatments of, 812–817
Eye contact, cultural diversity and, 96–98
Eye disease, 313–314, 314b, 314t
  tests and procedures for, 314b
Eye muscle, 312, 313f, 313t
Eye treatments
  instillation of, 817, 818b–819b
  irrigation of, 812–817, 815b–816b
Eyeball, 311–312, 312f
Eyebrows, 312–313
Eyelashes, 312–313
Eyelids, 312–313
Eyepiece, 901
Eyes, nonverbal communication and, 106

F

F. See Fahrenheit
Facial bones, 330f, 331–332
Facial expression muscles, 359t–360t
Facial, Arm, Speech, Time (FAST), 1137b
Facilities management, 439–441, 457
  requirements of ADA for, 440b
Fad diet, 147, 149
Fahrenheit (F), 690
Fainting, 1134–1136, 1135f, 1148
  guidelines for, 1136, 1136f
Fair Debt Collection Act of 1977, 569
Fair Debt Collection Practices Act, 58
Fair Labor Standards Act, 571–572, 580
Fallopian tubes, 386
False imprisonment, intentional torts and, 53
False ribs, 332
Familial, 722
  inherited disorders and, 180
Family and Medical Leave Act (FMLA), 60
Family history, medical history and, 720b, 722
Family history (FH), 728
Family nurse practitioner (FNP), 40
Family practitioner, 37, 42–43

Fantasy, 81t, 83–84
Farsightedness. See Hyperopia
Fascia, 354
FAST. See Facial, Arm, Speech, Time
Fasting blood sugar (FBS), 411b, 987, 1000
Fat-soluble vitamins, 138
Fats, 141–142, 142b, 148, 269f
Fatty acids, 141, 142b, 270t
Fatty casts, 972t
Fax machine (facsimile), 114, 114b, 442–443, 442f, 444b–445b
  HIPPA privacy rules and, 442b
FBS. See Fasting blood sugar
Fear, 77–80, 83, 98–99, 98f
Febrile, 690
FECA. See Federal Employee Compensation Act
Fecal, 267
Fecal occult blood test, 877, 877f, 881b–882b, 892
  documentation for, 878b
Fecal occult blood test documentation for, 878b
Feces, 267, 269f
Federal Employee Compensation Act (FECA), 614
Federal Employees' Compensation Act, 575
Federal Health Care Financing Administration (HCFA), 897
Federal Income Tax, 572–575
Federal Insurance Contributions Act (FICA), 572
Federal Register, conversion factor and, 610
Federal Trade Commission (FTC), 610
Federal Truth in Lending Act, 569, 569f
Federal Unemployment Tax Act (FUTA), 575, 580
Fee adjustment, 568
Fee policy, 567–568
  procedures for, 567b
Fee schedule, 549
Fee structure, methods of, 609–610
Fee-for-service plan. See Indemnity plan
Feedback
  communication evaluation and, 105
  instructors and, 18
  learning from, 18
  messages and, 109
  self-monitoring and, 18
Felony, 49b
Femoral artery, 702–703, 702f
Femur (thighbone), 334
Fertility, 66
Fertilization, 393, 400
Fetus, 393, 400
FFDM. See Full-field digital mammography
FH. See Family history
Fiberglass cast, 844
  application of, 849b–850b
Fibrin, 226
Fibrinogen, 226
Fibrocartilage, 188t–189t, 190
Fibromyalgia, 364t
Fibromyositis, 363b
Fibrous cartilage, 326
Fibrous tissue, 187–190, 188t–189t
Fibula, 334, 337f
FICA. See Federal Insurance Contributions Act
Fiduciary, 51
Fight or flight response, 292

Fight-flight-fright, 77
Figure-eight turn, 817–822
File folders, 532
Filing
  document preparation for, 538
  equipment for, 529–532, 530t–531t, 541
  guides for, 532
  methods of, 533–537
  procedures for, 537–540
Filing systems
  plan for, 541
  selection of, 528–533
  supplies for, 532–533
Film-screen radiography, 795–798, 795f–796f
  chest radiography and, 797–798
  digital radiography and, 796–797
  mammography and, 798
Filter paper, 929–930
Filter paper method, 929–930, 929f, 933b–935b
Filtration, 368, 370–371
  passive transport systems and, 177–178
Final diagnosis, 723b
Financial management, 543
Financial statements, 548, 548f
Fine focus adjustment knob, 901–902
First (primary) intention healing, 1114, 1116f, 1128
First Aid, 28b–29b, 1130–1132, 1131b–1132b, 1132t
  standard precautions and, 1132, 1132f, 1148
First morning specimen, 912, 959
First trimester, 393, 400
First-degree atrioventricular block, conduction system disorders and, 204b
First-degree burn, 428–429, 1139b
Fiscal intermediary, 611–612
Fissure, 287, 327t, 330f, 424–425, 430b, 435
Fixative, slide preparation and, 861
Fixator, prime mover muscle and, 356
Flaccid, 353–354
Flagella, 177t, 178f
Flash drive, 463
Flash sterilized, 657
Flashcards, 11–14, 17
Flat bones, 327–328, 348
Flatulence, 272b
Flexion, 337, 348
Flexors, 357
Floating ribs, 332
Floppy disk, 463
Fluorescein angiography, 314b
Fluorescein staining, 314b
Fluoroscopic imaging, 798–799
  contrast media and, 799
Fluoroscopy. See Fluoroscopic imaging
Flutter, conduction system disorders and, 204
FNP. See Family nurse practitioner
Foam, urine appearance and, 959
FOBT. See Fecal occult blood test
Focusing, 901–902, 903b–904b
  positive communication techniques and, 120t
Follicle, 422
Follicle-stimulating hormone (FSH), 389, 399, 405t, 406
Font, 467
Fontanel (soft spot), 327t, 328–331, 331f
Food, cultural differences and, 96–98

Food and Drug Administration (FDA), 134, 1007–1008, 1007b
Food guide pyramid, 132, 132t, 133f, 148
    ethnic food and, 132b, 134f
Food labels, 134, 135f, 136b
Food-drug interaction, 1016, 1016b
Foot, 334–335, 338f
    muscles of, 359t–360t
Foramen, 327t, 331f
Foramen magnum, 329–331
Foramen ovale, 206
Foramina, 329–331
Forced vital capacity (FVC), 883
Forceps, 1101–1103, 1102f–1103f, 1127
Forearm (Lofstrand) crutches, 838, 838f
Forensic, 918
Foreskin, 385
Form W-4. *See* Employee's Withholding Allowance Certificate (Form W-4)
Format
    full-block, 501f–502f, 504
    modified-block, 501f–502f, 504
    of text, 10
    source-oriented, 524
    Source-oriented format, 524
Format guidelines, for medical record, 524–527
Formed elements, 222–223, 224f
    blood and, 222, 223f
Fossa, 327t, 335f
Four 'Ds," of lawsuits, 53
Four-point gait, 842, 842f–843f
Fovea centralis, 311–312
Fowler's position, 738–747, 746b–747b, 758
Fracture, 345, 346t–347t, 349, 1142, 1142f, 1149
    repair of, 1142, 1143f
Fraud
    health insurance and, 604
    intentional torts and, 53
Free edge, 423
Frenulum, 264
FREPS, urinary function acronym, 368
Frequency, 318, 373b
Frontal (coronal) plane, 168–169, 193
Frontal bone, 329–331
Frontal lobe, 287, 288t, 289f
Frontal sinus, 329–331
Frostbite, 1142, 1149. *See also* Hypothermia
FSH. *See* Follicle-stimulating hormone
FTC. *See* Federal Trade Commission
Full-block format, 504
Full-field digital mammography (FFDM), 798
Full-liquid diet, 145
Full-thickness burn, 428–429, 1139b
Functional resumé, 1154b, 1155f, 1164
Fundus, 265, 277, 386–387
Fungal infections, 432t–433t
Fungi, 638–639, 639t, 667
Funny bone. *See* Olecranon process
Furuncle, 430b
FUTA. *See* Federal Unemployment Tax Act
FVC. *See* Forced vital capacity

G

GAFs. *See* Geographic adjusted factors (GAFs)
Gait, 298t–299t
    walking and, 182t–183t
Gait pattern, 838–842
Galactosemia, 960

Gallbladder, 268, 269f, 271
    disease of, 273t–276t
Galvanometer, 765–768
Gametes, 179, 383
Ganglion, 283
Gardnerella, 861, 870, 892
Gastric gland, 270t
Gastric ulcer, 273t–276t
Gastrin, 265–266
Gastritis, 273t–276t
Gastroenteritis, 265–266
Gastroesophageal reflux disease (GERD), 273t–276t
Gastrointestinal (GI) tract, 263
Gastrointestinal system *See* Digestive system
Gatekeeper, 607
Gauge
    of needles, 1039
Gel caps, 1024–1025
General anesthetics, 1113, 1128
Genes, 176, 194
Genetic counseling, 181
Genetic disorders, 180–181, 182t–183t, 194
Genetic engineering, 66–68
Genetic immunity, 237
Genetic information, 179
Genitalia
    external (female), 386, 389, 389f
    external (male), 385
Genitourinary tract, 383
Genomics, 66–68
Geographic adjusted factors (GAFs), 610
Geographic Practice Cost Indices (GPCI), 610
GERD. *See* Gastroesophageal reflux disease
Gestation, 391–393
Gestational diabetes, 872
Gestures
    cultural differences and, 113
    nonverbal, 108b
GHb *See* Glycosylated hemoglobin (GHb) test
GHRH. *See* Growth hormone-releasing hormone
GI. *See* Gastrointestinal (GI) tract
Gigantism, 412t–414t
Gingivitis, 273t–276t, 756t–757t
Glands
    epithelial cells and, 181
    skin and, 422–423, 425f
Glans penis, 385
Glass slides, 929–930
Glaucoma, 315t–316t
Glial cells, 190, 284, 285f
    types of, 284
Gliding joint, 337
Glomerulonephritis, 374t–375t
Glomerulus, 370–372
Glossitis, 139t, 273t–276t
Gloves, 651, 652b–653b, 667, 1107f
    and infection control, 651
    in the examination room, 673
Glucagon, 408, 409f
Glucocorticoids, 407–408
Glucometer, 987
Glucose, 961
    reagent tablets and, 966–968
Glucose reagent strip, 987, 987f
Glucose testing, 987–991, 989b–990b
    error in reading of, 987b

Glucose tolerance test (GTT), 411b, 907, 918, 987, 1000
Glycemic index, 145, 146b
Glycerol, 141, 270t
Glycosuria, 373b, 961
Glycosylated hemoglobin (GHb) test, 991, 991f
Glycosylated hemoglobin A_{1c}, 411b–412b
GnRH. *See* Gonadotropin-releasing hormone
Goals
    accomplishment of, 3–9, 19
    choosing of, 4b
    setting of, 4, 4b
Goiter, 140t, 411b, 412t–414t
Golgi apparatus, 177t, 178f
Gonad, 384f, 399, 408
Gonadotropin-releasing hormone (GnRH), 389
Gonadotropins, 405t
Gonads, 383
Goniometer, 756t–757t, 838
Gonioscopy, 314b
Good Samaritan Act, 51–52, 69, 1148
Goose flesh (cutis anserina), 421
Gout. *See* Arthritis, gouty
Government names, indexing of, 536, 536t
Government-sponsored programs, 604
Gowers' sign, muscular dystrophy and, 182t–183t
Gown, patient, 735–736, 758
GPCI. *See* Geographic Practice Cost Indices
Graafian follicle, 386, 389
Gram stain, 992, 995f, 996t, 997f, 1000
Grammar, 110
    written communication and, 109
Granular casts, 972t
Granulation phase
    of healing, 428
    of wound healing, 428
Granulocytes, 225, 227t
Grasping instruments, surgery and, 1089–1101
Graves disease, 412t–414t, 415f
Greatest specificity, 584
    CPT coding and, 594, 595b
Greenstick fracture, 345, 346t–347t, 1142
Grief, stages of, 82
Gross negligence, 51–53
Gross wages, 575, 575b, 580
Group policy, 611, 633
Group practice, 37, 37t, 42
Group practice association
    HMO's and, 607
Growth charts, 684–690, 688f–689f, 712
Growth hormone-releasing hormone (GHRH), 406b
Growth plate. *See* Epiphyseal plate
GTT. *See* Glucose tolerance test
Guaiac test. *See* Fecal occult blood test
Guarantor, 469
Guarding, 272b
Guidelines
    CPT manual and, 592
    of insurance carrier, 622
Gustatory receptors, 309, 311f
Gynecological examination
    prenatal care and, 857–861
    reproductive disorders and, 861–870

Gynecologist, 856
Gynecology, 856
Gyri, 287

H

H&P. *See* History and Physical report
Habit
   21-day, 8b
   development of, 8, 8b
   establishment of, 8–9
Hair, 422
Hallucination, 303b
Hammer. *See* Malleus
Hamstring, 354
Hand, 333
Hand hygiene, 648, 654b, 667–668
Hand rubs, 650–651, 651b
Hand signals, surgery and, 1107t–1108t
Hands, nonverbal communication and, 106
Hands-Only CPR, 1149
   guidelines for ECC and, 1146
Handwashing, 643–648, 649b–650b, 651, 651f, 1088–1089
   and infection control, 643–648
Hard drive, 463
Hard palate, 331–332
Hardware, 462
Haversian system, 326, 326f
Hazardous Chemical Standards, 58
   requirements of, 58
Hb. *See* Hemaglobin
HBV. *See* Hepatitis B virus
HCFA. *See* Health Care Financing Administration
hCG. *See* Human chorionic gonadotropin
HCPCS. *See* Healthcare Common Procedure Coding System
Hct. *See* Hematocrit
HDL. *See* High-density lipoprotein
Head muscles, 357, 359t–360t
Headache, 296b
   types of, 296f
Heading, of resume, 1154–1155, 1164
Health, 9, 75–80, 632
Health care delivery settings, 42
Health Care Financing Administration (HCFA), 583–584, 611
Health care reform, 604
Health care system, cultural perceptions of, 122
Health care team, 39–41, 40f
   physician's role in, 605
Health history form, 516–518, 520f
   subjective information and, 517
Health insurance
   choices of, 604–605
   cost and availability of, 603–604
   definitions and purpose of, 601, 603
   health care reform and, 604
   history of, 603, 632
   overview of, 603–604
   patient and provider roles in, 604–605
Health insurance policies, 606–610
   types of, 606
Health Insurance Portability and Accountability Act (HIPPA)
   appointment reminders and, 493
   confidentiality and, 63b

Health Insurance Portability and Accountability Act (HIPPA) *(Continued)*
   CPT codes and, 591
   documentation and, 524b
   electronic guidelines for, 620
   office maintenance and, 439, 457–458, 604, 632
   patient privacy, 725
   record retention, 539
   records ownership, 524b–525b
   Title I and, 60
Health Maintenance Organization (HMO), 604, 607, 632
   types of, 607
Healthcare Common Procedure Coding System (HCPCS), 626b–628b
Hearing
   disabilities and, 123, 127
   impairment of, 314–318
   loss of, 318b
Hearing acuity tests, 889–891, 893
Heart
   chambers of, 200, 202f
   circulatory system and, 200–205, 218
   conduction system of, 764f
   diseases of, 206–211, 218
   ECG leads and, 770f
   fetal circulation of, 206, 218
   function of, 200–201
   location of, 200, 201f
   mediastinum and, 171
   muscles of, 202f
   structure of, 200–201
   surfaces of, 770, 770b
   thoracic cavity and, 169–171
Heart attack, 1148. *See also* Chest pain
Heart block
   conduction system disorders and, 204
Heart coverings, 200
Heart system, 191t–193t
Heart valves, 200–201
Heartbeat, 202–203, 217
Heat burns, 1138–1141
Heat exhaustion, 1141, 1149
Heat stroke, 1141, 1149
Heat therapy, 825–831
Heating pad, 825–831, 832b–833b
HEENT, 756t–757t
Hegar uterine dilator, dilating instruments and, 1089–1101
Height
   adult measurement of, 681, 684f
   child measurement of, 683, 684f, 684t, 685b–686b
Heimlich maneuver, 1145, 1149. *See also* Choking
Hemaglobin (Hb), 999
Hematemesis, 272b
Hematocrit (Hct), 975–977, 975f, 975t, 999
Hematology, 904, 941, 972–983, 999
Hematology tests, 904, 923
Hematopoiesis, 222–223, 325
Hematuria, 373b, 961
Hemiparesis, 298t–299t
Hemiplegia, 296b
Hemoconcentration, 935b–940b
HemoCue, 975, 999
Hemodialysis, 376b–377b

Hemoglobin (Hb), 223, 226f, 975, 975t, 976b–977b
Hemoglobinuria, 961
Hemolysis, 223–224, 228, 952, 954b
Hemolyze
   hypotonic IV solutions and, 177
   red blood cells and, 968
Hemophilia, 182t–183t
   inherited disorders and, 180
Hemoptysis, 253b
Hemorrhagic shock, 1137t
Hemorrhoids, 273t–276t
Hemostasis, 225, 228f
Hemostatic forceps, 1101–1103
Hemostats. *See* Hemostatic forceps
Hemothorax, 253b, 257f
Heparin, 929–930
Heparin lock, 1080
Hepatic duct, 271
Hepatic portal system, 206, 218, 266
Hepatitis A, 273t–276t
Hepatitis B, 273t–276t
Hepatitis B vaccination
   declination of, 58
   new employee and, 60b
Hepatitis B virus (HBV), 58–60
Hepatitis C, 273t–276t
Herbal medicine, cultural differences and, 96–98, 96f
Hereditary, 722
   genetic disorders and, 180
Heredity, 86
Hernia, 362
Herpes simplex, 432t–433t, 435f
Herpes simplex 1, 756t–757t
Herpes zoster. *See* Shingles
Hiatal hernia, 273t–276t
High-calorie, high-protein diet, 146
High-complexity test, 897
High-density lipoprotein (HDL), 141, 983–987
High-fiber diet, 147
High-power field (HPF), 968, 971
Hilum, 248
   kidneys and, 371
Hinge joint, 337, 340f
HIPPA. *See* Health Insurance Portability and Accountability Act
Hirschsprung disease, 273t–276t
Hirsutism, 411b
Histamines, 237
History, of E/M service, 596
History and Physical (H&P) report, 504–505, 506f, 512, 516–518
History of present illness (HPI), 596
Histrionic, 304b
HIV. *See* Human immunodeficiency virus
HMO. *See* Health Maintenance Organization
Hodgkin's disease, 235t
Holistic health care, 119, 127
Holter monitor, 782–784, 783f, 784t, 785b–787b
Home health care agency, 42
Homeostasis, 74, 281, 292, 403–404
   feedback and, 417
Homonym, 163–164
Hordeolum (stye), 315t–316t, 316f

Horizontal recumbent position, 738, 740b–741b, 758
Hormonal method, 870, 892
Hormone level test, 411b
Hormone regulation, feedback and, 410
Hormones
 characteristics of, 403, 404b
 endocrine system and, 402
 functions of, 405t
 of reproduction, 389–390
 regulation of, 410
Hospice care, 42, 82
Hospitals, 42
Host, 465
Hot flashes, 389
Hot water bag, 825, 830b–831b
HPF. See High-power field
HPI. See History of present illness
HPV. See Human papillomavirus test
http (hypertest transfer protocol), 466
Hub, needle parts and, 1048–1059
Human behavior, labels and, 75–76
Human body
 areas of, 173–174, 174f
 as system, 166
 description of, 168–174
Human chorionic gonadotropin (hCG), 390, 393, 871–872, 972
Human development, 86–94, 391–396
Human immunodeficiency virus (HIV), special considerations for, 237
 nutrition and, 144, 148
 record retention and, 539
Human needs, 74–75
Human papillomavirus test (HPV), 860
Human relations, 28b–29b
Humerus, 332
Huntington chorea, 182t–183t
Hyaline cartilage, 190, 326
 connective tissue types and, 188t–189t
Hyaline casts, 972t
Hydrating solutions, 1080, 1080t
Hydrocele, 383, 387t
Hydrogenated fats, 141
Hyoid bone, 328
Hypercalcemia, 411b
Hypercholesterolemia, 142
Hyperglycemia, 411b
 diabetic ketoacidosis and, 1144
Hyperkalemia, 411b
Hypernatremia, 411b
Hyperopia (farsightedness), 315t–316t, 317f
Hypersecretion, 410
Hypertension, 707
Hyperthermia, 1141, 1141b
Hypertonic, IV solutions and, 177, 180f
Hypertonic solutions, 1080, 1080t
Hypertrophy, 200–201
Hypocalcemia, 411b
Hypoglycemia, 411b, 412t–414t, 1134, 1144
Hypokalemia, 411b
Hyponatremia, 411b
Hypophysis. See Pituitary gland
Hyposecretion, 410
Hypotension, 707
Hypothalamus, 287–289, 291f
Hypothermia, 1131–1132, 1142b

Hypotonic
 concentrated urine and, 968
 dilute urine and, 968
 IV solutions and, 177, 180f
Hypoxia, 208t–209t, 253b
Hysterosalpingography, 391b

I

I&D. See Incision and drainage
ICD-9-Clinical Modification (ICD-9-CM), 583, 598
 codes of, 584
 format and structure of, 598–599
 Part B Medicare claim and, 583–584
 system of, 584, 598
 users of, 584, 598
ICD-9-CM manual, 584–588, 598–599
 conventions and terminology of, 585–586
 instructional terminology of, 586, 586b
 introduction to, 584–586
 overview of, 591t
 print type for, 586
 Volume 3 of, 589–590
 volumes of, 584, 599
Ice bag, 825, 826b–827b
Ichthyosis, 430b, 458
ID. See Intradermal (ID) injection
Id, 73, 83
Identical names, indexing of, 535–536, 535t–536t
Idiopathic, 273t–276t
Idiopathic disorders, 432t–433t
Ileocecal valve, 266
Ileum, 266, 269f, 277, 333–334
Illness, response to, 98–99, 100b
IM. See Intramuscular (IM) injection
Immobilization, bandage use for, 817
Immobilizer, 844, 848f
Immune system, 235, 240
 diseases of, 237–240, 238t
Immunity, 236, 240. See also Immune system
 types of, 237, 237f
Immunization, 1018–1024, 1021t, 1022f–1023f, 1033
 documentation of, 1019b, 1024b
Immunoassay, 991–992, 991f
Immunological testing, 991–992
Immunology, 991–992
Impacted fracture, 345, 346t–347t
Impetigo, 432t–433t, 433f
Implementation, teaching process and, 126
Implied contract, 51, 69, 603
Impotence, 385
In vitro fertilization, 66
Inactive file, 539, 542
Incident, definition of, 1132
Incident report, 1132–1133, 1148
Incision, 428
Incision and drainage (I&D), 1101
Incisors, 264
Income statement, 548, 578
Incoming calls, 480
 multiline system and, 481b–483b
 placing on hold, 480, 481b–483b
Incoming mail, 495, 495b, 511
Incontinence, 373b
Incus (anvil), 314
Indemnity plan, 606–607, 632

Indenting
 indented codes and, 593, 594b
 stand-alone codes and, 593, 594b
Independent practice association (IPA)
 HMO's and, 607
Index to Diseases and Injuries, Section 1 of, 586, 586b
Indexing, 521b–523b, 533–534, 541, 583
Indirect contact, 642, 667
Indirect filing, 536
Indirect pressure, bleeding and, 1138, 1140f
Individual policy, 605, 611, 633
Induration, 1060, 1065b, 1065f
Infancy, 86–88, 87b–88b, 100. See also Infants
Infants. See also Infancy
 body measurements of, 683, 687b
 capillary puncture and, 928f
 chest circumference and, 684
 drug dosage calculation for, 1016–1018
 head circumference and, 684
 intramuscular injection and, 1071b–1073b
 nutrition and, 143
Infarction, 205
Infection control, 637–643
 OSHA and, 640–643
Infectious mononucleosis, 235t
Inferior body plane, 168–169, 193–194
Inferior vena cava, 200–201, 202f–203f
Infertility, 381, 390–391
Inflammatory phase
 healing and, 428
 of wound healing, 428
Influenza, 254t–256t
Information release guidelines, confidentiality and, 63b
Informed consent, 1127
 surgery form and, 52f, 69, 1086–1088, 1087f
Infraction, 49b
Ingestion, 263
Inhalation, 249, 251f
Inhalation drug administration, 1042–1045, 1083
 metered-dose and, 1045
 nebulizer and, 1042–1045
Initial dose, 1007b
Initialized, 463
Initials, indexing of, 534–535, 534t
Injection
 intradermal type of, 1040
 intramuscular type of, 1065
 sites of, 1059t
 subcutaneous type of, 1065
 tissue depth and, 1060b, 1060f
Injection equipment, 1047b
Ink-jet printer, 464
Inpatient, E/M coding and, 596
Input, 461
Inscription, 1028–1029
Insemination, 385
Insertion, of muscle end point, 356
Insidious, 298t–299t
 Huntington Chorea and, 182t–183t
Inspection, 747, 748f, 748t, 756t–757t, 758
Inspiration, 245, 250f, 705
Instillation
 ear and, 812, 813b–814b
 of the eye, 810, 818b–819b

Instructional terms, 586b
 ICD-9-CM manual and, 586
Instruments, 28b–29b
Insulin, 271, 408, 409f, 987
Insulin shock, 1144, 1149
Insurance
 basic, 606
 definition of, 603
 major medical, 606
Insurance claim cycle, 620, 620b, 633
Insurance claims register, 625–629, 629f, 634
Integrative neuron (interneuron), 283
Integrity, 23–24
 ethical questions of, 61
Integumentary system, 191t–193t, 197, 419, 431
 function and structure of, 420–423
Integumentary system diseases, 430–431, 430b–431b, 430t, 432t–433t
Intellectualization, 81t
Intelligence, special needs patients and, 123–124
Intercellular body tissue, 181
Intercostal muscle, 249
Interface, 465
Interferons, 236, 236f
Interjection, correct use of, 110t
Internal respiration, 249, 258
International Classification of Diseases 9th revision (ICD-9 code), 551, 598
International law, 48
Internet access, 466b
Internet job search, 1153
Internet research, 467b
Internet service provider (ISP), 465
Internet use, 465–466, 465f
Interneuron. See Integrative neuron
Internist, 206
Interoffice mail, 495
Interrogatory, lawsuit information and, 55t
Interstitial cystitis, 374t–375t
Interstitial fluid, lymph function and, 232
Interval, 763
Intervertebral disc, 332
Interviewing skills, 721–723
 PQRST technique and, 723, 728
Intestine, small, 266, 267f, 270t, 277
 diseases of, 273t–276t
Intradermal (ID) injection, 1059–1065, 1061f, 1062b–1064b
Intramuscular (IM) injection, 1065–1074, 1075b–1077b
 Z-track method of, 1074
Intranet, 465, 471
Intrauterine device (IUD), 870, 892
Intravenous (IV) therapy, 1074–1082
Intravenous fluids (IV), 1080, 1080t
 therapeutic uses of, 1080b
Intravenous line, 1081–1082, 1082f
Intravenous pyelography (IVP), 374b, 799t
Intravenous solutions (IV), 177, 180f, 1083
Intrinsic muscle, 312, 313t
Intussusception, 273t–276t, 276f
Inventory control system, 458
Inventory records, 447, 458
Inversion, 338
Invoice, 451
Involuntary muscle, 186, 355–356
IPA. See Independent practice association

Iris, 311
Iris diaphragm, 901
Irregular bones, 327–328, 348
Irrigation
 of the ear, 809, 810b–812b
 of the eye, 812–817, 815b–816b
Irritability, 356
Ischemia, 205, 762–763
Ischium, 333–334
Ishihara color vision plates, 741, 750f, 752b–753b
Islets of Langerhans, 408, 409f. See also Pancreas
Isoelectric line. See Baseline
Isotonic contraction, 354, 355f
Isotonic solutions, 180f, 1080, 1080t
ISP. See Internet service provider
Itinerary, 454, 458
IUD. See Intrauterine device
IV. See Intravenous (IV) therapy; Intravenous fluids
IVP. See Intravenous pyelography

J

Jaeger reading card, 750–755, 754b–755b
Jaundice, 272b, 756t–757t
Jaws, surgical clamp and, 1089–1101, 1101f
JCAHO. See Joint Commission on Accreditation of Health Care Organizations
Jejunum, 266, 269f, 277
Job application, 1158–1160, 1159f–1160f, 1165
 guidelines for, 1159b
Job interview, 1160–1163, 1161b–1163b, 1164f, 1165
 guidelines during, 1161f–1162f
 question responses and, 1162
Job search
 materials for, 1153–1156
 resources for, 1152–1153
Jock itch. See Tinea cruris
Joint
 components of, 336–337
 connective tissue and, 337
 moveable, 336–337, 348
 movement of, 337–338, 344f
 parts of, 348
 types of, 337, 339f, 348
Joint Commission on Accreditation of Health Care Organizations (JCAHO), 42
Joints, 325, 341t–343t
 structure and function of, 335–336

K

Kaiser Family Foundation, 601, 603
Kelly forceps, suturing instruments and, 1089–1101
Keloid, 430b
Keratin, 421
Kernig sign, 298t–299t
Ketones, 961
 reagent tablets and, 968, 968f
Ketonuria, 373b, 961
Kevorkian, Jack, 66, 82
Key components, E/M service and, 596, 599
Key unit, 534
Keyboard, 463, 463b
 function keys of, 464b

Kidney, 369–372, 370f, 378
 ureter and bladder (KUB) test, 374b, 1004
 urine and, 961
Kidney transplant, 376b–377b
Klinefelter syndrome, 180–181, 182t–183t
Kling-type bandage, 817
Knee joint muscles, 359t–360t
Knee-chest position, 738, 745b, 758
Knee-jerk response. See Patellar reflex
Kneecap. See Patella
KOH. See Potassium hydroxide
KUB. See Kidney, ureter and bladder (KUB) test
Kübler-Ross, Elisabeth, 82
Kussmaul breathing, 1144–1145
KWL strategy, 10–11, 11f
Kyphosis, 345f

L

Label, mental health, 75–76
Labels, office supply, 532, 533f, 905
 color-coded system of, 532–533, 533f
Labia majora, 389
Labia minora, 389
Labor, 394, 396, 410. See also Parturition
Laboratory equipment, 898
Laboratory procedure, 28b–29b
Laboratory regulations, 897–898, 897t
 CLIA-waived tests, 897
Laboratory reports, 907–911, 910f, 924
Laboratory requisition, 905, 905b–907b, 905f, 923
Laboratory safety, 898, 900b, 900f, 923
Laboratory tests, 904–911
 documentation for, 912b
Labyrinth, 314–318
Laceration, 428
Laceration repair, 1113, 1128
Lacrimal apparatus, 312–313
Lacrimal bones, 331–332
Lacrimal cavity, 172
Lactase, 266
Lacteals, 266
Lactic acid, 354
Lactiferous duct, 389
Lactose intolerance, 266
Lamellae, 325–326
LAN. See Local area network
Lancet, 928, 928f, 931b–932b, 954
Laparoscopy, 272b
Large intestine, 266–267, 268f–269f, 270t, 273t–276t
 subdivisions of, 277
Laryngitis, 254t–256t
Laryngopharynx, 247
Larynx, 247, 247b, 258
Laser, 1114, 1128
Laser printer, 464, 464f
Laser therapy, 838
Last menstrual period (LMP), 391–393, 756t–757t, 872
Laughter, 80f
Lawsuits, 53–54, 55t
 causes for, 53
Layered tablets, 1025b
LDL. See Low-density lipoprotein
Lead codes, 778, 778t, 779f
Lead shields, 795

Lead time, 450
Leads, 765–768, 778
 placement of, 770–777, 776f
Learning
 active, 14–16
 definition of, 2–3
 responsibility for, 2–3
 styles of, 125–126
 ways of, 2
Learning log, 15, 15f
Ledger card, 551, 553f, 566–567, 608f
Left hypochondriac, 264
Left lower quadrant (LLQ), 171–172, 171f
Left upper quadrant (LUQ), 171–172, 171f
Legal chart, 518. See also Patient file
Legal concepts, 27b
Legislation, 604, 632
Lens, 311, 900
LES. See Lower esophageal sphincter
Lesion
 high-grade, 869t
 low-grade, 869t
Lethal dose, 1007b, 1033
Leukemia, 231t–232t
Leukocyte esterase, 966
Leukocytes, 222–225, 224f, 227t
Leukocytosis, 225
Leukopenia, 225
Levators, 357
LH. See Luteinizing hormone
Liability, 48, 69, 545, 578
 types of, 548
Libel
 defamation and, 53
License
 suspension of, 47, 47b, 68–69
Licensed Practical Nurse (LPN), 40–41
Licensed Vocational Nurse (LVN), 40–41
Licensure, 46, 68
Life mission, 4b, 19
Life support, 1145–1146
Ligament, 337, 348, 362–363
Ligate, 1114–1116
Light source, 901
Limbic system, 287
Limits, setting of, 5–6
Linear, 287
Lingual tonsils, 234
Liniments, 1024
Lipase, 265–266, 269f, 270t
Liquid diet, 145
Liquid drug forms, 1024, 1033, 1038b–1040b
 oral administration of, 1037–1040
Liquid matrix. See Plasma
Listening, 107–109, 108f, 115
Lithotomy position, 738, 741b–742b, 758, 857–860
Lithotripsy, 377f
Litigation, 121–122
Liver, 269f, 270–271, 270t, 273t–276t, 277–278
 serum cholesterol and, 983–987
Living will, 56, 69
 characteristics of, 56
LLQ. See Left lower quadrant
LMP. See Last menstrual period
LMRPs. See Local Medicare Review Policies
Local
 drug effect, 1025

Local anesthetics, 1113, 1128
Local area network (LAN), 465, 471
Local Medicare Review Policies (LMRPs), 612
Lockjaw. See Tetanus
Lofstrand crutches. See Forearm crutches
Logistical planning
 meetings and, 454, 458
 travel and, 454
Logistics officer, disaster planning and, 1147
Long bones, 327–328, 348
Long term stress, 79, 79t
Long-term care facility, 42
Long-term goals, 5
Long-term memory, 2, 10
Longitudinal arch, 334–335, 338f
Longitudinal fracture, 346t–347t
Loop of Henle, 371–372
Lordosis, 341t–343t, 345f
Lotion, 1024, 1042
Lou Gehrig disease. See Amyotrophic lateral sclerosis
Low-calorie diet, calorie-controlled diet and, 146
Low-cholesterol, low-fat diet, 146, 146b
Low-density lipoprotein (LDL), 141, 983–987
Low fiber diet, 147
Low-power field (LPF), 968, 971
Lower arm, 333
Lower esophageal sphincter (LES), 264–265
Lower extremity, 348
 muscles of, 359t–360t, 362
Lower gastrointestinal series (lower GI), 799t
Lower respiratory tract, 245, 245f, 247–248, 254t–256t, 258, 260
Loyalty, 23
Lozenges, 1024–1025
LPF. See Low-power field
LPN. See Licensed Practical Nurse
Lubb-dubb sound, 703–705
Lubricant, 673
Lumbar
 spinal column divisions and, 172–173, 173f
Lumbar puncture, 296b, 297f
Lumbar vertebrae, 332
Lumen, 971
 of needles, 1039
Lung cancer, 254t–256t
Lung scan, 254b
Lungs, 201f, 204, 249f, 258
 pleural cavity and, 169–171
Lunula, 423
Lupus erythematosus, 238t
LUQ. See Left upper quadrant
Luteinizing hormone (LH), 389, 399
LVN. See Licensed Vocational Nurse
Lyme disease, 432t–433t
Lymph, 232
 circulation of, 233, 233f
Lymph nodes, 233, 234f
Lymphatic system, 191t–193t, 196, 229–236, 232b, 240
 diseases of, 235–236, 235t
Lymphatic vessels, 232–233
Lymphatics, 233, 233f
Lymphedema. See Elephantiasis
Lymphocytes, 227t
Lymphoid organs, 233–235, 234f

Lysis, 991–992, 1000
Lysosomes, 177t, 178f
Lysozyme, 312–313

M

Macrophages, 223–224
Macrotia, 756t–757t
Macula lutea, 311
Macular degeneration, 315t–316t
Macule, 424–425, 435
Magnetic resonance imaging (MRI), 254b, 296b, 363b, 411b, 800–801
 body measurements for, 681
Magnification, 901, 901t, 923
Mail
 classifications of, 495, 495b, 511
 handling of, 493–498, 496b, 511
Mailing equipment, 447
Main term, 599
 ICD-9 coding and, 585
Maintenance agreement, 448
Maintenance dose, 1007b
Maintenance solution, 1080, 1080t
Major medical insurance, 606
Majority opinion. See Consensus
Malabsorption, 144
Malaria, 231t–232t
Malfeasance, nonintentional torts and, 53, 69
Malignant tumors, 179b
Malleus (hammer), 314
Malnutrition, 142b
Malpractice
 avoidance of, 53, 54b, 69
 tort law and, 51
Mammary gland, 389
Mammogram, 390–391, 798
Mammography, 391b, 798, 798f
 patient preparation for, 798
Managed care, 607
 policy and procedures of, 618b
Managed care plan, 607
 network and, 607
Management service organization (MSO), 37
Mandates, of health insurance, 603
Mandible, 264, 331–332, 357
Manipulation, 747
Mantoux test, 1060–1065
Manual medical record, 516
Manubrium, 332
Manuscript, 504
Marginal artery, 205
Maslow's hierarchy of needs, 74–75, 74f, 83, 119b
 self-actualized person and, 75b
Maslow, Abraham, 74
Mastectomy, 235t
Master's of Science in Nursing (MSN), 40
Mastication, 264
 muscles of, 357, 359t–360t
Mastoiditis, 319t
Material safety data sheet (MSDS), 58, 646b, 647f–648f, 668
Matrix, 14f
 body tissue and, 187–190
 of appointment book, 485f, 486, 486b–488b, 511
Maturation
 delayed patients and, 125

Maturation phase
  of healing, 428
  of wound healing, 428
Maxilla, 264
Maxillae, 331–332
Maxillary sinus, 331–332
Maximum dose, 1007b
Mayo-Hegar needle holder, suturing instruments and, 1089–1101
McBurney's point, 273t–276t
MCH. *See* Mean cell hemoglobin
MCHC. *See* Mean cell hemoglobin concentration
MCV. *See* Mean cell volume
MD. *See* Doctor of Medicine
MDI. *See* Metered-dose inhaler
Mean cell hemoglobin (MCH), 974
Mean cell hemoglobin concentration (MCHC), 974
Mean cell volume (MCV), 974
Measurements, converting, 1016, 1017f, 1017t
Meatus, 373
Mechanical stage control knobs, 901
Medi-Medi, 615, 633
Media, 992, 997t
Mediastinum, 171–172, 200
Medicaid, 612–613, 613f
  guidelines for eligibility, 612, 613b
Medical asepsis, 643–651, 647b, 668, 1088, 1088t, 1127
Medical assistant. *See also* Professional medical assistant
  completion of training and, 1163
  credentialing and, 47
  law and, 30b
  lawsuit process and, 55t
  medical terms and, 152, 153b
  patient questioning and, 803–804
  role of, 40f–41f, 41, 41b, 46–47, 119–122
  tasks of, 28b–29b
Medical decision making, E/M service and, 597, 599
  types of, 597
Medical emergencies, 1130
Medical history
  chief complaint of, 716
  diagnostic coding and, 588
  sections of, 728
Medical insurance
  See Health insurance
Medical law, medical assistant and, 28b–29b, 48–54, 69
  health care professionals and, 58–60
Medical necessity, 584, 605
Medical office
  maintenance of, 441, 441b
  OSHA requirements for, 441
  reception area of, 440–441, 441f, 458
  success of, 438
  verbal directions to, 477b
Medical practice
  law and, 46–47
  licensure and, 46–47
  settings of, 37, 37f, 42
Medical Practice Acts, 46, 68
Medical practice information booklet, 475–476

Medical record
  documentation for, 516, 516b, 1034
  legal protection and, 540
  ownership of, 524b
  purpose of, 515–527
Medical record systems, types of, 516–527
Medical report, 504–508
  types of, 504, 512
Medical Reserve Corp (MRC), 1147
Medical savings account (MSA), 604–605
Medical secretary-receptionist, 28b–29b
Medical specialties, 37–38
  fields of, 37, 38t
Medical suffix, 159t, 161f
Medical supplemental insurance. *See* Medigap
Medical terminology, 151–153
  pronunciation of, 156–161
Medical transcription, 509–510
Medicare, 604, 611–612, 633
  allowable charges formula and, 610
Medicare Advantage. *See* Medicare Part C
Medicare Catastrophic Coverage Act, 583–584
Medicare Part A, 612
Medicare Part B, 612
Medicare Part B News, 612
Medicare Part C, 612
Medicare Part D, 612
Medicare secondary payer (MSP), 615, 616t, 633
Medicare tax, 572, 580
Medicare-Medicaid Crossover Program. *See* Medi-Medi
Medication administration
  documenting of, 1040b
  inhalation, 1042–1045
  intravenous therapy, 1074–1082
  parenteral, 1045–1082
  topical, 1041–1042
  vaginal/rectal, 1042
Medication log, 516–518, 524
Medication record, 1031, 1032f
Medications, 1002, 1036. *See also* Drugs
Medigap, 605, 615, 633
  plan types of, 615
Medulla, 371
Medulla oblongata, 251, 288f, 289, 291f
Medullary cavity, 325, 326f
Meeting
  minutes of, 454
  planning of, 458
Meiosis, 179
Melanin, 407–408, 420–421, 424f
Melanoma, malignant, 425–427, 427f, 427t, 435
Melatonin, 410
Melena, 272b
Membrane, 169–173
Memo, 504, 512
  heading of, 504
Menarche, 389
Ménière disease, 319t
Meninges, 172, 285, 287f, 305
  brain and, 285–286
Meningitis, 298t–299t
Meniscus, 1040–1041
Menopause, 389, 399, 411b
Menorrhagia, 390b
Menses, 389
  urine and, 961

Menstrual cycle, 389, 390f, 399
  abnormalities of, 390b
Mensuration, 680
Mental growth, 86, 100
Mental health, 302–303
Mental health disorders
  diagnostic tests and procedures for, 303b
  drug classifications of, 303t
  signs and symptoms of, 303b
  types of, 304b
Mental impairment, 124–125
Menus, 465
Mercury free thermometer, 691, 691b–693b, 691f, 712–713
Mesentery, 171–172, 264
Message
  analyzing of, 108–109, 115
  conditions of, 108
  listening to, 108, 108f
Message taking, incoming calls and, 480, 481b–483b, 510
Metabolic shock, 1137t
Metabolism, 223, 261, 271
  definition of, 278
Metacarpal, 333
Metaphysis, 328
Metastasis, 179b, 425
Metatarsal, 334–335, 338f
Metered-dose inhaler (MDI), 1045, 1045f, 1046b–1047b
Method of transmission
  infection chain and, 642
Metrorrhagia, 390b
MI. *See* Myocardial infarction
Microbiology, 904, 923, 992–999
Microcontainers, 929–930
Microfiche, 539
Microglia cells, 284
Microhematocrit centrifuge, 902, 902f
Microorganism, 638–639, 639f, 639t, 667
  and infection control, 637–638
Microprocessor, 462
Microscope, 898–902, 901f, 903b–904b, 923
Microtia, 756t–757t
Micturition, 372–373
Micturition reflex, 372–373
Midbrain, 289, 291f
Middle ear, 314
Midline, body planes and, 168–169
Midsagittal (median) plane, 168–169
Midstream clean-catch urine specimen, 912–918, 919b–920b
Mind map, 10
Mineralocorticoids, 408
Minerals, 140
  major, 140, 140t
Minimum dose, 1007b
Miscarriage, 394
Misdemeanor, 49b
Misfeasance, nonintentional torts and, 53, 69
Mission statement, personal, 4b
Mitch wound clips, suturing instruments and, 1089–1101
Mitochondria, 177t, 178f
Mitosis, 177t, 179, 181f
Mitral (bicuspid) valve, 200–201, 202f, 217
Mnemonic device, 11–14, 20

INDEX 1241

Modem, 464
Moderate-complexity tests, 897
Modified wave scheduling, 492, 511
Modified-block format, 504
Modified-wave scheduling, 492
Modifiers, 594, 594b
Molars, 264
Molasses, blackstrap, 137b
Molecules, 174
Monitor, 464
Monocular, 900
Monocytes, 227t
Monounsaturated fats, 141
Mons pubis, 389
Morbidity rates, 583
Morning-after pill, 870, 892
Mortality, 583
Motherboard, 463
Motion sickness, 318
Motor neuron, 283, 293f
Mouse, 463
Mouth, 264–268, 273t–276t, 277
    nonverbal communication and, 106
MRC. See Medical Reserve Corp
MRI. See Magnetic resonance imaging
MS. See Multiple sclerosis
MSA. See Medical savings account
MSD. See Musculoskeletal disorder
MSDS. See Material safety data sheet
MSN. See Master's of Science in Nursing
MSO. See Management service organization
MSP. See Medicare Secondary Payer
Mucous threads, 971–972
Multichannel electrocardiograph, 765, 768, 775b
Multiple sclerosis (MS), 298t–299t
Multisample needles, 942, 942f
Mumps, 264
Munchausen syndrome, 304b
Murmur, of the heart, 202–203
Muscle, 352
    fiber direction of, 357
    heat production and, 354
    size of, 356
    structure of, 364
    types of, 355–356, 364
Muscle biopsy, 363b
Muscle contraction, 354–355, 364
    types of, 354–355
Muscle disease
    drug classifications for, 363, 363t
    signs and symptoms of, 363b
    test and procedures for, 363b, 365
Muscle fiber, 186
Muscle injury, 362–363
Muscle strain, 362–363
Muscle tissue, 181, 186–187, 187b, 365
    types of, 186, 186t, 365
Muscle tone, 353–354
Muscular dystrophy, 182t–183t, 185f, 364t
Muscular system, 191t–193t, 196
    diseases and disorders of, 362–363, 364t
Musculoskeletal disorder (MSD), computers and, 447b
Musculoskeletal injury, 1142–1143
Mutated disease. See Single-cell diseases
Mutation, genetic disorders and, 180, 194
Mutual agreement. See Compromise

Myalgia, 362, 363b
Myasthenia gravis, 364t
Myelin sheath, 283
Myelogram, 340b
Myelography, 296b
Myocardial infarction (MI), 762–763
Myocardium, 186, 199–200, 202f
Myoglobin, 354
Myoglobinuria, 961
Myometrium, 387
Myopia (nearsightedness), 315t–316t, 317f
Myositis, 363b
Myxedema, 412t–414t

N

Nägele's rule, 872, 872b, 892
Nail body, 423, 471, 796b
Nail root, 423
Nails, fingers and, 423, 425f
Narcissistic, 283, 290, 304b
Nares. See Nostrils
Nasal bones, 331–332
Nasal cavity, 172, 173f
Nasal conchae, 331–332
Nasal septum, 246
Nasopharynx, 247
National Child Vaccine Injury Act (NCVIA), 1018
National Council Licensure Examination (NCLEX-RN), 40, 134
National Formulary (USP/NF), 1006–1007, 1010
National Provider Identifier (NPI), 626b–628b
Natural acquired immunity, 237
Nausea, 272b
Navicular, 334
NCLEX-RN. See National Council Licensure Examination
NCVIA. See National Child Vaccine Injury Act
Nearsightedness. See Myopia
Nebulizer, 1042–1045, 1044f–1045f, 1083
Neck muscles, 357, 359t–360t
Necropsy, 508
Needle holder, 1089–1103, 1116–1117, 1118f
Needles, 1048–1059, 1058f–1059f
    selection of, 1059, 1059t
Needlesticks
    immunization and, 1024b
    prevention of, 1059b
Negative feedback, 410
Negative stress, 9
Neglect, abuse and, 56b
Negligence
    lawsuits and, 53
    types of, 53, 69
Neoplasm, cell growth and, 179b
Nephrologist, 373
Nephron, 371–372, 372f, 378, 971
    structure and function of, 379
Nerve, 283
Nerve cells, 283–284
Nerve conduction studies, 296b
Nerve fibers, 283
    types of, 286, 301
Nerve impulse, 284, 285f
Nerve supply, of the heart, 203–204
Nerve tissue, 181, 190, 190f, 194, 286b

Nervous system
    aging and, 302b
    body systems and, 191t–193t, 281
    diagnostic tests for, 296b
    diseases and disorders of, 294–302, 296b, 298t–299t
    divisions of, 284–294, 287f
    drug classifications of, 295t
    organization of, 304
    structure and function of, 283–294
Net income, 548
Net loss, 548
Net pay, 580
Network, 465, 471
    security and, 466b, 471
Networking, 1153, 1164
Neurilemma, 283
Neurogenic shock, 1137t
Neuroglia, 284
Neuroglial cells, 285f, 304
Neurologist, 294–295
Neuromuscular junction, 354
Neuron
    nerve cell clusters and, 190, 283
    types of, 283
Neurotransmitters, 284, 286f
Neutrophils, 225, 225b, 227t
Nevus, 425
New patient
    appointments for, 488, 490b–491b, 511
    E/M coding and, 595–596
    greeting of, 475–476
    medical practice information booklet, 475–476
    medical records of, 540
    patient information brochure, 475–476, 476b, 477f
New patient file, 521b–522b
Newspaper classifieds, 1152, 1164
    abbreviations used in, 1153b
Night blindness, 138t
Nipple, 389
Nipple discharge, types of, 857b
Nitrates, 966
Nitrites, 966
NLEA. See Nutrition Labeling and Education Act
No food or water (NPO), 1113
Nocturia, 373b
Nodes of Ranvier, 283
Nomogram, 1018
Non-Hodgkin's lymphoma, 235t
Non-PAR. See Non-participating provider
Non-participating provider (Non-PAR), 606, 606b, 632
Noncapital goods, 450, 458
Noncompliance, 50, 69
Nondisplaced fracture, 346t–347t
Nonessential nutrients, 138, 148
Nonfeasance, nonintentional torts and, 53, 69
Nonpathogens, 638, 638b, 667
Nonspecific immunity, 236, 236f
Nonstriated muscle, 186, 187b
Nonsufficient funds (NSF), 568
Nonverbal communication
    behavioral styles of, 107t, 108b, 115
    cultural differences and, 122
    effective communication and, 105–107
    other considerations of, 107, 115

Norepinephrine, 408
Normal flora, 638, 668
Normal sinus rhythm (NSR), 763
Nose, 246, 258, 311f, 320
Nosebleed. *See* Epistaxis
Nosepiece, 901
Nosocomial infections, 636
Nostrils, 246
Notebook computer, 447
Noun, 153, 162, 164
    correct use of, 110t
NP. *See* Nurse practitioner
NPI. *See* National Provider Identifier
NPO. *See* No food or water
NSF. *See* Nonsufficient funds
NSR. *See* Normal sinus rhythm
Nuclear medicine, 796
Nucleolus, 176, 177t, 178f
Nucleus, 176, 177t, 178f, 194
Numbers
    indexing of, 535, 535t
    writing of, 111b
Numbness, 296b
Numerical filing system, 536–537, 539b, 541
Nurse, 39–41
Nurse practitioner (NP), 40, 41f
Nutrients, 138–142, 148
Nutrition, 148
    dietary guidelines and, 131, 131t
    principles of, 134–138, 148
Nutrition Labeling and Education Act (NLEA), 134, 148
Nutritional fact panel, 134
Nystagmus, 315t–316t

O

O_2. *See* Oxygen
Obese, 136–137
Object chart, 749–750, 750f
Objective information, 524–527, 728
Objective lens, 901
Objective symptoms, 716, 720b
Objectives, 901
Oblique, 312
Oblique fracture, 346t–347t
Observations, charting of, 727, 729
Obsessive-compulsive disorder (OCD), 304b
Obstetrical examination, 870–872
    postpartum care and, 872
Obstetrics, 870
Occipital bone, 329–331
Occipital lobe, 287, 288f, 290f
Occlusion, 208t–209t
Occupational Exposure to Bloodborne Pathogens Standard (1992), OSHA standards and, 643, 646b
Occupational Safety and Health Act, 58, 105
    needlestick injuries and, 1048
Occupational Safety and Health Administration (OSHA)
    and needlesticks, 1048
    standards enforcement and, 60, 640–643
    biohazard symbols and, 641f
    examination room maintenance and, 675
    guidelines for laboratory safety and, 900b, 900f
    Standard Precautions and, 640
OCD. *See* Obsessive-compulsive disorder

OCR. *See* Optical character recognition
Ocular lens, 901
Office emergencies, 1133–1145
Office equipment, 442–448, 458
Office management, 451–454
Oil-immersion lens, 901
Ointment, 1025, 1042
    for eye, 817
Old eyes. *See* Presbyopia
Olecranon process (funny bone), 332
Olfaction, 309
Oligodendroglia cells, 284
Oliguria, 373b
Omentum, 264
Oncology, cancerous tumors and, 179b
One-write system, 549. *See also* Pegboard system
Onychomycosis, 432t–433t
Opaque, 311
Open MRI, 801
Open reduction, 338
Open technique, gloving and, 1089
Open wound, 1114, 1128
Open-ended questions, 105, 725–727, 727b
Open-hour scheduling, 492, 511
Opened wound, 428, 428f, 435–436
Operating scissors, 1103
Operational functions, 27b
Operations officer, disaster planning and, 1147
Operative report, 505–506, 507f, 512, 524
Operative suffix, 160t, 161f–162f
Ophthalmologist, 313
Ophthalmoscope, 311, 672–673, 672t, 673f, 749, 749f, 759
Optic disc (blind spot), 311–312
Optic nerve, 311
Optical character recognition (OCR), 464, 497, 625, 634
Oral cavity, 265f. *See also* Mouth
Oral contract, 51
Oral drug administration, 1037–1041, 1038b–1040b, 1082
    guidelines for, 1041b, 1041f
Oral temperature, 690, 691t
Oral thermometer, 693, 701b, 712
Orbital cavity, 172, 173f
Orchitis, 383
Order of draw, 941–942, 942f, 954
Order quantity, 450
Organ of Corti, 318
Organelles, 175, 178f
Organic, 138b
Organism, 174, 176f
Organizations, indexing of, 535, 535t
Organize, 11–14
    verbal communication and, 104, 115
Organizing, memory storage and, 11–14
Organs, of the body, 190
Origin, muscle attachment and, 356
Oropharynx, 247
Orthopedic, 338
Orthopedist, 362, 844
Os, 860–861
OSHA. *See* Occupational Safety and Health Administration
Osmosis, passive transport systems and, 177, 180f
Ossicles, 314

Ossification, 325, 345b, 347
Ostealgia, 340b
Osteitis, 340b
Osteoarthritis, 341t–343t
Osteoblasts, 325
Osteoclasts, 325
Osteocytes, 325
Osteomalacia, 138t, 341t–343t
Osteomas, 341t–343t
Osteomyelitis, 341t–343t
Osteonecrosis, 340b
Osteoporosis, 341t–343t
Otalgia, 318b
OTC. *See* Over-the-counter
Otitis externa (swimmer's ear), 319t
Otitis media, 319t
Otolaryngologist, 318
Otorrhea, 318b
Otosclerosis, 319t
Otoscope, 672–673, 672f–673f, 672t, 755, 755f, 759
Otoscopy, 318b
Out guide, 516–518, 517b, 532, 532f
Outer (external) ear, 314
Outgoing calls, 480–485, 510
    telephone directory and, 480–485
Outgoing mail, 495–498
    handling methods for, 496b
Outpatient
    E/M coding and, 596
Output, 461
Outsourced, 454
Ova, 386
Ova and parasite collection, 918, 922f
Oval window, 314
Ovarian cyst, 392t–393t
Ovaries, 386, 388f, 405t, 408, 417
Over-the-counter (OTC) drugs, 518, 522f, 861, 1007–1008
Overcompensation, 81t, 83–84
Overpayment, adjustment of, 568
Ovulation, 389
Ovum, 387
Owner's equity, 545, 570
Oximetry sensor, 888, 888f
Oxygen (O_2), 243, 245, 818b–819b
    circulatory system and, 199
Oxytocin, 287–289, 390, 394, 399, 406

P

P wave, 763–765, 764t, 766f–767f
PA. *See* Physician assistant
PAC. *See* Premature atrial contraction
Pacemaker, 782, 782f
Packing slip, 451
Paget disease, 341t–343t
Pain, 296b
Palate, hard, 331
Palatine bones, 331–332
Palatine tonsils, 234, 247
Palliative care, 341t–343t
    sickle cell anemia and, 182t–183t
Pallor, 756t–757t
    sickle cell anemia and, 182t–183t
Palpation, 747, 748f, 756t–757t, 758
Pancreas, 270t, 271, 405t, 408. *See also* Islets of Langerhans
    diseases of, 273t–276t

Pancreatin, 271
Pancreatitis, 273t–276t
Pap smear, 391b, 860, 892
Papanicolaou test. *See* Pap smear
Papillae, 309, 320
Papule, 424–425, 435
PAR. *See* Participating provider
Paralysis, 296b
Paranasal sinus, 246, 247f, 258, 328
Paranoid, 304b
Parasites, 638
 urine and, 971–972
Parasitic diseases, 432t–433t
Parasympathetic division
 ANS and, 203–204
Parasympathetic nervous system (PNS), 287, 292t, 294f
 functions of, 305
Parathyroid gland, 405t, 406–407, 407f
Parathyroid hormone (PTH), 325, 345–347, 406–407, 410
Parenteral
 ampule for, 1048
 drug route for, 1015–1016
 equipment for, 1045–1050, 1047t
 guidelines for, 1060b, 1061t
 injection types and, 1059–1074
 needles and, 1048–1059
Parenteral medications, administration of, 1045–1083, 1060b
Paresthesia, 411b
Parietal bones, 329–331
Parietal lobe, 287, 288f, 290f
Parietal membrane, 169
Parietal pericardial membrane, 171
Parietal pleura, 169–171
Parkinson disease, 298t–299t
Parotid gland, 264
Paroxysmal atrial tachycardia (PAT), 781, 781f
Part B Medicare claim, ICD-9-CM coding and, 583–584
Partial disability, 614
Partial thromboplastin times (PTT), 983
Partial-thickness burn, 428–429, 436, 1139b
Participating provider (PAR), 606–607, 632
Partnered reading, 15–16
Partnership, 37, 37t, 42
Parturition, 394, 872. *See also* Labor
Passive immunity, 237
Passive listening, 108, 115
Passive transport method, cell systems and, 194
Password, 465
Past history, medical history and, 720b, 722
Past history (PH), 722, 728
PAT. *See* Paroxysmal atrial tachycardia
Patella (kneecap), 334, 337f
Patellar reflex, 294, 295f
Patency, 784
Patent, 756t–757t, 812
Pathogens, 236, 638, 638b, 667
Pathological fracture, 346t–347t
Patient
 as customer, 604–605, 632
 care of, 27b
 drug administration and, 1011
 education of, 27b–29b, 125–126, 128, 147
 greeting of, 475–479, 510
Patient Bill of Rights, 67b, 604

Patient Care Partnership, 66, 70, 632
 AHA and, 604
Patient communication
 improvement of, 119–120, 120t, 127
 role of medical assistant and, 119–122, 127
Patient complaint
 guidelines for, 121–122
 handling of, 121–122, 127
 types of, 121
Patient consent form, confidentiality and, 64f–65f
Patient file
 color codes for, 521b–522b
 legal issues and, 518
 service documentation and, 541
Patient information brochure, 475–476, 476b, 477f, 478b
Patient instruction, for minor surgery, 1126
Patient preparation
 for capillary puncture, 930
 for electrocardiogram (ECG), 769
 for fecal occult blood test, 877–878, 879b–880b
 for Holter monitor, 783, 783b
 for laboratory tests, 905, 923
 for MRI, 800–801
 for physical examination, 732–736, 733b–735b
 for sigmoidoscopy, 878–883, 884b–885b
 for venipuncture, 930–940, 940t
 medical assistant and, 804
Patient privacy, and interviewing skills, 725
Patient registration form, 516–518
Patient rights, 62–66
Patient Self-Determination Act of 1990, 56–58, 69
 advanced directives and, 56
Patient statements, charting of, 725–727, 725b, 729
Patient teaching, 121b, 121f
Payable, 548
Payee, 557, 579
Payer, 557, 579
Payments
 by credit card, 551
 by mail, 551
 by third-party payers, 551
 posting of, 551, 554b–557b
Payroll, 571
 processing of, 571–577
Payroll checks, 577, 577f
Payroll register, 576–577, 576f
PCP. *See* Primary care physician
PDA. *See* Personal digital assistant
PDR. *See* Physician's Desk Reference
Peak flow meter (PFM), 883, 883f, 887b–888b
Pectoral girdle, 332
Pediculosis, 432t–433t
Pegboard system, 549–551, 549f, 578
Pellagra, 139t
Pelvic cavity, 171–172
Pelvic examination, 857–860, 860f, 892
Pelvic girdle, 333–334, 336f
Pelvic inflammatory disease (PID), 392t–393t
Pelvimetry, 391b, 872
Penis, 385
Penlight, 672–673, 672f, 672t
Pepsin, 265–266, 269f

Peptidase, 266
Perception, 76
Percussion, 747, 748f–749f, 758
Percussion hammer, 672–673, 672f, 672t, 674f
Percutaneous, 1003
Perforation, of ears, 756t–757t
Pericardial membrane, 171
Pericardium, 200, 202f
Perimetrium, 387
Perineum, 389
Periosteum, 328
Peripheral nervous system (PNS), 283, 290–294, 305
Peripherals, computers and, 462
Peristalsis, 264
Peritoneal dialysis, 376b–377b
Peritoneum, 264, 277
 abdominal cavity membrane and, 171–172
Permanent teeth, 264
Pernicious anemia, 139t
PERRLA, 756t–757t
Personal appearance, 25f, 26t
Personal data, medical history in, 716, 720b
Personal digital assistant (PDA), 447, 464–465
Personal Health Records (PHR). *See* Electronic medical record
Personal mission statement, 4
Personal protective equipment (PPE), 643, 646b, 667, 898, 1147
Personality, 83
 pshycology and, 73–74
Pertinent past, family, and social history (PFSH), 596
Pertussis, 254t–256t
PET scan. *See* Positron emission tomography
Petechiae, 231t–232t, 430b
Petri dish, 992
Petty cash, 546, 546b–547b, 546f, 578
PFM. *See* Peak flow meter
PFSH. *See* Pertinent past, family, and social history (PFSH)
PFT. *See* Pulmonary function tests (PFTs)
PH. *See* Past history
pH, 270t
Phagocytes
Phagocytosis, 178, 224–225
Phalanges, 333
Pharmacodynamics, 1003, 1032
Pharmacokinetics, 1003, 1004f, 1032
Pharmacology, 1003–1006, 1032
 clinical, 28b–29b
Pharyngeal tonsils, 234. *See also* Adenoids
Pharyngitis, 254t–256t
Pharynx, 234, 246–247, 247b, 258, 264, 265f
 digestive role of, 277
Phenylketonuria (PKU), 182t–183t, 295
 blood collection for, 929–930, 933b–935b
PHI. *See* Protected Health Information (PHI)
Phlebitis, 215t–216t
Phlebotomy, 926, 930
Phobias, 77–78, 77t, 83
 types of, 78b
Photocopy machine, 443
Photodetector, 888, 890b
Phrenic nerve, 249
Physiatrist, 362
Physical abuse, signs of, 56b

Physical examination
　medical assistant role in, 731
　medical assistants role in, 758
　overview of, 756t–757t
　purpose of, 731
Physical growth, 86, 100
Physical needs, 74–75
Physical well-being, distracters and, 105
Physician, 39
　licensure and, 47, 47b, 68
Physician assistant (PA), 39, 465, 477f
Physician office laboratory (POL), 895–897, 923
Physician's Desk Reference (PDR), 1011, 1012f–1014f
　drug references and, 1010
Physician-patient contract, requirements of, 50, 69
Physiological, 76
Physiological influences, 76, 83
Physiology
　body function and, 166, 168
　medical assistant knowledge of, 28b–29b
PI. *See* Present illness
Pia mater, 285, 287f
Pick-ups. *See* Thumb forceps
PID. *See* Pelvic inflammatory disease
Pimple, 422–423
Pineal gland, 410
Pinkeye. *See* Conjunctivitis
Pinna (auricle), 314
Pinocytosis, 178
Pipette, 952
Pitch, 318
Pituitary gland, 287–289, 291f, 329–331, 404–406, 405t, 406f
Pivot joint, 337
Placement services, 1152, 1164
Placenta, 393, 872
Placenta abruptio, 397t
Placenta previa, 397t
Plan of action, 524–527
Planning, 6–8
　teaching process and, 126
Plantar reflex, 294
Plaque, 273t–276t, 991b
Plasma
　blood and, 222, 223f, 223t, 239
　centrifuge and, 902
　order of draw and, 942
　separation of, 952–954, 952f
Plasma membrane, 177t, 178f
Plaster cast, 844
Platelet counts, 974
Platelets. *See also* Thrombocytes
　complete blood count and, 975t
　diseases of, 231t–232t
　thrombocytes and, 224f, 225
Platform crutches, 838, 842f
Pleura, 248
Pleural cavity, 169–171
Pleurisy, 254t–256t
Plexus, 290
Plural, 162
　guidelines for, 162
PMS *See* Premenstrual syndrome
Pneumonia, 254t–256t
Pneumothorax, 253b
PNS. *See* Peripheral nervous system

POCT. *See* Point-of-care-testing
Point, 467
Point-of-care-testing (POCT), 926–927, 983
Point-of-service (POS) plan, 607, 632
Poison, 1143–1144, 1143b
　ingested, 1149
　　emergency care for, 1143
　inhaled, 1143–1144, 1149
　injected, 1144, 1144t
POL. *See* Physician office laboratory
Polarization, 763, 765f
Policy manual, 454–455
　HIPPA regulation and, 455b
Polycystic kidney, 374t–375t, 378f
Polycythemia, 231t–232t
Polydipsia, 373b, 411b
Polyp, 272b, 424–425, 435
Polyphagia, 411b
Polyunsaturated fats, 141
Polyuria, 373b, 411b
POMR. *See* Problem-oriented medical record
Pons, 251, 289, 291f
Popliteal artery, 702–703, 702f
Pore, 422
Portal vein, 206
Positioning, patient, 737–747, 737b, 758
Positive feedback, 410
Positron emission, 803
Positron emission tomography (PET scan), 303b, 803
　patient preparation for, 803
Post-traumatic stress disorder (PTSD), 304b
Postage meter, 447
Postdated, 557
Posterior body plane, 168–169
Posterior cavity, 311–312, 312f
Posterior descending artery, 205, 207f
Posterior lobe, 405t, 406, 406f
Posterior tibial artery, 702–703
Postpartum, 394, 872, 892
Postprandial specimen, 918
Postprandial test, 2-hour, 987
Posture, nonverbal communication and, 107
Potassium hydroxide (KOH), 869
Powders, 1024–1025
Power notes, 11–14, 14f, 17–18
PPD. *See* Purified-protein derivative
PPE. *See* Personal protective equipment
PPO. *See* Preferred provider organization
PR interval, 764t, 765
PR segment, 764t, 765
Practice management, 461
Practice management software
　installation of, 472
　insurance processing and, 470f
　new patient entry and, 469
　report generation and, 470, 470f
　scheduling and, 469, 469f–470f
Pratt rectal probe, probing instruments and, 1089–1101
Pre-filled cartridge unit, 1048, 1048f
　TUBEX type and, 1056f
Preauthorization, 616, 617f, 633
Precertification, 616–618, 618b
Precipitates, 991–992, 1000
Precordial leads. *See* Chest leads
Predisposing factor
　genetic disorders and, 180

Preexisting condition, 604
Preferred provider organization (PPO), 607, 632
Prefilled cartridge unit, 1048, 1048f
Prefix
　and indexing, 535t
　descriptive use of, 158t
　indexing of, 535, 535t
　representing number and quantity, 156t
　representing position and direction, 157t
　representing size and amount, 156t
　word parts and, 153
Pregnancy, 391–393, 871–872
　disorders of, 394, 397t
　ectopic, 386, 397t
　family and family history form and, 873f
　flow sheet and, 874f
　follow-up prenatal exam, 872, 875b–877b, 877f
　full term, 391–393
　nutrition and, 143
　obstetrical examination and, 871–872
Pregnancy test, urine analysis and, 972
Pregnancy-induced hypertension (PIH), 397t. *See also* Toxemia
Prejudice, 108
Premature atrial contraction (PAC), 781, 781f
Premature ventricular contraction (PVC), 781–782, 781f
Premenstrual syndrome (PMS), 392t–393t
Premiums, health insurance, 604, 632
Prenatal care, 871, 892
Prenatal development, 394, 394f
　stages of, 391–394
Preoperative instructions, 1086
Preposition
　correct use of, 110t
　indexing of, 534
Prepuce, 385. *See also* Penis
Presbycusis, 319t, 755
Presbyopia (old eyes), 315t–316t, 749
Preschool, 89, 90b, 90f
Prescribe, 1007b
Prescription, 1006b, 1028–1030, 1028t, 1030f, 1032, 1034
　sections of, 1028–1029
Present illness, of medical history, 716
Present illness (PI), 716, 728
Presenting problem, 597, 597b
Pressure ulcer, 838
Primary care physician (PCP), 607
Primary diagnosis, 588–589, 589f, 599
Prime mover, 356
Principle diagnosis, 588–589, 599
Principles, ethical standards and, 61
Printer, 464
Priorities, 5–6
　consequences and, 5, 5b
　setting of, 5
　verbal communication and, 104
Prioritizing, 1, 5–6, 9f
Privacy, patient, 62
　consent form and, 64f–65f
　information release guidelines and, 63b
　invasion of, 53
Private. *See* Confidential
Private law, 49f, 69

Probes, 1103, 1127
Probing instruments, surgery and, 1089–1101
Problem list, 524–527, 526f
Problem-oriented medical record (POMR), 524–527, 540
    stages of, 524–527
Problem-oriented record, 524–527, 540
Procedural coding. *See also* CPT codes; *Current Procedural Terminology* (CPT)
    category III codes and, 594
    code numbers and, 591–598
    CPT manual and, 591–592
    process of, 593–594, 593f, 599
Procedure consent form, 736, 736f, 758
Procedures manual, 454, 458
Process
    bone projection as, 332
Professional discounts, 568
Professional medical assistant, 25–34, 28b–29b. *See also* Medical assistant
Professional qualities, 23–25, 26t
Professional responsibilities, 61, 62b
Professional Service Corporation (PSA), 37
Progesterone, 386, 390, 408
    function of, 399
Progress notes, 508, 524, 720b
Projection, 81t, 83–84
Prolactin, 390, 399
Prompt, 465
Pronation, 338
Prone position, 193–194, 738, 744b, 758
Pronoun, correct use of, 110t
Pronunciation
    medical terminology and, 156–161, 161t, 164
    unusual, 161, 161t
Proofreading, 512
    key points of, 500t, 503b
Prophylactic, 208t–209t
Prophylactic drug, 1004
Proprioception, 309
Prostaglandins, 409, 417
Prostate gland, 384
Prostatitis, 387t
Protected Health Information (PHI), 524b
Protein, 136b, 142, 269f, 270t, 961–966
    sources of, 142b
Proteinuria, 959, 961–966
Prothrombin, 226
ProTimes (PT), 983
Protozoa, 231t–232t, 639, 639t, 667, 869–870, 869f–870f
Provider, 515
Pruritus, 430b
PSA. *See* Professional Service Corporation
Psoriasis, 432t–433t, 434f
Psychiatry, 73, 302
Psychogenic shock, 1137t
Psychological influences, 76, 83
Psychology, 73–74
Psychomotor learning, 126
Psychosis, 303b
Psychosocial growth, 86, 100
Psychosocial restrictions, 126
Psychosomatic disorders, 79
PT. *See* ProTimes
PTH. *See* Parathyroid hormone
Ptosis, 315t–316t, 316f

PTST. *See* Post-traumatic stress disorder
PTT. *See* Partial thromboplastin times
Ptyalin, 264
Pubis, 333–334
Public law, 48, 48f, 69
Puerperium, 870
Pulmonary artery, 200–201, 202f–203f, 205f
Pulmonary circulation, 204, 205f
Pulmonary edema, 253b
Pulmonary embolism, 254t–256t
Pulmonary function tests (PFTs), 251, 252t, 258, 883
Pulmonary semilunar valve, 200–201, 217
Pulmonary veins, 200–201, 202f
Pulse, 702–705, 702f, 702t, 713
    documentation of, 703b
Pulse deficit, 703–705
Pulse oximetry, 254b, 888–889, 893
Pulse pressure, 707
Pulse rate, 702, 702t, 713
Pulse rhythm, 702, 713
Pulse volume, 702, 713
Punctuality, 23
Punctuation
    indexing of, 334, 334t
    written communication and, 111, 112t, 116
Puncture, 428
Punitive damages, lawsuit damages and, 54t
Pupil, 311
Purchase order, 451
Purge, filing and, 539, 542
Purified-protein derivative (PPD), 1060–1065
Purkinje fibers, 203, 203f–204f, 764f, 765
Purpura, 430b
Purulent, wound drainage and, 1123
Pustule, 424–425, 435
PVC. *See* Premature ventricular contraction
Pyelonephritis, 374t–375t
Pyloric sphincter, 265
Pyloric stenosis, 273t–276t
Pyloris, 265
Pylorus, 265
Pyramids, 371
Pyuria, 373b

Q

QA. *See* Quality assurance
QC. *See* Quality control
QNS. *See* Quantity not sufficient
QRS complex, 763, 764t, 765, 766f–767f
QT interval, 764t, 765
Quad cane, 844
Quadrants
    abdominopelvic cavity and, 171–172, 171f, 194
    regions and, 171–172, 171f, 194
Qualified endorsement, 559
Qualitative, pregnancy test and, 972
Quality assurance (QA), 897–898, 923
Quality control (QC), 898, 923
    urine collection and, 912
Quantitative, blood chemistry and, 983
Quantity not sufficient (QNS), 943b
Questions
    multiple-choice, 17b
    open-ended, 105
    prediction, 15–16
Quid pro quo, 60

R

RA. *See* Rheumatoid arthritis
Radial artery, 702–703, 702f
Radial pulse, measurement of, 703, 704b
Radiation, 428, 654b
Radioactive iodine (RAI) uptake scan, 411b
Radiograph, 795–796, 796f
    procedures for, 796b
Radiography, 340b, 411b, 793–795
    medical assistant role in, 803–804
Radioimmunoassay (RIA), 411b
Radiology report, 506, 508f, 512, 720b
Radiopaque, contrast media and, 799
Radius, 333
RAI. *See* Radioactive iodine (RAI) uptake scan
Rales, 253b, 707, 713, 756t–757t
Random urine specimen, 912, 924, 959
    for infant, 912, 916b–917b
Random-access memory (RAM), 462
Range of motion (ROM), 747
Rapid screening test, 912, 913b–915b
Rapport, human behavior and, 119
Ratchet, surgical clamp and, 1089–1101, 1101f
Rationalization, 81t
RBCs. *See* Red blood cells
RBRVS. *See* Resource based relative value scale
RDAs. *See* Recommended dietary allowances
RDS. *See* Respiratory distress syndrome
Reabsorption, 368
Reactions, cultural differences and, 96–98
Read-only memory (ROM), 462–463
Reading, study strategies and, 10–11, 14–15
Reagent strip, 960–966, 960f–961f, 999
    use of, 962t, 963b–965b
Reagent tablet, 960, 960f, 966–968, 999
Reagents, 898, 898b
Receipt-charge slip, 551, 553f
Receiving, 452b–453b
Receptors, 284
Recessive genes, 179
Recipient
    blood types and, 227
    universal, 227
Reciprocity, licensure and, 46
Recommended dietary allowances (RDAs), 131–132
Reconciled bank statements, 560, 564f
    procedure for, 565b–566b
Rectal drug administration, 1042
Rectal temperature, 690, 691t
Rectum, 267, 269f, 277
    diseases of, 273t–276t
Rectus, 312
Recurrent turn, 817–822, 822f
Red blood cells (RBCs). *See also* Erythrocytes
    bilirubin and, 270
    complete blood count and, 975t
    diseases of, 231t–232t
    erythrocytes and, 223
    urine and, 968
Red cell indices, 974
References
    employer checking and, 1156b
    resumé and, 1154–1155, 1156t
Referral, E/M coding and, 596
Reflecting, positive communication techniques and, 120t
Reflex, types of, 305

Refraction, 311
Regional anesthesia, 1113
Regional Health Information Organizations (RHIO), 516
Regions
 of abdominal cavity, 171
 of abdominopelvic area and, 172, 172f, 172t, 194
Registered mail, 496b
Registered Medical Assistant (RMA), 30, 32t–33t, 41
 credentials of, 31–32, 31f
 testing for, 31
Registered Nurse (RN), 40
Regression, 81t
Regular diet, 145
Regurgitation, 200–201, 272b
Rejecting, communication barrier and, 121t
Relative value scale (RVS), 609–610, 632–633
Relative value units (RVUs), 610
Release of information (ROI), 620, 622, 622f, 633, 716, 722f
Releasing, 538
 of medical records, 541
Reliability, 23
Renal artery, 370–371
Renal calculi, 372, 372f, 374t–375t
Renal computed tomography, 374b
Renal epithelial cells, 971
Renal failure, 370, 374t–375t
 diet for, 147
Renal pelvis, 371, 372f
Renal ptosis, 370
Renin, 368, 370
Reorder point, 450
Reorganization, 14
Replacement drug, 1004
Repolarization, 763, 764t, 765, 765f
Reporting requirements, 56
 CDC and, 56
Repression, 81t
Reproductive cycle, 389–390
Reproductive organs (female), 386–389
Reproductive system, 191t–193t, 381, 391b
 female, 386–391
 function of, 383
 male, 383, 383f
Reproductive system diseases (female), 390–391, 392t–393t
 drug classifications for, 391t
Reproductive system diseases (male)
 drug classifications for, 385t
 tests and procedures for, 386b
Res ipsa loquitur
 dereliction of duty and, 53
 lawsuit information and, 55t
Reservoir host, 642, 667
Resident flora, 638
Residual disability, 614
Resistance, 237
Resource allocation, 68
Resource-based relative value scale (RBRVS), 610, 632–633
Respiration, 243, 245, 258, 705
 regulation of, 251
Respiratory arrest, 1145–1146
Respiratory depth, 707

Respiratory distress syndrome (RDS), 248
Respiratory drugs, classifications of, 253t
Respiratory measurement, 251–252
Respiratory rate, 705–707, 713
 documentation of, 705b
 measuring of, 708b
Respiratory rhythm, 707
Respiratory system
 diagnostic tests and procedures of, 252t, 254b
 diseases and disorders of, 253b, 254t–256t
 function of, 245, 258
 signs and symptoms of, 253b
 structure of, 244–245, 245f
 the body and, 191t–193t
Respondeat superior, 47
Rest, Ice, Compress, Elevate (RICE), 1143
Restating, positive communication techniques and, 120t
Restrictive endorsement, 559, 579
Resumé, 34, 1154–1156, 1154b–1156b
Retention, 373b
Reticular tissue, 188t–189t, 189
 matrix and, 187–190
Reticulocyte, 223–224
Retina, 311
Retracting instruments, surgery and, 1089–1101
Retractors, 1127
 surgical instruments and, 1103, 1104f
Retroperitoneal, 369–370
Revalidation, continuing education and, 33
Review of systems, 722–723, 723t, 724f
Review of systems (ROS), 596, 722–723, 723t, 724f, 728
RF. *See* Rheumatoid factor (RF) test
Rh factor, 226–228, 230f, 240
Rhesus factor. *See* Rh factor
Rheumatoid arthritis (RA), 341t–343t, 345f
Rheumatoid factor (RF) test, 340b
Rheumatologist, 362
Rhinitis, 254t–256t
RHIO. *See* Regional Health Information Organizations
Rhonchi, 253b, 707, 713, 756t–757t
Rhythm, 702, 713
Rhythm strip, 775
RIA. *See* Radioimmunoassay
Ribonucleic acid (RNA), 176
Ribosomes, 176, 177t, 178f
Ribs, 332
RICE. *See* Rest, Ice, Compress, Elevate
Rickets, 138t, 341t–343t
Rickettsiae, 638, 639t, 667
Riders, 611
Right lower quadrant (RLQ), 171–172, 171f
Right to Die issues, 66
Right upper quadrant (RUQ), 171–172, 171f
Right-to-know law, 646b, 668
Rigidity, 272b
Ringworm. *See* Tinea corporis
Rinne test, 318b, 673, 756t–757t, 889, 889f
Risk management, 53, 54b
 lawsuits and, 53
RLQ. *See* Right lower quadrant

RMA. *See* Registered Medical Assistant
RN. *See* Registered nurse
Rods, 311
Roe v. Wade, 66
ROI. *See* Release of information
ROM. *See* Range of motion
Roosevelt, Eleanor, 76
Root, of hair, 422
Root word, 153–156, 154t
 chemical elements and, 155t
 color and, 155t
 tissues and, 155t
ROS. *See* Review of systems
Rotating E chart, 749–750, 750f
Rotation, 338
Rotators, 357
Round window, 314
Route of entry, 642, 667
Route of exit, 642
Rugae, 265–266, 372
Rule of nines, 429, 429f, 436, 1139b, 1149
RUQ. *See* Right upper quadrant
RVS. *See* Relative value scale
RVUs. *See* Relative value units

S

SA. *See* Sinoatrial node
Sacral, spinal column divisions and, 172–173, 173f
Sacrum, 332
Saddle joint, 337
Safety, examination room and, 672
Safety and security needs, 74
Safety officer, disaster planning and, 1147
Safety stock, 450
Sagittal (lateral) plane, 168–169, 193
Salary, 575
Saliva, 264, 269f
Salivary gland, 268, 270t
Salivary gland ducts, 264, 265f
Sanguineous, wound drainage and, 1123
Sanitization, 654, 654f, 655b–656b, 668
Sarcoma, 341t–343t
Sarcopenia, 362b
SARS. *See* Severe acute respiratory syndrome
Saturated fats, 141, 142b
Saying 'No', 6 6b
Scabies, 432t–433t
Scalpel, 1101, 1102f, 1127
Scanner, 464
Scapulae, 332
Scheduling appointments, 485–493. *See also* Appointments
Schizoid, 304b
Schizophrenia, 304b
School age, 91, 91f
School mission, 4b
Scissors, 1127
 surgical instruments and, 1102f, 1103
Sclera, 311
Scleroderma, 432t–433t
Scoliosis, 341t–343t, 345f
Scored tablets, 1025b
Scrotum, 383, 384f
Scurvy, 139t
Search engine, 466, 467b, 471
Sebaceous gland, 422–423
Sebum, 422–423

Second (secondary) intention healing, 1114, 1116f, 1128
Second trimester, 393–394, 400
Second-degree burn, 428–429, 1139b
Secondary condition, 588–589, 599
Secretin, 268
Sediment, 968, 969f
Segment, 763
Segs. *See* Neutrophils
Seizure, 296b, 1137–1138, 1149
  types of, 301b
Self-actualization, 75
  Maslow's characteristics of, 75b
Self-esteem, 75–77
  cultural differences and, 122
Sella turcica, 329–331, 404
Semen, 373, 385
  purpose of, 399
Semicircular canal, 318
Seminal vesicles, 385
Seminiferous tubules, 383
Semipermeable cell membrane, 175
Semisolid drug forms, 1025, 1033
Sensitive tape thermometer, 693, 697f
Sensitivity test, 998
Sensory neuron, 283, 293f
Sensory system, 309–318, 310b, 310f, 313t, 320
  purpose of, 320
Sentence, 110
  structure of, 110b
Septic shock, 1137t
Septicemia, 231t–232t
Septum (septa), 200, 202f
Sequela, 208t–209t
Sequencing order, 534, 534t
Serological testing, 991–992, 991b
  viewable reactions of, 991–992, 993f
Serology, 904, 941, 991–992, 999–1000
Serology tests, 904, 923
Serosanguineous
  wound drainage and, 1123
Serous
  wound drainage and, 1123
Serous membrane, 169, 200
Serum, 231t–232t, 902, 942
  separation of, 952–954, 952f, 953b
Serum calcium (Ca), 340b
Serum cholesterol, 983–987
  measurement of, 983–987
Serum pregnancy test, 871–872
Service agreements, 448
Seven Rights, 1033
  of drug administration, 1011
Severe acute respiratory syndrome (SARS), 253, 257b
Sex characteristics
  female, 386, 409b
  male, 384, 399, 409b
Sexual abuse, signs of, 56b
Sexual harassment, 60
  definition of, 60
Sexually transmitted diseases (STDs), 396, 398t, 400, 870, 892
SH. *See* Social history
Shaft
  needle parts and, 1048–1059
  of hair, 422

Shank, 1089–1101
Sheath, 283
Shingles (herpes zoster), 298t–299t, 302f
Shock, 1137, 1149
  guidelines for, 1137
  types of, 1137t
Short bones, 327–328, 348
Short term stress, 79, 79t
Short-term care facility, 42
Short-term goals, 4b, 5
Short-term memory, 2, 10b, 19
  successful studying and, 9–10
Shortness of breath (SOB), 1136
Shoulder, 332, 335f
  muscles of, 359t–360t
Sickle cell anemia, 182t–183t, 185f
Side effects, 1028, 1033–1034
SIDS. *See* Sudden infant death syndrome
Sig, signature, 1028–1029, 1031t
Sigmoid colon, 261, 267, 277
Sigmoidoscope, 878, 878f
Sigmoidoscopy, 272b, 878–883, 892
  assisting with, 883
Signs, of chief complaint, 716
Silence, positive communication techniques and, 120t
Simple carbohydrates, 140
Simple fracture, 345, 346t–347t
Simple proteins, 142
Sims' position, 738, 742b–743b, 758
Single-cell diseases, 180–181
Single-channel electrocardiograph, 765, 768, 771b–774b
Single-sample needles, 942
Sinoatrial (SA) node, 203, 203f–204f, 217, 763b, 764f
Sinus, 246, 327t
Sinus arrhythmia, 780–781
Sinus bradycardia, 780, 781f
  conduction system disorders and, 204b
Sinus tachycardia, 780–781, 781f
  conduction system disorders and, 204b
Sinusitis, 254t–256t
Sitting position, 737–738, 739b, 758
Skeletal disorders
  drug classifications of, 340t
  signs and symptoms of, 340b
  tests and procedures for, 340b
Skeletal muscle, 186, 186t, 355–362, 359t–360t
Skeletal system, 191t–193t, 196, 322, 324–325, 347
  diseases and disorders of, 338–345, 341t–343t
Skin
  age and, 430b
  damage to, 423–429
  elasticity and color variations of, 748t
  function of, 420–421, 435
  integumentary system and, 419
  layers of, 435
  life cycle of, 421t
  structure of, 421–423, 423f
  substructures of, 421–423, 435
Skin biopsy, 420t
Skin closures, 1117f, 1123, 1123f, 1124b–1126b

Skin lesion, 424–425, 426f, 1113, 1128
  malignant, 425–428
  therapy for, 427–428
  precancerous, 425
Skin lesions, 435
Skin test, 420t
Skull, 328–332, 331f, 348
Slander, defamation and, 53
Slide, 892
  preparation of, 861, 892
Slit-lamp examination, 314b, 315t–316t
Slough, surgical glue and, 1122
SMART way, goal setting and, 4b
Smell, 309–311, 311f
Smooth muscle, 186, 186t, 355–356
Snellen eye chart, 758–759
  alphabet chart and, 749–750, 750f, 758
  object chart and, 749–750, 750f, 759
  rotating E chart and, 749–750, 750f, 759
  vision testing and, 749–750
Soak, hot, 831, 835b–836b
SOAP, 524–527, 526f, 541
SOB. *See* Shortness of breath
Social history, medical history and, 720b, 722
Social history (SH), 722, 728
Social needs, 74–75
Social roles, 76, 83
Social Security Act, Title 19, 612
Social Security Disability Income Insurance (SSDI), 615
Social Security Tax, 572, 580
Sodium, nutritional principles and, 137–138
Sodium-restricted diet, 146–147
Soft diet, 145
Soft spot. *See* Fontanel
Software, 462
Software program
  choosing of, 468
  installation and setup of, 468–469
  tasks of, 469–470
Sole proprietorship, 37, 37t, 42
Solid drug forms, 1024–1025, 1025f, 1033, 1038b–1040b
  oral administration of, 1037–1040
Solutes, 371–372, 371f, 902, 1024
Solutions, liquid drug forms and, 1024
Solvent, liquid drug forms and, 1024
Somatic cells, 179
Somatic nervous system, 290, 292–294
Somatic tremor, 779–780, 780f
Sorting, 541
Sound, 318
Sound card, 463
Source-oriented record, 524, 540
Space, physical
  cultural differences and, 96–98
  distance and, 107
  nonverbal communication and, 107
Spacer, 1045, 1045f
Spansules, 1024–1025
Spasms, 363b
Spatial, 287
Special endorsement, 559
Special needs patient, 123–125
Specialist, 37
Specialization, 37, 38b, 38t

Specialty boards, 37–38
Specialty certification, 37–38
Specific gravity, urine and, 961
Specific immunity, 237
Specimen, 673, 860–861
Specimen adequacy, Bethesda System and, 861
Specimen collection, 861f–862f, 905–907, 924
  containers for, 673
Specimen transport, 907, 907f, 908b–909b
Speculum, 672–673, 892
Speech, parts of, 110, 110t, 116
Spelling, 111, 111b
Sperm, 383, 384f, 385b, 399
  pathway of, 385b
Spermatozoa. See also Sperm
  urine and, 971–972
Sphenoid bone, 329–331
Sphincter, 264–265, 277, 357
Sphygmomanometers, 707, 709f
Spina bifida, 341t–343t
Spinal cavity, 172–173, 194
Spinal column, 285, 332, 348
Spinal cord, 173, 281, 286b, 289–290, 292f, 297f
Spinal nerve, 290, 293f, 305
Spinal tap. See Lumbar puncture
Spinous process, 332, 333f
Spiral fracture, 345, 346t–347t
Spiral reverse turn, 817–822, 821f
Spiral turn, 817–822, 821f
Spirilla, 638
Spirometer, 883
Spirometry, 253f, 258, 883, 885b–887b, 893
  body measurements for, 681
Spleen, 233–234, 234f
Splint, fractures and, 1142
Splinter forceps, 1101–1103
Sponge forceps, 1101–1103
Sponsor, 613–614
Spores, 638
Sprain, 345, 349, 362–363, 1143
Spreadsheet, 468, 472
Sputum, 257b
Sputum collection, 922, 922f, 924
SQ3R, 10
Squamous, epithelial tissue classification and, 184t
Squamous epithelial cells, 968–971
SSDI. See Social Security Disability Income Insurance
SSI. See Supplemental Security Income
ST segment, 764t, 765
Stage, 901
Standard limb leads, 770–775
  frontal plane activity and, 770
Standard mail, employer contact and, 1158, 1165
Standard Precautions, 640, 641f, 642b–643b, 667, 899b
Standardization, of ECG machines, 768–769, 768f–769f
Standardization mark, 769
Standing position, 756, 758
Stapes (stirrup), 314
Staphylococci, 638
Staples, 1117–1122, 1118f, 1119b–1122b, 1122f

Stark anti-referral rule, 516
State Unemployment Tax Act (SUTA), 575
State workers' compensation program, 614
Statement, of account, 451, 566–567, 571b, 579
Statement of owner's equity, 548
Statement-receipt. See Receipt-charge slip
Statute of limitations, 53
Statutes, 46
STDs. See Sexually transmitted diseases
Steam sterilization, 657
Stem cells, 222–223, 225f, 325
Stenosis, 208t–209t
Stereotyping, 108
Sterile, 654
Sterile dressing, 1128
  changing of, 1119b–1122b, 1123f, 1126
Sterile solution, 1106b
Sterile technique. See Surgical asepsis
Sterility (male), 383
Sterilization, 28b–29b, 654–657, 658b–659b, 668, 870
  methods of, 654b
Sterilization strip, 648, 661f, 668
Sternum (breastbone), 200, 332, 334f, 348
Sternum body, 265, 332
Steroids, 407, 407b
  side effects of, 408b
Stethoscope, 202–203, 705, 705f, 713
Stillbirth, 394
Stimulus, 284
Stirrup. See Stapes
Stockinette, 848
Stomach, 264–266, 269f, 277
  diseases of, 273t–276t
  sections of, 265
Stomatitis, 273t–276t
Stool, 267, 269f. See also Feces
Stool collection, 908b–909b, 918, 924
Storage
  of computer data, 461
  sterilized items and, 661, 661t, 668
Storage control, 451, 453f
Storage devices (computer), 463
Strabismus (cross-eye), 315t–316t, 316f
Straight-number filing, 536, 541
Strain, 345, 363b
  first aid and, 1143
Streak, 1000
  culture medium and, 998, 998f
Streaming scheduling, 492, 511
Streptococci, 638
Stress, 8–9, 9f, 16–17, 77–80, 80b
  symptoms of, 79t–80t
  types of, 9, 20
Striated muscle, 186, 187f, 355
Stridor, 253b, 707, 713
Stroke, 1136–1137, 1137b, 1148–1149. See also
  Cerebrovascular accident (CVA)
Stroke volume, 203
Study habits, 3
Study strategies, 9–16
Stye. See Hordeolum
Stylus, 765–768
Subarachnoid space, 286
Subconscious, 73
Subcutaneous (SubQ) injection, 1065, 1066f
  sites of, 1066f

Subcutaneous layer, 421
Subdural space, 286
Subject, parts of speech and, 110
Subject filing, 537, 541
Subject filing methods, 537
Subjective data, 525–527
Subjective findings, 596
Subjective information, 517, 728
Subjective symptoms, 716, 720b
Sublimation, 81t
Sublingual, 1037–1040
Sublingual gland, 264
Sublingual tablets, 1025b
Subluxation, 345, 349
Submandibular gland, 264
Subpoena
  lawsuit information and, 55t
Subpoena duces tecum, lawsuit information and, 55t
SubQ. See Subcutaneous (SubQ) injection
Subscriber, 603
Subscription, 1028–1029
Success, steps of, 9f
Sudden infant death syndrome (SIDS), 254t–256t
Sudoriferous gland (sweat glands), 422
Suffix, 153–156, 158t
Sugar, 269f
  nutritional principles and, 137
Suicide, physician assisted, 66
Sulcus, 287, 288f
Summarizing, positive communication techniques and, 120t
Summons, lawsuit process and, 55t
Sunstroke. See Heat stroke
Superbill/routing form. See Encounter form
Superego, 73, 83
Superficial wound, 1114
Superior body plane, 168–169, 193–194
Superior vena cava, 200–201, 201f–202f
Supernatant, 968
Superscription, 1028–1029
Supination, 338
Supine position, 168, 193–194. See also
  Horizontal recumbent position
Supplemental Security Income (SSI), 615
Supplies
  for manual filing, 541
  for medical office, 450–451
  for the examination room, 673–675, 673t, 677
  ordering of, 450f, 452b–453b
Supply inventory, 450–451
Suppository, 1025, 1042
Surfactant, 248, 250f
Surgery, minor
  assisting with, 1105–1114, 1105b–1106b, 1107t–1108t, 1109b–1113b
  decontamination and, 1114
  documentation of, 1105b, 1107f
  informed consent for, 1086–1088, 1087f, 1127
  preoperative instruction for, 1086, 1087b, 1127
Surgical asepsis, 654–661, 668, 1088–1089, 1088t, 1127
  guidelines for, 1088b
  sterile supplies for, 1089, 1099b–1100b, 1101f

INDEX

Surgical glue, 1122
Surgical handwash, 648
Surgical handwashing, 1088–1089, 1090b–1092b
Surgical instruments, 1089–1104, 1127
   guidelines for, 1102b
Surgical methods, alternative, 1114
Susceptible host, infection chain and, 642
Suspension, liquid drug forms and, 1024
Suspensory ligament, 313t
SUTA. *See* State Unemployment Tax Act (SUTA)
Suture scissors, 1103
Sutures
   cranial joints and, 328–331
   removal of, 1117, 1119b–1122b
   shapes of, 1086, 1118f
   sizes of, 1116, 1117f
Suturing instruments, surgery and, 1089–1101
Swab-transport media system, 911, 912f
Sweat glands. *See* Sudoriferous gland
Swimmer's ear. *See* Otitis externa
Swing-through gait, 842f–843f, 844
Symbols
   CPT manual and, 591–592, 592b
   indexing of, 534, 534t
Symmetry, 738
Sympathetic division
   ANS and, 203–204
Sympathetic nervous system, 292, 292t, 294f
   functions of, 305
Sympathy, 82
Symptom
   chief complaint and, 716
   definition of, 181
Symptomatic suffix, 159t
Synapse, 284, 304, 354
Synarthroses, 336
Syncope, 208t–209t. *See also* Fainting
Synergist, prime mover muscle and, 356
Synergistic, 353
Synergy, disaster preparedness and, 1146–1147
Synonym, 103–104
Synovial cavity, 336–337
Synovial fluid, 336–337, 348
Synthesize, 142
Synthetic cast, 844, 848f
Syringe, 1048
   safety and, 1059b
   types of, 1048b, 1057f
Syringe method, 943, 944b–947b
Syrups, 1024
Systemic, drug effects and, 1025
Systemic circulation, 204–205, 206f
Systole (S_1), 202
Systolic pressure, 707, 713

T

T lymphocytes, 234–235
T wave, 763, 764t, 765, 766f–767f
T-account, 545–546, 545b, 545f
Table of Hypertension, 586
Table of Neoplasms, 586
Tablet
   solid drug form and, 1024–1025, 1025f
   types of, 1025b

Tabular List of Diseases, 589, 598–599
   chapter structure of, 586–587, 587f
   ICD-9-CM, Vol. 1 and, 586–588, 587t
   supplementary classifications of, 587–588
Tabular List of Procedures, CPT manual and, 592
Tachycardia, 702, 713
Tact. *See* Diplomacy
Tactful, 24
Tactile, 309
Tailbone. *See* Coccyx
Talipes, 341t–343t, 345f
Talkativeness, response to illness and, 99
Talus, 334
Tape backup, 463
Tape measure, 672–673, 672f, 672t
Target organ, 403–404, 411b
Tarsal, 334, 338f
Tasks, office management software and, 472
Taste, 309, 311f
Taste buds, 264, 311f
   kinds of, 309
Tax Payment Act, 572, 580
Tay-Sachs disease
   single-cell diseases and, 180–181, 182t–183t
TBS. *See* Total body surface
Teaching process, patient education and, 126
Team members, 24b
   dying and, 82–83, 82f
   loyalty and, 23
   response to illness and, 98
Technique, drug administration and, 1016
Teeth, 264, 265f
Telephone
   employer contact and, 1158, 1165
   management of, 479–485
Telephone equipment, 443–445, 445f
   headset and, 445f
Telephone etiquette, 479–480, 480b, 510
Telephone system, multiline, answering of, 444b–445b, 452–453
Telephone voice, 479
Temperature, 690–693, 712
   documentation of, 691b
Temporal artery, 702–703, 702f
Temporal bone, 329–331
Temporal lobe, 287, 288f, 290f
Tendon, 337, 348, 354, 364
Tendonitis, computers and, 447b
Terminal-digit filing, 536–537, 541
Terminology, medical, 151
   guidelines for, 156–163
Test card, 877–878
Test taking, 16–19, 17b
   certification and, 32
Testes, 383–384, 386, 405t, 408
Testicular self-examination (TSE), 756t–757t, 857b
Testimony, lawsuit information and, 55t
Testosterone, 383–384, 385t, 407b, 408
   function of, 399
Tests, feedback and, 18
Tetanus (lockjaw), 362–363
Tetany, 354–355, 406–407, 411b
TFT. *See* Thyroid function test
Thalamus, 287, 291f
Thalassemia, 182t–183t
Therapeutic diet, 145, 149

Therapeutic drug, 1004
Therapeutic modalities, 28b–29b
Therapeutic procedures, 808
   documentation of, 812b
Thermal burns, 1149. *See also* Heat burns
Thermometer, types of, 712
Thighbone. *See* Femur
Third party, 603
Third trimester, 394, 400
Third-degree burn, 429, 436, 1139b
Third-party insurance, 610–618
   government payers and, 611–614
   private carriers and, 610–611
Third-party liability, 611, 611f, 633
Third-party payer, 607
Thoracic, 247–248
   spinal column divisions and, 172–173, 173f
Thoracic cavity, 169–171, 194
Thoracic vertebrae, 200, 332
Thoracic wall muscles, 359t–360t
Thorax (chest), 173, 173f, 332
Thoughtful. *See* Tactful
Three-point gait, 842f–843f, 843
Thrill, 756t–757t
Throat. *See* Pharynx
Thrombin, 226
Thrombocytes, 222–223, 225–226
Thrombocytopenia, 231t–232t
Thrombus, 215t–216t
Thrush, 273t–276t
Thumb forceps, 1089–1103
Thymosin, 234–235, 410
Thymus, 405t, 410
Thymus gland, 234–235, 410
Thyroid function test (TFT), 411b
Thyroid gland, 405t, 406
Thyroid-stimulating hormone (TSH), 405t, 406
Thyroxine, 406
TIA. *See* Transient ischemic attack
Tibia, 334, 337f
Tic douloureux (trigeminal neuralgia), 298t–299t
Tickler file, 537
Tidal volume, 251
Time
   cultural differences and, 96–98
   E/M service and, 597, 600
Time management, 5f, 6, 9f, 19
Time zone, 480, 483f
Time-specified scheduling, 489, 511
Timed specimen, 918, 957
Tinctures, 1024
Tinea, 432t–433t
Tinea capitis, 432t–433t, 434f
Tinea corporis (ringworm), 432t–433t, 434f
Tinea cruris (jock itch), 432t–433t, 434f
Tinea faciei, 432t–433t, 434f
Tinea pedis (athlete's foot), 432t–433t, 434f
Tinea unguium (onychomycosis), 432t–433t
Tinnitus, 318b, 319t, 755
Tissue, 194, 196, 673
Tissue forceps, 1101–1103
Tissue scrapings, 420t
Titer, 872
Title VII of the Civil Rights Act of 1964, 60
Titles, indexing of, 535, 535t
To-do list, 6, 6f

Toddler, 88, 88f
  nutrition and, 143
Toggle key, 463
Tomography, 801–802
Tongue, 264
Tongue depressor, 673
Tonometry, 314b, 315t–316t
Tonsils, 234, 234f
Tonus, 353–354
Tophi, 341t–343t
Topical anesthetics, 1113, 1128
Topical chemotherapy, 428
Topical drug administration, 1041–1042, 1082
  application of, 1042
Torso
  axial area and, 173, 175f
Tort, 51–53, 51f
Tort law, 51–53
  medical professional liability and, 51
Torticollis (wryneck), 362, 363f
Total body surface (TBS), 429
Total calcium, 411b
Total cholesterol, 983–987
Total disability, 614
Touch, nonverbal communication and, 106–107, 106f
Touch pad, 463
Touch screen, 464
Towel clamp, 1101–1103
Toxemia, 397t. *See also* Pregnancy-induced hypertension
Toxic dose, 1007b
Toxic shock syndrome (TSS), 392t–393t
Toxicity, 1028, 1033–1034
Trace minerals, 140, 141t
Tracer
  PET scan and, 803
Trachea, 247–248, 248f, 258
Tracing, cardiac cycles and, 763
Trackball, 463
Training programs, professional, 29
Trans-fatty acids, polyunsaturated fats and, 141
Transactions, 544–545
Transcriptionist, 509
Transdermal patch, 1025, 1042, 1042f, 1043b–1044b
Transducer, 799–800
Transformer cabinet, x-ray room and, 795
Transfusions, 227
Transient flora, 643, 668
Transient ischemic attack (TIA), 298t–299t
Transitional epithelial cells, 971
Transmit, verbal communication and, 104–105, 104f
Transverse (cross-sectional) plane, 168–169, 193
Transverse arch, 334–335
Transverse colon, 261, 267, 277
Transverse fracture, 346t–347t
Treadmill test, 784
Trench mouth. *See* Vincent's infection
Trend analysis, 1133
Trendelenburg's position, 747, 758
Trial, lawsuit process and, 55t
TRICARE, 604, 613–614, 633
  options of, 613–614
Trichinosis, 362–363

Trichomoniasis, 869–870, 892
Tricuspid valve, 200–201, 202f, 205f, 217
Trigeminal neuralgia. *See* Tic douloureux
Triglycerides, 141
Trigone, 372–373
Triiodothyronine, 406
Trimesters, pregnancy and, 391–393
Trochanters, 334
Troches. *See* Lozenges
True ribs, 332
Trunk, 328
Trypsin, 266
TSE. *See* Testicular self-examination (TSE)
TSH. *See* Thyroid-stimulating hormone
TSS. *See* Toxic shock syndrome
Tuberculosis, 254t–256t, 341t–343t
Tuberosity, 327t, 337f
Tubular gauze bandage, 817
Tumor, cell growth and, 179b
Tuning fork, 672–673, 672f, 672t, 675f, 889
Turbid, urine appearance and, 959
Turgor, 419, 748t, 756t–757t
Turner syndrome, chromosomal disease and, 180–181, 182t–183t
Tutorial, 465
Twitch, 354–355
Two-hour postprandial test, 987, 1000
Two-point gait, 842–843, 842f–843f
Tympanic membrane (eardrum), 312–313
Tympanic temperature, 690, 691t
Tympanic thermometer, 693, 697f, 699b–700b, 712
Tympanogram, 889, 891
Tympanometer, 891
Tympanometry, 889
Type and crossmatch, 227
Tzanck test, 420t

U

U wave, 763, 765, 999
U.S. Drug Enforcement Agency (DEA), 47
U.S. National Center for Health Statistics (NCHS), 583
UB-04 claim form, 580
UCR. *See* Usual, customary, and reasonable
Ulcer, 424–425, 430b, 435
Ulna, 333
Ultrasonography, 254b, 391b, 411b, 799–803
  patient preparation for, 800, 800t
Ultrasound, 799–800
Ultrasound therapy, 831, 836b–837b
Ultraviolet rays (UV), 420–421, 427, 654b
Umbilical, 264
Umbilical cord, 393
Umbilicus, 171–172
Unconscious, 1133
  patient condition as, 1133
Underarms (axilla), 422
Uniform Anatomical Gift Act of 1968, 58, 69
Unipolar lead. *See* Augmented lead
Unit dose, 1007b
Unit/floor time, E/M service and, 597
United States Adopted Name Council (USAN), 1004–1005
United States Pharmacopeia, 1004–1007, 1010
United States Postal Service (USPS), 447, 493–495
Universal donor, 227

Universal recipient, 227
Universal Serial Bus (USB), 463
Unsaturated fats, 141–142
Upper arm, 332
Upper extremity, 332–333, 348
  muscles of, 359t–360t, 362
Upper gastrointestinal series (upper GI), 799t
Upper GI. *See* Upper gastrointestinal series
Upper respiratory infection (URI), 252, 254t–256t
Upper respiratory tract, 245–247, 245f–246f, 254t–256t, 258, 260
Urea, 370
Uremia, 369, 373b
Ureter, 369f, 372, 373b
  structure and function of, 379
Urethra, 373, 373b, 379, 384
  structure and function of, 379
Urgency, 373b
URI. *See* Upper respiratory infection
Urinalysis, 912b, 958–972, 958f
  laboratory tests and, 904
Urinary bladder, 369f, 372–373, 379
  structure and function of, 379
Urinary disease
  diagnostic tests for, 374b
  signs and symptoms of, 373b
Urinary reflux, 372
Urinary system, 191t–193t, 196, 367
  aging and, 378b
  diseases and disorders of, 373–378, 374t–375t
Urinary tract infection (UTI), 373, 373t–375t
  nitrites and, 966
Urination, 372–373
Urine, 367, 378–379, 998–999
  structures of, 999
Urine collection, 912–918
Urine glucose, 411b
Urine ketones, 411b
Urine sediment, microscopic examination of, 968–972, 969f, 970b–971b, 999
Urine specimen, 24-hour, 918, 929b, 933b
URL, 465–466
Urobilinogen, 966
Urochrome, 958–959, 998
Urologist, 373, 385
Urticaria, 237, 430b
USAN. *See* United States Adopted Name Council
USB. *See* Universal Serial Bus
User ID, 465
USP/NF. See National Formulary
USPS. *See* United States Postal Service
Usual, customary, and reasonable (UCR), 609, 609b, 632–633
Uterine fibroids, 392t–393t
Uterus, 386–387
  prolapse of, 392t–393t
Uterus body, 389
UTI. *See* Urinary tract infection
UV. *See* Ultraviolet rays
Uvula, 264

V

V codes, 587–588, 588b
V fib. *See* Ventricular fibrillation

INDEX 1251

V leads. *See* Chest leads
V tach. *See* Ventricular tachycardia
Vaccination, 237
Vaccine, 1018
Vaccine Adverse Event Reporting System (VAERS), 1018
Vaccine Information Statement (VIS), 1018
Vacutainer, 941–943
Vacuum tube, 940
VAERS. *See* Vaccine Adverse Event Reporting System
Vagina, 386–389
Vaginal drug administration, 1042, 1082
Vaginal irrigation, 870
Vaginal speculum, 857–860
Vaginitis, 861–870, 892
Vagus nerve, 265–266
Valve, 200–201, 217. *See also* Heart valves
Valvular insufficiency, 200–201
Varices, 213
Variety, nutritional principles and, 134
Varix. *See* Varices
Vas deferens, 384, 384f
Vasoconstrict, 211
Vasodilate, 211
Vastus lateralis muscle
　intramuscular injection and, 1069, 1070f
　pediatric injection and, 1071b–1073b
VC. *See* Vital capacity
Vein, 213
Vein damage, bleeding and, 1138
Venae cavae, 200–201, 205f
Vendor, 451
Venipuncture, 930–954
　blood collection and, 930–954
　definition of, 927
　equipment for, 942–943, 942f–943f
　failed draws of, 943, 943b, 951b, 951f, 954
　procedures for, 935b–940b
　sites for, 930, 930t, 954
　tourniquet application and, 930, 935b–940b
Venn diagram, 11–14, 13f
Ventilation process, 240–251
Ventral, anterior body planes and, 168–169, 193–194
Ventral cavity, 169–172, 170f, 171t, 194
Ventricles, 202–203, 287, 291f
　of heart chambers, 200
Ventricular arrhythmia, 781–782
Ventricular depolarization, 764t
Ventricular fibrillation (V fib), 782, 782f
Ventricular tachycardia (V tach), 782, 782f
Ventrogluteal muscle, intramuscular injection and, 1069, 1073f
Venules, 213
Verb, 153
　correct use of, 110t
Verbal communication, 104–105
　cultural differences and, 122
Vermiform appendix, 267
Verrucae. *See* Warts
Vertebrae, 286b, 332, 333f–334f
Vertebral arteries, 205–206, 218
Vertebral column, 332, 334f
Vertigo, 296b, 318b, 755
Vesicle, 424–425, 435

Vestibular apparatus, 318
Vestibule, 318, 389
Veteran, CHAMPVA and, 614
Viable, cell transportation and, 176
Vial, 1045–1048, 1047f
Vicarious liability, 47b
Villi, 266, 267f, 269f
Vincent's infection, 273t–276t
Viral infection, 432t–433t
Virus, 639, 639f, 639t, 667
VIS. See Vaccine Information Statement (VIS)
Viscera, 289
　body cavities and, 169
Visceral layer, 200
Visceral membrane, 169
Visceral pleura, 169–171
Viscosity, 982–983
Vision, 311–314
Vision testing, 749–755, 749t, 751b–752b
　documentation of, 749b
Visual accessory organs, 312–313
Visual acuity, 749
Visual defects, correctable, 749, 749t, 759
Visual impairment, disabilities and, 123, 127
Vital capacity (VC), 883
Vital signs
　accuracy in, 690
　blood pressure, 707–709
　pulse, 702–705
　respiratory rate, 705–707
　temperature, 690–693
Vital signs/mensuration, 28b–29b
Vital statistics, reporting requirements and, 56, 56b
Vitamin D, 328, 420, 430b
Vitamin K deficiency, 231t–232t
Vitamins, 138–140
Vitamins B-complex, 139t
Vitiligo, 430b, 748t
Vitreous humor, 312f
Voice box. *See* Larynx
Voice mail system, 446
　electronic messaging and, 112–114
Voiding, 372–373
Volkmann finger retractor, retracting instruments and, 1089–1101
Volume, 702, 713
Voluntary muscle, 186, 355
Volvulus, 273t–276t, 276f
Vomer bone, 331–332
Vomiting, 272b
Voucher, 546, 546f
Vowel
　medical terminology and, 156–157
　phonetic symbols and, 157t
Vulva, 389, 389f

W

W-2 form, 575
Wages, 575
Waiver, 612–613
Walk-in. *See* Ambulatory
Walker, 844
　instructions for, 845b
Walther female urethral dilator, dilating instruments and, 1089–1101
WAN. *See* Wide area network
Wandering baseline, 780, 780f

Warm boot, 462–463
Warranties, 448
Warranty card, 439
Warts (verrucae), 432t–433t, 435f
Water, 142, 148
Water-soluble vitamins, 138–140, 138t
Wave scheduling, 489–492, 511
Waves, 763
Waxy casts, 972t
WBCs. *See* White blood cells
Weber test, 318b, 673, 756t–757t, 889, 889f
Website
　electronic messaging and, 114
　employer contact and, 1157–1158
Weight
　child measurement of, 683
　measurement of, 681, 681f, 712
Weight management, nutritional principles and, 134–137
Westergren method, 977, 980b–981b, 982t
Wet mount, 869, 870f
Wheal, 424–425, 435, 1060, 1065f
Wheezes, 253b, 707, 713
White blood cells (WBCs), 224–225. *See also* Leukocytes
　complete blood count and, 975t
　types of, 225
White coat syndrome, 99b
Whitehead. *See* Comedo, pustular
WHO. *See* World Health Organization (WHO)
Whorls, 421
Wide area network (WAN), 465, 471
Williams lacrimal probe, probing instruments and, 1089–1101
Windpipe. *See* Trachea
Winged infusion needle, 1080, 1081f
Winged infusion set, 943
Wintrobe method, 977–981, 982f, 982t
Withdrawal, 81t
　response to illness and, 99
Withholdings, required, 575–576, 576b, 580
Within normal limits (WNL), 861, 1144
Wizards, 465
WNL, *See* Within normal limits
Wood's light examination, 120t
Word choice, written communication and, 111, 113t
Word map, 16–17
Word origins, 152, 152t
Word parts, 153–156, 153t, 164
　integumentary system, 197
Word processing, 472
　envelope or label function in, 497
Words
　forming plurals of, 162
　origins of, 152
　sound-alike, 113t, 116
Work practice controls, 643, 646b
Work-related injury, 518
Workers' compensation insurance, 60, 575, 580, 614, 633
World Health Organization (WHO), 583, 598
Wound, 428
　types of, 1114, 1115f–1116f
Wound drainage, 1123, 1123f
Wrist, 333
Write-off, 568

Writing, active, 15
Wryneck. *See* Torticollis
www (World Wide Web), 466

X

X-ray film, 794
X-ray machine, 794, 796
    operator duties of, 793
X-ray room, 794–795
X-ray tube, 794
Xerophthalmia, 314b
Xiphoid process, 332

Y

Yeasts, urine and, 971–972

Z

Z-track method
    administration of, 1074, 1078b–1079b
    intramuscular injections and, 1074
Zip drive, 463
Zygomatic bones (cheekbones), 331–332
Zygote, 393, 400

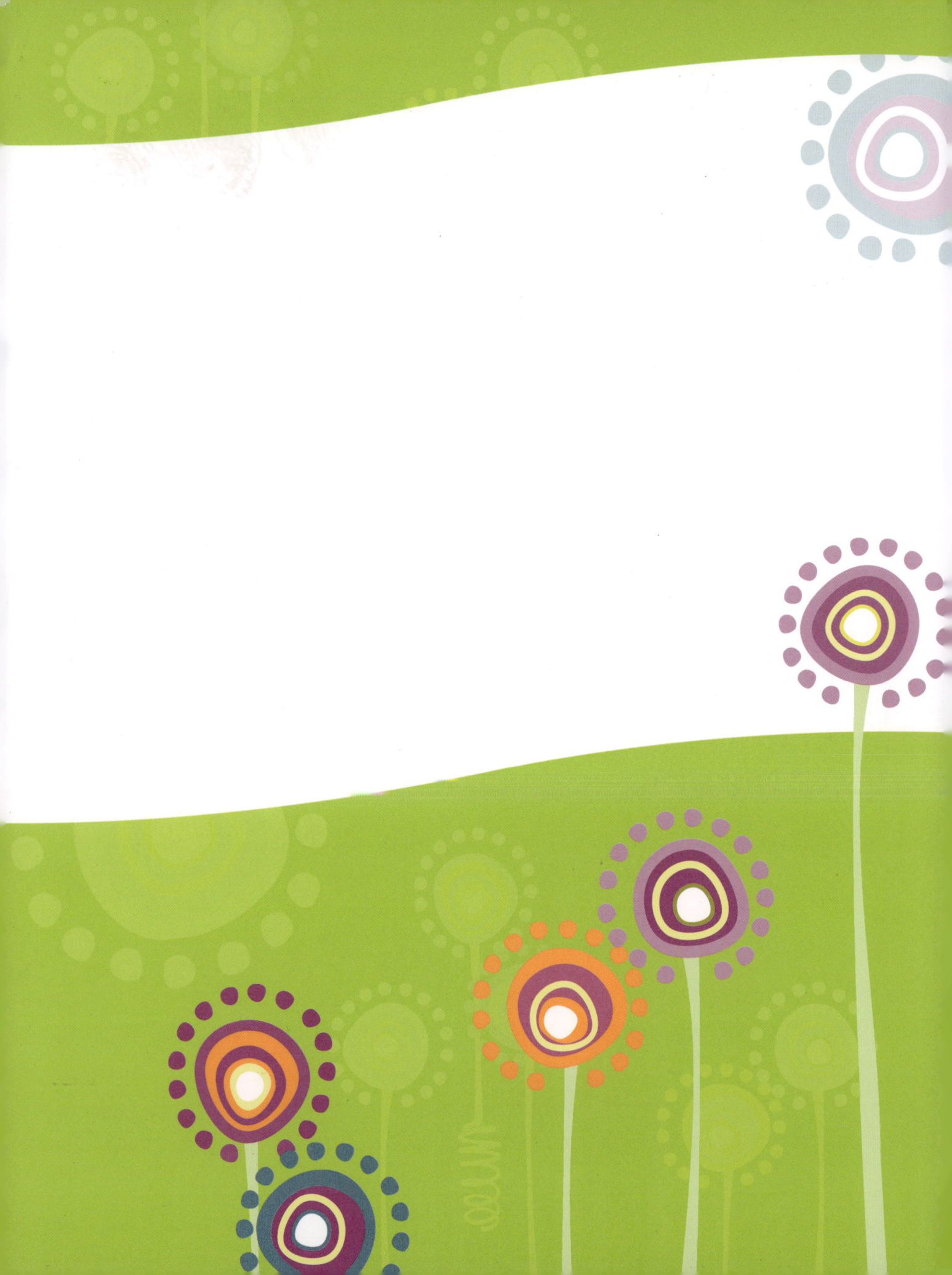